PEARSON

COMPREHENSIVE REVIEW FOR NCLEX-RN®

THIRD EDITION

REVIEWS & RATIONALES

MaryAnn Hogan, PhD(c), MSN, RN, CNE
Clinical Assistant Professor
University of Massachusetts–Amherst
Amherst, Massachusetts

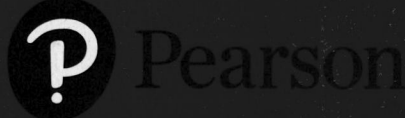

Pearson

330 Hudson Street, New York, NY 10013

Publisher: Julie Alexander
Portfolio Manager: Hilarie Surrena
Editorial Assistant: Bianca Sepulveda
Managing Content Producer: Melissa Bashe
Content Producer: Michael Giacobbe
Development Editor: Rachel Bedard
Design Coordinator: Mary Siener
Vice President of Sales and Marketing: David Gesell
Vice President, Director of Marketing: Margaret Waples
Senior Product Marketing Manager: Phoenix Harvey
Director, Digital Studio: Amy Peltier
Digital Project Manager: Jeff Henn
Full-Service Vendor: SPi Global
Full-Service Project Management: Karen Berry, SPi Global

Library of Congress Cataloging-in-Publication Data

Names: Hogan, Mary Ann (Nurse), author.
Title: Comprehensive review for NCLEX-RN / Mary Ann Hogan.
Other titles: Pearson nursing reviews & rationales series.
Description: Third edition. | New York, NY : Pearson, [2017] | Series: Reviews & rationales | Includes bibliographical references and index.
Identifiers: LCCN 2016040044| ISBN 9780134376325 | ISBN 0134376323
Subjects: | MESH: Nursing Care | Nursing Process | Licensure, Nursing | Examination Questions
Classification: LCC RT62 | NLM WY 18.2 | DDC 610.73076—dc23
LC record available at https://lccn.loc.gov/2016040044

1 17

Pearson

ISBN-13: 978-0-13-437632-5
ISBN-10: 0-13-437632-3

Contents

Preface

PEARSON COMPREHENSIVE REVIEW FOR NCLEX-RN®, THIRD EDITION

This volume of the popular *Pearson Nursing Reviews & Rationales* series is designed to serve as the ultimate study guide to prepare you for the NCLEX-RN® exam. It provides a comprehensive outline review of the essential content areas tested on the NCLEX-RN® exam, including critical areas such as management, delegation, leadership, decision-making, pharmacology, and emergency care. This book incorporates these topics throughout, and provides practice questions simulating the level of difficulty on the actual NCLEX-RN® exam.

The NCLEX-RN® exam is organized according to the categories and subcategories of client needs, integrating the concepts you learned in nursing school. While most other books provide a review of nursing concepts by course area, we integrate these concepts into the categories of client needs as they would be found on the actual NCLEX-RN® exam.

For example, in ***Pearson Comprehensive Review for NCLEX-RN®***, all of the concepts related to health problems commonly encountered in both medical–surgical and pediatric nursing are brought together in the body systems chapters in Section 9 on Physiological Adaptation. Similarly, the important concepts while working with healthy individuals (such as growth and development, lifestyle management, health screening, age-related changes, nutrition, and healthy mothers and newborns) are brought together in the chapters in Section 4 on Health Promotion and Maintenance. This unique organization allows you to study for specific sections of the test based on the results of any predictor tests for the NCLEX-RN® exam that you have taken.

WHAT'S NEW IN THIS EDITION

- Completely updated practice exam reflecting the 2016 NCLEX-RN® Test Plan.
- Access to a NEW web-based app that provides students with thousands of practice questions in preparation for the NCLEX experience.
- 5600 updated or brand-new NCLEX®-style practice test questions.
- New alternate-item format questions.
- The latest test prep advice from MaryAnn Hogan, trusted expert in what nursing students need to know.

WHAT YOU NEED TO KNOW ABOUT THE NCLEX-RN® EXAMINATION

Upon graduation from a nursing program, successful completion of the NCLEX-RN® licensing examination is required to begin professional nursing practice. The NCLEX-RN® exam is a Computer Adaptive Test (CAT) that ranges in length from 75 to 265 individual (stand-alone) test items, depending on your performance during the examination. The blueprint for the exam is reviewed and revised every three years by the National Council of State Boards of Nursing using results of a job analysis study of new graduate nurses practicing within the first six months after graduation. Each question on the exam is coded to a *Client Need Category* and an *Integrated Process.*

Client Need Categories

There are four categories of client needs, and each exam will contain a minimum and maximum percent of questions from each category. The *Client Needs* categories according to the NCLEX-RN® Test Plan effective April 2016 are as follows:

- **Safe and Effective Care Environment**
  - Management of Care (17–23%)
  - Safety and Infection Control (9–15%)
- **Health Promotion and Maintenance (6–12%)**
- **Psychosocial Integrity (6–12%)**
- **Physiological Integrity**
  - Basic Care and Comfort (6–12%)
  - Pharmacological and Parenteral Therapies (12–18%)
  - Reduction of Risk Potential (9–15%)
  - Physiological Adaptation (11–17%)

Integrated Processes

The integrated processes identified on the NCLEX-RN® Test Plan with condensed definitions, are as follows:

- **Nursing Process:** a scientific problem-solving approach used in nursing practice; consisting of assessment, analysis, planning, implementation, and evaluation
- **Caring:** client–nurse interaction(s) characterized by mutual respect and trust, which are directed toward achieving desired client outcomes
- **Communication and Documentation:** verbal and/or nonverbal interactions between nurse and others (client, family, healthcare team); a written or electronic recording of activities or events that occur during client care
- **Teaching and Learning:** facilitation of client's acquisition of knowledge, skills, and attitudes that lead to behavior change
- **Culture and Spirituality:** client-nurse interactions that consider individual and unique self-reported client preferences for care, in addition to standards of care and legal requirements

More detailed information about this examination may be obtained by visiting the National Council of State Boards of Nursing website and viewing the 2016 *NCLEX-RN® Examination Detailed Test Plan for the National Council Licensure Examination for Registered Nurses.*[1]

PREPARING FOR THE NCLEX-RN® EXAMINATION

Study Tips

Using this book should help simplify your review. To make the most of your valuable study time, also follow these simple but important suggestions:

1. **Use a weekly calendar to schedule study sessions.**
   - Outline timeframes for all of your activities (home, school, appointments, etc.) on a weekly calendar.
   - Find the "holes" in your calendar—the times when you can plan to study. Add study sessions to the calendar at times when you can expect to be mentally alert, and then follow your plan!

[1] National Council of State Boards of Nursing, Inc. NCLEX Examination Test Plan for National Council Licensure Examination for Registered Nurses. Effective April, 2016. Document retrieved from the World Wide Web at https://www.ncsbn.org/testplans.htm

2. Create the optimal study environment.
- Eliminate external sources of distraction, such as television, cell phone, etc.
- Eliminate internal sources of distraction, such as hunger, thirst, or dwelling on items or problems that cannot be worked on at the moment.
- Take a break for 10 minutes or so after each hour of concentrated study both as a reward and an incentive to keep studying.

3. Use pre-reading strategies to increase comprehension of chapter material.
- Skim read the headings in the chapter; they identify chapter content.
- Read the definitions of key terms, which will help you learn new words to comprehend chapter information.
- Review all graphic aids (figures, tables, boxes, memory aids); they are often used to explain important points in the chapter.

4. Read the chapter thoroughly but at a reasonable speed.
- Comprehension and retention are actually enhanced by not reading too slowly.
- Do take the time to reread any section that is unclear to you.

5. Summarize what you have learned.
- Use the accompanying web-based app to test yourself with thousands of NCLEX®-style practice questions.
- Review again any sections that correspond to questions you answered incorrectly or incompletely.

Test-Taking Strategies

Every question in the book and on the accompanying web-based app provides test-taking strategies that enable you to select the correct answer by breaking down the question, even if you don't know the correct response. Use the following strategies to increase your success in testing situations:

- Get sufficient sleep and have something to eat before taking a test. Take deep breaths during the test as needed. Remember, the brain requires oxygen and glucose as fuel. Avoid concentrated sweets before a test, however, to avoid rapid upward and then downward surges in blood glucose levels.
- Read each question carefully, identifying the stem, all options, and any critical words or phrases in either the stem or options.
  - Critical words in the stem such as "most important" indicate the need to set priorities, as more than one option is likely to contain a statement that is technically correct.
  - Remember that the presence of absolute words such as "never" or "only" in an answer option is more likely to make that option incorrect.
- Determine who is the client in the question; often this is the person with the health problem, but it may also be a significant other, relative, friend, or another nurse.
- Decide whether the stem is a true response stem or a false response stem. With a true response stem, the correct answer will be a true statement, and vice versa.
- Determine what the question is really asking, sometimes referred to as the core issue of the question. Evaluate all answer options in relation to the core issue, and not strictly in relation to the "correctness" of the statement in each individual option.
- Eliminate options that are obviously incorrect, then go back and reread the stem. Evaluate only those remaining options against the stem once more to make a final selection.
- If two answers seem similar and correct, try to decide whether one of them is more global or comprehensive. If one option includes the alternative option within it, it is likely that the more global option is the correct answer.

HOW YOUR BOOK PREPARES YOU FOR SUCCESS ON THE NCLEX-RN® EXAMINATION

Pearson's Comprehensive Review for NCLEX-RN®, 3e, helps you prepare for the NCLEX-RN® exam in three ways:

1. Highlights critical concepts on the NCLEX-RN® Exam

One key to your success on the NCLEX-RN® exam will be focusing your review on nursing concepts and interventions typically incorporated into test questions. Your book has a few devices to help familiarize you with these topics so you can better manage your review time.

Memory Aid

Moving from left to right and top to bottom (as when reading), remember location of valvular heart sounds with All Patients Take Meds (Aortic, Pulmonic, Tricuspid, Mitral). These sounds are best heard "downstream" from actual blood flow through valve, giving their unique auscultatory locations.

A. Anger and alienation of substance-using family member
B. Teach disease dynamics
1. Family rules and communication
2. Family members' dysfunctional behaviors and denial about addiction of family member

NCLEX® **C. Explore problematic coping skills, codependency, and low self-esteem**
D. Learn and practice recovery dynamics and skills
1. Include self-love and self-care
2. Utilize support groups (i.e., Al-Anon)
3. Establish healthy relationships and boundaries
4. Engage in daily meditation or prayer

NCLEX® 5. Improve coping and problem-solving skills
NCLEX® 6. Learn to ask for help
7. Confront dysfunctional beliefs and learn how to change them
8. Use affirmations, slogans, serenity prayer

E. Processing anger, losses, and memories
1. Confront substance user about consequences of use and effect on family
2. Process emotional distance between family members

NCLEX® 3. Process loss of "helper/competent" role now that recovering family member is taking back some of his or her lost family roles

Check Your NCLEX-RN® Exam I.Q. *You are ready for testing on this content if you can:*
- Assess a client's coping mechanisms.
- Help a client to use and enhance coping mechanisms.
- Assess a client experiencing a crisis.
- Help a client to process the experience of a crisis.
- Explore social supports to aid a client in recovery from a crisis.
- Assess a client's risk of self-harm.
- Provide care to reduce a client's risk of harm to self or others.

- **Memory Aid boxes** tie specific content from the review outline to the Test Plan. These boxes provide you with hints or suggestions about how to remember these concepts for easy recall during testing.
- **NCLEX® Alert** identifies concepts that are likely to be tested on the NCLEX-RN® exam. Be sure to learn the information highlighted wherever you see this icon.
- **Check Your NCLEX-RN® Exam I.Q.,** found at the end of each chapter, provides an opportunity for you to assess your readiness for the NCLEX-RN® exam on the topics covered in the chapter.

2. Provides practice opportunities

Most faculty tell students they must practice thousands of questions before taking the NCLEX-RN® exam. This book and the online Nursing Reviews & Rationales™ provide you with thousands of questions including the alternate item type questions found on the NCLEX® exam so you can approach your practice review in a variety of ways.

PRACTICE TEST

1. Which assessment data would prohibit the use of imagery with a client?
   1. No previous history of using imagery techniques
   2. States anxiety level of 6 on a 0–10 scale
   3. Client feels reluctant to close eyes for the imagery session
   4. Client has a history of psychosis
2. The nurse has determined that music therapy may be appropriate for use with a client. Which strategies should the nurse consider when choosing the music? Select all that apply.
   1. Choose only music with words.
   2. Choose music that is 5–7 minutes in duration.
   3. Allow the client to choose music of his or her choice.
   4. Encourage the client to respond to the music.
   5. Ask the client not to analyze the music.

- **Practice Test** sections provide a quiz at the end of each chapter to test your mastery of the concepts in that chapter.
- **Comprehensive Exam** at the end of the book contains 265 questions. This exam helps you build your endurance in case you have to answer questions for an extended time in the real exam.

Comprehensive Exam

1. A client exposed to *Mycobacterium tuberculosis* starts on chemoprophylaxis. The nurse provides which instruction to the client?
   1. "You will take a single drug such as isoniazid by mouth every day for 6–12 months."
   2. "You will be on at least two drugs effective against the tubercle bacillus for three months."
   3. "You will be on combination therapy in order to prevent development of drug resistance."
   4. "You will need to learn to give yourself subcutaneous injections."
2. The nurse delegates an unlicensed assistive person (UAP) to assist a client with a clean urinary catheterization procedure. The client was formerly able to perform the procedure alone but because of arthritis, he is no longer able to do so. Although the UAP has done this procedure before, which direction is most important for the nurse to emphasize to the UAP?
   1. Let the client do most of the procedure and report the expected output.
   2. Report immediately any unusual observations, such as bleeding.
   3. Complete in proper order the steps of the procedure.
   4. Perform health teaching while performing the procedure.
3. The surgical unit nurse is assigned to the care of a client who returned from surgery 8 hours ago. Which assessment is of highest priority at this time?
   1. Client remembers how to use incentive spirometer.
   2. Client remains free of nausea and vomiting.
   3. Client has active bowel sounds.
   4. Client has been able to void.
4. The clinic nurse is conducting health screenings. Which client assessment findings indicate the need for health education about reducing risk factors for stroke? Select all that apply.
   1. Weight 205 lbs and height 5 feet 4 inches
   2. Blood pressure 164/92 mmHg
   3. Eats bran for breakfast daily
   4. Smokes ½ pack of cigarettes per day
   5. Serum cholesterol level is 172 mg/dL
5. Which action should the nurse take to maintain medical asepsis when caring for a hospitalized client with diabetes mellitus who requires irrigation of a leg ulcer and insulin injections? Select all that apply.
   1. Wash hands before and after performing client care.
   2. Wear personal protective equipment during the dressing change.
   3. Recap the needle after administering insulin injection.
   4. Use sterile gloves to change the dressing for the leg ulcer.
   5. Wipe the rubber stopper on the insulin vial before withdrawing dose.
6. Hematologic laboratory test results indicate a client with cancer is in the nadir period following the latest round of chemotherapy. Which drug should the nurse avoid administering to this client at this time?
   1. Acetaminophen
   2. Ibuprofen
   3. Diphenhydramine
   4. Guaifenesin

1274

- **NEW web-based app** accompanying this book contains all 1600 questions from the book, PLUS an additional 4000 questions, to give you ample opportunities to practice NCLEX®-style questions and assess your readiness for the actual exam.

3. Hones your test-taking skills

An important part of preparing for the NCLEX-RN® exam is understanding the questions asked and knowing how best to answer them. This book provides you with feedback to build these important skills.

- **Answers & Rationales** are provided following the Practice Test at the end of each chapter and on the Nursing Reviews & Rationales™ website. For every question, you will see a comprehensive rationale for the correct and incorrect choices, because it is important for you to understand why an answer option is correct or incorrect.

- **Test-Taking Strategies** are highlighted in the Answers & Rationales section of the book and on the Nursing Reviews & Rationales™ website. Because you cannot skip questions on the NCLEX-RN® exam, you need to learn how to select the correct answer even if you don't recognize it immediately. These strategies break down each question and show you how to select the correct choice.

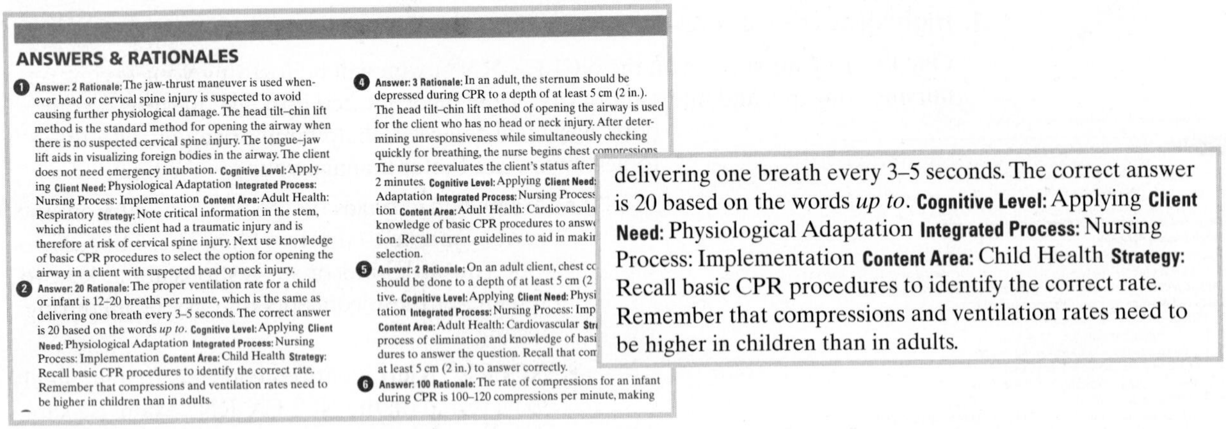

ANSWERS & RATIONALES

1 **Answer: 2 Rationale:** The jaw-thrust maneuver is used whenever head or cervical spine injury is suspected to avoid causing further physiological damage. The head tilt–chin lift method is the standard method for opening the airway when there is no suspected cervical spine injury. The tongue–jaw lift aids in visualizing foreign bodies in the airway. The client does not need emergency intubation. **Cognitive Level:** Applying **Client Need:** Physiological Adaptation **Integrated Process:** Nursing Process: Implementation **Content Area:** Adult Health: Respiratory **Strategy:** Note critical information in the stem, which indicates the client had a traumatic injury and is therefore at risk of cervical spine injury. Next use knowledge of basic CPR procedures to select the option for opening the airway in a client with suspected head or neck injury.

2 **Answer: 20 Rationale:** The proper ventilation rate for a child or infant is 12–20 breaths per minute, which is the same as delivering one breath every 3–5 seconds. The correct answer is 20 based on the words *up to*. **Cognitive Level:** Applying **Client Need:** Physiological Adaptation **Integrated Process:** Nursing Process: Implementation **Content Area:** Child Health **Strategy:** Recall basic CPR procedures to identify the correct rate. Remember that compressions and ventilation rates need to be higher in children than in adults.

4 **Answer: 3 Rationale:** In an adult, the sternum should be depressed during CPR to a depth of at least 5 cm (2 in.). The head tilt–chin lift method of opening the airway is used for the client who has no head or neck injury. After determining unresponsiveness while simultaneously checking quickly for breathing, the nurse begins chest compressions. The nurse reevaluates the client's status after 2 minutes. **Cognitive Level:** Applying **Client Need:** Adaptation **Integrated Process:** Nursing Process tion **Content Area:** Adult Health: Cardiovascula knowledge of basic CPR procedures to answ tion. Recall current guidelines to aid in makir selection.

5 **Answer: 2 Rationale:** On an adult client, chest cc should be done to a depth of at least 5 cm (2 tive. **Cognitive Level:** Applying **Client Need:** Physi tation **Integrated Process:** Nursing Process: Imp **Content Area:** Adult Health: Cardiovascular Str process of elimination and knowledge of basi dures to answer the question. Recall that com at least 5 cm (2 in.) to answer correctly.

6 **Answer: 100 Rationale:** The rate of compressions for an infant during CPR is 100–120 compressions per minute, making

delivering one breath every 3–5 seconds. The correct answer is 20 based on the words *up to*. **Cognitive Level:** Applying **Client Need:** Physiological Adaptation **Integrated Process:** Nursing Process: Implementation **Content Area:** Child Health **Strategy:** Recall basic CPR procedures to identify the correct rate. Remember that compressions and ventilation rates need to be higher in children than in adults.

Pearson NursingNotes offer a quick review of testing strategies and frequently used information organized by the categories of client needs. This appendix is designed to be useful also in the clinical setting, when quick and easy access to information is so important.

Nursing Reviews & Rationales™

For those who want to prepare for the NCLEX-RN®, taking multiple practice tests online will help you become more familiar with the web-based testing experience. With this new edition, use the web-based app to study on the go and access more than 5600 practice questions, including NCLEX®-style formats. This includes the practice questions found in all chapters of the book as well as the comprehensive exam questions. Plus, it contains 4000 newly updated questions to help you further evaluate your readiness for the exam and hone your test-taking skills. Nursing Reviews & Rationales™ allows you to choose two ways to prepare for the NCLEX-RN®. Both approaches personalize your practice experience according to what stage you are in your NCLEX® preparation:

Nursing Topics Review allows you to select which specific nursing topic areas you would like to review and test yourself. After a brief pretest, you receive a personalized study plan referring you to the eText for areas where you need additional review.

Integrated Process Review gives you focused practice tests according to each of the Integrated Processes from the NCLEX-RN® Test Plan, including the Nursing Process, Caring, Communication and Documentation, Teaching and Learning, and Culture and Spirituality.

PEARSON NURSING REVIEWS & RATIONALES

This popular series is the complete foundation for success within the classroom, in clinical settings, and on the NCLEX-RN® exam. Each topical volume offers a concentrated review of core content from across the nursing curriculum, while providing hundreds of practice questions and comprehensive rationales. The complete series includes the following volumes:

- Nursing Fundamentals
- Fluids, Electrolytes, & Acid–Base Balance
- Medical-Surgical Nursing
- Pathophysiology
- Pharmacology
- Maternal-Newborn Nursing
- Child Health Nursing
- Mental Health Nursing
- Comprehensive Review for NCLEX-RN®

Acknowledgments

It truly "takes a village" to create a publication. Without the contributions of many individuals, this book and Nursing Reviews & Rationales™ would not have been possible.

I owe a special debt of gratitude to the wonderful team at Pearson for their enthusiasm for this project, as well as their good humor, expertise, and encouragement during development of the third edition. Hilarie Surrena, Portfolio Manager, was unending in her support and encouragement for this edition. Rachel Bedard, Developmental Editor, devoted many long hours to coordinating different facets of this project, and tirelessly and cheerfully encouraged our efforts as well. Her high standards and attention to detail contributed greatly to the final "look" of this book. Product Manager Travis Moses-Westphal and Media Production Manager Rachel Collett were extremely helpful in developing Nursing Reviews & Rationales™ Online and the accompanying eText online. Editorial Assistant Bianca Sepulveda helped to keep the project moving forward on a day-to-day basis, and I am grateful for her efforts as well. A very special thank you goes to design coordinator Mary Siener and the production team, Managing Content Producer Melissa Bashe and Content Producer Michael Giacobbe, who brought the ideas and manuscript into final form.

Thank you to the team at SPi Global, led by Project Manager Karen Berry, for the detail-oriented work of revising this book. I greatly appreciate their hard work, attention to detail, and spirit of collaboration.

Thank you to Maura Connor, formerly of Pearson, for her creativity, talent, and knowledgeable assistance during all previous editions of Reviews and Rationales™ series books. I am grateful for the enduring friendship that we have developed over the last 15 years.

Thank you to all my nursing students, past and present, who continually search for knowledge to provide the best care possible to patients. Your work, today and in the future, is of the most important kind! Finally, I would like to acknowledge and gratefully thank my family, Michael, Michael Jr., Kathryn, Kristen, and William, whose love and support keep me energized and focused. You are at the heart of whatever I do!

MaryAnn Hogan

About the Author

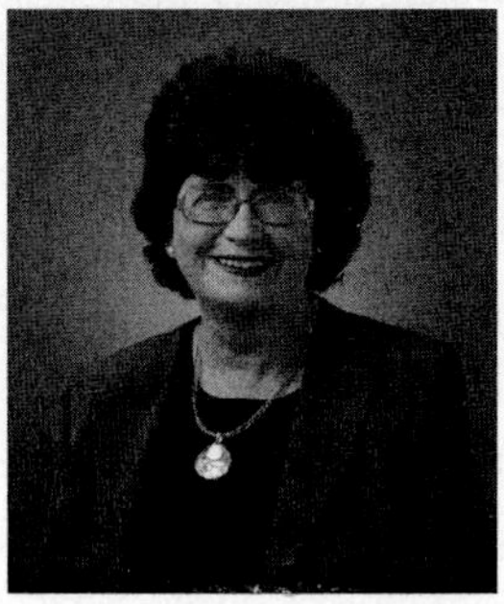

MaryAnn Hogan, PhD(c), MSN, RN, CNE, has been a nurse educator for more than 30 years, currently as a Clinical Assistant Professor at the University of Massachusetts, Amherst. She has taught in diploma, associate degree, and baccalaureate nursing programs. A former item writer for the CAT NCLEX-RN® exam, Ms. Hogan has been teaching review courses throughout New England for the past 25 years. She also has contributed to a number of publications in the areas of adult health, pharmacology, and fundamentals of nursing. She is a member of the American Nurses Association, ANA Massachusetts, Sigma Theta Tau International, Eastern Nursing Research Society, National League for Nursing, and International Network for Doctoral Education in Nursing (INDEN).

We wish to acknowledge the nurse educators around the country who contributed to the first two editions of this review book.

Kim Attwood, MSN, Moravian University, Bethlehem, PA

Sharon Beasley, MSN, RN, Technical College of the Lowcountry, Beaufort, SC

Denise Blais, MSN, St. Joseph's College, Rensselaer, IN

Barbara Carranti, MS, RN, CNS, Le Moyne College, Syracuse, NY

Jo Anne Carrick, MSN, RN, CEN, The Pennsylvania State University, Sharon, PA

Maureen Clusky, DNSc, RN, Bradley University, Peoria, IL

Julie Eggert, MSN, PhD, Clemson University, Clemson, SC

Latrell Fowler, RN, PhD, Florence Darlington Technical College, Florence, SC

Rebecca Gesler, MSN, RN, Spalding University, Louisville, KY

Margaret Gingrich, RN, MSN, Harrisburg Area Community College, Harrisburg, PA

Marilyn Greer, MS, RN, Rockford College, Rockford, IL

Kathleen Haubrich, PhD, RN, Miami University, Hamilton, OH

Judith Herrman, PhD, RN, University of Delaware, Newark, DE

Kathy Keister, PhD, RN, Miami University, Middletown, OH

Virginia Lester, RN, MSN, Angelo State University, San Angelo, TX

Donna M. Nickitas, RN, PhD, CNAA, BC, Hunter College, New York, NY

Lilli Raffeldt, RN, MA, Three Rivers Community College, Norwich, CT

Samir Samour, MSN, RN, Midlands Technical College, Columbia, SC

Kim Serroka, MSN, RN, Youngstown State University, Youngstown, OH

Priscilla Simmons, EdD, APRN, BC, Eastern Mennonite University, Lancaster, PA

Nancy Wagner, MSN, RN, Youngstown State University, Youngstown, OH

We also wish to express our gratitude to the reviewers for all editions of this book.

Mike Aldridge, MSN, RN, CCRN, CNS, The University of Texas at Austin, Austin, TX

Louise A. Aurilio, RNC, Ph.D., CNA, Youngstown State University, Youngstown, OH

Tatayana Bogopolskiy, ANRP, Florida International University, Miami, FL

Mary T. Boylston, RN, EdD, Eastern University, St. Davids, PA

Vera C. Brancato, EdD, MSN, RN, BC, Kutztown University, Kutztown, PA

Tracey Carlson, MSN, RNC, Kent State University, Kent, OH

Fang-yu Chou, RN, PhD, San Francisco State University, San Francisco, CA

Harvey "Skip" Davis, RN, PhD, CARN, PHN, San Francisco State University, San Francisco, CA

Peggy Davis, MSN, RN, CNS, The University of Tennessee at Martin, Martin, TN

Letty Chan Domingo, MSN, RN, CRNP, CEN Temple University, Philadelphia, PA

Mary L. Dowell, PhD, RNC, University of Mary Hardin-Baylor, Belton, TX

Marilyn S. Fetter, PhD, RN, CS, Villanova University, Villanova, PA

Julie Pearson Floyd, APRN, BC, The University of Tennessee at Martin, Martin, TN

Joni C. Goldwasser, RN, MSN, CEN, Radford University, Radford, VA

Rebecca Crews Gruener, RN, MS, Louisiana State University at Alexandria, Alexandria, LA

Sandra Gustafson, MA, RN, Hibbing Community College, Hibbing, MN

Patricia K. Hawley, MEd, Ferris State University, Mecosta Osceola Career Center, Big Rapids, MI

Susan P. Holmes, RN, MSN, CRNP, Auburn University, Auburn, AL

Katherine M. Howard, MS, RN, BC, Raritan Bay Medical Center, Perth Amboy, NJ

Barbara Konopka, MSN, RN, CCRN, CEN, Penn State University, Dunmore, PA

Darcus Margarette Kottwitz, MSN, RN, Fort Scott Community College, Fort Scott, KS

Sandra S. Meeker, RN, MSN, Central Texas College, Killeen, TX

Mary Pihlak, PhD, RN, University of Mary Hardin-Baylor, Belton, TX

Beth Hogan Quigley, RN, MSN, CRNP, University of Pennsylvania, Philadelphia, PA

Linda L. Rather, RN, MSN, MS, Neosho County Community College, Chanute, KS

Anita K. Reed, MSN, RN, Saint Joseph's College Lafayette, IN

Linda Snell, DNS, WHNP-C, SUNY College at Brockport, Brockport, NY

Marianne F. Swihart, RN, MEd, MSN, Pasco-Hernando Community College, New Port Richey, FL

Patricia R. Teasley, APRN, BC, Central Texas College, Killeen, TX

Loretta Wack, RN, BSN, MSN, Blue Ridge Community College, Weyers Cave, VA

Gerry Walker, MSN, RN, Park University Parkville, MO

Leanne M. Waterman, MS, APRN, BC, FNP Onondaga Community College, Syracuse, NY

Dorothy Williams, MSN, RN, Baptist Health System, San Antonio, TX

Linda S. Williams, MSN, RNBC, Jackson Community College, Jackson, MI

Kim C. Wright, MSN, RN, Amarillo College Amarillo, TX

The NCLEX-RN® Licensing Examination 1

In this chapter

The Pearson *Comprehensive Review for the NCLEX-RN®* is purposefully designed according to the NCLEX-RN® test plan so that you are able to gauge your preparation and readiness for the licensing examination during your course of study in your nursing program and immediately after graduation. The National Council Licensure Examination for Registered Nurses (NCLEX-RN®) is the final milestone you will need to achieve to begin your career as a professional nurse. Congratulations—you are well on your way! Although most students and new graduates are nervous about taking this test, remember that its purpose is to safeguard the public trust by ensuring that entry-level nurses are minimally competent and safe for practice. Diligent study during your nursing program and using this book effectively will help to empower you for success.

Becoming knowledgeable about the test plan and testing procedures should be part of your overall preparation to take the NCLEX-RN® exam. This knowledge will help you identify areas of strength and areas for further study before taking the exam. It may also help ease test anxiety by reducing fear of the unknown. This chapter is aimed at helping you to better understand the NCLEX-RN® exam developed by the National Council of State Boards of Nursing (NCSBN). Chapter 2 provides more information about how to manage test anxiety and use effective test-taking strategies.

COMPUTERIZED ADAPTIVE TESTING: WHAT IS IT?

Computerized adaptive testing (CAT) is a method of test administration in which a computer randomly generates a test question from the test item pool and, after the first question, selects the next question based on your ability to answer the previous one. If the question is answered correctly, the next question is at a similar or higher level of difficulty. If the question is answered incorrectly, the next question is at a similar or lower level of difficulty. This process continues with each subsequent question. Because the selection of questions is tailored to the individual, no two test takers will receive the same test. CAT also assures that anyone who takes the exam more than once never receives the same question twice within a defined period of time.

CAT explains why some people are able to answer the minimum number of questions (75) whereas others must take up to the maximum (265). In essence, successful test takers who can answer more difficult questions will have a shorter test, while those who can answer easier questions correctly can expect a longer test.

A key difference between a traditional paper-and-pencil test and CAT is that, with CAT, each question must be answered in the order presented before the test taker can proceed to the next question. Thus, questions cannot be "skipped" to be returned to later. Although being "forced" to answer a question may be uncomfortable if you typically skip questions on tests, it is actually beneficial. Why? Because in skipping and returning to questions, you could also return to questions already answered, and possibly change a correct answer to an incorrect one. This would not be to the advantage of any test taker.

The overall goal of CAT is to evaluate your ability to remain consistently above or below a predetermined passing standard. The computer will continue to select test items from the test bank until:

- The requirements of the test plan have been met (see next section) and
- The computer has determined with 95% confidence statistically that your ability is either clearly above or clearly below the passing standard, or
- The maximum 265 questions have been answered, or
- The maximum time limit (6 hours) has been reached.

At this point, the computer stops and an "examination is ended" message appears on the screen. Many test takers have mixed feelings at this time. Some are glad it is over, while others wish the computer would keep generating questions.

AN OVERVIEW OF THE NCLEX-RN® TEST PLAN

The test plan is designed to measure the knowledge, abilities, and skills needed by an entry-level nurse in order to practice safely and effectively (NCSBN, 2015c). Each question in the test bank is written according to a two-part framework: *Client Needs* and *Integrated Processes*. Each question is also written at a specific level of cognitive ability.

Cognitive Ability Level

Bloom's taxonomy for the cognitive domain of learning (Anderson & Krathwohl, 2001) is used when designing an individual test item and coding its difficulty level. Because nursing is an applied human discipline that requires critical thinking and clinical decision making, most questions on the NCLEX-RN® exam are written at the "applying" level or higher (see Box 1–1 and Box 1–2 for samples). Thus, these questions are often more difficult than test questions on teacher-generated tests, which are more likely to contain a greater number of questions at lower cognitive levels, such as the "remembering" and "understanding" levels.

Box 1–1

Sample Question Illustrating "Applying" Cognitive Level

The nurse has a prescription to administer a daily dose of sodium warfarin 5 mg by mouth. Prior to preparing this medication, the nurse should make note of which laboratory test result drawn at 0600 today?

___ **1.** Hematocrit (Hct) 42%

___ **2.** Hemoglobin (Hgb) 12.8 mg/dL

___ **3.** Partial thromboplastin time (PTT) 49 seconds

___ **4.** International normalized ratio (INR) 2.6

Answer: 4

A question written at the "applying" level of difficulty requires you to consider nursing knowledge that is relevant to the question and use it to make a nursing judgment. In this question, the relevant nursing knowledge is that effectiveness of warfarin is evaluated by noting the results of the INR or prothrombin time (PT, which is not an answer choice in this question).

Box 1–2

Sample Question Illustrating "Analyzing" Cognitive Level

The nurse on a medical nursing unit has been notified of an external disaster with an estimated 30 clients being brought to the emergency department. The nurse is asked to develop a list of clients on the unit that could be discharged. Which client should the nurse place at the top of the triage list for discharge?

___ **1.** A 39-year-old client who underwent laparoscopic cholecystectomy 24 hours ago and reports right shoulder pain rated as a 4 on a scale of 0 to 10.

___ **2.** A 54-year-old client with a draining venous leg ulcer and a new temperature of 100.8°F (38.2°C) who is alert and oriented.

___ **3.** A 76-year-old client with chronic obstructive pulmonary disease with an oxygen saturation of 89% while wearing oxygen at 2 liters/minute.

___ **4.** An 82-year-old client who underwent pacemaker insertion 4 hours ago and whose cardiac monitor shows ventricular paced rhythm with capture.

Answer: 1

A question written at the "analyzing" level of difficulty generally requires you to:

- ➤ Consider multiple sets of information to make a nursing decision, and/or
- ➤ Make nursing judgments using ordinary nursing knowledge in unusual circumstances.

In this question, the nurse needs to use knowledge about which client is the most stable in order to make a decision. The situation is also unusual because nurses are not frequently involved in disasters in everyday nursing practice. Considering stability, you would not discharge first the client in option 3 (airway) or the client in option 2 (risk of infection). The client in option 4 still has potential for developing complications postprocedure, so you would discharge first the client in option 1 who had surgery 24 hours ago. Because it is a laparoscopic procedure, referred shoulder pain is expected, and the client could be taught effective pain management strategies.

Client Needs

The framework for the test plan must identify nursing competencies that apply to all clients across all care settings. With this in mind, the NCSBN developed the test framework of Client Needs. There are four categories of Client Needs: *Safe and Effective Care Environment*, *Health Promotion and Maintenance*, *Psychosocial Integrity*, and *Physiological Integrity*. Two categories—Safe and Effective Care Environment and Physiological Integrity—are further divided into subcategories on the test plan. All test takers receive the same percentage of questions from each category or subcategory in the test plan, regardless of the length of an individual test (see Table 1–1). These percentages are in effect from April 1, 2016, to March 31, 2019.

Table 1–1 Overview of the 2016 NCLEX-RN® Test Plan

Client Need Category/Subcategory	Percentage of Questions
Safe and Effective Care Environment	
Management of Care	17–23%
Safety and Infection Control	9–15%
Health Promotion and Maintenance	6–12%
Psychosocial Integrity	6–12%
Physiological Integrity	
Basic Care and Comfort	6–12%
Pharmacological and Parenteral Therapies	12–18%
Reduction of Risk Potential	9–15%
Physiological Adaptation	11–17%

Safe and Effective Care Environment

This category contains two subcategories: *Management of Care* and *Safety and Infection Control*. The *Management of Care* subcategory contains questions that evaluate your ability to provide and/or direct nursing care in a manner that enhances the care delivery setting and protects not only clients, but also healthcare personnel (NCSBN, 2015c, p. 11). The *Safety and Infection Control* subcategory contains questions that evaluate your ability to protect the client and healthcare personnel from a variety of health and environmental hazards (NCSBN, 2015c, p.12). The topics included in each of these subcategories are outlined in Box 1–3.

Box 1–3

Sample Topics for Safe and Effective Care Environment

Management of Care

- Advance directives/self-determination/life planning
- Advocacy
- Assignment, delegation, and supervision
- Case management
- Client rights
- Collaboration with interdisciplinary team
- Concepts of management
- Confidentiality/information security
- Continuity of care
- Establishing priorities
- Ethical practice
- Information technology
- Informed consent
- Legal rights and responsibilities
- Organ donation
- Performance improvement (quality improvement)
- Referrals

Safety and Infection Control

- Accident/error/injury prevention
- Emergency response plan
- Ergonomic principles
- Handling hazardous and infectious materials
- Home safety
- Reporting of incident/event/irregular occurrence/variance
- Safe use of equipment
- Security plan
- Standard precautions/transmission-based precautions/surgical asepsis
- Use of restraints/safety devices

Health Promotion and Maintenance

This category has no subcategories in the test plan. It contains questions that evaluate your ability to apply knowledge of growth and development to care of clients, to provide and direct care for prevention or early detection of health problems, and to incorporate knowledge of strategies to promote optimal health (NCSBN, 2015c, p. 23). The topics included in this category are outlined in Box 1–4.

Box 1–4

Sample Topics for Health Promotion and Maintenance

- Aging process
- Ante/intra/postpartum and newborn care
- Developmental stages and transitions
- Health promotion/disease prevention
- Health screening
- High-risk behaviors
- Lifestyle choices
- Self-care
- Techniques of physical assessment

Psychosocial Integrity

This category also has no subcategories. It contains questions that evaluate your ability to provide or direct care to clients with either acute or chronic mental illness and to provide care that supports the emotional and psychosocial well-being of clients experiencing stressful events (NCSBN, 2015c, p. 27). The topics included in this category are outlined in Box 1–5.

Box 1–5

Sample Topics for Psychosocial Integrity

- Abuse/neglect
- Behavioral interventions
- Chemical and other dependencies/substance use disorder
- Coping mechanisms
- Crisis intervention
- Cultural awareness/cultural influences on health
- End-of-life care
- Family dynamics
- Grief and loss
- Mental health concepts
- Religious and spiritual influences on health
- Sensory/perceptual alterations
- Stress management
- Support systems
- Therapeutic communication
- Therapeutic environment

Physiological Integrity

This category has four subcategories: *Basic Care and Comfort*, *Pharmacological and Parenteral Therapies*, *Reduction of Risk Potential*, and *Physiological Adaptation*. The *Basic Care and Comfort* subcategory contains questions that evaluate your knowledge and ability to provide comfort and assistance during activities of daily living (NCSBN, 2015c, p. 27). The *Pharmacological and Parenteral Therapies* subcategory addresses your knowledge and ability to administer medications and parenteral therapies (e.g., intravenous therapy or blood transfusion therapy) (NCSBN, 2015c, p. 31). The *Reduction of Risk Potential* subcategory addresses your ability to take action to reduce risk for clients to develop a complication or health problem because of existing conditions, treatments, or procedures (NCSBN, 2015c, p. 35). The *Physiological Adaptation* subcategory addresses your ability to manage and provide care to clients who have acute, chronic, or life-threatening physical health problems (NCSBN, 2015c, p. 39). Topics included in each of these subcategories are outlined in Box 1–6.

Integrated Processes

The *Integrated Processes* category forms the second part of the framework of the NCLEX-RN® examination test plan. The five integrated processes are the five-step nursing process (assessment, analysis, planning, implementation, and evaluation), caring, communication and documentation, teaching/learning, and culture and spirituality. Because these processes are considered foundational to nursing practice, they are integrated throughout the *Client Need* categories; however, there are no specific percentages attached to each *Integrated Process* in the test plan.

Box 1–6

Sample Topics for Physiological Integrity

Basic Care and Comfort

Assistive devices

Elimination

Mobility/immobility

Nonpharmacological comfort interventions

Nutrition and oral hydration

Personal hygiene

Rest and sleep

Pharmacologic and Parenteral Therapies

Adverse effects/contraindications/side effects/interactions

Blood and blood products

Central venous access devices

Dosage calculation

Expected actions/outcomes

Medication administration

Parenteral/intravenous therapies

Pharmacologic pain management

Total parenteral nutrition

Reduction of Risk Potential

Changes/abnormalities in vital signs

Diagnostic tests

Laboratory values

Potential for alterations in body systems

Potential for complications of diagnostic tests/treatments/procedures

Potential for complications from surgical procedures and health alterations

System-specific assessments

Therapeutic procedures

Physiological Adaptation

Alterations in body systems

Fluid and electrolyte imbalances

Hemodynamics

Illness management

Medical emergencies

Pathophysiology

Unexpected response to therapies

QUESTION TYPES: MULTIPLE-CHOICE AND ALTERNATE-ITEM FORMATS

Early versions of the NCLEX-RN® exam consisted solely of multiple-choice questions. As you know, a multiple-choice question contains client information in the stem and poses a question to be answered. There are four answer options, one of which is correct. Alternate-item formats (AIFs) were introduced to provide ways, other than standard multiple-choice questions, to measure candidate ability level (NCSBN, 2015c). As part of its own ongoing quality improvement program, NCSBN continually looks to the future to design, field-test, and implement innovative methods for assessing entry-level nurse competence. In so doing, NCSBN holds itself to the same high professional standards as other health-oriented organizations that hold the public trust. Alternate-item format questions may include the following:

- Hot spot (candidate clicks on a specific area of an image or graphic to answer the question)
- Fill-in-the-blank (candidate types in a number after performing a calculation using directions in the tutorial or question for rounding)
- Multiple response (candidate clicks on as many responses as apply to the question, which will be more than one but fewer than the total number of options available)
- Chart/exhibit (candidate clicks on three tabs or buttons to view additional information needed to answer the question)
- Ordered response (candidate uses the mouse to "drag" unordered answer options on the left side of the screen and "drop" them in order on the right, according to sequence or priority)
- Audio (candidate dons a headset, clicks a sound icon, and listens to a sound prior to answering the question; volume button can be adjusted as needed)
- Graphic option (candidate answers a multiple-choice question by clicking on a graphic or picture as the answer)

It is important to note that standard multiple-choice items can also contain graphics such as images, charts, or tables. The inclusion of such materials does not automatically classify the question as an AIF. All questions, whether multiple choice or AIF, are scored as either correct or incorrect. No partial credit is given for answers. More information about AIF questions can be found on the National Council of State Boards of Nursing website (see References). At least 1,000 alternate-item format questions can be found in this book and accompanying online materials to provide you with ample opportunity to practice these types of questions.

BEHIND THE SCENES: THE TEST DEVELOPMENT PROCESS

The test plan for the NCLEX-RN® exam is developed considering the legal scope of practice according to the Nurse Practice Acts in the various U.S. states and territories and the rules and regulations of the various boards of nursing. A practice analysis study is also conducted every 3 years with newly licensed registered nurses to assess what activities entry-level nurses perform in the clinical setting, including their frequency and importance (NCSBN, 2015a). The sample includes graduates of all types of basic nursing education programs. The results are analyzed by a panel of content experts at NCSBN and used to make decisions about the framework of the test plan. A similar process is used to develop the Canadian version of the NCLEX-RN® exam (NCSBN, 2015a).

In a separate process, the passing standard for the examination is also reviewed on a 3-year cycle in the same year that the revised test plan is approved. In April 2013, the passing standard was raised from a level of −0.21 logit to 0 logit, and remains at 0 for the 2016 test plan. The passing standard is a mathematical "line" above which the test taker's estimated ability level must remain to pass the exam. As an example, test takers who can answer difficult questions correctly remain easily above the line (and will thereby also take a shorter test). Those who can answer easier questions correctly can also pass as long as they remain above the line, but they must answer more questions to do so. The most important point is that as long as the computer is generating questions, it has *not* determined failure, so answer each question thoughtfully and carefully.

To ensure that the exam reflects current clinical practice, new test questions are continually added to the test bank, and outdated questions are discarded or modified. After a question is written and reviewed, it is pilot-tested during actual examinations. For this reason, 15 of the first 75 questions on any licensing examination do not factor into the passing score. Because you will not know which questions they are, it is critical to answer all questions carefully.

New test items are written by a pool of volunteer item writers. Item writers are extensively screened by the NCSBN and are registered nurses who hold a master's degree or higher; often they are nurse educators. A review panel (consisting of content experts who work in clinical settings) also looks at all questions developed by item writers to ensure they reflect current nursing practice before being included in the test item pool.

REGISTERING FOR THE EXAM

The Registration Process

To take the NCLEX-RN® examination following graduation, you must complete two processes, which can be started concurrently. Be sure to download the *NCLEX-RN® Examination Candidate Bulletin* from the NCSBN website (see References) which has the information you need to register for and schedule your exam. The first process is to apply for licensure to the Board of Nursing (BON) in the state or territory in which you seek licensure. The second is to register for the NCLEX-RN® exam with the test service vendor, Pearson VUE. There is a separate registration process and fee to take this exam. You can register on the NCLEX® Candidate website (see References) or by telephone using the directions in the *NCLEX-RN® Examination Candidate Bulletin*. By initiating both processes simultaneously, your registration to take the exam will be in the Pearson VUE system once the BON verifies your eligibility to test.

Fill out the state licensure application completely and carefully, and submit the correct application fee (varies from state to state) using an approved form of payment. If the form is completed incorrectly, or if the proper fee is not enclosed using an approved form of payment, the application will be returned to you, which will delay your ability to take the licensing examination. After receiving your application, the BON will determine your eligibility for licensure (based on state law) and notify Pearson VUE once you are authorized to take the NCLEX-RN® exam. You will also receive an authorization to test (ATT) form, which allows you to schedule a date to take the NCLEX-RN® exam. If you do not receive an ATT within 4 weeks of registration, or if you lose the ATT once it is sent, report this to the NCLEX® Candidate Test Service according to the directions in the *NCLEX® Examination Candidate Bulletin*.

Scheduling an Examination Appointment

After receiving the ATT, note the validity dates (determined by the BON in which you seek licensure; average is 90 days). The ATT also contains other important information, including your candidate identification number and test authorization number. Keep the ATT in a safe place because you will need to present it on test day in order to take the exam. Schedule the appointment promptly, even if you do not plan to take the exam immediately. Doing so will provide you with the best selection of test dates and times from which to choose.

Remember that postgraduation, there are many people seeking to fill the appointment slots, so popular time slots fill up quickly. Also, if you wait until your ATT is almost ready to expire, the test center may not be as able to seat you easily. First-time applicants must be offered an appointment within 30 days of telephoning or e-mailing the test service; repeat candidates can be offered an appointment in 45 days. If you make the appointment by phone, mark your calendar with the date of your call and the expected test date in case there is need for follow-up. Finally, when you choose your test date, be sure you have 6 hours available (the maximum length of the test). You will receive a confirmation of your appointment (date and time) and directions to the test center you registered for.

If you need to change your appointment for any reason, you must make the change online or call the test center at least 24 hours (1 full business day) in advance. If you do not arrive for a scheduled appointment or have a late cancellation, your ATT is invalidated and you forfeit the testing fee. The BON is notified to provide you with a new ATT, and you must register and pay for the test a second time.

EXAM DAY: WHAT TO EXPECT

Getting to the Test Center

Before the day of your appointment, take a test drive to the test center to become familiar with the route and parking availability. Do this at the same time of day you will be driving to your exam, to give you an idea of traffic conditions and road construction or other delays that may occur at that time of day.

Be sure to arrive at the test center at least 30 minutes prior to your appointment. If you are late, you may have to forfeit your appointment and reschedule it at a later date for an additional fee. The test service will report to the appropriate Board of Nursing any candidate who does not test on the date and time scheduled (due to late arrival or absence). Do not bring textbooks or other study materials into the test center; these are prohibited and could lead to dismissal from the test center or cancellation of your results.

Test Center Procedures

On arrival, you must present your ATT and valid identification (government-issued, nonexpired, and contains your name, photograph, and signature). Go to the NCSBN website (see References) for more detailed information. You will be photographed and provide a digital fingerprint and palm vein scan as additional identity protection measures.

A small storage locker will be provided for your use for personal belongings (such as coats, scarves, watches, large jewelry, and other accessories). All electronic devices must be placed in a Pearson VUE–provided sealable bag and stored in a locker. These may not be accessed at any time during the examination, including breaks. Any tampering with the bag could trigger an incident report and your test results could be cancelled. Do not bring books or study materials with you for the same reason. It may be helpful to bring a small snack and/or drink in case you need to take a break during the test, but you may not bring them into the actual testing area. If family or friends accompany you to the test center (not recommended), they cannot wait in the test center while you take the exam.

The test administrator (TA) will escort you to a computer terminal after completion of admission procedures and a short orientation. The TA will give you an erasable note board for your use during the test. It must remain in the room and will be collected after the test. All test sessions are audio- and videotaped. If you are distracted by noise from keyboards in adjacent computer terminals, raise your hand and ask for ear plugs. You also must raise your hand to notify the TA if you need additional note boards, have a problem with the computer, need a break, have completed the exam, or need the TA for any other reason.

The Actual NCLEX-RN® Examination

General Information and Pacing Yourself

The examination has a minimum of 75 questions and a maximum of 265 questions. Fifteen of the first 75 questions of the examination are being pretested (pilot-tested) and do not factor into a pass/fail decision. The exam may take up to 6 hours to complete. This includes time needed for a short tutorial, a preprogrammed optional break after 2 hours, a second preprogrammed optional break after 3.5 hours, and any unscheduled breaks that you choose. The computer alerts you when the preprogrammed breaks begin. If you take any break, you must leave the testing area; NCSBN strongly advises examinees not to leave the test center during breaks (NCSBN, 2015b). You will have your identity verified by fingerprint and palm vein scan upon readmission. All breaks count against your testing time. There is no minimum or maximum time that you must spend on each question, but maintaining a steady pace (1–2 minutes per question, and averaging about one question every 80 seconds) will help ensure that you do not run out of time. Note that this is just an average; you may be able to answer some questions more quickly, and some may take longer. It is most important to do the best you can with each question that appears on the screen. Remember that as long as the computer is generating questions, you are in a position to pass! Maintain concentration and give each question your full and thoughtful attention.

Some examinees worry they will select an incorrect answer accidentally during the exam, but this is an unnecessary concern. Once you select an answer, the computer requires you to click to confirm your answer before generating another question. Until you confirm, you are able to change your answer as many times as you wish. A word of caution here: It is far more common to change the correct answer to an incorrect one because of self-doubt than the reverse. Change answers thoughtfully and only for a good reason!

Pass or Fail Decisions

The exam will continue until a pass or fail decision is reached. Pass or fail decisions are governed by three scenarios:

- *95% Confidence Interval Rule.* This applies to most candidates; the exam ends when there is 95% certainty that your ability is clearly above or below the passing standard.
- *Maximum Length Exam.* The confidence rule is discarded and your final ability estimate is considered. If the final ability estimate is above the passing standard, you pass; if it is at or below the passing standard, you fail.
- *Run-Out-of-Time Rule (ROOT).* If you run out of time, alternate scoring criteria are used. If you did not answer the minimum number of questions, you fail. If the minimum number of questions are completed and your ability estimates for the last 60 questions are consistently above the passing standard, you pass. If your ability estimate falls to or below the passing standard even once over the last 60 questions, you fail (NCSBN, 2015c).

Finishing the Exam

Once your exam ends, a brief computer survey about the testing experience will appear on the screen. When you finish this survey, raise your hand; the TA will collect the note board(s) and escort you from the testing area.

GETTING THE RESULTS: WHAT NEXT?

You did it! You've taken the test, and you are probably both relieved and nervous at the same time. Your examination is scored twice (for quality control), once by computer at the test site and again after the examination record has been transmitted to Pearson VUE. Official results are mailed from the BON to candidates, often in about 4 weeks, but this may take longer in some jurisdictions.

In most states and jurisdictions, an unofficial report of your result may be obtained for a fee on the Pearson VUE website 48 business hours after the exam. Check the NCSBN website (see References) for a listing of states and jurisdictions that participate in this service. Note this service is not available for candidates being licensed in Canada. The unofficial results do not authorize you to practice as a registered nurse. Only the official results from the BON allow you to begin practice.

What if you did not pass? Maintain your inner resilience and determination! The BON will send you a Candidate Performance Report, indicating whether you scored above, near, or below the passing standard on each area of the test plan. This information will be useful in formulating a study plan before retesting. Enlist the aid of former faculty or talk to a trusted mentor (who is familiar with the NCLEX-RN® exam) to help you develop this plan. Some excellent practicing nurses did not pass on the first try, so stay focused on your goal.

How long will you have to wait to retest? The NCSBN allows retakes 45 days after the previous exam, but individual jurisdictions (states) can require a longer wait period, such as 90 days. Check with your BON as needed to verify the retake policy.

References

Anderson, L., & Krathwohl, D. (Eds.). (2001). *A taxonomy for learning, teaching, and assessing. A revision of Bloom's taxonomy of educational objectives.* New York, NY: Addison-Wesley Longman.

National Council of State Boards of Nursing. (2015a). *2014 RN practice analysis: Linking the NCLEX-RN® Examination to practice. U.S. and Canada.* Chicago: Author.

National Council of State Boards of Nursing. (2015b). *2016 NCLEX® Examination Candidate Bulletin.* Chicago: Author.

National Council of State Boards of Nursing. (2015c). *NCLEX-RN® Examination: Detailed test plan for the National Council Licensure Examination for Registered Nurses. Item Writer/Item Reviewer/Nurse Educator Version.* Chicago: Author.

National Council of State Boards of Nursing, Inc. Website: http://www.ncsbn.org

Pearson VUE. NCLEX® Candidate website: http://www.pearsonvue.com/nclex

Test Yourself

Are you ready for the NCLEX-RN® or course exams? Access the NEW web-based app that provides students with thousands of practice questions in preparation for the NCLEX experience.

Test Preparation and Test-Taking Strategies 2

In this chapter

By successfully passing the courses in your nursing program, you have already shown that you have acquired a set of test-taking skills. Some of you may say, "Yes, that's true for me," while others may say, "Well, I did pass, but I tend to struggle with tests. I'm not looking forward to the NCLEX-RN® exam!" This chapter helps you use the test-taking skills you currently have and build on them to increase your success on the NCLEX-RN® licensing examination.

PHYSICAL AND PSYCHOLOGICAL PREPARATION FOR TEST TAKING

Many nurses say that life during nursing school was a constant balancing act—juggling school schedules, study times, work responsibilities, and family and personal needs. However, life after graduation but prior to licensure does not automatically get simpler. The school schedule is gone, but work schedules, study time, and family and personal needs are still part of your life.

One critical difference, though, is that you have graduated! You have demonstrated you have what it takes, and you must now focus on your final preparation for the licensing exam. A critical step in your preparation is to focus on physical and mental self-care. Physical self-care means focusing on diet, rest and sleep, and exercise. Mental self-care is fostered by creating a schedule in which you spend the right amount of energy at the right times doing the right things.

Diet

It's easy to give lip service to good nutrition, but it's another thing to follow through. Take time now to pay attention to what you eat and how you plan meals. Get back to the basics of eating regular, balanced meals and nutritious snacks. Three small, light, and nutrient-packed meals are much better than one large meal at the end of the day (when you're famished and more likely to eat almost anything). Choose low-fat and low-calorie snacks. Make sure you have enough whole grains and fiber, and drink six to eight glasses of water per day. Cut back on caffeine and drinks with sugar, and keep alcohol intake low. Even after a few days, you should feel a difference in both your energy level and your ability to focus.

Rest and Sleep

This is another area that probably got short-changed during nursing school. Most people know how many hours of sleep they need to feel rested, usually between 6 and 8 hours per night. Find out what is right for you, and get the sleep you need. Again, you will quickly reap the rewards of increased stamina, energy, and ability to concentrate.

Exercise and Diversional Activity

Most people have some form of physical activity or exercise that they enjoy. Exercise is not only good for the body, it's a stress reliever as well. Pick an activity that you enjoy (aerobic is great!) and do it regularly. Aerobic exercise will increase your energy, provide a break from studying, and generally benefit your overall health. If you don't like vigorous exercise, try walking. It's healthy and can be adjusted to any time and distance, depending on the schedule of your day.

Sometimes we all need mental relaxation, which is where diversional activities come into play. As you prepare for the licensing exam, take time to see a movie, go out to eat, visit with friends, or do something else that is fun and makes you happy. This gives you a mental as well as a physical break from studying. Again, when you don't feel short-changed in another area of your life, you are more likely to focus better during your study time.

GENERAL STUDY AND PREPARATION TIPS

The Importance of Self-Assessment

There are two areas of self-assessment that will help you succeed on the NCLEX-RN® licensing examination. The first is to understand your preferred learning style(s), and the second is to understand your relative strengths and areas of the test plan that need further development before you take the examination.

How Do You Learn Best?

The literature abounds with research about various learning styles, but this discussion focuses on how you use your senses for learning. If you are a visual learner (i.e., you learn best by seeing things), then form a mental picture of what you are studying or the scenario presented in the test question. Look carefully at pictures and diagrams. You may also enjoy reviewing materials on videotape. If you are an auditory learner, then use audiotapes, an MP3 player, or read material out loud as you do your review. Keep in mind, though, that you will not be able to read questions aloud during the exam. If you are a kinesthetic learner, then you learn best by doing. You might find it helpful to write things down as you study. For example, you might make flash cards with hard-to-remember facts. The act of writing may help you to retain the information better. The flash cards will also be handy to review when you have unexpected spare minutes in your schedule.

What Are Your Relative Strengths and Weaknesses?

Before you make a formal plan for NCLEX-RN® examination preparation, take a few minutes for an honest appraisal of your areas of relative strength. Write down in order from lowest to highest your nursing content areas of strength. Examples are maternity, child health, psychiatric–mental health, medical surgical, and leadership. If you took any standardized tests that provided results according to the Client Needs subcategory of the NCLEX-RN® Test Plan (National Council of State Boards of Nursing, 2015), write down the *Client Needs* areas from lowest score to highest score. An example might be *Pharmacological and Parenteral Therapies*, *Reduction of Risk Potential*, *Health Promotion and Maintenance*, *Psychosocial Integrity*, *Physiological Adaptation*, *Basic Care and Comfort*, *Management of Care*, and *Safety and Infection Control*. This information will form the basis for a formal study plan.

Develop a Study Plan

To make an effective study plan, first determine a target date for testing. Then calculate the number of weeks you have for preparation. Many students take anywhere from 4 to 8 weeks to prepare, but this varies depending on personal ability, perceived need for study, and availability of appointments near the target test date.

Create a calendar for those weeks that you plan to study. Block off one day per week that you will *not* devote at all to exam preparation. This will help ensure you keep that mental balance we discussed. Next, block off work schedules, appointments, and other commitments you may have. The holes remaining in your calendar are the times that you have available for review and study. Plan to review approximately 2 hours per day or longer if you have the stamina and feel that you need the extra time. Actual preparation time may vary widely among graduates.

Map out what areas you will review each week according to the lists you developed. Write into the calendar the areas to review, beginning with the areas in which you scored lowest and spacing the material out over the weeks you have available. Allow more time to review weaker areas, and less time for areas of identified strength. This will allow you to concentrate your efforts most on areas that need development, and if you run short on time, your areas of strength are the ones that have the least review.

Use this book to guide your review. This book was specifically designed to help you understand how the content blocks that you learned in school fit into the structure of *Client Needs* in the NCLEX-RN® Test Plan. On average, you should spend approximately one-third of your time initially reviewing content in the various chapters, with the other two-thirds of the time devoted to answering questions. For areas that are more difficult, it may be closer to half and half for review and questions. As a rule, do not use class notes or reread your textbooks. Refer back to them only to clarify residual areas of confusion or difficulty. Carefully read the answer rationales as well as the test-taking strategies to increase your retention and fine-tune your test-taking abilities. As you progress, you will spend less time on review and more on questions. Try to plan your review sessions for hours that you are normally alert.

Practice tests will also be an important part of your preparation. These are best scheduled on your days off when you have additional study time. In nursing school, your average tests were probably 50–100 questions in length. For the NCLEX-RN® exam, you may need to answer up to 265 questions. Because you can pass the exam answering the maximum number of questions, it is important to maintain your stamina to answer each question well. To build your test-taking concentration and endurance, integrate a comprehensive review test once per week into your plan, increasing the number of questions each time. Try to work your way from 100 to 125, then to 150, and so on. Try to answer 265 consecutive questions at least once or twice before your test date. Tests you took in nursing school prepared you to "sprint to the bus stop," but the licensing exam might be more like "running a marathon." You need to be able to stay strong and concentrate through the whole test. Be ready to go the distance! A sample calendar for exam preparation over a 6-week period of time might look like the plan outlined in Table 2–1.

Table 2–1 Sample 6-Week Exam Preparation Calendar

Sunday	Monday	Tuesday	Wednesday	Thursday	Friday	Saturday
6/5 Relax	6/6 (Work) Pharm	6/7 Pharm	6/8 (Work) Pharm	6/9 (Work) Pharm	6/10 (Work) Pharm	6/11 Pharm
6/12 Relax	6/13 (Work) Management of Care	6/14 (Work) Management of Care	6/15 Management of Care	6/16 (Work) Management of Care	6/17 (Work) Management of Care	6/18 Wedding
6/19 Relax	6/20 (Work) Health Promotion and Maintenance	6/21 (Work) Health Promotion and Maintenance	6/22 (Work) Health Promotion and Maintenance	6/23 (Work) Birthday party in evening!	6/24 Basic Care and Comfort	6/25 Basic Care and Comfort
6/26 Relax	6/27 (Work) Safety and Infection Control	6/28 (Work) Safety and Infection Control	6/29 Reduction of Risk Potential	6/30 (Work) Reduction of Risk Potential	7/1 (Work) Reduction of Risk Potential	7/2 (Work) Psych
7/3 Relax	7/4 (Work) Psych	7/5 Physiological Adaptation	7/6 (Work) Physiological Adaptation	7/7 (Work) Physiological Adaptation	7/8 (Work) Physiological Adaptation	7/9 Physiological Adaptation
7/10 Relax	7/11 (Work) 150-question comprehensive test and review wrong answers	7/12 (Work) 200-question comprehensive test and review wrong answers	7/13 (Work) 265-question comprehensive test and review wrong answers	7/14 Relax; no review!	7/15 NCLEX-RN exam date	7/16 Relax and celebrate

Comprehensive = all test plan areas; Pharm = Pharmacological and Parenteral Therapies; Psych = Psychosocial Integrity

Create a Study Environment

Find a household area that is relatively free of foot traffic and distractions such as television, music, and the like. Set this area up as your temporary study center. Turn off the telephone and cell phone if you need to. Also turn off other programs on your computer to avoid the distractions of social media and computer pop-ups.

Before you begin a review session, make sure you have created an optimal "internal" study environment as well. Make sure you are not hungry or thirsty. Take a few minutes to relax and take a deep breath to clear your mind; this will help you gather your attention for the task at hand and erase any issues that you cannot deal with right now. Get focused and go to work! Plan to take a 10-minute break after each 50–60 minutes of concentrated review. This will serve both as a reward and as an incentive to go back to studying.

Stick to the Plan and What to Do When You Don't

Try hard to stick to your plan. If you get behind, it's not the end of the world, but review your calendar to analyze the problem. Was the calendar unrealistic, or did you not follow it? Rearrange your calendar as needed. If procrastination is the problem, implement measures you have used in the past when this has become a problem. Remember, this period of time is an investment in yourself; do not use it poorly or throw it away! If you get very far behind, consider whether rescheduling the test is in your best interest.

TEST-TAKING STRATEGIES

Read the Entire Question but Only the Question

Every test question contains all the information you need to know to answer the question. Each question contains three parts:

- The first part presents case-related information about the client in a few sentences or less.
- The second part asks you a specific question about the case provided; these first two parts may be collectively called the question stem, although technically the second part is the stem.

- The third part consists of the answer options. In a standard multiple-choice question there are four options labeled 1 through 4, and you must select one as the answer. In an alternate-format question the third part may require typing in numbers, clicking on a diagram, arranging priorities, or selecting more than one option.

Read every word in the question, one at a time. Do not speed-read the question, and do not read into the question anything that is not there. It is easy to read into questions based on your personal experience or the experience of others. Resist the urge to choose your answer based on specific real-world experiences. This exam represents the ideal world, and the case situation in the question may or may not closely resemble the one with which you have experience. For each question you answer, remember the client in the question is your only client and you have all the supplies and materials you need to deliver care.

Reinterpret the Question to Identify the Core Issue

After you read the question stem but before you read the options, take a moment to reword the question in your head to help you identify the core issue of the question. The core issue is the specific skill, ability, or point of knowledge that is needed to make the correct answer selection. Identifying the core issue may prevent you from choosing incorrect options (called distracters). See Box 2–1 for an example of a reworded stem.

Focus on the Client in the Question

In most questions, the actual client presented is the subject of the question, but sometimes the question focuses on a significant other, family member or friend, or even another health team member. As you read each question, deliberately determine who is the real client in the question, and choose the option that helps you to answer accordingly.

Find Critical Words in the Question

Critical words in the question help you to discriminate what you need to focus on while answering the question because they put the question into a specific context. The critical words may relate to time, probability, and priority setting (or sequencing of actions), as shown in Box 2–2. Notice these words as you read because they will help you to eliminate options that are incorrect answer choices.

Box 2–1

The Core Issue of the Question

Sample question stem:
A 39-year-old female client is scheduled for discharge following right mastectomy with breast reconstruction. The nurse places highest priority on teaching the client which point before discharge?

Sample reworded question stem:
What is the most important client teaching point for a client going home after mastectomy and breast reconstruction?

Box 2–2

Examples of Critical Words in a Question

Time: early, late, the day before, the day of, the day after, just prior to, immediately following, 1 hour after (or *x* hours after)

Probability: most likely, least likely, at highest risk, at lowest risk

Priority setting (or sequencing): best, essential, initial, primary, first, last, immediately, highest (or lowest) priority, most (or least) appropriate

Be Alert for Words That Are Red Flags

We do not live in an all-or-nothing world, and nursing practice is not an all-or-nothing endeavor. Watch for words that oversimplify the decision-making process in nursing practice. Examples of these words are *all*, *every*, *none*, *never*, *always*, *cannot*, *must not*, and *only*. You may recognize these words more quickly and easily as you practice answering questions.

On the other hand, words that are not so extreme could indicate the option is correct. Options that contain words such as *often*, *usually*, *likely to*, and *probably* warrant closer examination because they could be part of a correct choice.

Identify Positive and Negative Words in Question Stems

Positive or negative words in the question stem help you decide whether to choose an option that is a true statement or one that is a false statement as it relates to the case situation. Many questions on the exam will be worded in the affirmative; fewer will use negative words. Consider the following examples, which ask about an identical core issue (discharge teaching information following tonsillectomy) but use positive and negative words that lead to entirely different answers:

- Positive: A 10-year-old child is being discharged to home following tonsillectomy. The nurse determines that the child's caregiver *understands* discharge teaching points after the caregiver makes which statement?

- Negative: A 10-year-old child is being discharged to home following tonsillectomy. The nurse determines that the child's caregiver *needs further instruction* related to discharge teaching after the caregiver makes which statement?

In the first example, the correct answer would be an option that is a true statement about a point of discharge teaching, while in the second, the correct answer would contain a false statement. Note how easy it could be to make an incorrect choice by missing the negative words "needs further instruction." Note also that the real client in this question is the child's caregiver, not the child who had surgery.

Eliminate Incorrect Options (Distracters)

Whenever you decide that an option is incorrect, immediately eliminate it as an answer choice. For some questions, you will easily recognize one or more options as distracters and eliminate them as possible choices. Each time you eliminate a distracter, you increase the probability of ultimately choosing the correct answer. For example, if you don't know an answer and randomly choose among four options, you have a 25% chance of answering correctly. If you can eliminate one (leaving three to choose from), your odds of success increase to 33%. If you can eliminate two distracters, you now have a 50% chance of making the correct choice. On the NCLEX-RN® exam, however, it is likely that more than one option or all of them may seem to be correct, so read on to the next section for more test-taking strategies.

Carefully Examine Options with Similarities

If you read a question to which you do not know the answer, look for similarities either between the stem and one option or between two of the options. Some possibilities are outlined below, with suggestions to guide your thought process.

Similarities between the Stem and an Option

If the stem of the question and one of the options contain a similar idea, action, word, or emotion, then that option could be the correct answer. Consider this option carefully as you read all the options and prepare to make a selection.

Similarities between Two or More Options in Standard Multiple Choice Questions

This could be a little trickier. If two or more options seem to have a similar idea, action, or response, examine them carefully. If they essentially say the same thing but use different words, then they cannot be correct and you must eliminate them both (or all). If, however, they seem to say similar things but one option is more encompassing or global than the other(s), the more encompassing option may be the correct answer. Recognize the encompassing option because it contains the main thought of the other option plus some others within it. Reread the question and all viable choices to determine if this should be your selection. Examples of topics to which this strategy could apply are communication processes, interdisciplinary care, or taking action in an emergency.

Recognize the Need to Prioritize

This is a very important test-taking strategy. Because many questions are written at the *analyzing* level of difficulty, expect to get a reasonable number of questions in which all of the options are technically correct actions or responses. You must decide what is the *best* action or response for that client and situation. Questions such as these require you to engage in priority setting. Universal strategies for prioritizing in nursing are outlined in the following sections.

Maslow's Hierarchy of Needs

Examine the question and analyze whether Maslow's hierarchy of needs theory applies. When Maslow's hierarchy seems relevant to a question, recall that physiological needs (air/oxygen, water, food, sleep) come first, followed by safety needs. Secondary or psychosocial needs are addressed only after physiological and safety needs are met.

The ABCs: Airway, Breathing, and Circulation

This strategy is very straightforward. Airway takes priority, followed by breathing and then circulation. Remember that oxygen saturation could refer to either airway or breathing and that hypovolemia and hemorrhage relate to circulation. You must know the one exception to ABCs. During cardiopulmonary resuscitation, the sequence changes to CAB (compressions, airway, breathing).

Least Stable or Most at Risk for Complications

When choosing between which client to visit, assess, or care for first, remember that the correct answer is most likely to be the client who is the least stable of all clients presented or, if all are stable, then the one who is most at risk for developing a serious complication. These questions can be difficult to answer. To make the correct choice for such a question, you must understand a variety of client health problems and their significance, and you must understand principles of clinical decision making or triage. For this reason, it is very important to review pathophysiology, nursing management, and client education for a wide variety of health problems.

Time/Scheduling

For some questions, priority setting may be guided by events that are time-bound. In questions that involve clients who have specific discharge times or have immediate preoperative or preprocedure status, consider whether the core issue of the question is caring for this client before other stable clients, using time as the priority.

What Can and Cannot Be Delegated

Some nursing activities cannot be delegated to other caregivers, such as licensed practical or vocational nurses (LPNs or LVNs) or unlicensed assistive personnel (UAPs)/unregulated care providers (UCPs). Priorities of care for the registered nurse (RN) include client education and all aspects of the nursing process except implementation. Examples of activities that can be delegated include carrying out simple procedures and making routine observations. Consider these principles when deciding priorities of care as they relate to delegation.

Use the Nursing Process Effectively

Assessment

Since assessment is the first step of the nursing process, consider whether the correct answer is focused on assessment. In general, when questions ask for your first nursing action, look to see how much data is presented in the case situation. If there is no data or just a single piece of data, the correct option is more likely to be one that gathers more subjective or objective assessment data. If, on the other hand, you have a complete set of data presented to you, an option that reflects further assessment or assessment of a low-priority item is not as likely to be correct.

Analysis

Analysis questions require critical thinking and clinical decision-making skills. These questions present physiological or psychosocial data in the case situation and ask you to interpret the information so you can take action based on the data or respond in some other therapeutic way. You need to be able to draw correct conclusions from the data in order to select the correct answer. Analysis questions are often difficult because they require interpretation of multiple pieces of data.

Planning

The planning step of the nursing process involves developing a plan of care, setting goals and/or establishing outcomes, and determining priorities of care. Actual problems are addressed before potential problems. Because the plan must be communicated to others on the healthcare team, these questions may also involve interdisciplinary communication and collaboration.

Implementation

Questions that address the implementation step of the nursing process are action-oriented. They may require you to do the following:

- Supervise and delegate care
- Manage care
- Carry out interventions
- Teach clients and families
- Provide counseling
- Communicate with clients, families, and interdisciplinary team members
- Document the outcomes of care

These types of questions are also often combined with priority setting, so again you need to use clinical decision-making skills in selecting an option.

Evaluation

Questions that address this step of the nursing process require you to determine whether a client has met the expected outcomes of care. They may require you to determine the following:

- Whether the client has adequate knowledge of the underlying health problem
- Whether the plan of care has been effective
- Whether a client has achieved the goals of care (returned to normal status or client's baseline)
- Whether revisions to the plan of care are necessary
- Whether a client or family member understands postdischarge care (diet, activity, medications, and follow-up care)
- Whether a health team member is performing care correctly

Because evaluation questions involve clinical judgment and decision making, they are also more likely to be written at an *analyzing* rather than an *applying* level of difficulty.

Strategies for Subsections of the Test Plan

Although there are many ways to write questions to address each part of the test plan, certain types of questions seem to align naturally with specific *Client Needs*. The types of questions that have such alignments involve use of communication, scientific principles, and pharmacology.

Communication

Questions addressing communication have a natural affinity for the *Psychosocial Integrity* category of *Client Needs*. These questions require you to apply therapeutic communication skills. The correct answer will contain the most therapeutic statement, focus on the client's feelings, and/or assist the client to work toward therapeutic goals. Although communication strategies and communication blocks were part of your foundational nursing coursework, they warrant review and practice. Questions related to communication may have several options that seem similar in some ways, but different in others. You must be able to choose which one is *most* therapeutic.

Scientific Principles

The use of everyday scientific principles is an all but unheard-of strategy for answering test questions. Yet, scientific principles play a key role in assisting you to answer some questions written to address the *Physiological Integrity* category of *Client Needs*. Consider, for example, how gravity may affect your answers to questions about positioning clients, troubleshooting IV flow rate problems, and monitoring various tubes and drains. Consider how concepts of pressure affect your answers to questions about flail chest, mechanical ventilation, intracranial pressure, the Valsalva maneuver, or stopping bleeding. If you visualize answer options in terms of how they are affected by pressure, you may be able to eliminate one or more of them.

Pharmacology

When answering questions related to pharmacology, look at the generic name provided. If you recognize the drug, use your knowledge about it to answer the question. If not, try next to determine what classification the medication belongs to by looking at the syllables in the name. For example, a medication that ends in *-mycin* is either an antibacterial agent or antitumor antibiotic. If you cannot determine the classification, try to look for hints in the case situation, such as the client's diagnosis. If these strategies do not work, look for other words in the question that provide clues. Discriminate among drug side effects, adverse effects, and toxic effects. Learn these effects for common medication classifications to answer pharmacology questions more easily.

Read the Memory Aid boxes contained in the pharmacology chapters in this book to learn common prefixes and suffixes that will help you recognize drugs more easily on sight. Also use general principles of medication administration, such as:

- Administer medications in the prescribed doses without changing the dose or discontinuing the medication; you *may* need to withhold a single dose for a specific reason, such as withholding digoxin for a pulse rate of 48, or withholding metoprolol for a blood pressure less than 90 systolic.
- Question a medication prescription if any part is missing or unclear, or is outside the safe dose range.
- Do not crush or break a sustained-release medication and do not allow the client to chew it.
- Do not take over-the-counter or herbal medications concurrently with a prescribed medication without checking with the prescriber first.
- Teach clients that taking an antacid with another medication may negatively affect absorption of that medication.
- Teach clients to avoid drinking alcohol while taking medications.

References

Katz, J., Carter, C., Kravits, S., Bishop, J., & Block, J. (2010). *Keys to nursing success* (3rd ed.). Upper Saddle River, NJ: Prentice Hall.

National Council of State Boards of Nursing. (2015). *NCLEX-RN® Examination: Detailed test plan for the National Council Licensure Examination for Registered Nurses. Item Writer/Item Reviewer/Nurse Educator Version.* Chicago: Author.

3 Test Preparation for Internationally Educated Nurses

In this chapter

Despite being an experienced practicing nurse in your home country, seeking licensure as a registered nurse in the United States is likely to be a new and unfamiliar process. There are two major areas on which to focus. The first is meeting the eligibility criteria for licensure in the United States. The second relates to preparing for and passing the NCLEX-RN® Licensing Examination. This chapter explores your unique concerns and explains how this book can assist you in preparing for the NCLEX-RN® exam.

ELIGIBILITY FOR LICENSURE

The National Council of State Boards of Nursing (NCSBN) has developed Uniform Licensure Requirements (URLs) that apply across every NCSBN jurisdiction. These requirements were developed to provide consistent standards for licensure across the U.S. states and territories. Beyond this, the Boards of Nursing (BONs) for individual states or territories do have variations in their requirements for licensure for internationally educated nurses. NCSBN does not maintain a list of these variations. Because of this, your first step should be to contact the BON from which you wish to seek licensure. You can do this efficiently by visiting the NCSBN website (see References), select the Boards and Regulation tab, and select Contact a Board of Nursing. Identify to the BON that you were educated outside of the United States and request an application for licensure and information about documents needed to determine your eligibility for licensure. Individual BONs may choose to either evaluate these documents themselves (in-house evaluation) or use the services of a credentialing agency, such as the Commission on Graduates of Foreign Nursing Schools (CGFNS). In general, these documents will include:

- Verification of graduation from a nursing program that is comparable to a program in the United States
- Official full academic transcripts
- Verification of licensure status in your country of origin
- Proof of English language proficiency
- Proof of citizenship or lawful alien status
- Criminal background check
- Photograph
- VisaScreen® certificate (a federal government screening program required to obtain an occupational [work] visa)
- Work visa; obtained from U.S. Citizenship and Immigration Services or services such as Immigration Direct (see References)

Official documents such as educational and licensure records should be sent directly from the appropriate agency in your home country. Once you are notified about eligibility for licensure, complete the licensure application and submit it to the BON with the appropriate fee. When you receive authorization to take the NCLEX-RN® exam, follow the procedures outlined in Chapter 1 of this book and the *Examination Candidate Bulletin* (NCSBN, 2015), available online from NCSBN.

NURSING IN THE UNITED STATES

Depending on the country in which you work as a nurse, your current nursing practice may be similar to or different from nursing practice in the United States. This section briefly highlights a few areas of practice that might be different from country to country.

Scope of Nursing Practice

Nurses belong to a profession that self-regulates its practice through a variety of nursing organizations and boards of nursing. There are well-defined standards of professional nursing practice for all areas of nursing. Nurses have a high level of accountability for their nursing practice.

Nurses meet the individualized needs of each patient or client. These needs may relate to physical care and monitoring or psychosocial support. Nurses must also know about the client's health problems and teach clients and their families how to manage these problems at home.

Nurses have an important voice as members of the healthcare team. Nurses routinely communicate with each other and with nursing supervisors, physicians, pharmacists, nutritionists and dietitians, respiratory therapists, physical and occupational therapists, social workers, and unlicensed assistive personnel. Communication is direct but respectful and includes acting as an advocate for the client if health needs are not being met by the current plan of care.

Nurses play a key role in helping clients to stay healthy, not just helping them to recover from disease, illness, or injury. Thus, health promotion (which commonly involves teaching) is also an important part of nursing practice.

Nurses are responsible for their own professional growth and seek opportunities to further their knowledge of nursing as it advances as a discipline through research. Nurses read books and journal articles, attend conferences, and use the Internet to help them to remain current in their nursing knowledge.

Working with a Variety of Cultures

Nurses work with people from many cultures. Part of the nurse's role is to deliver culturally relevant care. This means not only respecting the culture of various clients but also understanding some of their key beliefs and changing the plan of care to accommodate culturally based customs and rituals when possible. Aspects of one's personal culture that tend to influence health include the amount of control one has over one's environment, physical and genetic differences, social environment, communication patterns, need for space, and orientation to time (Giger, 2017). See Chapter 19 in this book for more information about delivering culturally relevant care.

Therapeutic Communication

One of the key tools used by nurses is communication. The special type of communication used in working with clients is called *therapeutic communication*. Nurses in the United States use eye contact while communicating with clients, which may be similar to or different from the practice in your home country. Facial expressions and body language are also used to enhance the client's understanding of communication.

Communication between nurses and clients is client-centered and relates to the steps of the nursing process. The focus may be on obtaining health information from clients (assessment), goal setting with clients about their care and its outcomes (planning), discussing how clients are experiencing or reacting to their care (implementation), or determining how effective the care was (evaluation). See Chapter 18 for more detailed information about therapeutic communication.

Pharmacology

Pharmacology may present special concerns for internationally educated nurses. The names of medications differ somewhat from country to country. In the United States, nurses must possess significant knowledge about client medications, how to safely administer them, and how to recognize and intervene if drug interactions or adverse effects occur. Nurses also teach clients about their medications and how to self-administer them. The body of knowledge for pharmacology is so large and keeps growing. See Chapters 29–45 for a review of pharmacology.

PREPARING FOR THE LICENSING EXAMINATION

The examination that you took to obtain your original nursing license may have been very different than the computerized adaptive test (CAT) used in the United States and Canada. If you are not familiar with this testing format, read Chapters 1 and 2 carefully. The NCLEX-RN® exam is difficult. The chapters of this book provide a thorough review of content that may be tested on the exam. Practice answering multiple-choice and alternate-item format questions to become comfortable with this type of testing. This book and the accompanying online resources provide you with over 5000 practice questions. Use all of the tips and strategies presented in this book.

Work with a mentor, if you have one, to help you succeed in the shortest possible time. Stay positive and focused on your goal, and continue to believe in yourself. I wish you great success in your pursuit of RN licensure in the United States.

References

CGFNS,, Inc. Commission on Graduates of Foreign Nursing Schools. Website: http://www.cgfns.org

Giger, J. (2017). *Transcultural nursing* (7th ed.). St. Louis, MO: Elsevier.

Immigration Direct website (www.immigrationdirect.com)

National Council of State Boards of Nursing. (2015). *2016 NCLEX® Examination Candidate Bulletin*. Chicago: Author.

National Council of State Boards of Nursing, Inc. Website: http://www.ncsbn.org

U.S. Citizenship and Immigration Services. Website: http://www.uscis.gov

Test Yourself

Are you ready for the NCLEX-RN® or course exams? Access the NEW web-based app that provides students with thousands of practice questions in preparation for the NCLEX experience.

Legal and Ethical Nursing Practice 4

In this chapter

Cross Reference

Other chapters relevant to this content area are

Nursing Leadership and Management **Chapter 5**

I. ETHICS, MORALS, AND VALUES

A. *Ethics*

1. A term with several meanings: method of inquiry about morality of human behavior, practices or beliefs of groups such as nurses or physicians (nursing or medical ethics), or expected standards of moral behavior defined in a group's code of professional ethics

NCLEX®

2. Professional codes of nursing ethics provide broad principles that guide nursing practice; they are not legally binding, although violation of ethical standards in some jurisdictions may result in a reprimand for unprofessional conduct by a board of nursing
   a. American Nurses Association (ANA) **Code of Ethics for Nurses** (see References)
   b. Canadian Nurses Association (CNA) Code of Ethics for Registered Nurses (see References)
   c. International Council of Nurses (ICN) Code of Ethics for Nurses (see References)

B. **Morals**

1. Private, personal standards of what is right or wrong in conduct, character, and attitude; usually incorporate personal or religious beliefs
2. Applying ethics is a practical way of putting morals into practice; it aids decision making and problem solving in nursing practice

C. **Values**

1. Enduring beliefs or attitudes about the worth of a person, idea, action, or object; personally and professionally developed
2. Organized into value systems, which define actions and reactions to issues and problems
3. Provide guidance in determining actions, especially actions that are based on decisions or choices

II. ETHICAL PRINCIPLES AND DECISION MAKING

NCLEX® A. **Ethical principles (see Table 4–1)**

Memory Aid

All interactions, even ordinary ones, between client and nurse utilize principles of ethical behavior. Learn these principles to be able to engage in effective decision making as a nursing professional.

Table 4–1 Ethical Principles Important in Nursing

Ethical Principle	Meaning
Autonomy	To respect a client's right to self-determination (making free and informed choices about own life)
Nonmaleficence	To do no harm, either intentional or unintentional
Beneficence	To do good to others; involves weighing risks and benefits of actions; includes client advocacy; a threat to beneficence is paternalism, in which healthcare providers make choices for clients without their input
Justice	Fair, equitable, and appropriate treatment; resources are distributed equally to all
Fidelity	Remaining faithful to ethical principles and professional Code of Ethics for Nurses; keeping commitments and promises
Veracity	To tell the truth, which has an added benefit of promoting trust between client and nurse
Accountability	Being answerable to self and others for own actions; includes responsibility, a specific type of **accountability** for duties performed in a specific role

B. Ethical decision making

1. Nursing is based on ethics of care, including medical indications, client preferences, quality of life, and contextual factors
2. Differences in clients' values, culture, and lifestyles may present healthcare providers with **ethical dilemmas** (situations in which ethical principles conflict) and a choice must be made between unsatisfactory alternatives
3. Ethics committees in healthcare agencies assist healthcare professionals to engage in group dialogue about specific client situations and develop policies and procedures aimed at preventing and resolving dilemmas as they arise

III. LEGAL PARAMETERS OF NURSING PRACTICE

A. Overview

1. Practice of nursing must be done within confines of law; nurses must know law and parameters of nursing license
2. *NCLEX®* Legal limits of nursing are dictated by state (U.S.), province (Canada), and federal law; a board of nursing in each state or province is responsible for enforcing these regulations (see Table 4–2)

B. Health Information Portability and Accountability Act (HIPAA)

1. Describes how personal health information (PHI) can be used and how clients can access this information; PHI includes client identifiable information related to health, treatment, and payment for services rendered
2. Healthcare agencies must maintain privacy of PHI, inform client of legal responsibilities about privacy, and explain client rights about PHI (including making a written request to view PHI, amend inaccurate PHI, or restrict how certain PHI may be shared regarding treatment or payment, unless needed to provide emergency care)

C. Good Samaritan laws

1. Designed to protect those who aid victims in emergencies; statutes vary among states and provinces
2. Care rendered must be free of charge and done in good faith; will not protect nurse if there is gross negligence; once aid is offered, must stay with victim until stable or another provider with equal or greater training takes over

D. Licensure

1. Credential determined by board of nursing (BON) of a state or province; qualifies a person to perform designated skills and services; requires person to complete a nursing curriculum successfully and pass a licensing examination
2. *NCLEX®* **Nurse Practice Act** (NPA) determines scope of practice for a professional nurse in a specific jurisdiction (state or province)
   a. Establishes guidelines by which nurses can perform skills or services
   b. A set of statutes (rules and regulations) addressing educational, examination, and behavioral standards for nurses that protect public
   c. A BON is authorized by NPA to oversee its implementation, maintain licensure requirements, and take disciplinary action against individual nurses for violations of NPA

Table 4–2 Selected Types of Laws Affecting Nurses

Type of Law	Examples
Constitutional law	Due process, equal protection
Statutory laws (legislative)	Nurse Practice Acts, guardianship codes, informed consent, advance directives, abuse reporting, sexual harassment, Good Samaritan laws
Criminal law (public)	Homicide (murder or manslaughter), theft, assault, illegal possession of controlled substance, active euthanasia
Contract law (private or civil)	Contracts between nurse and client, nurse and employer, nurse and insurance, employer and union, and client and agency
Tort law (private or civil)	Negligence/malpractice, defamation (slander, libel), invasion of privacy, false imprisonment, assault and battery

E. Sanctions against nursing license

1. A jurisdiction's BON can deny, suspend, or revoke license to practice as registered nurse on basis of authority granted in statute of state or province

NCLEX® 2. Possible reasons for disciplinary action or sanction
   - a. Unprofessional conduct
   - b. Conduct that could negatively affect public health and welfare
   - c. Accepting and carrying out assignments incorrectly or with insufficient preparation
   - d. Physical or verbal abuse of client
   - e. Breach of confidentiality
   - f. Improper delegation of care that places client at risk for harm
   - g. Failure to maintain accurate client record or falsifying client record
   - h. Abandonment (leaving an assignment without proper notification and approval)
   - i. Failure to engage in continuing education activities as required by statute

IV. LIABILITY IN NURSING PRACTICE

A. Liability: nurses are responsible and accountable for incorrect or inappropriate actions or inactions

NCLEX® **B. *Negligence*:** taking actions that fail to maintain a standard of care and that result in injury to another; elements of proof include:

1. Duty: at time of injury, nurse had responsibility for care of client as a component of employment; indicates legal relationship between client and nurse
2. Breach of duty: nurse failed to complete duty; can include acts of commission (activities nurse did) or omission (activities nurse failed to do)
3. Harm: client sustained injury, damage, or harm (must document physical injury, medical costs, loss of wages, pain and suffering as examples)
4. Proximate cause: there is a reasonably close causal connection between nurse's conduct and resulting injury

C. *Malpractice*: negligence by a professional; professional failure to carry out or perform duties that result in injury to another; acting outside one's scope of practice

1. Boundaries of malpractice are defined by statute, rules, and educational requirement
2. Malpractice is usually filed as a civil tort; a court finding of guilty usually results in restitution
3. Nurses may carry personal malpractice insurance to provide for restitution if malpractice occurs
4. Rarely are malpractice charges filed as criminal charges (in which a guilty verdict results in punishment, either jail or capital punishment)

D. Miscellaneous legal charges

1. Assault: threat of harm or unwanted contact with client that causes the client fear
2. Battery: a purposeful touching of client without that client's consent
3. Invasion of privacy: can result from violations of confidentiality
4. Fraud: deliberately deceiving client for purpose of unlawful gains
5. Defamation of character: sharing client information with a third party that results in damage to client's reputation; can occur in the form of slander (oral) or libel (in writing)
6. False imprisonment
   - a. Prohibiting a client from leaving a healthcare facility with no legal justification
   - b. Using chemical or physical restraints without satisfactory clinical evidence of need

NCLEX® **E. Nursing activities to reduce risk of liability**

1. Practice within provisions of NPA
2. Follow Code of Ethics for Nurses and standards of professional practice
3. Treat every client with kindness and respect
4. Maintain confidentiality by not sharing client information with a third party without client's consent; do not share chart or medical record information without written client consent and then do so only in accordance with agency policy; see also next item
5. Avoid violations of client privacy and HIPAA
   a. Protect client's personal identifying information (such as name, Social Security number, date of birth) and information about diagnosis or treatment
   b. Share information only with individuals involved directly in client's care, payment for care, and/or management of client's care
   c. Verify identity of persons asking for client information
   d. Dispose of confidential documents in accordance with agency policy (such as shredder, locked recycle bin)
   e. Keep contents of medical record (including computer screens showing electronic health record) out of public view
   f. Discuss client's care only in areas where conversation cannot be overheard
   g. Refrain from sharing client information or photographs of client, including on social networking sites
   h. Avoid situations that violate privacy (interviewing client in areas where conversation can be overheard, such as in an area that has only a curtain for separation; leaving door or curtain open during procedure; allowing others to observe treatment or procedure without client consent)
6. Document client assessments, interventions, and events factually and timely in medical record
7. Document on appropriate "against medical advice" forms when a competent client refuses care despite explanations about the benefits of that care
8. Maintain skills and knowledge base by completing continuing education programs
9. Recognize personal strengths and weaknesses; seek help when facing new experiences and job requirements

V. SAFEGUARDING CLIENT RIGHTS

A. Client rights

1. Patient's Bill of Rights communicates to clients and healthcare workers that clients are entitled to specific rights during care
2. Key rights include confidentiality (see previous discussion), informed consent, and others listed in following text that affect client self-determination

NCLEX® **B. Informed consent**

1. A legal protection of client's right to choose type of care desired and make own decisions about healthcare
2. A release (consent) is required before care is provided except in an emergency situation or when client is unresponsive (assumption is that client would consent if able); a client can withdraw consent at any time
3. Must meet specific requirements: client is of legal age (18 years or older) and has mental capacity to consent; consent is voluntarily given; and client understands information about treatment presented by provider
4. Information shared to obtain consent consists of condition requiring treatment, purpose of proposed treatment, procedure, surgery, or other care; associated risks and benefits; alternatives to treatment including their advantages and disadvantages; and name of provider performing surgery or procedure; client has opportunity to ask questions and hear answers
5. Obtaining informed consent is responsibility of healthcare provider performing treatment, procedure, or surgery
6. Nurses may witness signature of client on appropriate consent form validating that client is signing the form and has no further questions; does not indicate provision of information by nurse or understanding by client
7. Occasionally clients do not want to hear details of planned procedures but do wish to consent to them; clients may waive right to informed consent, but waiver must be documented in medical record
8. Special considerations in informed consent
   a. If client is declared incompetent to make informed decisions about healthcare, client's next of kin, durable power of attorney, or a court-appointed guardian has legal authority to make these decisions
   b. Informed consent for minors is obtained from parent or legal guardian except in emergency situations, when minor is married or emancipated from parents, or with special needs for care, such as with sexually transmitted infection or pregnancy

Memory Aid

The medical record of a hospitalized client could contain several consents: general admission consent for treatment, consent for surgery or other invasive procedure, consent for anesthesia, consent to receive blood products, consent for immunizations, consent to be a research participant, and special consents (such as photographs, disposal of body parts during surgery, and autopsy).

C. Privileged communication versus duty to disclose

1. Communications between clients and healthcare workers cannot be shared with others outside healthcare team (such as in court of law) unless client consents
2. Duty to disclose is healthcare professional's obligation to warn identified individuals if a client has made a credible threat to harm such individuals

NCLEX® **D. Advance directives**

1. Are authorized by Client Self-Determination Act; two common forms of advance directives are a living will or durable power of attorney for healthcare
   a. Living will outlines medical treatment client wishes to refuse or omit (e.g., intubation) if client becomes unable to make decisions
   b. Durable power of attorney for healthcare (healthcare proxy) identifies person (usually family or trusted friend) appointed by client to make healthcare decisions if client is unable to do so
   c. Some forms combine living will and durable healthcare power of attorney into one document, which is witnessed by two people or notarized
   d. A do-not-resuscitate (DNR) order is recorded by a healthcare provider when a client wishes to be allowed to die if respiratory or cardiac arrest occurs; protocols vary depending on jurisdiction; DNR orders must be clearly written (what treatments continue and what should not be initiated); they are reviewed regularly and communicated to all involved in client's care; if DNR status is not known, client must be resuscitated
2. Existence of an advance directive is questioned on admission to healthcare facility; a copy of existing advance directive or one completed at time of admission must be included in medical record
3. Healthcare provider is notified so that treatment is consistent with advance directive; all personnel should follow directive to safeguard against liability

NCLEX® **E. Organ/tissue donation**

1. Clients 18 years of age or older may choose to donate organs
2. Consent can be given through will, advance directive, or donor card
3. Decision can be made in advance when client is alive and competent or by family at time of death
4. All 50 states utilize Uniform Anatomical Gift Act to procure cadaver organs for transplant when there is either brain death (for heart, liver, or lungs) or clinical death (for several other organs and tissues)
5. Transplant considerations
   a. Bereaved family must be approached with compassion by defined personnel in requesting a discussion on organ donation
   b. Goal is to assist those in need of transplant with organ necessary to prolong life
   c. Brain death is defined as having no brain waves, no spontaneous breathing, and no superficial or deep reflexes; clinical death is cessation of all body functions, including brain activity, breathing, and heartbeat
   d. Transplant team recovers organs after consent is obtained; family does not incur additional costs because of organ donation

VI. SAFEGUARDING LEGAL PROFESSIONAL PRACTICE

A. Healthcare provider prescriptions

1. Include prescriptions for care such as medications, diet, activity, diagnostic and laboratory testing, and procedures or treatments
2. Nurses must legally carry out these prescriptions unless they are believed to be incorrect
3. Nurses are obligated to question or clarify prescriptions that are illegible, unclear, or possibly inappropriate or inaccurate
4. Nurses may be legally responsible for client harm sustained from implementing incorrect prescriptions

NCLEX® **B. Incident reports**

1. Each agency develops a policy or protocol for reporting accidents, unusual occurrences, or other incidents involving clients that are not in keeping with usual agency operation

2. Incident reports are communication tools that provide information to risk managers and administration about potential areas of exposure to liability; they may be used in legal cases
3. Incident reports are used to identify problems and develop solutions to prevent same incident from happening again
4. *NCLEX®* When completing an incident report, fill out form in accurate, complete, and factual manner; include client name and other identifying information, date/time/place of incident, facts (no opinions or conclusions), client's account of incident using quotation marks, witnesses, and, if applicable, equipment number or medication name and dosage
5. *NCLEX®* Do not place copy in client record or make reference to incident report in client record
6. *NCLEX®* Do record facts of incident in medical record

C. Risk management

1. A program designed to protect client and nurse from harm and protect organization from liability related to harm
2. A comprehensive risk management program includes organizational commitment to employee health and safety, a comprehensive worksite risk analysis, employee participation, and hazard prevention and control, including waste management

D. Reporting to external authorities or governing bodies

1. *NCLEX®* Nurses and healthcare providers are required to report specific communicable diseases to public health department
2. *NCLEX®* They are also required to report evidence of crimes (such as homicide, suicide, inflicted injury such as stab or gunshot wounds, and abuse) to appropriate authorities
3. *NCLEX®* Nurses need to confidentially report suspected chemical abuse by a co-worker to supervisor; administration will notify state board of nursing for investigation; priority issue in this type of case is treatment
4. Under protection of law, nurses as well as any other employee can report sexual harassment to supervisor or higher administration; consists of any unwelcome statements or behavior of a sexual nature
5. Unsafe working conditions can be reported confidentially under Occupational Safety and Health Act (OSHA) regulations; an employee cannot be retaliated against by employer for reporting unsafe working conditions

VII. SPECIAL ETHICAL AND LEGAL CONSIDERATIONS IN PSYCHIATRIC MENTAL HEALTH SETTINGS

A. Client autonomy and liberty

1. Must be ensured by treatment in least restrictive setting by active client participation in treatment
2. Voluntary admission occurs when a client consents to confinement in hospital and signs a document indicating as much
3. Commitment, or involuntary admission, may be done if client is a danger to self or others; some jurisdictions also have criterion of preventing significant physical or mental deterioration for involuntary admission

B. Competency

1. A legal determination that a client can make reasonable judgments and decisions about treatment and other significant areas of personal life
2. An adult is considered competent unless a *court* rules client incompetent; in such cases, a guardian is appointed to make decisions on client's behalf
3. Clients who are committed are still capable of participating in healthcare decisions

NCLEX® **C. Informed consent:** clients in mental health settings do not relinquish right to informed consent upon admission; may still accept or refuse specific aspects of treatment or care

D. Confidentiality: extremely important also in psychiatric mental health nursing

1. Federal rules apply to confidentiality regarding chemical dependence; staff cannot disclose admission or discharge information
2. Some states require written consent before human immunodeficiency virus (HIV) tests may be performed; states have laws regarding when HIV test results or diagnosis of acquired immunodeficiency syndrome (AIDS) may be disclosed; this occurs regardless of psychiatric or nonpsychiatric healthcare setting

Check Your NCLEX–RN® Exam I.Q.

You are ready for testing on this content if you can:

- Articulate ethical and legal issues in nursing practice that affect clients or families.
- Identify appropriate actions to promote ethical and legal nursing care.
- Evaluate the outcomes of interventions used to promote ethical and legal nursing care.
- Apply principles of confidentiality to client care situations.
- Identify actions to uphold client rights.
- Provide information to clients and families about advance directives.

PRACTICE TEST

PRACTICE TEST

1 A client is referred to a surgeon by the healthcare provider. After meeting the surgeon, the client decides to consult with a different surgeon about treatment options. The nurse supports the client's action, utilizing which ethical principle?

1. Beneficence
2. Veracity
3. Autonomy
4. Privacy

2 A nurse forgets to administer a dose of a client's diuretic drug and the client experiences an episode of pulmonary edema. The nurse should consider that this error constitutes negligence because the situation contains which element?

1. Purposeful failure to perform a healthcare procedure
2. Unintentional failure to perform a healthcare procedure
3. Act of substituting a different medication for the one prescribed
4. Failure to follow a healthcare provider's prescription

3 A client asks why a diagnostic test has been prescribed and the nurse replies, "I'm unsure but will find out for you." When the nurse later returns and provides an explanation, the nurse is acting under which principle?

1. Nonmaleficence
2. Veracity
3. Beneficence
4. Fidelity

fidelity = faithful to promises

4 An individual falls and fractures a hip while walking down the street. A companion notices a nurse drive past without stopping to assist. The individual sues the nurse for negligence but fails to win a judgment for which reason?

1. The nurse had no duty to the individual.
2. The nurse did what most nurses would do in the same circumstance.
3. The nurse did not cause the client's injuries.
4. The nurse was off-duty at that time.

5 A client who takes warfarin is given aspirin for a headache while visiting a neighbor, who is a nurse. The client subsequently has a bleeding episode caused by interaction of these drugs. The legal nurse consultant interprets which necessary elements of malpractice are missing from this case? Select all that apply.

1. Breach of duty
2. Duty owed
3. Injury experienced
4. Causation between nurse's action and injury
5. Intent to cause harm or injury

6 A client with cancer has decided to discontinue further treatment. Although the nurse would like the client to continue treatment, the nurse recognizes the client is competent and supports the client's decision using which ethical principle?

1. Justice
2. Fidelity
3. Autonomy
4. Confidentiality

7 The healthcare provider prescribes a medication in a dose that is considered toxic. The nurse administers the medication to the client, who later suffers a cardiac arrest and dies. What consequence can the nurse expect from this situation? Select all that apply.

1. The healthcare provider who prescribed the drug can be charged with negligence.
2. As the employing agency, only the hospital can be charged with negligence.
3. The nurse and prescriber may be terminated from employment to prevent a charge of negligence to the hospital.
4. Negligence will not be charged, as this event could happen to any reasonable person.
5. The nurse can be charged with negligence for administering the toxic dose.

8 A nurse and teacher are discussing legal issues related to the practice of their professions. The teacher asks about the functions of the Nurse Practice Act (NPA). The nurse should include which elements in a response? Select all that apply.

1. Accredit schools of nursing
2. Enforce ethical standards of behavior
3. Protect the public
4. Define the scope of nursing practice
5. Determine liability insurance rates

9 A staff nurse concerned about maintaining client confidentiality would take which action while carrying out assigned duties?

1. Read nonassigned client records to become more familiar with disease processes.
2. Share client information with nurses from the unit to which the client may eventually be transferred.
3. Allow the family to review the client's health record to obtain answers to their questions.
4. Share information about the client with those directly involved in that client's care.

10 The nurse working in an acute care environment would utilize which strategies to reduce the risk of malpractice litigation? Select all that apply.

1. Discuss any errors with the client and family in detail.
2. Keep incident reports on file.
3. Maintain expertise in practice.
4. Offer opinions to clients when the situation warrants.
5. Report unsafe staffing levels to supervisor.

ANSWERS & RATIONALES

1 **Answer: 3 Rationale:** Autonomy is the right of individuals to take action for themselves. Beneficence is an ethical principle to do good and applies when the nurse has a duty to help others by doing what is best for them. Veracity refers to truthfulness. Privacy is the nondisclosure of information by the healthcare team. **Cognitive Level:** Applying **Client Need:** Management of Care **Integrated Process:** Nursing Process: Implementation **Content Area:** Fundamentals **Strategy:** The core issue of the question is the ability to interpret which ethical principle is operating in a specific situation. Eliminate privacy because it does not apply to the situation as described. Eliminate beneficence and veracity next because they focus on the obligation of the nurse rather than on a right of the client.

2 **Answer: 2 Rationale:** Negligence is the unintentional failure of an individual to perform or not perform an act that a reasonable person would or would not do in the same or similar circumstances. A purposeful failure to perform a procedure would be the opposite of negligence, which is unintentional. Substituting a different medication does not fit the description of the situation in the question. Failure to follow a direct order does not fit the description in the situation in the question. **Cognitive Level:** Applying **Client Need:** Management of Care **Integrated Process:** Nursing Process: Assessment **Content Area:** Fundamentals **Strategy:** Two options are opposites, which is a clue that one of them may be correct. Choose unintentional failure to carry out a procedure over purposeful failure because it matches the definition of negligence.

3 **Answer: 4 Rationale:** Fidelity means being faithful to agreements and promises. This nurse is acting on the client's behalf to obtain needed information and report it back to the client. Nonmaleficence is the duty to do no harm. Veracity refers to telling the truth, for example, not lying to a client about a serious prognosis. Beneficence means doing good, such as by implementing actions (e.g., keeping a salt shaker out of sight) that benefit a client (heart condition requiring sodium-restricted

diet). **Cognitive Level:** Understanding **Client Need:** Management of Care **Integrated Process:** Nursing Process: Implementation **Content Area:** Fundamentals **Strategy:** Use the process of elimination. The correct answer is the one that matches the description in the stem; that is, the nurse made a promise to a client and kept it, which constitutes fidelity.

4 **Answer: 1 Rationale:** To be guilty of negligence, the nurse must have a relationship with the client that involves a duty to provide care. The relationship is usually a component of employment. The nurse did not necessarily do what others would do in this situation. Although the nurse did not cause the client's injuries, it does not prevent the nurse from assisting in this situation. Although the nurse was off-duty, the nurse could have assisted if motivated to do so. **Cognitive Level:** Understanding **Client Need:** Management of Care **Integrated Process:** Nursing Process: Implementation **Content Area:** Fundamentals **Strategy:** Use the process of elimination and nursing knowledge. The correct answer is the one that recognizes that the nurse was not in the role of employee at the time of the incident, removing the requirement of acting on the client's behalf.

5 **Answer: 2, 5 Rationale:** There was no nurse–client relationship because the nurse was acting as a neighbor and not in an employment capacity. Thus, there can be no duty owed. Intent is not a necessary element of malpractice because malpractice can occur because of unintended actions as well. There was no breach of duty because there was no official nurse–client relationship, which accompanies an employment situation. There was injury experienced because of this event. The bleeding was caused by the interaction of the aspirin with the anticoagulant. **Cognitive Level:** Analyzing **Client Need:** Management of Care **Integrated Process:** Nursing Process: Evaluation **Content Area:** Fundamentals **Strategy:** Use the process of elimination. The wording of the question indicates more than one option is correct, and the focus is on *necessary elements* that must be present. First, eliminate *intent to cause harm or injury*, since this is not necessary to a charge of malpractice. Next, note that there is no duty owed, and because of this, there can be no breach of duty, to choose these two options as the necessary missing elements.

6 **Answer: 3 Rationale:** Autonomy refers to the right to make one's own decisions, which is the principle supported in this situation. Justice refers to fairness. Fidelity refers to trust and loyalty. Confidentiality refers to the right to privacy of personal health information. **Cognitive Level:** Understanding **Client Need:** Management of Care **Integrated Process:** Nursing Process: Implementation **Content Area:** Fundamentals **Strategy:** Use the process of elimination. The wording of the question indicates that only one option is correct and that you need to select the principle that is consistent with the circumstances in the question.

7 **Answer: 1, 5 Rationale:** Healthcare providers who prescribe incorrect dosages of medications are liable for their errors. The nurse is open to a charge of negligency for failing to verify and question the incorrect dose. The hospital can be sued as the responsible employing agency, but the healthcare provider and the nurse can also be charged with negligence. Terminating the healthcare provider and nurse from employment would not stop a lawsuit charging negligence for employee actions that have already taken place. Prescribing and administering incorrect doses are not considered events that routinely happen to a "reasonable person." **Cognitive Level:** Applying **Client Need:** Management of Care **Integrated Process:** Nursing Process: Implementation **Content Area:** Fundamentals **Strategy:** The wording of the question indicates that more than one option is correct. Choose the responses that hold both individuals accountable, since the nurse failed to question an incorrect dose and the healthcare provider prescribed the incorrect dose.

8 **Answer: 3, 4 Rationale:** An NPA serves to protect the public by setting minimum qualifications for nursing in relation to skills and competencies. One way it fulfills responsibility to protect the public is by defining the scope of nursing practice in that state or province. The board of nursing approves schools to operate but does not accredit them. The board of nursing does not enforce ethical standards. An NPA has no role in setting liability insurance rates for nurses. **Cognitive Level:** Applying **Client Need:** Management of Care **Integrated Process:** Nursing Process: Implementation **Content Area:** Fundamentals **Strategy:** Use the process of elimination and basic nursing knowledge to answer the question. The wording of the question indicates that more than one option is correct and that the correct responses are worded as true statements.

9 **Answer: 4 Rationale:** Client confidentiality is maintained when the nurse shares client information only with those currently involved in the plan of care. Staff should only access information about clients currently assigned to their care. They should not access information about other clients on the unit not assigned to them. Client information should not be shared with nurses who are not currently working with the client. Family members would need approval from the client and the healthcare provider prior to reviewing a medical record. **Cognitive Level:** Applying **Client Need:** Management of Care **Integrated Process:** Communication and Documentation **Content Area:** Fundamentals **Strategy:** Select the response that protects the client's information, but allows communication necessary for the delivery of quality care.

10 **Answer: 3, 5 Rationale:** Maintaining expertise in practice by maintaining up to date knowledge and skills aids in reducing the risk of malpractice claims by fostering continued competence in practice. Unsafe staffing levels can result in a higher incidence rate of errors, which could later lead to charges of malpractice. Thus, reporting such situations so they can be prevented should be beneficial. Discussing errors in detail with the client and family does not reduce the risk of a malpractice claim. Incident reports are filed with agency but do not decrease the risk of malpractice litigation. The nurse should not offer opinions at any time as this is not part of therapeutic communication. **Cognitive Level:** Applying **Client Need:** Management of Care **Integrated Process:** Nursing Process: Implementation **Content Area:** Fundamentals **Strategy:** Focus on malpractice as the concept being tested. Recall that maintaining expertise is the best way to reduce personal risk and that reporting unsafe staffing situations may help reduce general agency risk by preventing omissions or errors due to insufficient numbers of caregivers to do the work required during the shift.

Key Terms to Review

accountability p. 20
Code of Ethics for Nurses p. 19
ethical dilemmas p. 20
ethics p. 19
malpractice p. 21
negligence p. 21
Nurse Practice Act p. 20

References

American Nurses Association (2015). *Code of ethics for nurses with interpretive statements.* Silver Spring, MD: Author. Available at http://www.nursingworld.org/DocumentVault/Ethics_1/Code-of-Ethics-for-Nurses.html.

Berman, A., Snyder, S., & Frandsen, G. (2016). *Kozier & Erb's fundamentals of nursing: Concepts, process, and practice* (10th ed.). New York, NY: Pearson Education.

Canadian Nurses Association (CNA). (2008). *Code of Ethics for Registered Nurses.* Available at http://cna-aiic.ca/~/media/cna/page-content/pdf-fr/code-of-ethics-for-registered-nurses.pdf.

Davis, A., Fowler, M., & Aroskar, M. (2010). *Ethical dilemmas and nursing practice* (5th ed.). Upper Saddle River, NJ: Pearson Education.

Guido, G. (2014). *Legal and ethical issues in nursing* (6th ed.). Upper Saddle River, NJ: Pearson Education.

International Council of Nurses. (2012). *The ICN code of ethics for nurses: Interpretation and application.* Geneva, Switzerland: Imprimerie Fornara. Available at http://www.icn.ch/about-icn/code-of-ethics-for-nurses/.

Test Yourself

Are you ready for the NCLEX-RN® or course exams? Access the NEW web-based app that provides students with thousands of practice questions in preparation for the NCLEX experience.

Nursing Leadership and Management

5

In this chapter

Cross Reference

Other chapters relevant to this content area are

Injury Prevention, Disaster Planning, and Protecting Client Safety	Chapter 6
Coping with Stressors	Chapter 20

I. HEALTHCARE SETTINGS AND MANAGEMENT

A. Types of healthcare settings and their management

1. Types of healthcare delivery settings include hospitals, extended care facilities (such as rehabilitation centers), skilled nursing facilities (for long-term care), ambulatory care settings (such as healthcare provider offices, outpatient clinics, urgent care centers, and same-day surgical centers), and home healthcare services (such as Visiting Nurse Associations)
2. Types of managed care organizations (systems that promote client health and self-health management, while focusing on reducing costs of care) include health maintenance organizations (HMOs), preferred provider organizations (PPOs), and point-of-service (POS) care

B. Health maintenance organizations (HMOs)

1. A configuration of healthcare agencies that provide health maintenance and treatment services to voluntary enrollees who prepay a fixed periodic fee without regard to either in-patient or out-patient services used
2. *NCLEX®* Geographically organized system that provides enrollees with an agreed-on package of health maintenance and treatment services

NCLEX® ***C. Managed care***

1. A healthcare plan that brings delivery and financing functions into one entity in contrast to a fee for service

Box 5–1

Key Objectives of Managed Care

Cost containment	Administrative efficiency
Some forms of rationing	Contracting efficiency
Efficiency of care	Managing care
Less duplication	Appropriateness of care

2. Objective is to enhance cost containment by decreasing unnecessary services, maintain quality, facilitate management of client care needs, and promote timely and appropriate care
3. Providers must submit written justification and request prior approval for diagnostic tests and interventions or to extend a client's length of stay
4. See Box 5–1, Key Objectives of Managed Care

NCLEX® **D. Case management**

1. Organizes client care by major diagnoses and focuses on attaining predetermined client outcomes within specific time frames
2. Advantages: all professionals are equal members of team; emphasis is on managing interdisciplinary outcomes; promotes continuity of care
3. Disadvantage: requires essential baseline data be available to team members; job descriptions of case managers vary among institutions

E. Nursing care delivery systems

1. Functional nursing
   - NCLEX® **a.** Represents a task approach to care that is coordinated by charge nurse; client needs are defined by activities delegated to registered nurses (RNs), licensed practical or vocational nurses (LPNs/LVNs), and unlicensed assistive personnel (UAPs) in U.S. or unregulated care providers (UCPs) in Canada
   - **b.** This system results in fragmentation of care and lack of a holistic view of client
2. Relationship-based nursing (primary nursing)
   - NCLEX® **a.** Primary nurse designs, implements, and is accountable for nursing care of clients from admission through discharge; care is carried out by associate nurses when primary nurse is off duty
   - **b.** Decentralizes nursing care decisions, authority, and responsibility to level of staff nurse; decreases number of unlicensed personnel; enhances family satisfaction with care; and maintains high level of accountability
   - **c.** Requires excellent communication between nurses; may be costly for institutions to hire highly skilled nurses
3. Team nursing
   - **a.** A team of nursing personnel provides total care to a group of clients; team is led by an RN (team leader) who assesses, makes nursing diagnoses, plans, implements, and evaluates care for clients on team
   - **b.** One variation based on physical layout of nursing unit is modular nursing, in which nurses care for clients in an assigned physical area or "pod"
   - **c.** Team leader creates work assignments based on job description, clinical expertise, and education of team members; team members retain accountability for client care and outcomes as provided by policy and law

F. *Shared governance* model of nursing practice

1. Principles of shared governance include partnerships, equity, accountability, and ownership; the structure demands participation in ownership
2. Characterized by decentralized power sharing and decision making; interdisciplinary team building; activities and conferences
3. Organizational priorities and issues and policy development are addressed through a series of committees (with one representative per committee from each nursing unit)
   - **a.** Nursing practice
   - **b.** Quality improvement
   - **c.** Education (ensures continuing education requirements and staff competency)
   - **d.** Management of service-specific areas such as general medical-surgical, maternal–child, critical care, intermediate care, and ancillary services such as employee and family health, radiology, and cardiac catherization

II. ORGANIZATIONAL SKILLS

A. *Time management*

1. A technique that encourages and supports effective and productive use of time; involves determining how best to prioritize client care, decide outcomes, and perform most important nursing interventions first
2. Requires ability to anticipate activities to be completed during work shift, consolidate nursing care activities when reasonable, resist being distracted by nonessential activities, and maintain flexibility when goals and outcomes need to change according to situation at hand
3. Poor time management can lead to inefficiency in completing work and inability to complete work on time

B. How to organize nursing care shift responsibilities and activities

1. Arrange nursing care environment with efficient access to supplies, equipment, and client designated areas
2. Use previous shift's report to determine priorities of care and importance of specific care activities to be completed during shift
3. Develop written action plan for shift work that includes nursing care activities/tasks and time frames for their completion, and that allows for all work to be accomplished during shift, including unexpected or unplanned work
4. Make assignments indicating who will perform specific interventions (involves delegation)
5. Implement shift action plan beginning with initial client care rounds and assessment of each assigned client
6. Plan for appropriate equipment and supplies to be available for care, and use them in a cost-effective manner
7. Maintain an hourly time log to provide visual structure of required nursing care activities; check off each activity at completion; and document pertinent results in client health record and on forms to be used for intershift report
8. Evaluate client outcomes and reexamine shift action plan at end of day to evaluate effectiveness of nurse's time management; plan to apply lessons learned to future shifts

III. ESTABLISHING PRIORITIES OF CARE

A. Frameworks for determining priorities of client care

1. Assist the nurse in determining which client needs require immediate action and which can be delayed to a later time according to urgency
2. *NCLEX®* Common frameworks for prioritizing include ABCs (airway, breathing, and circulation), Maslow's hierarchy of needs, agency policies and procedures, time, client and family preferences, care related to clinical condition, and priorities in medication therapy (see Table 5–1); note that CAB (compressions, airway, breathing), not ABC, is used for a client in cardiopulmonary arrest

B. Stability of client's condition

1. Attend to most unstable client first (whose condition is changing or deteriorating)
2. Clients who become unstable may have dramatic signs (such as bleeding, shock, or cardiopulmonary arrest) or may exhibit more subtle signs; watch for gradual trends in data, such as deteriorating vital signs (VS), declining urine output, decreasing level of consciousness (LOC)
3. When all clients are stable, attend first to client most likely to become unstable or who is at risk for most serious complications because of disease process

NCLEX® C. General client problems that usually indicate priority

1. Fresh postoperative clients (newly arrived on nursing unit from post-anesthesia care)
2. Clients whose status has deteriorated from baseline (VS, LOC, neurovascular status)
3. Clients exhibiting signs of shock (hypovolemic, hemorrhagic, cardiogenic, distributive)
4. Clients who have allergic reactions
5. Clients who have chest pain
6. Clients who have returned from diagnostic procedures and require temporary, more intensive monitoring, including assessing for complications
7. Clients who verbalize unexpected or unusual symptoms (such as new or suddenly increased acute pain, blurred vision, sudden weakness or paralysis)
8. Clients who have equipment or tubing malfunction or accident (such as disconnection of IV line, central line, chest tube or alarms ringing on mechanical ventilator or cardiac monitor)
9. Lower-priority clients are often those whose main needs include teaching, which is not as time-bound unless individual circumstances indicate otherwise

Table 5–1 Strategies for Priority Setting in Clinical Practice

Guiding Principles	First Priority	Second Priority	Third Priority
ABCs	Airway, breathing and circulation; exception is CAB for CPR	—	—
Maslow's hierarchy of needs theory	Physiological (primary) needs: air, breathing, circulation, water, food (oxygen therapy, circulatory support, IV hydration, nutrition, critical lab values, treatment of pain)	Safety and security (primary) needs: prevention of falls, re-orientation to surroundings, abnormally high or low values that are not critical; may include some client teaching (e.g., insulin administration)	Secondary needs: activities and care that support "love and belonging," self-esteem (includes ability for self-care and self-management of health problem), and self-actualization; includes routine client teaching and psychosocial support
Policies and procedures	Activities governed by agency policy or procedure that involve strict timelines (e.g., restraints, falls, stat medications)	Activities governed by policy or procedure that directly affect client care (e.g., nonstat, regularly scheduled medications, dressings)	Activities not affecting client care or that might be delegated to another (e.g., checking temperature of unit refrigerator, code cart check, emptying laundry bags)
Time	Clients with highly time-bound therapies (e.g., OR, stat x-ray); tasks that can be fully completed in less than 2 minutes if no competing priority present; necessary time-bound care for admission or discharge clients	Clients with scheduled therapies that need to be completed within a 2- to 4-hour window; routine client teaching	Clients with scheduled therapies that need to be completed once during the shift
Client and family preferences	Clients or families in physical or psychological distress	Clients or families with concerns about status or nursing care	Routine client and family psychological preferences or requests
Care activities related to clinical condition of client	Life-threatening or potentially life-threatening occurrences (adverse changes in VS, change in LOC, potential for respiratory or circulatory collapse); often unanticipated	Activities essential to safety: life-saving medications and equipment that protect clients from infections or falls	Activities essential to the plan of care leading to outcomes of symptom relief or healing (that if omitted would slow client recovery; e.g., nutrition, positioning, ambulation)
Medication or IV therapy priorities	Medications that prevent or treat physiological distress (e.g., analgesics, updrafts, or inhalers); medications prescribed more often (e.g., every 4 hours) because late medication delivery could affect next dose; IV therapy for hydration in clients who are NPO because of nonfunctional GI tract	Medications that prevent reoccurrences of symptoms of disease processes (e.g., digoxin, antibiotics); medications prescribed once per shift; routine maintenance of IV therapy or heparin/saline lock care	Medications that maintain normal organ system functioning (e.g., stool softener); medications prescribed daily or twice daily; site and dressing changes for IV therapy

IV. DELEGATION AND SUPERVISION

A. Overview of supervision

NCLEX®

1. A **supervisor** is an individual having authority from employer to hire, transfer, suspend, lay off, recall, assign, reward, or discipline other employees
2. Supervisors are responsible for:
   a. A thorough scope of technical knowledge of supervised work
   b. Clear directions, communication, and active listening skills
   c. Timely follow-up to ensure prompt execution of delegated activities
   d. Demonstrating fairness and respect toward all
   e. Feedback for work well done and resolution of problems and conflicts
3. **Supervision** is the provision of guidance or direction, evaluation, and follow-up of nursing personnel for accomplishment of a delegated nursing task; staff nurses are responsible for supervision of care they delegate to other nursing team members; nurses also need to recognize situations in which there is a need to contact shift supervisor for assistance

NCLEX® **B. Overview of delegation**

NCLEX®

1. National Council of State Boards of Nursing (NCSBN) defines **delegation** as transferring to a competent individual authority to perform a selected nursing task in a selected situation

NCLEX® **2.** Nurses delegate nursing care activities based on competency of delegatee, including educational knowledge and skill levels, and maintain ultimate accountability for care that is delegated to others

3. See Box 5–2 for suggestions on how to delegate effectively

4. It is important to clearly identify outcomes or expectations of each assigned nursing task or activity, including:

- **a.** Standard of care
- **b.** Time frame for assignment completion
- **c.** Limitations regarding performance of task

NCLEX® **5.** Activities that relate to implementation step of nursing process may be delegated

NCLEX® **6.** Activities that may not be delegated include client teaching and activities relating to any other step of nursing process (assessment, nursing diagnosis, planning, and evaluation)

7. Nursing care tasks may be delegated to unlicensed assistants (UAPs/UCPs) for clients who are in stable condition and when task has a predictable outcome; see Box 5–3 for tasks that may, in general, be delegated to UAPs/UCPs

8. LPNs/LVNs can perform, in general, all nursing care activities that UAPs/UCPs perform, plus more complicated or invasive nursing procedures such as medication administration (except IV push and certain IV piggyback medications according to laws of jurisdiction and job description), dressing changes, suctioning, and urinary catheterization (as examples); LPN/LVN can also reinforce client teaching that has been initiated by an RN

NCLEX® **C. Principles of delegation**

1. For delegation to occur, three elements must be present: delegator, delegatee, and task or activity to be accomplished
2. Only authority, but not ultimate responsibility, can be delegated
3. All delegated tasks must be clearly assigned and continuously clarified
4. Nurse must know staff job responsibilities and what can and cannot be delegated
5. Nurse sets clear parameters around how much authority is needed to accomplish assigned task successfully
6. Delegation requires ongoing follow-up and evaluation; obtain feedback on assigned tasks upon completion
7. Nurse retains responsibility for outcomes of delegated care activities

NCLEX® **D. The delegation process**

1. Determine and identify task and level of responsibility of each task
2. Evaluate delegatee's fit with assigned task
3. Decide what level of supervision is needed and describe expectations
4. Reach agreement on performance and outcome
5. Provide continuous feedback—monitor performance and adjust accordingly

Box 5–2

How to Delegate

- ➤ Identify a suitable person for the task who has the appropriate skill set.
- ➤ Prepare the person. Explain the task clearly. Make sure that you are understood.
- ➤ Make sure the person has the necessary authority to do the job properly.
- ➤ Keep in touch with the person for support and to monitor progress while allowing sufficient time and opportunity to complete the task.
- ➤ Retain responsibility for knowing the outcome of the delegation.
- ➤ Praise and acknowledge a job well done.

Box 5–3

Tasks That May Be Delegated to UAPs or UCPs

Bathing

Feeding

Ambulating clients

Attending to client safety

Measuring intake and output

Measuring vital signs

Performing simple dressing changes

Performing postmortem care

Range-of-motion exercises

Transferring clients, such as from bed to chair

Weighing clients

Performing cardiopulmonary resuscitation (if certified)

E. Barriers to delegation (see Table 5–2)

F. Inappropriate delegation

NCLEX®
1. **Underdelegation**: delegator does not think that team members can perform or complete an assignment or does not transfer full authority
   a. It is crucial to develop team members who can provide complete and comprehensive client care
   b. If unable to perform tasks, team members must be directed and trained to reach appropriate skill level
2. **Reverse delegation**
   a. Team member requests that nurse complete task because of inability or unwillingness to perform designated task or procedure
   b. Minimize reverse delegation with use of competency-based orientation programs and in-service or staff development classes

NCLEX®
3. **Overdelegation**: delegator becomes overwhelmed by situation and loses control by delegating authority and responsibility to delegate
   a. Tasks are delegated inappropriately; nurse cannot successfully achieve work-related goals if overwhelmed by numerous requests
   b. Tasks that are beyond their scope of practice should not be delegated to UAPs/UCPs

NCLEX®
G. Essential rights of delegation
1. NCSBN outlines five rights of delegation (see Box 5–4, The Essential Rights of Delegation)
2. Registered nurses (RNs) retain responsibility for caring for clients who require skilled assessment, whose status is changing or at risk for changing, and who require teaching

Table 5–2 Barriers to Delegation

Type of Barrier	Description	Possible Reasons
Delegator	Nurse will not delegate	"Do-it-myself" attitude or inability to ask others Inability to organize and manage Feelings of uncertainty Fear of competition Fear of liability or loss of control Fear of decreased job satisfaction
Delegatee	Delegate may resist accepting delegated tasks	Inexperience Incompetence Disorganization Irresponsibility
Situational	Workplace may be a barrier to delegation	Inadequate support Hurried atmosphere Hostile work environment

Box 5–4

The Essential Rights of Delegation

- **Right Task:** Nurses determine those activities team members may perform. For each situation, nurse must consider stability of client's condition, complexity and safety of activity, UAP's capabilities, and amount of supervision nurse can provide.
- **Right Circumstances:** Nurse evaluates individual clients and UAPs and matches the two. Nurse assesses client's needs, looks at care plan, considers the setting, and ensures that UAPs have proper resources, equipment, and supervision to work safely.
- **Right Person:** Nurse follows organizational policies, which are congruent with state law, in determining appropriate staff to which to delegate a nursing activity.
- **Right Direction and Communication:** Nurse needs to clearly understand organization's policies and procedures to carry out effective delegation. (Nurse needs to direct UAPs' actions and communicate clearly about each delegated task, being specific about how and when UAPs should report back to them.) Nurse should feel comfortable asking, *Do you know how to do this? Where did you learn? How many times have you done it in the past? Where is your experience documented?*
- **Right Supervision and Evaluation:** Nurse managers ensure that each unit has adequate staffing and time, identify tasks inherent to each staff role, and evaluate impact of organization's nursing service on the community. Delegating nurse must supervise, guide, and evaluate UAPs' task implementation, ensure that UAPs meet expectations, and intervene if not performing well.

3. LPNs or LVNs may be delegated care of clients who are stable, but have higher levels of acuity or require performance of skills beyond UAP/UPC training
4. LPNs and LVNs may collect data to report to RN but are not responsible for same level of client assessment that RN conducts
5. Routine nursing care and basic nursing procedures may be delegated to UAPs/UCPs; nursing care activities that require ongoing assessment, interpretation, or clinical decision making that cannot be separated from the activity itself should not be delegated to a UAP/UCP

V. ASSIGNMENT-MAKING

NCLEX®

A. **Assignment-making** is a process that transfers performance of client care activities from an assigning nurse to specific nursing unit personnel; responsibilities of nurse making an assignment include:
  1. Give clear, concise directions
  2. Delegate responsibility and authority for performance of care
  3. Retain accountability for assignment
  4. Ensure that education, skill, knowledge, and judgment levels of personnel are appropriate for assignment; for example, an RN who is "floating" from a childbirth unit to a surgical unit for the shift should be experienced in the care of surgical clients because of familiarity with cesarean births

B. **Assignment-making outcomes:** once an assignment is made, RN must specify:
  1. Expected outcome of assignment
  2. Time frame for completion
  3. Limitations on assignment
  4. Feedback at completion of assignment

VI. INTERDISCIPLINARY CONSULTATION AND REFERRALS

A. ***Interdisciplinary* consultation and referral** describes situations in which various disciplines are involved in reaching a common goal; each representative of a discipline brings own expertise to situation

NCLEX®

B. **Interdisciplinary consultation requires:**
  1. Cooperation, integration, and modification of efforts by contributing disciplines
  2. Acknowledgment by participants to take into account contributions of other team members in making their own contribution
  3. Understanding of intersecting lines of communication and collaboration that may emerge from these contributions

C. **Interdisciplinary care team: works together with client/family** in planning client care from each team member's discipline-specific perspective
  1. Discipline-specific perspectives are shared through staff conferencing and consultation
  2. Collaboration helps team members gain new insights for addressing problems and promotes development of a holistic plan for client

D. **Key components of interdisciplinary care team**
  1. Team members understand, appreciate, and collaborate with other disciplines and providers
  2. Team members make decisions about services in collaboration with client and other discipline(s) rather than dividing care decisions by discipline or setting
  3. Team members have a thorough understanding of their own profession

E. ***Consultation* involves communication** with another nurse or other healthcare professional (e.g., dietitian, pharmacist) about an aspect of client care
  1. Consultation is facilitated in agencies where employees enjoy collaborative work relationships with other health team members
  2. Nursing units that use interdisciplinary rounds on clients have created an environment that fosters consultation
  3. Health team members that may be involved in client care include healthcare provider, healthcare provider assistant (also called physician assistant), nurse practitioner, rehabilitative personnel (physical, occupational, and speech and language pathology therapists), respiratory therapist, nutritionist or dietitian, nurse case manager, continuing care nurse, pharmacist, medical social worker, and spiritual services provider (chaplain)

F. **Referrals:** often nurses are integral in assisting and coordinating client care that requires referrals
  1. A referral may be either a formal or informal process of sending a client from one healthcare provider to another for consultation, diagnostic intervention, and/or treatment; health plans may require primary care provider to authorize referrals for specialty services in order to be reimbursed

2. In an acute care setting, nurses may have authority to refer clients for consultation by specific departments, such as dietary or wound care specialist; always follow agency policy for scope of RN referral ability in specific agencies

VII. LEADERSHIP

A. Overview of leadership

1. Contemporary nursing **leadership** is about engaging people, building relationships, and influencing change
2. The terms leader and manager are sometimes used interchangeably; they are different but complementary
   NCLEX®
   a. A **leader** is a person who possesses personal traits that enable her or him to personally move others constructively and ethically to positively impact client/family care or to achieve an organizational goal or vision
   b. A **manager** accomplishes organizational goals either through personal action or directing the actions of others
3. Qualities of effective leaders include being able to think critically, take action, take calculated risks, communicate effectively, and be believable and persuasive
4. Behaviors of effective leaders include creating trust; inspiring and motivating employees to achieve goals; being visible to employees; treating employees with dignity and respect as unique individuals; providing guidance, assistance, and feedback to employees; and empowering employees
5. For followers to grow and flourish, nurse leaders must provide:
   a. Personal attention: support and guidance in foreseeing problems and challenges
   b. Role modeling: encouragement of self-management, assessment, openness, and forthrightness
   c. Precepting: to assist, approach, and coach in a timely and appropriate manner
   d. Mentoring: to invest by sharing expertise and experience with others

B. Formal versus informal leadership

NCLEX®
1. **Formal leadership** is bestowed by employing organization and described in a job description; it provides for influence through legitimate authority, power of position, and ability to reward and punish

NCLEX®
2. **Informal leadership** does not provide an official organizational title but informal leader can substantially influence others through thoughtful and convincing ideas, knowledge, status, and personal skills

C. A nurse leader's first objective is to assist and support professional clinical practice environment for nurses by:

1. Putting clients first
2. Focusing on client safety
3. Enhancing care quality
4. Improving client care outcomes

D. Theories of leadership and management

1. Behavioral theories: focus on abilities and behaviors of leaders
   a. Personal traits provide only a portion of leader capacity
   b. Leadership evolves through education, training, and life experiences
   c. **Autocratic leadership**: based on belief that individuals are motivated by power, authority, and need for approval; an autocratic leader makes all decisions, uses coercion and punishment, and is uncollegial
   d. **Democratic leadership**: based on belief that individuals are motivated by internal drives and impulses, desire active participation in decisions, and desire to get tasks done; democratic leadership promotes participation and majority rule for goal setting
   e. **Laissez-faire leadership**: based on belief that individuals are motivated by internal drives and impulses; need to be left alone to make decisions about how to complete work; leader provides no direction or facilitation
   f. **Bureaucratic leadership**: based on belief that individuals are motivated by external forces; leader trusts either followers or self to make decisions; relies on organizational policies and rules to identify goals and direct work flow
   g. Behavioral theory involves initiating structured behaviors that managers use to organize and define work goals, work patterns and methods, channels of communication, and roles
   h. Behavioral theory includes consideration of behaviors that show mutual trust, respect, friendship, warmth, and rapport between leader and followers

2. The managerial grid leadership theory plots leadership styles into four quadrants of a two-dimensional grid (visualize a box with four squares in it) that illustrates leader's concern for production or task (called structure) on one axis and concern for people (called consideration) on other axis; results in five leadership styles
   a. Impoverished: low concern for tasks or people
   b. Authority: high concern for tasks, low concern for people
   c. Country club: high concern for people, low concern for tasks
   d. Middle of the road: moderate concern for both tasks and people
   e. Team: high concern for both tasks and people
3. Contingency theories
   a. Leaders adapt their style according to the situation
   b. Leader behavior ranges accordingly, from authoritarian to permissive: crisis situations often require an authoritarian style to maintain command and control; problem solving and consensus building call for a participatory style that encourages respect for followers' ideas and input and gains their commitment to the team
   c. Leaders who base their leadership style upon the organizational environment, task to be achieved, and characteristics of their followers tend to be most effective; this is because their planned flexibility allows them to change styles as needed by the work environment
4. Situational leadership theory considers followers' readiness and willingness to perform a designated task; leadership styles can be categorized according to readiness and ability of follower to perform task
   a. Telling style (S1—high task, low relationship): used for followers who are unable, unwilling, or insecure about performing assigned task
   b. Selling style (S2—high task, high relationship): used for followers who are unable but who are willing or confident about performing task
   c. Participating style (S3—low task, high relationship): used for followers who are able, willing, and confident about performing task
5. Quantum leadership theory: leader is viewed as an influential facilitator and followers assume active role in decision making; is a contemporary theory
   a. Evolves from concepts of chaos theory; reality is constantly shifting; levels of complexity are constantly changing; movement reverberates throughout system; roles are fluid and outcome-oriented
   b. Leadership is a shared activity and information is freely disseminated to others
   c. Leaders are expected to be expert communicators and possess strong interpersonal skills
   d. Followers are equitable and accountable partners in client care outcomes
6. Charismatic leadership: based on personal beliefs and characteristics
   a. Leaders possess powerful personal qualities, such as charm, persuasiveness, personal power, self-confidence, extraordinary ideas, and strong convictions
   b. Leader's personality arouses affection and emotional commitment, and drives and advances vision, mission, and goals
7. **Transactional leadership:** built on principles of social exchange, in which individuals expect to give and receive rewards
   a. Exchange process between leaders and followers is economic, where workers perform according to policy and procedures to maximize self-interests and rewards
   b. Leaders are most successful when they understand and meet followers' needs
   c. Exchange between leader and follower continues until exchange of performance and incentive or reward is no longer valuable
   d. Aims at maintaining equilibrium or status quo and fosters interpersonal dependence
8. **Transformational leadership**: based on commitment to agency's vision and focuses on promoting change; not concerned with status quo
   a. Emphasizes interpersonal relationships and inspires followers
   b. Focuses on merging leader and follower motives and values to generate followers' commitment to leader's vision
   c. Encourages followers to exercise leadership abilities
   d. Uses power to instill a belief that followers can accomplish exceptional things
9. Relational leadership: acknowledges importance of relationships as cornerstone of effective leadership
   a. Connective relationships allow for better coordinated and integrated client care services in a caring, noncompetitive manner
   b. Connective leaders encourage collaboration and interpersonal skills to broker alliances

10. Shared leadership
    a. Founded on principles of empowerment, participation, and transformational leadership
    b. No one person or leader possesses all knowledge and abilities
    c. Elements of shared leadership include relationships, dialogues, partnerships, and understanding boundaries
    d. Shared leadership allows for appropriate leadership to emerge as problems and issues arise (different issues call for different responses)
11. **Servant leadership**: focuses on desire to serve others; based on principles of caring
    a. In the desire to serve, one can be called upon to lead—hence the name servant leadership
    b. A servant leader seeks to address others' needs as priority
    c. Nurse leaders provide care and compassionate service to others

E. Desired leadership traits and competencies

1. Action orientation
    a. Seizes opportunities when they arise; mobilizes resources; removes barriers
    b. Proceeds with extraordinary persistence and determination
    c. Champions initiatives beyond scope of own work
2. Team spirit focus
    a. Leverages team's synergy to create a common culture and get results
    b. Manages tensions inherent in group process to forge innovative solutions
    c. Establishes a positive work climate—through personal actions, policies, and consistent signals—that nurtures enthusiasm and commitment to team's mission
3. Command skills
    a. Inspires a high level of dedication to mission and maintains focus on goals
    b. Flexible in developing alternative methods of achieving goals
    c. Brings clarity and decisiveness in a crisis
4. Ethics and integrity
    a. Viewed as a highly credible and trustworthy person; creates and instills strong values and ethics within organization
    b. Stands up for what is right despite potential personal or business consequences
5. Interpersonal savvy
    a. Anticipates others' thoughts and reactions and responds accordingly
    b. Uses conflict as an advantage to create innovative solutions
    c. Forges opportunities to build long-term productive relationships
    d. Enhances workgroup dynamics through subtle methods of influencing
6. Ability to motivate and inspire others to see and achieve group's vision

NCLEX®

7. Problem-solving skills
    a. Makes breakthrough decisions based on analysis, wisdom, experience, and judgment
    b. Frequently sought out by other nurses for advice and solutions
    c. Suggests highly creative solutions to difficult problems
    d. Considers impact of global, cultural, geographic, political, and regulatory factors in making decisions
8. Results orientation
    a. Goes beyond what is expected to achieve objectives
    b. Anticipates potential problems and develops contingency plans to overcome them
    c. Demonstrates strong commitment and drive to achieve results
    d. Delivers results that consistently improve client care outcomes
9. Strategic agility
    a. Adapts strategies and plans to address impact of healthcare trends and issues on team or organization
    b. Sees connections and patterns often not recognized as important by others

VIII. MANAGEMENT CONCEPTS AND SKILLS

NCLEX®

A. Management process involves a variety of responsibilities

1. Effectively accomplishing goals of organization
2. Coordinating tasks and integrating resources
3. Using functions of planning, organizing, supervising, staffing, evaluating, and negotiating
4. Clarifying organizational structure
5. Evaluating client care outcomes and providing feedback
6. Coping with complexity

NCLEX® **B. Functions of management process: planning, organizing, leading, and controlling**

1. Planning and setting a direction
   - **a.** Sets goals and decides course of action through an inductive process
   - **b.** Gathers data and looks for patterns
   - **c.** Builds relationships and links to help explain issues, goals, expectations, and so on
   - **d.** Creates visions and strategies for organization's future
2. Organizing and aligning people
   - **a.** Identifies work to be accomplished and goals to be achieved
   - **b.** Hires right person for right work and coordinates work of others
   - **c.** Creates interdependence by getting people to move in same direction
   - **d.** Delegates authority by talking to those who can help implement a vision and those who can block implementation
3. Leading and getting others to believe the message
   - **a.** Influences others to get job done
   - **b.** Keeps message clear and communicates with integrity and trustworthiness
   - **c.** Molds the culture and maintains morale
   - **d.** Insists on consistency between words and deeds
4. Controlling
   - **a.** Sets standards for accomplishing organization's goals and activities
   - **b.** Determines means to measure performance and makes sure that quality lapses are spotted immediately
   - **c.** Evaluates performance and provides feedback

IX. MANAGING CHANGE

NCLEX® **A. Change is making something different than it was;** in many instances, the outcome remains the same, but the process is changed

NCLEX® **B. Types of change**

1. Personal change: voluntary change with a goal of self-improvement
2. Professional change: deliberate change with a goal of improving professional ability, status, or both
3. Organizational change: mandated change with a goal of improving efficiency

NCLEX® **C. Change process: *planned change* involves a natural process** that should be used as a guide for implementing change

1. Assessment: identifying problem or opportunity that necessitates change
2. Data collection and analysis: gathering structural, technological, and personnel information and documenting effects of these elements on the process
3. Strategic determination: identifying possible solutions, barriers, strategies
4. Change is often purposeful and usually is implemented to solve problems that affect nurses at work
5. Change is used to alter behavior of individuals and groups within an organization

NCLEX® **D. Forces of change**

1. Driving: those forces that facilitate change because they push toward a desired direction
2. Restraining: those forces that impede change because they push in an opposite direction
3. Change occurs because these forces shift the balance
4. Three-step process
   - **a.** Unfreezing: reasons for making a change are presented in a way to make change desirable
   - **b.** Moving: planned change is put into action
   - **c.** Refreezing: new goal becomes established as an expected outcome
5. Attention is aimed at increasing driving forces, decreasing restraining forces, or both

E. Planned change is for low-level complexity change

1. It is not a coercive act or an accident
2. Planned change is structured, more stable in nature, happens in increments, and proceeds sequentially and directionally
3. In contrast, high-level change is more fluid, more complex, and occurs in rapidly changing environments

NCLEX® **F. Recognizing resistance**

1. Individuals are often resistant to change because they are afraid of disorder, upset by interruption of daily routine, or fearful of losing job, power, or resources
2. Positive aspects of resistance
   - **a.** Change agent must be focused, ready to clarify information, and able to keep interest high
   - **b.** Resistance creates energy and movement

3. Negative aspects of resistance
   a. Wears down supporters
   b. Hard to stay focused among constant challenges

NCLEX® **G. Handling resistance**

1. Be sure to communicate—often; maintain close contact and keep resisters involved
2. Be clear, accurate, open, and flexible; promote trust, support, and confidence
3. Acknowledge negative consequences of resistance and positive consequences of change
4. Keep energy moving—create disturbances
5. Monitor politics of change
6. Develop good diagnostic skills; adapt leadership style to situation and the change
   a. Allow participants to verbalize their concerns
   b. Explain rationale for change
   c. Allow emotions to be expressed
   d. Give information frequently
   e. Help individuals cope with change

X. MANAGING CONFLICT

NCLEX® **A. Sources and types of conflict**

1. Conflict can occur when there are perceived differences or incompatibilities regarding goals, priorities, beliefs, or values
2. Types of conflict are labeled as intrapersonal (within a person), interpersonal (between individuals, such as clients, nurses, other healthcare team members), or organizational (between individual and organizational policies and procedures)

B. Traditional approaches for resolving conflict

1. Avoidance: postpones dealing with issue; engaged in by those who do not pursue own goals and needs, and do not assist others
2. Accommodation: meets or satisfies needs or goals of others while ignoring own; may lead to resentment and disappointment over time
3. Competition: allows one to pursue own needs and goals (possibly at expense of others) but can also lead to defense of important principles
4. Compromise: relies on assertiveness, cooperation, and working creatively to find solutions that are most satisfactory to all parties

C. Interest-based relational approach to resolving conflict

NCLEX®
1. Make it a priority to keep good relationships, treating others with respect and courtesy and engaging in constructive discussion
2. Distinguish between "people" and "problems," recognizing that valid differences can lie behind conflicting positions
3. Listen carefully to different points of view to gain a better idea of why people have adopted their position
4. Listen to what other person is saying before defending own position, which might result in a change of mind
5. Decide with other person about observable facts that might impact your decision, together
6. Explore options together, being open to possibility that other options may exist that could be reached jointly

XI. QUALITY IMPROVEMENT (QI)

NCLEX® **A. Overview**

1. **Quality improvement (QI):** a set of systematic and continuous actions that improve the health status of targeted client groups and delivery of healthcare services
2. Quality management: focuses on evaluating care delivery processes in order to correct problems or prevent errors in treatment to uphold client safety in a cost-effective manner
3. Overall, quality in healthcare refers to meeting or exceeding expectations of clients, meeting or exceeding standards of care or benchmarks for performance, and achieving planned outcomes for clients and organization
4. Performance improvement is a term used when QI is linked to performance of an individual, team, unit, or organization
5. Other terms associated with concept of quality improvement are continuous quality improvement (CQI), total quality management (TQM), and quality assurance

Box 5–5

Ways Nurses Can Enhance Quality Nursing Care

- **Seek to provide nursing care with the outcome of a continuous healing relationship.** Nursing care is responsive at all times (24 hours a day, every day), and access to nursing care should be provided over the Internet, by telephone, and by other means in addition to face-to-face visits.
- **Provide nursing care based on client needs and values.** Nursing care should be designed to meet the most common types of needs as well as to respond to individual client choices and preferences.
- **Remember that the client is the source of information.** Clients are given the necessary information and the opportunity to exercise the degree of control they choose over healthcare decisions that affect them.
- **Nursing care requires shared knowledge and the free flow of information.** Clients have access to their own nursing and medical information and to clinical knowledge. The health team communicates effectively and shares information with clients and their families.
- **Nurses use evidence-based decision making.** Clients receive care based on the best available scientific knowledge.
- **Safety is a key feature in all aspects of nursing care.** Clients are kept safe and are protected from injury caused by the care system. Reducing risk and ensuring safety requires all team members to pay greater attention to systems that help prevent errors.
- **Nurses anticipate client needs.** Nursing staff anticipate client needs rather than simply react to events.
- **Nurses understand the essential need to cooperate with other clinicians.** Nurses and other clinicians actively collaborate and communicate to ensure an appropriate exchange of information and coordination of care.

6. QI involves all employees of an organization in improvement process
7. Healthcare agencies attempt to engage employees in QI by adopting a "blame-free environment" (focus on problem, not an individual) or a "just culture" (balances blame-free environment with appropriate personal accountability; differentiates between human error, at-risk behavior, and reckless behavior)
8. *NCLEX®* See Box 5–5 for ways to enhance quality nursing care

B. Tools for assessment of quality in healthcare

1. Peer review: professional critique of a colleague's work based on predetermined standards in a safe and nonpunitive environment
2. Audits: an examination of records of one or a group of clients; can focus on one discipline (such as nurses) or multiple disciplines (such as nurses and providers); types of audits are
   a. Retrospective: performed after client discharge to evaluate care provided
   b. Concurrent: performed before discharge while client is still receiving care to evaluate adequacy of care and whether desired outcomes are met
3. Utilization review: analyzes use of healthcare agency resources to identify areas of overuse, misuse, or underuse; protects agency from unnecessary and inappropriate use of resources
4. *NCLEX®* Outcomes management: uses client experiences to improve care by providing a link between medical interventions to health outcomes and between health outcomes and cost of care
5. Benchmarking: a method of comparing performance of an individual or healthcare organization to industry standards; standards that can be benchmarked are structure standards (e.g., material resources and human resources needed to deliver care on a nursing unit), process standards (e.g., activities carried out in caring for clients), and outcome standards (client's status at a defined time following care interventions)

NCLEX® **C. Measuring outcomes**

1. **Indicators** are a measurement or flag used as a guide to monitor, assess, and improve quality of client care, support services, and organizational functions affecting client outcomes
2. Nurse-sensitive indicators are measurements of client care that are sensitive to nursing interventions, such as:
   a. Maintenance of skin integrity (pressure ulcer prevalence rate)
   b. Fall injury rate
   c. Medication error rate

d. Restraint utilization rate
e. Healthcare-associated infection rates (catheter-associated UTI, central line–associated bloodstream infections, ventilator-associated pneumonia)
f. Client satisfaction with pain management
g. Client satisfaction with overall nursing care
h. Nurse satisfaction
i. Incidence of episodes of failure to rescue

XII. RESOURCE MANAGEMENT

A. **Resource management determines best use of human and physical resources;** key activities include:
1. Recruiting, hiring, and training the best employees to meet specified needs
2. Ensuring employees are high performers and dealing with performance issues
3. Ensuring that personnel and management practices and policies (including compensation, benefits, employee records) conform to various regulations

B. **Staffing is a critical aspect of resource management**
1. Staffing is a process that involves deciding what human resources are needed and considers the knowledge, skills, and abilities needed to perform specified roles, jobs, and tasks (roles should be defined in job descriptions and/or competencies)
2. Staffing is a standard measure that quantifies nursing time and is measured by nursing care hours per day (nursing time available daily to each client)
3. Terms associated with staffing
a. Full-time equivalent (FTE): a label for the work-time commitment of an employee; a full-time nurse who works 40 hours a week has a 1.0 FTE position; a nurse who works 24 hours per week has a 0.6 FTE position
b. Productive hours: hours worked and available for nursing care; nonproductive hours are designated as benefit time and include vacation, sick time, and educational time
c. Client classification system: a measurement tool used to describe nursing workload for specific clients or a group of clients over hours worked
d. Staffing pattern: a plan that identifies numbers and types of staff needed by shift and by nursing unit

C. **Cost containment and cost effectiveness in resource management**
1. Controlling costs requires sound management practices, which include effective and efficient decision making based on standardized, accurate, and timely operational information (such as that provided by management information systems [MIS] and workload measurement systems [WMS])
2. MIS Guidelines are national standards used to support collection, reporting, and use of financial and statistical data that is used by managers for planning, budgeting, monitoring, and evaluation
3. The WMS are a key component of MIS Guidelines that quantify the volume of activity provided by a specific service
a. WMS identify all activities of a nursing unit associated with clinical and nonclinical activities and collect service activity statistics (e.g., in-patient days, visits) and caseload status statistics (e.g., new referrals, in-patient admissions, discharges)
b. Measuring workload, service activity, and caseload status statistics gives a good indication of the amount and kind of service provided by a specific unit
c. Data collected from WMS are used to develop indicators (ratios of financial and statistical data), which allow nurse managers to monitor variances between budgeted and actual results, determine causes, and decide on corrective action
d. Indicators enable nurse managers to explain utilization of human and financial resources in quantifiable terms (e.g., cost of nursing care per in-patient day, workload units per visit, etc.)

D. **Safety and quality of care**
1. These are directly related to numbers and mix of direct care nursing staff
2. Nurse staffing levels and skill mix make a difference in client outcomes; when there are more nurses, there are lower mortality rates, shorter lengths of stay, better care planning, lower costs, and fewer incidents
3. Increased registered nurse staffing is directly related to improved post-surgical outcomes, decreased incidences of shock and upper gastrointestinal bleeding, decreased hospital length of stay, and fewer hospital-acquired infections such as urinary tract infections and pneumonia

Check Your NCLEX-RN® Exam I.Q.

You are ready for testing on this content if you can:

- Describe the various healthcare settings.
- Monitor time management priorities.
- Assist in assignment-making.
- Request interdisciplinary consultation and referrals.
- Provide effective leadership and management to nursing care personnel.
- Demonstrate effective leadership strategies.
- Describe the management process.
- Effectively delegate nursing activities.
- Apply the principles of change.
- Incorporate performance improvement into clinical nursing practice.
- Apply cost-effective measures to nursing practice.

PRACTICE TEST

PRACTICE TEST

1 The registered nurse (RN) must delegate aspects of care for an assigned client to an unlicensed assistant (UAP/UCP) for the shift. Which client would be best to delegate to the UAP/UCP?

1. A client who would benefit from talking about the recent death of her husband
2. A client with a urinary drainage catheter and nasogastric feedings who is on bedrest
3. A client with an ostomy who has persistent problems with leakage
4. A client who was transferred from the critical care unit 3 days ago and is ambulatory

2 Which task would not be appropriate for the registered nurse (RN) to delegate to a licensed practical/vocational nurse (LPN/LVN) or unlicensed assistant (UAP/UCP)?

1. Instructing the LPN/LVN to reinforce teaching of the RN's assigned clients prior to discharge
2. Assigning UAPs/UCPs to complete vital signs and document and report changes to the RN
3. Asking the UAP/UCP to assess and evaluate the client response to IV pain medication
4. Instructing the LPN/LVN to remove a dressing from a postoperative client's abdominal wound

3 The charge nurse on the night shift reports that the narcotic count is incorrect. The nurse has spoken to the responsible staff nurse and believes that substance abuse by the nurse is the cause. If substance abuse proves to be the cause of the incorrect count, what is the most appropriate next step?

1. Recount the narcotics with the staff nurse and take disciplinary action
2. Ask the staff nurse to leave the unit and report the incident to the American Nurses Association
3. Complete an incident report and report findings to the pharmacy and nursing administration
4. Submit the findings to the Council on Nursing Practice

4 A quarterly audit is now due to evaluate implementation of an electronic medical record system on the nursing unit. As the unit representative who supervised the adaptation of this documentation system, how can the nurse best determine if nursing staff have accepted this change?

1. Nursing staff uses the electronic medical record daily in routine documentation
2. Nursing staff verbalizes the need for the electronic record but still hand-write nursing notes into the clients' charts
3. Nursing staff uses the electronic record sporadically to monitor clients' progress
4. Nursing staff likes the electronic record because they believe it saves them time

5 The nurse on the hospital quality improvement team has been asked to evaluate nursing care on the nurse's assigned unit. After deciding to ask the nursing staff for assistance in this effort, what would be most appropriate for the nurse to initially ask the staff to do?

1. Track the number of supplies used by clients on the unit
2. Document the time spent on direct client care
3. Administer a client and family satisfaction survey
4. Assess clients and report acuity daily

6 An RN is about to make first rounds after receiving an intershift report at 3:00 p.m. In what order should the RN see the following clients? Place the options in order. All options must be used.

correct:
35142

1. A 54-year-old client 4 hours post–cardiac catheterization who has mild discomfort at the access site
2. A client newly diagnosed with diabetes mellitus who needs reinforcement of sick-day management guidelines
3. A client who arrived 30 minutes ago from the postanesthesia care unit
4. A client who is ready for discharge but will not have available transportation home until 5:00 p.m.
5. A client with pneumonia who has received two doses of IV antibiotics and has an oxygen saturation of 93%

Fill in your answer below:

Answer: 5 3 1 2 4

7 A client is experiencing respiratory distress. Respirations are 32 breaths/min and shallow. The client is positioned in an orthopneic position, with a heart rate of 118/min and a blood pressure of 90/40 mmHg. The client is pale and confused. Which task should the nurse delegate to the charge nurse?

1. Head-to-toe assessment
2. Placement of a second IV site
3. Application of oxygen
4. Overhead page the respiratory therapist (RT)

8 A nurse is assisting a client in room 1 with lunch. The charge nurse calls the nurse and states the client in room 3 is reporting pain and requests pain medication. What is the nurse's best and first action?

1. Finish feeding the client in room 1, then medicate the client in room 3 for pain.
2. Stop feeding the client in room 1, and medicate the client in room 3 for pain.
3. Finish feeding the client in room 1, and ask the charge nurse to medicate the client in room 3.
4. Ask the charge nurse to feed the client in room 1 while the nurse medicates the client in room 3 for pain.

9 After receiving the intershift report, the registered nurse (RN) has many tasks to complete during the next 12 hours. Which tasks should the nurse delegate to an unlicensed assistant (UAP/UCP)? Select all that apply.

1. Flushing a nasogastric tube on a client who has had a colectomy
2. Irrigating a clogged urinary catheter on an older adult client
3. Rechecking vital signs on a 30-year-old client with a BP of 100/60
4. Changing a dressing on a client with an infected diabetic foot ulcer
5. Measuring and recording hourly urine output for a client who underwent nephrectomy

10 The registered nurse (RN) is assigned to five clients for the shift. Which tasks are best delegated to the licensed practical/vocational nurse (LPN/LVN)? Select all that apply.

1. Repositioning a nasogastric tube on a client who has had a small bowel resection
2. Irrigating a urinary catheter on a client admitted from a skilled nursing facility
3. Rechecking vital signs on a 40-year-old asymptomatic client with a BP of 100/64
4. Changing a dressing on a client with a diabetic foot ulcer in the metatarsal area
5. Administering red blood cells to a client with a hemoglobin of 10.2 grams/dL

11 The delivery of care system on a medical floor is team nursing. On wing A, there is a registered nurse (RN), licensed practical/vocational nurse (LPN/LVN), and an unlicensed assistant (UAP/UCP) to care for eight clients. Which tasks would be best delegated to the LPN/LVN?

1. Vital signs and assessment of a newly postoperative client
2. Wound care and oral medications for all clients
3. Vital signs and bed baths on all eight clients
4. Physical assessments on two young, stable clients

12 A nurse is delegating care of clients to an unlicensed assistant (UAP/UCP) and licensed practical/vocational nurse (LPN/LVN). Which tasks should the nurse give the UAP/UCP and LPN/LVN?

1. UAP/UCP: Measure vital signs; LPN/LVN: Give oral medications on assigned clients
2. UAP/UCP: Change a noninfected dressing; LPN/LVN: Administer IV piggyback medications
3. UAP/UCP: Ambulate a client who had a CVA; LPN/LVN: Assess two clients
4. UAP/UCP: Measure vital signs; LPN/LVN: Complete a head-to-toe assessment on a newly admitted client

13 A nurse is preparing for the shift, and makes a list of delegated tasks for the unlicensed assistant (UAP/UCP). Which task should the nurse delegate to the UAP/UCP?

1. Feeding a client who was admitted with dysphagia from cerebrovascular accident
2. Monitoring drainage from a chest tube on a client with a hemothorax
3. Rechecking vital signs on a client whose blood pressure is 190/102
4. Repositioning a client with severe weakness caused by multiple sclerosis

14 A registered nurse (RN) who is the charge nurse for the shift is making assignments for the day. Which client should be assigned to the licensed practical/vocational nurse (LPN/LVN)?

1. A client with sickle-cell anemia requiring pain medications every 3 hours
2. A 3-day postoperative client who will be discharged tomorrow morning
3. A 76-year-old client newly admitted with pneumonia and type 2 diabetes mellitus
4. A client who received chemotherapy for leukemia and has a hemoglobin of 6.4 grams/Dl

15 The staff nurse who is in charge of the medical-surgical unit for the shift is receiving four admissions. The emergency department is sending a client with hypertension and an exacerbation of heart failure, and a client who has pneumonia and a history of diabetes mellitus. The postanesthesia care unit (PACU) is transferring a client who had a total abdominal hysterectomy and a client who underwent hip replacement. If the staff consists of two RNs (one on orientation) and two LPNs/LVNs, what assignment would be appropriate?

1. The RN on orientation will be assigned the postoperative client who underwent hip replacement.
2. The experienced RN will be assigned the postoperative client who underwent hip replacement.
3. An LPN/LVN will be assigned the client with pneumonia and history of diabetes.
4. An LPN/LVN will be assigned the client with the abdominal hysterectomy.

16 An obstetric nurse is floated to a medical unit to care for a group of acutely ill clients. The charge nurse should assign which group of clients to the float nurse?

1. A client with a 3-day-old total knee replacement, a client who is postoperative for colectomy, and a client who is postoperative for hysterectomy
2. An older adult client with dehydration, a client with atrial fibrillation, and a client just admitted with hip fracture
3. A client with an old cerebrovascular accident, a client with a 3-day-old hip replacement, and a client with diabetic ketoacidosis
4. An older adult client with pneumonia, a client with an exacerbation of asthma, and a client who has below-knee amputation

17 A nurse plans to delegate some responsibilities of client care to a licensed practical nurse (LPN/LVN). Which task should the nurse delegate to the LPN/LVN?

1. Assessment of a newly admitted client
2. Admission of a postoperative client
3. Dressing changes for a client with wounds
4. Assist a client with ambulation and AM care

PRACTICE TEST

18 A nurse has delegated a venipuncture to an unlicensed assistant (UAP/UCP) who has been off orientation for 5 days. The UAP/UCP reports, "This client has a large, raised red area where the needle was inserted." The nurse's subsequent assessment reveals a hematoma in the venipuncture area. What elements of delegation have been breached? Select all that apply.

1. Task
2. Circumstance
3. Communication
4. Supervision
5. Skill

19 Upon calling the healthcare provider regarding a client with "heartburn," diaphoresis, and irregular pulse, the nurse receives stat orders for the following: electrocardiogram, cardiac panel, morphine 2 mg IV push, nitroglycerin 0.4 mg sublingual, and aspirin 325 mg p.o. chew and swallow. Which tasks should the nurse delegate? Select all that apply.

1. Administration of medications
2. Reassessment of the client's condition
3. Venipuncture for cardiac panel
4. Electrocardiogram
5. Oxygen saturation

20 A registered nurse (RN) working on the medical unit arrives at work 15 minutes late. The nurse is assigned five clients, and an admission is on the way. Place in order of priority how the nurse should complete the following activities at the beginning of the work shift. Place the options in order. All options must be used.

1. Listen to report
2. Check the medication administration record (MAR)
3. Check on the status of all clients
4. Review morning lab results, including glucose monitoring

Fill in your answer below:

Answer: 1 3 4 2

21 A nurse is preparing for a busy day on a medical nursing unit. Prioritize the tasks and place the options in order. All options must be used.

1. Irrigate a nasogastric tube on a client who had a colectomy the previous day.
2. Flush a poorly draining urinary catheter on an older adult client.
3. Check vital signs on a 30-year-old client with a BP of 114/68 and heart rate of 94.
4. Change a dressing on a client with an infected diabetic foot ulcer.
5. Begin a unit of packed red blood cells for a client with a hematocrit of 23.2%.

Fill in your answer below:

Answer: ______________________

ANSWERS & RATIONALES

1 **Answer: 4 Rationale:** Factors to consider when delegating care include complexity of task, problem-solving innovation required, unpredictability, and level of client interaction. The ambulatory client is best to delegate because this client is likely to be stable with a low level of unpredictability. The client who recently lost her husband would benefit from professional communication with the RN and requires a high level of client interaction. The client receiving enteral feedings and is immobilized represents a more complex client, who is better assigned to a licensed nurse. The client with a leaking ostomy would benefit from problem-solving innovation and is best cared for by the RN. **Cognitive Level:** Analyzing **Client Need:** Management of Care **Integrated Process:** Nursing Process: Planning **Content Area:** Leadership and Management **Strategy:** The core issue of the question is basic concepts that are useful when considering delegation to a UAP/UCP. Use this knowledge and the process of elimination to make a selection.

2 **Answer: 3 Rationale:** The decision to delegate should be consistent with the nursing process (appropriate assessment, planning, implementation, and evaluation). The person responsible for client assessment, diagnosis, care planning, and evaluation is the registered nurse. The LPN/LVN can reinforce teaching previously performed by the RN. Assistive personnel may perform simple nursing interventions, but the RN remains responsible for analyzing the data and the client outcome. The LPN/LVN can change a dressing. **Cognitive Level:** Applying **Client Need:** Management of Care **Integrated Process:** Nursing Process: Implementation **Content Area:** Leadership and Management **Strategy:** The core issue of the question is the knowledge related to delegation of nursing tasks. Recall that UAPs/UCPs cannot practice nursing; they cannot be delegated to assess or evaluate responses to treatment.

3 **Answer: 3 Rationale:** An incident report must be completed because of the inaccurate narcotic count. Narcotics are controlled substances and fall under federal law and regulation. Both the pharmacy and nursing administration must be notified. If the staff nurse is found to be using a controlled substance, this finding must be reported to the state board of nursing. Individual state boards of nursing identify the legal boundaries of nursing practice, including disciplinary action, through nurse practice acts (which differ among the states). The American Nurses Association, through the Code of Ethics for Nurses, provides guidance to nurses and protection for clients and their families but does not have the authority to discipline nurses. **Cognitive Level:** Applying **Client Need:** Management of Care **Integrated Process:** Nursing Process: Planning **Content Area:** Leadership and Management **Strategy:** Agency policies and procedures and state nurse practice acts dictate the course of action for drug diversion by nurses. Recall that nursing administration would communicate with outside agencies to aid in eliminating incorrect options.

4 **Answer: 1 Rationale:** When people accept change, they integrate it into their daily routines and the change is maintained. Nurses who manually write nurses notes have not accepted the change. Sporadic use does not indicate full acceptance of the change. While statements that staff like the system is a positive indicator, it is not the same as use of the system, which is a better indicator of acceptance. **Cognitive Level:** Applying **Client Need:** Management of Care **Integrated Process:** Nursing Process: Implementation **Content Area:** Leadership and Management **Strategy:** Resistance to a major change is expected. Consider that the best way to know whether change has occurred is to witness it.

5 **Answer: 3 Rationale:** Client satisfaction surveys are an important tool to monitor and evaluate client and family needs. This information helps healthcare organizations meet those needs. Tracking the number of supplies used by clients on the unit, documenting the time spent on direct client care, and performing daily client assessments with acuity reporting can provide useful information for preparing a budget or unit staffing requirements. **Cognitive Level:** Applying **Client Need:** Management of Care **Integrated Process:** Nursing Process: Planning **Content Area:** Leadership and Management **Strategy:** The core issue of the question is quality management. The purpose of quality management is to improve performance and meet client needs. Consider that the best way to assess client satisfaction with care is to ask the client directly.

6 **Answer: 3, 5, 1, 4, 2 Rationale:** Priority setting can be implemented using a variety of models. The client who is postoperative should be seen first because the client is newly arrived on the unit and is at greatest risk of becoming unstable or experiencing a change in clinical condition. The client with pneumonia should be seen next because the infection involves the airway, although oxygen saturation levels are higher than the critical value of 90% or less. The client who is 4 hours post–cardiac catheterization should be seen next to evaluate the site and conduct general assessment of the affected extremity. The client who will be discharged should be seen next to determine that there are no last-minute needs or issues. The client who needs teaching should be seen last because this is not a physiological need. **Cognitive Level:** Analyzing **Client Need:** Management of Care **Integrated Process:** Nursing Process: Planning **Content Area:** Leadership and Management **Strategy:** Determine which client is at greatest risk of becoming unstable to choose the postanesthesia client, followed by assessing the client whose airway is potentially at risk. The client who had cardiac catheterization could become unstable but has been on the unit for 4 hours, so this client can be seen third. The client scheduled for discharge should be checked fourth because it will not take long to complete the discharge procedure and address any remaining issues or concerns. The client needing teaching will need the most time and can be planned for last.

7 **Answer: 2 Rationale:** The charge nurse should be used to complete a task within the RN's scope of practice, such as starting an intravenous line, while leaving client assessment to the assigned nurse. The assigned nurse should complete a head-to-toe assessment. The nurse assigned to the client knows more about the client than other nurses on the unit do, and can determine a change in the client's status. The application of oxygen is a task for the nurse assigned to the client. Given the information provided in the scenario, the nurse should apply the oxygen immediately to rectify low oxygen levels. The unit secretary could page RT to the room stat for assistance **Cognitive Level:** Applying **Client Need:** Management of Care **Integrated Process:** Nursing Process: Planning **Content Area:** Leadership and Management **Strategy:** Use knowledge of scope of practice and delegation to select the correct answer.

8 **Answer: 2 Rationale:** The nurse should stop feeding the client in room 1, and medicate the client in room 3 as the priority action. While eating is a priority, it does not take precedence over an individual with pain. The client in pain is experiencing discomfort that should be addressed immediately. While medicating the client is important, the charge nurse is busy overseeing the functions on the unit. The task of feeding the client in room 1 can be delegated, but it should be delegated to an appropriate person, such as a nursing assistant. **Cognitive Level:** Analyzing **Client Need:** Management of Care **Integrated Process:** Nursing Process: Implementation **Content Area:** Leadership and Management **Strategy:** Use knowledge of prioritization and delegation to select the correct answer.

9 **Answer: 3, 5 Rationale:** The UAP/UCP can measure vital signs and report the findings to the RN. The UAP/UCP can measure and record the urine output, although the RN would need to make further assessments about the client's status. The RN should irrigate the nasogastric tube and irrigate the urinary catheter as these are not in the UAP's/UCP's scope of practice and job description. A client with an infected wound should have the dressing changed by the RN for assessment of effectiveness of wound therapy and complications. **Cognitive Level:** Applying **Client Need:** Management of Care **Integrated Process:** Nursing Process: Planning **Content Area:** Leadership and Management **Strategy:** Use knowledge of delegation and the process of elimination to select the correct answers. Recall that the RN makes client assessments, engages in problem solving, and does client teaching as key roles.

10 **Answer: 2, 4 Rationale:** The scope of practice for LPNs/LVNs allows them to irrigate urinary catheters and change dressings on diabetic ulcers. While LPNs/LVNs are allowed to irrigate nasogastric tubes, the RN should reposition the tube if it is necessary. The routine measurement of a client with a BP of 100/64 does not require the skills of an LPN/LVN; a UAP/UCP could do this instead. Blood administration should not be delegated to an LPN/LVN due to the complications that could arise during the transfusion; rather, it is within the scope of practice of the RN. **Cognitive Level:** Applying **Client Need:** Management of Care **Integrated Process:** Nursing Process: Planning **Content Area:** Leadership and Management **Strategy:** The wording of the question indicates that more than one

option is correct. Use knowledge of delegation and scope of practice to select the correct answers.

11 **Answer: 2 Rationale:** The LPN/LVN may check vitals and give bed baths, but the skill set of the LPN/LVN is better utilized in providing wound care and medications for the clients. Due to scope of practice the RN should check vital signs and perform assessment of the postoperative client. The scope of practice of a UAP/UCP involves completion of tasks, so the UAP/UCP should check vital signs and complete bed baths on the clients. Physical assessment is within the scope of practice of the RN. **Cognitive Level:** Applying **Client Need:** Management of Care **Integrated Process:** Nursing Process: Planning **Content Area:** Leadership and Management **Strategy:** Use knowledge of delegation and scope of practice to choose the correct answer.

12 **Answer: 1 Rationale:** The scope of practice and most job descriptions for UAP/UCPs include vital signs. It is within the scope of practice for the LPN/LVN to administer oral medications. In some facilities, UAP/UCPs are allowed to change dressings; however, the scope of practice for LPNs/LVNs does not allow them to administer IV medications. UAP/UCPs are allowed to ambulate clients; however, LPNs/LVNs should not assess clients. UAP/UCPs are able to measure vital signs but LPNs/LVNs do not complete admissions because it involves assessment. **Cognitive Level:** Applying **Client Need:** Management of Care **Integrated Process:** Nursing Process: Planning **Content Area:** Leadership and Management **Strategy:** Use knowledge of delegation and scope of practice to select the correct answer.

13 **Answer: 4 Rationale:** The UAP/UCP is qualified to reposition a client with multiple sclerosis who has severe weakness. Due to the risk for aspiration, the nurse should feed the client with dysphagia. The nurse should monitor drainage from a chest tube for characteristics of exudate being removed from the client's thoracic cavity. When a client has an elevated or low blood pressure, the nurse should recheck and assess the client for validity of information and changes in status. **Cognitive Level:** Analyzing **Client Need:** Management of Care **Integrated Process:** Nursing Process: Planning **Content Area:** Leadership and Management **Strategy:** Use knowledge of delegation and the process of elimination to select the correct answer.

14 **Answer: 2 Rationale:** The 3-day postoperative client who will be discharged tomorrow is stable. The client's outcomes are almost met. The LPN/LVN could provide the care for this client. A client with sickle-cell anemia who requires pain medications every 3 hours would need frequent observations and assessments. Because of the RN's ability to problem-solve and think critically, this client should be assigned to a registered nurse. A 76-year-old client who is newly admitted with a chronic condition (type 2 diabetes) exacerbated by an acute condition (pneumonia) is at risk for changes in status and requires frequent assessment. A client with leukemia who has a hemoglobin of 6.4 grams/dL might need a blood transfusion and has unpredictable outcomes. The RN should care for clients with unpredictable outcomes. **Cognitive Level:** Applying **Client Need:** Management of Care **Integrated Process:** Nursing Process: Planning **Content Area:** Leadership and Management **Strategy:** Use knowledge of delegation and the process of elimination to select the correct answer.

15 **Answer: 2 Rationale:** Of the answer options, the best option is that the skilled RN should get the postoperative client with the hip replacement and the abdominal hysterectomy. Postoperative clients are critical clients due to the risk for hypovolemia and shock. The experienced nurse should receive the surgical clients. The RN on orientation should care for the clients with medical conditions such as CHF, hypertension, and diabetes. In this case, the LPNs/LVNs should assume duties such as vital signs and assisting with ADLs. **Cognitive Level:** Analyzing **Client Need:** Management of Care **Integrated Process:** Nursing Process: Planning **Content Area:** Leadership and Management **Strategy:** Use nursing knowledge and knowledge of principles for delegation of client assignments to select the correct response.

16 **Answer: 1 Rationale:** The float nurse from the obstetrics unit can be assigned clients who have abdominal surgery, since the nurse likely has experience working with clients having cesarean section. The nurse can also be assigned clients whose conditions are relatively stable. Clients who have acute conditions compounded by chronic health problems are more complicated, and are better assigned to nurses with experience on the medical-surgical unit. Also, older adult clients can have fluctuations in status, placing them at higher risk for complications, which is not an ideal situation for the float nurse. **Cognitive Level:** Applying **Client Need:** Management of Care **Integrated Process:** Nursing Process: Planning **Content Area:** Leadership and Management **Strategy:** Use knowledge of delegation and the process of elimination to select the correct answer.

17 **Answer: 3 Rationale:** The best choice is to assign the LPN/LVN to change the client's dressing. The RN should perform all assessments. The RN is skilled in assessment and in providing care to those with unpredictable outcomes. The nursing assistant may ambulate the client and provide AM care. **Cognitive Level:** Applying **Client Need:** Management of Care **Integrated Process:** Nursing Process: Planning **Content Area:** Leadership and Management **Strategy:** Use knowledge of delegation and the process of elimination to select the correct answer.

18 **Answer: 1, 4, 5 Rationale:** The nurse assigned a task at which the UAP/UCP evidently was weak, and did not provide supervision. The nurse has delegated a venipuncture to a UAP/UCP who may or may not be comfortable providing the skill. Though the task is permissible in general, venipuncture is not the right task for this UAP/UCP. **Cognitive Level:** Applying **Client Need:** Management of Care **Integrated Process:** Nursing Process: Evaluation **Content Area:** Leadership and Management **Strategy:** Use knowledge of delegation and the process of elimination to select the correct answer.

19 **Answer: 3, 4, 5 Rationale:** The nurse should delegate the venipuncture, electrocardiogram, and oxygen saturation to nursing unit staff or ancillary personnel. The nurse caring for the client should administer the medications and continue to assess the client. The nurse assigned to the client has a baseline of the client's condition, and can attest to changes in status. **Cognitive Level:** Applying **Client Need:** Management of Care **Integrated Process:** Nursing Process: Planning **Content Area:** Leadership and Management **Strategy:** Use knowledge of delegation and the process of elimination to select the correct answers.

20 **Answer: 1, 3, 4, 2 Rationale:** The nurse should start the day by listening to report. This allows the nurse to receive information about the status of each client. The next action is to check the clients. The nurse should check on each assigned client to determine the current status of each client. The goal of checking each client at the beginning of the shift is to make sure distress is not present. Once the nurse has checked each client, the nurse should review AM labs. This information gives

ANSWERS & RATIONALES

the nurse pertinent information that helps plan the day and detect subtle changes in the client's status, which allows earlier treatment and preventative interventions. Lastly, the nurse should review the MAR to detect priority medications. The laboratory results can impact the medications given, which is why they need to be checked before the MAR. **Cognitive Level:** Analyzing **Client Need:** Management of Care **Integrated Process:** Nursing Process: Planning **Content Area:** Leadership and Management **Strategy:** Use knowledge of time management and the process of elimination to make the correct selection.

21 **Answer: 5, 1, 2, 4, 3 Rationale:** The first priority is the administration of a blood product to the anemic client because this client is at risk for decreased tissue perfusion. The nurse then should check the postoperative client with the nasogastric tube and irrigate the tube to ensure it is functioning properly. The urinary catheter should be flushed next; while urine will collect in the bladder at first, it will back up into the renal pelvis and kidney if not treated. The nurse then should proceed to the client with the diabetic foot ulcer because dressing changes, while not urgent, are scheduled treatments. Finally, the nurse would recheck the normal vital signs on the 30-year-old or delegate them to an unlicensed assistant. **Cognitive Level:** Analyzing **Client Need:** Management of Care **Integrated Process:** Nursing Process: Implementation **Content Area:** Leadership and Management **Strategy:** Use nursing knowledge and strategies for prioritization to make the correct selection.

Key Terms to Review

autocratic leadership p. 36
bureaucratic leadership p. 36
consultation p. 35
delegation p. 32
democratic leadership p. 36
formal leadership p. 36
health maintenance organization (HMO) p. 29
indicators p. 41
informal leadership p. 36
interdisciplinary p. 35
laissez-faire leadership p. 36
leader p. 36
leadership p. 36
managed care p. 29
manager p. 36
overdelegation p. 34
planned change p. 39
quality improvement (QI) p. 40
reverse delegation p. 34
servant leadership p. 38
shared governance p. 30
supervision p. 32
supervisor p. 32
time management p. 31
transactional leadership p. 37
transformational leadership p. 37
underdelegation p. 34

References

Amer, K. (2013). *Quality and safety for transforming nursing: Core competencies.* Upper Saddle River, NJ: Pearson Education.

Berman, A., Snyder, S., & Frandsen, G. (2016). *Kozier & Erb's fundamentals of nursing: Concepts, process, and practice* (10th ed.). New York, NY: Pearson Education.

Blais, K. K., & Hayes, J. S. (2016). *Professional nursing practice: Concepts and perspectives* (7th ed.). New York, NY: Pearson Education.

Finkelman, A. W. (2016). *Leadership and management for nurses: Core competencies for quality care* (3rd ed.). New York, NY: Pearson Education.

Grohar-Murray, M. E., DiCroce, H. R., & Langan, J. (2011). *Leadership and management in nursing* (4th ed.). Upper Saddle River, NJ: Pearson Education.

Hansten, R. I., & Jackson, M. (2009). *Clinical delegation skills: A handbook for professional practice* (4th ed.). Sudbury, MA: Jones & Bartlett.

Motacki, K., & Burke, K. (2016). *Nursing delegation and management of patient care* (2nd ed.). St. Louis, MO: Elsevier.

National Council of State Boards of Nursing. (n.d.). Joint statement on delegation. Available at https://www.ncsbn.org/Delegation_joint_statement_NCSBN-ANA.pdf.

National Council of State Boards of Nursing. (1995). *Delegation: Concepts and decision making process* (Position paper). Chicago, IL: Author.

Sullivan, E. J. (2013). *Effective leadership and management in nursing* (8th ed.). Upper Saddle River, NJ: Pearson Education.

Yoder-Wise, P. *Leading and managing in nursing* (6th ed.). St. Louis, MO: Elsevier.

Test Yourself

6 Injury Prevention, Disaster Planning, and Protecting Client Safety

In this chapter

Cross Reference

Other chapters relevant to this content area are

Preventing and Controlling Infection — Chapter 7

I. ACCIDENT PREVENTION ACROSS THE LIFESPAN

NCLEX®

A. **Infant safety depends on actions of parents and infant caretakers;** anticipatory guidance at well-baby checkups is an opportunity for nurse to educate parents

1. Place infants on back after eating and while sleeping; this will not increase risk of aspiration and will reduce risk of sudden infant death syndrome (SIDS)
2. Rapid changes in development and acquisition of new motor skills put infants at increased risk for injury from falls from tables, beds, high chairs, infant seats, and so on
3. Place infants riding in a car in a rear-facing car restraint system in back seat; use a rear-facing restraint system until child is 2 years old or has reached maximum height and weight for seat (American Academy of Pediatrics)
4. Because of their inability to communicate, infants are at risk for burns from applications of heat to skin, such as from a hot water bottle or other heated device
5. Carefully select infant furniture, paying special attention to current safety standards
   a. Infants may be trapped by crib slats spaced too far apart
   b. Infants or young children may be poisoned by lead paint on antique furniture (normal serum lead level is < 10 mg/dL; lead level 10–19 mg requires environmental history; higher levels require treatment to reduce or prevent neurologic deficits)

NCLEX®

B. **Toddlers are most frequently prone to accidents and injury** due to increased physical mobility and intellectual curiosity

1. Store medications, cleaning supplies, and poisons in locked cabinets to prevent poisonings in a curious toddler; have poison control phone number readily available to caregiver and posted on telephone
2. Place car restraint systems for toddlers in back seat and may be forward-facing after toddler has reached 2 years of age or exceeds weight limits of seat; use forward-facing car restraint systems that have a harness until child's shoulders are above the harness or ears have reached top of seat; when a child outgrows system, a booster seat with a lap/shoulder belt is required
3. Toddlers explore all objects with their mouths; assess toys for small parts; avoid giving foods such as hard candy, peanuts, and chewing gum to prevent choking and aspiration

4. Burns in toddlers occur because of chewing on electrical wires, pulling hot liquids from tables or stove tops, and touching space heaters; keep electrical outlets covered and keep handles of pans on stove tops facing inward
5. Drowning is a leading cause of death in toddlers; accompany children at all times when in and around water in bathtub, wading pool, or swimming pool

NCLEX® **C. School-age children are at risk for injury at home and in community** because a school-age child spends increased time away from parent or caregiver

1. Teach and model pedestrian and bicycle safety to children at this age; bicycle helmets can prevent head injury to children biking, rollerblading, or skateboarding
2. Place children under 1.4 m (4 ft 9 in.) in rear seat of a car with a booster seat and lap/shoulder seatbelt (often until 8–12 years of age); never allow children to ride in the bed of a pickup truck or open, unsecured area of an automobile, such as a station wagon or van
3. Teach school-age children principles of fire safety; injury can occur from experimentation with matches, lighters, and fireworks; school-age children can participate in implementing a school or home fire escape plan; teach to "stop, drop, and roll" if clothing catches fire
4. Teach school-age children principles of water safety; swimming lessons and life jackets are necessary for boating and swimming; children should never swim without adult supervision
5. Include in safety education for children to play in safe areas, avoid strangers, recognize unwelcome touch, and obey traffic signals

NCLEX® **D. Adolescent injury and death may be very violent in nature;** newly found independence, feelings of invincibility and immortality, and access to motor vehicles can lead to accidents with injury

1. Encourage courses in driver's education; children 13 years and older may ride in front seat of vehicle while wearing a seatbelt; seatbelt regulations should be role modeled and enforced by parents
2. Teach adolescents dangers of alcohol and substance use
3. Adolescents may be injured in sports-related accidents; encourage protective sporting gear for organized and impromptu sporting events
4. Review water safety principles because adolescents can overestimate endurance when swimming
5. Adolescents benefit from information about sexual health, including information about sexually transmitted infections and pregnancy prevention (birth control)

E. Adult safety concerns can be related to home, workplace, and leisure activities

1. Encourage working adults to participate in occupational health programs offered in workplace; musculoskeletal injury is most frequent workplace injury
2. Hazardous conditions and toxic substances may occur in workplace; educate employees in **OSHA** (Occupational Safety and Health Administration) regulations and guidelines for use of safety devices and handling hazardous substances
3. Alcohol consumption is involved in 40% of deaths from motor vehicle accidents, making it important to have community education programs about hazards of drinking and driving; other drugs that cause impairment pose similar risks
4. NCLEX® Firearms in the home may lead to accidental injury or death; encourage owners to attend firearm safety class and store all firearms and ammunition in a locked cabinet
5. Residents in some neighborhoods may be at risk for crime and injury; assess for access to police and fire services
6. NCLEX® Residential fires account for the majority of fire-related injuries; teach that homes should have smoke detectors, a fire extinguisher in the kitchen, and a fire evacuation plan

F. Older adults may experience a decrease in strength, vision, hearing, and cognitive ability that could lead to accidents or injury; evaluate homes for safety hazards

1. NCLEX® Falls are the leading cause of accidents in older adults
   a. Stairwells should be well lit
   b. Small scatter rugs, runners, and mats should not be used
   c. Bathrooms and showers/tubs should have grab bars
   d. Furniture, floors, and passageways should be free of clutter
2. Home modifications may be necessary to accommodate safe use of wheelchairs or walkers
3. Clients taking some medications may have decreased cognitive abilities or impaired judgment; encourage them to ask for assistance with activities of daily living
4. NCLEX® Neighbors, police, and fire officials should be made aware of older adults with disabilities living alone
5. Decrease in temperature regulation may increase risk of hyperthermia or hypothermia; be careful with use of space heaters; be sure older adults have fans or air conditioners in summer heat

6. Older adults may be prey to strangers and criminals who can inflict physical and financial injury; caution them against letting strangers into their homes or responding to telephone calls, e-mails, or letters asking for money or personal information
7. Motor vehicle accidents are of concern for older adults; frequent assessment of driving ability is required; loss of driving privileges can mean a loss of independence

II. ERROR PREVENTION IN HEALTHCARE SETTINGS

A. Medication errors are most frequent type of medical error in hospital setting

1. Types of untoward medication events
    a. Medication error involves wrong client, medication, dose, time, or route
    b. **Adverse reaction** is an undesired effect of a prescribed medication, whether a severe side effect or a toxicity
    c. **Toxic reaction** occurs when prescribed medication dosage is excessive or poisonous to an individual; this may be due to client's size, health condition, or other medications being taken
    d. Side effects are actions or effects of drugs other than that desired
    e. **Idiosyncratic reaction** is an unusual response to a drug that may be unrelated to dose; reaction may or may not reoccur if medication is given again
    f. Hypersensitivity or allergic reactions may range from mild rashes to life-threatening anaphylaxis; this reaction will recur and could get worse with each subsequent exposure

NCLEX®
2. Nursing interventions to prevent medication errors (see Box 6–1)

Box 6–1

Nursing Interventions to Prevent Medication Errors

- Know agency medication administration system; follow protocols
- Be familiar with medication resources at agency
- Ensure client information (e.g., height, weight, allergies) is accessible to healthcare providers, clinicians, and pharmacists
- Verify medication prescriptions; do not transcribe prescriptions that contain unapproved or nonstandard abbreviations until clarified
- Use standard hours and times for medication administration
- Be familiar with drug side effects or possible adverse reactions; observe for these on an ongoing basis
- Ask a nurse colleague to double-check complex dosage calculations
- Do not interrupt nurses giving medications because this can lead to errors during administration
- Check client identification bracelet before administering medication; ask client to verbalize name and date of birth (or other method of checking two unique identifiers) according to agency policy; additional measures are needed with blood administration (see Chapter 32)
- Stop and double-check medication if client questions appearance or dose
- Report and document any error or variation in medication administration process

B. Allergies or an allergic response to an allergen can be life-threatening

NCLEX®
1. Include allergies in all health histories; ask about allergies to medications, food, tape, latex, or soap; document type and severity of reaction to allergen
2. Allergies to iodine indicate a need for use of hypoallergenic (rather than iodine-based) dyes in radiologic procedures
3. Document all allergies on medical records, lab records, pharmacy records, and client identification bracelet

III. INJURY PREVENTION IN HEALTHCARE SETTINGS

NCLEX®
A. Client safety can be at risk when admitted to a healthcare agency; assess risk factors for each client upon admission and identify methods to reduce possibility of injury

B. Risk for falls is most common in infants and older adult clients; implement a fall prevention program for those at risk (see Box 6–2, Nursing Interventions to Reduce Risk for Falls)

Box 6–2

Nursing Interventions to Reduce Risk for Falls

- Familiarize client with environment on admission and as needed
- Perform falls risk assessment (most tools assess age, number of health problems, medications, environment, physical ability, vision, and history of falls) on admission or with change in condition
- Assess ability to ambulate and transfer
- Orient client to nurse call system and have client "teach back" its use
- Be sure nurse call system is within reach at all times
- Keep personal possessions and bedside table within safe reach
- Keep hospital bed in low position with brakes locked when client is in bed
- Use a bed or chair exit safety monitoring device for clients at risk for falls
- Assess need for constant companion for confused clients
- Keep crib side-rails up when child is unattended
- Encourage use of nonskid footwear
- Keep room tidy and free of clutter and keep floor surfaces clean and dry (clean spills promptly)
- Perform "scheduled" rounding hourly to assist clients in meeting their needs (many falls occur when clients go to bathroom)

C. *Restraints* are protective devices used to limit client mobility

1. Restraints can be physical (limiting physical activity) or chemical (medications given to inhibit a specific movement or behavior)
2. Purposes of restraints
   a. Reduce risk of client injury from falls
   b. Prevent interruption of therapy such as traction or IV infusions
   c. Prevent a confused or agitated client from removing life support
   d. Reduce risk of injury to others by an agitated client
3. When possible, use alternatives to restraint, such as bed or chair alarm safety devices
4. Explain reason for restraint as a safety device to client and family; obtain their permission whenever possible

NCLEX®

5. There are legal implications with use of restraints because they limit client freedom
   a. A written prescription is needed to restrain a client
   b. Prescription must include type of restraint, reason for restraint, and time period limits for use; PRN (as needed) restraint prescriptions are prohibited
   c. A nurse may apply physical restraints; however, healthcare provider must evaluate client within an agency-prescribed time period, which may be as soon as 1 hour; verify hospital policy and follow it

NCLEX®

6. Assess neurovascular status and skin integrity every 30 minutes and document; remove restraint at least every 2 hours according to agency policy to promote circulation and muscle movement
7. Bed side-rails
   a. Considered restraints

NCLEX®

   b. Half or three-quarter rails are better than full-length rails for confused or agitated clients who may be injured climbing over rail; instead, consider use of alternative safety devices to prevent risk for falls

NCLEX®

8. Jacket, belt, or extremity restraints
   a. Apply only as specified by manufacturer; never tie them to a movable part of a bed or chair; allow enough slack on straps to allow some movement
   b. Use a half-bow knot for easy release when attaching restraint to bed or chair
   c. Check for adequate circulation when using restraints; maintain two finger widths between client and restraint
9. Try creative nursing measures to prevent use of physical or chemical restraints
   a. Orient client to surroundings
   b. Encourage family, friends, or a sitter to stay with client
   c. Keep confused clients near nursing station
   d. Provide confused clients with diversionary activities

e. Maintain frequent toileting routine
f. Reposition or ambulate frequently, if appropriate
g. Evaluate client medications for undesirable effects
h. Use relaxation techniques such as music, aromatherapy, and books on tape

D. Seizure precautions protect client from injury in case of seizure activity

1. Explain purpose of seizure precautions
2. *NCLEX®* Pad head and side-rails of bed to prevent injury
3. Keep suction and oxygen equipment near bed; use oxygen mask after seizure activity has ceased
4. Do not attempt to insert anything into mouth of client during seizure (bitestick, airway)
5. Do not attempt to restrain or limit movement during a seizure; instead, remove objects that could lead to client harm

E. Fire safety

1. Preventive measures for hospital or agency
   a. Know locations of exits, fire alarms, and distinguishers, and telephone number to call to report fire
   b. Keep hallways and other open areas free of clutter (beds, stretchers, wheelchairs, etc.)
   c. Know categories of fire and correct type of extinguisher to use for each
   d. *NCLEX®* Participate in practice fire drills and evacuation procedures
2. Actions to take during an actual fire
   a. Use the acronym RACE to recall what to do in an actual fire:

Memory Aid

Use the mnemonic RACE to remember in order the four steps to maintain client safety during a fire:
Remove clients from danger.
Activate the fire alarm.
Contain the fire.
Evacuate the area (horizontal evacuation should be done before vertical evacuation, if possible).

   b. Turn off oxygen and any electrical appliances in use near fire
   c. Avoid using elevator during a fire
   d. Direct clients who can walk to a specific area that is deemed safe; horizontal evacuation (on the same floor or level) is done before vertical evacuation (stairs)
   e. Clients who are bed-bound are evacuated from area by bed, stretcher, or wheelchair
   f. Clients on mechanical ventilation must be manually ventilated with a manual resuscitation (Ambu) bag until they are moved to a safe area where they can be placed again on ventilator
3. Preventive measures for home
   a. Focus on teaching emergency phone numbers, maintaining smoke alarms and fire extinguishers, importance of family fire drills, careful disposal of burning cigarettes and use of matches, grease-fire prevention
   b. Teach precautions during an actual fire: Close windows and doors to contain fire, cover nose and mouth with damp cloth when leaving a smoke-filled area, and stay as close as possible to ground

NCLEX® **F. Electrical safety**

1. Each employee is responsible for ensuring that electrical equipment is in proper working order
2. Inspect all electrical equipment used in client care for damaged cords, frayed or exposed wires, or other damage; remove damaged equipment from service and label with a tag for repair; notify appropriate department (such as biomedical engineering)
3. Have any electrical equipment brought into hospital checked for electrical safety before use
4. Implement basic electrical safety measures such as reading instructions for use on unfamiliar electrical equipment, using three-pronged (grounded) electrical plugs, plugging equipment into appropriate wall electrical outlets, avoiding overload of electrical circuit, grasping plug instead of pulling on cord to remove cord from outlet, and unplugging equipment before cleaning
5. If a client receives an electrical shock, do not touch client until electricity has been shut off or has already been removed from contact with electrical current

6. Teach clients additional electrical safety measures for use in home such as using electrical extension cords only when necessary, taping them to floor to prevent falls or damage to cord, avoiding running cords under carpeting, placing protective covers on wall outlets to protect small children, and avoiding use of electrical equipment near water (sinks, bathtub, shower, pool, etc.)

G. Radiation safety

1. Become familiar with and adhere to agency policies and procedures for radiation safety
2. Recognize label indicating radioactivity placed on bags containing radioactive materials and doors at entry to areas where radioactive substances may be stored (such as nuclear medicine)
3. Minimize personal exposure to radiation by limiting *time* spent near source, ensuring adequate *distance*, and using proper *shielding* (such as a lead apron) per agency policy
4. When caring for client with an implanted radiation device, wear dosimeter badge to monitor cumulative exposure to radiation, ensure client is admitted to a private room, avoid touching dislodged radiation implants, and follow other specified agency procedures

H. Employee safety

1. Occupational Safety and Health Administration (OSHA), a federal agency, regulates workplaces to protect health of employees
2. **Bloodborne pathogen** exposure is a health hazard for many employees in a healthcare setting; OSHA standards include recommendations from Centers for Disease Control and Prevention (**CDC**) regarding standard precautions (see also Chapter 7 on preventing and controlling infections)
   a. Standard precautions are techniques used with all clients to decrease risk of exposure to pathogens
   b. Gloves and face and eye protection help protect healthcare workers from bloodborne pathogens
   c. Nurses may be required to have a vaccine for hepatitis B or influenza, or sign a declination refusing vaccines
3. Needlestick precautions, when properly used, protect healthcare workers
   NCLEX® a. Do not recap needles and do not bend or break needles before disposal
   NCLEX® b. Ensure that sharps containers are in each client room and medication area
   c. Needle-free technology should be provided by employers
   d. Each health agency must have a needle/sharps injury protocol in case of injury; report all injuries and follow protocol for self-protection
   e. Many institutions now use needleless devices or syringes with needles that retract after use to prevent exposure
4. Environmental infection control can protect employees and clients from exposure to pathogens; CDC sets infection control standards for healthcare agencies
   a. Employees may be annually tested for tuberculosis
   b. Laundry and medical waste are regulated by environmental infection control guidelines; laundry and items soiled with blood or body fluids must be identified by biohazard markers such as red bags
5. NCLEX® Latex allergy is an actual or potential hazard for healthcare workers and clients
   a. Latex rubber is used in many medical products but healthcare agencies are increasingly using products that do not contain latex
   b. Always ask clients about latex allergies; be sure latex-free gloves are available
   c. Provide a latex-free cart that includes latex-free tourniquets, IV tubing and IV supplies, and other items for clients with a latex allergy
6. NCLEX® Hazardous chemicals pose a safety threat in many areas of a healthcare setting
   a. Material Safety Data Sheets (**MSDS**) are OSHA-required informational handouts that describe any and all chemical agents in an employment setting
   b. Employees are required to be trained in use of MSDS
   c. All chemicals must be properly labeled and have a corresponding MSDS
   d. Read and be aware of all information related to chemicals before handling or cleaning spills; a few examples of chemicals in healthcare settings are antineoplastic (chemotherapy) drugs, cleaning supplies, and pesticides
   NCLEX® e. In case of a chemotherapy drug spill, restrict access to area of spill and contact environmental services or other department per protocol; if nurse must clean spill, refer to MSDS protocol on unit (see Box 6–3)

Box 6–3

Procedure for Chemotherapy Drug Spill

1. Restrict access to area of the spill.
2. Obtain a chemotherapy spill kit (gloves, gown, goggles, detergent, sponges, labeled container for disposal).
3. Use absorbent sponges to absorb spill.
4. Clean surface with designated cleanser.
5. Dispose of all supplies in approved container.
6. Wash hands.
7. Cleanse all skin exposed to chemotherapy agent—both client and staff.
8. Document the occurrence.

IV. INCIDENT REPORTS

A. Overview

1. An agency record of an accident or other event in a healthcare agency that is not consistent with hospital policy; may also be called unusual occurrence report or variance report
2. Agencies have specific forms to report these events, such as accidents, falls, needlesticks, client infections, medication errors, or missing personal property
3. Agencies may use one type of form for patients and visitors and another for employees
4. For the protection of client and nurse, it is vital to report all incidents

NCLEX®

B. Procedure for responding to and reporting an incident

1. Prevent further injury and provide care for client, visitor, or employee
2. Notify healthcare provider immediately and implement prescriptions for interventions that may limit further harm
3. File report as soon as possible; person filing report may or may not be same person responsible for or involved in incident
4. Identify client, visitor, employee, and all witnesses to event
5. State objective facts of incident; do not draw conclusions or lay blame
6. Be specific—list name of medication or equipment involved
7. Also document facts of incident in client's record; do not document in client record that an incident report was filed (an incident report is a risk management tool); do not put a copy of incident report in client record
8. The policy for incident reporting is unique to each healthcare agency; review and follow specific agency policy for incident reporting

V. DISASTER PLANNING AND EMERGENCY RESPONSE

A. Disasters and emergencies are traumatic events that can affect an individual, family, community, or nation; nurses and healthcare providers are instrumental in disaster preparedness, disaster response, and client care in community and hospital settings

1. Disasters may be natural or man-made; disasters vary by predictability, frequency, preventability, imminence, and destructive potential
2. Natural disasters such as hurricanes and floods generally allow time for planning and evacuation; disasters such as earthquakes and tornadoes do not but are predictable in certain areas of the country; residents and healthcare providers should be encouraged to prepare
3. Man-made disasters are usually less predictable; explosions, fires, airline accidents, radiation emergencies, bioterrorism, and toxic chemical releases occur randomly; however, plans can be made by healthcare providers and emergency response personnel to have trained resources to take action
4. The Federal Emergency Management Agency (FEMA) is a government agency that has a National Response Plan; it provides states and local communities guidelines for reporting threats and incidents and for assessment, response, and recovery during disasters; nurses are part of disaster planning and response at federal, state, and local levels
5. Purpose of disaster planning is to decrease community vulnerability and to assure available resources if a disaster occurs

B. **Planning for any type of disaster must start with individuals and families;** one community health nurse role is to educate and guide citizens in preparedness
   1. Families must have a communication plan; emergency phone numbers should be carried by all family members; establish a place to meet in an emergency
   2. Be prepared to shut off all utilities in home; water may be precious after a disaster; electricity and natural gas may pose a safety threat
   3. A package of vital records should be readily available when evacuating a home; identification, health and immunization records, insurance policies, deeds, and cash or traveler's checks would be needed during and after an evacuation
   4. *NCLEX®* Identify special family needs; make an emergency kit; have extra medications and food items for dietary requirements; have extra batteries for medical devices
   5. Make plans for homebound pets; pets are not usually allowed in shelters; leave food and water; attach proper pet identification
   6. Encourage family members to learn CPR and first aid

C. ***The Joint Commission* requires hospitals to have a disaster plan** and to periodically practice response to plan
   1. Plan should include policy and procedures for administration, nursing and patient service, medical staff, security, medical records, engineering, laboratory, radiology, as well as the following:
      a. Notification and communication of disaster
      b. Assessment of hospital resources
      c. Personnel recall system/transportation plan
      d. Establishment of a facility control center
      e. Maintenance of accurate records
      f. Communication and public relations
      g. Equipment and resupply
   2. Nurses are responsible for knowing their role in disaster response and are part of committees that design and evaluate hospital plan; nursing tasks during a disaster may include the following:
      a. Assess nursing unit for resources—staff, beds, and equipment
      b. *NCLEX®* Assess current clients for discharge in case of increased need of hospital/nursing services by high-acuity/injured clients
      c. Activate staff recall plan
      d. Communicate with hospital disaster control center
      e. *NCLEX®* Assess disaster victims for extent of injury; this is called **triage**
      f. Render first aid
      g. Provide treatment based on protocols

D. **Triage is a French word meaning "to sort";** in case of emergency, nurses may be asked to triage injured or ill clients to identify those in need of emergent, urgent, or nonurgent care
   1. Primary survey focuses on airway, breathing, circulation, and neurologic disability/deficits (ABCD)
      a. Clear and open the airway
      b. Assess for respiratory distress
      c. Assess quality of ventilation (rate, color, breath sounds)
      d. Check pulses for quality and rate
      e. Assess for external bleeding
      f. Take blood pressure
      g. Assess level of consciousness and pupillary response, weakness or paralysis of extremities

Memory Aid

Remember ABCD to recall the components of the primary survey for a victim of trauma: airway, breathing, circulation, disability (deficits).

   2. The secondary survey is initiated after initiating life-saving interventions
      a. Measure and record a full set of vital signs
      b. Remove all of client's clothing
      c. Do a complete health history and physical examination
      d. Identify family members
      e. Administer comfort measures or pain medication, if appropriate

3. After initial assessment, identify and label victims according to triage acuity system
   a. Priority I or emergent care: victims who need immediate treatment, such as those with cardiac or respiratory distress, trauma and bleeding, or neurologic deficits; these victims should be labeled with a red tag
   b. Priority II or urgent care: victims who need treatment within 2 hours, such as clients with simple fractures, lacerations, or fevers; these victims should be labeled with a yellow tag and reevaluated every 30–60 minutes
   c. Priority III or nonurgent care: victims who need treatment that can wait for hours; those with sprains, rashes, and minor pain should be labeled with a green tag and reevaluated every 1–2 hours; an orange tag indicates a client who has a nonemergent psychiatric condition
   d. Victims who are deceased should be labeled with a black tag and transported to designated temporary morgue
4. It is common to use terms *emergent*, *urgent*, and *nonurgent* to describe a client's triage status if situation is not part of a disaster

Check Your NCLEX–RN® Exam I.Q. *You are ready for testing on this content if you can:*

- Identify client developmental and environmental factors that may lead to accidents or injury.
- Provide care and teaching to the client at risk for accident or injury.
- Protect the client who is at risk for injury.
- Utilize restraints safely, effectively, and only when necessary, such as when less restrictive measures are unsuccessful.
- Accurately identify situations requiring completion of an incident or unusual occurrence report.
- Explain personal and professional actions to take for disaster preparedness.
- Effectively utilize triage concepts in an emergency or disaster situation.

PRACTICE TEST

1 The nurse determines a new mother is in greatest need of more education about infant care and safety when the mother makes which statement?

1. "I am pretty sure that I am going to breastfeed my baby."
2. "After feeding, I should put my baby on her tummy to prevent choking."
3. "Solid foods are unnecessary during the baby's first 4–6 months."
4. "I should wake my baby up every 3–4 hours for feeding."

2 The result of a toddler's lead screening is 12 mg/dL. What would the nurse say to the mother at this time?

1. "His lab values are just fine."
2. "Have you noticed any blood in his stools?"
3. "When were his last immunizations?"
4. "Tell me about where you live."

3 A newborn is scheduled for discharge from the birthing center tomorrow. When teaching the new parents about car seats, which characteristics of infant restraint systems would the nurse include as essential for the newborn? Select all that apply.

1. Forward-facing
2. Rear-facing
3. In the back seat
4. In the front seat
5. Of a solid and neutral color

4 Which snack would the nurse appropriately offer the hospitalized toddler?

1. Crackers
2. Peanuts
3. Grapes
4. Cereal bar

5 What is the best method for the nurse to use to encourage the use of bicycle helmets by school-age children?

1. Advocate for legislation on helmet laws.
2. Teach parents to role-model helmet use while riding bicycles.
3. Verbally reprimand children who report not wearing helmets while riding.
4. Recommend the parents purchase stylish helmets to increase compliance.

6 A school nurse is planning a health class on accidents and injuries for high school students. Which topic is most important to include?

1. Occupational-related injuries at work
2. Motor vehicle–related injuries
3. Fall-related injuries
4. Injury due to residential fires

7 The home health nurse is visiting an older adult client with diabetes mellitus. The nurse becomes concerned and implements safety education when which of the following occurs?

1. Neighbors bring a warm lunch to client
2. Children install air conditioners in kitchen and bedroom
3. Grandchildren place baskets of folded laundry by bedroom door
4. Client stores diabetic testing supplies on kitchen table

8 The nurse preceptor observes the new RN administering medications. The preceptor concludes there is a risk for medication error when the new RN takes which action?

1. Answers a healthcare provider's page while passing medications
2. Uses military time for documentation
3. Asks for help with a dosage calculation
4. Does not give a medication that the client questions

9 The nurse would ask a client scheduled for a venogram about allergy to which substance before the procedure?

1. Peanuts
2. Iodine
3. Eggs
4. Meat tenderizer

10 Which of the following medication prescriptions should the nurse question?

1. Morphine sulfate 4 mg IV every 3–4 hours as needed for pain
2. Ceftriaxone IVPB every 8 hours
3. Furosemide 40 mg po daily
4. Metoprolol 50 mg po twice a day

11 The nurse has applied elbow splints on a confused client to prevent the client from removing the intravenous (IV) line. Which of the following interventions is required?

1. Document appearance of client's IV site every hour.
2. Remove elbow splints every 8 hours.
3. Ask for renewal of prescription for restraint every 72 hours.
4. Assess and document client's condition at least every hour.

12 A Code Red (fire) has been announced on the hospital unit. What is the nurse's first response?

1. Remove clients in danger from the fire.
2. Contain the fire.
3. Report fire to other staff.
4. Extinguish the fire.

13 A client on the hospital unit has fallen. Place the nursing interventions in order of priority. All options must be used.

1. Identify all witnesses.
2. Call the healthcare provider.
3. Assess and provide urgent care.
4. Notify the charge nurse.
5. Fill out the incident report.

Fill in your answer below:

Answer: ______________________________

14 Which information would the nurse omit from written documentation when a reportable incident has occurred?

1. Names of witnesses on incident report
2. Nursing interventions in medical record
3. Time healthcare provider was called about incident report
4. That an incident report was submitted in medical record

15 Public health nurses have been activated to open a shelter due to an approaching hurricane. What most important items should families be encouraged to take to the emergency shelter?

1. Food and extra clothing
2. Cats and small dogs
3. Medication and vital records
4. Radios and small personal electronics

16 A major portion of a construction project has collapsed. The emergency department (ED) has been notified that numerous victims are being transported to the ED. What should be the first action of the ED nurses?

1. Assess department for resources—staff, beds, equipment.
2. Implement personnel recall system.
3. Discharge stable clients.
4. Set up a temporary morgue.

17 A young man is brought to the emergency department as a victim of a multivehicle accident that caused multiple casualties. The man is awake and alert. He has a fracture of his right tibia and several small lacerations on his face. How will the triage nurse categorize this client?

1. Priority 1 (red tag)
2. Priority 2 (yellow tag)
3. Priority 3 (green tag)
4. Priority 4 (black tag)

18 The nurse should explain to the mother of a 10-month-old infant that a rear-facing car safety seat should continue to be used until the child exceeds the weight limit or is ____ months of age. Record your answer rounding to the nearest whole number.

Fill in your answer below:

____ months

19 The nurse is treating a client who continues to return to a violent relationship saying, "There is nothing I can do." What is the nurse's best response?

1. "You do have some choices; let's sit together and explore them."
2. "If you return you are at risk for further abuse."
3. "Here is the number of the crisis hotline."
4. "Do you have family or friends who can help?"

20 The nurse is assessing a school-age child. Which finding by the nurse may indicate physical neglect?

1. Not following instructions well
2. Boisterous activity
3. Stealing or hoarding food
4. Sudden onset of enuresis

21 The nurse admits a female client to the emergency department who arrives with a black eye and reports of headache, chronic pain, GI problems, menstrual irregularities, and anxiety. A previous physical workup was negative. The nurse should assess the client for which priority problems? Select all that apply.

1. Premenstrual syndrome
2. Physical or sexual abuse
3. Irritable bowel syndrome
4. Self-destructive potential
5. Migraine headache

ANSWERS & RATIONALES

1 **Answer:** 2 **Rationale:** Infants should always be put to sleep on the back, indicating the need for further teaching about newborn care and safety. Breastfeeding is a nutrition choice. Solid foods are not needed in the first 4–6 months of infancy. Newborns do sleep frequently and should be awakened every 3–4 hours for feeding. **Cognitive Level:** Analyzing **Client Need:** Safety and Infection Control **Integrated Process:** Nursing Process: Evaluation **Content Area:** Maternal-Newborn **Strategy:** The wording of the question guides you to look for a false statement as the correct response. Use the process of elimination and nursing knowledge.

2 **Answer:** 4 **Rationale:** The lead value of 12 mg/dL is high. Lead levels below 10 mg/dL are acceptable. Levels of 10–19 mg/dL require an environmental history. Levels above 20 mg/dL

require a full medical evaluation. Asking about the child's home is the first step in evaluating the environment. Older homes may have lead paint and lead in the plumbing. Blood in the stool and immunization status are unrelated to lead poisoning. **Cognitive Level:** Applying **Client Need:** Safety and Infection Control **Integrated Process:** Nursing Process: Assessment **Content Area:** Child Health **Strategy:** To answer the question it is required to know acceptable lead values. Notice that option 4 is related to an environmental assessment.

3 **Answer: 2, 3 Rationale:** An infant child restraint system should always be in the back seat and rear-facing. After a child is 2 years of age and has reached the manufacturer's weight limit, the seat may be in the rear and front-facing. Although bright colors are stimulating to an infant, the color of the system does not matter. **Cognitive Level:** Applying **Client Need:** Safety and Infection Control **Integrated Process:** Teaching and Learning **Content Area:** Child Health **Strategy:** Choose between opposites, since usually one of each is correct. Use the process of elimination and nursing knowledge of infant safety measures to make appropriate selections.

4 **Answer: 1 Rationale:** Crackers are of a soft consistency when chewed and swallowed. Toddlers can easily choke on small foods such as peanuts, popcorn, and grapes and firm-consistency foods such as cereal bars. **Cognitive Level:** Applying **Client Need:** Safety and Infection Control **Integrated Process:** Nursing Process: Implementation **Content Area:** Child Health **Strategy:** Note that the question is determining risk for choking and select the option that has a food that will dissolve easily in the mouth.

5 **Answer: 2 Rationale:** Parent role models of behavior are most effective in fostering good habits in children. Legislative action provides legal support for helmet use, but this is not a direct motivator for children. Reprimands for lack of use may be effective on a case-by-case basis, but make less of an impression than positive role modeling. Stylish helmets may be effective on a case-by-case basis, but make less of an impression than positive role modeling. **Cognitive Level:** Applying **Client Need:** Safety and Infection Control **Integrated Process:** Nursing Process: Planning **Content Area:** Child Health **Strategy:** Note the critical word *best*, indicating that all answers could be correct, but one is better than the others. Consider that legislation is a positive step but may not change behaviors. Reprimanding is a negative behavior. The style of helmet may be effective but may not be realistic for all families depending on financial circumstances.

6 **Answer: 2 Rationale:** Driving a car and having the independence to ride with friends are important milestones for high school–age adolescents. Some adolescents experiment with alcohol and drugs, putting them at increased risk for motor vehicle accidents, in addition to inexperience. Occupational injury is a risk for the working adult. Falls are risk factors for the older adult. Residential fires can affect any age. **Cognitive Level:** Analyzing **Client Need:** Safety and Infection Control **Integrated Process:** Nursing Process: Planning **Content Area:** Child Health **Strategy:** Use knowledge of the principles of growth and development to aid in answering this question.

7 **Answer: 3 Rationale:** Laundry baskets that are set on the floor will pose a risk for falling for the older client. All hallways, floors, stairways, and furniture should be free of clutter. Neighbors bringing lunch for the elderly client is a good safety intervention. Family controlling the climate for the elderly client is a good safety intervention. Keeping diabetic supplies on a kitchen table with easy access will facilitate diabetic testing. **Cognitive Level:** Applying **Client Need:** Safety and Infection Control **Integrated Process:** Nursing Process: Assessment **Content Area:** Fundamentals **Strategy:** Focus on the critical word *safety* and choose the option that poses a risk to the client. Recall that older adults are at increased risk for falls, so this should guide your thought process as you make a selection.

8 **Answer: 1 Rationale:** The nurse should never interrupt the medication administration process because this increases the risk for errors. Military time is frequently used by institutions for documentation. The nurse should always ask for assistance with dosage calculations when in doubt. The nurse should never give a medication that a client questions; instead, recheck the prescription, dosage, and medication, and give the client an explanation. **Cognitive Level:** Analyzing **Client Need:** Safety and Infection Control **Integrated Process:** Nursing Process: Diagnosis **Content Area:** Fundamentals **Strategy:** Focus on the risk for error and select the option that poses a threat to the safe administration of medications.

9 **Answer: 2 Rationale:** Iodine is used in many radiological procedures. Peanuts, eggs, and meat tenderizer do not pose a risk of cross-sensitivity to iodine. **Cognitive Level:** Applying **Client Need:** Safety and Infection Control **Integrated Process:** Nursing Process: Assessment **Content Area:** Fundamentals **Strategy:** Knowledge of radiological procedures must be applied. In addition, recall that allergy to iodine commonly applies to radiological procedures.

10 **Answer: 2 Rationale:** The ceftriaxone prescription does not have a medication dosage listed. The prescriptions for morphine sulfate, furosemide, and metoprolol have the required information for dispensing medications. **Cognitive Level:** Applying **Client Need:** Safety and Infection Control **Integrated Process:** Nursing Process: Planning **Content Area:** Fundamentals **Strategy:** Read all options carefully. Apply the five rights of medication administration.

11 **Answer: 4 Rationale:** The client should be checked at least hourly, and the nurse must document client status. The IV site should be checked every hour, but documentation may be done only once per shift unless a problem occurs. Because restraints may impede circulation, they should be removed according to agency policy, which is generally every 1–2 hours rather than every 8 hours. Physical restraints impede a client's freedom; their use needs to be prescribed every 24 hours. **Cognitive Level:** Applying **Client Need:** Safety and Infection Control **Integrated Process:** Nursing Process: Implementation **Content Area:** Fundamentals **Strategy:** Utilize knowledge of common policy and procedures for use of physical restraints. Always consider an answer that contains assessment as an option.

12 **Answer: 1 Rationale:** The primary responsibility of the nurse is client safety. Removing a client from danger should be the priority. Next, the alarm should be sounded. The nurse and others can then contain and possibly extinguish the fire. **Cognitive Level:** Analyzing **Client Need:** Safety and Infection Control **Integrated Process:** Nursing Process: Implementation **Content Area:** Fundamentals **Strategy:** Option one is client-focused. The other options are fire-focused. Remember the mneumonic RACE (remove, alarm, contain, extinguish).

13 **Answer: 3, 4, 2, 1, 5 Rationale:** The primary actions of the nurse are emergency assessment and first aid. If the nurse notifies the charge nurse, there will be nursing help to contact the healthcare provider and speak with witnesses. After caring

ANSWERS & RATIONALES

for the client and assessing the situation, the nurse is prepared to fill out the incident report. **Cognitive Level:** Analyzing **Client Need:** Safety and Infection Control **Integrated Process:** Nursing Process: Implementation **Content Area:** Fundamentals **Strategy:** Focus on the client first. Then obtain additional help, collect data, and do the paperwork last.

14 **Answer: 4 Rationale:** The medical record belongs to the client and should contain all facts related to the client and the incident. The incident report belongs to the hospital and should contain all facts and supportive data related to the client and the incident. The medical record should not refer to the incident report. **Cognitive Level:** Applying **Client Need:** Safety and Infection Control **Integrated Process:** Nursing Process: Implementation **Content Area:** Fundamentals **Strategy:** Use knowledge of policy and procedure regarding incident reports to analyze this situation.

15 **Answer: 3 Rationale:** Client medications and vital records are needed for a short or extended stay at an emergency shelter. Because space is very limited, there is no provision for storing food, and animals are not allowed. Loud electronic devices may cause disturbance between families or individuals. Electricity may or may not be available. **Cognitive Level:** Analyzing **Client Need:** Safety and Infection Control **Integrated Process:** Nursing Process: Planning **Content Area:** Fundamentals **Strategy:** Focus on the required items for a stay in the emergency shelter. A client's medications are the only provisions listed that emergency personnel may not be able to provide.

16 **Answer: 1 Rationale:** The nurses must first assess current ED resources. No decisions can be made without a comprehensive assessment of staff, beds, and equipment. Implementing a personnel recall system, discharging stable clients, and setting up a temporary morgue are specific interventions that may be needed during the response, but a comprehensive assessment is needed first when there is a possible impending disaster. **Cognitive Level:** Analyzing **Client Need:** Safety and Infection Control **Integrated Process:** Nursing Process: Assessment **Content Area:** Fundamentals **Strategy:** Choose the option that is the most comprehensive or global of the option choices.

17 **Answer: 2 Rationale:** The client is awake and alert. He does not have overt signs of cardiac or respiratory distress. This client can wait for treatment for 1–2 hours, indicating priority 2 (yellow tag). The nurse should check on his status every 30–60 minutes. A client with priority 1 (red tag) status requires treatment immediately. A client with priority 3 (green tag) most likely has minor injuries and can wait for a number of hours as long as reassessment is done every 1–2 hours. Clients who have a black tag do not have a priority rating; they are deceased and should be transported to a temporary morgue. **Cognitive Level:** Applying **Client Need:** Safety and Infection Control **Integrated Process:** Nursing Process: Implementation **Content Area:** Adult Health **Strategy:** Recall the principles and protocols of triage. Eliminate priority 1, which is always life-threatening, and option 4, which indicates death. Choose priority 2 over 3 because fractures need attention within a few hours to reduce risk of complications.

18 **Answer: 24 Rationale:** As long as the infant does not exceed the weight limit for the safety seat, the child should remain in a rear-facing car safety seat until the child is 2 years old, which is the same as 24 months. **Cognitive Level:** Applying **Client Need:** Safety and Infection Control **Integrated Process:** Teaching and Learning **Content Area:** Child Health **Strategy:** Because this item is a standard, it is necessary to commit this information to memory.

19 **Answer: 1 Rationale:** Helping the client to explore alternatives helps empower this client, who is feeling powerless. Powerlessness is common in victims of ongoing violence, as the emotional component of the violence instills terror and helplessness. The client is ashamed and demoralized, criticized and controlled by the perpetrator, who often makes numerous serious threats and convinces the victim that there is no hope of escape. Teaching about further risk of violence and providing and/or mobilizing resources are appropriate interventions, but they will not be effective if the client feels powerless to act. **Cognitive Level:** Analyzing **Client Need:** Psychosocial Integrity **Integrated Process:** Communication and Documentation **Content Area:** Mental Health **Strategy:** Recognize the powerlessness of the client and choose an option that will allow the client to take action to combat this feeling and achieve a feeling of competence and control.

20 **Answer: 3 Rationale:** Children who are physically neglected will often steal and hoard food because of inadequate nutrition. The child's level of physical activity and response to discipline may be indicators of emotional or physical abuse. A sudden onset of enuresis is one possible indication of sexual abuse. **Cognitive Level:** Applying **Client Need:** Safety and Infection Control **Integrated Process:** Nursing Process: Assessment **Content Area:** Child Health **Strategy:** Look carefully at the options. Identify the one that has to do with meeting basic needs. This child has been neglected and is trying to cope with that and provide for own basic needs.

21 **Answer: 2, 4 Rationale:** Physical or sexual abuse and self-destructive potential are the priority assessments at this time. Anxiety, a black eye, and various somatic complaints, when combined, suggest unacknowledged violence against the client. The client's safety should be a priority. In situations where violence might have or actually has occurred, people can feel so trapped and desperate that suicide (or homicide) may seem the only way out of the situation. Providing for the client's safety includes assessing for suicidal and/or homicidal potential. After assessing for abuse and the risk of harm toward self or others, the nurse can then assess for other physical causes, such as premenstrual syndrome, migraine headache, and irritable bowel syndrome. **Cognitive Level:** Analyzing **Client Need:** Safety and Infection Control **Integrated Process:** Nursing Process: Assessment **Content Area:** Mental Health **Strategy:** Look beyond the physical and think what might, in the absence of physical explanations, be causing the client's symptoms. Remember that violence occurs in all strata of society.

ANSWERS & RATIONALES

Key Terms to Review

adverse reaction p. 52
bloodborne pathogen p. 55
CDC p. 55
idiosyncratic reaction p. 52
MSDS p. 55
OSHA p. 51
restraints p. 53
The Joint Commission p. 57
toxic reaction p. 52
triage p. 57

References

Adams, M., Holland, L., & Urban, C. (2017). *Pharmacology for nurses: A pathophysiologic approach* (5th ed.). New York, NY: Pearson Education.

Adams, M., & Urban, C. (2016). *Pharmacology: Connections to nursing practice* (3rd ed.). New York, NY: Pearson Education.

Berman, A., Snyder, S., & Frandsen, G. (2016). *Kozier & Erb's fundamentals of nursing: Concepts, process, and practice* (10th ed.). New York, NY: Pearson Education.

LeMone, P., Burke, K., Bauldoff, G., & Gubrud, P. (2015). *Medical surgical nursing: Clinical reasoning in patient care* (6th ed.). Hoboken, NJ: Pearson Education.

Lewis, S., Dirksen, S., Heitkemper, M., & Bucher, L. (2014). *Medical surgical nursing: Assessment and management of clinical problems* (9th ed.). St. Louis, MO: Elsevier Science.

Test Yourself

7 Preventing and Controlling Infection

In this chapter

Cross Reference

Other chapters relevant to this content area are

I. STANDARD PRECAUTIONS

NCLEX®

A. *Chain of infection* comprises six elements that must occur for infection to develop

1. Etiologic agent: any pathogen capable of causing infection; causative agents include bacteria, virus, fungi, protozoa, rickettsiae, and helminths
2. Reservoir: favorable environment in which infectious organism grows and reproduces; reservoir may be animate (humans, animals, insects) or inanimate (food, water, soil, equipment); blood and respiratory, gastrointestinal (GI), reproductive, and urinary tracts serve as reservoirs in humans
3. Portal of exit from reservoir: route by which microorganism leaves reservoir; portal of exit can be breaks in skin, the blood, and respiratory, GI, reproductive, and urinary tracts in humans
4. Method of transmission: mode by which microorganism is transferred from reservoir to host; transfer occurs by three mechanisms: direct, indirect, and airborne transmission
   a. Direct contact involves physical transfer of causative agent from person to person; routes of direct transmission include touching, kissing, biting, and sexual intercourse; transmission can also occur through droplets when person talks, coughs, sneezes, or spits, but only when source is within about 1 m (3 ft) of susceptible host
   b. Indirect contact involves transfer from reservoir to susceptible host via either a vehicle or a vector; vehicle-borne transmission requires inanimate object to serve as mode of transmission; intermediary agent, such as an animal or insect, is required in vector-borne transmission
   c. Airborne transmission involves transport of droplet nuclei or dust bearing infectious agent by air currents
5. Portal of entry to susceptible host: route by which infectious agent enters susceptible host; examples include breaks in skin and respiratory, GI, reproductive, and urinary tracts
6. Susceptible host: individual at increased risk for infection; infection occurs when infectious agent overwhelms host's defenses against infection (Figure 7–1)

NCLEX®

B. *Standard precautions*

1. Represent first tier of Centers for Disease Control and Prevention (CDC) guidelines for isolation precautions

NCLEX®

2. Reduce risk of transmission of infection, protecting both healthcare providers and clients from recognized and unrecognized sources

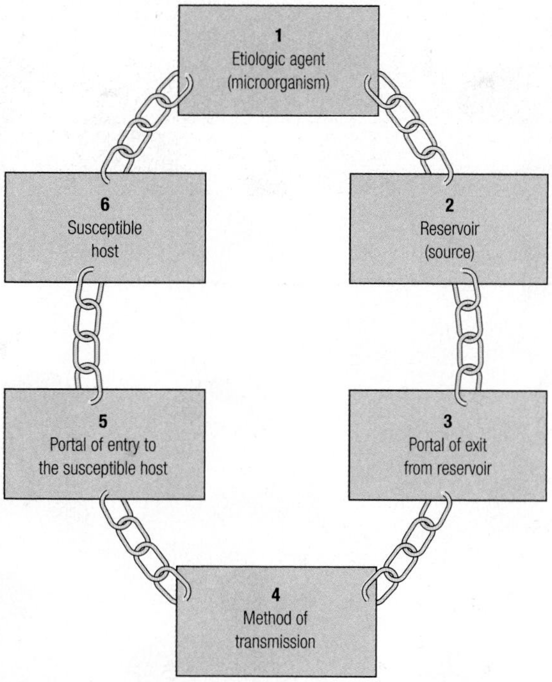

Figure 7–1

Links in the chain of infection.

NCLEX® 3. Are used in providing care to all clients regardless of medical diagnosis or setting
4. Applies to blood, all body fluids, excretions, and secretions except sweat regardless of whether blood is visible or whether skin and mucous membranes are not intact

C. Standard precautions include hand hygiene and use of *personal protective equipment (PPE)*

1. Hand hygiene: most effective way to prevent spread of microorganisms; perform before and after each client contact, immediately following exposure to blood and/or other body fluids and contaminated items, and before and after donning gloves; wash hands with plain (nonantimicrobial) soap and water or use waterless alcohol-based hand rub
2. PPE is equipment worn by healthcare providers to prevent transmission of microorganisms
   a. Gloves (clean, nonsterile): worn to protect hands when exposure to blood, body fluids, secretions, excretions, and contaminated items is likely; used for touching mucous membranes and nonintact skin; change gloves if they become torn or heavily soiled and between procedures on same client; avoid adjusting PPE or touching noncontaminated items with contaminated gloves; remove promptly after use and wash hands
   b. Gown: worn to protect healthcare provider's skin and clothing; used during procedures and care activities when splashing or spraying of blood, body fluids, secretions, and excretions is possible
   c. Mask: worn to protect mucous membranes of nose and mouth; should fully cover nose and mouth; used during care activities when splashes or sprays of blood, body fluids, secretions, and excretions can be expected
   d. Eye protection: goggles are worn to protect eyes; do not use personal glasses as a substitute for goggles; face shield is worn to protect face, including eyes, nose, and mouth, and should cover forehead, extending below chin and wrapping around each side of face; eye protection is used during care activities when splashes or sprays of blood, body fluids, secretions, and excretions are likely

D. Procedures for using PPE

NCLEX® 1. Donning PPE: perform hand hygiene immediately before donning PPE; don PPE before coming in contact with client, usually outside client's room; don gown first, followed by mask, then eye protection (if separate from mask), then gloves

NCLEX® 2. Removing PPE: remove carefully at doorway of client's room; remove gloves first and perform hand hygiene, followed by eye protection (if separate from mask), then gown, then mask (see Figure 7–2, p. 66); discard contaminated PPE in appropriate container; perform hand hygiene again immediately after removing PPE

II. MEDICAL ASEPSIS

NCLEX® **A. General principles**

1. **Medical asepsis** involves practices, such as hand hygiene and use of PPE, to reduce the number and limit the spread of microorganisms

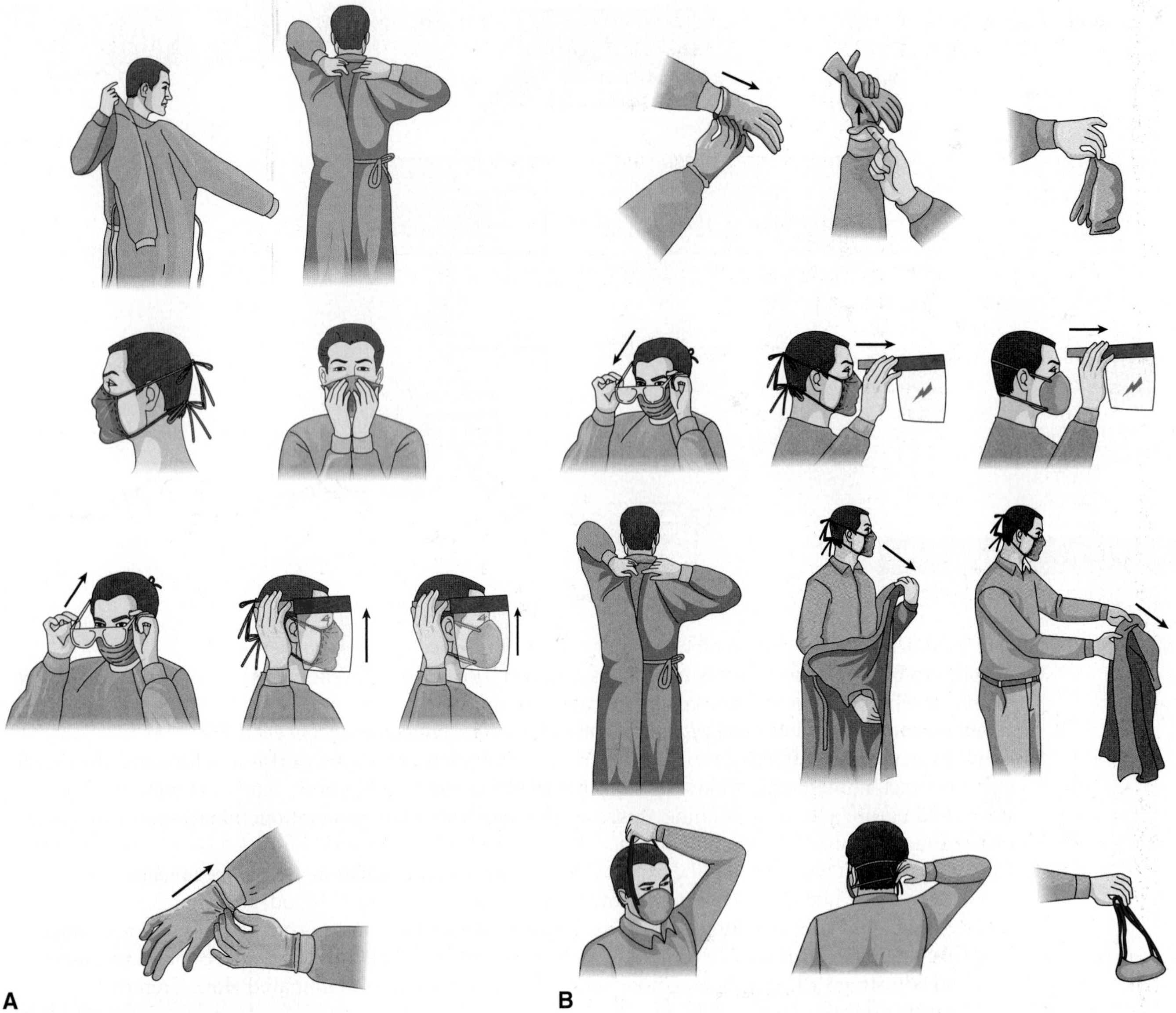

Figure 7–2 Donning and removal of PPE. A. Correct order for putting on PPE. B. Correct order for removal of PPE.

2. Also known as clean technique; objects are designated as "clean" (nearly free of microorganisms) or "dirty" (contaminated)
3. Used in implementing nonsterile procedures, such as taking vital signs, nasogastric tube insertion, and tube feeding administration

B. Disposal of contaminated equipment and supplies is conducted in accordance with institution policies and procedures

1. Linens: handle soiled linen as little as possible in a manner that prevents exposure to own skin, mucous membranes, and clothing; contain soiled linens in a bag before removal from client's room
2. Dishes: no special considerations are needed; some facilities may use disposable dishes for convenience
3. Syringes, needles, and sharps: avoid recapping needles or detaching needles from syringes; dispose of items in a rigid, puncture-resistant container immediately after use
4. Equipment (thermometers, blood pressure equipment): dedicated equipment is used for clients with transmission-based precautions; discard single-use (disposable) items immediately after use in an appropriate manner; reusable (nondisposable) equipment must be cleaned and decontaminated before use with other clients

NCLEX®

5. Lab specimens: place specimen in a leak-proof container with a biohazard label; then place container in a sealed plastic bag

NCLEX®

6. Transportation of clients with infections: avoid transporting clients with infections to other areas of hospital; if transportation is necessary, take precautions to prevent spread of infection to others; a client with respiratory infection should wear a mask; a client with an infected wound should have wound covered; notify personnel in receiving department of client's infection

III. SURGICAL ASEPSIS

A. General principles

1. **Surgical asepsis** involves practices to maintain objects and areas free of microorganisms
2. Also known as sterile technique; objects are designated as "sterile" (completely free of microorganisms) or "nonsterile" (contaminated)

NCLEX®

3. Used in implementing sterile procedures, such as intravenous therapy and urinary catheterization

B. Principles and practices of surgical asepsis are listed in Table 7–1

Table 7–1 Principles and Practices of Surgical Asepsis

Principles	Practices
All objects used in a sterile field must be sterile.	All articles are sterilized appropriately by dry or moist heat, chemicals, or radiation before use. Always check a package containing a sterile object for intactness, dryness, and expiration date. Sterile articles can be stored for only a prescribed time, after which they are considered unsterile. Consider as unsterile any package that appears already open, torn, punctured, or wet. Storage areas should be clean, dry, off the floor, and away from sinks. Check package for chemical indicator of sterilization, which is often a tape used to fasten the package or contained inside the package (indicator changes color during sterilization). If the color change is not evident consider the package unsterile. Commercially prepared sterile packages that do not have indicators are marked with the word *sterile*.
Sterile objects become unsterile when touched by unsterile objects.	Handle sterile objects that will touch open wounds or enter body cavities only with sterile forceps or sterile gloved hands. Discard or resterilize objects that come into contact with unsterile objects. Whenever sterility of an object is questionable, assume the article is unsterile.
Sterile items that are out of sight or below waist or table level are considered unsterile.	Once left unattended, a sterile field is considered unsterile. Always keep sterile objects in view. Nurses do not turn their backs on a sterile field. Only the front part of a sterile gown from shoulder to waist (or table height, whichever is higher) and cuff of the sleeves to 5 cm (2 in.) above the elbows are considered sterile. Always keep sterile gloved hands in sight and above waist level; touch only objects that are sterile. Sterile draped tables in the operating room or elsewhere are considered sterile only at surface level.
Sterile objects can become unsterile by prolonged exposure to airborne microorganisms.	Keep doors closed and traffic to a minimum in areas where a sterile procedure is being performed because moving air can carry dust and microorganisms. Keep areas in which sterile procedures are carried out as clean as possible by frequent damp cleaning with detergent germicides to minimize contaminants in the area. Keep hair clean and short or enclose it in a net to prevent hair from falling on sterile objects. Microorganisms on the hair can make a sterile field unsterile. Wear surgical caps in operating rooms, delivery rooms, and burn units. Refrain from sneezing or coughing over a sterile field. This can make it unsterile because droplets containing microorganisms from the respiratory tract can travel 1 m (3 ft 3 in.). Some agencies recommend that masks covering the mouth and the nose should be worn by anyone working over a sterile field or an open wound. When working over a sterile field, keep talking to a minimum. Avert the head from the field if talking is necessary. To prevent microorganisms from falling over a sterile field, refrain from reaching over a sterile field unless sterile gloves are worn and refrain from moving unsterile objects over a sterile field.

Table 7–1 Principles and Practices of Surgical Asepsis *(continued)*

Principles	Practices
Fluids flow in the direction of gravity.	Unless gloves are worn, always hold wet forceps with the tips below the handles. When tips are held higher than the handles, fluid can flow onto the handle and become contaminated by the hands. When the forceps are again pointed downward, the fluid flows back down and contaminates the tips. During a surgical hand wash, hold the hands higher than the elbows to prevent contaminants from the forearms from reaching the hands.
Moisture that passes through a sterile object draws microorganisms from unsterile surfaces above or below to the sterile surface by capillary action.	Sterile, moisture-proof barriers are used beneath sterile objects. Liquids (sterile saline or antiseptics) are frequently poured into containers on a sterile field. If they are spilled onto the sterile field, the barrier keeps the liquid from seeping beneath it. Keep the sterile covers on sterile equipment dry. Damp surfaces can attract microorganisms in the air. Replace sterile drapes that do not have a sterile barrier underneath when they become moist.
The edges of a sterile field are considered unsterile.	A 2.5 cm (1 in.) margin at each edge of an opened drape is considered unsterile because the edges are in contact with unsterile surfaces. Place all sterile objects more than 2.5 cm (1 in.) inside the edges of a sterile field. Any article that falls outside the edges of a sterile field is considered unsterile.
The skin cannot be sterilized and is unsterile.	Use sterile gloves or sterile forceps to handle sterile items. Prior to a surgical aseptic procedure, wash hands to reduce the number of microorganisms on them.
Conscientiousness, alertness, and honesty are essential qualities in maintaining surgical asepsis.	When a sterile object becomes unsterile, it does not necessarily change in appearance. The person who sees a sterile object become contaminated must correct or report the situation. Do not set up a sterile field ahead of time for future use.

Source: Berman, A., Snyder, S., & Frandsen, G. (2016). *Kozier & Erb's fundamentals of nursing: Concepts, process, and practice* (10th ed.). New York, NY: Pearson Education, p. 627.

IV. TRANSMISSION-BASED PRECAUTIONS

A. *Transmission-based precautions* are measures to limit spread of pathogenic microorganisms

NCLEX® **B. *Airborne precautions***

1. Involves spread of infection through airborne droplet nuclei smaller than 5 microns, evaporated droplets that remain suspended in air for long periods of time, or dust particles containing infectious agent
2. Because microorganisms can be widely spread by air currents, special air handling and ventilation are needed
3. Examples of diseases include rubeola (measles), varicella (chicken pox), and tuberculosis
4. Use standard precautions and mask; use other PPE as appropriate for expected risk of exposure
   a. For tuberculosis, wear particulate respirator mask that is fit-tested to individual nurse
   b. For other airborne diseases such as rubeola or varicella, susceptible persons should not enter client's room; if entry is unavoidable, respiratory protection must be worn
   c. Individuals immune to rubeola or varicella do not need to wear respiratory protection
5. Place client in private, negative–air pressure room with 6 (older construction) to 12 (renovations or new construction) air exchanges per hour; air is exhausted directly to outdoors or recirculated through HEPA filtration before return
6. If private room is not possible, client may be placed in room with another client (cohorted) who has an infection with same microorganism but no other infection
7. Client should remain in room with door closed
8. If transportation of client to other hospital departments is unavoidable, client should wear surgical mask
9. Visitors should wear mask appropriate to type of infection at all times

NCLEX® **C. Droplet precautions**

1. Involves spread of infection by particle droplets larger than 5 microns that can be generated when client coughs, sneezes, talks, laughs, and so on
2. Examples of diseases include diphtheria (pharyngeal), mycoplasma pneumonia, rubella, pertussis, mumps, streptococcal pharyngitis, pneumonia, and scarlet fever

3. Use standard precautions; mask is required when providing care or if within about 1 m (3 ft) of client; use other PPE as appropriate
4. Place client in private room; if private room is not possible, client may be cohorted with another client who has same infection but no additional infections
5. Client should remain in room; if transportation of client to other hospital departments is unavoidable, client should wear surgical mask; notify personnel in receiving department of client's infection
6. Door to room may remain open
7. Visitors should wear mask if within about 1 m (3 ft) of client and should try to maintain distance of about 1 m (3 ft) whenever possible

NCLEX®

D. Contact precautions

1. Involves spread of infection by contact with client or contact with items in client's environment
2. Examples of diseases include skin infections (scabies, pediculosis, herpes simplex or zoster), hepatitis A, and wound, GI, or urinary infections, including those with multidrug-resistant organisms, such as **methicillin-resistant *Staphylococcus aureus* (MRSA)** and **vancomycin-resistant enterococcus (VRE)**
3. Use standard precautions; gloves are required; wear gown when contact with infected secretions is expected; use other PPE as appropriate for expected risk of exposure gloves gown
4. Place client in private room; if private room is not possible, client may be cohorted with another client who has same infection
5. Door to room may remain open
6. Limit transportation of client to other hospital departments; infected wound should be securely covered; notify personnel in receiving department of client's infection
7. Dedicate equipment for client care (such as stethoscope or sphygmomanometer) to a single client or cohort of clients; if such items must be used to care for other clients, adequately clean and disinfect them first

E. Multiple precautions

1. A client is not limited to one set of transmission-based precautions; rather, precautions are implemented based on specific need
2. For example, a client with measles who has a wound infected with MRSA would require both airborne and contact precautions
3. Clients with severe acute respiratory syndrome (SARS) require the use of both airborne and contact precautions; SARS is a highly infectious viral infection that is transmitted by airborne respiratory droplets and by touching surfaces and objects contaminated with infectious droplets

Check Your NCLEX–RN® Exam I.Q.

You are ready for testing on this content if you can:

- Describe the chain of infection.
- Explain the principles of standard precautions.
- Correctly don and remove personal protective equipment.
- Distinguish between medical and surgical asepsis.
- Explain principles of medical and surgical asepsis.
- Compare and contrast transmission-based airborne, droplet, and contact precautions.
- Identify infectious diseases that require transmission-based precautions.

PRACTICE TEST

1 The nurse would perform which action when washing hands as part of medical asepsis before caring for a client in an outpatient clinic? Select all that apply.

1. Wash hands with the hands held higher than the elbows.
2. Adjust temperature of water to the hottest possible.
3. Scrub hands and nails with a scrub brush for 5 minutes.
4. Use a clean paper towel to turn water off.
5. Rub vigorously using firm circular motions.

2 The nurse's forearm becomes splattered with blood while inserting an intravenous catheter. What action should the nurse take?

1. Wash blood away with isopropyl alcohol.
2. Wipe blood away with a tissue.
3. Flush forearm with hot water, letting water flow from elbow toward fingers.
4. Wash forearm with soap and water.

PRACTICE TEST

3 The nurse would take which action to protect the client from infection at the portal of entry?

1. Place sputum specimen in a biohazard bag for transport to the lab.
2. Empty Jackson-Pratt drain using sterile technique.
3. Dispose of soiled gloves in waste container.
4. Wash hands after providing client care.

4 Which actions by the nurse comply with core principles of surgical asepsis? Select all that apply.

1. Wash hands before and after client care.
2. Keep sterile field in view at all times.
3. Wear personal protective equipment.
4. Add contents to sterile field holding package 15 cm (6 in.) above field.
5. Consider outer 3.8 cm (1.5 in.) of sterile field as contaminated.

5 Which precaution would the nurse implement when admitting a client with herpes zoster to the nursing unit?

zoster = airbone

1. Airborne precautions
2. Contact precautions
3. Droplet precautions
4. Neutropenic precautions

6 A client with tuberculosis asks the nurse if visitors will need to wear masks. What response by the nurse is most accurate?

1. "Everyone who enters your room must wear a mask to protect themselves from tuberculosis."
2. "Masks would not be necessary for visitors who have had tuberculosis before."
3. "It is less important for your family to wear masks, since they live in close contact with you."
4. "Only visitors who are at risk for tuberculosis need to wear a mask."

7 The nurse is leaving the room of a client who has methicillin-resistant *Staphylococcus aureus* (MRSA) microorganisms in a wound and the urine. Place the following personal protective equipment in order of removal.

1. Eye protection
2. Gloves
3. Mask
4. Gown

Fill in your answer below:

Answer: 2143

8 A client with suspected severe acute respiratory syndrome (SARS) arrives at the emergency department. Which healthcare provider prescription should the nurse implement first?

1. Airborne and contact precautions
2. IV D_5NS at 100 mL/hr
3. Nasopharyngeal culture for reverse-transcriptase polymerase chain reaction
4. Sputum for enzyme immunoassay testing

9 A client with vancomycin-intermediate-resistant *Staphylococcus aureus* (VISA) is admitted to the nursing unit. What type of precautions should the nurse institute?

1. Standard precautions
2. Neutropenic precautions
3. Droplet precautions
4. Contact precautions

10 The nurse would implement which of the following as a requirement of care specific to the client who has tuberculosis?

1. Disposal of needles and syringes in a rigid, puncture-proof container
2. Handwashing after removing contaminated gloves
3. Wearing a gown if splashing is possible
4. A private room with negative air flow

PRACTICE TEST

11 The nurse would expect to institute transmission-based precautions for a client with which infection?

1. Pneumonia caused by *Pseudomonas aeruginosa*
2. *Pneumocystis jiroveci* pneumonia
3. A sacral wound contaminated by *Escherichia coli*
4. A draining leg wound with methicillin-resistant *Staphylococcus aureus*

12 A client asks, "How did I get scarlet fever?" What would be the nurse's best response?

1. "Scarlet fever is transmitted through sexual intercourse."
2. "You can get scarlet fever if you share contaminated needles or get a blood transfusion."
3. "Most people get it by eating contaminated food."
4. "You inhaled infected droplets in the air."

13 The nurse is assisting a client who has methicillin-resistant *Staphylococcus aureus* in the urine to collect a clean-catch urine specimen. Which protective equipment is unnecessary?

1. N95 particulate respirator
2. Gown
3. Eye protection
4. Clean gloves

14 The nurse is preparing to irrigate a wound infected with vancomycin-resistant enterococci. What personal protective equipment (PPE) would the nurse wear?

1. Gloves, gown, and particulate respirator
2. Gloves and surgical mask
3. Gloves, eye protection, and shoe covers
4. Gloves, gown, eye protection, and surgical mask

15 The nurse assigned to the respiratory care unit is working with four clients who have pneumonia. The nurse should assign the only remaining private room on the nursing unit to the client infected with which organism?

1. Penicillin-resistant *Streptococcus pneumoniae* pneumonia
2. *Pseudomonas aeruginosa* pneumonia
3. *Pneumocystis jiroveci* pneumonia
4. *Legionella pneumophila* pneumonia

16 The nurse is caring for a client with hepatitis A. Which client statements indicate that teaching conducted by the nurse about disease transmission was effective? Select all that apply.

1. "We must avoid kissing."
2. "We can use the same bath towels."
3. "We must avoid eating with the same utensils."
4. "We must wear masks."
5. "No special precautions are needed."

17 The nurse would take which actions to comply with principles of medical asepsis? Select all that apply.

1. Wash hands before and after assisting client with personal hygiene.
2. Wear gown and gloves when working with client on contact precautions.
3. Recap needle after administering insulin.
4. Insert needle into rubber port of a previously used multidose vial without swabbing it with alcohol.
5. Use surgical facemask while working with client who has tuberculosis.

18 The nurse is preparing to enter the room of a client with pneumonia caused by penicillin-resistant *Streptococcus pneumoniae* (PRSP). The client has a tracheostomy and requires suctioning. Put the following personal protective equipment in order of donning.

1. Eye protection
2. Gloves
3. Mask
4. Gown

Fill in your answer below:

Answer: ____________

PRACTICE TEST

19 The nurse is performing a wound irrigation and sterile dressing change for a client with an open infected abdominal incision. Which actions should the nurse take when completing this procedure? Select all that apply.

1. Keep hands in sight and above the knee level of the nurse.
2. Turn head to the side when talking to avoid speaking over the sterile field.
3. Replace a sterile cloth drape that became wet when wound irrigant spilled.
4. Place sterile dressing sponges 1.2 cm (0.5 in.) inside the edge of the sterile field.
5. Use sterile gloves or sterile forceps when applying dressing sponges to wound.

20 The nurse is restarting an IV line on a client known to have hepatitis B. Which precautions should the nurse use to protect against exposure? Select all that apply.

1. Handwashing
2. Gloves
3. Mask
4. Face shield
5. Gown

ANSWERS & RATIONALES

1 **Answer: 4, 5 Rationale:** A paper towel is used to shut off the faucet because the faucet is considered contaminated. Rubbing vigorously using firm circular motions creates friction on the skin to assist in cleansing. The hands are considered to be more contaminated than the elbows, and the hands should be held down so water flows from least contaminated to most contaminated. Hot water can result in burns to the nurse. Warm water protects from burns and removes less protective skin oil than hot water. A surgical scrub is performed over 5 minutes while in medical asepsis hands are washed for at least 10–15 seconds. **Cognitive Level:** Applying **Client Need:** Safety and Infection Control **Integrated Process:** Nursing Process: Implementation **Content Area:** Fundamentals **Strategy:** The core issue of the question is utilization of medical asepsis. Recall basic principles of care and use the process of elimination to make a selection.

2 **Answer: 4 Rationale:** Washing the skin with the combination of soap and water will remove the blood through mechanical friction. While alcohol can kill bacteria, it cannot kill viruses and fungi. Tissues would not adequately remove the blood. Hot water can burn the nurse. Water alone is inadequate in removing the blood. **Cognitive Level:** Applying **Client Need:** Safety and Infection Control **Integrated Process:** Nursing Process: Implementation **Content Area:** Fundamentals **Strategy:** The core issue of the question is the most effective means of reducing the risk of bloodborne disease transmission after contact with the skin. Recall principles of medical asepsis and use the process of elimination to make a selection.

3 **Answer: 2 Rationale:** Using sterile technique to empty wound drains is aimed at interrupting the portal-of-entry link in the chain of infection. By using sterile technique, the nurse reduces the risk of introducing pathogens into the client's wound via the drain. Proper handling of specimens interrupts the chain of infection at the reservoir link. Disposing of gloves properly and washing hands after providing care break the chain of infection at the mode of transmission link. **Cognitive Level:** Applying **Client Need:** Safety and Infection Control **Integrated Process:** Nursing Process: Implementation **Content Area:** Fundamentals **Strategy:** Knowledge of the chain of infection is required. The portal of entry has to be a route whereby microorganisms can enter the client, so select the option that is directly in contact with the client.

4 **Answer: 2, 4 Rationale:** Keeping the sterile field in view and holding items 15 cm (6 in.) above the sterile field are core principles of surgical asepsis. Washing hands after providing care and wearing personal protective equipment are core principles of medical asepsis. The outer 1 inch of a sterile field is considered contaminated, not 3.8 cm (1.5 in.). **Cognitive Level:** Analyzing **Client Need:** Safety and Infection Control **Integrated Process:** Nursing Process: Implementation **Content Area:** Fundamentals **Strategy:** The core issue of the question is the ability to discriminate between medical and surgical asepsis and to choose correct interventions that support surgical asepsis. Use these principles and the process of elimination to make a selection.

5 **Answer: 1 Rationale:** Herpes zoster is caused by the herpes virus varicella zoster. It can be transmitted by the airborne route until lesions have crusted over. Contact precautions are implemented when the nurse may come into contact with microorganisms during care. Herpes zoster is not transmitted by droplets. Neutropenic precautions are not indicated because the client is not at risk for contracting an infection from the nurse or other individuals. **Cognitive Level:** Applying **Client Need:** Safety and Infection Control **Integrated Process:** Nursing Process: Implementation **Content Area:** Fundamentals **Strategy:** Herpes zoster is a viral skin infection. Specific knowledge of the types of transmission-based precautions is needed to select the correct answer. Eliminate airborne and droplet precautions because herpes zoster is not transmitted on air currents. Next eliminate neutropenic precautions, which are are used with immunocompromised clients.

6 **Answer: 1 Rationale:** Tuberculosis is highly contagious and spread by inhalation of airborne droplets. Airborne precautions would be initiated, requiring everyone to wear a special particulate respirator fit-tested mask. Individuals who have had tuberculosis in the past can be re-exposed and develop the active form of the disease again. It is just as important

ANSWERS & RATIONALES

for family to wear the appropriate type of mask. The need to wear masks applies to all visitors, not just those at risk for developing tuberculosis. **Cognitive Level:** Applying **Client Need:** Safety and Infection Control **Integrated Process:** Communication and Documentation **Content Area:** Fundamentals **Strategy:** Look for similarities among the options in order to eliminate choices. In this case, the incorrect options are similar in that they suggest certain individuals would not be required to wear masks.

7 **Answer: 2, 1, 4, 3 Rationale:** Gloves are removed first because they would be most contaminated. Eye protection would be removed next, followed by the gown. The mask is removed last, followed by washing the hands. **Cognitive Level:** Analyzing **Client Need:** Safety and Infection Control **Integrated Process:** Nursing Process: Implementation **Content Area:** Fundamentals **Strategy:** Remember that removal of PPE should occur in order of most contaminated to least contaminated items.

8 **Answer: 1 Rationale:** SARS is a highly contagious viral respiratory illness that is spread by close person-to-person contact. SARS is transmitted by airborne respiratory route and by touching surfaces and objects contaminated with the virus, necessitating initiation of airborne and contact precautions as the first priority of the nurse. This action would protect both healthcare workers and other clients in the emergency department. Specific activities for the client's care, such as instituting IV therapy, obtaining nasopharyngeal culture, and obtaining sputum sample, can be done once all clients and personnel are protected from disease transmission. **Cognitive Level:** Analyzing **Client Need:** Safety and Infection Control **Integrated Process:** Nursing Process: Implementation **Content Area:** Fundamentals **Strategy:** The critical word *first* indicates all of the answers are correct and the nurse needs to set priorities. The first priority is to implement measures that protect the client and/or nurse—instituting airborne and contact precautions.

9 **Answer: 4 Rationale:** Clients with antibiotic-resistant microorganisms must be isolated with transmission-based precautions. The organism is transmitted via close person-to-person direct contact and by touching contaminated surfaces and objects. Standard precautions are used with all clients, regardless of medical diagnosis. Reverse isolation is instituted for immunocompromised clients. This organism is not transmitted via droplet nuclei. **Cognitive Level:** Applying **Client Need:** Safety and Infection Control **Integrated Process:** Nursing Process: Implementation **Content Area:** Fundamentals **Strategy:** The critical words *vancomycin-intermediate-resistant* suggest the microorganism is difficult to eradicate, indicating it is highly contagious. Eliminate standard and neutropenic, as they are not disease-specific precautions. Select contact over droplet, recalling that *Staphylococcus aureus* is a microorganism that is commonly found on skin.

10 **Answer: 4 Rationale:** The client with tuberculosis can spread the infection by breathing, and so requires a private room and airborne precautions. Proper equipment disposal, handwashing, and wearing protective equipment as indicated are precautions that would be implemented with any client, regardless of medical diagnosis. **Cognitive Level:** Applying **Client Need:** Safe, Effective Care Environment **Integrated Process:** Nursing Process: Implementation **Content Area:** Fundamentals **Strategy:** The critical word *specific* suggests that the correct option must apply to a client with tuberculosis and is not a general measure used for all clients. Next, consider that this is transmitted by the airborne route to make the correct selection.

11 **Answer: 4 Rationale:** A client who has a draining leg wound with methicillin-resistant *Staphylococcus aureus* requires implementation of transmission-based precautions. Such precautions are required for all antibiotic-resistant microorganisms. Pneumonia caused by *Pseudomonas aeruginosa* or *Pneumocystis jiroveci* would not require transmission-based precautions. A sacral wound contaminated by *Escherichia coli* would not require transmission-based precautions. **Cognitive Level:** Analyzing **Client Need:** Safety and Infection Control **Integrated Process:** Nursing Process: Planning **Content Area:** Fundamentals **Strategy:** The critical words *methicillin-resistant* indicate a microorganism that is difficult to eradicate. Eliminate each of the incorrect options after visualizing each situation because they can be managed by use of standard precautions.

12 **Answer: 4 Rationale:** Scarlet fever is transmitted by particle droplets larger than 5 microns. Scarlet fever is not transmitted through sexual intercourse or the blood, or by consuming contaminated food. **Cognitive Level:** Applying **Client Need:** Safety and Infection Control **Integrated Process:** Communication and Documentation **Content Area:** Fundamentals **Strategy:** Begin by recalling that scarlet fever is transmitted by droplets. With this in mind, use the process of elimination to select the client situation that is compatible with the mode of transmission.

13 **Answer: 4 Rationale:** N95 respirators are needed when caring for the client with tuberculosis, so it is inappropriate for this scenario. Methicillin-resistant *Staphylococcus aureus* requires transmission-based contact precautions. Eye protection would be worn to protect the mucous membranes of the eyes when splatters of body fluids or excretions are possible. A gown would be worn when the nurse is in direct contact with the client. Contact precautions require gloves. **Cognitive Level:** Applying **Client Need:** Safety and Infection Control **Integrated Process:** Nursing Process: Planning **Content Area:** Fundamentals **Strategy:** The critical word *unnecessary* suggests that all but one of the answers are correct. Using the process of elimination, look for the choice that identifies personal protective equipment that is not needed for contact precautions.

14 **Answer: 4 Rationale:** An infection with vancomycin-resistant enterococci requires transmission-based contact precautions. Since the nurse will be irrigating the wound and splatters of body fluids or exudates are possible, eye protection and surgical mask should be worn to protect the mucous membranes of the eyes, nose, and mouth. A gown would be worn when the nurse is in direct contact with the client. Contact precautions require gloves. Shoe covers are unnecessary. **Cognitive Level:** Applying **Client Need:** Safety and Infection Control **Integrated Process:** Nursing Process: Implementation **Content Area:** Fundamentals **Strategy:** Wound infections require contact precautions. Look for the option that identifies the correct PPE to be used with contact precautions. Eliminate options with particulate respirator and shoe covers, since these are unnecessary. Choose the option containing eye protection because the risk for splatters exists.

15 **Answer: 1 Rationale:** While each option contains "pneumonia," the causative agent is different for each. An organism that is "resistant" (penicillin-resistant *Streptococcus pneumoniae* pneumonia) is a pathogenic microorganism that is difficult to treat and requires droplet precautions. *Pseudomonas aeruginosa* pneumonia, *Pneumocystis jiroveci* pneumonia, and *Legionella pneumophila* pneumonia do not require the

use of transmission-based precautions. **Cognitive Level:** Applying **Client Need:** Safety and Infection Control **Integrated Process:** Nursing Process: Implementation **Content Area:** Fundamentals **Strategy:** Note the critical word *resistant* in the correct option. This provides a clue that the infection is difficult to treat and requires specific additional infection control practices, in this instance droplet precautions. The pneumonias in the other options do not require transmission-based precautions.

16 **Answer: 1, 3 Rationale:** Hepatitis A is an infectious disease transmitted by the fecal–oral route. Standard precautions are mandatory. Contact precautions are instituted if the client is incontinent of stool. Family members should avoid close contact with the client. They should not kiss the client or use the same eating utensils and bath towels. Masks are not necessary because the disease is not transmitted by the respiratory tract. **Cognitive Level:** Applying **Client Need:** Safety and Infection Control **Integrated Process:** Nursing Process: Planning **Content Area:** Fundamentals **Strategy:** The critical words *methicillin-resistant* indicate a microorganism that is difficult to eradicate. Eliminate each of the incorrect options after visualizing each situation because they can be managed by use of standard precautions.

17 **Answer: 1, 2 Rationale:** Washing hands before and after assisting a client with personal hygiene, and wearing a gown and gloves when working with a client on contact precautions are core principles of medical asepsis. Recapping the needle after administering insulin violates principles of medical asepsis. Inserting a needle into the rubber port of a previously used multidose vial without swabbing it with alcohol violates principles of medical asepsis. Using a surgical face mask while working with a client who has tuberculosis violates principles of transmission-based precautions for a client with tuberculosis. The nurse should wear an N95 (fit-tested) mask instead of a simple surgical mask. **Cognitive Level:** Analyzing **Client Need:** Safety and Infection Control **Integrated Process:** Nursing Process: Implementation **Content Area:** Fundamentals **Strategy:** Knowledge of medical versus surgical asepsis is essential to answer this question. Note that hand hygiene, gown, and gloves use medical aseptic technique. Recall also that recapping a needle and failure to wipe a port are not consistent with medical asepsis principles. Also discard surgical face mask because it addresses transmission-based precautions and is an incorrect statement.

18 **Answer: 4, 3, 1, 2 Rationale:** The gown is applied first, as it takes the most time to don. The mask is donned next, followed by eye protection. These items can be more securely applied with ungloved hands. Gloves are donned last, so the gloves can be pulled up to cover the cuffs of the gown. **Cognitive Level:** Applying **Client Need:** Safety and Infection Control **Integrated Process:** Nursing Process: Implementation **Content Area:** Fundamentals **Strategy:** Rationalize the ordering based on nursing knowledge of standard precautions and surgical asepsis. Visualize the procedure to aid in choosing correctly.

19 **Answer: 2, 3, 5 Rationale:** The nurse should turn the head to the side when talking to reduce the risk of directing microorganisms over the sterile field from air movement. The nurse should replace a sterile cloth drape that became wet because microorganisms can penetrate the field by capillary action. The nurse should use sterile gloves or sterile forceps when applying dressing sponges to a wound to avoid introducing new microorganisms into the wound. Hands should be kept in sight but they should be kept above waist level, not knee level. The nurse should place sterile dressing sponges 2.5 cm (1 in.) inside the edge of the sterile field (not 1.2 cm [0.5 in.]). **Cognitive Level:** Analyzing **Client Need:** Safety and Infection Control **Integrated Process:** Nursing Process: Implementation **Content Area:** Fundamentals **Strategy:** When more than one option is correct, consider each option as a true–false statement and select the options that are true statements because of the wording of the question.

20 **Answer: 1, 2 Rationale:** Handwashing and gloves are the only precautions needed for starting an IV. Masks, face shields, and gowns are appropriate for procedures that may result in splashing of body fluids. **Cognitive Level:** Analyzing **Client Need:** Safety and Infection Control **Integrated Process:** Nursing Process: Planning **Content Area:** Fundamentals **Strategy:** Recall standard precautions and infectious disease precautions. Handwashing and use of gloves are appropriate for any procedure.

Key Terms to Review

airborne precautions p. 68
chain of infection p. 64
medical asepsis p. 65
methicillin-resistant *Staphylococcus aureus* (MRSA) p. 69
personal protective equipment (PPE) p. 65
standard precautions p. 64
surgical asepsis p. 67
transmission-based precautions p. 68
vancomycin-resistant enterococcus (VRE) p. 69

References

Berman, A., Snyder, S., & Frandsen, G. (2016). *Kozier & Erb's fundamentals of nursing: Concepts, process, and practice* (10th ed.). New York, NY: Pearson Education.

LeMone, P., Burke, K., Bauldoff, G., & Gubrud, P. (2015). *Medical surgical nursing: Clinical reasoning in patient care* (6th ed.). Hoboken, NJ: Pearson Education.

Lewis, S., Dirksen, S., Heitkemper, M., & Bucher, L. (2014). *Medical surgical nursing: Assessment and management of clinical problems* (9th ed.). St. Louis, MO: Elsevier Science.

Smith, S., Duell, D., Martin, B., Aebersold, M., & Gonzalez, L. (2017). *Clinical nursing skills: Basic to advanced skills* (10th ed.). New York, NY: Pearson Education.

Reproduction, Family Planning, and Infertility

8

In this chapter

Cross Reference

Other chapters relevant to this content area are

Uncomplicated Antenatal Assessment and Care	Chapter 9
Uncomplicated Labor and Delivery Care	Chapter 10
Uncomplicated Postpartum Assessment and Care	Chapter 11
Uncomplicated Newborn Care	Chapter 12
Complicated Antenatal Care	Chapter 49
Complicated Labor and Delivery Care	Chapter 50
Complicated Postpartum Care	Chapter 51
Complicated Newborn Care	Chapter 52

I. THE MALE AND FEMALE REPRODUCTIVE SYSTEMS

A. Female internal structures

1. Vagina: muscular, membranous tube that connects external genitalia with cervix; provides passageway for sperm, menstrual flow, and delivery of fetus
2. Uterus: hollow muscular organ that sheds endometrium with menstrual cycles and holds fetus during pregnancy; consists of fundus, body, and cervix
3. Fallopian tubes: connect each ovary to uterus; ciliated to transport ovum or zygote; parts are isthmus, ampulla, and infundibulum
4. Ovaries: almond-sized glands that secrete estrogen and progesterone; release one mature follicle and ovum per menstrual cycle from menarche to menopause, except during pregnancy

B. Functions of female structures

NCLEX®

1. Oogenesis: oocyte matures to ovum via meiosis under influence of follicle-stimulating hormone (FSH); luteinizing hormone (LH) transforms follicle into corpus luteum, which produces progesterone to maintain pregnancy; ovaries produce estrogen and progesterone in pregnant and nonpregnant states
2. Menstruation occurs when ovum is not fertilized and corpus luteum disintegrates; endometrium becomes ischemic as progesterone and estrogen levels drop, leading to sloughing of myometrium
3. Conception occurs in fallopian tube when a 23-chromosome-containing spermatozoon enters a 23-chromosome-containing ovum and produces a 23-chromosome-pair-containing diploid zygote
4. Pregnancy: cleavage (rapid mitotic division of zygote) creates a blastocyst, which becomes a multi-cellular solid ball of 16 cells (morula); further division leads to trophoblast stage, when it implants within endometrium
5. Secretion production: cervical secretions become elastic and stretchy during ovulation to facilitate sperm transport toward ovum; are rich in glycogen to nourish developing embryo until placental circulation is in place

C. Age-related changes of female reproductive system

1. Menses begin during puberty, stimulated by estrogen and progesterone
2. Menopause is characterized by 1 year of amenorrhea and occurs on average at age 50; postmenopausal reproductive changes include thinning and atrophy of external and internal structures

NCLEX®

D. Male internal structures

1. Testes: two lobular, oval glands located within scrotum where spermatogenesis takes place via meiosis
2. Epididymis: tubelike duct arising from top of each testis and ending in vas deferens
3. Vas deferens: connects epididymis to prostate gland
4. Prostate gland: encircles urethra just below bladder; produces alkaline fluid released during ejaculation
5. Seminal vesicles: lobular glands located just above prostate; produce seminal fluid (secreted during ejaculation to support sperm metabolism, motility)
6. Urethra: passes through prostate; connects bladder and urethral meatus and is passage for ejaculate
7. Semen: male ejaculate containing spermatozoa and glandular secretions; milky white in color; average volume from 2 to 5 mL

E. Functions of male structures

NCLEX®

1. Spermatogenesis takes place in testes; spermatozoa proceed through epididymal tubules where motility and fertility develop and are stored in reservoir of epididymis
2. Ejaculation is a series of muscular contractions that release spermatozoa and seminal fluid through penis
3. Urination also takes place through urethra in penis
4. Secretion production: prostate and seminal glands create a milky-white fluid that nourishes spermatozoa during and after ejaculation

F. Age-related changes of male reproductive system

1. Puberty: serum testosterone levels increase, which stimulates elongation and thickening of penile shaft, spermatozoa production, and enlargement of testes and scrotum
2. Spermatozoa count, motility, and morphology begin to decrease in middle age
3. External organs atrophy in older adults

II. FERTILITY

A. Female components

NCLEX®

1. Primary infertility occurs before ever conceiving; secondary infertility occurs after a pregnancy
2. Menstrual cycle: follicular phase is days 1–14 of cycle, incorporating menstrual phase (menses) and proliferative phase (beginning of endometrial thickening); variations in menstrual cycle length are caused by variations in follicular phase; luteal phase is days 15–28 of cycle and includes secretory phase (endometrium secretes glycogen to prepare for fertilized ovum) and ischemic phase (begins endometrial breakdown after no fertilization); luteal phase is always 12–14 days long

NCLEX®

3. Ovulation: ovum begins to mature during follicular phase (FSH); at onset of luteal phase, a graafian follicle appears and enlarges on ovary surface under influence of FSH and LH; ovum oozes out of follicle; ruptured follicle becomes corpus luteum, which disintegrates if fertilization does not occur or creates progesterone if fertilization does occur; 14% or more body fat is needed to support ovulation (estrogen is stored in body fat); less than 14% body fat results in irregular menses or amenorrhea
4. Cervical mucus: becomes more plentiful, thinner, and more stretchy; forms columns to facilitate transport of sperm into uterus during ovulation

5. Uterine structure: abnormalities result in unhealthy myometrium and fewer healthy places for successful embryo implantation; abnormalities include a septum (fibrous, vertical, wall-like structure in center of uterine body), a unicornate uterus (one-sided, banana-shaped uterus), or a bicornate uterus (two banana-shaped uteri side by side)
6. Hormones

NCLEX®

   a. Estrogen: produced by ovaries; responsible for development of secondary sex characteristics at puberty; peaks in follicular phase of menstrual cycle; inhibits FSH and LH production
   b. Progesterone: secreted by corpus luteum; peaks during luteal phase; stimulates FSH and LH secretion; responsible for endometrial thickening
   c. FSH: anterior pituitary hormone that matures one ovarian follicle each cycle
   d. LH: anterior pituitary hormone that completes maturation of ovarian follicle; ovulation occurs 10–12 hours after LH peaks
7. Fallopian tube: must be patent for sperm to reach ovum and for fertilized ovum to reach uterus; scarring can occur from an infection, such as a ruptured appendix or **pelvic inflammatory disease (PID)**, an infection of uterus and fallopian tubes; cilia in fallopian tubes (which propel ovum toward sperm) have decreased motility in cigarette smokers, thus decreasing fertility

B. Male components

1. Sperm production: at least 50% of sperm must have normal form and motion patterns for optimal fertility; decreased sperm count and motility can be caused by increased scrotal temperature (from frequent hot tub or sauna use, tight clothing, or varicocele); heavy alcohol, marijuana, or cocaine use; scrotal trauma; mumps during adulthood; developmental factors; and cigarette smoking
2. Testosterone is primary hormone responsible for libido, sperm production, ability to achieve and maintain erection, and ejaculation
3. Erections must be maintained long enough for ejaculation to occur in vagina and near cervix for optimal fertility
4. Ejaculation must occur and contain sufficient numbers of healthy sperm to achieve fertility

III. INFERTILITY

A. Common diagnostic studies for infertility

NCLEX®

1. **Basal body temperature (BBT)** or resting body temperature: obtained by taking oral temperature daily prior to arising from bed and graphing results on a month-long graph; a sudden dip occurs on day before ovulation and is followed by a rise of 0.5–1.0°F (0.3–0.6°C), which indicates ovulation; this rise remains until menstruation begins; **fertility awareness** includes monitoring BBT and cervical mucus changes to detect ovulation
2. Serum hormone testing: venous blood levels of FSH and LH in infertile women indicate ovarian function
3. Postcoital exam: couple has intercourse 8 to 12 hours prior to exam, 1 or 2 days before expected ovulation; a 10-mL syringe with catheter attached is used to collect a specimen of vaginal secretions, which are examined for signs of infection, number of active and nonmotile spermatozoa, sperm–mucus interaction, and consistency of cervical mucus
4. **Endometrial biopsy**: used to obtain an endometrial tissue sample; client is positioned on exam table in lithotomy position; provider inserts vaginal speculum to visualize cervix; a paracervical block is first administered to decrease cramping and pain; a sample of endometrium is obtained to check for a luteal-phase defect (lack of progesterone)
   a. Preprocedure care includes assisting client onto exam table and advising client that she will feel crampy discomfort both during paracervical block administration and during aspiration
   b. Postprocedure care includes providing sanitary napkins for client (vaginal bleeding will occur) and assessing for a vasovagal response (sudden fainting caused by hypotension induced by vagus nerve stimulation) prior to arising from exam table
5. Hysterosalpingogram (HSG): detects uterine anomalies (septate, unicornate, or bicornate structures) and tubal anomalies or blockage; after client is sedated or anesthetized, iodine-based radiopaque dye is instilled via catheter into uterus and tube and x-rays are taken
6. Laparoscopy: carried out under general or epidural anesthesia; three-puncture approach (umbilicus and suprapubic areas) often used to introduce laparoscope into abdomen, insufflate it with carbon dioxide, and view pelvic structures or perform surgical procedures
7. Male semen analysis: client ejaculates into specimen container, and ejaculate is examined microscopically for number, morphology, and motility of sperm
8. Male and female partner: antisperm antibody evaluation of cervical mucus and ejaculate are tested for agglutination (indicates occurrence of immunological reactions between cervical mucus and spermatozoa)

B. Psychological factors associated with infertility

NCLEX® 1. Many couples experience shame, guilt, blame, or grief stages during diagnosis and treatment of infertility

NCLEX® 2. Nurse should facilitate communication between couple and provide information on resources for coping with infertility (such as support groups, professional counseling)

C. Collaborative management of infertility

1. Educational needs of infertile couple often pertain to various procedures (e.g., semen collection or postcoital exam), understanding test results, self-monitoring during medication administration, and understanding how assisted reproductive technologies (ART) are performed
2. Hormone therapy is used to induce ovulation prior to in vitro fertilization; client and/or partner must learn subcutaneous and/or intramuscular injection techniques
3. Medications such as clomiphene citrate and gonadotropins may be used to induce ovulation in cases of anovulatory menstrual cycles or to achieve multiple ova prior to in vitro fertilization; risks of ovulation induction include multiple births and ovarian hyperstimulation, which can result in enlarged ovaries, abdominal distention, pain, and occasionally ovarian cysts
4. Sperm washing for intrauterine insemination (IUI): client's ejaculate is centrifuged to concentrate spermatozoa, rinsed in saline to remove seminal fluid, centrifuged again, and used for either in vitro or intrauterine artificial insemination

NCLEX® 5. Intrauterine insemination is a form of **artificial insemination** whereby
   a. Sperm collected within 3 hours of ejaculation are inserted via catheter into uterus
   b. Donor sperm may be used if male partner's sperm count or motility is low or for single women who desire pregnancy; sperm donor identity is kept confidential

6. **In vitro fertilization (IVF)**: multiple ova are harvested via large-bore needle and syringe transvaginally under ultrasound guidance; ova are mixed with spermatozoa, and up to four resultant embryos are returned to uterus 2–3 days later; side effects include ovarian cysts, multiple births, and ovarian hyperstimulation
   a. Preprocedure care: instruct client to give synthetic FSH injections subcutaneously to stimulate ova production for 5–6 days preprocedure; give sedation for ova retrieval procedure; observe client for 2 hours after egg retrieval, and instruct to limit activity for next 24 hours
   b. Postprocedure care following embryo placement in uterus includes minimal client activity for 24 hours; progesterone supplementation is commonly prescribed

IV. GENERAL CONSIDERATIONS IN FAMILY PLANNING AND CONTRACEPTION

A. Overview

1. Family planning assists clients with reproductive decision making by enabling client to prevent pregnancy, limit number of children, space time between children, and/or voluntarily interrupt pregnancy as desired

NCLEX® 2. Factors to discuss with a client who is choosing a contraceptive method include client preferences, client age and future childbearing plans, possible contraindications to specific methods, safety and effectiveness of method(s) under consideration (including protection against sexually transmitted infections [STIs]), and partner support and willingness to cooperate

B. Methods: natural, fertility awareness, barrier, hormonal, and operative sterilization; choice may be influenced by cultural practices, religious beliefs, and other personal preferences and attitudes

V. NATURAL METHODS OF FAMILY PLANNING

A. Natural methods are safe, situational methods requiring self-awareness and self-control to be effective

B. Types of natural family planning methods

1. Abstinence: avoiding sexual intercourse

NCLEX® a. Advantages: safe, free, and available to all; 100% effective in preventing pregnancy and STIs when practiced consistently; can be initiated at any time; encourages communication between partners
   b. Disadvantage: both partners must practice self-control
   c. Client education: teach alternative methods of obtaining sexual pleasure; provide positive feedback to clients who desire and maintain abstinence

2. Coitus interruptus (withdrawal)
   a. Requires male to withdraw penis from vagina when urge to ejaculate occurs and ejaculate away from external female genitalia
   b. Clients must use self-control because most pleasurable moment during intercourse may coincide with time to withdraw penis

c. Advantages: can be practiced at any time during menstrual cycle; cost free
d. Disadvantages: least reliable contraceptive method; some pre-ejaculatory fluid (which may contain sperm) may escape from penis; at peak sexual excitement, exercising self-control may be difficult
e. Client education: before intercourse male should urinate and wipe off tip of penis to decrease risk of sperm entering vagina; conception may occur if pre-ejaculatory fluid containing sperm enters introitus; spermicide or postcoital contraceptive may be needed if female partner is exposed to sperm

VI. FERTILITY AWARENESS METHODS OF FAMILY PLANNING

A. Overview

1. These methods are based on an understanding of woman's ovulation cycle and timing of sexual intercourse
2. All methods attempt to identify period of female fertility and avoid unprotected intercourse during that time
3. Advantages: free, safe, and acceptable to couples whose religious beliefs prohibit other methods; encourages couple communication; can prevent or plan a pregnancy
4. Disadvantages: requires extensive initial counseling and education; may interfere with sexual spontaneity; may be difficult or impossible for women with irregular menstrual cycles; requires extensive record-keeping; offers no protection against STIs if used alone; is theoretically reliable but less effective in actual use

B. *Calendar method*

1. Also known as rhythm method; based on assumptions that ovulation occurs 14 days (plus or minus 2 days) prior to next menses, sperm are viable for up to 7 days, and ovum is viable for up to 3 days
2. Client education: teach woman to first keep a menstrual calendar for 6–8 months to identify shortest and longest cycles; using first day of menses as first day of cycle, calculate fertile period by subtracting 18 days from length of shortest cycle through length of longest cycle minus 11 days; counsel to avoid intercourse during fertile period

C. Basal body temperature (BBT) method

1. Based on thermal shift in menstrual cycle; temperature drops just prior to ovulation, rises and fluctuates at a higher level until 2 to 4 days prior to next menses, then falls if no conception
2. Client education
   a. Teach client to measure temperature with a BBT thermometer, which shows tenths of a degree, and record findings on a temperature chart (see Figure 8–1)
   b. *NCLEX®* Teach client to take temperature each morning prior to arising or beginning activity
   c. Counsel to avoid intercourse on day temperature drops and for 3 days after temperature rises
   d. Inform client that reliability can be affected by a decrease in BBT too small to detect, factors that raise or lower BBT (such as illness, stress, fatigue, consuming alcohol the prior evening, or sleeping in a heated waterbed), and that intercourse just prior to drop in BBT may result in pregnancy

D. Cervical mucus method

1. Also known as ovulation or Billings method; based on cervical mucus changes that occur during menstrual cycle; effectiveness same as BBT method
2. Client education
   a. Teach client to assess cervical mucus daily for amount, color, consistency, and viscosity
   b. *NCLEX®* Counsel to avoid intercourse when client first notices cervical mucus becoming more clear, elastic, and slippery and for about 4 days after

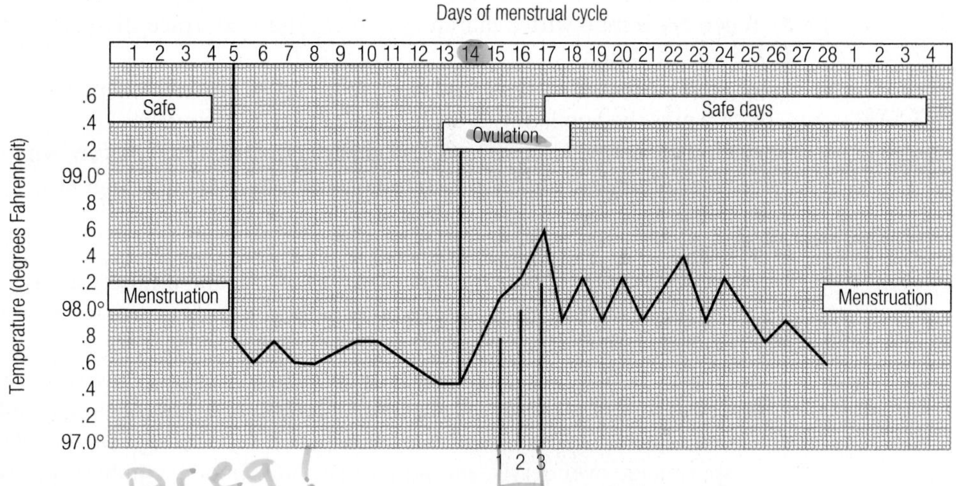

Figure 8–1
Sample basal body temperature chart.

c. Convey sensitivity as women who are uncomfortable touching their genitals may find this method unacceptable
d. Instruct client that cervical mucus can be affected by douches and vaginal deodorants, semen, blood and discharge from vaginal infections, antihistamine drugs, and contraceptive gels, foams, film, or suppositories

E. ***Symptothermal method***
1. The symptothermal method involves assessing multiple indicators of ovulation, recording findings and coital history on a menstrual calendar, then abstaining from intercourse during fertile period; provides no protection against STIs
2. Client education
a. Instruct client to assess and record BBT and condition of cervical mucus as primary indicators of ovulation
b. Teach client to recognize and record secondary indicators of ovulation: increased libido, abdominal bloating, midcycle abdominal pain (Mittelschmerz), breast or pelvic tenderness, pelvic or vulvar fullness, slight dilatation of cervical os, and softer cervix located higher in vagina

VII. BARRIER METHODS OF CONTRACEPTION

A. Overview
1. Provide a physical or chemical barrier to block sperm from entering cervix
2. Some barrier devices are made from latex and should be avoided by those with latex allergies
3. All barrier methods have advantages and disadvantages (see Table 8–1)

B. ***Male condom***
1. A sheath made of latex, plastic, or natural membranes that is placed over erect penis to collect semen
2. Client education
a. Check package expiration date, and if past date, use another condom
NCLEX® b. Avoid using oil-based lubricants, but contraceptive foam or water-based lubricants may be used
c. Put on condom by placing it on tip of erect penis, leaving enough room at tip to collect sperm, then unrolling condom from tip to base of erect penis
NCLEX® d. After intercourse, client should hold rim of condom while withdrawing erect penis from vagina to prevent leakage
e. Inspect used condom for tears or holes because these will decrease effectiveness
f. Discard used condom in a disposable waste container; do not flush in toilet

C. ***Female condom***
1. A thin, polyurethane sheath with flexible rings at each end, which covers cervix, lines vagina, and partially shields perineum
2. Client education
a. Insert closed end of condom into vagina so ring fits loosely against cervix
b. Have partner insert penis into open end leaving approximately 2.5 cm (1 in.) of sheath from flexible ring outside of introitus
NCLEX® c. After intercourse, before woman stands up, remove condom by squeezing and twisting outer ring to close sheath while gently pulling it from vagina

D. ***Spermicide***
1. The approved spermicidal agent in U.S. is nonoxynol-9 (N9); allergic response is possible
2. Forms a chemical barrier preventing pregnancy by killing sperm or neutralizing vaginal secretions; is available as a cream, jelly, foam, vaginal film, and suppository
3. When N9 is used with a diaphragm or condom, contraceptive and antimicrobial benefits increase
4. Client education
a. Apply N9 inside vagina and close to cervix before placing penis near introitus
NCLEX® b. N9 must be applied with each act of sexual intercourse
NCLEX® c. Contraceptive foam, cream, and gel are effective immediately, while contraceptive film and suppository are effective 15 minutes after insertion into vagina
d. When used alone effectiveness is no longer than 1 hour

E. ***Diaphragm***
1. A dome-shaped appliance made of latex (or silicone if latex allergy) with a flexible rim that fits over cervix, used with spermicidal cream or jelly, prevents sperm from entering cervix
2. Client education
a. Utilize models and visual aids to demonstrate insertion and removal
b. Teach proper insertion: apply about a teaspoon of spermicidal cream or jelly around rim and inside cup; squeeze sides of diaphragm together, insert through vagina, place side of device containing spermicide over cervix, and push upper edge under symphysis pubis

Table 8–1 Advantages and Disadvantages of Barrier Contraceptives

Barrier Method	Advantages	Disadvantages
Male condom	Males can participate in contraception Sexual intercourse may be prolonged Low cost and available in a variety of sizes and styles Partners can participate in placing condom to enhance enjoyment All condoms except those made of natural skins offer protection against both pregnancy and STIs	Penis must be erect before placing condom To prevent spillage of semen, male must withdraw after ejaculating, while penis is still erect Condoms can rupture or leak, increasing potential for semen to escape into vagina Oil-based lubricants can decrease effectiveness Condoms are for single use only Misplacement, perineal/vaginal irritation, or dulled penile sensation may occur Natural skin condoms have pores that can allow passage of viruses and do not protect against STIs
Female condom	May be inserted up to 8 hours before intercourse Clients who are sensitive to latex can use female condom Both partners are protected against STIs during intercourse Are available without a prescription Use of lubricants will not decrease effectiveness Breastfeeding women can safely use condoms	May twist or slip during intercourse If penis is placed outside of condom, effectiveness is jeopardized Improper removal results in risk of ejaculate leaking out of condom Outer ring may irritate external genitalia High cost, noise produced with intercourse, or altered sensation are unacceptable for some couples Initially, insertion may be difficult or awkward
Spermicide	No prescription is required May be used alone, with a diaphragm, or with a condom Foam, gel, and suppository may add additional lubrication and moisture Penis can remain in vagina following ejaculation Method is safe for breastfeeding women A variety of forms offers clients additional choices	May be irritating to one or both clients or be perceived as messy May interfere with spontaneity, as it is inserted before each act of intercourse and may require an interval of time before onset of action Does not protect against STIs if used alone without additional barrier method
Diaphragm	Gives woman control Provides some protection against STIs A partner may insert diaphragm if client has trouble with placement or as part of foreplay Contains no hormones and is safe for breastfeeding client Penis can remain inside vagina after ejaculation	Must be fitted by a qualified healthcare provider and replaced annually Refitting may be needed following pregnancy or 4.5–6.8 kg (10–15 lb) weight gain or loss Some clients may have difficulty learning to place diaphragm correctly
Cervical cap	Similar to those of diaphragm	May be more difficult to fit because of limited sizes; some clients may have difficulty with insertion and removal Must be fitted by a qualified healthcare provider and should be replaced annually Clients must be rechecked for fit following pregnancy or 4.5–6.8 kg (10–15 lb) weight gain or loss Effectiveness is reduced for parous women
Vaginal contraceptive sponge	Same as for diaphragm, plus low cost and no prescription	Some clients perceive sponge as bulky or awkward when in place, or uncomfortable during intercourse Effectiveness is reduced for parous women
Intrauterine device	High rate of effectiveness Provides continuous contraceptive protection No coitus-related activity required Is relatively inexpensive over time	May cause discomfort, bleeding, and cramping during and between menses Uterus may perforate during insertion May be expelled spontaneously Increased risk of pelvic infection up to 3 weeks after insertion

c. Teach proper removal by grasping rim to dislodge from cervix and pulling down to remove through vagina
d. Encourage client to practice insertion and removal when healthcare provider is present to check for proper placement in vagina

NCLEX® e. Diaphragm should be left in place at least 6 hours after coitus

NCLEX® f. If diaphragm is placed more than 4 hours prior to intercourse or if coitus is desired again within 6 hours, a condom should be used or additional spermicide should be used without disturbing diaphragm

NCLEX® g. Remove at least once during a 24-hour period to decrease risk of toxic shock syndrome
h. Clean diaphragm with mild soap and water and inspect for tears, punctures, and thinning; avoid oil-based lubricants, which weaken the latex; replace diaphragm if any damage is observed
i. Air-dry device thoroughly and store in carrying case away from light and heat
j. Avoid use during menses or when abnormal vaginal discharge is present to decrease risk of toxic shock syndrome

NCLEX® k. Contact healthcare provider for any warning signs listed in Table 8–2

NCLEX® 3. Contraindications
a. A history of urinary tract infections (pressure of diaphragm on urethra may interfere with complete bladder emptying and increase risk of infection from urine stasis)
b. A history of toxic shock syndrome (if left in place for a long period of time, diaphragm may increase risk of infection)

Table 8–2 Warning Signs and Symptoms Associated with Various Methods of Contraception

Method	Warning Signs and Symptoms
Cervical cap, diaphragm, and contraceptive sponge	Toxic shock syndrome: elevation of temperature >101.4°F (38.6°C), diarrhea and vomiting, weakness and faintness, muscle aches, sore throat, sunburn-type rash Difficult or painful urination Abdominal or pelvic fullness Foul-smelling vaginal discharge
IUD	Acronym **PAINS** **P**—Period late (pregnancy), abnormal spotting or bleeding **A**—Abdominal pain, pain with intercourse **I**—Infection exposure (STI), abnormal vaginal discharge **N**—Not feeling well, fever >100.4°F (38°C), chills **S**—String missing, shorter or longer than usually felt
Oral contraceptives	Acronym **ACHES** **A**—Abdominal pain **C**—Chest pain, cough, and/or shortness of breath **H**—Headaches, dizziness, weakness, or numbness **E**—Eye problems (blurring or change in vision) and speech problems **S**—Severe leg, calf, and/or thigh pain
Vasectomy	Fever >100.4°F (38°C); excessive pain Difficulty urinating Redness, swelling, bruising, drainage, or skin edges of the incision that are not closed Bleeding at the site
Tubal ligation	Fever >100.4°F (38°C); excessive pain Difficulty with defecation or urination Nausea or vomiting Redness, swelling, bruising, drainage, or skin edges of the incision that are not closed

F. *Cervical cap*

1. A small, cup-shaped device that fits over cervix; held in place by suction; acts as a barrier between sperm and cervix; has many similarities to diaphragm
2. Client education
   a. Teach client to apply spermicide inside cap
   NCLEX® b. Insert cap at least 20 minutes but not longer than 4 hours prior to intercourse
   c. May be left in place up to 48 hours
   NCLEX® d. Reapplication of spermicide with repeated intercourse is not needed
   e. Do not use cap during menses or if abnormal vaginal discharge is present
   NCLEX® f. Contact healthcare provider for warning signs described in Table 8–2

G. *Vaginal contraceptive sponge*

1. A small, round synthetic sponge with nonoxynol-9 spermicide; has a concave or cupped area on cervical side and a loop for easy removal on other
2. Client education
   a. Moisten sponge with water prior to insertion to activate spermicide
   b. Place concave side of sponge next to cervix
   c. Leave sponge in place for at least 6 hours after intercourse
   d. Remove by pulling polyester loop on convex side of sponge downward and out of vagina
   e. The sponge provides protection up to 24 hours and for repeated acts of intercourse; remove by 24-hour time limit to reduce risk of toxic shock syndrome
   f. Contact healthcare provider for warning signs listed in Table 8–2

H. *Intrauterine device (IUD)*

1. Produces local inflammatory effects on endometrium that prevents fertilization
2. Types of IUDs available in United States
   NCLEX® a. Copper T380A (ParaGard) can be left in place for 10 years 10 yr!
   b. Levonorgestrel-releasing intrauterine system (LNG-IUS or Mirena) can be left in place up to 5 years
   c. Preferred candidates for use include women in a stable monogamous relationship (low risk for STI) with no history of pelvic inflammatory disease (PID) and with healthy uterine anatomy
   d. Placement of Copper T IUD within 5 days after unprotected intercourse may also reduce pregnancy risk by up to 99%
3. Client education
   a. Cramping or intermittent bleeding may occur for 2–6 weeks after insertion
   b. After placement, first few menses may be irregular
   c. Follow-up examination is suggested in 4–8 weeks
   NCLEX® d. Check for presence of string protruding through cervix by inserting a finger into vagina once a week for first month and then after each menses
   NCLEX® e. Counsel client to contact healthcare provider if exposed to STI or warning signs known as PAINS develop, as listed in Table 8–2

Memory Aid

Use the mnemonics in Table 8–2 to remember the warning signs for complications of selected contraceptive methods.

VIII. HORMONAL METHODS OF CONTRACEPTION

A. *Combined oral contraceptives* (COCs or birth control pills)

1. Act by inhibiting release of an ovum, blocking cyclical release of gonadotropin-releasing hormone, and changing cervical mucus
2. Typical COCs contain both estrogen and progestin and are available in packages with 21 pills or 28 pills (seven are "blank" pills)
3. Newer COCs with very low estrogen are supplied as 24/4 formulations (only four "blank" pills) to suppress chance of ovulation better than formulations providing seven hormone-free days
4. Extended oral contraceptives are 91-day regimens; client takes active pill daily for 84 days, followed by inactive pill for 7 days, during which client has menses

5. Contraindications
   a. Absolute contraindications: pregnancy, history of thrombophlebitis or thromboembolic disease, presence of estrogen-dependent neoplasms, undiagnosed uterine bleeding, heavy smoking, cholestatic liver disease or gallbladder disease, hypertension, diabetes, and lyperlipidemia; women over age 35 who smoke
   b. Relative contraindications: epilepsy, depression, oligomenorrhea and amenorrhea, and breastfeeding for less than 30 days
6. Client education
   a. When starting oral contraceptives, begin pills on first Sunday after onset of menses and take one pill at same time each day
   b. If a 28-day pack is prescribed, don't skip days between packages
   c. Clients using a 21-day pack should wait 7 days before starting next cycle of pills
   d. *NCLEX®* If one or more doses are missed, follow directions on product; may include taking pill immediately (one dose missed); if two or more doses are missed, directions differ according to product, but may include a method to "catch up" and generally include a recommendation to use backup contraception
   e. *NCLEX®* Observe for side effects of oral contraceptives, which can be estrogen related (such as headache, fluid retention, breast tenderness, nausea, and thromboembolic disease) or progestin related (including acne, increased LDL and decreased HDL cholesterol levels, depression, fatigue, hirsutism, increased appetite and weight gain, oligomenorrhea or amenorrhea)
   f. *NCLEX®* Contact healthcare provider immediately if warning signs develop, which are remembered using the mnemonic ACHES; see Table 8–2
7. Advantages
   a. Use of method is not directly related to act of sexual intercourse
   b. Menstrual cycle is more regular with reduced flow and cramping
   c. Safe during reproductive years for women who do not smoke
   d. Noncontraceptive benefits include a decrease in menstrual migraines, iron-deficiency anemia, pelvic pain from endometriosis, perimenopausal "hot flashes," and ovarian, endometrial, and colorectal cancers; improvement of bone mineral density and acne
8. Disadvantages
   a. COCs offer no protection against STIs
   b. Clients need to remember to take pill at same time each day
   c. *NCLEX®* Clients with preexisting medical problems may not be candidates for this method
   d. COCs may decrease effectiveness of insulin and oral anticoagulants such as warfarin
   e. *NCLEX®* Effectiveness may be decreased when taken with other drugs, making it important to share information about COC use with healthcare provider

B. Other combined hormonal methods

1. Contraceptive skin patch (Ortho Evra): applied weekly to one of four sites (abdomen, buttocks, upper outer arm, or trunk but not breasts); during week 4 no patch is worn and menses occurs
2. Vaginal contraceptive ring (Nuvaring) is a soft flexible ring inserted into vagina for 3 weeks and delivers low-dose, sustained-release contraceptive hormone; removed for week 4 and menses occurs

C. Progestin contraceptives (oral, implant, and injection)

1. Progestin-only pill, also known as a mini-pill, does not contain estrogen, contains less progestin than COCs
   a. May be used by lactating women and those who have contraindications to estrogen component of COCs
   b. *NCLEX®* Client teaching involves taking a dose immediately if missed and to use an additional method of contraception through end of that cycle
   c. Disadvantages include increased risk of ectopic pregnancy, irregular bleeding, or amenorrhea
2. Progestin-only **subdermal implant**
   a. A long-acting single-capsule implant (Implanon) is inserted subdermally into upper inner arm during first 7 days of menstrual cycle; prevents ovulation and stimulates production of thick cervical mucus, preventing penetration by sperm
   b. Client education: signs and symptoms of postprocedure infection to report to healthcare provider; possible side effects such as spotting, irregular bleeding, amenorrhea, weight gain, headache, fluid retention, mood changes, and depression
   c. Advantages: provides continuous contraception not related to sexual intercourse; does not contain estrogen; effective within 24 hours and for up to 3 years
   d. Disadvantages: requires minor surgery to insert and remove implant; cost may be prohibitive; offers no protection against STIs

3. Long-acting progestin injection
   a. Medroxyprogesterone acetate is a long-acting progestin that blocks luteinizing hormone surge, suppresses ovulation, and thickens cervical mucus to prevent penetration of sperm
   b. Client education: side effects (menstrual irregularities, headache, weight gain, breast tenderness, and depression), need for follow-up injections every 3 months (10–14 weeks), need to take 1200 mg calcium daily to offset bone demineralization, and need to watch for warning signs of ACHES identified in Table 8–2
   c. Advantages: safe for lactating women; does not contain estrogen; requires administration only every 3 months
   d. Disadvantages: must comply with need for follow-up injections to maintain effectiveness; return of fertility may be delayed up to 1 year after stopping method

D. *Emergency contraception*

1. Indicated when there is concern about pregnancy because of unprotected intercourse, rape, or possible contraceptive failure
2. Are available over-the-counter to women age 17 years or older
3. Should be initiated as soon as possible after intercourse (but not longer than 72 hours later), with second dose 12 hours later if two-step method used)
4. A prescription-only version may be taken up to 5 days after unprotected intercourse

IX. OPERATIVE STERILIZATION

A. Overview

1. Surgical contraceptive methods result in voluntary sterilization of male or female
2. Surgical consent is obtained after risks and benefits of specific method are explained

B. *Vasectomy*

1. A form of sterilization for males in which vas deferens is resected through small incisions made in each side of scrotum
2. Client education
   a. Procedure takes about 15–20 minutes and can be performed in a clinic setting under local anesthesia
   b. Client should not drive immediately after procedure; should have someone drive him home after discharge and remain with him for 24 hours postprocedure

   NCLEX®

   c. Rest after procedure with minimal activity for 48 hours and avoid strenuous activity for 1 week, avoid tub baths for 48 hours, and increase comfort by wearing a scrotal support for comfort, using ice packs intermittently, and taking sitz baths after 24 hours

   NCLEX®

   d. Contact healthcare provider if warning signs develop, as listed in Table 8–2
   e. Possible side effects of vasectomy include pain, infection, hematoma, sperm granulomas, and spontaneous reconnection
   f. Sterility is not achieved until semen is free of sperm, about 4–6 weeks or 6–36 ejaculations; until then, use another contraceptive method and bring in two or three semen samples for sperm count
   g. Semen should be rechecked at 6 and 12 months to verify sterility has been maintained
3. Although reversal may be possible, this method is considered permanent; restored fertility is about 60% using subsequent pregnancy as a guide, but this decreases over time because of secondary obstruction of epididymis

C. *Tubal ligation*

1. Fallopian tubes are accessed via a small subumbilical incision or laparoscopic technique, then cut, tied, cauterized, or banded to block passage of sperm and prevent ovum from becoming fertilized

NCLEX®

2. Client education
   a. Outpatient procedure takes about 30 minutes; performed under regional or general anesthesia
   b. May need to restrict food and fluid intake for several hours prior to procedure, especially if general anesthesia is planned
   c. May experience pain for several days after procedure
   d. Avoid tub baths for 48 hours and driving, lifting, and strenuous activity for 1 week
   e. Contact healthcare provider if warning signs develop, as listed in Table 8–2
3. Advantages: permanent and effective in preventing pregnancy; may be performed at any time (immediately after childbirth is optimal because uterus is enlarged and fallopian tubes are easy to identify); sexual function and spontaneity are not affected
4. Disadvantages: potential complications are adverse reaction to anesthesia, infection, and bleeding; if pregnancy occurs after tubal ligation, reversal of procedure may not be possible

Check Your NCLEX–RN® Exam I.Q.

You are ready for testing on this content if you can:

- Provide support to a client and partner during infertility assessment and treatment.
- Use knowledge from biologic and social sciences in discussions with clients contemplating contraception and family planning.
- Assess the client's readiness to use contraception.
- Determine the client's preferences for contraceptive methods.
- Describe risks and contraindications to selected contraceptive methods.

PRACTICE TEST

PRACTICE TEST

1 Which statement indicates to the nurse that a couple is coping with the stress of infertility treatment?

1. "We are trying to maintain a little romance in our relationship."
2. "My wife was so upset she threw a syringe at me yesterday."
3. "My husband couldn't have an erection when he was supposed to."
4. "We have two or glasses of wine each night to help us relax."

2 The client has been diagnosed with Trichomonas vaginitis. The nurse explains during client teaching that this infection can affect fertility by which mechanism?

1. Using glycogen in vaginal secretions, leaving no nutrition for spermatozoa
2. Blocking fallopian tubes, which prohibits spermatozoa from reaching an ovum
3. Decreasing pH of vaginal secretions, thus destroying most spermatozoa
4. Increasing temperature inside the vagina, which decreases sperm motility

3 The nurse is concerned that which viral infection, if experienced by an adult male, may cause infertility?

1. Varicella zoster
2. Rubella
3. Influenza
4. Mumps

4 Which statement by a client being treated for infertility indicates an understanding of treatment?

1. "I should come back for a postcoital test 1–2 days before I expect to ovulate."
2. "I should schedule my hysterosalpingogram for the week after ovulation."
3. "We should abstain for 2–7 days prior to coming back for the sperm penetration test."
4. "I should schedule my endometrial biopsy for the last week of my menstrual cycle."

5 What information would the nurse gather before scheduling a client's endometrial biopsy?

1. Usual length of menstrual cycle
2. Blood type and Rh factor
3. Presence of any metal implants
4. Last type of birth control used

6 The nurse is teaching a class in the community on common myths regarding fertility and infertility. Which statement made by a class participant indicates teaching has been successful?

1. "If my husband works out everyday, he won't be able to make a baby."
2. "If we have intercourse standing up, we won't be able to conceive."
3. "If we have intercourse on the even days after ovulation, we will conceive a girl."
4. "If my husband sits in the hot tub every night, his sperm count will decrease."

7 The client couple is planning intracytoplasmic sperm injection, followed by intrauterine embryo transfer. Which statement indicates the nurse's teaching was effective?

1. "His sperm swim too fast for me to become pregnant."
2. "My eggs have thick walls and don't let his sperm in."
3. "Any extra embryos can be frozen for implantation later."
4. "We will have to wait several weeks to see if any eggs get fertilized."

8 The clinic nurse is interviewing a client couple for an initial infertility workup. Which priority topic would the nurse plan to address?

1. Whether or not the couple has medical insurance
2. How infertility is affecting their lives
3. Whether the man has iodine allergies
4. Whether the woman works outside the home

9 The client is unable to become pregnant after she has had one full-term pregnancy. The nurse should develop a plan of care for which health problem?

1. Primary infertility
2. Secondary infertility
3. Unexplained infertility
4. Combined-factor infertility

10 The client has an obstruction between the uterus and fallopian tubes. In obtaining a health history, the nurse collects information about which possible etiology?

1. Rubella infection prior to adolescence
2. Pelvic inflammatory disease caused by gonorrhea
3. Smoking two packs of cigarettes per day
4. Ingestion of 2 ounces of alcohol daily

11 Which statement by a client could indicate a potential problem for a couple planning to use coitus interruptus?

1. "I really don't want to get pregnant right now, so we need a very effective method."
2. "I think I can always pull out before I ejaculate."
3. "We don't have any other sex partners."
4. "We want a contraceptive method that is inexpensive and completely natural."

12 Which client statement indicates that teaching about cervical mucus changes as an indicator of ovulation has been understood?

thin + clear = ovulation

1. "If my cervical mucus is yellowish and thick, I am probably fertile."
2. "The thin, clear mucus will block sperm from getting to my cervix."
3. "If my cervical mucus is thick and white, I will need to avoid intercourse or use a backup method of contraception."
4. "If my cervical mucus is thin and stretchable, I am probably fertile."

13 The client, who is married and has three children, has come to the family planning clinic asking about a birth control method that is most effective and sanctioned by the Roman Catholic Church. What would be the nurse's best recommendation?

1. Billings or cervical assessment method
2. Ovulation testing kit
3. Symptothermal method
4. Basal body temperature (BBT) method

14 The client is interested in using female condoms and wants to know if there are any disadvantages. What is the nurse's best response?

1. "The female condom provides good protection against pregnancy but not against sexually transmitted infections (STIs)."
2. "The female condom may be difficult to insert and may be uncomfortable to both partners."
3. "The female condom is very effective; let me arrange to get you a prescription."
4. "The female condom is made of latex and should not be used by those with latex allergies."

PRACTICE TEST

15 Which client being seen in the outpatient clinic would be the best candidate for insertion of an intrauterine device (IUD)?

1. A client who is married, has one child, and wants to get pregnant in about 6 months
2. A client who is unmarried, has no children, and has numerous sexual partners
3. A client who is married, has two children, and does not want more children for at least 3 years
4. A client who is unmarried, has one child, and has a history of pelvic inflammatory disease (PID)

16 In planning care for the infertile client, the nurse should take which actions? Select all that apply.

1. Encourage client to seek additional formal education.
2. Restrict the amount of information given so as not to overwhelm client.
3. Facilitate client's self-esteem through use of careful wording and avoiding blame.
4. Aid client in finding a relaxing vacation spot to improve the chances of conception.
5. Explain that fertility testing process is lengthy and results will not be instantaneous.

17 A client who has a complete bicornuate uterus with two vaginas is considering getting pregnant. The nurse would include in discussions with the client which associated concerns? Select all that apply.

1. Inability to ever achieve pregnancy
2. Increased risk for preterm labor
3. Need for artificial insemination to conceive
4. Need for cesarean delivery
5. Risk for multiple pregnancy loss

18 The client brings her basal body temperature (BBT) chart to the clinic. In evaluating the chart, the nurse suspects that ovulation has occurred. Indicate the area on the chart shown that supports the nurse's judgment.

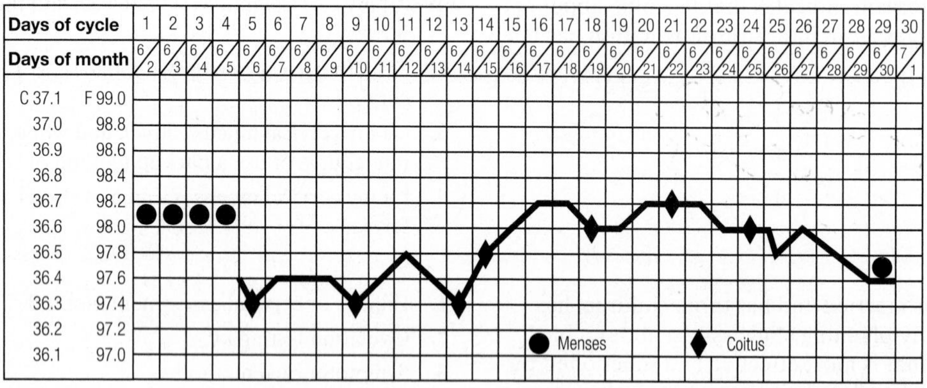

19 The nurse working in an infertility clinic explains to an infertile couple that they will likely have which tests ordered? Select all that apply.

1. Semen analysis
2. Papanicolaou smear
3. Colposcopy with endocervical biopsy
4. Sexually transmitted infection testing
5. Hysterosalpingogram

20 The women's health clinic nurse determines that which clients would be appropriate candidates for use of emergency postcoital contraception? Select all that apply.

1. Had unprotected intercourse 4 days ago
2. Took her oral contraceptive 7 hours late
3. Removed her cervical cap 40 hours after intercourse
4. Had her last Depo-Provera injection 4 months ago
5. Had been sexually assaulted the previous day

21 Which statements indicate to the nurse that a male client understands how to correctly apply a condom? Select all that apply.

1. "I need to put it on before the penis is erect."
2. "I should unroll the condom, then place it on the penis."
3. "When putting on the condom, I need to leave some space at the tip to collect the sperm."
4. "I can use oil-based lubricants if needed."
5. "I can use a water-based lubricant if needed."

ANSWERS & RATIONALES

1 **Answer:** 1 **Rationale:** Maintaining a healthy relationship, such as romance, is important during infertility treatments, which can be very stressful. Emotional outbursts, decreased libido, and regular use of alcohol to relax warrant further investigation as possible signs of excess stress. **Cognitive Level:** Analyzing **Client Need:** Health Promotion and Maintenance **Integrated Process:** Nursing Process: Evaluation **Content Area:** Adult Health: Reproductive **Strategy:** Note a critical word in the question is *coping*. Look for the option that indicates effective functioning or therapeutic communication with questions such as these.

2 **Answer:** 3 **Rationale:** Vaginal fluid pH is slightly alkaline, as is semen. Spermatozoa cannot survive in an acidic environment. Trichomonas vaginitis increases the acidity of the vaginal and cervical secretions, thus reducing the number of viable sperm. **Cognitive Level:** Applying **Client Need:** Health Promotion and Maintenance **Integrated Process:** Teaching and Learning **Content Area:** Adult Health: Reproductive **Strategy:** Look for the option that is a true statement and use knowledge of pathophysiology to eliminate incorrect distractors.

3 **Answer:** 4 **Rationale:** Mumps in adult males can cause permanent blockage of the vas deferens, contributing to or resulting in infertility. Varicella, rubella, and influenza do not have this effect. **Cognitive Level:** Applying **Client Need:** Health Promotion and Maintenance **Integrated Process:** Nursing Process: Diagnosis **Content Area:** Adult Health: Reproductive **Strategy:** Look for the option that exerts this effect and use knowledge of pathophysiology to eliminate incorrect distractors.

4 **Answer:** 3 **Rationale:** The sperm penetration test, which tests for the ability of sperm to penetrate an egg, should be performed after 2–7 days of abstinence. Having a postcoital test before ovulation is not useful. A hypersalpingogram would be scheduled in the proliferative phase before ovulation to avoid early pregnancy or secretory changes in endometrium after ovulation, which could obstruct dye passage. Endometrial biopsy should not be scheduled earlier than 10–12 days after ovulation to accurately detect effects of progesterone and endometrial sensitivity. **Cognitive Level:** Applying **Client Need:** Health Promotion and Maintenance **Integrated Process:** Nursing Process: Evaluation **Content Area:** Adult Health: Reproductive **Strategy:** The wording of this question indicates an incorrect statement is the correct answer to the question. Evaluate each option as to whether it is true or false, and select the false statement.

5 **Answer:** 1 **Rationale:** The nurse assesses the first day of the last normal menstrual period and the menstrual cycle length. Endometrial biopsy is performed on day 21–27 of the menstrual cycle to assess endometrial response to progesterone and development of luteal-phase endometrium. It is unnecessary to assess for blood type and Rh factor, metal implants, or most recent type of birth control used. **Cognitive Level:** Applying **Client Need:** Health Promotion and Maintenance **Integrated Process:** Nursing Process: Assessment **Content Area:** Adult Health: Reproductive **Strategy:** Eliminate implants first as irrelevant and then blood type because excessive bleeding requiring transfusion is not expected. Recall the relationship between the menstrual cycle and biopsy procedure to choose length of cycle over birth control method.

6 **Answer:** 4 **Rationale:** Hot tubs, saunas, and tight underwear can raise the temperature of the testes too high for efficient spermatogenesis and lead to decreased sperm numbers and motility. Exercise by the male partner does not affect fertility. A standing position does not prevent conception. Sex of a fetus is not affected by whether intercourse occurs on an odd or even day. **Cognitive Level:** Analyzing **Client Need:** Health Promotion and Maintenance **Integrated Process:** Nursing Process: Evaluation **Content Area:** Adult Health: Reproductive **Strategy:** The wording of this question indicates a correct statement is the answer to the question. Evaluate each option as to whether it is true or false, then select the true statement.

7 **Answer:** 3 **Rationale:** In vitro fertilization usually creates multiple embryos, of which up to four are implanted. Cryopreservation of excess embryos is common, and they can be implanted at a later date. Slow sperm motility could adversely affect fertilization. The thickness of the wall of the egg does not impede sperm penetration. It does not take several weeks to determine whether eggs are fertilized with intracytoplasmic sperm injection. **Cognitive Level:** Analyzing **Client Need:** Health Promotion and Maintenance **Integrated Process:** Nursing Process: Evaluation **Content Area:** Adult Health: Reproductive **Strategy:** The wording of this question indicates a correct statement is the answer to the question. Evaluate whether each option is true or false, then select the true statement.

8 **Answer:** 2 **Rationale:** The psychological, cultural, and social ramifications of infertility can be extensive. These areas are assessed to determine if the couple needs assistance in coping with infertility and treatment. Payment for infertility workup is an area of concern, but is not the priority of the nurse when interviewing the couple. Iodine allergies of the man are not of concern, although they may be of concern for the woman if having tests that involve dye injection. Working outside the home is not a priority concern of the nurse during the interview. **Cognitive Level:** Applying **Client Need:** Health Promotion and Maintenance **Integrated Process:** Nursing Process: Planning **Content Area:** Adult Health: Reproductive **Strategy:** Note the critical word *infertility* and note also that this is a nursing assessment. With this in mind, eliminate medical insurance and working outside the home as irrelevant, and allergies as not directly related to the topic.

9 **Answer: 2 Rationale:** Secondary infertility is the term for couples who have had one pregnancy but are unable to conceive again. Primary infertility describes the inability to conceive even once. Unexplained and combined-factor infertility are not terms used when discussing fertility. **Cognitive Level:** Analyzing **Client Need:** Health Promotion and Maintenance **Integrated Process:** Nursing Process: Diagnosis **Content Area:** Adult Health: Reproductive **Strategy:** First eliminate terms that are not used, then choose secondary over primary because the couple has had one successful pregnancy.

10 **Answer: 2 Rationale:** Infectious processes of the reproductive tract such as PID may result in tubal scarring and therefore tubal blockage. Rubella infection in childhood usually results in the development of active immunity to the disease. Smoking and alcohol present health risks to the woman but are not related to tubal patency. **Cognitive Level:** Analyzing **Client Need:** Health Promotion and Maintenance **Integrated Process:** Nursing Process: Diagnosis **Content Area:** Adult Health: Reproductive **Strategy:** Look for an association between blockage in the reproductive system and a condition that is causally related to this. Recall that inflammation and infection can lead to scarring and obstruction in the body. Choose PID over rubella because of its association with inflammation.

11 **Answer: 1 Rationale:** Because some semen is released before ejaculation, coitus interruptus has an 18% failure rate and would not be considered a very effective method for a couple wanting to avoid pregnancy. An ability to withdraw before ejaculation is necessary for coitus interruptus to be effective, so the client's statement would be consistent with successful use of this method. Not having other sex partners has no effect on choice of coitus interruptus as a contraceptive method. Coitus interruptus has no cost and is completely natural. **Cognitive Level:** Analyzing **Client Need:** Health Promotion and Maintenance **Integrated Process:** Nursing Process: Assessment **Content Area:** Adult Health: Reproductive **Strategy:** The critical words in the question are *potential problem*, guiding you to look for a statement that corresponds to a negative aspect of coitus interruptus. With this in mind, each incorrect option can be systematically eliminated.

12 **Answer: 4 Rationale:** Thin and clear cervical mucus indicates a rising level of estrogen and impending ovulation. Stretchability of the cervical mucus, or spinnbarkeit, is indicative of the fertile period and promotes motility of the sperm. Thick cervical mucus occurs during the infertile period when sexual intercourse is unlikely to result in pregnancy. **Cognitive Level:** Analyzing **Client Need:** Health Promotion and Maintenance **Integrated Process:** Nursing Process: Evaluation **Content Area:** Adult Health: Reproductive **Strategy:** The critical word *understood* indicates the correct option is also a correct statement. Use knowledge of physical changes during ovulation to make a selection, or use logic to reason that sperm are more motile through thinner liquids than thicker liquids.

13 **Answer: 3 Rationale:** The symptothermal method combines cervical mucus and BBT measurements and results in a lower failure rate than either BBT or cervical mucus as a single assessment of the fertile period. This method is completely natural and congruent with beliefs of this religious group. Ovulation testing kits do not give enough warning of ovulation to prevent pregnancy. **Cognitive Level:** Analyzing **Client Need:** Health Promotion and Maintenance **Integrated Process:** Nursing Process: Planning **Content Area:** Adult Health: Reproductive **Strategy:** Note the word *best*, which indicates more than one option could be true. In this question, eliminate ovulation testing first as least timely, and choose symptothermal method over Billings and BBT methods because the symptothermal method is comprehensive and includes these other options.

14 **Answer: 2 Rationale:** The female condom may be difficult to insert and may cause discomfort. It protects against both pregnancy and STIs. The female condom does not require a prescription. It is made of polyurethane, not latex. **Cognitive Level:** Applying **Client Need:** Health Promotion and Maintenance **Integrated Process:** Communication and Documentation **Content Area:** Adult Health: Reproductive **Strategy:** Note the critical word *disadvantages* to focus your selection. Eliminate first the option referring to a prescription because a prescription is not necessary. Eliminate the option that says it is only good at protecting against pregnancy next because it is an effective barrier against STIs, and eliminate the option containing latex as a false statement.

15 **Answer: 3 Rationale:** An IUD is a long-term method of contraception usually recommended for women who have been pregnant and are in a monogamous relationship so that they are at a low risk for sexually transmitted infection. A client who wants to get pregnant in about 6 months is not a good candidate for a long-term contraceptive method. A client who has numerous sexual partners is at increased risk for STIs, making an IUD a less suitable method. A client who has a history of pelvic inflammatory disease (PID) is not a good candidate for an IUD because of the increased risk of infection. **Cognitive Level:** Analyzing **Client Need:** Health Promotion and Maintenance **Integrated Process:** Nursing Process: Planning **Content Area:** Adult Health: Reproductive **Strategy:** Use knowledge of advantages and disadvantages of this birth control method to evaluate the options. Eliminate the options with PID and many sexual partners because of the risk for infection, and choose the client desiring pregnancy in 3 years instead of 6 months because the method is for long-term, not short-term, use.

16 **Answer: 3, 5 Rationale:** Self-esteem can be threatened by the inability to conceive a child. Care must be taken to avoid placing blame on the person whose body is not functioning as expected. Fertility testing takes a long time and therefore results are not instantaneous. The amount of formal education does not affect fertility or treatments for infertility. Information should be given when appropriate and not limited or withheld. The need to take a relaxing vacation to conceive is a potentially expensive myth. **Cognitive Level:** Applying **Client Need:** Psychosocial Integrity **Integrated Process:** Nursing Process: Implementation **Content Area:** Adult Health: Reproductive **Strategy:** The core issue of the question is the care of a client experiencing infertility. Eliminate the options referring to formal education, as this does not affect fertility. Next, eliminate the options that withhold information because it should be given when appropriate. Finally, eliminate the option about taking a vacation because it is not true.

17 **Answer: 2, 5 Rationale:** A complete bicornuate uterus is two complete and separate unicornuate uteri. Because the uteri are long and narrow (instead of pear-shaped), the maximum uterine volume is often less than that of a normally shaped uterus. Risks of bicornuate uterus include multiple pregnancy losses, preterm labor, and breech presentation. Becoming pregnant is not an issue; carrying the pregnancy to term is the problem. **Cognitive Level:** Applying

Client Need: Physiological Adaptation **Integrated Process:** Nursing Process: Diagnosis **Content Area:** Maternal–Newborn **Strategy:** The critical words are *bicornuate uterus*. Recall anatomical differences between the normal uterus and bicornuate uterus, keeping in mind that the risks involve carrying a pregnancy due to altered anatomy.

18 **Answer:**

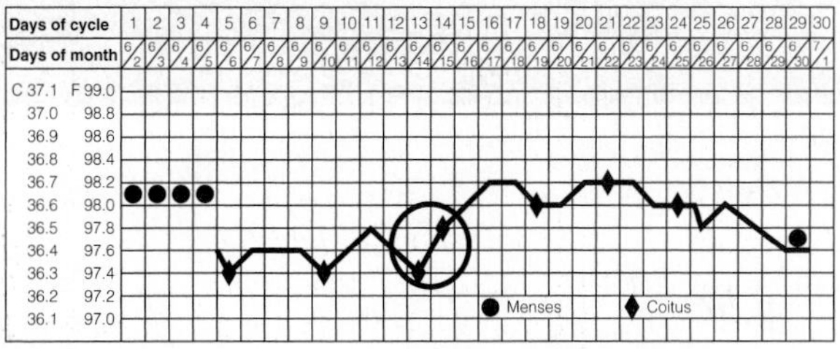

Rationale: An ovulatory cycle is biphasic. The BBT drops slightly, then rises 0.5–1.0°F (0.3–0.6°C) 24–48 hours after ovulation. Progesterone is thermogenic (heat-producing), thereby maintaining the temperature increase during the second half of the menstrual cycle. **Cognitive Level:** Analyzing **Client Need:** Health Promotion and Maintenance **Integrated Process:** Nursing Process: Assessment **Content Area:** Maternal–Newborn **Strategy:** Recall the timing of ovulation at about the midpoint of the menstrual cycle to help choose correctly.

19 **Answer: 1, 5 Rationale:** The most common causes of infertility are inadequate number or motility of sperm and tubal anomaly or blockage. Semen analysis will provide information on number of and motility of sperm. Hysterosalpingogram will detect uterine or tubal anomalies or blockage. A Papanicolaou smear tests for abnormal cervical cells. Colposcopy and testing for sexually transmitted infections will not directly test for causes of infertility. **Cognitive Level:** Applying **Client Need:** Health Promotion and Maintenance **Integrated Process:** Nursing Process: Planning **Content Area:** Adult Health: Reproductive **Strategy:** Critical words are *infertile* and *tests*, which eliminate those tests not pertinent to infertility diagnosis. The focus of the question is testing for the couple, so the correct responses will include tests for both the male and the female.

20 **Answer: 4, 5 Rationale:** Emergency contraception must be initiated within 72 hours of unprotected intercourse, rape, or method failure. Oral contraceptives may be taken up to 12 hours late. Cervical caps may be left in up to 48 hours without compromising safety. Depo-Provera is given every 80–90 days, after which a repeat dose is needed or emergency contraceptive protection is indicated. **Cognitive Level:** Analyzing **Client Need:** Health Promotion and Maintenance **Integrated Process:** Nursing Process: Assessment **Content Area:** Maternal–Newborn **Strategy:** Critical words are *candidate* and *emergency postcoital contraception*. Knowledge of emergency postcoital indications is necessary to answer the question correctly.

21 **Answer: 3, 5 Rationale:** The male condom is placed when the penis is erect, then rolled down. Leaving space at the end of the condom to collect semen can prevent breakage or spillage after ejaculation. Water-based lubricants can be used to provide additional comfort, if needed. Oil-based lubricants are contraindicated. **Cognitive Level:** Analyzing **Client Need:** Health Promotion and Maintenance **Integrated Process:** Teaching and Learning **Content Area:** Maternal–Newborn **Strategy:** The wording of the question is positive, indicating that the correct options are true statements about points of client education. Use nursing knowledge to select these options.

Key Terms to Review

References

Davidson, M., London, M., & Ladewig, P. (2016). *Olds' maternal newborn nursing and women's health across the lifespan* (10th ed.). New York, NY: Pearson Education.

Ladewig, P., London, M., & Davidson, M. (2014). *Contemporary maternal–newborn nursing care* (8th ed.). Upper Saddle River, NJ: Pearson Education.

London, M., Ladewig, P., Davidson, M., Ball, J., Bindler, R., & Cowen, K. (2014). *Maternal and child nursing care* (4th ed.). Upper Saddle River, NJ: Pearson Education.

Lowdermilk, D., Perry, S., Cashion, M., & Alden, K. (2016) *Maternity and women's health care* (11th ed.). St. Louis, MO: Elsevier.

9 Uncomplicated Antenatal Assessment and Care

In this chapter

Cross Reference

Other chapters relevant to this content area are

I. ESSENTIAL CONCEPTS OF PREGNANCY

A. *Estimated date of birth (EDB)*, or due date can be determined by several methods

NCLEX®

1. **Naegele's rule**: take first day of last menstrual period, subtract 3 months, and add 7 days; most accurate when able to recall last menstrual period and menses occurs every 28 days
2. **McDonald's method** uses uterine size (**fundal height**), measured from symphysis pubis to top of uterine fundus in centimeters (cm), to indicate gestational age
   a. This distance, fundal height, correlates well with number of weeks' gestation between 22 and 34 weeks
   b. Formula for calculating gestational age based on fundal height:

$$\frac{\text{distance in centimeters} \times 8}{7} = \text{total weeks of gestation}$$

   c. Prediction of EDB using this method can be affected by maternal height, irregular fetal growth, multiple gestation, and abnormal amounts of amniotic fluid

NCLEX®

3. **Quickening**, feeling of fetal movement by mother, usually occurs between 16 and 18 weeks; because of wide range of times, this method gives a less accurate EDB

4. Fetal heart rate (FHR) can be auscultated as early as 8 weeks' gestation using an ultrasonic Doppler device but is more common between 10 and 12 weeks; this variation can reduce accuracy
5. Ultrasound estimates EDB when date of last menstrual period is unknown or uterine size is inconsistent with EDB calculated with other methods

NCLEX®

B. *Gravida* and *para*

1. Gravida is a pregnant woman; gravidity refers to number of pregnancies
2. Common terms include *nulligravida* (never been pregnant), *primigravida* (first pregnancy), and *multigravida* (two or more pregnancies)
3. Para is number of infants delivered after 20 weeks' gestation, born dead or alive; multiple births count as one delivery regardless of number of infants delivered
4. TPAL is a more detailed description of para

Memory Aid

Use the mnemonic GTPAL to remember detailed description of gravidity and parity (para)
G number assigned to **G**ravidity (number of pregnancies)
T number of **T**erm infants born after 37 completed weeks
P number of **P**reterm infants born between 20 and 37 weeks
A number of pregnancies ending in spontaneous or therapeutic **A**bortion before 20 weeks
L number of **L**iving children

II. SIGNS AND SYMPTOMS OF PREGNANCY

NCLEX®

A. *Presumptive signs of pregnancy*

1. Subjective signs and symptoms that the woman reports (see Table 9–1)
2. May or may not be associated with pregnancy

NCLEX®

B. *Probable signs of pregnancy*

1. Objective signs and symptoms noted by examiner (see Table 9–1)
2. May or may not be associated with pregnancy

C. *Positive signs of pregnancy*

1. Diagnostic signs and symptoms noted by examiner (see Table 9–1)
2. Can only be associated with pregnancy

III. NURSING CARE DURING FIRST PRENATAL VISIT

A. First prenatal visit

1. Determine why woman is seeking care; perform complete health history and physical examination
2. History taking should include:
   a. Weight, nutrition, and exercise pattern
   b. Over-the-counter (OTC), prescription, and illicit drug use
   c. Allergies and potential teratogens
   d. History of surgery or present disease states, especially those that have implications for pregnancy, such as viral infections, diabetes, hypertension, bleeding disorders, and cardiovascular, renal, or thyroid disease
   e. Gynecologic history including date of last Papanicolaou (Pap) smear, previous infections, age at menarche, and menstrual, contraceptive, and obstetric histories
3. Physical assessment

NCLEX®

   a. **Fetal heart rate** (FHR): fetal heart beats per minute, assessed by fetoscope (at 17–20 weeks) or by Doppler (at 10–12 weeks); useful in determining gestational age and fetal well-being; normally ranges from 110 to 160 beats per minute

Table 9–1 Signs and Symptoms of Pregnancy

Category	Signs and Symptoms
Presumptive signs	Amenorrhea, nausea and vomiting, fatigue, urinary frequency, breast changes, quickening (first perception of fetal movement at about 16–20 weeks)
Probable signs	Hegar's sign (softening of lower uterine segment at 6 weeks), McDonald's sign (softening of cervix at beginning of second month), Chadwick's sign (bluish, purple, or deep red coloration of cervix, vagina, and vulva at about 4 weeks), enlargement of abdomen, pigmentation changes, abdominal striae, ballottement (rebounding of fetus against examiner's fingers on palpation), positive pregnancy test, palpation of fetal outline
Positive signs	Fetal heartbeat, fetal movement palpable by examiner, visualization of fetus by ultrasound

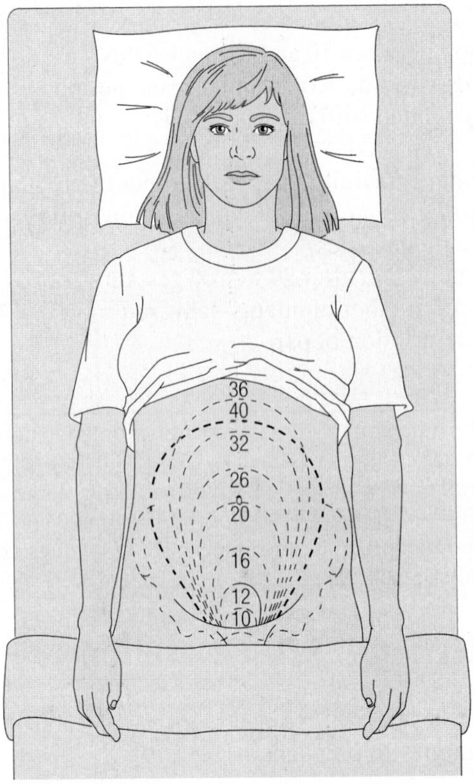

Figure 9–1

Fundal height changes during pregnancy.

NCLEX®
b. Fundal height helps estimate gestational age and fetal growth (see Figure 9–1)

NCLEX®
c. Complete maternal physical exam includes vital signs; height and weight; thyroid function; heart and lung sounds; and reproductive organs (size of uterus, pelvic musculature, adequacy of pelvis for delivery)

d. Laboratory assessment includes hematocrit and hemoglobin, blood type, Rh and irregular antibody, rubella titer, tuberculin skin test, renal function tests, urinalysis and culture, screening for sexually transmitted infections (STIs), and Pap test; offer of HIV test (see section that follows)

NCLEX®
4. Psychosocial assessment
   a. Emotions such as excitement, anxiety, and/or ambivalence about pregnancy
   b. Available support systems
   c. Stability and functional level of client's immediate and extended family
   d. Economic support adequate for housing, daily needs, and medical expenses
   e. Cultural preferences including practices to be used or avoided during pregnancy, preference of caregiver gender, and preferred support person(s)
5. Collaborative management
   a. Prepare client for physical exam by stating what to expect
   b. Provide information about prenatal care program, setting, and personnel

NCLEX®
   c. Provide information about physiologic changes to be expected in pregnancy as well as danger signs to report

B. Laboratory and diagnostic testing during first prenatal visit

1. Complete blood count (CBC): provides information on hematologic and other body systems; for individual tests, normal results, and changes in pregnancy, see Table 9–2

NCLEX®
2. Blood group and Rh typing: identifies maternal blood type (ABO antigen system) and Rh status; Rh-negative status (absence of rhesus antigen) indicates need for repeat antibody screens and injection of $Rh_0(D)$ immune globulin at 28 weeks' gestation
3. Urinalysis and urine culture
   a. Color should be pale yellow to amber depending on foods ingested and concentration

NCLEX®
   b. Glucose: should be tested at each prenatal visit; reabsorption is impaired in pregnancy, resulting glycosuria at serum glucose level of 160 mg/dL; persistent glycosuria may indicate gestational diabetes

NCLEX®
   c. Protein: should be tested at each prenatal visit; is normally found in urine during pregnancy at a level of trace to +1 using dipstick method; increased protein may indicate infection or preeclampsia

NCLEX®
   d. White blood cells (WBCs) or nitrites can indicate possible urinary tract infection, which can place client at risk for preterm labor

Table 9–2 Complete Blood Count

Test	Normal Results	Changes in Pregnancy
Red blood cell count	4.2–5.4 million/mm^3	5–6.25 million/mm^3
Hemoglobin	12–16 grams/dL	>11 grams/dL
Hematocrit	37–47%	>33%
White blood cell (WBC) count	5,000–10,000/mm^3	5,000–15,000/mm^3
Polymorphonuclear cells	55–70% of WBCs	60–85% of WBCs
Lymphocytes	20–40% of WBCs	15–40% of WBCs
Platelet count	150,000–400,000/mm^3	None until 3–5 days after delivery

e. Casts (clumps of materials or cells in renal distal and collecting tubules) form when urine is acidic and concentrated; can be associated with proteinuria and stasis in renal tubules

NCLEX® f. Ketonuria: may indicate diabetes mellitus and hyperglycemia

g. Urine culture: can identify asymptomatic bacteriuria or urinary tract infection (greater than 10,000 bacteria/mL urine)

h. Urine toxicology can screen for illicit drug use

C. Screening for TORCH infections

1. **TORCH infections**: a group of infections caused by viruses and protozoa that cause serious fetal problems when contracted by mother during pregnancy; each letter represents a different infection: **T**oxoplasmosis, **O**ther infections (usually hepatitis), **R**ubella, **C**ytomegalovirus, and **H**erpes simplex virus; see sections that follow
2. Toxoplasmosis: caused by toxoplasmosis protozoa and transmitted by eating infested undercooked meat and poor handwashing after handling cat litter; fetal infection can occur via placenta
   a. Diagnosis: made by serologic testing; indirect fluorescent antibody test is most commonly used; IgG titers greater than 1:256 suggest a recent infection, whereas IgM titers greater than 1:256 indicate an acute infection
   b. Maternal effects: flulike symptoms in acute phase
   c. Fetal/neonatal effects: spontaneous abortion is likely in early pregnancy; in neonates central nervous system (CNS) lesions can result in hydrocephaly, microcephaly, chronic retinitis, and seizures
3. Other infections, usually hepatitis A virus (HAV) or hepatitis B virus (HBV); HBV is most common in fetus
   a. Transmission: HAV is spread by droplets or hands and is associated with poor handwashing after defecation; transmission to fetus is rare but can occur; HBV transmission to fetus can occur via placenta, but usually occurs when infant is exposed to blood and genital secretions during labor and delivery
   b. Diagnosis: radioimmunoassay and enzyme-linked immunosorbent assay methods are used to detect HAV antibodies; elevated IgM with normal IgG antibody indicates probable acute hepatitis; elevated IgG with normal IgM indicates a convalescent or chronic stage of HAV; HBV is detected through hepatitis B surface antigen (HbsAg)
   c. Maternal effects: fever, malaise, nausea, and abdominal discomfort; may be associated with liver failure
   NCLEX® d. Fetal/neonatal effects: preterm birth, hepatitis infection, and intrauterine fetal death
4. *NCLEX®* Rubella (sometimes called German measles or 3-day measles): caused by infection with rubella virus and transmitted by droplets
   a. Diagnosis: IgG antibodies to rubella are measured to determine rubella immunity status; a titer of 1:8 or less indicates minimal or no immunity and client should receive rubella vaccine in postpartum period and wait 1–3 months before becoming pregnant again
   b. Maternal effects: fever, rash, and mild lymphedema
   NCLEX® c. Fetal/neonatal effects: congenital defects of eyes, heart, ears, and brain and death
5. *NCLEX®* Cytomegalovirus (CMV): caused by exposure to CMV through respiratory droplets (most common), semen, cervical and vaginal secretions, breast milk, placental tissue, urine, feces, and banked blood
   a. Diagnosis: a viral culture is most definitive; CMV antibodies indicate a recent infection; a fourfold increase in CMV titer in paired sera drawn 10–14 days apart usually indicates an acute infection
   b. Maternal effects: asymptomatic illness, cervical discharge, and mononucleosis-like syndrome
   NCLEX® c. Fetal/neonatal effects: fetal death or severe generalized disease with hemolytic anemia and jaundice, hydrocephaly or microcephaly, pneumonitis, hepatosplenomegaly, and deafness

NCLEX®

6. Herpes simplex virus (HSV): caused by exposure to HSV from vesicular lesions on male or female genitalia; infant infection results from exposure to lesion in birth canal or ascending infection after rupture of membranes
   a. Diagnosis: viral culture is used for definitive diagnosis; serologic tests have a lower accuracy
   b. Maternal effects: blisters, rash, fever, malaise, nausea, and headache
   c. Fetal/neonatal effects: spontaneous abortion, preterm labor, or stillbirth; transplacental infection is rare but can cause skin lesions, intrauterine growth restriction (IUGR), mental retardation, and microcephaly (NCLEX®)
   d. Implications: vaginal delivery is possible if client has no visible lesions in birth canal or if lesions are limited to anal, perineal, or inner thigh area (strict precautions are taken to protect fetus); if visible lesions are present in birth canal, cesarean delivery is indicated

D. Screening for sexually transmitted infections

1. **Sexually transmitted infections (STIs)** are caused by bacteria, viruses, protozoa, or ectoparasites and include human papillomavirus (HPV), human immunodeficiency virus (HIV), group B streptococcus (GBS), syphilis, gonorrhea, and chlamydia; all sexual partners of clients with STIs should be contacted and treated, as indicated; see sections that follow
2. HPV: sometimes called genital warts; spread through sexual contact; neonates can acquire infection during birth; can now be prevented by vaccine (NCLEX®)
   a. Diagnosis: direct visualization of warts and confirmation by biopsy
   b. Maternal effects: symptoms depend on viral strain but can include genital lesions, chronic vaginal discharge, pruritis, and cervical dysplasia; some strains are asymptomatic
   c. Fetal/neonatal effects: juvenile laryngeal papillomata
3. HIV: transmitted primarily through exchange of body fluids (semen, blood, or vaginal secretions); neonatal transmission can occur transplacentally (is less likely if mother receives treatment during pregnancy); transmission can also occur via contact at time of delivery or through breast milk (NCLEX®)
   a. Diagnosis: if a reactive enzyme-linked immunofluorescence assay (ELISA) is positive twice, HIV infection is confirmed with a positive Western blot or immunofluorescence assay (IFA); viral cultures provide best diagnostic tool for neonates but are expensive and require 4–6 weeks for results
   b. Maternal effects: general symptoms associated with HIV infection; opportunistic diseases including *Pneumocystis jiroveci* pneumonia, candida esophagitis, and wasting syndrome; increased risk for intrapartum or postpartum hemorrhage, postpartum infection, poor wound healing, and infections of genitourinary tract
   c. Fetal/neonatal effects: asymptomatic at birth followed by opportunistic infections, failure to thrive, lymphadenopathy, hepatosplenomegaly, fever, chronic diarrhea, dermatitis, thrush, and death (NCLEX®)
   d. Implications: avoid risk of perinatal transmission (amniocentesis, fetal scalp sampling, internal scalp electrodes, episiotomy, oxytocin [strong contractions increase risk of vaginal tears]) and minimize neonatal exposure to maternal blood and body fluids at delivery; administer zidovudine to mother during labor and delivery; avoid breastfeeding
4. Group B streptococcus (GBS): considered normal vaginal flora (found in 10–30% of healthy pregnant women); transmitted vertically from birth canal of infected mother to fetus; treated with antibiotic therapy (mother and neonate)
   a. Diagnosis: routine screening with GBS culture 36–37 weeks' gestation; presence of GBS in urine at any time during pregnancy is considered diagnostic (NCLEX®)
   b. Maternal effects: preterm labor, chorioamnionitis, premature rupture of membranes, urinary tract infections, and postpartum infections
   c. Fetal/neonatal effects: neonatal meningitis, sepsis, and septic shock; early-onset GBS has a significant infant mortality rate
5. Syphilis: caused by spirochete *Treponema pallidum*; transmitted by contact with syphilitic lesions (often found on skin, mucous membranes of mouth, and genitals); transmission to fetus can occur via placenta during pregnancy (NCLEX®)
   a. Diagnosis: women should be screened at first prenatal visit and possibly at 36 weeks' gestation with VDRL (Venereal Disease Research Laboratories) or RPR (rapid plasma reagin) test; positive result indicates need for treatment with antibiotic therapy
   b. Maternal effects: during primary (acute) stage, a chancre develops on skin near infection; second stage (6 weeks to 6 months after primary stage) is marked by lymphadenopathy and rash on palms of hands and soles of feet; tertiary stage (10–30 years after untreated primary lesion) involves CNS problems such as progressive deterioration of mental status, ataxia, meningitis, general paresis, and disease of aorta and cardiac valves; can cause spontaneous abortion or premature labor
   c. Fetal/neonatal effects: CNS damage, hearing loss, or death (NCLEX®)

6. Gonorrhea: caused by *Neisseria gonorrhoeae* bacteria; transmitted by sexual contact; neonates can acquire infection by exposure to bacteria in birth canal
   - NCLEX® a. Diagnosis: screen all pregnant women at initial prenatal visit and at-risk women again at 36 weeks' gestation
   - b. Maternal effects: often asymptomatic but can cause purulent vaginal discharge, pelvic or lower abdominal pain, and premature rupture of membranes
   - NCLEX® c. Fetal/neonatal effects: preterm birth, neonatal sepsis, IUGR, and ophthalmia neonatorum, which can cause blindness
7. Chlamydia: caused by *Chlamydia trachomatis* bacteria; transmitted through sexual contact; Centers for Disease Control and Prevention (CDC) recommends screening of asymptomatic, high-risk women
   - a. Diagnosis: by vaginal culture
   - b. Maternal effects: usually asymptomatic; bleeding, mucoid or purulent cervical discharge, dysuria, pelvic pain
   - NCLEX® c. Fetal/neonatal effects: conjunctivitis, pneumonia, and ophthalmia neonatorum
   - d. Implications: treated with antibiotic therapy followed by repeat culture; sexual partner needs to be treated as well

IV. NURSING CARE DURING SUBSEQUENT PRENATAL VISITS

NCLEX® **A. Frequency of follow-up prenatal visits**

1. Every 4 weeks during first 28 weeks' gestation
2. Every 2 weeks until 36 weeks
3. Every week until delivery

q month until 28
q 2 wk until 36
q 1 wk 36 - birth.

B. Collaborative management

1. Visits should include teaching and assessment of maternal and fetal well-being
2. Instruct mother concerning physical changes associated with pregnancy, such as quickening (first fetal movements felt), Braxton Hicks contractions (irregular, often painless contractions occurring intermittently throughout pregnancy), and colostrum production, as well as danger signs of pregnancy, presented in Table 9–3
3. NCLEX® Assess for acceptance of pregnancy and adjustment to maternal role, changes from baseline vital signs, weight gain, nutritional status, and presence of glucose and/or protein in urine
4. Collect clean-catch urine specimen at each visit to assess for glucose (diabetes mellitus), protein (preeclampsia), and nitrites and leukocytes (urinary infection)
5. Assess maternal hemoglobin monthly for iron-deficiency anemia
6. NCLEX® Assess fetus at each visit for growth as measured by fundal height, movement, and heart rate

C. Diagnostic screening tests during subsequent prenatal visits

1. **Quadruple screening test** includes serum measurement of **alpha-fetoprotein (AFP)**, human chorionic gonadotropin (hCG), unconjugated estriol (uE3), and inhibin A
   - a. During pregnancy, AFP leaks from fetus's body into amniotic fluid and is absorbed into maternal circulation; hCG, uE3, and inhibin A are placental hormones

Table 9–3 Danger Signs in Pregnancy

Danger Sign	Possible Cause
Gush of fluid from vagina	Rupture of membranes
Vaginal bleeding	Abruptio placentae, placenta previa, bloody show
Abdominal pain	Premature labor, abruptio placentae
Temperature > 101°F (38.3°C)	Infection
Persistent vomiting	Hyperemesis gravidarum
Visual disturbances	Hypertension, preeclampsia
Edema of hands and face	Hypertension, preeclampsia
Severe headache	Hypertension, preeclampsia
Epigastric pain	Preeclampsia
Dysuria	Urinary tract infection
Decreased fetal movement	Compromised fetal well-being

NCLEX® **b.** Usually performed between 15 and 22 weeks' gestation but is most accurate at 16–18 weeks

NCLEX® **c.** Findings: increased maternal AFP levels may indicate neural tube defects or other body wall defects, threatened abortion, fetal distress, or death; decreased maternal AFP levels may indicate trisomy 21 (Down syndrome) or fetal wastage; changes in hormonal levels can support AFP

d. Interfering factors: multiple pregnancy, incorrect estimate of gestational age

e. Follow-up: abnormal levels may indicate a need for a repeat test, ultrasound, or assessment of amniotic fluid using amniocentesis

2. **Triple-screen test** includes AFP, hCG, and uE3, but does not include inhibin A

NCLEX® 3. **Glucose tolerance test (GTT)** to screen pregnant clients for gestational diabetes; generally completed between 24 and 28 weeks' gestation

a. Test procedure: a 50-gram oral glucose load is ingested (time of day or time since last meal is not a factor); plasma glucose level is measured 1 hour after glucose load

NCLEX® **b.** Findings: a level greater than 130–140 mg/dL (depending on lab) after 1 hour is considered abnormal

c. Follow-up: clients with an abnormal GTT result should have a 3-hour, 100-gram oral GTT to diagnose gestational diabetes (see Table 9–4)

d. Note about variation in procedure: American Diabetes Association recommends a 75-gram 2-hour oral GTT after an overnight fast, with blood glucose levels collected in fasting state and at 1 and 2 hours

4. **Ultrasound**: uses sound waves to produce a three-dimensional view and pictorial image to identify maternal and fetal tissues, bones, and fluids; screen for anomalies, assess fetal well-being, and establish gestational age; results can be used to decide whether to continue pregnancy or terminate because of fetal abnormalities

NCLEX® **a.** Transvaginal ultrasound used primarily during first trimester; eliminates need for full bladder and gives clearer images in obese clients; some clients are embarrassed or uncomfortable with vaginal insertion of probe

NCLEX® **b.** Abdominal ultrasound provides a safe, noninvasive fetal assessment, but is best done when client's bladder is full; can result in discomfort

c. Viability is determined by assessment of fetal heart activity; possible at 6–7 weeks' gestation with real-time echo scan; fetal death can be determined by absence of heart activity as well as scalp edema and maceration

d. Gestational age is best established during first 20 weeks' gestation because fetal growth rate is fairly consistent during this time; body part assessed is based on development (gestational sac at 5–6 weeks after LMP; crown-rump length at 6–10 weeks' gestation; biparietal diameter (BPD) and femur length at 13–40 weeks' gestation)

e. Fetal growth is assessed by serial measurements of BPD and femur length; assists healthcare provider to distinguish between IUGR and inaccurate dating of pregnancy

D. Childbirth education

1. Childbirth classes provide information on pregnancy and childbirth to facilitate families in optimal decision making; topics are timed during pregnancy; see Table 9–5
2. Classes can be planned for special groups such as grandparents, siblings, adolescents, and clients who will deliver by cesarean method
3. Exercise is an important topic for childbirth education; encourage women to participate in regular (three times per week) exercise during pregnancy

a. Benefits of exercise include maintaining muscle tone and bowel function and having fewer complications during labor and delivery

NCLEX® **b.** Exercises especially helpful for childbirth include pelvic tilt, partial sit-ups, Kegel exercises, and exercises to stretch inner thigh muscles

Table 9–4 Abnormal Oral Glucose Tolerance Test Results

Time	Abnormal Result
Fasting	Greater than 95 mg/dL
1 hour	Greater than 180 mg/dL
2 hours	Greater than 155 mg/dL
3 hours	Greater than 140 mg/dL

Table 9–5 Childbirth Education Topics by Trimester

Trimester	Educational Topic
First	Physical and psychosocial changes of pregnancy Self-care in pregnancy Protecting and nurturing the fetus Choosing a care provider and birth setting Prenatal exercise Relief of common early-pregnancy discomforts
Second	Planning for breastfeeding Sexuality in pregnancy Relief of common later-pregnancy discomforts
Third	Preparation for childbirth Development of a birth plan

Table 9–6 Comparison of Common Birthing Methods

Method	Characteristics	Breathing techniques
Lamaze	Uses education about fetal growth and changes associated with pregnancy along with training in exercises that strengthen muscles used during labor and delivery to decrease fear and help mother cope with pain of labor	Patterned, paced
Bradley	Relies on partner or husband to coach laboring woman; promotes relaxation through abdominal breathing and exercises	Primarily abdominal
Kitzinger	Prepares woman for birth through use of sensory memory and relaxation	Chest breathing with abdominal relaxation

4. Classes on preparation for birth process provide information on selection of birthing method and relaxation techniques
   a. Commonly taught birthing methods: Lamaze, Kitzinger, and Bradley methods of prepared childbirth; see Table 9–6

   NCLEX®

   b. Relaxation techniques commonly taught for use in labor include touch, breathing, disassociation, and progressive relaxation
5. Classes focused on knowledge needed postdelivery include postpartum self-care, newborn care, infant stimulation, and infant safety needs

E. Management of common discomforts of pregnancy

1. Discomforts occur because of physiologic or anatomic changes of pregnancy; differ from trimester to trimester

NCLEX®

2. While not dangerous, discomforts constitute a significant problem for client and present an opportunity for nursing intervention (see Table 9–7, page 100)

V. PHYSIOLOGICAL CHANGES OF PREGNANCY

A. Reproductive

1. Uterus: takes on an ovoid shape and increases in capacity from 10 mL to 5 L; primarily caused by increased size of cells (hypertrophy) in response to estrogen and distention from growing fetus; by end of pregnancy, uterus and its contents require up to one-sixth of total maternal blood flow

NCLEX®

2. Cervix: under influence of estrogen, secretes mucus that forms a plug at opening of endocervical canal to limit bacteria entering uterus; increased blood flow to cervix results in **Goodell's sign** (softening of cervix) and **Chadwick's sign** (bluish, purple, or deep red color of cervix during pregnancy)
3. Vagina: under influence of estrogen, vaginal mucosa thickens and connective tissue relaxes; vaginal secretions thicken and increase in amount; pH is acidic, 3.6–6.0
4. Breasts: increase in size and number of glands (from estrogen and progesterone); **colostrum** (thin bluish-white fluid high in protein and immune properties) is produced and may be expressed during last trimester

Table 9–7 Management of Discomforts in Pregnancy

Discomfort	Management
	Early Pregnancy
Nausea and vomiting	Avoid strong odors; drink carbonated beverages; avoid drinking while eating; eat crackers or toast before getting out of bed; eat small, frequent meals; avoid spicy or greasy foods
Breast tenderness	Wear a well-fitting, supportive bra
Urinary frequency	Increase daytime fluid intake; decrease evening fluid intake; empty bladder as soon as urge is felt
Fatigue	Plan rest period or nap during day; go to bed as early as possible
Ptyalism	Use gum, mints, hard candy, or mouthwash
Nasal stuffiness/bleeding	Use cool air vaporizer
	Late Pregnancy
Heartburn	Eat small, frequent meals; avoid spicy or greasy foods; refrain from lying down immediately after eating; use low-sodium antacids
Constipation	Increase fluid and fiber intake; exercise regularly; develop regular bowel habits; use stool softeners as needed
Hemorrhoids	Avoid constipation; apply topical anesthetics, ointments, or ice packs; use sitz baths or warm soaks; reinsert into rectum, if necessary
Backache	Practice good body mechanics; practice pelvic tilt exercise; avoid high heels, heavy lifting, overfatigue, and excessive bending or reaching
Leg cramps	Dorsiflex feet; apply heat to affected muscle; evaluate calcium-to-phosphorus ratio in diet
Varicose veins	Elevate legs; wear support hose; avoid crossing legs at the knee, restrictive clothing, and standing for long periods of time
Ankle edema	Practice frequent dorsiflexion of feet; avoid standing for long periods of time; elevate legs when sitting or resting
Faintness	Arise slowly; avoid prolonged standing; maintain hematocrit and hemoglobin
Flatulence	Avoid gas-forming foods; chew food thoroughly; establish regular bowel habits

B. Cardiovascular
1. Cardiac output increases 30–40% over nonpregnant output with an increase in pulse of 10–15 beats/minute
2. Peak time for cardiac problems occurs around 28 weeks
3. Pulmonary and peripheral vascular resistance decreases 40–50%, resulting in decreased BP in first two trimesters; in third trimester, begins to increase to prepregnant levels; postural hypotension can occur if pregnant uterus presses on pelvic and femoral vessels, limiting blood return to heart
4. *NCLEX®* Vena cava syndrome results as gravid uterus compresses vena cava, causing decreased blood flow to right atrium and decreased BP
   a. Symptoms include pallor, dizziness, and clammy skin
   b. Prevent or treat by positioning woman on left side or with a pillow under right hip
5. Blood volume increases 45% over prepregnant levels
   a. Red blood cells (RBCs) increase 18–30% depending on amount of iron supplementation
   b. Plasma volume increases 50%
   c. The greater increase in plasma over RBCs results in physiologic anemia and is seen as a 7% decrease in hematocrit

C. Respiratory
1. Volume of air breathed increases 30–40% because of decreased airway resistance that occurs in response to progesterone
2. Intrathoracic volume remains unchanged even though enlarged uterus presses up on diaphragm because rib cage flares and chest circumference increases

D. Neurologic: no known changes

E. Musculoskeletal
1. Relaxation of pelvic joints results in classic "waddling" gait often seen in pregnancy
2. *NCLEX®* Physiologic lordosis develops as curvature of lumbar spine increases to compensate for weight of gravid uterus; can result in low back pain
3. Diastasis recti, separation of rectus abdominis muscle, can result as uterus enlarges

F. Gastrointestinal (GI)

1. During first trimester, human chorionic gonadotropin (hCG) increases and can cause nausea and vomiting
2. *NCLEX®* Increased progesterone levels relax smooth muscles, resulting in decreased peristalsis as noted by bloating, gastric reflux, and constipation; these worsen as gravid uterus presses on intestines
3. Constipation and increased pressure on blood vessels in rectum can lead to hemorrhoids

G. Renal

1. In first trimester, gravid uterus presses on bladder, causing urinary frequency; relieved in second trimester (uterus moves up into abdomen); frequency returns in third trimester as presenting part presses on bladder
2. Glomerular filtration increases 50% during second trimester and remains elevated until delivery; kidneys may not be able to reabsorb all filtered glucose, resulting in glycosuria

H. Integumentary

1. Increased estrogen levels may lead to areas of increased skin pigmentation, especially in areas already highly pigmented such as areola, nipples, and vulva
   - a. **Chloasma**, mask of pregnancy, is an increase in pigmentation on forehead and around eyes; is seen most often in women of color and is aggravated by sun exposure
   - b. **Linea nigra** is a darkly pigmented line that extends from umbilicus to pubic area
   - c. **Striae gravidarum** (stretch marks) appear as reddish streaks on trunk and thighs from stretching of connective tissue (caused by increased adrenal steroid levels); generally become thinner with a shiny gray-white color after delivery but do not disappear
2. Sweat and sebaceous gland activity increases during pregnancy

I. Endocrine

1. Metabolism: water retention occurs because of increased sex hormones and decreased serum protein; basal metabolic rate increases; see nutrition section that follows for weight gain during pregnancy
2. Hormones in pregnancy
   - a. hCG is secreted by trophoblast early in pregnancy and stimulates progesterone and estrogen production; it is thought to support pregnancy and cause nausea and vomiting in first trimester
   - b. Human placental lactogen (hPL), also known as chorionic somatomammotropin, is an insulin antagonist that promotes lipolysis, increasing circulating free fatty acids for maternal metabolic use
   - c. Estrogen and progesterone are produced by corpus luteum for first 7 weeks of pregnancy and then by placenta; estrogen stimulates uterine development to support fetal growth and stimulates ductal system of breast for lactation; progesterone maintains endometrium, decreases uterine contractility, stimulates development of breast acini and lobules, and causes relaxation of smooth muscle
   - d. Relaxin, primarily made by corpus luteum, decreases uterine contractility, contributes to softening of cervix, and has long-term effects on collagen
   - e. Prostaglandins, lipids that are found throughout female reproductive system, contribute to decrease seen in placental vascular system, and probably contribute to onset of labor

VI. NUTRITIONAL NEEDS

A. Factors affecting maternal nutrition requirements

1. Prepregnancy nutritional status: women who are underweight or overweight may need more or less calories, respectively, for adequate fetal weight gain
2. Maternal age: adolescents may need increased caloric intake for both maternal and fetal growth
3. Maternal parity: number of pregnancies and interval between them can affect nutritional needs

B. General principles of maternal nutrition

1. *NCLEX®* Healthy pregnant woman requires an additional 300 calories per day and lactating women require an additional 500 calories per day
2. *NCLEX®* Other nutritional requirements increase during pregnancy, including protein, vitamins (especially folic acid), minerals, and trace elements; many healthcare providers recommend taking a prenatal vitamin supplement to ensure adequate intake and reduce risk of birth defects associated with folic acid deficiency
3. *NCLEX®* Fluid intake should consist of at least 8–10 (8-oz) glasses per day, with 4–6 glasses being water
4. Sodium restriction is not necessary unless recommended by healthcare provider
5. Recommended weight gain during pregnancy depends on pre-pregnancy weight status
   - a. Normal weight before pregnancy: 11.5–16 kg (25–35 lb)
   - b. Overweight before pregnancy: 6.8–11.5 kg (15–25 lb)
   - c. Obese before pregnancy: 5–9 kg (11–20 lb)
   - d. Underweight before pregnancy: 12.7–18.1 kg (28–40 lb)

norm wt ↑ = 25-35 lbs!

C. Lactose intolerance

1. Results from insufficient levels of lactase, an enzyme that breaks down lactose in dairy products into glucose and galactose (simple sugars)
2. *NCLEX®* Leads to nausea and vomiting, epigastric discomfort, abdominal cramping and distention, and loose stools when foods containing lactose are ingested
3. *NCLEX®* Lactase may be replaced by adding it as a liquid to milk or by chewing a tablet before ingesting milk products; lactose-free products are also available
4. Dairy products that may be better tolerated include cheese and yogurt, or milk products in cooked form
5. Pregnant women need to ensure that other sources of calcium are substituted for dairy products in diet

D. Vegetarianism

1. A vegetarian diet commonly includes unrefined grains, legumes, nuts, seeds, fruits, vegetables, sprouts, tofu, tempeh, and soy products (including soy milk)
2. *NCLEX®* All clients adhering to a vegetarian diet should eat sufficient foods of various types to meet daily nutritional needs
3. *NCLEX®* Strict vegetarians (vegans) need to eat adequate amounts and combinations of complementary proteins to have all essential amino acids; combinations should include whole-grain foods and legumes, nuts and legumes, and nuts and whole-grain foods
4. Ovovegetarians may add eggs to diet to help meet protein requirement
5. Lacto-ovovegetarians may use milk and eggs
6. A vegetarian diet may result in deficiencies of protein, omega-3 fatty acids, vitamin B_{12}, vitamin D, and micronutrients (such as calcium, iron, and zinc); clients should consider whether they may benefit from vitamin and mineral supplementation

E. Pica

1. A condition of unknown etiology that leads client to eat nonfood items or those having no nutritional value
2. Can lead to iron-deficiency anemia
3. Commonly ingested substances are clay, dirt, and ice
4. Explore cultural beliefs about effect of ingested substance on mother or fetus if pica affects pregnant client

VII. PSYCHOSOCIAL NEEDS OF PREGNANCY

A. Role changes: occur as decisions are made as to whether mother will continue or return to work and who will meet household responsibilities

B. Anxieties: related to birthing process, well-being of mother and baby, and finances

C. Family strengths in coping with psychosocial changes of pregnancy

1. Communication skills
2. Ability to resolve conflict and reach compromise
3. Willingness to seek and utilize support systems

D. Collaborative management

1. Discuss with client psychosocial processes that occur during pregnancy, such as role changes, anxieties related to well-being of mother and infant, and additional financial responsibilities
2. Explore family coping mechanisms, communication skills, and support systems

Check Your NCLEX–RN® Exam I.Q.

You are ready for testing on this content if you can:

- Assess the physiological status of a pregnant client.
- Calculate an expected delivery date.
- Assess the psychosocial needs of a pregnant client.
- Assess results of maternal and fetal diagnostic tests.
- Provide antenatal care to a client.
- Provide instructions about self-care during the antenatal period.

PRACTICE TEST

1 The client has come to the clinic for her first prenatal visit. During the pelvic examination, the examiner indicates that the vaginal mucosa has a bluish color. The nurse should document which assessment as positive?

1. Hegar's sign
2. Goodell's sign
3. McDonald's sign
4. Chadwick's sign

2 With regard to normal changes in the reproductive system during pregnancy, the nurse should teach the pregnant client about which of the following?

1. Vaginal secretions will increase and thicken.
2. Uterus will grow by adding many new cells.
3. Breasts will become red and hard.
4. Cervix will begin to dilate during the second trimester.

3 What should the nurse include when teaching a pregnant client about normal changes in the cardiovascular system during pregnancy?

1. Her pulse rate will decrease.
2. She may experience dizziness if she lays on her back.
3. She will have a decrease in red blood cells.
4. She may experience a feeling of fullness in her chest.

4 During a prenatal visit in the second trimester, which item reported by the client should be a cause for concern?

1. Thirst and urinary frequency
2. +1 deep tendon reflexes
3. Constipation
4. Backache in the lower sacral area

5 The nurse is examining a client who is at 12 weeks' gestation. The examiner would expect to find the fundus at which location at this time?

1. 3 cm below the sternum
2. The level of the umbilicus
3. The level of the symphysis pubis
4. 3 cm below the umbilicus

6 What should the prenatal clinic nurse conclude to be a contraindication for maternal serum alpha-fetoprotein (AFP) testing for a pregnant client?

1. Being at 25 weeks' gestation
2. Client would not consider termination of pregnancy
3. Client has no family history of neural tube defects
4. Client had ultrasound at 8 weeks' gestation

7 The nurse should focus on which wellness-oriented nursing concept for a client in the second trimester of pregnancy?

1. Anxiety about inadequate understanding about early prenatal physical changes
2. Attachment of mother to fetus related to statements about perceived fetal movement
3. Client safety focused on fall prevention
4. Inadequate knowledge of how best to prepare for labor and delivery

8 At the first prenatal visit, the client reveals that her last menstrual period began March 18 (03.18). The nurse calculates her estimated date of delivery to be _________. Provide a numerical answer using format month.day (e.g., July 10 = 07.10).

Fill in your answer below:

Answer: ____________

9 The nurse concludes by which client statement that the pregnant client understands prenatal nutrition education?

1. "I understand that if I don't eat foods with folic acid, my baby will have birth defects."
2. "I understand that eating fruits, especially apples, will help me meet my need for folic acid."
3. "I understand that if my level of folic acid is low, it could cause my baby to have a neural tube defect."
4. "I understand that I should limit my intake of folic acid because it can build up in the liver and cause birth defects."

10 A pregnant client who is a vegetarian is concerned about her folic acid intake and asks the nurse to recommend some foods that she should include in her diet. Which foods should the nurse recommend?

1. Peanuts
2. Hamburger
3. Bananas
4. Pineapple juice

11 The pregnant client has been started on an iron supplement. What information should be included by the nurse as a priority in prenatal teaching about the iron supplement?

1. It should be taken 30 minutes after eating a full meal.
2. It is better absorbed if taken with a liquid containing vitamin C.
3. It will eliminate the need for prenatal vitamins.
4. It should be taken at the same time as the prenatal vitamin.

12 The pregnant client tells the nurse that she is lactose-intolerant. When considering the recommendation of a calcium supplement, what assessment should the nurse make?

1. History of kidney stones
2. Presence of leg cramps
3. Color of mucous membranes and conjunctiva
4. Resting heart rate

13 During the first prenatal assessment, the nurse discovers that the client has not had a second vaccination for measles, mumps, and rubella. What is the best plan for this client?

1. Administer the vaccine during this visit
2. Wait until the third trimester to administer the vaccine
3. Administer the vaccine following delivery
4. Omit the vaccine because these are childhood diseases not acquired by adults

14 The pregnant client, who is at 34 weeks' gestation, calls the prenatal clinic reporting cramping pain in her abdomen. After the diagnosis of Braxton Hicks contractions is made, the nurse should give the client which recommendation?

1. "Go to bed and wait for your real labor to begin."
2. "Empty your bladder frequently and change positions if these contractions are bothering you."
3. "Avoid using your Lamaze breathing with these contractions because it might precipitate preterm labor."
4. "Just ignore these contractions; we will let you know if there is a problem."

15 The client who is at 37 weeks' gestation reports joint pain, especially in the lower back and pelvic area. What is the best reply by the nurse?

1. "I'm afraid you are just going to have to put up with that for a few more weeks."
2. "Sleeping flat on your back may help with the pain."
3. "Aspirin taken every 3–4 hours will be the best thing to relieve this pain."
4. "It may help to apply a heating pad to the painful area for 15–20 minutes."

16 In reviewing the chart of a prenatal client, which client finding would be considered by the nurse to be a probable sign of pregnancy?

1. Fetal heartbeat on ultrasound
2. Amenorrhea
3. Positive pregnancy test
4. Chloasma

17 The client is planning to breastfeed and asks the nurse what she should do to prepare. The nurse should advise the client to do which of the following?

1. Wash her nipples with water daily
2. Apply lanolin daily in the last trimester
3. Rub the nipples briskly with a towel twice a day
4. Perform the pinch test daily

18 The client has come to the clinic for her first prenatal visit and tells the nurse that she eats only vegetables. To assess for a problem related to this information, the nurse should assess what part of the complete blood count (CBC)?

1. Hemoglobin
2. Lymphocytes
3. Polymorphonuclear cell count
4. Platelet count

19 What information, if revealed to the nurse in a prenatal interview, would indicate an increased risk for exposure to cytomegalovirus?

1. Caring for a cat and litter box
2. Working at a daycare center
3. Using IV drugs several years ago
4. Giving blood twice yearly

20 Which of the following, if found by the nurse, would indicate a need for a pregnant client to have a cesarean delivery?

1. Positive herpes culture at the first prenatal visit; client asymptomatic at the time of delivery
2. History of genital herpes lesions; few vaginal lesions present at time of delivery
3. Oral fever blisters at the time of delivery; no prodromal symptoms
4. Genital herpes lesion 1 month prior to delivery; no symptoms at the time of delivery

21 What should the nurse anticipate as follow-up in the plan of care for a pregnant client who is diagnosed with a sexually transmitted infection?

1. Contacting and treating all sexual partners
2. Delivery by cesarean section
3. Amniocentesis for assessment of genetic damage
4. Close monitoring of hematocrit and hemoglobin throughout pregnancy

22 The nurse should plan for Group B streptococcus screening if the pregnant client meets what criteria?

1. History of a sexually transmitted infection
2. 36–37 weeks' gestation
3. Has come in for her initial prenatal visit
4. Rash noted in the vaginal area

23 Which of the following, if reported to the nurse by a pregnant client prior to collection of a gonorrhea culture, would result in postponing specimen collection?

1. Recent diagnosis and treatment for herpes
2. Persistent vaginal discharge
3. Douching 3 days ago
4. Is currently menstruating

24 The client has come to the prenatal clinic reporting repeated nausea and vomiting. The nurse should look to which laboratory finding for the best information about the client's hydration status?

1. Hematocrit
2. Platelet count
3. Urine specific gravity
4. IgG level

25 In interviewing a pregnant client concerning sexually transmitted infections, the nurse should recognize which approach as a barrier to client disclosure?

1. Nurse's use of a nonjudgmental attitude
2. Collecting information while the woman is still dressed
3. Frequent use of yes-or-no questions
4. Use of a culturally sensitive approach

26 Which of the following statements by the pregnant client indicates to the nurse an understanding of the client's nutritional needs during the second and third trimester? Select all that apply.

1. "I will need to increase my intake of protein."
2. "I will need to increase my daily intake by 500–600 calories per day."
3. "I will need to increase my intake of calcium so that it is double my phosphorus intake."
4. "I will need to decrease my intake of iodine."
5. "I will need to increase my iron and may even need a prenatal iron supplement."

27 The nurse is planning an educational program for clients in the third trimester of pregnancy. Which childbirth education topics would be most appropriate? Select all that apply.

1. Childbirth healthcare provider selection
2. Morning sickness management
3. Nutritional needs during pregnancy
4. Pain relief during labor and delivery
5. Care of the newborn

28 A client comes to the clinic for her first prenatal visit and reports that July 10 was the first day of her last menstrual period. Using Naegele's rule, the nurse calculates the estimated date of birth for the client to be ____________. Provide a numerical answer using format month.day (i.e., July 10 = 07.10).

Fill in your answer below:

Answer: ____________

29 The client, who is at 36 weeks' gestation, calls the prenatal clinic because she is concerned about a thin, bluish-white fluid leaking from her breasts. What is an appropriate response by the nurse? Select all that apply.

1. "This probably indicates an infection in your breasts. You will need to come into the office."
2. "This usually happens when you are going into premature labor. You should go to the hospital."
3. "This normally occurs as your breasts prepare for breastfeeding. You should continue to wear a good-fitting bra."
4. "This is an indication that you may have some problems with breastfeeding. I will have the lactation consultant call you."
5. "The fluid is colostrum and normally leaks from the breast during the last trimester of pregnancy."

ANSWERS & RATIONALES

1 **Answer: 4 Rationale:** Beginning around the fourth week of pregnancy, vasocongestion in the pelvic area results in a bluish color to the vulva, vagina, and cervix, known as Chadwick's sign. Hegar's sign is a softening of the lower uterine segment. Goodell's sign is a softening of the cervix. McDonald's sign is an ease in flexing the body of the uterus against the cervix. **Cognitive Level:** Analyzing **Client Need:** Health Promotion and Maintenance **Integrated Process:** Nursing Process: Assessment **Content Area:** Maternal–Newborn **Strategy:** The critical words in the question are *first prenatal visit* and *bluish color*. Use the process of elimination and knowledge of the changes in cervical mucosa in early pregnancy to make your selection.

2 **Answer: 1 Rationale:** During pregnancy, increased estrogen production results in an increased amount and thickening of vaginal secretions. The uterus grows by cell hypertrophy, not by adding more cells. Red and hard breasts or a cervix dilating during the second trimester are not normal findings. **Cognitive Level:** Applying **Client Need:** Health Promotion and Maintenance **Integrated Process:** Teaching and Learning **Content Area:** Maternal–Newborn **Strategy:** Note the critical words *normal changes during pregnancy*. Eliminate cervical dilation and reddened breasts first because they are abnormal. Use concepts of physiology to choose vaginal secretions over new uterine cells.

3 **Answer: 2 Rationale:** Pressure on the vena cava from the gravid uterus may cause a decrease in blood flow to the right atrium and result in a decrease in blood pressure. Dizziness is a symptom of hypotension. The pulse rate could stay the same or increase as the workload of the heart increases during the course of pregnancy. There is an increase in the number of red blood cells to meet physiological demand. A feeling of fullness in the chest is not a cardiovascular change during pregnancy, although abdominal fullness occurs as the pregnancy progresses. **Cognitive Level:** Applying **Client Need:** Health Promotion and Maintenance **Integrated Process:** Teaching and Learning **Content Area:** Maternal–Newborn **Strategy:** Note the critical words *normal changes*, *cardiovascular*, and *pregnancy*. With these in mind, eliminate both decreased pulse rate and RBCs as incorrect. Choose dizziness over chest fullness by recalling concepts of maternal and fetal circulation.

4 **Answer: 1 Rationale:** Urinary frequency usually disappears in the second trimester. Thirst and urinary frequency may be signs of developing gestational diabetes and warrant further investigation. Deep tendon reflexes are assessed during a physical examination and are not reported to a healthcare provider by the client. Constipation is a typical finding because of the pressure exerted by the growing fetus. Backache in the lower sacral area can occur because of changing posture associated with the growing fetus. **Cognitive Level:** Analyzing **Client Need:** Health Promotion and Maintenance **Integrated Process:** Nursing Process: Assessment **Content Area:** Maternal–Newborn **Strategy:** Note the critical words *cause for concern*, which indicates the correct answer is an option that is an abnormal finding. Eliminate constipation and backache first, since they are typical symptoms that may be associated with pregnancy. Choose thirst and urinary frequency over deep tendon reflexes because these symptoms are clearly abnormal and are also subjective data that are reported by the client.

5 **Answer: 3 Rationale:** By the 12th week of gestation, the uterus should have increased in size to be palpable at the symphysis pubis. Factors affecting this finding include abnormal fetal growth or the presence of a multiple gestation. It is too early in the pregnancy for the fundus to rise close to the sternum. The fundus is at the level of the umbilicus at about 20 weeks' gestation. The fundus should be 3 cm below the umbilicus at some time earlier than 20 weeks' gestation. **Cognitive Level:** Analyzing **Client Need:** Health Promotion and Maintenance **Integrated Process:** Nursing Process: Assessment **Content Area:** Maternal–Newborn **Strategy:** To answer this question correctly, recall the expected physiological changes during pregnancy. Use nursing knowledge and the process of elimination to make your selection.

6 **Answer: 1 Rationale:** Measurement of maternal serum AFP is most sensitive between 16 and 18 weeks' gestation, but can be performed at up to 22 weeks' gestation. This client has a gestational age of 25 weeks, which is too late. Knowledge of fetal anomalies can help a client determine need for added services after delivery if pregnancy termination would not be considered. A negative family history for neural tube defects is not a contraindication for AFP testing. Having an ultrasound at 8 weeks' gestation is unrelated to AFP testing. **Cognitive Level:** Analyzing **Client Need:** Health Promotion and Maintenance **Integrated Process:** Nursing Process: Planning **Content Area:** Maternal–Newborn **Strategy:** Note the critical word *contraindication*. This means the correct answer is an option that is a false statement. Use knowledge of the purpose of the test to eliminate each of the incorrect options.

7 **Answer: 2 Rationale:** Quickening usually begins around 16 weeks and results in enhanced attachment as the fetus becomes more real. Anxiety about early-pregnancy changes would be more appropriate for the client in the first trimester. Inadequate knowledge of labor and delivery is appropriate during the third trimester. Promoting client safety is not specific to falls or the second trimester. **Cognitive Level:** Analyzing **Client Need:** Health Promotion and Maintenance **Integrated Process:** Nursing Process: Diagnosis **Content Area:** Maternal–Newborn **Strategy:** Note the critical words *wellness-oriented nursing diagnosis* and *second trimester*. Eliminate Anxiety and Knowledge Deficit because they are not wellness-oriented, then eliminate Promoting Client Safety because it is a nursing goal rather than a nursing diagnosis and risk for falls is not high.

8 **Answer: 12.25 Rationale:** According to Naegele's rule, the estimated date of birth can be calculated by subtracting 3 months from the beginning date of the last menstrual period (LMP) and then adding 7 days to that date. December is 3 months earlier than March. Adding 7 days to 18 (the beginning date of the LMP) equals 25. Thus, the due date is estimated as December 25 (12.25). **Cognitive Level:** Applying **Client Need:** Health Promotion and Maintenance **Integrated Process:** Nursing Process: Diagnosis **Content Area:** Maternal–Newborn **Strategy:** Specific knowledge of Naegele's rule is needed to answer the question. Use knowledge of this rule and mathematical/calculating ability to determine the appropriate due date.

9 **Answer: 3 Rationale:** Maternal folic acid deficiency has been linked to infant neural tube defects. Folic acid may be obtained from prenatal vitamin supplements as well as foods. Apples are not high in folic acid. Foods that are high in folic acid include dark leafy greens, asparagus, broccoli, citrus fruits, and beans, peas, and lentils. Folic acid does not build up in the liver to cause birth defects; insufficient folic acid can lead to neural tube defects. **Cognitive Level:** Analyzing **Client Need:** Health Promotion and Maintenance **Integrated Process:** Nursing Process: Evaluation **Content Area:** Maternal–Newborn **Strategy:** Note the critical word *understands*, which indicates that the correct answer is also a correct statement. First eliminate the option that indicates water-soluble vitamins will accumulate in the liver. Next eliminate the option that indicates birth defects will occur because that level of certainty is unrealistic. Choose correctly between the remaining options recalling either that neural tube defects are associated with low folic acid or because oranges are not an especially good source of folic acid.

10 **Answer: 1 Rationale:** Both peanuts and hamburger are good sources of folic acid, but since the client is a vegetarian, peanuts are a better recommendation. Bananas and pineapple juice do not contain significant amounts of folic acid. **Cognitive Level:** Applying **Client Need:** Health Promotion and Maintenance **Integrated Process:** Nursing Process: Implementation **Content Area:** Maternal–Newborn **Strategy:** Use the process of elimination and knowledge of nutrition to answer this question. Eliminate hamburger first because the client is a vegetarian, and eliminate bananas and apple juice because they are fruit or fruit products. Nuts are better sources of folic acid.

11 **Answer: 2 Rationale:** Iron is better absorbed if taken with a source of vitamin C. Iron is absorbed best on an empty stomach (not after a full meal). Iron does not replace the need for other vitamins. Iron does not have to be taken at the same time as other vitamin supplementation. **Cognitive Level:** Applying **Client Need:** Health Promotion and Maintenance **Integrated Process:** Nursing Process: Planning **Content Area:** Maternal–Newborn **Strategy:** First, recall that iron intake does not eliminate the need for other vitamins. Next, recall that a full meal may decrease iron absorption. Choose between the remaining two options by recalling the beneficial effect of vitamin C on iron absorption.

12 **Answer: 1 Rationale:** Increased calcium intake can lead to formation of kidney stones. A calcium supplement is not expected to affect leg cramps, color of mucous membranes and conjunctiva, or resting heart rate. **Cognitive Level:** Analyzing **Client Need:** Health Promotion and Maintenance **Integrated Process:** Nursing Process: Assessment **Content Area:** Maternal–Newborn **Strategy:** Recall that calcium is a salt,

and use this information to recall that salts can form crystals, which can in turn lead to kidney stones.

13 **Answer: 3 Rationale:** The measles, mumps, and rubella vaccine contains live, attenuated virus and could cause disease and harm to the fetus during pregnancy. It should be given after delivery, and the woman should avoid conceiving for 3 months. The client should not receive the vaccine during this prenatal visit. The client should not receive the vaccine during the third trimester. The vaccine should not be omitted because an adult can become infected with measles, mumps, or rubella. **Cognitive Level:** Analyzing **Client Need:** Health Promotion and Maintenance **Integrated Process:** Nursing Process: Planning **Content Area:** Maternal–Newborn **Strategy:** The issue in this question is immunization safety during pregnancy. The vaccine does need to be administered, so choose the option that considers the live attenuated viral nature of the vaccine.

14 **Answer: 2 Rationale:** Braxton Hicks contractions are probably caused by stretching of the myometrium. They are usually relieved by position changes, frequent emptying of the bladder, resting in a lateral recumbent position, and walking or light exercise. Continuous bedrest until true labor begins is not necessary. Lamaze breathing is helpful for some women in managing discomfort that can be associated with Braxton Hicks contractions. Clients are not advised to ignore symptoms; instead, the nurse should focus on teaching the client how to recognize true labor. **Cognitive Level:** Applying **Client Need:** Health Promotion and Maintenance **Integrated Process:** Communication and Documentation **Content Area:** Maternal-Newborn **Strategy:** The question addresses the issue of client teaching about Braxton Hicks contractions. The wording of the question indicates the correct answer is a true statement. Recall that emptying the bladder and position changes help to relieve this discomfort.

15 **Answer: 4 Rationale:** Heat may relieve pain caused by increased joint mobility resulting from hormonal changes. Aspirin should be avoided in the last trimester because it increases bleeding time. Telling the client to just put up with it is not a therapeutic communication. Sleeping flat on the back may not be helpful for maternal–fetal circulation because the gravid uterus may cause pressure on the great vessels in the abdomen. The client should lie on one side; often the left is advised. **Cognitive Level:** Applying **Client Need:** Health Promotion and Maintenance **Integrated Process:** Communication and Documentation **Content Area:** Maternal–Newborn **Strategy:** Recall principles of heat and cold therapy and therapeutic communication to choose correctly.

16 **Answer: 3 Rationale:** Probable signs of pregnancy are those that are detected by the examiner and are usually related to the physical signs of pregnancy. Amenorrhea and chloasma are reported by the client (presumptive signs) and can be caused by conditions other than pregnancy. Fetal heartbeat on ultrasound is a positive sign of pregnancy. **Cognitive Level:** Analyzing **Client Need:** Health Promotion and Maintenance **Integrated Process:** Nursing Process: Assessment **Content Area:** Maternal–Newborn **Strategy:** Specific knowledge of the different classifications of signs of pregnancy is needed to answer this question. If you recall that *probable* is the middle category, it may help you to eliminate positive and possible signs.

17 **Answer: 1 Rationale:** The use of water to wash the nipples can help avoid irritation that could lead to nipple cracking or trauma. Daily use of lanolin on the nipples during the last trimester is unnecessary. Rubbing the nipples briskly could cause trauma. The pinch test is to determine if nipples are inverted and need only be done one time. **Cognitive Level:** Applying **Client Need:** Health Promotion and Maintenance **Integrated Process:** Nursing Process: Implementation **Content Area:** Maternal–Newborn **Strategy:** Use nursing knowledge to answer the question. It may also be helpful to recall general principles of skin care and avoidance of skin trauma, which helps eliminate each of the incorrect options.

18 **Answer: 1 Rationale:** The client who is not eating meat may have a problem with decreased iron intake, which could impact her hemoglobin level. Polymorphonuclear cells, lymphocytes, and platelets are unrelated to iron intake. **Cognitive Level:** Applying **Client Need:** Health Promotion and Maintenance **Integrated Process:** Nursing Process: Assessment **Content Area:** Maternal–Newborn **Strategy:** Recall that meat is rich in iron, which is needed for RBC production. Then recall that the hemoglobin level is affected by iron intake and iron stores. As an alternate strategy, eliminate each of the other options because they do not identify RBCs.

19 **Answer: 2 Rationale:** Daycare workers are frequently exposed to the virus. Exposure to cat litter can result in toxoplasmosis. IV drug use increases the risk for HIV or hepatitis. Giving blood does not increase the client's risk. **Cognitive Level:** Analyzing **Client Need:** Health Promotion and Maintenance **Integrated Process:** Nursing Process: Diagnosis **Content Area:** Maternal–Newborn **Strategy:** Use the process of elimination and knowledge of transmission of viral infections to answer this question. Eliminate giving blood first as unrelated to acquiring infection. Eliminate the option with cat litter next because the organism in toxoplasmosis is not a virus. Choose working in a daycare center over past use of IV drugs because there is more risk of exposure.

20 **Answer: 2 Rationale:** Indications for cesarean delivery are presence of one or more herpes lesions in the birth canal (vaginal area) at the time of labor and delivery. A positive herpes culture at first prenatal visit is not sufficient for cesarean delivery. Oral fever blisters (oral herpes) would not pose a risk to vaginal delivery. If there are no herpes lesions at the time of delivery, a vaginal birth is recommended. **Cognitive Level:** Analyzing **Client Need:** Health Promotion and Maintenance **Integrated Process:** Nursing Process: Diagnosis **Content Area:** Maternal–Newborn **Strategy:** Specific knowledge related to risk of delivery with herpes infection is needed to answer the question. Use concepts of time and direct contact with lesions to eliminate the incorrect options.

21 **Answer: 1 Rationale:** All partners have been exposed and should be made aware, tested, and treated as indicated. Cesarean delivery would be appropriate only if there were symptoms of a herpes lesion or prodromal symptoms. Genetic assessment and more-than-routine assessment of hematocrit and hemoglobin are not indicated. **Cognitive Level:** Applying **Client Need:** Health Promotion and Maintenance **Integrated Process:** Nursing Process: Implementation **Content Area:** Maternal–Newborn **Strategy:** Use knowledge of principles of communicable disease transmission to answer the question. The client in the question is actually the sexual partner(s), not the fetus.

22 **Answer: 2 Rationale:** Carrier status of Group B streptococcus is variable, so identification several weeks before delivery may not identify a woman who is positive at the time of delivery. The current recommendation is screening during the 36–37th week of gestation. Rash and history of STI do not alter this recommendation. **Cognitive Level:** Applying **Client Need:** Health

Promotion and Maintenance **Integrated Process:** Nursing Process: Planning **Content Area:** Maternal–Newborn **Strategy:** Specific knowledge of the timing of prenatal assessments is needed to answer this question. Eliminate the option that identifies history, which does not necessarily imply a risk for an active problem. Next, eliminate vaginal rash as unrelated to Group B streptococcus. Choose among the other options considering the risk for exposure at the time of delivery.

23 **Answer: 4 Rationale:** Menstrual blood can affect the results of a gonorrheal culture. Recent diagnosis and treatment for herpes would not affect the results of a gonorrhea culture. Persistent vaginal discharge may be an indication for a gonorrhea culture, rather than a reason to postpone specimen collection. Douching within 24 hours can affect results, but douching 3 days earlier should not affect the culture results. **Cognitive Level:** Applying **Client Need:** Health Promotion and Maintenance **Integrated Process:** Nursing Process: Planning **Content Area:** Maternal–Newborn **Strategy:** Use general knowledge of specimen collection procedures to answer the question. Visualize each option and choose the one that could physically alter the test results.

24 **Answer: 3 Rationale:** Urine specific gravity is a measure of the concentration of particles in the urine. Urine specific gravity rises when the client is dehydrated. Hematocrit would also rise when the client is dehydrated, but is an indirect measure. Hemoglobin measurements are not as greatly affected. Platelet count and IgG levels are not affected. **Cognitive Level:** Applying **Client Need:** Health Promotion and Maintenance **Integrated Process:** Nursing Process: Assessment **Content Area:** Maternal–Newborn **Strategy:** Note the critical word *best* in the question, which means that more than one value could be affected. Use knowledge of laboratory indicators of dehydration to eliminate platelet count and IgG level. Then choose urine specific gravity over hematocrit because it is a more direct measurement of fluid balance.

25 **Answer: 3 Rationale:** Closed-ended questions (requiring yes or no answers) are a barrier to communication in many nurse–client interactions. They are best used when trying to elicit very specific pieces of assessment data. A nonjudgmental approach tends to establish a trusting and open relationship with the client and enhance client disclosure. Conducting the interview with the client dressed may increase overall client comfort and aid in client disclosure. Questions that are framed using a culturally sensitive approach tend to establish a trusting relationship with the client and enhance client disclosure. **Cognitive Level:** Applying **Client Need:** Health Promotion and Maintenance **Integrated Process:** Communication and Documentation **Content Area:** Maternal–Newborn **Strategy:** Use general principles related to communication and history taking to answer this question. Application of these principles will help to eliminate each incorrect option.

26 **Answer: 1, 5 Rationale:** Protein and iron intake in pregnancy must increase to meet the needs of the growing fetus. Calcium requirements increase at the same rate as phosphorus. Caloric needs increase, but only about 300 calories per day. Iodine requirements increase during pregnancy. **Cognitive Level:** Applying **Client Need:** Health Promotion and Maintenance **Integrated Process:** Teaching and Learning **Content Area:** Maternal–Newborn **Strategy:** Recall specific concepts of nutrients needed during pregnancy to help answer the question correctly.

27 **Answer: 4, 5 Rationale:** Childbirth education should be geared to the trimester of pregnancy. In the third trimester, the pregnant woman begins to focus on aspects of labor and delivery, including need for pain relief. In the third trimester, the pregnant woman is likely to be concerned about learning to care for the newborn. The healthcare provider should have been selected at the time pregnancy was discovered. Morning sickness management and nutritional needs during pregnancy are topics that are appropriate for the first trimester of pregnancy. **Cognitive Level:** Analyzing **Client Need:** Health Promotion and Maintenance **Integrated Process:** Teaching and Learning **Content Area:** Maternal–Newborn **Strategy:** Critical words are *third trimester* and *childbirth education topics*. Recall childbirth education topics associated with the various trimesters and select the information that corresponds to the third trimester. This question is time-sensitive.

28 **Answer: 04.17 Rationale:** According to Naegele's rule, the estimated date of birth can be calculated by subtracting 3 months from the beginning date of the last menstrual period (LMP) and then adding 7 days to that date. April is 3 months earlier than July. Adding 7 days to 10 (the beginning date of the LMP) equals 17. Thus, the due date is estimated as April 17 (04.17). **Cognitive Level:** Analyzing **Client Need:** Health Promotion and Maintenance **Integrated Process:** Nursing Process: Diagnosis **Content Area:** Maternal–Newborn **Strategy:** Recall Naegele's rule to calculate the answer to this question.

29 **Answer: 3, 5 Rationale:** The fluid leaking from the pregnant client's breasts is colostrum. It normally leaks from the breasts during the last trimester. The client should wear a supportive bra. Leakage of colostrum does not indicate an infection. Premature labor is not associated with leakage of colostrum. Leakage of colostrum is normal and does not predict problems with breastfeeding. **Cognitive Level:** Analyzing **Client Need:** Health Promotion and Maintenance **Integrated Process:** Teaching and Learning **Content Area:** Maternal–Newborn **Strategy:** Recall normal changes to the breast during pregnancy and associated teaching needs to help to answer this question.

Key Terms to Review

References

Davidson, M., London, M., & Ladewig, P. (2016). *Olds' maternal newborn nursing and women's health across the lifespan* (10th ed.). New York, NY: Pearson Education.

Kee, J. (2017). *Pearson's handbook of laboratory and diagnostic tests* (8th ed.). New York, NY: Pearson Education.

Ladewig, P., London, M., & Davidson, M. (2014). *Contemporary maternal–newborn nursing care* (8th ed.). Upper Saddle River, NJ: Pearson Education.

London, M., Ladewig, P., Davidson, M., Ball, J., Bindler, R., & Cowen, K. (2014). *Maternal and child nursing care* (4th ed.). Upper Saddle River, NJ: Pearson Education.

Lowdermilk, D., Perry, S., Cashion, M., & Alden, K. (2016). *Maternity and women's health care* (11th ed.). St. Louis, MO: Elsevier.

Test Yourself

Are you ready for the NCLEX-RN® or course exams? Access the NEW web-based app that provides students with thousands of practice questions in preparation for the NCLEX experience.

Uncomplicated Labor and Delivery Care 10

In this chapter

Cross Reference

Other chapters relevant to this content area are

Reproduction, Family Planning, and Infertility	**Chapter 8**
Uncomplicated Antenatal Assessment and Care	**Chapter 9**
Uncomplicated Postpartum Assessment and Care	**Chapter 11**
Uncomplicated Newborn Care	**Chapter 12**
Complicated Antenatal Care	**Chapter 49**
Complicated Labor and Delivery Care	**Chapter 50**
Complicated Postpartum Care	**Chapter 51**
Complicated Newborn Care	**Chapter 52**

I. NURSING CARE OF THE LABOR AND DELIVERY CLIENT

A. Physiological safety and psychological safety

1. The laboring client is actually two clients—mother and newborn
2. Nursing care that focuses on physiological safety is concerned with both clients
3. Nursing care to address psychological safety focuses on mother and includes fear, comfort, partner involvement, attachment to newborn, and past experiences
4. Primigravida women experience fear of unknown and often have longer labors
5. Multigravida women can have a shorter labor with subsequent pregnancies but may have mixed memories of good and bad experiences from previous births
6. Assess for history of abuse, assault, and violence because such experiences often manifest as extreme fear and tension during labor process or vaginal examinations

B. Cultural background

1. Must be assessed and understood to provide a safe and acceptable birthing environment for childbearing family
2. Some common nursing actions may be cultural taboos for a particular client and affect parents' view of child throughout life

C. Educational preparation for labor by client and her support person(s)

1. Varies from formal prenatal classes to information passed through generations
2. Address any misconceptions about birthing process or sensations to expect during birth in a nonjudgmental manner that informs and supports birthing family

D. Electronic fetal monitoring

1. Provides computer-assisted auditory and visual assessment of fetal heart rate (FHR) and uterine contractions (UC)
2. *NCLEX®* FHR monitoring continuously records FHR on upper portion of monitor strip; measured in beats per minute (bpm); normal range: 110–160; bradycardia: <110; tachycardia: >160
3. *NCLEX®* External monitoring: ultrasound transducer is placed over fetal back and detects movements of fetal heart; fetal or maternal movement and maternal obesity may interfere with obtaining a continuous reading
4. Internal monitoring
   a. An **internal fetal scalp electrode** is inserted through cervix (must be at least 2 cm dilated with ruptured membranes) and attached to epidermis of presenting part, providing a direct electrocardiogram (ECG) of fetal heart
   b. Unaffected by maternal obesity, maternal or fetal movement; thick fetal hair may prevent adequate insertion on a cephalic presentation
5. *NCLEX®* **Baseline variability**: fluctuations in baseline FHR of two cycles per minute or greater that is irregular in frequency and amplitude; measured on fetal tracing as peak and trough levels
   a. Creates a jaggedness or zigzag appearance in baseline FHR
   b. Determined by interplay between fetal sympathetic and parasympathetic nervous systems
   c. Defined as absent (amplitude undetectable), minimal (amplitude detectable but less than 5 bpm), moderate (amplitude 6–25 bpm; normal), marked (amplitude greater than 25 bpm)
   d. Reduced variability is caused by fetal sleep, fetal tachycardia, prematurity, and fetal heart and CNS anomalies
   e. *NCLEX®* Reduced variability is single best predictor of fetal compromise if not associated with fetal sleep
   f. Marked variability can be caused by early mild hypoxia (variability increases to compensate), fetal stimulation or activity, fetal breathing movements, and advancing gestational age (over 30 weeks)
6. *NCLEX®* **Accelerations**: transient increases in FHR of at least 15 beats/min from baseline and lasting 15 seconds or longer
   a. Nonperiodic (spontaneous): symmetric, uniform, not related to contractions, occur in response to fetal movement and indicate fetal well-being
   b. Periodic: occur with contractions and may indicate decreased amniotic fluid or mild umbilical cord compression
7. Decelerations are categorized as early, late, or variable
8. *NCLEX®* **Early deceleration**: decrease in FHR beginning at onset of contraction and returning to baseline by end of contraction; FHR at lowest point remains above 100 bpm
   a. Uniform shape inversely mirrors contraction
   b. Caused by fetal head compression; usually benign
   c. Nursing interventions: possible vaginal examination to determine dilatation and whether fetus is descending in pelvis
9. *NCLEX®* **Late deceleration** begins after contraction starts, with lowest FHR occurring after peak of contraction and returning to baseline after end of contraction
   a. Smooth, uniform shape that inversely mirrors contractions but late in onset and recovery
   b. Caused by uteroplacental insufficiency; always considered nonreassuring
   c. Nursing interventions focus on maintaining oxygenation: reposition client to left lateral, administer oxygen by mask at 7–10 L/min, correct hypotension by increasing IV fluid rate or administering medications, discontinue oxytocin if being administered, assess cervical status, and report to healthcare provider
10. **Variable deceleration** occurs suddenly, varies in duration and intensity, varies in relation to contractions, and resolves abruptly
    a. Variable shape, usually U or V, with steep sides; may or may not be associated with contractions
    b. Caused by compression of umbilical cord
    c. Categorized as mild, moderate, or severe based on lowest FHR reading and duration of deceleration; repetitive, prolonged, or more severe decelerations with a slow return or overshoot to baseline are ominous and indicate fetal asphyxia
    d. Nursing interventions: relieve cord compression by repositioning client until improvement occurs, perform vaginal exam to detect prolapsed cord, give oxygen if decelerations are severe or uncorrectable, and discontinue oxytocin infusion if present
    e. Amnio-infusion (instillation of warmed normal saline through an intrauterine pressure catheter) may be done to recreate cushioning effect on umbilical cord during contractions that is normally provided by amniotic fluid

11. Uterine contraction monitoring documents contraction frequency, duration, and intensity on lower half of monitor strip
    a. External monitoring: tocodynamometer is placed on maternal abdomen near fundus and held in place with elastic belt; documents contraction frequency and duration, but not intensity; affected by fetal or maternal movement, transverse or oblique lie, and maternal abdominal fat
    b. Internal monitoring is accomplished through an **intrauterine pressure catheter (IUPC)**, a wire with pressure gauge on one end or a saline-filled tube, which is inserted through cervix and past presenting part into amniotic fluid in uterus; increase in intrauterine pressure reflects intensity of contraction; cervix must be at least 2–3 cm dilated with ruptured membranes before an IUPC can be inserted; nurse should continue to evaluate labor status by palpating intensity and resting tone of uterine fundus during contractions

II. THE LABOR PROCESS

A. **Initiation of labor:** comes about from an interplay of factors, including distension of uterus causing irritability and contractility, and hormonal influence of prostaglandins, oxytocin, fetal cortisol, estrogen, and progesterone

NCLEX® B. **True versus false labor:** differentiated by cervical change: effacement and dilatation

C. **Factors of labor:** passageway, passenger, powers, and psyche (4 Ps)
1. *Passageway* is maternal bony pelvis comprised of innominate bones (ilium, ischium, and pubis), sacrum, and coccyx
    a. False pelvis lies above pelvic brim, supports increasing weight of enlarging pregnant uterus, and directs presenting part into true pelvis below
    b. True pelvis consists of inlet, midpelvis, and outlet and represents bony limits of birth canal; adequacy of each part, measured as transverse and anterior–posterior (AP) diameters, must be sufficient to allow passage of fetus
    c. Four pelvic types are gynecoid, android, anthropoid, and platypelloid (see Table 10–1); type and diameters of pelvis influence fetal descent, progression of labor, and type of delivery
2. *Passenger* refers to fetus

NCLEX® a. **Attitude** is relationship of fetal parts to one another; normal attitude is flexion of neck, arms, and legs

NCLEX® b. **Lie** is relationship of cephalocaudal axis of fetus to cephalocaudal axis of mother; is either longitudinal (or vertical, most common) or transverse (lateral)

NCLEX® c. **Presentation** is fetal part entering pelvis first; most common is cephalic—head first (with subcategories of vertex, military, brow, or face presentation), but breech—buttocks first (subtypes of complete, frank, or footling) and shoulder (also called transverse lie) can also occur

NCLEX® d. **Position** is relationship of fetal presenting part to maternal pelvis; a three-letter notation describes fetal position: see memory aid box; most common positions at delivery are ROA (right occiput anterior) and LOA (left occiput anterior)

Table 10–1 Pelvic Types

Pelvic Type	Inlet	Midpelvis	Outlet	Implications for Birth
Gynecoid	Round, adequate diameters	Round, adequate diameters	Wide transverse, long anterior–posterior (AP) diameters	Occiput anterior most common, most favorable for vaginal birth
Android	Heart-shaped, angulated	Short AP diameter	Short AP diameter	Slow descent, arrest of labor, not favorable for vaginal birth
Anthropoid	Ovoid, long AP diameter	Rounded, adequate diameters	Narrow transverse diameter	Occiput anterior or posterior, favorable for vaginal birth
Platypelloid	Ovoid, wide transverse diameter	Rounded, wide transverse diameter	Wide transverse, short AP diameter	Occiput posterior more common, not favorable for vaginal birth

Memory Aid

Use the mnemonics in 2 and 3 to help remember fetal position:
1. **R or L:** right or left; direction that presenting part of fetus faces
2. **AMOS:** **a**cromion process, **m**entum, **o**cciput, **s**acrum; the landmark of the fetal presenting part
3. **PAT:** **p**osterior, **a**nterior, **t**ransverse; the relationship of the landmark of the presenting part to the front, back, or side of pelvis

occiput = head
acromion : shoulder
mentum = chin
sacrum = butt

where back faces

Post = back is in the back
ant = front

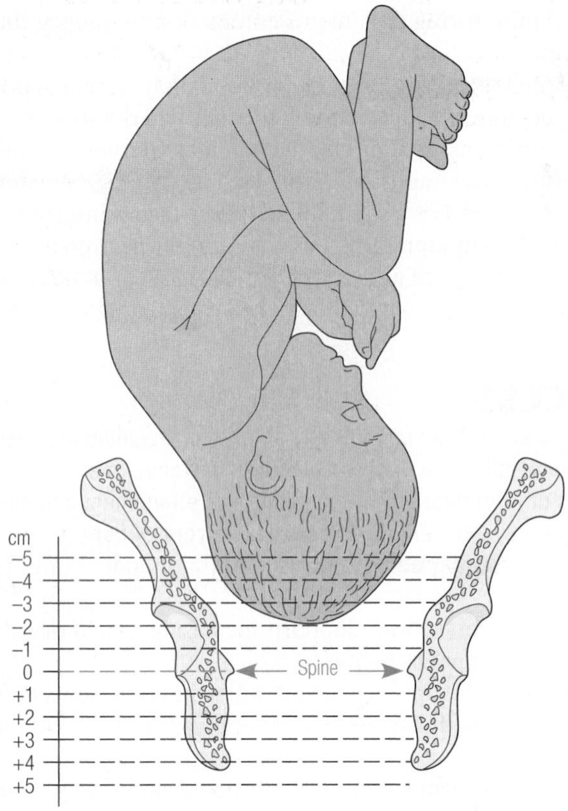

Figure 10–1

Stations of fetal descent measured in centimeters.

D. *Leopold's maneuvers* are methods of palpation used to monitor fetal presentation and position

1. If fetal head is positioned in fundus, it is palpated as a hard, round, and movable object
2. Fetal buttocks feel soft, are irregular in shape, and move less easily
3. Fetal back is firm and smooth, and should be felt on one side of abdomen; while fetal hands, feet, elbows, and knees may be palpated as irregular bumps on opposite side of abdomen

NCLEX®
   a. **Engagement** occurs when largest diameter of presenting part reaches pelvic inlet and can be detected by vaginal exam; termed *floating* if it is directed toward pelvis but can easily be moved out of inlet; termed *ballotable* when presenting part dips into inlet but can be displaced with upward pressure by examiner's fingers; termed *engaged* if fixed in pelvic inlet and cannot be displaced
   b. **Station** is relationship of presenting part to pelvic ischial spines; measured in centimeters (cm) above (−1 to −5 station), at (0 station), or below (+1 to +4 station) ischial spines (see Figure 10–1)
4. *Powers* include primary and secondary forces of labor
   a. Primary forces: involuntary contractions of uterine muscle fibers, which are stimulated by a pacemaker located in upper uterine segment
   b. Phases of contractions: increment (building-up), acme (peak), and decrement (letting-up) followed by a resting phase (nadir) to facilitate uteroplacental–fetal reoxygenation

NCLEX®
   c. Frequency of contractions: time in seconds or minutes from onset of one contraction to onset of next

NCLEX®
   d. Intensity: strength of contraction at peak, which can be palpated as mild, moderate, or strong; detected with a fetal monitor externally or measured internally in mmHg

NCLEX®
   e. Duration: length of contraction measured in seconds from beginning of increment to end of decrement
   f. With each contraction, muscles of upper uterine segment shorten and exert longitudinal traction on cervix, causing **effacement** (thinning and drawing-up of internal os and cervical canal into uterine side walls); measured from 0 to 100%; in primigravidas, effacement usually precedes dilatation; in multigravidas, they normally occur simultaneously
   g. As uterus elongates with contractions, fetal body straightens and exerts pressure against lower uterine segment and cervix; **dilatation** or opening of cervix results; measured from 0 to 10 cm; allows for birth of fetus
   h. Secondary powers: voluntary use of abdominal muscles during second stage of labor to facilitate descent and delivery of fetus

5. *Psyche*: psychological component of childbearing; excitement, fear, perceived loss of control, anxiety are common emotions during labor and delivery
   a. Extreme emotions such as fear result in muscular tension, which can create more pain from friction between working uterus and tense abdominal muscles or impede descent of fetus when pelvic and perineal muscles are tense rather than relaxed when pushing
   b. Psyche can also manifest physiologically because maternal blood pressure (BP), pulse, and respiratory rate can increase with fear, excitement, and anxiety
   c. Lack of knowledge and preparation for childbirth can negatively affect psyche

III. THE STAGES OF LABOR

A. First stage

1. Extends from onset of true labor to complete dilatation of cervix (0–10 cm) and is divided into three phases: latent, active, and transition; a labor curve, often referred to as a Friedman curve, can be used to track progression of cervical dilation and also station of fetal head

NCLEX®

2. Latent phase
   a. 0–3 centimeters dilated; little descent occurs
   b. Contractions usually begin irregularly and become more regular, with increasing frequency (every 10–30 min), duration (up to 30 sec), and intensity (from mild to moderate)
   c. Client is usually relieved labor has started; can recognize and express anxiety; may be happy, excited, and talkative; changes position without reminder
   d. Average duration is 8.6 hours for nulliparas and 5.3 hours for multiparas

NCLEX®

3. Active phase
   a. 4–7 centimeters dilated; effacement and descent are progressive
   b. Contractions usually every 2–5 minutes, 40–60 seconds in duration, and moderate to strong intensity
   c. Client is usually serious, intense, has a need for increased concentration, answers questions in short phrases between contractions; fatigue increases and woman becomes more dependent; pain increases, relaxation is more difficult, and woman may need reminders to change positions
   d. Average duration is 4.6 hours for nulliparas and 2.4 hours for multiparas

NCLEX®

4. Transition phase
   a. 8–10 centimeters dilated; effacement is complete (100%) and descent increases
   b. Contractions every 1½–2 minutes, lasting 60–90 seconds, and strong intensity
   c. Client is working hard with intense concentration; gives one-word answers to questions only between contractions; anxiety increases, fears loss of control and abandonment, senses helplessness; relaxation is difficult as contraction time exceeds resting phase; may experience intense low abdominal, pelvic, and rectal discomfort from fetal descent; nausea and vomiting are common; may need reminders to empty bladder and change position
   d. Average duration is 3 hours for nulliparas and less than 1 hour for multiparas
5. Assessment upon admission: review medical, obstetric and prenatal history; labor status (contractions, vaginal examination if indicated), fetal status (FHR, variability, periodic changes), status of membranes (intact or if ruptured, length of time and amount, color, odor), maternal vital signs, laboratory testing if prescribed (Hgb and UA), desired birth plan including cultural considerations, preparation for childbirth, level of comfort and coping, and support system

NCLEX®

6. Nursing assessments during first stage of labor
   a. Latent phase: BP, pulse, respirations q1h if normal; temperature q4h if normal or membranes intact and q2h if abnormal or membranes ruptured; contractions q30 min; FHR q1hr for low-risk women or q30min for high-risk women or nonreassuring pattern
   b. Active phase: BP, pulse, respirations, temperature, contractions same as latent phase; FHR q30min for low-risk women or q15min for high-risk women or nonreassuring pattern; look for bloody mucus or "show" from cervical dilatation as active labor progresses toward transition
   c. Transition phase: BP, pulse, respirations q30min; temperature same as latent phase; contractions q15min, FHR q15min
7. Collaborative management
   a. Orient to environment, expected assessments, and procedures
   b. Encourage ambulation (if presenting part is engaged) unless contraindicated

NCLEX®

   c. Provide comfort through frequent position change, effleurage, focal point, hydrotherapy, caregiver presence, therapeutic touch, sacral pressure, back rub, or administration of analgesia as requested by client and prescribed by healthcare provider
   d. Encourage voiding q2h

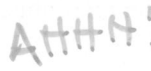

e. Monitor labor progress and fetal well-being

NCLEX® f. Provide ice chips and clear liquids to prevent dehydration

g. Teach, reinforce, or support use of relaxation, visualization, or breathing patterns

NCLEX® h. Encourage rest between contractions

i. Document and provide continuing status reports to healthcare provider

B. Second stage

NCLEX® 1. Extends from complete dilatation of cervix to delivery of fetus; accompanied by involuntary efforts to expel fetus and low-pitched, guttural, grunting sounds

2. Many women initially feel renewed energy because they can voluntarily work with contractions to push out fetus; over time can be exhausting work

3. Normal duration is up to 3 hours for nulliparas and less than 1 hour (average 15 mins) for multiparas

4. **Cardinal movements**: adaptations that fetus undertakes to maneuver through pelvis during labor and birth; in most common presentation, occiput, movements occur in the following order (see Memory Aid):

a. *Engagement* of presenting part occurs

b. *Descent* of fetus into pelvis

c. *Flexion* of fetal head; (descent and flexion often occur simultaneously)

d. *Internal Rotation* of fetal head takes place to accommodate maternal pelvis so that anterior–posterior (AP) diameter of fetal head (largest diameter of fetus) aligns with AP dimension of maternal pelvis

e. *Extension* of fetal head occurs as it comes under maternal symphysis pubis and emerges from vagina

f. *Restitution* occurs as fetal head turns 45 degrees to untwist neck after head has delivered

g. *External Rotation* is viewed as head turns an additional 45 degrees as second-largest fetal diameter (lateral diameter of fetal shoulders) rotates into alignment with AP dimension of maternal pelvis

h. *Expulsion* occurs as anterior shoulder slips beneath symphysis pubis, which facilitates delivery of body

Memory Aid

Use the following mnemonic phrase to assist in remembering the cardinal movements, using the first letter of each cardinal movement to begin a word: *Every darn fool in Rotterdam eats rotten egg rolls everyday.*

5. **Crowning**: outward perineal bulging and thinning and opening of vagina that occurs as fetal presenting part presses downward onto perineum and becomes visible prior to delivery; process is slower in nulliparous client than multiparous client

NCLEX® 6. Nursing assessment

a. BP, pulse, and respirations q5–q15min

b. Contractions palpated continuously

c. FHR q15min if low risk, q5min if high risk, and if nonreassuring pattern, monitor continuously

d. Monitor fetal descent, cardinal fetal movements, and crowning

NCLEX® 7. Collaborative management

a. Position comfortably for pushing and birth; encourage rest and relaxation between contractions

b. Comfort measures: cool cloth to forehead, support legs while pushing, provide encouragement to push

c. Ice chips and clear fluids to prevent dehydration

d. Empty bladder, straight catheter if bladder distended or unable to void

e. Local infiltration of anesthetic agent for birth by healthcare provider

NCLEX® f. **Episiotomy**: surgical incision into perineum to enlarge vaginal opening; usually done during or just prior to crowning; medically indicated in presence of fetal distress, but often performed to prevent tearing of perineal tissues because lacerations have irregular edges and are more difficult to repair

g. Types of episiotomy: midline (1- to 3-cm incision straight back from vagina toward rectum), mediolateral (4- to 5-cm incision from vagina obliquely toward one buttock)

h. Lacerations to perineum or surrounding tissues may occur during childbirth; see Box 10–1 for degrees of laceration; 3rd- and 4th-degree lacerations most commonly occur after midline episiotomy is performed

i. Document in client record: time of birth, gender, position, nuchal cord if present, and medications administered

C. Third stage

1. Extends from birth of newborn to delivery of placenta; average duration is 30 minutes for nulliparas and multiparas

Box 10–1

Degrees of Laceration

1st degree: involves only epidermal layers; if no bleeding, may not need repair

2nd degree: epidermal and muscle/fascia involvement, which requires suturing

3rd degree: extends into rectal sphincter

4th degree: extends through rectal mucosa

2. Maternal assessment

NCLEX®

a. BP, pulse, and respirations q5min
b. Uterine fundus maintains tone and contraction pattern to deliver placenta by decreasing surface volume of uterus and shearing placenta from uterine wall
c. Monitor for signs of placental separation: uterus rises up in abdomen; uterine volume shrinks as a result of contractions, creating a gush of blood vaginally as uterine contents are expelled; and as placenta is separating and beginning to be expelled, umbilical cord protrudes further from vagina and appears to lengthen

3. Fetal assessment
a. **Apgar score**: quick method to assess fetal adaptation to extrauterine life; five criteria are scored at 1 and 5 minutes after birth with 0, 1, or 2 points given for each criteria (see Table 10–2); Apgar scores of 8 or greater indicate need for minimal intervention (nasopharyngeal suction and oxygen near face, called "blow-by" oxygen); scores of 4–7 indicate need for oropharyngeal suctioning, tactile stimulation, and oxygen administration; scores of 3 or less indicate need for resuscitation; if Apgar is less than 7 at 5 minutes, scoring should be repeated every 5 minutes for up to 20 minutes
b. Respirations: normally 30–60, may be irregular
c. Apical pulse: 110–160, may be irregular and may be as high as 180 when crying
d. Temperature (skin): above 97.8°F (36.5°C)
e. Umbilical cord: normally two arteries and one vein
f. Gestational age assessment: consistent with expected date of delivery
g. Physical assessment: abbreviated exam done to detect visible congenital anomalies

4. Collaborative management
a. Encourage mother to rest and relax while awaiting delivery of placenta

NCLEX®

b. Immediate care of newborn: place in a modified Trendelenburg position, suction nose and oropharynx (bulb syringe or DeLee mucus trap), provide and maintain warmth (dry immediately with warm blankets, skin-to-skin contact with mother covered with warm blankets, radiant heat source, cap)
c. Assist parents in seeing and holding newborn to begin attachment
d. Document time of placental delivery, appearance and intactness of placenta, mechanism of placental expulsion, and estimated delivery blood loss (averages 250–500 mL)
e. Administer oxytocic agent as prescribed
f. Consider cultural practices in disposal of placenta

D. Fourth stage (immediate recovery phase)

1. Includes first 1–4 hours after delivery; actually part of postpartal period

NCLEX®

2. Assessment: BP, pulse, respirations, fundus, lochia, and perineum per agency protocol; usually q15min for 1 hour; q30min for 2 hours; q60min for 1 hour
3. Collaborative management
a. Episiotomy or lacerations are repaired
b. Provide comfort: clean gown, warm blanket, position of comfort, ice to perineum if sutures or edema present, analgesia as requested and prescribed

NCLEX®

c. Help parents to explore newborn and initiate breastfeeding if desired and if mother and baby are stable
d. Provide fluids and regular diet as tolerated; consider cultural preferences

Table 10–2 Apgar Scoring

	Color (Appearance)	Heart Rate (Pulse)	Reflex Irritability (Grimace)	Muscle Tone (Activity)	Respiratory Effort (Respirations)
0 points	Blue, pale	Absent	Absent	Absent	Absent
1 point	Blue extremities, pink body	<100	Grimace	Some flexion of extremities	Slow, irregular
2 points	Completely pink	≥100	Vigorous cry	Active motion	Good cry

Color HR Irritable Tone Resp. Effort

4. Outcome is that maternal and newborn well-being are maintained; family unit is supported and participates in birth process as desired

IV. PAIN MANAGEMENT DURING BIRTH

A. **Analgesia and anesthesia:** can decrease or eliminate pain during birthing process when nonpharmacologic methods of pain relief are ineffective

B. **Type of analgesia or anesthesia**
1. Determined by obstetric history of client, stage and phase of labor, rate of progression in labor, and preferences of client and healthcare provider
2. Regional differences in use of particular methods or medications exist

NCLEX®

C. **Nonpharmacologic methods of pain relief**
1. Position changes to decrease weight of fetus on area of most intense pain
2. Hydrotherapy by standing or sitting in a warm shower or reclining in a tub
3. Breathing techniques to prevent breath-holding and facilitate oxygen and carbon dioxide exchange; use of a focal point for concentration
4. Relaxation through verbal instruction, massage, soft music, or therapeutic touch

D. **Pharmacologic methods of pain relief**
1. Analgesics decrease perception of pain; goal is maximum pain relief with minimal risk; must consider effect on woman, fetus, and contractions (see also Table 10–3 for advantages, disadvantages, and nursing implications of various pain relief methods)

Table 10–3 Pharmacologic Pain Relief Methods During Labor

Pharmacologic Pain Relief Method	Advantages	Disadvantages	Nursing Implications
Intravenous opioids	RN administration, rapid onset of pain relief, easy to administer, relatively short duration	May ↓ contraction frequency and intensity, crosses placenta resulting in neonatal respiratory depression, short duration may not give adequate pain control during first or prolonged labor	Do not give opioid agonist-antagonist if opioid dependency, as immediate withdrawal will occur that can lead to seizures
Intrathecal opioids	Excellent pain control occurring within several minutes, lasts several hours, rarely results in neonatal respiratory depression, easier and faster than epidural for both provider and client	Undesirable for rapidly progressing labor or transition phase; may stop urge to push; must be injected by anesthesia personnel and is uncomfortable; client must hold still during injections; spinal headache may occur if CSF leaks through dura at injection site	Monitor for common side effects, including nausea, pruritus, urinary retention, muscle spasms at site of injection
Lumbar epidural block	Excellent pain relief, redosing possible, no neonatal respiratory depression results, may provide a few hours of postpartum pain relief as well as during labor and delivery	Undesirable for rapidly progressing labor or transition phase; must be inserted by anesthesia personnel; usually causes numbness of lower extremities, limiting mobility; ↓ contraction frequency and intensity; ↓ or eliminates urge to push; relaxation of musculature below site of injection often results in failure of fetus to accomplish internal rotation, necessitating an operative birth	Monitor urine output because retention requiring indwelling urinary catheter may result Monitor BP because maternal hypotension commonly results from vasodilation; avoid supine position
Paracervical block	Rapid onset of pain relief, no neonatal respiratory depression, can be given during transition, relatively easy to administer	Systemic absorption of drug through vascular cervix, excessive bleeding from cervix, ↓ or absent urge to push	FHR drop (bradycardia) can result from systemic absorption
Pudendal block	Provides excellent anesthesia of perineum, rarely needs second dose, provides a few hours of postpartum pain relief	Must inject along presenting part, creating ↓ vaginal pressure and discomfort for client; eliminates urge to push	Monitor client safety because ↓ sensation in lower extremities affects mobility
Local tissue infiltration	Easy to administer, provides a few hours of postpartum pain relief	Reinjection may be needed to obtain complete anesthesia with extensive lacerations or large episiotomies	Loss of sensation may ↓ urge or ability to urinate

NCLEX®

2. All systemic drugs cross placental barrier in varying amounts; analgesia given too early may prolong labor and depress fetus; analgesia given too late may cause neonatal respiratory depression with no benefit to woman
3. Intravenous synthetic agonist-antagonist opioids: nalbuphine and butorphanol tartrate most commonly used in active phase of first stage of labor
4. Intrathecal opioids: morphine sulfate or fentanyl citrate injected into L4–L5 or L5–S1 subarachnoid space
5. Lumbar **epidural block**: provides temporary and reversible loss of sensation by injection into area with direct contact to nerve tissue; needle and catheter introduced at L4–L5 or L5–S1 level; local anesthetics such as bupivacaine hydrochloride or lidocaine hydrochloride injected; provides either regional analgesia or anesthesia depending on dose injected
6. **Paracervical block**: a type of regional anesthesia; local anesthetic agent injected into lateral aspects of cervix during active or transition phases
7. **Pudendal block**: local anesthetic agent injected into lateral vaginal walls near ischial spines to anesthetize pudendal nerve; administered during second stage in preparation for cutting and repairing an episiotomy
8. Local infiltration: local anesthetic agents are injected into tissues of perineum to provide anesthesia for episiotomy incision or repair and suturing of lacerations

PRACTICE TEST

Check Your NCLEX–RN® Exam I.Q.

You are ready for testing on this content if you can:

- Monitor the physiological status of a client in labor.
- Teach relaxation methods during labor.
- Assess fetal heart rate.
- Assist in delivery of a newborn.
- Provide effective support, teaching, and nursing care to a client in labor.

PRACTICE TEST

1 After walking for 30 minutes, the laboring client now has blood-tinged mucus on her underpad. Which of the following is the most appropriate interpretation by the nurse?

1. The fetus has had a bowel movement.
2. The amniotic sac has ruptured.
3. The client has fallen while walking and sustained internal injury.
4. The cervix is opening more rapidly.

2 After administration of an epidural block for labor analgesia, the client's blood pressure decreases from 130/75 to 90/50. The nurse should assist the woman to do which of the following?

1. Lie in a supine position
2. Assume a semi-Fowler's position
3. Empty her bladder
4. Turn to the side to a left lateral position

3 The client is in active labor and the nurse receives a prescription for an opioid analgesic from the healthcare provider. The nurse verifies that the prescription is for which priority route for administration?

1. Intramuscular (IM)
2. Oral (PO)
3. Intravenous (IV)
4. Rectal (PR)

4 A laboring client has recently had an intrathecal narcotic administered for relief of labor pain. The nurse determines that teaching has been effective when the client makes which statement?

1. "If I stay on the bedpan a little longer, I think I can urinate."
2. "I know my itching is from the intrathecal medication."
3. "The baby won't move as much now that I've had the intrathecal medication."
4. "I wouldn't be nauseated if I had received the intrathecal medication earlier."

5 The nurse concludes that the use of nonpharmacologic pain management techniques have been helpful to the client after noting which assessment data?

1. Decreased short-term variability in the fetal heart rate
2. Increased maternal blood pressure and pulse
3. Decreased muscle tension in the arms and face
4. Increased frequency of contractions

PRACTICE TEST

6 The nurse's plan of care for the pain of a laboring client should incorporate which concept?

1. Childbirth pain is caused only by physical factors.
2. The expression of pain is universal.
3. Having the presence of a supportive partner eliminates pain.
4. Labor pain has physiologic and psychologic components.

7 The therapeutic plan of care for a client with a prolonged latent phase of labor should include which intervention as a priority measure?

1. Encouraging rest and relaxation through the playing of soft music
2. IV hydration with either lactated Ringer's solution or 5 percent dextrose
3. Continuous internal fetal monitoring of the fetal response to contractions
4. Measuring maternal blood pressure, temperature, and pulse every 15 minutes

8 The client's fetal heart rate (FHR) is 150 before a contraction begins. During the contraction, the FHR falls to 110 and returns to baseline 30 seconds after the contraction ends. What is the priority nursing action in response to this finding?

1. Place the client into a semi-Fowler's position.
2. Administer oxygen by nasal cannula at 2 liters per minute.
3. Insert a Foley catheter and measure urinary output.
4. Place the client in left lateral position.

9 The fetal heart rate (FHR) baseline is 145 beats per minute with short-term variability of 12 beats per minute. The nurse should take which action at this time?

1. Notify client's healthcare provider immediately.
2. Obtain prescription to start IV of lactated Ringer's solution.
3. Reposition client on her hands and knees.
4. Encourage continued use of breathing and relaxation techniques.

10 The fetal heart rate (FHR) shows variable decelerations. Which activity carried out by the nurse could decrease or eliminate this pattern?

1. Encourage woman to relax in a warm shower.
2. Apply a fetal scalp electrode.
3. Assist client into a supine position.
4. Begin amnio-infusion of normal saline.

11 The laboring client is 8 centimeters dilated, 100% effaced, with vertex presenting at +2 station. The fetal heart rate gradually slows during each contraction, returning to baseline by the end of the contraction. The nurse should draw which conclusion from this data?

1. The umbilical cord is becoming compressed.
2. There is uteroplacental insufficiency.
3. The fetal head is becoming compressed.
4. The fetus is moving between contractions.

12 A woman is admitted to the birth unit. She is bearing down uncontrollably with contractions and says, "The baby is coming!" What should be the priority action of the nurse?

1. Telephone the healthcare provider.
2. Put on gloves and prepare for immediate birth.
3. Obtain a medical and obstetric history.
4. Assess maternal vital signs and fetal heart rate.

13 The laboring client has begun to make guttural, grunting sounds during contractions. The nursing plan of care should now include which nursing intervention?

1. Inspect the perineum to see if it is bulging outward.
2. Encourage the client's husband to go and eat now.
3. Teach the client about breastfeeding soon after delivery.
4. Assess the client's blood pressure and temperature.

14 A primigravida client is in the second stage of labor. The nurse determines that teaching has been effective when the client makes which statement?

1. "I'll push two or three times and the baby will be born."
2. "It's not the baby, I have to have a bowel movement."
3. "I know I'll have to push a while. This is hard work."
4. "My doctor will come and pull the baby out now."

15 The newly delivered infant has been placed on the mother's abdomen. What is the nurse's priority nursing intervention for the newborn?

1. Dry off the infant with blankets or towels.
2. Apply identification bracelets and obtain footprints.
3. Conduct a gestational age assessment.
4. Use the bulb syringe to clear the mouth and nose of mucus.

16 A laboring client's membranes spontaneously rupture. What should the nurse's first action be?

1. Assess the fetal heart rate.
2. Encourage the woman to ambulate.
3. Document the color, odor, and amount of amniotic fluid.
4. Prepare for imminent delivery of the newborn.

17 The nurse should include which elements in a psychosocial assessment of the laboring client? Select all that apply.

1. Cultural assessment
2. Plans for naming the child
3. Fetal heart rate assessment
4. Socioeconomic status of the family
5. Expectations of the experience

18 The nurse is teaching a group of expectant parents about cardinal movements, or changes in position, that occur as the fetus with a cephalic presentation passes through the birth canal. Order the cardinal movements in proper sequence for the nurse's presentation. All options must be used.

1. Expulsion 3
2. External rotation 4
3. Flexion 5
4. Internal rotation 2
5. Restitution 1

19 The nurse should implement which interventions for a client with an episiotomy in the fourth stage of labor? Select all that apply.

1. Application of ice beginning 4 hours after delivery
2. Ice pack to the perineum for up to 60 minutes per application
3. Inspection every 15 minutes during the first hour after birth
4. Instructions to avoid intercourse for at least 12 weeks
5. Ice packs to be applied for 20–30 minutes and removed for at least 20 minutes

20 The neonate is crying, pink except for blue extremities, has flexed arms with clenched hands, a heart rate of 154, and gags when the bulb suction is used. What should the nurse record for an Apgar score? Record an answer using a whole number.

Fill in your answer below:
Answer: 9/10

21 The nurse notes that earlier in the shift, the fetal heart rate (FHR) was 140 beats/minute and the baseline has now risen to 170. The nurse should investigate which factors as possible causes for the higher baseline readings? Select all that apply.

1. Maternal fever
2. Narcotic administration
3. Fetal movement
4. Uteroplacental insufficiency
5. Fetal distress

ANSWERS & RATIONALES

1 **Answer: 4 Rationale:** Bloody mucus is often called bloody show and becomes more profuse during the late active phase and into the transition phase of the first stage of labor and during the second stage of labor. Fetal bowel movements are not blood-tinged. Rupture of the amniotic sac would produce a clear, watery fluid. There is no correlation of blood-tinged mucus during labor with injury sustained through walking. **Cognitive Level:** Analyzing **Client Need:** Health Promotion and Maintenance **Integrated Process:** Nursing Process: Diagnosis **Content Area:** Maternal–Newborn **Strategy:** Note the critical word *blood-tinged* and associate this with progression in labor. Recall that exercise such as walking hastens labor. Both of these concepts should guide you to select cervical dilation as the answer.

2 **Answer: 4 Rationale:** Vasodilation occurs with epidural analgesia and anesthesia, which can result in hypotension. The client who is hypotensive after epidural administration should be turned to a left lateral position and have the IV fluid rate increased to increase the circulation to the fetus and increase circulating volume, respectively. Lying supine allows the gravid uterus to place pressure on the aorta and can reduce the circulation to the fetus further. A semi-Fowler's position could worsen the hypotension. Emptying the bladder will not alleviate the hypotension. **Cognitive Level:** Applying **Client Need:** Health Promotion and Maintenance **Integrated Process:** Nursing Process: Implementation **Content Area:** Maternal–Newborn **Strategy:** The issue of the question is the appropriate action that counteracts a side effect of epidural analgesia. Recall that opioid analgesics often cause vasodilation, which can be counteracted by proper positioning.

3 **Answer: 3 Rationale:** Opioid analgesics given for pain relief during labor are most often given by the IV route so that the medication will have a rapid onset and a relatively short half-life. This desired drug profile will provide maternal benefit while preventing neonatal respiratory depression. The IM and oral routes require medication absorption before the drug takes effect and thus have a slower onset of action. The rectal route is not the route of choice for analgesia during labor. **Cognitive Level:** Applying **Client Need:** Health Promotion and Maintenance **Integrated Process:** Nursing Process: Planning **Content Area:** Maternal–Newborn **Strategy:** Use the process of elimination, choosing the route that will work rapidly but that hastens metabolism and excretion for the benefit of the fetus. With this in mind, choose the IV route as the one that works most rapidly and also hastens biotransformation (metabolism) and excretion.

4 **Answer: 2 Rationale:** Women receiving intrathecal opioids for labor analgesia often experience adverse effects of pruritus (itching). An indwelling urinary catheter is routinely used to allow for urinary elimination because of urinary retention caused by opioids. Fetal movement is not affected by intrathecal opioids. Nausea and vomiting are side effects of opioids regardless of the timing of the dose. **Cognitive Level:** Analyzing **Client Need:** Health Promotion and Maintenance **Integrated Process:** Teaching and Learning **Content Area:** Maternal–Newborn **Strategy:** Note the issue of the question, which is knowledge of adverse effects of intrathecal opioids during labor. The word *effective* in the question tells you the correct answer is a true statement.

5 **Answer: 3 Rationale:** Objective signs of pain relief include decreased muscle tension as evidenced by unclenched fists, relaxed facial muscles, and decreased grimacing, frowning, or creasing of the brow. Pain relief would not cause a reduction in short-term variability in fetal heart rate. Pain relief should lead to slightly lower, rather than higher, maternal blood pressure and pulse rate. Frequency of uterine contractions would not be affected by relieving pain through nonpharmacological methods. **Cognitive Level:** Analyzing **Client Need:** Health Promotion and Maintenance **Integrated Process:** Nursing Process: Evaluation **Content Area:** Maternal–Newborn **Strategy:** The issue of the question is a satisfactory outcome of nonpharmacologic methods of pain relief. With this in mind, use knowledge of general signs of pain relief to make your selection. Eliminate short-term variability and contractions first because they are not evidence of pain relief, then eliminate maternal blood pressure and pulse because they would decrease rather than increase with pain relief.

6 **Answer: 4 Rationale:** The pain of labor and childbirth has both physiological and psychological components. Childbirth pain is not limited to a physiological component. A support person's presence has been shown to decrease the perceived pain of childbearing. However, the expression of pain through nonverbal cues or verbalizations is highly culturally based (not universal), having been learned in early childhood. **Cognitive Level:** Applying **Client Need:** Health Promotion and Maintenance **Integrated Process:** Nursing Process: Planning **Content Area:** Maternal–Newborn **Strategy:** Note that two are essentially the opposite of each other. When two options are opposites, often one of them is correct. Choose the more comprehensive option as the correct answer.

7 **Answer: 1 Rationale:** Prolonged latent phase of labor is defined as greater than 20 hours in primigravida women and greater than 14 hours in multigravida women. Encouraging rest and relaxation during this phase will help the client have enough energy to push effectively during the second stage of labor. Music is often used effectively to induce relaxation. Encouraging a well-rested client to ambulate will also facilitate the latent phase. Intravenous hydration is given to women who are unable to take oral fluids. Internal monitoring is indicated if labor is being augmented or induced, the amniotic fluid is meconium-stained, or there is evidence of fetal distress by external monitoring. During the first stage of labor, maternal vital signs are obtained every hour. **Cognitive Level:** Applying **Client Need:** Health Promotion and Maintenance **Integrated Process:** Nursing Process: Planning **Content Area:** Maternal–Newborn **Strategy:** Note the critical word *priority* in the question. This tells you some or all options may be partially or totally correct, but one is most important. First eliminate maternal vital signs every 15 minutes as unnecessary. Then eliminate internal fetal monitoring because external monitoring may be equally effective. Choose correctly between the remaining options because there is no indication that the client cannot tolerate fluids and also because of the words *prolonged latent phase* in the question.

8 **Answer: 4 Rationale:** Late decelerations are caused by uteroplacental insufficiency and are always ominous. To optimize uteroplacental blood flow and therefore fetal oxygenation, the client should be positioned on her left side. The client is not placed in a semi-Fowler's position. Oxygen is appropriate but would be administered via mask at 7–10 liters per minute. A Foley catheter is unrelated to the fetus's needs at this time. **Cognitive Level:** Applying **Client Need:** Health Promotion and Maintenance **Integrated Process:** Nursing Process: Implementation **Content Area:** Maternal–Newborn **Strategy:** Determine what the question is testing, which is uteroplacental insufficiency. With this mind, reposition the client because it is more effective in increasing delivery of oxygen and blood flow to the fetus.

9 **Answer: 4 Rationale:** Normal FHR baseline is 110–160 beats per minute. Normal short-term variability is 6–25 beats per minute. This is a normal FHR tracing and requires continued support and assessment by the nurse. There is no indication to contact the healthcare provider, provide intravenous fluids, or position the client on her hands and knees. **Cognitive Level:** Applying **Client Need:** Health Promotion and Maintenance **Integrated Process:** Nursing Process: Implementation **Content Area:** Maternal–Newborn **Strategy:** The issue of the question is the ability to recognize a normal FHR and variability on fetal monitoring. Recall that a normal fetal heart rate is 110–160 to determine that at least the fetal heart rate is normal. Next, recall that a variability of 12 beats is acceptable to help you choose correctly.

10 **Answer: 4 Rationale:** Variable decelerations are caused by compression of the umbilical cord. The treatment for variable decelerations focuses on relieving the cord compression, which can be accomplished by either infusing saline into the uterus via an intrauterine pressure catheter or by repositioning the client to get the weight of the fetus off the portion of cord that is being compressed. Taking a warm shower would be unlikely to affect fetal heart rate directly. Pregnant women are never placed in a supine position because the fetus will compress the vena cava, thus decreasing uterine blood flow. **Cognitive Level:** Applying **Client Need:** Health Promotion and Maintenance **Integrated Process:** Nursing Process: Implementation **Content Area:** Maternal–Newborn **Strategy:** Specific knowledge of the meaning of variable decelerations is needed to answer this question. Choose an option that could help relieve pressure on the umbilical cord to choose correctly.

11 **Answer: 3 Rationale:** Gradual decelerations that begin and end with contractions are early decelerations and are caused by fetal head compression. Variable decelerations result from umbilical cord compression and are characterized by a sudden drop from baseline during contractions with a sudden return to baseline as the contraction ends. Late decelerations are caused by uteroplacental insufficiency and are characterized by gradual decrease in the fetal heart rate after the contraction begins, and gradual return to baseline after the contraction has ended. Fetal movement usually results in fetal heart rate accelerations. **Cognitive Level:** Applying **Client Need:** Health Promotion and Maintenance **Integrated Process:** Nursing Process: Diagnosis **Content Area:** Maternal–Newborn **Strategy:** Specific knowledge of the relationship between fetal monitoring results and the effect on the fetus is needed to answer this question. Note that the data indicate the changes are occurring during contractions, when the head would be compressed against the lower pelvic structures.

12 **Answer: 2 Rationale:** Delivery appears imminent and priority should be given to the safety of the woman and her newborn. The nurse should apply gloves and prepare for a controlled and attended birth. Another person can be summoned to contact the healthcare provider and perform assessments. The history provides helpful information but should be deferred until a later time in this situation. Assessing maternal vital signs and fetal heart rate are routine activities that can be performed by another nurse or provider; the nurse's priority is the imminent delivery. **Cognitive Level:** Applying **Client Need:** Health Promotion and Maintenance **Integrated Process:** Nursing Process: Implementation **Content Area:** Maternal–Newborn **Strategy:** The situation in the question is urgent and requires immediate action by the nurse. Eliminate options that are assessments, and choose the option that addresses the immediate physiological and safety needs of the mother and fetus.

13 **Answer: 1 Rationale:** The second stage of labor begins when the cervix is completely dilated and pushing begins. Most women make a low-pitched, guttural, grunting sound when they push spontaneously. The nurse should immediately inspect the perineum for bulging and the appearance of the presenting part. If neither of these is occurring, the nurse should perform a vaginal examination to assess for complete dilatation of the cervix. Because delivery is more imminent once the second stage of labor begins, it would be better for the client if the husband does not leave at this time. The focus of the nurse at this time is the client's progress toward delivery, not teaching. There is no specific need to assess blood pressure or temperature at this time. **Cognitive Level:** Applying **Client Need:** Health Promotion and Maintenance **Integrated Process:** Nursing Process: Planning **Content Area:** Maternal–Newborn **Strategy:** The issue of this question is accurate interpretation of onset of the second stage of labor. Knowing that pushing is characteristic of this stage, recall it is important for the husband to be present at this time. Eliminate the option with teaching next because it is not timely. Choose inspection of the perineum as the appropriate assessment because it addresses the status of the fetus during the pushing stage.

14 **Answer: 3 Rationale:** The average duration of the second stage of labor for primigravidas is 2 hours. It is unrealistic for the primigravida client to believe that delivery will occur after two or three pushes. Many women feel rectal pressure, as if they were having a bowel movement, as the baby descends deeper into the pelvis. The use of vacuum extraction or forceps to assist delivery is not routine. **Cognitive Level:** Applying **Client Need:** Health Promotion and Maintenance **Integrated Process:** Teaching and Learning **Content Area:** Maternal–Newborn **Strategy:** The wording of the question indicates that the correct answer is a statement that is true. Use knowledge of the second stage of labor to systematically eliminate each of the incorrect options.

15 **Answer: 4 Rationale:** Although all of the nursing actions presented are important after delivery, clearing the airway of mucus is the highest physiological need and ensures safe adaptation to the extrauterine environment. While drying the newborn is important, it is also important for the newborn to have "skin-to-skin" time with the mother after delivery. While applying identification bracelets and obtaining footprints are important procedures, the newborn's airway takes priority. A gestational age assessment can be conducted once the newborn's airway is attended to. **Cognitive Level:** Applying **Client Need:** Health Promotion and Maintenance **Integrated Process:** Nursing Process: Implementation **Content Area:** Maternal–Newborn **Strategy:** The critical word in the question is *priority*, which indicates that one intervention is more important than the others to be completed first. Recall that physiological needs take priority over psychosocial needs, and make a final selection that addresses the airway.

16 **Answer: 1 Rationale:** The nurse should immediately assess the fetal heart rate to detect changes, which may be associated with prolapse of the umbilical cord. Ambulation is appropriate if the fetal heart is determined to be within normal parameters and the presenting part is engaged. Documentation is important but is not the priority intervention. The membranes may rupture at any time during labor; preparing for delivery may not be indicated at this time. **Cognitive Level:** Analyzing **Client Need:** Health Promotion and Maintenance **Integrated Process:** Nursing Process: Planning **Content Area:** Maternal–Newborn **Strategy:** The critical word in the question is *first*, which indicates that one intervention is more important than the others at this time. Choose the option that protects the fetus after membrane rupture, and recall that this does not mean that delivery is imminent.

17 **Answer: 1, 5 Rationale:** Knowing what culture the client comes from, and how traditional she is with her cultural beliefs and practices, is important to understand, as it may dictate labor and birthing practices that the client will want to follow, as well as the client's response to pain. The expectations of the experience are important in order to try to integrate realistic ones into the labor plan or help to establish realistic ones that can be explored. FHR assessment is not part of the psychosocial assessment. Plans to name the child and the socioeconomic status of the family are not relevant at this time. **Cognitive Level:** Analyzing **Client Need:** Health Promotion and Maintenance **Integrated Process:** Nursing Process: Assessment **Content Area:** Maternal–Newborn **Strategy:** Eliminate naming the child first because this does not directly relate to psychosocial assessment. Eliminate fetal heart rate because it does not focus on psychosocial assessment and socioeconomic status because financial resources do not provide insight into beliefs, practices, or coping strategies at the time of birth.

18 **Answer: 3, 4, 5, 2, 1 Rationale:** In order, the cardinal movements (position changes) of the fetus are engagement, descent, flexion, internal rotation, extension, restitution, external rotation, and expulsion. These movements represent the

normal adaptation of the fetus in a cephalic presentation to the maternal pelvis and facilitate vaginal birth. **Cognitive Level:** Analyzing **Client Need:** Health Promotion and Maintenance **Integrated Process:** Nursing Process: Planning **Content Area:** Maternal–Newborn **Strategy:** Recall the memory aid *Every darn fool in Rotterdam eats rotten egg rolls everyday*. The first letters of each word in the memory aid represent the first letter of each of the cardinal movements of the fetus in a cephalic position.

19 **Answer: 3, 5 Rationale:** Frequent inspection for redness, swelling, tenderness, and hematoma is essential to fourth-stage nursing care. Pain relief begins with immediate application of ice. Ice packs should be applied for 20–30 minutes and removed for at least 20 minutes. If ice is applied for more than 30 minutes, vasodilation and edema may occur. Clients are usually advised to wait until bleeding stops and stitches heal (about 3 weeks) before resuming sexual activity, but this teaching would be part of the client's discharge instructions, and is not appropriate during the fourth stage of labor. **Cognitive Level:** Applying **Client Need:** Health Promotion and Maintenance **Integrated Process:** Nursing Process: Implementation **Content Area:** Maternal–Newborn **Strategy:** The critical issue in this question is time-related. The fourth stage of labor is a time of critical physiologic adaptation and requires frequent assessment. The correct answers are the options that include a true statement about nursing actions at this time.

20 **Answer: 9 Rationale:** Apgar scores are based on 0, 1, or 2 points in each of five categories: respiratory effort, color, muscle tone, heart rate, and reflexes. This neonate would score 2 points in each category except color, where the presence of acrocyanosis would warrant a score of 1 point. **Cognitive Level:** Applying **Client Need:** Health Promotion and Maintenance **Integrated Process:** Nursing Process: Assessment **Content Area:** Maternal–Newborn **Strategy:** Recall that the Apgar score includes 0–2 points on five criteria. The data given in the question include one exception statement, making a perfect score of 10 unlikely and leading you to subtract one point.

21 **Answer: 1, 5 Rationale:** An increase in fetal heart rate baseline can be an indication of fetal distress, as well as maternal fever. Narcotics may decrease the short-term variability but do not affect the baseline. Fetal movement will create an acceleration of the fetal heart rate. Uteroplacental insufficiency causes late decelerations. **Cognitive Level:** Analyzing **Client Need:** Physiological Adaptation **Integrated Process:** Nursing Process: Diagnosis **Content Area:** Maternal–Newborn **Strategy:** Eliminate options that are obviously incorrect; narcotics are CNS depressants, movement temporarily increases heart rate, and uteroplacental insufficiency causes periodic late decelerations.

Key Terms to Review

accelerations p. 112
Apgar score p. 117
attitude p. 113
baseline variability p. 112
cardinal movements p. 116
crowning p. 116
dilatation p. 114
early deceleration p. 112
effacement p. 114
engagement p. 114
epidural block p. 119
episiotomy p. 116
internal fetal scalp electrode p. 112
intrauterine pressure catheter (IUPC) p. 113
late deceleration p. 112
Leopold's maneuvers p. 114
lie p. 113
paracervical block p. 119
position p. 113
presentation p. 113
pudendal block p. 119
station p. 114
variable deceleration p. 112

References

Adams, M., & Urban, C. (2016). *Pharmacology: Connections to nursing practice* (3rd ed.). New York, NY: Pearson Education.

Davidson, M., London, M., & Ladewig, P. (2016). *Olds' maternal newborn nursing and women's health across the lifespan* (10th ed.). New York, NY: Pearson Education.

Kee, J. (2017). *Pearson's handbook of laboratory and diagnostic tests* (8th ed.). New York, NY: Pearson Education.

Ladewig, P., London, M., & Davidson, M. (2014). *Contemporary maternal–newborn nursing care* (8th ed.). Upper Saddle River, NJ: Pearson Education.

London, M., Ladewig, P., Davidson, M., Ball, J., Bindler, R., & Cowen, K. (2014). *Maternal and child nursing care* (4th ed.). Upper Saddle River, NJ: Pearson Education.

Lowdermilk, D., Perry, S., Cashion, M., & Alden, K. (2016). *Maternity and women's health care* (11th ed.). St. Louis, MO: Elsevier.

Uncomplicated Postpartum Assessment and Care

11

In this chapter

Cross Reference

Other chapters relevant to this content area are

Reproduction, Family Planning, and Infertility Chapter 8
Uncomplicated Antenatal Assessment and Care Chapter 9
Uncomplicated Labor and Delivery Care Chapter 10
Uncomplicated Newborn Care Chapter 12
Complicated Antenatal Care Chapter 49
Complicated Labor and Delivery Care Chapter 50
Complicated Postpartum Care Chapter 51
Complicated Newborn Care Chapter 52

I. PHYSICAL CHANGES DURING POSTPARTUM PERIOD

A. *Involution*
1. Reduction in uterine size after delivery to prepregnant size, caused by uterine contractions that constrict and occlude underlying blood vessels at placental site
2. NCLEX® Table 11–1 presents factors that slow or hasten this process during **puerperium**, the 6-week period after delivery

B. *Fundus*
1. Top portion of uterus is a palpable indicator of involution
2. If contractions of uterine muscle are interrupted, a **boggy uterus** (one that is soft, relaxed) results and is likely to cause hemorrhage

C. Lochia
1. NCLEX® Discharge of blood and debris after delivery; types include **lochia rubra**, **lochia serosa**, and **lochia alba**
2. Characteristics of lochia are shown in Table 11–2
3. Should not contain large clots
4. Total volume is 240–270 mL, and daily volume gradually decreases
5. NCLEX® Amount may be increased by exertion or breastfeeding
6. Pooling in uterus or vagina may occur while reclining, causing increased bleeding upon arising
7. NCLEX® Unexplained increase in amount or reappearance of lochia rubra is abnormal

Table 11–1 Factors That Influence Involution

Factors That Enhance Involution	Factors That Slow Involution
Uncomplicated labor and delivery	Prolonged labor and difficult delivery
Breastfeeding	Anesthesia
Early ambulation	Grand multiparity
Complete expulsion of placenta and membranes	Retained placental fragments or membranes
	Full urinary bladder
	Overdistention or infection of the uterus

D. *Afterpains*

NCLEX®

1. Caused by intermittent uterine contractions following delivery
2. Occur in all women but are more painful in multiparous and breastfeeding women

E. Cervix

1. Soft, irregular, and edematous; may appear bruised with multiple small lacerations
2. Closes to 2–3 cm after several days, admits a fingertip after 1 week
3. Shape permanently changes after first delivery from round, dimple-like os of nullipara to lateral slit-like os of multiparous woman

F. Vagina

1. Smooth walls, edematous with multiple small lacerations; muscle tone never fully returns to pre-pregnant state
2. Client should be free from perineal pain within 2 weeks

NCLEX®

3. Low estrogen levels postpartum lead to decreased vaginal lubrication and vasocongestion for 6–10 weeks, which can result in painful intercourse

G. Abdominal wall

1. Abdominal wall soft and flabby with decreased muscle tone
2. Striae, or stretch marks, that were red during pregnancy will fade to silver or white in Caucasian women; darker-skinned women will have darker striae
3. **Diastasis recti**, separation of rectus muscles of abdomen, may improve postpartum depending on physical condition, number of pregnancies, and type and amount of exercise

H. Breasts

1. Colostrum is secreted up to 72 hours postdelivery
2. Estrogen and progesterone levels drop after delivery, stimulating secretion of prolactin, which stimulates milk production in breasts
3. Milk production leads to breast distention on or about third postpartum day
4. Milk production can lead to breast engorgement in breastfeeding and bottle-feeding mothers by fourth postpartum day; usually resolves in 24–36 hours
5. Breastfeeding relieves engorgement; nonbreastfeeding mothers can relieve engorgement by avoiding nipple stimulation and by use of breast binder, snug-fitting bra, ice packs, and mild analgesics

Table 11–2 Characteristics of Lochia

Type	Occurrence	Appearance	Composition
Lochia rubra	1–3 days	Dark red, bloody; fleshy, musty, stale odor that is nonoffensive; may have clots smaller than a nickel	Blood with small amounts of mucus, shreds of decidua, epithelial cells, leukocytes; may contain fetal meconium, lanugo, or vernix caseosa
Lochia serosa	4–10 days	Pink or brownish; watery; odorless	Serum, erythrocytes, shreds of degenerating decidua, leukocytes, cervical mucus, numerous bacteria
Lochia alba	11–21 days, up to 6 weeks if lactating	Yellow to white; may have slightly stale odor	Leukocytes, decidual cells, epithelial cells, fat, cervical mucus, cholesterol, bacteria

I. Cardiovascular

1. Returns to prepregnant state within 2 weeks
2. The 40% increase in blood volume during pregnancy is lost primarily by diuresis
3. NCLEX® First 48 hours postpartum pose greatest risk of complications for clients with heart disease
4. Blood pressure should remain consistent with pregnancy baseline
5. Bradycardia of 50–70 beats per minute is common during first 6–10 days; tachycardia would occur with increased blood loss, temperature elevation, or difficult, prolonged labor and birth
6. Increased fibrinogen continues for 1 week with increased erythrocyte sedimentation rate (ESR) and risk for thrombophlebitis
7. NCLEX® Increased white blood cells (WBCs) up to 30,000/mm^3 does not necessarily mean infection or may indicate a masked infection; an increase of more than 30% in 6 hours indicates pathology
8. Decreased hemoglobin is related to amount of blood lost during delivery; should return to prelabor value in 2–6 weeks depending on degree of decrease
9. Hematocrit increases by third to fifth day postpartum related to diuresis; a drop indicates abnormal blood loss

J. Urinary

1. Increased bladder capacity and decreased bladder tone lead to decreased sensation and increased risk of urinary retention and infection
2. NCLEX® Postpartum diuresis of 2–3 L increases output in first 12–24 hours after delivery and accounts for a 2.3-kg (5-lb) weight loss
3. Increased glomerular filtration rate assists in diuresis
4. NCLEX® A full bladder displaces uterus, increasing risk of uterine atony and postpartum hemorrhage
5. Fluids are also lost through diaphoresis, with increased perspiration most commonly occurring at night

K. Gastrointestinal

1. Hunger and thirst are common following birth
2. NCLEX® Risk for constipation increases because of decreased peristalsis, use of opioid analgesics, dehydration and decreased mobility during labor, and fear of pain with defecation
3. Risk for hemorrhoids increases due to pressure from pushing during second stage of labor

L. Endocrine

1. Estrogen and progesterone levels drop rapidly after delivery of placenta
2. Menstruation usually resumes at 7–9 weeks for nonlactating women, with 90% experiencing a menstrual period by 12 weeks; first cycle is usually anovulatory
3. NCLEX® Ovulation and menstruation return time is prolonged in lactating women and affected by length of time the woman breastfeeds and whether formula supplements are used; may vary from 2 to 18 months
4. Lactation
   a. Nipple stimulation leads to oxytocin release from pituitary gland; this stimulates release of prolactin from pituitary gland, which causes production of milk and the **let-down reflex**, release of milk by contractions of alveoli of breast
   b. **Colostrum** is first milk secreted and is rich in protein and immunoglobulins
   c. NCLEX® Primary **engorgement** occurs on second or third day as supply of blood and lymph in the breast is increased and transitional milk is produced
   d. NCLEX® Mature milk is produced after 2 weeks and appears watery and slightly bluish in color, similar to skim milk

II. PSYCHOSOCIAL CHANGES DURING POSTPARTUM PERIOD

A. Phases of maternal adjustment

1. Taking-in phase: first 3 days postpartum; needs to discuss labor and delivery; preoccupied with own needs; passive and dependent; touches and explores infant
2. Taking-hold phase: third to tenth day postpartum: obsessed with body functions; rapid mood swings; anticipatory guidance most effective now
3. Letting-go phase: 10 days to 6 weeks postpartum; mothering functions established; sees infant as a unique person

NCLEX® **B. *Bonding* (also known as attachment)**

1. Process by which parents form an emotional relationship with their infant over time
2. Mother explores infant first with fingertips, then palms, and finally enfolding newborn with whole hands and arms

3. Holds infant in **en face** position, face-to-face position, about 20 cm apart and on same plane
4. Uses a soft, high-pitched tone of voice
5. **Engrossment** is father's absorption, preoccupation, and interest in infant shortly after birth, which can be stimulated by witnessing birth

NCLEX® C. ***Postpartum blues***: a maternal adjustment reaction
1. Transient depression usually occurs between second and third postpartum days and/or within first 2 weeks' postpartum
2. Probably related to changes in hormone levels, fatigue, and psychological stress related to infant dependency
3. Experienced to some degree by a majority of women
4. Characterized by mood swings, anger, tearfulness, feeling let down, anorexia, and insomnia
5. Usually resolves spontaneously; may need evaluation for postpartum depression if symptoms persist or are severe

III. NURSING CARE OF POSTPARTUM CLIENT

A. General considerations with postpartum assessment
1. Evaluate prenatal and intrapartal history for risk factors
2. Provide privacy and encourage client to void prior to assessment
3. Position client in bed with head flat for most accurate findings (NCLEX®)
4. Proceed in a head-to-toe direction
5. Measure vital signs with woman at rest for better accuracy; will determine need or priority for other assessments
   a. Temperature: above 100.4°F (38°C) after first 24 hours may indicate an infection; may be elevated initially after delivery related to dehydration (NCLEX®)
   b. Pulse: normal range postpartum is 50–80 beats per minute; report a rate greater than 100 to healthcare provider (NCLEX®)
   c. Respirations: normal range is 16–24 breaths/min
   d. Blood pressure: assess for orthostatic hypotension; monitor more closely if client has a history of preeclampsia (NCLEX®)
6. Women who experience operative procedures, cesarean delivery, or tubal ligation have postpartum needs similar to those with vaginal births and of postoperative clients; monitor breath sounds and have client cough and breathe deeply

B. Postpartum assessment: use memory aids to remember nine components of assessment
1. Breasts
   a. Determine if mother is breast- or bottle-feeding
   b. Palpate for engorgement or tenderness
   c. Inspect nipples for redness, cracks, and erectility if nursing
2. Uterus (see Figure 11–1)
   a. Gently place nondominant hand on lower uterine segment just above symphysis pubis; dominant hand palpates top of fundus
   b. Determine uterine firmness, height of fundus, and position of fundus in relation to midline of abdomen (NCLEX®)
   c. Correlate fundal location with expected descent of 1 cm each postpartum day
   d. Inspect any abdominal incisions (cesarean delivery or tubal ligation) for REEDA: redness, edema, ecchymosis, discharge, and approximation of skin edges (NCLEX®)

Memory Aid

Use the mnemonic BUBBLE-HEB to aid in remembering the nine components of postpartum assessment:

B—Breasts
U—Uterus
B—Bladder
B—Bowel
L—Lochia
E—Episiotomy or perineal lacerations
H—Homans sign
E—Emotional status
B—Bonding

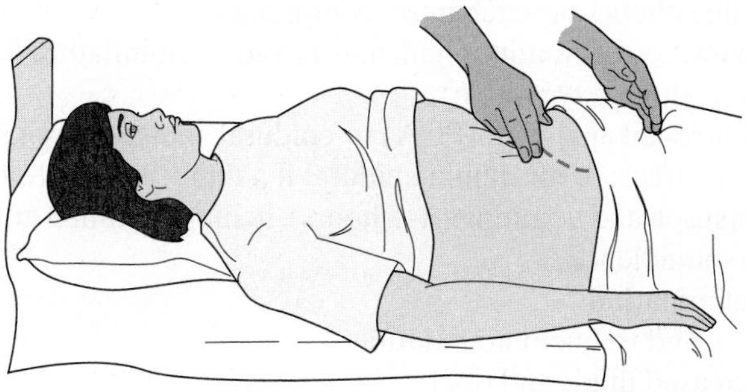

Figure 11–1
Measuring the descent of the fundus.

Memory Aid

Use the mnemonic REEDA to remember components of episiotomy/wound assessment:
R—Redness
E—Edema
E—Ecchymosis
D—Discharge
A—Approximation of skin edges

3. Bladder
   NCLEX®
   a. Client should void within 6–8 hours after delivery
   b. Assess frequency, burning, or urgency (could indicate urinary tract infection)
   c. Evaluate ability to completely empty bladder
   d. Palpate for bladder distention if questionable ability to void or completely empty bladder
4. Bowel
   a. Assess for passage of flatus
   b. Inspect for distention
   c. Auscultate bowel sounds in all four quadrants for postoperative clients
5. Lochia *NCLEX®*
   a. Inspect type, quantity, amount, and odor
   b. Correlate findings with expected characteristics of bleeding
   c. Cesarean-delivered women may have less lochia
6. Episiotomy or perineal lacerations *NCLEX®*
   a. Inspect perineum for REEDA (redness, edema, ecchymosis, discharge, approximation of skin edges)
   b. Inspect for hemorrhoids
7. **Homans sign**
   NCLEX®
   a. Pain in calf when client dorsiflexes foot is a positive sign and may indicate thrombophlebitis
   b. Inspect for pedal edema, redness, or warmth; if abnormal changes are present, assess pedal pulse
8. Emotional status
   a. Assess whether emotions are appropriate for situation
   b. Determine phase of postpartum psychological adjustment
   c. Assess for signs of postpartum blues
9. Bonding: describe how parents interact with infant

C. Collaborative management

1. Prevent hemorrhage
   a. Assess for risk factors
   b. Keep bladder empty
   NCLEX®
   c. Gently massage fundus if boggy; teach self-massage of uterus
   d. Administer oxytocic medications if ordered: oxytocin, methylergonovine maleate, ergonovine maleate
   e. Monitor for side effects of oxytocics if administered; hypotension with rapid IV bolus of oxytocin, hypertension with methylergonovine and ergonovine
2. Promote comfort
   NCLEX®
   a. Apply ice to perineum 20 min on/10 min off for first 24 hours
   NCLEX®
   b. Encourage sitz bath, warm or cool, three times a day and prn (as needed) after first 12–24 hours
   NCLEX®
   c. Teach client to perform perineal care after every elimination: squirt or pour warm water over perineum; blot dry from front to back to prevent tissue trauma and contamination from anal area; apply clean perineal pad from front to back without touching surface in contact with client
   d. Teach client to tighten buttocks, then sit and relax muscles

e. Apply topical anesthetics or witch hazel compresses
f. Administer analgesics; acetaminophen, nonsteroidal antiinflammatory agents (ibuprofen), opioids (codeine, hydrocodone, oxycodone)
g. Use patient-controlled analgesia (PCA) or epidural analgesia as needed for cesarean births
NCLEX® h. Monitor for side effects of morphine epidural if administered: late-onset respiratory depression (8–12 hours), nausea and vomiting (4–7 hours), itching (within 3 and up to 10 hours), urinary retention, and somnolence

NCLEX® 3. Promote bowel elimination
a. Encourage early and frequent ambulation
b. Encourage increased fluids and fiber
c. Administer stool softeners as ordered; suppositories are contraindicated if client has a third- or fourth-degree perineal laceration involving rectum
d. Teach client to avoid straining; normal bowel pattern returns in 2–3 weeks

4. Urinary elimination
a. Encourage voiding every 2–3 hours even if no urge is felt
b. Catheterize as ordered for urinary retention; indwelling urinary catheter for 12–24 hours after cesarean delivery

5. Promote successful establishment of lactation and breastfeeding if desired
a. Utilize well-fitting bra for continuous support of breasts
b. Teach breast care, including no use of soap and air-drying nipples after feedings
NCLEX® c. Encourage nursing on demand every 2–4 hours, awakening infant during day and allowing to sleep at night
NCLEX® d. Advise mother to nurse 10–15 minutes on first breast and until infant lets go of second; alternate breast used first and rotate positions
e. Suggest football hold or side-lying position for mothers with cesarean delivery or tubal ligation to avoid discomfort caused by weight of infant on abdominal incision
f. Provide help with positioning, latching on, and breaking suction after nursing, especially with multiple births

6. Promote successful suppression of lactation and successful bottle-feeding
a. Utilize snug bra or breast binder continuously for 5–7 days to prevent engorgement
b. Avoid heat and stimulation of breasts
c. Apply ice packs for 20 min four times a day if engorgement occurs
NCLEX® d. Encourage demand feedings every 3–4 hours, awakening infant during day and allowing to sleep at night

7. Explore impact of culture on feeding practices and support family choices as illustrated in Table 11–3
a. Amount of contact and degree of closeness between mother and newborn is often culturally determined
b. Culture may influence how long breastfeeding continues
c. Feeding practices vary across cultures

8. Promote rest and gradual return to activity
a. Organize nursing care to avoid frequent interruptions
b. Plan maternal rest periods when infant is expected to sleep
c. Teach client to resume activity gradually over 4–5 weeks; avoid lifting, stair-climbing, and strenuous activity
d. Encourage simple postpartum exercises, per orders, to strengthen muscles affected by childbearing; Kegel exercises tighten perineum by alternately stopping and starting flow of urine; strengthen abdomen by raising chin to chest while on back and by doing knee rolls and buttocks lifts
e. Increased lochia or pain indicates overexertion; modify exercise plan

Table 11–3 Cultural Influences on Infant Feeding

Cultural Group	Infant Feeding Practice
North American and European	Exposing the breast is indecent; weaning is a sign of infant development
Hmong (southeast Asian)	Breast- and bottle-feeding may be combined; expressing or pumping breast milk is unacceptable
Mexican American, Filipino, Navajo, Vietnamese	Colostrum is not offered to newborn
African American	Plentiful feeding is emphasized; solids are introduced early
Muslim	Breastfeeding is encouraged to 2 years of age

NCLEX®

9. Promote adequate nutritional intake
   a. Encourage lactating mothers to add 500 kcal/day to prepregnancy diet; bottle-feeding mothers should return to prepregnancy diet
   b. Encourage fluid intake of 2,000 mL/day
   c. Continue administration of prenatal vitamins and iron, as ordered; iron is best absorbed in presence of vitamin C and may increase constipation

10. Promote psychological well-being
   a. Plan nursing care based on phase of psychological adjustment and degree of dependence/independence; provide choices whenever possible
   b. Encourage and support expression of feelings, positive and negative, without guilt
   c. Encourage client to tell story of her labor and birth to integrate expectations and fantasies with reality
   NCLEX® **d.** Provide recognition and praise for self- and infant-care activities

11. Promote family well-being
   a. Provide an environment that supports family unity and promotes attachment to newborn
   NCLEX® **b.** Encourage rooming-in, presence of family members
   c. Assist parents in preparing siblings with realistic expectations of newborn; involve siblings in infant care
   d. Teach parents that sibling regression is common
   NCLEX® **e.** Advise couple to resume sexual activity after episiotomy has healed and lochia has stopped, about 3 weeks after delivery; level of sexual interest and activity may vary, additional water-soluble lubrication may be needed, and breast milk may be released with orgasm
   f. Counsel couples regarding contraception before discharge, assist couple to select a method compatible with health needs and individual preferences; a diaphragm or cervical cap must be refitted after delivery; oral contraceptives containing estrogen may interfere with lactation

NCLEX® **12.** Give $Rh_0(D)$ gamma globulin if needed to prevent Rh sensitization and future hemolytic disease of newborn
   a. Confirm woman is a candidate: Rh-negative mother not sensitized (negative indirect Coombs test), Rh-positive newborn not sensitized (negative direct Coombs test), and no known maternal allergy to globulin preparations
   b. Administer 300 mcg IM within 72 hours of delivery

NCLEX® **13.** Give rubella vaccine to provide active immunity for mother and avoid fetal malformations if disease is contracted during a future pregnancy
   a. Confirm woman is a candidate: titer of less than 1:8 (not immune); no known allergy to neomycin
   b. Administer 0.5 mL subcutaneously prior to discharge
   c. If woman is a candidate for both $Rh_0(D)$ gamma globulin and rubella vaccine, delay rubella vaccine at least 6 weeks, and preferably 3 months, to avoid drug interaction and reduced rubella immunity
   d. Teach client to avoid pregnancy for at least 3 months following vaccination; vaccine contains live virus and can adversely affect fetus; side effects include burning and stinging at injection site, warmth and redness, mild symptoms of disease

NCLEX® **14.** Teach client postpartum warning signs to report
   a. Bright red bleeding saturating more than one pad per hour or passing large clots
   b. Temperature greater than 100.4°F (38°C)
   c. Chills
   d. Excessive pain
   e. Reddened or warm areas of breast
   f. Reddened or gaping episiotomy, foul-smelling lochia
   g. Inability to urinate; burning, frequency, or urgency with urination
   h. Calf pain, tenderness, redness, or swelling

Check Your NCLEX–RN® Exam I.Q.

You are ready for testing on this content if you can:

- Perform a postpartum assessment.
- Assess the client for postpartum complications.
- Perform postpartum care.
- Provide postpartum discharge instructions.
- Incorporate cultural considerations into postpartum care.

PRACTICE TEST

PRACTICE TEST

1. A goal on the nursing care plan is "to facilitate parent–infant bonding." Which nursing intervention should take priority in order to attain this goal?
   1. Provide assistance and encouragement with rooming-in.
   2. Encourage the parents to join a new parent support group.
   3. Keep the newborn in the nursery at night to allow the parents to rest.
   4. Teach the parents infant-care skills to increase their confidence.

2. A postpartum client who delivered 3 hours ago states, "I feel all wet underneath." What should be the initial action of the nurse?
   1. Determine when she last voided.
   2. Ask the client to rate her discomfort on a 0–10 scale.
   3. Perform perineal care.
   4. Have the client roll over to assess her lochia flow.

3. After delivering a 4355-gram (9-lb, 10-oz) baby, a client who is a gravida 5, para 5 is admitted to the postpartum unit. What should be a priority in delivering nursing care to this client?

   ↑gravida ↑bb size = atony

   1. Palpate the fundus because she is at risk for uterine atony.
   2. Offer fluids, since multiparas generally dehydrate faster during labor.
   3. Perform passive range of motion on extremities because she is at risk for thromboembolism.
   4. Assess client's diet because she is at risk for anemia.

4. Although a client initially wanted to breastfeed, she has now decided to bottle-feed her newborn. The nurse concludes that teaching about breast care for this client has been effective when the client makes which statement?
   1. "I'll pump two to three times each day until my milk supply decreases."
   2. "I'll rub lotion on my breasts if they are sore."
   3. "I'll soak my breasts in a warm tub twice daily for the first week."
   4. "I'll wear a snug bra continuously until my breasts are soft again."

5. When teaching a new mother how to breastfeed, the nurse should include which instruction?
   1. Wash the nipples with soap and water twice daily.
   2. Begin nursing with the right breast at each feeding.
   3. Slide a finger into the baby's mouth to break suction before removing from the breast.
   4. Supplement the baby with formula every 12 hours until the milk supply is established.

6. The nurse is caring for an Rh-negative client who delivered vaginally 2 hours ago. The client's fundus is firm at 1 centimeter below the umbilicus and vital signs are stable. She received morphine IV 4 hours ago for labor pain. The nurse should question which new prescription from the healthcare provider?
   1. Sitz bath 20 minutes TID
   2. Bathroom privileges
   3. Regular diet
   4. $Rh_0(D)$ gamma globulin

7. The nurse should notify the healthcare provider immediately of which assessment finding?
   1. Three pea-sized clots passed 4 hours after delivery
   2. Musty odor to lochia 48 hours postpartum
   3. Scant amount of rubra lochia after cesarean delivery
   4. Firm uterus with steady trickle of blood 2 hours after delivery

8. Three hours after a vaginal delivery, the client reports increased perineal pain. What should the nurse do first?
   1. Assess the perineum
   2. Administer analgesia as ordered
   3. Apply ice to the perineum
   4. Perform perineal care

9 The nurse notes that the postpartum client is Rh-negative and her baby is Rh-positive. Which maternal laboratory result should the nurse review next in determining if the client is a candidate for $Rh_0(D)$ gamma globulin?

1. Hemoglobin
2. Direct Coombs' test
3. Indirect Coombs' test
4. Bilirubin

10 A postpartum client's hemoglobin is 9.2 mg/dL after delivery, and she has been instructed to take an iron supplement at home. The nurse should include which instruction when teaching the client about this medication?

1. Call the healthcare provider if your stools become black.
2. Take your iron with a glass of orange juice.
3. Don't drive a car while taking this medication.
4. Diarrhea is a common side effect of iron pills.

11 The nurse is teaching a new mother how to breastfeed her infant. Which intervention should be included in the teaching plan?

1. Place pillows under the baby's buttocks to elevate the hips while nursing.
2. Reposition the baby with the hips rotated away from the mother's abdomen.
3. Encourage the mother to use the football hold exclusively.
4. Provide positive feedback to the mother for correctly positioning the infant at the breast.

12 A new mother calls the clinic 4 days after delivery. She is breastfeeding and is concerned that her baby is not getting enough milk. What is the most important question for the nurse to ask this mother?

1. "How many wet diapers has your baby had in the last 24 hours?"
2. "Do you have any red or tender areas on the breasts?"
3. "Are your nipples sore or bleeding?"
4. "Do your breasts tingle when you begin nursing?"

13 A nurse is teaching a new mother how to care for herself after delivery. Which statement should the nurse make during this discussion?

1. "Call your healthcare provider if you experience night sweats."
2. "Wait 1 week before resuming sexual intercourse."
3. "Change your perineal pad twice daily."
4. "Your diaphragm will need to be refitted."

14 A postpartum client's hemoglobin is 10.5 mg/dL. The nurse should encourage the client to include which food item in her diet?

1. Whole-wheat bread
2. Red meat
3. Yellow vegetables
4. Skim milk

15 A postpartum client asks the nurse how to strengthen her perineal muscles. The nurse teaches the client which strengthening technique?

1. Try to start and stop the flow of urine.
2. Bear down as though having a bowel movement.
3. Gently squeeze the uterus while pushing downward on the fundus.
4. Straighten the leg and point the toes toward the head.

16 In planning care for a postpartum client who delivered 2 days ago, the nurse should expect the client to do which of the following?

1. Ask questions about infant care.
2. Hesitate in making decisions.
3. Need help with hygiene and ambulation.
4. Request the baby be fed in the nursery at night.

17 What interventions should be included in the care plan when caring for a client who has a midline episiotomy with a third-degree laceration? Select all that apply.

1. Increase fiber in diet.
2. Administer bisacodyl suppository prn.
3. Increase fluid intake.
4. Administer an oral stool softener.
5. Administer an enema.

18 The nurse palpates the uterus of a client immediately after delivery. Where does the nurse expect to feel the fundus? Draw an "X" in the correct area on the image shown.

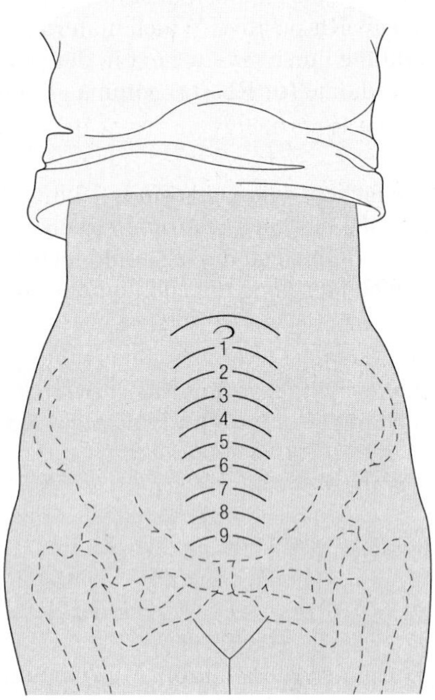

19 The nurse is preparing to instruct a new mother on resuming sexual intercourse postpartum. What items should the nurse include in the teaching plan? Select all that apply.

1. Use petroleum jelly for vaginal lubrication.
2. An intrauterine device (IUD) is appropriate for birth control in the early postpartum period.
3. Wait until episiotomy has healed and lochia has stopped before resuming intercourse.
4. Refrain from intercourse until first menstrual period after delivery is completed.
5. A water-soluble lubricant may be used if necessary.

20 The nurse is caring for a client who has decided not to breastfeed. What elements should the nurse include in client teaching to promote suppression of lactation? Select all that apply.

1. Applying warm compresses
2. Pumping the breasts
3. Applying ice bags
4. Using medication to suppress lactation
5. Binding the breasts, either with a snug bra or binder

ANSWERS & RATIONALES

1 **Answer: 1 Rationale:** Bonding occurs best when parents have direct and prolonged contact with their newborn in a supportive environment. There is not enough information to know whether the client may benefit from a new parent support group. Keeping the newborn in the nursery at night does allow the parents to rest but does not facilitate bonding. Teaching infant-care skills is an important part of care but does not facilitate bonding. **Cognitive Level:** Applying **Client Need:** Health Promotion and Maintenance **Integrated Process:** Nursing Process: Implementation **Content Area:** Maternal–Newborn **Strategy:** The word *priority* in the question indicates that more than one or all options may be partially or totally correct. Identify the critical issue as parent–infant bonding. Compare each option in terms of its ability to stimulate attachment, and then use the process of elimination to make a final selection.

2 **Answer: 4 Rationale:** It is possible that a significant amount of lochia could pool beneath the client after delivery. The highest priority at this time is risk for hemorrhage, and this should be the initial assessment. Assessing time of last voiding and perineal care could then follow. Rating discomfort is irrelevant to the question as stated. **Cognitive Level:** Analyzing **Client Need:** Health Promotion and Maintenance **Integrated Process:** Nursing Process: Assessment **Content Area:** Maternal–Newborn **Strategy:** The critical word *initial* in the question indicates that more than one or all actions are potentially correct, but one is better than the others. Focus on the ABCs (airway, breathing, and circulation) and on risk of hemorrhage to make your selection.

3 **Answer: 1 Rationale:** Uterine atony is the most common cause of early postpartum hemorrhage. This client is at greater risk for hemorrhage because she had an overdistended uterus with a large baby, and she is a grand multipara. Parity does not influence dehydration. The client may be at risk for thromboembolism, but there is no indication passive range of motion should be implemented rather than early ambulation. Nutritional assessment is important, but there is no indication the client is anemic and this action is not the priority for the client. **Cognitive Level:** Applying **Client Need:** Health Promotion and Maintenance **Integrated Process:** Nursing Process: Implementation **Content Area:** Maternal–Newborn **Strategy:** The critical word *priority* in the question indicates that more than one or all actions are potentially correct, but one is better than the others. Consider that the core issue of the question is uterine atony and associated risk of hemorrhage. Then focus on the ABCs (airway, breathing, and circulation) and on the risk of hemorrhage to make your selection.

4 **Answer: 4 Rationale:** Mothers who are bottle-feeding should be encouraged to suppress milk production by wearing a snug bra or breast binder, applying cold compresses, and avoiding breast stimulation until primary engorgement subsides. Pumping the breasts and applying lotion to them are forms of breast stimulation that should be avoided. Applying heat via a warm bath will also stimulate the breasts and should not be done. **Cognitive Level:** Analyzing **Client Need:** Health Promotion and Maintenance **Integrated Process:** Nursing Process: Evaluation **Content Area:** Maternal–Newborn **Strategy:** The core issue of the question is measures that will reduce breast stimulation and milk production. With this in mind, eliminate options that contain mechanical or thermal stimulants.

5 **Answer: 3 Rationale:** It is important for a breastfeeding mother to break the infant's suction on the nipple before removing the baby from the breast. This will help prevent the nipples from becoming sore and the skin from cracking. The nipples should be cleansed with water after each feeding, but soaps can be harsh or irritating. The client should alternate between the right and left breasts for first use at each feeding. Milk production and supply is enhanced when no supplementation is used. **Cognitive Level:** Applying **Client Need:** Health Promotion and Maintenance **Integrated Process:** Nursing Process: Implementation **Content Area:** Maternal–Newborn **Strategy:** The wording of the question indicates that there is one clearly correct answer. Use nursing knowledge to systematically eliminate each incorrect option based on appropriate breastfeeding techniques.

6 **Answer: 1 Rationale:** Application of heat (sitz bath) to the perineum 2 hours after delivery will cause vasodilation and increase the client's risk of edema and hematoma formation. Instead, ice should be applied for the first 24 hours. The client may have bathroom privileges. The client should be allowed to eat a regular diet. An Rh-negative mother would need $Rh_0(D)$ gamma globulin after delivery. Other interventions presented are appropriate. **Cognitive Level:** Analyzing **Client Need:** Health Promotion and Maintenance **Integrated Process:** Nursing Process: Implementation **Content Area:** Maternal–Newborn **Strategy:** The core issue of the question is knowledge of the effects of heat and cold on a client who is newly postpartum. Note the critical word *question*, which tells you the correct answer is an incorrect item. Eliminate each item that is an acceptable part of care and choose the option that increases the client's risk through application of heat instead of cold.

7 **Answer: 4 Rationale:** A steady trickle of blood in the presence of a firm uterus could indicate the presence of a vaginal or cervical laceration. The healthcare provider should be notified immediately so further evaluation can be initiated. There is no cause for concern about three pea-sized clots passed 4 hours after delivery; they are small in size and number. Lochia is expected to have a musty odor 48 hours after delivery. A scant amount of rubra lochia after cesarean delivery is no cause for concern. **Cognitive Level:** Analyzing **Client Need:** Health Promotion and Maintenance **Integrated Process:** Nursing Process: Diagnosis **Content Area:** Maternal–Newborn **Strategy:** The critical words *notify . . . immediately* indicate the correct answer is an abnormal finding. Use nursing knowledge and the process of elimination to make a selection. The words *steady trickle of blood* are also a strong clue that this is the correct answer.

8 **Answer: 1 Rationale:** Increased perineal pain in a client with a vaginal delivery could be normal as anesthetics wear off or could indicate a problem, such as development of a hematoma. Assessment of this client is needed prior to intervention. Analgesics may be needed once the nurse has conducted an assessment of the client. Ice tends to reduce swelling and promote comfort, but the nurse should assess the client first. Performing perineal care is a routine measure that does not address the client's discomfort. **Cognitive Level:** Analyzing **Client Need:** Health Promotion and Maintenance **Integrated Process:** Nursing Process: Assessment **Content Area:** Maternal–Newborn **Strategy:** Analyze the question to determine that there is not enough information to guide nursing intervention. When more information is needed, an option that provides for further assessment is a good choice.

9 **Answer: 3 Rationale:** An indirect Coombs' test assesses for the presence of Rh antibodies in the maternal blood. Direct Coombs' test and bilirubin tests are conducted on the newborn. Hemoglobin is not a determinant for the administration of $Rh_0(D)$ gamma globulin. **Cognitive Level:** Analyzing **Client Need:** Health Promotion and Maintenance **Integrated Process:** Nursing Process: Diagnosis **Content Area:** Maternal–Newborn **Strategy:** The core issue of the question is the effect of an Rh-positive newborn on an Rh-negative mother. Use nursing knowledge to select the laboratory test that will directly evaluate the mother rather than the newborn.

10 **Answer: 2 Rationale:** Iron absorption is enhanced when taken with vitamin C, and orange juice is a good source of vitamin C. Darker-colored stools is a common side effect of iron. Constipation (not diarrhea) can be a side effect of iron administration. Iron should not cause impaired judgment or dizziness that would impair safety while driving. **Cognitive Level:** Applying **Client Need:** Health Promotion and Maintenance **Integrated Process:** Nursing Process: Implementation **Content Area:** Maternal–Newborn **Strategy:** The core issue of the question is knowledge of administration and effects of iron as a supplement. Use the process of elimination and knowledge of basic mineral supplements to make the selection.

11 **Answer: 4 Rationale:** The baby should be positioned with the head midline and with the abdomen toward the mother's abdomen. Positive reinforcement will facilitate the development of maternal competence and confidence in infant care. It is not appropriate to place pillows under the baby's buttocks to elevate the hips while nursing. The infant's hips should not be rotated away from the mother for feeding. There is no reason to use one position, such as the football hold, exclusively. **Cognitive Level:** Applying **Client Need:** Health Promotion and Maintenance **Integrated Process:** Nursing Process: Planning **Content Area:** Maternal–Newborn **Strategy:** The core issue of this question is proper breastfeeding techniques. Use factual

information to systematically eliminate each incorrect option. The wording of the question tells you that only one option contains a true statement.

12 **Answer: 1 Rationale:** Once the mother's milk comes in, typically after the third postpartum day, breastfed babies should have six to eight wet diapers each day. This would indicate the baby is getting enough milk. The other options address the mother, not the intake of the newborn. Red, tender areas on the breasts could make breastfeeding uncomfortable for the mother, but this assessment does not focus on the newborn's status. Sore, bleeding nipples can contribute to infection such as mastitis. Tingling is often used to describe the feeling mothers experience with the letdown reflex. **Cognitive Level:** Analyzing **Client Need:** Health Promotion and Maintenance **Integrated Process:** Nursing Process: Assessment **Content Area:** Maternal–Newborn **Strategy:** Analyze the question and determine that the core issue is how to evaluate whether an infant is getting sufficient milk intake while breastfeeding. Then systematically eliminate any option that focuses on the mother instead of the infant.

13 **Answer: 4 Rationale:** Diaphragms need to be refitted after each delivery and a change in body weight of greater than 4.5–6.8 kg (10–15 lb). Night sweats are common and need not be reported. Sexual intercourse can be safely resumed once the episiotomy is healed and the lochia stops in about 3 weeks. Perineal pads should be changed after each elimination. **Cognitive Level:** Applying **Client Need:** Health Promotion and Maintenance **Integrated Process:** Communication and Documentation **Content Area:** Maternal–Newborn **Strategy:** The core issue of this question is self-care and self-management following delivery. The wording of the question indicates the correct answer is a true statement. Use nursing knowledge to systematically eliminate each incorrect option.

14 **Answer: 2 Rationale:** A hemoglobin level of 10.5 is low and indicates anemia. Because of this, the client should eat foods high in iron, such as red meat. Whole-wheat bread is a good source of fiber, which helps prevent constipation. Yellow vegetables are rich in vitamins and are part of an overall healthy diet. Skim milk is low in fat, but is not rich in iron. **Cognitive Level:** Analyzing **Client Need:** Health Promotion and Maintenance **Integrated Process:** Nursing Process: Implementation **Content Area:** Maternal–Newborn **Strategy:** The core issues of the question are laboratory indicators of anemia and dietary treatment. Knowledge of both concepts is needed to answer the question. As a strategy, however, recall that hemoglobin contains iron; use this knowledge to make a dietary selection from the options presented.

15 **Answer: 1 Rationale:** Kegel exercises are designed to strengthen the muscles of the perineum. By alternately tensing and releasing the muscles of the perineum, as if to start and stop the flow of urine, muscle tone and strength are enhanced. Bearing down is the opposite type of exercise for this set of muscles. Squeezing the uterus while pushing on the fundus and straightening the leg and pointing the toes toward the head are incorrect statements of technique. **Cognitive Level:** Applying **Client Need:** Health Promotion and Maintenance **Integrated Process:** Nursing Process: Implementation **Content Area:** Maternal–Newborn **Strategy:** The core issue of the question is specific knowledge of Kegel exercises. As a strategy, however, choose the option that helps to tighten the perineal floor, which is weakened by pregnancy and childbirth.

16 **Answer: 1 Rationale:** By the second or third postpartum day, mothers are moving into the taking-hold phase of adjustment and are eager to care for the baby and self independently. Being hesitant in making decisions, needing help with hygiene and ambulation, and requesting the baby be fed in the nursery at night are characteristics of the taking-in phase, which occurs earlier and reflects greater dependence on the part of the mother. **Cognitive Level:** Analyzing **Client Need:** Health Promotion and Maintenance **Integrated Process:** Nursing Process: Planning **Content Area:** Maternal–Newborn **Strategy:** The core issue of this question is the progression of maternal behaviors in the days following delivery. The wording of the question indicates the correct option is an expected behavior for that time period. Use nursing knowledge to make a selection.

17 **Answer: 1, 3, 4 Rationale:** A third- or fourth-degree perineal laceration involves the rectal sphincter, therefore suppositories, enemas, and rectal exams are contraindicated until the rectum heals. Increased fiber in the diet will promote bowel elimination, which could be painful in a client with a perineal laceration. Increased fluid intake is helpful to keep stool soft, thus making it less uncomfortable to have a bowel movement. A stool softener will prevent the stool from being hard, which would cause pain for a client with a perineal laceration. A third- or fourth-degree perineal laceration involves the rectal sphincter, so suppositories should not be used until the rectum heals. Enemas should not be used to promote bowel elimination until the rectum heals, and fluids or use of stool softeners is appropriate to promote bowel elimination in all postpartum clients. **Cognitive Level:** Applying **Client Need:** Physiological Adaptation **Integrated Process:** Nursing Process: Implementation **Content Area:** Maternal–Newborn **Strategy:** The wording of the question indicates the correct option(s) are also appropriate interventions. Incorrect options would contain inaccurate nursing actions or jeopardize client safety and restoration of health. Use knowledge of management of a third- or fourth-degree laceration to make your selection(s).

18 **Answer:**

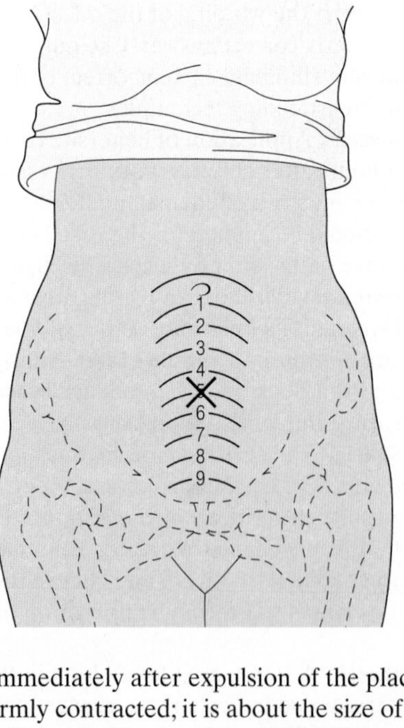

Rationale: Immediately after expulsion of the placenta, the uterus is firmly contracted; it is about the size of a grapefruit. The fundus is located in the abdominal midline halfway

ANSWERS & RATIONALES

between the symphysis pubis and umbilicus. Within 6–12 hours after delivery, the fundus rises to the level of the umbilicus. The top of the fundus then descends the width of a fingerbreadth (1 cm) each day until it descends into the pelvis by about 2 weeks, when it is no longer palpable. **Cognitive Level:** Applying **Client Need:** Physiological Adaptation **Integrated Process:** Nursing Process: Implementation **Content Area:** Maternal–Newborn **Strategy:** Recall the physiologic process of uterine involution and the changes in fundal position after delivery.

19 **Answer: 3, 5 Rationale:** The client should not have sexual intercourse before the episiotomy is healed or the lochia has stopped because this can increase the risk of infection. Water-soluble lubricants can be used, if necessary, for vaginal lubrication. Petroleum jelly is an oil-based product and should not be used for vaginal lubrication. An IUD is contraindicated during the early postpartum period. The timing of when a client resumes menstruation after delivery can be influenced by factors such as breastfeeding, so waiting until after the first menstrual period to resume intercourse could be too soon for some clients, and too long for others. **Cognitive Level:** Applying **Client Need:** Health Promotion and Maintenance **Integrated Process:** Teaching and Learning **Content Area:** Maternal–Newborn **Strategy:** Use the process of elimination and look for a statement that is true. Knowledge of client teaching for resumption of sexual activity after delivery will help to answer the question correctly.

20 **Answer: 3, 5 Rationale:** Applying cold therapy, such as ice bags, to the breasts of a postpartum woman will help to suppress lactation. Binding the breasts, either with a snug bra or binder, will help suppress lactation. Applying warm compresses to the breasts will stimulate the milk supply. Pumping the breasts to express milk will help to promote a continued milk supply. Medications to suppress lactation are not recommended. **Cognitive Level:** Applying **Client Need:** Health Promotion and Maintenance **Integrated Process:** Teaching and Learning **Content Area:** Maternal–Newborn **Strategy:** Knowledge of the ways to suppress lactation in the nonbreastfeeding mother will help to answer the question correctly. Correct answers are options that include a true statement about a point of client education.

Key Terms for Review

afterpains p. 126
boggy uterus p. 125
bonding p. 127
colostrum p. 127
diastasis recti p. 126
en face p. 128
engorgement p. 127
engrossment p. 128
fundus p. 125
Homans sign p. 129
involution p. 125
let-down reflex p. 127
lochia alba p. 125
lochia rubra p. 125
lochia serosa p. 125
postpartum blues p. 128
puerperium p. 125

References

Adams, M., & Urban, C. (2016). *Pharmacology: Connections to nursing practice* (3rd ed.). New York, NY: Pearson Education.

Davidson, M., London, M., & Ladewig, P. (2016). *Olds' maternal newborn nursing and women's health across the lifespan* (10th ed.). New York, NY: Pearson Education.

Kee, J. (2017). *Pearson's handbook of laboratory and diagnostic tests* (8th ed.). New York, NY: Pearson Education.

Ladewig, P., London, M., & Davidson, M. (2014). *Contemporary maternal–newborn nursing care* (8th ed.). Upper Saddle River, NJ: Pearson Education.

London, M., Ladewig, P., Davidson, M., Ball, J., Bindler, R., & Cowen, K. (2014). *Maternal and child nursing care* (4th ed.). Upper Saddle River, NJ: Pearson Education.

Lowdermilk, D., Perry, S., Cashion, M., & Alden, K. (2016). *Maternity and women's health care* (11th ed.). St. Louis, MO: Elsevier.

12 Uncomplicated Newborn Care

In this chapter

Cross Reference

Other chapters relevant to this content area are

Reproduction, Family Planning, and Infertility	Chapter 8
Uncomplicated Antenatal Assessment and Care	Chapter 9
Uncomplicated Labor and Delivery Care	Chapter 10
Uncomplicated Postpartum Assessment and Care	Chapter 11
Complicated Antenatal Care	Chapter 49
Complicated Labor and Delivery Care	Chapter 50
Complicated Postpartum Care	Chapter 51
Complicated Newborn Care	Chapter 52

I. ASSESSMENT OF HEALTHY NEWBORN

A. Physical assessment

NCLEX®

1. Vital signs and newborn measurement (see Table 12–1)
2. Pain assessment: intermittent crying not lasting more than 60 seconds, not high-pitched, quiets easily, and no tears noted
3. Collaborative management

NCLEX®

   a. Maintain newborn on radiant warmer or in isolette with servocontrol to maintain skin temperature 97.5–98.6°F (36.4–37°C)
   b. Allow infant to assume a flexed position to decrease skin surface area exposed to environment (reduces heat loss)
   c. Monitor axillary and skin probe temperature per institution's protocol

NCLEX®

   d. Monitor respirations for tachypnea and skin color changes for mottling; use bulb syringe or suction device as appropriate to remove secretions from nose and/or mouth
4. Outcomes: at 2 hours of age newborn maintains axillary temperature of 97.5–98.6°F (36.4–37°C), heart rate of 110–160/min, respirations 30–60/min with no distress, has pink skin color, and remains in flexed position

B. General assessment (performed in cephalocaudal or head-to-toe manner within 4 hours of birth)

1. Head
   a. One-quarter of body size, molding of fontanels and suture spaces, round, and moves easily from left to right and up to down

Table 12–1 Newborn Vital Signs and Measurements

Vital Sign or Measurement	Normal Range	Comments
Heart rate	110–160 beats/min	Irregular, especially when crying, and possible functional murmur; may be as high as 170 when crying or as low as 100 when sleeping; count apical pulse for one full minute
Respirations	30–60 breaths/min	May have short periods of apnea, irregular; cry is vigorous and loud; may elevate slightly when crying, but report respirations over 60/min (tachypnea) 2 hours after delivery or under 30/min (bradypnea); count for one full minute
Temperature	97.5–98.6°F (36.4–37°C) axillary	Stabilizes about 8–10 hours after birth; poor thermostability results from heat loss via *convection* (loss to cooler air currents), *radiation* (indirect heat transfer from body to cooler surfaces), *evaporation* (from wet skin), and *conduction* (direct heat loss to cooler objects)
Blood pressure	90–60/50–40 mm Hg	Varies with changes in activity and blood volume; more accurate when newborn is resting; increases to 100/50 by day 10
Weight	2500–4500 grams (5 lb, 8 oz–8 lb, 13 oz)	Average 3405 grams (7 lb, 8 ounces [oz]); influenced by race and maternal size and age; expect physiologic weight loss of 5–10% for term newborns and up to 15% if preterm
Length	46–56 cm (18–22 in)	Average 50 cm (20 in); place newborn flat on back with legs extended to measure; normal newborn legs are flexed and tense
Head circumference	32–37 cm (12.5–14.5 in)	Average 33–35 cm (13–14 in); is about 2 cm (0.8 in) larger than chest circumference; place measuring tape over most prominent part of occiput and bring forward just above eyebrows
Chest circumference	30–35 cm (12–14 in)	Average 32 cm (12.5 in); place measuring tape at lower edge of scapulas and bring forward across nipple line

   b. Symmetric exception may be caused by birth trauma—that is, **caput succedaneum** (swelling of soft tissue under scalp that subsides within a few days) or **cephalohematoma** (collection of blood between cranial bone and periosteum; absorbs spontaneously in about 6 weeks)
   c. Anterior and posterior fontanels should be open, with posterior closing sooner (8–12 weeks) than anterior (by 18 months)
2. Hair: smooth with texture variations per ethnic background, grows toward face, high above eyebrow
3. Face: symmetric features and movement; eyebrows and eyelashes present
4. Eyes
   a. Clear blue or slate blue-gray in color
   b. Pupils equal and reactive to light, blink reflex present, sclera is bluish white
   c. May have subconjunctival hemorrhage (small, broken capillaries on sclera, will disappear in few weeks)
   d. Edematous eyelids
   e. Lacrimal structures (tearing) functions at about 2 months
5. Nose: patent nares bilaterally, no discharge, may have flat bridge, sneezing done to clear nostrils
6. Mouth
   a. Symmetrical when cries, hard palate intact, uvula midline, reflexes present
   NCLEX®
   b. **Rooting reflex** (infant turns to side stimulated and opens mouth to suck); **sucking reflex** (when object placed in mouth or touches lips)
   c. May have **Epstein's pearls** (small white specks, inclusion cysts, on gum ridges), tongue not protruding
7. Ears: well-formed notch of ear on straight line with outer canthus of eye
8. Neck: short, freely movable, has **tonic neck reflex** or fencer position (when head is turned to one side, extremities on same side extend and extremities on opposite side flex)
9. Chest
   a. Clavicles straight and intact, barrel-shaped chest with bilateral expansion on inspiration
   b. Breath sounds clear

c. Heart rate auscultated at border of left sternum extending left to midclavicle; regular rate and rhythm
d. Point of maximum impulse (PMI) lateral to midclavicular line at third to fourth intercostal space

NCLEX®
10. Breasts: nipples symmetrical, may have whitish discharge or supernumerary (extra small) nipples on chest surface
11. Abdomen
a. Soft, dome-shaped, round, some laxness of muscles, moves with respirations
b. Bowel sounds when relaxed
c. Umbilical cord is white, gelatinous with two arteries and one vein, clamped with no foul odor
d. Femoral pulses palpable and equal, no bulges or nodes along bilateral inguinal areas
12. Genitalia
a. Male: pendulous scrotum with rugae, testes descended into scrotum, penis with urinary meatus at tip of glans on ventral surface of penile shaft

NCLEX®
b. Female: labia minora may have **vernix caseosa** (white, cheesy protective covering that decreases as gestational age increases) and smegma increases, labia majora normally covers labia minora and clitoris, discharge (blood-tinged mucus) may be present because of maternal hormones
13. Extremities and trunk
a. Trunk: short, flexed, synchronized movement
b. **Trunk incurvation** (Galant reflex): newborn lies prone, and when side is stroked, pelvis turns to stimulated side
c. Hips: stable with no clicks or snaps upon movement
d. To assess hip dislocation, **Barlow's maneuver** adducts legs over hips and a snap is felt as femur leaves the acetabulum; with **Ortolani's maneuver**, the hip joint is abducted and lifted, and a click is felt as femur enters acetabulum
e. Arms: equal in length with symmetrical movement; **grasp reflex** present, newborn grasps when object is placed in hand; nonmovement may indicate **Erb-Duchenne paralysis** or **Erb's palsy**; newborn inability to move upper arms or asymmetric Moro response may be caused by damage to fifth and sixth cervical roots of brachial plexus; five digits on each hand with normal palmar creases, nails present
f. Legs: equal length, bowed, well flexed, symmetric skin folds, peripheral pulses present

NCLEX®
g. Feet: creases on soles, may have "positional" clubfoot caused by intrauterine position but should be able to turn toward midline; **plantar grasp**—pressure on soles of feet elicits curling of toes; **Babinski reflex**—stroking sole upward and across ball of foot elicits fanning and extension of toes, disappears at 12 months

NCLEX®
h. Back: spine straight and flexible, may have small **pilonidal dimple**, a small dimple at base of spine but without connection to spinal cord
i. Anus: patent, well placed, may have meconium stool
14. Skin
a. Color consistent with ethnic background, pink-tinged

NCLEX®
b. **Acrocyanosis**: bluish discoloration of hands and feet may be present
c. May have mottling: lacy pattern of dilated blood vessels under skin caused by fluctuation of general circulation

NCLEX®
d. May have **milia**—obstructed secretions of sebaceous glands
e. May have **Mongolian spots**—bluish pigmented areas on dorsal area of buttocks; most common in Asian, African, or Hispanic descent
f. May have **lanugo**—downy, fine hair of fetus between 20 weeks and birth, noticeably found on shoulders, forehead, and cheeks
g. May have Harlequin's sign—a deep red color over one side of body while other side remains pale; results from vasomotor disturbance

C. Gestational age assessment using Ballard tool
1. Evaluates six neuromuscular and six physical characteristics during first few hours after birth
2. A score of 1–5 is assigned to each characteristic and total score correlates to gestational age: that is, a term newborn given a score of 3 for each characteristic scores 18 for neuromuscular assessment and 18 for physical characteristics; total of 36 points correlates to 38+ weeks' gestation
3. Rating is marked on a graph with newborn's birth weight, length, and head circumference to classify newborn based on maturity and intrauterine growth
4. An overall rating below 10th percentile indicates infant is *small for gestational age (SGA)*; between 10th and 90th percentile is *appropriate for gestational age (AGA)*; above 90th percentile is *large for gestational age (LGA)*

5. Determining ratings for each of the subscores
   a. Wear gloves when assessing newborn after birth prior to first bath
   b. First evaluate observable characteristics without disturbing newborn, then proceed to characteristics that require more handling of infant
   c. Maternal conditions such as gestational hypertension, diabetes, and maternal analgesia and anesthesia in intrapartal period may affect some gestational age components
   d. Neuromuscular maturity: during first 24 hours, newborn nervous system is unstable; reflexes and assessments depend on brain centers; results may be unreliable and need to be repeated in 24 hours
   e. Physical maturity: not influenced by labor and birth and do not change significantly within first 24 hours after birth
   f. Skin: opaque texture, few distinct larger veins, dry, some peeling
   g. Lanugo: minimal, decreases as gestational age increases
   h. Plantar surface: a reliable indicator of gestational age in first 12 hours of life; beginning at top of foot, creases should cover at least two-thirds of entire foot surface
   i. Breast: using forefinger and middle finger, gently measure breast tissue diameter in millimeters (mm); should be 5–10 mm at term; nipple should be raised above skin level
   j. Eye/ear: eyes are open and clear; ears—when top and bottom of pinna are folded over each other, pinna will spring back quickly when released; upper two-thirds of pinna incurves
   k. Male genitalia: testes descended, scrotum pendulous and covered with rugae
   l. Female genitalia: labia majora increases with gestation and nearly covers clitoris at 36–40 weeks; at 40 weeks, majora cover labia minora and clitoris

II. PHYSIOLOGICAL CHANGES AFTER BIRTH

A. Cardiovascular

1. Expansion of lungs occurs with first breath; increases pulmonary blood flow and decreases pulmonary vascular resistance
2. Increased aortic pressure and decreased venous pressure present: clamping of umbilical cord increases vascular resistance, and aortic blood pressure increases
3. Increased systemic pressure and decreased pulmonary artery pressure occur because of loss of placenta; lung expansion increases pulmonary blood flow and dilates pulmonary vessels; pulmonary vascular beds open and perfuse other body systems
4. The **foramen ovale** (opening that previously connected right and left atria), functionally closes in about 1–2 hours and anatomically closes in a few weeks to 1 year, increasing left atrial pressure; some shunting may occur early in transition and with crying
5. The **ductus arteriosus** (in fetal circulation, an anatomic shunt between pulmonary artery and arch of aorta) closes, reversing blood flow, so now blood flows from aorta to pulmonary artery because of increased left arterial pressure
6. The **ductus venosus** closes (in fetal circulation, shunts arterial blood into inferior vena cava); results in redistribution of blood and cardiac output; closure forces perfusion of liver

B. Respiratory

1. Initial respirations are triggered by physical, sensory, and chemical factors
   a. Physical: effort is required to expand lungs and fill collapsed alveoli; changes in pressure gradient
   b. Sensory: temperature, noise, light, sound
   c. Chemical: changes in blood (decreased O_2 level, increased CO_2 level, decreased pH) as a result of transitory asphyxia during delivery

NCLEX®
2. Newborn is an obligatory nose-breather, and any obstruction will cause respiratory distress; ability to maintain respiratory function is influenced by a large heart that reduces lung space and weak intercostal muscles, horizontal ribs and high diaphragm, which restrict space available for lung expansion
3. Collaborative care
   a. Monitor respirations for any signs of respiratory distress (increased rate, audible grunting, nasal flaring, retractions) per institutional protocol; normal limits are 30–60/min

   NCLEX®
   b. Monitor color of skin, oral area, and extremities for any signs of hypoxia
   c. Keep newborn on warmer for closer observation

   NCLEX®
   d. Keep infant NPO if respirations are above 60/min
   e. Maintain oral area free from mucus or emesis
4. Outcomes: newborn's respirations are within normal limits, color is pink, temperature stable with no signs of respiratory distress

C. Neurologic

1. Newborn's brain is 25% of adult size and nerve fiber myelination is incomplete
2. Newborn exhibits uncoordinated movements, labile temperature regulation, poor control over musculature, easy startling, and tremors of extremities
3. Newborn reflexes are important indicators of development; include **Moro reflex** (elicit by startling newborn; thighs and knees flex and fingers fan and then clench as arms are thrown out then brought together) and previously discussed Babinski grasp, plantar grasp, sucking, and tonic neck reflexes
4. Periods of reactivity: pattern of behavior during first several hours after birth

NCLEX®
   a. First period of reactivity: lasts approximately 30 minutes after birth; awake and alert; may display strong sucking reflex and attachment behaviors with random diffuse movements
   b. Period of inactivity to sleep phase: activity diminishes, heart and respiratory rates decrease, and newborn enters sleep phase lasting from a few minutes to 2–4 hours; will be difficult to awaken
   c. Second period of reactivity: awakes from deep sleep, lasts 4–6 hours; heart and respiratory rates increase; observe for apneic periods, which could cause heart rate and oxygen saturation to drop; observe for changes in color if these occur

D. Thermoregulation

1. Newborn cannot shiver to produce heat
2. Newborn does have brown fat deposits to produce heat

NCLEX®
3. Focus in newborn period is keeping infant warm and preventing cold stress

E. Musculoskeletal

1. Newborn should have full range of motion—when extremities are fully extended, they should return to a flexed position
2. Any variations should be further investigated

F. Gastrointestinal

1. Digestive enzymes are active at birth and can support extrauterine life by 36–38 weeks' gestation
2. Necessary muscular and reflex developments for transporting food are present at birth
3. Digestion of protein and carbohydrates is easily accomplished, but fat digestion and absorption are poor due to absence of pancreatic enzymes
4. Little saliva is manufactured until 3 months
5. An immature lower esophageal sphincter often leads to regurgitation or spitting up

NCLEX®
6. **Meconium**, stool that contains bile, epithelial cells, and amniotic cells, is excreted within 24 hours in 90% of healthy newborns
7. Wide variations occur among newborns regarding interest in feeding

G. Genitourinary

1. Functioning nephrons are complete by 34–36 weeks' gestation
2. Glomerular filtration rate (reabsorption and filtration) is low; therefore, newborn may tend to reabsorb sodium and excrete large amounts of water

NCLEX®
3. Decreased ability to excrete drugs and excessive fluid loss can lead to acidosis and fluid imbalance; uric acid crystals may cause a reddish stain in diaper

H. Hepatic

1. If mother's iron intake has been adequate, iron stores are sufficient through fifth month of extrauterine life; iron supplements may be given after this age
2. Liver controls amount of circulating unconjugated bilirubin, a pigment derived from hemoglobin that is released with breakdown of red blood cells

NCLEX®
3. Unconjugated bilirubin can leave vascular system and permeate other extravascular tissues (e.g., skin, sclera, oral mucous membranes), causing a yellow color termed *jaundice* or *icterus*
4. Because unconjugated bilirubin binds to albumin (protein) and is eliminated in stools, early and increased feeding may be encouraged to promote increased excretion of stool
5. Collaborative care
   a. Record intake (oral and parental) and output (weigh diapers) every 2–4 hours
   b. Monitor for adequate hydration; skin turgor, specific gravity with each voiding, noting quality and characteristics of urine
   c. Phototherapy; maintain "bili-mask" over eyes, check eyes for pressure from mask

NCLEX®
   d. Monitor diaper area for skin breakdown and rash
6. Outcomes: newborn feeds every 2–3 hours with balanced intake and output; skin is elastic; oral mucous membranes are moist; urine is clear, straw-colored, and has six to eight wet diapers in 24 hours; bili-mask positioned over eyes if used; diaper area is clean with no skin breakdown

I. Integumentary

1. Maturity of skin increases with gestational age; mature skin helps protect newborn from heat loss and infection
2. Skin color depends on activity level, temperature, hematocrit levels, and ethnicity
3. Plethora is a ruddy (red) appearance and usually indicates a hematocrit greater than 65% and should be evaluated; monitor a polycythemic infant closely for cyanosis, respiratory distress, hypoglycemia, and jaundice

NCLEX®

4. When infant cries, skin becomes bright red because of immature capillary system; acrocyanosis is common

J. Immune system

1. Of three major types of immunoglobulins (IgG, IgA, and IgM), only IgG crosses placenta; therefore, infants receive passive immunity from mother in form of IgG near end of gestation, or passive acquired immunity
2. Infants eventually produce antibodies (active acquired immunity) beginning at about 3 months, but IgA is missing from respiratory, urinary, and GI tract until approximately 4–6 months of age unless newborn is breastfed or until infant produces own antibodies
3. Breastfed infants receive antibodies from breast milk for as long as breastfeeding continues, and thereby receive protection from many infectious diseases, including influenza, mumps, and chickenpox
4. Use standard precautions and aseptic technique when caring for newborn; wear gown during care and don't assign caregivers with infections to newborns

III. NEWBORN NUTRITION

A. Nutrition guidelines

1. A healthy newborn needs 90–120 kcal/24 hr of nutrition and 140–160 mL/kg/24 hr of fluid intake
2. Weight gain is 4–8 oz/week; weight doubles by 6 months of age and triples by 1 year

B. Teaching guidelines for formula/bottle-feeding

1. Formula meets energy and nutrient requirements of newborns/infants, but does not have immunologic properties and digestibility of human milk
2. Standard formulas are available in three types
   a. Concentrated liquid: dilute with water at a 1:1 ratio
   b. Powder: mix with water, usually 1 scoop to 60 mL water
   c. Ready-to-feed: can be poured directly into a bottle; refrigerate once opened and discard after 24 hours
   d. The American Academy of Pediatrics (AAP) recommends that infants be given formula or breast milk until 12 months of age

NCLEX®

   e. Soy formulas are available if infant cannot tolerate cow's milk protein and lactose, and hypoallergenic (hydrolysate) formulas are available for infants with an allergic response to standard formulas
3. Preparation of formula
   a. Aseptic sterilization: supplies are sterilized separately from formula by boiling in water for 20 minutes
   b. Terminal sterilization: formula is poured into unsterilized bottles and sterilized together for 25 minutes
   c. With sanitary conditions, bottles and formula are not routinely sterilized, but all equipment is cleaned thoroughly, including top of can of formula
   d. Formula may be warmed to room temperature in a container of warm water; never warm bottles in a microwave; hot spots may develop and burn infant's mouth or throat; heating also changes nutritional composition of formula

NCLEX®

4. Feeding techniques
   a. Hold infant close with head elevated
   b. Keep bottle tipped so that nipple remains full of formula
   c. Never prop bottle or put infant to bed with a bottle in mouth; propping can cause aspiration and middle ear infections
   d. Discard any formula left in bottle because of risk of bacterial growth

C. Teaching guidelines for breastfeeding

1. Influences on supply and demand (infant need)
   a. Maternal supply is related to frequency of feedings until about 3–4 weeks when the milk supply is well established; thereafter, critical factor for supply to meet demand is breast emptying
   b. Infants self-regulate their intake and control breast milk production by degree to which they "empty" breast; a lactating breast is never "emptied" completely

NCLEX® 2. The suckling sequence and proper **latch-on**
   a. Nipple and areola are drawn into mouth enough for lips to cover 1–1.5 inches of areola
   b. Jaw should move up and down in a rhythmic motion during milk transfer; ears may wiggle; cheeks should be full and rounded, not sucked in
   c. Upper and lower lips should be flanged
   d. Tongue should be troughed—cup-shaped, beginning at bottom of mouth and extending over lower alveolar ridge; tongue draws nipple in and presses it against hard palate, forming a teat; tongue moves from back to front of areola in a rolling movement for milk transfer

NCLEX® 3. Frequency of feedings: increasing frequency will not increase supply unless transfer of milk is successfully occurring; audible swallowing is best indicator of milk transfer; swallowing is more frequent as more milk is transferred
   a. Schedules should not be imposed on breastfeeding newborns because they have a stomach capacity of about 30 mL, and breast milk is more easily digested than artificial milk (formula)
   b. Breastfeeding infants should be fed when hunger cues (rooting, sucking on fists) are displayed, which may be 90 mins to 3 hrs after last feeding; crying is last sign of hunger
   c. Night feedings are necessary during first 6–8 weeks; fat content of breast milk is high in evening, which may help infant to consume more calories and feel more satiated; infants who consume more calories during day may have longer stretches of sleep at night

4. Duration of feedings
   a. Limiting time at breast will not minimize or prevent sore nipples; sore nipples are almost always caused by incorrect positioning at breast or poor latch-on
   b. Mothers should watch infant, not the clock; what infant is doing at breast is a better indicator of milk transfer than time spent there
   c. Newborns/infants with different sucking styles take different amounts of time to complete a feeding, anywhere from 10 to 30 minutes; foremilk is milk that is produced and stored between feedings, looks like skim milk—bluish in tint—and usually has less fat content than hindmilk, which is produced during and released at end of a feeding and looks much richer, with a yellowish tint
   d. Signs of satiation are slowing of audible swallowing; pauses between sucking bursts; infant takes self off breast; hunger cues disappear; infant is relaxed, drowsy, sleeping

NCLEX® 5. Good positioning for feeding is critical for proper latch-on and effective suckling
   a. Maternal body position starts with good posture: straight back, pillows under arms (and under infant), feet touching floor or a footstool beneath feet
   b. Hand position: in early weeks, breast should be supported using C-hold or scissor-hold hand position; use caution that fingers do not cover lactiferous sinuses or areola that infant needs to take into mouth; later on, infant will be able to support breast after initial latch-on
   c. Cradle hold: infant is in chest-to-chest position, facing breast close enough to touch with nose and chin, with shoulder resting slightly lower on mother's forearm; mother's hand supports infant's buttocks, opposite hand supports breast
   d. Side-lying position: infant lies alongside mother with a rolled-up blanket behind infant and a pillow behind mother to maintain position; suggested for nighttime feedings and after cesarean delivery
   e. Football or clutch position: infant is positioned in mother's arm with head, back, and shoulders in palm of hand; infant is tucked up under mother's arm, lining up infant's lips with nipple

6. Breastfeeding support is necessary for beginning and continuing breastfeeding
   a. Encourage use of breastfeeding support groups or telephone hotlines at hospitals
   b. Lactation consultants are trained and certified to provide assistance to breastfeeding mothers who experience problems
   c. La Leche League is an international breastfeeding support and information group, with local groups often meeting in neighborhoods

NCLEX® d. Hospitals and birthing centers that subscribe to World Health Organization's (WHO) Baby Friendly Hospital promote "ten steps to successful breastfeeding" and stop distribution of breast milk substitutes (Box 12–1)

D. Outcomes

1. Infant gains 14–28 grams (0.5–1 oz) per day, doubles weight by age 6 months and triples weight by 1 year
2. Infant has 8–10 wet or soiled diapers per day and is alert and responsive

Box 12–1

Ten Steps to Successful Breastfeeding

Every facility providing maternity services and care for newborn infants should:

- Have a written breastfeeding policy routinely communicated to all healthcare staff.
- Train all healthcare staff in the skills necessary to implement this policy.
- Inform all pregnant women about the benefits and management of breastfeeding.
- Help mothers initiate breastfeeding within a half-hour of birth.
- Show mothers how to breastfeed and how to maintain lactation even if they are separated from their infants.
- Give newborn infants no food or drink other than breast milk unless it is medically indicated.
- Practice rooming-in—allow mothers and infants to stay together—24 hours a day.
- Encourage breastfeeding on demand.
- Give no artificial teats or pacifiers (also called dummies or soothers) to breastfeeding infants.
- Foster the establishment of breastfeeding support groups and refer mothers to them upon discharge from the hospital or clinic.

IV. NURSING CARE OF HEALTHY NEWBORN

A. Eye prophylaxis after birth

1. May be done immediately after birth or delayed up to 1 hour (to allow eye contact that facilitates parent–newborn bonding); prevents ophthamalia neonatorum, caused by *Neiserria gonorrhoeae* and *Chlamydia trachomatis*
2. Commonly used solutions are erythromycin (0.5%) and tetracycline (1%) ophthalmic ointment
3. Eye prophylaxis can cause chemical conjunctivitis with possible edema, inflammation, and discharge; clears within 24–48 hours

B. Preventing hemorrhagic disorders after birth

1. Newborn cannot synthesize own vitamin K_1 phytonadione until intestinal bacteria are present
2. Give prescribed vitamin K_1 phytonadione 0.5–1.0 mg IM in middle third of vastus lateralis muscle (lateral aspect) as a one-time dose

C. Screening for phenylketonuria (PKU)

1. Instruct that screening is done before hospital discharge; if initial specimen obtained before infant is 24 hours old, a second screening should be done before 5 days of age; some states require a second test
2. *NCLEX®* Newborn should be taking breast milk or formula for 24 hours prior to screening so that there is sufficient protein intake; early specimen collection could yield inaccurate results

D. Protecting thermoregulation

1. Take axillary temperature every hour for first 4 hours of life, then every 4 hours until 24 hours old, then per agency routine
2. Keep room temperature warm
3. Prevent heat loss in newborn from evaporation, radiation, convection, and conduction
   a. Evaporation: keep newborn dry; wrap newborn in blanket
   b. Radiation: position infant away from cold surfaces, such as cold objects and exterior walls or windows
   c. Convection: protect infant from drafts; placing infant in an isolette helps maintain infant temperature while undressed
   d. Conduction: perform infant care and procedures on warm, padded surfaces

E. Bathing

1. Teach parent to use mild soap and to give sponge bath every other day or twice weekly for first 2 weeks; prevents skin dryness and allows time for umbilical cord to fall off and for umbilicus to heal
2. Demonstrate bath and provide ample time for new parents to practice skills
3. Plan bath for a time prior to feeding and ensure a warm room temperature
4. Principle of care is to bathe from cleanest area to dirtiest
   a. Clean eyes from inner to outer canthus to reduce risk of clogging at tear duct, followed by ears, rest of face, neck, chest, back, arms, legs, and finally perineum
   b. Use care when cleaning areas with skinfolds, such as neck, axillae, genitals, and peri area

5. Explain that bath time provides excellent opportunity for parent–infant interaction
6. Once tub bathing begins, only 7.6–10.1 cm (3–4 in) of water is needed; teach parents to be cautious because infant skin is slippery when wet

F. Cord care

1. Keep cord clean and dry; cord clamp may be removed after 24 hours
2. Assess cord for yellowish discharge, odor, or swelling and report if noted
3. Perform cord care in hospital according to agency protocol; many variations of care exist, including air-drying or applying triple-dye, antimicrobial agent such as bacitracin or 70% alcohol to cord stump
4. Before discharge teach parents to clean base of cord stump with cotton balls two to three times daily during diaper change; do not apply unclean substances to cord; air-drying results in faster cord separation than other measures
5. *NCLEX®* Fold diaper down below cord stump to avoid covering it, prevent soiling of area, and enhance drying
6. Instruct to use sponge baths and avoid submerging cord in water until it falls off (in 7–14 days)
7. Assess for cultural practices related to umbilical cord care, such as binding of abdomen; if such a practice is necessary, recommend sanitary method such as use of clean gauze

G. Circumcision care

1. Assess circumcision for signs of hemorrhage every 30 mins for 2 hrs after procedure
2. Observe first voiding to assess urinary obstruction from penile edema or injury
3. Apply petrolatum and gauze following procedure and for first few diaper changes to reduce further bleeding unless Plastibell is used
4. Plastibell remains in place and should fall off within 8 days; no ointments or creams are used while in place, but may be used after it falls off; consult healthcare provider if it remains in place after 8 days
5. For either type of circumcision, a yellowish film indicates presence of normal granulation tissue
6. Use hygiene measures to reduce risk of infection; report signs of infection such as increased swelling, drainage, or absence of urine flow

H. Care of uncircumcised penis

1. Foreskin and glans are two layers of cells that separate fully between 3 and 5 years of age
2. Teach mother not to force foreskin back over glans for cleansing
3. Explain that when separation does occur, foreskin may be gently retracted daily for gentle cleansing with soap and water

I. Clothing

1. Instruct how to swaddle (wrap) an infant to maintain body temperature, provide a sense of closeness and security, and perhaps quiet a crying infant
2. Dress infant in layers to avoid overheating or chilling
3. Cover infant's head in cool/cold weather to minimize heat loss when outdoors
4. Wash baby clothing with mild soap or detergent separate from other laundry; rinse clothing twice to remove soap and residue and reduce risk of rash

J. Newborn safety (see Box 12–2)

Box 12–2

Maintaining Newborn Safety in Hospital

- Compare names and numbers on identification bracelets of mother and newborn before giving newborn to parent.
- Allow only people with proper birthing unit picture identification to bring and remove newborn from hospital room. If parents do not know staff person, call nurse for assistance.
- Teach parents to:
  - Report any suspicious people on birthing unit to staff.
  - Avoid leaving newborn alone in room, such as during showering or walking in hall; have a family member watch newborn or return newborn to nursery.
  - Avoid lifting newborn if weak, faint, or unsteady on feet; call for assistance.
  - Watch and keep hand on newborn whenever out of crib.
- To protect against infection, do not allow visitors who have a cold, contagious illness, discharge from sores, or diarrhea.
- At discharge, place infant in rear-facing, federally approved infant car seat in back seat of car.

Check Your NCLEX–RN® Exam I.Q.

You are ready for testing on this content if you can:

- Assess the healthy newborn.
- Provide care to the healthy newborn.
- Assist the client in learning skills needed to perform newborn care.
- Evaluate client's ability to care for newborn.
- Provide discharge teaching about newborn care.
- Appreciate cultural differences related to aspects of newborn care.

PRACTICE TEST

1 A 6-hour-old infant passes an unformed, black, tarlike stool. What conclusion should the nurse draw from this finding?

1. It is meconium stool that is expected at this time.
2. It is meconium stool expected at the time of birth.
3. It is a transitional stool expected at this time.
4. It is a transitional stool that is expected later.

2 Following delivery, the nurse should first assess which two newborn body systems that must undergo the most rapid changes to support extrauterine life?

1. Gastrointestinal and hepatic
2. Urinary and hematologic
3. Neurologic and temperature control
4. Respiratory and cardiovascular

3 A newborn's father expresses concern that his baby does not have good control of his hands and arms. The nurse should explain which concept in response to the client, using wording that the client can understand?

1. Neurologic function progresses in a head-to-toe, proximal-to-distal fashion.
2. Purposeful, uncoordinated movements of the arms are abnormal.
3. Mild hypotonia is expected in the upper extremities.
4. Asymmetric muscle tone is not unusual.

4 When caring for a newborn, the nurse must be alert for what potential sign of cold stress?

1. Decreased activity level
2. Increased respiratory rate
3. Hyperglycemia
4. Shivering

5 Which physical assessment finding should the nurse record as part of a newborn's gestational age assessment?

1. Umbilical cord moist to touch
2. Anterior and posterior fontanels nonbulging
3. Plantar creases present on anterior two-thirds of sole
4. Milia present on bridge of nose

6 When planning client instruction on breastfeeding, the nurse should include that the amount of breastmilk the mother produces is directly related to which factor?

1. Her newborn's sucking stimulus
2. Her breast size
3. Her newborn's weight
4. Her nipple erectility

7 Which action by a new postpartum client indicates to the nurse the need for further instruction in breastfeeding technique?

1. Holds the breast with four fingers along the bottom and thumb on top
2. Leans forward to bring her breast toward the baby
3. Stimulates the rooting reflex, then inserts the nipple and areola into the newborn's mouth
4. Checks the placement of the newborn's tongue before breastfeeding

8 A mother is anxious about her newborn. She asks the nurse why there are no tears when her baby is crying. The nurse's response incorporates an understanding of which concept?

1. The lacrimal ducts must be punctured to initiate tear flow.
2. Antibiotic instillation at birth reduces tear formation for several days.
3. Exposure to rubella *in utero* can result in lacrimal duct stenosis.
4. Lacrimal ducts are nonfunctional until 2 months of age.

9 The nurse observes that when a newborn is supine and the head is turned to one side, the extremities straighten to that side while the opposite extremities flex. How should the nurse document this finding?

1. Tonic neck reflex
2. Moro reflex
3. Cremasteric reflex
4. Babinski reflex

10 The nurse anticipates that a newborn male, estimated to be 39 weeks' gestation, should exhibit which characteristic?

1. Extended posture when at rest
2. Testes descended into the scrotum
3. Abundant lanugo over his entire body
4. The ability to move his elbow past his sternum

11 If a newborn does not pass meconium during the first 36 hours of life, what is the priority action by the nurse?

1. Observe the anal area for fissures.
2. Notify the healthcare provider.
3. Increase the amount of oral feedings.
4. Measure the abdominal girth.

12 During a physical assessment, the nurse palpates the newborn's hard and soft palate with a gloved index finger. The infant's mother asks the nurse to explain what is being done. The nurse replies that this assessment is done to detect which possible problem?

1. A shortened frenulum
2. Openings in the palate
3. A thrush infection
4. Adequacy of saliva production

13 A new mother overhears a nurse mention "first period of reactivity" and asks the nurse for an explanation of the term. Which statement would be best to include in a response?

1. "The period begins when the infant awakens from a deep sleep."
2. "The period is an excellent time to acquaint the parents with the newborn."
3. "The period is an excellent time for the mother to sleep and recover from labor and delivery."
4. "The period ends when the amount of respiratory mucus has decreased."

14 Which suggestion should the nurse make to the mother of a breastfeeding newborn as the best treatment for physiologic jaundice?

1. Switching permanently to formula
2. Giving supplemental water feedings
3. Increasing the frequency of breastfeeding sessions
4. Feeding the newborn nothing by mouth

15 In providing guidelines to follow when using concentrated formula for bottle-feeding, the nurse should give which instruction to new parents?

1. Wash the top of the can and can opener with soap and water before opening the can.
2. Adjust the amount of water added according to the weight-gain pattern of the newborn.
3. Make sure the newborn takes all the formula measured into each bottle.
4. Warm the formula in a microwave oven for a few minutes before feeding.

16 A new mother who is breast-feeding her infant asks the nurse, "What kind of stools will my baby have, and how many will there be during the next month?" What would be the best response by the nurse?

1. "One or two well-formed yellow-orange stools per day."
2. "As many as 6–10 small, loose, yellow stools per day."
3. "A well-formed brown stool at least every other day."
4. "Frequent loose, green stools."

17 During a physical exam of a newborn with developmental hip dysplasia, which assessment findings should the nurse expect to obtain? Select all that apply.

1. Symmetrical gluteal folds
2. Limited adduction of the affected leg
3. Absent femoral pulse when the hip is flexed and the leg is abducted
4. Limited abduction of the affected leg
5. Asymmetrical gluteal folds

18 The nurse conducts a neurological assessment of the newborn. What findings indicate the need for further evaluation? Select all that apply.

1. Asymmetrical fine jumping movements of the leg and arm muscles
2. Fanning and hyperextension of the toes when the sole is stroked upward from the heel
3. Grasping a finger placed in the neonate's palm
4. Muscle flaccidity not relieved by holding the newborn
5. Weak but effective sucking movements

19 A postpartum client is bottle-feeding her newborn. What should the nurse teach the client about regurgitation of small amounts of formula? Select all that apply.

1. Take a rectal temperature to check for fever.
2. Recognize this as a normal occurrence.
3. Discontinue feedings for 6–8 hours.
4. Report this promptly to the healthcare provider.
5. Understand that this may result from overfeeding.

20 The nurse concludes that a postpartum client is using appropriate bottle-feeding technique after observing which behavior? Select all that apply.

1. Keeps the nipple full of formula throughout the feeding
2. Props the bottle on a rolled towel
3. Points the bottle at the infant's tongue
4. Enlarges the nipple hole to allow for a steady stream of formula to flow
5. Keeps the infant close with head elevated

PRACTICE TEST

ANSWERS & RATIONALES

ANSWERS & RATIONALES

1 **Answer: 1 Rationale:** Meconium stools are tarry, black, or dark green, and are usually passed within 8–24 hours of birth. It is unusual to pass meconium at birth, unless there has been hypoxia or trauma. Transitional stools are thinner in consistency, with a brown-to-green appearance, and consist of part meconium and part fecal material. Transitional stools are expected a few days later, after food has been digested. Transitional stools do not have the appearance of meconium stool. **Cognitive Level:** Analyzing **Client Need:** Health Promotion and Maintenance **Integrated Process:** Nursing Process: Diagnosis **Content Area:** Maternal–Newborn **Strategy:** The core issues of the question are recognition and identification of meconium stool. The wording of the question indicates that only one option is correct. Use nursing knowledge to make a selection.

2 **Answer: 4 Rationale:** To begin life, the infant must make the adaptations to establish respirations and circulation. These two changes are crucial to life. The gastrointestinal and hepatic systems become established over a longer period of time. The urinary and hematologic systems become established over a longer period of time. The neurologic and temperature control systems become established over a longer period of time. **Cognitive Level:** Analyzing **Client Need:** Health Promotion and Maintenance **Integrated Process:** Nursing Process: Assessment **Content Area:** Maternal–Newborn **Strategy:** A critical word in the question is *first*, which indicates more than one option might be partially or totally correct. The question requires you to set priorities for assessment. Use nursing knowledge and the ABCs to make your selection.

3 **Answer: 1 Rationale:** The newborn body grows in a head-to-toe and proximal-to-distal fashion. Purposeful but uncoordinated movements of the hands and arms are expected, rather than abnormal. Mild hypertonia might be noted, but not hypotonia. Muscle tone should be symmetric. Diminished tone or asymmetric movement could indicate neurological dysfunction. **Cognitive Level:** Analyzing **Client Need:** Health Promotion and Maintenance **Integrated Process:** Nursing Process: Planning **Content Area:** Maternal–Newborn

Strategy: The core issue of the question is discriminating between normal and abnormal motor movements of a newborn. Use knowledge of growth and development to make your selection.

4 **Answer: 2 Rationale:** When an infant is stressed by cold, oxygen consumption increases, and the increased respiratory rate is a response to the need of oxygen. Cold stress would lead to increased activity rather than decreased activity. Hypoglycemia would occur instead of hyperglycemia because the newborn's glucose stores become depleted. Newborns are unable to shiver as a means to increase heat production.**Cognitive Level:** Analyzing**Client Need:** Health Promotion and Maintenance**Integrated Process:** Nursing Process: Assessment**Content Area:** Maternal–Newborn**Strategy:** This question is eliciting knowledge of manifestations for cold stress. Make a connection between increased metabolic need (oxygen) without shivering and increased supply of oxygen (increased respiratory rate) to make a correct choice.

5 **Answer: 3 Rationale:** Plantar creases are part of the physical maturity rating on the gestational age assessment. Umbilical cord, fontanels, and milia may be observed but are not part of the gestational age assessment.**Cognitive Level:** Applying **Client Need:** Health Promotion and Maintenance**Integrated Process:** Nursing Process: Assessment**Content Area:** Maternal–Newborn**Strategy:** The critical words in the question are *gestational age*. Eliminate umbilical cord and fontanels, which should be typical findings for all infants. From this point, use the process of elimination and nursing knowledge to eliminate milia.

6 **Answer: 1 Rationale:** Prolactin and oxytocin, two hormones necessary for breast milk production and letdown, are released from the stimulus of the newborn suckling. The mammary gland of each breast is composed of 15–20 lobes (where milk is produced and travels to the nipple) arranged around the nipple. Breast size is related to adipose tissue. Neither newborn weight nor nipple erectility is directly related to breast milk production.**Cognitive Level:** Applying **Client Need:** Health Promotion and Maintenance**Integrated Process:** Nursing Process: Evaluation**Content Area:** Maternal–Newborn**Strategy:** The wording of this question is straightforward and direct. Use nursing knowledge and the process of elimination to make a selection.

7 **Answer: 2 Rationale:** The newborn should be brought to the breast, not the breast to the newborn; therefore, the mother would need further demonstration and teaching to correct this ineffective action. Holding the breast with four fingers along the bottom and the thumb on top, checking for rooting reflex, and checking the newborn's tongue position are correct actions for successful breastfeeding.**Cognitive Level:** Applying **Client Need:** Health Promotion and Maintenance**Integrated Process:** Nursing Process: Implementation**Content Area:** Maternal–Newborn**Strategy:** Note the critical words *further instruction*, which indicates the correct answer has incorrect information in it. Evaluate the truth of each option presented, and select the option that contains false information.

8 **Answer: 4 Rationale:** The cry of the newborn is tearless because the lacrimal ducts are not usually functioning until the second month of life. Lacrimal ducts are naturally patent, and not punctured. Antibiotics will not reduce tear formation. Exposure to rubella is not known to cause stenosis of the lacrimal duct.**Cognitive Level:** Applying**Client Need:** Health Promotion and Maintenance**Integrated Process:** Nursing Process: Assessment**Content Area:** Maternal–Newborn**Strategy:** The core issue of this question is physical growth and development of the newborn. The wording of the question indicates the correct option is also a true statement.

9 **Answer: 1 Rationale:** The tonic neck reflex, or fencing position, refers to the position the newborn assumes when supine with the head turned to one side. The extremities on that side will extend, and the extremities on the opposite side will flex. The Moro reflex occurs when the newborn is startled and responds by abducting and extending arms, with fingers fanning out and the arms forming a "C." The cremasteric reflex refers to retraction of the testes when chilled, or when the inner thigh is stroked. The Babinski reflex refers to the flaring of the toes when the sole of the foot is stroked upward.**Cognitive Level:** Applying**Client Need:** Health Promotion and Maintenance**Integrated Process:** Nursing Process: Assessment**Content Area:** Maternal–Newborn**Strategy:** The core issue of this question is knowledge of the normal reflexes of a newborn. Use knowledge of growth and development, and the process of elimination, to make a selection.

10 **Answer: 2 Rationale:** A full-term male infant will have both testes in his scrotum, with rugae present. Good muscle tone results in a more flexed posture, not extended posture, when at rest. Only a moderate amount of lanugo is present, usually on the shoulders and back. The tendency toward a flexed posture would result in an inability of the newborn to move his elbow past midline to cross the sternum.**Cognitive Level:** Applying**Client Need:** Health Promotion and Maintenance **Integrated Process:** Nursing Process: Assessment**Content Area:** Maternal–Newborn**Strategy:** The core issue of this question is knowledge of physical findings of an infant according to gestational age. Use knowledge of physical growth and development of the newborn to eliminate each of the incorrect options.

11 **Answer: 4 Rationale:** The first meconium stool should be passed within the first 24 hours after birth; if not, the abdominal girth should be measured to evaluate distention and the possibility of obstruction. The presence of anal fissures will not prevent the passage of a meconium stool. Notifying the healthcare provider will not provide more information. Increasing the amount of feedings will not provide more information, and if there is an obstruction, will complicate the problem.**Cognitive Level:** Analyzing**Client Need:** Health Promotion and Maintenance**Integrated Process:** Nursing Process: Implementation**Content Area:** Maternal–Newborn **Strategy:** Note the critical words *not* and *first 36 hours*. This tells you that there is a problem with the infant's gastrointestinal status. When the nurse has only one piece of assessment data, often it is important to gather more assessment data unless the situation represents an emergency, which is not the case in this question.

12 **Answer: 2 Rationale:** The hard and soft palates are examined to feel for any openings, or clefts. The frenulum is a ridge of tissue found under the tongue and usually does not affect sucking. A thrush infection is usually visible as white patches adhering to the mucous membranes and does not need to be felt. Saliva is normally scant and can be observed.**Cognitive Level:** Applying**Client Need:** Health Promotion and Maintenance**Integrated Process:** Nursing Process: Assessment **Content Area:** Maternal–Newborn**Strategy:** The focus of the question is knowledge of the underlying rationales for

newborn assessment. Use knowledge of physical assessment to eliminate incorrect options to make a final selection, noting the correlation between the word *palate* in both the stem of the question and the correct option.

13 **Answer: 2 Rationale:** The first period of reactivity lasts up to 30 minutes after birth. The newborn is alert, and it is a good time for the newborn to interact with parents. The second period of reactivity begins when the newborn awakens from a deep sleep. The amount of respiratory mucus may still be noted during this period. Mothers may sleep and recover during the newborn's sleep state. **Cognitive Level:** Applying **Client Need:** Health Promotion and Maintenance **Integrated Process:** Communication and Documentation **Content Area:** Maternal–Newborn **Strategy:** Note the critical words *first* and *reactivity* in the stem of the question. This leads you to interpret that this will be the first time the infant is quite alert, which could then lead you to select the option that maximizes interaction between mother and infant after birth.

14 **Answer: 3 Rationale:** Physiologic jaundice is best treated by more frequent feedings to increase stooling and the excretion of bilirubin. Switching to formula undermines the mother's feeling of her ability to provide nutrition for the newborn and may result in too-early weaning. Supplemental water may lead the infant to take less breast milk, delay the breast milk supply, and cause the bilirubin level to increase. Withholding food from the newborn will provide inadequate nutrition and cause bilirubin levels to increase. **Cognitive Level:** Applying **Client Need:** Health Promotion and Maintenance **Integrated Process:** Nursing Process: Implementation **Content Area:** Maternal–Newborn **Strategy:** The core issue of the question is what interventions a new mother can use to decrease physiologic jaundice. Eliminate options that contain the extreme words *permanently* and *nothing*. Choose the option that provides nutrition, not just hydration, for the newborn infant.

15 **Answer: 1 Rationale:** The top of the can and can opener should be washed with soap and water to remove microorganisms. The concentrate is mixed with an equal amount of water. Forcing an infant to finish a bottle after he seems satisfied may cause regurgitation and lead to infant obesity. Warming the bottle in the microwave can cause "hot spots" and burn the infant's mouth. **Cognitive Level:** Applying **Client Need:** Health Promotion and Maintenance **Integrated Process:** Nursing Process: Implementation **Content Area:** Maternal–Newborn **Strategy:** The core issue of the question is proper methods and techniques for bottle-feeding an infant. Note the words *to instruct*, which tells you that the correct option is also a true statement. Use the process of elimination and nursing knowledge to make a final selection.

16 **Answer: 2 Rationale:** Breastfed infants will have 6–10 small, loose yellow stools per day during the first few months. They are not brown, green, or well formed. Meconium may have a greenish color to it, but it is not a permanent color. **Cognitive Level:** Applying **Client Need:** Health Promotion and Maintenance **Integrated Process:** Communication and Documentation **Content Area:** Maternal–Newborn **Strategy:** The core issue of the question is normal bowel elimination patterns for a newborn infant who is breastfeeding. A simple way to remember this is to remember that they are yellow, liquid, and frequent.

17 **Answer: 3, 4, 5 Rationale:** Abduction is limited in the affected leg. The nurse would expect an absent femoral pulse when the affected leg is abducted. The nurse should expect limited abduction (movement away from the center) in the affected leg. The nurse would expect to find asymmetrical gluteal folds in an infant with hip dysplasia. An infant with hip dysplasia would not have symmetrical gluteal folds. An infant with hip dysplasia would not have limitations in adduction (movement toward the center) of the affected leg. **Cognitive Level:** Analyzing **Client Need:** Physiological Adaptation **Integrated Process:** Nursing Process: Assessment **Content Area:** Maternal–Newborn **Strategy:** The core issue of the question is abnormal assessment findings associated with hip dysplasia. Eliminate normal findings and discriminate between abduction and adduction to make your selections.

18 **Answer: 1, 4 Rationale:** The usual position of the infant is partially flexed, and all movements should be symmetrical. Any absent, asymmetrical, or fine jumping movements suggest nervous system disorders and should be evaluated further. Muscle tone should increase when the newborn is stimulated by being held. A weak sucking effort in the newborn would be considered adequate as long as it is effective. The Babinski or plantar reflex (fanning and hyperextension of the toes when the sole is stroked upward from the heel toward the ball of the foot) is normal in the newborn. The grasping reflex (in which a newborn grasps onto an object placed in the palm of the hand) is normal in the newborn. **Cognitive Level:** Applying **Client Need:** Health Promotion and Maintenance **Integrated Process:** Nursing Process: Assessment **Content Area:** Maternal–Newborn **Strategy:** This question is worded as a negative statement. The correct answer would be the options that contain abnormal assessment findings that warrant further investigation.

19 **Answer: 2, 5 Rationale:** Regurgitation of small amounts of formula is common in the newborn. Regurgitation may be caused by "overfeeding" or occur because the newborn has an immature cardiac sphincter. There is no reason to measure the newborn's temperature at this time. Feedings should not be discontinued for 6–8 hours; the newborn needs nutrition and hydration. There is no need to notify the healthcare provider. **Cognitive Level:** Applying **Client Need:** Health Promotion and Maintenance **Integrated Process:** Nursing Process: Planning **Content Area:** Maternal–Newborn **Strategy:** Because the wording in the stem of the question is positive, the correct option(s) will all be true statements. Knowledge of normal newborn care related to bottle-feeding will aid in answering this question correctly.

20 **Answer: 1, 5 Rationale:** Keeping the nipple full of formula prevents the infant from sucking air. Keeping the infant close with head elevated is an optimal position for bottle-feeding. Propping the bottle increases the risk of aspiration of formula. Pointing the bottle at the infant's tongue could cause the infant to gag and vomit. Enlarging the nipple opening can allow too much formula to enter the mouth, leading to vomiting and possible aspiration. **Cognitive Level:** Analyzing **Client Need:** Health Promotion and Maintenance **Integrated Process:** Nursing Process: Evaluation **Content Area:** Maternal–Newborn **Strategy:** The question is worded positively, indicating that the correct options are also correct actions. Use principles related to prevention of aspiration to help make your selections.

Key Terms to Review

acrocyanosis p. 140
Babinski reflex p. 140
Barlow's maneuver p. 140
caput succedaneum p. 139
cephalohematoma p. 139
ductus arteriosus p. 141
ductus venosus p. 141
Epstein's pearls p. 139
Erb-Duchenne paralysis (Erb's palsy) p. 140
foramen ovale p. 141
grasp reflex p. 140
lanugo p. 140
latch-on p. 144
meconium p. 142
milia p. 140
Mongolian spots p. 140
Moro reflex p. 142
Ortolani's maneuver p. 140
pilonidal dimple p. 140
plantar grasp p. 140
rooting reflex p. 139
sucking reflex p. 139
tonic neck reflex p. 139
trunk incurvation p. 140
vernix caseosa p. 140

References

Davidson, M., London, M., & Ladewig, P. (2016). *Olds' maternal newborn nursing and women's health across the lifespan* (10th ed.). New York, NY: Pearson Education.

Ladewig, P., London, M., & Davidson, M. (2014). *Contemporary maternal–newborn nursing care* (8th ed.). Upper Saddle River, NJ: Pearson Education.

London, M., Ladewig, P., Davidson, M., Ball, J., Bindler, R., & Cowen, K. (2014). *Maternal and child nursing care* (4th ed.). Upper Saddle River, NJ: Pearson Education.

Lowdermilk, D., Perry, S., Cashion, M., & Alden, K. (2016). *Maternity and women's health care* (11th ed.). St. Louis, MO: Elsevier.

Test Yourself

Are you ready for the NCLEX-RN® or course exams? Access the NEW web-based app that provides students with thousands of practice questions in preparation for the NCLEX experience.

Lifespan Growth and Development 13

In this chapter

Cross Reference

Other chapters relevant to this content area are

Providing Immunizations	Chapter 14
Promoting Healthy Lifestyle Choices	Chapter 16
Age-Related Care of Older Adults	Chapter 17
End-of-Life Care	Chapter 24
Pediatric Dosage Calculation and Medications	Chapter 30
Maternal and Newborn Medications	Chapter 34

I. INTRODUCTION TO GROWTH AND DEVELOPMENT

A. Patterns of growth and development

1. Each person displays definite predictable patterns of growth and development that are universal and basic to all human beings
2. Individual differences: although sequence is predictable, variations exist in rates of growth at which people reach developmental milestones
3. Directional trends: growth and development follow a specific pattern
   a. **Cephalocaudal development**: proceeds from head downward through body toward feet (head to tail)
   b. **Proximodistal development**: proceeds from center of body outward to extremities (near to far)
   c. **Differentiation**: development from simple operations to more complex activities and functions
4. Sequential trends: orderly; each person normally passes through every stage
   a. Each stage is affected by preceding stage and affects stages that follow
   b. **Critical periods**: time period in which person is especially responsive to certain environmental effects; sometimes called sensitive periods
   c. Positive and negative stimuli enhance or defer achievement of a skill or function

B. Factors influencing development (see Table 13–1)

Table 13–1 Factors Influencing Development

Factor	Influence
Genetics	A family history of diseases may be inherited by unique genes linked to specific disorders; chromosomes carry genes that determine physical characteristics, intellectual potential, and personality
Nutrition	Greatest influence on physical growth and intellectual development; adequate nutrition provides essentials for physiologic needs, which promote health and prevent illness
Prenatal and environmental factors	Nutritional status in utero and exposures in utero such as alcohol, smoking, infections, drugs; also environmental exposures, such as radiation and chemicals
Family and community	A stimulating family environment helps individual reach his or her potential; family structure and community support services influence environment and thereby growth and development
Cultural factors	Customs, traditions, and attitudes of cultural groups influence growth and development regarding physical health, social interaction, and assumed roles

II. GROWTH AND DEVELOPMENT THEORIES

NCLEX® **A. Stages of Piaget's theory of cognitive development (see Table 13–2)**

Table 13–2 Stages of Piaget's Theory of Cognitive Development

Stage	Characteristics
Sensorimotor (birth to 2 years)	1. Infant learns about world through senses and motor activity 2. Progresses from reflex activity through simple repetitive behaviors to imitative behaviors 3. Develops a sense of "cause and effect" 4. Language enables child to better understand the world 5. Curiosity, experimentation, and exploration result in the learning process 6. Object permanence is fully developed
Preoperational (2–7 years)	1. Forms symbolic thought 2. Exhibits egocentrism—inability to understand another's position or put him- or herself in the place of another 3. Unable to understand conservation (e.g., clay shapes, glasses of liquid) 4. Increasing ability to use language 5. Play becomes more socialized 6. Can concentrate on only one characteristic of an object at a time (centration)
Concrete operational (7–11 years)	1. Thoughts become increasingly logical and coherent 2. Able to shift attention from one perceptual attribute to another (decentration) 3. Concrete thinkers: view things as black or white, right or wrong, no in between or gray areas 4. Able to classify and sort facts, do problem solving 5. Acquires conservation skills
Formal operations (11 years to death)	1. Able to manipulate abstract and unobservable concepts logically 2. Adaptable and flexible 3. Able to deal with contradictions 4. Uses scientific approach to problem solve 5. Able to conceive the distant future

NCLEX® **B. Stages of Erikson's theory of psychosocial development (see Table 13–3)**

Table 13–3 Stages of Erikson's Theory of Psychosocial Development

Stage	Characteristics
Trust vs. mistrust (birth to 1 year)	1. Task of first year of life is to establish trust in people providing care 2. Mistrust develops if basic needs are inconsistently or inadequately met
Autonomy vs. shame and doubt (1–3 years)	1. Increased ability to control self and environment 2. Practices and attains new physical skills, developing autonomy 3. Symbolizes independence by controlling body secretions, saying "no" when asked to do something, and directing motor activity 4. If successful, develops self-confidence and willpower; if criticized or unsuccessful, develops a sense of shame and doubt about own abilities
Initiative vs. guilt (3–6 years)	1. Explores physical world with all senses, initiates new activities, and considers new ideas 2. Initiative is demonstrated when child is able to formulate and carry out a plan of action 3. Develops a conscience 4. If successful, develops direction and purpose; if criticized, leads to feelings of guilt and a lack of purpose
Industry vs. inferiority (6–12 years)	1. Middle years of childhood; displays development of new interests and involvement in activities 2. Learns to follow rules 3. Acquires reading, writing, math, and social skills 4. If successful, develops confidence and enjoys learning about new things; if compared to others, may develop feeling of inadequacy; inferiority may develop if too much is expected
Identity vs. role confusion (12–18 years)	1. Rapid and marked physical changes 2. Preoccupation with physical appearance 3. Examines and redefines self, family, peer group, and community 4. Experiments with different roles 5. Peer group very important 6. If successful, develops confidence in self-identity and optimism; if unable to establish meaningful definition of self, develops role confusion
Intimacy vs. isolation (early adulthood)	1. Depends on strong sense of self-accomplishment in adolescence 2. Extends beyond sexual relations to broader view of psychosocial intimacy with a partner, parents, children, or friends 3. Searches for continuity, regularity, or unity in meaningful relationships rather than for relationships with little commitment
Generativity vs. stagnation (middle adulthood)	1. Includes a sense of productivity 2. Reaches and attains goals 3. Engages in critical self-review 4. Lack of achievement of developmental goal leads to stagnation and self-absorption
Ego integrity vs. despair (older adulthood)	1. Honest acceptance of life that has passed and current stage of life 2. At peace with self 3. Includes achieving an identity apart from work, acceptance of bodily changes without preoccupation, and acceptance of death

III. PRENATAL DEVELOPMENT

NCLEX® **A. Physical growth and development (see Table 13–4)**

Table 13–4 Overview of Fetal Development by Gestational Age in Weeks

Weeks	Length and Weight	Neurological and Musculoskeletal Systems	Cardiovascular and Respiratory Systems	Gastrointestinal and Genitourinary Systems	Endocrine, Integumentary, and Immune Systems, Eye/Ear
2–3	2 mm crown-to-rump (C-R)	Groove forms along middle back; neural tube forms from closure of groove	Blood circulation begins; tubular heart begins to form in 3rd week; nasal pits form	Liver begins to function; kidneys begin to form	***Endo:*** thyroid tissue forms ***Eyes:*** optic cup and lens pit form; pigment in eyes ***Ears:*** auditory pit closes
4	4–6 mm C-R; 0.4 grams	Anterior neural tube closes to form brain; posterior closure forms spinal cord; limb buds noted	Tubular heart beats (28 days); primitive RBCs circulate	Oral cavity forms; primitive jaws present; esophagus and trachea begin to divide; stomach forms; esophagus and intestine become tubular; pancreatic/liver ducts form	***Eyes:*** primitive eye is present ***Ears:*** primitive ear is present
6–7	**6 wks:** 12 mm C-R **7 wks:** 18 mm C-R	**6 wks:** Brain becomes differentiated with cranial nerves present at week 5; bone rudiments present; primitive skeleton forms; muscle mass begins to develop; skull and jaw ossification begins	**6 wks:** Heart chambers present (atrial division at 5 weeks); blood cell groups identifiable; trachea, bronchi, lung buds present **7 wks:** Fetal heartbeats detectable; diaphragm separates abdominal/thoracic cavities	**6 wks:** Oral/nasal cavities and upper lip form; liver starts to form RBCs; embryonic sex glands appear **7 wks:** Tongue separates; palate folds; stomach in final form; bladder and urethra separate from rectum; sex glands become testes or ovaries	**6 wks:** ***Ear:*** formation of external, middle, and inner ear continues **7 wks:** ***Eyes:*** optic nerve forms, eyelids present, lens thickens
8	2.5–3 cm C-R; 2 grams	Digits form; skeletal cells differentiate further; ossification begins in cartilaginous bones; muscle development in head, trunk, and limbs allows some movement	Development of heart and fetal circulation complete	Lip fusion complete; rotation in midgut; anal membrane has perforated; external male and female genitalia appear similar until end of 9th week	***Ear:*** external, middle, and inner ear assuming final forms
10	5–6 cm crown-to-heel (C-H); 14 grams	Neurons appear at caudal end of spinal cord; brain has basic divisions; nail growth begins in fingers/toes	By 9th week RBCs produce in liver	Lips separate from jaw; palate folds fuse; developing intestines are enclosed in abdomen; bladder sac forms; testosterone physical characteristics at 8–12 wks (males)	***Endo:*** Islets of Langerhans differentiated ***Eyes:*** lids fuse closed
12	8 cm C-R; 11.5 cm C-H; 45 grams	Clear outline of miniature bones (12–20 wks); process of ossification establishes; involuntary muscles in viscera appear	Lungs acquire definitive shape	Mouth palate complete; muscles in gut appear; bile secretion begins; liver produces most of RBCs	***Skin:*** delicate, pink ***Endo:*** thyroid secretes hormones; insulin present in pancreas ***Immune:*** lymphoid tissue in thymus gland

Table 13–4 Overview of Fetal Development by Gestational Age in Weeks (*continued*)

Weeks	Length and Weight	Neurological and Musculoskeletal Systems	Cardiovascular and Respiratory Systems	Gastrointestinal and Genitourinary Systems	Endocrine, Integumentary, and Immune Systems, Eye/Ear
16	13.5 cm C-R; 15 cm C-H; 200 grams	Teeth begin to form hard tissue for central incisors	Fetal heart tones audible with fetoscope at 16–20 weeks	Hard and soft palate differentiate; gastric and intestinal glands develop; intestines start to collect meconium; kidneys assume shape and organization; able to note sex	***Skin:*** scalp hair appears; body has lanugo; visible blood vessels beneath transparent skin; sweat glands develop ***Eyes, ears, nose:*** fully form
20	25 cm C-H; 435 grams (6% fat)	Spinal cord myelination begins; teeth begin to form hard tissue for canine and first molar (lateral incisors at 18 wks); lower limbs have final relative proportions	Fetal heart tones audible; primitive respiratory-like movements begin; iron is stored in blood; bone marrow important	Fetus sucks and swallows amniotic fluid; peristalsis begins	***Skin:*** lanugo covers entire body; brown fat and vernix caseosa begin to form ***Endo:*** iron is stored; bone marrow functioning, fetal antibodies detectable ***Immune:*** fetal IgG levels detectable
24	28 cm C-H; 780 grams	Brain appears mature; teeth begin to form 2nd molars	Respiratory movements occur (24–40 wks); nostrils reopen; alveoli appear and begin to produce surfactant; gas exchange possible	Testes descend into inguinal ring (males)	***Skin:*** reddish and wrinkled ***Immune:*** IgG at mature levels ***Eyes:*** structurally complete
28–32	**28 wks:** 35 cm C-H; 1200–1250 grams **32 wks:** 38–43 cm C-H; 2000 grams	**28 wks:** Nervous system begins regulation of some bodily processes **32 wks:** More reflexes present	Viability is reached at 26–27 weeks; if born now, intensive care is needed to support respirations	Testes descend into inguinal canal and upper scrotum (males)	**28 wks: *Eyes:*** eyelids open ***Skin:*** adipose tissue begins to accumulate; eyebrows and eyelashes develop
36–40	**36 wks:** 42–48 cm C-H; 2500–2750 grams **40 wks:** 48–52 cm C-H; 3200+ grams (16% fat)	**36 wks:** Ossification centers present in distal femur	**38 wks:** Lecithin-sphingomyelin (L/S) ratio approaches 2:1 (less risk of respiratory distress from inadequate surfactant if born)	**36 wks:** small scrotum with few rugae (males); final descent of testes into upper scrotum (36–40 wks); labia majora/minora equally prominent (females) **40 wks:** rugous scrotum (males); labia majora well developed and cover the smaller labia minora and clitoris (females)	**36 wks: *Skin:*** pale, lanugo disappearing, hair fuzzy/wooly, few sole creases, increased vernix caseosa (36–40 wks) ***Ears:*** lobes soft with little cartilage **40 wks: *Skin:*** smooth, pink; vernix in skinfolds, silky hair, lanugo on shoulders and upper back, nails extend to tips of digits, creases cover sole ***Ears:*** lobes firmer, increased cartilage

NCLEX® **B. Highlights of development of concern to parents**

1. Fetal heart begins to beat at 4 weeks
2. All body organs formed by 8 weeks
3. Fetal heart sounds heard by Doppler device at 8–12 weeks
4. Gender can be seen and has appearance of baby at 16 weeks
5. Heartbeat heard with a fetoscope and mother feels movement (quickening); assumes a favorite position in utero; head hair, eyebrows, and eyelashes present at 20 weeks
6. Weighs approximately 726 grams (1 lb, 10 oz) and activity is increasing; fetal respiratory movements begin at 24 weeks
7. Surfactant needed for breathing at birth is formed, and baby is two-thirds final size at 28 weeks
8. Fingernails and toenails formed and subcutaneous fat appears; baby appears less red and wrinkled at 32 weeks
9. Baby fills uterus and gets antibodies from mother at 38–40 weeks

IV. INFANT GROWTH AND DEVELOPMENT

A. Neonatal period (birth to 1 month)

1. General appearance: newborn's head is one quarter of body length; is top heavy with short lower extremities
2. NCLEX® Weight: 2.7–3.6 kg (6–8 lb); gains 142–198 grams (5–7 oz) weekly for first 6 months
3. Height: 50 cm (20 in.); grows 2.5 cm (1 in.) monthly for first 6 months
4. Head circumference: 33–35 cm (13–14 in.); head circumference is greater than chest circumference

B. Growth during infancy (1–12 months)

1. NCLEX® Weight: doubles birth weight in 6 months; triples birth weight in 1 year
2. Height: increases 50% by 1 year
3. Head growth is rapid; brain increases in weight 2.5 times by 1 year
   a. Head circumference exceeds chest circumference
   b. NCLEX® Posterior fontanel closes at 2–3 months
   c. Anterior fontanel closes by 12–18 months
4. NCLEX® Reflexes present at birth
   a. Moro: startle reflex elicited by loud noise or sudden change in position
   b. Tonic neck: elicted when infant lies supine and head is turned to one side; infant will assume a "fencing position"
   c. Gag, cough, blink, pupillary: protective reflexes
   d. Grasp: infant's hands and feet will grasp when hand or foot is stimulated
   e. Rooting: elicited when side of mouth is touched, causing infant to turn to that side
   f. Babinski: fanning of toes when sole of foot is stroked upward
5. Reflexes that appear during infancy
   a. Parachute: involves extension of arms when suspended in prone position and lowered suddenly
   b. Landau: when infant is suspended horizontally, head is raised
   c. Labyrinth righting: provides orientation of head in space
   d. Body righting: when caregiver turns hips to the side, the body follows
6. NCLEX® Gross motor development: developmental maturation in posture, head balance, sitting, creeping, standing, and walking
   a. Gains head control by 4 months
   b. Rolls from back to side by 4 months
   c. Rolls from abdomen to back by 5 months
   d. Rolls from back to abdomen by 6 months
   e. Sits alone without support by 8 months
   f. Stands holding furniture by 9 months
   g. Crawls (may go backward initially) by 10 months
   h. Creeps with abdomen off floor by 11 months
   i. Cruises (walking upright while holding furniture) by 10–12 months
   j. Can sit down from upright position by 10–12 months
   k. Walks well with one hand held by 12 months
7. NCLEX® Fine motor development: use of hands and fingers to grasp objects
   a. Hand predominantly closed at 1 month
   b. Desires to grasp at 3 months
   c. Two-handed, voluntary grasp at 5 months

d. Holds bottle, grasps feet at 6 months
e. Transfers from hand to hand by 7 months
f. Pincer grasp established by 10 months
g. Neat pincer grasp (e.g., picks up raisin) with thumb and finger by 12 months

8. Sensory development
a. Hearing and touch well developed at birth
b. Sight not fully developed until 6 years; differentiates light and dark at birth; prefers human face; smiles at 2 months
c. Usually searches and turns head to locate sounds by 2 months
d. Has taste preferences by 6 months
e. Responds to own name by 7 months
f. Able to follow moving objects; visual acuity 20/50 or better; amblyopia ("lazy eye") may develop by 12 months
NCLEX® g. Can vocalize four words by 1 year

9. Nutrition
a. Human breast milk is easily digested and most complete
b. Iron-fortified commercial formulas used for bottle feeding closely resemble nutritional content of human milk; recommended for first 12 months
NCLEX® c. Solids are introduced no sooner than 6 months to avoid exposure to allergens
d. Iron-fortified rice cereal is introduced first because of its low allergenic potential
e. Deciduous "baby" teeth erupt by 5–6 months; lateral incisors erupt first; increase in drooling and saliva; may be accompanied by slight elevated temperature
f. Gradual weaning from breast to bottle to cup during second 6 months of infancy
g. Juices may be introduced, diluted 1:1 at 6 months; preferably given by a cup
h. Introduction of fruits, vegetables, and meats (one food each week is recommended to identify any allergy)
i. Junior foods or chopped table foods introduced by 12 months
NCLEX® j. Limit intake of formula to no more than 907 grams (32 oz) per 24 hours to avoid iron-deficiency anemia

NCLEX® 10. Safety
a. Infants up to 9 kg (20 lb) and age 1 year should be restrained in a rear-facing car seat in middle of back seat of car; they may continue to be placed in a rear-facing direction until they reach the maximum height and weight allowed by car seat manufacturer
b. Keep side-rails of crib up
c. Never leave infant unattended on table or bed or in bathtub
d. Check temperature of bath water, formula, foods
e. Avoid giving bottles at naps or bedtime (may cause dental caries)
f. Parents should learn injury prevention, including aspiration of foreign objects (buttons, toys, peanuts, hot dogs), suffocation (plastic bags, strangulation), falls, poisonings, and burns (electric cords, wall outlets, radiators, pots and pans on stoves)

NCLEX® 11. Play (solitary)
a. Provide black/white contrasts for premature and newborn infants
b. Hang mobile 20–25 cm (8–10 in.) from infant's face
c. Provide sensory stimuli (bath water) and tactile stimuli (feel of various shapes of objects), large toys, balls
d. Expose to environmental sounds: rattles, musical toys
e. Use variety of primary-colored objects during infancy
f. Place unbreakable mirror in crib for infants to focus on own face
g. Provide toys that let infants practice skills to grasp and manipulate objects
h. Vocalization provides pleasure in relationships with people (smiling, cooing, laughing)

V. TODDLER GROWTH AND DEVELOPMENT

A. Period from 1 to 3 years of age

B. Weight: growth rate slows considerably; weight is four times the birth weight by 2½ years

C. Height: at 2 years, height is 50% of future adult height

D. Head circumference: 49–50 cm (19.5–20 in.) by 2 years; increases only 3 cm (1.2 in.) second year; achieves 90% of adult-sized brain by 2 years

NCLEX® **E. Anterior fontanel closes by 18 months**

NCLEX® **F. Gross motor development:** still clumsy at this age
1. Walks without help (usually by 15 months)
2. Jumps in place by 18 months
3. Goes up stairs (with 2 feet on each step) by 24 months
4. Runs fairly well (wide stance) by 24 months

NCLEX® **G. Fine motor development**
1. Uses cup well by 15 months
2. Builds a tower of two cubes by 15 months
3. Holds crayon with fingers by 24–30 months
4. Good hand–finger coordination by 30 months
5. Copies a circle by 3 years

H. Sensory development
1. Binocular vision well developed by 15 months
2. Knows own name by 12 months; refers to self
3. Identifies geometric forms by 18 months
4. Uses short sentences by 18 months to 2 years
5. Follows simple directions by 2 years
6. Able to speak 300 words by 2 years
7. Remembers and repeats three numbers by 3 years

I. *Object permanence* is knowledge that an object or person continues to exist when not seen, heard, or felt

J. Ritualistic behavior is exhibited during toddler period; *ritualism* is toddler's need to maintain sameness and reliability; provides sense of comfort

NCLEX® **K. Nutrition**
1. Growth slows at age 12–18 months; thus, appetite and need for intake decrease
2. Toddlers are picky, ritualistic eaters
3. Avoid more than 32 oz formula or milk/day to prevent iron-deficiency anemia
4. Avoid large pieces of food such as hot dogs, grapes, cherries, peanuts
5. Able to feed self completely by 3 years
6. Deciduous teeth (approx. 20) are present by 2½–3 years
7. Teach good dental practices (brushing, fluoride)

NCLEX® **L. Safety**
1. Continue to use car seat properly; children 20–40 lb (9–18 kg) should be in a forward-facing position in back seat of car, once they exceed car seat manufacturer height and weight limits for rear-facing seat; harness straps should be placed at or above shoulders
2. Supervise indoor play and outdoor activities
3. Teach that use of ipecac for accidental ingestions is no longer recommended
4. Teach injury prevention
   a. Childproof home environment: stairways, cupboards, medicine cabinet, outlets
   b. Suffocation: plastic bags, pacifier, toys, unused refrigerators
   c. Burns: ovens, heaters, sunburns; check water and food temperature
   d. Falls: stairs, windows, balconies, walkers
   e. Aspiration/poisonings: medications, cleaners, chemicals; store harmful substances out of reach

NCLEX® **M. Play (parallel)**
1. Begins as imaginative and make-believe play; may imitate adult in play
2. Provide blocks, wheel toys, push toys, puzzles, crayons to develop motor and coordination abilities
3. Toddlers enjoy repetitive stories and short songs with rhythm

VI. PRESCHOOL GROWTH AND DEVELOPMENT

A. Period from 3 to 5 years of age

B. Weight: growth is slow and steady; gains 1.8–2.3 kg (4–5 lb) per year

C. Height: increases 5–7.5 cm (2–3 in.) per year

D. Motor
1. Rides tricycle by 3 years
2. Skips and hops on one foot by 4 years
3. Throws and catches ball well by 5 years
4. Balances on alternate feet by 5 years
5. Knows 2,100 words by 5 years
6. NCLEX® Increased strength and refinement of fine and gross motor abilities

E. Nutrition
1. Similar to toddlers' eating patterns
2. Demonstrates food preferences: likes and dislikes
3. Influenced by others' eating habits
4. Caloric requirement: 90 kcal/kg/day
5. Reinforce good dental hygiene: regular exams, brushing, fluoride, less concentrated sugar

NCLEX® **F. Safety**
1. Belt–positioning booster seat can provide safety when child reaches 18 kg (40 lb) weight; should include use of lap and shoulder belts
2. Able to learn safety habits
3. Teach injury prevention such as traffic safety, risks with strangers, fire prevention/safety, water safety/drowning

NCLEX® **G. Play (associative)**
1. Enjoys imitative and dramatic play (imitates same-sex role in play)
2. Provide toys to develop motor and coordination skills (tricycle, clay, paints, swings, sliding board)
3. Parental supervision of television
4. Enjoys sing-along songs with rhythm

VII. SCHOOL-AGE GROWTH AND DEVELOPMENT

A. Period from 6 to 12 years of age
B. Weight: steady, slow growth; gains approximately 2.3 kg (5 lb.)/yr
C. Height: increases 2.5–5 cm (1–2 in.) per year; boys and girls differ little at first, but by end of period girls gain more weight and height compared to boys
D. Motor/sensory develop
1. Bones grow faster than muscles and ligaments develop
2. Susceptible to greenstick fractures
3. Movements become more limber, graceful, and coordinated
4. Have greater stamina and energy
5. Vision 20/20 by 6–7 years; myopia may appear by 8 years

E. Nutrition
1. Risk of obesity in this age group
2. NCLEX® Identify those above 95th and below 5th percentiles in weight and height on plotted growth charts
3. Requirement of 85 kcal/kg/day
4. Tendency to eat "junk" food, empty calories
5. Secondary sex characteristics begin at 10 years in girls; 12 years in boys
6. Loses first deciduous teeth at age 6; by age 12 has all permanent teeth, except final molars

NCLEX® **F. Safety**
1. Incidence of accidents/injuries less likely
2. Teach proper use of sports equipment
3. Discourage risk-taking behaviors (smoking, alcohol, drugs, sex)
4. Introduce sex education
5. Teach injury prevention: bicycle safety, firearms, smoking education, hobbies/handicrafts

NCLEX® **G. Play (cooperative)**
1. Comprehends rules and rituals of games
2. Enjoys team play, which helps instill values and develop sense of accomplishment
3. Enjoys athletic activities such as swimming, soccer, hiking, bicycling, basketball, baseball, football
4. Provide construction toys: puzzles, erector sets, small interlocking blocks
5. Good hand–eye coordination: interested in video and computer games (needs monitoring and time limits)
6. Enjoys music, adventure stories, competitive activities

VIII. ADOLESCENT GROWTH AND DEVELOPMENT

A. Period from 13 to 18 years of age
B. Weight: rapid period of growth causes anxiety; girls gain 7–25 kg (15–55 lb); boys gain 7–29 kg (15–65 lb)
C. Height: attain final 20% of mature height; girls: height increases 7.6 cm (3 in.) per year, slows at menarche, stops at 16 years; boys: height increases 10 cm (4 in.) per year, growth spurt approximately at 13 years, slows in late teens

NCLEX® **D. Puberty**
1. Related to hormonal changes
2. Apocrine glands become active; adolescent may develop body odor

3. Appearance of acne on face, back, trunk
4. Development of secondary sex characteristics: girls experience breast development, menarche (average age 12½ yrs), pubic hair; boys experience enlargement of testes (13 years), increase in scrotum and penis size, nocturnal emission, pubic hair, vocal changes, possibly gynecomastia

E. Nutrition

1. **Growth spurt**: brief period of rapid increase in growth
2. "Hollow leg stage": appetite increases
3. Nutrition requirements: 60–80 kcal/kg/day (approximately 1,500–3,000 kcal/day at 11–14 years) and 2,100–3,900 kcal/day at 15–18 years)
4. At risk for fad diets; food choices influenced by peers
5. Require increased calcium for skeletal growth
6. Continue emphasis on prevention of caries and good dental hygiene
7. Final molars erupt at end of adolescence; orthodontia common dental need

NCLEX® **F. Safety**

1. Accidents: leading cause of death (motor vehicle accidents, sports, firearms)
2. Provide drug and alcohol education
3. Provide sex education
4. Discourage risk-taking activities
5. Adolescents may display lack of impulse control, reckless behaviors, sense of invulnerability
6. Teach health promotion: breast self-exam (BSE), testicular self-exam (TSE)
7. Teach injury prevention
   a. Proper use of sports equipment (protective gear)
   b. Diving, drowning
   c. Provide driver's education
   d. Use of seat belts
   e. Violence prevention
   f. Crisis intervention (stress, depression, eating disorders)
   g. Provide information about the risks of body piercing
8. Reinforce rules when necessary

NCLEX® **G. Play/activities**

1. Enjoy sports, school and peer group activities (movies, dances, eating out, music, videos, computers)
2. Interest in heterosexual relationships common

IX. ADULT GROWTH AND DEVELOPMENT

A. Consists of young adulthood (18–35 years), middle adulthood (36–64 years), and older adulthood (65 years and older)

B. See Chapter 17 for discussion of needs of older adults

NCLEX® **C. Weight:** stabilizes in adulthood, although risks of overweight and obesity may apply based on lifestyle and eating habits

D. Height: stabilized

E. Young adulthood generally considered to be healthiest time of life

F. Physical strength, coordination, endurance, and speed of response are at maximal levels

G. Nutrition

1. Nutrient needs influenced by activity level and body size
2. Nutritional needs increase during pregnancy and lactation
3. Decreased fat intake, and increased intake of fruits, vegetables, and fiber recommended to promote healthy lifestyle (see Chapter 16)

NCLEX® **H. Safety**

1. Accidents, injuries, and acts of violence are frequent causes of death
2. Injury prevention methods similar to adolescence: proper use of safety and sports equipment, seat belts, and reduction of personal risk behaviors

NCLEX® **I. Leisure activities**

1. Should include healthy form of exercise most days of week (see Chapter 16)
2. May take a wide variety of forms depending on personal interests
3. Leisure activities should be encouraged for personal enjoyment and as means to reduce stress

X. CHILD'S REACTION TO ILLNESS AND HOSPITALIZATION

A. Infants and toddlers

1. Parent–child relationship is disturbed
2. Unpredictable routine of hospital promotes feelings of distrust

3. Infants and toddlers experience **separation anxiety**, which is distress behavior observed between ages 6 and 30 months when separated from familiar caregivers; it peaks around 15 months
4. Stages of separation anxiety include protest (child appears sad, agitated, angry, inconsolable, watches desperately for parents to return), despair (child appears sad, hopeless, withdrawn; acts ambivalent when parents return), and detachment (child appears happy, interested in environment, becomes attached to staff members; may ignore parents)

NCLEX®

5. Goal of nursing interventions is to preserve child's trust
   a. Reassure child that parents will return
   b. Provide "rooming in" to encourage parent–child attachment
   c. Have parents leave a personal article, picture, or favorite toy with child
   d. Maintain usual routine and rituals, whenever possible
   e. Allow choices, whenever possible, to return control to parent and child

NCLEX®

6. Responses to pain
   a. Infants will have increases in blood pressure and heart rate and decrease in arterial oxygen saturation
   b. Harsh, tense, or loud crying
   c. Facial grimacing, flinching, thrashing of extremities
   d. Toddlers will verbally indicate discomfort ("no," "ouch," "hurts")
   e. Generalized restlessness, uncooperative, clings to family member

NCLEX®

7. **Regression:** use of behavior representative of an earlier stage of development, often used to cope with stress or anxiety
   a. Result is lack of control, frustration, possible return to bottle-feeding, temper tantrums, incontinence
   b. Help parents to understand changes in behavior; avoid punishment

B. Preschoolers

1. Major fears
   a. Mutilation: have general lack of understanding of body integrity
   b. Intrusive procedures: will misinterpret words; have active imagination
2. Very egocentric and present-oriented
3. Perceive illness as punishment; associate own actions with disease; may believe hospitalization is punishment for bad behavior

NCLEX®

4. Some degree of separation anxiety still exists; may become uncooperative, develop nightmares, become withdrawn or aggressive

NCLEX®

5. Nursing interventions
   a. Encourage parents to participate in childcare
   b. Allow child to express feelings
   c. Give simple explanations; avoid medical terminology
   d. Provide **therapeutic play** (planned play techniques that provide an opportunity for children to deal with fears and concerns about illness or hospitalization)
   e. Allow child to manipulate and play with equipment
   f. Maintain trusting relationship with parents and child; allow time for questions
   g. Praise child, focus on the desired behavior, give rewards (stickers)
6. May show signs of regression to toddlerhood (such as loss of bowel/bladder control)

NCLEX®

7. Response to pain
   a. All children have a major fear of needles; preschoolers will deny pain to avoid an injection
   b. Restless, irritable, cries, kicks with experiences of pain
   c. Able to describe location and intensity of pain

C. School-age children

1. Major fears
   a. Pain and bodily injury
   b. Loss of control
   c. Fears often related to school, peers, and family
2. Ask relevant questions, want to know reasons for procedures, tests
3. Have a more realistic understanding of disease
4. Become distressed over separation from family and peers

NCLEX®

5. Nursing interventions
   a. Communicate openly and honestly; explain rules
   b. Clarify any misconceptions
   c. Encourage participation in care to maintain sense of control and independence
   d. Provide visiting for siblings and peers

e. Use age-appropriate therapeutic play to provide an opportunity for children to deal with fears and concerns about illness or hospitalization
f. Art therapy to assist child to express feelings
g. Provide explanations; use visual aids such as diagrams, models, and body outlines
h. Praise child; focus on desired behavior

NCLEX® 6. Response to pain
a. Able to describe pain; concerned with disability and death
b. Girls express pain more often than boys do
c. Demonstrate overt behaviors: biting, kicking, crying, and bargaining
d. Cues to pain: facial expression, silence, false sense of being "okay"

D. Adolescents

1. Major fears: loss of independence and/or identity, body image disturbance, rejection by others
2. Separation from peers is a source of anxiety
3. Physical appearance has major influence on how adolescents perceive themselves
4. Behaviors seen with loss of control: anger, withdrawal, uncooperative, power struggles
5. Reluctant to ask questions; question competency of others, verify answers with more than one person to determine if others are truthful
6. Often believe they are invincible, nothing can hurt them, resulting in risk-taking and noncompliant behaviors

NCLEX® 7. Nursing interventions
a. Involve adolescent in plan of care
b. Support relationships with family and peers
c. Provide consistent and truthful explanations; can use abstract terms
d. Accept emotional outburts
e. Promote communication between adolescents and parents

NCLEX® 8. Response to pain
a. Associate pain with being different from peers
b. May exhibit projected confidence, conceited attitude; withdraws, rejects others
c. Increased muscle tension and body control
d. Understand cause and effect; able to describe pain

XI. CHILD'S REACTION TO DEATH AND DYING

A. Infants and toddlers

1. Both lack an understanding of concept of death

NCLEX® 2. Infants react to loss of caregiver with behaviors such as crying, sleeping more, and eating less
3. Aware someone is missing; may experience separation anxiety

NCLEX® 4. Toddlers may develop fearfulness, become more attached to remaining parent, cease walking and talking

B. Preschoolers

1. View death as temporary and reversible
2. Magical thinking and **egocentricity** (preoccupied with own interests and needs; self-centered) lead to belief that dead person will come back
3. View death as a punishment; believe bad thoughts and actions cause death
4. First exposure to death is frequently death of a pet

NCLEX® 5. Common behaviors: nightmares, bowel and bladder problems, crying, anger, out-of-control behaviors

NCLEX® 6. Preschoolers will ask a lot of questions, may display fascination with death

C. School-age children

1. View death as irreversible, but not necessarily inevitable
2. By age 10, understand death is universal and will happen to them
3. May believe death serves as a punishment for wrongdoing
4. May deny sadness, attempt to act like an adult

NCLEX® 5. Common behaviors: difficulty with concentration in school, psychosomatic complaints, acting-out behaviors

D. Adolescents

1. View death as irreversible, universal, and inevitable
2. Seen as a personal but distant event
3. Develop a better understanding between illness and death

NCLEX® 4. Sense of invincibility conflicts with fear of death

NCLEX®

5. Common behaviors: feelings of loneliness, sadness, fear, depression; acting-out behaviors may include risk-taking, delinquency, suicide attempts, promiscuity

E. Adults (see Chapter 24, "End-of-Life Care")

Check Your NCLEX–RN® Exam I.Q.

You are ready for testing on this content if you can:

- Describe expected physical, cognitive, psychosocial, and moral stages of development.
- Assess the developmental stage of a client.
- Plan appropriate nursing care based on client's developmental stage.
- Modify nursing care based on developmental stage of client.
- Evaluate achievement of developmental milestones.

PRACTICE TEST

PRACTICE TEST

1 The charge nurse is developing plans to reduce the stress of a hospitalized, chronically ill 8-year-old child. Which approach by the nurse is most likely to improve the child's coping ability? Select all that apply.

1. Allow 24-hour open visitation with peers.
2. Provide care specifically designed for a school-age child.
3. Have tutoring postponed until discharge.
4. Caution against making any decisions while hospitalized.
5. Offer the child some choices for activities such as bathing or ambulating.

2 A mother brings her 15-month-old son to the clinic. During the nursing assessment, the mother makes the following comments. Which comment merits further investigation?

1. "My son cries at times when I leave him at his grandparents' house."
2. "My son always takes his blanket with him."
3. "My son is not crawling yet."
4. "My son likes to eat mashed potatoes."

3 An inexperienced mother is playing with her 8-month-old in the playroom. The nurse has taught the mother about toys that are developmentally appropriate for the child. The nurse will conclude that teaching has been successful when the mother selects which type of toy? Select all that apply.

1. A set of blocks
2. A wagon
3. A puzzle with large pieces
4. A rattle — too little / for yunger
5. A soft ball

4 The nurse is caring for a 7-year-old child scheduled for surgery in the morning. While conducting preoperative teaching, the nurse would choose which aid to enhance the child's learning about the perioperative experience?

1. Videotape
2. Colorful brochure
3. Doll or puppet
4. A visit from the surgeon

5 A mother has brought her 4-year-old child for Denver II testing for routine assessment of social and physical abilities. The child refuses to complete the testing. What should the nurse do?

1. Refer the child to a specialist.
2. Explain that the child is developmentally delayed.
3. Complete the test as scheduled.
4. Reschedule the testing for another day.

6 The parents of a 16-month-old ask when they should begin toilet training. What information should the nurse include in a response? Select all that apply.

1. When the child walks well
2. When the child is able to sit alone without support
3. When the child enters preschool
4. When the child has a dry diaper throughout the night
5. When the child can pull pants up and down

7. The grandparents of a 2½-year-old ask what would be an appropriate toy to buy their grandson. Which toy should the nurse recommend? Select all that apply.

1. A play telephone
2. A 54-piece puzzle
3. A paint-by-number set
4. ~~A musical mobile~~
5. A small tricycle

8. The pediatric nurse should avoid using therapeutic play with a hospitalized 6-year-old at which times? Select all that apply.

1. During preoperative teaching
2. At bedtime
3. Before a diagnostic test
4. During a bedside procedure
5. When the child is stressed

9. The nurse discusses the risk of aspiration with the parents of an 18-month-old. To minimize this risk, the nurse recommends the parents avoid giving their child which food items?

1. Orange slices, crackers, and applesauce
2. Apple slices, fruit juice, and raisins
3. Cherries, peanuts, and hard candy
4. Cheerios, toast, and bananas

10. The pediatric nurse is a guest speaker for general health teaching in a prenatal class with young adults. The nurse should stress which factor that is most important to promote positive fetal growth and development?

1. Nutrition
2. Financial income
3. Exposure to secondary smoke
4. Ethnic background

11. The nurse working in a sexually transmitted infection (STI) clinic of the city health department gives a tour to a group of student nurses. A student notes that the clinic population consists largely of teenagers. The nurse should explain that adolescents are at a greater risk for contracting STIs because of which factor?

1. The immune system of an adolescent is immature.
2. Untreated urinary tract infections will develop into an STI.
3. Adolescents are risk-takers and believe they are invincible.
4. Adolescents often lack parental supervision.

12. The nurse working in a sexually transmitted infection (STI) clinic uses communication skills to assess clients and to provide health education. When developing rapport with a new adolescent client, it is important for the nurse to use which approach?

1. Consistently give honest information.
2. Have the parents present if at all possible.
3. Use jargon when communicating with the adolescent.
4. Allow the adolescent to smoke if desired during the conversation.

13. Results of a Denver Developmental Screening Test reveal that a 6-month-old infant is delayed in gross motor development. What activities by the nurse would best help the child reach the expected developmental level? Select all that apply.

1. Encouraging the child to stand
2. Talking to the child
3. Propping the child in a sitting position
4. Encouraging the child to hold a rattle
5. Pulling the child to a sitting position

14. A 4-year-old child is delayed in language skills. In developing a care plan, what would be the most appropriate nursing concept for the nurse to focus on for this child?

1. Social isolation
2. Parenting skills
3. Verbal communication
4. Auditory sensory perception

15. The nurse needs to obtain a height on a 3-year-old child as a part of routine health screening. To obtain an accurate measurement, the nurse should instruct the child to perform which action?

1. Lie down in a supine position.
2. Remove shoes and stand upright with head erect.
3. Stand with his or her feet wide apart.
4. Face the wall while being measured.

16 The nurse admitting four children to the hospital unit learns that none of the parents will be staying with the children. The nurse would be most concerned with adjustment to hospitalization and separation from parents in the infant or child of which age?

1. 2 months old
2. 13 months old
3. 8 years old
4. 14 years old

17 A toddler is admitted for severe anemia, which is found to be dietary in nature. What recommendation should the nurse make to the parents to enhance dietary iron intake to promote healthy growth and development?

1. Limit milk to no more than 907 grams (32 oz) per day.
2. Increase fat-soluble vitamins in the diet.
3. Include grains and legumes in the daily intake.
4. Limit foods that are high in protein in the daily caloric requirement.

18 The mother of a neonate states she is concerned about her relationship with the infant. She says the baby goes to anyone and doesn't seem to care if she is present or not. The nurse explains that prior to developing a dependence on the mother, the infant must develop which of the following?

1. Ritualistic behavior
2. Egocentrism
3. Conservation
4. Object permanence

19 The nurse discusses swimming pool safety with the parents of 4-year-old twins. Which statement identifies that additional instruction is needed? Select all that apply.

1. "We remove all toys from the pool area when not in use."
2. "The twins wear flotation devices when they are in the pool by themselves."
3. "We never go in the house for more than a minute when the twins are in the pool."
4. "We always tell the twins not to run by the pool."
5. "Our children are enrolled in swimming classes."

20 The nurse prepares to transport a sedated 2-year-old from the pediatric unit to the endoscopy department. Taking into consideration the child's developmental stage and safety, what should the nurse use to transport the child to the area?

1. Padded wagon
2. Small wheelchair
3. High-top crib
4. Gurney (stretcher)

ANSWERS & RATIONALES

1 **Answer: 2, 5 Rationale:** Age-specific care is care that better meets the developmental needs of the hospitalized child. Providing opportunity for choices is beneficial for the child to achieve some sense of control while being hospitalized. Although visitation of peers is important, open visitation is usually recommended only for family members. Depending on the status of the child's illness and resources available, tutoring may be recommended. Mutual decision making is beneficial for the child and family. **Cognitive Level:** Applying **Client Need:** Health Promotion and Maintenance **Integrated Process:** Nursing Process: Planning **Content Area:** Foundational Sciences **Strategy:** Use the process of elimination. Critical words in the question are *8-year-old*, which leads you to look for an option that matches the needs of a child of this age group.

2 **Answer: 3 Rationale:** Infants crawl or pull their body along the floor using their arms by age 8–10 months, which is a growth and developmental milestone. An inability to crawl by age 15 months is an abnormal finding, and should be referred to the healthcare provider for follow-up. It is a normal response for a 15-month-old to cry when left with others. Infants and toddlers are often attached to security items, such as a blanket. Toddlers begin to display food preferences. **Cognitive Level:** Analyzing **Client Need:** Health Promotion and Maintenance **Integrated Process:** Nursing Process: Diagnosis **Content Area:** Foundational Sciences **Strategy:** Use the process of elimination and knowledge of growth and development to answer the question. The wording of the question indicates the correct option is one in which the child is not meeting developmental milestones.

3 **Answer: 1, 5 Rationale:** Objects that can be grasped and banged together, such as blocks, develop manipulation skills and are most appropriate for an 8-month-old infant. Pleasure is experienced from the feel and sounds of these activities. Throwing or rolling a ball helps the infant to develop gross motor skills and is appropriate for this age. A wagon may be used by preschoolers and toddlers. A large-piece puzzle may be used by preschoolers and toddlers. Rattles are recommended for infants ages 1–6 months. **Cognitive Level:** Applying **Client Need:** Health Promotion and Maintenance **Integrated Process:** Nursing Process: Evaluation **Content Area:** Foundational Sciences **Strategy:** Use the process of elimination and knowledge of growth and development to answer the question. The question indicates that more than one option may be correct. The correct answers match the physical development level of the child with the skills ability needed to use the toy.

4 **Answer: 3 Rationale:** The use of a doll or puppet may decrease a 7-year-old child's anxiety and fear if the nurse uses such aids to explain what is expected. Videotapes are useful with explanations to adolescents. Brochures are useful with explanations to adolescents. A visit from the surgeon is informative primarily with the parents. **Cognitive Level:** Applying **Client Need:** Health Promotion and Maintenance **Integrated Process:** Nursing Process: Implementation **Content Area:** Foundational Sciences **Strategy:** Use the process of elimination and knowledge of growth and development to answer the question. The core issue of the question is the most effective method of teaching to use with a school-age child.

5 **Answer: 4 Rationale:** There are many reasons why a child would be uncooperative, including fatigue, illness, and fear. To get accurate results, the test should be rescheduled for another day. There is no evidence at this time that the child needs a specialist. The child's behavior does not indicate developmental delay. The child should not be forced to undergo testing that day. **Cognitive Level:** Analyzing **Client Need:** Health Promotion and Maintenance **Integrated Process:** Nursing Process: Implementation **Content Area:** Foundational Sciences **Strategy:** Use the process of elimination and knowledge of growth and development. Recalling that a 4-year-old may be trying to assert independence and control, each incorrect option may be eliminated as a less than optimal response by the nurse.

6 **Answer: 1, 5 Rationale:** Children must have the physical and developmental capabilities to begin toilet training. They should be able to stand and walk well, pull pants up and down, recognize the urge to urinate or defecate, and be able to wait until they reach the potty chair. **Cognitive Level:** Analyzing **Client Need:** Health Promotion and Maintenance **Integrated Process:** Nursing Process: Planning **Content Area:** Foundational Sciences **Strategy:** Use the process of elimination and knowledge of growth and development. The core issue of the question is physical and mental readiness for toilet training. The wording of the question indicates more than one option is likely to be correct.

7 **Answer: 1, 5 Rationale:** Toddlers enjoy such toys as a play telephone, which allows them to practice imitative behaviors and fine motor skills. Manipulation of toys such as a tricycle develops gross motor abilities in toddlers. More complex puzzles, such as those with 54 pieces, are recommended for school-age children. Paint-by-number sets are recommended for school-age children. Musical mobiles are appropriate for infants. **Cognitive Level:** Applying **Client Need:** Health Promotion and Maintenance **Integrated Process:** Nursing Process: Implementation **Content Area:** Foundational Sciences **Strategy:** Use the process of elimination and knowledge of growth and development. The core issue of the question is knowledge of appropriate play items for a toddler.

8 **Answer: 2, 4 Rationale:** Play is not recommended at bedtime to maintain a restful environment, or when the child needs to remain quiet, such as during a procedure. A quiet and calm environment will promote sleep. Play is a very effective teaching intervention. It is often used before surgery and diagnostic tests to aid understanding of these events. Play is therapeutic to help the child express feelings during stressful times. **Cognitive Level:** Applying **Client Need:** Health Promotion and Maintenance **Integrated Process:** Teaching and Learning **Content Area:** Foundational Sciences **Strategy:** Use the process of elimination and knowledge of growth and development. The core issue of the question is that therapeutic play must be used at appropriate times and in appropriate ways to be effective.

9 **Answer: 3 Rationale:** Toddlers chew well but may have difficulty swallowing large pieces of food. Young children cannot discard pits (such as from cherries). Firm foods such as peanuts and hard candies are easily aspirated. Orange slices, crackers, and applesauce have a soft consistency that can be swallowed easily by a toddler. Apple slices, fruit juice, and raisins can be easily swallowed by toddlers after chewing. Cheerios, toast, and bananas are either soft or become soft with action of saliva and are easily swallowed by toddlers. **Cognitive Level:** Applying **Client Need:** Health Promotion and Maintenance **Integrated Process:** Teaching and Learning **Content Area:** Foundational Sciences **Strategy:** Use the process of elimination and knowledge of growth and development. The core issue of the question is knowledge of the physical abilities of the child to swallow foods at various ages.

10 **Answer: 1 Rationale:** Nutrition is the greatest influence on growth and development because diet supplies the nutrients needed to sustain physiological needs and for bodily growth, which then influences overall development. Insufficient income could indirectly affect growth and development, but this depends on how income is used in providing nutritious foods for the body. Exposure to secondary smoke can indirectly affect health but does not exert the greatest influence on growth and development. Ethnic background has significant influence on culturally based habits but not necessarily on biological growth and development. **Cognitive Level:** Analyzing **Client Need:** Health Promotion and Maintenance **Integrated Process:** Nursing Process: Implementation **Content Area:** Foundational Sciences **Strategy:** Use the process of elimination and knowledge of growth and development to answer the question. The core issue of the question is knowledge of priority factors affecting overall growth and development.

11 **Answer: 3 Rationale:** Adolescents often think no harm can come to them, which places them at high risk for injury or disease from dangerous behaviors. The adolescent's immune system is well developed. Urinary tract infections do not cause STIs. Not all adolescents lack parental supervision. **Cognitive Level:** Analyzing **Client Need:** Health Promotion and Maintenance **Integrated Process:** Nursing Process: Implementation **Content Area:** Foundational Sciences **Strategy:** Use the process of elimination and knowledge of growth and development to answer the question. The core issue of the question is characteristics of adolescent growth and development that can increase risk of illness or injury to an adolescent.

12 **Answer: 1 Rationale:** Nurses are credible sources of information, support, and encouragement that can help adolescents

cope with challenges. To develop trust, honest and accurate information must be given to the client. The adolescent should be given the choice to have parents present because of the nature of the health problem, but treatment for STIs can be given without parental consent. The nurse should use appropriate language rather than jargon when communicating with clients. The client should not smoke during discussions with the nurse for general health reasons. **Cognitive Level:** Applying **Client Need:** Health Promotion and Maintenance **Integrated Process:** Communication and Documentation **Content Area:** Foundational Sciences **Strategy:** Use the process of elimination and knowledge of growth and development. The core issue of the question is knowledge that honest communication builds trust in a therapeutic relationship, regardless of age. A concept that also applies is knowledge related to issues of informed consent for an adolescent.

13 **Answer: 3, 5 Rationale:** Propping the child in a sitting position helps to develop self-righting behaviors. Pulling the child to a sitting position allows neck muscles to support the head and also aids with sitting. It is too early to begin assistance with standing. Talking to the child promotes language development. Handling a rattle involves fine-motor behavior. **Cognitive Level:** Analyzing **Client Need:** Health Promotion and Maintenance **Integrated Process:** Nursing Process: Planning **Content Area:** Foundational Sciences **Strategy:** Use the process of elimination and knowledge of growth and development to answer the question. The core issue of the question is the abilities of a 6-month-old infant.

14 **Answer: 3 Rationale:** The best concept to focus on is impaired verbal communication because it directly relates to the lack of language skills and gives the best guidance for appropriate nursing interventions. There is no information to determine whether social isolation is occurring because of the language delay. There is no information to support a focus on parenting skills. With the data presented in the question, there is no evidence of hearing disability. **Cognitive Level:** Analyzing **Client Need:** Health Promotion and Maintenance **Integrated Process:** Nursing Process: Diagnosis **Content Area:** Foundational Sciences **Strategy:** Use the process of elimination and knowledge of growth and development to answer the question. Note the linkage between language in the stem of the question and verbal communication in the correct answer.

15 **Answer: 2 Rationale:** It is recommended that the child's height be measured with a stadiometer. The correct procedure is to have the child remove his or her shoes and stand upright with the head erect. An infant would be weighed by laying the infant on an infant scale. The shoulders, buttocks, and heels should touch the back of the wall, so the feet would be close together, not wide apart. The child faces the examiner, not the wall. **Cognitive Level:** Applying **Client Need:** Health Promotion and Maintenance **Integrated Process:** Nursing Process: Implementation **Content Area:** Foundational Sciences **Strategy:** Use the process of elimination and knowledge of growth and development to answer the question. The correct answer is the one that incorporates proper technique based on the child's developmental level.

16 **Answer: 2 Rationale:** The 13-month-old will experience toddler hospitalization reaction, which is primarily related to separation from the parents. The 2-month-old has not recognized object permanence and will not suffer from the hospitalization as long as his or her needs are met in a consistent fashion. The 8-year-old and the 14-year-old are accustomed to separation from parents and working with new adults. **Cognitive Level:** Analyzing **Client Need:** Health Promotion and Maintenance **Integrated Process:** Nursing Process: Assessment **Content Area:** Foundational Sciences **Strategy:** Use the process of elimination and knowledge of growth and development to answer the question. The core issue of the question is recognition of the client that is most at risk for separation anxiety from parents during hospitalization.

17 **Answer: 1 Rationale:** Excessive milk consumption should be discouraged, especially more than 1 liter/day (32 oz), since it is a poor source of iron. Fat-soluble vitamins will not increase absorption or utilization of iron. Although grains and legumes are good sources of nutrients, they are not especially high in iron. Foods high in protein should be encouraged, especially food proteins of animal origin and organ meats, such as liver. **Cognitive Level:** Applying **Client Need:** Health Promotion and Maintenance **Integrated Process:** Teaching and Learning **Content Area:** Foundational Sciences **Strategy:** Use the process of elimination and knowledge of nutrition, growth, and development to answer the question. The correct answer is the one that would either decrease the intake of iron-poor foods or increase the intake of iron-rich foods.

18 **Answer: 4 Rationale:** Object permanence is the knowledge that an object or person continues to exist when not seen, heard, or felt. The baby will not attach to a single person, even the mother, until he or she is aware of the mother's existence. Ritualistic behavior, egocentrism, and conservation do not address this phenomenon. **Cognitive Level:** Applying **Client Need:** Health Promotion and Maintenance **Integrated Process:** Teaching and Learning **Content Area:** Foundational Sciences **Strategy:** Use the process of elimination and knowledge of growth and development to answer the question. The core issue of the question is knowledge that a young infant has not developed an awareness of object permanence.

19 **Answer: 2, 3 Rationale:** Flotation devices are not a substitute for supervision by an adult. Young children should never be left unattended in a swimming pool, even for a minute. Removing toys from the pool area when not in use helps prevent falls and supports safety. It is appropriate to advise children not to run near a pool. Enrolling children in swimming classes helps support their safety around and in water. **Cognitive Level:** Analyzing **Client Need:** Health Promotion and Maintenance **Integrated Process:** Nursing Process: Evaluation **Content Area:** Foundational Sciences **Strategy:** Use the process of elimination and knowledge of growth and development. The critical words *need further instruction* guide you to choose options that represent safety hazards to 4-year-olds using a pool.

20 **Answer: 3 Rationale:** Toddlers should be transported in a high-top crib with side rails up to ensure safety. The sedated toddler is at risk for falls. A wagon, wheelchair, or gurney will not eliminate the risk of fall injury to a sedated toddler. **Cognitive Level:** Applying **Client Need:** Safety and Infection Control **Integrated Process:** Nursing Process: Planning **Content Area:** Foundational Sciences **Strategy:** Use the process of elimination and knowledge of growth and development. The correct option is one that prevents the child from slipping out of the transport device while under sedation.

Key Terms to Review

cephalocaudal development p. 153
critical periods p. 153
differentiation p. 153
egocentricity p. 164
growth spurt p. 162
object permanence p. 160
proximodistal development p. 153
regression p. 163
ritualism p. 160
separation anxiety p. 163
therapeutic play p. 163

References

Ball, J., Bindler, R., & Cowen, K. (2014). *Child nursing: Partnering with children and families* (3rd ed.). Upper Saddle River, NJ: Pearson Education.

D'Amico, D., & Barbarito, C. (2016). *Health and physical assessment in nursing* (3rd ed.). New York, NY: Pearson Education.

Jarvis, C. (2016). *Physical examination and health assessment* (7th ed.). St. Louis, MO: Elsevier Science.

Hockenberry-Eaton, M., & Wilson, D. (2015). *Wong's nursing care of infants and children* (10th ed.). St. Louis, MO: Elsevier Science.

Test Yourself

Are you ready for the NCLEX-RN® or course exams? Access the NEW web-based app that provides students with thousands of practice questions in preparation for the NCLEX experience.

Providing Immunizations 14

In this chapter

Cross Reference

Other chapters relevant to this content area are

Preventing and Controlling Infection	Chapter 7
Uncomplicated Newborn Care	Chapter 12
Lifespan Growth and Development	Chapter 13
Promoting Healthy Lifestyle Choices	Chapter 16
Maternal and Newborn Medications	Chapter 34
Communicable or Infectious Diseases	Chapter 67

I. OVERVIEW OF IMMUNIZATIONS

A. Overview

1. A **vaccine** is a suspension of live, usually **attenuated** (less virulent) microorganisms (e.g., bacteria, viruses, or rickettisiae) or fractions of microorganisms administered as an antigen to induce immunity through antibody formation
2. A vaccine produces **active immunity** (antibody production is stimulated without causing clinical disease)
3. **Passive immunity** can be conferred using immune globulins, in which antibodies to offending organism are already formed; it is also conferred via breast milk to breast-fed infants

B. Information resources

NCLEX®

1. Centers for Disease Control and Prevention (CDC)
   a. Recommended Immunization Schedule for Persons Aged 0 Through 18 Years, United States, 2016
   b. Recommended Adult Immunization Schedule—United States, 2016
   c. CDC website updates immunization lists for children, adolescents, and adults yearly

2. American Academy of Pediatrics (AAP) Red Book: Report of the Committee of Infectious Diseases (updated each year)
3. Advisory Committee on Immunization Priorities (ACIP)

C. General nursing guidelines for vaccine administration

1. Provide a written vaccine information statement to client or caregiver and obtain written consent prior to administration
2. *NCLEX®* Before administering any vaccine, assess for allergy to vaccine or any of its components
3. Strictly follow manufacturer's directions for storing, reconstituting, and administering any vaccine
4. *NCLEX®* Store vaccine in center shelf of refrigerator (not in door) at 35–46°F (2–8°C) to maintain stable temperature and vaccine potency; do not freeze
5. Check expiration date prior to administration; if a multidose vial is used, follow manufacturer's directions; some vials may be used for 30 days after initial use but must be relabeled with newer expiration date; follow agency policy and vaccine directions
6. *NCLEX®* If more than one vaccine is given at one time, draw up in different syringes and administer in different sites
7. *NCLEX®* See Box 14–1 for suggestions to reduce discomfort in a child receiving an immunization
8. *NCLEX®* Administer intramuscular (IM) vaccines into vastus lateralis muscle (optimally) in newborns and in deltoid muscle of arm for children and older infants; avoid using dorsogluteal site (buttocks)
9. Inject subcutaneous injection into fatty area in lateral upper arm or anterior thigh
10. *NCLEX®* Document on immunization record the day, month, and year of administration; vaccine manufacturer, lot number, and expiration date; route and site of administration; and name, title, and work address of person administering dose
11. Advise parent or caregiver that mild side effects include fever and soreness, swelling, or redness at site; local symptoms may be treated with cool compresses (first 24 hours) or either warm or cool compresses (after first 24 hours); acetaminophen or ibuprofen may be used if recommended by healthcare provider
12. If an adverse reaction occurs, complete a Vaccine Adverse Event Report (VAER) form and report severe reactions to health department or other agencies as designated by law

II. HEPATITIS B VACCINE

A. Hepatitis B virus (HBV)

1. Hepatitis B is a liver infection caused by HBV, which is transmitted in blood or body secretions
2. A series of three (3) injections prevent HBV infection

B. Administration technique (see Table 14–1)

1. Ask if there have been any previous immunization reactions
2. Vaccine will appear cloudy; shake prior to withdrawing
3. *NCLEX®* An infant born from a HbsAg+ mother should also receive hepatitis B immune globulin (HBIG) at same time in a different site using new needle and syringe

Box 14–1

Reducing Discomfort from Immunizations

Reduce pain and anxiety associated with injections by using the following techniques:

- Determine feasibility of parent or caregiver applying topical anesthetic to site an hour before injection to numb area.
- Consider giving infants up to 4 months of age 24% sucrose water just prior to injection (has been shown to reduce pain in newborns and young infants).
- Apply site pressure for 10 seconds before injection.
- Use a vapocoolant spray immediately before injection.
- Distract child using age-appropriate measure (have child select distraction method if feasible).
- Communicate honestly about discomfort associated with injection and that it is OK to cry.
- Encourage parent or caregiver to hold child and explain how child can cooperate.
- Promote coping by allowing child to choose which arm or leg will be used.
- Obtain assistance of another provider and give two injections simultaneously in different extremities (reduces time child has to be anxious).

Adapted from Ball, J., Bindler, R., & Cowen, K. (2016). *Child health nursing: Partnering with children and families* (3rd ed.). New York, NY: Pearson Education, pp. 619, 623.

Table 14-1 Hepatitis B Vaccine

Recommended Age	Route
For infant whose mother is HbsAg+	IM
Within 12 hours of birth, 1–2 months, 6 months	
For infant whose mother is HbsAg−	IM
Before hospital discharge, 1–2 months, 6–18 months	
For older child, adolescent, or adult	IM
First dose anytime, second dose 1–2 months after first, third dose 4–6 months after first	
or	
Adolescents 11–15 years may only need two (2) doses separated by 4–6 months (consult healthcare provider)	IM

Note: For more detailed information and for catch-up immunization schedule, see CDC website.

Box 14-2

Actions to Take for Anaphylaxis

To be prepared for potential vaccine-induced anaphylaxis:

- Keep epinephrine 1:1000 and resuscitation equipment immediately available.
- Administer weight-based dose of epinephrine once prescription obtained from healthcare provider; dose may be repeated according to agency protocol and severity of symptoms.
- For very mild reactions that do not compromise airway, respirations, or circulation, an antihistamine such as diphendydramine may be prescribed, with or without a prescription for epinephrine.
- For more severe reactions, prepare to establish an airway, elevate the head of bed to support respirations, use supportive measures as prescribed including oxygen, fluid resuscitation, vasopressors, and CPR if indicated.

C. Precautions

1. Give second dose at least 4 weeks after first dose
2. Give third dose at least 8 weeks after second dose and at least 16 weeks after first
3. Do not give third dose to infants younger than 6 months of age because this could reduce long-term protection
4. Reschedule dose to a later date if person is moderately or severely ill when scheduled to receive vaccine

NCLEX® **D. Contraindications**

1. Life-threatening allergic reaction to baker's yeast (yeast used for baking bread)
2. Serious reaction to a previous dose of hepatitis B vaccine including anaphylaxis
3. Liver abnormalities

NCLEX® **E. Side effects/adverse reactions**

1. Common side effects: pain or redness at injection site; fever; headache; photophobia; elevated liver enzymes
2. Rare serious side effect: anaphylaxis; see Box 14–2 for treatment

III. DIPHTHERIA, TETANUS, AND PERTUSSIS VACCINES

A. Diphtheria, tetanus, and pertussis

1. Diphtheria is an acute, contagious infection that can cause respiratory obstruction
2. Tetanus (lockjaw) can cause muscle spasms and rigidity over entire body; ultimately obstructs breathing, and can be fatal
3. Pertussis (whooping cough) can lead to respiratory distress, pneumonia, seizures, brain damage, or death
4. Diphtheria, tetanus **toxoid**, and pertussis vaccines are examples of **inactivated vaccines** (or **killed vaccines**), which confer a weaker response than a live virus and require regular booster injections
5. Current available vaccines include DTaP (tetanus, diphtheria, and acellular pertussis) for children receiving initial five-dose immunization series from ages 2 months to 4–6 years, Tdap (tetanus, diphtheria, and acellular pertussis) booster one time only for adolescents ages 11–18 years, and Td (tetanus, diphtheria) booster every 10 years thereafter (does not protect against pertussis)

Table 14–2 Diphtheria, Tetanus, and Pertussis Vaccines

Vaccine	Recommended Age	Route
DTaP	2, 4, 6, and 15–18 months, then at 4–6 years	IM
Tdap	11–12 years 13–18 years for 1 dose if received Td at age 11–12 19–64 years for 1 dose if received Td for all previous boosters	IM
Td	Every 10 years	IM

Note: For catch-up immunization schedule and variations based on specific cases, see CDC website.

B. Administration technique (see Table 14–2)

1. It may be given at same time as other vaccines; ask about previous reactions to immunizations
2. Preferably administer in vastus lateralis muscle for nonwalking infants

C. Precautions

1. Anyone who is moderately or severely ill at time of vaccine should wait until they recover; people with minor illnesses, such as a cold, may be vaccinated
2. Aspirin-free pain reliever is recommended if fever or pain at injection site occurred after previous dose of DTaP; administer for a period of 24 hours according to advice from healthcare provider
3. Delay for 1 month after immunosuppressive therapy or if immune serum globulin has been administered within 90 days

NCLEX® **D. Contraindications**

1. Life-threatening reaction to a previous dose of DTaP
2. Seizure, inconsolable crying for 3 hours or more, or fever above 105°F (40.6°C) after previous dose

NCLEX® **E. Side effects/adverse reactions**

1. Serious: anaphylaxis, seizure, inconsolable crying for 3 hours or more, fever greater than 105°F (40.6°C); decreased level of consciousness; and permanent brain damage (rare)
2. Common: redness, pain, swelling, and nodule at injection site; fever up to 101°F (38.3°C); drowsiness and fussiness; anorexia within 2 days of injection

IV. *HAEMOPHILUS INFLUENZAE* TYPE B (HIB) VACCINE

A. Haemophilis influenzae

1. *H. influenzae* type B was most common cause of meningitis in children over 1 month of age
2. Hib conjugate vaccine protects against a number of serious diseases such as bacterial meningitis, epiglottitis, bacterial pneumonia, sepsis, and septic arthritis

B. Administration technique (see Table 14–3)

1. It may be given at same time as other vaccines
2. Depending on brand of Hib used, child may not need 6-month dose; consult healthcare provider
3. Encourage use of same brand for all doses (some brands require three doses while others require four doses)

Table 14–3 Other Vaccines Started in Infancy or Early Childhood

Vaccine	Recommended Age(s)	Route
Haemophilus influenzae type B (Hib)	2, 4, 6, and 12–15 months	IM
Inactivated polio vaccine (IPV)	2, 4, 6–18 months, and 4–6 years	Subcut
Measles, mumps, rubella (MMR) vaccine	12–15 months, 4–6 years	Subcut
Varicella vaccine (VAR)	12–18 months, 4–6 years	Subcut
Pneumococcal conjugate vaccine (PCV13)	2, 4, 6, and 12–15 months	IM
Rotavirus vaccine (RV1 or RV5)	2, 4 months (RV1) 2, 4, 6 months (RV5)	Oral Oral
Hepatitis A	12–23 months Second dose 6–18 months later	IM

Note: For catch-up immunization schedules and variations based on specific cases, see CDC website.

4. Ask about previous reactions to immunizations
5. Preferably administer in vastus lateralis muscle

C. Precautions
1. Children with minor illnesses may receive immunization
2. Moderately or severely ill children should not be immunized until they recover from illness

NCLEX® **D. Contraindications:** prior anaphylactic reaction or severe reaction to previous dose (rare)

NCLEX® **E. Side effects/adverse reactions:** pain, redness, or swelling at site; anaphylaxis (rare)

V. INACTIVATED POLIO VIRUS (IPV) VACCINE

A. Poliomyelitis
1. A disease caused by a virus that affects central nervous system (CNS); may not cause serious illness, but can cause paralysis, respiratory complications, and death
2. IPV is a trivalent vaccine that contains all three forms of polio; given subcutaneously (subcut)
3. IPV is an inactivated vaccine, or killed vaccine, which confers a weaker response than a live vaccine, necessitating frequent boosters

B. Administration (see Table 14–3): clear, colorless suspension; do not use if contains particulate matter, becomes cloudy, or changes colors

C. Precautions: prior to immunization, assess for allergies to formalin, neomycin, streptomycin, or polymyxin B

NCLEX® **D. Contraindications**
1. Anaphylactic reaction
2. Anyone who is moderately or severely ill at time of vaccination should wait until recovered; people with minor illnesses, such as a cold, may be vaccinated

NCLEX® **E. Side effects/adverse reactions**
1. Serious: anaphylaxis
2. Common: elevated temperature 1–2 weeks after immunization; redness or pain at injection site; noncontagious rash; joint pain; irritability

VI. MEASLES, MUMPS, RUBELLA (MMR) VACCINE

A. Measles (rubeola), mumps (parotitis), rubella (German measles)
1. Infectious and communicable diseases in children that are vaccine-preventable; rubella is generally a mild disease but presents a major risk of spontaneous abortion, stillbirth, fetal death, and other anomalies for fetus during first trimester of pregnancy
2. MMR vaccine is a **live, attenuated vaccine** created from a live organism grown under suboptimal conditions to produce a live vaccine with reduced virulence

B. Administration (see again Table 14–3)
1. Reconstituted solution is clear yellow; keep refrigerated and away from light; discard if unused within 8 hours
2. Table 14–3 lists recommended ages; however, second dose can be given at any age as long as it is at least 4 weeks after first dose

C. Precautions
1. College students are at greater risk due to increased exposure; ensure they have received a second MMR dose
2. NCLEX® Caution females to avoid pregnancy for at least 3 months after immunization
3. Wait at least 3–6 months after administration of immune serum globulin before giving MMR vaccine (immunoglobulin can interfere with immune system response to MMR)
4. Thrombocytopenia or history of thrombocytopenic purpura

NCLEX® **D. Contraindications**
1. Allergy to neomycin, gelatin, or eggs
2. Severely impaired immune system due to malignancy, immune deficiency disease, immunosuppressive therapy
3. Avoid administering a live-virus immunization during pregnancy and to women likely to become pregnant within 3 months

NCLEX® **E. Side effects/adverse reactions**
1. Serious: anaphylaxis; encephalopathy; thrombocytopenic purpura; chronic arthritis
2. Common: elevated temperature 1–2 weeks after immunization; redness or pain at injection site; noncontagious rash; joint pain

VII. VARICELLA VACCINE (VAR)

A. *Varicella* (chickenpox)

1. A common childhood disease, usually mild, that can lead to severe skin infection, scars, pneumonia, brain damage, or death
2. Varicella immunization is a live, attenuated vaccine used to stimulate immunity
3. Vaccine generally prevents chickenpox, but if child has been vaccinated and gets infected, disease will be usually very mild, resulting in faster recovery

B. Administration (see again Table 14–3)

1. Individuals 13 years or older who have not had the disease require two doses 4–8 weeks apart
2. May use as postexposure prophylaxis if given within 3–5 days

C. Precautions

NCLEX® 1. Instruct females of childbearing age to avoid pregnancy for 3 months after immunization
2. Varicella vaccine is *not* recommended for those infected with HIV
3. Wait at least 3–11 months after administration of immune serum globulin before giving varicella vaccine

NCLEX® **D. Contraindications**

1. Allergy to neomycin or gelatin
2. Active, untreated TB
3. Pregnancy
4. Immunodeficiency or receiving immunosuppression therapy
5. Moderate or severe febrile illness

NCLEX® **E. Side effects/adverse reactions**

1. Serious: anaphylaxis
2. Common: pain or redness at injection site; fever up to 102°F (38.8°C) in children, up to 100°F (37.7°C) in adults, lasting for 1 week; varicella-like rash at injection site; irritability

VIII. PNEUMOCOCCAL CONJUGATE VACCINE (PCV)

A. Pneumoccocal infections

1. Pneumococcal infection caused by *Streptococcus pneumoniae* is a leading cause of bacterial meningitis
2. Other pneumococcal infections include otitis media, sinusitis, pneumonia, and septicemia

B. Administration (see again Table 14–3): is a clear, colorless, or slightly opalescent liquid

C. Precautions

1. It is highly recommended for children in daycare (close contact with others)
2. Also recommended for children with immunosuppression, pulmonary or cardiac illness, diabetes, sickle-cell disease, or asplenia

NCLEX® **D. Contraindications:** hypersensitivity to diphtheria toxoid or severe illness and anaphylaxis to a previous dose

NCLEX® **E. Side effects/adverse reactions**

1. Severe: anaphylaxis
2. Common: soreness, swelling, redness at injection site; mild to moderate fever; irritability; drowsiness; restlessness; sleep; decreased appetite; vomiting and diarrhea; rash or hives

IX. ROTAVIRUS VACCINE

A. Rotavirus infection

1. A leading cause of severe acute gastroenteritis (vomiting and diarrhea) among children worldwide; is often accompanied by fever
2. Two rotavirus vaccines are approved for use in infants in United States: RV1 (two-dose series) and RV5 (three-dose series)

B. Administration (see Table 14–3): given as a liquid oral dose; vaccine replicates in gut

C. Precautions

1. Delay dose for infant currently experiencing vomiting and/or diarrhea, but administer soon after recovery
2. Do not begin first dose before age 6 weeks and finish final dose by age 8 months

D. Contraindications

1. Hypersensitivity to vaccine or any component of vaccine
2. History of severe combined immunodeficiency disease (SCID)

E. Side effects/adverse reactions

1. Severe: seizures, bronchiolitis, gastroenteritis, pneumonia, fever, urinary tract infection
2. Common: vomiting, diarrhea, irritability

X. HEPATITIS A (HEP A) VACCINE

A. Hepatitis A

1. Hepatitis A virus (HAV), which is found in stool of infected persons, causes serious liver disease; usually spread by close personal contact and sometimes eating food or drinking water contaminated by HAV
2. Hep A vaccine, an inactivated or killed vaccine, can be given for postexposure prophylaxis against hepatitis A
3. Immune globulin and Hep A vaccine can be given at same time in different sites

B. Administration (see Table 14–3 again)

1. Do not restart series no matter how long since previous dose
2. May give at same time as all other vaccines

C. Precautions

1. Safety of hepatitis A vaccine for pregnant women is not yet known; risk is thought to be low
2. NCLEX® Moderate to severe acute illness with or without fever warrants delay of vaccination

NCLEX® **D. Contraindications**

1. Known hypersensitivity to any component of vaccine, including neomycin
2. Anaphylactic reaction to prior vaccine dose

NCLEX® **E. Side effects/adverse effects**

1. Serious: anaphylaxis (rare)
2. Common: soreness at injection site, headache, loss of appetite, fatigue

XI. INFLUENZA VACCINE

A. Influenza

1. Is a highly contagious viral infection that affects respiratory system
2. Influenza vaccine, also referred to as flu shot, provides protection against strains of influenza; protection begins 2 weeks after administration and lasts 1 year
3. Injection is available as an inactivated or killed vaccine (IIV), but a live attenuated (LAIV) form is available for use by intranasal route

B. Administration (see Table 14–4)

1. Administer in autumn and repeat yearly
2. Give two doses 4 weeks apart for children under age 8 years; one dose for those over 8 years

C. Precautions: LAIV form should not be given to pregnant women, immunosuppressed individuals, and children receiving aspirin products; see CDC website for additional precautions to take depending on type of vaccine

NCLEX® **D. Contraindications**

1. Allergy to eggs
2. Anaphylaxis

NCLEX® **E. Side effects/adverse reactions**

1. Serious: allergic reaction (rare)
2. Common: redness, soreness, swelling at injection site; fever; aching

XII. MENINGOCOCCAL VACCINES

A. Meningococcal infection

1. A serious respiratory infection that can lead to critical illness such as meningitis, disseminated intravascular coagulopathy (DIC), shock, or death
2. This vaccine provides protection against *Neisseria meningitidis*

B. Administration

1. Recommended for children 2 years and older with anatomic or functional asplenia (including sickle-cell disease) and persistent complement component deficiencies
2. Recommended for 11- to 12-year-olds with a booster dose at age 16 years, unvaccinated freshman college students, military recruits, and those traveling to certain countries where there is added risk for exposure

Table 14–4 Influenza Vaccine

Vaccine	Recommended Age	Route
Inactivated influenza vaccine (IIV)	6–23 months of age ≥ 2 years of age with risk factors	IM
Live attenuated influenza vaccine (LAIV)	≥ 2 years	Intranasal

3. See CDC website for formulations of vaccine and recommended administration schedules based on risk factors
4. Administer subcutaneous injection in anterolateral fat of thigh in young children or posterolateral fat of upper arm for older children and adults; administer IM injection in large muscle

C. **Precautions:** duration of protection is uncertain; safety in pregnancy not established

D. **Contraindications:** prior sensitivity to vaccine component; history of Guillain-Barré syndrome unless at high risk for meningococcal infection

E. **Side effects/adverse reactions**

1. Serious: anaphylaxis
2. Common: redness or tenderness at site

XIII. HUMAN PAPILLOMAVIRUS (HPV) VACCINE

A. **Human papillomavirus infection**

1. Clinical infection seen as clustered or single warts in genital area (on vulva, perineal area, vagina, or cervix in females; on penis, scrotal skin near base of penis or near anus in males)
2. Subclinical infection in females can be diagnosed on Papanicolaou (Pap) smear
3. Specific types of HPV infection are responsible for more than 99% of female cervical cancers

B. **Administration (see Table 14–5)**

1. Vaccines to protect against HPV infection include 2vHPV, 4vHPV, and 9vHPV; are administered in a three-dose series
2. Solution is white and cloudy; shake before use; protect vaccine from light to protect potency

C. **Precautions**

1. Delay dose if moderate to severe illness with or without fever; can give if mild acute illness present
2. Use cautiously in lactating women; unknown if vaccine is excreted in human milk

D. **Contraindications**

1. Severe allergic reaction to prior dose or hypersensitivity to any vaccine component (e.g., yeast)
2. Pregnancy or bleeding disorder

E. **Side effects/adverse reactions**

1. Severe: bronchospasm, asthma, arthritis, and possibly headache or gastroenteritis, fainting or syncope
2. Common: pain, swelling, erythema at injection site, pruritus, fever

Table 14–5 **Human Papillomavirus (HPV) Vaccine**

Vaccine	Recommended Age(s)	Route
2HPV	Females only; 11–12 years, second and third doses 2 and 6 months after first	IM
4HPV or 9HPV	Males and females; 11–12 years, second and third doses 2 and 6 months after first	IM

Check Your NCLEX-RN® Exam I.Q.

You are ready for testing on this content if you can:

- Assess a client's or family's knowledge of immunization schedules.
- Assess a client's or family's immunization status.
- Administer prescribed immunizations correctly.
- Teach a client or family about prescribed immunizations.
- Identify contraindications to immunizations and other precautions.
- Respond appropriately when a client experiences side effects, adverse effects, or allergy to an immunization.

PRACTICE TEST

PRACTICE TEST

1 A newly adopted 8-year-old child is brought to the pediatric immunization clinic to begin the hepatitis B immunization series. Before providing the immunization, the nurse inquires about any known history of allergy to which item?

1. Aminoglycoside antibiotics
2. Mold
3. Baker's yeast
4. Egg yolks

2 A mother brings her infant to the immunization clinic for the final hepatitis B vaccine. After picking up the vial of vaccine to draw up the dose, the nurse notes that it is cloudy. What action should the nurse take?

1. Warm the vaccine under running water.
2. Discard the vaccine and contact the supplier of the vaccine.
3. Agitate the vial gently and draw up the vaccine.
4. Calculate the pediatric dosage, since it is intended for adult use.

3 A nurse preparing to draw up a dose of vaccine notices that a vial of DTaP vaccine on the countertop does not have a date recorded for when it was opened. What action should the nurse take?

1. Use the vaccine but explain to the caregiver that the site may be quite tender.
2. Discard the vaccine according to agency's policy.
3. Contact the supervisor because this is reportable to the state Board of Public Health.
4. Use the vaccine just for the day and then discard it.

4 A parent brings a 3-year-old child to the immunization clinic for a DTaP vaccine. During the interview, the mother indicates the child is just finishing a tapered dose of prednisone for a chronic respiratory problem. Which action should the nurse take at this time?

1. Delay the vaccine administration for 1 month after the medication is completed.
2. Provide the child with the vaccine as scheduled.
3. Cleanse the injection site with sterile saline instead of alcohol and administer the vaccine.
4. Keep the child in the clinic for 30 minutes after administration to assess the child's response.

5 A child is brought to the pediatric ambulatory clinic with a runny nose and a low-grade fever. He is scheduled to receive the MMR (measles, mumps, and rubella) and DTaP (diphtheria, pertussis, and tetanus toxoid) vaccines. What should the nurse do at this time?

1. Get special permission from the healthcare provider to administer the vaccine.
2. Defer both vaccines until the child is well.
3. Administer the vaccines as scheduled.
4. Administer the DTaP vaccine but defer the MMR.

6 A pediatric client is scheduled to receive a dose of MMR (measles, mumps, rubella) vaccine. The nurse would question the order to give the dose at this time if which data was obtained during the short intake history?

1. Recent upper respiratory infection
2. Weight loss of 3 pounds during the last month
3. History of allergy to neomycin or gelatin
4. Local reaction to previous dose

7 The mother of a child who has been exposed to chickenpox telephones the pediatric clinic for advice. The triage nurse asks about which of the following before responding to the mother's request for information?

1. The child's exposure and immune status
2. Whether the child has had a rubella vaccination
3. The age, height, and weight of the child
4. The relationship of the person to whom the child was exposed

8 A 9-year-old client is brought to the pediatrician's office for a varicella virus vaccine. Before preparing the dose of the vaccine, the nurse would determine the child's status regarding what health history item?

1. Recent blood product transfusion
2. Allergy to milk
3. Allergy to penicillin
4. History of splenectomy

9 A child stepped on a rusty nail and is brought to the emergency department. The child's electronic health record indicates the child has not been adequately immunized against tetanus according to the immunization schedule. What would the emergency department nurse expect to be ordered for this child?

1. Diphtheria, tetanus, and pertussis vaccine
2. Tetanus immune globulin
3. A broad-spectrum antibiotic
4. Tetanus toxoid

10 A 2-month-old client is seen in the pediatric clinic for a well-baby checkup. The nurse anticipates which routine immunizations will be administered at this time? Select all that apply.

1. Inactivated poliovirus vaccine (IPV)
2. Diphtheria, tetanus and acellular pertussis (DTaP)
3. *Haemophilus influenzae* B conjugate vaccine (Hib)
4. Measles, mumps, and rubella vaccine (MMR)
5. Varicella zoster vaccine (VAR)

11 A nurse is preparing to draw up a dose of *Haemophilus influenzae* type B (Hib) vaccine for a pediatric client. The nurse concludes that the vial is acceptable to use after noting which expected coloration of the fluid in the vial?

1. Pale yellow
2. Light pink
3. Clear
4. Slightly brown tinged

12 The pediatric clinic nurse has just administered a dose of *Haemophilus influenzae* type B (Hib) vaccine to a child. The nurse explains to the parents that they can expect which type of local reaction following the injection?

1. Mild to moderate fever
2. Pain or redness at site
3. Irritability
4. Decreased appetite

13 The nurse has an order to give an infant a dose of inactivated poliovirus vaccine (IPV). The nurse would take which action before administering the medication to ensure the dose is safe and effective?

1. Take dose that has not expired from a box on the shelf in the medication room.
2. Assess prior to dose for allergy to neomycin, streptomycin, or polymixin B.
3. Gently agitate the cloudy white solution before drawing up.
4. Select a proper-sized muscle for injection.

14 The neonatal nurse is providing anticipatory guidance to the mother of a newborn infant. When discussing immunization schedules, the nurse explains that the first dose of inactivated poliovirus vaccine (IPV) is given at what age?

1. 1 week
2. 1 month
3. 2 months
4. 4 months

15 A pediatric client has received a dose of heptavalent pneumococcal conjugate vaccine (PCV). The nurse evaluates that the parents understand postvaccination instructions if they state that which symptom is most important to report promptly to the healthcare provider?

1. Mild fever
2. Drowsiness
3. Decreased appetite
4. Rash with hives

16 A child with cardiac disease is recommended to receive the yearly influenza vaccine. The nurse would schedule the child to receive the vaccine at the routine visit scheduled in which month?

1. January
2. April
3. July
4. October

17 A 6-year-old child with asplenia is receiving the meningococcal vaccine. The nurse explains to the child's mother that the vaccine should be effective for how many years?

1. 1
2. 2
3. 5
4. 10

18 A nurse working in an immunization clinic ensures at the beginning of each workday that which priority medication is available and within the expiration date?

1. Lidocaine
2. Epinephrine
3. Acetaminophen
4. Ibuprofen

19 The pediatric nurse is seeing a 2-month-old infant in the outpatient clinic for routine immunizations. The nurse should select which immunization teaching sheets to give to the mother before preparing the immunizations appropriate for this visit? Select all that apply.

1. Varicella
2. Diphtheria, tetanus, and acellular pertussis (DTaP)
3. Measles, mumps, and rubella (MMR)
4. *Haemophilus influenzae* type b (Hib)
5. Inactivated polio (IPV)

20 What should the nurse tell a mother whose child is receiving the immunizations required at 1 year of age? Select all that apply.

1. "You can give your child acetaminophen if he develops a mild fever."
2. "We give all these immunizations at the same time because they are more effective if given together."
3. "If your child develops a mild fever, you need to call the healthcare provider."
4. "You can expect your child not to feel well for a couple of days."
5. "Some children develop itching or a rash after immunizations are given. This can be treated at home with an antihistamine."

21 The mother of a 15-month-old child is anxious about the immunizations her child is about to receive. What information should the nurse provide to the mother about immunizations? Select all that apply.

1. Possible localized reactions to injection sites
2. Administration of acetaminophen as needed after vaccine administration
3. Informed consent or refusal form for mother to sign
4. Administration of aspirin every 4 hours post–vaccine administration
5. Symptoms of anaphylaxis reaction with immediate access to emergency care

PRACTICE TEST

ANSWERS & RATIONALES

ANSWERS & RATIONALES

1 **Answer: 3 Rationale:** A history of an allergic reaction to baker's yeast would be a contraindication to receiving this series of immunizations. Aminoglycoside antibiotics, mold, and egg yolks do not pose any risk to the client for allergy to the vaccine. **Cognitive Level:** Analyzing **Client Need:** Health Promotion and Maintenance **Integrated Process:** Nursing Process: Assessment **Content Area:** Pharmacology **Strategy:** Specific knowledge of contraindications to hepatitis B vaccine is needed to answer this question. Use the process of elimination, and review this content area if needed.

2 **Answer: 3 Rationale:** It is normal for the solution in the vial to appear cloudy. The nurse should gently agitate the vaccine and then draw it up for administration. It is unnecessary to discard it or to notify the manufacturer. Warming the solution will not affect the cloudiness. **Cognitive Level:** Applying **Client Need:** Health Promotion and Maintenance **Integrated Process:** Nursing Process: Implementation **Content Area:** Pharmacology **Strategy:** Specific knowledge of the nursing considerations for hepatitis B vaccine is needed to answer this question. Use the process of elimination, and review this content area if needed.

3 **Answer: 2 Rationale:** The vial should be discarded according to agency policy. Giving the vaccine with follow-up teaching about site tenderness does not protect the client's safety. Using the vaccine for just that day and then discarding it does not protect the safety of clients. It is unnecessary for administration to report this incident to the state Board of Public Health. **Cognitive Level:** Applying **Client Need:** Health Promotion and Maintenance **Integrated Process:** Nursing Process: Implementation **Content Area:** Pharmacology **Strategy:** The core issue of this question is safe handling of vaccinations. Use principles of general medication preparation to make a selection.

4 **Answer: 1 Rationale:** The dose should be delayed for 1 month following any type of immunosuppressive therapy, such as prednisone. The child should not receive the vaccine as scheduled. Cleaning the injection site with sterile saline instead of alcohol is not related to safe administration. Monitoring the child for 30 minutes after the dose is a routine nursing action to assess for possible allergic reaction, but it does not uphold safe administration procedures for this immunization. **Cognitive Level:** Applying **Client Need:**

Health Promotion and Maintenance **Integrated Process:** Nursing Process: Implementation **Content Area:** Pharmacology **Strategy:** Use the process of elimination. Recall that immunizations affect the immune system and that steroids such as prednisone suppress the immune system to make the correct selection.

5 **Answer: 3 Rationale:** The immunizations should be administered as scheduled. They would be withheld for clients who are immunosuppressed or have moderate to severe febrile illnesses. The presence of a runny nose and low-grade fever is not a contraindication according to the literature. **Cognitive Level:** Applying **Client Need:** Health Promotion and Maintenance **Integrated Process:** Nursing Process: Implementation **Content Area:** Pharmacology **Strategy:** The core issue of the question is contraindications to administering scheduled immunizations. Use the process of elimination, and take time to review these immunizations as needed.

6 **Answer: 3 Rationale:** A contraindication to MMR vaccine is a history of allergic reaction to neomycin or gelatin. Minor illnesses and history of local reaction to a previous dose are not contraindications. Weight loss is irrelevant to the question. **Cognitive Level:** Applying **Client Need:** Health Promotion and Maintenance **Integrated Process:** Nursing Process: Implementation **Content Area:** Pharmacology **Strategy:** The core issue of the question is knowledge of contraindications to MMR vaccine. Use the process of elimination, keeping in mind that both neomycin and gelatin are reasons to withhold the dose.

7 **Answer: 1 Rationale:** The nurse would inquire about the nature of the exposure and the client's immune status. Chickenpox can be fatal in immunocompromised children, such as those who are undergoing steroid therapy, chemotherapy, and those with other illnesses. If warranted, the varicella zoster immune globulin can be given up to 4 days after exposure to those with no history of chickenpox or prior exposure. Exposure to rubella (a different disease), height and weight of the child, and the person to whom the child was exposed are irrelevant as priority items in protecting the health of this child. **Cognitive Level:** Analyzing **Client Need:** Health Promotion and Maintenance **Integrated Process:** Nursing Process: Assessment **Content Area:** Pharmacology **Strategy:** The core issue of the question is knowledge of indications for use of varicella zoster immune globulin. Use the process of elimination and general concepts of immunity to answer the question.

8 **Answer: 1 Rationale:** Contraindications to varicella virus vaccine include allergy to neomycin or gelatin, immunosuppression, or administration of immune serum globulin or blood products in the last 3–11 months. An allergy to milk or penicillin is irrelevant to safe vaccine administration. A history of splenectomy is irrelevant to safe use of this vaccine. **Cognitive Level:** Applying **Client Need:** Health Promotion and Maintenance **Integrated Process:** Nursing Process: Assessment **Content Area:** Pharmacology **Strategy:** The core issue of the question is knowledge of contraindications for use of varicella vaccine. Use the process of elimination and general concepts of immunity to make a selection.

9 **Answer: 2 Rationale:** When there is accidental exposure and inadequate vaccination, passive immunity with tetanus immune globulin is indicated for immediate protection from the bacterial spores in the nail. DTaP is a vaccine provided on an administration schedule and provides active immunity to diphtheria, tetanus, and pertussis. Tetanus toxoid would provide active immunity but this client needs immediate protection that can be provided with passive immunity. A broad-spectrum antibiotic is inadequate. **Cognitive Level:** Applying **Client Need:** Health Promotion and Maintenance **Integrated Process:** Nursing Process: Planning **Content Area:** Pharmacology **Strategy:** The core issue of the question is the ability to discriminate situations requiring active immunity and those requiring passive immunity. Use the process of elimination, and take time to review this information if needed.

10 **Answer: 1, 2, 3 Rationale:** The IPV, DTaP, Hib, and PCV vaccines are all scheduled to be given at 2 months of age. The MMR is given at 12–15 months, and again at 4–6 years. The varicella zoster vaccine is given at 12–18 months. **Cognitive Level:** Applying **Client Need:** Health Promotion and Maintenance **Integrated Process:** Nursing Process: Planning **Content Area:** Pharmacology **Strategy:** The core issue of the question is knowledge of routine immunization schedules for a 2-month-old infant. Use general knowledge of immunization schedules and the process of elimination to make your selections.

11 **Answer: 3 Rationale:** The solution used for Hib vaccine is clear and colorless. MMR and varicella vaccines are a clear yellow in color. No vaccines are pale pink or brown, although some are cloudy. **Cognitive Level:** Applying **Client Need:** Health Promotion and Maintenance **Integrated Process:** Nursing Process: Diagnosis **Content Area:** Pharmacology **Strategy:** The core issue of this question is the ability to determine safe appearance of vaccines before administration. Use nursing knowledge and the process of elimination to make a selection.

12 **Answer: 2 Rationale:** The parents should be taught to expect pain and redness at the site as possible local reactions to the Hib vaccine. Fever, irritability, and decreased appetite are common side effects of the heptavalent pneumococcal conjugate vaccine (PCV). **Cognitive Level:** Applying **Client Need:** Health Promotion and Maintenance **Integrated Process:** Teaching and Learning **Content Area:** Pharmacology **Strategy:** Use the process of elimination. One strategy to determine local reaction is to evaluate the options in terms of how confined they are to the site of injection. The incorrect responses are systemic in nature.

13 **Answer: 2 Rationale:** Before administering a dose of IPV, the nurse should assess for allergy to neomycin, streptomycin, or polymixin B. The solution should be kept in the refrigerator. The solution administered should be clear and colorless. The dose is administered by the subcutaneous route. **Cognitive Level:** Applying **Client Need:** Health Promotion and Maintenance **Integrated Process:** Nursing Process: Implementation **Content Area:** Pharmacology **Strategy:** The core issue of this question is the ability to administer IPV safely. Use nursing knowledge and the process of elimination to make a selection.

14 **Answer: 3 Rationale:** The first dose of IPV is given at 2 months with subsequent doses at 4 months, 12–18 months, and 4–6 years, for a total of four doses. Giving a dose of IPV at the age of 1 week is too early. Giving a dose of IPV at 1 month of age is too early. The infant should be receiving the second dose at 4 months. **Cognitive Level:** Applying **Client Need:** Health

Promotion and Maintenance **Integrated Process:** Nursing Process: Implementation **Content Area:** Pharmacology **Strategy:** The core issue of this question is the ability to administer IPV safely according to its recommended schedule. Use nursing knowledge and the process of elimination to make a selection.

15 **Answer: 4 Rationale:** The development of hives is likely to indicate an allergic reaction, which could progress to anaphylaxis if left untreated. The healthcare provider should be notified. Mild fever is a side effect of PCV that is easily managed at home. Drowsiness is an expected mild side effect of PCV vaccine. Decreased appetite is a temporary and mild side effect of PCV vaccine. **Cognitive Level:** Analyzing **Client Need:** Health Promotion and Maintenance **Integrated Process:** Nursing Process: Evaluation **Content Area:** Pharmacology **Strategy:** The core issue of this question is the highest-priority teaching regarding PCV. The critical words in the question are *most important* and *promptly*, which tells you that one is more serious than the others. Use nursing knowledge, the ABCs, and the process of elimination to make a selection.

16 **Answer: 4 Rationale:** The influenza vaccine is administered annually in the autumn, especially during October, November, and into December to provide protection during the winter months of flu season. Administering the vaccine in January would be too late to provide significant protection during the current flu season. The flu season has generally ended by April. July is a summer month in which influenza is not a concern. **Cognitive Level:** Applying **Client Need:** Health Promotion and Maintenance **Integrated Process:** Nursing Process: Planning **Content Area:** Pharmacology **Strategy:** The core issue of the question is the timing of the annual dosage of influenza vaccine. Use knowledge of the epidemiology of the disease to choose the month prior to when flu season occurs.

17 **Answer: 3 Rationale:** Meningococcal vaccine is indicated for children older than 2 years with asplenia. The vaccine duration is 5 years if the client is older than 4 years at the time of immunization. If the client is younger than 4 at the time of initial immunization, it should be repeated after 1 year. The duration of protection for meningococcal vaccine is not 2 years or 10 years. **Cognitive Level:** Applying **Client Need:** Health Promotion and Maintenance **Integrated Process:** Teaching and Learning **Content Area:** Pharmacology **Strategy:** Specific knowledge related to the meningococcal vaccine is needed to answer the question. Take time to review this material if needed, and use the process of elimination in making a selection.

18 **Answer: 2 Rationale:** Epinephrine is the priority medication to have on hand if a client should experience hypersensitivity reaction/anaphylaxis following a dose of an immunization. Lidocaine is given for cardiac dysrhythmias. Acetaminophen is an analgesic and antipyretic agent. Ibuprofen is a nonsteroidal anti-inflammatory agent. **Cognitive Level:** Analyzing **Client Need:** Health Promotion and Maintenance **Integrated Process:** Nursing Process: Planning **Content Area:** Pharmacology **Strategy:** The core issue of the question is knowledge that anaphylaxis is a potentially life-threatening consequence of immunization. Use the process of elimination, choosing the answer that is an emergency drug associated with reducing allergic response.

19 **Answer: 2, 4, 5 Rationale:** Diphtheria, tetanus, and acellular pertussis (DTaP), *Haemophilus influenzae* type b (Hib), inactivated polio vaccine (IPV), and the pneumococcal conjugate vaccine (PCV) are the routine immunizations scheduled for the 2-month well-child visit. The MMR is given first at 12–15 months, and the varicella can be given at or anytime after 12 months. **Cognitive Level:** Analyzing **Client Need:** Health Promotion and Maintenance **Integrated Process:** Nursing Process: Implementation **Content Area:** Pharmacology **Strategy:** The core issue of the question is knowledge of vaccinations that are due at a 2-month well-child visit. Use the process of elimination, recalling that MMR and varicella cannot be given before 12 months of age.

20 **Answer: 1, 4 Rationale:** A mild fever can be treated safely and effectively with acetaminophen. Sometimes children act as if they do not feel well because of mild discomfort after receiving immunizations. Immunizations are given according to an administration timetable, not because they are more effective if given together. The healthcare provider does not need to be called unless the fever is high. Itching or rash are of concern because they could indicate hypersensitivity, and needs to be addressed rather than treated at home. **Cognitive Level:** Analyzing **Client Need:** Health Promotion and Maintenance **Integrated Process:** Communication and Documentation **Content Area:** Child Health **Strategy:** Differentiate between mild and severe adverse reactions to immunizations, and use the process of elimination to make the correct selections.

21 **Answer: 1, 2, 3, 5 Rationale:** The nurse should provide information about localized reactions that can occur at the injection site of vaccines. Acetaminophen is often effective in relieving discomfort associated with vaccine administration. Before administering a vaccine, the mother must sign a consent form. If the mother refuses the vaccine, a refusal form needs to be signed. The use of aspirin is contraindicated due to the risk of Reye syndrome. The mother needs to be informed of the symptoms of anaphylaxis and the need for emergency follow-up care if they occur. **Cognitive Level:** Applying **Client Need:** Safety and Infection Control **Integrated Process:** Nursing Process: Implementation **Content Area:** Child Health **Strategy:** Recall general information about immunizations, and use this information to recognize the common teaching points. Recall also that aspirin is contraindicated in children to prevent the risk of Reye syndrome to eliminate this as a possible answer choice.

Key Terms to Review

References

American Academy of Family Physicians. www.aafp.org

American Academy of Pediatrics. www.aap.org

Centers for Disease Control and Prevention. (2016). *Recommended immunization schedules for persons aged 0 through 18 years—United States 2016.* Available at www.cdc.gov/vaccines/schedules/downloads/child/0-18yrs-child-combined-schedule.pdf.

Centers for Disease Control and Prevention. (2016). *Recommended adult immunization schedule—United States 2016.* Available at www.cdc.gov/vaccines/schedules/downloads/adult/adult-combined-schedule.pdf.

Davidson, M., London, M., & Ladewig, P. (2016). *Olds' maternal newborn nursing and women's health across the lifespan* (10th ed.). New York, NY: Pearson Education.

Ladewig, P., London, M., & Davidson, M. (2014). *Contemporary maternal-newborn nursing care* (8th ed.). Upper Saddle River, NJ: Pearson Education.

London, M., Ladewig, P., Davidson, M., Ball, J., Bindler, R., & Cowen, K. (2014). *Maternal and child nursing care* (4th ed.). Upper Saddle River, NJ: Pearson Education.

Lowdermilk, D., Perry, S., Cashion, M., & Alden, K. (2016). *Maternity and women's health care* (11th ed.). St. Louis, MO: Elsevier.

Test Yourself

Are you ready for the NCLEX-RN® or course exams? Access the NEW web-based app that provides students with thousands of practice questions in preparation for the NCLEX experience.

Health and Physical Assessment 15

In this chapter

Cross Reference

Other chapters relevant to this content area are

Lifespan Growth and Development — Chapter 13

I. HEALTH HISTORY OF ADULT

A. Overview

1. A **health history** is a collection of data about a client's present and past health status obtained using communication skills and interviewing techniques; provides **subjective data** while allowing opportunity to develop a therapeutic relationship with client
2. Sources of data
   a. Primary: client (best source of data unless confused, too young, or too ill to participate)
   b. Secondary: family members, caregivers, support people; old health records; and results of laboratory and diagnostic tests
3. Principles of history taking
   a. Provide privacy and maintain confidentiality
   b. If client is tired or ill, ask most critical questions first
   c. Immediately document data in chart; do not keep data on loose pieces of paper
   d. Plan an appropriate time frame: may require up to 1 hour or longer; allot enough time to take health history to avoid missing pertinent data; pace interview so as not to overtire client
   e. Gain trust: approach client and family in a professional manner; explain rationale for interview; tell client to immediately report if he or she becomes ill during interview; use therapeutic communication skills

   NCLEX®

   f. Note nonverbal cues about client's demeanor, posture, and overall appearance: physical indicators include cleanliness, body odor, personal grooming, hygiene, client's eye contact; signs of physical discomfort include diaphoresis, tremors, grimaces, and continual changes in position; signs of client stress include tears, skin blotching, nervous movements, inability to concentrate, arms folded, diaphoresis; if client wants to end interview, respect this request
   g. Assess client's reliability: can use proper terminology or words that indicate an understanding of health status; offers pertinent information about health status; does not change data reported; refers to previous health problems and treatment associated with them; is oriented to person, place, time, and event; family members present concur that data is accurate

h. Use an interpreter if there is a language barrier
i. Conduct interview in a logical, orderly manner; ask open-ended questions first regarding most important issues, then ask pertinent follow-up questions; use closed-ended questions (yes–no responses) to clarify previous statements or to ask for specific additional information; clarify any discrepancies

B. Health history components

1. Format used may vary slightly depending on client's age, developmental considerations, and reason for visit (routine care or an acute problem)
2. Biographical data includes name, address, telephone number, gender, marital status, religion, occupation, health insurance information, and possibly name and contact information for primary healthcare provider
3. Chief complaint (current problem or reason for which client is seeking care)

NCLEX®

4. Symptom analysis, getting data about each of the following:
   a. Location: be as specific as possible regarding part(s) of body involved
   b. Quantity: sometimes referred to as *severity* or *intensity*; whenever possible, use a numerical rating scale (0 to 10) or some type of visual analog scale; examples of symptoms frequently assessed this way are pain and dyspnea
   c. Quality: description of symptoms using various adjectives such as *burning*, *stabbing*, *pressure*; some disorders tend to be described in similar ways by clients, which can aid in diagnosing problem
   d. Setting: location of client when symptom(s) began and a description of events going on at that time
   e. Timing or chronology: notation of when symptom first began; slow onset versus sudden; constant versus intermittent; whether symptom disturbs sleep
   f. Aggravating or alleviating factors: practices that make symptom worse or better (such as eating, resting, use of medication, among others)
   g. Associated factors: other symptoms that accompany primary symptom (such as diaphoresis or shortness of breath with chest pain)
5. Previous state of health and physical capabilities and how current symptoms have impacted physical, emotional, and psychosocial functioning

NCLEX®

6. History of present illness (useful if problem has occurred more than once)
   a. When symptoms originally started
   b. How frequently exacerbations occur and whether onset is gradual or sudden
   c. Medications and/or other therapies used and extent to which they were successful
7. Past health history: also called *past history* or *medical history*; includes the following:
   a. Other possible health problems; some agencies use a checklist to obtain this information; focused (more detailed) assessment can be done on areas currently problematic; clients commonly seek treatment for one health problem while having an active history of others (called comorbidities) that require ongoing management

NCLEX®

   b. Childhood and adult immunizations, date of last tetanus prophylaxis and influenza vaccine
   c. Childhood illnesses such as measles, mumps, rubella (German measles), rubeola, chickenpox, rheumatic fever, scarlet fever, streptococcal infections, or other major illnesses
   d. Prior hospitalizations, including dates, reasons (accidents, injuries, and illnesses), surgeries, outcomes, and any complications (such as reactions to anesthesia or blood products)

NCLEX®

   e. Allergies: medication (reaction and symptoms, includes prescription, over-the-counter, and herbal products), food, seasonal (and their treatment), allergy to dyes used in diagnostic procedures (often assessed by asking about allergy to iodine)
   f. Pregnancy history and menstrual history as appropriate for female clients

NCLEX®

   g. Current medications: prescribed dose, rationale, and duration of therapy; date and time of last dose; over-the-counter and herbal products; home remedies; complementary or adjunctive healthcare (if so, have client explain remedies used and effects)
8. Family health history
   a. Overall state of health of parents and relatives: any significant and chronic illnesses, cause of death, and age at time of death
   b. Can highlight genetically transmitted traits or disorders; ethnic background also plays a role in risk of developing certain disorders

c. Establish any history of hereditary disorders such as coronary heart disease, diabetes mellitus, stroke, high blood pressure, cancer, obesity, arthritis, bleeding disorders, or mental health disorders

NCLEX® d. Helps to prioritize efforts on disease prevention and health promotion to lessen client's risk in an area; for example, cardiac health and healthy living

9. Personal/social history: includes social data and lifestyle assessment

NCLEX® a. Diet: foods eaten on a typical day; number of meals and snacks; who shops and cooks; food preferences including patterns based on culture and/or religion; usual fluid intake; caffeine intake (e.g., coffee, tea, cola)

NCLEX® b. Activity and exercise: type, frequency, and duration; ability to perform activities of daily living (ADLs) (eating, bathing, elimination, dressing, grooming); ability to move about at will

c. Sleep and rest: usual number of hours of sleep, sleep problems, and effectiveness of any remedies used

NCLEX® d. Tobacco use: number of packs per day (cigarettes) and years of smoking; type, frequency, and duration of use for other tobacco products

e. Substance use: amount, frequency, and duration of alcohol or recreational drug use

f. Living arrangements: location, type of dwelling, number of stairs to climb, home safety information, ability to access neighborhood or community resources

g. Family relationships or friendships: who is/are support person(s) in times of need; effects of illness on client and family roles and relationships (dynamics); identification of next of kin

h. Psychological data: major lifestyle changes or stressors experienced and how client dealt with them; usual coping patterns; general communication style and ability; appropriateness of verbal and nonverbal behavior; whether client is receiving mental health services; significance of current illness to client; effect of current illness on self-esteem or body image

i. Occupation: presence of occupational hazards, such as exposure to carcinogens (e.g., asbestos, other chemicals); distance and time for commute to work and associated concerns; amount of time missed from work due to illness; history of a need to change jobs because of illness

j. Travel: out of country, when and length of time; military service abroad

k. Current and past health resources used: all healthcare providers, dentists, folk healers; satisfaction with and accessibility of care

10. Review of systems (ROS): used to obtain subjective data in a medical model; nursing assessments may use a nursing model (Gordon's 11 functional health patterns as one example); healthcare agencies generally have a specific form to gather this data; forms may blend gathering of subjective data (history) and **objective data** (physical assessment or examination)

a. Skin: skin disease (eczema, psoriasis, hives), changes in moles, skin dryness or moisture, itching, bruising, rashes or other lesions, changes in hair or nails, sun exposure

b. Head: headaches, dizziness (vertigo) or fainting (syncope), head injury

c. Eyes: vision problems (blurring, blind spots, reduced acuity), double vision (diplopia), glaucoma, cataracts, eye pain, redness, discharge or watering, swelling, method of vision correction being used

d. Ears: hearing loss, hearing aid use, tinnitus, vertigo, earaches, infections, discharge, and characteristics

e. Nose/sinuses: frequency and severity of colds, sinus pain or obstruction, discharge, nosebleeds, allergies, reduced sense of smell

f. Mouth/throat: pain or lesions in mouth (or tongue), toothaches, change in taste, frequency of sore throats, bleeding gums, dysphagia, hoarseness, history of tonsillectomy, frequency of dental care, presence of dental prostheses

g. Neck: pain, mobility, enlarged or tender lymph nodes, goiter, lumps or other swelling

NCLEX® h. Breasts: history of breast disease or surgery, pain, lumps, rashes, nipple discharge, knowledge and performance of breast self-examination (BSE); date of last mammogram

i. Axilla: rash, lumps, tenderness, or swelling

NCLEX® j. Respiratory: history of lung disease (tuberculosis, pneumonia, asthma, bronchitis, emphysema), shortness of breath (amount and triggering factors, such as activity level), wheezes/other noises associated with respiration, cough, sputum production (color, amount, and, if relevant, timing), pain associated with breathing, hemoptysis, and exposure to pollutants or other inhaled toxins

NCLEX® k. Cardiovascular: history of heart disease, murmur, hypertension, or anemia; chest pain (precordial or retrosternal, radiation, and other pain characteristics); dyspnea on exertion (specify amount); orthopnea, paroxysmal nocturnal dyspnea (PND); edema, nocturia

l. Peripheral vascular: discoloration of extremities (especially feet and ankles; note whether associated with activity); coolness, numbness, or tingling of lower limbs (note relationship to activity and time of day); history of intermittent claudication, ulcerations, thrombophlebitis, or varicose veins
m. Gastrointestinal (GI): appetite, nausea and vomiting, constipation or diarrhea, frequency and recent changes in bowel movements, tarry or bloody stools, rectal conditions (such as hemorrhoids), food intolerances, dysphagia, heartburn, pyrosis (upper-GI burning with sour eructation), indigestion, abdominal pain (with or without eating), history of GI disorder, antacid use, and prescribed diet
n. Urinary: frequency, urgency, or dysuria; nocturia; polyuria or oliguria; characteristics of stream (narrowed, hesitancy, straining); cloudy urine or hematuria; incontinence; history of urinary disorder (renal disease or calculi, urinary tract infections); pain in back, flank, suprapubic area, or groin
o. Male genital: lumps, hernia, penile lesions or discharge, pain in testicles or penis, knowledge and performance of testicular self-examination (TSE), sexual health practices (contraception and prevention of sexually transmitted infections)
p. Female genital: menstrual history (age of menarche, last monthly period, duration of cycle, premenstrual pain, intermenstrual spotting or metrorrhagia, dysmenorrhea, amenorrhea, menorrhagia), vaginal itching or discharge, age at menopause, menopausal manifestations, postmenopausal bleeding, last Papanicolaou (Pap) test and gynecological exam, sexual health practices
q. Musculoskeletal: joint pain, stiffness, or swelling; history of arthritis or gout; limited movement, noise with joint movement, obvious deformity; muscle pain, weakness, or cramping; difficulty with gait or activities; back pain or stiffness, history of back pain or disease; use of mobility aids and satisfaction with ability to perform ADLs

NCLEX®
r. Neurologic: weakness, tics or tremors, paralysis, problems with coordination, paresthesias (numbness and tingling), recent or distant memory disorder, nervousness, mood changes, history of depression or other mental health problem, hallucinations, history of stroke, fainting or blackouts, seizure disorder
s. Hematologic: easy bruising or bleeding, swollen lymph nodes, history of blood transfusion and reactions, exposure to radiation or other toxins

NCLEX®
t. Endocrine: history of diabetes, thyroid or adrenal disease, abnormal hair distribution, change in skin (pigmentation, texture), excess sweating, relationship between appetite and weight, hormone therapy

II. HEALTH HISTORY OF CHILD

A. Overview
1. Provides opportunity to observe parent–child interactions
2. Principles are same as for an adult health history

B. Demographic and biographical information: similar to adult with addition of child's nickname, ages of child, siblings, and parents

C. Reason for seeking care
1. Sometimes called *chief complaint*; may be wellness- or illness-oriented
2. Record in words of informant, parent, or child

D. History of present illness

NCLEX®
1. Symptom analysis as previously described for adult client
2. Parents' perceptions of illness versus child's perception, if applicable

E. Past medical history
1. Birth history
   a. Length of pregnancy and mother's health and access to prenatal care
   b. Medications taken during pregnancy and any alcohol, tobacco, or street-drug use
   c. Duration of labor and type of delivery and Apgar scores, if known
   d. Birth weight, length, head circumference
   e. Postnatal health problems
   f. Feeding: formula, including type, or breastfed, including length of time
2. Past illnesses and hospitalizations, injuries, accidents, or surgeries

NCLEX®
3. Allergies: medication, food, or environmental, including symptoms experienced

NCLEX®
4. Immunizations including boosters

NCLEX®
5. Habits and behaviors: sleep; discipline; socialization; exercise or activity; behavior issues; wellness behaviors; use of alcohol, drugs, nicotine, or caffeine; sexuality issues

6. Medications taken regularly: prescription, over-the-counter, herbal, home or folk remedies
7. Developmental data
   a. Age at which child achieved specific developmental milestones, including first held head erect, first rolled over, first sat unsupported, first steps, first used words appropriately, bowel and bladder control
   b. Current developmental performance measured by a screening tool such as Denver II, if known
   c. Academic performance if in school
8. Nutritional data

NCLEX®

   a. Timing and frequency of meals and snacks, consider adequacy in terms of age
   b. Ethnic or cultural considerations in food choices
   c. Use a 24-hour diet recall or food frequency record to assess adequacy of diet
9. Family history

NCLEX®

   a. Primarily to discover potential or actual hereditary diseases in child or parents
   b. Includes a **genogram** (pictorial representation of family tree) that includes hereditary diseases, ages and causes of death, and chronic conditions (see Figure 15–1)
   c. Family structure: immediate and extended members of family; previous marriages, divorces, separations, or deaths of spouses
   d. Home and community environment: type of dwelling, sleeping arrangements, safety features, relationships with neighbors
   e. Occupations and education of family members, including work schedules
   f. Cultural and religious traditions, including language spoken at home
   g. Family function: interactions and roles; power, decision making, and problem solving; communication; and expression of feelings and individuality
10. Review of systems (a specific review of each body system)
   a. Begin with a broad question about child's overall health
   b. Integument: pruritus, rashes (including location), acne, bruising, hair growth or loss, disorders or deformities of nails
   c. Head: headaches, dizziness, or injuries
   d. Eyes: visual problems (bumping into things, squinting, blurred vision, holding books close or sitting close to television or computer), rubbing eyes, eye infections, glasses or contact lenses
   e. Ears: earaches (frequency and treatment), evidence of hearing loss (needing to repeat requests, loud voice), previous hearing test results
   f. Nose: history of nosebleeds, constant or frequent runny or stuffy nose, problems with sense of smell
   g. Mouth: mouth breathing, dental visits, tooth-care habits (brushing, flossing), toothaches
   h. Throat: sore throats, difficulty swallowing, choking, hoarseness or voice problems
   i. Neck: stiffness or problems moving; difficulty in holding head erect
   j. Chest: breast enlargement or development, breast self-examination for adolescents
   k. Respiratory: frequency of colds, coughing or wheezing, difficulty breathing, sputum production, history of pneumonia or tuberculosis (TB), last TB test date

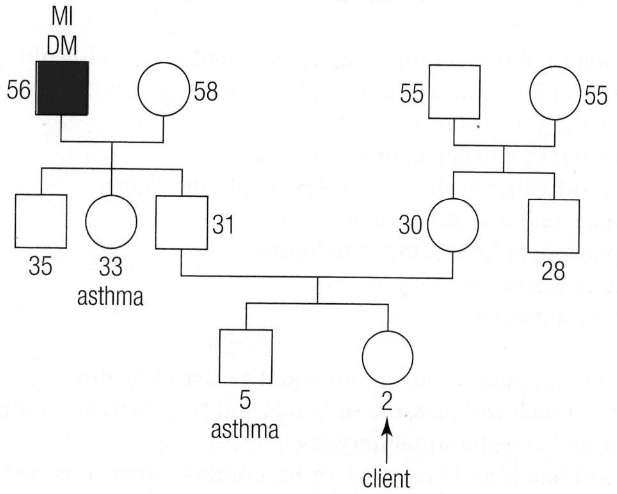

Figure 15–1

Sample genogram for a female child. The child's brother has asthma, a paternal aunt has asthma, and the paternal grandfather died having myocardial infarction (MI) and diabetes mellitus (DM).

NCLEX®
l. Cardiovascular: cyanosis or fatigue on exertion; history of heart murmurs, anemia, or rheumatic fever; blood type if known

NCLEX®
m. Gastrointestinal: nausea or vomiting, jaundice, change in bowel habits, diarrhea, constipation
n. Genitourinary: pain on urination, unpleasant odor to urine, enuresis, testicular self-examination for adolescents, condom use if sexually active
o. Gynecological: date or age of menarche, date of last menstrual period, pain on menstruation, vaginal discharge, last Pap smear and contraceptive use if sexually active
p. Musculoskeletal: weakness, clumsiness or lack of coordination, back or joint pain, muscle pain or cramps, abnormal gait or posturing or spasticity, history of fractures or sprains, usual activity level
q. Neurologic: history of seizures, speech problems, nightmares or fears, dizziness or tremors, learning disabilities or problems with attention at home or at school

NCLEX®
11. Review of psychosocial systems
   a. Family composition: family members in home and relationship to child, marital status of parents, parents' educational level, persons participating in care of child, recent changes or crises in family
   b. Financial resources: family members' employment status or occupation, health insurance coverage
   c. Home environment: safe play area; water supply; availability of heat, electricity, and so on; transportation; neighborhood safety issues
   d. Childcare arrangements: daycare resources needed/available, school attended
   e. Daily living habits: peer relationships; sleep, rest, activity patterns; social activities; self-esteem and body image
   f. Child's temperament

III. PREPARING FOR PHYSICAL EXAMINATION

A. Equipment needed

1. Basic equipment for a brief physical exam includes blood pressure equipment, clean disposable gloves, drape, penlight, stethoscope, tape measure, thermometer, watch with a second hand, and weight scale
2. Additional equipment for a complete physical exam includes cotton ball, doppler, goniometer, lubricant, nasal speculum, near vision charts, neurologic hammer, ophthalmoscope, otoscope, reflex hammer, skin calipers, Snellen visual acuity chart, strabismoscope, tongue depressor/blade, tuning fork, tympanometer, and vaginal speculum; a nurse generalist may not conduct these aspects of exam but may need to set up exam room

B. Promoting comfort during physical assessment

1. Provide a comfortable room and minimize distractions
2. Ensure client privacy
3. Provide adequate lighting and normalize room temperature

IV. TECHNIQUES OF PHYSICAL EXAMINATION

A. *Inspection*

1. Uses observation to obtain information about client's state of health; also includes smell
2. Ensure adequate lighting (artificial or sunlight) to inspect body without distortions or shadows
3. Items to assess using skill of inspection
   a. Overall appearance and demeanor, eye contact
   b. Interactions with other healthcare professionals and family

NCLEX®
   c. Skin color, hair, nail beds, skeletal deformities
   d. Clothing appropriate for weather conditions
   e. Congruence of verbal and nonverbal behavior
   f. Sense of smell: any odors

B. *Palpation*

1. Uses touch to obtain information about client's state of health
2. Use sensation of touch and pressure of hands and fingers to determine masses, elevations, temperature, organ position, and any abnormal findings

NCLEX®
3. Ulnar surfaces of hands and fingers are most common areas used for palpation; hands should be warm and gentle; wear gloves if there will be contact with body fluids, open skin areas, or mucosa

Table 15–1 Percussion Notes

Tone	Quality	Pitch	Example
Tympany	Drumlike	High	Gastric bubble
Resonance	Hollow	Low	Healthy lungs
Hyperresonance	Booming	Very loud	Emphysemic lung tissue
Flatness	Very dull	High	Muscle, bone
Dullness	Thudlike	Soft to moderate	Liver, spleen, heart

4. Can be light (1 cm in depth) or deep (4 cm in depth) depending on area being examined; nurse controls amount of pressure; deep palpation should occur after light palpation; most nurses use light palpation during physical exam, while deep palpation is used during a complete physical exam by healthcare provider

C. ***Percussion***

1. A skill in which finger of one hand touches or taps a finger of other hand to generate vibration to produce a specific, diagnostic sound; sound changes as examiner moves from area to area
2. Sounds can be classified as tympanic, hyperresonant, resonant, dull, or flat; further description and examples of percussion notes can be found in Table 15–1

D. ***Auscultation***

NCLEX® 1. Place stethoscope over bare skin to eliminate change in sound caused by clothing
2. Listen to sound, duration, pitch, and intensity
NCLEX® 3. Must isolate sounds; if client has a large amount of chest or back hair, wet hair to flatten it and diminish extra sounds
4. Allot enough time to listen carefully to sounds; if in doubt, consult another healthcare professional

V. PHYSICAL EXAMINATION OF ADULT

A. Various purposes of physical assessment

1. Full exam by healthcare provider as part of wellness screening (annually or as recommended)
2. Full history and physical assessment done at time of hospital admission
3. Head-to-toe assessment at beginning of shift for hospitalized clients
4. Focused or body system–specific assessments that may be done frequently (more than once per shift, such as every 4 hours)

B. Vital signs

1. Temperature: average is 98.6°F or 37°C (normal range 96.4°F–99.1°F or 35.8°C–37.3°C); varies slightly depending on age, time of day, phase of menstrual cycle, exercise level, and method of measurement (rectal measures 1° higher than oral; axillary measures 1° lower than oral); measure using oral, rectal, axillary, or otic (tympanic membrane) route
2. Pulse: average is 68–78 beats per minute (bpm) in adult with a range of 60–100
   a. Radial: count rate and note rhythm and amplitude
   b. Apical: listen for a full minute and compare to radial pulse; place stethoscope on chest at fifth intercostal space, midclavicular line (5ICS, MCL)
   c. Rhythm should be regular; if pulse is irregular, assess whether rhythm is regularly irregular or irregularly irregular and alert healthcare provider
3. Respiration: normal range in adult is 12–20 breaths/minute; count rate, rhythm, and depth of respiration; note comfort level as client breathes; normal respirations are relaxed, silent, automatic, and regular
4. Blood pressure (BP): normal adult range is 100/60 mmHg to 130/85 mmHg; varies with age, gender, weight, exercise, emotion/stress, and diurnal rhythm (early-morning low and late-afternoon high)
   a. Have person sit or lie down with arm supported at heart level; allow a 5-minute rest period with no activity, smoking, eating, or drinking before measuring BP
   NCLEX® b. If BP is questionable, wait 1–2 minutes before taking it again to avoid false high diastolic reading

c. If unable to hear BP, palpate BP by placing index finger over brachial artery, inflate cuff, deflate cuff while palpating, and note when pulsation disappears; only systolic pressure is noted and recorded as palpated
d. If client has poor circulation, BP may be faint; in this case or if BP cannot even be palpated, use a Doppler to hear sounds; note systolic pressure only and record as a Doppler BP

C. Height and weight

1. Height: using a balance scale, raise headpiece on measuring pole; align it with top of head while client is shoeless, standing erect, and looking forward
2. Weight: use platform scale if client can stand without assistance; special electronic scales and bed scales are also available if needed
3. *NCLEX®* Use professionally authorized charts to determine if height and weight fall within normal age limits; also compare readings to client's previous measurements

D. General appearance

1. Includes client's grooming and attire and personal hygiene
2. Includes gait and posture, general body build, and behavior

E. Mental status

1. A short mental status exam is often done during health history interview; assess client for overt signs of mental distress, crying, sullen demeanor, appropriate comments for situation
2. *NCLEX®* Four key areas of functioning
   a. Appearance: as noted in previous section
   b. Behavior: level of consciousness (LOC), awake, alert, aware of and responding to internal and external stimuli; lethargic and drowsy, stuporous, or unresponsive (use Glasgow coma scale as needed); facial expression, speech (quality, pace, articulation of words, word choice); aphasia (receptive/Wernicke's, motor/expressive/Broca's, global), mood and affect
   c. Cognition: orientation (to time, place, person, events), attention span, recent memory, remote memory, new learning (four unrelated words test), judgment
   d. Thought processes: thought content (logical, consistent), client's perceptions (reality based, congruent with others), and absence/presence of suicidal thoughts/ideation

Memory Aid

Remember the four key areas of mental status (appearance, behavior, cognition, and thought processes) by using the abbreviation ABCT.

   e. The Mini-Mental State Exam (Folstein, Folstein, & McHugh, 1975) may be used to gather this data; requires 5–10 minutes to administer; highest score is 30 (average people score 27)
   f. A full mental status exam may be done if indicated, and other tests can be added if problems exist (brain lesions or stroke, aphasia, mental illness, memory changes, alcoholism, and others)

F. Integument

1. Skin provides first layer of protection for body against infection, trauma, and fluid loss; it regulates body temperature, provides sensory perception, produces vitamin D, excretes sweat and impurities, and is a barometer of emotions
2. Inspection of skin
   a. Assess skin for color; compare areas exposed to sun with those that are not
   b. *NCLEX®* Daylight is best light to detect jaundice (yellowing of skin, sclera); use good lighting for best illumination; flashlights/penlights are also helpful for general inspection
   c. Scan body for color, texture, tone, distribution of lesions, skin symmetry, differences between body areas, evidence of rashes or eruptions, hygiene
   d. Assess moles (pigmented nevi) for defining features such as symmetry, elevation, color, and texture
   e. Normal findings: range of skin color varies from person to person; color should be uniform; sun-exposed areas will be darker; calluses appear yellow; nevi (moles) can be normal findings
   f. *NCLEX®* Abnormal findings: color changes in moles (may be cancerous changes); pale, shiny skin of lower extremities (possible decreased peripheral circulation or diabetes mellitus); localized hemorrhages into skin (petechiae less than 0.5 cm in diameter or purpura more than 0.5 cm in diameter) that appear purple-red (could indicate injury, steroid use, or vasculitis)
3. Palpation of skin
   a. Feel skin for moisture, temperature, texture, turgor, and mobility; gently pinch skin to test turgor; skin should immediately return to normal but will be delayed if edema or dehydration is present

b. Normal findings: cool to warm, dry, and smooth under normal conditions; in stressful situations, skin may feel cool and clammy; assess skin by touching bilaterally with dorsum of hands and comparing findings

NCLEX®

c. Abnormal findings: lesions (descriptions of size, shape, color, texture, elevation/depression, pedunculation, exudates, configuration, location, and distribution)

4. Inspection of nails
   a. Inspect for color, contour, texture, configuration, symmetry, and cleanliness
   b. Note whether clean and well-manicured, bitten down, yellow and tobacco-stained; color should be pink with a brisk capillary refill (less than 3 seconds) when depressed (blanch test)
   c. Normal findings: nail plate is smooth and flat or slightly convex; nail base angle is 160 degrees
   d. Abnormal findings: white bands (melanoma); white spots (cuticle manipulation or trauma); yellow (psoriasis, fungal infections, and chronic respiratory diseases); diffuse darkening (malaria medication, candidal infection, hyperbilirubinemia, or chronic trauma); a green-black color (pseudomonas infection or nail bed trauma [subungual hematoma])
5. Palpation of nails: should be hard and smooth with uniform thickness
   a. Squeeze nail; if it separates from nail bed, can indicate psoriasis or trauma
   b. A clubbed boggy nail can indicate infection with candida or pseudomonas

G. Head and neck

1. Inspection
   a. Head should be erect and still with symmetrical facial features
   b. Assess structure, conjunctiva, sclera, cornea, and iris of each eye
   c. Assess position, alignment, skin condition, and external meatus of ear
   d. Inspect external nose
   e. Inspect inside of mouth and throat (mucosa, tongue, teeth and gums, floor of mouth, palate, uvula)
   f. Assess for tics, spasms, lesions, and facial paralysis
   g. Neck should be symmetrical without masses
2. Palpation: palpate from front to back for smoothness and symmetry of cranium, scalp, and hair; palpate salivary glands; palpate temporal artery and temporomandibular joint; palpate maxillary and frontal sinuses; push on tragus of ear for tenderness; palpate thyroid gland (size, shape, tenderness, and presence of nodules)—stand behind client and use two fingers of each hand on sides of trachea, then displace trachea to left and ask client to swallow (thyroid should feel smooth, small, and free of nodules); palpate for midline position of trachea
3. Inspect and palpate cervical lymph nodes
4. Special testing

NCLEX®

   a. Eyes: test visual fields (confrontation), extraocular movements (EOMs), pupil size, equality, roundness, and response to light and accommodation (PERRLA); check ocular fundus (with ophthalmoscope) for red reflex, condition of optic disc, blood vessels and background of retina; may be documented under neurologic exam
   b. Ears: use an otoscope to inspect ear canal and tympanic membrane (movable, intact, and pearly white-gray in color); use tuning fork to do Rinne and Weber tests to check for bone and air conduction in hearing (see also section on neurologic exam); may be documented under neurologic exam
   c. Nose: use a nasal speculum to check nasal mucosa, septum, and turbinates

H. Breasts and axillae

1. With client in a sitting position, inspect breasts for symmetry, contour, and shape; should be rounded, generally symmetrical
2. Look for areas of discoloration, hyperpigmentation, dimpling or retraction, swelling or edema; should be uniform in color, smooth, and elastic
3. Detect areas of retraction by asking client to do three maneuvers: raise arms above head, push hands together with elbows flexed, and press hands down on hips
4. Observe areola for size, shape, symmetry, color, general surface characteristics, lesions or masses; should be round or oval; color may vary among individuals from light pink to dark brown
5. Inspect nipples for size, shape, position, color, and presence of any discharge or lesions; should be round, everted, and equal in size
6. Palpate axillary, subclavicular, and supraclavicular lymph nodes using palmar surface of fingertips in four areas: edge of greater pectoral muscle in anterior axillary line, thoracic wall in midaxilla, upper portion of humerus, and anterior edge of latissimus dorsi muscle in posterior axillary line

7. Palpate breast for masses and tenderness, using one of three patterns: hands-of-the-clock, spokes-on-a-wheel, concentric circles; there should be no masses or tenderness
8. Palpate areola and nipples for masses; there should be none

I. Chest

1. Lungs
   a. Use standard thoracic landmarks when performing respiratory assessment

NCLEX®

   b. Inspection: overall appearance, nutritional status (dyspnea can impair oral intake), ability to breathe, respirations (rate, shortness of breath, dyspnea), contour and movement of chest (should be symmetrical); presence of retractions (abnormal); color of skin, nail beds, and lips (oxygenation)
   c. Palpation: assess posterior aspect of chest for masses, bulges, muscle tone, subcutaneous emphysema (crepitus), and areas of tenderness
   d. Palpation: assess respiratory expansion by placing hands on eighth to tenth ribs (posterior); place thumbs close to vertebrae; slide hand medially and grasp a small fold of skin between thumbs; ask client to take a deep breath; thumbs should move evenly away from vertebrae during inspiration; note any delay in expansion
   e. Palpation: assess tactile fremitus (a palpable vibration that transmits sounds via patent bronchi to lung parenchyma and chest wall) by placing ulnar surface of hand or balls of fingers (palmar base) on outer chest wall; ask client to speak words "ninety-nine" or "blue moon"; begin palpating at lung apices and work from one side to other, moving down posterior chest (but not over scapula); vibration should be equal on both sides in any location; decreased fremitus occurs with conditions that obstruct transmission of vibrations (pleural effusion, pneumothorax, and others); increased fremitus occurs with consolidation or compression of lung tissue (such as in extensive lobar pneumonia with patent bronchus)
   f. Percussion: have client lean forward slightly; begin percussion over apex of left lung; then move hands systematically and compare percussion notes lobe to lobe and side to side; to determine excursion, locate 7th intercostal space and percuss downward along scapular line to diaphragm; mark line where resonance changes to dullness; have client take a deep breath and hold; mark second line; distance should be between 3 and 6 cm

NCLEX®

   g. Auscultation: use flat diaphragm of stethoscope to listen systematically to chest; begin posteriorly and listen from apices (at C7 level) to bases (at about T10), and laterally from axilla to 7th or 8th rib; normal sounds include bronchial, bronchovesicular, and vesicular; compare findings side to side while working downward over posterior chest (see Table 15–2 for description of various adventitious breath sounds); note location, quality, and time of occurrence during respiratory cycle
   h. Other abnormal findings during auscultation include bronchophony (ask client to repeat words "ninety-nine"; if heard clearly, indicates lung density in that area); egophony (ask client to say "ee-ee-ee-ee" during auscultation; sound changes to a long "aaaa" sound in areas of consolidation or compression); whispered pectoriloquy (ask client to whisper "one-two-three" during auscultation; sound will be faint yet clear and distinct with small amounts of consolidation); pleural friction rub (grating, creaking, or groaning noise, often more noticeable on inspiration, and may be heard over inflamed areas of parietal and visceral pleura)
   i. Repeat entire assessment process with anterior chest

NCLEX®

2. Neck vessels
   a. Inspect carotid arteries for visible pulsation with head of exam table raised to 45 degrees

Table 15–2 Adventitious Breath Sounds

Sound	Characteristics	Timing and Occurrence
Crackles (coarse)	Popping, frying sound; moist, low-pitched	Inspiration, some expiration
Crackles (medium)	Not as loud as coarse crackles	Middle of inspiration
Crackles (fine)	Noncontinuous, popping, high-pitched	End of inspiration
Rhonchi or gurgles	Continuous, low-pitched, prolonged	Expiration
Wheezes	Continuous, high-pitched, musical	Inspiration and/or expiration
Pleural friction rub	Low-pitched, dry, grating	Inspiration and/or expiration

b. Palpate carotid arteries *one at a time* in area medial to sternocleidomastoid muscle; avoid area higher in neck (could stimulate baroreceptors and trigger bradycardia from vagus nerve stimulation); note pulse contour and amplitude and compare findings side to side
c. Auscultate over carotid arteries for bruits using bell of stethoscope; sound should be absent; if bruit present, note type of sound (buzzing, swishing, or blowing); bruit indicates turbulent blood flow from obstruction (i.e., atherosclerotic narrowing)
d. Assess jugular vein distention (head elevated 45 degrees); turn head slightly away; highest pulsation should be no more than 3.8 cm (1.5 in.) above sternal notch

3. Heart
a. Inspection: general appearance and color of skin and nail beds; observe for symmetry of movement, anatomical defects, retractions, pulsations, and heaves; locate point of maximal impulse (PMI) if visible (usually at apex, 5ICS, MCL)
b. Palpate PMI (not visible in all clients) with ball of hand, then fingertips; next assess for abnormal pulsations in sternoclavicular, aortic, pulmonic, tricuspid, and epigastric areas; palpate for thrills (over areas of turbulent blood flow)

NCLEX®

c. Auscultate in predetermined sequence (see Figure 15–2 and Memory Aid) for S1, S2, extra heart sounds (S3 and S4), and murmurs; see Table 15–3 for heart sounds; place client in three positions for complete assessment: lying on back with head elevated 30 degrees, sitting up, and lying on left side; use diaphragm of stethoscope (higher-pitched sounds) and then bell (lower-pitched sounds)

Memory Aid

Moving from left to right and top to bottom (as when reading), remember location of valvular heart sounds with **A**ll **P**atients **T**ake **M**eds (**A**ortic, **P**ulmonic, **T**ricuspid, **M**itral). These sounds are best heard "downstream" from actual blood flow through valve, giving their unique auscultatory locations.

d. Percussion: can locate cardiac border (sound changes from resonance to dullness); rarely done because chest x-ray determines cardiac size

Figure 15–2

Sites for auscultation of the heart. Aortic valve area: right sternal border (RSB), 2nd ICS; pulmonic valve area: left sternal border (LSB), 2nd ICS; tricuspid valve area: left lateral sternal border (LLSB), 4th ICS; mitral valve area: left midclavicular line (MCL), 5th ICS.

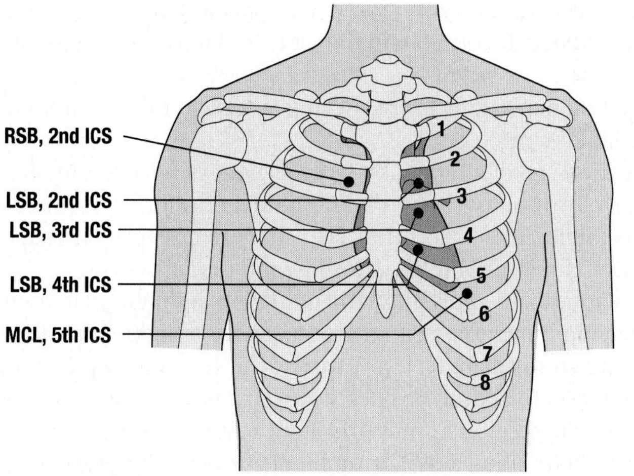

Table 15–3 **Heart Sounds**

Sound	Location	Description	Character	Significance
S1	Apex	Lub	Low-pitched and dull	Closure of mitral and tricuspid valves
S2	Base	Dub	Shorter, more high-pitched than S1	Closure of pulmonic and aortic valves
S3	Apex	"Ken-tuck-y"	Low-pitched	Ventricles filling rapidly
S4	Tricuspid or mitral areas	"Ten-ness-ee"	Occurs just before S1 after atrial contraction	Increased resistance to ventricular filling
Pericardial friction rub	Left sternal border	Grating, leathery	Muffled, high-pitched, and transient	Pericardial inflammation

J. Abdomen

1. Preparation: ask client to empty bladder; position client supine with a small pillow under head; bend or place a pillow under client's knees; expose abdomen fully; place client's arms at sides or across chest (not over head because it tenses abdominal muscles); warm examiner's hands and stethoscope and ensure that fingernails are short; keep room warm to prevent chilling; use distraction techniques as needed
2. Inspection: assess four quadrants for contour, symmetry, bumps, bulges, or masses; note skin color (redness, jaundice) and condition (striae, scars), umbilicus, hair distribution, and any pulsations or movements of abdomen
   - NCLEX® **a.** A bulge may indicate a distended bladder or hernia; look at shape and contour
   - **b.** Midline umbilicus: to assess for umbilical hernia, have client lift arms over head; if umbilicus protrudes, hernia may be present
   - **c.** Abdominal movements: slight, wavelike movements are normal, especially in a thin person; visible rippling waves may indicate obstruction
3. NCLEX® Auscultation: perform before palpation and percussion to avoid increasing frequency of bowel sounds
   - **a.** Place diaphragm of stethoscope lightly against skin in right lower quadrant, where bowel sounds are most frequent (location of ileocecal valve)
   - **b.** Listen in a clockwise fashion for at least 2 minutes
   - **c.** Note character and quality; normal sounds are high-pitched, gurgling, at rate of 5–34 per min
   - **d.** Sounds are classified as normal, hypoactive (heard infrequently), or hyperactive (loud, high-pitched, more frequent than normal)
   - **e.** Use bell of stethoscope to hear vascular sounds over iliac, aortic, renal, and femoral arteries; listen for bruits, venous hums, and friction rubs
4. Percussion: detects size and location of abdominal organs in all four quadrants
   - NCLEX® **a.** Do not percuss if abdominal aortic aneurysm is present or suspected
   - **b.** Tympany indicates an area of empty stomach or bowel
   - **c.** Dullness is normally heard over liver, kidney, full bladder, and feces-filled intestines
5. Palpation: with warm hands, palpate lightly (about 1 cm deep with four fingers positioned close together) using a rotary motion in all areas to assess skin surface and superficial musculature; then repeat sequence deeply (about 4–6 cm) to determine size, shape, position, and tenderness of organs
   - **a.** Light palpation helps detect superficial masses and fluid accumulation; a normal finding is a soft, nontender abdomen
   - **b.** Deep palpation can identify masses, tenderness, pulsations, organ enlargement (liver, spleen, kidneys); usually done by primary care provider or advanced practice nurse
   - **c.** If a mass is found, note its location, size, shape, consistency (hard, firm, or soft), type of surface (smooth or nodular), mobility, pulsatility, and tenderness
   - NCLEX® **d.** If a mass is noted to be pulsatile, stop palpating in that area to avoid rupture
   - NCLEX® **e.** Identify rebound tenderness: if an area is tender to light palpation or if client reports pain in an area, move hand to an area away from painful site, and position hand perpendicular (at a 90-degree angle) in relation to abdomen; push down slowly and deeply and then lift up quickly; normally there is no pain or tenderness, but if present (often severe and accompanied by muscle rigidity), it indicates peritoneal inflammation, possibly appendicitis or peritonitis from another disorder
   - **f.** Abdominal pain: indicates possible ulcers, intestinal obstruction, cholecystitis, peritonitis
   - **g.** Ascites: use a tape measure at fullest site on abdomen, usually at or just above umbilicus, to determine changes in girth caused by fluid retention
   - **h.** Inguinal area: palpate each groin for femoral pulse and inguinal nodes

K. Extremities

1. NCLEX® Inspect bilaterally for symmetry, skin characteristics, and hair distribution; hair loss, thin shiny skin, and thickened toenails in older adults are called trophic changes and are often caused by decreased circulation from peripheral arterial disease secondary to atherosclerosis
2. Palpate peripheral pulses; in upper extremities, includes radial and ulnar pulses; in lower extremities, includes popliteal, dorsalis pedis (DP), and posterior tibial (PT) pulses
3. NCLEX® Palpate skin for pretibial or other edema; note temperature and compare side-to-side bilaterally
4. Separate toes and inspect them

L. Musculoskeletal

1. Inspect each joint for size, contour, masses, and deformity; measure discrepancies in leg length
2. Palpate joints for musculature, bony articulations, crepitation, heat, swelling, tenderness
3. Test range of motion (ROM) of joints of upper extremities (shoulders, elbows, wrists, and fingers) and lower extremities (hips, knees, ankles, and toes); describe any physical limitations; if less than full ROM is present, a goniometer may be used in a full exam to measure joint angles more precisely
4. Note size, tone, and any involuntary movements of major muscle groups; compare findings bilaterally
5. Test strength of major muscle groups that control joints in upper and lower extremities by asking client to resist attempts to put joint through ROM; grading scale ranges from grade 0, no contraction to grade 5, full ROM against gravity and full resistance
6. *NCLEX®* Test ROM in spine by asking client to bend forward and touch toes (flexion should be 75–90 degrees with no curvature side to side; if curvature present, suspect and further assess for scoliosis), bend sideways (35 degrees of flexion normal), bend backward (hyperextension of 30 degrees normal), and twist shoulders from one side to other (rotation of 30 degrees bilaterally normal)
7. *NCLEX®* Straight leg-raising (with knee straight) should not be painful; if it is, suspect herniated nucleus pulposus (in intervertebral disk)
8. Note any musculoskeletal pain present during assessment; pain description should be very specific
   a. Bone pain: pain unrelated to movement unless fracture is present, deep, aching, and continuous; it also causes insomnia
   b. Muscle pain: cramps or spasms with possible relationship to posture or movement; tremors, twitches, or weakness may be manifested; muscle tension may produce referred pain
   c. Joint pain: joint may be tender to palpation; referred pain can be present; nerve root irritation may produce radiculitis (pain is distal); mechanical joint pain is worse with movement and worsens throughout day

M. Neurologic

1. Assess cranial nerves; see Table 15–4 for a summary of normal and abnormal findings
   a. Olfactory nerve (CN I): not tested routinely but use items with different smells (alcohol, coffee, vanilla, peppermint, etc.) to detect abnormalities in sense of smell; test one nostril at a time if performed; sense of smell generally diminishes with age
   b. Optic nerve (CN II): test visual acuity with Snellen chart, test visual fields by confrontation, and use an ophthalmoscope to examine fundus of eye (refer back to section G on head and neck)
   c. Oculomotor, trochlear, and abducens nerves (CN III, IV, VI): assess pupils for size (in mm), equality, roundness, reactivity to light, and accommodation (PERRLA); assess EOMs by asking client to visually follow a finger through cardinal fields of gaze; observe for nystagmus (rapid back-and-forth oscillating movements of eyes in a horizontal or vertical plane, rotary direction, or combination)
   d. Trigeminal nerve (CN V): assess motor function by palpating temporal and masseter muscles, ask client to clench teeth and try to separate jaws by pushing down on chin; assess sensory function by touching client's face bilaterally in three divisions of nerve (ophthalmic, maxillary, and mandibular) and ask client to say "now" when face is touched with a wisp of cotton; test corneal reflex if necessary (may be omitted in a screening exam) by lightly touching cornea with a wisp of cotton brought in from side of client's face
   e. Facial nerve (CN VII): test motor function by asking client to smile, frown, close eyes tightly (while examiner tries to keep them open), lift eyebrows, puff cheeks, and show teeth; test sensory function (not done routinely) by asking client to identify salty, sweet, or sour solutions applied to tongue
   f. Acoustic or vestibulocochlear nerve (CN VIII): use voice test (whispered words from 0.3 to 0.6 meters [1–2 ft] away) to determine hearing ability; do Weber test (place a vibrating tuning fork on midline of skull and ask whether sound is heard equally in both ears or better in one ear); do Rinne test (place a vibrating tuning fork on mastoid process and ask client to indicate when sound disappears); quickly invert tuning fork and place vibrating end near ear canal and ask client to indicate when sound is no longer heard
   g. Glossopharyngeal and vagus nerves (CN IX and X): using a tongue blade, note pharyngeal movement when client says "ahh" or yawns; watch for uvula and soft palate to rise in midline and for tonsillar pillars to move medially; test gag reflex by touching posterior pharyngeal wall with tongue blade; note voice quality (should be smooth with no straining)

Table 15–4 Cranial Nerve Assessment

Cranial Nerve(s)	Assessment	Normal	Abnormal
CN I	Smell	Can identify common substances	Difficulty detecting common substances
CN II	Visual acuity	Able to read; visual fields intact	Visual field defects
CN III, IV, VI	EOMs, elevation of eyelids, pupil constriction	Can elevate eyes, PERRLA, eyeball movement present	Drooping of eyelid (ptosis), unequal pupils
CN V	Sensory: corneas, nasal and oral mucosa, facial skin Motor: jaw and chewing muscles	Sensory: able to detect both sharp and dull sensations when face touched with pointed or blunt object Motor: clenches teeth while palpating temporal and masseter muscles	Inability to feel or identify facial stimuli; muscle weakness Pertinent disorder: trigeminal neuralgia
CN VII	Sensory: taste on anterior portion of tongue Motor: facial muscles	Sensory: can discriminate sweet, sour, and salty tastes Motor: facial symmetry present at rest and when frowning and smiling	If neurologic impairment, entire side of face could be immobile Pertinent disorders: Bell's palsy, stroke
CN VIII	Hearing and equilibrium	Cochlear (hearing): • Whisper test: client can repeat what was said • Weber test: sound lateralizes equally • Rinne test: sound heard normally twice as long by air conduction (AC) as bone conduction (BC) Vestibular (equilibrium): normal balance, absence of nystagmus	Whisper: sensorineural hearing loss Weber: Sound lateralizes to bad ear with conductive hearing loss or to good ear with sensorineural hearing loss Rinne: AC equal to or less than BC with conductive hearing loss; AC-to-BC ratio normal but reduced overall with sensorineural hearing loss Vestibular: problems with gait or balance; presence of nystagmus
CN IX, X	Swallowing, salivating, taste perception, voice quality	Client swallows; gag reflex present; with tongue depressor against posterior pharynx, client says *ahh*; movement of soft palate and uvula present	Soft palate does not rise; deviation of soft palate and uvula, no gag reflex, dysphagia, hoarseness, taste abnormalities
CN XI	Strength of sternocleidomastoid muscles and upper portion of trapezius	Client shrugs shoulders with equal strength bilaterally	Drooping shoulders, asymmetric muscle contraction
CN XII	Tongue movement in swallowing and speech	Tongue protrudes in midline; client pushes tongue into cheek against resistance from examiner	Tongue atrophy and fasciculation, deviation

h. Spinal accessory nerve (CN XI): ask client to rotate head forcibly against resistance applied to other side of chin; ask client to shrug shoulders against resistance (all findings should be equal bilaterally); examine sternocleidomastoid and trapezius muscles for size

i. Hypoglossal nerve (CN XII): inspect tongue; ask client to protrude tongue (should stay in midline); ask client to say words such as "light, dynamite, tight" to determine that lingual speech (letters *l*, *t*, *d*, *n*) is clear

2. Assess motor system: inspect and palpate muscles as described in previous section

3. Assess cerebellar function

a. Observe gait after asking client to walk 3–6 meters (10–20 ft), turn, and return to starting point; efforts should be rhythmic, smooth, and without effort; step length should be about 37.5 cm (15 in.) heel to heel; next ask client to walk heel-to-toe in a straight line (should be able to do this and maintain balance)

NCLEX®

b. Romberg test: ask client to stand with feet together and arms at sides, close eyes, and hold this position for 20 seconds (should be able to maintain posture with minimal to no swaying, but stand close by to support client if client starts to fall)

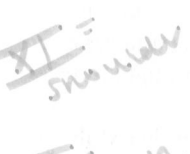

c. Other tests of cerebellar function include hopping on one leg; rapid alternating movements test (patting knees with palms of hands and then back of hands quickly or touching each finger to thumb, one hand at a time), finger-to-finger test (touching examiner's finger and then own nose); finger-to-nose test (touching own nose with eyes closed after stretching out arm); and heel-to-shin test (placing heel of one foot on other knee and running it down leg to heel); these movements should be done smoothly or in a straight line, depending on test

4. Assess sensory system
   a. Requires client to be alert, cooperative, have an adequate attention span, and be in a comfortable position
   b. Test client's ability to discriminate light pain (with sharp object such as a pin) and touch (with dull object such as cotton wisp or pencil eraser), to detect temperature (warm water versus cold), vibration (placement of vibrating tuning fork on various points of body), stereognosis (recognition of objects placed in hand while eyes are closed), graphesthesia (ability to determine number traced on palm of hand) with eyes closed, two-point discrimination (ability to detect two separate stimuli, generally varies depending on area of body; fingertips are most sensitive at 2–8 mm; upper arms, thighs, and back are least sensitive at 40–75 mm)
5. Assess deep tendon reflexes using a reflex hammer
   a. Have limb relaxed and muscle partly stretched; strike reflex hammer on insertion tendon of biceps (C5 to C6), triceps (C7 to C8), brachioradialis (C5 to C6), quadriceps or "knee jerk" (L2 to L4), and Achilles or "ankle jerk" (S1 to S2)
   b. Reflexes are graded on a scale of 0 to 4, with 0 being absent and 4 being brisk or hyperactive; a rating of 2 is normal
6. Assess superficial reflexes
   a. Abdominal (upper T8 to T10; lower T10 to T12): stroke skin with a smooth object from one side of abdomen toward midline; abdominal muscle contracts on side of stimulus (ipsilateral response) and umbilicus deviates toward stroke; perform at both upper and lower end of abdomen
   b. Cremasteric reflex (L1 to L2): lightly stroke inner aspect of thigh of a male client with a reflex hammer or tongue blade and watch for elevation of ipsilateral testicle

   NCLEX®

   c. Plantar reflex or Babinski reflex (L4 to S2): use same object to stroke upward on lateral sole of foot and across ball of foot; normal (negative) response in adult is flexion of toes and possibly foot; an abnormal or positive response (but normal in infants) is dorsiflexion of big toe and fanning of other toes

N. Genitals/rectum

1. Perianal region
   a. Don gloves and spread buttocks to visualize site
   b. Inspect for hemorrhoids, blood, fissures, scars, lesions, rectal prolapse, discharge
   c. Palpation: rectal exam is done by an experienced or advanced practice nurse; purpose is to palpate for rectal masses and assess stool for blood
2. Male genitalia
   a. Inspection: hair distribution in pubic region; penis (note presence of dorsal vein; urethral meatus appears slitlike; note bumps, blisters, redness, lesions, and masses; assess underlying skin after moving pubic hair); scrotum should be loose, wrinkled, with deeply pigmented pouch at base of penis; two compartments house testicles (oval, rubbery, suspended vertically and slightly forward in scrotum); may appear asymmetrical because left testicle has a longer spermatic cord
   b. Palpation: use thumb and first two fingers; area is sensitive to gentle compression; penis should feel smooth, semifirm, and nontender; testicles should feel smooth, rubbery, and moveable with no nodules, lumps, swelling, soreness, masses, or lesions
3. Female genitalia
   a. Inspect external genitalia: mons pubis, labia majora, labia minora, clitoris, vagina, and urethra; with gloved hands, spread labia and assess urethral meatus; should be a pink, slitlike midline opening; labia majora and minora should be moist and free from swelling, lesions, discharge, and unusual odors
   b. Palpate external genitalia: spread labia and palpate; should feel smooth
   c. Internal genitalia examination and rectovaginal palpation are usually done by an advanced practice nurse, not a nurse generalist

O. Postexamination responsibilities

1. Provide tissues or assist client to cleanse lubricant/secretions as needed
2. Remove drape
3. Allow client opportunity or assistance to get dressed
4. Leave client in comfortable position

NCLEX®

5. Document data clearly and immediately; compare findings to established norms and to previous findings; note specimens obtained during exam

NCLEX®

6. Handle collected specimens in a manner consistent with standard precautions; label specimens completely and send to laboratory with requisition attached according to agency policy

VI. PHYSICAL EXAMINATION OF CHILD

A. General considerations

1. Developmental level is most important consideration for a successful assessment (see Table 15–5)
2. NCLEX® Use terms understandable to and appropriate for child and parents; encourage active participation of all when possible; reassure child throughout exam
3. Allow child to become familiar with examiner prior to beginning exam
4. NCLEX® Save distressful or intrusive parts of exam for last
5. NCLEX® Prepare child and parents for new or painful procedures
6. Examine child in a comfortable and secure position

B. Methods of restraint NCLEX®

1. May be necessary with infants, toddlers, or uncooperative children
2. When examining eyes, ears, nose, or throat, examiner may need to have a parent or other adult hold child supine with arms extended alongside head
3. "Hug" method has child sit on parent's lap with legs to one side and one arm tucked under parent's arm while parent holds other arm securely; child's legs may need to be held between parent's legs to prevent kicking
4. Ask another adult for assistance if parent is distressed and cannot help

C. Growth measurements

1. Plot results on growth charts; length/height to age, weight to age, length to weight
2. NCLEX® Overall pattern of growth is more important than any single measurement
3. Use 5th and 95th percentiles to determine measurements outside normal limits
4. NCLEX® Length/height
   a. Recumbent length (birth up to 36 months) with child supine and legs extended; use a horizontal measuring board; avoid using a tape measure because readings are often inaccurate; extend an infant's legs to obtain true length because infants tend to flex legs while at rest
   b. Use crown-to-heel measurement
   c. Children older than 2 or 3 years may stand shoeless as straight as possible
   d. A wall-mounted ruler can be used to measure height of small children who have difficulty standing erect on a scale

Table 15–5 Age-Specific Approaches to Physical Examination

Age	Approach
Infant	Child lying flat or held in parent's arms Use distraction with older infant Assess heart, pulse, lungs, respirations while quiet, then head to toe Eyes, ears, and mouth near end Check reflexes as body parts are examined Moro reflex last
Toddler	Minimal contact initially Allow to inspect equipment Assess heart and lungs while quiet, then head to toe Eyes, ears, and mouth last
Preschool	Allow to inspect equipment Head to toe if cooperative Same as toddler if uncooperative
School age	Respect privacy and explain procedures Head to toe with genitalia last
Adolescent	Explain proceedings and proceed as for school-age child

5. Weight
   a. Weigh naked infant lying or sitting; measure infants on a platform-type balance scale; ensure calibration by noting that beam is balanced when weight is set to zero
   b. Weigh older children on upright scale dressed only in underpants or light gown
6. Head circumference
   NCLEX® a. Measure at every physical assessment for infants and toddlers under 2 years; always measure if neurologic problem or developmental delay is suspected
   b. Best indication of brain growth
   c. Place measuring tape (paper or nonstretching tape) over most prominent part of occiput and just above supraorbital ridges
   NCLEX® d. Make three measurements and take average as number to record
   e. Percentiles should be comparable to child's height and weight
   f. Head circumference exceeds chest circumference until between 1 and 2 years of age
7. Chest circumference
   a. Usually measured at birth and during early infancy
   NCLEX® b. Place measuring tape at nipple level with child supine
   c. Take measurement midway between inspiration and expiration
   d. Head and chest circumference should be approximately equal between 1 and 2 years of age
   e. During childhood, chest circumference exceeds head circumference by 5–7.5 cm (2–3 in.)

D. Vital signs (see Table 15–6)

1. Temperature
   NCLEX® a. Rectal, axillary, skin, or tympanic when assessing infants
   b. Oral route may be used in children over 4 years of age
   NCLEX® c. Use rectal only when necessary because of discomfort and intrusiveness
   d. May be altered by exercise, crying, stress, or environmental conditions
2. Pulse
   a. Newborn average is 110–160 bpm (range of 100–180) and decreases with increasing age
   NCLEX® b. Try to measure with child at rest, sleeping, or lying quietly
   c. Take an apical pulse for child younger than 2 years and a radial pulse in child over 2 years of age
   NCLEX® d. Count for one full minute
   e. May be altered by anxiety, activity, pain, crying, medications, or disease
   f. Record rate, rhythm, quality, and amplitude
3. Respirations
   NCLEX® a. Try to measure while child is at rest, sleeping, or lying quietly
   b. Measure in infants and young children by observing abdominal movements; measure in older children by observing rise and fall of chest
   c. Record rate, rhythm, and quality
   d. May be altered by anxiety, activity, medications, fever, or disease
4. Blood pressure
   NCLEX® a. Measure annually in children over 3 years of age
   b. Select cuff width that covers 75% of length of upper arm
   c. Cuff should encircle arm circumference without overlapping

Table 15–6 Normal Vital Signs for Infants and Children

Age	Pulse Rate Range	Respiratory Rate Range	Blood Pressure Range
Newborn	90–160	30–50	60–90/40–60
1–11 months	85–170	24–45	94–104/50–60
1–2 years	70–150	22–38	98–109/56–63
3–5 years	72–140	21–30	100–115/59–71
6–10 years	68–130	18–24	105–123/67–80
11–14 years	65–120	14–20	110–130/64–84
15 years and older	55–100	14–20	113–130/50–84

d. Use Doppler or electronic device for infants
e. May be altered by anxiety, activity, crying, medications, or disease

E. General appearance

1. Cumulative, subjective impression of a child's physical appearance, nutrition status, behavior, hygiene, personality, posture and body movement, interactions with parents and nurse, speech and development
2. Observe **facies** (facial expression and appearance) for clues about illness, pain, fear, and so on

F. Skin, hair, and nails

1. Inspect and palpate
2. Skin: note color, texture, temperature, moisture, turgor, edema, rashes, or lesions
   a. **Mongolian spots**: bluish-colored areas common on buttocks or lower back of dark-skinned infants; they disappear with age
   b. Storkbites, café au lait stains, or port-wine stains are common birthmarks
   NCLEX® c. Bruises in various stages or unusual locations or circular burn areas may indicate child abuse
   d. Acne vulgaris may be present in adolescents
3. Hair: observe for color, distribution, characteristics, quality, infestations, and texture
4. Nails: note color, texture, shape, and condition; clubbing frequently indicates pulmonary disease

G. Head, neck, and cervical lymph nodes

1. Inspect and palpate head, neck, and lymph nodes
2. Head: note shape and symmetry Ant 12-18
   NCLEX® a. Anterior fontanel: closes by 12–18 months
   NCLEX® b. Posterior fontanel: closes by 2 months Post 2
   c. Infant should be able to hold head erect by 4 months of age
   d. Newborn skull may show molding from birth process or flattening from repeated lying in same position
   e. Note symmetry by having older child make faces
3. Neck and lymph nodes: note size, mobility, swelling, temperature, and tenderness
   a. Thyroid is difficult to palpate in infants because of thick neck
   b. Palpate submaxillary, sublingual, and parotid glands
   c. Observe trachea for midline placement
   d. Determine mobility of neck

H. Mouth, throat, nose, and sinuses

1. Inspect mouth, nose, and throat, and palpate sinuses
2. Mouth and throat
   a. Examine last in young children; intrusive and may provoke fear
   b. Note tooth eruption, condition of gums, lips, teeth, palates, tonsils, tongue, and buccal mucosa
   NCLEX® c. Deciduous teeth erupt by about 6 months of age; all 20 appear by about 30 months
   NCLEX® d. Teeth begin to fall out at about 6 years when permanent teeth erupt; this progresses until all 32 teeth erupt by late adolescence
   e. Tonsils may normally be enlarged, atrophying to stable adult size by late adolescence
3. Nose and sinuses
   a. Inspect structure, patency of nares, discharge, tenderness, and any color or swelling of turbinates
   b. Percuss and palpate sinuses of children over age 3; not palpable at younger ages

I. Eyes

1. Inspect external eye
   a. Note position, slant, epicanthal folds, eyelid placement, swelling, discharge, color of sclera and conjunctiva, redness, eyebrows, and lashes
   b. Epicanthal folds are normal in Asian children, suggestive of Down syndrome in others
   NCLEX® c. Outer canthus should be in line with tip of pinna
2. Visual acuity tests
   a. Include Snellen letter chart for school-age children, Snellen symbol chart (E chart) for preschool age, Faye symbol chart (pictures) for preschool age
   b. Visual acuity is difficult to assess in infants; test by observing infant's ability to fixate and follow objects
   c. Should be able to differentiate colors by 5 years
3. Extraocular muscle tests
   a. Cover–uncover test: cover one eye and have child look at object; observe uncovered eye for movement; remove cover and observe that eye for movement

NCLEX® b. Eye movement during cover–uncover test may indicate **strabismus** (lack of eye muscle coordination), which can lead to **amblyopia** (blindness caused by weak eye muscle)
c. Hirschberg test: shine light on cornea while child looks straight ahead; light should reflect symmetrically in center of both pupils
d. Unequal reflection may indicate strabismus

4. Ophthalmoscopic examination
a. Same procedure as for adults but save until last; may require restraint or distraction; done by primary care provider or advanced practice nurse
b. Expected finding: pupils equal, round, and reactive to light and accommodation (PERRLA); red reflex should be present
NCLEX® c. Permanent eye color by 9 months

J. Ears

1. Inspect and palpate external ear for placement, discharge, and lesions
2. Inspect internal ear with otoscope
a. Save until last; this usually requires restraint in infants and young children
NCLEX® b. With infants, pull pinna down and back because canal is short and straight; with older child and adult, pull pinna upward and back
c. Observe for **cerumen** (earwax), foreign bodies, or discharge
d. Tympanic membrane should be pearly gray to light pink with landmarks visible
NCLEX® e. Tympanic membranes redden during crying
f. May assess mobility of tympanic membrane with pneumatic otoscope
3. Hearing acuity
a. Tested in infants by noting reaction to loud noise
b. Newborns exhibit Moro (startle) reflex and blink eyes
c. Older children may be tested with whispered voice
NCLEX® d. Audiometry testing of all children should be done before they enter school

K. Thorax and lungs

1. Inspect shape of thorax and respiratory rate, depth (deep or shallow), quality (effortless, difficult, or labored), and rhythm (regular or irregular)
2. Palpate back or chest for respiratory movement and **fremitus** (conduction of voice sounds through respiratory tract)
3. Percuss lungs; hyperresonance is normal in infants and young children because of thin chest wall; begin with anterior lung from apex to base with child lying or sitting
4. Auscultate lungs
NCLEX® a. Encourage deep breathing in children by having them blow a pinwheel, cotton ball, or other readily available object
b. Breath sounds may seem louder or harsher because of thin chest wall
c. Use bell and diaphragm of stethoscope to hear both low- and high-pitched sounds
d. Evaluate breath sounds for noise, grunting, snoring, and so on
5. Inspect and palpate breasts
a. Newborns may have enlarged or engorged breasts due to maternal hormones
NCLEX® b. Breast exam and teaching of breast self-exam for adolescents

L. Heart

1. Inspect and palpate precordium for heaves and apical impulse
2. Perform early in exam because quiet child and environment are essential
NCLEX® a. Apical pulse at 4th ICS until age 7; then apical pulse at 5th ICS after age 7
b. Apical pulse to left of MCL until age 4; just lateral to left MCL from 4 to 6 years; and at left MCL by age 7
3. Auscultate heart sounds
a. Rate (should be regular and same as radial pulse), rhythm (should be even and regular); note quality (should be clear, not muffled) and intensity (should not be heavy or pounding)
NCLEX® b. Sinus arrhythmia (rate speeds up with inspiration and slows with expiration) is common in children
c. Evaluate for presence of murmurs
d. Sounds are louder, higher pitched, and of shorter duration in infants and children

NCLEX® **M. Abdomen**

1. To promote relaxation and cooperation, have child place one hand beneath examiner's, use age-appropriate distraction, or use conversation focused on topic of interest to child; inspect shape
   a. Abdomen is prominent when standing and supine in infants and children until age 4; abdomen is somewhat prominent when standing but flat when supine after age 4
   b. Scaphoid abdomen indicates malnutrition or dehydration
   c. Umbilicus should be pink without redness or discharge
   d. Umbilical hernias fairly common, especially in African American children
2. Auscultate bowel sounds in same manner as for adults
3. Palpate for masses or tenderness; principles are same as for adults; advanced practice nurses are more likely to do deep palpation to outline organs; palpate for inguinal or femoral hernias

N. Genitalia

1. Always wear gloves during examination
2. Assess development of secondary sexual characteristics with Tanner's Sexual Maturity Rating Scale
3. Male
   a. Inspect penis and urinary meatus; foreskin should be retractable by 3 months
   b. Redness, discharge, or lacerations in young children may indicate abuse
   c. Inspect and palpate scrotum and testes to determine if both are descended
   d. In young children, testicle may withdraw into inguinal canal because of cremasteric reflex; block cremasteric reflex in infants by beginning palpation at inguinal ring and moving down to scrotum
   e. Check for inguinal hernias by having child blow or bear down
4. Female
   a. Inspect external genitalia for discharge or redness; may indicate abuse in young children
   NCLEX® b. Internal examination for sexually active adolescents, or at age 16–18

O. Anus and rectum

1. Inspect for patency in infants
2. Skin should be smooth and free of lesions
3. Internal exam not done unless symptoms suggest a problem

P. Musculoskeletal

1. Inspect neck, extremities, hips, and spine for symmetry, increased or decreased mobility, and anatomical defects
   a. Extremities should be warm and mobile, with pulses strong and equal bilaterally
   NCLEX® b. Newborn's feet may be turned in but can be manipulated to normal position without resistance
   c. True deformities do not return to normal position with manipulation and include metatarsus varus (forefoot turned in), talipes varus (adduction of forefoot and inversion of entire foot), talipes equinovarus or clubfoot (adduction of forefoot, inversion of entire foot, and pointing downward of entire foot), medial tibial torsion (entire foot turned in while knee remains straight), medial femoral torsion (entire leg turned in with foot)
2. NCLEX® Assess for congenital hip dislocation until about 1 year of age
   a. Use Ortolani's maneuver (with infant supine, flex infant's knees while holding your thumbs on mid-thighs and fingers over greater trochanters; abduct legs, moving knees outward and down toward table); note click if dislocation present
   b. Use Barlow's maneuver (with infant supine, flex infant's knees while holding your thumbs on mid-thighs and fingers over greater trochanters; adduct legs until thumbs touch)
   c. Gluteal folds should be equal, hips abduct easily, and legs should be of same length
3. Assess spine and posture
   a. Newborn spine is flexible and rounded
   b. Cervical curve develops by 3–4 months; lumbar curve develops by 12–18 months
   c. Healthy toddler has **lordosis** (exaggerated curvature of lumbar spine)
   NCLEX® d. Check for **scoliosis** (lateral curvature of spine) in adolescent girls by looking at spine as child is bent over with knees straight
4. Assess gait, joints, and muscles
   a. Observe unobtrusively during history; joints should have full range of motion, and muscles should be equally strong bilaterally
   b. Toddlers have wide-based gait and are usually bowlegged
   c. Children ages 2–7 are often mildly knock-kneed
   NCLEX® d. Scissoring gait in which thighs cross over each other with each step is common in cerebral palsy

PRACTICE TEST

Table 15–7 Autonomic Infant Reflexes

Type of Reflex	Description
Rooting reflex	Touch infant's lip or cheek; infant should turn head toward stimulation and open mouth; should disappear by 3–4 months
Sucking reflex	Infant should suck vigorously when gloved finger inserted into mouth; disappears by 10–12 months
Palmar grasp reflex	Pressing fingers against palmar surface of infant's hand produces grasp strong enough to pull infant to sitting position; disappears by 3–4 months
Plantar grasp reflex	Touching ball of foot causes toes to curl downward tightly; disappears by 8–10 months
Tonic neck reflex	With infant supine, turn head to one side; arm and leg on side to which head is turned will extend and opposite extremities will flex; appears at about 2 months and disappears by 4–6 months
Moro (startle) reflex	Upon hearing a loud noise, infant flexes and abducts legs, laterally extends arms, forms a "C" with thumb and forefinger, and fans other fingers; is immediately followed by anterior flexion and adduction of arms; disappears by 3 months
Babinski reflex	While holding infant's foot, stroke up lateral edge across ball; positive reflex is fanning of toes; some infants have normal adult response of flexion of toes; either response should be symmetrical bilaterally; disappears within 2 years
Stepping reflex	Holding infant upright with support under arms, let feet touch a surface and infant appears to take steps in a walking motion; disappears by 2 months

Q. Neurologic

1. Integrate into overall assessment as much as possible; assess child over 2 years the same as adult
2. Newborn and infant assessment
   a. Observe symmetry of spontaneous movements, appearance, positioning, posture, and responsiveness to parents and environment
   b. Assess level of consciousness, behavior, adaptation, and speech
3. Autonomic infant reflexes (see Table 15–7)
4. *NCLEX®* Presence of reflexes beyond expected times indicates CNS problem
5. Cranial nerves and deep tendon reflexes are same as for adults
6. *NCLEX®* Hand preference develops during preschool years
7. Observe for "soft" neurologic signs (gray area between normal and abnormal); may change with age
   a. Short attention span, easy distractibility
   b. Impulsiveness
   c. Poor coordination
   d. Language and articulation problems
   e. Problems with learning, especially reading, writing, and arithmetic

Check Your NCLEX–RN® Exam I.Q. *You are ready for testing on this content if you can:*

- Assess a client's perception of health.
- Describe expected physiological status based on age.
- Conduct a physical assessment appropriate to the age of the client.
- Use critical thinking when interpreting data gathered during health and physical assessment.

PRACTICE TEST

1 While palpating a client's thorax, the nurse notes a crackling, popping noise under the skin. Upon auscultation, an additional finding is a sound similar to when hair is rubbed between the fingers. The nurse concludes that what problem is probably responsible for this finding?

1. Pneumocystis pneumonia
2. Pneumothorax
3. Hemothorax
4. Hemodilution

PRACTICE TEST

2 After assessing the client's pupils with a penlight for reaction, roundness, symmetry, and accommodation, the nurse would document normal findings using which acceptable notation?

1. PARL
2. PERRLA
3. PRLE
4. PLRAE

3 The nurse would use which test to evaluate a client's motor ability and function as part of a neurologic assessment?

1. Glasgow coma scale
2. Abdominal reflex
3. Babinski test
4. Romberg test

4 The nurse notes unexpectedly during a routine screening examination that the client has a thready pulse. In what other way could this finding be documented?

1. A 2+ pulse
2. Pulse rate irregular and forceful
3. Pulse difficult to palpate and easy to obliterate
4. Pressure with the index finger causes pulsation

5 To assess the intensity of a client's pain during a health history, the nurse could ask the client to do which of the following?

1. Identify the location.
2. Rate the pain on a scale of 0 to 10.
3. Identify the methods the client uses to control the pain.
4. Disclose how long the pain has persisted.

6 The nurse performing the Rinne test during a physical examination expects to gather data that could support which identified client problem?

1. Impaired physical mobility
2. Impaired thought processes
3. Impaired swallowing
4. Altered sensory/perception: auditory

7 The nurse would take which action as a high priority during a routine health assessment?

1. Teach the client about ways to maintain health and wellness.
2. Identify all areas of pathology.
3. Use humor if the client is anxious.
4. Explore the client's family relationships.

8 The nurse plans to do which of the following using the skill of inspection during a health assessment on an adult?

1. Use eyes, ears, and sense of smell to make observations.
2. Look at one side of the body first, then the other.
3. Leave all prepared supplies on a nearby table.
4. Spend a significant amount of time completing this portion of the exam.

9 A client tells the nurse during the health history, "I feel jumpy all over since using my new respiratory inhaler." Which question would be most appropriate for the nurse to ask next?

1. "Do you also feel sweaty when this happens?"
2. "Why are you using a respiratory inhaler?"
3. "Can you tell me what you mean by jumpy?"
4. "What helps you to get over this feeling?"

10 When asking a client newly admitted to the hospital about dietary history, which question by the nurse would be most important?

1. "What time of day do you eat each meal?"
2. "Do you eat alone or with family members?"
3. "How often do you eat meals at restaurants?"
4. "Do you have any dietary restrictions?"

11 An older adult client has experienced Wernicke's aphasia following a cerebrovascular accident (CVA). The nurse assessing this client would expect the client to have difficulty with which activity?

1. Reading the newspaper
2. Reciting the alphabet
3. Spelling his or her last name
4. Chewing solid food

12 What data regarding the family history of an adult client is most important for the nurse to obtain during an initial interview?

1. Quality of emotional support provided by family
2. Dates of immunizations and vaccines received
3. Number and ages of client's siblings
4. Major diseases of close family members

13 When assessing a preschool-age child's mouth, how many deciduous teeth should the nurse expect to find?

1. Up to 10
2. 11–15
3. 16–20
4. Up to 32

14 When assessing a child for strabismus, the nurse should use which eye test?

1. The Snellen eye chart
2. The cover–uncover test
3. An ophthalmoscope exam
4. Test of pupillary reaction

15 When assessing the heart sounds of a 10-year-old, the nurse notices that the rate varies with inspiration and expiration. The nurse concludes that which action is most appropriate?

1. Discuss a referral to a cardiologist for further workup.
2. Question the child about caffeine intake.
3. Do nothing, as this is a normal finding.
4. Schedule an electrocardiogram following the exam.

16 When preparing to assess the vital signs of an infant, the nurse should make a decision to use which sequence?

1. Measure temperature, pulse, and respirations at the end of the exam.
2. Measure respirations, pulse, and temperature in that order.
3. Measure vital signs after the infant becomes familiar with the nurse.
4. Measure blood pressure before other vital signs.

17 When assessing a 1-month-old infant, the nurse finds a head circumference of 32 cm and a chest circumference of 30 cm. The nurse should draw which conclusion about this data?

1. Consider this normal.
2. Reevaluate the findings in 2 weeks.
3. Expect the chest circumference to be larger than the head circumference.
4. Report the finding to the healthcare provider.

18 The nurse is completing an assessment of a child in the clinic. Which items should be documented in the child's health history? Select all that apply.

1. The child was born by cesarean delivery
2. Mother states child has a rash
3. Child appears feverish
4. Diminished reflexes
5. Older sister had the chickenpox recently

19 When using the otoscope to examine the ears of a 2-year-old child, the nurse should pull the pinna in which direction? Select an arrow in the picture shown.

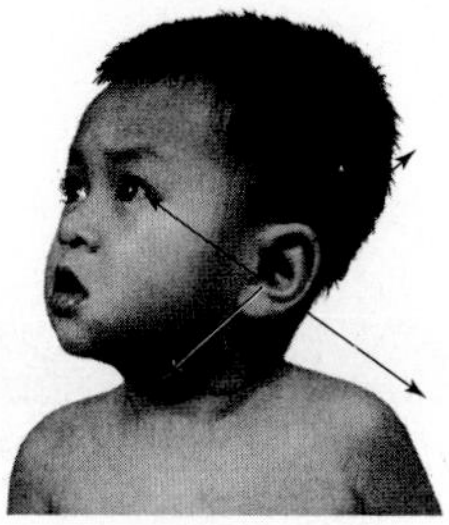

20 The pediatric nurse would perform abdominal percussion to assess which of the following? Select all that apply.

1. Generalized tenderness
2. Local inflammation
3. Density of tissues and organs
4. Size and placement of liver
5. Borders and size of abdominal organs

21 The nurse is assessing a newborn while the mother watches. While assessing the fontanel, the nurse explains that the posterior fontanel will close by how many months of age? Record your answer using a whole number.

Fill in your answer below:

Answer: ______________________

22 A 7-month-old infant has acquired all of the following abilities. The nurse expects that these skills were acquired in which order from earliest to most recent? Place the options in the correct order. All options must be used.

1. Smiling at self in a mirror
2. Transferring a rattle from one hand to the other
3. Rolling from back to abdomen
4. Pulling feet to mouth

Fill in your answer below:

Answer: ______________________

23 While taking the family history of a child, the mother states that her brother had been diagnosed with diabetes mellitus. Mark the affected individual on the genogram shown.

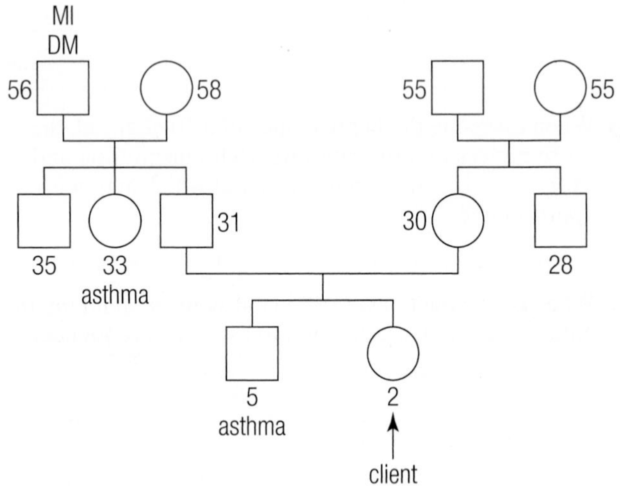

24 In what order should the nurse perform the steps of a physical assessment on a sleeping 8-month-old baby? Place the options in the correct order. All options must be used.

1. Measure the occipital-frontal head circumference.
2. Auscultate the heart and lungs.
3. Check the eyes for the red reflex.
4. Inspect the genitalia.

Fill in your answer below:

Answer:______________________

25 When preparing to examine a preschool child, the nurse should take which actions? Select all that apply.

1. Give detailed explanations to alleviate the child's anxiety.
2. Give reassurance and feedback to the child during the examination.
3. Suggest that the child act like the "big kids" when he or she is examined.
4. Say that the shirt is the only clothing that must be removed.
5. Ask if the child prefers to sit on the parent's lap to be examined.

ANSWERS & RATIONALES

1 **Answer: 2 Rationale:** Subcutaneous emphysema or crepitus is caused by pneumothorax. This condition consists of air introduced into the tissue from another condition, such as pneumothorax. Pneumocystis pneumonia is an opportunistic infection often experienced by individuals who are HIV-positive. Hemothorax refers to blood in the chest. Hemodilution is associated with fluid overload of the vascular system. **Cognitive Level:** Analyzing **Client Need:** Health Promotion and Maintenance **Integrated Process:** Nursing Process: Diagnosis **Content Area:** Fundamentals **Strategy:** The core issue of the question is identification of subcutaneous emphysema and the ability to correlate this finding with common causes. Rely on knowledge of abnormal physical assessment findings and associated pathophysiological conditions to eliminate the incorrect options.

2 **Answer: 2 Rationale:** The correct abbreviation for pupils that are equal, round, and responsive to light and accommodation is PERRLA. PARL, PRLE, and PLRAE are incorrect abbreviations. It is important for nurses to document using agency-approved abbreviations to avoid misinterpretations and to enhance communication among caregivers. **Cognitive Level:** Applying **Client Need:** Health Promotion and Maintenance **Integrated Process:** Communication and Documentation **Content Area:** Fundamentals **Strategy:** Use knowledge of physical assessment techniques of the eye to answer the question. Recall that the first observation is whether pupils are equal (symmetry), which will help you to choose the option that has an E near the beginning of the abbreviation.

3 **Answer: 4 Rationale:** The Romberg test is done when the nurse asks the client to stand with eyes closed and feet together. There should be minimal swaying for up to 20 seconds. The Glasgow coma scale assesses level of consciousness. The abdominal reflex, if absent, may indicate a disease of the upper and lower motor neurons. A positive Babinski test in adults indicates upper motor neuron disease of the pyramidal tract. **Cognitive Level:** Applying **Client Need:** Health Promotion and Maintenance **Integrated Process:** Nursing Process: Assessment **Content Area:** Fundamentals **Strategy:** The core issue of the question is basic knowledge of physical examination techniques. Use this knowledge and the process of elimination to make a selection.

4 **Answer: 3 Rationale:** A weak, thready pulse is one that is difficult to palpate and easy to obliterate by slight pressure. A 2+ pulse is one that is easily palpable and normal. A pulse that is forceful, regardless of whether it is regular or irregular, may be labeled as "full" or "bounding." A pulsation that is felt with pressure from the index finger may be labeled as "full" or "bounding." **Cognitive Level:** Applying **Client Need:** Health Promotion and Maintenance **Integrated Process:** Nursing Process: Implementation **Content Area:** Fundamentals **Strategy:** The core issue of this question is knowledge of how to document an abnormal finding in a clear and objective manner. First eliminate +2 pulse, which is a normal finding. Use the process of elimination to select the option that most clearly matches the data in the question.

5 **Answer: 2 Rationale:** The nurse seeks to identify the intensity of the pain by asking the client to rate the pain on a scale of 0 to 10, with 0 indicating no pain and 10 indicating the worst pain. The location is identified by asking the client to identify the area where the pain is felt. Methods used to control the pain are called alleviating factors. Asking how long the pain has persisted refers to duration of pain. **Cognitive Level:** Applying **Client Need:** Health Promotion and Maintenance **Integrated Process:** Nursing Process: Assessment **Content Area:** Fundamentals **Strategy:** The critical word in the question is *intensity*. Correlate this word with the degree or strength of the pain to choose the rating scale as the answer.

6 **Answer: 4 Rationale:** The Rinne test involves use of a tuning fork to compare air conduction– to bone conduction–related sound transmission. Impaired physical mobility would be assessed by observing the client ambulate. Impaired thought processes would be assessed by a mental status exam. Impaired swallowing is detected through cranial nerve assessment (includes asking client to swallow). Mobility, thought processes, and swallowing are not assessed with this examination. **Cognitive Level:** Applying **Client Need:** Health Promotion and Maintenance **Integrated Process:** Nursing Process: Assessment **Content Area:** Fundamentals **Strategy:** The core issue of this question is the ability to correlate the Rinne test with the ear, and then to choose the nursing diagnosis that relates to hearing or balance (functions of the ear). Use the process of elimination to make your selection.

7 **Answer: 1 Rationale:** As the nurse performs the health assessment and focuses on various systems, time can be spent educating the client about achieving and maintaining wellness. The nurse should use a professional, caring approach. An in-depth focus on pathology is not needed during a routine screening. The focus of routine examinations is not to explore client–family relationships. **Cognitive Level:** Applying **Client Need:** Health Promotion and Maintenance **Integrated Process:** Nursing Process: Assessment **Content Area:** Fundamentals **Strategy:** Note the critical words *high priority*. This means that some or all options may be partially or totally correct, and you must choose the most important item. Note also the critical word *routine*, which implies the client is healthy. With this in mind, the highest priority is to maintain and promote health and wellness.

8 **Answer: 1 Rationale:** Inspection of a client can offer many clues about the overall state of health and can include all data gathered through the senses. The nurse should compare each side of the body for symmetry prior to inspecting the next system. Equipment such as a tongue blade, otoscope, or tape measure can be used during inspection but does not necessarily need to be prepared ahead of time. The time required depends on the client's condition and the nurse's skill level. **Cognitive Level:** Applying **Client Need:** Health Promotion and Maintenance **Integrated Process:** Nursing Process: Assessment **Content Area:** Fundamentals **Strategy:** The core issue of the question is the skill of inspection. Choose the option that reflects principles of visual assessment.

9 **Answer: 3 Rationale:** The nurse should use the communication technique of clarifying to fully understand the client's subjective complaint. Asking about associated symptoms such as sweating would be appropriate after exploring the current symptom further. The reason for use of an inhaler is part of routine assessment but not directly related to the client's current concern. Asking about alleviating factors would be appropriate after obtaining further information to clarify the client's current symptom. **Cognitive Level:** Analyzing **Client Need:** Health Promotion and Maintenance **Integrated Process:** Communication and Documentation **Content Area:** Fundamentals **Strategy:** The core issue of this question is appropriate use of therapeutic communication techniques. Note the word *next* in the question that tells you that all questions may be asked, but one is more important to determine first. With this in mind, choose the option that obtains more information about the client's symptom.

10 **Answer: 4 Rationale:** Noting dietary restrictions based on a medical condition (e.g., low sodium for heart disease), food allergies, or religious convictions (e.g., abstaining from pork if Jewish or Muslim) helps to provide safe and appropriate care for the client. The timing of client meals may be of interest, but mealtimes in hospitals are based on a unit schedule, not client preference. Asking about whether a client eats alone or with others provides data about family or other dynamics, but is not the priority at this time. The frequency of dining in restaurants may become important if the nurse conducts dietary teaching with the client.

Cognitive Level: Analyzing **Client Need:** Health Promotion and Maintenance **Integrated Process:** Nursing Process: Assessment **Content Area:** Fundamentals **Strategy:** Note the critical words in the question are *dietary history* and *most important*. These tell you that the answer is the option that has a high priority, although some or all of the questions may be asked of the client. Select the option that impacts the diet the client will receive in the hospital. The others could be asked based on need or as the basis for later dietary teaching.

11 **Answer: 1 Rationale:** Wernicke's aphasia is the inability to understand verbal or written words. Impairment is located in the posterior speech cortex in the temporal and parietal lobes. Difficulty in reciting the alphabet would be consistent with expressive aphasia (Broca's or motor aphasia). An ability to spell the last name may depend on the ability to speak or ability to recall information. The ability to chew solid food is influenced by having specific intact cranial nerves. **Cognitive Level:** Applying **Client Need:** Health Promotion and Maintenance **Integrated Process:** Nursing Process: Diagnosis **Content Area:** Fundamentals **Strategy:** Specific knowledge of the types of aphasia is needed to answer this question. Use nursing knowledge and the process of elimination to make a selection.

12 **Answer: 4 Rationale:** Major diseases such as diabetes, hypertension, arteriosclerosis, and cancer often have a genetic disposition and put the client at greater risk for developing them. The number and ages of siblings is a component of the family history. Inquiring about the client's support network would be part of psychosocial assessment. Vaccines and immunizations would be covered in the section known as past history. **Cognitive Level:** Applying **Client Need:** Health Promotion and Maintenance **Integrated Process:** Nursing Process: Assessment **Content Area:** Fundamentals **Strategy:** Note the words *most important* in the question. This indicates that some or all options are data that you might wish to obtain but you must prioritize to choose the most essential piece of data. First eliminate immunization status because it does not relate to the family. Choose family history of diseases over emotional support and numbers and ages of family members because it has the greatest potential impact on physiological health status.

13 **Answer: 3 Rationale:** Children get the first of 20 deciduous teeth between the ages of 6 months and 5 years. A child who is of preschool age should have between 16 and 20 deciduous teeth. An infant or early toddler may have up to 10 teeth. A toddler would be more likely to have 11–15 deciduous teeth. Permanent teeth begin to erupt at about the age of 6 as deciduous teeth fall out. All 32 permanent teeth are usually erupted by late adolescence. **Cognitive Level:** Applying **Client Need:** Health Promotion and Maintenance **Integrated Process:** Nursing Process: Assessment **Content Area:** Fundamentals **Strategy:** Specific knowledge of physical growth and development is needed to answer this question. Use nursing knowledge and the process of elimination to make a selection.

14 **Answer: 2 Rationale:** The cover–uncover test assesses coordination of eye muscle movement. In strabismus, one muscle is weaker and the eye wanders rather than focusing forward. Undetected and untreated strabismus can lead to amblyopia. A Snellen eye chart is used to determine visual acuity. An ophthalmoscopic exam detects problems with interior structures of the eye. Pupillary reaction is the ability of the pupils to constrict in response to light. **Cognitive Level:** Applying **Client Need:** Health Promotion and Maintenance **Integrated Process:** Nursing Process: Assessment **Content Area:** Fundamentals **Strategy:** The core issue of the question is assessment of strabismus. Use specific knowledge of physical assessment procedures and the process of elimination to make a selection.

15 **Answer: 3 Rationale:** An irregular heart rate that increases with inspiration and decreases with expiration is a sinus arrhythmia, which is common in children. It requires no action on the part of the nurse. There is no need for a referral to a cardiologist. An assessment of caffeine (such as in carbonated beverages) is not indicated. There is no need to schedule an electrocardiogram following the exam. **Cognitive Level:** Analyzing **Client Need:** Health Promotion and Maintenance **Integrated Process:** Nursing Process: Implementation **Content Area:** Fundamentals **Strategy:** Note that a core issue of the question is the age of the child, which is 10 years. With this in mind, correlate the heart sounds described with normal growth and development findings. After determining that this is a normal finding, eliminate each of the incorrect options.

16 **Answer: 2 Rationale:** Vital signs in an infant are best taken when the infant is quiet early in the exam. Counting respirations by observing the abdomen is least intrusive of the vital signs. Vital signs are more accurately measured early in the exam before the infant begins to cry, which could interfere with respirations. There is no need to delay vital sign measurements until the infant becomes familiar with the nurse. Respirations and pulse should be measured before blood pressure. **Cognitive Level:** Analyzing **Client Need:** Health Promotion and Maintenance **Integrated Process:** Nursing Process: Assessment **Content Area:** Fundamentals **Strategy:** Note that the client in the question is an infant. Recall that vital signs may be affected by activity such as crying. With this in mind, select the order or sequence that creates minimal disturbance for the infant.

17 **Answer: 1 Rationale:** The normal head circumference of a full-term infant is 32–38 cm, about 2 cm greater than the chest circumference. There is no need to reevaluate the findings in 2 weeks. In the toddler, both measures are about equal; after the age of 2, the chest circumference exceeds that of the head. There is no need to report the finding to the healthcare provider. **Cognitive Level:** Analyzing **Client Need:** Health Promotion and Maintenance **Integrated Process:** Nursing Process: Assessment **Content Area:** Fundamentals **Strategy:** Use specific knowledge of growth and development of the infant to systematically eliminate incorrect options. Recall that the measurements "cross over" at about age 2 when the head becomes smaller in circumference than the chest.

18 **Answer: 1, 2, 5 Rationale:** The history deals with subjective data, which is reported by the parents or other caregivers. A report of cesarean delivery is part of the child's health history. A report of a rash by the mother is a subjective report that is part of the health history. "Appearing feverish" is vague and represents a conclusion drawn from unidentified data; the nurse should record the actual data. Diminished reflexes would be obtained by physical exam, not health history. Information about an older sister's communicable disease may be important data, but it is not part of the child's health history. **Cognitive Level:** Applying **Client Need:** Health Promotion and Maintenance **Integrated Process:** Nursing Process: Assessment **Content Area:** Child Health **Strategy:** The core concept is the term "nursing history." To answer the question, it is necessary to differentiate history from physical findings.

19 **Answer:**

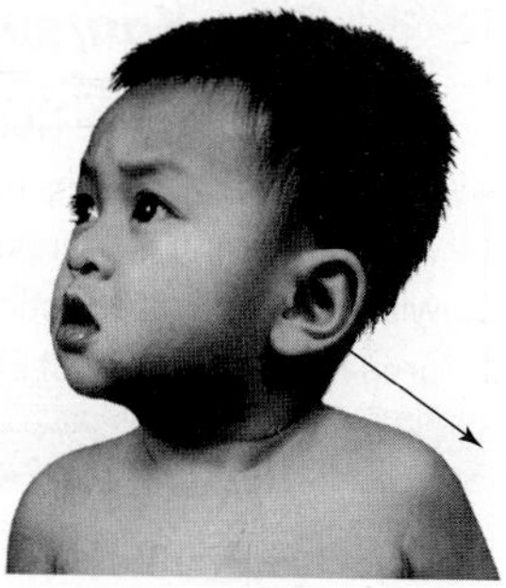

Rationale: The ear canal in infants and young children is shorter, wider, and more horizontally positioned than in older children. To adequately examine the tympanic membrane in young children, the pinna must be pulled back and down. **Cognitive Level:** Applying **Client Need:** Health Promotion and Maintenance **Integrated Process:** Nursing Process: Assessment **Content Area:** Child Health **Strategy:** Critical words are *using the otoscope* and *2-year-old*. Recall normal anatomy and physiology of the ear canal to answer the question correctly.

20 **Answer: 3, 5 Rationale:** Indirect percussion can be used to evaluate borders and sizes of abdominal organs and masses. Percussion produces sounds of varying loudness and pitch, and these sounds help to identify the density of organs and tissues. The nurse assesses the liver with palpation and percussion, but not for placement. Inflammation is assessed with inspection. Tenderness is assessed with palpation. **Cognitive Level:** Analyzing **Client Need:** Health Promotion and Maintenance **Integrated Process:** Nursing Process: Assessment **Content Area:** Child Health **Strategy:** The core issue of the question is the ability to differentiate between palpation, auscultation, and percussion assessments. Use knowledge of physical assessment skills to choose correctly.

21 **Answer: 2 Rationale:** The posterior fontanel closes by 2 months of age, while the anterior fontanel closes by 18 months of age. **Cognitive Level:** Applying **Client Need:** Health Promotion and Maintenance **Integrated Process:** Teaching and Learning **Content Area:** Child Health **Strategy:** The core concept is normal growth and development of the head. Specific knowledge is needed to answer the question.

22 **Answer: 4, 1, 3, 2 Rationale:** Pulling feet to mouth begins at about 4 months. Smiling at self begins at about 5 months. Rolling over begins at about 6 months of age. An infant of 7 months just begins to transfer objects from one hand to the other. **Cognitive Level:** Analyzing **Client Need:** Health Promotion and Maintenance **Integrated Process:** Nursing Process: Assessment **Content Area:** Child Health **Strategy:** Understand that the core concept being tested is normal growth and development and order of skill development. Begin with simple skills and progress to those that are more complex.

23 **Answer:**

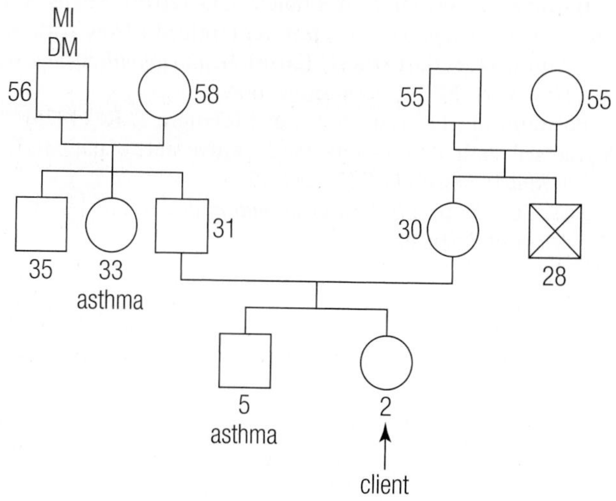

Rationale: Females are indicated by circles and males by squares. Numbers indicate age in years. The child is indicated so the individual will be one generation up on the mother's side. The mother is indicated as number 30. Therefore, the uncle of the child is number 28. **Cognitive Level:** Applying **Client Need:** Health Promotion and Maintenance **Integrated Process:** Nursing Process: Assessment **Content Area:** Child Health **Strategy:** Start with the client and go up one generation.

24 **Answer: 2, 1, 4, 3 Rationale:** Auscultation is always easiest in a sleeping or quiet baby. Checking the eyes is considered invasive and should be saved for the end of the examination. Otherwise, the examination should proceed in an orderly fashion from head to foot. **Cognitive Level:** Applying **Client Need:** Health Promotion and Maintenance **Integrated Process:** Nursing Process: Assessment **Content Area:** Child Health **Strategy:** This question asks for ordering the procedure. The core concept is cooperation from the baby.

25 **Answer: 2, 5 Rationale:** Because the preschooler may be somewhat anxious, the nurse should give feedback and reassurance about what will be done during the exam. Younger children often prefer to sit on the parent's lap to be examined. Children do not need detailed explanations. In potentially stressful situations, children should not be pressured to act older than they are. Most children at this age are willing to remove clothing. **Cognitive Level:** Applying **Client Need:** Health Promotion and Maintenance **Integrated Process:** Nursing Process: Implementation **Content Area:** Child Health **Strategy:** Critical words are to *examine a preschool child*. Use knowledge of physical assessment of the preschooler to make a selection.

Key Terms to Review

amblyopia p. 203
auscultation p. 191
cerumen p. 203
facies p. 202
fremitus p. 203
genogram p. 189
health history p. 185
inspection p. 190
lordosis p. 204
Mongolian spots p. 202
objective data p. 187
palpation p. 190
percussion p. 191
scoliosis p. 204
strabismus p. 203
subjective data p. 185

References

Berman, A., Snyder, S., & Frandsen, G. (2016). *Kozier & Erb's fundamentals of nursing: Concepts, process, and practice* (10th ed.). New York, NY: Pearson Education.

D'Amico, D., & Barbarito, C. (2016). *Health and physical assessment in nursing* (3rd ed.). New York, NY: Pearson Education.

Folstein, M., Folstein, S. E., & McHugh, P. R. (1975). "Mini-Mental State." A practical method for grading the cognitive state of patients for the clinician. *Journal of Psychiatric Research, 12*(3), 189–198.

Jarvis, C. (2016). *Physical examination and health assessment* (7th ed.). St. Louis, MO: Elsevier Science.

Test Yourself

Are you ready for the NCLEX-RN® or course exams? Access the NEW web-based app that provides students with thousands of practice questions in preparation for the NCLEX experience.

Promoting Healthy Lifestyle Choices 16

In this chapter

Cross Reference

Other chapters relevant to this content area are

Meeting Nutritional Needs **Chapter 25**

I. SUN EXPOSURE AND SKIN INTEGRITY

A. Sun exposure damages skin

NCLEX®
1. Most harmful ultraviolet rays occur between 10:00 a.m. and 4:00 p.m.
2. Whether sunny or overcast, daylight allows damaging rays to affect skin
3. Ultraviolet rays can penetrate loosely woven fabrics and harm skin
4. Individuals who are outside almost daily are particularly at risk for sun damage to skin: farmers, carpenters, fishermen, golfers
5. Exposure to chemicals may increase risk of skin damage

B. Important points in health education to prevent skin cancer

1. Infants and children under age 6 and those with light complexions are at highest risk for skin damage
2. Immunosuppressed clients have increased risk for skin cancers
3. There is a genetic link to melanoma
4. Limit sun exposure during middle of day
5. NCLEX® Use sunscreen with solar protection factor (SPF) of 15 and higher
6. NCLEX® Apply sunscreen 30 minutes before sun exposure and reapply every 2–3 hours thereafter while outside
7. Daily use of sunscreen on exposed face, ears, and hands decreases risk
8. NCLEX® Wide-brimmed hats offer extra protection to head and neck
9. Apply sunscreen liberally to scarred skin, which is more vulnerable to damage
10. Preventing severe sunburns in early childhood is key to reducing risk of skin cancer later in life
11. Skin cancers can occur and recur in adults at any age, so inspect bare skin using two mirrors to inspect front and back of body to allow for early discovery

II. BREAST SELF-EXAMINATION

A. General concepts

1. Both men and women can get breast cancer
2. It is important to perform breast self-examination (BSE) monthly (both males and females)
3. Clients need to see healthcare provider for regular checkups

NCLEX® 4. Women should have the choice to begin annual mammography screening at ages 40–44, should have annual mammograms at ages 45–54, and annual or biannual (every other year) screening at ages 55 years and older

NCLEX® 5. Although research evidence is mixed, females are encouraged to begin BSE at time of first gynecologic exam, about age 18 or 20

6. Nurse's role is pivotal in educating females and males that BSE is important

NCLEX® **B. Procedure**

1. Focus on palpating consistency of breast tissue
2. Perform procedure 5–7 days after menses for female; for men and postmenopausal women, perform exam on same day of each month; associate it with a specific date, such as the first of the month
3. Look at breasts in mirror, arms by side, over head, and on hips
4. Lie down and palpate each breast with opposite hand while other arm is under head, flattening out breast tissue
5. Palpate under axilla as well as nipple region (both males and females)
6. Feel breasts by pressing tissue firmly against chest wall, each region from outer to inner, with a circular or "corn-rows" approach
7. Once a baseline of "normal" is felt, each client will better understand changes to report to practitioner; report changes from personal baseline immediately for further evaluation
8. Menses, breastfeeding, and pregnancy enlarge the breast tissue naturally, and tissue feels more lobular
9. Clients who have cysts in breasts must carefully perform BSE to detect changes from personal baseline, which need to be reported

III. TESTICULAR SELF-EXAMINATION

A. General concepts

1. Normal testicle is smooth and uniform in consistency
2. One testis is often larger and hangs lower in scrotum

NCLEX® **B. Procedure**

1. Once monthly, males should perform testicular self-examination (TSE), preferably during a warm shower when testicles are relaxed and may be soapy
2. Using one hand to displace penis, grasp testis with dominant hand, placing fingers beneath and thumb on top of testis to palpate it
3. Roll gently between thumb and fingers, feeling for any abnormality
4. Palpate testis, epididymis, and spermatic cord on each side
5. Report any nodules or lumps to healthcare provider as soon as possible
6. NCLEX® Report symptoms of testicular swelling, painless testicular swelling, or dragging sensation in scrotum

IV. EXERCISE

NCLEX® **A. Introduction**

1. Regular **aerobic exercise**, such as walking, jogging, or cycling, on most days of the week, is important to cardiovascular, respiratory, and musculoskeletal systems
2. Aerobic exercise is rhythmic, uses major muscle groups, and is maintained for 20–30 minutes or more

Memory Aid

Choose aerobic exercise over other forms when the goal is general health, because it increases circulation and respiration and burns calories for better weight control.

B. Client can monitor most appropriate level of exercise by monitoring pulse and speaking ability

1. Exercise is too vigorous if individual cannot speak without breathlessness
2. Exercising to specific target heart rates may be prescribed as part of a health-promoting exercise plan
3. To calculate target heart rate, first determine maximum heart rate by subtracting client's age from 220; then calculate target heart rate by subtracting client's resting heart rate from his or her maximum heart rate

C. Principles for instruction in exercise to promote good health and deter progressive complications of heart and musculoskeletal diseases

1. NCLEX® Fast walking to target heart rate is an effective aerobic exercise that strengthens all muscles (including heart) and keeps bones strong, with less stress on knees than jogging
2. Inability to talk due to shortness of breath can mean excessively strenuous exercise

3. Current Centers for Disease Control and Prevention (CDC) *2008 Physical Activity Guidelines for Americans* recommend that adults exercise with moderate intensity for 30 minutes or more five times weekly (150 minutes) and perform muscle strengthening activities (that work all major muscle groups) twice weekly
4. Whenever teaching parents of young children, stress importance of regular exercise as a lifelong habit
5. Children ages 6–17 should exercise for at least 60 minutes daily with most time being for aerobic activity; muscle strengthening (gymnastics, push-ups) and bone strengthening (jumping rope, running) activities should also be done three times per week as part of 60 minutes of activity
6. Walking or weight-bearing exercises help to prevent osteoporosis by increasing force exerted on long bones

NCLEX®

7. Anyone with a chronic illness such as diabetes or hypertension should consult a healthcare provider before beginning a rigorous exercise routine
8. Cautions for clients with health problems should include start slowly, monitor body's response to exercise, and take medication and fluids before exercise

V. NUTRITION

A. General concepts

1. Nutrition is an essential parameter of health and helps prevent some diseases and their complications
2. Nutritional intake is foundational for body's development, growth, and all healing processes

NCLEX®

3. A balanced diet for adults and children using MyPlate consists of protein, vegetables, fruits, grains, and dairy, with little fat (see Figure 16–1)

Memory Aid

To easily remember the components of a balanced diet, visualize a lunch plate divided into quadrants (fourths). Put fruits and vegetables in two, protein in one, and grains in one. Add milk and the meal is balanced!

4. Eating a variety of foods helps ensure all essential vitamins and nutrients in a balanced proportion

NCLEX®

5. Sodium intake should be limited to 2 grams daily
   a. Cooking with other seasonings such as lemon, liquid smoke, pepper, and other spices helps to limit sodium intake
   b. Limit salt to what is naturally found in foods, especially for clients with hypertension or cardiac and renal disease
   c. Canned vegetables, soups, and tomato sauces may contain almost 1 gram of sodium per serving
   d. Do not assume that salt substitutes are acceptable; these are often high in potassium, which could pose risk to clients with renal disease or who take potassium-sparing diuretics; clients should consult a healthcare provider before using them

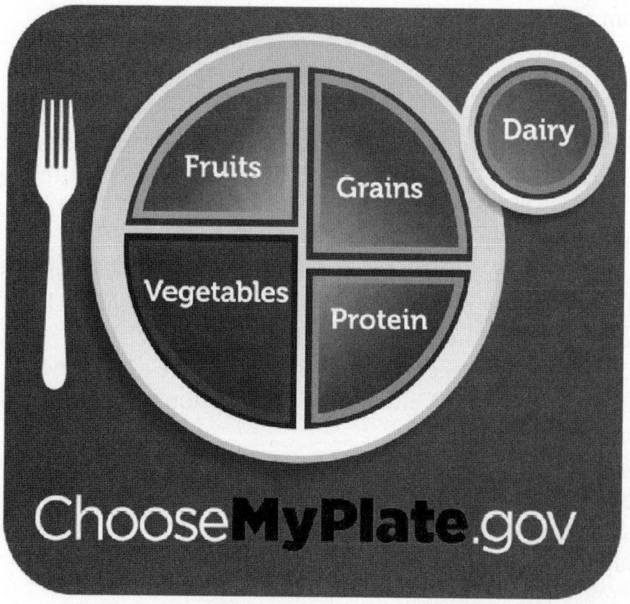

Figure 16–1
Recommended balance of foods from myplate.gov.

6. Fresh and frozen vegetables and fruits have more available nutrients than canned and highly processed foods
7. Color indicates freshness and usually more available nutrients, so recommend undercooking and retaining color, not overcooking vegetables
8. See also Chapter 25 for detailed information about nutritional needs of clients

B. Principles to guide nutrition instructions for disease prevention

NCLEX®
1. Heart-healthy eating refers to consuming a low-fat, low-sugar, and balanced diet, which includes more than five fruits and vegetables daily and limits red meats
2. The American Diabetes Association diet is recommended for clients with diabetes or with hypoglycemia because it controls insulin release by limiting glucose
3. Quick, accessible foods usually have more fat and sugar than adults can use in a day, and they add excess calories, which becomes fat
4. Sweets, like fats, should be limited in quantity for all ages; sugary foods provide ready glucose, increase insulin production, but do not sustain the body's energy

NCLEX®
5. Vegetarians may choose to eat dairy products; strict vegetarians may not eat any eggs, cheese, or dairy products; alternative protein sources include soy milk, tofu, dry beans, and nuts; watch for vitamin B_{12} deficiency in those who avoid all meats

NCLEX®
6. Many colorful orange and green vegetables have vitamins A, C, D, E, and K and serve as anti-aging antioxidants to body cells, especially skin
7. Eating leafy green vegetables interferes with anticoagulant therapy by increasing vitamins D or K
8. Eating more frequent and smaller meals or snacks, such as three meals and two snacks, is healthier for most adults than eating three large meals

NCLEX®
9. Water is needed to move nutrients through and flush waste products from body; about 8 glasses daily promotes hydration, prevents constipation, and aids in digestion; as a general rule, drink 1 milliliter (mL) for each calorie consumed, so for a 2,000-calorie diet, drink at least 2000 mL water daily
10. Folic acid is an important element to childbearing-age female

NCLEX®
11. Extra iron is needed during pregnancy and is usually added in a daily vitamin

NCLEX®
12. Females need additional calcium after menopause

NCLEX®
13. Daily calcium intake is important, especially for women and children; calcium is essential for bone growth; women who are prone to osteoporosis should supplement calcium according to healthcare provider recommendations
14. Foods high in calcium include dairy products, green vegetables, salmon canned with bones, sardines, tofu, and molasses

C. See also Chapter 25 for additional information on meeting client's nutritional needs

VI. ALTERNATIVE HEALTHCARE PRACTICES

A. General concepts

1. Herbs should be used with medical supervision
2. Alternative and homeopathic healthcare practices can help relieve symptoms and aid healing with guidance from a trained practitioner
3. Caution clients not to abandon traditional prescription medicines or replace medicines with herbs without guidance and monitoring of a healthcare provider

NCLEX®
4. Individuals taking warfarin or any other anticoagulants must avoid use of over-the-counter herbs such as garlic, ginseng, ginger, primrose oil, dong quai, and grape seed extract because of interactive effects
5. Certain vitamins—A, D, E, K—are fat-soluble and require healthy liver function to use; otherwise toxicity can result

B. Summary of specific key points

1. Echinacea is used to increase immunity and to treat colds and infections, but it is not intended or effective for daily use over long periods of time; persons with AIDS, lupus, arthritis, or any autoimmune disorders should not take echinacea
2. Individuals need to consult healthcare provider before adding herbal supplements such as St. John's wort to treat depression when already on prescription medications; such therapy is generally contraindicated

NCLEX®
3. Ginseng and ginkgo are commonly taken by those who wish to improve cognition, and both cause drug interactions; monitor clients who take these herbs regularly for drug interactions, cross-toxicity, and altered bleeding times
4. See also Chapter 28 on integrative and complementary therapies for detailed discussion of specific herbs

VII. HEALTH SCREENING

A. Overview

1. Routine health screenings are recommended for early detection of disease; in addition, health screenings provide an opportunity to do health-related preventive teaching
2. NCLEX® General guidelines for health screenings for adults are presented in Table 16–1 and for children in Table 16–2

B. Specific points related to health screening

1. Children should be screened at least annually for first 6 years of life; nurses can monitor growth patterns, emotional and social skills, and motor and sensory (eye and ear) functions during routine physical exams and interactions with child and parent or caregiver
2. Premature infants need screening exams for deficits earlier and are more likely to experience developmental delays and motor and visual deficits
3. At age 4, arrange for child to begin 6-month dental checks and to have a baseline eye exam
4. The Denver Development Assessment is commonly used annually from infancy to age 6
5. NCLEX® Height and weight are charted annually and serve as screening for obesity
6. If muscle function, vision, or hearing is abnormal, exams may be done during infancy and several times yearly for follow-up and intervention
7. NCLEX® Hemoglobin assessment at any age is a common screening blood test for nutrition and general health

Table 16–1 Unified Screening Recommendations for Adults*

Target Group	Type of Screening	Beginning Age	Frequency
Men and women	Blood pressure measurement	20	Each regular healthcare visit, at least every 2 years
	Body mass index (BMI) measurement	20	Each regular healthcare visit
	Blood cholesterol test	20	At least every 5 years
	Blood glucose (sugar) test	45	Every 3 years
	Colorectal screening	50	Every 1–10 years depending on test used
Women	Clinical breast exam (CBE)	20	Every 3 years; yearly after age 40; may be modified by individual provider according to risk
	Mammography	45	Yearly; may start age 40
	Papanicolaou test	21	Every 3 years
		30	Every 5 years with added HPV test
Men	Prostate-specific antigen (PSA) test and digital rectal exam	50	Variable according to individual risk and pros and cons of testing

*Developed collaboratively by the American Cancer Society, American Diabetes Association, and American Heart Association.

Table 16–2 Health Screening Recommendations for Children*

Type of Health Screening	Frequency
Well-child exam	Birth, 1, 2, 4, 6, 9, 12, and 15–18 months, age 2, 3, 4, 5, 6, 8, and annually age 10–21 years
Blood pressure	Age 3, 4, 5, 6, 8, and annually age 10–21 years
Vision	Age 3, 4, 5, 6, 8, 10, 12, 15 years
Hearing	Age 4, 5, 6, 8, 10, 12, 15 years
Hereditary metabolic screening	Birth to 1 month
Lead screening	As needed
Hemoglobin and hematocrit	12 months and as indicated; may be annually for females during adolescence
Urinalysis	Age 5, in adolescence, and when indicated

*Summary of recommendations from U.S. Preventative Services Task Force, American Academy of Pediatrics, American Academy of Family Physicians, and Centers for Disease Control and Prevention.

8. A complete blood count (CBC) gives information about development of all blood cells
9. Urinalysis and blood glucose testing is advised for obese children
10. Adolescents need to be screened for sexually transmitted infection if sexually active
11. Other health screening to include for adolescents: blood pressure (BP), heart murmurs, Pap smears for females who are sexually active, testicular exams for males, eyes, dental, hemoglobin testing
12. NCLEX® Height and weight should be documented annually for adolescents, and they should be monitored for obesity or anorexia
13. Chest x-rays may be necessary for smokers to establish lung function
14. Young adults who are college-bound (especially 20–30 years of age) need to continue with updating immunizations: tetanus, hepatitis, meningitis, tuberculosis, and possibly pertussis; contact with larger numbers of people and possibly more crowded living conditions increases risk
15. Screenings for young adults include Pap smears for abnormal cell growth, height and weight to monitor for obesity, blood testing for normal blood cells and glucose, BP, chest x-rays, and female mammograms
16. NCLEX® Adults over age 40 need to have annual screenings or self-exams to detect heart disease, cancer, hypertension, or risks for other chronic diseases such as diabetes
17. If at higher than normal risk for breast or colon cancer, begin annual screening exams earlier than for general population and adhere to recommended frequency of exam
18. If at average risk and over age 40, screen for cancer every 2 years with mammograms, and at every visit check feces for occult blood; consider a colon or sigmoid endoscopy exam every 5 years for polyps leading to colon cancer as recommended by healthcare provider
19. After age 60, screening should address changes related to aging: skin changes, bone density and osteoporosis, height (decreases due to bone loss), motor function, and balance
20. Emotional well-being should be addressed as retirement and lifestyle changes occur
21. Health screening throughout life should include
    a. Hearing, vision, and all sensory functions
    b. Safety for living and functioning in home/work environment
    c. Emotional adjustments to life stage and world surroundings
    d. Nutritional status, excess or deficits
    e. Ability to seek help and manage health; independence

VIII. GENETIC TESTING

A. Purposes of genetic testing

1. Diagnose, rule out, or confirm specific genetic or chromosomal conditions, such as sickle-cell disease or polycystic kidney disease; determine carrier status of specific genes; and detect genetic mutations that may lead to disorders later in life (such as Huntington's disease)
2. Provide information about health problems *in utero* (such as Down syndrome) or in newborn (such as cystic fibrosis, phenylketonuria)
3. Identify mutations that increase risk of developing specific cancers, such as breast or ovarian cancer, to aid in decision making about prophylactic measures (such as mastectomy, oophorectomy)

B. Generic nurses' role in genetic counseling

1. Advocate for clients and families by facilitating access to resources for genetic testing
2. Explain that genetic testing might not be covered by health insurance plans, so clients should ask their insurance providers
3. Tailor client teaching according to client's culture, religion, preferred language, knowledge, and health literacy level
4. Be aware that new information about genetic predispositions may be unwelcome or rejected at first
5. NCLEX® Maintain confidentiality and respect client's values and beliefs, realizing that genetic information could have significant health and social implications
6. Be aware that many psychological, emotional, and ethical concerns can arise (e.g., disclose or not disclose, become pregnant or not, have children tested or not)
7. Share information about Genetic Information Nondiscrimination Act, which protects against discrimination by employers and health insurers
8. NCLEX® Offer support to clients and families throughout genetic testing process, and refer to genetic counselors and other local and national resources, including online resources

Check Your NCLEX–RN® Exam I.Q.

You are ready for testing on this content if you can:

- Identify health-promotion activities for individuals relative to nutrition and exercise.
- Describe risks, screening, and prevention measures for skin cancer, breast cancer, and testicular cancer.
- Explain importance of assessing use of herbal remedies and alternative therapies.
- Utilize health education principles that guide client teaching about health management.

PRACTICE TEST

1 The nurse makes which dietary menu selection for a client with iron-deficiency anemia?

1. Salad with lettuce, fruit, and nuts
2. Roast beef and broccoli
3. Lasagna with tomato sauce and steamed carrots
4. Mixed greens salad topped with tuna fish

2 The nurse is most concerned with providing further teaching for the client with diabetes who has which dietary habit?

1. Drinks orange juice each morning
2. Eats an apple and cheese before going to bed
3. Buys canned fruit instead of fresh because it is cheaper
4. Eats six meals per day

3 The nurse explains to a client who has had all molars removed that he will likely be allowed to have which foods added to the diet by the third postoperative day?

1. Bacon and eggs
2. Pancakes and eggs
3. Cereal flakes and milk
4. Gelatin and applesauce

4 When the nurse assesses the intake of a vegetarian client's health and dietary patterns, which finding does the nurse conclude is most likely to negatively affect health status?

1. Use of vitamin B_{12} supplements
2. Intake of milk and dairy products
3. Genetic tendency toward lactose intolerance
4. Reports of problems with vision

5 The nurse should interpret that which client is most at risk for developing skin cancer?

1. An 80-year-old farmer who wears a cap when working
2. A 20-year-old lifeguard at the lake who wears sunscreen
3. A baby underneath a large beach umbrella
4. A teenager who wears a ski outfit when skiing

6 During a health fair at a public recreational park, the nurse providing cancer health risk information answers several questions for clients who use tanning salons. Which item of information is most important to include?

1. Tanning from ultraviolet light is safer than sunshine
2. Skin damage from ultraviolet light is more likely than from indirect sunlight
3. Using sunscreen will prevent skin cancers, even in tanning beds
4. Using tanning beds without clothing contaminates skin and leads to infections

7 When giving postoperative care to a 30-year-old male client, the nurse discusses cancer risks. The client states, "I have never heard of testicular exams." The nurse should include which priority intervention in the plan of care?

1. Teach the client to see a healthcare provider for a yearly testicular examination
2. Assist the client to set up a calendar of dates to perform self-testicular exams
3. Allow the client to verbalize fears related to cancer risk
4. Encourage a high-fiber diet to decrease the risk of testicular cancer

8 When a client comes into the emergency department (ED) reporting constipation and abdominal pain, what would be the most common risk factors for constipation for the nurse to assess for?

1. History of diverticulitis or diverticulosis
2. Dietary and exercise patterns
3. Nutritional intake of proteins and fatty acids
4. Level of nutrition understanding and laxative abuse

9 When teaching a 30-year-old male about testicular self-examination (TSE), the nurse recognizes more education is needed when the client makes which statement?

1. "I will perform TSE monthly and see my practitioner yearly."
2. "In the morning after a shower is the best time for TSE."
3. "The testicle and spermatic cords can be easily felt."
4. "One testicle may ride up into my lower abdomen during sleep, but I need to do TSE when it is descended."

10 The ambulatory care nurse working with adolescent male clients determines that which client is most at risk for testicular cancer?

1. Client whose father had colon cancer
2. Baseball catcher who wears supportive gear during sports activities
3. Teenager who swims daily on a swim team
4. Twenty-year-old with one undescended testicle

11 The nurse is participating in a health promotion fair. When discussing aerobic exercise, the nurse should include which point?

1. Exercise should be done 7 days per week
2. Fast walking is a good form of aerobic exercise
3. If one cannot talk when exercising, then the appropriate level of energy is being used
4. Each exercise session should last for at least 45 minutes, and preferably 60

12 A postmenopausal client is just learning to do breast self-examination (BSE). To aid in remembering to perform the procedure, at which time should the nurse recommend that the client perform BSE?

1. Weekly just before grocery shopping
2. On a random day once each month according to convenience
3. Once a month on a standard day that the client can remember
4. Just prior to each 6-month checkup for another identified health problem

13 A school nurse has finished conducting a teaching session with high school students about breast self-examination (BSE). The nurse concludes that the information was learned correctly when a female student states to do the exam at which time?

1. Once per month when the client thinks she is ovulating
2. On the first day of each month
3. Seven days after menstruation begins
4. On the first day of the menstrual cycle

14 An older adult female client has osteoporosis. In counseling the client about the best form of exercise, what exercise would the nurse recommend?

1. Swimming
2. Jogging
3. Cycling on a stationary bicycle
4. Walking

15 The nurse working in a prenatal clinic concludes that genetic counseling would be most important for the client who has a family history of which disorder?

1. Coronary heart disease
2. Sickle-cell disease
3. Type 2 diabetes mellitus
4. Hypertension

16 A 20-year-old female sees a healthcare provider for her first adult physical examination. The nurse anticipates which screening measures will be done at this visit as baseline for further reference? Select all that apply.

1. Body mass index (BMI) measurement
2. Blood glucose level
3. Clinical breast exam (CBE)
4. Mammography
5. Serum cholesterol level

17 A 4-year-old client is coming to the healthcare provider's office for a well-child visit. For which routine screenings does the nurse plan? Select all that apply.

1. Blood pressure
2. Vision
3. Urinalysis
4. Lead screening
5. Hearing

18 When teaching a male client about testicular cancer, which manifestations would the nurse include that are important? Select all that apply.

1. Painless swelling of scrotum
2. Dull pain in scrotum
3. Nodules in between testes and cord
4. Dragging sensation in scrotum
5. Reddened rash over affected testicle

19 The ambulatory pediatric nurse explains to the mother of a 4-year-old that a routine health screening would include which items? Select all that apply.

1. Reading an eye chart
2. Standing on one foot
3. Urinalysis
4. Measuring height and weight
5. Testing of all cranial nerves

20 What statement made by a client indicates to the nurse an understanding of genetic testing? Select all that apply.

1. "My nutritional intake will be recorded."
2. "Medicine will be prescribed for me."
3. "Blood may be drawn from my spouse and I, as well as our children."
4. "Counseling will be provided at a follow-up appointment."
5. "I need to keep a diary of my activities during the week of the screening."

ANSWERS & RATIONALES

1 **Answer: 2 Rationale:** With iron-deficiency anemia, it is important to select dietary items that are high in iron to counteract the deficit. Red meat tends to be high in iron, as do some green leafy vegetables. Although some options contain salad (and therefore green leafy vegetables), the other components of these meals are not as high in iron. Lasagna and carrots are not as high in iron as the other choices. **Cognitive Level:** Analyzing **Client Need:** Health Promotion and Maintenance **Integrated Process:** Teaching and Learning **Content Area:** Foundational Sciences: Nutrition **Strategy:** The critical words *most appropriate* indicate that more than one option may contain iron, but you must pick the total meal selection that is best. Recall that iron is found in red blood cells to help focus on a dietary item such as red meat. Recall that green vegetables are also helpful to confirm your selection. Thus, the best option is the one that contains two good sources of dietary iron.

2 **Answer: 4 Rationale:** The client who has diabetes needs to have regular meals that are evenly spaced throughout the day and may need to supplement meals with snacks. Eating six meals per day is excessive and could lead to inadequate glucose control. Drinking orange juice and eating apples and cheese pose no risk as long as they are in the client's meal pattern. Canned fruit is acceptable as long as it is packed in 100% juice or water instead of syrup. **Cognitive Level:** Analyzing **Client Need:** Health Promotion and Maintenance **Integrated Process:** Nursing Process: Planning **Content Area:** Foundational Sciences: Nutrition **Strategy:** Use principles of general dietary planning and calorie control to answer the question. Remember not to "read in" information into the question or the options.

3 **Answer: 2 Rationale:** By the third postoperative day, the suture lines from the teeth extraction should be beginning to heal, and the client should be able to manage soft foods. Pancakes and eggs provide the client with carbohydrates and a protein source for healing in a soft form. Bacon and cereal could be scratchy and irritate the suture lines. Gelatin and applesauce would be appropriate the day after surgery while the suture lines are still new. **Cognitive Level:** Applying **Client Need:** Health Promotion and Maintenance **Integrated Process:** Nursing Process: Implementation **Content Area:** Foundational Sciences: Nutrition **Strategy:** Keep in mind principles of healing and principles of nutrition needed for healing to make a selection. The correct option is the one that combines appropriate nutrients and a soft form that can be tolerated by the client.

4 **Answer: 4 Rationale:** Problems with vision may be attributed to vitamin deficiency, especially vitamin A. This finding could adversely affect the client's health status and requires follow-up by the nurse. Vitamin B supplements and milk

and dairy products will not adversely affect health status. Risk of lactose intolerance has a lesser chance of adversely affecting health status, since it is a familial risk and not a personally identified problem. **Cognitive Level:** Analyzing **Client Need:** Health Promotion and Maintenance **Integrated Process:** Nursing Process: Assessment **Content Area:** Foundational Sciences: Nutrition **Strategy:** Use knowledge of components of a balanced diet to eliminate the options with vitamin supplements and dairy products. Choose vision problems over familial tendency toward lactose intolerance because actual problems take priority over potential problems.

5 **Answer: 1 Rationale:** The older adult client has more years of living to increase risk of skin cancer from exposure to the sun. In addition, the farmer wears a cap, but no mention is made of protectant sunscreens or long-sleeved shirts and pants. Wearing sunscreen is a protective factor against skin cancer. The infant is less at risk because of age and protection against ultraviolet rays by the beach umbrella. Wearing a ski outfit while skiing protects against the sun's rays as well as against the cold. **Cognitive Level:** Analyzing **Client Need:** Health Promotion and Maintenance **Integrated Process:** Nursing Process: Assessment **Content Area:** Adult Health: Integumentary **Strategy:** First recall that exposure to ultraviolet light is a risk for skin cancer. Use the process of elimination while considering which option provides the least sufficient barrier to exposure to ultraviolet light to make your selection.

6 **Answer: 2 Rationale:** Ultraviolet light exposure greatly increases risk of skin cancer, both basal cell and melanoma types. While direct sunshine contains ultraviolet light, the amount is decreased in indirect light. The use of sunscreen can reduce the risk of cancer but not "prevent" it. Risk of infection from tanning beds may or may not be significant depending on the disinfectant methods used. **Cognitive Level:** Analyzing **Client Need:** Health Promotion and Maintenance **Integrated Process:** Nursing Process: Implementation **Content Area:** Adult Health: Integumentary **Strategy:** The core issue of the question is which option provides the most accurate and important information about ultraviolet light exposure. First eliminate statements that are not necessarily correct all of the time, then choose the true statement over the false statement because of the wording of the question.

7 **Answer: 2 Rationale:** The priority for this client is to learn and begin to perform testicular self-exam on a monthly basis. A yearly exam is insufficient in time frame, and a healthcare provider does not need to perform the screening. A high-fiber diet is a general health measure but is not specific to testicular cancer. Encouraging the client to verbalize fears is generally a helpful strategy but does not target the client's immediate need for information about detecting testicular cancer. **Cognitive Level:** Applying **Client Need:** Health Promotion and Maintenance **Integrated Process:** Nursing Process: Planning **Content Area:** Adult Health: Oncology **Strategy:** Use the process of elimination and knowledge of cancer risk to make a selection. Note that the question and the options with healthcare provider and dates refer to testicular examination, which gives a clue that one of them may be correct. Choose correctly after noting the frequency and accuracy of the statement.

8 **Answer: 2 Rationale:** Two common and key factors that increase risk of constipation are a diet low in fiber and fluids and inadequate exercise to stimulate bowel motility, which could lead to impaction and abdominal pain. Diverticulitis is something to assess for but is not as frequently an etiology as inadequate exercise and a low-fiber diet. In addition, diverticulosis does not give rise to signs and symptoms. Intake of protein and fatty acids are irrelevant to the client's complaint. Nutrition intake and laxative abuse are too vague to be correct. **Cognitive Level:** Analyzing **Client Need:** Health Promotion and Maintenance **Integrated Process:** Nursing Process: Assessment **Content Area:** Adult Health: Gastrointestinal **Strategy:** Note the critical words *most significant* in the stem of the question. This tells you that more than one option is likely to be correct and that you must choose the best option, which in this case is the most frequent cause.

9 **Answer: 4 Rationale:** Testicles should remain in a descended position (in the scrotal sac). The client needs to see a healthcare provider for this health problem. The client should perform TSE monthly and see a healthcare provider yearly. The best time to conduct TSE is in the morning after a shower. It should be easy to feel the testicle and spermatic cords. **Cognitive Level:** Analyzing **Client Need:** Health Promotion and Maintenance **Integrated Process:** Nursing Process: Evaluation **Content Area:** Adult Health: Oncology **Strategy:** The critical words in the stem of the question are *more education is needed*, which tells you that the correct answer is an incorrect statement. Use the process of elimination and knowledge of TSE.

10 **Answer: 4 Rationale:** Testicular cancer is most likely to affect late-adolescent and young adult males. An undescended testicle is one risk for testicular cancer. A familial history of colon cancer does not increase specific risk of testicular cancer because colon cancer occurs at a different site. A client who wears protective gear is not at increased risk for testicular cancer. A client who swims is not at increased risk of testicular cancer. **Cognitive Level:** Analyzing **Client Need:** Health Promotion and Maintenance **Integrated Process:** Nursing Process: Diagnosis **Content Area:** Adult Health: Oncology **Strategy:** Use the process of elimination, focusing on the core issue of the question, which is risk factors for testicular cancer.

11 **Answer: 2 Rationale:** The latest recommendations indicate that clients should exercise most days of the week. Fast walking is a good form of aerobic exercise. If one cannot speak when exercising, it is too strenuous and should be decreased in speed or amount. Exercising for a minimum of 30 minutes is sufficient to be effective; it is unnecessary to have 45 or 60 minutes as the minimum time frame. **Cognitive Level:** Applying **Client Need:** Health Promotion and Maintenance **Integrated Process:** Teaching and Learning **Content Area:** Adult Health: Cardiovascular **Strategy:** The core issue of the question is characteristics of effective aerobic exercise. Remember guidelines have changed to include most days of the week, to rule out some distracters. Then choose walking as an extremely effective exercise as the correct answer.

12 **Answer: 3 Rationale:** The client needs to perform BSE once per month, on the same day each month. It is excessive to perform BSE weekly. Choosing a day randomly each month does not guarantee regularity in BSE. Performing BSE just prior to a 6-month checkup is not frequent enough. **Cognitive Level:** Applying **Client Need:** Health Promotion and Maintenance **Integrated Process:** Teaching and Learning **Content Area:** Adult Health: Oncology **Strategy:** Use the process of elimination and note that the core issue of the question is frequency and timing of BSE. Because the client

is postmenopausal, look for the monthly option that is not associated with menses (as none are in this question).

13 **Answer: 3 Rationale:** BSE should be performed once per month, 1 week after beginning menstruation. At this time, the breasts are least likely to be tender and/or swollen from the effects of hormones. At ovulation and menstruation, hormonal changes are likely to interfere with accurate palpation of breast tissue. Performing the exam on the first of the month is recommended for postmenopausal women who are not concerned with hormone level changes associated with the menstrual cycle. **Cognitive Level:** Analyzing **Client Need:** Health Promotion and Maintenance **Integrated Process:** Teaching and Learning **Content Area:** Adult Health: Oncology **Strategy:** The core issue of the question is knowledge that accurate BSE results depend on the exam being done without the interference of hormonal factors that could alter the results or make the BSE difficult to perform. With this in mind, each of the incorrect options can be eliminated using the influence of hormones as a guide.

14 **Answer: 4 Rationale:** Although all exercises listed are aerobic and therefore beneficial, the older adult client with osteoporosis benefits from an exercise that has a weight-bearing component and does not stress the joints. Such an activity helps to retain calcium in bone and reduce the rate of bone loss. Walking is an aerobic exercise that does not stress the knee and ankle joints. Swimming is not a weight-bearing exercise. Stationary cycling is not a weight-bearing exercise. Jogging could harm the knee and ankle joints and is not a preferred method of exercise for this client. **Cognitive Level:** Applying **Client Need:** Health Promotion and Maintenance **Integrated Process:** Nursing Process: Implementation **Content Area:** Adult Health: Musculoskeletal **Strategy:** The core issue of the question is the type of exercise that is appropriate for a client with osteoporosis and who is an older adult. With this in mind, eliminate swimming and stationary cycling as non-weight-bearing, and eliminate jogging as increasing stress on joints in the leg.

15 **Answer: 2 Rationale:** Sickle-cell disease has an onset in childhood. This makes it the priority for genetic counseling. Coronary heart disease, type 2 diabetes mellitus, and hypertension are adult-onset problems and therefore have lower priority. **Cognitive Level:** Analyzing **Client Need:** Health Promotion and Maintenance **Integrated Process:** Nursing Process: Diagnosis **Content Area:** Child Health **Strategy:** Note that the stem of the question contains the critical words *most important*. This means that all options may represent conditions for which some genetic counseling may be useful, but you must select the option that has highest priority. Use age at onset as a means of making your selection.

16 **Answer: 1, 3, 5 Rationale:** A body mass index (BMI) measurement is done at age 20 and at each health visit. Clinical breast exam is done starting at age 20 and may be done every 3 years or more frequently depending on risk. Serum cholesterol levels are started at age 20 and are recommended every 5 years. Blood glucose screening is recommended to begin at age 45 unless there is evidence of higher risk for diabetes. Mammography is done yearly starting at age 40. **Cognitive Level:** Analyzing **Client Need:** Health Promotion and Maintenance **Integrated Process:** Nursing Process: Diagnosis **Content Area:** Adult Health: Cardiovascular **Strategy:** Specific knowledge of frequency of recommended health screenings is needed to answer the question. Use the process of elimination, and review this content area if needed.

17 **Answer: 1, 2, 5 Rationale:** Blood pressure screening is started at age 3 and continues with each visit. Vision screening is started at age 3 and continues with each visit. Hearing screening begins at age 4. Urinalysis is done at age 5, in adolescence, and otherwise only as indicated. Lead screening would only be done on an as-needed basis for a 4-year-old. **Cognitive Level:** Applying **Client Need:** Health Promotion and Maintenance **Integrated Process:** Nursing Process: Diagnosis **Content Area:** Child Health **Strategy:** Specific knowledge of frequency of recommended health screenings is needed to answer the question. Use the process of elimination, and review this content area if needed.

18 **Answer: 1, 2, 3, 4 Rationale:** Painless swelling of scrotum, dull pain in scrotum, nodules between testes and cord, and dragging sensation in scrotum are signs of testicular cancer. A reddened rash in the area is not applicable to this diagnosis but should be followed up for general health reasons. **Cognitive Level:** Analyzing **Client Need:** Health Promotion and Maintenance **Integrated Process:** Nursing Process: Assessment **Content Area:** Adult Health: Oncology **Strategy:** Specific knowledge of manifestations of testicular cancer is needed to answer the question. Use the process of elimination and review this content area if needed.

19 **Answer: 1, 2, 4 Rationale:** A routine health screening for a child who is 4 years old would include a vision screen, such as reading an eye chart. Routine assessment of growth and development, such as with the Denver II screening exam, is appropriate and would include activities such as standing on one foot. A routine urinalysis could be done at age 5. Measuring height and weight is part of a routine health screening for a 4-year-old child. Cranial nerve testing is unnecessary at age 4. **Cognitive Level:** Applying **Client Need:** Health Promotion and Maintenance **Integrated Process:** Teaching and Learning **Content Area:** Foundational Sciences: Growth and Development **Strategy:** The critical word in the question is *routine*. Consider that an incorrect option would be more likely to be one that is excessively in-depth or one that is done to detect specific disorders.

20 **Answer: 3, 4 Rationale:** Genetic testing may involve obtaining blood samples of parents and children to analyze genetic makeup. Counseling is provided at a follow-up appointment. It is unnecessary to record nutritional intake. It is unnecessary to take prescribed medications. The client does not need to keep a diary during the week that the screening is conducted. **Cognitive Level:** Analyzing **Client Need:** Health Promotion and Maintenance **Integrated Process:** Nursing Process: Evaluation **Content Area:** Adult Health: Hematological **Strategy:** Use the process of elimination and principles of genetics to make a selection.

ANSWERS & RATIONALES

Key Term to Review

aerobic exercise p. 214

References

Agency for Healthcare Research and Quality. (2014). *Guide to clinical preventive services 2014. Recommendations of the U.S. Preventive Services Task Force.* Available at www.ahrq.gov/professionals/clinicians-providers/guidelines-recommendations/guide/index.html.

American Cancer Society. (2015). *Guidelines for the early detection of cancer.* Available at www.cancer.org/healthy/findcancerearly/cancerscreeningguidelines/american-cancer-society-guidelines-for-the-early-detection-of-cancer.

American Cancer Society, American Diabetes Association, & American Heart Association. (2009). What health tests do you need for cancer, diabetes, heart disease and stroke? Available at www.everydaychoices.org/wp-content/uploads/2014/10/4804.00_Pad-2012.pdf.

Ball, J., Bindler, R., & Cowen, K. (2014). *Child nursing: Partnering with children and families* (3rd ed.). Upper Saddle River, NJ: Pearson Education.

Berman, A., Snyder, S., & Frandsen, G. (2016). *Kozier & Erb's fundamentals of nursing: Concepts, process, and practice* (10th ed.). New York, NY: Pearson Education.

Centers for Disease Control and Prevention. (n.d.). *Physical activity for everyone.* Retrieved June 15, 2010, from www.cdc.gov/physicalactivity/everyone/-guidelines/children.html.

LeMone, P., Burke, K., Bauldoff, G., & Gubrud, P. (2015). *Medical surgical nursing: Clinical reasoning in patient care* (6th ed.). Hoboken, NJ: Pearson Education.

Lewis, S., Dirksen, S., Heitkemper, M., & Bucher, L. (2014). *Medical surgical nursing: Assessment and management of clinical problems* (9th ed.). St. Louis, MO: Elsevier Science.

Office of Disease Prevention and Health Promotion. (n.d.). *Physical activity guidelines.* Available at http://health.gov/PAGuidelines/?_ga=1.134809073.1863886276.1459339804.

The Skin Cancer Foundation. (n.d.). *Skin cancer prevention guidelines.* Available at www.skincancer.org/Guidelines/.

Test Yourself

Are you ready for the NCLEX-RN® or course exams? Access the NEW web-based app that provides students with thousands of practice questions in preparation for the NCLEX experience.

Age-Related Care of Older Adults

17

In this chapter

Cross Reference

Other chapters relevant to this content area are

I. NEED FOR CARE

A. **Age ranges for subgroups of older adults have been identified;** each subgroup has its own needs
   1. Young-old: 65–74 years
   2. Old-old: 75–100 years
   3. Centenarians: over 100 years

B. **Most older adults live in some type of community setting;** only 4% live in a skilled nursing facility

C. **Threats to health and need for assistance with daily needs** increase with increasing age

D. **Biological aging occurs at a loss of about 0.5% of maximum function per year, starting at age 35;** most organ systems have large reserves, so detrimental effects are not noticed

E. **Chronic illnesses occur frequently in older adults (see Box 17–1)**

F. **Disuse is a core problem;** 2% of decline per year may be accounted for by simple disuse: "use it or lose it"

G. **Aging process can be slowed using preventative strategies** related to health practices, nutritional intake, and exercise (see also Chapter 16)

NCLEX® H. **Healthcare providers need skill to assist clients in promoting healthy lifestyle choices** and to differentiate between "normal aging" and indicators of underlying health problems

Box 17–1

Most Frequently Occurring Conditions in Adults 65 Years and Older

Hypertension (or taking antihypertensive): 71%	Cancer (any): 25%
Diagnosed arthritis: 49%	Diagnosed diabetes: 21%
Heart disease: 31%	

From U.S. Department of Health and Human Services, Administration for Community Living. *Portfolio of Older Americans 2014.*

II. AGE-RELATED PHYSIOLOGICAL CHANGES

A. Basic principles of physical aging

1. Rates of aging among people vary; not year-specific
2. Each organ ages at a different rate within same person
3. Toxic compounds called free radicals damage cellular proteins and eventually cause cell mutation and senescence
4. Physical aging presents differently in different cultures and environments
5. Aging process can be slowed
6. It is important to differentiate normal aging from illness

B. Specific system changes and related health promotion activity

1. Skin changes
   - NCLEX® **a.** Subcutaneous tissue loss and dermal thinning leads to a loss of moisture, wrinkles, sagging, decreased perspiration, increased risk of heat stroke, inability to respond to heat and cold rapidly, skin pallor, and slowed healing processes
   - **b.** Increase in **lentigines** (brown age spots)
   - **c.** Hair thins and loses pigment on scalp, pubic, and ancillary areas but increases in male ears and female upper lip areas
   - **d.** Nail growth slows and nails may become thicker
   - NCLEX® **e.** Skin tissue is more fragile, with fewer elastic fibers, decreasing skin turgor and increasing vulnerability to tears and pressure ulcers; caution clients about effects of sun
   - NCLEX® **f.** Use mucous membranes to assess potential anemia and fluid volume deficit
   - **g.** Sebaceous glands secrete less sebum, causing dryness and itching
2. Sensory and perceptual changes
   - **a.** Visual acuity changes; ocular changes in cornea, pupil, and lens lead to farsightedness and inability of lens to accommodate (**presbyopia**)
   - **b.** There is increased sensitivity to glare and decreased ability to adjust to light or darkness (slower constriction and dilation of pupils); it is also more difficult to differentiate colors because of changes in rods and cones
   - NCLEX® **c.** There is an increased need for light and use of glasses; nightlights may be needed; driving at night may be difficult
   - NCLEX® **d.** Because decreased vision increases risk of falls, high-gloss wax should not be used on floors; safety strips should be placed at least on first and last steps
   - **e.** Cataracts may develop; eyelids lose elasticity
   - **f.** Arcus senilis often occurs because of deposits of calcium salts and cholesterol; appears as a gray-white ring or partial ring surrounding limbus or outer edge of iris
   - **g.** Dry eyes often develop because of inability of goblet cells in conjunctiva to secrete mucin
   - **h.** Clients need to have regular ophthalmic exams
   - NCLEX® **i.** Auditory acuity changes; ear canal narrows with calcification of ossicles and increased cerumen, resulting in progressive hearing loss (**presbycusis**)
   - NCLEX® **j.** Older adults have particular difficulty hearing high-pitched tones and words that begin with consonants, especially *sh, th, wh*; they might not hear "Swish this around your mouth" accurately if they cannot see speaker's face; shouting does not help clients to hear
   - **k.** Ears should be cleaned of cerumen; if hearing aids are used, check batteries and use regularly
   - NCLEX® **l.** Olfactory bulb decreases, leading to inability to smell and discriminate odors (**anosomia**); housing for older adults should include working smoke alarms to detect fires
   - NCLEX® **m.** Gustatory buds decrease on tongue, causing decline in ability to taste; sweet sensation is especially affected; avoid use of extra sugar and salt to satisfy desire; explore alternatives
   - NCLEX® **n.** Touch sensation changes with reduced ability to sense heat and cold; monitor temperature of liquids to avoid injuries, monitor extremities for wounds that may go unnoticed because of decreased sensation, and beware of myth that older adults do not experience pain
3. Neurological changes
   - **a.** Conduction speeds of neuron firing and transmission decrease; decreased sensation and slowed response time may impact safety, driving, and decision making
   - **b.** Active participation in mind exercises (learning new things, crossword puzzles, reading) has been shown to slow changes; assist client to incorporate exercise into lifestyle
   - NCLEX® **c.** Memory retrieval is slower; short-term memory may decline but long-term memory is more intact (information is encoded); older adults are capable of learning new health-related information, but may need more processing time

d. Sleep stage 2–4 will shorten, leading to a reduced deep sleep and less physiologic and psychological rejuvenation; monitor perception of sleep, immune system, and mood/cognition state; promote healthy sleep rituals (e.g., quiet, restful environment; no stimulants before bedtime; go to bed only when tired)

NCLEX® e. **Proprioception** (sensation about body's movement and position) decreases, so achieving balance or changing position may be difficult; demonstrate safe changes of position; incorporate safety devices and clear walkways in living spaces

4. Musculoskeletal changes
   a. Muscles **atrophy** (decrease in size and physiologic activity) leading to decreased strength and stamina; legs lose more strength than arms; encourage regular exercise
   b. Joints stiffen because of deterioration of joint cartilage
   NCLEX® c. Intervertebral disks atrophy, resulting in a loss of height of 1–3 inches; bone demineralization may lead to **osteoporosis** and increased risk of fractures
   NCLEX® d. Encourage weight-bearing exercise, intake of calcium and vitamin D; walking is beneficial
   e. Monitor functional activity levels
5. Pulmonary changes
   a. Chest wall becomes rigid, thoracic muscles weaken, and ciliary activity decreases, leading to less efficient lung expansion, exchange of oxygen/carbon dioxide, coughing effectiveness, and foreign body capture
   NCLEX® b. Teach effective coughing and deep breathing techniques
   c. Practice healthy hygiene because of increased susceptibility to infection; encourage appropriate vaccine administration; sputum specimen collection may require suction technique
   NCLEX® d. Delivery and diffusion of oxygen to tissues decreases so that dyspnea can occur after moderate, stressful activity; teach pacing of activities between periods of rest and throughout day instead of clustered together
6. Cardiovascular changes
   a. Heart size remains same unless there is pathology
   NCLEX® b. Cardiac output and stroke volume decrease, especially during time of increased demands, so there is a decreased stress response
   c. Shortness of breath on exertion and pooling of blood in extremities may occur
   d. Help client to pace self during activities of daily living (ADLs) and instrumental activities of daily living (IADLs)
   e. Valves stiffen so that murmurs may be heard; know baseline so that disease-related abnormalities can be detected
   f. Conductivity is altered, so there are more ectopic beats; assess apical heart rhythm and rate for a full minute
   NCLEX® g. Vessels are less elastic, resulting in higher blood pressure; orthostatic hypotension may occur, and there is decreased perfusion to vital organs
   NCLEX® h. Monitor client BP according to latest guidelines; assess perfusion to and resulting function of vital organs
   i. Palpate peripheral pulses; use Doppler for measurement if needed
   NCLEX® j. Instruct not to make sudden position changes to avoid orthostatic hypotension because of altered physiology or effect of many medications taken for chronic health problems, such as hypertension
7. Renal changes
   a. Nephrons decrease in function because of aging and decreased arterial blood flow; monitor for output of at least 30 mL/hr (0.5 mg/kg/hr)
   b. Glomerular filtration rate (GFR) decreases, which may decrease rate of excretion of drug metabolites
   NCLEX® c. Creatinine clearance decreases; monitor for nephrotoxic medication adverse effects
   d. Ability to concentrate urine and conserve water is decreased; urinary urgency and frequency may occur from enlarged prostate in men or decreased perineal muscle support and urinary sphincter strength in women
   e. Bladder capacity decreases
   NCLEX® f. Incontinence is *not* part of normal aging; it occurs because of pathology
   g. Residual urine and nocturnal frequency may occur; teach client to apply suprapubic pressure to bladder after voiding (Credé maneuver)
   NCLEX® h. Monitor for urinary infection (new-onset confusion may be sign in older adults) and for restful nights (lack of nocturia); refer for treatment if needed

8. Gastrointestinal (GI)

NCLEX®

a. Thirst sensation decreases; monitor intake to prevent fluid deficit, especially if taking diuretics or environment is hot
b. GI system usually stays healthy overall but generates most complaints from older adults
c. Swallowing time is delayed, and epiglottis does not completely cover trachea unless older adult is in a 90-degree position
d. Monitor swallowing; have client sit upright when eating or drinking; gag reflex may diminish
e. Gingivitis/periodontal disease often leads to loss of teeth and is caused by poor nutrition and inadequate oral care
f. Saliva secretions lessen, so breakdown of carbohydrates may be decreased
g. Intra-abdominal strength decreases; gastric acid and enzymes decrease, and absorption time is slower; monitor for reflux and vitamin deficiencies

NCLEX®

h. Intestinal walls weaken, and there is a slower neural transmission and resulting decrease in peristalsis; observe for constipation and incontinence; caution against inappropriate use of laxatives because of risk of dependence

9. Endocrine
a. Thyroid-stimulating hormone (TSH) and thyroxin are reduced; slowed basal metabolism, dry skin, and thin hair are characteristic of hypothyroidism in young adults but are normal age-related changes in older adults with no history of disease
b. Insulin levels increase, but insulin sensitivity decreases; observe for hypoglycemia or hyperglycemia, depending on client condition
c. Alteration in hormone regulation decreases ability to respond to stress

10. Genital

NCLEX®

a. Prostate enlarges in men (often benign); decreased sperm production occurs; encourage regular health checkups and prostate-specific antigen (PSA) testing

NCLEX®

b. Vaginal changes in women occur because of diminished secretion of hormones; alkaline pH leads to vaginal dryness and atrophy; there may be a need for increased foreplay and use of a water-soluble lubricant; encourage regular gynecologic exams; monitor menopausal changes; estrogen is not routinely prescribed
c. For both genders, assess sexual activity and safe sex practices

11. Immune
a. Thymus has decrease in cell production with decreases in cell-mediated immunity and T-cell functioning

NCLEX®

b. Monitor for signs and symptoms of infection and/or altered cell production

NCLEX®

c. First sign of infection in an older adult may be a fall; temperature pattern may be lower than for younger adult with the same infection
d. Autoimmune response may not be associated with disease; monitor for changes in soaps or detergents if older adult develops unknown allergic rash

NCLEX®

e. Outbreaks of shingles occur if varicella virus is reactivated during times when older adult's immune system is weakened, *not* if they come in contact with new cases of chickenpox

III. AGE-RELATED PSYCHOSOCIAL CHANGES

A. Role and relationship transitions occur; adaptation is critical to positive aging

NCLEX®

B. Maintain independence in as many activities as possible

C. According to Erikson, everyone has specific developmental stages and tasks to fulfill; in 8th (last) stage of life, older adults review their life to establish beliefs of integrity or despair

1. Discrete tasks must be addressed to establish integrity:
a. Ego differentiation versus work-role preoccupation; adults are no longer defined by work; satisfaction is found in other activities
b. Body transcendence versus body preoccupation; adults care for themselves but do not spend all their energy caring for body; they see meaning in illness and death
c. Ego transcendence versus ego preoccupation; adults focus on humanity outside of themselves; "I" is not as important; volunteerism for a greater good may be seen
2. Erikson's reframed work: ego integrity is tinged with some regrets, wisdom is balanced with frivolity, and letting go is balanced with hanging on; an adult comes to terms with life as it was lived and derives sustenance from past but is active in present and plans for future; reminiscence and life review are effective tools to encourage ego integrity

D. Other key changes

NCLEX® **1.** Balance is found in solitude and social interactions; adults who adapt develop a capacity for aloneness and ability to enjoy own company (not to exclusion of significant others but in preparation for loss and death); old and new friendships are still valued; communication problems (vision, hearing, and withdrawal) may detract from finding this balance

2. Grandparenting has become an important role; some grandparents are the primary caregivers; communication clarification is important

NCLEX® **3.** Retirement may be unattainable for some and undesirable for others; financial needs, resources, and loss of health insurance benefits may deter retirement, as may perceived loss of prestige, friends, and self-satisfaction; number of retirement years is increasing, so transition counseling or mentoring may be useful

4. Widowhood is more difficult for young-old during adaptation process; transitions for all include stages that span 5 years

- **a.** First stage (reactionary): early responses of disbelief, anger, inability to communicate, searching for mate; interventions: support, reduce expectations
- **b.** Second stage (withdrawal): occurs in first few months with depression, physiological vulnerability, insomnia, unpredictable waves of grief; interventions: protect against suicide and encourage involvement in support groups
- **c.** Third stage (recuperation): occurs in second 6 months with periods of depression and feelings of personal control beginning to return; interventions: support usual lifestyle patterns while assisting to explore new possibilities
- **d.** Fourth stage (exploration): occurs in second year with new ventures but vulnerability during holidays, anniversaries, birthdays; interventions: prepare widow or widower for feelings during special times; support new roles
- **e.** Fifth stage (integration): occurs in fifth year with a healthy resolution of grief; interventions: assist individual to share own pattern of growth

E. Stressors of aging

NCLEX® **1.** Include loss of people or pets or driver license, abandonment, acute and chronic pain, sensory changes, medications, caregiving for spouse with dementia, illness, hospitalization, lack of protection when frail, abuse and neglect, housing and home maintenance, relocation, institutionalization, fear of loss of independence, and fear of death or dying alone

2. Encourage recognition of fears and reinforce positive coping methods; monitor for inappropriate coping: alcoholism, withdrawal, contemplation of suicide

3. Role transitions from worker to retiree/volunteer and spouse to widow(er) require looking at former roles differently; to the extent these are accepted and "at the right time," older adults can transition smoothly

F. Intimacy and sexuality

1. Continue to be critical at any age; touch is important to all; watch for touch deprivation; use of therapeutic touch and massage may enhance health

NCLEX® **2.** Sexually transmitted infections are not exclusively young people's diseases; safe sex practices should be followed

3. Sexual dysfunction counseling, if needed, is multidimensional; use of medications to promote erections requires education related to safety

4. Privacy is needed in residential settings for marital sexual relations; healthcare workers need to evaluate own feelings regarding sexuality in older adults

G. Many organizations promote positive aging adaptation, including American Association of Retired Persons (AARP), local senior centers, area councils/agencies on aging, churches, and groups such as Meals on Wheels

IV. MEDICATION CONSIDERATIONS

A. Issues with medications in older adults

1. Medication (drug) use is affected by finances, ability to acquire drugs, advertisements, and client's motivation and health

2. Fragmented care and lack of communication among prescribers can lead to **polypharmacy** (prescriptions for multiple drugs written by multiple prescribers and possibly filled at multiple pharmacies); this can lead to adverse drug interactions and possible toxicity

NCLEX® **3.** Nurse may be only caregiver who knows all prescribed and over-the-counter (OTC) drugs and herbs used by client, making it critical for nurses to administer, educate, monitor for therapeutic effects and adverse effects, prevent and treat toxic effects, and advocate for appropriate and affordable medication use

NCLEX® **B. Pharmacokinetics determines concentration of drug in body**

1. Absorption: aging alone affects oral drug absorption minimally but may be reduced with intramuscular (IM) delivery
2. NCLEX® Distribution: decreased circulation to skin, muscles, and fat results in slower and lower concentrations in these tissues; increased overall body fat and decreased lean body mass and water may also affect movement of drug; healthy older adults show little change in plasma binding proteins; however, lowered albumin levels in disease states can result in increased intended and adverse effects; note that some disease states (cancer, arthritis) that elevate protein binding capacity decrease effectiveness of some drugs
3. NCLEX® Metabolism/biotransformation: liver size and hepatic blood flow decrease with advanced age so drugs that undergo a first-pass effect in liver are affected by age; drugs such as propranolol exhibit decreased metabolism and increased bioavailability, leading to risk of toxicity
4. NCLEX® Excretion: aging reduces renal drug excretion because of decreased glomerular filtration rate, renal plasma flow, tubular function, and reabsorptive capacity; creatinine clearance rates are calculated and some drug dosages are calculated by lean body weight versus ideal body weight

C. Pharmacodynamics

1. NCLEX® Aging changes some receptor sites, which increases susceptibility to some adverse effects; older adults are very sensitive to anticholinergic side effects of drugs as well as orthostatic hypotension
2. Older adults tend to have more adverse effects related to a greater number of chronic problems and drugs taken

D. Medication usage

1. Older adults may require lower drug dosages especially when starting a drug regimen; therapeutic window narrows with age; "start low, go slow" is a common adage
2. NCLEX® Adverse effects are often atypical and may include falls, incontinence, **delirium** (a reversible, acute confusional state that must be evaluated), depression, sedation, urinary retention
3. NCLEX® Use brown bag method to take adequate history of medications taken
4. Review whether medications are taken as prescribed
5. Confirm that clients can see what they are taking
6. Remind clients that pills should not be crushed if enteric coated
7. Antihypertensive should be taken as ordered even if blood pressure is within normal range
8. NCLEX® Diuretics should be taken during early waking hours so that effective sleep can occur
9. NCLEX® Drugs that have hypotensive or sedative effects may be best taken at bedtime, especially if single daily dose
10. Review all prescriptions if client takes more than five to eight drugs; primary prescriber reviews necessity of all drugs
11. NCLEX® Altered electrolytes such as potassium or sodium may exacerbate imbalance and adverse drug effects; if a client is taking spironolactone and a diet high in potassium, toxic potassium levels could occur
12. NCLEX® Mental status changes may be a drug side effect; diazepam, clonidine, digoxin, levodopa, and isoniazid cause delirium and confusion in many older adults
13. NCLEX® Monitor for oto- and nephrotoxicity; assess urine output and ringing in ears, especially in older adults receiving aminoglycosides or high doses of aspirin
14. NCLEX® Monitor for sexual changes; decreased sexual desire is seen with antipsychotics, SSRI type of antidepressants, ketoconazole; priapism (prolonged painful erection) is a surgical emergency associated with sildenafil, alprostadil, trazodone, and antipsychotics
15. NCLEX® Drug allergies may occur; take history especially of antibiotics (penicillin, cephalosporin, erythromycin, gentamicin, sulfa), nonsteroidal anti-inflammatory drugs, opiates, anesthetics, and contrast media; assess their usage and reactions
16. NCLEX® Changes in diet can impact medication; increased green vegetables counteract anticoagulant effects of warfarin; iron is not absorbed when calcium is taken at same time; decreased fluid intake, especially during hot weather, may lead to fluid volume deficit and increased sensitivity to orthostatic effects of beta blockers
17. NCLEX® Food–drug interactions must be reviewed; do not give dairy products with ciprofloxacin or tetracycline because drug will chelate with food; grapefruit juice can interact with many drugs, causing either increased or decreased drug action
18. Monitor where medications are stored; store nitrates in a dry, dark area; adhere to expiration dates

E. Common medications considered inappropriate for older adults

1. Analgesics: propoxyphene and combination products, meperidine
2. Hypnotics: diazepam, barbiturates except phenobarbital

3. Antiplatelet: dipyridamole
4. Anticoagulant: ticlopidine
5. Antihypertensive: methyldopa
6. Any medication with a highly anticholinergic profile
7. Garlic and ginkgo may increase risk of bleeding

V. OLDER ADULT ABUSE AND NEGLECT

A. Abuse is willful infliction of pain or injury physically, psychologically, financially, or socially

1. Examples include confinement, willful deprivation of services, verbal assault, theft, mismanagement of belongings, demand to perform undesirable tasks, and physically injurious acts
2. Exploitation is illegal or improper use of an older adult's resources
3. *NCLEX®* Individuals at risk are those who are dependent because of health issues such as altered mental status, sensory deficits, or immobility
4. History of family violence and caregiver stress also increase risk of abuse

B. Neglect is lack of provision of services necessary for health

1. Self-neglect occurs when older adult chooses not to uses services that would promote health
2. If legally competent, an older adult has the right to refuse care

NCLEX® **C. Assessment of abuse and neglect may reveal**

1. Bruises, cuts, burns
2. Sprains, fractures, dislocations
3. Inconsistent history about injuries
4. Untreated medical problems
5. Improper use of medication
6. Malnutrition, dehydration, or both
7. Inappropriate dress, hygiene, drowsiness, or social interactions
8. Pulling away or expression of fear when touched
9. Excessive attachment to caregiver

D. Care includes

1. Continued assessment
2. *NCLEX®* Reporting to appropriate agencies as mandated by each state
3. Involvement with protective services
4. Referral to appropriate resources and treatment for dysfunctional families

VI. COMMON PROBLEMS IN OLDER ADULTS

A. Nutrition

1. Assessment
   a. Food patterns and preferences
   b. Symbolism of food: sociability, security, and reward
   c. Health screen for malnutrition
   d. Dentition efficiency and oral hygiene
   e. Taste and sensory changes influence choices; taste bud receptors decrease, especially for sweet and salt; olfactory receptors atrophy, decreasing taste ability further; visual changes affect presentation, while touch proprioception is altered also
   f. Decreased thirst sensation and satiety
   g. BMI, height and weight, ideal body weight; a BMI of 20 to 24.9 is considered healthy
   h. Labwork: related to potassium levels, hemoglobin and hematocrit ranges, prealbumin and albumin values
   i. *NCLEX®* Disease and functional profile: any disease can cause poor food intake and weight loss for older adults; lactose intolerance is becoming more prevalent; arthritis may prevent use of regular forks, spoons, knives, and cups
   j. Common nutritional problems include hypercholesterolemia, weight loss, protein malnutrition, osteoporosis (low bone density), obesity; see also Chapter 25
   k. Income and food acquisition patterns may change
   l. *NCLEX®* Clients at highest risk for decreased nutritional health: live alone, have many medications, have a history of dementia or depression, are institutionalized
2. Plan/implementation
   a. Decrease total fats and saturated transfat
   b. Control calories

c. Increase fluids to 30mL/kg body weight or up to 2 liters per day if not on fluid restriction
d. Increase whole grains and fiber intake
NCLEX® e. Limit intake of sodium and sugar; 2300 mg or 1 teaspoon per day (current recommendation for sodium); canned and processed foods contain large amounts of sodium; use substitute flavor enhancers but beware of potassium content of salt substitutes if client takes potassium-sparing diuretics or has renal disease
f. Use supplements if vitamins or minerals are needed to get 100% of RDA if client has difficulty eating or an illness that reduces absorption, is on a restricted diet, or takes medications that reduce appetite or nutrient absorption; assess calcium, iron, zinc, folic acid, and vitamins A, B_6, C, and E (frequently inadequate in older adults' diet)
g. Promote enjoyment of food by setting different table areas and eating with another; learn to savor foods; if alcohol is used, do so in moderation; include cultural preferences in diet
NCLEX® h. Increase physical activity; walking is an efficient exercise, but increased exercise can be done in a chair, too
i. Refer to a nutritionist if BMI is below 20 or above 25, food intake is limited in quality or quantity for prolonged time, or there is a limited knowledge of and motivation to comply with diet
j. Refer to a nutritionist and specialist for disorders requiring nutritional intervention: elevated lipid profile, osteoporosis, malabsorption, uncontrolled diabetes, obesity, congestive heart failure and other cardiac conditions, advanced renal or liver disease, prolonged high doses of chemotherapy or radiation
k. Refer to Meals on Wheels if preparation and acquisition of food is not easily done
NCLEX® l. Teach sources of nutrients (fat, protein, carbohydrate) and potassium (potato, banana, fortified orange juice) and reinforce with written or pictorial materials
m. Investigate food storage practices for hygienic safety; recommend nonperishable food items such as boxes of dry skim milk, peanut butter, canned tuna, dried fruit, fresh seasonal fruit, tea if refrigeration is limited
n. In healthcare settings, screen for nutritional risk; provide intervention and counseling, food and nutrition products, prescribed nutritional supplements; and monitor client response

B. Urinary incontinence

NCLEX® 1. Incontinence is not part of normal aging but a disease process or functional change
2. Assessment is critical so that treatment can be started
NCLEX® 3. Continence requires functional status in lower urinary tract, cognitive ability, dexterity in mobility, usable toileting environment, and motivation
4. Causes of transient incontinence include delirium; restricted mobility, retention; infection, inflammation, impaction; polyuria, pharmaceuticals; use the pneumonic DRIP to remember these causes

Memory Aid

Use DRIP to recall causes of transient incontinence:
D—delirium
R—restricted mobility, retention
I—infection, inflammation, impaction
P—polyuria, pharmaceuticals

5. Adverse effects of urinary incontinence
a. Physical: odor, discomfort, skin problems, urinary tract infections, falls
b. Psychosocial: embarrassment, isolation, depression, need for nursing home care
c. Economic: skilled nursing facility costs and national effect on Medicare and Medicaid
6. Types of persistent urinary incontinence include stress, urge, overflow, functional, and neurogenic
7. Treat according to cause and promote regular toileting schedules (such as every 2 hours), spacing fluids over day but not at night to avoid nocturia, and administering diuretics during early part of day

C. Constipation versus diarrhea

NCLEX® 1. Older adults are at risk for constipation if they use laxatives excessively, have reduced fiber in diet, or ingest insufficient fluids
NCLEX® 2. A brown liquid ring on sheets may be a sign of impaction, not diarrhea

D. Vision and hearing

1. Visual problems associated with aging include presbyopia, dry eye, cataracts, glaucoma, diabetic retinopathy, and macular degeneration; see Chapter 63 for a discussion of these health problems
2. Hearing problems associated with aging include presbycusis, cerumen impaction, and possibly tinnitus; see Chapter 63 for a discussion of these health problems

E. Impaired skin integrity

1. Skin loses elasticity with aging process
2. Decreased mobility also increases risk of pressure ulcer development (see also Chapters 26 and 62 for skin-related health problems)

F. Impaired mobility

1. Can occur with chronic health problems such as arthritis, neuromuscular disorders, or osteoporosis leading to fractures, or because of acute illness, injury, or surgery (such as hip and knee replacement)
2. Can occur because client is afraid of falling; impaired mobility can lead to increased risk for falls; see Table 17–1 for risk factors for falls in older adults
3. May require use of assistive devices (mobility aids) such as a cane or walker

G. Dehydration

1. Assessment is critical because older adults are at risk for dehydration
2. *NCLEX®* Mucous membranes provide indication of hydration
3. *NCLEX®* Use abdomen or forehead to assess for skin turgor; tenting is a normal, age-related change on hand and is not a reliable indicator of dehydration
4. Delirium (acute confusion) is frequently caused by dehydration and may accompany urinary tract infection; it often goes undiagnosed in older adults, and client is labeled cognitively impaired
5. See Chapter 53 for a detailed discussion of dehydration or deficient fluid volume

H. Depression

1. *NCLEX®* Older adults are at risk for depression related to multiple losses in their lives
2. *NCLEX®* Differentiate between depression, delirium, and **dementia** (impairments in memory, abstract thinking, judgment, and personality); see Table 17–2
3. For a detailed discussion, see Chapter 21 on mental health disorders

Table 17–1 Fall Risk Factors

Etiology of Risk	Examples of Type of Factor
Intrinsic age-related changes	Gait (step length and height, symmetry and path); balance when sitting, standing or turning; stability; cognition
Intrinsic disease-related changes	Orthostatic hypotension, dehydration, cardiac dysrhythmias and anemias, urinary tract and other infections, osteoporosis and fractures, hypoglycemia, seizures, transient ischemic attacks (TIAs), stroke, adverse effects of medication, delirium
Extrinsic risk factors	Clutter, high-heeled shoes, bathrooms without grab bars and shower seats, dim light or bright light with glare, curbing and other edges without contrasting colors, uneven steps, no hand rails, problems with floor surface (waxed, scatter rugs, tears in carpet)

Table 17–2 Comparisons of Delirium, Dementia, and Depression in Older Adults

	Delirium	Dementia	Depression
Onset	Acute	Gradual	Sudden or gradual
Duration	Brief, resolve underlying cause	Years	Weeks to years
State of consciousness	Disoriented	Alert	Self-absorbed
Behavior	Difficulty with attention and concentration	Personality changes, labile, easily agitated	Apathetic, feelings of worthlessness, vague somatic complaints
Ability to follow instructions	Unable to do tasks	Tries hard to follow and do with gradual loss of abilities	Able to, but does not do tasks
Mental ability	Fluctuations in memory and orientation, disorganized thinking	Impaired memory, gradual loss of knowledge, language, and judgment	Selective memory loss
Ability to cure	Reversible	Irreversible	Reversible

PRACTICE TEST

Check Your NCLEX–RN® Exam I.Q.

You are ready for testing on this content if you can:

- State basic principles related to aging.
- List physical changes of aging and implied health promotion activities.
- Differentiate normal physical aging changes from indicators of illness.
- Discuss psychosocial issues of aging and how to promote healthy adaptation.
- Identify common problems, safety issues, and required health promotion teaching.

PRACTICE TEST

1 A nurse is teaching a class about aging at a senior citizen center. Which client statement suggests that the client needs further instruction?

1. "Through nutrition and exercise, we can modify the rate of aging."
2. "Free radicals influence the quality of growing old."
3. "Some of the physical changes within our bodies are the result of disuse."
4. "Deterioration of body systems occurs at the same rate."

2 The nurse assesses that a 75-year-old client has lentigines and presbycusis. Which action should the nurse take when planning care for this client?

presbycusis = hearing loss

1. Refer client to an oncologist and an ophthalmologist.
2. Ask a unlicensed assistive person (UAP) to use water-soluble creams on client's skin.
3. Look at the client while speaking, so that client can see the nurse's lips.
4. Adjust temperature and lighting of the room.

3 The nurse prepares to teach a class about normal aging changes to a group of UAP. Which teaching technique would be most appropriate?

1. Demonstrate use of incontinence pads for clients who become incontinent of urine.
2. Teach crutch walking because of high risk for falls and fractures in older adults.
3. Discuss a case study in which an older adult with an infection had a temperature of 98°F (36.7°C).
4. Show how to use a blood glucose monitoring device and how to disinfect it because of increased incidence of diabetes.

4 A nurse evaluates that a teaching plan related to normal physiological changes of aging has been effective for a 70-year-old client if he makes which statement?

1. "I have more sebaceous gland activity."
2. "I have lost some of my social support systems."
3. "I have an increased need for sleep."
4. "I have less joint cartilage than I used to."

5 After conducting a physical assessment, the nurse would conclude that a 75-year-old client's ability to maintain personal safety would be most adversely affected by declining function in which body system?

1. Cardiovascular
2. Respiratory
3. Sensory
4. Integumentary

6 A 75-year-old woman with a pathologic fracture of the arm asks, "How did I get a broken bone?" The nurse most appropriately responds by stating that which problem is most likely to be responsible for the fracture?

1. Decreased mobility
2. Osteoarthritis
3. Scoliosis
4. Osteoporosis

7 Which nursing intervention would be most appropriate to meet safety needs when caring for an older adult with sensory changes?

1. Assist in preparing a bath because the client may be less able to feel intensity of heat.
2. Use care when administering an injection because older adults experience more pain.
3. Massage with additional pressure because tactile perception of older adults is diminished.
4. Use minimal touch with an older adult because touch will feel uncomfortable.

8 When explaining the needs of older adults to children of aging parents, which element should the nurse include?

1. They require help making important decisions.
2. They like an active family role and need to be with grandchildren often.
3. When feasible they should be supported in their desire to remain independent.
4. They must be protected from injury at all times.

9 After reviewing driving safety education principles with an older adult, a nurse should recognize which behavior as evidence of a favorable response by an older adult when driving?

1. Keeping car interior warm at all times because of loss of subcutaneous fat with decreased tolerance to cold
2. Not turning the head to look to the left or the right because the older adult's response time is slower
3. Driving at a speed that matches the flow of traffic to facilitate increased response time
4. Driving during the day to maximize vision capabilities

10 A nurse teaches an older adult client about misuse of medications. Which subsequent behavior by the client indicates that the instruction was effective?

1. Combining prescribed medications with over-the-counter ones
2. Having prescriptions from several healthcare providers
3. Using someone else's medications
4. Taking medications on time and, if a dose is missed, taking the next one on time

11 Which instruction, if included by the nurse in the care plan for an older adult who has "leaking urine," would be most effective in strengthening pelvic muscles?

1. When coughing, bear down in the standing position.
2. Percuss the lower abdomen for dull sounds, indicating a distended bladder.
3. Observe for bladder fullness immediately after voiding.
4. Stop the stream of urine during the middle of urination.

12 Which clinical manifestation would be most significant and require further investigation when assessing the skin of an 85-year-old client?

1. Ecchymoses on both forearms
2. Cherry hemangiomas across the anterior and posterior trunk
3. Tenting of the skin on the back of the hands
4. Nevi on the neck and forehead

13 An older adult client is admitted to an extended care facility for continuing care after a total hip replacement. The nurse assesses a BMI of 20, lackluster hair, and pallor. Which laboratory assessments will the nurse review to obtain the most sensitive information about the client's current nutritional status?

1. Serum albumin
2. Total cholesterol
3. Prealbumin
4. Complete blood cell count (CBC)

14 On admission, a 78-year-old client states he uses laxatives three times a week for constipation. What is the nurse's best response?

1. "As people age, they need laxatives to stimulate defecation."
2. "Eat a balanced diet if you use laxatives."
3. "Long-term use of laxatives can actually lead to constipation."
4. "Please use laxatives two times a week at night."

15 The care plan for a client who has severe osteoporosis should include which intervention to prevent injury?

1. Administer vitamin D and calcium as ordered.
2. Use a lift sheet to reposition the client.
3. Place the client in a high Fowler's position to promote lung expansion.
4. Position pillows on the client's left side when in the side-lying position.

16 Which assessment finding in an older adult client should alert the nurse to an increased risk of falls?

1. Decreased bone density
2. Increased bone prominence
3. Kyphotic posture
4. Cartilage deterioration

17 The nurse is irrigating the ears of an older adult man with a cerumen impaction. At what point would the nurse stop the procedure?

1. If the client became nauseated
2. If the irrigating fluid did not return
3. If the cerumen became softer
4. If the client says he can't hear as well

18 An older adult client is receiving the third unit of packed red blood cells in the last 8 hours. One hour into the third transfusion, the nurse observes distended neck veins in the client. What action would the nurse take next?

1. Document the observation.
2. Measure the volume left in the bag.
3. Slow the rate of the infusion.
4. Assess the client's pulse and blood pressure.

19 The nurse explains to a group at a senior citizen center that older adults may be predisposed to fluid imbalances for which reasons? Select all that apply.

1. They might not pay attention to thirst or may experience less thirst.
2. They might fear too much fluid if they have a tendency for ankles to swell.
3. They might not drink fluids if it is difficult to go to the bathroom.
4. They eat only canned and prepackaged food.
5. They tend to dislike the taste of water.

20 A nurse is instructing an older adult client about cataract prevention. The nurse will instruct the client that which factors increase the incidence of cataract development? Select all that apply.

1. Ultraviolet light
2. Injury
3. Vitamin A
4. Viral infections
5. Eyestrain

ANSWERS & RATIONALES

1 **Answer: 4 Rationale:** Each physiological system of a person ages at a different rate. Proper diet and regular exercise can be beneficial in slowing the rate of the aging process. Free radicals do influence the aging process. Physical changes within the body can occur as a result of disuse. **Cognitive Level:** Applying **Client Need:** Health Promotion and Maintenance **Integrated Process:** Nursing Process: Implementation **Content Area:** Foundational Sciences: Growth and Development **Strategy:** Note that the question has negative wording in the stem, which indicates the correct answer is an incorrect statement. Consider that tissues do not age at precisely the same rate to choose correctly.

2 **Answer: 3 Rationale:** When presbycusis (age-related sensorineural hearing loss) exists, it is helpful to look at the affected client while speaking so client can see speaker's lips. Lentigines (brown age or liver spots) represent normal aging of the skin and do not require referral to an oncologist or ophthalmologist. These changes do not require use of water-soluble creams on the client's skin. There is no indication for altering the temperature or lighting of the client's room because of presbycusis or lentigines. **Cognitive Level:** Applying **Client Need:** Health Promotion and Maintenance **Integrated Process:** Nursing Process: Planning **Content Area:** Foundational Sciences: Growth and Development **Strategy:** When answering questions, look for all parts of the answer to be correct.

3 **Answer: 3 Rationale:** A normal body temperature of an older adult person may range from 96.5–99°F (35.9°C to 37.3°C). Therefore, a temperature of 98.6°F (37°C) may signify a fever in an older person. Incontinence is not a normal age-related change. Not all older adults have altered mobility

needs, and those who do are more likely to use a cane or walker than crutches (which are used for injury). Use of blood glucose devices is generic or related to a diagnosis of diabetes and is not specifically related to normal aging changes. **Cognitive Level:** Analyzing **Client Need:** Health Promotion and Maintenance **Integrated Process:** Nursing Process: Planning **Content Area:** Foundational Sciences: Growth and Development **Strategy:** Eliminate choices that do not correlate to all parts of the question as well as those choices that have incorrect information.

4 **Answer: 4 Rationale:** With normal aging, there is loss of cartilage and joint fluid. Overall wear and tear does occur. Sebaceous glands are less active, and older adults sweat less. Social support may decrease with deaths and fewer resources but does not relate to the question of physiological needs. There is a decreased need for sleep, with shorter REM and non-REM sleep cycles. **Cognitive Level:** Analyzing **Client Need:** Health Promotion and Maintenance **Integrated Process:** Nursing Process: Implementation **Content Area:** Foundational Sciences: Growth and Development **Strategy:** Read all options and use concepts of the normal aging process to eliminate those that are incorrect.

5 **Answer: 3 Rationale:** With normal aging changes, there is a decrease in the senses of vision, hearing, touch, smell, and taste. These changes can lead to falls, inability to leave a situation when called to do so, inability to distinguish temperature with resulting burns, inability to smell smoke in a fire, and inability to taste contaminated food. Cardiovascular changes could lead to safety risks if the client was taking medication that has a side effect of orthostatic hypotension, but this is not specified in the question. Age-related respiratory changes are not necessarily associated with safety risks. Integumentary changes do not pose a threat to client safety. **Cognitive Level:** Analyzing **Client Need:** Safety and Infection Control **Integrated Process:** Nursing Process: Planning **Content Area:** Foundational Sciences: Growth and Development **Strategy:** When answering questions related to development and aging, distinguish between normal development, which affects all, and illness, which affects some.

6 **Answer: 4 Rationale:** Osteoporosis, a decrease in bone density, makes the older adult more prone to pathologic fractures. Decreased mobility can have several adverse effects on the body, including bone demineralization, but this does not necessarily lead to pathologic fractures. Osteoarthritis is likely to lead to joint stiffness and pain. Scoliosis is a curvature of the spine, usually diagnosed in adolescents. **Cognitive Level:** Applying **Client Need:** Physiological Adaptation **Integrated Process:** Nursing Process: Implementation **Content Area:** Foundational Sciences: Growth and Development **Strategy:** Consider the etiology of pathologic fractures and correlate the best reason with the correct answer choice.

7 **Answer: 1 Rationale:** Because of loss of skin receptors, the older adult has an increased threshold to pain, touch, and temperature. When feeding or bathing, remember that the older adult may be unable to distinguish hot or cold or to determine the intensity of heat. The older adult may feel less pain than younger adults and report only pressure or a minor sensation. The older adult, however, is the only one who can identify whether he or she has pain. An older client's sensory perception is less acute than that of younger adults, so when giving a massage, less pressure is needed. Everyone, and especially the older adult, needs touch. **Cognitive Level:** Analyzing **Client Need:** Safety and Infection Control **Integrated Process:** Nursing Process: Planning **Content Area:** Foundational Sciences: Growth and Development **Strategy:** Imagine giving the stated care to assist in choosing the correct answer.

8 **Answer: 3 Rationale:** Remaining independent is important for older adults. Older adults prefer to make their own decisions and do not appreciate others making decisions for them. Although some older adults cherish a family role, this is not necessarily the wish of every older adult. Excessive protection from injury is unnecessary and inappropriate. **Cognitive Level:** Applying **Client Need:** Psychosocial Integrity **Integrated Process:** Nursing Process: Implementation **Content Area:** Foundational Sciences: Growth and Development **Strategy:** Recognize that usually the word *all* denotes an incorrect choice.

9 **Answer: 4 Rationale:** Driving at night requires caution because accommodation of the eye to light is impaired and peripheral vision is diminished. Keeping the inside of the car warm at all times is not a significant issue when driving in warm climates or during warm seasons. Peripheral vision is diminished, so it is important to look to the left and right. Reflexes are slowed for older adults; thus, caution about speed while driving should be emphasized. **Cognitive Level:** Analyzing **Client Need:** Health Promotion and Maintenance **Integrated Process:** Nursing Process: Evaluation **Content Area:** Foundational Sciences: Growth and Development **Strategy:** The phrase *favorable response* cues you to look for the desired outcome.

10 **Answer: 4 Rationale:** Proper self-administration of medications includes taking medications on time and, if a dose is missed, taking the next one on time. Misuse of medications by older adults includes behaviors such as combining prescribed and over-the-counter medications. Obtaining prescriptions from different healthcare providers can result in polypharmacy, which can pose a risk to medication safety. Using someone else's medications may lead to adverse health effects. **Cognitive Level:** Analyzing **Client Need:** Health Promotion and Maintenance **Integrated Process:** Nursing Process: Evaluation **Content Area:** Foundational Sciences: Growth and Development **Strategy:** The phrase *indicates that the instruction was effective*, means the choices will have three incorrect outcomes and one desired outcome, which will be the correct choice.

11 **Answer: 4 Rationale:** Interrupting the flow of urine assists the external urethra to contract and strengthens pelvic floor muscles. Coughing and bearing down will worsen urinary incontinence, regardless of whether the client is standing or sitting. Percussion is an assessment technique and does not constitute an intervention for incontinence. Observing for bladder fullness after voiding is an assessment technique, not an intervention. **Cognitive Level:** Applying **Client Need:** Physiological Adaptation **Integrated Process:** Nursing Process: Planning **Content Area:** Foundational Sciences: Growth and Development **Strategy:** Distinguish between assessments and interventions, and then choose the intervention that will reduce urinary incontinence rather than worsen it.

12 **Answer: 1 Rationale:** Ecchymoses are not the result of aging and should be investigated to determine whether the client is sustaining injury or taking anticoagulant therapy. Cherry hemangiomas do not require further investigation as to cause. Tenting of the skin is a normal, age-related change in an older adult. Nevi on the neck and forehead are not

significant age-related findings. **Cognitive Level:** Applying **Client Need:** Health Promotion and Maintenance **Integrated Process:** Nursing Process: Assessment **Content Area:** Foundational Sciences: Growth and Development **Strategy:** The critical phrase *most significant* leads you to look for an option that is not an age-related change or a benign skin condition.

13 **Answer: 3 Rationale:** Prealbumin is a sensitive indicator of changes in nutritional protein status and can also alert the nurse to clients at risk for pressure ulcer development. Serum albumin can provide data about visceral protein stores but has a relatively long half-life and may not accurately reflect recent protein losses. Total cholesterol would be assessed as a risk factor for cardiovascular disease. CBC is a hematology test commonly used for screening purposes, although decreased red blood cell count would indicate anemia. **Cognitive Level:** Applying **Client Need:** Reduction of Risk Potential **Integrated Process:** Nursing Process: Assessment **Content Area:** Foundational Sciences: Growth and Development **Strategy:** Eliminate total cholesterol and CBC first as general screening measures, then choose prealbumin over albumin because the value changes more rapidly in response to nutritional intake.

14 **Answer: 3 Rationale:** Prolonged use of laxatives can lead to dependence on them for stimulation of defecation and can actually lead to uncontrollable defecation. Laxatives are not necessarily required to stimulate defecation in older adults. A proper diet, adequate fluid intake, and sufficient activity will help to maintain normal bowel function during later years. A balanced diet is important even if not using laxatives. Laxatives should be used only as needed. **Cognitive Level:** Applying **Client Need:** Pharmacological and Parenteral Therapies **Integrated Process:** Nursing Process: Implementation **Content Area:** Foundational Sciences: Growth and Development **Strategy:** Choose the response that represents factual scientific information and teaches the client about risks associated with laxative use.

15 **Answer: 2 Rationale:** Severe osteoporosis causes bone density loss, which can result in pathologic fractures when the client is moved. A lift sheet can reduce the risk. Vitamin D and calcium are necessary to prevent further bone loss but will not prevent injury. Use of high Fowler's position will not reduce risk for pathologic fractures, although it would be of use with respiratory problems. Positioning on the side will not be of use to prevent pathologic fractures. **Cognitive Level:** Applying **Client Need:** Health Promotion and Maintenance **Integrated Process:** Nursing Process: Implementation **Content Area:** Foundational Sciences: Growth and Development **Strategy:** Note the critical words *severe osteoporosis* and *prevent injury*. Then consider that osteoporosis can lead to pathologic fractures to help select the option that will reduce this risk.

16 **Answer: 3 Rationale:** Posture changes (such as kyphotic posture) shift the center of gravity in an older adult client and put the client at risk for falls. Decreased bone density can increase the risk of injury if a fall occurs but not the risk of falling. Increased bone prominence does not put the client at risk for falls. Cartilage is a soft tissue, not bone, and its deterioration does not increase the risk of falls. **Cognitive Level:** Applying **Client Need:** Safety and Infection Control **Integrated Process:** Nursing Process: Assessment **Content Area:** Foundational Sciences: Growth and Development **Strategy:** Read the question carefully and use similarities in the question stem and the answer to make a selection.

17 **Answer: 1 Rationale:** Motion receptors can be stimulated with instillation of large amounts of fluid. Nausea or vomiting can result and relief will occur if the irrigation procedure is stopped. If the irrigant did not return, the nurse should reposition the head. If the cerumen becomes softer, it indicates partial success of the procedure and the irrigation should continue. A temporary reduction in hearing is expected during the procedure in the affected ear and is not a cause for concern. **Cognitive Level:** Applying **Client Need:** Physiological Adaptation **Integrated Process:** Nursing Process: Implementation **Content Area:** Adult Health: Eye and Ear **Strategy:** The correct choice is the only answer that does not involve the ear or irrigation procedure directly.

18 **Answer: 3 Rationale:** Older adult clients are at risk for developing fluid overload during fluid and blood component therapy. The infusion rate should be slowed to prevent worsening of the problem. Documentation is a routine function that should be completed once the client has received care. Noting the volume remaining in the bag is a useful assessment but is not the highest priority. The vital signs should be assessed once an intervention is completed that will assist the client. **Cognitive Level:** Analyzing **Client Need:** Reduction of Risk Potential **Integrated Process:** Nursing Process: Implementation **Content Area:** Adult Health: Cardiovascular **Strategy:** Visualize care to determine first, second, third, and fourth action order.

19 **Answer: 1, 2, 3 Rationale:** Older adults may be at higher risk for fluid imbalances because of decreased thirst or oral intake, diagnosed health conditions that affect fluid balance, and difficulty with mobility to use the bathroom. It is not necessarily true that older adults eat only canned or prepackaged foods, or that they dislike water. **Cognitive Level:** Analyzing **Client Need:** Physiological Adaptation **Integrated Process:** Nursing Process: Evaluation **Content Area:** Adult Health: Endocrine and Metabolic **Strategy:** Consider age-related changes (decreased thirst and mobility) and health problems that affect fluid balance (such as heart failure or renal insufficiency) to aid in making selections. Note the wording of the question indicates that more than one option is correct.

20 **Answer: 1, 2, 4 Rationale:** Ultraviolet light, injury, and viral infections increase the incidence of cataract development. The nurse recommends the use of sunglasses, eye protection, and safety throughout the lifespan. Vitamin A and eyestrain do not increase the risk of cataract development. **Cognitive Level:** Applying **Client Need:** Health Promotion and Maintenance **Integrated Process:** Nursing Process: Assessment **Content Area:** Adult Health: Eye and Ear **Strategy:** Specific information is needed to answer the question. Consider that risk factors have the ability to cause damage to the eye.

Key Terms to Review

anosomia p. 226
atrophy p. 227
delirium p. 230
dementia p. 233
lentigines p. 226
osteoporosis p. 227
polypharmacy p. 229
presbycusis p. 226
presbyopia p. 226
proprioception p. 227

ANSWERS & RATIONALES

References

Adams, M., & Urban, C. (2016). *Pharmacology: Connections to nursing practice* (3rd ed.). New York, NY: Pearson Education.

Berman, A., Snyder, S., & Frandsen, G. (2016). *Kozier & Erb's fundamentals of nursing: Concepts, process, and practice* (10th ed.). New York, NY: Pearson Education.

Lehne, R. (2016). *Pharmacology for nursing care* (9th ed.). St. Louis, MO: Saunders.

Touhy, T., & Jett, K. (2015). *Ebersole & Hess' toward healthy aging: Human needs and nursing response* (9th ed.). St. Louis, MO: Elsevier.

U.S. Dept. of Health and Human Services, Administration on Aging. (2014). *A profile of older Americans: 2014*. Available at www.aoa.gov/Aging_Statistics/Profile/2014/14.aspx.

18 Therapeutic Communication and Environment

In this chapter

Cross Reference

Other chapters relevant to this content area are

Culturally Relevant Care	Chapter 19
Mental Health Disorders	Chapter 21

I. OVERVIEW OF COMMUNICATION

A. Characteristics of effective *communication*

1. An exchange of information, ideas, attitudes, and emotions occurs; message intended is message received
2. A basic skill in providing healthcare to clients; occurs between nurse and clients and between nurse and other healthcare providers

B. Elements of communication (see Box 18–1): can either promote or inhibit flow of accurate communication

C. Levels of communication

1. Intrapersonal: occurs within oneself and happens constantly; involves thinking about a message before it is sent, interpreting it, and evaluating it (self-talk)
2. Interpersonal: occurs between people and involves sending and receiving a message and **feedback**
3. Public communication: involves sending a message to a group of people for dissemination of information; it generally does not require feedback

D. Forms of communication

1. Communication occurs both verbally and nonverbally in a therapeutic relationship; purposeful communication between nurse and client is often termed **therapeutic communication**
2. *NCLEX®* Be aware of communication chosen to ensure message sent is message received; be aware of own nonverbal body language and physical boundaries, such as client's personal space
3. *NCLEX®* **Verbal communication**: use of spoken or written words
   a. Therapeutic rapport: verbal communication is facilitated by a trusting nurse–client relationship (client believes nurse cares about client's well-being and wants to assist in meeting health-related client goals)
   b. Pacing: rhythm and speed with which verbal message is sent; pace of a message may indicate interest, disinterest, or anxiety, among other emotions
   c. Intonation: pattern of pauses and accents or stresses when sending a message can reflect an underlying mood of sender, such as anger, boredom, excitement
   d. Clarity and brevity: clear, brief messages are more likely to be interpreted correctly than vague and lengthy messages; clarity is influenced by congruence between verbal and nonverbal behavior
   e. Timing and relevance: messages should contain content of interest to client and be delivered when client is interested in receiving it

Box 18–1

Elements of Communication

Sender: initiates communication to convey information, thoughts, ideas, or feelings to another; encodes information by selecting signs and symbols used (language, word selection, voice intonations, gestures, etc.)

Message: information to be communicated; includes codings (vocabulary, tone of voice, body language, and way the message is transmitted); effective communication occurs when message intended is message received

Channel: vehicle used to convey message using any of five senses; for example, written documentation (sight), oral communication (hearing), and therapeutic touch; use correct medium to send message, such as writing a message for a hearing-impaired client to ensure message intended is message received

Receiver: person or group that message is intended for, also called *decoder* of message; perceives or interprets message

Environment: physical, cultural, and social conditions in which information is transmitted; sometimes called *context* of communication

Feedback: sometimes called *response*; requires that receiver respond to message communicated by sender; may be verbal or nonverbal and helps to determine whether communication was effective or ineffective

NCLEX®

4. **Nonverbal communication**: occurs without words; often called body language
   a. Facial expression: can either convey or mask emotions; cautiously interpret eye and facial movements and validate impressions with further assessment; some facial expressions are universal, such as a smile for happiness and a frown for displeasure
   b. Eye contact: can be influenced by cultural norms; avoiding eye contact may be culturally appropriate or can indicate other feelings, such as embarrassment or lack of interest in communicating
   c. Gestures: can convey urgency of message or be a coping response when client cannot express an urgent message quickly enough using words; some gestures (such as a hand wave) have almost universal meanings, while others are culture-specific; can also be used as signals when unable to communicate with words
   d. Posture and gait: can indicate physical well-being, self-concept, and mood; an erect posture and a steady purposeful gait generally indicate a sense of well-being; slouching or a shuffling, slow gait may indicate depressed mood, presence of Parkinson's disease, or being tired or uncomfortable; validate with client any impressions gained from observing posture and gait
   e. Territoriality and personal space: all people have a physical zone around body considered to be an extension of self that should not be entered by others; size of space can vary considerably among cultures and individuals; type of relationship also affects desired personal space; body language is often used to signal when someone has violated personal space (such as taking a step back)
   f. Personal appearance: can be a general indicator of self-esteem, social status, emotional status, culture or other group association; selection of clothing is often highly personal; hygiene may be influenced by physical ability, emotional status, mental illness, energy level, and time; be careful not to judge clients based on personal appearance

NCLEX®

E. Effective communication techniques (see Box 18–2)

1. Maintain appropriate boundaries as part of therapeutic communication
2. Understand that one cannot always know how others perceive or misperceive messages sent; developing a sense of self-awareness and checking client's understanding of messages is critical to good communication

Memory Aid

The answers to communication questions are those that utilize therapeutic communication techniques while avoiding the use of communication blocks.

NCLEX®

F. Communication techniques (blocks) to avoid (see Box 18–3)

1. Avoid statements that discourage further communication from client to nurse and/or place client's feelings on hold
2. Such communications are disruptive to nurse–client relationship

G. Communicating with clients who have special needs (see Box 18–4)

Box 18–2

Effective Communication Techniques

Acknowledging: gives nonjudgmental recognition to a client for a certain behavior or contribution, or indicates attention to and care of client

Clarifying: asks for additional information to ensure understanding of message sent; a statement like "Would you tell me more about what you have just said?" conveys client's message is important to the nurse

Focusing: focuses client on pertinent information and helps client expand on that information; directs client toward information that is important

Giving information: provides specific information to a client either with or without client's request

Offering self: offers nurse's presence without attaching any expectations or conditions on client's behavior during that time

Restating or paraphrasing: ensures nurse understands message sent; utilizing this technique, nurse repeats main thought of message sent

Reflecting: redirects content of a client's message back to client for further thought or consideration

Summarizing: may be used at end of an interaction to identify material discussed; helps to sort out relevant from irrelevant information

Using silence: allows for quiet time without conversation for several seconds or minutes to allow for reflection about discussion that just occurred, to reduce tension, or to gather thoughts about how to proceed

Box 18–3

Communication Blocks to Avoid

Self-disclosure: communicates personal experience to client that focuses relationship on nurse instead of client; is not client-centered or goal-directed

Inattentive listening: blocks communication by indicating that client's needs are not important

Overuse of medical jargon: confuses client and indicates nurse is not interested in ensuring healthcare information is understood

Giving personal opinions (approval, disapproval) or offering advice: may give impression that a person is closed to new ideas or to open discussion

Prying or probing techniques: if not used to seek specific health-related information or to clarify a client's statement, this is a nontherapeutic technique; in such instances, client may provide information to satisfy nurse's curiosity and nurse's questions are inappropriate and may violate client's right to privacy

Changing the subject: blocks therapeutic communication by indicating that client should not continue to talk about previous topic; leads conversation to only those areas that nurse wants to discuss

Challenging the client or being defensive: creates a power struggle between client and nurse and does not foster open and honest communication (asking "why?")

Providing false reassurance: does not contribute to open and honest communication and can break bond of trust between client and nurse

Box 18–4

Communication with Clients with Special Needs

Difficulty hearing

- To ensure that effective communication occurs with a client who is hearing impaired, stand or sit near client and speak clearly and slowly using a low-pitched voice.
- Ensure environment has adequate lighting and is quiet and free from distractions.
- Use therapeutic communication techniques to ensure that message sent is message received.
- Use writing, if necessary, to enhance communication with a client who is hearing impaired.
- Avoid using a loud voice when speaking to a client who is hearing impaired.

Difficulty seeing

- Ensure environment has adequate light.
- Ensure that quality of spoken word matches message communicated.
- Remember a visually impaired person may not be able to use nonverbal cues to help interpret message.

Mute or unable to speak clearly

- When communicating with a client who is unable to speak clearly, has an artificial airway, or is mute, encourage client to write a response or utilize word boards or pictures to ensure effective communication.
- Utilize therapeutic technique of clarification or paraphrasing as needed to assist in communication.

Cognitively impaired

- Ensure language is simple, concise, and spoken slowly and calmly.
- Allow adequate time for client to process information.
- Use environmental cues to convey message to client; for instance, hold a toothbrush in view while asking if client would like to brush teeth.

Unresponsive

- Use touch along with spoken word and try to elicit a response from client.
- Ask a closed question such as "Can you hear me?" and observe for nonverbal cues that may indicate client has received message to try to obtain a response.
- Speak to client in a manner that assumes client can hear every spoken word; avoid having conversations about client's status or that are irrelevant to client at the bedside.

Non-English-speaking clients

- Seek an interpreter fluent in client's primary language if client does not speak English; until an interpreter is available, communication must take place through nonverbal means.
- Use pictures, environmental cues, and body language to communicate with a client who speaks a different language.

II. THERAPEUTIC NURSE–CLIENT RELATIONSHIPS

A. A *therapeutic relationship* is a nurse–client interaction that focuses on client needs and is goal-specific, theory-based, and open to observation or scrutiny by other healthcare team members

B. Phases of therapeutic relationship

1. Preinteraction phase
   a. Occurs prior to initial contact with a person and is similar to planning stage before an interview
   b. Any available client information is organized and analyzed prior to contact with client; during this phase, nurse prepares for initial contact

NCLEX®

2. Orientation phase
   a. May also be called introductory phase or prehelping phase
   b. Nurse and client get to know one another and develop a degree of trust
   c. Three processes occur during this phase: opening the relationship, clarifying the problem, and structuring and formulating the contract for what will be accomplished during the relationship

NCLEX®

3. Working phase
   a. Includes exploring and understanding thoughts and feelings, along with facilitating client's work and taking action
   b. Skills required during this phase are empathetic listening and understanding, respect, genuineness, concreteness, and confrontation
   c. Client **transference**, an unconscious process of displacing feelings for significant people in past onto nurse in present relationship, can occur in this phase; **countertransference** is nurse's emotional reaction to clients based on feelings for significant people in past
   d. At completion of this phase, client makes decisions and takes action, while nurse provides information and collaborates with and supports client

NCLEX®

4. Termination phase
   a. Primary goal of termination phase of therapeutic relationship is to review client's progress and plans for immediate future after reaching goals
   b. May be difficult for both nurse and client; to reduce feelings of loss and ambivalence, it may be helpful for nurse to summarize relationship and make follow-up phone calls to help client transition to independence
   c. Nurse should prepare client for termination phase early in relationship

C. Components of a therapeutic relationship

1. Physical component of relationship includes all procedures and technical skills that nurses provide for clients
2. Psychosocial component involves qualities such as positive regard, nonjudgmental attitude, acceptance, warmth, empathy, and authenticity
3. Spiritual component is feeling of connectedness with clients and respect for diversity of spiritual needs among clients
4. Power component includes beliefs about external and internal locus of control
   a. Clients who have a strong **internal locus of control** tend to believe that they are able to make their own decisions and influence their own health; these clients may experience more positive health outcomes
   b. Clients who have a strong **external locus of control** tend to believe that other people and events heavily affect their decisions and lives, and may perceive themselves as somewhat powerless; these clients may have less positive health outcomes unless appropriate support people and services are in place

D. Nurse's responsibilities in a therapeutic relationship

1. Deliver care that is holistic and comprehensive of current client needs and priorities
2. Respect client's uniqueness, with consideration given to cultural and spiritual beliefs, values, and practices that provide comfort, support, and hope during illness
3. Foster open and honest communication that focuses on client's needs and feelings
4. Value empathy, respect, and genuineness in interactions with client
5. Set limits when necessary to foster client progress and growth
6. Promote client independence by assisting client to utilize internal resources (such as personal strengths, problem-solving skills) and community resources

III. TEACHING AND LEARNING AS THERAPEUTIC COMMUNICATION

A. Purposes of client teaching

1. Health promotion and maintenance and prevention of illness
   a. Examples include providing information about immunization requirements, nutrition, and exercise; offering parenting and prenatal classes
   b. Generally these programs are aimed toward groups of people with a healthcare need and disseminate information and skills needed for clients to develop positive health practices
2. Restoration of health
   a. Teaching is intended for clients with an active health problem and focuses on cause, condition, and treatment
   b. An example of this type of client teaching is insulin administration for a client who has new-onset type 1 diabetes mellitus
3. Coping with impaired functioning
   a. Teaching centers around providing instruction to a client who has not made or cannot make a complete recovery
   b. An example is a client who modifies activities of daily living because of a lower limb amputation

B. Domains of learning

1. Cognitive learning involves acquiring and using knowledge; for example, when teaching a parenting class, nurse provides information on developmental stages of children; when applying that knowledge to toilet training a child, parent is learning in **cognitive domain**
2. Affective learning occurs when a client changes unhealthy attitudes or feelings and values; a parent who accepts and understands that children have specific developmental stages and may not become toilet-trained until after age 2 is learning in **affective domain**
3. Psychomotor: psychomotor learning is learning how to complete a physical act; for example, nurse may show a parent how to properly administer ear drops for a toddler with otitis media; this is learning in the **psychomotor domain**

C. Factors that influence client learning

1. Motivation: desire to learn
   a. Important for client to recognize the need to learn a new behavior
   b. Nurses can assist a client in solving problems and identifying needs that may increase desire to learn
2. *NCLEX®* Health beliefs
   a. Must be assessed to develop beneficial teaching plan; client's health beliefs may or may not be congruent with information to be taught
   b. Assist a client by showing a cause-and-effect relationship between positive and negative health practices; for example, if client does not believe that smoking will affect his or her cardiac status, individual is unlikely to change behavior
   c. Be aware that a client's healthcare beliefs may not change, despite concentrated efforts, because of multiple psychological, cultural, and environmental factors
3. Psychosocial adaptation to illness
   a. Describes transition from a healthy, independent state to an illness state
   b. Successful adaptation or acculturation to illness depends on client's emotional makeup
   c. *NCLEX®* Understand that a client is unlikely to learn new health-related behaviors if not ready or motivated to learn or is experiencing problems unrelated to health
   d. Regularly assess how a client is adapting
4. Active participation
   a. Active participation by client in teaching and learning process makes learning more meaningful
   b. *NCLEX®* Assess a client's learning needs and involve client in learning process to encourage active participation
5. Literacy level and educational level: ability of client to read materials provided and understand spoken word
6. Developmental level affects ability to understand health problem and learn information needed for self-management
7. Individual learning style: learning is enhanced when nurse uses instructional methods that match client's preferred learning style

D. Basic teaching principles

1. *NCLEX®* Set priorities: rank client's learning needs according to importance; involve client in ranking needs because learning is more likely to occur when client's perceived needs are met
2. *NCLEX®* Use appropriate timing; for example, a client with diabetes is more likely to successfully self-administer insulin immediately after watching a video than the next morning
3. Organize materials: learning occurs from simple to complex; organize material in this manner to allow learner to assimilate information more readily
4. Promote and maintain learner attention and participation: keep environment physically comfortable and free from distractions; involve client actively in learning process; ensure that information is personally relevant to client; provide opportunity for client feedback
5. Build on existing knowledge: assess client's knowledge of subject before teaching to make material more personal to client and enhance learner's confidence in material
6. Select appropriate teaching methods
   a. Discussion: one-on-one formal or informal instruction allows client to set pace of learning and engage in verbal exchange with nurse; promotes customized learning
   b. Question and answer: meets needs of clients for specific pieces of information as requested by client; often beneficial as a follow-up to other teaching methods
   c. Role-play, discovery: allows client to simulate real-life situations and apply new knowledge or skills in an artificial or "safe" setting; helps to build client's confidence in newly acquired knowledge and skills once feelings of shyness, embarrassment, or awkwardness are worked through

d. Computerized instruction: allows client to regulate pace of instruction and possibly direct nature of material presented next (interactive programs)

7. To supplement instruction use teaching aids that are well selected according to content, health literacy level, and client's learning style
   a. May include visual aids (drawings, charts, models, printed materials), audiotapes, films or videotapes, programmed instruction, games, and others
   NCLEX® b. Written teaching aids should support health literacy: using language at or below sixth-grade level, written in client's own language, containing simple words and short sentences, using at least 14-point type size (to help readability), stating important points first, and focusing on desired behaviors rather than facts
8. Provide content of teaching related to developmental level
   NCLEX® a. Infant: immunizations, infant safety, nutrition, rest/sleep patterns, and sensory stimulation; assess parents' learning needs and provide instruction accordingly; complete client teaching when infant is calm and happy to minimize parents' distraction
   NCLEX® b. Toddler: accident prevention, toilet training, dental hygiene, and appropriate play activities; toddlers fear pain and separation from parents; parent teaching for a hospitalized toddler includes participation in care, purpose of care plans, and developmental regression that can occur because of hospitalization
   NCLEX® c. Preschooler: accident prevention, dental health, nutrition, cognitive stimulation, and sleep patterns; assist hospitalized preschooler by using visual, tactile, and auditory images to decrease fear of procedures; therapeutic play or using dolls or puppets to demonstrate procedures before they are done is also helpful
   NCLEX® d. School-age child: dental hygiene, safety measures, promotion of physical fitness, and hygiene measures to prevent spread of infection; provide concrete examples and explanations of procedures to help child understand healthcare; encourage child to identify own learning needs; therapeutic play may assist child to learn
   NCLEX® e. Adolescent: effects of drugs and alcohol, sexually transmitted infections, reducing risk of injury (e.g., motor vehicle accidents, sports), and nutrition information; actively involve adolescent in learning to aid assimilation of information provided; client contracting and peer education also promote learning
   NCLEX® f. Young to middle-aged adult: importance of routine health tests and screening, sun protection measures, nutrition (especially adequate protein and calcium intake), and exercise to maintain health; evaluate client's learning needs and determine those that client believes are important to maintaining health
   NCLEX® g. Older adult: importance of exercise in maintaining joint mobility, nutrition (including caloric and fluid requirements), and fall prevention information; ensure there is adequate lighting and use large print if necessary for visually impaired client; for hearing-impaired client, use written teaching materials and visual aids
9. NCLEX® Evaluate client understanding of teaching using "teach-back" technique (in which nurse asks client to state in own words what is important to know or do) or "show back" technique (for return demonstration of a skill)

IV. THERAPEUTIC ENVIRONMENTS

A. Overview

1. A therapeutic environment is one that is manipulated or created to help restore or promote physical and mental health
2. See Box 18–5 for practice settings in which therapeutic environments are integral to care
3. Physical space may be designed with attention to color, layout (such as circular halls for clients with Alzheimer's disease), and aesthetic appeal, including artwork
4. Aids to memory or cognition, such as clock and white boards in room identifying names of caregivers for day, may be used in hospital or long-term care environments

B. Nursing interventions commonly used during care in a therapeutic environment

1. Health promotion and maintenance
2. Assessment and evaluation
3. Case management
4. Provision of a therapeutic milieu
5. Client education about factors that influence mental health and mental illness
6. Promotion of self-care and independence

Box 18–5

Practice Settings That Utilize a Therapeutic Environment

Psychiatric hospitals

Community mental health centers

General hospitals

Community health agencies (e.g., home health, primary-care centers, homeless clinics)

Outpatient services

Senior centers and daycare centers

Schools

Prisons

Emergency and crisis centers

7. Administration and monitoring of psychobiological treatment regimens
8. Crisis intervention and counseling
9. Engaging in social and community mental health efforts

C. *Milieu* therapy

1. Provides a therapeutic and safe environment in which client is free to express thoughts and feelings; this is particularly employed in mental health settings (see also Chapter 21)
2. Clients interact, share frustrations, and learn to relate to others in honest and constructive ways under supervision and assistance of mental health professionals
3. There are norms for client behavior on unit to foster safety of all clients and staff and are shared with clients; when client behavior violates these norms, such as being verbally or physically aggressive with other clients or staff, staff sets limits with client and may enforce sanctions that are discussed in advance
4. Individual client growth is often achieved through group meetings in which focus may be learning social skills, problem solving, goal setting, or otherwise effecting positive self-change
5. A prime tenet of group therapy is that all group members are valued and contribute to overall functioning of group

Check Your NCLEX–RN® Exam I.Q. *You are ready for testing on this content if you can:*

- Utilize communication techniques appropriately and effectively.
- Determine accurately the components of a therapeutic relationship and how to maintain one.
- Create an environment conducive to client teaching, including preparation of the teaching plan.

PRACTICE TEST

1 The nurse has explained a therapeutic diet to a client. To ensure that learning has occurred, which follow-up action should the nurse take?

1. Repeat details of the diet once or twice more.
2. Listen to comments from client.
3. Ask another nurse to verify client understands the diet.
4. Refer client to a nutritionist.

2 A nurse is trying to establish whether a client who appears unconscious can communicate. What would be the best approach for the nurse to use?

1. Ask open-ended questions.
2. Ask client to blink once or twice in response to questions.
3. Observe for facial grimaces during verbal stimuli from the nurse.
4. Assess for response to painful stimuli.

PRACTICE TEST

3 A client who is legally blind has been admitted to the cardiac unit. Which action by the nurse would be best to promote adjustment to the environment?

1. Speak slowly and in a low-pitched voice while facing the client.
2. Post a sign on the door indicating the client is blind.
3. Explain unit noises and physical surroundings.
4. Give clear, concise, simple instructions to the client.

4 The home care nurse has asked the client to demonstrate self-injection technique. In doing so, the nurse is primarily attempting to determine which of the following?

1. Number of home visits that will be required
2. Other support services the client will need
3. Quality of the client teaching plan
4. Client's ability to perform the skill

5 Which of the following would be the most appropriate time for a nurse to use confrontation as a therapeutic technique in communication with an assigned client?

1. When a good relationship exists and client's anxiety level is low
2. During periods when client is noncompliant
3. After client has had time to reflect on his or her behavior
4. Immediately after a negative behavior has occurred

6 Which teaching strategy should the nurse choose as being most likely to be effective when providing health instruction to an adolescent client?

1. Lecture format
2. Professionally made videos
3. Client contracting
4. Role-play

7 A nurse is evaluating a client's ability to change the surgical dressing before discharge. During the demonstration, the nurse notices the client has not performed the procedure correctly. What is the most appropriate action of the nurse at this time?

1. Immediately change dressing again to demonstrate correct technique.
2. Praise client for aspects of the procedure done accurately and correct the client's mistakes.
3. Praise client for steps completed correctly and refer the client to home care for follow-up.
4. Explain kindly that the procedure was performed incorrectly and have client repeat the procedure.

8 When beginning to present information about heart disease to a newly diagnosed client, what is most important for the nurse to do first?

1. Find out what client knows or has heard about the disorder.
2. Consult with healthcare provider to determine content based on individual severity of disease.
3. Have family member or significant other present who can reinforce diet and exercise tips.
4. Proceed from simple to complex concepts when discussing pathophysiology.

9 During a nursing assessment of an older adult female client, the nurse would enhance communication by taking which action?

1. Speaking loudly and using many gestures
2. Interviewing client quickly to conserve the client's energy
3. Interviewing client with family present to verify responses to questions
4. Restating terms or phrases in different ways if the client does not understand

10. Which statement by the nurse best encourages a client to express feelings and allows the nurse to genuinely respond to those feelings?

1. "You mentioned that you broke your leg last year. Can you tell me more about how that happened?"
2. "You shared with me much information about your history of depression. It sounds as if medication alone may not be controlling your symptoms as you hoped."
3. "You said your back pain has not gone away since surgery. How difficult has it been to adapt to having pain during everyday activities?"
4. "You said you have had asthma since you were 11 years old and that medication therapy requires adjustment every 8 to 10 months or so. Is that right?"

11. What would be the best approach for a nurse to use to encourage a client with psychological distress to develop an awareness of feelings and express them effectively?

1. Challenge the client.
2. Offer reassurance.
3. Suggest coping strategies.
4. Offer empathy.

12. While talking with the nurse, a client says, "You are just like my mother; you don't trust me or like me. You and she wish I were dead." The nurse interprets this statement as indicating which process?

1. Psychosis
2. Countertransference
3. Transference
4. Projection

13. The nurse is preparing to explain an upcoming procedure to a 72-year-old, English-speaking Latino client. The nurse determines that which approach is best to communicate verbally with this client?

1. Speak quickly and avoid eye contact, which could be perceived as threatening.
2. Speak slowly and provide brief and simple explanations.
3. Get an interpreter or family member to interpret for the nurse as needed.
4. Give very complete explanations of all information.

14. The nurse observes a client who is fidgeting, wringing the hands, and has body tenseness and a wrinkled brow. What is the best response to the client by the nurse?

1. "You look tense. Can you tell me if something is making you afraid or nervous?"
2. "You look upset. Would you like some medication to help you become more calm?"
3. "You look worried. Is something bothering you?"
4. "Why are you so nervous and jumpy?"

15. A nurse floating to the surgical nursing unit learns during intershift report that a client suffered disfiguring injuries in an accident a week ago. What is the best way for the nurse to prepare for the first encounter with this client?

1. Learn about client's support systems (family, friends, religion).
2. Obtain specifics of the disfigurement to better control first reactions by the nurse.
3. Review all medications and treatment procedures prior to meeting the client.
4. Have all supplies and equipment ready to be able to provide efficient care.

16. The nurse enters a client's room to obtain an admission history, moves the chair to the top of the bed by the client's head, and sits down to better hear the client. The client draws back and moves to the opposite side of the bed. What is the best response by the nurse?

1. Move the chair a foot or two away from the bed and observe the client's response.
2. Say, "I will come back later when you are ready to talk to me."
3. Ignore the behavior and continue with the interview, observing the client for depression.
4. Lean over and touch the client to convey reassurance.

17 The nurse, who has a heavy work assignment for the shift due to high client census, sees that a client is crying. What would be the best way for the nurse to convey a willingness to be with the client for support?

1. State, "Let's talk while I change your colostomy bag."
2. Ask, "Would you like to talk?" from the doorway, and go in if the client says yes.
3. Pull up a chair, sit down, and state, "I see something is bothering you. Do you want to talk?"
4. State, "I'll be back later and we can talk about what is troubling you at the moment."

18 A client asks about a new diagnostic test with which the nurse is unfamiliar. What is the best response by the nurse?

1. "I don't know much about that procedure, but I will find out and bring you information about it."
2. "The technicians in the radiology department will explain the procedure to you when you go for the test."
3. "It is your healthcare provider's responsibility to explain the procedure. Would you like me to telephone your provider?"
4. "I can't explain that now, but I'll get back to you later after all the morning medications are distributed."

19 A client can understand only minimal English, and no interpreter is available. What alternative measures can the nurse use to enhance communication?

1. Speak loudly to the client.
2. Provide a paper and pencil to write questions and information.
3. Use pictures and nonverbal cues to communicate.
4. Speak more slowly and face the client.

20 A client has been on the nursing unit for a few weeks because of surgical complications requiring extensive wound care. During the last dressing change before discharge to home with home health services, the client becomes angry with the nurse and says, "You don't have to be so careful. I'm being sent home anyway!" Which response by the nurse would be therapeutic? Select all that apply.

1. "I hear frustration or perhaps anger in your voice. Can you tell me more about how you are feeling right now?"
2. "Many people who have been in the hospital for an extended period have mixed feelings about going home. Can you tell me how you are feeling about discharge?"
3. "It sounds as though you are nervous about going home, but the wound care nurse who will see you also uses excellent technique. I'm sure your wound will continue to heal."
4. "Just because you are going home doesn't mean that your wound doesn't still require strict technique during a dressing change. Do you have any questions about your wound care after discharge?"
5. "Do you have any concerns about what will happen after discharge that you would like to talk about?"

ANSWERS & RATIONALES

1 **Answer: 2 Rationale:** It is important for the nurse to listen to the feedback given by the client to ensure the message sent was the message received. Repetition is important in the teaching process but does not evaluate clients' understanding. Asking another nurse to verify teaching is unnecessary. Referral to a nutritionist is not necessary as part of evaluation of nursing instruction. **Cognitive Level:** Applying **Client Need:** Psychosocial Integrity **Integrated Process:** Communication and Documentation **Content Area:** Fundamentals **Strategy:** The core issue of the question is determining the client response to teaching. In evaluation questions such as these, the correct option is likely to be one that focuses directly on the client.

2 **Answer: 2 Rationale:** To evaluate an unresponsive client's ability to communicate, it is best for the nurse to ask questions that will elicit a single act or response by the client. Asking open-ended questions is not appropriate for the client's condition. Facial grimacing may occur during neurological assessment in response to unpleasant stimuli. Assessing for response to pain may be noted during neurological assessment but does not relate to communication. **Cognitive Level:** Analyzing **Client Need:** Psychosocial Integrity **Integrated Process:** Communication and Documentation **Content Area:** Fundamentals **Strategy:** In communication questions such as these, the correct option is client-focused and relates directly to communication. With this in mind, eliminate facial grimaces and painful stimuli immediately, and choose the option to blink because of its simplicity.

3 **Answer: 3 Rationale:** A client who is blind does not have the benefit of nonverbal cues to facilitate communication and understanding of the environment. It is important for the nurse to explain physical surroundings and noises because

the client cannot determine these without the added benefit of sight. Speaking slowly and in a low-pitched voice while facing the client is useful when communicating with a client who has hearing impairment. Placing a sign on the client's door regarding blindness encroaches on the client's right to privacy. Giving simple explanations is a useful approach when speaking with a client who is hearing impaired. **Cognitive Level:** Analyzing **Client Need:** Psychosocial Integrity **Integrated Process:** Communication and Documentation **Content Area:** Fundamentals **Strategy:** In communication questions with a client who has loss of vision, the correct option is one that supplements vision impairment with verbal communication. Note the critical word *best* in the stem of the question, which indicates more than one response may be partially or totally correct.

4 **Answer: 4 Rationale:** A return demonstration specifically identifies the client's ability to perform a skill. The success of the return demonstration may or may not affect the number of home visits that will be required, depending on the client's overall health status. Other support services that the client may need would be determined by a systematic assessment of the client's ability to perform direct and indirect activities of daily living. The client's skill level may be influenced by the quality of the teaching plan but this is not the primary reason for return demonstration of a skill. **Cognitive Level:** Analyzing **Client Need:** Psychosocial Integrity **Integrated Process:** Communication and Documentation **Content Area:** Fundamentals **Strategy:** Recall that to evaluate learning of a skill, which is in the psychomotor domain, the best option is the one that utilizes return demonstration. In this way, the nurse can verify that the client can perform the skill and also has an opportunity to provide additional feedback.

5 **Answer: 1 Rationale:** Confrontation should not be used as a therapeutic communication technique unless trust has been established in the nurse–client relationship. Because confrontation can be uncomfortable for the client, it is important for the nurse and client to have a trusting relationship as a foundation. The nurse should assess for barriers to a client's noncompliance with a therapeutic plan of care, rather than being confrontational. Client reflection does not necessarily indicate that confrontation would be a timely technique to use. The nurse might like to use confrontation after a negative behavior has occurred but this would not be the appropriate time for this communication technique. **Cognitive Level:** Applying **Client Need:** Psychosocial Integrity **Integrated Process:** Communication and Documentation **Content Area:** Fundamentals **Strategy:** Note the critical words *most appropriate* in the stem of the question. This tells you that more than one option will be plausible and that you must choose one over the others based on what is most therapeutic for the client.

6 **Answer: 3 Rationale:** Client contracting provides adolescents with the ability to be involved in their care. Adolescents should be involved in planning and decision making regarding their need for information about their own health issues. A lecture format does not allow opportunity for feedback or involvement. Viewing a video may be visually interesting but is not designed for interactivity or feedback. Role-play may be a useful strategy in selected instances if the client is learning new ways of interacting with others, but it is not a strategy that would be widely applicable. **Cognitive Level:** Analyzing **Client Need:** Psychosocial Integrity **Integrated Process:** Communication and Documentation **Content Area:** Fundamentals **Strategy:** In teaching and learning questions in which communication is key, choose the option that provides for two-way communication between the client and nurse. Note the critical words *most likely to be effective* in the stem of the question, which tells you that more than one option is plausible and that you must choose based on knowledge of communication theory.

7 **Answer: 2 Rationale:** Praising the client for steps performed correctly provides positive reinforcement. In addition, explaining the client's mistakes reinforces the correct way to perform the procedure. Redoing the dressing decreases the client's confidence and is not useful. Praising the client without correcting the mistakes gives feedback that the procedure was done correctly. Having the client repeat the procedure and stating it was done correctly without further guidance does not reinforce or assist learning. **Cognitive Level:** Analyzing **Client Need:** Psychosocial Integrity **Integrated Process:** Communication and Documentation **Content Area:** Fundamentals **Strategy:** Note the critical words *most appropriate* in the stem of the question. This tells you that more than one option is plausible and that you must choose based on knowledge of communication theory.

8 **Answer: 1 Rationale:** When presenting information to a client, it is important that the nurse find out what the client already knows, and then build on existing knowledge. It is not necessary to consult with a healthcare provider. It may be helpful to have family members present, but it is not the priority at the time of initial teaching. It is important when teaching to begin with basic concepts and progress to the complex after determining current client knowledge. **Cognitive Level:** Analyzing **Client Need:** Psychosocial Integrity **Integrated Process:** Communication and Documentation **Content Area:** Fundamentals **Strategy:** Focus on the critical word *first* in the stem of the question. This indicates that more than one option may be correct and that a time sequence is involved. Recalling that assessment is the first step of the nursing process, choose an option that assesses the client's current level of knowledge before beginning instruction.

9 **Answer: 4 Rationale:** Restating the information using different words or phrases as needed may assist the older adult client's understanding. Increasing speech volume is unnecessary and the use of gestures is helpful only if the client has a hearing deficit. Older adults do better with a slower-paced interview with frequent breaks to decrease fatigue. Relying on family to verify responses is not respectful of the older adult's autonomy. **Cognitive Level:** Applying **Client Need:** Psychosocial Integrity **Integrated Process:** Communication and Documentation **Content Area:** Fundamentals **Strategy:** The core issue of the question is how to communicate most effectively with an older adult client. The correct option is the one that focuses on the client, incorporates age-related needs, and does not incorporate ageism into the response.

10 **Answer: 3 Rationale:** The communication technique of reflection occurs when the nurse directs feelings and questions back to the client to encourage elaboration. The nurse uses the technique of focusing by asking questions to help the client focus on a specific area of concern. With the use of summarizing, the nurse highlights important points of the conversation. The nurse uses restating by repeating back to clients the main points or content of the conversation. **Cognitive Level:** Analyzing **Client Need:** Psychosocial Integrity **Integrated Process:** Communication and Documentation **Content Area:** Fundamentals **Strategy:** The core issue of the

question is knowledge of various types of therapeutic techniques, specifically one that utilizes reflection as a means of encouraging continued communication. Use this knowledge and the process of elimination to make a selection.

11 **Answer: 4 Rationale:** Empathy is the ability of the nurse to see the client's perception of the world, which aids in therapeutic communication and the nurse–client relationship. Challenging clients is not helpful and often triggers them to defend themselves from what appears to be an attack by the nurse. False reassurance can be seen as a way to encourage clients how to feel and ignores their distress. Advising occurs when the nurse tells clients what to do, preventing them from exploring problems and using the problem-solving process to find solutions. **Cognitive Level:** Applying **Client Need:** Psychosocial Integrity **Integrated Process:** Communication and Documentation **Content Area:** Fundamentals **Strategy:** The core issue of the question is knowledge of the purpose and use of therapeutic communication techniques. Use this knowledge and the process of elimination to make a selection.

12 **Answer: 3 Rationale:** Transference is the unconscious process of displaying feelings for significant people in the client's past onto the nurse in the present relationship. Psychosis is a state in which a client is unable to comprehend reality and has difficulty relating to others. Countertransference is the nurse's emotional reaction to clients based on feelings for significant people in the nurse's past. Projection is a defense mechanism in which blame for unacceptable desires, thoughts, shortcomings, and mistakes is attached to others in the environment. **Cognitive Level:** Analyzing **Client Need:** Psychosocial Integrity **Integrated Process:** Communication and Documentation **Content Area:** Fundamentals **Strategy:** The core issue of the question is knowledge of various processes that can occur during therapeutic communication. Eliminate psychosis (a disorder) and projection (a defense mechanism) first. Choose transference over countertransferance because it is the client who has made the transference, not the nurse.

13 **Answer: 2 Rationale:** Taking into account the age and ethnicity of the client, it is helpful to speak slowly and provide short and simple explanations. Speaking quickly does not help the client understand the information presented. Eye contact is acceptable. There is no need for an interpreter based on the information in the question. Simple explanations are more effective than lengthy ones. **Cognitive Level:** Applying **Client Need:** Psychosocial Integrity **Integrated Process:** Communication and Documentation **Content Area:** Fundamentals **Strategy:** Note that some options have more than one part to them. In such questions, all parts must be correct for the option to be correct. Eliminate incorrect options using principles of therapeutic communication and information presented in the question.

14 **Answer: 1 Rationale:** After noting the client's nonverbal behavior, the best response is one that will elicit further data from the client, which is accomplished by providing a broad opening for the client. Asking whether the client would like medication to become calm places a judgment on the client's behavior. By asking, "Is something bothering you?" after acknowledging the client's feelings, the nurse risks placing the client on the defensive. Asking a question using the word "why" is a block to communication and likely to make the client defensive. **Cognitive Level:** Analyzing **Client Need:** Psychosocial Integrity **Integrated Process:** Communication and Documentation **Content Area:** Fundamentals **Strategy:** The core issue of the question is how to apply general principles of therapeutic communication. In this question, the correct option is the one that is nonjudgmental, uses therapeutic communication techniques, and avoids communication blocks.

15 **Answer: 2 Rationale:** The nurse is more likely to exhibit therapeutic verbal and nonverbal communication by being aware of the extent of the client's disfiguring injuries. This will reduce the likelihood of surprise that can be seen in nonverbal behavior. Learning about clients' support systems (family, friends, religion) is a general nursing action that is not specific to this client. Reviewing all medications and treatment procedures should be done before caring for any client. Having equipment and supplies ready assists the nurse to provide efficient care, but does not prepare the nurse for the first interaction with this client. **Cognitive Level:** Analyzing **Client Need:** Psychosocial Integrity **Integrated Process:** Communication and Documentation **Content Area:** Fundamentals **Strategy:** The critical phrases in the stem of the question are *best way* and *first encounter*. The phrase *best way* indicates that more than one option is a true statement and more than one option may compete for priority. The phrase *first encounter* assists you to focus on the real core issue of the question, which relates to communication.

16 **Answer: 1 Rationale:** The client may have a need for increased personal space, which may account for moving to the other side of the bed. However, cultural considerations cannot be ruled out by the information in this stem. Thus, the correct action is to validate the reason for the client's behavior. This is what moving the chair represents, an attempt to determine whether increased need for personal space is the reason for the behavior. Leaving the client punishes the client for the behavior. Ignoring the behavior is inappropriate because it does not acknowledge an unspoken need by the client. Touching the client would further invade personal space and is inappropriate until further data is gathered. **Cognitive Level:** Analyzing **Client Need:** Psychosocial Integrity **Integrated Process:** Communication and Documentation **Content Area:** Fundamentals **Strategy:** The core issue of the question is how to respond to a client's nonverbal behavior in a therapeutic manner. Eliminate options that are nontherapeutic or that could worsen the situation.

17 **Answer: 1 Rationale:** The nurse has two competing priorities: the need to accomplish work on a busy shift and the need to address the psychosocial needs of a client in distress. Talking while working takes into consideration both of these factors. Asking a question from the doorway creates psychological as well as physical distance between the nurse and the client. Immediately sitting down ignores the other workload of the nurse. Stating the nurse will come back later puts the client's feelings on hold. **Cognitive Level:** Analyzing **Client Need:** Psychosocial Integrity **Integrated Process:** Communication and Documentation **Content Area:** Fundamentals **Strategy:** The core issue of the question is the most therapeutic response to a client in distress. Note that the question also contains the critical words *best way*, which implies that the options will have greater or lesser degrees of correctness and that you must choose between them. Use the process of elimination and choose the option that takes into account all of the relevant information in the stem of the question.

18 **Answer: 1 Rationale:** Stating lack of knowledge and intent to find out demonstrates honesty and openness between the

client and the nurse. It also addresses the client's need for information. Deferring the client's questions to personnel in the radiology department puts the client's information needs on hold. Deferring the client's questions to the healthcare provider is not a candid response by the nurse. Putting off a response until after medications are distributed implies that the client's questions are less important to the nurse than other care activities. **Cognitive Level:** Analyzing **Client Need:** Psychosocial Integrity **Integrated Process:** Communication and Documentation **Content Area:** Fundamentals **Strategy:** The correct answer to communication questions is the one that best acknowledges the client and utilizes therapeutic communication techniques. First eliminate options that are similar by putting the client's request on hold and divert the responsibility to someone else. Next eliminate the option that is not a totally candid response. Alternatively, choose correctly by selecting the response that incorporates all the information in the question regarding the nurse's level of knowledge and the client's need to know.

19 **Answer: 3 Rationale:** Because the client does not speak English, the nurse must utilize nonverbal communication. With this in mind, use of pictures and nonverbal cues takes this need into account. Speaking loudly or more slowly while facing the client are helpful when client is hearing impaired. Using paper and pencil would be useful for the aphasic client who has use of the dominant hand, such as after a CVA. **Cognitive Level:** Applying **Client Need:** Psychosocial Integrity **Integrated Process:** Communication and Documentation **Content Area:** Fundamentals **Strategy:** The core issue of the question is the best method for communicating with a client when there is a language barrier. Eliminate the options that are similar with respect to the spoken word. Eliminate the option that also relies on words that may not be in the client's vocabulary.

20 **Answer: 1, 2, 5 Rationale:** The correct answers to communication questions are those that utilize therapeutic communication techniques and avoid communication blocks. Options that focus on the client's feelings utilize these techniques, while incorrect options use the communication blocks of false reassurance and challenging the client. **Cognitive Level:** Analyzing **Client Need:** Psychosocial Integrity **Integrated Process:** Communication and Documentation **Content Area:** Fundamentals **Strategy:** Analyze each statement in terms of being a communication enhancer or blocker. Choose the ones that incorporate therapeutic communication techniques without having any components of communication blocks.

Key Terms to Review

References

Berman, A., Snyder, S., & Frandsen, G. (2016). *Kozier & Erb's fundamentals of nursing: Concepts, process, and practice* (10th ed.). New York, NY: Pearson Education.

Craven, R., & Hirnle, C., & Henshaw, C. (2017). *Fundamentals of nursing: Human health and function* (8th ed.). Philadelphia: Wolters-Kluwer.

Potter, P., Perry, A., Stockert, P., Hall, A. (2017). *Fundamentals of nursing* (9th ed.). St. Louis, MO: Mosby.

19 Culturally Relevant Care

In this chapter

Cross Reference

Other chapters relevant to this content area are

Reproduction, Family Planning, and Infertility	Chapter 8
Uncomplicated Antenatal Assessment and Care	Chapter 9
Uncomplicated Postpartum Assessment and Care	Chapter 11
Alternative and Complementary Therapies	Chapter 28
Blood and Blood Component Therapy	Chapter 32

I. CULTURALLY RELEVANT CARE OVERVIEW

A. *Culture* defined

1. A complex whole, encompassing knowledge, beliefs, values, practices, customs, and any habits acquired by members of society
2. Represents ways of perceiving, behaving, and evaluating world

B. Culture and nursing care

1. Leininger's *theory of culture care diversity and universality* includes concepts of culture care delineated as preservation/maintenance, accommodation/negotiation, and repatterning/restructuring
2. The *health traditions model* explores what one does to maintain, protect, and restore health (physical, mental, and spiritual) within a framework of one's ethnoreligious cultural heritage

NCLEX®

3. Cultural phenomena that can affect health include environmental control (health practices and remedies), biological variations (physical and genetic), social organization (holidays, special events such as births and funerals), communication (greetings, gestures, smiling, eye contact), personal space (body language and distance), and time orientation (punctuality, announced versus surprise visits from family and friends)
4. Prerequisites to delivering culturally competent care are understanding one's personal cultural values and health beliefs, being respectful and understanding of client's culture, and becoming familiar with health beliefs and practices held by commonly encountered groups in healthcare agency's service area

NCLEX®

5. Use purposeful strategies to aid communication with clients of various cultures
   a. Assess fluency in English and make arrangements for an interpreter if needed; speak directly to client even if using an interpreter
   b. Use language that is free of slang or currently popular jargon; use simple, straightforward sentences or questions and rephrase if client does not understand

c. Be attentive to body language that might offend client
d. Learn and follow how client wishes to be addressed
e. Provide an environment for communication that respects habits regarding eye contact and amount of personal space
f. Prior to giving written health teaching materials, even if written in client's primary language, assess reading ability; health literacy can affect ability to learn health information regardless of cultural background

6. Religious laws may influence dietary practices, which in turn may influence nursing care during illness (see Table 19–1); common restrictions include pork and alcohol; fasting may be done on certain religious holidays; children, pregnant women, and those who are ill are usually exempt from fasting
7. Religious beliefs may also influence views on health-related issues and events (see Table 19–2)
8. Culturally based dietary preferences are lifelong habits and can significantly influence health as well as compliance with medically recommended dietary changes (see Table 19–3)
9. Cultural beliefs about maintaining or restoring health may clash with those of healthcare provider; remain nonjudgmental and work with client to incorporate client's cultural health practices while assisting client to meet health goals
10. Avoid generalizing and **stereotyping** (an expectation that all people within same ethnic or cultural group are alike and share same beliefs and attitudes)

Table 19–1 Dietary Practices of Selected Religions

Religion	Dietary Restrictions or Practices
Orthodox Judaism	Kosher dietary laws allow fish that have scales and fins, cloven-hoofed animals, and animals that eat vegetables or are ritually slaughtered. Milk and meat may not be combined in any way. Fasting during Yom Kippur (24 hours). Pregnant women, children, and those who are ill do not need to fast. During Passover, only unleavened bread may be eaten.
Roman Catholicism	Meat is prohibited on Ash Wednesday and Fridays during Lent. Fasting is done on Ash Wednesday and Good Friday, is optional during rest of Lent. Fasting is not required for children, pregnant women, and those who are ill.
Eastern Orthodox	Meat and dairy products are prohibited on Wednesdays, Fridays, and during Lent. Fasting occurs during Advent. Fasting is not required for pregnant women and those who are ill; some children may also be exempt.
Buddhism	Vegetarianism for some sects, often lacto-ovo-vegetarian diet. Some eat fish; others avoid beef only. Alcohol and drug use is not favored.
Hinduism	Vegetarianism for some; beef and veal prohibited for all. Fasting rituals vary depending on god worshiped. Children do not fast.
Islam	Prohibited meats include pork, birds of prey, and meats not slaughtered as part of ritual. Drug and alcohol use prohibited. Fasting occurs during daylight hours during month of Ramadan; pregnant women and selected others may be exempt from fasting.
Jehovah's Witness	Meats that are allowed have been drained of blood; no foods to which blood has been added are allowed.
Church of Jesus Christ of Latter Day Saints (Mormon)	Alcohol and sources of caffeine (coffee and tea) are often prohibited. There is limited consumption of meat. Fasting is optional on the first Sunday of the month.
Pentecostal (Assembly of God)	No foods to which blood has been added are allowed. Some avoid pork. Alcohol is often prohibited.
Seventh-Day Adventist (Church of God)	Ingestion of alcohol and caffeinated beverages is not allowed. Dietary moderation is practiced; meals are spaced at least 5 hours apart with no snacking between meals. Those who eat meat avoid pork; many are lacto-ovo-vegetarians.

Table 19–2 Religious Influence on Common Health Issues and Events

Religion	Abortion	Autopsy	Birth Control	Blood/Blood Products	Medication Use	Organ Donation
Baha'i	Not allowed	Allowed with medical or legal need	Allowed	Allowed	Narcotics with prescription; vaccines allowed	Allowed
Buddhist	Mother's condition determines	Allowed	Allowed	Allowed	Allowed	Act of mercy
Roman Catholic	Not allowed	Allowed	Natural means only	Allowed	Use if benefits outweigh risks	Allowed
Christian Science	Not allowed	Not usual; family decides	Allowed	Usually not used	None except vaccines to comply with law	Individual choice
Hindu	No policy	Allowed	Allowed	Allowed	Allowed	Allowed
Islam	Not allowed	Allowed with medical or legal need	Allowed	Allowed	Allowed	Controversial; discuss with family
Jehovah's Witness	Not allowed	Allowed with legal need	Allowed except for sterilization	Forbidden	Allowed unless derived from blood products	Forbidden
Judaism	Therapeutic allowed, otherwise varies within groups	Allowed under some conditions; all body parts buried together	Allowed except for Orthodox Jews	Allowed	Allowed	Complex issue; consult rabbi
Mennonite	Therapeutic only	Allowed	Allowed	Allowed	Allowed	Allowed
Mormon	Not allowed	Allowed with next of kin consent	Incompatible with beliefs	Allowed	Allowed	Allowed
Seventh-Day Adventist	Therapeutic only	Allowed	Allowed	Allowed	Allowed	Allowed
Unitarian/ Universalist	Allowed	Recommended	Allowed	Allowed	Allowed	Allowed

Table 19–3 Preferred Foods of Various Cultures

Cultural Group	Preferred Foods
Mexican Americans	Corn, dried beans, and chili peppers are basic foods. Tortillas are used for bread (corn, sometimes wheat). Relatively small amounts of meat are used. Fruits such as papaya and mango are used in varying amounts (based on availability and price).
Hispanic/Latino Americans	Similar food pattern to Mexican diet. Rice and beans are basic foods. Dried codfish is a staple, but meat, milk, green and yellow vegetables are used less often. Viandas (starchy vegetables and fruits such as plantains and green bananas) are used, but other fruits are used in limited amounts.
Native American and Alaska Natives	Variable depending on region and local crops or game. Fish (Alaskan) and meat (Navajo), including game, chicken, pork, mutton are daily staples. Other staples are bread (tortillas or fry bread, blue corn bread, cornmeal mush), eggs, vegetables (corn, potatoes, green beans, tomatoes), and some fruit.
African Americans	Breads and cereals include biscuits, cornmeal mush or muffins or cornbread, cooked cereals with corn and oats. Eggs and cheese are used, but milk is not as popular (perhaps because lactose intolerance has greater prevalence). Preferred vegetables include leafy greens, okra, sweet potatoes, potatoes, corn, and a variety of beans, often served with rice. Pork, poultry, fish, and organ meats are often more popular than beef. Fried foods are popular.
Asian Americans	Varies to some extent based on region. Chinese: rice, vegetables cooked in wok, eggs, soybean products (tofu), small amounts of meat, green tea Japanese: rice, soy products, and green tea (similar to Chinese); seafood, sushi, steamed vegetables, fresh fruit Southeast Asian: rice, fresh fruits and vegetables, seafood, chicken, duck, pork, nuts, and legumes
European Americans	Varies somewhat by country of origin but tends to include more red meat and carbohydrates as well as vegetables and fruits.

II. CULTURAL CONSIDERATIONS FOR AFRICAN AMERICANS

NCLEX®

A. Communication and personal space

1. African Americans live in United States but have ancestral origins in any African country
2. English is primary language; may use African American Vernacular English (AAVE)
3. Prolonged direct eye contact may be considered inappropriate (aggressive or rude)
4. May use oculistics (eye rolling) or silence in response to communications deemed inappropriate
5. Verbal and nonverbal communication is integral in communication process
6. Close personal space may be shared with family and friends during interactions

B. Time orientation

1. Varies with age, subculture, and socioeconomic status; members may be past, present, or future oriented
2. May not be punctual for appointments if needs of family or friends require immediate attention

C. Social roles

1. Extended family is important; tend to have large family support systems
2. Strong sense of obligation to relatives and friendships are valued
3. Many single-parent families, typically headed by females
4. Religious affiliation is common; tend to be part of social and/or religious organizations within local community

NCLEX®

D. Views of health and illness

1. Body, mind, and spirit are integrated
2. Religious beliefs influence ideas about health and illness
3. Illness may be a punishment from God or related to one's harmony with nature
4. Emotional or personal problems can be resolved through use of a spiritualist who is called by God to heal
5. Voodoo may be considered a powerful cultural healer
6. Practitioners who use roots, herbs, oils, candles, and ointments may be used in healing process

E. Health risks

1. Lactose intolerance and lactase deficiency
2. Hypertension and coronary heart disease
3. Obesity
4. Sickle-cell anemia
5. Cancers, including breast, colorectal, esophageal, stomach, cervical, uterine, and prostate
6. Diabetes mellitus

NCLEX®

F. Nursing considerations

1. Include family in medical care if desired by client
2. Allow for flexibility in scheduling appointments
3. Be open to use of herbs, prayer, and laying-on of hands as complementary healing therapies
4. Encourage family to bring traditional diet if medically acceptable

III. CULTURAL CONSIDERATIONS FOR ASIAN AMERICANS

NCLEX®

A. Communication and personal space

1. Because Asian Americans have ancestral origins in China, Japan, Vietnam, Korea, and the Philippines, primary languages (other than English) include Chinese, Japanese, Vietnamese, Korean, and Filipino
2. May use silence to demonstrate respect for elders
3. If direct eye contact is considered impolite or aggressive, may look away as nurse attempts to make direct eye contact
4. Unlikely to criticize or disagree with others verbally; consider word "no" to be disrespectful
5. Nodding head or smiling does not always mean agreement
6. Personal space is valued but may be shared with family and close friends
7. Touching does not occur during conversation and may be unacceptable in some groups between members of opposite sex; touching on head may be considered disrespectful

B. Time orientation: tend to be present oriented while highly regarding past

C. Social roles

1. Family bonds are important; large extended family networks exist with devotion to tradition and respect for aging members
2. Daughters and daughters-in-law may be expected to care for older family members as their health declines
3. Structured and hierarchical family unit, with men having power and authority; women are expected to be subservient to men

4. Loyalty to family members is expected and highly regarded
5. Education is highly valued
6. Religious affiliation common, including Taoism, Islam, Buddhism, Hinduism, Confucianism, Shintoism, Islam, and Christianity

NCLEX® **D. Views of health and illness**

1. Health results from harmony with nature, both physically and spiritually, and from balance between yin and yang (positive and negative energy forces)
2. Illness is a state of disharmony or imbalance of yin and yang
3. Foods are associated with concept of yin and yang; for example, yin foods are cold, whereas yang foods are hot; cold foods and beverages are consumed for hot illnesses, and hot food and beverages are consumed for cold illnesses
4. Illnesses may be attributed to overexertion or to prolonged sitting or lying

E. Health risks

1. Thalassemia
2. Lactase deficiency (lactose intolerance)
3. G6PD deficiency
4. Hypertension
5. Cancer, with stomach and liver more common sites

NCLEX® **F. Nursing considerations**

1. Clients might be quiet and compliant during illness, thus placing them at risk for not having needs met
2. Clients may wish to take medications with certain foods or beverages believed to promote correct balance for health
3. Clients may not trust healthcare providers and wish to include traditional healers along with Western medicine practices
4. Limit eye contact and request permission before physically touching client; touch a client's head only with permission from client or parent
5. Encourage and facilitate family involvement in care
6. Female clients may prefer female care providers
7. Complementary therapies such as acupuncture, massage, and herbal remedies are widely used

IV. CULTURAL CONSIDERATIONS FOR LATINO/HISPANIC AMERICANS

NCLEX® **A. Communication and personal space**

1. Latino or Hispanic Americans have origins in Cuba, Puerto Rico, Central America, and upper South America; primary languages include Spanish, Portuguese, and English
2. *Simpatia*, a desire for smooth or harmonious interpersonal relationships, is demonstrated by courtesy, respect, and absence of critical or confrontational behavior; confrontational interaction is avoided
3. In nurse–client relationship, eye contact may be expected of nurse, although client may avoid eye contact to signal respect and attentiveness when interacting with people having authority
4. Tend to be verbally expressive; use of gestures and facial expressions are important as forms of nonverbal communication during assessment and care
5. May engage in "small talk" or general conversation as a method of establishing rapport
6. May be comfortable sharing personal space with family, friends, and acquaintances; may use handshakes and embraces freely (tactile communication); tend to value physical presence of others

B. Time orientation: tend to be present oriented, but varies according to age, subculture, and socioeconomic status

C. Social roles

1. Family is most valued institution and is a primary source of personal identification
2. Both nuclear families and large extended family networks are common
3. Father is likely to assume head of household role and may make decisions for family depending on age and other factors
4. Collective family needs tend to take priority over individual family member needs
5. Religion is important; Catholicism is prevalent but may vary depending on geographic origin
6. Tend to be part of social organizations within local community

NCLEX® **D. Views of health and illness**

1. Health may be viewed as a gift from God or the result of good fortune; illness may be viewed by some as punishment for past actions
2. *Curanderos*, folk healers, may be consulted

3. Health may represent a state of equilibrium in world, which is characterized by balance of hot, cold, wet, and dry; when an imbalance exists, treatment focuses on application of opposite quality

E. Health risks

1. Diabetes mellitus
2. Hypertension and heart disease
3. Obesity
4. Pernicious anemia
5. Parasite infections

NCLEX® **F. Nursing considerations**

1. Clients may seek guidance from within family network rather than from healthcare providers; include family members in health-related discussions when appropriate
2. Male family member may be decision maker for client
3. Modesty is important, and measures should be taken to protect clients' privacy at all times; clients may prefer to have a healthcare provider of same gender
4. Use of alternative therapies is prevalent and should be explored when client enters healthcare system; if possible, facilitate continuation of such services, which may include herbs, use of hot and cold foods, prayer, use of religious artifacts (such as medals), and consultation with folk healers
5. It is important to request permission before touching children during assessment or care; touching a child while looking at child is believed by some to prevent "mal de ojo" or "evil eye" that could result from looking at child
6. Encourage family to bring traditional diet if medically acceptable

V. CULTURAL CONSIDERATIONS FOR INDIGENOUS PEOPLES

NCLEX® **A. Communication**

1. Indigenous peoples include American Indians, Alaskan natives (Eskimos/Aleuts), Hawaiian Islanders, and in Canada they include Canadian Indians (First Nations), Metis, and Inuit; native languages vary widely among subgroups; official languages include English (United States and Canada) or French (Canada)
2. Words may be spoken using low tone of voice; body language may also be important
3. May appear silent and reserved upon meeting strangers; when shaking hands, may tend to extend a hand and lightly touch hand of person they are greeting
4. May expect others to listen attentively during communication
5. Eye contact may be a sign of disrespect for some groups
6. Maintaining personal space is important

B. Time orientation

1. Time exists in a three-point range, including past, present, and future
2. Viewed as being primarily present oriented, with some members being both past and present oriented

C. Social roles

1. Family oriented, with biological family being central social organization; family members work collaboratively to ensure success of family unit
2. Family includes all members of extended family
3. Grandparents may be considered family leaders in some groups; elders are respected and honored
4. Male family members work outside home and may make decisions for family; females tend to be responsible for domestic activities
5. Extended family may care for hospitalized relative for duration of hospital stay
6. Many groups practice some form of Christianity, and for others, religion may be guided by sacred myths and legends

NCLEX® **D. Views of health and illness**

1. Desire to be in harmony with environment and family
2. Health is not limited to body; includes harmony with family, environment, livestock, supernatural forces, and community
3. Health and religion are considered to be connected; healing ceremonies are common; magic, religion, and folk medicine may all be used for healing; healers may be men or women

E. Health risks

1. Alcohol abuse and chronic liver disease
2. Obesity
3. Arthritis
4. Chronic lower respiratory diseases and tuberculosis

5. Diabetes mellitus
6. Hypertension and heart disease
7. Lactose intolerance
8. Malnutrition secondary to high rates of poverty
9. Increased risk of suicide

NCLEX®

F. Nursing considerations

1. Because of wide variation among individuals and subgroups, assess each client's preferences carefully
2. Respect client's desire to be in harmony with environment whenever possible
3. Incorporate complementary modalities into client's plan of care when possible, including herbs and use of healers from own cultural group
4. Encourage active participation of family in client's care
5. Encourage family to bring personal items of client to hospital to personalize space
6. Perform home assessment including availability of running water; modify care practices and health teaching as appropriate

VI. CULTURAL CONSIDERATIONS FOR WHITE/EUROPEAN AMERICANS

A. Communication and personal space

1. English is primary language but often also includes a language of origin
2. Eye contact is valued and shows interest and respect
3. Body language and facial expression are important in communication process
4. Handshake is utilized for formal greetings
5. Personal space tends to be required during communication

B. Time orientation

1. Many are considered to be future oriented
2. Time is of value; adhere to schedules and time frames

C. Social roles

1. Nuclear family is predominant, although extended family plays important role
2. Religion is important, with a variety of denominations existing
3. Encourage children to develop their personal sense of identity
4. Subscribe to Protestant work ethic values, which stress importance of planning for future
5. Individual goals may take precedence over those of family

D. Views of health and illness: health is considered absence of disease or illness; utilize Western healthcare system; concept of health promotion becoming increasingly important

E. Health risks

1. Hypertension and heart disease
2. Obesity
3. Diabetes mellitus
4. A variety of cancers

F. Nursing considerations

1. Respect client's need for autonomy and personal space
2. Maintain eye contact with client
3. Include family members in healthcare decisions when appropriate and with client's approval
4. Respect a resurgence in interest in homeopathic medicine

Check Your NCLEX–RN® Exam I.Q.

You are ready for testing on this content if you can:

- Be respectful, interested in, and understanding of other cultures without being judgmental.
- Assess the impact of clients' culture or ethnicity when planning, implementing, and evaluating nursing care.
- Determine level of fluency in English and need for interpreter to aid in planning care effectively for clients with a language barrier.
- Consider client's culture when providing client teaching.
- Demonstrate cultural sensitivity when communicating with clients.
- Evaluate client understanding and acceptance of health-related recommendations.

PRACTICE TEST

1 While conducting an initial assessment of an infant, a home health nurse notices that the infant is wearing a soiled piece of braided yarn around the neck. Which action by the nurse is most appropriate?

1. Leave the yarn in place but wash it with a cloth and mild soap.
2. Ask about its significance and suggest that it be placed more safely on the body.
3. Explain that the yarn offers no benefit and ask the parents to remove it.
4. Remove the yarn because it is soiled and could lead to strangulation.

2 A Native American client who has a low-grade fever tells the nurse on the reservation that he will only use a sweat lodge to treat his illness. Which approach by the nurse would be most therapeutic?

1. Explain to the client that the sweat lodge is likely to worsen the fever.
2. Request that the healthcare provider talk to the tribe's healer.
3. Continue to monitor the client's status.
4. Ask the client's family to convince him not to use the sweat lodge.

3 A male nurse needs to check the vital signs and oxygen saturation level of a female client from a different culture. As the nurse approaches, the client moves to the other side of the bed and draws up the blanket. What is the best nursing action at this time?

1. Invite a family member to be present and to assist with the oxygen saturation reading.
2. Ask a female nurse to perform the procedures.
3. Perform the assessments without acknowledging her reaction because she will adjust over time to hospital procedures.
4. Before touching the client, explain the procedure and ask for permission to continue.

4 A nurse is caring for two clients who have had abdominal surgery. One client is of Hispanic heritage, who withdraws in pain and moans when touched. The other is a client of Asian descent, who appears calm and rarely verbalizes pain or discomfort. The nurse appropriately draws which conclusion from these observations?

1. Hispanic client is exaggerating his pain.
2. Asian client is not experiencing pain.
3. Two clients have different culturally influenced ways of coping with pain.
4. Hispanic client may be exhibiting drug-seeking behavior.

5 A hospice nurse in a small Appalachian community is caring for a client at home who is an active member of the community church. As death nears, the minister and several members of the congregation come together in the home for a "death watch." Which action by the nurse is most therapeutic?

1. Ask the minister to have church members come in scheduled time blocks to avoid overcrowding.
2. Observe client's religious beliefs and allow family and minister unlimited access to the client.
3. Allow family and three other visitors at a time to stay with the client, but keep everyone else in the next room.
4. Explain that the watch will not be a problem as long as it does not conflict with medical care.

6 A home health nurse is assigned to an Asian American client who refuses to take the blood pressure medication prescribed by the healthcare provider. The client is using acupuncture treatments and does not believe in taking pills. How can the nurse best help this client?

1. Notify healthcare provider of the client's health practices, and monitor the condition for an impending crisis.
2. Ask supervisor to transfer the client to an Asian American primary nurse.
3. Advocate for client's decision, and explain that pills may not help based on the client's beliefs.
4. Discharge client and advise client to call if he or she wishes to obtain home care services at a later date.

PRACTICE TEST

7 The nurse is checking the dietary trays that have been delivered to the nursing unit. A client of Orthodox Jewish faith has received a tray containing a chicken dinner with vegetables, tea, and a carton of 2% milk. What action by the nurse is best?

1. Instruct nursing assistant to deliver the meal tray after removing the tea.
2. Remove the chicken from the dietary tray.
3. Have dietary department replace the entire meal tray.
4. Ask client if lactose-free milk would be preferred.

8 The nurse is caring for a Native American woman who has given birth. The nurse anticipates that the couple will make which request regarding the umbilical cord?

1. Have it burned.
2. Have the blood drained from it.
3. Take it home.
4. Inspect it.

9 The nurse has taken a position in an ambulatory clinic in a Hispanic neighborhood. The nurse would use knowledge of which practices to provide culturally sensitive care to this population? Select all that apply.

1. Herbal medicines are believed to be as important as Western medicines in treating illness.
2. Mourners are likely to be hired by a family to demonstrate grief after a death.
3. Staring at a client who is a child will help to prevent or ward off the "evil eye."
4. Depending on the specific illness, hot or cold foods would be used in treatment.
5. The client may want a caregiver of the same gender to enhance privacy.

10 The nurse working with a client who immigrated from Mexico should consider during care which cultural characteristics typically associated with Mexican American culture? Select all that apply.

1. Value extended family.
2. Have patriarchal outlook.
3. Value independence and autonomy.
4. Respect authority.
5. Oppose the status quo.

11 A Chinese American client is menstruating, a condition considered to be yin (cold). The nurse anticipates which type of food would be eaten by the client who is striving to promote balance? Select all that apply.

1. Beef
2. Eggs
3. Fried foods
4. Honey
5. Broccoli

12 When teaching an in-service on culturally competent care, the nurse should explain which cultural values tend to be associated with Anglo-American culture? Select all that apply.

1. Interdependence
2. Materialism
3. Youth
4. Competition
5. Harmony

13 While realizing that all clients are unique, the nurse would tend to associate which cultural values with clients of African American descent? Select all that apply.

1. Extended family
2. Religion
3. Long-term goals
4. Interdependence
5. Seclusion

ANSWERS & RATIONALES

1 **Answer: 2 Rationale:** The action that demonstrates cultural sensitivity is the one that inquires about the significance of the braided necklace while taking into account issues of client safety (in this case risk of strangulation). Washing the yarn addresses risk of infection but not safety. Forcing the nurse's beliefs about the yarn's lack of benefit is not consistent with cultural sensitivity. Removing the yarn without communication with the family is disrespectful of the client's culture. **Cognitive Level:** Applying **Client Need:** Psychosocial Integrity **Integrated Process:** Culture and Spirituality **Content Area:** Fundamentals **Strategy:** Use the process of elimination and basic principles of culturally sensitive communication to make a selection. Eliminate options that remove the yarn as least respectful, and choose the correct option because it addresses the priority need of safety.

2 **Answer: 3 Rationale:** The nurse should continue to monitor the client's status because the fever is low grade and treatment consistent with the client's beliefs will probably be the most successful. It is inappropriate to state that the sweat lodge would worsen the fever. The healthcare provider does not need to consult with the tribe's healer. Asking the client's family to reject a culturally based treatment does not demonstrate cultural sensitivity. **Cognitive Level:** Applying **Client Need:** Psychosocial Integrity **Integrated Process:** Culture and Spirituality **Content Area:** Fundamentals **Strategy:** Use basic principles of therapeutic communication, client autonomy, and cultural sensitivity to make a selection. The critical words in the stem are *low-grade fever*, which tells you that the situation is not life-threatening or even an emergency. Avoid alerting the healthcare provider because it does not keep the responsibility with the nurse and engaging the family because this action would violate a client's right to self-determination.

3 **Answer: 4 Rationale:** The response that shows cultural sensitivity is one that respects the personal boundaries of the client and asks permission to engage in care activities. There is no need for a family member to assist with noninvasive procedures such as measuring vital signs or oxygen saturation. The nature of the nursing activities does not require a nurse of the same sex as the client. The nurse should not ignore the nonverbal communication being sent by the client; this would not be therapeutic. **Cognitive Level:** Applying **Client Need:** Psychosocial Integrity **Integrated Process:** Culture and Spirituality **Content Area:** Fundamentals **Strategy:** Use basic principles of therapeutic communication, client autonomy, and cultural sensitivity to make a selection. First note that the nature of the nursing care activities involved indicate that this is not a situation that requires assistance from family or other nurses. Choose an option that focuses directly on the client.

4 **Answer: 3 Rationale:** Pain is an experience that is more likely to be culturally influenced for clients. Hispanic or Latino clients are more likely to externalize their pain, while Asian clients and some European American clients tend to show few external signs. The nurse should not conclude that a client who vocalizes pain is exaggerating the pain experience. The nurse should not conclude that a client is free of pain based on nonverbal cues. A client who is demonstrating pain should not be labeled as drug seeking. **Cognitive Level:** Analyzing **Client Need:** Psychosocial Integrity **Integrated Process:** Culture and Spirituality **Content Area:** Fundamentals **Strategy:** Use principles of therapeutic, helping relationships and cultural sensitivity to evaluate each option. Keep in mind that the correct option will also be the one that is most respectful of the client.

5 **Answer: 2 Rationale:** Cultural practices near the time of death are important for clients and their families. The nurse should respect the client and family wishes. Scheduling blocks of time for visitors is not helpful at this time. Limiting non-family visitors to three at a time is arbitrary and serves no useful purpose. Medical care is ineffective at this point in time and should not interfere with cultural practices near the end of life. **Cognitive Level:** Applying **Client Need:** Psychosocial Integrity **Integrated Process:** Culture and Spirituality **Content Area:** Fundamentals **Strategy:** Recall that practices related to birth and death are highly culturally influenced. With this in mind, select the option that provides the greatest respect for the client and significant people in his life.

6 **Answer: 1 Rationale:** The nurse should notify the healthcare provider of the client's practices and should continue to monitor the client to promote safe management of the health problem. It is unnecessary to ask for a nurse of the same culture to be assigned. The nurse should not state that the medication would not work because of health beliefs. It would be punitive to discharge the client from services because of culturally based health practices. **Cognitive Level:** Applying **Client Need:** Psychosocial Integrity **Integrated Process:** Culture and Spirituality **Content Area:** Fundamentals **Strategy:** First eliminate options that imply punishment or abandonment of the client. Then choose correctly by eliminating the option that represents a false statement.

7 **Answer: 3 Rationale:** The Jewish religion prohibits the ingestion of meat and dairy products during the same meal. The nurse should ask that the entire meal tray be replaced by the dietary department. Removing the tea does not address the culturally based dietary issue. Removing the chicken from the dietary tray is not sufficient because Kosher law says meat and dairy cannot be combined in any way, which would include being on the same meal tray. The use of lactose-free milk will not resolve the dietary issue. **Cognitive Level:** Applying **Client Need:** Psychosocial Integrity **Integrated Process:** Culture and Spirituality **Content Area:** Fundamentals **Strategy:** The core issue of this question is that milk and meat products cannot be consumed during the same meal or combined in any way for clients of the Orthodox Jewish faith. Use knowledge of culturally based dietary practices to make a selection.

8 **Answer: 3 Rationale:** Following birth, the umbilical cord may be buried near a place or an object that symbolizes the parents' hope for the child's future. For this reason, the parents of the newborn are likely to request to take it home. Having the cord burned, having the blood drained from it, and inspecting the cord are not consistent with the cultural beliefs of Native Americans regarding the significance of the umbilical cord after birth. **Cognitive Level:** Analyzing **Client Need:** Psychosocial Integrity **Integrated Process:** Culture and Spirituality **Content Area:** Fundamentals **Strategy:** Use the process of elimination and knowledge of the cultural

practices surrounding childbirth to make a selection. If needed, take time to review key cultural practices of Native American clients.

9 **Answer: 1, 4, 5 Rationale:** In the Latino culture, herbal medicines are just as important as Western medicines in treating illness. Cold foods would be used to treat an illness that is considered hot, while hot foods would be used to treat an illness that is considered to be cold. Depending on the client, a caregiver of the same gender may be preferred to enhance privacy. Mourners would not be hired by a family to demonstrate grief after a death (that practice could occur in Korean culture). Staring at a child could cause the "evil eye" because of their inexperienced and vulnerable spirits. **Cognitive Level:** Applying **Client Need:** Psychosocial Integrity **Integrated Process:** Culture and Spirituality **Content Area:** Fundamentals **Strategy:** The wording of the question tells you that the correct options will also be correct statements about the Latino American culture. Use knowledge of specific Hispanic cultural practices to make a selection.

10 **Answer: 1, 2, 4 Rationale:** Mexican American culture is associated with placing a high value on extended family relationships. Mexican American culture is associated with being patriarchal (machismo). Mexican American culture is associated with having respect for authority. Mexican American culture does not value independence and autonomy. Rather, interdependence is valued. Mexican American culture is not associated with defying the status quo. **Cognitive Level:** Applying **Client Need:** Psychosocial Integrity **Integrated Process:** Culture and Spirituality **Content Area:** Fundamentals **Strategy:** Recall more common characteristics of Mexican American culture to correctly answer the question. Note the wording of the question suggests that more than one option is likely to be correct.

11 **Answer: 1, 2, 3 Rationale:** Beef, eggs, and fried food are considered warm foods, and, as such, would be a treatment for yin (cold) conditions. Honey and broccoli are considered cold foods, and would not be consumed with a cold condition. **Cognitive Level:** Applying **Client Need:** Psychosocial Integrity **Integrated Process:** Culture and Spirituality **Content Area:** Foundational Sciences: Nutrition **Strategy:** Recall yin/yang principles, including foods categorized in each group, to make the correct choices. Note the wording of the question indicates that more than one option is likely to be correct.

12 **Answer: 2, 3, 4 Rationale:** Anglo-American culture values materialism (such as money and belongings), youth, and beauty. Competition is valued over harmony. Independence is valued over interdependence. **Cognitive Level:** Applying **Client Need:** Psychosocial Integrity **Integrated Process:** Culture and Spirituality **Content Area:** Fundamentals **Strategy:** Recall the more common characteristics of Anglo-American culture to correctly identify the best responses. Note the question indicates that more than one option is likely to be correct.

13 **Answer: 1, 2, 4 Rationale:** African American culture typically values extended family, religion, and interdependence. Long-term goals and seclusion are not typically associated with African American culture. **Cognitive Level:** Applying **Client Need:** Psychosocial Integrity **Integrated Process:** Culture and Spirituality **Content Area:** Fundamentals **Strategy:** Recall characteristics that are commonly associated with African American culture to identify the correct responses. The wording of the question indicates more than one option is likely to be correct.

Key Terms to Review

culture p. 254

stereotyping p. 255

References

Berman, A., Snyder, S., & Frandsen, G. (2016). *Kozier & Erb's fundamentals of nursing: Concepts, process, and practice* (10th ed.). New York, NY: Pearson Education.

Giger, J. (2016). *Transcultural nursing: Assessment and intervention* (7th ed.). St. Louis, MO: Elsevier.

McFarland, M. R., & Wehbe-Alamah, H. B. (2014). *Leininger's culture care diversity and universality: A worldwide nursing theory* (3rd ed.). Burlington, MA: Jones & Bartlett Learning.

Potter, P., Perry, A., Stockert, P., Hall, A. (2017). *Fundamentals of nursing* (9th ed.). St. Louis, MO: Mosby.

Purnell, L. (2014). *Transcultural health care: A culturally competent approach* (4th ed.). Philadelphia: F. A. Davis.

Spector, R. (2013). *Cultural diversity in health and illness* (8th ed.). Upper Saddle River, NJ: Pearson Education.

Coping with Stressors 20

In this chapter

Cross Reference

Other chapters relevant to this content area are

I. COPING AND DEFENSE MECHANISMS

A. Coping behaviors

1. Constitute a client's response to a stressful event that causes anxiety
2. **Coping** involves cognitive, physical, or emotional attempts to manage anxiety and manage stressful situation effectively; both adaptive (constructive) and maladaptive (destructive) coping behaviors may be manifested
3. Cognitive attempts at coping involve problem solving or diminishing the problem's meaning, while emotional coping engages use of defense mechanisms as a means of self-protection

Memory Aid

All clients attempt to exhibit coping behaviors. The nurse's key role is to determine whether they are healthy (adaptive) or unhealthy (maladaptive) and to support healthy ones.

NCLEX® **B. Defense mechanisms (see Table 20–1)**

1. Strategies that assist client to protect own ego and reduce anxiety
2. Nurse's role is to assist client in identifying source of anxiety, determine effectiveness of currently used defense mechanisms in facilitating client's coping, and to support appropriate use of defense mechanisms
3. NCLEX® It is important not to attempt to break down inappropriate defense mechanisms until client has learned other, more effective coping strategies

Table 20–1 Common Defense Mechanisms

Defense Mechanism	Description
Compensation	Taking action to make up for real or imagined weaknesses in one area
Conversion	Manifesting physical symptoms as an unconscious means to manage anxiety that accompanies emotional conflict
Denial	Refusing to acknowledge thoughts, impulses, or feelings that are unacceptable to self
Displacement	Directing feelings about a person who is threatening to self to another person who is less threatening to self
Fantasy	Attaining symbolic satisfaction through use of nonrational thought, wishful thinking, and imaginary achievements
Identification	Attempting to change oneself unconsciously to resemble someone who is admired or to assume similarity between self and that person
Intellectualization	Using excessive cognitive reasoning to minimize or avoid feelings associated with distressing events or occurrences
Introjection	Incorporating the values and characteristics of another into oneself
Minimization	Refusing to acknowledge importance or significance of one's behavior
Projection	Transferring unacceptable desires, thoughts, or internal feelings to another
Rationalization	Justifying unacceptable feelings or behavior by using faulty logic or applying false but socially acceptable motives to behavior
Reaction formation	Behaving or displaying attitudes that are exactly opposite of those that are felt when real feelings are deemed unacceptable
Regression	Reverting back to an earlier developmental stage to deal with an uncomfortable reality
Repression	Using an unconscious process to block threatening or unacceptable thoughts, feelings, or desires to keep them from becoming conscious
Sublimation	Displacing energy associated with unacceptable needs or drives into more socially acceptable activities
Substitution	Replacing a highly valued but unobtainable or unacceptable object with a less satisfying but acceptable and available one
Suppression	Keeping unacceptable thoughts and feelings out of awareness consciously
Undoing	Using words or actions to cancel out previous unacceptable thoughts or behaviors in an attempt to relieve guilt by making reparation

II. COPING WITH ABUSE OR NEGLECT

A. Vulnerable individuals (victims)

1. Describe feelings of powerlessness, dependency, or a sense of being trapped
2. Often present with depression and diminished self-esteem with chronic abuse
3. NCLEX® May not recognize that they are victims and may believe they are to blame for abuse

B. Abusers

1. Also have low self-esteem; tend to be self-absorbed, suspicious, and highly dependent on victim
2. Depersonalize victims so as to feel entitled to engage in abuse
3. May have been abused themselves during childhood

C. Types of abuse/violence

1. Partner abuse: cycle of physical or emotional threats and assaults by abuser followed by abuser remorse or attempts to make peace
2. Child abuse: may be physical, emotional, or sexual; includes shaken baby syndrome (characterized by full bulging fontanels, unexpectedly large head circumference, retinal hemorrhage with ophthalmic exam, and absence of external trauma)
3. Older adult: may be physical, emotional, sexual; another issue is financial exploitation (may be recognized when a cognitively intact client displays lack of knowledge of finances and inability to pay

bills, and/or when others taking funds or possessions against client's wishes or without client knowledge)

4. Abuse versus neglect: neglect is passive in nature because of a failure to act, while abuse is active and purposeful

NCLEX®

D. Assessment

1. Neglect: intentional or unintentional failure to meet client's physical needs (nutrition, fluids, healthcare, and medications), developmental needs (inadequate cognitive or physical stimulation to meet growth and development milestones), or educational neglect
2. Abuse: can be physical, emotional, or sexual in nature (see Table 20–2)
3. Assessment questions to determine risk for abuse
   a. Children: who child does and does not play with, types of games child enjoys or dislikes, whether anyone is hurting child, whether child is touched in a way that makes child feel uncomfortable
   b. Older adults: whether client has experienced degrading or threatening comments by others, whether client has basic services and assistance needed at home, whether client has food or fluids withheld, or has sustained pain or injury caused by another

E. General principles of collaborative management (see also Chapter 5)

NCLEX®

1. Report suspected abuse cases according to agency and state guidelines as part of mandatory reporting laws
2. Provide safe, nonthreatening environment for care using an empathetic and nonjudgmental approach; interview client without abuser present whenever possible
3. Support client during physical assessment and treatment of physical injuries

Memory Aid

Safety is always a key concern for victims of abuse and neglect.

NCLEX®

4. Document assessments and client-reported events in an objective manner
5. Do not leave victim alone with suspected abuser

NCLEX®

6. Support client's coping mechanisms and problem-solving abilities
7. Encourage therapy for abuser, victim, and appropriate others (family)

Table 20–2 Signs of Neglect and Abuse

	Child	Older Adult
Signs of Neglect	Poor hygiene, presence of chronic hunger and inadequate weight gain, chronic fatigue, excessive school absences, and inadequate or lack of supervision	Poor hygiene and unkempt appearance, inadequate dress, absence of necessary physical aids (dentures, glasses, hearing aids), malnutrition, dehydration, skin tears
Signs of Abuse Physical	Unexplained physical or thermal injuries Unusual apprehension, aggression, or withdrawal Withdraws from or is fearful of parents Does not cry when approached by strangers/caregivers	Skin tears Bruises that are multiple or in patterns (finger or hand prints) Burn injuries Lacerations or punctures Bone fractures
Emotional	Presence of repetitive motion habits such as sucking or rocking Psychoneurotic reactions Disorders of speech Difficulty with concentration or learning Suicidal behavior	Confusion Fear and apprehension Agitation Withdrawal from social activities Loss of interest in self Decreased appetite and weight
Sexual	Difficulty in sitting or walking Torn, stained, or bloody undergarments Pain, swelling, bruising, or bleeding in area of genitalia Change in usual routine, such as disruptive behavior or disrupted sleep Changes in school behavior, such as withdrawal from peers, truancy, or refusal to undress/change clothes for physical education classes	Difficulty in sitting or walking New-onset genital infection Pain or bleeding in area of genitalia Torn, stained, or bloody undergarments

NCLEX®
8. Assess support systems of victim and abuser
9. Refer to appropriate community agencies for support
10. Assist with legal procedures as appropriate (police reports, restraining order/order of protection)

NCLEX®
F. Interventions specific to care of child
1. Avoid loud noises and make no sudden movements
2. Position self to be at eye level with child when speaking
3. Place child in safe environment that prevents further injury
4. Support child during physical assessment and treatment
5. Reassure child that he or she is not to blame for abusive behavior

NCLEX®
G. Interventions specific to older adults
1. Recognize older adults who are at increased risk for abuse, including those with increased dependency on others because of altered mental status, decreased mobility, or chronic debilitating illness
2. Assess for caregiver role strain as possible contributing factor for neglect or abuse, and facilitate access to respite care and counseling as needed
3. Take action to separate client from abusive environment by referring to case worker, social services, or adult protective services as required by law
4. Explore alternative housing that provides greatest freedom to client and least amount of disruption to routine
5. Assist with exploring protection of finances and any other legal matters

III. OVERVIEW OF PSYCHOLOGICAL ASPECTS OF MEDICAL ILLNESS

A. Factors influencing response to medical illness include developmental level, personality type/behaviors, coping behaviors, precipitating stressors, support systems, and nature of illness

NCLEX®
B. Developmental/lifespan issues: developmental stage at time of diagnosis of medical illness influences client's response to illness; in addition, illness can affect client mastery of a developmental level, which further affects how client responds to illness
1. Early to middle adulthood
   a. Medical illnesses during early to middle adulthood can interfere with intimacy, sexuality, and career goals
   b. An adolescent with a chronic illness is at high risk, and this may result in severe emotional stress, depression, anxiety, and possible suicidal ideation (see also Chapter 21)
2. Older adulthood: medical illnesses that occur during older adulthood can interfere with self-care and daily functioning, which may result in severe emotional stress

C. Personality traits: predictable pattern of response to events; can be used to predict how client may respond to medical diagnosis, which then assists with planning care
1. Type A personality trait behaviors: might increase unhealthy responses to medical illness; these traits include rapid speech, irritability, rapid movements, time consciousness, difficulty relaxing, internalization of feelings, excessive dependence on approval of others, and low self-esteem
2. Type B personality trait behaviors: may contribute to healthy responses to medical illness and include easygoing manner, relaxed and goal-directed behaviors
3. Behaviors that increase likelihood of occurrence of medical illness include pessimism, repression, limited/guarded social interactions, hostility, and despair
4. Behaviors that decrease likelihood of occurrence of medical illness include behaviors that are self-healing, energetic, questioning, humorous, inspirational, and that demonstrate good interpersonal skills

D. *Precipitating stressors*
1. Defined as events occurring prior to a medical illness that initiated a stress response consisting of physiological and psychological alterations
2. These can influence a client's response to medical illness because client may already be in an emotionally compromised state prior to diagnosis of medical illness

E. Support systems: presence or absence of strong support systems influences response to medical illness; strong family, friend, and community support systems can result in positive or negative responses

F. Nature of illness: response to medical illness can depend on whether illness is an acute (or short-lasting), chronic (long-lasting), or terminal, life-ending type
1. Acute illness: sudden onset, may be caused by injury or fast-onset illness
   a. Often results in crisis for client and family; **crisis** refers to an event in which client's regular coping mechanisms are inadequate

NCLEX®
   b. Client may demonstrate a short attention span and a tendency to be unproductive and impulsive

NCLEX® 2. Chronic illness: client must cope with illness that may be long-standing and debilitating in nature; often results in ongoing stress for client and family; client often feels frustrated, hopeless, and fatigued

3. Terminal illness: may place client and family in a crisis mode
   a. Extremely disruptive to client and family functioning
   b. NCLEX® Client often exhibits signs of anger, hopelessness/helplessness, and despair

IV. ASSOCIATED COMMON PSYCHOLOGICAL SYMPTOMS

A. Anger

1. Clients with medical illness may demonstrate behaviors indicative of anger
2. These behaviors reflect feelings of helplessness and frustration about illness and effects it has on daily functioning
3. NCLEX® Common behaviors include demanding types of action, loud verbalization, slamming of items, and social withdrawal

B. Depression

1. Clients with medical illness may demonstrate symptoms of depression related to disruption of daily functioning
2. Signs of depression include feelings of helplessness/hopelessness, flat affect, poor eye contact, disrupted eating/sleeping patterns, absence of motivation and compliance, and a decreased energy level

C. Anxiety

1. Clients with medical illness may demonstrate feelings and behaviors of anxiety
2. Anxious behavior reflects feelings of real or imagined threat to body image
3. NCLEX® Anxiety results in stimulation of autonomic nervous system (increased heart rate, respirations, and visual acuity, diaphoresis, shortness of breath, and restlessness)

D. Helplessness/hopelessness

1. Clients with medical diagnoses may demonstrate feelings of helplessness/hopelessness
2. NCLEX® Helplessness relates to feelings of powerlessness associated with being unable to change what is happening, while hopelessness relates to feelings of despondency and loss of optimism
3. This is reflected in feelings of loss of **control** (feeling that an event can be managed), loss of individuality, and increased dependency on others

V. MEDICAL CONDITIONS CONTRIBUTING TO PSYCHOLOGICAL SYMPTOMS

A. Critical/acute illness: may occur without warning and immediately affect a client's daily functioning; clients typically experience feelings of loss of control, anxiety, helplessness, and anger

1. Cardiovascular illnesses
   a. Have been linked to occurrence of stress
   b. Include myocardial infarction, stroke, and hypertension
   c. Stress levels can influence course and/or outcomes of medical illness
2. Trauma
   a. May result from an accident or crime
   b. Behavioral and physiological responses occur and are demonstrated in client through social isolation, agitation, nightmares, and numbness
   c. Client typically struggles to control episodes of anxiety related to traumatic event
3. Surgery performed because of a critical or acute medical condition may be disfiguring or incapacitating, and result in changes in client daily functioning and self-image
4. Pain can accompany many acute illnesses; client's response is based on a need to protect oneself from harm

B. Chronic illness: produces long-term effects that can be unpredictable in nature and require ongoing use of adaptive coping behaviors; lower socioeconomic status increases risk for multiple ongoing health problems, reduced access to healthcare, and insufficient finances to adhere to treatment plans

1. Pulmonary diseases
   a. Include disorders such as chronic obstructive pulmonary disease (COPD) and asthma
   b. NCLEX® Higher stress levels lead to increased secretions and airway spasms and result in more frequent episodes of breathing difficulties

2. Gastrointestinal (GI) diseases
   a. Irritable bowel syndrome, peptic ulcer, and ulcerative colitis are stress-influenced illnesses
   b. GI tract and autonomic nervous system are involved; during periods of stress, symptoms are exacerbated by increased stomach acid secretion and increased parasympathetic stimulation of lower bowel

NCLEX® 3. Medical illnesses that result in chronic pain can have profound effect on clients' coping behaviors (adaptive and maladaptive); clients respond to pain in a psychological and physiological manner that requires them to continually attempt to adapt

C. Life-ending illnesses (see also Chapter 24)
1. Client who is dying may experience feelings of depression, anger, hostility, helplessness, and hopelessness
2. Client's response to a life-ending illness is affected by coping skills, developmental level, and spiritual, cultural, biological, and psychosocial factors
3. Interventions include use of empathy and compassion; a focus on positive aspects of client's life; spirituality assessment and reinforcement; support of family and significant others; allowing client dignity and control; and managing pain

VI. ASSOCIATED PSYCHIATRIC SYMPTOMS

A. Psychosis is a disorder of organic or emotional origin characterized by gross impairment in reality testing

B. Psychotic symptoms that may be demonstrated in clients with selected medical illness diagnoses include evidence of delusions and hallucinations, thought-process disruption, and difficulty in caring for oneself (see also Chapter 21)
1. Delusions may be persistent and recurrent; they are beliefs that are false but cannot be altered by reason or evidence
2. Hallucinations may be persistent and recurrent; they are defined as occurrences of a sight, sound, smell, taste, or touch when there is no external stimulus to corresponding sensory organ

VII. ASSESSMENT

A. Use various resources to collect psychological, biological, and social data, considering subjective and objective symptoms, family/significant other reports, and diagnostic reports in assessment phase

B. Psychological assessment
1. Elicits client's emotional reaction to medical illness diagnosis, coping abilities, and support resources
2. Perform a stress appraisal to identify source, number, and duration of stressors
3. Complete a full mental status exam if client exhibits severe symptoms induced by stress

NCLEX® 4. Complete a depression symptom assessment, noting time of initial symptoms, duration of symptoms, and physical appearance

NCLEX® 5. Identify coping behaviors, including adaptive and maladaptive behaviors that reflect client's ability to identify problems and analyze feelings

6. Assess substance abuse/dependence, which is crucial in assessment phase because it can contribute to symptoms of depression, anxiety, hopelessness, helplessness, and eating/sleeping disruptions
7. Theoretical emotional stages of medical illness include the following (individual clients may move forward and backward through these stages to some degree):
   a. Denial of medical illness and associated limitations
   b. Anger at loss of control and associated limitations
   c. Bargaining, with a plea for another chance and seeking new answers/treatments
   d. Depression when grieving occurs due to loss or anticipated loss
   e. Acceptance/adaptation when conflicts are resolved and client participates in care
8. Identify emotional stage of medical illness; plan interventions accordingly

C. Biological assessment
1. Done to assess how stress might alter a client's internal body functioning
2. Biological changes can assist nurse with determining severity of an illness
3. Assess recent and past health conditions that may contribute to current level of physical and psychological functioning; recent and chronic illnesses alter client's immune system and raise susceptibility to additional health problems
4. Conduct complete physical exam to reveal any physical conditions contributing to psychological symptoms; some medical illnesses can cause client to exhibit psychological symptoms that may be misdiagnosed as a mental health disorder

5. Complete a thorough neurological status exam to reveal current neurological state and any changes; findings will provide baseline level of functioning and may alert nurse to medical problems
6. Analyze laboratory results, which can provide insight into occurrence of psychological symptoms
7. *NCLEX®* Assess client's current abilities with physical functioning, activities, and exercise to identify baseline information from which to develop plan of care
8. *NCLEX®* Investigate sleep patterns, noting disruptions such as inability to fall asleep, stay asleep, or a desire to sleep constantly; sleep disruptions may indicate either physiological or psychological problems
9. *NCLEX®* Complete a nutritional pattern assessment, noting disruptions such as lack of appetite, failure to enjoy previously enjoyable food, and overeating; eating disruptions can indicate either physiological or psychological stress
10. *NCLEX®* Complete a pharmacological assessment, noting current medications that could account for level of physical and psychological functioning

D. Social assessment

1. Explore family history, client lifestyle, life-changing events, and social support systems (either negative or positive)
2. Explore recent life-changing events that may impact adaptation to current illness
3. Discuss client's lifestyle patterns and potential impact of lifestyle choices on development and progression of disease
4. *NCLEX®* Note cultural practices for unique aspects that may indicate specific responses or need for special interventions
5. *NCLEX®* Assess family communication patterns, level of cohesion, flexibility, functioning, and general support
6. Explore community and support resources for availability of home services, mental health services, and other related services
7. Assess spiritual concerns; note traditional patterns or rituals, and inquire about other forms of spirituality that may be important to the client
8. Do an occupational assessment to determine whether client can continue in current occupation, either at present time or in future
9. Determine economic status, specifically whether finances will support current and future expenses

VIII. EMPOWERING STRATEGIES

A. Interventions

1. Collaborate with client and family to develop a plan of care in which client response can be monitored; counseling and possibly psychotherapy may be appropriate
2. Interventions serve as foundation for all client care and are subject to change as client's condition changes
3. *NCLEX®* Specific interventions that exemplify empowering strategies
   a. Increase client control; provide opportunities for client decision making regarding care
   b. Engage in therapeutic interactions—empathetic listening
   c. Assist with stress management—teach relaxation methods, imagery, biofeedback, exercise
   d. Reinforce current positive, adaptive coping behaviors
   e. Promote comfort and healing
   f. Utilize spiritual resources—provide opportunities for client to engage in spiritual traditions or rituals; offer resources related to complementary medicine if desired

B. Differential interventions for critical/acute versus chronic illnesses

1. *NCLEX®* Critical/acute illnesses typically result in abrupt interruption of a client's usual daily activities; this can precipitate a crisis stage if client perceives events as a threat to safety, self-esteem, or self-image
   a. Seek immediate ways to increase client's control
   b. Engage in therapeutic interactions with client and family; encourage verbalization of feelings
   c. Assist with immediate anxiety reduction through use of relaxation techniques
   d. Use firm, direct limit-setting to assist client with staying focused
2. *NCLEX®* Chronic illnesses typically require ongoing adaptation because long-term effects are unpredictable; they often deplete energy levels, support systems, coping reserves, and economic abilities, and may lead to suicidal ideation
   a. Increase self-care responsibilities as appropriate to preserve or facilitate functioning, self-esteem, and self-image
   b. Reward positive adaptive coping behaviors
   c. Reinforce existing support network and assist client with creating new links to support; identify support groups, self-help groups, and special interest groups

IX. EVALUATION/OUTCOMES

A. Preservation of healthy physiological function

1. Client learns about illness and ways to decrease disease process, such as diet, exercise, and stress-reduction activities
2. Client participates in treatment/rehabilitation process to achieve optimal level of functioning and independence in self-care

B. Development and use of adaptive coping behaviors

1. Client expresses feelings about medical diagnosis and effects of illness
2. Client develops functional support systems, such as family, friends, and community services as needed
3. Client demonstrates decreased anxiety

C. Evidence of an internal locus of control

1. Clients who believe they are able to decrease likelihood or effects of illness have an internal locus of control and are less likely to experience symptoms of distress
2. In contrast, clients who have an external locus of control, who believe that forces outside them determine their lives, are less likely to believe they can control illness or manage stressors

Check Your NCLEX–RN® Exam I.Q.

You are ready for testing on this content if you can:

- Assess clients experiencing stress.
- Support appropriate use of coping strategies and defense mechanisms for clients experiencing stress.
- Provide care to the abused client and family.
- Identify common clinical symptoms of psychotic disorders due to medical illness.
- Differentiate intervention strategies for clients experiencing critical acute illness and chronic illness.

PRACTICE TEST

1 A client diagnosed with a terminal illness states, "What's left for me? I feel hopeless." The nurse determines that which of the following would be the best response?

1. "It makes me feel sad that you feel hopeless."
2. "Sometimes people in your situation get depressed, which makes them feel hopeless."
3. "It must be difficult feeling as though there is no hope."
4. "Can you think of one or two reasons to not feel so bad?"

2 The nurse observes that a client hospitalized with newly diagnosed heart disease is frequently crying and stays in the room. The nurse should interpret these actions to be examples of what type(s) of behaviors? Select all that apply.

1. Inappropriate
2. Psychiatric
3. Psychotic
4. Coping
5. Expected

3 The nurse would plan to include which of the following in a biological assessment of a client? Select all that apply.

1. Laboratory test results
2. Feelings of anxiety about illness
3. Spiritual needs during illness
4. Prognosis
5. Sleep patterns

4 A client with a terminal illness states, "If I could only live until I can walk my daughter down the aisle at her wedding, I will donate all of my money to research." The nurse reports that the client is in which phase of the grief process?

1. Denial
2. Seeking
3. Bargaining
4. Acceptance

5. A client diagnosed with a medical illness states, "I don't enjoy my food anymore." The nurse notes during the assessment phase that this statement indicates what kind of nutritional pattern?
   1. Eating disruption
   2. Eating disorder
   3. Bulimia
   4. Compulsive disorder

6. As part of the admission process, the nurse is conducting a social assessment of a client. Which question should the nurse ask during this part of the assessment?
   1. "What medications are you currently taking?"
   2. "Can you tell me what illnesses you have had in the past?"
   3. "Do you have any culturally based practices that you would like to continue in the hospital?"
   4. "Do your brothers or sisters have any chronic illnesses?"

7. A client who has a diagnosis of a chronic illness states, "I'm so tired. I can't keep on like this every day." The nurse interprets that the feeling the client is expressing can be described as which of the following?
   1. Atypical
   2. Expected
   3. Pathological
   4. Resentful

8. The client hospitalized for 5 days with a medical illness says loudly, "Bring me my pain pills now!" Which initial interpretation of the client's statement should the nurse make?
   1. This is a common response to feeling lack of situational control.
   2. This response by the client is inappropriate.
   3. This indicates a problem with care delivery to the client.
   4. This response reflects the client's feeling of anger at the self.

9. The nurse notices that a client admitted with chronic obstructive pulmonary disease has poor eye contact and has not been eating well. The nurse then looks for additional data consistent with which potential problem?
   1. Hopefulness
   2. An eating disorder
   3. Anxiety
   4. Depression

10. What item should the nurse assess during a biological assessment to determine susceptibility to additional health problems in a client who has a medical illness? Select all that apply.
    1. Past medications
    2. Recent illnesses
    3. Spiritual needs
    4. Cultural background
    5. Functional abilities

11. A client with a recent onset of multiple sclerosis is observed taking part in self-care. The nurse interprets this behavior to be consistent with which stage of adaptation?
    1. Acceptance
    2. Denial
    3. Compensation
    4. Indulgence

12. A client who underwent surgery for removal of a bowel tumor is exhibiting new onset of verbal outbursts and speaks aloud when no one is in the room. What should the nurse conclude that the client would benefit from next?
    1. Psychiatric workup
    2. Physical exam
    3. Counseling session
    4. Teaching session about the illness

13. The nurse is assessing a client's coping behaviors during a psychological assessment and wishes to address factors that can contribute to depression. The nurse would ask the client about which priority items? Select all that apply.
    1. Occupation
    2. Substance abuse
    3. Number of siblings
    4. Level of income
    5. Recent losses

PRACTICE TEST

14 In a client newly diagnosed with amyotrophic lateral sclerosis, an illness that leads to progressive loss of ability to perform activities of daily living, which initial coping strategy should the nurse anticipate the client may use in reacting to the diagnosis?

1. Denial
2. Gambling
3. Exercise
4. Verbal abuse

15 The nurse observes a client and family interaction. Observed behaviors include anger, rigidity, and lack of support for one another. The nurse should consider this interaction as an assessment of which family characteristic?

1. Recent life-changing events
2. Communication patterns
3. Lifestyle patterns
4. Community resources

16 A client with a medical illness tells the nurse that going to church is not a priority. Based on this information, what should the nurse do at this time?

1. Not mention religion again
2. Conclude that the client does not believe in God
3. Ask the client to go to church
4. Explore other spiritual patterns or rituals with the client

17 A client who was paralyzed from severe injuries sustained during an automobile accident continually attempts to do activities beyond capabilities. What would be the most appropriate clinical problem to address?

1. Inadequate adjustment
2. Anxiety
3. Anger
4. Breaks in skin integrity

18 A client tells the nurse that acupuncture helps ease the pain of a terminal illness. How should the nurse react to this statement?

1. Tell the client to stop the acupuncture.
2. Tell the client that it is illegal.
3. Understand that it is an appropriate intervention.
4. Understand that the client is not thinking clearly.

19 A client with inflammatory bowel disease has exacerbations when job responsibilities become heavy or when family conflicts occur at home. The nurse determines that this client would benefit from instruction that focuses on which of the following?

1. How to keep feelings inside
2. Communication strategies
3. How to ignore stress
4. Stress management techniques

20 A client with chronic obstructive pulmonary disease has given up smoking and spaces out activities over the course of the day. The nurse should respond by doing which of the following?

1. Say nothing about the behavior to avoid refocusing the client on the disease process.
2. Ignore the maladaptive behaviors.
3. Reward the adaptive coping behaviors.
4. Tell the client that adjustment was bound to occur over time.

ANSWERS & RATIONALES

1 **Answer: 3 Rationale:** Use of empathy toward what the client is sharing communicates understanding and allows the client to explore inner feelings of hopelessness. Stating that the nurse feels sad draws attention to the nurse rather than the client. Focusing on depression as the first response limits further exploration of the client's feelings. Intellectualizing the client statement, such as asking to think of reasons not to feel hopeless, does not encourage the client to further explore feelings with the nurse. **Cognitive Level:** Applying **Client Need:** Psychosocial Integrity **Integrated Process:** Communication and Documentation **Content Area:** Mental Health **Strategy:** For questions involving nurse–client communication, choose the answer that provides the broadest opening in promoting further communication and sharing of client's feelings.

2 **Answer: 4, 5 Rationale:** Crying and remaining in the room are client behaviors that indicate the client is attempting to cope with the situation in some way. Crying and withdrawal are expected reactions while the client tries to assimilate information about a new chronic illness. The client's reaction is appropriate rather than inappropriate. The label of psychiatric does not apply to this situation. The client shows no signs or symptoms of psychosis. **Cognitive Level:** Applying **Client Need:** Psychosocial Integrity **Integrated Process:** Nursing Process: Assessment **Content Area:** Mental Health **Strategy:** Consider that the client has just learned about diagnosis of

a chronic illness. Reason that the client may engage in any number of behaviors, such as crying, to cope with the initial diagnosis.

3 **Answer: 1, 5 Rationale:** Laboratory test results and sleep patterns are part of biological assessment and may provide insight into the occurrence of psychological symptoms. Spiritual needs are part of the social assessment. Anxiety is part of the psychological assessment. Prognosis is a prediction about the outcome of illness rather than an assessment. **Cognitive Level:** Applying **Client Need:** Psychosocial Integrity **Integrated Process:** Nursing Process: Assessment **Content Area:** Mental Health **Strategy:** The critical word in the stem of the question is *biological*. With this in mind, select the option that deals most directly with physiological needs or parameters.

4 **Answer: 3 Rationale:** Bargaining is the stage in which the client attempts to barter for more time. Denial indicates the stage in which the client denies that he or she is terminally ill. Seeking reflects the stage in which a client seeks more answers and cures. Acceptance is the stage in which the client has come to terms with the illness. **Cognitive Level:** Applying **Client Need:** Psychosocial Integrity **Integrated Process:** Communication and Documentation **Content Area:** Mental Health **Strategy:** The core issue of the question is ability to analyze a stage of grief by interpreting client comments. Use nursing knowledge and the process of elimination to make a selection.

5 **Answer: 1 Rationale:** The client's statement indicates an eating disruption in that the client's normal eating pattern has been disturbed in some way. An eating disorder is a specific, possibly severe disruption in eating pattern, and is a specific diagnosis. Bulimia is a more severe, true eating disorder characterized by binge eating and vomiting and is not merely lack of enjoyment of food. A compulsive disorder would be one in which the client feels the need to carry out certain behaviors. **Cognitive Level:** Analyzing **Client Need:** Psychosocial Integrity **Integrated Process:** Nursing Process: Assessment **Content Area:** Mental Health **Strategy:** The core issue of the question is the ability to associate medical illness with the appropriate alteration in eating pattern. Use the process of elimination and nursing knowledge to make a selection.

6 **Answer: 3 Rationale:** Culturally based practices are part of a social assessment and provide information about how a client might respond to the illness based on cultural background. A medication history is part of a biological assessment. History of past illnesses is part of a biological assessment. Family history of illness is part of a biological assessment. **Cognitive Level:** Analyzing **Client Need:** Psychosocial Integrity **Integrated Process:** Nursing Process: Assessment **Content Area:** Mental Health **Strategy:** The core issue of the question is knowledge of the components of a social assessment. Use the process of elimination and focus on the option that takes into account the social habits or expectations of a client.

7 **Answer: 2 Rationale:** It is typical of clients with a chronic illness to become tired and feel as though they can't continue on in this way, making this behavior expected. If the client's behavior is expected, it cannot be atypical. Since chronic illness often leads to fatigue, it is inappropriate to label this symptom as pathological. The client's statement does not reflect a state of being resentful. **Cognitive Level:** Analyzing **Client Need:** Psychosocial Integrity **Integrated Process:** Nursing Process: Diagnosis **Content Area:** Mental Health **Strategy:** The core issue of the question is the nurse's ability to draw accurate conclusions about client statements in terms of coping with chronic illness. Use nursing knowledge and the process of elimination to make a selection.

8 **Answer: 1 Rationale:** Hospitalized clients often feel that their situation is out of their control and their frustration rises. Although the behavior might not be appropriate if it is disruptive, the nurse should first recognize that it is a common response. There is not enough data to support a problem with care delivery to the client. There is no evidence that the client's anger is directed toward the self. **Cognitive Level:** Analyzing **Client Need:** Psychosocial Integrity **Integrated Process:** Nursing Process: Assessment **Content Area:** Mental Health **Strategy:** The core issue of the question is the recognition that clients who are hospitalized may feel out of control and may express this feeling in ways that are not socially acceptable. Note the critical word *initially*, which indicates that more than one option may be partially correct but that one conclusion is more appropriate to draw first.

9 **Answer: 4 Rationale:** The symptoms are indicative of possible depression and require further assessment. The observed behaviors do not indicate hopefulness, an eating disorder, or anxiety. **Cognitive Level:** Analyzing **Client Need:** Psychosocial Integrity **Integrated Process:** Nursing Process: Assessment **Content Area:** Mental Health **Strategy:** The core issue of the question is the ability to recognize signs of depression in a client. Use nursing knowledge and the process of elimination to make a selection.

10 **Answer: 2, 5 Rationale:** Recent illnesses should be considered when conducting a biological assessment to determine impact on current illness. Functional abilities (ability to perform activities of daily living) may impact on the client's ability to adhere to therapy for the current illness. Past medications are not a primary concern related to biological assessment, although current medications would be. Spiritual needs and cultural background are a part of social assessment. **Cognitive Level:** Analyzing **Client Need:** Psychosocial Integrity **Integrated Process:** Nursing Process: Assessment **Content Area:** Mental Health **Strategy:** The core issue of the question is the ability to determine what elements to include in a biological assessment of a client. Use nursing knowledge and the process of elimination to make a selection.

11 **Answer: 1 Rationale:** Acceptance indicates that the client is accepting limitations imposed by the illness and is attempting to help self as much as possible. A client would not be helping self if the stage was denial because there would be no awareness of need in the denial stage. Compensation and indulgence are not stages related to helping the self during medical illness. **Cognitive Level:** Analyzing **Client Need:** Psychosocial Integrity **Integrated Process:** Nursing Process: Evaluation **Content Area:** Mental Health **Strategy:** The core issue of the question is the ability to determine the client's stage of adaptation to a chronic illness. Use nursing knowledge and the process of elimination to make a selection.

12 **Answer: 2 Rationale:** Physical illnesses can create psychiatric symptoms and a physical examination would help to identify or rule out a physiological basis for the symptoms. A psychiatric workup represents a conclusion that the origin of the client's symptoms is psychiatric in nature, which is premature. A counseling session may be useful if the cause of the symptoms is determined to be psychological in nature. Teaching when the client is in distress may not be

appropriate as it may not lead to retention of information. **Cognitive Level:** Applying **Client Need:** Psychosocial Integrity **Integrated Process:** Nursing Process: Planning **Content Area:** Mental Health **Strategy:** The core issue of the question is recognition that psychiatric symptoms may have a medical basis in a hospitalized client. Note the critical word *next*, which indicates that one action should be taken before some others.

13 **Answer: 2, 5 Rationale:** Substance abuse is of primary interest as a maladaptive coping strategy and is also associated with depression. One or more recent losses can also increase the client's risk for developing depression. Number of siblings, income level, and occupation are general factors related to lifestyle but do not directly relate to risk of developing depression. **Cognitive Level:** Analyzing **Client Need:** Psychosocial Integrity **Integrated Process:** Nursing Process: Assessment **Content Area:** Mental Health **Strategy:** Note the critical word *depression* in the question. The wording of the question indicates that more than one option may be correct. Review each option and choose those that correlate best with depression, which are substance abuse and recent losses.

14 **Answer: 1 Rationale:** Denial is most accurate because it is a typical and initial stage of grief related to loss. Gambling, exercise, and verbal abuse are isolated responses that could possibly occur but would be based on individual client characteristics rather than anticipated general patterns of response. **Cognitive Level:** Analyzing **Client Need:** Psychosocial Integrity **Integrated Process:** Nursing Process: Diagnosis **Content Area:** Mental Health **Strategy:** Note that the correct answer is a more comprehensive and global option, while the others refer to specific behaviors. This makes the correct option different from the others; also recall that a global option is often correct.

15 **Answer: 2 Rationale:** Communication patterns within the family should be assessed for flexibility and support. Recent life-changing events, lifestyle patterns, and community resources would not directly relate to this observed pattern of family interaction. **Cognitive Level:** Analyzing **Client Need:** Psychosocial Integrity **Integrated Process:** Nursing Process: Assessment **Content Area:** Mental Health **Strategy:** The core issue of the question is the nurse's ability to observe family behavior and interpret it correctly. Note the critical word *interaction* in the stem of the question and the word *communication* in the correct response.

16 **Answer: 4 Rationale:** Exploring other spiritual patterns or rituals is therapeutic because it broadens the definition of spirituality and what this might mean to the client. Not mentioning religion again implies that communication should be closed. There is not enough data to conclude the client does not believe in God. Asking the client to go to church is inappropriate as it imposes the nurse's values on the client. **Cognitive Level:** Applying **Client Need:** Psychosocial Integrity **Integrated Process:** Culture and Spirituality **Content Area:** Mental Health **Strategy:** The core issue of the question is the ability of the nurse to assess the spiritual needs of a client. Use nursing knowledge and the process of elimination to choose the option that asks a follow-up question during the interview process.

17 **Answer: 1 Rationale:** Inadequate adjustment refers to difficulty with adapting to the current situation. Although anxiety and anger might be present, it is not evident by the scenario described. There is no information in the question to support a break in skin integrity. **Cognitive Level:** Applying **Client Need:** Psychosocial Integrity **Integrated Process:** Nursing Process: Diagnosis **Content Area:** Mental Health **Strategy:** The core issue of the question is the ability of the nurse to critically analyze data and select the appropriate clinical concept on which to focus. Use nursing knowledge and the process of elimination to make a selection.

18 **Answer: 3 Rationale:** Acupuncture as a complementary therapy can be very helpful in coping with illness. Understanding its appropriateness supports the client's right to autonomy and self-determination. There is no rationale for telling the client to stop acupuncture. Acupuncture is not illegal. Believing the client is not thinking clearly is a false assumption. **Cognitive Level:** Applying **Client Need:** Psychosocial Integrity **Integrated Process:** Nursing Process: Implementation **Content Area:** Mental Health **Strategy:** The core issue of the question is the appropriate response to a client's choices about managing symptoms of chronic or terminal illness. The correct answer is the one that provides the greatest support to the client.

19 **Answer: 4 Rationale:** Stress management techniques assist the client with ways to effectively cope with stress, which may limit exacerbations of the disease. Keeping feelings inside is not a healthy way to cope with stress. Focusing on communication strategies is not indicated based on the information provided. Ignoring stress is not a healthy way to cope with stress. **Cognitive Level:** Applying **Client Need:** Psychosocial Integrity **Integrated Process:** Nursing Process: Planning **Content Area:** Mental Health **Strategy:** The core issue of the question is the ability to recognize the association between client stressors and exacerbation of the disease. First eliminate ignoring stress and keeping feelings inside as inappropriate, then choose stress management techniques because of the association between client stressors in the stem and the words *stress reduction* in the correct option.

20 **Answer: 3 Rationale:** A client's appropriate behavior should be acknowledged and reinforced. Saying nothing is incorrect because the client is already living with the disease process and an attempt to avoid drawing attention to it is not reasonable. The client's adjustment is not maladaptive. Saying the adjustment was bound to occur over time is incorrect because it patronizes the client. **Cognitive Level:** Applying **Client Need:** Psychosocial Integrity **Integrated Process:** Communication and Documentation **Content Area:** Mental Health **Strategy:** Use principles of communication to answer the question. The core issue of the question is recognition that the client has made an adaptation to medical illness and that this adaptation should be positively reinforced with the client.

Key Terms to Review

control p. 269
coping p. 265
crisis p. 268
precipitating stressors p. 268

References

Boyd, M. (2015). *Psychiatric nursing: Contemporary practice. Enhanced update.* (5th ed.). Philadelphia: Wolters Kluwer Health.

Potter, M., & Moller, M. (2016). *Psychiatric-mental health nursing: From suffering to hope.* New York, NY: Pearson Education.

Stuart, G. (2013). *Principles and practice of psychiatric nursing* (10th ed.). St. Louis, MO: Elsevier Science.

Townsend, M. (2015). *Psychiatric mental health nursing: Concepts of care in evidence-based practice* (8th ed.). Philadelphia: F. A. Davis.

Varcarolis, E. (2014). *Foundations of psychiatric mental health nursing: A clinical approach* (6th ed.). St. Louis, MO: Saunders.

21 Mental Health Disorders

In this chapter

Cross Reference

Other chapters relevant to this content area are

Therapeutic Communication and Environment	Chapter 18
Coping with Stressors	Chapter 20
Substance Use and Addictive Disorders	Chapter 22
Crisis Intervention and Suicide	Chapter 23
Psychiatric Medications	Chapter 35
Perioperative Care	Chapter 48
Neurologic Disorders	Chapter 57

I. OVERVIEW OF MENTAL HEALTH CONCEPTS

NCLEX® **A. Assessment**

1. Appearance, behavior, and mood: grooming, relaxed state, confidence
2. Level of consciousness/sensorium: oriented to time, place, person; memory intact; able to think abstractly
3. Speech, content/thought processes, insight and judgment, self-perception
4. Stage of growth and development
5. Satisfaction of Maslow's hierarchy of needs (see Figure 21–1)
6. Interactions with others: satisfying interpersonal relationships, ability to cope with stress, ability to trust
7. Risk factors for mental health problems: family history of mental illness, stressful life events, hormonal influence, weak or ineffective mental defense mechanisms
8. Inadequate support systems

B. Therapeutic management

1. Therapeutic communication techniques (see Chapter 18)
2. Therapeutic milieu *NCLEX®*
   a. Provides a safe physical and social environment while client is receiving treatment
   b. Treatment team focuses on providing consistent "therapeutic" encounters with client during one-to-one interactions to promote successful achievement of individualized treatment outcomes, and acquisition of adaptive coping skills and relationship skills

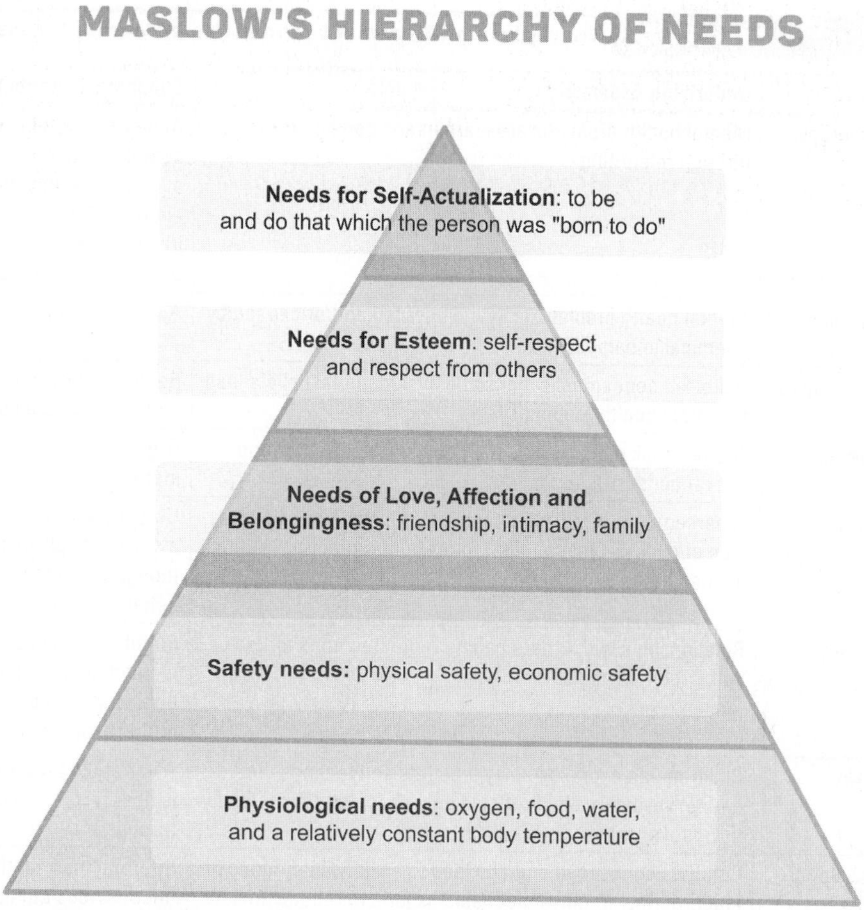

Figure 21–1

Maslow's hierarchy of needs.

Source: helgaknut/Fotolia.

c. Treatment team members include registered nurse, advanced practice nurse, psychologist, psychiatrist, social worker, occupational therapist, exercise therapist, and recreational therapist
d. Individual staff–client relationships, use of therapeutic groups (social skills group, physical activity group, activity groups), and community meetings assist client to reflect on and modify own feelings, interactions, and behaviors

3. Treatment modalities (see Table 21–1)

II. ANXIETY DISORDERS

A. Overview of Anxiety

1. **Anxiety**: an emotional, subjective state of apprehension, dread, uneasiness, or uncertainty that is experienced at times by all human beings
   a. May be triggered by misperception or misinterpretation of a possible threat to self or self-esteem, real or perceived threat to personal values, or anticipation of new experiences
   b. Acute anxiety (state anxiety) occurs with an imminent event or loss that threatens personal sense of security; chronic anxiety (trait anxiety) occurs as a persistent response to regular events or activities
2. Fear: a reaction to a specific danger
3. Stress: a state of imbalance between demands placed on a person and his or her ability to deal with these demands
4. Stressor: an internal or external event or situation that leads to feelings of anxiety
   a. Physical illness, hospitalizations, and medical treatment
   b. Person's perception of stressor leads to anxiety
   c. People evaluate stressors based on past experiences, social influences, and current resources
5. Burnout: a state of mental and/or physical exhaustion caused by excessive, prolonged stress
6. Anxiety can be a healthy adaptive reaction if it alerts client to impending threats
7. Anxiety is considered pathological when it is disproportionate to risks, continues after threat no longer exists, and/or interferes with functioning

Table 21–1 Therapies and Treatment Modalities in Mental Illness

Type of Therapy	Underlying Assumptions	Summary of Treatment
Behavior therapy	Mental health problems are learned and can be corrected through relearning	Aimed at changing undesirable behaviors; operant conditioning (rewarding positive behavior to reinforce it); aversion therapy (pairing stimulus perceived positively by client with negative consequence to negatively reinforce it); desensitization for phobias; modeling of positive behaviors by therapist so client learns through imitation
Biologically based therapies	Mental health problems may be inherited and/or caused by chemical imbalances	A variety of medications; electroconvulsive therapy (ECT)
Cognitive therapies	Distorted conceptualizations and dysfunctional beliefs lead to mental health problems	Reality testing; correcting distorted conceptualizations and dysfunctional beliefs by reinterpreting them
Activity therapy	A group task can set the stage to allow important group interactions to occur	Organized group activities that promote socialization and increase self-esteem
Family therapy	A person's emotional symptoms or problems are an expression of family's emotional symptoms or problems; a change in one person leads to changes in other members	Unit of therapy is entire family; each member develops a sense of self; members learn to identify and express thoughts and feelings, gain new insights and coping behaviors, and learn new ways of interacting and behaving
Group therapy	Relationships with others can be recreated and worked on with group members	Regular meetings are held with a therapist and five to eight members to form a stable group; members learn new behaviors and coping skills with feedback and support during group work to achieve individual goals
Play therapy	Children can express in play thoughts and feelings they cannot verbalize; child reflects his or her situation in family using toys, colors, activities (drawing)	A variety of toys are provided to facilitate interaction; play is observed; child is helped to work through problems through play
Psychotherapy	Conflicts between id and ego lead to anxiety; ineffective or inappropriate defense mechanisms form to reduce anxiety	Interactions with therapist assist client to recognize unconscious thoughts, feelings, anxieties, and defenses (supportive therapy), enter into a contract to learn new ways of perceiving and behaving in a planned systematic way (reeducative therapy), or use psychoanalysis to achieve emotional and cognitive restructuring (reconstructive therapy)

NCLEX®

B. Levels of anxiety (see Table 21–2)

C. General adaptation syndrome: an automatic physical reaction to stress mediated by sympathetic nervous system (SNS); three distinct stages are alarm, resistance, and exhaustion

1. Stress is viewed as a nonspecific body response to any demand
2. Alarm is initial response to a stressor
   a. Hormonal activity triggers a fight-or-flight reaction (an automatic psychological state of high anxiety mediated by SNS), causing increased alertness that is focused on immediate task or threat
   b. Level of anxiety is mild to moderate

Table 21–2 Responses to Varying Levels of Anxiety

	Cognitive and Perceptual Response	Physiological Response	Emotional Response
Mild	Alert, increased perceptual field, with positive effect on motivation, creativity, and learning	Normal physiological response to ordinary life stressors	Positive affect
Moderate	Perceptual field is narrowed, focus is on immediate concerns, selective inattention occurs but learning and problem solving can still occur	Low-level sympathetic nervous system arousal occurs	Tension and fear are experienced
Severe	Perceptual field greatly reduced, focus is on small or scattered details, learning and problem solving cannot occur, behavior is directed toward relief of anxiety	Sympathetic nervous system is aroused	Severe emotional distress is experienced
Panic	Details are exaggerated, personality disorganization occurs, rational thought is lost, perceptions are distorted, person fails to function	Physiological arousal interferes with motor activities	Dread and terror, possible regression to primitive or childish behaviors

3. Resistance occurs when body mobilizes resources to combat stress
   a. Body stabilizes and adapts to stress but functions below optimal level
   b. Coping (efforts to manage specific demands that are appraised as threatening) and defense mechanisms (unconscious psychological responses designed to diminish or delay anxiety and protect client) are used
   c. Psychosomatic symptoms begin to develop
   d. Level of anxiety is moderate to severe
4. Exhaustion occurs when adaptational resources are depleted
   a. Results from inability to cope with overwhelming or long-lasting stress
   b. Thinking becomes disorganized and illogical; may experience sensory misperceptions, delusions, hallucinations, and/or reduced orientation to reality
   c. Level of anxiety is severe to panic
   d. Physical illness and even death can occur if period of exhaustion is prolonged

D. Assessment

1. Because anxiety can contribute to organic illness, and organic illness can lead to anxiety, include physical assessment when assessing anxious individuals
2. Shame and fear may prevent individuals from disclosing anxiety
3. Assess anxiety using direct and specific questions (consider cognitive ability, literacy level, and primary language)
4. *NCLEX®* Assess physical, affective, cognitive, social, and spiritual symptoms of anxiety (see Table 21–3)

E. Therapeutic management

1. Tailor interventions to client's level of anxiety
   a. For mild to moderate anxiety, assist client to identify source of anxiety, talk about feelings and issues of concern, examine what occurred before anxiety began (including thoughts and feelings), coach with problem solving and encourage gross motor activity
   b. For moderate to severe anxiety, stay with client and interact in a calm manner using low-pitched voice and clear, simple statements; reduce anxiety quickly, administering medications as prescribed and provide gross motor activity for client
2. Assist in developing mental coping strategies
   a. Include methods such as breathing exercises, guided imagery, meditation, listening to music, progressive muscle relaxation, recreational activities, crying, exercising, laughing, sleeping, diet and fluid intake, time management
   b. *NCLEX®* Encourage problem-focused coping (task-oriented): assessing facts, developing a goal, determining alternatives for coping, identifying risks and benefits of each alternative, selecting an alternative, implementing alternative, evaluating outcome, and modifying actions based on evaluation
   c. Emotion-focused coping requires client to reinterpret meaning of situation and explore defense mechanisms (see Chapter 20)
3. Psychopharmacology
   a. Common anti-anxiety agents (also called anxiolytics) used to treat anxiety are listed in Table 21–4 and are discussed in Chapter 35
   b. Benzodiazepines are commonly used, but prolonged use can lead to dependency
   c. Nonbenzodiazepine sedative-hypnotics are used for short-term treatment of insomnia associated with anxiety
   d. Buspirone is a serotonin and dopamine agonist used in short-term treatment of anxiety

Table 21–3 Manifestations of Anxiety

Category	Specific Manifestations
Physical signs	↑ blood pressure, respiration, and heart rate; diaphoresis; dilated pupils; dyspnea or hyperventilation; vertigo or lightheadedness; blurred vision; urinary frequency; headache; sleep disturbance; muscle weakness or tension; anorexia, nausea and vomiting
Affective symptoms	Depression; irritability; apathy; crying; hypercriticism; feelings of guilt, grief, anger, worthlessness, apprehension, and helplessness
Cognitive symptoms	Inability to concentrate, indecisiveness, inability to think and reason, lack of interest, and forgetfulness
Social symptoms	Refusal to communicate or excessive communication, self-isolation, social withdrawal, and possibly suicidal ideation
Spiritual symptoms	Feelings of hopelessness and despair, fear of death, and inability to find life meaningful

Table 21–4 Medications Used to Treat Anxiety

Class	Specific Medications
Benzodiazepine	Alprazolam, chlordiazepoxide, clonazepam, clorazepate, diazepam, lorazepam, oxazepam
Nonbenzodiazepine anxiolytics	Buspirone, eszopiclone, ramelteon, zaleplon, zolpidem
Antidepressants (approved for anxiety and insomnia)	Duloxetine, escitoprolam, fluoxetine, fluvoxamine, paroxetine, sertraline, venlafaxine

e. Beta blockers have a calming effect on central nervous system (CNS): propranolol may be used to treat physical symptoms of anxiety, such as tremors and tachycardia
f. Antidepressants may be used to treat coexisting depression and insomnia associated with anxiety

4. Individual and **group therapy** (see again Table 21–1)
   a. Helps clients to discuss feelings and problems and develop insight regarding anxiety
   NCLEX® b. See Box 21–1 for intervention strategies to assist anxious clients
   c. Client education is an important intervention for anxious clients
5. Other useful therapies
   a. Cognitive-behavior therapy helps clients learn to identify stressors and plan responses to stressors
   NCLEX® b. Cognitive restructuring assists clients to examine involuntary negative thoughts and to replace negative self-talk with more positive thoughts
   c. Response prevention (a form of behavior modification) teaches clients with obsessive–compulsive disorder how to prevent compulsive behaviors associated with obsessive thoughts
   d. Systematic desensitization is a form of behavior modification used to treat anxiety
   e. Flooding (implosion therapy) exposes client to imaginary or real-life stress-provoking stimuli for an extended period of time, and session is terminated when client's anxiety decreases
   f. Thought-stopping involves such techniques as instructing client to shout "Stop!" or snap a rubber band placed on wrist when unwelcome thoughts occur
   g. Other useful behavior-modification techniques for anxiety include modeling, shaping, token economy, role-playing, social skill training, aversion therapy, response prevention, and contingency contracting

F. Phobic disorders

1. A **phobia** (persistent, irrational fear of specific object or situation) develops when an unconscious conflict is repressed and then displaced onto an external object or situation related symbolically to conflict
2. Avoidance of feared stimulus drastically interferes with routine activities, and panic-level anxiety can result if stimulus cannot be avoided

Box 21–1

Therapeutic Nursing Interventions to Assist Anxious Clients

- Use a quiet, calm approach to reduce interpersonal transmission of anxiety.
- Establish a trusting relationship; protect and reassure client.
- Structure environment to eliminate stressors; stay with client who has severe or panic level of anxiety and place in a smaller, less stimulating environment.
- Provide ongoing assessment of client's anxiety.
- Assess client's use of caffeine, nicotine, and other stimulants.
- Assess client for signs of depression and suicidal ideations.
- Help client to identify stressors, express feelings, and explore sources of feelings.
- Help client to examine cognitive processes and encourage positive self-talk.
- Help client to maintain hope and find meaning in life.
- Support use of effective coping mechanisms.
- Teach new coping behaviors and provide opportunities for client to practice them.
- Teach client relaxation techniques and provide opportunity to practice them.
- Encourage appropriate grooming, sleep, diet, recreational activity, and exercise.
- Facilitate client's interactions with supportive significant others.
- Use role-playing to help client rehearse appropriate reactions to stressors.
- Refer client to community resources as indicated.

3. Phobias
   a. Common phobias include **agoraphobia** (fear of being in a public place or open space), acrophobia (fear of heights), claustrophobia (fear of closed spaces), hematophobia (fear of blood), hydrophobia (fear of water), pyrophobia (fear of fire), xenophobia (fear of strangers), and zoophobia (fear of animals)
   b. Social phobia is excessive fear of embarrassment and humiliation in public settings
4. Treatments include cognitive therapy and graduated exposure or desensitization; anti-anxiety medications may provide short-term relief of phobic anxiety
5. NCLEX® Nursing care includes accepting but not supporting phobia, exploring client's perceptions of threats, discussing feelings that may contribute to irrational fears, and identifying strategies for change

G. Generalized anxiety disorder (GAD)
1. Characterized by pervasive, persistent anxiety over time about everyday concerns and not associated with panic attacks, phobias, obsessions, or compulsions
2. Anxiety leads to symptoms such as restlessness, irritability, fatigue, depression, difficulty concentrating, muscle tension, sleep disturbance, and feeling helpless; these interfere with normal daily activities
3. GAD has been successfully treated by combined cognitive therapy and relaxation training
4. NCLEX® Encourage clients with GAD to rethink perceptions of stressor, recognize that some anxiety is a normal part of life, and learn new coping mechanisms
5. Use nursing interventions previously identified in Box 21–1 as needed and administer anti-anxiety medications if prescribed

H. Panic disorder
1. Characterized by recurrent panic attacks; between panic attacks, client may have little or no debilitating anxiety or may have chronic worry about future panic attacks
2. Onset of a panic attack is sudden, and source of anxiety may not be identifiable; clients frequently associate their symptoms with physical illness and are concerned about death
3. NCLEX® Symptoms of panic attacks include a desire to escape, chest pain, chills or hot flashes, choking sensations, depersonalization, dizziness, nausea, palpitations, shortness of breath, sweating, trembling, and fear of loss of control and mental illness
4. Feelings of hopelessness, helplessness, and despair may lead to suicidal ideations
5. NCLEX® During panic attacks, remain calm, stay with client, offer reassurance, use short, clear sentences, and reduce environmental stimuli
6. When level of anxiety is mild or moderate, explore possible causes of anxiety, teach signs and symptoms of escalating anxiety, and teach and reinforce appropriate coping mechanisms and strategies
7. Benzodiazepines and antidepressants are used to treat panic disorders

I. Obsessive–compulsive disorder (OCD)
1. Characterized by recurrent irrational obsessive thoughts and uncontrollable compulsive behaviors; control of self, others, and environment is an important issue
2. Common **obsessions** (unwanted, persistent thoughts that cannot be removed from consciousness without anxiety or distress) often include thoughts about specific objects, contamination, orderliness, sexual behavior, aggression or violence, or religion
3. Common **compulsions** (persistent unwanted urges to perform acts to relieve severe tension associated with obsession) include such behaviors as counting, handwashing, repeating words, checking doors or locks, and dressing and undressing rituals
4. NCLEX® Anxiety increases if obsessive thoughts and compulsive behaviors are interrupted; defense mechanisms employed may be repression, displacement, and undoing
5. Treatments include relaxation and cognitive-behavioral techniques such as flooding and thought-stopping
6. NCLEX® Assist clients to identify situations that increase anxiety, explore meaning and purpose of thoughts and behavior, and support client attempts to decrease obsessions and compulsions
7. NCLEX® Assist client to meet basic human needs (food, grooming, sleep) as needed; do not interrupt compulsive behaviors as long as they do not pose a threat to safety of client or others
8. Assist client to develop a schedule that allows time to perform compulsive behavior but also provides for distraction with other activities or tasks
9. Conduct teaching immediately after completion of a ritual when client is least anxious
10. Selective serotonin reuptake inhibitors (SSRIs) are most effective somatic treatment for OCD; electroconvulsive therapy (ECT) has been used to treat depressive symptoms associated with OCD

J. Posttraumatic stress disorder (PTSD)

1. Associated with recurrent experiencing of a psychologically traumatic event through dreams and flashbacks; may include military combat, terrorist attack, natural disaster, traumatic accident, crime (rape, assault, kidnapping, torture), and abuse (physical, emotional, sexual)

NCLEX® 2. Symptoms
   a. Apathy, social withdrawal and isolation, loss of interest in activities, poor concentration, and possible depression and hopelessness
   b. Restlessness, irritability, intrusive and unwanted memories of traumatic event, amnesia for certain aspects of trauma, nightmares or sleep disturbances, flashbacks, hypervigilance, survivor guilt, and avoidance of activities that trigger memory of event

3. Denial, repression, and suppression are used as coping mechanisms; treatments may include progressive review of trauma, systematic desensitization, hypnotherapy, and/or support groups may helpful

NCLEX® 4. Provide a nonthreatening and nonjudgmental supportive environment; reassure client that this reaction is normal; encourage client to discuss traumatic event and associated feelings; assess and acknowledge feelings of guilt, grief, anger, and shame

NCLEX® 5. Encourage and reinforce appropriate coping strategies and relaxation techniques, and assist client in resuming regular activities and relationships

6. SSRIs, especially sertraline, seem to have some effect in treating PTSD

III. MOOD DISORDERS

A. Overview

1. **Mood**: a prolonged emotional state that affects a person's life and personality
2. Change of mood and a range of emotions (such as happiness, sadness, depression, anger, and fear) are normal and expected during life
3. **Affect**: a person's present feelings and moods with verbal and nonverbal behavioral cues
4. *Mood disorders* are characterized by changes in mood that range from depression to elation
   a. **Major depression**: a loss of interest in life and a mild to severe depressed mood that lasts at least 2 weeks; if uncontrolled, interferes with eating, sleeping, and functioning at work, home, and/or school; withdrawal and decreased sociability; possible delusions and/or hallucinations with psychotic features if disorder progresses to severe depression; 15% of clients die by suicide
   b. **Dysthymic disorder**: a chronic disorder in which depressed mood fluctuates with normal mood; symptoms are less severe than in major depression
   c. **Bipolar disorder** (also called manic-depressive disorder): alternation of depression and elation; categorized as bipolar I disorder (one or more manic episodes and one or more depressive episodes) or bipolar II disorder (one or more *hypomanic* or mild manic episodes and one or more depressive episodes)
   d. **Cyclothymic disorder**: mood changes between moderate depression and hypomania; lasts for at least 2 years; usually no sign of a normal range
   e. **Seasonal affective disorder (SAD)**: depressed mood occurs during fall and winter when there are fewer hours of daylight (direct correlation of light with melatonin production)
   f. **Schizoaffective disorder**: a combination of manifestations of schizophrenia and mood disorders; delusions, hallucinations, disorganized speech and behavior, communication difficulties, poor abstractions, passive social withdrawal, poor grooming and hygiene, poor rapport, and major depressive or manic symptoms or mixed symptoms, and possibly other physical or psychological disorders

B. Assessment

NCLEX® 1. Conduct intake assessment in 15- to 20-minute segments at one time; clients with depression may not have enough energy to talk or focus attention for extended periods of time, while clients with mania may not be able to sit still and concentrate because of elevated mood and flight of ideas

2. Bipolar disorders
   a. Characterized by moods alternating between episodes of depression and episodes of mania or hypomania
   b. Manic episodes are periods of elation during which there is an abnormally and persistently elevated, expansive, or irritable mood for at least 1 week and also includes at least three of the following: inflated self-esteem, decreased need for sleep, more than usual talkativeness, racing thoughts, distractibility, increase in goal-directed activity, and excessive involvement in pleasurable activities
   c. Hypomania is described as an elevation in mood with increases in activity but not as severe elation as in mania

3. Major depression
    a. Loss of interest in life and a depressed mood is present for most of day, nearly every day (for at least 2 weeks), as indicated by client's subjective report or objective data (facial expression, appears tearful)
    b. Markedly diminished interest or pleasure in almost all activities for most activities nearly every day
    c. Significant weight loss or gain
    d. Insomnia or hypersomnia
    e. Psychomotor agitation or retardation nearly every day
    f. Fatigue or loss of energy nearly every day
    g. Diminished ability to think or concentrate, or indecisiveness, nearly every day
    h. Social withdrawal
    i. Recurrent thoughts of death; suicidal ideation with or without a specific plan or a suicide attempt
4. Dysthymic disorder is a chronic, low-level depression; must have depressed mood and at least three symptoms of depression for most of day, nearly every day, for at least 2 years: poor appetite or overeating; insomnia or hypersomnia; low energy; low self-esteem; poor concentration and difficulty making decisions; and feelings of hopelessness
5. Key characteristic differences between depressive disorder and bipolar disorders are noted in Table 21–5

C. Therapeutic management

1. Address risk for threats to safety of client or others as first priority; provide a safe environment, removing objects and barriers to prevent accidental or purposeful injury to self or others
    a. Danger for self-harm is more prominent as client begins to regain strength and hope; frequently assess for levels of hopefulness or hopelessness and self-esteem, and be alert for signs of thoughts or plan for suicide

NCLEX®

Table 21–5 Assessment Findings in Depression Disorder and Bipolar Disorders

	Depression Disorder	Bipolar Disorders
Behavior	Progression from a decreased desire to engage in social, work, and school activities to lack of participation in common ADLs; progressive loss of self-esteem, feelings of incompetence, decreased motivation; statements such as "Why bother, I can't anyway" are common	Initial high energy and productivity with positive reinforcement from others; reduced ability to concentrate, make judgments, or engage in activities; increasing frustration and irritability, shortened attention span, unrealistic self-confidence, and poor judgment (spending sprees, risky financial investments, high-risk lifestyle changes)
Relationships	Withdrawal from personal and social activities and events	Unable to set boundaries; incessant talkativeness and gregarious behaviors that are often embarrassing upon return to normal range of mood
Affective characteristics	Sense of sadness that becomes increasingly pronounced; guilt that may be expressed as a vague concern or a specific issue: "I have so much to be thankful for, I shouldn't feel this way"; loss of emotional attachment with expressions of indifference toward family and friends; anhedonia, or a lack of pleasure	Mood ranges between cheerful and euphoric; if there is an external negative stimulus, can become irritable, argumentative, hostile, and combative, then return to euphoria when stimulus is removed; absent sense of guilt; responds to others' feelings of hurt or anger with anger, laughter, or indifference; tries to participate in every available activity or event
Cognitive characteristics	Personal worth: presents self as a failure and incompetent; personalizes comments by others; is self-critical and perfectionistic; anticipates disapproval; while in a depressed state: • Exhibits decreased ability or inability to make decisions • Has decreased rate and number of thoughts • Perceives self as unattractive • Has somatic delusions • Has hallucinations (15–25% of cases)	Personal worth: very grandiose belief about self; exhibits unwarranted positive expectations, is unable to see potential negative outcomes, and is irate if criticized by others; while in manic state: • Is easily distractible and impulsive • Has flight of ideas • Believes self to be very attractive • Exhibits delusions of grandeur • Exhibits hallucinations in approximately 15–25% of cases
Physiological characteristics	Increased or decreased appetite; when severely depressed, a decrease in appetite usually occurs; constipation; increased or decreased sleep in mild to moderate depression; usually decreased sleep in severe depression; loss of desire in sexual activities	Difficulty eating because of the inability to physically slow down or sit still; constipation; usually only 1 or 2 hours of sleep per night and hyperactivity during activities; increased sexual activity, even promiscuity
Physical appearance	Unkempt appearance with little to no attention to hygiene	Bright clothes, frequent clothing changes, exaggerated presentation of physical self

b. History of violence is *always* important in determining seriousness of client's present risk for harm to self or others
c. Client often displays ambivalence or expresses sadness, dejection, hopelessness, or loss of pleasure or purpose in life
d. Assess for and prevent overt attempts to harm self (e.g., hoards medications, performs self-mutilation, attempts to hang self)
NCLEX® e. Assess for overt signs of hopelessness: refusal to eat, withdrawal from milieu, resistance to or refusal of medications; inability to see future for self; sudden giving away of possessions; refusal to sign a no-self-harm contract
f. Encourage client to sign a no-self-harm contract, check on client frequently (not left alone for long periods) and use one-to-one supervision as appropriate
g. Assess client's ability to tolerate frustration in individual situations; poor impulse control and labile affect can increase risk of injury to others
h. To reduce risk of injury to others, encourage client during calm moments to recognize and identify factors leading to agitation and loss of control and alternative behaviors that are acceptable to client and staff
NCLEX® i. Decrease environmental stimuli when client is agitated; gradually increase environmental stimulation after agitation subsides
j. Communicate with respect and nonjudgmental tone; offer alternatives when available (e.g., "There is no coffee available; how about a glass of juice?")

2. Support coping, which may be impaired because of lack of energy and inability to concentrate or make decisions
a. Maintain activities of daily living (ADLs) and safe environment
b. Use a problem-solving approach
c. Encourage client to focus on strengths rather than weaknesses and identify people and systems that can support client
d. Help client to learn strategies that will effect more positive thinking (cognitive, behavioral, imagery)
NCLEX® e. Encourage client to express feelings and needs
f. Teach family and friends that client may direct anger toward them but that client is learning more effective coping skills to deal with feelings
NCLEX® g. Help client to gradually become involved with activities on unit and to socialize as tolerated with staff, other clients on unit, and family members in a structured environment

3. Support adequate nutrition
a. Assess client for lack of interest in eating/food or choosing nutritional foods, aversion to eating, or dysfunctional eating pattern (e.g., eating in response to internal cues other than hunger)
b. Clients with depression may have a nutritional pattern that relates more to their depressed mood, including disinterest in eating, poor or no appetite, aversion to food, dysfunctional eating patterns, poor food choices, recent weight loss or gain, poor muscle tone, pale conjunctivae and mucous membranes
NCLEX® c. Note common findings in manic states, including weight loss; easy distraction from eating; inability to sit through routine meals; wary or frightened appearance when offered food; physical signs of poor nutrition, dehydration, and electrolyte imbalances; hyperactive bowel sounds
NCLEX® d. Offer small, frequent feedings and high-calorie, protein-rich snacks and fluids throughout day; remain with client during meals
NCLEX® e. Offer nutritious finger foods and sandwiches and easy-to-carry drinks that are high in vitamins, minerals, and electrolytes
NCLEX® f. Determine client's daily caloric intake needs; monitor and record daily intake and output; monitor body weight
g. Assess daily bowel movements for frequency and consistency (risk of constipation with depression) and administer high-fiber foods unless contraindicated
h. Explain to client importance of maintaining adequate intake of food and fluids to prevent malnutrition
i. Monitor laboratory study results (such as serum prealbumin, albumin, glucose, electrolytes, nitrogen balance)

4. Support adequate sleep, which can be interrupted by biochemical alterations (decreased serotonin) or psychological stress, lack of recognition of fatigue or need to sleep, hyperactivity
a. Sleep disturbances associated with mania include denial of need for sleep, changes in behavior and performance, increasing irritability, restlessness, and dark circles under eyes

b. Identify environmental factors that might prevent or interrupt sleep

NCLEX®

c. Identify variations from usual sleep pattern (difficulty falling asleep, remaining asleep, or waking early and unable to return to sleep)

d. Restrict caffeine; offer small snack or warm milk at bedtime or when client is awake during night

NCLEX®

e. Encourage activities in morning and early afternoon, and reduce environmental stimuli during evening and prior to bedtime

f. Encourage routine bedtime relaxation techniques; identify previously effective nighttime rituals and reestablish when possible

g. Administer medications as indicated

h. Restrict evening fluids, and have client void before retiring

5. Support clients experiencing spiritual distress (sense of no purpose or joy in life; lack of connectedness to others; misperceived shame and guilt)

NCLEX®

a. Allow client to express feelings and thoughts about religious doubt or fears of abandonment

b. Explore with client alternative or past effective religious or spiritual practice or ritual as an illness-prevention measure

c. Encourage client to discuss thoughts and feelings with clergy or chaplain as desired

6. Electroconvulsive therapy (ECT) as treatment

a. Useful for clients with severe depression, bipolar depressive disorder, mania, or depression with psychotic symptoms, especially when resistant to other treatments, including medications such as TCAs and MAOIs

b. Involves delivery of electricity through electrodes attached to forehead and temporal area of scalp sufficient to cause a brief seizure; carried out after providing premedication to relax muscles, so only slight movement of hands, feet, or digits is seen

c. A series of 6–12 ECT treatments is usually carried out at a rate of two to three per week; may be repeated once monthly to reduce relapse rate for recurrent depression

NCLEX®

d. Side effects seem to be limited to disorientation, confusion, and short-term memory deficits that may last as long as 6 months; risks related to anesthesia or premedication are also present

NCLEX®

e. Preprocedure care involves same principles as those used for client undergoing surgery or moderate (conscious) sedation: ensure informed consent, maintain NPO status as prescribed (after midnight or 4 hours prior), record baseline vital signs and have client void; remove jewelry, contact lenses, dentures, and hair pins; administer any prescribed preprocedure medications

f. During procedure, attach blood pressure cuff to one arm and pulse oximeter probe to one finger for continuous monitoring; attach electrocardiographic and encephalographic electrodes; begin intravenous line; place airway or bite stick to prevent client from biting tongue during procedure; administer 100% oxygen and protect client's airway; provide for safety after administration of short-acting anesthetic and muscle relaxant

g. Postprocedure care is identical to postanesthesia care (see Chapter 48); reorient and reassure client as needed because of confusion, monitor vital signs; transfer client back to unit when vital signs are stable, oxygen saturation is maintained at 90% or higher, and client has stable mental status; withhold food and fluid until protective airway reflexes (cough, gag, and swallow reflexes) have returned

7. Medication therapy for mood disorders includes TCAs, SSRIs, MAOIs, atypical antidepressants, and mood stabilizers (see Chapter 35 for full discussion of medications to treat depression and bipolar disorders)

8. Group and individual therapies may help, including cognitive therapy, behavioral therapy, and interpersonal therapy for mild to moderate depression

NCLEX®

9. Phototherapy may be a useful adjunct treatment for recurrent SAD during fall and winter months

a. Healthcare provider prescribes a minimum amount of light (usually 2,500 lux) on waking in morning; clients can be exposed for 30 minutes to several hours, depending on strength of light source

b. An antidepressant effect is usually seen within 2–4 days and is complete after 2 weeks; maintenance therapy is usually 30 mins of exposure each day; side effects are usually minimal

10. Evaluate goal achievement for clients with mood disorders: remaining safe; absence of suicidal or homicidal intent or plan; establishing effective pattern of activity and sleep to meet self-care needs and role function; and demonstrating understanding of disorder, including triggers for relapse, measures to prevent relapse, and medications to control symptoms

IV. SCHIZOPHRENIA AND OTHER PSYCHOTIC DISORDERS

A. Types of psychotic disorders

1. **Schizophrenia**: a mental health disorder characterized by disturbances in thought processes and decision making, perceptual disturbances, behavioral abnormalities, affective disruptions, and difficulty in maintaining interpersonal relationships
2. Schizoaffective disorder: having clinical manifestations characteristic of both schizophrenia and a mood disorder, such as depression, mania, or a mixed episode
3. Schizophreniform disorder: essential features of schizophrenia are present with the exception that duration is at least 1 month but less than 6 months
4. Other psychotic disorders
   a. Delusional disorder: presence of nonbizarre delusions (delusions that could possibly occur in reality) that persist for at least 1 month with no other manifestations of psychosis
   b. Brief psychotic disorder: presence of at least one positive symptom of schizophrenia lasting 1 day to 1 month, with or without an identified stressor
   c. Shared psychotic disorder (*folie a deux*): a delusional system that develops in context of a close relationship between two people who share a similar delusion
   d. Substance-induced psychotic disorder: presence of hallucinations and delusions that result directly from physiological effects of a substance
   e. Psychotic disorder (presence of hallucinations and delusions) due to a general medical condition

B. Overview of schizophrenia

NCLEX®

1. Generally, client exhibits normal behavior early in life, has subtle changes after puberty, and severe symptoms in late teens to mid-30s
2. Most clients develop disorder in early 20s (men) or late 20s (women), with only 10% first diagnosed after age 45
3. Subtypes of schizophrenia include paranoid, catatonic, residual, disorganized, and undifferentiated schizophrenia; see Table 21–6 for critical essential features of each subtype
4. Psychiatric rehabilitation emphasizes development of skills and supports; considers client to be in control; and promotes choices, self-determination, and individual responsibility

C. Assessment

1. Symptoms of schizophrenia are labeled as positive or negative symptoms

   NCLEX®

   a. Positive symptoms: presence of behaviors not normally seen, such as **delusions** (false beliefs occurring without appropriate external stimulation and inconsistent with logic or evidence), **hallucinations** (false sensory perceptions that may involve any of five senses [auditory, visual, tactile, olfactory, and gustatory]), disorganized speech patterns, and disorganized or bizarre behavior (pacing, touching objects) or abnormal motor behavior

   NCLEX®

   b. Negative symptoms: a loss or absence of healthy behaviors that develop over time and hinder client's ability to complete life tasks; may include flat affect, apathy, anhedonia (decreased ability to experience pleasure), avolition (inability to pursue goal-directed behavior), alogia (poverty of speech), anergia (lack of energy), ambivalence (inability to make a decision because of conflicting emotions), minimal self-care, ineffective social skills with social withdrawal, and isolation and concrete thinking
2. Types of delusions
   a. Persecution: client believes others or a powerful force is harassing or threatening client; behavior may be hostile, suspicious, and aggressive

Table 21–6 Essential Features of Subtypes of Schizophrenia

Subtype	Features
Paranoid	Auditory hallucinations, preoccupation with one or more delusions usually of a persecutory nature, may appear hostile or angry
Catatonic	Stupor (state of daze or unconsciousness) or extreme motor agitation, excessive negativism, inappropriate or bizarre body postures, *echolalia* (an involuntary, parrot-like repetition of words spoken by others), *echopraxia* (a meaningless imitation of motions made by others), or *waxy flexibility* (placing one's arms or legs in a specific position and maintaining that position for hours)
Residual	Absence of prominent psychotic symptoms, social withdrawal and inappropriate affect, eccentric behavior, past history of at least one episode of schizophrenia
Disorganized	Disorganized speech or behavior, inappropriate or flat affect
Undifferentiated	Disorganized behaviors, psychotic symptoms (including delusions and hallucinations)

b. Grandeur: client has exaggerated feelings of importance and power over others or in relation to universe
c. Somatic type: client believes there are unusual changes in body that have no basis or evidence in reality
d. Loss of reference: client believes external events or interactions somehow relate directly to self

3. Other abnormal thought processes
a. May have fragmentation of thoughts, loose associations, magical thinking, inability to differentiate reality from internal personal perceptions (impaired reality testing), distortions in perception of environment, and inability to organize thoughts and facts
b. Thought broadcasting: client believes that others can hear his or her thoughts
c. Thought insertion: client believes that others have ability to put thoughts in his or her mind against client's will
d. Thought control: client believes that others can control his or her thoughts against client's will
e. Thought blocking: client forgets a thought while speaking and is unable to continue the thought; may shift to new thoughts unrelated to old topic

4. **Illusion:** inaccurate perception or misinterpretation of sensory cues, usually brief in nature
5. Hallucinations: false perception can affect any of five senses but are usually auditory; visual is second-most common type
6. **Psychosis:** a disorderly mental state in which client has difficulty distinguishing reality from his or her own internal perceptions
7. Appearance and motor behavior
a. May neglect hygiene (unkempt appearance) and need for food and fluids, sleep, and elimination
b. May report somatic symptoms or have distorted body image
c. May exhibit total immobilization and be unable to initiate activity; may have repetitive movements, catatonic posturing (see Table 21–6 again) or motor agitation (pacing, impulsive behavior, inability to eat or sleep)
d. May fail to respond to directions or alternatively may only respond to directions to do something

8. Affective manifestations
a. Blunted or flat affect; may also have inappropriate affect
b. May mistrust others (including healthcare personnel) and view world as a dangerous and unsafe place
c. May exhibit a range of emotions related to diagnosis and presence of delusions and hallucinations, such as anxiety, helplessness, anger, grief, guilt, and depression

9. Speech and language disturbances
a. Echolalia (involuntary, parrot-like repetition of words spoken by others)
b. **Clang associations**: rhyming words in a sentence that makes no sense
c. **Neologisms**: inventing new words that are meaningful only to that person; often associated with delusions
d. **Word salad**: combining in a sentence words that have no connection and make no sense
e. Mutism: lack of production of verbal speech
f. Pressured speech: rapid speech produced with a sense of urgency
g. Verbigeration: repetition of words or phrases that serves no purpose

D. Psychopharmacology (see Chapter 35): includes typical (traditional) antipsychotics, atypical antipsychotics, and antiparkinsonian agents (anticholinergics)

E. Therapeutic management

NCLEX®

1. Nursing interventions to manage delusions and hallucinations
a. Establish a trusting, therapeutic relationship with client by being honest, supportive, and consistent; this helps reduce suspicion on client's part
b. Assess for signs of delusions or hallucinations (cues and content)
c. Encourage description of delusion or hallucination and expression of feelings about it
d. Interact with client on a one-on-one basis
e. Communicate with client using clear, direct statements
f. Provide an environment that is free from excessive stimulation but provides structure to support easy accomplishment of routine activities of daily living
g. Acknowledge client's belief about delusion or hallucination experience but do not share in it; do not argue with client; instead, encourage expression of feelings associated with delusion or hallucination
h. Focus on reality-based topics rather than delusion or hallucination; set limits on time spent talking about delusion if client obsesses about it
i. If client has visual hallucinations, provide a room with adequate lighting
j. Do not touch a client who is experiencing a hallucination

k. Substitute food from home or prepackaged foods if needed for client with delusion about poisoning during hospital stay
l. Monitor for increasing anxiety or agitation as indicators of reoccurring or worsening hallucination
2. General nursing interventions for client with schizophrenia
NCLEX® a. Provide an environment that is safe for client and others and reassure client about safety; assess for self-destructive behaviors or behaviors harmful to others (such as command hallucinations) and provide needed precautions
NCLEX® b. Avoid physical contact or touching of client
c. Assess client's physiological needs and assist with grooming and other self-care needs until client is able to meet them
d. Communicate therapeutically with client to reduce sense of threat; use simple, direct, and concise speech; use a neutral rather than an overly warm approach; use therapeutic silence as needed when sitting with client
e. Be honest with client; refrain from supporting delusions or hallucinations; avoid making promises that can't be kept; and acknowledge if client says something that is not understood
f. Initiate frequent contact with client for short periods rather than extended in time to keep client at ease; however, stay with client if client is frightened; tell client when leaving room
g. Assist client with determining what is real and what is not; reorient as needed; monitor for altered thought processes, including delusions and hallucinations
h. Assist client to establish daily routine and offer simple activities (such as puzzles) for diversion; provide opportunities for socialization to decrease isolation; may begin with one-on-one contact and progress to small groups
i. Involve client in setting realistic goals in treatment plan; explore with client other ways to express feelings, such as through use of art, writing, or music
NCLEX® j. Set limits on client's behavior if it becomes disruptive or affects others; remove client from group setting if dangerous or disturbing to other clients in therapeutic milieu

F. **Evaluation of client outcomes:** freedom from harm, absence of violence toward others, cessation of hallucinations or delusions, increased socialization skills, decreased isolative behavior, appropriate affect, improved thought processes, improved speech patterns and congruent communication, adherence to medication schedule, and effective use of coping skills and community resources

G. **Evaluation of family outcomes:** can identify early signs and symptoms of disease exacerbation, implications of schizophrenia as a chronic illness, medication regimen, and how and when to access emergency services

V. PERSONALITY DISORDERS

A. Overview

1. **Personality traits** are enduring patterns that determine how individuals perceive, relate to, and think about environment and themselves; they are reflected in how people cope with feelings and impulses, respond to their surroundings, and find meaning in relationships
2. **Personality disorders** are diagnosed when resulting behavior patterns are inflexible, enduring, pervasive, maladaptive, and cause significant functional impairment or subjective distress
   a. Result in problems in living rather than in clinical symptoms because behavior patterns reflect inner experience and do not fit with cultural expectations
   b. Clients frequently experience their personality patterns as natural or comfortable (**egosyntonic**) rather than painful or uncomfortable (**egodystonic**)
   c. Frequently overlap: clients may exhibit patterns or traits associated with more than one personality disorder
   d. Client tends to lack insight into own behavior but is usually in touch with reality; in severe states, disorder may deteriorate and include elements of psychosis
   e. Are organized into three diagnostic clusters (see Table 21–7)
3. Manifestations of personality disorders adversely affect four areas of function:
   a. Behavioral: client exhibits poor impulse control; may act out with physical and verbal aggression, manipulation of others, or preoccupation with self, sexual behaviors, or religion; these behaviors are likely to be attempts to manage internal pain
   b. Affective: may exhibit a range of emotions, from emptiness, depression, and feelings of abandonment, to guilt, fear, and rage; emotions may be labile and inappropriate to situation; may project own feelings onto others
   c. Cognitive: client experiences differences in how self, others, and events are interpreted; may have distorted sense of reality and of self (resulting in idealization of self or self-hate); may be unable to

Table 21–7 Personality Disorder Clusters

Cluster	Specific Type of Personality Disorder
Cluster A disorders: characterized by odd or eccentric behavior	*Paranoid:* distrust and suspiciousness; others' motives are interpreted as malevolent *Schizoid:* detached from social relationships, lack of interest in others, restricted range of emotions *Schizotypal:* acute discomfort in close relationships, cognitive or perceptual distortions, and eccentricities of behavior
Cluster B disorders: characterized by dramatic and erratic behavior	*Antisocial:* disregard for and violation of rights of others *Borderline:* instability in interpersonal relationships, self-image, and affect and marked impulsivity *Histrionic:* excessive emotionality and attention-seeking *Narcissistic:* grandiosity and self-importance, need for admiration, lack of empathy
Cluster C disorders: characterized by anxious and fearful behavior	*Avoidant:* social inhibition, feelings of inadequacy, and hypersensitivity to negative evaluation *Dependent:* submissive and clinging behavior related to a need to be taken care of *Obsessive–compulsive:* preoccupation with orderliness, control, and perfectionism

anticipate consequences of own actions; judgment may be impaired, leading to less effective problem solving; may have difficulty with concentration, attention span, and memory, and may exhibit either diffuse or concrete thought patterns

d. Sociocultural: interpersonal functioning may be impaired if rigid and inflexible behavior or poor impulse control causes strain on relationships with others, especially intimate relationships

B. Assessment guidelines

1. Since client may not perceive that a problem exists or believes that problem is related to behavior of others, maintain sensitivity during interview process so client does not become guarded or defensive
2. Use professional judgment to protect client rights and maintain confidentiality
3. NCLEX® Assess client's level of function in areas of affect, cognition, behavior (including impulse control), and sociocultural adaptation (interpersonal relationships)

C. Basic principles of nursing intervention

1. NCLEX® Help clients to see how behavior affects their lives to motivate them to develop a more adaptive lifestyle
2. Assist and encourage client to discuss feelings instead of acting on them; keeping a daily journal may help client focus on feelings
3. Because personality traits are too ingrained to expect radical, long-term behavioral change, plan interventions to meet short-term goals and focus on small steps to improve role function
4. Explain behavioral expectations of client and consequences that will result from acting-out behaviors
5. Implement standard safety interventions such as behavioral contracts to avoid self-harm, harm to others, or damage to property
6. NCLEX® Identify own emotional responses when caring for clients diagnosed with a personality disorder
7. Praise appropriate social behaviors and limit manipulative behaviors; remove client from groups when attention-seeking behavior occurs

D. Specific nursing management strategies: cluster-specific nursing interventions can be individualized for each client

1. NCLEX® Cluster A personality disorders (paranoid, schizoid, and schizotypal)
   a. Approach client in a gentle, interested, but nonintrusive manner
   b. Respect client's needs for distance and privacy
   c. Be mindful of own nonverbal communication (client may perceive others as threatening)
   d. Gradually encourage interaction with others, if appropriate
2. NCLEX® Cluster B personality disorders (antisocial, borderline, histrionic, narcissistic)
   a. Be patient when client displays emotional and erratic behavior
   b. Provide a consistent and structured milieu to avoid manipulation and power struggles
   c. Safety is always first priority of care—protect clients from suicide and self-mutilation until they can protect themselves
   d. Set limits as necessary to help client maintain impulse control to protect client and others from injury
   e. Engage in frequent staff conferences to prevent client's ability to play one staff member against another
   f. Help client recognize and discuss fear of abandonment

g. Help client recognize presence of dichotomous thinking or splitting, in which self and others are perceived as all good or all bad
h. Encourage direct communication to minimize attention-seeking through use of dramatic or seductive behavior
i. Help client who displays a sense of entitlement to acknowledge needs of others

NCLEX®

3. Cluster C personality disorders (avoidant, dependent, and obsessive–compulsive)
   a. Point out avoidance behaviors and related losses and secondary gains
   b. Provide problem-solving and assertiveness training to increase self-confidence and independence
   c. Encourage expression of feelings to decrease rigidity and need for control
   d. Help client recognize any impairment or distress related to need for perfection and control
   e. Help client acknowledge and discuss sense of inadequacy and fear of rejection

E. **Psychopharmacology:** may include short-term antipsychotic agents to alleviate psychotic symptoms (schizotypal or borderline personality disorders); SSRIs to diminish rapid mood swings and impulsive, aggressive, self-destructive behavior (borderline personality disorder) and to treat obsessive thoughts associated with certain personality disorders (see Chapter 35)

F. **Individual and group therapy**
1. May be recommended based on a client's level of function and specific needs
2. Self-help groups may increase self-awareness and assist clients in coping with problems in living

G. **Behavioral therapy**
1. Impulse-control training supports client safety by decreasing risk of suicide or self-mutilation through use of antiharm contracts, staff and client (self) monitoring, identifying triggers and patterns related to self-destructive behavior, and identifying alternative coping strategies

NCLEX®

2. Setting limits discourages tendency to test and manipulate others
   a. Involves establishing a structured environment with clear ground rules
   b. Setting limits reflects three principles: limits must be clearly stated, necessary, and enforceable
3. Behavioral modification: social skills for clients who are helpless and dependent; goal is to increase coping skills and independent functioning
   a. Assist clients to acknowledge feelings of helplessness and fear of becoming more independent
   b. Explore clients' dichotomous thinking or tendency to see themselves as totally dependent or totally independent
   c. Help clients identify what they would gain and lose by becoming less helpless
   d. Engage clients in problem-solving exercises to increase self-confidence
   e. Provide assertiveness training
   f. Take care not to be seen as a rescuer
4. Behavioral modification: social skills for clients who are socially isolative related to a fear of rejection; goal is to increase self-confidence
   a. Help clients acknowledge their fear of criticism and rejection
   b. Help clients identify what they would gain and lose by risking criticism and rejection
   c. Help clients identify interpersonal effects of social isolation and feelings associated with it
   d. Engage clients in problem-solving exercises to increase self-confidence
   e. Provide assertiveness training
5. For clients who are socially isolated because of suspicion and mistrust of others, respect their need to be isolative while gradually encouraging interaction with others; if appropriate, help clients identify interpersonal effects of social isolation and feelings associated with them
6. For clients who seek out relationships with others through behavior that is attention-seeking (dramatic, seductive) but superficial, help them to interact in a more direct fashion; help clients identify what they would gain and lose by communicating more directly
7. For clients whose relationships are based on manipulation, focus on their attempts at manipulation and help them to identify ways to interact in a more collaborative and less power-based manner; help clients identify what they would gain and lose by becoming less manipulative

H. **Psychological comfort promotion—anxiety reduction**
1. Encourage decision making to support a sense of competence and an internal locus of control
2. Some clients become perfectionistic to guard against anxiety of feeling inferior; explore their fear
3. Anxiety prevents some clients from asking for help because they fear rejection; help clients identify what they would gain and lose by asking for help

I. **Evaluation and client outcomes**
1. Be aware that realistic goals must reflect small steps to improve function and decrease subjective distress
2. Evaluate effectiveness of nursing interventions in relation to stated outcomes

VI. DISSOCIATIVE DISORDERS

A. Overview

1. In dissociative disorders, there is a sudden disruption in client's consciousness, identity, or memory
2. Possible etiologies include traumatic experience (commonly accidents, natural disasters, assault) or severe physical, sexual, or emotional abuse
3. Defense mechanisms of dissociation and repression are used, although these processes are not used consciously

B. Specific dissociative disorders

1. **Dissociative amnesia**: client cannot remember important personal information, and memory loss cannot be accounted for by ordinary forgetfulness
   a. Client suddenly cannot recall memories: *localized amnesia* is loss of memory of a short time period (hours) after a disturbing event; *selective amnesia* is loss of memory of some, but not all, events; *generalized amnesia* is loss of memory of a whole lifetime of experiences (very rare); *continuous amnesia* is inability to remember successive events as they occur
   b. Client with amnesia can recall other information, learn, and function coherently
   c. More common during wars and natural disasters
   d. **Primary gain**: symbolic resolution of unconscious conflict that decreases anxiety and keeps conflict from awareness
   e. **Secondary gain**: receipt of extra support and caring when experiencing an illness
   f. Usually terminates abruptly
   g. Special therapies: survivor support groups; gradual reconstruction of events through talking, listening, and reading others' accounts of the trauma
2. **Dissociative fugue**: client suddenly leaves usual environment with no memory of some or all of past; assumes complete new identity but does not recognize old identity has been forgotten
   a. Usually lasts from hours to days, rarely months; is often a response to psychological stressors (marital, family, war)
   b. Client has no memory of events during fugue after returning to prefugue state
   c. Special interventions: hypnosis, possible drug-facilitated interviews, support groups
3. **Dissociative identity disorder (DID)**: presence of two or more distinct personalities or identities (*alters*) in one person; also called multiple personality disorder
   a. **Host personality** is primary identity, while alters are other personalities that intermittently take full control of behavior of client; host is typically unaware of alters but alters may be aware of host and of other alters
   b. Alters communicate with one another through "executive" alter
   c. "Switching" (transition from one personality to another) is sudden and usually occurs in response to stress or trauma (dissociation is an unconscious self-protective mechanism); behaviors during switching may include blinking, eye rolls, headaches, covering or hiding face, and twitches
   d. Client (host) "loses time" and cannot recall important information during time that alter is present; may appear forgetful or be accused of lying
   e. Client may have impaired insight; may appear anxious or depressed; may have marked variation in appearance or speech from time to time

NCLEX®

   f. Special interventions: institute no-harm contract and environmental safety if client is suicidal or self-mutilating; meet and recognize alters and their unique experiences and needs; "map" personality system, noting characteristics of alters and co-consciousness; create emotionally safe environment for all alters; individualize psychotherapy to integrate personalities
4. Depersonalization disorder
   a. **Depersonalization**: feeling of detachment or separation from one's self, as if being in a dreamlike state; client is able to function during experience (intact reality testing)
   b. Client may report distress about experiences and become depressed and anxious; feelings may be accompanied by **derealization**, a feeling that external world is unreal or strange
   c. Precipitated by stress and anxiety

NCLEX®

   d. Special interventions: problem solving to reduce stress in general; stress-management techniques; "grounding" or focus on external environment

C. Assessment

1. Recounts trauma and/or severe stress, often in childhood
   a. Symptoms appear in adulthood after stressful event(s)
   b. Symptoms appear immediately or may be delayed for years

2. Extent of symptoms of dissociation or amnesia varies widely with different dissociative disorders
   a. **Dissociation** is a defense mechanism in which experiences are blocked from consciousness so that affect, behavior, identity, memories, and/or thoughts are not integrated
   b. **Repression** is a defense mechanism in which thoughts and feelings are kept from consciousness
3. May report symptoms of depression or anxiety
4. Physical symptoms: headaches common with DID, but other dissociative disorders have no associated physical symptoms

NCLEX®
5. Mental status examination
   a. Appearance: facial expressions and mannerisms may vary widely within one session or appearance may vary widely from day to day (DID)
   b. Mood: anxious, depressed; some clients have little mood change
   c. Memory: amnesia for events (variable extent)
   d. Perception: feelings of detachment from self or environment, feeling of physical change in body
   e. Insight: impaired, unaware of memory impairment

NCLEX®
D. Nursing intervention strategies
1. Create safe, calm environment; prevent stressors that could elicit dissociation; mutually develop plan of care
2. Discuss and explore with client anxieties, concerns, sources of conflict, and painful experiences (especially those that can lead to dissociation)
3. Identify client's strengths and current methods of coping
4. Teach stress management and coping techniques
   a. Progressive muscle relaxation
   b. Physical exercise
   c. "Grounding," or focus on external environment (what client can see and hear) rather than on internal feelings, thoughts, or sensations that can lead to feelings that distance self from world
   d. Problem-solving strategies
   e. Distraction
5. Assist client to progress at own pace to avoid increasing anxiety
6. Teach client, family, and significant others about specific dissociative disorder and relationship between anxiety and dissociation
7. Implement simple routines that are not demanding and plan for use of leisure time (anxiety often increases when alone without activities)

E. Psychopharmacology: anti-anxiety agents; antidepressants for depression and antipsychotics for extreme agitation (if present)

F. Individual and group therapy
1. Hypnosis therapy assists client to recover memories
2. Individual psychotherapy focuses on emotional responses to trauma or stressors and helps client work through unacceptable impulses or behavior verbally
3. Family therapy may benefit client, partner, and children
4. Behavior modification focuses on cognitive techniques to promote positive self-statements and reinforce stress management and coping strategies rather than dissociation
5. Support groups may be useful, such as parenting or occupational support groups, or "survivor" groups (particularly for natural disasters or abuse)

G. Evaluation and client outcomes
1. Client explains relationship between trauma, stress, anxiety, and dissociation and can recall stressors and traumatic events with congruency
2. Client employs stress-management and positive coping behaviors and actively seeks to solve problems
3. Client assumes or resumes social and occupational roles and uses leisure time constructively

VII. SOMATOFORM DISORDERS

A. Overview
1. **Somatoform disorders** are characterized by client's subjective concerns about a physiological illness or condition that has no associated physical findings; they constitute a defense against anxiety
   a. A person expresses conflict and resultant anxiety through physical symptoms (physical illness is socially acceptable); client receives help and nurturance and has dependency needs met
   b. May consciously seek relief from physical symptoms or may unconsciously not want to give up symptoms because they decrease anxiety or assist with control over others
   c. Family may provide secondary gain (increased attention, decreased responsibility, stabilized relationships)

NCLEX®
2. Physical symptoms have no *organic basis*; that is, objective diagnostic tests usually do not reveal structural or functional changes

B. Specific disorders

1. Somatization disorder
    a. Multiple physical complaints that involve several body systems
    b. New symptoms often arise with increased emotional distress
    c. Client seeks treatment for physical symptoms, usually pain, and occasionally for psychological concerns (fear or anxiety that may be accompanied by low self-esteem)
    d. Special interventions: long-term medical management; treat physical symptoms conservatively, "matter-of-fact" approach; antidepressants if depressive symptoms present but no drug therapy for anxiety symptoms
2. **Conversion disorder**
    a. A somatoform disorder with sudden onset of a physical symptom about which client is usually unconcerned or indifferent ("la belle indifference")
    b. Symptoms do not have an underlying organic cause but instead express a psychological need or conflict (anxiety, frustration, guilt, anger, inadequacy, low self-esteem)
    c. Symptoms may affect motor function (mutism, paralysis, tremors). sensory function (blindness, deafness, numbness,) or be visceral in nature (urinary retention, breathing difficulties, headaches)
    d. Physical symptoms are not consciously controlled by client but they do lead to secondary gain
    NCLEX® e. Special interventions: treat symptom as "real" because client experiences it; use problem-solving approaches for dealing with conflicts and stressors
3. **Hypochondriasis**
    a. A disorder in which physical symptoms are interpreted as severe or life-threatening, resulting in exaggerated worry and preoccupation
    b. Physical symptoms are varied and range over time; may begin with sensitivity to vague physical sensations or mild physical symptoms that most people would not notice
    c. Concern persists despite negative findings and clinician reassurances
    d. History of multiple visits to multiple practitioners, use of over-the-counter medications and home remedies
    e. Accompanied by significant anxiety that impairs social and occupational function
    NCLEX® f. Special interventions: teach rational interpretation of body sensations; assist resolution of family conflict about medical treatment and client distress; nonpharmacological treatment of anxiety
4. **Body dysmorphic disorder**
    a. A somatoform disorder characterized by preoccupation with or excessive concern and embarrassment about an imagined or minor defect in appearance
    b. Causes significant distress or impairment in role function
    c. May involve perceived flaws of face or head (complexion, hair thinning, asymmetry), abdomen, extremities, or body shape/size
    d. Client may frequently check defects, avoid reminders (removing mirrors), seek reassurances from others, or repeatedly attempt to improve defect (exercise, surgery, cosmetics)
    e. Often leads to social isolation; emotional distress may be severe enough to lead to depression and suicidal ideation
    NCLEX® f. Special interventions: respect preoccupation; avoid challenging validity of client perceptions; focus on coping techniques; contract with client to increase social activities and relationships

C. Assessment

1. Client sees problem as "physical" and denies psychological influences on symptoms
2. Client has seen multiple care providers without relief of symptoms
3. Involves primary gain (relief from responsibilities) and secondary gain (dependency needs are met)
4. Over time, client is increasingly socially isolated and physically inactive
5. Family may insist on client seeking assistance due to altered role performance
6. Mental status variations depend on type of disorder
    a. Appearance: ranges from deeply anguished to indifferent; may assume antalgic position
    b. Mood: depressed, anxious, or unaffected or labile
    c. Thought: usually preoccupied with symptoms
    d. Insight: highly impaired, usually denying any stressors or minimizing reactions to stressful events; not "psychologically minded"
7. Evaluate physical symptoms respectfully and objectively, with supportive laboratory and diagnostic studies to support or rule out physical illness; see Table 21–8 for specific symptoms

Table 21–8 Specific Symptoms in Somatoform Disorders

Organ System	Specific Symptom
Cardiovascular	Fainting, hypertension, migraine headache, tachycardia
Musculoskeletal	Back pain, fatigue, tension headache, tremor
Respiratory	Bronchospasm, dyspnea, hyperventilation
Integumentary	Pruritis
Genitourinary	Difficulties in micturation, menstrual disturbances, sexual dysfunction

D. Specific nursing intervention strategies

NCLEX®

1. Establish trusting, therapeutic relationship
   a. Avoid describing physical symptoms as "in client's head"
   b. Note that symptoms are not an attempt to get attention
   c. Recall that client does not create symptoms consciously or purposefully
   d. Accept reality of symptoms as client presents them, avoiding dispute

NCLEX®

2. Client education
   a. Explain symptoms on a physiological level, using simple and acceptable language
   b. Present current knowledge of mind–body interaction, emphasizing how stress and anxiety affect physiological functioning
   c. Teach methods to reduce physiological arousal, including relaxation techniques, visual imagery, self-talk strategies, and physical exercise (see Box 21–2)
3. Encourage verbalization of thoughts and feelings, life events, and stressors
4. Assist in problem solving specific conflicts or situations
5. Self-care strategies
   a. Modify exercise/activity plan to fit client's physical status
   b. Promote sleep and rest
   c. Promote healthy nutritional practices
   d. Teach day-to-day client management of symptoms
6. Encourage client to gradually resume expected work, family, and community roles commensurate with physical capabilities

E. Psychopharmacology: no specific psychotropic medications used; possible use of antidepressants with or anxiolytics for comorbid anxiety or depression; medications to treat physical symptoms may be prescribed

F. Individual and group treatment

1. Cognitive-behavioral approaches assist with identification of beliefs and assumptions about stress, anxiety, and sick role; challenge irrational beliefs; provide accurate data to counter misinformation; and encourage positive coping strategies
2. Groups for clients and families provide forum for discussion and encourage client to talk out problems as a deterrent to physical symptoms, correct misinformation about origin of somatoform disorders, and provide support for families and/or clients as roles shift during recovery

Box 21–2

Tips for Teaching Relaxation Training

- Emphasize the relationship between stress and physiological arousal/symptoms.
- Note that relaxation techniques work by focusing attention to relaxation task, thus interrupting the preoccupation with symptoms and decreasing physiological arousal, which negates physical symptoms of anxiety.
- To promote a sense of control, remind the client that he or she (not the technique) effects the change.
- Promote a daily return to physiological and psychological baseline to calm the mind and body through relaxation techniques, thus keeping general arousal low.
- Note that daily practice rather than episodic use builds skill level.
- Suggest additional techniques for use when client anticipates a stressful situation or finds him- or herself becoming anxious.
- Explain and teach a variety of techniques so that client can choose a technique that is acceptable and can be used in specific client environments.

3. Supportive approaches include conveying respect and empathy without reinforcing symptoms and exploring ways to decrease isolation, improve role performance, and enhance self-esteem
4. Behavior modification teaches client to self-reward for engagement in treatment plan and teaches family members to reinforce verbalization of stressors rather than symptoms

G. Evaluation and client outcomes

1. Identifies interaction of mind and body and effects of stress
2. Increases ability to verbalize thoughts and feelings and conflicts and/or problems in situations and relationships
3. Employs self-help strategies: challenges irrational thoughts, corrects own misinformation, uses positive coping statements, engages in physical activity on regular basis; employs relaxation techniques or visual imagery; demonstrates sound nutritional practices, and resumes appropriate roles

VIII. COGNITIVE IMPAIRMENT DISORDERS

A. Autism (see Chapter 57)

B. Attention-deficit/hyperactivity disorder (see Chapter 57)

C. *Delirium*

1. An acute, abrupt-onset confusional state characterized by disorientation, disturbed perception, vivid dreams, frightening hallucinations, agitated behavior, inability to sleep at night with daytime napping, and emotional disturbances
   - NCLEX® **a.** Develops over a short period of time (usually hours to days) and tends to fluctuate during course of day
   - **b.** Has an identifiable cause that can include direct physiological consequences of a general medical condition, substance intoxication, substance withdrawal, or multiple etiologies
2. NCLEX® Presenting signs and symptoms of delirium
   - **a.** Cyclic alternating periods of coherence with periods of confusion, specifically with disorientation that worsens at end of day, often referred to as **sundown syndrome**
   - **b.** Alternating patterns of hyperactivity (typical of drug withdrawal) to hypoactivity (typical of metabolic imbalance)
   - **c.** Hyperactive behaviors: rambling, bizarre, incoherent, rapid, pressured, or loud speech; restlessness, picking at clothes or bed linens, irritability, euphoria; calling out for help, striking out at others, bizarre and destructive behavior, combativeness, anger, profanity
   - **d.** Hypoactive behaviors: limited, dull patterns of speech; lethargy, apathy, withdrawn behavior; reduced alertness or awareness of environment
   - **e.** Cognitive changes: disorganized thinking; diminished ability to focus attention, easily distracted; disorientation to time and place; impairment in recent and remote memory; visual or auditory hallucinations, frightening delusions
   - **f.** Sleep pattern disturbances, including vivid and terrifying dreams or nightmares
   - **g.** Predominant emotion is fear with a high level of anxiety
3. Identify and treat underlying cause and rule out other reasons for delirium (depression, anxiety, dementia, or personality disorder)

D. Dementia and Alzheimer's disease

1. **Dementia**: a chronic, irreversible syndrome characterized by progressive deterioration in memory, cognition (abstract thinking, judgment, insight, problem-solving ability), executive functioning (planning, organizing, sequencing, abstracting), and behavior
   - NCLEX® **a.** Both long-term and short-term memory are affected
   - **b.** Course is insidious and progressive, characterized by gradual onset and continuing cognitive decline
   - **c.** Cognitive deficits cause significant impairment in social or occupational functioning and self-care deficits
   - **d.** Can be classified as vascular dementia, dementia due to other general medical conditions, substance-induced persisting dementia, or Alzheimer's disease (most common type)
2. Alzheimer's disease is an irreversible form of dementia caused by deterioration of brain cells and is characterized by formation of amyloid plaques and neurofibrillatory tangles
   - **a.** It can be divided into four stages: 1 (mild; client is forgetful), 2 (moderate: client has confusion), 3 (severe; client has ambulatory dementia), and 4 (late; client is end stage)
   - **b.** Functional changes lead to specific deficits including **aphasia** (inability to understand or use language), **apraxia** (inability to carry out skilled and purposeful movement or to use objects properly, although

motor function is intact), **agnosia** (inability to recognize familiar situations, people, or stimuli although sensory function is intact), and amnesia (loss of memory)

c. During later stages, client may require specialized care in a long-term skilled nursing facility

E. Screening tools

1. Folstein Mini-Mental State Examination: an organic screening tool useful for differentiating dementia from functional states; total score 30 points (9–12 score indicates high likelihood of organic illness)
2. Cognitive Performance Scale: a subscale from nursing home Minimum Data Set (MDS); scores range from 0 (cognitively intact) to 6 (very severe cognitive impairment)
3. Geriatric Depression Screening Scale (GDSS): specifically developed for older adults to screen for possible depression (which can mimic dementia); results indicate absence of or mild depression (0–10), moderate depression (11–20), or severe depression (21–30) using the 30-item questionnaire

F. Differentiating between delirium and dementia

1. Delirium may coexist with dementia, making accurate assessment and appropriate treatment difficult; Table 21–9 compares delirium and dementia
2. Most prevalent primary dementia is Alzheimer's type, (occurs in 50% of older adults); others include vascular dementia (from narrowing of arteries), degenerative nervous system disorders (e.g., Parkinson's disease), and other pathological processes (e.g., AIDS dementia complex)

G. Nursing interventions: see Box 21–3 for general nursing interventions that are useful when caring for clients with dementia

H. Specific treatment modalities

NCLEX®

1. Psychopharmacology: commonly used medications include donepezil (cholinesterase inhibitor) to slow rate of decline in mild to moderate dementia and memantine (NMDA receptor antagonist) for abnormal glutamate activity that may contribute to Alzheimer's disease; others may include anti-anxiety agents (lorazepam, trazodone, buspirone), SSRIs (fluoxetine, paroxetine, sertraline, nefazadone), which are better tolerated than TCAs in older adults, and atypical antipsychotics (olanzapine, quetiapine, and risperidone); use of haloperidol, a potent neuroleptic, is controversial because it has caused tardive dyskinesia in older adults; small doses (0.5 mg) may help to regulate sleep

NCLEX®

2. Group and individual therapies
   a. "Review of life" therapy: discuss specific life transitions and events, pets, music, and special foods to evoke memories from client's past; share positive and negative feelings
   b. Validation therapy: interact with clients on a topic they initiate, in a place and time where they feel most secure; reflect underlying feelings of concern (e.g., "You miss your husband. You must be feeling lonely here"); reality orientation is geared to person and place rather than to time
3. **Milieu therapy**
   a. Special care unit (SCU): environmentally designed and specifically programmed to serve needs of residents with Alzheimer's disease and related dementias

Table 21–9 Comparisons Between Delirium and Dementia

Delirium	Dementia
Onset is usually sudden (acute)	Onset is insidious and progressive (chronic)
Temporary, reversible disturbance in brain function	Irreversible alteration of brain function
Duration: hours to days	Duration: months to years
EEG: diffuse slowing of fast cycles related to state of excitement	EEG: normal or mildly slow
Disturbed attention, learning, and thinking, poor perception	Disorientation, impairments in judgment, abstract thinking, and learning
Impaired memory, both recent and remote	Impaired memory (recent affected before remote)
Orientation: fluctuates throughout day; periods of lucidity; sundown syndrome (worsens at night)	Progressively loses orientation to time, then place, then person; sundown syndrome
Hallucinations, delusions, illusions	Change in personality; normal peculiarities are exaggerated: suspicious–paranoid, compulsive–rigid, orderliness
Labile affect	Labile affect; prone to apathy, depression, withdrawal, stubbornness in attempt to cope with surroundings and decreased abilities

Box 21–3

Nursing Interventions for Clients with Dementia

- Provide a simple, structured environment with consistent personnel to minimize confusion and provide a sense of security and stability.
- Reorient client to environment and personnel as needed. Use clock and calendar as aids.
- Identify client's current skill level and reinforce current abilities to maintain independence.
- Allow client to have familiar objects and furnishings to maintain reality orientation and enhance self-worth and dignity.
- Consider special interventions to maintain safety such as sufficient lighting, removing obstacles from path while walking, reduced hot water temperature, and removal of electrical appliances as warranted.
- Acknowledge client's feelings and frustrations regarding memory loss and declining abilities.
- Provide cognitive stimulation to client with simple activities or games (but avoid activities that tax client's memory).
- Stand in front of client when speaking, use a low-pitched voice, and maintain eye contact.
- Ask client only one question at a time and provide time for client to respond. If question needs to be repeated, use same words and add gestures as needed.
- Provide simple, clear instructions focusing on one task at a time. Break tasks into very small steps and allow client extended time to complete them.
- Monitor and assist client to have sufficient exercise, such as walking, but provide supervision for safety.
- Manage wandering behaviors by providing client with a safe environment that is free of obstacles, observing client, closing doors (such as at exits and stairs), and using electronic surveillance technology in addition to identification bracelet.
- Discuss topics that are meaningful to the client, such as significant life events, family, work, hobbies, and pets.
- Encourage reminiscence and discussion of life review by sharing picture albums.
- Discuss family traditions and holidays, memories of school, courtship, dating rituals, favorite pets, and other past events.
- Foster adequate sleep by allowing wandering so client becomes tired, using indirect light to prevent shadows that might frighten client, and use sleep aids carefully to prevent additive confusion.
- Manage agitation by assessing for precipitating factor(s), approaching client from the front, using calm voice and gentle slow movements and touch, reducing excess stimuli, and moving client to a quieter environment.
- Encourage family/caregivers to express feelings, such as frustration and anger, and concerns about caregiving.
- Provide a list of community resources and support groups available to assist in decreasing stress and role strain for the family/caregiver.

NCLEX®

b. SCU is designed as a safe, secure, specially adapted physical environment to accommodate wandering behavior inside and outside (circular design, secure walkway and patio); personalized rooms with own furniture and familiar belongings; clean, well-maintained, well-lit environment with windows; stimuli from birdcage, fish aquarium, or other pets; possible location adjacent to child daycare programs for multigenerational interaction

c. Structured programs and activities provide quality interaction between staff, residents, and families

I. Evaluation and client outcomes

1. Client remains free of injury (no falls, fractures, bruises, contusions, burns)
2. Client participates in self-care with appropriate supervision and guidance
3. Client communicates basic needs using visual and verbal clues as necessary and has minimal level of response to frustrating situations
4. Client sleeps 5–7 hours per night and naps 1–2 hours per day, and maintains stable vital signs and weight
5. Caregivers demonstrate adaptive coping strategies for caregiver role stress

IX. EATING DISORDERS

A. Overview of eating disorders

1. Eating disorders are manifested by gross disturbance in a client's eating patterns
2. People with anorexia lose weight by dramatically decreasing food intake and sharply increasing amount of physical exercise
3. People with bulimia nervosa remain at near-normal weight and develop a cycle of binge-eating and then purging

B. Anorexia nervosa

1. Overview
   a. Life-threatening health problem because of fluid and electrolyte imbalance, starvation, cardiac abnormalities, or suicide
   b. Client is preoccupied with food intake, fears obesity, and often has a disturbed body image and self-concept
   c. Client eats minimal amounts of food, often in a rigid and regimented manner, such as eating only three bites of carrots or two mouthfuls of cereal; denies hunger
   d. Onset is often in teens and frequently associated with a major stressful life event
   e. Client is often an overachiever, seeks perfection, and experiences feelings of lack of control

NCLEX®

2. Physical assessment findings
   a. Weight loss
   b. Electrolyte imbalances
   c. Vital signs: decreased body temperature, pulse, and blood pressure; cyanosis of extremities
   d. Gastrointestinal (GI): constipation, tooth and gum degeneration
   e. Skin: dry, scaly
   f. Neuromuscular/skeletal: numbness of extremities, bone deterioration
   g. Amenorrhea for at least three cycles
   h. Reports of sleep disturbances

C. Bulimia nervosa

1. Overview
   a. Client is preoccupied with food intake and body size and appearance; may believe that conflict related to eating dominates lifestyle
   b. Associated with low self-esteem and poor relationships with others
   c. Client engages in cycles of binge-eating (consuming large amounts of high-calorie foods, often in secret) followed by purging behaviors (vomiting, laxatives, enemas, diuretics, or amphetamines)
   d. Client experiences conflict between perceived loss of control and need for control, as well as guilt from binge–purge cycles; may exhibit mood swings

NCLEX®

2. Physical assessment findings
   a. Weight is often normal or near-normal
   b. Other symptoms are similar to anorexia nervosa with addition of possible esophageal varices from induced vomiting

NCLEX®

D. Specific nursing intervention strategies

1. Clients with anorexia nervosa are typically treated in an eating disorders unit
2. Develop a therapeutic, nonjudgmental relationship with client to foster sharing of precipitating factors to eating disorder and feelings about it
3. Support client during behavior modification, psychotherapy, support groups; encourage client to take any prescribed medications, such as antidepressants
4. Perform baseline and periodic assessments of nutritional status, including fluid and electrolyte balance and daily intake of food
5. With severe malnutrition, refeeding protocols and tube feedings may be used
6. Form a contract with client regarding daily intake of food
7. Set a time limit for meals
8. Provide a pleasant environment for meals and observe client at mealtimes and following meals
9. Provide positive feedback for appropriate eating behaviors and goal attainment; token rewards system may be used
10. Record intake and output and daily weight (postvoid, same clothing, same time, same scale)
11. Monitor elimination patterns
12. Monitor and limit activity level (anorexia and bulimia)
13. Assess risk of suicide and implement suicide precautions as necessary

E. Evaluation and client outcomes: client has normal or near-normal nutritional status, gains 0.5–1 kg (1–2 pounds) of weight per week (anorexia nervosa), uses newly learned eating behaviors regularly, is free of complications of eating disorder, and identifies and uses available support programs or services

Check Your NCLEX–RN® Exam I.Q.

You are ready for testing on this content if you can:

- Assess for alteration in mood, judgment, and cognition in clients with a mental health problem.
- Assess for signs and symptoms of specific mental health problems.
- Assess the client's and family's reaction to diagnosis of an acute or chronic mental health problem.
- Help a client to adhere to the treatment plan for a mental health problem.
- Assess for change in a client's mental status and impaired cognition.
- Plan care for the client with an acute or chronic mental health problem.
- Provide client and family education about an acute or chronic mental health problem.
- Provide appropriate nursing care to a client undergoing electroconvulsive therapy.

PRACTICE TEST

1 A nurse has been told that a client's anxiety is at the panic level. The nurse would assess the client for which manifestations expected at this level of anxiety?

1. Dizziness, palpitations, and nausea
2. Feelings of "butterflies" in the stomach
3. Feelings of fatigue and inability to remain awake
4. Obsessive thoughts and compulsive behavior

2 The nurse concludes that a client has agoraphobia after the client states a fear of which of the following?

1. Spiders
2. Being embarrassed in public
3. Leaving the home
4. Losing control

3 A nurse asks a client, "Have you ever felt a sudden, intense fear for no apparent reason?" When the client responds "yes," the nurse would assess the client for other symptoms compatible with which problem?

1. Agoraphobia
2. Obsessive–compulsive disorder
3. Panic disorder
4. Posttraumatic stress disorder

4 A client has just been told that a second operation must be performed to correct a physical health problem. The client begins to cry and says, "I just can't take it anymore. Everything has gone wrong. I can't even think straight anymore." The nurse interprets that the client is in which stage of anxiety?

1. Alarm
2. Exhaustion
3. Fight-or-flight
4. Resistance

5 A counselor working with an extremely anxious client reports feeling short of breath, tense, restless, apprehensive, and nervous. The nurse would most appropriately draw which conclusion?

1. The client's anxious feelings have been transmitted to the counselor.
2. The client is probably becoming angry with the counselor.
3. The client should be reassigned to a different counselor.
4. The counselor is probably new to the position.

6 A client will begin electroconvulsive therapy (ECT) after being diagnosed with major depression. The nurse prepares a teaching plan, keeping in mind that which attribute is characteristic of clients with major depression?

1. Clients need to be treated with respect and dignity.
2. Clients need to be brought to the treatment suite on a stretcher.
3. Clients should have the procedure explained many times because of inability to retain information.
4. Clients should not receive ECT.

7 The nurse is making a postoperative home visit to a 52-year-old male client. During his presurgical physical assessment, the client was diagnosed with type 2 diabetes mellitus, reported he was not sleeping well, had a decreased appetite, and stated he was angry because he lost his job of 34 years 3 weeks prior. At this time, the nurse performs a follow-up assessment by asking questions to detect which possible mood disorder?

1. Hypomania
2. Major depression
3. Cyclothymia
4. Dysthymia

8 The nurse concludes that which living environment would be safest for a client who inflicted harm on a family member earlier in the day? Select all that apply.

1. In a local respite home
2. In a locked unit
3. In an open-door seclusion room
4. In a closed-door seclusion room
5. With a family member in another state

9 Part of a discharge plan for a client on a psychiatric inpatient unit includes walking for half an hour 5 days per week to maintain cardiovascular health and decrease stress levels. The nurse includes this in the care plan as what optimal type of nursing intervention?

1. Active
2. Performance
3. Preventive
4. Physical

10 The nurse is evaluating a client diagnosed with bipolar disorder in the home environment following discharge 2 weeks ago from an inpatient unit. The nurse assesses the client for which behaviors that are expected at this time?

1. Euphoric and talkative presentation with nurse
2. Gregarious interactions with significant others
3. Quiet and evasive presentation
4. Calm, focused exchange of self-care information with nurse

11 A 21-year-old male college student who has become increasingly suspicious of others has accused a professor of conspiring with two other classmates to get him expelled from school. The client is admitted to a psychiatric unit after telephoning and threatening to kill the professor and his classmates. The client states, "They are all out to get me expelled. I think they are even trying to kill me. I have to stop them!" What would be a therapeutic-appropriate response by the nurse? Select all that apply.

1. "Why do you think they are out to get you expelled or to kill you?"
2. "It is difficult to believe that your professor and classmates are out to get you expelled or to kill you."
3. "It's not right to kill others even if they are out to get you expelled or want to kill you."
4. "Your professor and classmates are not out to get you expelled or to kill you. Let's look at the facts."
5. "It must be frightening to think that others are out to kill you or cause you some type of harm."

12 A client with schizophrenia is exhibiting delusions, hallucinations, minimal self-care, and hyperactive behavior. Which of these observations would the nurse document as a negative symptom of schizophrenia?

1. Minimal self-care
2. Delusions
3. Hallucinations
4. Inappropriate affect

13 A client hears voices telling him that he is a terrible person who would be better off dead. What would be a priority problem for the nurse to address in the client's plan of care?

1. Inadequate communication
2. Risk for suicide
3. Impaired sensory perceptions
4. Impaired social interactions

14 A client living in an assisted-living facility is taking conventional antipsychotic medications. One evening the nurse notices that the client is experiencing muscle rigidity, confusion, delirium, and has a temperature of 104°F (40°C). The nurse interprets these as symptoms of which adverse drug effect?

1. Dystonia
2. Akathisia
3. Neuroleptic malignant syndrome
4. Tardive dyskinesia

15 A client states that he is able to receive radio waves from aliens because they placed a computer chip in his brain. The nurse would document this behavior as which of the following in the medical record?

1. A hallucination
2. Reality-oriented
3. An illusion
4. A delusion

16 What would the nurse formulate as the most appropriate outcome of care when initiating a care plan for a male client who has experienced a dissociative fugue?

1. Remember what occurred during his fugue state.
2. Gain additional coping skills to deal with his current problems.
3. Report no feelings of being detached from his body.
4. State three positive aspects about himself.

17 A female client with dissociative identity disorder (DID) who has just been admitted with several new burns on her ankles and wrists is refusing to attend group therapy. Which client problem identified by the nurse would have highest priority?

1. Inadequate ability to care out self-care activities
2. Impaired sensory perceptions
3. Risk for self-harm
4. Nonadherence to the treatment plan

18 A client reports depersonalization experiences that have been frightening to him. Which response by the nurse would be therapeutic? Select all that apply.

1. "It must be very scary for you to have these experiences."
2. "Don't worry, you will always come back together."
3. "Being in the hospital must be very frightening."
4. "Let's focus on the stressors in your life."
5. "Can you tell me more about how these experiences occur?"

19 Which of the following behaviors would indicate to the nurse that care for a client who dissociates has been most effective?

1. Client reports dissociative episodes to the nurse.
2. Client seeks out social relationships.
3. Client demonstrates three stress management techniques.
4. Client is free from injury.

20 A client with amnesia is hospitalized. What might the nurse expect to find during the initial assessment?

1. Confabulation of historical information
2. Gradual loss of memory over months
3. Disheveled appearance
4. History of severe stress

21 The nurse would look for which characteristics in the behavior of a client diagnosed with obsessive–compulsive disorder (OCD)? Select all that apply.

1. Dramatic
2. Eccentric
3. Anxious
4. Ritualistic
5. Erratic

22 The nurse places highest priority on which nursing intervention when caring for a client diagnosed with antisocial personality disorder?

1. Supporting the development of insight
2. Encouraging socialization
3. Maintaining consistent limits
4. Monitoring for suicidal ideation

23 The nurse looks for which characteristic that is expected in a client diagnosed with a personality disorder?

1. Flexibility and adaptability to stress
2. A tendency to evoke some form of interpersonal conflict
3. A concurrent physical disorder
4. A desire for interpersonal relationships

24. Which belief by the nurse as a member of the interdisciplinary team is most important to remember when developing a care plan for a client diagnosed with antisocial personality disorder?

1. Everyone involved in the client's care must agree with the diagnosis, goals, and plan.
2. The team leader must determine the diagnosis and treatment plan to ensure accuracy.
3. The involvement of all team members in developing a nursing care plan is not necessary.
4. An unstructured treatment approach is usually beneficial.

25. The nurse assessing a client with obsessive–compulsive disorder (OCD) anticipates that most of the client's cognitive content will be centered around which of the following?

1. The importance of rules and regulations
2. Global approaches to problem solving
3. Relationships with others
4. Preferred leisure activities

26. A client continues to have pain despite negative neurological and diagnostic findings. The nurse concludes that such pain is likely to continue because of which factor?

1. Secondary gain
2. High endorphin levels
3. Structural changes of tissue
4. Derealization

27. On the morning of his wedding, a male client is suddenly unable to move his left hand, which is the hand that would wear the wedding ring. Upon diagnosis with conversion disorder, what would the nurse expect to find in the mental status examination?

1. Mood: depressed
2. Mood: anxious
3. Mood: blunted
4. Mood: indifferent

28. A female client with hypochondriasis discloses she may leave the psychiatric facility without completing her treatment and seek exploratory surgery. What is the nurse's *best* response to the client?

1. "If you decide to leave now, you will be committed against your will."
2. "You should not go until your doctor releases you. She knows what you need."
3. "Tell me more about your decision."
4. "Your surgery will probably prove useless. Please stay."

29. A client who had several physical illnesses in the past few years is no longer employed, rarely shops or does housework, and states, "I just can't seem to do anything." Which client problem identified by the nurse should take priority?

1. Inability to maintain home environment
2. Fatigue that prevents daily activities
3. Powerlessness in managing daily living
4. Altered body image caused by illness

30. The nurse evaluates that the plan of care for a client who suddenly lost her hearing (diagnosed as a conversion disorder) was effective after noting which client behavior?

1. Resumed normal hearing
2. Began learning sign language
3. Was fitted for a hearing aid
4. Agreed to have a stapedectomy

31. Which of the following approaches would be best for the nurse who is communicating with the cognitively impaired client? Select all that apply.

1. Loud
2. Concise
3. Clear
4. Nonverbal
5. Unhurried

32. To which evaluation criterion should the nurse give first priority to when planning the care of a client with dementia?

1. Preventing further deterioration
2. Finding a suitable long-term care placement
3. Supporting family caregivers
4. Preventing injury

33 A client with suspected Alzheimer's disease is undergoing diagnostic workup. When the family asks the nurse the reasons for the "tests," the nurse responds that the diagnosis of Alzheimer's disease is usually based on which of the following?

1. Laboratory test findings
2. A definitive CT scan
3. Physiological findings
4. Ruling out other causes for symptoms

34 The nurse writing a care plan for a client with dementia would include which goal as the overall goal of nursing care?

1. Reorient the client to reality.
2. Keep the loss of capacity for self-care to a minimum.
3. Assist the client with tasks of daily living.
4. Maintain adequate hydration and nutrition.

35 Which intervention would the nurse perform to support optimal memory function for a client with dementia?

1. Develop stimulating and meaningful therapeutic activities
2. Remind the client of forgotten events
3. Orient the client to reality
4. Restrain the client when agitated

36 The nurse would conclude that a client with schizophrenia is exhibiting positive symptoms of the disorder after noting that the client does which of the following? Select all that apply.

1. Exhibits lack of energy
2. States he is a king
3. Repeats words the nurse says
4. Has a flat affect
5. Withdraws from other people

ANSWERS & RATIONALES

1 **Answer: 1 Rationale:** Subjective complaints of panic level of anxiety include choking or smothering sensation, dizziness, chest pain or pressure, and fear of loss of control and death. Feelings of stomach "butterflies" are seen in the fight-or-flight response. Feelings of fatigue and inability to remain awake may be seen in the exhaustion stage of the general adaptation syndrome. Obsessive thoughts and compulsive behaviors are common in obsessive–compulsive disorder. **Cognitive Level:** Applying **Client Need:** Psychosocial Integrity **Integrated Process:** Nursing Process: Assessment **Content Area:** Mental Health **Strategy:** The core issue of the question is an ability to identify signs of panic in a client with anxiety. Use nursing knowledge and the process of elimination to make a selection.

2 **Answer: 3 Rationale:** Agoraphobia involves fear of being away from home and being alone in public places. A specific phobia involves unrealistic fear of a particular situation or object, such as a spider (arachnophobia). Social phobia is excessive fear of embarrassment and humiliation in public settings. Fear of loss of control is common in most phobias and thus is not useful in identifying a single phobia. **Cognitive Level:** Applying **Client Need:** Psychosocial Integrity **Integrated Process:** Nursing Process: Assessment **Content Area:** Mental Health **Strategy:** The core issue of the question is an ability to identify signs of agoraphobia in a client. Use nursing knowledge and the process of elimination to make a selection.

3 **Answer: 3 Rationale:** The onset of a panic attack is sudden, and the client may not be aware of the source of the anxiety. The nurse should assess for other associated symptoms of panic disorder that would occur at the onset of the fear. Agoraphobia is fear of being incapacitated by being trapped in an unbearable situation from which there is no escape. Obsessive–compulsive disorder is characterized by obsessive thoughts and compulsive behaviors. Posttraumatic stress disorder is associated with exposure to an extremely traumatic, menacing event. **Cognitive Level:** Applying **Client Need:** Psychosocial Integrity **Integrated Process:** Nursing Process: Assessment **Content Area:** Mental Health **Strategy:** The core issue of the question is an ability to identify signs of panic disorder. Use nursing knowledge and the process of elimination to make a selection.

4 **Answer: 2 Rationale:** Because coping resources are depleted, the client can no longer deal with stressors and is in the stage of exhaustion. The stage of alarm is characterized by the fight-or-flight response, and increased alertness is focused on the immediate task or threat. The stage of resistance occurs when the body mobilizes resources to combat stress. **Cognitive Level:** Applying **Client Need:** Psychosocial Integrity **Integrated Process:** Nursing Process: Assessment **Content Area:** Mental Health **Strategy:** The core issue of the question is an ability to differentiate stages of anxiety based on client presentation. Use nursing knowledge and the process of elimination to make a selection.

5 **Answer: 1 Rationale:** Anxiety in a client may be empathetically experienced by the counselor. It is imperative that these symptoms be recognized. There is not enough data to support the client being angry. Reassigning the client may not be therapeutic. Even those with work experience may develop anxiety empathetically. **Cognitive Level:** Analyzing **Client Need:** Psychosocial Integrity **Integrated Process:** Nursing Process: Assessment **Content Area:** Mental Health **Strategy:** The core issue of the question is the ability to determine the

effect that an anxious client can have on healthcare workers. Use nursing knowledge and the process of elimination to make a selection.

6 **Answer: 1 Rationale:** Clients always need to be treated with dignity and respect. There is no reason to bring the client to the treatment suite on a stretcher. The client does not need to have a procedure explained many times. Explanations are reinforced as needed, which would be done for a client with any diagnosis. The client with major depression can receive ECT if medication therapy is not effective. **Cognitive Level:** Understanding **Client Need:** Psychosocial Integrity **Integrated Process:** Nursing Process: Diagnosis **Content Area:** Mental Health **Strategy:** The core issue of the question is the right of every client to be treated in a respectful manner. Use nursing knowledge and the process of elimination to make a selection.

7 **Answer: 2 Rationale:** The client's symptoms are consistent with major depression, and the nurse should provide a follow-up assessment to detect symptoms of depression, and also whether the prior symptoms (not able to sleep and decreased appetite) have persisted. Hypomania is characterized by a mood of elation. Cyclothymia is a disorder ofat least 2 years' duration with episodes of hypomania. Dysthymia is a depressive disorder of at least 2 years' duration. **Cognitive Level:** Analyzing **Client Need:** Psychosocial Integrity **Integrated Process:** Nursing Process: Diagnosis **Content Area:** Mental Health **Strategy:** The core issue of the question is an ability to identify clients at risk for various forms of depression. Use nursing knowledge and the process of elimination to make a selection.

8 **Answer: 2, 4 Rationale:** Admission to a locked unit would be a safe option for this client. The client would be safe in a closed-door seclusion room. The client would not have the necessary continuous monitored care if he were in a respite home. In an open-door seclusion room, the client could leave the area and harm others if there were distractions to the staff on the unit. The client would have less safety or care in the home of a relative in another state than is needed at this time. **Cognitive Level:** Analyzing **Client Need:** Psychosocial Integrity **Integrated Process:** Nursing Process: Planning **Content Area:** Mental Health **Strategy:** The core issue of the question is placement of a client who has harmed another. Use nursing knowledge and the process of elimination to make a selection. Keep in mind that the safety of the client and others around him or her is the first priority.

9 **Answer: 3 Rationale:** The term *preventive* is the most correct terminology for the nursing intervention described because it will help prevent increased anxiety and stress. *Active* is a term that can be associated with exercise, but is not the intended term in this context. All behavior constitutes some type of *performance*. *Physical* may be an adjective to differentiate bodily exercise from mental exercise, but it is not the intended term in this context. **Cognitive Level:** Applying **Client Need:** Psychosocial Integrity **Integrated Process:** Nursing Process: Planning **Content Area:** Mental Health **Strategy:** The core issue of the question is the ability to determine various types of nursing interventions needed by a hospitalized client with a mental health problem. Use nursing knowledge and the process of elimination to make a selection.

10 **Answer: 4 Rationale:** A client who demonstrates a calm, focused exchange of information and self-care information would demonstrate control of the disorder, which is expected following discharge from an inpatient setting. A client in a manic state would present with euphoria and be talkative. A client who is in a manic state or a client who is very outgoing could have gregarious interactions with significant others. A client with depression would be more likely to have a quiet and evasive presentation. **Cognitive Level:** Applying **Client Need:** Psychosocial Integrity **Integrated Process:** Nursing Process: Assessment **Content Area:** Mental Health **Strategy:** The core issue of the question is appropriate behavior exhibited by a client with bipolar disorder after treatment. Use nursing knowledge and the process of elimination to make a selection.

11 **Answer: 2, 5 Rationale:** Voicing doubt about the delusion is a therapeutic intervention. This reinforces reality with the client. Statements that reflect the underlying feelings of the client are therapeutic and may enhance a therapeutic relationship with the client. "Why" statements may put the client on the defensive. The client will continue to voice a delusion even if there is no evidence of its truth or if evidence suggests the delusion is false. A paranoid client cannot use logic to dispel delusions. A statement based on logic challenges the client's belief instead of voicing doubt. Providing evidence will not usually sway a paranoid client. **Cognitive Level:** Analyzing **Client Need:** Psychosocial Integrity **Integrated Process:** Communication and Documentation **Content Area:** Mental Health **Strategy:** The core issue of the question is appropriate therapeutic communication techniques to use with a client who exhibits paranoia. Use nursing knowledge and the process of elimination to make a selection.

12 **Answer: 1 Rationale:** Minimal self-care is a negative behavioral symptom of schizophrenia. A delusion is a positive cognitive symptom. A hallucination is a positive perceptual symptom. An inappropriate affect is a positive affective symptom. **Cognitive Level:** Applying **Client Need:** Psychosocial Integrity **Integrated Process:** Communication and Documentation **Content Area:** Mental Health **Strategy:** The core issue of the question is an ability to discriminate between positive and negative signs of schizophrenia. Use nursing knowledge and the process of elimination to make a selection.

13 **Answer: 2 Rationale:** Risk for suicide is a priority because the voices the client hears could lead the client to attempt suicide. While hearing voices (hallucination) is a sensory-perceptual alteration, safety is the priority. There is no indication that the client has inadequate communication. There is no information regarding the client's social interactions with others. **Cognitive Level:** Analyzing **Client Need:** Psychosocial Integrity **Integrated Process:** Nursing Process: Diagnosis **Content Area:** Mental Health **Strategy:** The core issue of the question is an ability to set priorities for a client who experiences auditory hallucinations. Look for the option that puts client safety first. Use nursing knowledge and the process of elimination to make a selection.

14 **Answer: 3 Rationale:** Neuroleptic malignant syndrome is a potentially fatal extrapyramidal symptom characterized by muscle rigidity, respiratory problems, and hyperpyrexia. Dystonia is an extrapyramidal symptom characterized by involuntary movements and prolonged muscle contraction, resulting in twisting body motions, possible tremors, and abnormal posture. Akathisia is an extrapyramidal symptom characterized by restlessness and an inability to sit still. Tardive dyskinesia symptoms include frowning, blinking, grimacing, puckering, blowing, smacking, licking, chewing, tongue protrusion, and spastic facial distortions, which can be socially disfiguring. **Cognitive Level:** Analyzing **Client Need:**

Psychosocial Integrity **Integrated Process:** Nursing Process: Assessment **Content Area:** Mental Health **Strategy:** The core issue of the question is an ability to identify signs of adverse medication effects in a client being treated for psychosis. Use nursing knowledge and the process of elimination to make a selection.

15 **Answer: 4 Rationale:** A delusion is a false belief that cannot be changed by logical reasoning or evidence. A hallucination is the occurrence of a sight, sound, touch, smell, or taste without any external stimulus to the corresponding sensory organ; however, it is real to the client. The client is not exhibiting reality orientation. An illusion is a sensory misperception of environmental stimuli. **Cognitive Level:** Applying **Client Need:** Psychosocial Integrity **Integrated Process:** Communication and Documentation **Content Area:** Mental Health **Strategy:** The core issue of the question is an ability to correctly identify the types of thought patterns expressed in a client's communications. Use nursing knowledge and the process of elimination to make a selection.

16 **Answer: 2 Rationale:** The client who gains coping skills reduces anxiety to a level at which dissociation is unlikely to recur. This is an appropriate outcome statement for the client. The client does not remember what occurred during the fugue state. Feelings of being detached from the body are consistent with depersonalization and would not be an appropriate outcome of care. Being able to state three positive aspects of self is useful but does not represent a reduction in anxiety, which is needed to avoid recurrence of a dissociative state. **Cognitive Level:** Analyzing **Client Need:** Psychosocial Integrity **Integrated Process:** Nursing Process: Planning **Content Area:** Mental Health **Strategy:** The core issue of the question is an appropriate outcome of care for a client who was in a dissociative fugue state. Use nursing knowledge and the process of elimination to make a selection, recalling that anxiety is usually the cause of the state, and therefore the answer points to an item that reduces anxiety.

17 **Answer: 3 Rationale:** Risk for self-harm (self-mutilation) is not uncommon with clients who have DID, and this is identified in the assessment. The client remains at risk for injuring herself, producing tissue damage that provides tension relief. Inadequate ability to carry out self-care activities is not specified in the situation, but would have lower priority if it occurred. There is no indication the client has impaired sensory perceptions. The client's refusal to attend group therapy constitutes nonadherence to the treatment plan, but is of lower priority than a risk for self-harm. **Cognitive Level:** Analyzing **Client Need:** Psychosocial Integrity **Integrated Process:** Nursing Process: Planning **Content Area:** Mental Health **Strategy:** The core issue of the question is a priority nursing diagnosis. Questions such as these are frequently focused on safety. Use nursing knowledge and the process of elimination to make a selection.

18 **Answer: 1, 5 Rationale:** Stating that the experiences must be frightening to the client demonstrates empathy. Asking the client to share more information about the experiences encourages elaboration and is therapeutic. Telling the client not to worry dismisses the affective component of the client's communication. Focusing on being in the hospital misses the point of the client's communication because it is the depersonalization that is frightening to the client. Focusing on stressors is ultimately helpful, but is not timely in response to the client's current concern. **Cognitive Level:** Applying **Client Need:** Psychosocial Integrity **Integrated Process:** Communication and Documentation **Content Area:** Mental Health **Strategy:** The core issue of the question is selection of therapeutic responses to a client who is experiencing depersonalizing events. Use nursing knowledge of therapeutic communication skills and use the process of elimination, noting that more than one option is likely to be correct.

19 **Answer: 3 Rationale:** The goal of care is to eliminate or reduce dissociative experiences, which are exacerbated by anxiety. The use of stress management techniques may reduce anxiety to a level that the client can cope with effectively without dissociation. Reporting dissociative experiences is useful but does not eliminate or reduce them, which would be the result of effective care. Seeking out social relationships can provide support systems to the client but are not directly related to reducing dissociation. Preventing injury is important in the care of all clients, but is not the most effective indicator of successful treatment of dissociation. **Cognitive Level:** Analyzing **Client Need:** Psychosocial Integrity **Integrated Process:** Nursing Process: Evaluation **Content Area:** Mental Health **Strategy:** The core issue of the question is the ability to determine an appropriate outcome of care for a client who dissociates. Recall that anxiety plays a role in dissociation and choose the option that reduces anxiety.

20 **Answer: 4 Rationale:** Amnesia is precipitated by stress related to trauma or conflict. The amnesia occurs abruptly and there is no attempt to cover the memory loss. Confabulation to fill in memory gaps occurs often in clients with dementia. Gradual loss of memory is a common trait of dementia. Disheveled appearance is common in clients experiencing dementia. **Cognitive Level:** Analyzing **Client Need:** Psychosocial Integrity **Integrated Process:** Nursing Process: Assessment **Content Area:** Mental Health **Strategy:** The core issue of the question is knowledge of expected assessment findings in a client with amnesia. Use nursing knowledge and the process of elimination to make a selection.

21 **Answer: 3, 4 Rationale:** A client with OCD, a Cluster C personality disorder, experiences anxiety and uses ritualistic compulsive behaviors to reduce this anxiety. Individuals with a Cluster A personality disorder appear odd or eccentric. Clients with a Cluster B personality disorder appear dramatic or erratic. **Cognitive Level:** Applying **Client Need:** Psychosocial Integrity **Integrated Process:** Nursing Process: Assessment **Content Area:** Mental Health **Strategy:** The core issue of the question is knowledge of expected behaviors that would be exhibited by a client with OCD. Recall that a client with this type of diagnosis is anxious and uses ritualistic behaviors to cope with anxiety. Note that the wording of the question indicates more than one option is likely to be correct.

22 **Answer: 3 Rationale:** In caring for clients diagnosed with antisocial personality disorder, it is important to maintain a structured and consistent environment to decrease their attempts to control the situation through manipulation. Clients diagnosed with antisocial personality disorder are unlikely to develop insight as the causes of problems in living are externalized. Clients diagnosed with antisocial personality disorder may tend to take advantage of others for personal profit, and socialization is not a priority. Suicidal ideation is not associated with this disorder. **Cognitive Level:** Analyzing **Client Need:** Psychosocial Integrity **Integrated Process:** Nursing Process: Implementation **Content Area:** Mental Health **Strategy:** The core issue of the question is an ability to set priorities for a client who has an antisocial

personality disorder. Use nursing knowledge and the process of elimination to make a selection.

23 **Answer: 2 Rationale:** Individuals diagnosed with personality disorders display either functional impairment or subjective distress. Frequently these problems in living are reflected in impaired interpersonal relationships. Flexibility and adaptability to stress are incongruent with a diagnosis of a personality disorder. The presence of a physical disorder has no relation to the diagnosis of a personality disorder. Individuals diagnosed with personality disorders may or may not desire interpersonal relationships. **Cognitive Level:** Applying **Client Need:** Psychosocial Integrity **Integrated Process:** Nursing Process: Assessment **Content Area:** Mental Health **Strategy:** The core issue of the question is knowledge of expected assessment findings regarding behavior style in a client with a personality disorder. Note that the type of disorder is not specified, so the answer is a global or general pattern. Use nursing knowledge and the process of elimination to make a selection.

24 **Answer: 1 Rationale:** Individuals diagnosed with antisocial personality disorder frequently try to play one staff member against the other in order to control their environment. It is imperative that staff present a unified and consistent approach to care to prevent this. The team leader is not responsible for determining the diagnosis and treatment plan. The entire team needs to be involved in developing the plan of care. The client benefits from a structured approach to care rather than an unstructured approach. **Cognitive Level:** Analyzing **Client Need:** Psychosocial Integrity **Integrated Process:** Nursing Process: Planning **Content Area:** Mental Health **Strategy:** The core issue of the question is core beliefs about the value and roles of the interdisciplinary team. Use nursing knowledge and the process of elimination to make a selection.

25 **Answer: 1 Rationale:** Individuals diagnosed with obsessive–compulsive personality disorder become overly involved in details such as rules and regulations related to a need to be perfect. As a result, they fail to see the "big picture." Their relationships with others and participation in leisure activities are less important than their devotion to work and productivity. **Cognitive Level:** Applying **Client Need:** Psychosocial Integrity **Integrated Process:** Nursing Process: Assessment **Content Area:** Mental Health **Strategy:** The core issue of the question is knowledge of expected behavior styles in a client with OCD. Use nursing knowledge and the process of elimination to make a selection.

26 **Answer: 1 Rationale:** The continuance of pain is related to reinforcement of the symptoms, such as the caring responses of others, which give the client benefits that otherwise might not occur. High endorphin levels are associated with feelings of euphoria. Structural changes of tissue would be detected by neurological and diagnostic testing. Derealization is not evident in the client's situation. **Cognitive Level:** Analyzing **Client Need:** Psychosocial Integrity **Integrated Process:** Nursing Process: Diagnosis **Content Area:** Mental Health **Strategy:** The core issue of the question is knowledge of possible explanations of causation of pain in a client with no physical basis for pain. Use nursing knowledge and the process of elimination to make a selection.

27 **Answer: 4 Rationale:** The client with a conversion disorder is characteristically indifferent to the symptoms (la belle indifference). A depressed mood is not associated with a conversion disorder. The client with a conversion disorder does not present with anxiety. Although the client may be indifferent to the symptom, the client does not have a blunted affect in general. **Cognitive Level:** Analyzing **Client Need:** Psychosocial Integrity **Integrated Process:** Nursing Process: Assessment **Content Area:** Mental Health **Strategy:** The core issue of the question is knowledge of expected assessment findings related to mood in a client with a conversion disorder. Use nursing knowledge and the process of elimination to make a selection.

28 **Answer: 3 Rationale:** The best response is nonjudgmental and affirms the client's personal power in the decision-making process. It also would help the client understand connections in her own decision-making process. The best responses would not threaten, judge, or disempower the client. **Cognitive Level:** Applying **Client Need:** Psychosocial Integrity **Integrated Process:** Caring **Content Area:** Mental Health **Strategy:** The core issue of the question is a therapeutic communication to a client with hypochondriasis. Use nursing knowledge of therapeutic communication skills and the process of elimination to make a selection.

29 **Answer: 3 Rationale:** Data indicates that the client perceives a lack of control over the situation, making powerlessness the most appropriate priority selection. Although the client is having difficulty in maintaining the home environment, this is only one part of the problem presented by the client. Fatigue may be present but does not represent the major etiology of the client's difficulties. There is no information to suggest that the client's illness has led to an altered body image. **Cognitive Level:** Analyzing **Client Need:** Psychosocial Integrity **Integrated Process:** Nursing Process: Diagnosis **Content Area:** Mental Health **Strategy:** The core issue of the question is the ability to form an appropriate nursing diagnosis based on client assessment data. Use nursing knowledge and the process of elimination to make a selection.

30 **Answer: 1 Rationale:** When stressors and anxiety are decreased, there remains no need for conversion symptoms, and normal function resumes. Because there is no organic basis for a conversion disorder, learning sign language, being fitted for a hearing aid or having a stapedectomy would not be effective methods for addressing the underlying problem. **Cognitive Level:** Analyzing **Client Need:** Psychosocial Integrity **Integrated Process:** Nursing Process: Evaluation **Content Area:** Mental Health **Strategy:** The core issue of the question is knowledge of appropriate outcomes of care for a client with a conversion disorder. Use nursing knowledge and the process of elimination to make a selection.

31 **Answer: 2, 3, 5 Rationale:** Verbal communication should be clear, concise, and unhurried. Loud communication (or shouting) may be interpreted as anger; therefore, a pleasant, calm, supportive tone of voice should be used. The use of mostly nonverbal gestures would be frustrating to the client who may not understand what is being said. **Cognitive Level:** Applying **Client Need:** Psychosocial Integrity **Integrated Process:** Caring **Content Area:** Mental Health **Strategy:** The core issue of the question is therapeutic communication to a client with a cognitive impairment. Use nursing knowledge of therapeutic communication skills and the process of elimination to make a selection.

32 **Answer: 4 Rationale:** The most important area of concern identified by both family and staff is the safety of clients with dementia. Because the risk for injury is always present in clients, the outcome of preventing injury has highest priority. Preventing further deterioration, supporting family caregivers, and possibly finding an appropriate skilled nursing facility placement are appropriate but are not the first priority. **Cognitive Level:** Applying **Client Need:** Psychosocial Integrity **Integrated Process:** Nursing Process: Planning **Content Area:** Mental Health **Strategy:** The core issue of the question is the ability to determine the appropriate priority of care for a client who has dementia. Focus on safety as an early priority whenever a client has a neurological impairment. Use nursing knowledge and the process of elimination to make a selection.

33 **Answer: 4 Rationale:** Alzheimer's disease is diagnosed by ruling out causes for the client's symptoms. Reviewing laboratory findings, CT scan results, and noting physiological findings all assist in ruling out other causes of the client's symptoms. **Cognitive Level:** Analyzing **Client Need:** Psychosocial Integrity **Integrated Process:** Nursing Process: Assessment **Content Area:** Mental Health **Strategy:** The core issue of the question is methods of diagnosis for Alzheimer's disease. Use nursing knowledge and the process of elimination to make a selection.

34 **Answer: 2 Rationale:** Dementia is a progressive disease that results in loss of ability to perform tasks that were once familiar and routine. Self-care deficits involving many functional abilities occur to varying degrees. The most effective and respectful goals are those that allow the client to carry out as much self-care as possible. A client with dementia will gradually lose orientation to time, place, and person, making reality orientation an unrealistic goal. The overall goal is to assist the client to remain as independent as possible, and assist with daily living activities only to the extent that is needed. Maintaining hydration and nutrition are important goals for the client, but are not global enough to represent the overall goal of nursing care. **Cognitive Level:** Applying **Client Need:** Psychosocial Integrity **Integrated Process:** Nursing Process: Planning **Content Area:** Mental Health **Strategy:** The core issue of the question is the ability to set goals of care for a client with dementia. Note the critical word *overall* in the question, which guides you to look for a global option that encompasses the others.

35 **Answer: 1 Rationale:** Cognitive function is supported by participation in meaningful activities that the client enjoys. Stimulating activities also promote self-esteem and encourage the client to attain the highest level of cognitive function possible. Reminding the client of forgotten events may be helpful momentarily but could also lead to frustration. Reorienting the client to reality will not support sustained memory function and while it might be helpful momentarily, it could also lead to frustration. Restraining a client who is agitated could increase agitation rather than decrease it. **Cognitive Level:** Applying **Client Need:** Psychosocial Integrity **Integrated Process:** Nursing Process: Implementation **Content Area:** Mental Health **Strategy:** The core issue of the question is planning for a client with dementia that supports remaining memory function. Use nursing knowledge and the process of elimination to make a selection.

36 **Answer: 2, 3 Rationale:** Positive symptoms of schizophrenia are those behaviors that a client would not usually exhibit in everyday life, including echolalia or a delusion of being a king. Negative symptoms of schizophrenia are those that reflect the absence of what is normally seen in a person's behavior. These would include anergy, flat affect, and social withdrawal. **Cognitive Level:** Applying **Client Need:** Psychosocial Integrity **Integrated Process:** Nursing Process: Assessment **Content Area:** Mental Health **Strategy:** The core issue of the question is the ability to discriminate between positive and negative symptoms of schizophrenia. Use nursing knowledge of these manifestations and the process of elimination to make a selection.

Key Terms to Review

affect p. 284
agnosia p. 298
agoraphobia p. 283
anxiety p. 279
aphasia p. 297
apraxia p. 297
bipolar disorder p. 284
body dysmorphic disorder p. 295
clang association p. 289
compulsions p. 283
conversion disorder p. 295
cyclothymic disorder p. 284
delirium p. 297
delusions p. 288
dementia p. 297
depersonalization p. 293
derealization p. 293
dissociation p. 294
dissociative amnesia p. 293
dissociative fugue p. 293
dissociative identity disorder (DID) p. 293
dysthymic disorder p. 284
egodystonic p. 290
egosyntonic p. 290
group therapy p. 282
hallucinations p. 288
host personality p. 293
hypochondriasis p. 295
illusion p. 289
major depression p. 284
milieu therapy p. 298
mood p. 284
neologisms p. 289
obsessions p. 283
personality disorder p. 290
personality traits p. 290
phobia p. 282
primary gain p. 293
psychosis p. 289
repression p. 294
schizoaffective disorder p. 284
schizophrenia p. 288
seasonal affective disorder (SAD) p. 284
secondary gain p. 293
somatoform disorders p. 294
sundown syndrome p. 297
word salad p. 289

References

Boyd, M. (2015). *Psychiatric nursing: Contemporary practice. Enhanced update.* (5th ed.). Philadelphia: Wolters Kluwer Health.

Potter, M., & Moller, M. (2016). *Psychiatric-mental health nursing: From suffering to hope*. New York, NY: Pearson Education.

Stuart, G. (2013). *Principles and practice of psychiatric nursing* (10th ed.). St. Louis, MO: Elsevier Science.

Townsend, M. (2015). *Psychiatric mental health nursing: Concepts of care in evidence-based practice* (8th ed.). Philadelphia: F. A. Davis.

Varcarolis, E. (2014). *Foundations of psychiatric mental health nursing: A clinical approach* (6th ed.). St. Louis, MO: Saunders.

Substance Use and Addictive Disorders

22

In this chapter

Cross Reference

Other chapters relevant to this content area are

Coping with Stressors **Chapter 20**
Mental Health Disorders **Chapter 21**
Psychiatric Medications **Chapter 35**

I. OVERVIEW OF SUBSTANCE USE AND ADDICTIVE DISORDERS

A. Commonly used terms

NCLEX® 1. **Substance:** any of several drug classes known to act on brain's reward system
2. **Substance use disorder:** purposeful but maladaptive substance use pattern despite negative physiological and psychological consequences
3. **Substance dependence:** physical need for a substance; is preceded by **tolerance** (needing increased amounts of substance to achieve desired effect); cessation of use leads to **withdrawal** (physiological, cognitive, and behavior changes associated with sudden discontinuation or rapid decrease in use of substance)

B. Types of addictive disorders

1. Substance use disorder and **process addiction** are characterized by preoccupation with and compulsion to engage in an activity
   a. Substances: depressants (opiate, opioids, sedatives, hypnotics), stimulants (cocaine, amphetamines), cannabinoids and hallucinogens, inhalants
   b. Process addictions: compulsive gambling or shopping/spending, compulsive sexual disorders, compulsive gaming or Internet use
   NCLEX® c. **Addiction:** chronic and relapsing disease characterized by compulsive and ongoing use despite harmful consequences, including neurochemical and molecular changes in brain; dysfunctional patterns include patterns of alcohol, drug, or tobacco use, excessive gambling or spending, and certain compulsive sexual disorders

NCLEX® 2. Treatment focus is **abstinence** (voluntarily going without drugs), medications as appropriate, education, lifestyle change, and increasing self-awareness and personal growth

C. Genetic/biologic risk

1. No one specific marker is responsible for substance use or addictive disorders—the more risk factors, the greater the risk for developing disease

NCLEX® 2. Genetics: clients who have biological relatives with substance problems are at increased risk; drug use negatively affects egg and sperm health

D. Psychosocial risk

1. Personality: clients with certain personality traits may be more susceptible to reinforcing effects of engaging in addictive behaviors
   a. Dominant and critical with underlying personal insecurity, low self-esteem and self-criticism
   b. Problems with sexual identification, difficulty with intimacy
   c. Rebellious toward authority, escapist or sensation-seeking tendencies, difficulty with impulse control
2. Developmental: clients who have lived with painful experiences are at risk to self-medicate or misuse medication
   a. Abuse survivors—may experience disturbances in sense of self
   b. Lack of nurturance in childhood—may lead to an inability to self-soothe
   c. Coping skills deficit—not sufficiently learned in person's family of origin
3. Social: clients can be at risk because of influence of family, role models, and peer pressure
   a. Engaging in addictive behavior is influenced by exposure to peer pressure or role models; may begin in adolescence
   b. Family or friends may indirectly enable substance use by allowing it in home, keeping secrets about use, or tolerating associated dangerous or intimidating behavior
   c. **Codependency** occurs when family or others fail to address substance use behaviors by caretaking (providing financial and other support) and shielding client's behavior from discovery and consequences of actions
4. Culture: use of addictive substances is influenced by culture; some substances, such as tobacco, alcohol, marijuana, opium, and peyote, may be more acceptable in some cultures than in others

NCLEX®

5. Profession: healthcare professionals (HCPs), including nurses, may be at risk to use addictive substances because of high-stress, high-pressure jobs and exposure to substances
   a. Risk factors for vulnerability: access to drugs, long hours, tremendous responsibility, job-related stress, family history of chemical dependence or mental health disorder

   NCLEX®

   b. Signs: increased irritability with clients and colleagues; mood swings; withdrawn or isolated; absent or late for work, often with elaborate excuses; decreased quality of work; a nurse-specific indicator is that nurse signs out more narcotics than others on unit; nurses have an ethical obligation to report impaired nurses
   c. System response: in most states, there is opportunity for supportive intervention rather than loss of license if impaired nurse seeks treatment and strictly follows treatment and monitoring recommendations from Board of Nursing; if noncompliant, may lose nursing license

E. Dual disorders risk

NCLEX®

1. Some clients with a mental health disorder also have addiction; initially drugs or alcohol may be used to compensate for lack of coping skills if client experiences depressive symptoms, anxiety, or recurrence of painful memories; with continued use, addiction develops for client at risk
2. Client with addiction may have or is at risk for developing a mental health disorder
   a. Substance use can induce development of a mental health disorder by affecting brain regulation of cognition, motivation, learning, and mood regulation
   b. Any one of a number of disorders can develop
3. Clients with addictive disorders may be misdiagnosed because some disorders (such as anxiety disorders, depression, and chronic pain) mask addiction

Memory Aid

When a client has a problem with substance use or addiction, screen carefully for other mental health disorders, which may be comorbidities.

NCLEX®

4. Clients with dual diagnoses and who are intoxicated are at increased risk of suicide
5. Treatment for dual diagnoses is more successful if both are treated concurrently

II. ASSESSMENT

A. Screening and assessment tools

1. CAGE: a positive answer for two of these screening questions indicates need for further assessment
   a. Have you ever felt you should *Cut down* on your drinking/substance use?
   b. Have people *Annoyed* you by comments criticizing your drinking/substance use?
   c. Have you ever felt bad or *Guilty* about your drinking/substance use?
   d. Have you ever had a drink (*Eye-opener*) first thing in the morning to steady your nerves or get rid of a hangover?

Memory Aid

Use the initials of the CAGE questionnaire to trigger the memory of what each question refers to.

NCLEX®

2. General screening questions should elicit information about substance use, time of last use, amount used, and route of self-administration; others include:
   a. Have you ever tried to stop using (alcohol or substance)?
   b. Are you able to identify any situations or feelings that trigger use of (alcohol or substance)?
   c. Have you ever been hospitalized for use of alcohol or drugs?
   d. How often do you use (alcohol or substance)?
   e. Have you ever been unable to recall what you did?
   f. Have you ever been arrested related to use of alcohol or drugs?

B. History and physical assessment/systems review

1. Blackout or lost consciousness: can be related to use of alcohol or other substances
2. Changes in bowel movement: changes range from diarrhea caused by drinking to constipation caused by pain medications; withdrawal from narcotics can cause diarrhea (NCLEX®)
3. Liver problems: include manifestations of Wernicke's encephalopathy or Korsakoff's psychosis
4. Weight loss or weight gain: regular alcohol or drug use may lead to weight loss or gain and/or poor nutritional balance (NCLEX®)
5. Stress: stressful situations can lead to increased drinking; stress can also result from drinking or using drugs regularly
6. Sleep disturbances: alcohol and/or drug use can lead to a variety of sleep disturbances; client may start using alcohol to promote sleep, but once tolerance develops, sleep is more difficult (NCLEX®)
7. Chronic pain: may lead to use of drugs and/or alcohol to self-medicate
8. Concern over substance use: if friends and relatives worry about substance use, it is generally because a genuine problem exists (NCLEX®)

Memory Aid

It is just as important to screen for psychosocial data as for physical assessment data during admission for treatment for addiction.

9. Genetic risk: persons with positive family history are at risk for developing a substance use or other addictive disorder
10. Specific substance use assessment: key elements (NCLEX®)
    a. Identify type of substance, amount, and pattern and frequency of use
    b. Age at onset and age of regular use
    c. Changes in use patterns
    d. Periods of abstinence in history
    e. Previous withdrawal symptoms
    f. Date of last substance use/compulsive behavior
    g. Ask about each substance or behavior separately
11. Medication assessment (NCLEX®)
    a. Use of pain relief medications, laxatives, cold medications, and medications to induce sleep, help client stay awake, and/or control anxiety
    b. Whether original dose is now not enough to control pain or anxiety even though it helped at first
    c. Whether client runs out of medication early and needs a refill early
    d. If pain medication intended for physical pain is now used for emotional pain
    e. If medication is used for dealing with "stress" or stressful events or more was taken than intended
    f. Whether laxatives are used regularly (because opioids cause constipation or client has difficulty having bowel movements without laxative use)
    g. If cold tablets or cough syrup are taken more frequently than expected
12. Over-the-counter (OTC) or nutritional supplement assessment: use of any herbal, vitamin, or OTC products to help with sleep, weight loss, staying awake, increasing energy, stabilizing and/or improving mood, or making client feel a certain way
13. Social history assessment: clients experiencing physical, sexual, or emotional abuse may medicate internal distress by using mood-altering substances

14. Laboratory assessment: blood alcohol content (BAC) 0.1% or higher for intoxication (legal BAC may vary among states or provinces); urine toxicology and blood screen for drugs of abuse

III. PLANNING AND IMPLEMENTATION

A. Care of client while intoxicated

1. Focus is on safety
2. Assess signs and symptoms of intoxication (see Table 22–1)
3. Interventions *NCLEX®*
   a. Maintain safe environment
   b. Orient to time, place, and person
   c. Maintain adequate nutrition and fluid balance
   d. Monitor for beginning of withdrawal signs and symptoms

Memory Aid

In general, drugs that are CNS depressants lead to signs of CNS excitation during withdrawal, and drugs that are CNS stimulants lead to CNS depression during withdrawal.

B. Care of client experiencing withdrawal: focus is on safe supervised withdrawal

1. Maintain safe and low-stimulation environment; initiate seizure precautions appropriate to substance; provide one-to-one observation as needed
2. Interact with client in a nonjudgmental manner
3. Monitor for withdrawal syndrome *NCLEX®*
   a. Monitor vital signs for hypertension, tachycardia, and tachypnea
   b. Monitor for other withdrawal symptoms, such as disorientation, nausea/vomiting, tremor, paroxysmal sweats, anxiety, agitation, or delirium tremens (visual, auditory, or tactile hallucinations); see Table 22–1 again
   c. Use appropriate withdrawal scales, such as Clinical Institute Withdrawal Assessment Scale for Alcohol (CIWA-Ar)

Table 22–1 Signs of Substance Intoxication and Withdrawal with Treatments

Type of Substance	Signs of Intoxication	Signs of Withdrawal	Treatment of Withdrawal
CNS depressants (alcohol, benzodiazepines, barbiturates)	Impaired memory, attention, judgment, or general functioning; drowsiness, slurred speech, irritability, hypotension	Nausea, vomiting, tachycardia, diaphoresis, abdominal cramping, insomnia, irritability, delirium, tremors, seizures	Seizure precautions Alcohol: chlordiazepoxide, thiamine, antiepileptics Benzodiazepines: flumazenil IV Barbiturates: phenobarbital or long-acting benzodiazepine
CNS stimulants (amphetamines, cocaine, crack)	Ataxia, fever, respiratory distress, seizures, coma, cerebrovascular accident, myocardial infarction, death	Apathy, extreme fatigue, lethargy, disorientation, anxiety, insomnia, agitation, depression, drug craving	Primarily supportive treatment Drug therapy: antidepressants, bromocriptine (dopamine agonist, off-label use)
Opioids (codeine, morphine, opium, heroin, meperidine, hydromorphone, methadone, fentanyl, oxycodone)	Euphoria, drowsiness, constricted pupils, hypotension, slurred speech, decreased respirations, and impaired movements, memory, attention, and judgment	Excessive sweating, restlessness, agitation, dilated pupils, piloerection, tremors, yawning, tachycardia, hypertension, abdominal cramps, muscle spasms	Methadone/buprenorphine Clonidine/lofexidine to reduce severity of withdrawal Oxazepam (muscle spasms and insomnia) Antiemetics (nausea and vomiting)
Hallucinogens (lysergic acid diethylamide [LSD]), mescaline (peyote), psilocybin (mushrooms), phencyclidine (PCP)	Agitation, bizarre or violent behavior, dilated pupils, blank stare, piloerection, tachycardia and hypertension, incoordination, muscle rigidity with jerking, paranoia, hallucinations, tremors or seizures	Depends on specific drug; possible anxiety, mental depression, lethargy, insomnia, paranoid delusions, panic attacks	Supportive care with low environmental stimuli Gastric lavage or acidification of urine with vitamin C or ammonium chloride to speed drug clearance (PCP)
Marijuana (cannabis sativa)	Relaxation, euphoria, detachment, more talkative, slowed perception of time, possible anxiety or paranoia	Irritability, restlessness, insomnia, tremors, chills, weight loss	Supportive care; no specific medications

4. Maintain adequate nutrition and fluid intake
5. Methadone is used to manage some clients who are opiate-dependent; may be initially prescribed for withdrawal but then client is maintained on certain daily dose

NCLEX®
6. Monitor for alcohol withdrawal delirium, psychotic symptoms, suicide risk, and seizure risk

NCLEX®
7. Administer medication to assist with withdrawal process: antiepileptics, benzodiazepines, sedatives, vitamins, or others as prescribed; thiamine helps to prevent confusion and other mental status changes (see again Table 22–1)
8. Various products are available to help with withdrawal from nicotine and cravings, including nicotine patches, inhaler, or gum, and bupropion if prescribed

NCLEX®
9. Maintain normal comfort measures
10. Monitor for covert substance use during detoxification period
11. Assist client to deal with emotions and provide emotional support to client and family
12. Provide reality orientation and address hallucinations in a therapeutic manner
13. Advise client of depressive uneasy feelings and fatigue that usually occur during withdrawal; set limits on any angry, manipulative, or abusive behavior
14. Begin to educate client about disease of addiction and initial treatment goal of abstinence

NCLEX®
15. Outcomes are safe withdrawal; client begins to develop motivation for and commitment to abstinence and **recovery** (abstinence plus engagement in a program of personal growth and self-discovery)

C. Nursing care during rehabilitative stages of abuse

1. Focus is on teaching about disease and recovery process and building on client's motivation for abstinence, lifestyle change, and recovery

NCLEX®
2. Assist client to complete detoxification from all psychoactive substances; monitor for suicide and/or seizure risk
3. Promote abstinence from all psychoactive substances
4. Administer medications to enhance abstinence or treat mood, anxiety, and/or thought disorders as applicable
5. Assist client in putting structure and discipline back into life
6. Assist client to identify strengths, methods for coping with stressors that trigger substance use or other addictive behavior
7. Assist client to develop goals and subgoals for behavior change; provide positive reinforcement for goals achieved
8. Explore how disease has impacted client and family roles and functions

NCLEX®
9. Provide therapeutic interaction/group counseling to process losses (i.e., loss of independence), discuss memories and flashback, address shame and guilt, educate about disease/recovery, and facilitate acceptance of illness

NCLEX®
10. Teach and encourage practice of recovery skills
    a. Encourage daily commitment to sobriety and recovery
    b. Build and utilize sober support networks (i.e., Alcoholics Anonymous or other 12-step groups)
    c. Encourage daily meditation or prayer
    d. Teach drink refusal skills and how to manage cravings
    e. Enhance coping, communication, and problem-solving skills
    f. Practice asking for help

NCLEX®
    g. Recognize signs of impending **relapse** (return to addictive behavior): being hungry, angry, lonely, or tired (acronym HALT); having thoughts about using but not telling anyone, slipping back into using old defensive mechanisms instead of honesty and openness

NCLEX®
11. Help client to develop an emergency plan (list of things client can do and people to call if he or she has urge to use or actually uses)

Memory Aid

Developing an emergency plan is high priority before discharge to home so that the client is better empowered to act on own behalf when the urge to use recurs.

12. Demonstrate how to use affirmations, slogans, and serenity prayer
13. Explain possible use of random breathalyzers and urine drug screens to objectively assess for sobriety/ substance use

NCLEX® 14. Clients with anorexia nervosa or bulimia need to work with dietitian and primary care provider about increasing or decreasing (as indicated) caloric intake and discontinuing laxative use; they will need to increase daily water and fiber intake

15. Clients with multiple relapses with severe addiction may not have a goal of immediate total abstinence; their goals may be to reduce number of drinks ingested or money gambled at one sitting (harm reduction model); while not an ideal goal, decreased engagement in use or behavior is a step in a positive direction

D. Treatment modalities and nursing interventions

1. Medical model: teach disease and recovery dynamics
2. Assist client in complying with treatment recommendations
3. Detoxification, abstinence medications
   - NCLEX® a. Disulfiram: prevents breakdown of alcohol; alcohol ingestion leads to flushing, weakness, nausea/vomiting, dizziness, tachycardia, and hypotension); teach about avoiding alcohol in any form (cough or cold products, mouthwash); can elevate liver enzymes
   - NCLEX® b. Naltrexone: prevents or diminishes cravings for substance use; can elevate liver enzymes
   - NCLEX® c. Antidepressant/anti-anxiety medications: enhance and stabilize mood and diminish anxiety; teach about decreased effectiveness of medication with use of psychoactive substances; medication should be discontinued gradually to prevent rebound effect or seizures
4. NCLEX® The 12-step model
   - a. Teach that there is no effective cure for addiction
   - b. Regular attendance at meetings diminishes ambivalence and promotes acceptance about never engaging in addictive behaviors again
   - c. Key elements of 12-step framework are acceptance, surrender, processing grief, higher power, and power of group
5. Cognitive behavioral model
   - a. Develop and use positive coping skills
   - NCLEX® b. Implement specific skill training: assertiveness, drink refusal, problem solving, cognitive restructuring, mood management, anger problems, social skills, listening and communication skills
   - c. Identify and change behaviors associated with addictive behaviors (i.e., going into liquor store to buy soft drinks)
6. Relapse prevention model
   - a. Identify situations and factors that contribute to relapse
   - NCLEX® b. Increase positive self-efficacy expectations about ability to achieve abstinence
7. Motivational enhancement and stages of change
   - NCLEX® a. Use various types of reflective listening and other specialized communication strategies to help build client's commitment to change
   - b. Express empathy; ambivalence is a normal part of change process
   - NCLEX® c. Help clients develop discrepancy between how they see themselves and how they really are
   - d. Change strategies if resistance is encountered; avoid arguments
   - NCLEX® e. Support client's self-efficacy
8. Assess client's stage of change and apply nursing interventions accordingly
   - a. Precontemplation: "We are blind to our problems"
   - b. Contemplation: "We are not ready to change"
   - c. Determination and preparation: "We are getting ready to change"
   - d. Action: "We are learning how to change; we are doing it"
   - e. Maintenance: "We make changes stick"

IV. EVALUATION/OUTCOMES

A. Completes withdrawal process safely

B. Makes a commitment to sobriety, participates in treatment process

C. Identifies consequences of substance use or addictive behaviors

D. Begins to practice some recovery behaviors while in treatment and identifies coping behaviors to address cravings, thoughts, and triggers to use or engage in addictive behaviors

V. DUAL DISORDER ISSUES

A. Focus is on recognition of each disorder as a unique illness that requires treatment and builds on client's motivation for abstinence, remissions of mental illness, lifestyle change, and recovery process

B. Additional interventions

1. Discuss physiological aspects of mental illness, substance abuse, and interaction effects
2. Teach that psychiatric medications are nonaddictive and can enhance recovery
3. Medication teaching includes emphasizing that drinking or drug use will interfere with efficacy of psychiatric medication and not to mix medication with other substances

VI. FAMILY ISSUES

A. Anger and alienation of substance-using family member

B. Teach disease dynamics

1. Family rules and communication
2. Family members' dysfunctional behaviors and denial about addiction of family member

NCLEX® **C. Explore problematic coping skills, codependency, and low self-esteem**

D. Learn and practice recovery dynamics and skills

1. Include self-love and self-care
2. Utilize support groups (i.e., Al-Anon)
3. Establish healthy relationships and boundaries
4. Engage in daily meditation or prayer
5. NCLEX® Improve coping and problem-solving skills
6. NCLEX® Learn to ask for help
7. Confront dysfunctional beliefs and learn how to change them
8. Use affirmations, slogans, serenity prayer

E. Processing anger, losses, and memories

1. Confront substance user about consequences of use and effect on family
2. Process emotional distance between family members
3. NCLEX® Process loss of "helper/competent" role now that recovering family member is taking back some of his or her lost family roles

Check Your NCLEX–RN® Exam I.Q.

You are ready for testing on this content if you can:

- Assess clients for signs of dependency or addiction.
- Assess reactions of clients and families to a diagnosis related to dependency or addiction.
- Counsel clients who have a substance-related disorder.
- Participate in providing therapy to a client with a disorder of dependency or addiction.
- Identify factors that could interfere with the recovery of a client from a substance-related disorder.
- Provide teaching about treatments, including support groups, for disorders of dependency or addiction.
- Assess and provide care to a client undergoing substance withdrawal or drug toxicity.

PRACTICE TEST

1 A client is transitioning to a less intensive level of outpatient treatment for addiction. The nurse concludes the client is most at risk for relapse after the client makes a statement reflecting which theme?

1. Dreaming about gambling
2. Not feeling happy in general
3. Feeling hungry or tired after a long day
4. Keeping thoughts of using opioids a secret

2 What statement made by the mother of a recovering compulsive Internet user would indicate the need for more teaching?

1. "My son is not going to enough 12-step meetings, and I don't think he is taking this seriously enough."
2. "My daughter and I are going to go to Al-Anon because we realize we have been affected by my son's addiction."
3. "I need to sign up for a meditation class for myself because I get too preoccupied with what my son is or is not doing."
4. "I still have a lot of anger about the relationship problems that occurred between me and my son as a result of his addiction."

PRACTICE TEST

3. The nurse observes a family visit on the unit and recognizes that the family is experiencing effects of addiction and codependence. What long-lasting interpersonal problems might the nurse expect family members to manifest?

1. Lowered self-esteem
2. Impatience
3. Frustration tolerance
4. Being argumentative

4. A mother brings her daughter to the emergency department. The daughter was at a dance party for the last few hours, but now she is sweating and does not look well. Assessment reveals temperature of 103°F (39.4°C), weight loss, and teeth grinding. What should be the nurse's greatest concern?

1. Poor nutrition from excessive alcohol consumption
2. Possible eating disorder
3. Dehydration and electrolyte imbalance
4. Influenza with accompanying high fever

5. The nurse is completing an admission for a client with alcohol dependence. During the admission process, the client acknowledges occasional sexual performance problems but says, "It's nothing a little alcohol can't fix." The nurse explains that regular alcohol use can have which effect on sexual functioning?

1. Increased desire and performance ability
2. Headaches and a "too tired syndrome"
3. Hyperarousal and confidence about sexual performance
4. Decreased desire and ability to perform

6. A healthcare provider has prescribed naltrexone for a client. What would be the greatest concern of the nurse while getting ready to administer this medication?

1. The medication blocks the euphoric feeling from narcotics and alcohol.
2. The healthcare provider may not have shared sufficient information about the medication.
3. The medication can precipitate withdrawal if the client is not completely detoxified.
4. The client will not be able to experience pleasurable sensations.

7. The nurse is conducting a daily nursing assessment on a client with gambling and alcohol addictions who is in an outpatient addiction program. Which client statement reflects a need for teaching?

1. "I am going to have a night out with some friends at a local night club."
2. "I felt like drinking, so I cleaned the house instead."
3. "It is hard for me to make phone calls if I feel like using, but I did it last night."
4. "I told my brother that I couldn't help him as much as I have in the past."

8. After completing a family session about addiction, a woman approaches the nurse and shares that she will always worry about her chemically dependent daughter, who could relapse at any time. What important information should the nurse share about family recovery from addiction?

1. Family recovery can begin when the addictive behavior ceases.
2. Family recovery can begin even if active use continues.
3. Family recovery will fail if the recovering addicted client relapses.
4. Family recovery will be enhanced if the recovering addict attends several Alcoholics Anonymous meetings.

9. A married client with heavy marijuana use has difficulty keeping her house clean because she spends hours playing games on the Internet. She also says that she waits until everyone goes to bed to write messages with sexual content online with another man. What is the nurse's greatest concern?

1. The Internet usage may lead to an extramarital affair.
2. Her children will stop bringing friends home because the house is messy.
3. She seems preoccupied with the Internet and is using poor judgment.
4. She is depressed and may find her marriage unfulfilling.

10 At a 6-week postpartum visit, a new mother who bottle-feeds her infant discusses feeling depressed and is prescribed an antidepressant. The nurse assesses the client's alcohol-use patterns and learns the client has one to two drinks once or twice a week. What explanation should the nurse provide for not using alcohol or drugs in this situation?

1. It will cause nausea and vomiting.
2. It will lead to excessive antidepressant effects.
3. It will decrease the effectiveness of the antidepressant.
4. It will cause increased blood pressure.

11 A cocaine-dependent client in recovery shares that she has been using an over-the-counter (OTC) sleep aid each night for the past 3 weeks. She becomes defensive when the nurse raises concerns, stating emphatically that it is not addictive. How should the nurse respond to the client? Select all that apply.

1. Validate how difficult it is to have trouble sleeping.
2. Acknowledge to the client that because the medication cannot be abused, it is not addictive.
3. Confront her firmly because there is increased risk for addiction if she uses this aid too often.
4. Suggest an herbal sleep aid such as valerian or melatonin, which cannot activate the brain reward system.
5. Explain that nonaddictive medication can be abused if taken in larger doses or more frequently than recommended.

12 As the nurse asks about sexuality during a nursing assessment, the client acknowledges that she has a masturbation compulsion and is trying to stop on her own but can't. She says she needs to know what she can do to stop. Based on her stage of change, the nurse should use which approach to care?

1. Help her to see that she has a serious problem.
2. Encourage her by stating she will feel better if she stops the compulsive sexual behavior.
3. Identify a date for her to stop her compulsive sexual behavior.
4. Review strategies to assist her to stop the compulsive sexual behavior.

13 The mental health nurse explains to clients who are learning about cross-addiction that there is a synergistic or additive effect from using various kinds of chemicals together. The nurse illustrates this point using which example of items that create this combined effect?

1. Drinking beer and smoking cigarettes
2. Drinking coffee and eating doughnuts
3. Drinking wine and taking a benzodiazepine
4. Drinking wine and coffee

14 A male client is saying he is "wired," feels like he is on "pins and needles," and is irritable. He says he stopped using alcohol abruptly. What is the nurse's next intervention in caring for this client?

1. Observe whether other symptoms occur in the next few hours and then report them to the healthcare provider.
2. Assess the time of his last drink and begin assessing for signs and symptoms of alcohol withdrawal.
3. Assess for all current substance-use patterns, including time of last use, and begin to assess for withdrawal.
4. Request a prescription for a stimulant medication to help prevent alcohol withdrawal delirium.

15 A booth at a church parish health fair addresses safe driving. The nurse at this booth explains that coordination and mental alertness are affected at a blood alcohol level (BAL) of 0.04, even though many states have a legal limit of intoxication of 0.08 or 0.1. When asked how many drinks per hour the average person needs to be close to the 0.08 BAL, the nurse should make which reply?

1. A 4-ounce glass of wine if the individual has eaten recently
2. A 4-ounce glass of wine on an empty stomach
3. Three to five 4-ounce glasses of wine, depending on how recently food was consumed
4. Seven to eight 4-ounce glasses of wine, depending on how recently food was consumed

16 A client who broke his ankle while drinking at a party questions whether his drinking is "okay." He has never been arrested for driving intoxicated, and has no health or relationship problems. He reports calling in sick to work once after drinking and drove intoxicated several times. Family information validates his self-report. The nurse concludes the client has an alcohol use disorder based on which characteristic?

1. Drinking more than two drinks per occasion
2. Inability to stop drinking despite negative consequences
3. Drinking that causes an individual to pass out or experience a blackout
4. Drinking too much and too often with using poor judgment, despite negative consequences

17 The nurse is conducting an education session about alcoholism. Which statement should the nurse include when explaining the concept of alcohol dependence? Select all that apply.

1. Continuing to drink despite critical alcohol-related problems
2. Drinking larger amounts or over a longer time than was intended
3. Drinking to the point of drunkenness on average of once per week
4. Experiencing a diminished effect with intake of the same amount of alcohol
5. Using confabulation as a defense mechanism

18 A client is in the rehabilitative stage of treatment for substance use disorder. When teaching the client relapse prevention skills, what should the nurse emphasize? Select all that apply.

1. Preventing fatigue
2. Maintaining physical health
3. Suppressing thoughts of returning to substance use
4. Reducing amount of solitary unstructured time
5. Reconnecting with the recent social network

19 Which comment by a client with substance use disorder should lead the nurse to conclude that the client is vulnerable for relapse? Select all that apply.

1. "I like being able to have a lot of free time."
2. "Going to a football game makes me want to use again."
3. "I've been sober for 2 years. I've got this problem under control."
4. "No one else seems to work as hard as I do."
5. "It's easy. I can go to a club and just drink soft drinks."

20 The nurse instructs the client about the disease of addiction. The nurse determines that the client understands the information given when the client uses which descriptions of addiction? Select all that apply.

1. "A moral weakness"
2. "A medical illness"
3. "A behavioral habit"
4. "An emotional attachment"
5. "A difficult problem to cure"

ANSWERS & RATIONALES

1 **Answer: 4 Rationale:** When keeping thoughts of using secret, the client is not telling the whole truth. Engaging in secrets is reminiscent of using behaviors and can trigger addiction behaviors. Feeling sad sometimes is natural and does not by itself indicate risk for relapse. Hunger and tiredness are natural sometimes, and they do not always indicate risk for relapse. Having thoughts of engaging in addictive behavior is normal, and this alone does not indicate risk for relapse. **Cognitive Level:** Applying **Client Need:** Psychosocial Integrity **Integrated Process:** Nursing Process: Evaluation **Content Area:** Mental Health **Strategy:** Use the process of elimination and nursing knowledge to answer the question. The wording of the question tells you that one answer is better than the others because it contains the critical word *best.*

2 **Answer: 1 Rationale:** Checking on the compliance of a family member is an example of codependent behavior. The nurse would focus the teaching on helping the mother detach from her son and his recovery program and focus on her own well-being. Learning meditation is a way to cope with feelings Expressing anger is a way to identify and deal with feelings. Attending Al-Anon is an obvious healthy behavior. **Cognitive Level:** Applying **Client Need:** Psychosocial Integrity **Integrated Process:** Nursing Process: Evaluation **Content Area:** Mental Health **Strategy:** The wording of the question tells you that only one answer is correct. Use knowledge of codependency to differentiate the problematic behavior from the other expected behaviors.

3 **Answer: 1 Rationale:** Three communication rules tend to be learned in families in which addiction is present: don't talk, don't trust, don't feel. While these experiences cause anger, anxiety, or maladaptive coping, they also contribute to development of shame, depression, and low self-esteem. Without family healing, these problems can create much pain and suffering for all involved. Impatience, frustration tolerance, and being argumentative are not hallmarks or features of long-term family interpersonal problems. **Cognitive Level:** Applying **Client Need:** Psychosocial Integrity **Integrated Process:** Nursing Process: Diagnosis **Content Area:** Mental Health **Strategy:** The core issue of the question is underlying consequences to families when addiction is present. Use nursing knowledge and the process of elimination to make a selection.

4 **Answer: 3 Rationale:** The client most likely has used one of the "club" or "rave" drugs (which are often are a cross between a stimulant and a hallucinogen). The stimulant effect of the drug causes users to grind their teeth. The combination of drugs, dancing, and dehydration leads to a dangerous body temperature increase, which must be addressed immediately. The weight loss might also be related to an eating disorder, but that would not be the nurse's primary concern. Poor nutrition due to alcohol consumption and flu are not issues of concern at this time. **Cognitive Level:** Applying **Client Need:** Psychosocial Integrity **Integrated Process:** Nursing Process: Diagnosis **Content Area:** Mental Health **Strategy:** Note the stem of the question contains the critical words *most concerned*. This tells you that more than one option may be partially correct and that you must prioritize an answer. Correlate elevated body temperature and weight loss with fluid balance to choose dehydration and electrolyte imbalance as correct.

5 **Answer: 4 Rationale:** While many individuals believe that alcohol enhances their sexual experience, the opposite is often true. Regular alcohol use can lead to decreased desire and an inability to perform. Regular alcohol use does not lead to increased desire and ability to perform sexually. Although a client might verbalize decreased desire as being "too tired," regular alcohol use does not cause headaches as an interfering factor for sexual activity. Hyperarousal is the opposite of what clients tend to experience, anxiety about performance (not confidence) tends to occur. **Cognitive Level:** Analyzing **Client Need:** Psychosocial Integrity **Integrated Process:** Teaching and Learning **Content Area:** Mental Health **Strategy:** The core issue of the question is the relationship between chronic substance abuse and sexual performance. Use the process of elimination and nursing knowledge to answer the question. The wording of the question tells you that only one option is correct.

6 **Answer: 3 Rationale:** If the client is not completely detoxified from opiates, the use of naltrexone can precipitate withdrawal. Clients should be opiate-free for 7–10 days before starting this medication. Naltrexone blocks the euphoric response if alcohol or opioids are ingested as an expected drug effect, but this is an expected action and not a reason for the nurse to be concerned. The nurse should routinely evaluate the client's understanding of prescribed medications and provide education as needed, but this is not the greatest concern at this time. Naltrexone does not interfere with the client being able to experience pleasurable sensations in general. **Cognitive Level:** Analyzing **Client Need:** Psychosocial Integrity **Integrated Process:** Nursing Process: Diagnosis **Content Area:** Mental Health **Strategy:** Note the critical words *greatest concern* in the question. This tells you that more than one option could be partially correct and that you must prioritize an answer. Use nursing knowledge of this medication to choose the option in which the client is at greatest risk.

7 **Answer: 1 Rationale:** Recovering clients may underestimate how difficult it will be to stay sober if they visit with friends who are still using or visit old "hangout" places where they used to engage in addictive behaviors. In early recovery, clients are encouraged to detach from people, places, and things associated with their addiction. As they gain sobriety and recovery, they may be able to re-engage, on a limited basis, with certain activities, such as being with friends who drink or celebrating an occasion at a bar. Physical activity is a positive coping measure. Use of support systems indicates positive coping. Limiting demands of others demonstrates positive coping measures and good management of potential triggers. **Cognitive Level:** Analyzing **Client Need:** Psychosocial Integrity **Integrated Process:** Nursing Process: Assessment **Content Area:** Mental Health **Strategy:** The wording of the question indicates the correct option is a statement that contains either a false statement or one that indicates the client is at risk. Choose the correct option over the others because it puts the client in an area where temptation is likely.

8 **Answer: 2 Rationale:** Addiction affects the entire family system: communication roles and boundaries. Family members may experience low self-esteem, guilt, shame, insecurity, and preoccupation with the chemically dependent family member. Families need treatment to facilitate their own healing. Programs such as a treatment facility–operated family program, a spiritually centered family recovery program, or any of the family 12-step programs may help active healing to take place, whether the addicted family member is using or not. Families can begin the recovery process even if the addicted family member is still using. Family recovery can continue even if the recovering addicted client relapses. If the family is not engaged in its own treatment, it may not make any difference how many meetings the addicted member attends. **Cognitive Level:** Analyzing **Client Need:** Psychosocial Integrity **Integrated Process:** Teaching and Learning **Content Area:** Mental Health **Strategy:** The core issue of the question is the family dynamics and impact on the family of a substance-using family member. Use nursing knowledge and the process of elimination to make a selection. The wording of the question indicates that only one answer is correct.

9 **Answer: 3 Rationale:** The client is spending excessive time on the Internet, which seems to interfere with her parental relationships but also the time spent with her husband. This constitutes poor judgment. There is no indication the client's behavior will lead to an extramarital affair. Whether or not children bring friends home because of a messy house is not of great concern. There is not enough data to determine if the client is depressed. **Cognitive Level:** Applying **Client Need:** Psychosocial Integrity **Integrated Process:** Nursing Process: Diagnosis **Content Area:** Mental Health **Strategy:** Use the process of elimination and critical thinking skills to answer the question. The correct answer is one that is most comprehensive of all aspects of the problem described and does not place judgment on the client.

10 **Answer: 3 Rationale:** Antidepressants regulate dysfunction in the neurotransmitter system, which results in mood equilibrium. Alcohol has depressant effects in the neurotransmitter system; it can cause depression and/or anxiety and decrease the effectiveness of the antidepressant drug. Use of alcohol or other mood-altering drugs while taking antidepressants is contraindicated. Combining alcohol or drugs with an antidepressant does not raise blood pressure. Combining alcohol or drugs with an antidepressant will not cause nausea or vomiting. Combining alcohol or drugs with an antidepressant does not lead to excessive antidepressant effects. **Cognitive Level:** Analyzing **Client Need:** Pharmacological and Parenteral Therapies **Integrated Process:** Teaching and Learning **Content Area:** Mental Health **Strategy:** The core issue of the question is the interaction of a prescribed antidepressant with alcohol use. Recall that alcohol is a CNS depressant, which has an opposite effect of antidepressants. Use the process of elimination and general knowledge of drug interactions to make a selection.

11 **Answer: 1, 5 Rationale:** Sleep difficulties are often a problem for people in early recovery. Clients can experience tolerance or tolerance-like symptoms in response to taking certain OTC medications. OTC sleep medications or psychoactive sleep medications are meant for short-term use, no longer than 1 week consecutively. Because the FDA does not regulate herbal products, it is difficult to know what dose to

recommend or how the product might interact with the client. An initial approach that is educational rather than confrontational is more likely to be effective. **Cognitive Level:** Applying **Client Need:** Psychosocial Integrity **Integrated Process:** Communication and Documentation **Content Area:** Mental Health **Strategy:** Use the process of elimination and nursing knowledge to answer the question. Eliminate incorrect options because of the presence of "red flag" words *cannot* in two options and *firmly* in another.

12 **Answer: 4 Rationale:** Because the client acknowledges the problem and has tried to stop on her own, she is in the action stage of change. The correct action of the nurse, then, is to assist the client to stop by reviewing strategies that may be helpful. Helping the client see she has a problem would be useful during the precontemplation stage of change. Encouraging the client that she will feel better by stopping the compulsion may be useful during the contemplation stage of change. Identifying a date to stop the behavior may be useful during the determination and preparation stage of change. **Cognitive Level:** Applying **Client Need:** Psychosocial Integrity **Integrated Process:** Nursing Process: Implementation **Content Area:** Mental Health **Strategy:** The critical words in the question are *stage of change*. This tells you that the correct answer is the one in which the action of the nurse matches the stage of change represented by the client statements. Use the process of elimination and nursing knowledge to make a selection.

13 **Answer: 3 Rationale:** Alcohol and benzodiazepines are both depressants. Persons often use two drugs within the same class to enhance their effects. The capacity of other psychoactive substances within the same class of drugs to enhance the effect of the primary drug is called cross-tolerance. Cigarettes are a stimulant while beer is a depressant, which have opposite effects rather than synergistic ones. Coffee is a stimulant while doughnuts have no direct effect on the central nervous system. Coffee is a stimulant while wine is a depressant, which have opposite effects rather than synergistic ones. **Cognitive Level:** Applying **Client Need:** Psychosocial Integrity **Integrated Process:** Nursing Process: Diagnosis **Content Area:** Mental Health **Strategy:** The core issue of the question is knowledge that cross-addiction occurs between drugs in the same class. Use the process of elimination and knowledge of the categories of the chemicals in the options to make a selection.

14 **Answer: 3 Rationale:** Tactile disturbances are a symptom of alcohol dependence, and if the client reports stopping alcohol use abruptly, he or she may be starting to experience withdrawal symptoms. However, the client may also have used and stopped other substances abruptly as well. The nurse must assess for other substances used. Multiple drug use is the rule more than the exception. Waiting to take action by only observing the client places the client at risk. The use of stimulants is not indicated. **Cognitive Level:** Applying **Client Need:** Psychosocial Integrity **Integrated Process:** Nursing Process: Implementation **Content Area:** Mental Health **Strategy:** The wording indicates that the core issue of the question is possible withdrawal. Choose the option that is most comprehensive in nature and takes into account the possibility of multiple drug use and cessation.

15 **Answer: 3 Rationale:** It takes the average person 1 hour to metabolize 1 ounce of alcohol or a 4-ounce glass of wine. If three to five glasses of wine are consumed within an hour, the average person reaches the legal intoxication level. A 4-ounce glass of wine is insufficient to lead to intoxication. Having an empty stomach does not influence the amount of alcohol ultimately absorbed into the system. Intake of seven to eight glasses of wine would far exceed the legal intoxication level. **Cognitive Level:** Analyzing **Client Need:** Psychosocial Integrity **Integrated Process:** Teaching and Learning **Content Area:** Mental Health **Strategy:** Use the process of elimination to answer the question. Recognize that the question has the critical words *average person* and *be close to*. First eliminate the options that have 4 ounces of wine, since there is no room for individual variation, and then choose the option that has three to five glasses of wine, since it is more moderate in amount than the option with seven to eight glasses.

16 **Answer: 4 Rationale:** The behavior of drinking and driving fits in the abuse category as "recurrent substance use in hazardous situations." Drinking more than two drinks per occasion is not sufficient to be classified as alcohol abuse. Being unable to stop drinking despite negative consequences demonstrates the category of dependence. There is no evidence that the client has tried to stop drinking. Passing out or experiencing a "blackout" is a symptom of intoxication. **Cognitive Level:** Analyzing **Client Need:** Psychosocial Integrity **Integrated Process:** Nursing Process: Assessment **Content Area:** Mental Health **Strategy:** Use the process of elimination to make a selection, matching the client statements in the question with the conclusions in the correct option. The wording of the question tells you that only one option contains a correct statement.

17 **Answer: 1, 2, 4 Rationale:** Continuing to drink despite critical alcohol-related problems occurs with alcohol dependence. Drinking larger amounts or over a longer time than intended is consistent with a state of alcohol dependence. Experiencing a diminished effect from the same amount of alcohol occurs with alcohol dependence. Drinking to the point of drunkenness on average of once per week is not consistent with the definition of alcohol dependence. The characteristic defense mechanisms used by a client who is dependent on alcohol are denial, rationalization, and projection, not confabulation. **Cognitive Level:** Analyzing **Client Need:** Psychosocial Integrity **Integrated Process:** Teaching and Learning **Content Area:** Mental Health **Strategy:** Review the definition and criteria for substance dependency. Specific information is needed to answer this question. Note the wording of the question indicates more than one option is likely to be correct.

18 **Answer: 1, 2, 4 Rationale:** Preventing fatigue is a useful relapse prevention skill. Maintaining health is a positive strategy to use in preventing relapse. Reducing the amount of unstructured time spent alone may help prevent or distract from urges to use alcohol. Suppressing thoughts of returning to substance use is incorrect as treatment programs emphasize the need to be open and honest about having urges to return to use of the substance. Suppressing feelings is considered to be an addictive behavior. Relapse prevention skills include developing a new social network of persons who will support efforts toward sobriety, not reconnecting with an old network that is likely comprised of other substance users. **Cognitive Level:** Applying **Client Need:** Health Promotion and Maintenance **Integrated Process:** Teaching and Learning **Content Area:** Mental Health **Strategy:** Recall information about usual behaviors and defense mechanisms associated with substance use. Recognize the importance of giving the client

specific guidance that will assist with learning more effective coping skills.

19 **Answer: 1, 3, 4, 5 Rationale:** Clients with substance dependence should be taught to have structure and routine in their lives, as well as to avoid boredom and loneliness, to reduce the risk of relapse. Stating the problem is under control suggests that the client feels overly confident, which can be lead to unwise behaviors that test the recovery. Stating that no one else seems to work as hard as the client indicates dissatisfaction and impatience with others and can lead the client to feel justified in returning to the "solace" of using a substance. An intention to go to a club but only buy soft drinks indicates that the client is putting him- or herself into a situation of high risk to return to alcohol use. Also, the client is showing complacency rather than cautiousness. Verbalizing knowledge of high-risk situations that could lead to relapse is healthy. After developing awareness, the client can make a conscious decision as to how to cope with the situation without using a substance. **Cognitive Level:** Analyzing **Client Need:** Psychosocial Integrity **Integrated Process:** Nursing Process: Diagnosis **Content Area:** Mental Health **Strategy:** Look for options that clearly indicate that the client is in a situation of risk. Notice that only one option shows insight, while the question is looking for risk of relapse.

20 **Answer: 2, 3, 4 Rationale:** Addiction is a medical disease and is therefore an illness. Addiction includes behavioral habits. Addiction includes a component of emotional attachment to the substance used. Although alcoholism has been recognized as a disease for many years, some people still view addiction as a moral weakness. Addiction experts do not consider that addiction can be cured; instead, they consider it a chronic medical disease that can be managed. **Cognitive Level:** Analyzing **Client Need:** Psychosocial Integrity **Integrated Process:** Teaching and Learning **Content Area:** Mental Health **Strategy:** Remember that treatment approaches for alcoholism include both biomedical and biosocial models.

Key Terms to Review

abstinence p. 311
addiction p. 311
codependency p. 312
process addiction p. 311
recovery p. 315
relapse p. 315
substance p. 311
substance dependence p. 311
substance use disorder p. 311
tolerance p. 311
withdrawal p. 311

References

Boyd, M. (2015). *Psychiatric nursing: Contemporary practice. Enhanced update.* (5th ed.). Philadelphia: Wolters Kluwer Health.

Potter, M., & Moller, M. (2016). *Psychiatric-mental health nursing: From suffering to hope*. New York, NY: Pearson Education.

Stuart, G. (2013). *Principles and practice of psychiatric nursing* (10th ed.). St. Louis, MO: Elsevier Science.

Townsend, M. (2015). *Psychiatric mental health nursing: Concepts of care in evidence-based practice* (8th ed.). Philadelphia: F. A. Davis.

Varcarolis, E. (2014). *Foundations of psychiatric mental health nursing: A clinical approach* (6th ed.). St. Louis, MO: Saunders.

Test Yourself

Are you ready for the NCLEX-RN® or course exams? Access the NEW web-based app that provides students with thousands of practice questions in preparation for the NCLEX experience.

23 Crisis Intervention and Suicide

In this chapter

Cross Reference

Other chapters relevant to this content area are

Coping with Stressors	Chapter 20
Mental Health Disorders	Chapter 21
Psychiatric Medications	Chapter 35

I. OVERVIEW OF CRISIS

A. Definition of *crisis*: experience of being confronted by a stressor with which client is unable to cope and cannot resolve

1. An external precipitating event threatens client's **equilibrium** (state of balance; a condition in which contending forces are equal) and creates anxiety and tension
2. Client may cope with precipitating event because of previous life experience and coping mechanisms, and resolve crisis immediately
3. If coping mechanisms fail or previous experience is insufficient, crisis can lead to cognitive disorganization, in which client's ability to make decisions and solve problems becomes inadequate
4. Physical symptoms and relationship problems can develop as a consequence of being in a state of crisis
5. External and internal resources must be mobilized to assist client to return client to at least a precrisis level of functioning

NCLEX®

6. Crises are generally time limited, lasting from 4 to 6 weeks; during this time there is potential for either increased psychological vulnerability or personal growth

Memory Aid

A crisis cannot go on for extended periods; it lasts generally for 4–6 weeks.

NCLEX®

B. Types of crisis (see Box 23–1)

C. Balancing factors determining client's response to crisis

1. Client's perception of event
2. Past experience in coping with stress and established coping strategies
3. Availability of support persons and other resources

Box 23–1

Types of Crises

- **Maturational crisis:** involves normal life transitions that evoke changes in client's self-perception in role, status, and integrity; examples include birth, graduation, marriage, or retirement
- **Situational crisis:** involves an external event that disturbs client's equilibrium (loss, change) and threatens consistency between self-behaviors and values or beliefs; examples include job loss or change, abortion, divorce, change in family composition, or sudden onset of severe illness
- **Adventitious crisis:** involves external events (natural disasters or other catastrophic events) that are unpredictable and often engender fear, confusion, and loss of consistency with internalized beliefs or values and behavior; these may also be called community crises

Memory Aid

The better a client's coping strategies are in general, the better the client will be prepared to cope with a crisis.

D. Client goals for treatment

1. Remain free of self-harm
2. Identify specific problem and verbalize feelings related to event
3. Analyze event or problem and express perceptions of it
4. Identify and seek help from support systems
5. Explore alternatives for coping with crisis
6. Participate in choosing an action plan and implement plan
7. Experience less anxiety and tension and verbalize enhanced self-esteem

II. NURSING PROCESS DURING CRISIS

A. Assessment

1. Identify history of presenting problem
   - *NCLEX®* **a.** Focus on immediate problem, not on past history
   - *NCLEX®* **b.** Determine client's perception of problem: how threatened is client?
   - **c.** Assess client's cognitive appraisal; identify any faulty thinking
2. Identify current feelings
   - **a.** Help client express current feelings
   - **b.** Validate current feelings and help client to accept them
   - **c.** Acknowledge that client ultimately makes own decisions
3. Assess coping mechanisms
4. Assess client's support systems
   - **a.** Identify available resources in whom client trusts
   - **b.** Identify spiritual and religious beliefs
5. *NCLEX®* Assess potential for self-harm
   - **a.** Ask directly if client has had any thoughts of hurting or killing him- or herself; some clients engage in self-mutilation and do not want to die but do inflict self-harm, such as with razor blades or glass
   - **b.** Use questions such as "Do you have thoughts of killing yourself?" and "Do you have thoughts of hurting yourself?"
   - **c.** If client has thoughts of self-harm, determine if client has made specific plans to accomplish this, which is a danger signal—the more specific the plan, the more likely it is that the client will carry it out
   - **d.** Determine if client has means to harm or kill self (guns in house, access to medications with potential for overdose)
   - **e.** Determine if client can contract with nurse to maintain safety; work with client to identify an action plan if suicidal ideation increases or client feels he or she will act on ideas to harm self

B. Planning and implementation for clients in crisis

1. Specific treatment modalities
   - **a.** Mutual goal planning; often nurse must use a directive approach
   - **b.** Goals are set based on assessment and nursing diagnoses

c. Overarching goals include establishing relationship with client, identifying problem, identifying and reducing client's perceptual distortions, enhancing self-esteem, alleviating anxiety, promoting use of support systems (family and friends), reinforcing healthy coping, and validating problem-solving ability

NCLEX® d. Examine client's feelings that may block ability to cope adaptively

NCLEX® e. Teach client how to ask for help from others

f. Identify previously acquired adaptive coping strategies and help client modify and expand these coping strategies to new stress

NCLEX® g. Teach and encourage use of expression of feelings, comfort strategies, and self-care activities

NCLEX® h. Focus on problem resolution in a step-by-step, concrete way, first focusing on alternatives and then selecting and acting on appropriate ones

Memory Aid

Clients in crisis tend to be disorganized in their thinking. Use simple words and sentences, and give concrete, step-by-step instructions to facilitate effective communication.

i. Consider involving client in a crisis group, which helps clients feel less isolated and engage in group problem solving to identify alternatives

j. Involve family in crisis intervention because other family members often experience crisis

C. Evaluation and outcomes for clients in crisis

NCLEX® 1. Client remains free of self-harm and clearly identifies problem
2. Client acknowledges need for help and asks for help; identifies and verbalizes feelings
3. Perceptual distortions are identified and resolved
4. Client demonstrates self-care behaviors
5. Client verbalizes a stable sense of self-esteem and ability to work on problem
6. Anxiety is reduced by implementing effective coping strategies; unhealthy coping mechanisms are identified and explored if client is willing
7. Client verbalizes an action plan and begins to implement action plan

D. Potential for growth

1. Client identifies and practices new coping skills that may be useful in future in dealing with stressful and potentially traumatic events
2. Client verbalizes a renewed or enhanced sense of self-worth

III. PSYCHOPHARMACOLOGY AS TREATMENT DURING CRISIS

A. General principles

NCLEX® 1. Drug therapy should not interfere with crisis intervention strategies; rather, they target symptoms that interfere with ability to function
2. A crisis is not a psychiatric illness nor a prolonged condition; therefore, pharmacologic interventions are not interventions of choice

B. Medications useful during crisis

1. Anxiolytics such as alprazolam, clonazepam, diazepam, and lorazepam may be used to treat anxiety, panic, and sleep disturbances during a crisis; emphasis is on short-term use because of risk of dependence
2. Sleep aids such as zolpidem and zaleplon may be used to manage insomnia
3. Neuroleptic medications: atypical agents, such as olanzapine, risperidone, and quetiapine, and typical agents such as haloperidol may be used to treat psychotic symptoms that may emerge if client has a preexisting psychotic disorder

IV. ANGER AND AGGRESSION

A. Assessment of other-directed violence

NCLEX® 1. Violence is frequently, although not always, preceded by specific behaviors

a. Increased activity or hyperactivity such as restlessness or pacing behaviors
b. Verbal abuse, instigation of arguments, and use of profanity
c. Change in amount of eye contact (greater or lesser)
d. Visible signs of tension such as clenched fists or jaws, rigid facial expression or posture, talking or muttering to self
e. Change in voice such as louder or softer, and possibly either faster or slower rate of speech

2. Key risk factors: client history of violent behavior and impulsivity
3. Precipitating events for violence in in-patient settings often include staff factors such as inexperience, controlling behavior, inability to set effective limits, and indiscrimate removal of unit privileges

B. Planning and implementation to deescalate violent client

1. Remain calm
2. Maintain client dignity and self-esteem
3. Identify client stressors and indications of stress presented by client
4. Assess what client considers to be his or her need
5. *NCLEX®* Use calm and clear tone of voice and nonaggressive body posture
6. *NCLEX®* Keep large personal space between self and client and assess for personal safety; always stay positioned facing client with an escape route to the back
7. *NCLEX®* Provide several options to client
8. Remain goal-oriented and avoid arguing with client
9. Use stepwise progression of interventions from least restrictive to more restrictive, according to client's behavior
10. *NCLEX®* Use time-outs when appropriate
11. *NCLEX®* Use seclusion and restraints as a last option when other interventions have failed; use least amount of restraint that is effective; if physical restraints are used, check circulation every 30 minutes and release one at a time every 2 hours and provide range of motion
12. Administer medications according to order or protocol
13. Provide debriefing session for staff to ventilate feelings immediately after event in which violence has occurred

C. Evaluation

1. Client is able to control own behavior
2. Safety of client, other clients, and staff is maintained

D. Bullying as a form of aggression

1. Bullying is a pattern of behavior toward a person consisting of repeated events of abuse or misuse of power
2. Although generally associated with children and adolescents, bullying can occur in other contexts, such as within a family, work setting, or social groups
3. Bullying can involve physical threats or harm, isolation and exclusion of target(s) of bullying, aggression within relationships
4. Verbal bullying can take the form of lies, insults, threats, harassment, or gossip, and take place through personal verbal exchange or via Internet (cyberbullying) through e-mails, text messages, social media, and distribution of photos
5. Can lead to bullied person's withdrawal, isolation, low self-esteem, depression, and possibly suicide or homicide
6. Nurse's role
   a. Educate parents, teachers, and school officials about bullying; teach them to respond actively to bullying behaviors
   b. Encourage adoption of policies against bullying in school and workplace
   c. Provide early intervention to decrease risk of adverse psychological effects
   d. Encourage parents to meet their children's friends
   e. Encourage, as needed, attendance at groups aimed at anger management, development of social skills, positive parenting, and reducing family violence

V. OVERVIEW OF SUICIDE

A. ***Suicide*****:** intentionally and voluntarily taking one's life

B. Risk factors and warning signs for suicide

1. Risk factors include history of previous suicide attempt, family history of suicide, adolescent or older adult age group, presence of mental health disorders (primarily depression, but possibly also psychosis, dementia, or other organic brain syndrome), substance use disorder in combination with other mental disorder, and diagnosis of terminal illness
2. *NCLEX®* Clients contemplating suicide often perceive themselves as physically or emotionally isolated from others; they often experience feelings of helplessness, loss of self-esteem with feelings of worthlessness, and hopelessness, the latter being most predictive of suicide
3. Often a desire to be free from pain or to be dead is accompanied by depression and anger
4. *NCLEX®* Warning signs include changes in personal habits such as appetite, sleep patterns, personal appearance, personality, use of alcohol and other drugs, as well as bodily complaints, self-deprecating comments, making or changing wills, taking out or increasing life insurance policies, and giving away personal belongings

NCLEX® 5. Academic and occupational warning signs include truancy and absenteeism, decline in academic or occupational performance, boredom, apathy, disruptive classroom or work behavior, and anger and hostility toward authority figures

NCLEX® 6. Family and social relationship warning signs include decreased interactions with peers and friends; a change in people with whom client spends time, and a decrease in or absence of romantic relationships

NCLEX® 7. The single-most predictive psychiatric disorder for suicide is presence of a mood disorder

Memory Aid

Do not ignore warning signs of suicide; take action to further assess and intervene immediately, seeking help from other healthcare professionals as well.

C. Conscious and unconscious suicidal intention

1. Conscious suicidal ideations include an awareness of potential outcomes or results of suicidal behavior, awareness of others' response to suicidal threats or attempts, awareness of lethality index of a chosen method, and awareness of rescue possibilities
2. Unconscious suicidal ideation may be more difficult to assess as it is beyond client's awareness
   a. Client may engage in high-risk behaviors as a way of acting out unconscious desire for self-harm (e.g., drinking and driving and engaging in potentially lethal activity)
   b. Pay careful attention to direct and indirect ways in which client may be communicating unconscious suicidal ideations

VI. NURSING PROCESS FOR SUICIDAL CLIENTS

A. Suicide assessment

NCLEX® 1. During initial assessment, question client about any thoughts or feelings related to self-harm; determine suicidal ideations, how client has sought help, what kind of plan client has made and client's mental status, available support systems, and lifestyle
   a. Ask questions such as, "Have you had any thoughts about life not being worth living?"
   b. Move from general to specific questions such as, "Have you had any ideas about killing yourself?"
   c. It is a false assumption that client will volunteer this information without being asked
   d. Be comfortable asking these questions directly and in a matter-of-fact way
   e. If client answers yes, ask client, "Have you thought of, or made any plans for, how you might harm or kill yourself?" (passive suicidal ideation is presence of suicidal thoughts without a plan, in contrast to suicidal ideation with a plan)
   f. Further assessment of level of lethality includes asking about access to means for self-harm (e.g., "Do you have a gun in your home?" "Do you know how to use it?") and evaluating lethality of means (e.g., guns vs. pills)
   g. Take a careful history of previous self-harming behaviors by asking client such questions as "Have you ever tried to harm or kill yourself in the past?"
   h. Assess also use of alcohol, drugs, and level of impulsivity
   i. Complete a mental status assessment to determine alterations in thought process, impulsiveness, perceptual distortions, insight, and judgment
   j. Inquire about currently available support systems

2. Many people experience ambivalence about committing suicide; assessment of ambivalent feelings is important
3. Initially, clients may lack emotional or psychic energy to act on suicidal ideations because of some negative or neurovegetative symptoms they experience

NCLEX® 4. Be aware that a sudden sense of peace or wellness reported by client may indicate that client has sufficient psychic energy to carry out a suicidal act; this risk increases as client stabilizes on antidepressant medications

B. Goals for clients at risk for suicide

1. Remain safe and free of self-harm
2. Verbalize suicidal ideations and discuss these with nursing staff
3. Develop a safety plan with nursing staff and other members of treatment team that identifies steps to keep self safe, and ask for help before acting out a suicidal or self-harm thought
4. Verbalize a decrease in or absence of suicidal ideations
5. Verbalize a desire to live and reasons for living

NCLEX® 6. Identify an aftercare plan following discharge from hospital that includes a commitment to follow-up treatment and adherence to medication therapy
7. Identify one or more support systems outside hospital

C. Nursing interventions to reduce risk of suicide

1. Inpatient treatment is indicated if client is assessed as high risk for self-directed or other-directed violence
2. Inpatient interventions include providing a safe milieu in which client's ability to act out on suicidal ideations or other-directed violence is minimized
   a. While client may be admitted to milieu voluntarily, unit is self-contained and doors are commonly locked; nursing staff regulate flow of traffic on and off unit
   NCLEX® b. Depending on degree of suicidal ideation and lethality assessed, place client on constant observation for first 24 hours or until degree of suicidal risk is lessened according to agency policy
   NCLEX® c. Place client on every-15-minute checks or every-30-minute thereafter, depending on agency policy
   d. Maintain constant awareness of client's whereabouts
   e. Develop rapport and foster a therapeutic relationship with client
   f. On admission to unit, assess client's belongings and remove items that could be used to harm self or others (drugs, potentially sharp objects, cords, shoelaces, belts, neck ties, lighters) and keep them in a safe place
   NCLEX® g. Keep unit free of materials that can be readily used by clients to harm themselves or others (e.g., metal or glass objects that may be altered to create a sharp edge, shoelaces, belts, electrical or call bell cords); keep windows locked and count silverware; check gifts and other items brought in by family members or friends for safety before they are given to client; let family members place belongings in locker before entering unit; scan all visitors with a metal detector prior to entering unit

Memory Aid

When a client is at risk for violence toward self or others, act to protect the safety of all: the client, other clients, and staff.

   h. Work with client to develop a safety plan, and assess client frequently
   i. Explore client's feelings and help client work toward reengagement with significant others and fulfilling life activities
   NCLEX® j. Give suicidal client a roommate to reduce opportunity for solitude
   k. Make sure that client swallows oral medications and is not holding medication in oral cavity (cheeking) to hoard for a later overdose
   l. Work with client to identify an aftercare plan that includes client commitment to attend aftercare appointments, maintain contact with social support systems, and identify a safety plan with emergency contact numbers and an action plan should suicidal ideations return
   m. Realize that despite precautions, a client may still take own life after hospitalization; an ultimate decision to live rests with client
   n. Initiate debriefing session for staff members after client's suicide or any violent behavior to provide forum for staff to ventilate feelings and evaluate event

NCLEX® **D. Evaluation and outcomes for clients contemplating suicide; the client**

1. Remains safe and free from self-harm
2. Verbalizes absence or decreased intensity and severity of suicidal ideations, with absence of plan and intent
3. Verbalizes a desire to live and state several reasons for living
4. Agrees to maintain a no-self-harm contract with nursing staff and other treatment staff for specified periods of time
5. Identifies a safety plan that provides for asking for help before acting out should suicidal ideations worsen, intent reemerge, or unsafe feelings occur
6. Meets other goals in treatment plan relative to other problems identified

VII. PSYCHOPHARMACOLOGY AS TREATMENT TO PREVENT SUICIDE

A. Description

1. Pharmacologic interventions used in presence of suicidal ideations are aimed at treating underlying mood disorder, or other psychiatric disorder(s); see Chapter 35 for detailed information on these medications

2. Because a high correlation exists between mood disorders and suicide, adequate treatment of a mood disorder is essential in overall treatment of client at risk for suicide

NCLEX® **B. Depressive disorders are treated with antidepressants**

1. Because of relatively low risk of lethal overdose and relatively low side-effect profiles with use of selective serotonin reuptake inhibitors (SSRIs), these agents are often first-line drugs to treat depression that could lead to suicide (see Table 23–1)

NCLEX® 2. While effective in treating depression, tricyclic antidepressants can be highly lethal in overdose and are not a first-line agent; when used, quantity dispensed at any one time should be kept to a minimum and may need to be managed by a family member (see again Table 23–1)

3. Other agents such as tetracyclics and atypical antidepressants are also helpful in treating depressive disorders (see again Table 23–1)

NCLEX® 4. Monoamine oxidase inhibitors (MAOIs) are useful occasionally in treating depressive disorders; however, serious drug and food interactions can occur; clients using MAOIs must comply with a low tyramine diet (noncompliance can lead to hypertensive crisis); see again Table 23–1

C. Bipolar disorders can be associated with suicide during depressive phase; treated with mood stabilizers such as lithium and valproic acid

D. Clients with other psychiatric disorders may also be at risk for suicide and may be treated with anxiolytics, neuroleptics, and other psychotropic agents

1. Any psychotropic medication can be dangerous in overdose, so careful assessment and sufficient client and family education are needed (see Section III, Psychopharmacology as Treatment during Crisis)

NCLEX® 2. Clients may be at increased risk of suicide once medication takes effect and client has sufficient energy to act on suicide plan; assess client carefully and provide protective measures as needed

Table 23–1 Drugs for Depression That Could Lead to Suicide

Type of Antidepressant	Specific Drug Names
Selective serotonin reuptake inhibitors	Citalopram, paroxetine, fluoxetine, sertraline, escitalopram
Tricyclic antidepressants	Amitriptyline, clomipramine, desipramine, doxepin, imipramine, nortriptyline, trimipramine
Tetracyclic and atypical antidepressants	Bupropion, nefazadone, trazadone, venlafaxine, mirtazipine, duloxetine
Monoamine oxidase inhibitors	Tranylcypromine, phenelzine, isocarboxazid

Check Your NCLEX–RN® Exam I.Q.

You are ready for testing on this content if you can:

- Assess a client's coping mechanisms.
- Help a client to use and enhance coping mechanisms.
- Assess a client experiencing a crisis.
- Help a client to process the experience of a crisis.
- Explore social supports to aid a client in recovery from a crisis.
- Assess a client's risk of self-harm.
- Provide care to reduce a client's risk of harm to self or others.

PRACTICE TEST

1 When conducting an assessment of a client admitted to the mental health unit to determine the potential for violent or aggressive behavior, what important communication strategy should the nurse use?

1. Reassure the client that everything will be all right, and the staff will make sure nothing untoward happens.
2. Reinforce that the client is solely responsible for his or her own actions and will experience the consequences of acting out.
3. Explain that violence is not acceptable, and the staff will not allow the client to act out.
4. Reassure the client that limited acting out will be allowed but only in a controlled setting.

2 When responding to a client who displays the potential for violence, the nurse would use which intervention as the most restrictive technique?

1. Meeting in a quiet room to reduce stimulation
2. Administering a PRN medication to reduce anxiety
3. Providing physical interventions, such as two-person escort out of a program area
4. Using restraints, such as a four-point restraint

3 What is the most important intervention by the nurse when a client does not respond to less restrictive interventions and is rapidly escalating toward violence?

1. Cease negotiation with client and implement plan of intervention to control client and provide safety.
2. Bargain with client to determine what can be done to prevent assaultive behavior.
3. Offer a PRN medication to reduce anxiety.
4. Ask client to move to a less stimulating, private area and spend some time alone.

4 After a staff member has been involved in a particularly violent episode with a client, when should the nurse plan for debriefing to occur?

1. After the staff has had an opportunity to become calm
2. Immediately to facilitate processing of feelings
3. Not until the staff requests such an intervention
4. After a 3-day time-off period

5 The nurse is working with a client in psychological distress. Which event experienced by the client would the nurse document as a situational crisis?

1. Approaching the age of retirement
2. Recently being involved in a severe motor vehicle accident
3. Being a survivor of a flood following a hurricane
4. Recently returning home from military duty after an armed conflict

6 Which coping behavior would the nurse expect to note in a client involved in a situation in which there is a significant psychological threat and great personal vulnerability?

1. Finding inner strength to get through the crisis
2. Being more oriented toward mastery
3. Acting in a more self-protective manner
4. Being totally immobilized

7 A nurse is planning an intervention for a client in crisis who witnessed a violent crime. What key component of crisis intervention should the nurse plan to use at this time?

1. Identify the client's maladaptive coping mechanisms.
2. Identify and support the client's coping patterns.
3. Assist the client in forgetting the crisis situation.
4. Teach the client to handle future crises.

8 The nurse developing a care plan for a client using crisis management principles would base interventions on which of the following primary tasks of crisis management? Select all that apply.

1. Provide support.
2. Relieve anxiety.
3. Provide encouragement.
4. Foster independence.
5. Provide guidance.

9 An adult client is having difficulty coping with a new diagnosis of colon cancer. The nurse contacts the healthcare provider for a medication prescription to assist the client during this crisis situation. The nurse anticipates a prescription for which medication?

1. Haloperidol
2. Amitriptyline
3. Lorazepam
4. Valproic acid

PRACTICE TEST

10 The family of a client with suicidal ideations asks the nurse if the medication the client is taking will prevent suicide. What would be the best response by the nurse?

1. "Clients who take their medication as prescribed are at decreased risk for suicide."
2. "Medication helps to treat an underlying mood disorder associated with suicidal thinking and therefore prevents suicide."
3. "Medication helps decrease the frequency and intensity of suicidal thoughts."
4. "The client has said that she would never try to hurt herself again. There is no need to worry."

11 A suicidal client with low self-esteem seems less lethargic today and agrees to participate in an occupational therapy program. To help make the session successful, the nurse should take which action?

1. Introduce the client to wood carving; show him how to safely use the carving and burning tools.
2. Stay away from the client in occupational therapy so that he is free to express himself.
3. Teach the client to macrame a plant hanger from jute rope and encourage him to work on it later in his room.
4. Structure his activity to help him complete one simple task, such as painting a picture.

12 A client has recently been admitted for depression and suicidal ideations with a plan to hang himself. The nurse assesses the client most carefully for risk for attempting suicide at which time?

1. When the client is silent and unlikely to tell anyone
2. When the client is ready to go home and afraid of leaving the hospital
3. When the client's family goes on vacation
4. When the client begins to demonstrate clinical improvement

13 Which of the following clients is at greatest risk for attempting suicide?

1. A 65-year-old African American male
2. A 70-year-old European American male
3. A 30-year-old Hispanic American female
4. A 16-year-old African American female

14 A client states that voices are telling him to hang himself. The nurse documents that the client is at risk for suicide on the basis of which of the following?

1. An intractable sense of hopelessness
2. Intolerable emotional pain
3. Delusions of grandeur
4. Command hallucinations

15 Which statement made by a client would indicate the highest risk for suicide?

1. "I know you've been worried about me. You won't have to worry too much longer."
2. "I think I've found a solution to my problem. I'm going to check it out with my doctor."
3. "I'm looking forward to having the children home for the holidays. They will be a good distraction."
4. "Over the past week I haven't been hearing voices tell me to hurt myself as often."

16 A client who became violent on the psychiatric unit had restraints applied at 0800. The nurse makes a note to release the restraints at no later than what time per protocol? Record your answer as a number.

Fill in your answer below:
Answer: ____________________

17 When interviewing a potentially violent or aggressive client, which environmental factor is most important for the nurse to consider?

1. The interview should take place in a calm and quiet area to reduce stimuli.
2. Care should be taken to make sure that other staff do not interrupt.
3. Restraint devices should be in full view of the client to reinforce consequences for violent behavior.
4. The client should be told that violent behavior will not be tolerated.

18 The nurse has been working with a teenage female client who was in crisis after being assaulted and robbed late one night when leaving a local mall. Which outcome indicates to the nurse that the client has achieved the expected benefit of treatment? Select all that apply.

1. The client can talk about the incident without excessive distress.
2. The client states she will never shop at the mall again.
3. The client states a plan to choose parking spaces that are close to building entrances when possible.
4. The client is enrolling in a local self-defense class for women.
5. The client states she will go shopping only when she has someone available to accompany her.

19 The client has suicidal ideation with a vague plan for suicide. When teaching the family how to care for the person at home, what should the nurse emphasize? Select all that apply.

1. Suicide occurring within the family environment indicates family dysfunction.
2. Warning signs, even if indirect, generally are present before a suicidal attempt.
3. When the client no longer talks about suicide, the risk of suicide has decreased.
4. Following a failed suicidal attempt, the risk for future attempts is increased.
5. Family members are responsible for preventing future suicidal attempts.

20 The client is in a crisis state. At the beginning of the initial assessment interview, what should the nurse assist the client to identify? Select all that apply.

1. Current feelings
2. The realistic nature of the event
3. Others who might be affected by the event
4. An immediate action plan
5. Past emotional traumas

21 A client with suicidal ideation and a specific lethal plan for self-harm was admitted to the hospital. The client's spouse died recently after a very brief illness. The client states, "There's no reason to go on living. We did everything together. Now I have no one to turn to or do things with." Which concepts should be a priority focus of the nurse? Select all that apply.

1. Client's helplessness
2. Decisional conflict
3. Increased risk for suicide
4. Possible social isolation
5. Disenfranchised grief

ANSWERS & RATIONALES

1 **Answer: 2 Rationale:** Clients need to have communicated to them that they are in control of their own behaviors and that "acting out" will result in consequences. Reassuring the client that the staff will make sure nothing happens takes away responsibility from the client. Just explaining that violence is unacceptable without explaining to the client that he or she is in control is nontherapeutic. Acting out is usually not allowed because of the risks to the safety of the client and others. **Cognitive Level:** Applying **Client Need:** Psychosocial Integrity **Integrated Process:** Nursing Process: Implementation **Content Area:** Mental Health **Strategy:** The core issue of the question is effective communication with a client at risk for acting out. Use the process of elimination and choose the option that provides accurate information to the client and holds the client accountable for his or her actions.

2 **Answer: 4 Rationale:** Preventing a client from free mobility, such as the use of restraints, is the most restrictive technique. Meeting in a quiet room is the least restrictive and most therapeutic. Chemical restraint with medication is restrictive but less so than full four-point restraints. Escorting a client is restrictive but less so than full four-point restraint. **Cognitive Level:** Analyzing **Client Need:** Psychosocial Integrity **Integrated Process:** Nursing Process: Implementation **Content Area:** Mental Health **Strategy:** Note the critical word *most* in the stem of the question. This tells you that ordering the interventions presented from least restrictive to most restrictive will assist you to choose correctly.

3 **Answer: 1 Rationale:** Once a client has escalated beyond least restrictive interventions, the nurse should plan for the next step. Bargaining with a client is counterproductive and positively reinforces behavior. Offering a PRN medication to reduce anxiety would occur after negotiation for least restrictive interventions is complete. Asking a client to take a time-out is a least restrictive intervention to which the client is not responding. **Cognitive Level:** Applying **Client Need:** Psychosocial Integrity **Integrated Process:** Nursing Process: Implementation **Content Area:** Mental Health **Strategy:** The wording of the question tells you that more than one option may be partially or totally correct and that you must prioritize your answer. Choose the option that best protects the safety of all people in the environment, including other clients and staff.

4 **Answer: 2 Rationale:** Debriefing allows the staff an opportunity to ventilate feelings. It should not wait until the staff has had opportunity to become calm because the process of ventilating will assist the staff to do this. The staff should not have to ask for a debriefing meeting. It should be done as soon as possible after the client and all others are safe, not 3 days later. **Cognitive Level:** Applying **Client Need:** Psychosocial Integrity **Integrated Process:** Nursing Process: Evaluation **Content Area:** Mental Health **Strategy:** The core issue of the question is the need for staff to process personal feelings after an episode of violence occurs with a client. Use the process of elimination and knowledge that staff can be traumatized by these events to choose the correct option.

5 **Answer: 2 Rationale:** A situational crisis is one that occurs from external life events, such as being involved in a severe motor vehicle accident. An event involving normal stages of development (such as aging) is a maturational crisis. A natural disaster such as a flood is an example of a community crisis. An armed conflict is an example of a community crisis. **Cognitive Level:** Analyzing **Client Need:** Psychosocial Integrity **Integrated Process:** Nursing Process: Assessment **Content Area:** Mental Health **Strategy:** Use the process of elimination. The core issue of the question is the ability to differentiate among various types of crises (maturational, situational, and community) and to document them appropriately.

6 **Answer: 3 Rationale:** When a person is threatened and perceives him- or herself to be vulnerable to a situation, coping behaviors are self-protective. Coping behaviors may be ineffective to provide strength. Coping during a crisis is oriented toward the immediate here-and-now, not mastery. A client who is immobilized is not displaying a specific coping behavior. **Cognitive Level:** Applying **Client Need:** Psychosocial Integrity **Integrated Process:** Nursing Process: Diagnosis **Content Area:** Mental Health **Strategy:** The core issue of the question is the expected response of a client to a threatening situation. Use knowledge of coping skills and the process of elimination to select the correct answer.

7 **Answer: 2 Rationale:** Assisting the client to identify coping patterns and then supporting them is essential to managing a crisis. Identifying the client's maladaptive coping mechanisms may be beneficial after identifying the client's strengths. Assisting the client to forget is not a therapeutic intervention for crisis management. Teaching a client to handle future crises is more appropriate once the current crisis has abated. **Cognitive Level:** Applying **Client Need:** Psychosocial Integrity **Integrated Process:** Nursing Process: Implementation **Content Area:** Mental Health **Strategy:** The critical words in the question are *at this time*. This tells you that more than one option may be correct, but one of them is more timely than the others. Use nursing knowledge and the process of elimination to make a selection.

8 **Answer: 1, 5 Rationale:** During a crisis a client requires support. Providing guidance is also important during a client's crisis. Anxiety may be useful to energize the client to cope with the crisis; the goal is to achieve a manageable level of anxiety. Providing encouragement is useful after the primary tasks of crisis management are complete. Fostering independence is important after the primary tasks of crisis management have been met. **Cognitive Level:** Applying **Client Need:** Psychosocial Integrity **Integrated Process:** Nursing Process: Planning **Content Area:** Mental Health **Strategy:** The critical word in the question is *primary*. This tells you that more than one option may be correct, but some of them are more important than the others. Use nursing knowledge and the process of elimination to make a selection.

9 **Answer: 3 Rationale:** A short-acting anti-anxiety agent such as lorazepam is most useful in helping a client to achieve an effective reduction in level of anxiety. Antipsychotics such as haloperidol are not helpful and should be avoided. An antidepressant such as amitriptyline requires some time to achieve therapeutic levels and is not useful in a crisis situation. Mood stabilizers such as valproic acid are not indicated. **Cognitive Level:** Applying **Client Need:** Psychosocial Integrity **Integrated Process:** Nursing Process: Diagnosis **Content Area:** Mental Health **Strategy:** The critical words in the question are *crisis situation*, which tell you that the correct answer is a medication with a rapid onset of action and will be effective in treating the client's reaction to the diagnosis. Use nursing knowledge and the process of elimination to make a selection.

10 **Answer: 3 Rationale:** Medication will help decrease the frequency and intensity of suicidal thoughts. Medication does not prevent suicide; in fact, many times when clients regain their energy from medications, they are at an increased risk for completing suicide. Medication may treat the underlying cause of the suicidal ideation but does not necessarily reduce the risk for completing suicide. A client may not be currently suicidal according to self-reports, but medications do not ensure that they will not be suicidal in the future. **Cognitive Level:** Applying **Client Need:** Psychosocial Integrity **Integrated Process:** Communication and Documentation **Content Area:** Mental Health **Strategy:** The critical word in the question is *best*. This tells you that more than one option may be partially correct, but one of them is better than the others. Use nursing knowledge and the process of elimination to make a selection.

11 **Answer: 4 Rationale:** A client who is just regaining his or her energy should be encouraged to do safe, simple tasks, which will also promote the client's self-esteem. Suicidal clients are most at danger when they are feeling better and regaining their energy. Introducing the client to wood carving places the client at risk for self-harm. The nurse should encourage the client to participate in occupational therapy for self-expression. Teaching the client how to make a plant hanger from jute rope places the client at risk for self-harm. **Cognitive Level:** Analyzing **Client Need:** Psychosocial Integrity **Integrated Process:** Nursing Process: Implementation **Content Area:** Mental Health **Strategy:** The core issue of the question is a safe activity for a client who is suicidal. The correct answer is the option that does not pose risk to the client or provide the client with the means to engage in self-harm.

12 **Answer: 4 Rationale:** Suicidal clients are at most risk when they begin to demonstrate improvement and have the energy to carry out suicide. A silent client who is not willing to share with others is at risk for suicide but may be placed on constant observation. Being afraid to go home may be a positive sign that the client is aware of the danger he or she may pose to him- or herself. Vacation is a stressful time, and being left alone would place the client at risk; however, it is well documented that clients are at greatest risk when showing signs of improvement. **Cognitive Level:** Applying **Client Need:** Psychosocial Integrity **Integrated Process:** Nursing Process: Planning **Content Area:** Mental Health **Strategy:** The core issue of the question is recognition that the risk of suicide increases when a client begins to feel better, since the client now may have the energy to carry out a suicide attempt. Use the process of elimination and this knowledge to make a selection. The wording of the question tells you that only one answer is correct.

13 **Answer: 2 Rationale:** The group at highest risk for successfully completing suicide attempts are European American males over the age of 50 (white, male, older adult). Older African American males, young adult Hispanic females, and teenage females are not in the highest risk groups because of age, gender, ethnicity, or a combination of those factors. **Cognitive Level:** Analyzing **Client Need:** Psychosocial Integrity **Integrated Process:** Nursing Process: Assessment **Content Area:** Mental Health **Strategy:** The core issue of the question is knowledge of high-risk groups for suicide. The wording of the question tells you only one answer is correct. Use nursing knowledge and the process of elimination to make a selection.

14 **Answer: 4 Rationale:** Voices telling a client to hurt himself or others are called *command hallucinations*. There is not enough data to support hopelessness, emotional pain, or delusions of grandeur. **Cognitive Level:** Applying **Client Need:** Psychosocial Integrity **Integrated Process:** Communication and Documentation **Content Area:** Mental Health **Strategy:** The core issue of the question is correct interpretation of a client's symptoms. The wording of the question tells you only one answer is correct. Use nursing knowledge and the process of elimination to make a selection.

15 **Answer: 1 Rationale:** The client is communicating that he or she may not be around for the nurse to worry about. Being able to find a solution, expressing hope for the future and making plans, and decreasing frequency of voices indicate that the client is experiencing a reduction in the risk for suicide. **Cognitive Level:** Analyzing **Client Need:** Psychosocial Integrity **Integrated Process:** Nursing Process: Evaluation **Content Area:** Mental Health **Strategy:** The critical words in the stem of the question are *highest risk*. This tells you that more than one option may indicate risk, but one is stronger than the others. Use nursing knowledge and the process of elimination to make a selection.

16 **Answer: 1000 Rationale:** Releasing restraints at least every 2 hours is a standard of care to prevent physical harm. In addition to this intervention, the client's circulation should be checked at least every 30 minutes. Ensuring the client's safety and well-being are of high priority. **Cognitive Level:** Applying **Client Need:** Safety and Infection Control **Integrated Process:** Nursing Process: Planning **Content Area:** Mental Health **Strategy:** The core issue of the question is knowledge of safe care to a client who is in restraints. Use nursing knowledge to formulate an answer, recalling that 2-hour release times are a standard of care.

17 **Answer: 1 Rationale:** The nurse should ensure that the interview be conducted in a quiet environment. Interruption should be kept to a minimum, but may not be possible to prevent. Keeping restraint devices in full view is intimidating to the client and should not be done. Telling the client that violent behavior will not be tolerated may be appropriate at some point, but this is not an environmental factor and could escalate aggression by the client if stated in an intimidating way. **Cognitive Level:** Applying **Client Need:** Psychosocial Integrity **Integrated Process:** Nursing Process: Implementation **Content Area:** Mental Health **Strategy:** The critical words in the stem of the question are *most important*. This is a clue that more than one option may be partially or totally correct, but one is more important than the others. Use nursing knowledge and the process of elimination to make a selection.

18 **Answer: 1, 3, 4 Rationale:** The client demonstrates effective coping by being able to discuss the incident without excessive distress. Planning to park near building entrances reduces environmental risk for the client. Taking a class in self-defense is proactive and may help reduce anxiety. Stating she will never shop at the mall again shows continued anxiety and does not indicate achievement of treatment goals. Stating she will shop only when accompanied shows unresolved anxiety and a nonadaptive approach that is likely to interfere with her lifestyle. **Cognitive Level:** Analyzing **Client Need:** Psychosocial Integrity **Integrated Process:** Nursing Process: Evaluation **Content Area:** Mental Health **Strategy:** The core issue of the question is knowledge of adaptive responses to crisis or near-crisis situations. Choose the options that demonstrate adequate coping, which are ones that are neither insufficient nor extreme in tone.

19 **Answer: 2, 4 Rationale:** Warning signs of suicide generally exist but they may not be recognized until after a suicidal attempt or suicidal death. Since almost all suicidal persons are ambivalent about dying, they either consciously or unconsciously communicate their intent to others hoping (knowingly or unknowingly) to be rescued from their own impulses. The nurse should recognize that the risk for future attempts always increases once a person has made an unsuccessful attempt. This means that the nurse should always inquire about past suicidal behaviors and attempts, including those that occurred in the distant past. Suicide is a very individual act that does not necessarily reflect negative relationships in the family. Sometimes the person does not talk about suicide because he or she has made a specific plan and has the means to carry it out. Not talking about suicide can be a warning sign, and the nurse and family members need to know this. Family members are not responsible for preventing future suicidal attempts. They should be encouraged to create safe interpersonal and physical environments, but in spite of their best efforts, they may not be able to prevent their family member from ultimate self-destruction. **Cognitive Level:** Analyzing **Client Need:** Safety and Infection Control **Integrated Process:** Nursing Process: Diagnosis **Content Area:** Mental Health **Strategy:** Look for myths and facts about suicide. Recognize the importance of teaching facts before dispelling myths.

20 **Answer: 1, 2 Rationale:** It is helpful for the client to identify and ventilate personal feelings being experienced. This relieves anxiety, allows the client to feel validated, and prepares the nurse and client to progress to other steps in crisis resolution. The nurse must have a clear idea of what the problem represents to the client and also be able to identify the current reality the crisis presents for the client. Then action plans can be developed. The focus of crisis intervention is on the individual who is experiencing the crisis response, not on others. The goal is to assist the person in crisis to reestablish equilibrium by using previously effective coping techniques. It is premature to develop an action plan at this time. Complete assessment and analysis of the problem must occur before proceeding to develop an action plan. Past emotional traumas are not explored in crisis intervention. Intervention should focus on the current problem and facilitating the client's coping so that a return to pre-crisis baseline may be accomplished. If past emotional traumas become apparent during a crisis, referral for counseling at a later time would be appropriate. **Cognitive Level:** Applying **Client Need:** Psychosocial Integrity **Integrated Process:** Nursing Process: Implementation **Content Area:** Mental Health **Strategy:** Remember that crisis intervention focuses on a current problem and the "here and now."

21 **Answer: 3, 4 Rationale:** The client's statement directly indicates feelings of hopelessness, as well as more indirect expressions of risk for suicide. The spouse's death has left the client without adequate interpersonal support to cope with and adjust to a significant loss. The client is experiencing a situational crisis and to cope effectively in a crisis, clients must identify and be able to rely on others to support them emotionally both during and after the crisis. While the client is lonely, there is no indication that the client is helpless. Additionally, the question does not indicate there was an actual suicide attempt, and additionally a suicidal attempt would not cause helplessness. The client's statements do not suggest difficulty with decision making, although this can be one of the manifestations of a crisis state. The client is experiencing acute grief that is normal. With disenfranchised grief, the client is unable to share expressions of grief because the grief is considered unacceptable. **Cognitive Level:** Analyzing **Client Need:** Psychosocial Integrity **Integrated Process:** Nursing Process: Diagnosis **Content Area:** Mental Health **Strategy:** Look carefully at what the client is saying. The client directly expresses feelings of being alone and isolated. Additionally, there is an indirect message that could indicate suicidal intent. Make sure that the concepts reflected in the answers are shown in the stem of the question.

Key Terms to Review

crisis p. 324 **equilibrium** p. 324 **suicide** p. 327

References

Boyd, M. (2015). *Psychiatric nursing: Contemporary practice. Enhanced update.* (5th ed.). Philadelphia: Wolters Kluwer Health.

Potter, M., & Moller, M. (2016). *Psychiatric-mental health nursing: From suffering to hope*. New York, NY: Pearson Education.

Stuart, G. (2013). *Principles and practice of psychiatric nursing* (10th ed.). St. Louis, MO: Elsevier Science.

Townsend, M. (2015). *Psychiatric mental health nursing: Concepts of care in evidence-based practice* (8th ed.). Philadelphia: F.A. Davis.

Varcarolis, E. (2014). *Foundations of psychiatric mental health nursing: A clinical approach* (6th ed.). St. Louis, MO: Saunders.

ANSWERS & RATIONALES

End-of-Life Care 24

In this chapter

Cross Reference

Other chapters related to this content are

Coping with Stressors **Chapter 20**

I. GENERAL NEEDS NEAR END OF LIFE

A. Quality end of life

1. Positive experience for client and family with accomplishment of personal goals, even with suffering and loss
2. Caregiver-led client advocacy with a meaningful and dignified death
3. Recognition that there is no typical death

NCLEX® **B. Core principles guiding clinical policy and professional practice for end-of-life care**

1. Respect dignity of both client and caregivers
2. Be sensitive to and respectful of client's and family's wishes
3. Use most appropriate measures that are consistent with client's choices
4. Make **palliation** (alleviation of pain and other physical symptoms) a high priority
5. Assess and manage psychological, social, and spiritual or religious problems
6. Offer continuity (client should be able to continue to be cared for, if so desired, by his or her primary care and specialist providers)
7. Provide access to any therapy that may realistically improve client's quality of life, including integrative therapies or nontraditional treatments; ensure clients are not abandoned because of their choice
8. Provide access to palliative care services and to hospice care (usually offered when clients have 6 months or less to live)
9. Respect right to refuse treatment, as expressed by client or authorized surrogate
10. Respect healthcare provider's professional judgment and recommendations with consideration for both client and family preferences
11. Recognize that dying is a profoundly personal experience and part of life cycle
12. Encourage healthcare professionals to help ensure that care environment provides quality care and accountability for performance
13. Promote clinical and evidence-based research on providing care at end of life

C. Issues of policy, ethics, and law

1. Ethical issues are influenced by personal values, religion, and culture
2. Principles of autonomy, privacy, and **veracity** (truthfulness) are foundations of nursing practice
3. **Beneficence** (doing good), **nonmaleficence** (doing no harm), and **justice** (being fair) are basic ethical principles for end-of-life care

4. An **advance directive (AD)** (a document outlining preferences for care when client is unable to do so) allows clients to make decisions in advance about end-of-life care should they become unable to communicate their desires
5. **Euthanasia** is a controversial intervention that offers a deliberate end to life for persons with a terminal illness or intolerable suffering; the Code for Nurses and American Nurses Association's position statements indicate nurses should not participate in euthanasia
6. A decision to withdraw food and fluids allows disease to progress to its natural end
7. Confidentiality allows client to feel secure in safely discussing sensitive matters regarding healthcare without fearing disclosure

II. PHYSIOLOGICAL CARE NEAR END OF LIFE

A. **Palliative care focuses on assessing and treating symptoms** that are distressing to a client whose disease is no longer responsive to curative treatment

B. **Symptom management is important at end of life;** nurses should focus on interventions that promote client advocacy, assess client needs, provide pharmacologic and nonpharmacologic treatments, and educate client and family

NCLEX® 1. Fatigue
   a. May be related to disease, stress, and/or treatment
   b. Treatment of disease-related causes, such as anemia, may alleviate fatigue
   c. Provide frequent rest periods, and balance activity with rest; modify client's environment to conserve energy

NCLEX® 2. Pain
   a. Nurses have an obligation to promote comfort and relief of pain for client and to provide support to clients, families, and their surrogates when a decision has been made to withhold further life-sustaining treatments
   b. Become comfortable with decision not to limit use of opioids and to provide pain relief without fear of respiratory depression
   c. Nonverbal signs of pain include grimaces, moans, irritability, or withdrawal; carefully monitor for these in noncommunicative clients
   NCLEX® d. Nonpharmacologic approaches include life review, grief or psychiatric counseling as indicated, and encouraging client to draw on previous successful coping mechanisms, such as use of faith

NCLEX® 3. Dyspnea
   a. Elevate head of bed for comfort and to maximize chest expansion
   b. Provide oxygen as prescribed and teach pursed lip breathing (to keep airways open longer) to possibly alleviate dyspnea

4. Nausea and vomiting (N/V)
   a. Identify underlying cause (medications, pain, decreased intestinal blood flow as death nears)
   NCLEX® b. Administer antiemetic or prokinetic drugs, seek to discontinue food or medications that trigger nausea, provide oral care every 2–4 hours, offer ice chips and clear liquids (avoid acidic beverages), serve meals at room temperature, and eliminate strong odors

5. Anorexia (loss of appetite) and cachexia (general wasting syndrome often seen with terminal illnesses)
   a. Possible causes include pain, medications, depression, anxiety, N/V, constipation, taste alterations from chemotherapy, and decreased blood flow to gastrointestinal (GI) tract
   b. Pharmacologic interventions include appetite stimulants or antiemetics
   NCLEX® c. Offer small portions at a time of client-preferred foods; do not force foods on client
   d. Offer small amounts of fluid at a time of beverages preferred by client to avoid dry mouth and dehydration
   e. Treat underlying cause of anorexia if known

6. GI alterations: constipation or diarrhea
   a. To prevent constipation encourage client to follow personal bowel regimen; encourage high-fiber intake with adequate fluids and stool softeners
   b. Differentiate between diarrhea caused by fecal impaction and anal incontinence; review medications to determine whether diarrhea is a drug side effect
   c. Malabsorption is associated with foul-smelling, fatty, pale stools
   NCLEX® d. Problems with skin integrity occur with diarrhea as peripheral circulation diminishes; encourage skin care with moisture barrier and position change at regular intervals

NCLEX® C. **Physical symptoms of nearing death**

1. Changes in neurologic function with decreased level of consciousness, confusion, disorientation, and/or delirium
2. Weakness and fatigue, which are enhanced by decline in food and fluid intake
3. Increased drowsiness and sleeping with diminished reaction

4. Decreased oral food and fluids; client rarely reports hunger as death approaches; may be difficult for family because feeding (including provision of fluids) is symbolic of nurturing
5. Dehydration, which can result in concerns for client comfort because of potential for "dry mouth"; dehydration can promote comfort of dying client because it increases release of endorphins (producing natural analgesic effect that aids in pain control) and ketone production (causing sleepiness)
6. Hypernatremia and uremia, resulting in clouding of consciousness
7. Noisy respirations because of stasis of lung secretions, decreased muscle tone, and decreased strength of swallow and cough reflexes
8. Possible surge of energy
9. Terminal restlessness and/or agitation, which may be due to metabolic alterations near end of life; these need to be distinguished from behavior change caused by untreated symptoms
10. Fever (may be influenced by dehydration)
11. Change in bowel elimination ranging from constipation to diarrhea
12. Incontinence of stool and/or urine

D. Imminent death

1. Monitor for signs and symptoms of imminent death
2. Teach family signs and symptoms so they understand client's impending death (see Box 24–1)

E. Postmortem care of body (see Box 24–2)

Box 24–1

Signs/Symptoms of Imminent Death

- Increasing periods of unresponsiveness or sleep
- Possible restlessness or disorientation
- Decreased urine output with darkening and/or colorations such as brown or red
- Drop in body temperature, with cool and mottled extremities
- Vital sign changes, including systolic blood pressure below 70 and diastolic below 50; pulse may be weak and difficult to locate
- Respiratory congestion, including respiratory bubbling with breathing pattern changes, with very rapid respirations and/or Cheyne-Stokes respirations
- Glassy eyes that are tearing and half open
- Decreased muscle tone, sagging mouth because of relaxed jaw muscles

Box 24–2

Care of the Body After Death

- Gather equipment needed: bath towels and washcloths, wash basin, bed linens, scissors, shroud kit with name tags, and documentation forms per agency policy
- Verify pronouncement of death, whether autopsy required, and organ donation status
- Identify client using two unique identifiers according to agency policy
- Elevate head of bed as soon as possible to reduce or prevent discoloration of face
- Collect any specimens that are ordered
- Remove tubes, indwelling lines, and other equipment except if they must remain in place because of autopsy or organ donation (follow agency policy)
- Close eyes by gently holding them shut and place dentures in mouth to maintain shape of face
- Clean body thoroughly, removing any mucus, wound drainage, and any urine or feces released at time of death
- Pad any drainage areas and pack anal orifice with gauze
- Align body with hands folded across chest or lap
- Pull a sheet up to neck to cover body and prepare environment for family to view body
- If family chooses to view body, offer to accompany them or other support person(s) they choose; provide privacy and unhurried atmosphere; encourage family to say good-bye in own way (rituals, prayers, singing, touch, etc.)
- Determine which personal belongings should stay with body (such as wedding ring) and document all belongings taken by family (document description of items and to whom they were given)
- Apply shroud after family leaves; keep ID band in place; attach two tags to toe and outside shroud, or according to agency policy
- Document in accordance with agency policy

III. PSYCHOSOCIAL SUPPORT NEAR END OF LIFE

A. Communication with dying clients and families

1. Goals of communication focus on individualized needs of client and family, keeping communication lines open, and ensuring nurse clearly understands expectations of clients, family, and plan developed by partners in care
2. NCLEX® Use active and sensitive listening skills
3. Sensitively address physical limitations due to age or disease treatment or progression
4. NCLEX® Be aware that a variety of death-related issues can create communication barriers at end of life; these can be due to lack of experience with topic, unresolved loss, concern about showing emotion or not knowing answers, and even worry that family/caregivers would be held responsible for client's death
5. Be truthful when reinforcing bad news previously given to client and family; build rapport, plan what to say in understandable terms, and continuously identify what client and family want and need to know
6. NCLEX® Realize that changes in roles of family members at end of life can cause altered family dynamics; family members may require assistance to work through these issues
7. NCLEX® Recall that beliefs about spirituality and organized religions are not necessarily the same; be sensitive to culture, ethnic values, and religion when discussing end-of-life concerns with clients and family members (see Box 24–3)
8. Communicate with interdisciplinary team to accurately implement client's desires and end-of-life goals for care using well-documented medical records and daily communication among multiple team members

Box 24–3

Religious Aspects of Care at End of Life

Christianity

Roman Catholic

- No specific restrictions on autopsy; many Catholic leaders accept medical definition of brain death and view organ donation as a final charitable act.
- Sacraments before death include Sacrament of the Sick (anointing and prayer) as well as Reconciliation and Holy Communion.
- Burial or cremation is allowed; if cremation is done, cremains (ashes) must remain together (not scattered).

Protestant

- Organ donation is allowed by many groups (sects).
- Some groups provide for anointing of the sick, while others do not.
- Many groups allow cremation, although some (such as Presbyterians) prefer burial (no clear commandment against cremation).

Jehovah's Witnesses

- Blood transfusion is not allowed, even to save a life; organ transplant may be allowed.
- Funerals are conducted according to scriptural guidelines and are simple and modest.

Latter-Day Saints (Mormons)

- Organ donation is acceptable.
- A sacrament may be administered upon request.
- There is no official church position on cremation; person is buried in his or her temple clothing.

Quakers (Religious Society of Friends)

- Organ donation and autopsy are allowed.
- Burial or cremation are allowed; remains are not present at funeral, which takes the form of a Quaker meeting.

Judaism

- Organ donation is acceptable; routine autopsy should not be done (seen as a desecration to body); if autopsy is required for legal reasons, rabbi should be present.
- A dying person should not be left alone (presence of rabbi desirable); body should not be left alone after death; a "shomer" (guardian) stays with body until time of burial.

- Cremation is not allowed for Orthodox and Conservative Jews, but is increasingly allowed for Reform Jews.

Islam

- Organ donation is generally allowed, but routine autopsies are not acceptable.
- Bed may be turned to face Mecca.
- Family and close friends gather near time of death to offer hope and show kindness.
- Upon death, eyes and lower jaw are closed; body is washed three times by same-gender Muslim (non-Muslims should wear gloves), and body is wrapped in clean sheets.
- Cremation is not allowed, and burial is done as soon as possible.

Buddhism

- Organ donation is allowed.
- Family members and close friends may gather to help dying person feel calm and peaceful.
- A small statue of Buddha may be placed by dying person's head, and protective verses may be chanted.
- Family and close friends clean and dress body after death.
- Either burial or cremation is acceptable; cremated remains may be kept by family, placed in columbarium wall or urn garden, or scattered at sea.

Hinduism

- A number of sects and subsects have differing beliefs; regional variations also occur.
- Organ donation is allowed.
- Near time of death, priest and family gather with dying person to chant mantras.
- At time of death, those gathered should avoid unnecessary touching of body (seen as impure).
- Traditionally, all Hindus are cremated (with exception of infants, children, and saints)

B. The dying child

1. End-of-life care provided by pediatric nurse includes working with dying child as well as with siblings, parents, and extended family and friends
2. Some families prefer not to tell a child that she or he has a terminal illness; however, children are often aware even if it is not openly discussed; they are sensitive to subtle changes in how staff and family members interact with them both interpersonally and during physical care
3. *NCLEX®* Respect parents' choices and decision making while assessing opportunities to encourage open communication between parents and child
4. Provide support and caring to client and family without taking away realistic need for hope
5. Be available to listen and talk, even if child chooses not to talk about disease
6. Consider child's developmental and educational level and interact accordingly
7. *NCLEX®* Be aware that a child may let nurse know he or she no longer wants to talk about a topic by walking away, changing subject, shifting posture, or with other verbal or nonverbal cues
8. Understand that nurse's presence can be meaningful to a child and/or parents
9. Encourage all family members to care for child
10. *NCLEX®* Siblings often feel left out as parents focus on dying child
    a. Assess all children in family for acting out, negative behavior, or "perfect child" behavior
    b. Encourage parents to find resources and support people to take siblings to their extracurricular activities
    c. Allow siblings to verbalize feelings in a safe place without their feeling as though they are making parents feel worse
11. Encourage a life review by getting family members and friends to discuss meaningful events (birthdays, vacations, anniversaries, and special events)
12. Provide support to other family members, including grandparents, extended families through divorce and remarriage, and classmates

C. The dying older adult

NCLEX® 1. Determine whether client has examined own mortality before learning of impending death; older adults may or may not easily accept idea of own death, although they may have less death anxiety with advancing age

2. Older adults may find it easier to face their mortality if they:
   a. Philosophically accept what their life had to offer
   b. Have numerous experiences with death, including parents, friends, spouse or partner, or children
   c. Learn to cope with personal losses
   d. Are able to recover emotionally between multiple deaths
   e. Believe death is a part of living
   f. Find support in religious beliefs and concept of life after death
3. Cultural aspects
   a. Many cultures view death and dying differently from the open and blunt European-American approach
   NCLEX® b. From a cultural perspective, it is important to talk with client and family about a designated decision maker, management of pain, and care of body after death (see again Box 24–3)

IV. FAMILY SUPPORT NEAR END OF LIFE

A. Concepts of loss and grief

1. **Loss**: new absence of someone or something previously available and desired; can be actual (objective and identifiable by others), perceived (known to individual but not verifiable by others), or anticipatory (perceived before actual event occurs)
2. **Grief**: an expected emotional response to loss that is resolved by moving through theoretical stages or tasks; types of grief include "normal" (involves emotional, physical, behavioral, or cognitive reactions that may take months or years to resolve), anticipatory (occurring before loss begins), disenfranchised (loss is outside defined societal norms so cannot be openly acknowledged), or dysfunctional (associated with prolonged emotional state of grief and inability to cope successfully with loss)

B. Models of theoretical tasks of grief that may assist nurses to work with clients and families experiencing grief and loss

1. Psychodynamic models (e.g., Freud) address complicating factors of grief, such as quality of relationship with deceased or mental health of any affected individuals
2. Stage models (Kübler-Ross) (see Table 24–1) suggest grief occurs within individuals and their families
3. Table 24–1 summarizes additional models of grief work

NCLEX® **C. Assessment of grief**

1. Distinguish between loss, grief, **mourning** (external social behaviors, rituals, and traditions associated with loss and grief), and **bereavement** (a combination of grief and mourning; includes inner feelings and outward expressions of loss)
2. Differentiate between anticipatory, normal, complicated, and disenfranchised grief
3. Identify grief reactions, including stage, task, and factors affecting grieving process
4. Perform careful review of caregiver survivor to determine if he or she is maintaining nutritional status and self-care, sleeping, ability to work, and is sustaining family roles and social networks

D. Interventions and resources

1. Working with dying clients may require nurse to move through five stages of adaptation: intellectualization, emotional survival, depression, emotional arrival, and deep compassion

Table 24–1 Theoretical Tasks of Grief

Model	Description
Kübler-Ross Stages of Grief	Denial, anger, bargaining, depression, acceptance
Bowlby and Parkes' Phases of Grief	Shock and numbness, yearning and searching, disorganization and despair, reorganization and recovery
Rando's Process of Bereavement	Recognition of loss/death, experiencing and expressing separation and pain, reminiscing, relinquishing old attachments, readjusting while maintaining memories, reinvesting
Wordon's Tasks of Grief	Acceptance of reality of loss, experience of pain of grief, adjustment to environment without deceased, withdrawal of emotional energy and reinvestment in another relationship

2. Education in end-of-life care provides nurse with tools to deliver competent and nurturing care to dying client and his or her family
3. Formal support systems need to be available to nurse for safe expression of feelings; these can include postclinical debriefing and ceremonies or programs that enable acknowledgment and expression of grief

E. **Diagnosis of staff grief**
1. Multiple losses within a brief period of time put staff at risk for "bereavement overload" and dysfunctional grieving
2. Focusing on only physical needs and care of clients, avoiding emotion-laden conversations, or talking only about topics of comfort are indications a nurse may be experiencing **death anxiety** (being overcome with fears about death)
3. Awareness of feelings, responses, and reactions to death allows a nurse to provide sensitive care to clients and families

Check Your NCLEX–RN® I.Q.

You are ready for testing on this content if you can:

- Monitor the physiological status of a dying client.
- Provide effective physical, psychological, and spiritual support; teaching; and nursing care to a dying client and his or her family members.
- Identify how culture impacts end-of-life care.
- Differentiate between the needs of the dying child and the dying adult.

PRACTICE TEST

1 While the nurse is discussing a client's likely death with family members, one of the adult children asks, "We plan on taking turns being here for now, but we all want to be here at the time of mother's death. How can we tell when that time is close?" What is the nurse's best response?

1. "Often, people become more lucid for a short time about an hour before death. They become more alert with clearer eyes and focus on faces. Call the others in at that time."
2. "I wish I could tell you that there was a way to know. It could be minutes from now or another 3 days. One just never knows."
3. "The arms and legs become cool and more bluish in color. Breathing becomes irregular and shallow, and you may hear mucus in the throat. Pulse and blood pressure will decrease."
4. "You can expect muscles to become rigid, with staring eyes and mouth closed. The head is pulled back with neck rigidity. Don't be alarmed if you hear a death rattle in the throat."

2 A 90-year-old client expresses a wish to die at home after being told that an esophageal stricture prevents swallowing. The client refuses a feeding tube. The family fully supports this decision. What would be the most appropriate resource for the nurse to call?

1. Hospice care
2. The rabbi
3. An attorney
4. The medical examiner's office

3 The nurse is providing postmortem care for a client. Which intervention would be appropriate prior to allowing the family to visit? Select all that apply.

1. Prepare the body to look as clean and natural as possible.
2. Keep the sheet over the client's face until the family is comfortably seated in the room.
3. Wear sterile gloves to pack the anal canal with gauze.
4. Remove the external tubes and drains.
5. Call the healthcare provider to verify time of death before taking the body to the morgue.

PRACTICE TEST

4 A dying client's partner is afraid to get a meal in the cafeteria for fear the client will die while she is gone. No other family members or visitors are present. The client is nonresponsive, has an irregular and slow pulse, and has Cheyne-Stokes respirations. What is the best course of action by the nurse?

1. Encourage the partner to eat in the cafeteria. The client is nonresponsive and won't know the partner is gone.
2. Make arrangements for the partner to receive a meal in the client's room.
3. Promise to call the partner if any changes occur and ask an unlicensed assistive person to sit with the client while the partner is away.
4. Refrain from saying anything that interferes with the partner's decision.

5 The family of a client diagnosed with cancer and entering hospice care has been informed the client is not expected to live more than 2 months. Which statement made by a family member indicates to the nurse that the family understands the role of hospice care?

1. "Hospice nurses are going to help care for him at home until he gets better."
2. "Hospice nurses are going to help care for him until we learn how to provide the care."
3. "Hospice nurses are going to help care for him until he can take care of himself."
4. "Hospice nurses are going to help care for him to make him more comfortable."

6 The nurse anticipates which client newly diagnosed with a terminal illness is least likely to have difficulty facing his or her mortality?

1. A 71-year-old female whose grandson, sister, and best friend died over the past 6 months
2. A 59-year-old male who never married, is an only child, and whose parents are both healthy
3. A 70-year-old male who planned his funeral and enjoys riding a motorcycle at high speed in the desert
4. A 68-year-old female who has been an atheist for most of her life

7 A client with lung cancer is receiving total brain radiation therapy to control hand tremors due to multiple metastatic lesions. The client says, "I'm hoping this treatment will let me see my first tomatoes near the Fourth of July. It makes me want to cry to think I won't make it till then." The nurse concludes that this statement contains elements of which of Kübler-Ross's stages of death and dying? Select all that apply.

1. Denial
2. Bargaining
3. Anger
4. Depression
5. Acceptance

8 The registered nurse (RN) would intervene after hearing a licensed practical/vocational nurse (LPN/LVN) make which statement about a client with severe arthritis who is also newly diagnosed as being terminally ill with rapidly growing colorectal cancer?

1. "Even though it hurts a bit, your arthritic joints will become less stiff with gentle exercise."
2. "If we give more pain medication, will it stop his breathing?"
3. "He has a living will that says he does not want to be resuscitated."
4. "You have on a diaper so it's OK if you do not make it to the bathroom."

9 The mental health nurse is counseling a client who is grieving his father's death. Based on Rando's Process of Bereavement, in what order would the mental health nurse expect a client to make the following statements as he moves through the bereavement process? Place the options in correct sequence.

1. "This is the second anniversary of my father's death."
2. "My father had alcoholism, so during the holidays I bring coffee and chocolates to local AA groups."
3. "It was so much fun to rummage through the antique stores together."
4. "Since I no longer have connections to my father's stepfamily, I visit friends on vacation."
5. "The homestead has run down since his death. It was hard to drive past and see the lack of care in his vegetable garden."

Fill in your answer below:

Answer: ________________

10 A 46-year-old female client with a history of head and neck cancer was recently told she has multiple metastatic sites in her lung. The nurse is discussing the situation with the client and her sister. Which statement during the conversation reflects the ethical principle of justice?

1. "The staff will do everything possible to make your sister comfortable while she is in hospice."
2. "The healthcare provider should not have forced her into taking experimental chemotherapy. Now she is dying."
3. "Why did I have to get this terrible disease? I just want my life back."
4. "We will care for her at home. She has always been brave so she will probably try to use little pain medication."

11 A 22-year-old hospitalized client with a recent diagnosis of acquired immunodeficiency syndrome (AIDS) says to the nurse, "The food on this breakfast tray is terrible. Why can't you people do even simple things well?" What is the nurse's best response?

1. "I know you are angry, but I cannot let you make me the object of your anger. I will send up the dietitian."
2. "This is not about breakfast. Tell me what you are really angry about."
3. "I understand you are angry. I'll shut the door and let you calm down and then we can talk again."
4. "I hear a lot of anger in your voice that is expected and healthy. Do you want a new breakfast or would you like something else?"

12 While talking to adult children of a dying man, the nurse finds them tearful, with ambivalent feelings toward the client. The client often expresses beliefs of a wasted life. The children say that their father often showed love but followed it with criticism, anger, and emotional abuse. Which intervention is most likely to be helpful at this time?

1. Suggest that the family listen to relaxation tapes before visiting each other. If negative feelings arise, listen to the tapes together.
2. Have a nurse stay in the room when a family member visits the client so the nurse can intervene with conflict resolution if problems arise.
3. Assure the client and children that what matters is the present and the future, not the past. Encourage the children to spend more time with their father.
4. Suggest they videotape each adult child speaking of a time when the father showed love, and tape the father telling of a special love for each child. Plan a time for them to watch the tape together.

13 A terminally ill client questions the nurse about the difference between a living will and power of attorney for healthcare. What is the nurse's best response?

1. "A living will allows you to indicate treatments to be omitted, while durable healthcare power of attorney legally appoints another to make those decisions on your behalf."
2. "A lawyer carries out a living will, while a designated family member or friend carries out advanced directives."
3. "In a living will, you specify treatments to be carried out if you become unable to make decisions. A durable healthcare power of attorney allows you to include both treatments to be carried out and those to be omitted."
4. "The living will indicates when you wish life support to be discontinued, while a durable healthcare power of attorney gives that power to someone else."

14 The nurse working with a terminally ill client wishes to support the client's decisions concerning end-of-life care. To do this appropriately, the nurse should plan which of the following?

1. Be comfortable in assisting the client with euthanasia when requested to do so.
2. Ask another nurse to provide care if the client has a belief system that differs from the nurse's belief system.
3. Respect the client's wishes about death to the extent possible by law.
4. Encourage the client to request a do-not-resuscitate order because of terminal illness.

15 The nurse concludes that which behaviors indicate grief resolution in a bereaved client whose husband died a year ago? Select all that apply.

1. Becoming future-oriented when discussing details of everyday life
2. Considering the opinions of the deceased before making decisions about everyday life
3. Experiencing occasional waves of grief triggered by pictures or events
4. Sharing stories of good times that the client and her husband shared over the years
5. Being unable to visit places that hold happy memories of times spent with her husband

16 Which nursing intervention would be most appropriate for the nurse to include in the care plan of a client who is experiencing anticipatory grieving?

1. Hope instillation
2. Forgiveness facilitation
3. Medication management
4. Hypnotherapy

17 A client is dying, is in great pain, and refuses anything for relief that alters his sensorium. The nurse checks the religion recorded in the medical record, after concluding that the client's behavior is consistent with the practices of which religion? Select all that apply.

1. Islam
2. Judaism
3. Buddhism
4. Catholicism
5. Hindu

18 Which manifestation indicates to the nurse that the pain of a terminally ill nonverbal client is not well managed?

1. Crackles in the lungs
2. Hyperactive bowel sounds
3. Unwillingness to eat without assistance
4. Constant restlessness and leg movement

19 The family of a dying client is concerned about making certain their mother is as comfortable as possible. Which statement indicates to the nurse that the family understands how lack of fluid and nutrition can promote comfort as a client dies? Select all that apply.

1. "There will be less nausea and vomiting, since gastrointestinal secretions will be decreased."
2. "Natural analgesia from the body's endorphin production will help with pain control."
3. "A dry mouth may be a problem without fluid intake."
4. "Coughing and mucus production decrease after fluids are discontinued."
5. "Swelling and edema might decrease once we stop giving fluids."

20 A newly hired nurse is beginning to work with dying clients in a hospice unit. In which order does the nurse expect to move through the stages of adaptation when working with this population? Place these stages in expected order of occurrence.

1. Deep compassion
2. Emotional survival
3. Depression
4. Intellectualization
5. Emotional arrival

Fill in your answer below:

Answer: ________________

ANSWERS & RATIONALES

1 **Answer: 3 Rationale:** Peripheral circulation decreases and shifts to vital organs. The vascular system collapses, causing decreasing pulse and blood pressure. The gag reflex is lost, and mucus accumulates in the back of the throat. Respirations decrease in rate and become irregular. Vision is blurred near the time of death. A lucid moment is not a pattern in death. It is difficult to pinpoint the exact time when death will occur, but the imminence of clinical death can be detected. Muscle rigidity typically occurs after death, not before. **Cognitive Level:** Applying **Client Need:** Psychosocial Integrity **Integrated Process:** Teaching and Learning **Content Area:** Mental Health **Strategy:** Note the issue of the question, which is knowledge of impending signs of death. The words *best response* in the question tell you it is a true statement and will be a priority in client care. Choose the option in which all information stated is true.

2 **Answer: 1 Rationale:** Hospice specializes in end-of-life care. A rabbi is an important person during the end of life, but there is not an immediate need to make this call. The need for an attorney would be determined by the client and family. A medical examiner would be called after death in situations where the death is of a suspicious nature. **Cognitive Level:** Applying **Client Need:** Psychosocial Integrity **Integrated Process:** Nursing Process: Planning **Content Area:** Mental Health **Strategy:** The core issue is that the client wishes to die at home. Recall that hospice care can be provided in the home at all times. The other options (the attorney, rabbi, or medical examiner) do not address the client's issue, which is 24-hour care in the home at the end of life.

3 **Answer: 1, 4 Rationale:** The body is to be handled with dignity. The body is cleaned and linens are freshened. All external tubes and drains are removed. A sheet is pulled up to cover the client's shoulders. While gloves should be worn during postmortem care, sterility is not an issue. State laws and policies differ regarding the nurse's ability to declare death. Even if a healthcare provider is required to declare death, verification of time of death is not required prior to the family being allowed to view the client after death. **Cognitive Level:** Applying **Client Need:** Psychosocial Integrity **Integrated Process:** Nursing Process: Implementation **Content Area:** Fundamentals **Strategy:** Use the process of elimination to identify the options that contain inaccurate information. Recall that if an option contains only partially correct information, then that option is then incorrect.

4 **Answer: 2 Rationale:** Obtaining a meal for the client's partner who remains at the bedside demonstrates knowledge of the dying process in addition to compassion and concern for the client and partner. The signs and symptoms listed indicate death will occur soon, so encouraging the partner to leave to eat does not address the fear of having the client die alone. The client is showing signs of dying and if there are further changes, there may not be time to reach the partner in the cafeteria before death occurs. Having the partner stay in the room without assisting in providing nourishment demonstrates lack of caring or compassion. **Cognitive Level:** Applying **Client Need:** Psychosocial Integrity **Integrated Process:** Nursing Process: Implementation **Content Area:** Mental Health **Strategy:** The focus of the question is the signs and symptoms of imminent death of the client and the partner's desire to be with the client at the time of death. Choose the option that minimizes the partner's anxiety and also shows support for the partner.

5 **Answer: 4 Rationale:** Hospice care is provided to those clients who have 6 months or less to live. Hospice nurses are skilled in pain and symptom management as well as in emotional support to the dying clients and their families. A client in need of hospice services cannot be expected to "get better." Hospice care does not terminate once families learn to provide care. A client in need of hospice services cannot be expected to resume self-care. **Cognitive Level:** Applying **Client Need:** Psychosocial Integrity **Integrated Process:** Nursing Process: Evaluation **Content Area:** Mental Health **Strategy:** The core issue of the question is knowledge of the purpose and goals of hospice care. The incorrect options indicate the family expects improvement in the client's condition, which is not realistic.

6 **Answer: 3 Rationale:** People cope better when they accept what their life has had to offer, have previously coped with personal losses, have the time and ability to recover emotionally between multiple deaths, believe that death is a part of living, and have religious beliefs. The 70-year-old client who planned for the future demonstrates the belief that death is part of living. The 71-year-old client who lost three people in the last 6 months may not cope with terminal illness as well because this client has not had time to recover from multiple losses. The 59-year-old male client shows dependence, having never moved out of the home of his parents, and has not had to cope with the personal loss of parents. The client who is an atheist may have difficulty facing mortality; individuals with religious beliefs are often found to cope better. **Cognitive Level:** Applying **Client Need:** Psychosocial Integrity **Integrated Process:** Culture and Spirituality **Content Area:** Mental Health **Strategy:** The focus of this question is knowledge of how older adults cope with a diagnosis of a life-threatening illness. With the criteria outlined in the rationale, use the process of elimination to make the correct choice.

7 **Answer: 2, 4 Rationale:** During bargaining, clients "negotiate" to meet a life goal, such as going through radiation to see one more crop of tomatoes bloom. Feelings of sadness evidenced by wanting to cry are consistent with the stage of depression. Denial would be evidenced by a refusal to accept the diagnosis of terminal cancer. There is no evidence in the client's words that he is feeling anger. Acceptance would be shown when the client has come to terms with the illness and anticipated death. **Cognitive Level:** Applying **Client Need:** Psychosocial Integrity **Integrated Process:** Communication and Documentation **Content Area:** Mental Health **Strategy:** This question focuses on Kübler-Ross's five stages of death and dying. Evaluate the content of the client's statements and match them to the stages of death and dying. Note the wording of the question indicates that more than one option is likely to be correct.

8 **Answer: 4 Rationale:** The statement about wearing a diaper does not treat the client with respect and sensitivity and therefore is an example of maleficence. The RN should intervene after hearing this communication. The statement about joints becoming less stiff with gentle exercise is therapeutic and does not require intervention by the RN. Being worried about the effects of analgesics on respirations shows client advocacy, and does not require the RN to intervene. The statement about the living will indicates client advocacy and does not require the RN to intervene. **Cognitive Level:** Applying **Client Need:** Psychosocial Integrity **Integrated Process:** Caring **Content Area:** Fundamentals **Strategy:** The critical word in the stem of the question is *intervene*, making the correct option the one that is physically or emotionally harmful. Eliminate the helpful options that are therapeutic or demonstrate client advocacy.

9 **Answer: 1, 5, 3, 4, 2 Rationale:** In Rando's process of bereavement, the first step is to recognize the loss and death. The second step is to react to the experience and express the separation and pain (such as difficulty seeing the homestead). The third step is to reminisce (such as times shared with the example of antique shopping). The fourth step is to relinquish old attachments (visiting friends instead of father's stepfamily). The fifth and sixth steps are to readjust while retaining memories and reinvest (bring coffee and chocolates to local AA groups). **Cognitive Level:** Analyzing **Client Need:** Psychosocial Integrity **Integrated Process:** Nursing Process: Evaluation **Content Area:** Mental Health **Strategy:** Remember the Six Rs of Rando: recognize, react, reminisce, relinquish, readjust, and reinvest. They all begin with *re* and then the letters *CAMLAI*. A helpful memory aid could be Chocolate Always Makes Lads Act Icky.

10 **Answer: 1 Rationale:** The definition for the ethical principle of justice is "fairness." The statement that the staff will do everything possible to maintain comfort is just and fair. The statement about forcing the client to have chemotherapy cannot be verified and reflects anger on the part of the family. The statement about getting "this terrible disease" reflects anger on the part of the client. The statement about taking little pain medication could represent a lack of beneficence if the client experiences great pain and the family believes she does not want to be medicated. **Cognitive Level:** Applying **Client Need:** Psychosocial Integrity **Integrated Process:** Communication and Documentation **Content Area:** Fundamentals **Strategy:** The core issue of the question is the ethical principle of justice. Evaluate each statement and eliminate all options that do not reflect a sense of "fairness."

11 **Answer: 4 Rationale:** Anger is a common element in all the theories of grief and stages of dying. It is important to acknowledge the client's anger, help him or her identify the source of the anger, and offer choices or control when possible. Taking the anger personally and deferring to the dietitian is not therapeutic. Being confrontational about the client's source of anger is not therapeutic. Leaving the room and closing the door ignores the client's issue and connotes a sense of punishment. **Cognitive Level:** Applying **Client Need:** Psychosocial Integrity **Integrated Process:** Nursing Process: Diagnosis **Content Area:** Mental Health **Strategy:** Use principles of therapeutic communication to answer the question. The correct option is the one that acknowledges the client's anger and helps the client to deal with it, while offering the client choices to maintain some control.

12 **Answer: 4 Rationale:** Open communication with concrete evidence of emotional attachments assists in coping at the end of life. A videotape provides concrete assurance in the presence of the loved ones. Relaxation tapes help with stress reduction but do not help with resolution of problems experienced by the family. Staffing patterns do not permit a nurse to be with one client continually, and families require privacy as well. Assurance that the past no longer matters is a nontherapeutic assurance. **Cognitive Level:** Applying **Client Need:** Psychosocial Integrity **Integrated Process:** Caring **Content Area:** Mental Health **Strategy:** Use the process of elimination and address the client in the question. In this case, both the client and the adult children are the affected clients, so the correct option is one that benefits all of them.

13 **Answer: 1 Rationale:** A living will is written by the client and includes desires for use of different types of treatment in case of a life-threatening illness. A durable healthcare power of attorney is a legal document designating an individual to make legal healthcare decisions if the client is unable to make choices independently. A lawyer does not have to be the person to carry out a living will. A living will allows for expression of what measures may and may not be used to sustain life. A durable healthcare power attorney is not designed to override the wishes expressed in a living will. **Cognitive Level:** Applying **Client Need:** Psychosocial Integrity **Integrated Process:** Teaching and Learning **Content Area:** Fundamentals **Strategy:** The core issue of the question is knowledge of a living will. The wording of the question indicates that the correct answer is a true statement. Systematically eliminate options containing incorrect statements.

14 **Answer: 3 Rationale:** To uphold client autonomy, the nurse needs to consider the client's wishes while also acting within the law. Euthanasia constitutes illegal nursing practice in the United States at this time. To act ethically, the nurse should provide care to clients according to need, regardless of belief systems. Clients who are diagnosed with terminal illness may or may not be ready for do-not-resuscitate status, depending on anticipated life expectancy, quality of current life, and psychosocial variables. **Cognitive Level:** Applying **Client Need:** Psychosocial Integrity **Integrated Process:** Nursing Process: Implementation **Content Area:** Fundamentals **Strategy:** Eliminate options that are illegal, fail to provide unbiased care, or may not consider the client's preference at this time.

15 **Answer: 1, 3, 4 Rationale:** Grief resolution requires letting go of the past and looking forward to the future. The client needs to be able to put the loss in perspective and engage fully and effectively in daily life as an independent person. Having occasional episodes of grief triggered by pictures or events is consistent with healthy grief resolution. Being able to share stories of good times indicates healthy grief resolution. If current decisions are being made based on preferences of the deceased, the client has not let go of the past and grief is not resolving. To be unable to visit places that she enjoyed with her husband a year ago indicates inadequate resolution of grief. **Cognitive Level:** Applying **Client Need:** Psychosocial Integrity **Integrated Process:** Nursing Process: Diagnosis **Content Area:** Mental Health **Strategy:** The focus of the question is on grief resolution, so eliminate options that do not show resolution 1 year later. The wording of the question indicates that more than one option is likely to be correct.

16 **Answer: 1 Rationale:** Hope instillation is often an effective intervention in dealing with anticipatory grieving. There is no evidence in the stem of the question to support the need for forgiveness facilitation. Medication management would address symptoms but not the actual problem of anticipatory grief. There is no evidence in the stem of the question to support the need for hypnotherapy. **Cognitive Level:** Applying **Client Need:** Psychosocial Integrity **Integrated Process:** Nursing Process: Planning **Content Area:** Mental Health **Strategy:** The

critical words in the question stem are *most appropriate* and *anticipatory grieving*. Use the process of elimination to select the option that best focuses on anticipated loss.

17 **Answer: 3, 5 Rationale:** The Hindu and Buddhist religions require believers to be alert and mindful as they leave life on Earth and transcend to their next life. A requirement to be alert and mindful is not found in Islam, Judaism, or Catholicism. **Cognitive Level:** Applying **Client Need:** Psychosocial Integrity **Integrated Process:** Culture and Spirituality **Content Area:** Fundamentals **Strategy:** Use the process of elimination. Select the religions that require a state of being *mindful* and *alert* as their faithful transcend from life into death. The wording of the question indicates there is more than one correct answer.

18 **Answer: 4 Rationale:** Constant restlessness and leg movement can be physiological indicators of pain. Crackles in the lungs indicate fluid overload or ineffective pumping action of the heart, but not pain. Hyperactive bowel sounds are more likely a reflection of gastrointestinal status than pain. Unwillingness to eat without assistance could indicate weakness, loneliness, or other factors but is not a manifestation of pain. **Cognitive Level:** Applying **Client Need:** Psychosocial Integrity **Integrated Process:** Nursing Process: Assessment **Content Area:** Fundamentals **Strategy:** First eliminate lung crackles and bowel sounds, which directly reflect functioning of the cardiopulmonary and gastrointestinal systems, respectively. Choose restlessness and leg movements over unwillingness to eat without assistance because unwillingness to eat could have psychosocial as well as physiological etiologies.

19 **Answer: 1, 2, 4, 5 Rationale:** Lack of fluids can promote comfort in the dying client by decreasing gastrointestinal secretions that can lead to nausea and vomiting. Dehydration can aid in natural analgesia because it leads to release of endorphins. Reduced fluid intake leads to decreased fluid accumulation in the peripheral tissues. Lack of fluids would contribute to the client's sense of dry mouth, which does not promote comfort. Decreased fluid intake would lead to reduced production of respiratory secretions. **Cognitive Level:** Applying **Client Need:** Basic Care and Comfort **Integrated Process:** Teaching and Learning **Content Area:** Fundamentals **Strategy:** Consider the possible physiological benefits of lack of fluids to a dying client. Note that the question indicates that more than one option is likely to be correct.

20 **Answer: 4, 2, 3, 5, 1 Rationale:** Recognizing the five stages of adaptation is important for nurses working with dying clients and their families. Intellectualization occurs first, where the nurse uses a cognitive approach to adaptation. Emotional survival occurs second as the nurse attempts to cope with death and dying during daily work. Depression occurs third as the emotional aspects are experienced by the nurse. Emotional arrival occurs fourth as the nurse copes with these losses. Deep compassion occurs last (fifth) as the nurse fully adapts to working with this population. **Cognitive Level:** Analyzing **Client Need:** Psychosocial Integrity **Process:** Nursing Process: Implementation **Content Area:** Mental Health **Strategy:** Think *"IS DAD" adapting?* It is an acronym for *I*ntellectualization, Emotional *S*urvival, *D*epression, Emotional *A*rrival, and *D*eep Compassion.

Key Terms to Review

advance directive (AD) p. 338
beneficence p. 337
bereavement p. 342
death anxiety p. 343
euthanasia p. 338
grief p. 342
justice p. 337
loss p. 342
mourning p. 342
nonmaleficence p. 337
palliation p. 337
veracity p. 337

References

American Nurses Association. (2010). Registered nurses' roles and responsibilities in providing expert care and counseling at the end of life (revised position statement). Available at www.nursingworld.org/MainMenuCategories/EthicsStandards/Ethics-Position-Statements/etpain14426.pdf.

American Nurses Association. (2013). Euthanasia, assisted suicide, and aid in dying (revised combined position statement). Available at www.nursingworld.org/MainMenuCategories/Policy-Advocacy/Positions-and-Resolutions/ANAPosition-Statements/Position-Statements-Alphabetically/Euthanasia-Assisted-Suicide-and-Aid-in-Dying.pdf.

Berman, A., Snyder, S., & Frandsen, G. (2016). *Kozier & Erb's fundamentals of nursing: Concepts, process, and practice* (10th ed.). New York, NY: Pearson Education.

LeMone, P., Burke, K., Bauldoff, G., & Gubrud, P. (2015). *Medical surgical nursing: Clinical reasoning in patient care* (6th ed.). Hoboken, NJ: Pearson Education.

Potter, P., Perry, A., Stockert, P., & Hall, A. (2017). *Fundamentals of nursing* (9th ed.). St. Louis, MO: Mosby.

25 Meeting Nutritional Needs

In this chapter

Cross Reference

Other chapters relevant to this content area are

Integrative Therapies Chapter 28
Total Parenteral Nutrition Chapter 33
Common Laboratory Tests Chapter 46

I. OVERVIEW OF NUTRIENTS

A. Proteins (macronutrients)

1. Composed of amino acids; required for growth and development; provide 4 calories/gram
2. Essential amino acids cannot be synthesized by body and must be obtained in diet
3. Proteins may be complete (contain all essential amino acids), incomplete, or complementary (provide all essential amino acids when eaten with certain other foods)
4. High-quality proteins are found in meat, fish, poultry, eggs, dairy products, and dried beans
5. Protein is needed for energy, growth, bodily repair, maintenance of fluid and electrolyte balance, and production of enzymes, hormones, and antibodies
6. Adult recommended daily allowance (RDA) for protein is 0.8 grams/kg/day (approximately 10% of total calories); additional protein may be needed by infants, children, and pregnant or lactating women
7. Insufficient protein intake can lead to protein energy malnutrition, characterized by muscle wasting

B. Carbohydrates (macronutrients)

1. Include starches, sugars (fructose, glucose, lactose, sucrose), and cellulose
2. Provide 4 calories/gram and are a key source of energy
3. Found in fruits, vegetables, milk, and grains
4. Promote normal metabolism, including fat metabolism, and prevent protein from being used for energy (protein sparing)
5. Insufficient intake results in protein and fat being used for energy

C. Fats (macronutrients)
1. Concentrated sources of energy, providing 9 calories/gram
2. Needed for proper absorption of fat-soluble vitamins
3. Stored in body to maintain body warmth and protect internal organs
4. Sources include animal products, egg yolks, organ meats (including liver), butter, cheeses, and various oils
5. Can be described by cholesterol content and as saturated, monounsaturated, or polyunsaturated; in general, the more solid the fat, the higher the saturated fat content
6. Can lead to obesity, heart disease, and some cancers if taken in excess of bodily needs
7. Insufficient intake can result in increased risk of infection, skin lesions, amenorrhea, and cold sensitivity (insufficient fat stores)

D. Minerals (micronutrients)
1. Part of bones, cells, and hormones; enhance cellular function; catalyze bodily processes
2. Widely abundant in foods
3. Major minerals include calcium, sodium, potassium, magnesium, chloride, and phosphorus
4. Trace elements that are also needed include iron, iodine, copper, zinc, selenium, manganese, fluoride, chromium, and molybdenum
5. Mineral intake can also be supplemented, often as part of a multivitamin

E. Vitamins (micronutrients)
1. Classified as water soluble (B and C vitamins), which are easily excreted from body, or fat soluble (vitamins A, D, E, K), which can be stored and cause toxicity if taken to excess
2. Used as catalysts of body functions, coenzymes in metabolic processes, for growth, collagen production, wound healing, hormone synthesis, and vision
3. See Table 25–1 for summary of vitamin functions, food sources, and signs of deficiency or excess states
4. Vitamins can be obtained by diet alone or by supplement, either with or without minerals

II. GENERAL DIETARY GUIDELINES

NCLEX® **A. Characteristics of healthy diet**
1. Focus on variety, amount, and choice of nutrient-dense foods
2. *NCLEX®* Daily diet is low in saturated fat (less than 10% of calories and less than 300 mg cholesterol) and trans fat, sodium (less than 2,300 mg or approximately one teaspoon), and added sugars (less than 10% of calories)
3. Begin by making small changes and build toward healthier food and beverage choices

B. Current dietary recommendations: MyPlate (USDA) (see Figure 25–1)
1. Eat correct number of calories based on age, sex, activity level, height, and weight
2. *NCLEX®* Choose from five food groups to obtain necessary nutrients
   a. Vegetables: all fresh, frozen, dried, or canned vegetables or vegetable juice; choose from all vegetable subgroups (dark green, orange, legumes, starchy vegetables, and other vegetables)
   b. Fruits: all fresh, frozen, dried, or canned fruits or fruit juices
   c. Grains: all foods made from wheat, rice, oats, cornmeal, and barley, such as bread, pasta, oatmeal, breakfast cereal, tortillas, and grits; at least one-half of grains should come from whole grains
   d. Protein: lean meat, poultry, fish, eggs, peanut butter, beans, nuts, and seeds
   e. Dairy: all fluid milk products and foods made from milk that retain calcium content (yogurt and cheese, but not cream cheese, cream, or butter, which do not have significant calcium content); drink milk that is low-fat (1%) or fat-free
3. Fill half of plate with vegetables and fruits; vary food selections
4. Make selections from dairy food group that are high in calcium
5. Choose fresh foods instead of frozen or canned foods when possible
6. *NCLEX®* Weight management
   a. Avoid eating oversized food portions
   b. Balance calories ingested from foods and beverages with calories expended
   c. Prevent gradual weight gain over time by making small decreases in calories and increasing physical activity
   d. Drink water instead of beverages that contain sugar

Table 25–1 Overview of Fat- and Water-Soluble Vitamins

Vitamin	Function	Food Sources	Signs of Deficiency or Excess
Thiamin (B_1)	Coenzyme in CHO and amino acid metabolism	Pork, wheat germ, black beans, black-eyed peas, fortified cereals	Deficiency: Beriberi disease, anorexia, weight loss, muscle weakness and wasting, peripheral neuropathy, Wernicke encephalopathy Toxicity: none reported (water-soluble vitamin)
Riboflavin (B_2)	Coenzyme in protein metabolism	Milk and dairy products, eggs, liver, fortified cereals	Deficiency: ariboflavinosis, lesions in mouth and on lips, dermatitis (seborrheic), anemia (normocytic, normochromic) Toxicity: none reported (water-soluble vitamin)
Niacin (B_3)	Coenzyme in energy production, aids in synthesis of fatty acids and steroid hormones	Tuna, liver, chicken, and other meats and poultry, whole or fortified grains	Deficiency: pellagra (3 Ds: dermatitis, diarrhea, dementia) Toxicity: flushing, liver damage if long term
Pyridoxine (B_6)	Coenzyme in amino acid metabolism	Sirloin steak, salmon, chicken breast, whole and fortified grains, bananas, nuts	Deficiency: mouth lesions, fatigue, anemia (microcytic, hypochromic), seizures in infants Toxicity: megadoses lead to sensory neuropathy and severe ataxia without weakness
Folic acid Folate	Formation of DNA, aids in formation of heme	Dried peas, beans, and lentils, dark green leafy vegetables, peanuts, fortified cereals and grains	Deficiency: megaloblastic anemia, neural tube defects, fatigue, weakness, shortness of breath, palpitations Toxicity: none reported (water-soluble vitamin)
Cyanocobalamin (B_{12})	Amino acid and fatty acid metabolism, synthesis of DNA and RNA, synthesis and maintenance of myelin	Meat, fish, poultry, eggs, milk, cheese, nutritional yeast, fortified soy milk or tofu	Deficiency: pernicious anemia from lack of intrinsic factor, fatigue, pallor, shortness of breath, palpitations, numbness and tingling of extremities, abnormal gait, possible memory loss, possible irreversible dementia Toxicity: none reported (water-soluble vitamin)
Ascorbic acid (vitamin C)	Antioxidant, collagen synthesis, iron absorption, adrenal hormone synthesis	Citrus fruits, broccoli and Brussels sprouts, green and red peppers, cantaloupe, kiwi, strawberries	Deficiency: scurvy, bleeding gums and mucous membranes, poor wound healing Toxicity: megadoses lead to nausea, abdominal cramps, and diarrhea
Vitamin A	Vision, bone and tissue growth, immune and reproductive function	Animal foods (liver, egg yolk), fruits, vegetables, fortified milk	Deficiency: night blindness, xerophthalmia (dry, thick outer covering of eye), sore throat, mouth abscesses Toxicity: headaches, blurred vision, bone and joint pain, dry skin
Vitamin D	Bone production, increases calcium absorption, decreased urinary excretion of calcium	Dairy products, herring, salmon, sardines, fortified food sources	Deficiency: rickets, osteomalacia Toxicity: anorexia, nausea, vomiting, polyuria, muscle weakness, constipation, hypercalcemia, calcium deposits in soft tissues
Vitamin E	Antioxidant, protects cell membranes	Vegetable oil, whole grains, nuts, fortified cereals, leafy vegetables	Hemolytic anemia, degenerative neurologic problems Toxicity: GI symptoms, muscle weakness, double vision, increased bleeding tendencies (interferes with vitamin K)
Vitamin K	Production of blood clotting factors, assists vitamin D to synthesize regulatory bone protein	Liver, spinach and salad greens, vegetables of cabbage family	Hemorrhagic disease of newborn, prolonged clotting time Toxicity: no adverse effects with naturally occurring forms of K_1 and K_2

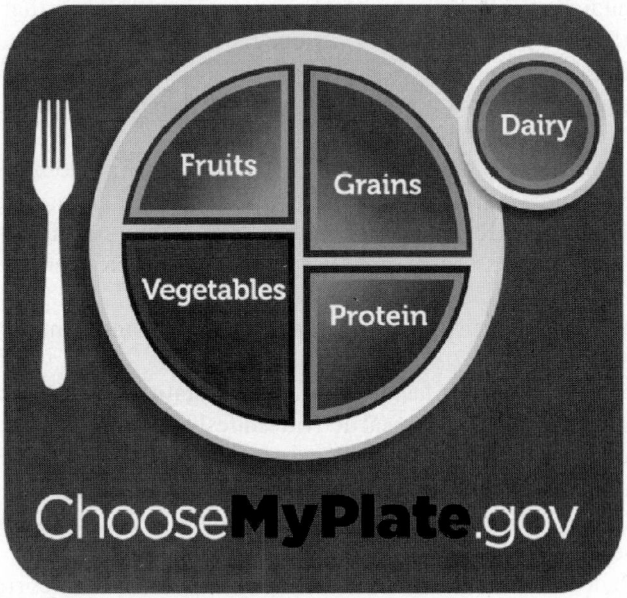

Figure 25–1

MyPlate. Emphasizes proportions of food groups per meal.

Source: USDA. Available at www.choosemyplate.gov.

III. ASSESSMENT OF NUTRITIONAL STATUS

A. Documented history

1. Food record: client records all foods and beverages ingested over several days (often 1 week); record is then analyzed for nutrient content
2. Diet recall (24-hour recall): all foods, liquids, and dietary supplements consumed in last 24 hours are recalled either verbally or in writing (includes time and location of intake, portion sizes, preparation methods, whether foods are fortified); greatly affected by changes in usual eating patterns and routines
3. Food frequency questionnaire: assesses intake of foods and food groups by day, week, or month; useful in capturing intake of nutrients that are not eaten daily
4. Review of systems: assesses each body system for symptoms of nutrition problems related to excess or deficiency (e.g., constipation as a result of low fiber and water intake)
5. After diet history is completed, nutrient content can be determined by comparing data collected with food composition tables or using a computerized diet analysis program

B. Anthropometric measurements

1. Height and weight are measured and recorded; a history of weight gain or loss is also assessed
2. BMI: assesses relative weight for height; calculated by dividing weight in kilograms (2.2 lb = 1 kg) by the square of height in meters (2.54 cm = 1 in.), or Weight ÷ $(\text{Height})^2$ = BMI; may be calculated using nomograms or online BMI calculators

NCLEX®

   a. Provides a range to evaluate a healthy body weight ("healthy" range: 18.5–24.9) and underweight, overweight, and obese status (see Table 25–2)

Table 25–2 Classifications of Body Mass Index for Adults

Classification	BMI Measurement
Severe malnutrition	Less than 16
Moderate malnutrition	16 to 16.99
Mild malnutrition	17 to 18.49
Normal	18.5 to 24.9
Overweight	25 to 29.9
Obesity Class I	30 to 34.9
Obesity Class II	35 to 39.9
Obesity Class III	40 or higher

b. BMI in children ages 2–20 years is tracked using growth charts that outline BMI-for-age in percentiles, with less than 5th percentile as risk for underweight and greater than 95th percentile as risk for overweight
c. BMI does not reflect body composition, and individuals with greater muscle mass may appear to be overweight and yet not have increased body fat
d. High or low BMIs may correlate with clinical or disease pathology

3. Basal metabolic rate (BMR): measures oxygen consumption and rate of calories burned during basic activities—a higher BMR indicates client can consume more calories without weight gain
   a. Lean muscle tissue mass most directly affects BMR; BMR decreases about 2% during each decade after maximum at age 30
   b. BMR increases with activity, stress, temperature, pregnancy, smoking, caffeine, stress, and during growth spurts
   c. BMR decreases with sleep, fasting, or starvation states and undernutrition
   d. *NCLEX®* Identification of BMR and typical activities/lifestyle is necessary to determine exact caloric requirements
4. *NCLEX®* Distribution of body fat aids assessment of health risk potential
   a. Central (truncal) **obesity** represents increased intra-abdominal fat and is associated with increased risk of disease
   b. Determination of waist circumference and/or hip–waist ratio correlates with "apple" versus "pear" body type and reflects risk pattern for disease ("apple" types are at greater risk than "pear" types)
5. Skinfold measurements using calipers are an objective measure of body fat stores and nutritional status
   a. Triceps skinfold (TSF) is most commonly performed; uses subscapular and suprailiac skinfolds
   b. Mid-arm circumference (MAC) provides information about muscle and fat stores; is used to calculate mid-arm muscle circumference (MAMC), which provides information about skeletal muscle mass and distinguishes differences in muscle and body fat

C. Laboratory and diagnostic measurements

1. *NCLEX®* Albumin level (normal: 3.5–5.5 g/dL): good overall indicator of nutritional status because of long half-life (18–20 days); body can store and maintain normal levels until chronic malnutrition occurs; low level indicates inadequate nutritional status
   a. *NCLEX®* Prealbumin levels are a more sensitive indicator of nutritional status because of shorter half-life and thus faster response to short-term changes in protein stores
   b. *NCLEX®* Transferrin levels identify iron stores, which reflect visceral body protein
   c. *NCLEX®* Albumin, prealbumin, and transferrin levels are used to evaluate clinical response of clients to total parenteral nutrition (TPN) and overall nutritional status in other clients
2. Total lymphocyte count (TLC) decreases as protein stores become depleted, which can negatively affect immune system function
3. *NCLEX®* Screening for specific nutrient deficiencies: hemoglobin levels reflect iron intake; transferrin transports iron from intestine into serum and drops more rapidly than albumin

IV. KEY NUTRITIONAL CONCERNS ACROSS THE LIFESPAN

A. Culture and religion influence food choices in times of health and illness; see Table 25–3

B. Pregnancy and lactation

1. *NCLEX®* Calorie needs increase during pregnancy by about 300 cal/day and during lactation by 500 cal/day
2. Intake of a balanced diet is important, with adequate intake of protein, magnesium, iron, calcium, vitamin C, and B-complex vitamins (especially folic acid to prevent neural tube defects)
3. *NCLEX®* Weight gain during pregnancy is based on prepregnancy weight using BMI as a reference point (note variation in underweight classification from nonpregnant state)
   a. Underweight clients (BMI < 19.8) should gain 12.5–18 kg (28–40 lb)
   b. Healthy-weight clients (BMI 19.8–24.9) should gain 11.5–16 kg (25–35 lb)
   c. Overweight clients (BMI 25–29) should gain 7–11.5 kg (15–25 lb)
   d. Obese clients (BMI > 29) should gain 6.8 kg (15 lb)
4. *NCLEX®* Common symptoms that may affect nutrition
   a. Nausea and vomiting: consume CHOs before getting out of bed in morning; eat small, frequent meals; avoid foods with offensive odors; do not drink fluids with meals; avoid coffee, tea, and spicy foods; limit high-fat foods
   b. Heartburn: interventions are similar to above; wait at least 1 hour before reclining after a meal

Table 25–3 Influence of Selected Cultures and Religions on Nutritional Status

Cultural or Religious Group	Practices and/or Issues*
	Cultural Group
Southern Black American	Traditional foods high in fat, cholesterol, sodium. Frying and adding fat to food is common. Popular foods may include pork, chicken, fish, rice, grits, okra, sweet potatoes, corn, black-eyed peas, peppers, green and lima beans, greens (collard, turnip, mustard), and specialty gravies. Obesity, cardiovascular disease, and diabetes are nutritionally related health risks.
Asian	Traditional diet varies by country and region, but tends to be plant-based: mushrooms, bean sprouts, bok choy, bamboo, alfalfa sprouts, tofu, rice, noodles; may include beef, poultry, and seafood. Diet tends to be low in fat, saturated fat, and cholesterol and rich in fiber and nutrients; may be high in sodium. High risk for osteoporosis.
Native American and First Nations	Diet varies with region. Some use corn and other cultivated crop staples; meats may include game and seafood. Vegetables and fruits may include wild berries, black cherries, rhubarb, wild mushrooms, roots, and Indian celery. Seeds and nuts are eaten according to region and availability. Diabetes and obesity are common.
Hispanic (Mexican origin)	Traditional diet includes tortillas, corn, potatoes, chili peppers, tomatoes, beets, onions, cabbage, pumpkins, meat, poultry, eggs, and beans (pinto, calico, garbanzo). Food preparation commonly uses fat. Obesity, diabetes, and high triglyceride levels are common.
	Religious Group
Christianity	Catholics eat no meat on Ash Wednesday or Fridays during Lent; fasting is common on some religious days. Eastern Orthodox practice some fasting. Mormons consume no coffee, tea, alcohol, or tobacco. Seventh-Day Adventists generally are lacto-ovovegetarians. No coffee, tea, alcohol, or strong seasonings are consumed. Meals are at least 4–5 hours apart with no snacking between meals.
Judaism (those following strict dietary rules)	Only kosher meat and poultry and fish with fins and scales are eaten (no pork or pork products, shellfish, or fishlike mammals). Consuming milk or dairy at same meal with meat or poultry is forbidden. Separate utensils are required for preparing and serving meat and dairy. Bakery products and prepared food mixtures must be made according to kosher standards. During Passover, leavened bread and cake are forbidden.
Seventh-Day Adventist	All pork or pork products, shellfish, blood, highly spiced foods, meat broths, all alcoholic beverages, coffee, and tea are not allowed. Some members do not eat flesh foods, dairy products, and eggs.
Islam	No pork or pork products, carnivorous animals, land animals without external ears, birds of prey, alcohol, tea, or coffee are consumed. Meat must be slaughtered according to ritual blood letting. Fasting is common during certain religious events.
Buddhism	All meat is prohibited.
Hinduism	Beef, pork, and some fowl are prohibited.

* Although identified by a specific ethnic or religious group, practices vary with area of origin and sect. Not all individuals within these groups follow these practices or have these issues.

c. Cravings and aversions: avoid non-nutritive substances (pica) that replace essential nutrients or interfere with their absorption; aversions are often self-limiting

d. Constipation: caused by iron intake, enlarging uterus, decreased physical activity, and possibly inadequate fiber and fluid; consume at least 8 glasses of water daily and increase fiber in diet

C. Infancy

1. Infants may be breast- or bottle-fed according to maternal preference; breastfeeding is accepted as preferred nutrition whenever possible
2. *NCLEX®* Weight doubles in first 6 months of life and triples by 1 year
3. *NCLEX®* Avoid giving cow's milk during first year (deficient in essential fatty acids, iron, zinc, vitamin E, and vitamin C); could lead to decrease in hemoglobin and hematocrit and possible intestinal bleeding
4. Fluoride supplements are generally prescribed for infants 6 months of age and older if water supply has less than 0.3 parts per million (ppm) fluoride
5. Do not add cereal to bottle because of risk of aspiration with stronger suck reflex needed
6. Do not give bottle containing milk, juice, or sweetened beverage before sleep to avoid nursing bottle syndrome (dental caries)
7. *NCLEX®* Start solid foods at 4–6 months of age to reduce risk of food allergies and because of immaturity of GI tract
8. *NCLEX®* Introduce one new food no more frequently than every 4–7 days to detect allergy; give only 1–2 teaspoons initially and increase over time
9. *NCLEX®* Cook foods well and cut or grind into tiny pieces to reduce risk of choking; supervise during meals and avoid giving hard round foods such as grapes, peanuts, popcorn, hotdogs, and others
10. Avoid using honey because of risk of infant botulism

D. Childhood

1. Dietary needs differ among toddlers, preschoolers, and school-age children; total energy needs increase with age, but calories per kilogram of weight decrease

NCLEX®
2. Toddlers and preschoolers may have erratic and ritualistic eating patterns and strong food preferences, including food jags (preferring one or a few types of foods over all others); these place child at risk for nutritional deficiencies; provide a balanced diet over time if not at each meal

NCLEX®
3. Facilitate nutrient intake in young children by not forcing child to eat, maintaining relaxed mealtimes, offering one new food with a favorite food, using child-sized portions, serving foods with mild flavors, and providing finger foods
4. Encourage school-age children not to skip breakfast; encourage regular meal patterns; nutrient stores for puberty are laid during this time
5. Encourage healthy after-school snacks rather than high-calorie and high-fat items found in fast foods; choose popcorn, fresh fruits and vegetables, peanut butter, cheese, nuts, eggs, and yogurt
6. Encourage adequate physical activity to reduce risk of childhood obesity
7. Daily intake of a multivitamin may reduce risk of vitamin deficiency from occasional erratic dietary patterns (such as from after-school and sports schedules)

E. Adolescence

1. Need for macro- and micronutrients significantly increases during this time
2. Male adolescent growth spurt begins at 12–13 years, peaks at 14, and continues until approximately 19 years
3. Female adolescent growth spurt begins at 10–11 years, peaks at 12, and continues until approximately 15 years
4. Adolescents frequently consume inadequate amounts of vitamin A, C, B_6, iron, calcium, zinc, and magnesium

NCLEX®
5. Adolescents frequently engage in dieting; follow fad or restrictive diets; skip meals; snack on high-calorie, high-fat, or high-sugar foods; and eat more meals outside home (including fast foods); these eating patterns increase risk of calorie and/or nutrient deficiencies

NCLEX®
6. Diet should be well balanced with sufficient calories but eliminating empty (non-nutritive) calories and high-fat foods; vitamin supplements may be helpful
7. Eating disorders (anorexia nervosa, bulimia nervosa) or obesity may be of concern; see Chapter 21 for discussion of eating disorders

F. Adulthood (age 18–64 years)

1. Dietary needs include balanced intake and maintaining ideal body weight
2. There is significant variation in metabolic needs based on age, weight, height, and physical activity; overall energy needs decrease during adulthood, although needs for selected nutrients may increase
3. Stress (which affects metabolic processes) and occupational influences (such as travel) may affect meal patterns and dietary intake
4. Poor nutritional habits during a lifetime increase risk of cardiovascular disease, diabetes mellitus, cancer, and obesity
5. Take multivitamin and mineral supplements as needed and follow balanced meal plan and possibly therapeutic diet based on identified health problem(s)
6. Lose weight if indicated to reduce further health risks

G. Older adulthood (age 65 and older)

1. Caloric requirements continue to decrease
2. Nutrient absorption may be adversely affected because of chewing difficulties (periodontal disease, loss of teeth, dysphagia due to stroke or other neuromuscular disease), decreased peristalsis, and reduced secretion of digestive enzymes
3. Therapeutic diets may affect intake of calories and specific nutrients

NCLEX®
4. Clients who have dysphagia from stroke will have dysphagia staged and appropriate diet prescribed
5. Prescribed medications may interact with specific foods or may cause side effects (nausea, vomiting, diarrhea, constipation, inactivation of nutrients) that affect nutritional health
6. Loss of family or friends may reduce socialization at mealtimes and provide for fewer opportunities for social eating
7. Those who have insufficient finances or rely on others to shop for food or prepare food are at risk for nutritional deficiencies

NCLEX®

8. Thirst response declines with age and can lead to dehydration and electrolyte imbalances
9. Common nutrient deficiencies in older adults include protein, fiber, total calories, iron, calcium, magnesium, and vitamins D, B_{12}, and B_6

V. PHYTOCHEMICALS AND NUTRITIONAL SUPPLEMENTS

A. *Phytochemicals*

1. Physiologically active food ingredients in plant sources that may correlate with health benefits in preventing or treating disease (also called functional foods)
2. Phytochemicals are found in plant sources (fruits and vegetables), whole grains, tea, and soy products; many foods contain several phytochemicals and therefore can exert multiple effects on many body systems (see Table 25–4)

NCLEX®

3. Health applications: phytochemicals function as antioxidants and may provide some protection against cancer, cardiovascular disease, and diabetes; dietitians can assist in selecting food products that contain phytochemicals

B. Nutritional supplements

1. Contain vitamins, minerals, herbs, botanicals, amino acids, enzymes, extracts, or combinations of these; must follow FDA guidelines to be labeled as such
2. Available in several forms including pills, liquids, powders, or are incorporated into foods (such as power bars or energy beverages)
3. Also included in this category are **ergogenic aids** that enhance body performance and work output
   a. Amino acids are often used to promote anabolism and maintain strength in the form of glutamine and branch-chain amino acids (BCAA); protein is increased often to the level of 1.3–2 grams/day
   b. CHO loading (glycogen loading) consists of high glucose ingestion before intense exercise in order to increase glycogen stores and delay onset of fatigue
   c. Metabolic end products are often used as ergogenic aids (creatine and steroids) in body

Table 25–4 Types of Phytochemicals

Phytochemical	General Information
Carotenoids	Found in colorful fruits and vegetables (green, orange, red, and yellow) Include beta-carotene and lycopene (found in tomato products, sauces, and ketchup); function as both pro-oxidant and antioxidant Health benefit claims: retinal protection; decreased risk of heart disease, lung, prostate, and breast cancers; enhanced immune effects in older adults
Indoles	Found in vegetables such as broccoli, cauliflower, cabbage, and kale Include organosulphur compounds; members of cruciferous vegetable family Health benefit claims: reducing estrogen effectiveness (decreasing risk of non-hormone-dependent breast cancer); influencing DNA enzyme activity to protect against cancer
Isoflavones	Found in soy foods (tofu, soy milk, and soybean products) and black and green tea Include phenylpropanoids that include flavonoid group (also found in nuts, wine, and oregano) Health benefit claims: inhibiting cancer cell growth (breast, prostate, and endometrial), alleviating menopausal symptoms, and preventing osteoporosis by increasing bone density
Phenolic acids	Found in coffee beans, fruits and vegetables, green tea, wine, and soybeans Include phenylpropanoids, which act as antioxidants and bind metals to promote excretion of carcinogenic substances Health benefit claims: decreased risk of skin, lung, and stomach cancers, controlling blood glucose
Terpones	Found in oil of citrus peel and menthol Chemical structure includes isoprenoid Health benefit claims: protection against carcinogens
Phytoestrogens	Found in vegetables, plants, soybean, and whole-grain fruits and berries Include phenylpropanoids that include isoflavones and lignans Health benefit claims: protection against cardiovascular disease, cancer (breast and prostate), and osteoporosis
Catechins	Found in teas Include phenylpropanoids that are rich in phenolic acid Health benefit claims: possible antioxidant activity, prevention of cancer, and antihypertensive effects

NCLEX® 4. Although many products claim to be ergogenic aids, clinical research does not support all claims; clients should consider each product's potential harm and/or available benefit prior to use

NCLEX® **C. Indications for use**

1. Decrease risk of disease, support increased needs during growth and periods of stress, and improve overall functioning
2. Support clients who are in at-risk categories due to life-cycle concerns (pregnancy, lactation, or children), underlying disease states (illness, stress, or malabsorption), inadequate intake of nutrients (strict vegans or constant dieters), and/or clinical intervention that requires therapy

VI. THERAPEUTIC DIETS WITH ALTERED CONSISTENCY

A. Clear liquid diet

1. Provides adequate fluid/water, 500–1,000 kcal of simple sugars and electrolytes but is fiber-free
2. Requires minimal digestion because there is no residue or fiber
3. Recommended for short-term use (1–2 days), before and after surgery or diagnostic procedures, during acute stages of illness, or as initial diet after significant period of GI inactivity/bowel rest
4. Consists of clear foods that are liquid at body temperature: gelatin, bouillon, clear broth, popsicles, apple or cranberry juice, clear carbonated beverages, tea or coffee with no added milk or milk product

B. Full liquid diet

1. Provides water, calories, protein, vitamins and minerals, and dairy products (contains lactose) and is considered to be low in residue
2. Indicated for some clients who have difficulty chewing or swallowing, but not indicated for a client following a stroke
3. Can be a transition diet (temporary diet as client progresses postoperatively or postprocedure from clear liquids to solids); deficient in many nutrients and calories
4. Consists of all foods found on a clear liquid diet and opaque liquids (milk, juices, pudding, ice cream, strained soups, yogurts, any prepared liquid formulas) and all foods that are liquid at body temperature
5. Clients who are lactose intolerant may require lactose-free supplements to prevent clinical symptoms

C. Pureed diet

1. Provides essential nutrients in a chopped, ground, or pureed form for clients who are unable to chew or swallow
2. Can be used as a long-term diet—preparation of food items is deciding factor
3. Use of seasoning depends on individual client preferences
4. Uses a blender or food processor to change foods into pureed or blended form
5. Certain foods such as raw eggs, nuts, whole breads, raw fruits and vegetables, and foods containing seeds are not allowed

D. Dysphagia diet

1. Uses foods with altered textures and thickened liquids (nectar, honey, or pudding consistency) for clients who have swallowing problems and are at risk for aspiration
2. Thickening agents can also be added to foods to maximize texture and aid swallowing process
3. Dysphagia diet can be prescribed at different levels; pureed foods (Level 1); minced foods, approximately 0.3-cm (⅛-in.) pieces (Level 2); ground foods, approximately 0.6-cm (¼-in.) pieces (Level 3); chopped foods, approximately 1.25-cm (½-in.) pieces (Level 4); or modified regular foods that are soft and moist with regular texture (Level 5)
4. Foods to avoid because of risk of aspiration include stringy, raw, dry, and fried foods, and those that are small in size or hand-held, such as popcorn, nuts, and small candies
5. NCLEX® Position client to at least 30- to 45-degree head elevation, use chin tuck (head and neck slightly flexed), and monitor feedings to decrease risk of aspiration and evaluate client's attempts at eating

E. Soft diet

1. Used for clients who have problems with chewing (dental problems, oral lesions, difficulty chewing or swallowing)
2. Includes food items that contain small amounts of seasoning and moderate fiber content but are easy to chew, digest, and absorb
3. Avoid highly seasoned, fried, and high-fiber foods; nuts; coconuts; and foods that contain seeds because they could cause GI upset
4. Can be used as a progressive or transition diet and is a modification of regular diet

F. Mechanical soft diet

1. Includes all foods and seasonings in a form that is easily handled by client
2. Soft textured, tender, and chopped foods are included in diet, while tough foods (seeds, nuts, and fruits with pits) are not
3. Can be used as a long-term diet or a transition diet
4. Modification of regular diet with attention to texture

G. Bland diet

1. Consists of foods that do not irritate GI tract, reduce gas formation, and reduce gastric acid stimulation
2. Avoids spicy or fried foods, pepper, alcohol, and caffeine–containing beverages
3. Is used for a wide variety of GI disorders, such as esophagitis, gastritis, inflammatory bowel disease

H. High-residue/high-fiber diet

1. Includes intake of 20–25 grams of fiber daily to add bulk to stool and speed rate of passage through GI tract
2. Used for clients with constipation, asymptomatic diverticular disease, and to treat alternating constipation and diarrhea of irritable bowel syndrome; stimulates peristalsis, promotes regularity, and maintains normal bowel function and elimination patterns
3. Fruits, vegetables, legumes, and whole grains are eaten in larger quantities or proportions
4. Additional benefits are reduced serum cholesterol and blood glucose, which is useful to clients with heart disease and diabetes mellitus

I. Low-residue/low-fiber diet

1. Includes foods such as white bread, cereals, and pasta (high CHO)
2. Avoids raw vegetables, fruits (bananas allowed), whole grains, plant fiber, and seeds; limits intake of dairy products to 2 servings daily
3. Fried foods, pepper, alcohol, and heavily seasoned foods are restricted because of possible GI upset
4. Used for conditions in which GI inflammation or scarring has narrowed bowel lumen and food intake could contribute to obstruction, such as inflammatory bowel disease, partial bowel obstruction, enteritis, and diarrhea

VII. RESTRICTED OR ENHANCED DIETS

A. Carbohydrate-controlled

1. Assists in regulating serum glucose levels in conditions such as diabetes mellitus, hypoglycemia, dumping syndrome, galactosemia, and obesity
2. Utilizes a dietary exchange system that groups foods according to protein, CHO, and fat content per specified food serving
3. Includes complex CHOs for 55–60%, proteins for 10–20%, and saturated fats for less than 10% of total daily calories; also includes recommended fiber intake of 20–35 grams/day
4. Gestational diabetes diet encourages adequate calories based on prepregnancy weight status, frequent small feedings, and snacks during day to normalize postprandial glucose levels, maintain euglycemia during pregnancy, and prevent ketosis
5. *NCLEX®* Hypoglycemic diet consists of small feedings at frequent intervals to help normalize blood glucose levels; when episodes of hypoglycemia occur, ingest 15-gram CHO snack, recheck glucose in 15 minutes, and repeat if necessary (15/15 rule)
6. Carbohydrate counting is a means of controlling CHO intake over a 24-hour period

B. Gastric bypass diet

1. *NCLEX®* Consists of eating small nutrient-dense meals several times a day, drinking liquids between meals, instead of with meals, and taking multivitamin supplements
2. Diet is low in fat and high in protein, with restrictions on carbonated beverages, simple CHOs, and foods high in fiber and residue

C. Fat-restricted diet

1. Used to manage malabsorption, chronic pancreatitis, and gallbladder disease
2. Medium-chain triglycerides (MCT) are used in diet because they are easily digested along with high intake of CHOs and protein
3. High-fat foods are limited or omitted (such as red meats and dairy products) and no additional fat is used in cooking process
4. Enzyme replacements and fat-soluble vitamin and mineral supplements may be needed
5. Foods high in oxalates (spinach, rhubarb, sweet potato, beet greens, nuts, wheat bran, tea, and chocolate) are limited to prevent risk of kidney stone formation

6. Fat restriction coupled with sodium restriction is referred to as a cardiac diet, which is indicated as a life-long diet for clients with atherosclerosis, heart disease, hyperlipidemia, and hypertension

D. **Protein-restricted diet**

NCLEX®
1. Used for clients with renal disease (renal failure, end-stage renal disease, dialysis, and transplant) or liver disease (liver failure, hepatic encephalopathy, cirrhosis, transplant, and hepatitis) who are unable to handle protein load
2. Provides protein needed to maintain nutritional status without causing excess wastes or metabolites of protein breakdown (usually 40–60 grams protein daily or 0.8 grams/kg of dry weight)
3. Depending on client's clinical condition, protein levels may be increased to account for metabolic response to dialysis and regeneration of liver tissue (1.5–2.0 grams/kg/day)
4. A minimum level of CHOs must be present in the diet (50–100 grams/day) in order to spare protein; protein intake must be high quality
5. Vitamin and mineral supplements may be prescribed for clients who have liver failure

NCLEX®
6. Restricts foods such as meat, fish, poultry, and dairy products; other foods need to be evaluated individually for protein content

E. **Food allergy diet**

1. Many foods, such as cow's milk, eggs, fish, shellfish, nuts, soybean, and wheat, have allergic potential
2. Primary therapy is avoidance of the particular food item
3. Egg-free diet is used for clients who have a known sensitivity to eggs and restricts use of eggs and egg products
4. Children often present with food allergies and certain diets (allergy I and allergy II) are used in sequence to identify potential food allergens by eliminating their intake in a controlled manner; these diets are used for a limited time frame because they are not nutritionally complete
5. Gluten-restricted diet (gluten gliaden–free diet) is used for clients who have celiac disease (malabsorption syndrome); see Box 25–1
   a. Clinical manifestations caused by inability to handle gluten protein (leading to reduced absorption of nutrients) are steatorrhea, diarrhea, weight loss, anemia, and edema formation
   b. Lactose-intolerant clients must follow additional diet restrictions
6. Lactose-restricted diet is used for clients who have lactose intolerance (lactase enzyme deficiency) and may require lactase enzymes in diet to tolerate dairy products (see Box 25–2)

Box 25–1

Gluten-Restricted Diet

- Foods included: cornmeal, corn flakes, popcorn, hominy, and potato chips
- Food substitutions: corn, potato, rice, and soybean flour and low-gluten wheat flour
- Foods to avoid: processed (commercially prepared) foods with wheat flour extenders, additives, or stabilizers; root beer, beer, and all products that contain identified grain sources (wheat, rye, barley, buckwheat, oats, and malt)

Box 25–2

Lactose-Restricted Diet

- Foods included: aged cheese (hard) rather than soft cheese because hard cheese is lower in lactose due to aging process
- Yogurt can be included because of its bacterial action, and frozen yogurt may have even less lactose due to bacterial action and freezing process
- OTC products such as Lactaid are specific formulations for those with identified lactase deficiency; these products are usually available in liquid or tablet form
- Special milk products formulated with Lactaid are available for use by lactose-intolerant clients (these products are usually sweeter than regular milk products)
- Individual tolerance varies, and client is best judge of how little or how much "lactose" can be ingested without onset of clinical symptoms
- Check food labels for milk, milk solids, casein, and whey, which are sometimes used as additives and stabilizers in processed food products
- Check medication ingredients because lactose can be used as binders or fillers in certain formulations
- Lactose-restricted diets are often low in calcium, vitamin B_2 (riboflavin), and vitamin D, so additional nutrient supplements may be needed

a. Primary lactose intolerance is more common among certain ethnic groups (African American, Asian, Hispanic, and Native American or First Nations)
b. Secondary lactose intolerance is caused by another established disease process (such as infection) or medication (such as chemo agents that inhibit cell growth) that affect GI tract's ability to produce lactase
c. Clinical symptoms affect GI tract, resulting in gas, bloating, and diarrhea

7. Restriction and/or avoidance therapy is used to minimize food allergies

F. Purine-controlled diet

1. Indicated for clients who have gout, tumor lysis syndrome, or multiple myeloma, all of which cause elevated uric acid levels
2. Excessive purine accumulation leads to an increase in uric acid (normal end product of purine catabolism); excess uric acid can be deposited in joints and tissues, and also lead to development of uric acid renal stones
3. *NCLEX®* Includes use of dairy products and restricts organ meats, anchovies, alcohol, and seafood

G. Sodium-controlled diet

1. Indicated for clients with hypertension, cardiovascular disease, heart failure, and conditions in which fluid restriction is beneficial (renal failure, cirrhosis, or liver failure)
2. Restriction ranges from mild (3,000–4,000 mg/day) to severe (500 mg/day)
3. *NCLEX®* It is important to evaluate food labels (sodium is a common preservative), medications, and restaurant dietary intake pattern for hidden sources of sodium
4. Clients using salt substitutes may be at risk for elevated potassium levels and should be evaluated for risk of hyperkalemia, especially if taking potassium-sparing diuretics, such as triamterene
5. *NCLEX®* Avoid table salt and using salt in cooking; meat and dairy products have physiologic saline, while fruits tend to be lowest overall in sodium
6. See Box 25–3 for examples of high-sodium foods to avoid

H. Tyramine- and dopamine-restricted diet

1. Indicated for clients taking monoamine oxidase inhibitor (MAOI) antidepressants; foods containing tyramine affect drug action by blocking enzyme pathways, which leads to norepinephrine release and hypertensive crisis
2. Tyramine is an intermediate product of amino acid metabolism formed in conversion of tyrosine to epinephrine and is found in many food items
3. Other amines, such as dopamine, are also restricted because excess accumulation can lead to similar hypertensive effects
4. *NCLEX®* Diet restrictions include aged cheese, chocolate, smoked fish, processed meats such as bologna, bananas, liver, fava beans, and large amounts of soy sauce
5. Foods that can be eaten are unfermented cheese (ricotta and cottage cheese) and small amounts of certain foods such as sour cream

I. Low-potassium diet

1. Used for clients who have renal failure or take potassium-sparing diuretics
2. Potassium is found in many foods, but avoid high-potassium foods in Box 25–4
3. Reduce potassium content of vegetables by cooking and then draining cooking water; however, this method also reduces vitamin content of foods
4. Avoid use of salt substitutes, which are high in potassium

Box 25–3

Foods High in Sodium

Condiments: pickles, olives, nuts, meat tenderizers, commercial salad dressings, ketchup, soy sauce, Worcestershire and other sauces, monosodium glutamate (MSG), commercial mustard, table salt, and seasoned or buttered salts

Breads: commercial breads with salt added, salted crackers, potato chips, popcorn, pretzels, other salted snacks

Meats: smoked, cured, or processed meats (ham, bacon, hot dogs, luncheon meat, canned meats); all cheeses except cottage cheese and low-sodium cheese

Soups: canned or dehydrated soups, bouillon

Vegetables: sauerkraut, pork and beans, canned tomato or vegetable juices, hominy

Beverages: commercial milk, instant drink mixes

Box 25–4

Foods High in Potassium

Apricots	Dried beans or peas	Potatoes (white or sweet)
Avocado	Dried fruits	Prune juice
Bananas	Melons	Spinach
Cantaloupe	Oranges and orange juice	Tomatoes and tomato products
Raw carrots	Peanuts	Winter squash

J. High-calcium diet

1. Indicated for client disease states that promote calcium loss and lead to bone demineralization (osteoporosis, osteopenia), endocrine abnormalities, and kidney failure

NCLEX® 2. Good sources of calcium include milk and other dairy products; green leafy vegetables are adequate sources

K. High-protein diet

1. The use of a high-protein diet has been indicated for burns, liver disease, and for athletes (1.2–1.6 grams/kg/day) to maximize endurance, according to current research evidence

NCLEX® 2. Includes meat, fish, poultry, and dairy products and protein supplements

L. High-calorie diet

1. Indicated for clients with debilitating disease or need for tissue repair, including cancer, burns, stress, acquired immunodeficiency disease (AIDS), and others
2. Should include added protein to preserve muscle mass
3. Includes nutritious snacks (milkshakes, puddings) between meals and added use of sugars and possibly fats to increase overall calories

M. High-iron diet

1. Indicated for clients with anemia

NCLEX® 2. Includes added sources of iron, such as meat (especially organ meats), egg yolks, leafy vegetables, whole wheat breads and products, legumes, and dried fruits

N. Vegetarian diets

1. Vegan (strict vegetarian): includes plant-based foods with no meat, fish, poultry, dairy products, or eggs
2. Ovo-vegetarian: no meat, fish, or poultry and no dairy products; eggs are allowed
3. Lacto-vegetarian: no meat, fish, poultry, or eggs; dairy products are allowed
4. Ovo-lacto-vegetarian: no meat, fish, or poultry; dairy products and eggs are allowed

VIII. ENTERAL NUTRITION

A. Overview

1. **Enteral nutrition** is a method of feeding clients who have a functioning GI tract but have chewing or swallowing difficulty or impaired upper GI tract function, leading to poor nutrient digestion, transport, and absorption
2. Liquid feedings can be administered for short-term use via nasogastric tubes or oral route, while clients requiring long-term use have an enterostomy placed surgically or percutaneously

B. Administration

1. Continuous feedings are given over a 24-hour period at a prescribed flow rate and a set total volume using an infusion pump
2. Intermittent feedings are given over 30 minutes or more (to mimic usual eating pattern) with a prescribed set total volume ranging from 250 to 400 mL using an infusion pump or gravity
3. **Cyclic feeding** occurs over a period of several hours (prescribed flow rate and a set total volume using an infusion pump), usually at night as a transitional approach to healthy GI functioning
4. **Bolus feeding** occurs when there is a rapid delivery of a large amount of formula in a short time frame (preset volume 250–300 mL in a preset time of 10 minutes or less)

C. Collaborative management

1. Formula selection
   a. Characteristics of formula include protein classification, nutrient density, and amounts of residue and fiber; different osmolality of formulas are available (isotonic and hypertonic)

b. Client's underlying clinical condition influences selection of formula
c. Older adults and newborns may be unable to tolerate large volume feedings and may need modified treatment regimens to meet nutritional needs

NCLEX® 2. Monitoring response to treatment
a. Document weight status; note trends and communicate to healthcare team
b. Monitor for expected weight gain and stabilization of visceral protein measurements (albumin, prealbumin, and transferrin), TLC, BUN, creatinine, and other pertinent serum chemistries during therapy
c. Dietitian will evaluate requirements for macronutrients and fluid requirements based on body-weight calculations

D. Nursing responsibilities

NCLEX® 1. Record baseline weight and then daily weights to evaluate response to therapy
2. Inspect tube insertion site for signs of potential irritation or infection
NCLEX® 3. Check tube placement prior to administering any feeding regimen or medications
a. Aspirate to check for gastric contents and measure pH of gastric aspirant
b. Use stethoscope to auscultate for "whoosh" caused by air placement in stomach if agency does not provide pH testing strips
NCLEX® 4. Check for residual on all tube feedings (based on rate per hour) to prevent complications, and document response to therapy
a. Residuals are often checked every 4 hours during continuous feedings
b. When feedings are intermittent, check residual prior to instituting next feeding
5. If residual amount is greater than expected, feeding will be withheld or rate will be decreased to prevent overload complications caused by inadequate digestion
a. In a continuous feeding checked every 4 hours, if residual is greater than or equal to the 1-hour rate, then feeding should be withheld and residual rechecked in 1 hour to determine if client is now able to tolerate feeding
b. If feeding is not on a continuous schedule, then if half of volume from previous feeding is remaining, feeding should be withheld and residual rechecked in 1 hour as with a continuous feeding
c. Adjustment of volume and/or method of feeding (bolus, continuous, cyclic, or intermittent) may be needed based on residual volume measured
d. Follow agency or provider guidelines if different from those listed above
6. Check pertinent labs, daily weight, and I&O to monitor response to clinical therapy
7. Communicate with other healthcare team members to meet specific client goals
NCLEX® 8. Refer to Box 25–5 for nursing interventions specific to enteral tube feedings
NCLEX® 9. Be aware of potential complications of tube feedings (Box 25–6)

Box 25–5

Interventions for Enteral Tube Feedings

- Inspect formula for particulate matter and unusual appearance that might suggest chemical breakdown
- Do not hang more formula than is allowed per shift according to hospital protocol to prevent bacterial overgrowth and chemical breakdown
- Change solution and tubing per hospital protocol to prevent risk of infection
- Check tube placement prior to any feeding, flush, or medication to ensure patency
- Flush tube with water per hospital protocol to prevent dehydration that can occur if formula feedings are used as the sole fluid replacement
- Include flush or irrigation used in the client's I&O
- Position client to ensure patency and maintain head of bed at 30 degrees prior to and during feeding
- Monitor pertinent labs per hospital protocol and document daily weights
- Work with healthcare team members (dietitian and enterostomal therapist) to maintain nutritional balance and skin integrity
- Address altered nutritional status and body image when developing plan of care

Box 25–6

Complications of Tube Feedings

- Mechanical complications include clogged tube, tube dislodgment, and malfunctioning infusion pump
- Metabolic complications include dehydration, electrolyte imbalances, and altered blood glucose levels (usually hyperglycemia)
- Complications related to formula selection and client tolerance include diarrhea, cramps, abdominal distention, constipation, nausea, and vomiting
- If client is experiencing diarrhea from enteral feedings, a decreased rate and volume of solution may be indicated; the feeding interval may need to be lengthened to allow client to digest and absorb feedings
- Check serum albumin levels because changes in colloid oncotic pressure can cause fluid shifting (greater amount of water in the bowel), which can also lead to diarrhea; low serum albumin levels also represent a malnourished state with decreased intestinal enzyme action that can increase incidence of diarrhea
- Formula may have to be switched to an isotonic formula or a less hypertonic formula to minimize risk of diarrhea from dumping syndrome
- Dermatologic complications include irritation at feeding tube site (enterostomy) caused by leakage of formula or in response to skin applications or dressings at site
- Potential complications from medication instillation via tube include clogging of tube from incorrect medication form or formula–drug interactions
- Monitor amount of feeding and fluid replacement (water) specified per shift and 24-hour totals to minimize risk of dehydration and maintain hydration
- Clients who have nasogastric tube feedings may be at risk for aspiration due to positioning or decreased gastric emptying; maintain adequate client position by elevating head of bed during feedings and check residuals

IX. PROBLEMS WITH WEIGHT CONTROL

A. Overview of obesity

1. Obesity: weight that is more than 20% above ideal body weight (IBW)
2. Caused by an excess of body fat; can exist in a person of normal weight
   a. Men: greater than 22% body fat in young men and greater than 25% body fat in older men
   b. Women: greater than 35% body fat
   c. Morbid obesity is generally more than 100% above ideal body weight and having an adverse effect on a person's health
3. Uncommon causes of obesity include genetic factors (Prader-Willi syndrome)
4. Neuroendocrine causes of obesity include Cushing's syndrome, polycystic ovarian syndrome, hypogonadism, insulinoma, and growth hormone insufficiency
5. Most common cause is dietary; associated with high-fat diet and sedentary lifestyle
6. Some drugs promote obesity, such as estrogens, corticosteroids, antidepressants, antiepileptics, antihypertensives, nonsteroidal anti-inflammatory drugs (NSAIDs), and phenothiazines
7. Social factors such as loneliness, stress, depression, guilt, and boredom, as well as cultural views of obesity as desirable and a sign of prosperity, influence eating habits and development of obesity
8. *NCLEX®* Complications of obesity include hypertension, hiatal hernia, diabetes mellitus, hyperlipidemia, coronary artery disease, sleep apnea, cholelithiasis, osteoarthritis, back pain, and increased susceptibility to infection

B. Nursing assessment of obesity

1. Measure height and weight and determine BMI; refer back to Table 25–2 for interpretation of BMI
2. Assess fat distribution profile: "apple" (intra-abdominal/truncal obesity) and "pear" (hips and thighs) waist-to-hip ratio (greater than 1.0 in males and 0.8 in females) can help establish a diagnosis of obesity
3. Examine body type: endomorph (stocky), ectomorph (tall), and mesomorph (middle range), along with upper body (android) and lower body (gynecoid) categories
4. Calculate body weight as a percentage of IBW, usual weight, and recent weight changes to assist in clinical diagnosis
5. Detect complications of obesity or comorbid conditions by measuring serum glucose, serum cholesterol and lipid profile, and by electrocardiogram (ECG)

NCLEX® 6. Obtain history of eating habits, duration of obesity, medications, cultural factors, 24-hour food recall, usual physical activity, and situations that trigger eating behavior
7. Assess methods used for previous attempts at weight loss

C. Therapeutic management of obesity

1. Diet therapy
    a. Developed collaboratively with client, healthcare provider, and dietitian
    b. Safe weight loss rate is 0.5–0.9 kg (1–2 lb) per week; results may be higher at first and then slow over time; FDA indicates weight loss is effective if maintained for 2 years
    c. Goals of diet therapy are aimed at decreasing weight to a healthy level based on client's BMI, activity status, and basal energy expenditure (BEE)
2. Behavioral therapy: helps client to change daily eating habits and includes keeping a food diary, establishing exercise patterns, controlling external cues to eating behavior, and switching focus from physical appearance to health
3. Surgery is an option for obese individuals who do not respond to other methods of weight loss and have a BMI above 35 with additional health risks, or for anyone with a BMI above 40; most common operative procedures include gastric banding and gastric bypass; pre- and postoperative care is similar to that for other gastric surgeries; acute complications of surgery include nausea, vomiting, heartburn, obstruction, and dumping syndrome
4. NCLEX® Exercise enhances weight loss; recommendations for a healthy lifestyle include at least 30 minutes aerobic activity on most days of week; walking is recommended; plan activity appropriate for client considering physical and environmental limitations
5. Provide information about support groups such as Overeaters Anonymous and Weight Watchers
6. Medication/pharmacological intervention
    a. Drug treatment is controversial and is usually only suggested with BMI above 30 (or >27 with comorbidities) and in conjunction with diet modifications and exercise
    b. Anorexic medications may be used to suppress appetite so client eats less and loses weight slowly over time; they are contraindicated during pregnancy and lactation and in clients with cardiac, hepatic, or renal disease
    c. Amphetamines and antidepressants are controversial because of reported cases of toxicity and dependency

D. Client teaching related to obesity

1. Prescribed diet therapy and exercise
2. Portion control with MyPlate (e.g., a serving of meat is 3 oz and is about the size of a deck of cards; a serving of dry breakfast cereal is 1 oz or 1 cup)
3. Symptoms of possible adverse effects of weight loss medications, such as chest pain, shortness of breath, insomnia, and nervousness

E. Overview of underweight status

1. An **underweight** client has a BMI below 18.5 with subsequent ill effects on health
2. Physical conditions caused by disease or medical treatments can lead to underweight status
3. Failure to thrive (FTT) infants do not meet expected growth curves and developmental milestones and are clinically malnourished; weight and height are below expected percentile; these infants start out underweight and become more underweight over time
4. Psychological conditions (anorexia, bulimia, and depression) can lead to decreased intake, poor nutrition, and underweight status
5. Loss of visceral protein stores (body storage) results in negative nitrogen balance
6. Underweight clients may have adverse health effects if further compromised by stress, injury, or infection

NCLEX® **F. Therapeutic management of underweight status**

1. Increase calories and reestablish regular meal pattern to promote weight gain
2. Increase intake of foods with high nutrient density (highest kcal/food)
3. Calculate ongoing nutrient needs based on BEE and evaluation of pertinent labwork (albumin, prealbumin, transferrin levels, and TLC) in collaboration with dietitian and healthcare provider
4. Refer to Box 25–7 for realistic eating plan to promote weight gain
5. Medication therapy: megestrol acetate and dronabinol as appetite stimulants (useful in clients with cancer, HIV, and AIDS)

G. Overview of malnutrition

1. State of poor nutrition from either undernutrition or overnutrition
2. Includes protein-calorie malnutrition (PCM) or protein-energy malnutrition (PEM)
3. Healing is adversely affected because of loss of protein stores and essential and nonessential nutrients that are coenzymes in metabolic processes

Box 25–7

Realistic Eating Plans for Underweight Client

- Do not skip meals; it is important to start an eating pattern based on eating all scheduled meals.
- Increase portion sizes and add nutrient-dense foods to eating plan; now is the time to add new foods, taste new foods, and sample old foods.
- Drink fluids and make sure to include them as sources of energy by using fruit juices and milkshakes to add to dietary intake.
- Incorporate physical activity to maintain muscle tone, gain strength, and promote endurance.
- Supplemental feedings may be required via enteral or parenteral route to realize dietary goals.
- Be aware of reasonable weight gain expectations and note that weight gained over time is more likely to stay on than weight gained through daily forced feeding.
- Medications may be prescribed to boost appetite and stimulate weight gain; if nausea or other GI symptoms occur, additional medications may be prescribed to minimize these symptoms and promote an adequate eating pattern.

4. Immune function is compromised because of insufficient nutrients
5. Fluid shifts due to low protein levels can lead to third spacing (ascites as in Kwashiorkor) and edema states (dependent and/or periorbital) because of electrolyte imbalances
6. Dermatologic changes include brittle hair that can fall out, nail changes (brittle with ridges), pruritus, and poor healing
7. Hormonal imbalances can develop, affecting neurologic status (irritability, paresthesias, decreased reflex response), musculoskeletal status (decreased muscle tone, cramping, deformities), and cardiac status (altered blood pressure, murmurs, possible cardiac enlargement)
8. Clinical evidence of malnutrition: mouth sores, oral cavity changes, and decreased hydration status

NCLEX® **H. Therapeutic management of malnutrition**

1. Nutrient calculation by dietitian uses BEE, BMI, activity level, and lab results
2. A significant increase in caloric intake is required to effect weight gain (3,500 calories per week for a 1-pound weight gain requires additional 500 calories per day)
3. Supervised program is needed to work toward achieving individual client goals
4. Supplemental feeding may be required via enteral or parenteral routes
5. Frequent feeding regimen may be utilized to prevent hypoglycemia and hypothermia, which can cause further tissue catabolism
6. Controlled regimen for children (not less than 80 calories/kg/day up to 100 or more) and for adults (30–40 kcal/kg/day) may be used to meet nutritional goals
7. Document and trend pertinent labs and weight status and correlate with client's underlying medical condition

I. Weight cycling

1. "Yo-yo" effect is a weight loss/weight gain pattern that can lead to a higher weight than when diet therapy was started; this usually occurs with unrealistic weight goals and/or altered dietary patterns without benefit of activity or lifestyle changes
2. *NCLEX®* For weight control to be effective, a combination of dietary, lifestyle, behavioral, and activity changes (not merely changes in food intake) are necessary

Check Your NCLEX–RN® Exam I.Q.

You are ready for testing on this content if you can:

- Apply knowledge of nursing procedures to the care of a client with nutritional needs.
- Assess nutritional status of client, including a diet history.
- Determine impact of illness on nutritional status.
- Provide a special diet based on health problem and nutritional needs of a client.
- Provide dietary teaching according to client need.
- Provide nutritional supplements to clients as needed.
- Promote independence in eating.
- Check placement and patency of a feeding tube.
- Assess for side effects of enteral nutrition.
- Evaluate effectiveness of diet therapy on weight and overall nutritional status.

PRACTICE TEST

1 The nurse is teaching an adolescent client who is preparing for a long-distance running event about eating for competition. The nurse explains that which type of meal is most appropriate before the competition?

1. Sausages, eggs, biscuits, and gravy
2. Pancakes with fresh strawberries, orange juice, wheat toast, and fresh melon
3. Yogurt, milk fortified with dry skim milk powder, and a protein bar
4. Cheese omelet, hash brown potatoes, bacon, and coffee

2 The nurse who has completed an assessment of a Hispanic client determines that some cultural food practices place the client at risk for cardiovascular disease. Which suggestion by the nurse is appropriate?

1. "Try to stop eating so many complex carbohydrates."
2. "Try to bake some foods instead of frying them."
3. "Lean meats should replace the beans and nuts in your diet."
4. "Do not stop stewing meat and vegetables together; it is a healthy cooking method."

3 Which dietary recommendation should the nurse include in discharge instructions for a client diagnosed with coronary heart disease?

1. Limit intake of whole grains.
2. Limit intake of tuna.
3. Limit intake of soybean products.
4. Limit intake of egg yolks.

4 The nurse is planning discharge teaching for the client with gastroesophageal reflux disease (GERD). What dietary modification should be included?

1. Eat three meals and a bedtime snack.
2. Avoid intake of caffeine and alcoholic beverages.
3. Drink 12–16 ounces of water with each meal.
4. Lie down for 15–20 minutes after eating.

5 The nurse concludes that which behavior by the client is consistent with adherence to a 2-gram sodium-restricted diet?

1. Using only the two packets of salt found on the meal tray
2. Limiting milk to one cup per day
3. Avoiding use of salt in cooking
4. Using salted butter with meals

6 The nurse determines that a hypertensive client understands the DASH diet (Dietary Approaches to Stop Hypertension) when the client chooses which items from a sample menu used in dietary teaching?

1. Caesar salad, bread sticks, frozen yogurt
2. Grilled chicken sandwich, strawberries, and lettuce salad
3. Grilled cheese sandwich, canned pineapple, brownie
4. Chicken and vegetable stir-fry, rice, egg roll

7 A client who is recovering from partial- and full-thickness burns has been advanced to a general diet. Which foods should the nurse encourage the client to eat most often?

1. Meats, citrus fruits, milk
2. Vegetables, cheese, pasta
3. Milkshakes, salads, soups
4. Breads, cereals, yogurt

8 Which client comment indicates to the nurse that more teaching is needed about measures to reduce dumping syndrome after gastric surgery?

1. "I should eat six small meals per day."
2. "I should not drink fluids with my meals."
3. "I should use honey or jelly instead of butter."
4. "I should lie down for 30–60 minutes after eating."

PRACTICE TEST

9. Which statement would the nurse make during dietary teaching to a client who has renal calculi?

1. "The presence of renal calculi is directly correlated to dietary intake."
2. "Decreasing calcium intake will prevent the formation of renal calculi."
3. "An increase in dietary protein can increase the likelihood of renal calculi."
4. "Reducing dietary intake of complex carbohydrates decreases formation of renal calculi."

10. A client with chronic obstructive pulmonary disease (COPD), who ingests more than 3,000 calories/day to gain weight, now reports increased breathing difficulty. The client states, "I thought that if I gained weight by eating more, I would feel better." How should the nurse respond to the client's concern?

1. "The increase in calories is not as important as an increase in the fat percentage in the diet."
2. "It is not necessary to increase caloric intake because medication therapy can be given to help with desired weight gain."
3. "An increase in both calories and carbohydrates can lead to increased respiratory effort and clinical symptoms that you are having."
4. "An increase in high-quality proteins will help correct the respiratory symptoms."

11. Which snack selection would be most appropriate for the nurse to make for a client with cancer who has stomatitis?

1. Peanut butter sandwich
2. Soft pretzels with salt
3. Tomato soup
4. Yogurt

12. A client who is lactose intolerant is recovering from a surgical procedure. What impact should the nurse expect this to have on progression of diet as tolerated?

1. The client will be able to progress from a clear to full liquid diet easily once bowel sounds and gag reflex return.
2. There is no impact with regard to diet progression because of lactose intolerance.
3. The client's diet can be progressed following a bowel movement indicating return of bowel activity.
4. The client's full liquid diet may have to be altered because this diet contains milk products.

13. A client is placed on enteral feedings via nasogastric tube to meet nutritional goals. Which intervention should the nurse include in the plan of care to help maintain fluid balance?

1. Assess the skin area around the tube site.
2. Weigh the client every other day.
3. Maintain strict I&O and flush the tube once a day to ensure patency.
4. Irrigate the tube with water as ordered and include this fluid in total I&O.

14. What information should the nurse provide when doing dietary teaching with a client placed on a fat-restricted diet because of significant cardiac history?

1. "This diet will be used temporarily to reduce saturated fat intake and cholesterol levels."
2. "All forms of fat should be restricted because of your significant cardiac history."
3. "No additional fat should be utilized when cooking or preparing foods."
4. "Ice cream can be included in the diet, although fat from butter and meat is excluded."

15 A client's mother wants to know why she should have her daughter follow an allergy I and II diet. How would the nurse reply to this mother's concern?

1. "This is a short-term therapy diet, and it will be over before you know it."
2. "This diet needs to be followed until your daughter grows out of her allergy phase."
3. "This diet sequence helps to both identify and eliminate potential allergens, making future diet selection choices easier."
4. "Allergy testing usually accompanies this type of diet pattern, and you should see an immunologist."

16 Which food item should the nurse encourage in the diet of a client diagnosed with celiac disease?

1. Oatmeal
2. Whole-wheat toast
3. Beef barley soup
4. Cornflakes

17 Which food item from the lunch menu should the nurse suggest to a client taking a monoamine oxidase inhibitor (MAOI)?

1. Smoked fish
2. Bologna sandwich
3. Cottage cheese
4. Salad with bleu cheese dressing

18 How should the nurse best respond to a client who states, "I am always dieting, but I never seem to be losing weight."

1. "Weight loss is only maintained if you really want to lose the weight."
2. "Dieting is a way of life, and compliance is required to maintain weight loss."
3. "By saying you are always dieting, it sounds like you need some assistance in attaining your weight-loss goals."
4. "I need to know which type of diet you are on because it may not be effective."

19 The nurse should encourage the client wishing to reduce risk of cancer to maintain adequate intake of which foods?

1. Meat and dairy products
2. Fruits and vegetables
3. Rice and beans
4. Milk and cheese

20 An athletic client states that he is thinking of using carbohydrate (CHO) loading to increase his performance. How should the nurse respond to this client?

1. Suggest the use of alternative ergogenic aids such as creatine because they provide better results.
2. Discuss foods that are high in CHOs to assist the client in meeting his desired goal.
3. Ask the client what type of sport activity he is doing to see if this method would help.
4. Refer the client to a sports/nutritional specialist or trainer so that he can be properly supervised.

21 The nurse should consult with the healthcare provider about either advancing the diet or instituting parenteral nutrition if the client has been on a clear liquid diet for the maximum how many days? Provide a numerical answer.

Fill in your answer below:
Answer: ______ days

ANSWERS & RATIONALES

1 **Answer: 2 Rationale:** The diet before competition should be high in complex carbohydrates and low in fat and protein. Pancakes and fruit reflect the best selection to meet this dietary balance. Sausage, eggs, and gravy are high in fat. Fortified yogurt and a protein bar are high in protein but low in carbohydrate. A cheese omelet and bacon is high in fat. **Cognitive Level:** Applying **Client Need:** Basic Care and Comfort **Process:** Nursing Process: Planning **Content Area:** Foundational Sciences: Nutrition **Strategy:** The core issue of the question is knowledge that complex carbohydrates are beneficial before lengthy exercise. Use nutrition knowledge and the process of elimination to make a selection.

2 **Answer: 2 Rationale:** One characteristic of Hispanic diets is the high-fat preparation method used in cooking. Suggesting a new preparation method for a familiar food item would best help the client to begin changing cooking habits. Complex carbohydrates should not be eliminated because they are components of a healthy diet. The Hispanic client would probably be unwilling to relinquish beans and nuts in the diet because these are considered staple food products. Stewing is considered a high-fat method of cooking because the fat from the meat does not drain off. **Cognitive Level:** Applying **Client Need:** Basic Care and Comfort **Integrated Process:** Culture and Spirituality **Content Area:** Foundational Sciences: Nutrition **Strategy:** The core issue of the question is knowledge of methods of reducing fat in the diet. Use nutrition knowledge and the process of elimination to make a selection.

3 **Answer: 4 Rationale:** Egg yolks are high in cholesterol and should be limited to two or three per week. Dietary fiber, fish, and soybean products have been shown to lower blood lipids. Dietary fiber is necessary in the body to promote regulation of elimination patterns and to help lower blood lipids. Soybean products are a source of phytoestrogens and have been shown to be cardioprotective. Tuna is an excellent source of omega-3 fatty acids, which are helpful in protecting cardiac function and decreasing clot formation. **Cognitive Level:** Applying **Client Need:** Basic Care and Comfort **Integrated Process:** Nursing Process: Planning **Content Area:** Foundational Sciences: Nutrition **Strategy:** The core issue of the question is knowledge of the components of a low-fat diet and that this is the diet required by clients with heart disease. Use nutrition knowledge and the process of elimination to make a selection.

4 **Answer: 2 Rationale:** Foods that decrease lower esophageal sphincter (LES) pressure should be avoided to reduce reflux symptoms; these include caffeine, alcohol, and chocolate. Clients should also avoid eating large meals and may benefit from eating smaller, more frequent meals. Fluids should be taken in between meals rather than with meals. Clients should remain upright for 1–2 hours after eating. **Cognitive Level:** Applying **Client Need:** Basic Care and Comfort **Integrated Process:** Nursing Process: Planning **Content Area:** Foundational Sciences: Nutrition **Strategy:** The core issue of the question is knowledge of foods that lower LES pressure and increase risk of reflux in GERD. Use nutrition knowledge and the process of elimination to make a selection.

5 **Answer: 3 Rationale:** A 2-gram sodium-restricted diet requires use of no salt in cooking, no salt added at the table, avoiding high-sodium foods, and limiting milk to two cups per day. No salt can be added in this restricted diet. Limiting milk to one cup per day is part of a 1-gram sodium-restricted diet. A better choice would be to use unsalted butter. **Cognitive Level:** Applying **Client Need:** Basic Care and Comfort **Integrated Process:** Nursing Process: Diagnosis **Content Area:** Foundational Sciences: Nutrition **Strategy:** The core issue of the question is knowledge of the various degrees of sodium restriction in the diet. Use nutrition knowledge and the process of elimination to make a selection.

6 **Answer: 2 Rationale:** The DASH diet increases daily servings of vegetables and fruits, and recommends low-fat dairy foods and less saturated fat and cholesterol. Caesar salad and bread sticks reflect increased fats. Cheese and a brownie represent increased fat, cholesterol, and sugar. Stir-fry and an egg roll reflect increased sodium content. **Cognitive Level:** Applying **Client Need:** Basic Care and Comfort **Integrated Process:** Nursing Process: Evaluation **Content Area:** Foundational Sciences: Nutrition **Strategy:** The core issue of the question is knowledge that hypertensive clients should lose weight if necessary and restrict dietary intake of sodium. Use nutrition knowledge and the process of elimination to make a selection.

7 **Answer: 1 Rationale:** The client with burns needs increased amounts of protein and vitamins C and D until the wounds are completely healed. Foods such as meats, citrus fruits, and milk represent a high-protein source, an antioxidant source, and fortified milk includes vitamin D and calcium. Foods such as vegetables and pasta are low in protein. Foods such as milkshakes, salads, and soups may not provide sufficient protein. Foods such as breads, cereals, and yogurt may not provide sufficient protein, vitamins, and minerals. **Cognitive Level:** Applying **Client Need:** Basic Care and Comfort **Integrated Process:** Nursing Process: Implementation **Content Area:** Foundational Sciences: Nutrition **Strategy:** The core issue of the question is knowledge that increased protein and vitamins are needed for wound healing. Use nutrition knowledge about food sources of protein and vitamins and the process of elimination to make a selection.

8 **Answer: 3 Rationale:** Simple sugars and carbohydrates, including honey and jelly, increase the osmolality of gastric contents and enhance movement of food out of the stomach. These should be avoided by the client at risk for dumping syndrome. Eating six small meals per day will help prevent dumping syndrome. Avoiding fluids with meals helps prevent excess stomach distention and thus may help prevent dumping syndrome. Lying down for 30–60 minutes after meals, rather than remaining upright, may help reduce the risk of dumping syndrome. **Cognitive Level:** Analyzing **Client Need:** Basic Care and Comfort **Integrated Process:** Nursing Process: Evaluation **Content Area:** Foundational Sciences: Nutrition **Strategy:** The stem of the question has negative wording, which tells you that the correct answer is an incorrect statement. Recall that sugars and concentrated carbohydrates should be avoided to help choose the statement that is incorrect.

9 **Answer: 3 Rationale:** Increased dietary protein can lead to increased uric acid formation, which in turn lowers urinary pH and causes precipitation of uric acid stones. Clients should not exceed protein intake of 100 grams per day and should monitor purine content of foods. Factors other than dietary intake can cause stone formation, specifically alterations in urinary pH and the presence of metabolic disease. There is no clinical evidence to suggest that decreasing calcium intake will prevent the formation of renal calculi; rather, research is showing that a high-calcium diet offers protection against stone formation. Even though most renal calculi are composed of calcium oxalate, it is the oxalate component that appears to cause the formation of stones. Increasing intake of complex carbohydrates is recommended to prevent renal calculi formation. **Cognitive Level:** Applying **Client Need:** Basic Care and Comfort **Integrated Process:** Nursing Process: Implementation **Content Area:** Foundational Sciences: Nutrition **Strategy:** The core issue of the question is knowledge that protein sources can lead to uric acid formation and subsequent stone formation. Use nutrition knowledge and the process of elimination to make a selection.

10 **Answer: 3 Rationale:** Clients with COPD who overeat, in addition to consuming excess carbohydrates, have increasing difficulty with breathing because of excessive CO_2 levels that place additional stress on the lungs. The client should eat a proper diet and correct percentages of macronutrients to maintain adequate weight. In addition, chronic COPD is associated with PEM (protein-energy malnutrition), infection, and unintentional weight loss. Increased calories alone can lead to increased work of breathing. The percentage of fat in the diet may also pose a problem if the client is experiencing contributory disease or malabsorption. Merely providing medication therapy to stimulate weight gain does not address the problem of the obvious excess of calories that the client is consuming or that the client is experiencing difficulty breathing. An increase in high-quality proteins will not help to correct the clinical symptoms. **Cognitive Level:** Analyzing **Client Need:** Basic Care and Comfort **Integrated Process:** Communication and Documentation **Content Area:** Foundational Sciences: Nutrition **Strategy:** The core issue of the question is knowledge that excessive carbohydrate intake results in excess carbon dioxide production, which can be harmful to the client with COPD. Use nutrition knowledge and the process of elimination to make a selection.

11 **Answer: 4 Rationale:** A client who has stomatitis will have pain upon ingestion of food caused by the inflammatory process. Cool foods are often tolerated better than hot foods, as are soft, creamy products, such as yogurt. Peanut butter is a thick, dense food that may irritate the mouth by sticking on mucous membranes and requiring more effort to swallow. Pretzels are high in salt, which may cause further irritation to the oral cavity. Tomatoes are high in ascorbic acid; even though they are in the form of a soup, they may cause irritation. **Cognitive Level:** Applying **Client Need:** Basic Care and Comfort **Integrated Process:** Nursing Process: Implementation **Content Area:** Foundational Sciences: Nutrition **Strategy:** The core issue of the question is knowledge that clients with stomatitis need foods that are soft, nonirritating, and not hot. Use nutrition knowledge and the process of elimination to make a selection.

12 **Answer: 4 Rationale:** A client who is lactose intolerant has difficulty handling milk and dairy products because of deficient lactase enzyme. Full liquid diets are likely to contain milk and dairy products, so lactose-reduced or lactose-free products will need to be substituted in the diet to prevent GI irritation. Focusing on the presence of bowel sounds and gag reflex does not reflect the added clinical condition of lactose intolerance. Lactose intolerance does have an impact on diet progression. Diet progression is based on both bowel sounds and tolerance of food intake, not merely on return of a bowel movement pattern. **Cognitive Level:** Analyzing **Client Need:** Basic Care and Comfort **Integrated Process:** Nursing Process: Planning **Content Area:** Foundational Sciences: Nutrition **Strategy:** The core issue of the question is knowledge of concepts related to lactose intolerance. Use nutrition knowledge and the process of elimination to make a selection.

13 **Answer: 4 Rationale:** A client who is receiving enteral feedings via nasogastric tube can be at risk for dehydration caused by inadequate fluid intake. It is therefore important to irrigate the tube with water as prescribed (before and after feedings or medication administration) and include these irrigations in the client's total I&O measurements. Although inspection of the skin surrounding the tube is necessary, it does not relate specifically to fluid balance. Clients are often weighed daily, not every other day. Feeding tubes are flushed at least once per shift, not only once a day. **Cognitive Level:** Applying **Client Need:** Basic Care and Comfort **Integrated Process:** Nursing Process: Planning **Content Area:** Foundational Sciences: Nutrition **Strategy:** The core issue of the question is knowledge that a client receiving enteral feedings is at risk for dehydration if there are no sources of free water provided. Use nutrition knowledge and the process of elimination to make a selection.

14 **Answer: 3 Rationale:** A client with a significant cardiac history on a fat-restricted diet should not use additional fat during the cooking or food preparation process. A client with a significant cardiac history will require lifelong (not temporary) fat restriction. To deprive a client of all fat sources can lead to a clinical deficiency of essential fatty acids that can cause further problems for the client. Ice cream is considered a high-fat product. The client could have low-fat ice cream, yogurt, or sherbet to satisfy dietary needs. **Cognitive Level:** Applying **Client Need:** Basic Care and Comfort **Integrated Process:** Teaching and Learning **Content Area:** Foundational Sciences: Nutrition **Strategy:** The core issue of the question is knowledge of aspects of a low-fat diet and that the diet needs to be lifelong. Use nutrition knowledge and the process of elimination to make a selection.

15 **Answer: 3 Rationale:** Allergy I and II diets are used in sequence to identify and eliminate potential food allergens. Even though the allergy I and II diet pattern is used over a short time period, this response does not address why it is necessary to follow the diet pattern. Implying the client will grow out of it provides inaccurate information. Referral to an immunologist for allergy testing is not a required accompaniment to this dietary pattern, but may eventually be indicated if the client is found to have a multiple allergy profile. **Cognitive Level:** Applying **Client Need:** Basic Care and Comfort **Integrated Process:** Communication and Documentation **Content Area:** Foundational Sciences: Nutrition **Strategy:** The core issue of the question is knowledge of the purposes of allergy I and II diets. Use nutrition knowledge and the process of elimination to make a selection.

16 **Answer: 4 Rationale:** Foods that contain gluten (wheat, oats, rye, and barley) are restricted for a client with celiac disease because of an inability to handle gluten protein. Cornflakes are an acceptable food choice because corn does not contain gluten. Oatmeal contains oats, which contain gluten. Whole-wheat toast contains wheat, which contains gluten. Beef barley soup contains barley, which contains gluten. **Cognitive Level:** Applying **Client Need:** Basic Care and Comfort **Integrated Process:** Nursing Process: Implementation **Content Area:** Foundational Sciences: Nutrition **Strategy:** The core issue of the question is knowledge that a food containing wheat, rye, oats, and barley are restricted in celiac disease. Use nutrition knowledge about foods containing these grains and the process of elimination to make a selection.

17 **Answer: 3 Rationale:** A client taking MAOIs has to avoid foods high in tyramine because it can lead to hypertensive crisis. Cottage cheese is an unfermented cheese and is acceptable; aged cheeses are not allowed in the diet. Smoked fish is high in tyramine and is prohibited. Bologna and other lunch meats contain tyramine and are prohibited. Although salad is acceptable, the bleu cheese dressing (made with an aged cheese) is high in tyramine. **Cognitive Level:** Analyzing **Client Need:** Basic Care and Comfort **Integrated Process:** Nursing Process: Planning **Content Area:** Foundational Sciences: Nutrition **Strategy:** The core issue of the question is knowledge that clients taking MAOIs require a low-tyramine diet. Use nutrition knowledge of low-tyramine foods and the process of elimination to make a selection.

18 **Answer: 3 Rationale:** The perception of being in a state of "always dieting" can be problematic in terms of compliance and goal attainment because it can be viewed either as a restriction or as a form of punishment. Compliance is not always the issue. Wanting to lose weight is not the only factor to consider; many other variables affect weight loss. While it is important to find out the type of the diet the client is on (or has been on), this knowledge doesn't address the main concern of the client regarding "always dieting" and the yo-yo effect (weight cycling). **Cognitive Level:** Applying **Client Need:** Basic Care and Comfort **Integrated Process:** Communication and Documentation **Content Area:** Foundational Sciences: Nutrition **Strategy:** The core issue of the question is identification of a client's need for assistance with weight control. Use nutrition knowledge and the process of elimination to make a selection.

19 **Answer: 2 Rationale:** Diets that are rich in fruits and vegetables have been proven to be effective in decreasing the risk of developing cancer because these foods contain phytochemicals. Meat and dairy products do not protect against cancer. Rice and beans do not offer protection against cancer. Milk and cheese are high in calcium but have not been shown to decrease the risk of cancer. **Cognitive Level:** Applying **Client Need:** Basic Care and Comfort **Integrated Process:** Nursing Process: Implementation **Content Area:** Foundational Sciences: Nutrition **Strategy:** The core issue of the question is knowledge of foods that contain protective chemicals against cancer development. Use nutrition knowledge and the process of elimination to make a selection.

20 **Answer: 4 Rationale:** When an athletic client is considering utilizing any ergogenic aid or supplement, trainers and/or nutritional specialists can monitor the client closely to establish a client baseline, provide education, and prevent potential complications related to therapy. A nurse should not suggest an alternative ergogenic aid. The client needs a proper referral to an expert in the field. Discussing foods that are high in CHO does not address the priority need—to make the referral. Although it is important to note what type of exercise the client practices, it is still more important to refer the client to the proper specialist who can assist in supervising an athletic treatment regimen. **Cognitive Level:** Applying **Client Need:** Management of Care **Integrated Process:** Nursing Process: Implementation **Content Area:** Foundational Sciences: Nutrition **Strategy:** The core issue of the question is appropriate anticipatory guidance to a client seeking to use nontraditional methods of nutrition for supplemental use. Use knowledge that this client requires special monitoring and the process of elimination to make a selection.

21 **Answer: 2 Rationale:** A clear liquid diet is recommended for short-term use (1–2 days). Therefore, the maximum time frame is 2 days. It can be used both before and after surgery or diagnostic procedures, during acute stages of illness, or as an initial diet after a significant period of GI inactivity or bowel rest. **Cognitive Level:** Applying **Client Need:** Basic Care and Comfort **Integrated Process:** Nursing Process: Implementation **Content Area:** Foundational Sciences: Nutrition **Strategy:** The core issue of the question is the length of time a clear liquid diet is appropriate. Use knowledge of clear liquid diet as a therapeutic diet to make a selection.

Key Terms to Review

bolus feeding p. 362
cyclic feeding p. 362
enteral nutrition p. 362
ergogenic aids p. 357
obesity p. 354
phytochemicals p. 357
underweight p. 365

ANSWERS & RATIONALES

References

Ball, J., & Bindler, R., & Cowen, K. (2015). *Principles of pediatric nursing: Caring for children* (6th ed.). Hoboken, NJ: Pearson Education.

Berman, A., Snyder, S., & Frandsen, G. (2016). *Kozier & Erb's fundamentals of nursing: Concepts, process, and practice* (10th ed.). New York, NY: Pearson Education.

Lutz, C. & Mazur, E. (2014). *Nutrition and diet therapy* (6th ed.). Philadelphia, PA: F. A. Davis.

Ross, A., Caballero, B., Cousins, R., Tucker, K., & Ziegler, T. (Eds.) (2014). *Modern nutrition in health and disease* (11th ed.). Philadelphia, PA: Lippincott, Williams, & Wilkins.

Smith, S., Duell, D., Martin, B., Aebersold, M., & Gonzalez, L. (2017). *Clinical nursing skills: Basic to advanced skills* (10th ed.). New York, NY: Pearson Education.

Tucker, S., & Dauffenbach, V. (2011). *Nutrition and diet therapy for nurses*. Upper Saddle River, NJ: Pearson Education.

U.S. Department of Agriculture (n.d.). *MyPlate.* Available at http://www.choosemyplate.gov.

U.S. Department of Health and Human Services (USDHHS) and U.S. Department of Agriculture (USDA). (n.d.). *Dietary guidelines for Americans 2015–2020* (8th ed.). Washington, DC: Author. Available at http://health.gov/dietaryguidelines/2015/guidelines/.

Test Yourself

Are you ready for the NCLEX-RN® or course exams? Access the NEW web-based app that provides students with thousands of practice questions in preparation for the NCLEX experience.

26 Meeting Basic Human Needs

In this chapter

Cross Reference

Other chapters relevant to this content area are

Meeting Nutritional Needs	Chapter 25
Maintaining the Function of Tubes and Drains	Chapter 27
Eye, Ear, Nose, and Throat Disorders	Chapter 63

I. HYGIENE NEEDS

A. Functions of skin

1. Protection against microorganisms
2. Sensation of pain, temperature, and pressure
3. Temperature regulation and excretion of water, electrolytes, and urea through sweat

B. Skin care

1. Developmental changes: age and ability influence skin care practices
   a. A newborn requires only sponge baths, not tub baths; dry newborn immediately and wrap to prevent heat loss; shivering in newborns starts at a lower body temperature than in adults, and infants have greater body surface area for heat loss compared to adults
   b. A toddler depends on caregiver to provide care but may want to perform tasks (such as brushing teeth) independently
   c. A frail older adult may require assistance but may still have skin care preferences; excessive bathing can contribute to dry skin
2. Cultural considerations
   a. Hygiene practices vary considerably among cultures; in some, daily bathing is a ritual, while in others, weekly is acceptable; other differences may be use of deodorants and preference for tub or shower
   b. Some cultures are concerned with hot/cold imbalances as a cause of illness
   c. Bathing may be avoided with some body conditions; for instance, some cultures avoid bathing during menstruation and childbirth

NCLEX®

3. Common skin problems requiring care
   a. Dryness: flaky, rough skin may crack; pruritus (itching) may occur
   b. Abrasions: epidermis (superficial layer of skin) rubbed or scraped off

Box 26–1

Care of an Eye Prosthesis

- Using gloves, exert slight pressure below eyelid and remove artificial eye.
- Clean eye socket and periorbital tissues with moistened washcloth.
- Clean artificial eye with warm normal saline and rinse.
- To reinsert prosthetic eye:
  - Retract eyelids and exert pressure on supraorbital and infraorbital bones.
  - Hold prosthetic eye with index finger and thumb of other hand and slip it gently into socket.

c. Ammonia dermatitis (diaper rash): reddened skin that may be excoriated, caused by skin bacteria reacting to urea in urine
d. Contact dermatitis: reddened skin accompanied by pruritus that may result in infection if scratched
e. Erythema: redness of skin associated with rashes, infections, and allergies
f. **Pressure injury**: an open skin lesion, often over bony prominences, caused by decreased circulation

C. Specific hygiene measures

1. May include complete bed bath, partial bed bath, perineal care to genitalia and rectal area, and/or nail and foot care
2. *NCLEX®* Document observations such as general skin condition, reddened areas over bony prominences, irritation, and inflammation
3. Oral care: brushing and flossing teeth and denture care; document abnormalities such as irritated mucous membranes and ill-fitting dentures
4. Hair and scalp care: includes brushing and shampooing hair; personal habits and cultural influences affect hair care practices; clean hair limits microbe count, and groomed hair can increase general comfort level
5. Care of eyes, ears, and nose
   a. *NCLEX®* Eye care: wipe from inner to outer canthus; for unconscious client, use artificial tears every 2 hours or as prescribed to reduce corneal injury
   b. Ear care: if cerumen (earwax) is visible, retract auricle downward, then remove with a damp washcloth
6. Care of removable prosthetic (artificial) eye: see Box 26–1
7. Promote client independence as much as possible during care
8. *NCLEX®* Document ability to bathe, feed, groom, and toilet self as indicators of functional ability; communicate this information to discharge planners, long-term or rehabilitation care centers, and home health nurses

D. Care of client's room environment

1. *NCLEX®* Keep area clutter-free
   a. Arrange furniture to avoid accidents; for example, no furniture in middle of room
   b. Remove unnecessary objects; keep obstacles out of walkways
2. Keep objects needed for activities of daily living within reach (e.g., eyeglasses, cane, fluids, and call bell)
3. Control odors: provide good ventilation, remove and dispose of offensive waste products, and use room deodorizers as needed

II. OXYGENATION NEEDS

A. Summary of physiology of cardiovascular and respiratory systems

1. Heart pumps blood through blood vessels to tissues and transports blood containing oxygen and nutrients to cells; wastes are collected for elimination
2. Respiratory system
   a. Pulmonary ventilation, or breathing: inspiration (inhalation)—air flows into lungs; expiration (exhalation)—air moves out of lungs
   b. Alveolar gas exchange: after alveoli are ventilated, diffusion of oxygen occurs from alveoli into pulmonary blood vessels
   c. Oxygen (O_2) is transported from lungs to tissues, and carbon dioxide (CO_2) is transported from tissues back to lungs; O_2 combines with hemoglobin in red blood cells (RBCs) and is carried to tissues as oxyhemoglobin

B. Factors affecting oxygenation

1. Environment
   a. Altitude: higher altitude increases respiratory rate and depth and heart rate (HR)
   b. Heat: causes peripheral vessel dilation, increased blood flow to skin, and decreased resistance to blood flow; cardiac output (CO) increases, raising blood pressure (BP); rate and depth of breathing also increase
   c. Cold: vasoconstriction occurs; slowed metabolism reduces need for O_2
   d. Air pollution: causes symptoms such as coughing, choking, and difficulty breathing
   e. Health status: healthy clients have sufficient O_2 to meet body's demands; in cardiovascular disease, O_2 transport is compromised; in respiratory disease, oxygenation of blood is affected

   NCLEX® f. Narcotics: opioids such as morphine decrease respiratory rate and depth by depressing respiratory center of medulla
2. Developmental factors

   NCLEX® a. Premature infants: inadequate respiratory status is caused by immature lungs; respiratory center of brain is immature; gag and cough reflexes are weak

   NCLEX® b. Infants and toddlers: smaller airway passages contribute to obstruction by foreign objects such as peanuts, coins, and small toys; diseases such as cystic fibrosis and asthma affect oxygenation

   c. Because of exposure to infectious agents at school and at play, upper respiratory problems are common in school-age children
   d. At puberty, heart and lungs increase considerably in size and heart rate drops
   e. Starting at age 35–40, aerobic capacity (ability to provide O_2 to body's organs) and CO show age-related changes during work or exercise; loss of blood vessel elasticity may contribute to hypertension, which affects oxygenation; atherosclerosis (plaque buildup in arterial walls) decreases blood flow

   NCLEX® f. In older adults, chest wall becomes more rigid and lungs are less elastic, so more air is retained in lungs at expiration; cough effectiveness decreases; protective cilia are less effective, increasing risk of upper respiratory infections; decreased respiratory reserve reduces exercise tolerance; blood flow may be impaired by hypertension, atherosclerosis, and obstructive lung disease
3. Lifestyle factors
   a. Nutrition: high fat and salt intake may increase risk for heart disease, and inadequate diet can lead to anemia (insufficient RBCs)
   b. Physical exercise: increases rate and depth of respirations and HR, thus increasing supply of oxygen in body

   NCLEX® c. Smoking: nicotine increases HR, BP, and peripheral resistance; vasoconstriction occurs and decreases oxygenation to tissues

   d. Substance use: alcohol is a respiratory depressant and slows respirations; long-term use increases BP and tendency for malnutrition and anemia

   NCLEX® e. Anxiety: when moderate or severe, client hyperventilates and arterial O_2 pressure rises and CO_2 pressure falls; client often reports lightheadedness, numbness of fingers and toes; epinephrine and norepinephrine released under stress increase BP and HR

C. Alterations in respiratory functioning

1. **Hyperventilation**: increased rate and depth of respirations; causes include stress and increased CO_2 retention; metabolic acidosis may cause Kussmaul breathing, a type of hyperventilation
2. **Hypoventilation**: decreased rate and/or depth of respirations leading to inadequate alveolar ventilation; causes include alveolar collapse, airway obstruction, and sedative or narcotic drug side effect; CO_2 retained in bloodstream; can lead to hypoxia

NCLEX® 3. Hypoxia: inadequate amount of O_2 transported to tissues
   a. Manifestations: rapid HR, rapid shallow respirations, **dyspnea** (difficulty breathing progressing to air hunger), flaring of nostrils, restlessness, substernal or intercostal retractions, and cyanosis; in chronic hypoxia, client may have fatigue, lethargy, and clubbing of digits
   b. Causes: anemia, pulmonary edema, heart failure; drugs such as anesthetics

Memory Aid

Early respiratory symptoms are mild in nature, such as increasing respiratory rate and mild dyspnea; later signs are more extreme, such as severe dyspnea and air hunger.

4. Cyanosis: bluish discoloration of skin, nail beds, and mucous membranes; very late indicator of hypoxia; causes include severe anemia, respiratory tract obstruction, heart disease, cold environment

Memory Aid

Cyanosis is always a late sign, regardless of what the health problem is!

5. Pain: chest pain can impair breathing patterns and respiratory functioning
   a. Manifestations: reports of pain that may be dull, aching, persistent, or localized and radiating; pallor; rapid or slowed breathing; anxiety; rapid HR
   b. Causes: respiratory diseases such as pneumonia, pulmonary embolism, advanced bronchogenic carcinoma; heart conditions, such as coronary artery disease and angina
6. **Orthopnea**: positional breathing discomfort associated with lying down; client needs to have head and chest elevated, sit, or stand to breathe comfortably; causes include respiratory and cardiac diseases, airway obstruction
7. Wheezing: high-pitched, continuous musical, rasping, or whistling sound heard during inspiration or expiration; does not clear with coughing; caused by severely narrowed bronchus or bronchioles
8. Cough: natural lung clearance mechanism to remove secretions through forced exhalation; causes include excessive sputum production, allergies, or pulmonary diseases
9. Hemoptysis: bright red, frothy blood mixed with sputum; initial symptoms include tickling in throat, salty taste, burning or bubbling sensation in chest; causes include lung infection, lung cancer, or heart or blood vessel abnormalities

D. Nursing interventions to promote oxygenation

1. Positioning: Fowler's position (head of bed elevation) promotes maximum chest expansion to ease dyspnea; reposition client side to side every 1–2 hours so alternate sides of chest can expand
2. Decrease anxiety: promote relaxation techniques, alleviate pain by using distraction or guided imagery
3. Deep breathing and coughing: helps to clear fluid from lungs and promote oxygenation
   a. Help client assume a comfortable position: sitting or lying position with knees flexed
   b. Place one hand on abdomen just below ribs
   c. With mouth closed, breathe in deeply through nose to count of three; concentrate on feeling abdomen rise
   d. Purse lips and breathe out slowly and gently; concentrate on feeling abdomen fall and tightening abdominal muscles; count to seven during exhalation
   e. Repeat several times (but avoid hyperventilation) and repeat 5–10 times hourly; a memory cue may be to do this during television commercials
   f. For coughing: inhale deeply and hold breath for a few seconds, lean forward, and cough rapidly using abdominal, thigh, and buttock muscles (coughing is contraindicated in postoperative eye, ear, neck, or brain surgery or in other clients at risk for increased intracranial pressure)

Memory Aid

Airway and breathing are the A and B of ABCs. Assessments and interventions to promote these are high priority using Maslow's hierarchy of needs theory for prioritizing care.

4. Suctioning: oro/nasopharyngeal, tracheal
   a. See Box 26–2 for procedure
   b. *NCLEX®* Limit suctioning time to 10 seconds (no O_2 exchange during this time); provide rest periods between suctioning to allow client to inhale oxygen
   c. *NCLEX®* Assess for dysrhythmias or cyanosis as grave indicators of inadequate oxygenation; hyperoxygenate before suctioning, between attempts, and when suctioning is complete
5. Chest physiotherapy: percussion, vibration, postural drainage (often done by respiratory therapist unless nurse is authorized and competent to perform)
   a. Percussion (clapping): cup the hands and alternately flex and extend wrists rapidly over affected lung segments for 1–2 minutes; yields a hollow sound if done correctly
   b. Vibration (vigorous or high-frequency quivering over chest wall) is done during exhalation only; tense hand and arm and, using mostly heel of hand, vibrate or shake hands against client's chest; perform five times over each lung segment; vibration may be done after percussion or may be alternated with percussion over affected lung segments

Box 26–2

Summary of Key Points for Suctioning with a Multiuse Catheter in Sleeve

- Prepare equipment: suction unit with tubing and collection container; sterile normal saline or water; clean gloves; water-soluble lubricant; Y-connector; sterile gauzes; disposal bag.
- Select appropriate sterile suction catheters, usually #12 to #18 for adults, #8 to #10 for children, and #5 to #8 for infants.
- Set pressure on wall suction gauge (adults: 100–120 mm Hg; children: 95–110; infants: 50–95).
- Explain procedure to client; place a conscious client in a semi-Fowler's or Fowler's position or an unconscious client in a lateral position with head turned toward nurse.
- Don personal protective equipment (protect against splash); apply gloves, hold catheter in protective covering, and attach end to suction tubing.
- Measure distance between client's nose and earlobe (approximately 13 cm or 5 in. for adult) and mark position with fingers of gloved hand; test pressure and patency by placing nodominant thumb or finger on port or open branch of Y-connector.
- Hyperoxygenate client with deep breaths or using resuscitator (Ambu) bag.
- Retract sleeve to lubricate catheter tip with sterile water or saline (or for nasopharyngeal suctioning, may use lubricant)
- Insert catheter while retracting protective sleeve without applying suction pressure.
  - For oropharyngeal suctioning: pull tongue forward with gauze; introduce and advance catheter along one side of mouth into oropharynx; it may be necessary to suction secretions that collect in buccal cavity.
  - For nasopharyngeal suctioning: introduce catheter through nostril (naris) and advance to recommended distance.
  - For tracheal suctioning: insert during inhalation because epiglottis is open; advance catheter to approximately 28 cm (11 in.), or 1 cm beyond end of tracheostomy or endotracheal tube; retract slightly if resistance is met (expect client to cough during insertion).
- Apply suction intermittently (place and release thumb over catheter suction port) and rotate catheter while retracting it into protective sleeve; limit suctioning to 10 seconds maximum for single pass of catheter.
- Allow 20- to 30-second interval of rest between each suction attempt; oxygenate client between attempts and at completion of procedure.
- Flush suction catheter and tubing with sterile saline or water and retract catheter into protective sleeve; keep sleeved catheter attached to suction tubing for repeated use up to 24 hrs (or per agency policy); note that a separate catheter must be used for suctioning pharynx.
- Provide nasal or oral hygiene; dispose of equipment.
- Assess effectiveness of suctioning: observe respiratory rate, skin color, dyspnea, and level of anxiety; document relevant information.

c. Postural drainage involves positioning client so that head is lower than chest (in prone or side-lying position) to promote drainage of secretions from affected lung segment(s); may be done during or after percussion and vibration

NCLEX®

6. Oxygen therapy: when oxygen therapy is used, follow safety precautions (see Box 26–3)

a. Check oxygen prescription and assess client's respiratory and cardiovascular status

b. Explain procedure and place client in a semi-sitting position

c. Set up O_2 equipment: attach flow meter to wall outlet or portable oxygen cylinder; fill humidifier with water and attach to base of flow meter

d. Attach delivery system and tubing to flow meter; turn on O_2 at prescribed rate; see Table 26–1 for types of O_2 delivery systems

e. Assess respiratory and cardiovascular status regularly; check nares for irritation if cannula is used, facial skin if face mask is used; document observations

f. Check flow of O_2 and level of water in humidifier regularly

Box 26–3

Safety Precautions During Oxygen Therapy

- Place cautionary signs reading, "No Smoking: Oxygen in Use" on client's door, at head or foot of bed, and near home use oxygen equipment.
- Instruct client and visitors about danger of smoking when oxygen is in use; if necessary, remove matches, lighters, and ashtrays.
- If oxygen therapy is used at home, instruct family members or caregivers to smoke only outside; if smoking is permitted, teach visitors to use smoking room.
- Avoid materials that generate static electricity, such as woolen blankets and synthetic fabrics; use cotton fabrics instead.
- Avoid use of volatile, flammable substances such as acetone in nail polish removers, alcohol, ether, and oils near clients using oxygen.
- Remove any friction-type or battery-operated gadgets, devices, or toys.
- Make sure electronic devices such as radios, televisions, and electric razors are in good working order to prevent short-circuit sparks.
- Ensure that electric monitoring equipment and machines used in client care are properly grounded; disconnect any ungrounded equipment.
- Know location and proper use of fire extinguishers; know location of oxygen meter turn-off lever.

Table 26–1 Types of Oxygen Delivery Systems

Type	Description
Nasal cannula (prongs)	Has double short prongs inserted into nostrils; most common device; does not interfere with ability to eat or talk. Reservoir cannulas are oxygen-conserving devices often used in home settings. Often uses flow of 1–6 L/min of a 23–42% O_2 concentration.
Oxygen mask	Most effective means of delivering O_2; types include simple, partial rebreather, nonrebreather, and Venturi masks (see below). Made of clear, pliable plastic that covers nose and mouth and is held in place with elastic band around head; many have a metal clip over nose to allow for snug fit.
Simple face mask	Useful for short-term therapy (i.e., early postoperative period or when intermittent O_2 therapy is required). Delivers O_2 concentration of 40–60% at a flow rate of 5–8 L/min.
Partial rebreather mask	Has a reservoir bag and a partial rebreathing valve. Delivers O_2 concentration of 40–60% at a flow rate of 6–10 L/min. On expiration, reservoir bag conserves approximately one-third of exhaled air, which allows client to inhale additional O_2 previously exhaled. To prevent rebreathing exhaled CO_2 reservoir bag should deflate only slightly on inhalation. If it fully deflates, increasing O_2 flow rate should correct problem.
Nonrebreather mask	Has a reservoir bag and one-way valves at sides of mask and between reservoir bag and mask. Delivers highest O_2 concentration of 95–100% by mask at a flow rate of 10–15 L/min adjusted to keep reservoir bag inflated. On inhalation, O_2 flows into bag and mask; one-way valves prevent exhaled air from reentering bag and mask. At times one side valve can be removed to allow client to breathe room air if O_2 supply is accidentally cut off. Used for short-term therapy, such as counteracting smoke inhalation.
Venturi mask	Has wide-bore tubing and color-coded jet adapters that allow for precise delivery of O_2 concentrations of 25–50% at matched flow rates of 4–10 L/min. Increasing flow rates alone will not increase O_2 concentration delivered to client because O_2 % is set by jet adapter.
Face tent	Useful when client cannot tolerate snug fit of face mask. Delivers varying O_2 concentration of about 30–50% because mask is open at a flow rate of 4–8 L/min.
Transtracheal catheter	Delivers humidified O_2 at greater than 1 L/min and up to 15–20 L/min. Tube is placed through surgically created tract that has matured (healed). Tube is held in place by securing faceplate around neck. Client removes and cleans catheter between two and four times per day.
Noninvasive positive pressure ventilation (NPPV)	Delivers air or oxygen under constant pressure without need for invasive tube. Useful for clients with acute or chronic respiratory failure, COPD, and obstructive sleep apnea. Continuous positive airway pressure (CPAP) can be delivered using a mask fitted over nose and secured with straps around head and under chin. Bilevel positive airway pressure (BiPAP), a variation of CPAP, delivers lower pressure on exhalation than on inhalation.

7. Incentive spirometer
   a. Check prescription; assist client to a sitting or Fowler's position and explain procedure
   b. Assemble equipment; set marker at recommended volume goal
   c. Instruct client to exhale and then place mouth tightly around mouthpiece
   d. Instruct client to inhale slowly and maintain a steady flow, like pulling through a straw; encourage client to raise and maintain flow rate indicator
   e. Instruct client to remove mouthpiece but hold breath for 2–3 seconds and then exhale slowly through pursed lips
   f. Have client repeat procedure a few times and then cough; encourage to use 5–10 times hourly; keep spirometer within reach of client

III. CLIENT'S NEED FOR SLEEP

A. Physiology of sleep

1. Circadian rhythm: rhythmic repetition of patterns each 24 hours; when client's biological clock coincides with sleep–wake patterns, client is in **circadian synchronization**
2. Sleep regulation: centers in lower portion of brain actively inhibit wakefulness, causing sleep
3. NREM (non–rapid eye movement): deep and restful sleep characterized by decrease in physiologic functions: BP and HR decrease, skeletal muscles relax, basal metabolic rate (BMR) decreases, brain waves become slower; there are four stages of NREM
   a. Stage I: very light sleep; sleeper is relaxed and drowsy and feels a floating sensation; eyes roll from side to side; lasts only a few minutes
   b. Stage II: light sleep; sleeper is easily roused; HR and respiratory rate (RR) decrease slightly; lasts 10–15 minutes
   c. Stage III: medium-depth sleep; sleeper is less easily aroused; HR, RR, BP, and temperature continue to fall; skeletal muscles are relaxed, reflexes are diminished; snoring may occur
   d. Stage IV: called delta sleep; deepest stage; sleeper is difficult to rouse and rarely moves; muscles are completely relaxed; dreaming may occur; may last about 30 minutes
4. REM (rapid eye movement) sleep: usually occurs every 90 minutes and lasts 5–30 minutes; active dreaming occurs and dreams are remembered; brain is highly active, and sleeper is difficult to rouse or may wake up spontaneously; REM and irregular muscle movements occur; muscle tone is depressed; HR and RR are irregular

B. Normal sleep requirements and patterns

1. Neonates: newborns sleep, on average, 16–18 hours per day, divided into about seven sleep periods; most NREM sleep is spent in stages III and IV, and nearly 50% is in REM sleep
2. Infants: range of sleep is 12–22 hours; periods of wakefulness increase with age; by 4 months, infants sleep through night and nap during day; at end of first year, they sleep about 14 of every 24 hours; half of time, infants have light sleep, and 20–30% is REM sleep
3. *NCLEX®* Toddlers: normal sleep–wake cycle established by 2–3 years; generally sleep for 10–12 hours, still require a midafternoon nap, but morning nap needs decrease; still 20–30% is REM sleep
4. Preschoolers: need 11–12 hours sleep but may fluctuate because of activity and growth spurts; older preschoolers do not need a nap; continue to have 20–30% REM sleep
5. School-age: most school-age children sleep 8–12 hours without daytime naps; REM sleep decreases to about 20%
6. Adolescents: amount of sleep time declines, but adolescents still need 8–10 hours of sleep; changes in pattern occur for adolescents who need daytime napping
7. Young adults: generally, young adults require 7–8 hours, but because of lifestyle changes, they may have erratic sleep patterns
8. Middle-aged adults: sleep pattern established earlier is maintained, and middle-aged adult sleeps 6–8 hours/night; about 20% is REM sleep; duration of stage IV NREM sleep decreases
9. *NCLEX®* Older adults: sleep about 6 hours a night with about 20–25% REM and a marked decrease in stage IV NREM sleep; they awaken more frequently and have difficulty returning to sleep, so they experience less restorative sleep

C. Factors affecting sleep

1. Illness: increases sleep requirement but may cause pain, breathing difficulty, or discomfort with movement that interferes with sleep; elevated body temperature can reduce stages III and IV NREM and REM sleep

2. Drugs and substances
   a. Excessive alcohol may accelerate onset of sleep but disrupts REM sleep; individuals with tolerance to alcohol may have difficulty with sleep, and when drug effects wear off, may have nightmares
   NCLEX® b. Caffeine and amphetamines are stimulants and interfere with sleep
   c. Nicotine has stimulating effect, and smokers may have more difficulty falling asleep
3. Lifestyle: shift work may interfere with ability to adjust sleeping patterns; inactivity or boredom may contribute to sleep problems
4. Usual sleep patterns and excessive daytime sleepiness: individuals often refer to themselves as morning or night people, which coincides with their wake and sleep patterns; excessive daytime sleepiness may be caused by nighttime sleep deprivation
5. Emotional stress: anxiety makes it difficult to fall asleep; depression may cause difficulty in falling asleep or premature awakening
6. Environment: any change in noise level may inhibit sleep—people are habituated to certain noises; ventilation and environmental temperature can affect sleep
7. NCLEX® Various prescribed drugs: decongestants, narcotics, sedatives, beta-blockers, and antidepressants may cause drowsiness and may disrupt REM sleep
8. Exercise and fatigue: moderate exercise is conducive to sleep but, if excessive, may delay sleep; moderate fatigue may lead to a restful sleep
9. Food/calorie intake: weight loss may be associated with reduced quantity of sleep, broken sleep, and earlier awakening; weight gain may be associated with increased total sleep time, less broken sleep, and later waking

D. Overview of sleep disorders

1. Insomnia: inability to obtain an adequate amount or quality of sleep
   a. Can be initial (difficulty falling asleep), middle or intermittent (difficulty maintaining sleep because of frequent or prolonged waking), or terminal (early or premature awakening), which may be associated with depression
   NCLEX® b. Treatment usually involves developing new sleep-inducing and sleep-maintaining behaviors such as modifying environment or relaxation techniques
2. Sleep apnea: periodic cessation of breathing during sleep; episode lasts from 10 seconds to 2 minutes, and incidence may range from 50 to 600 per night
   a. Suspected when person snores loudly, has frequent nocturnal awakening, and experiences excessive daytime sleepiness, fatigue, irritability, and personality changes caused by disrupted sleep
   b. Incidence of sleep apnea is higher in older adult men and with obesity
   c. Complications of prolonged sleep apnea may be increased BP, cardiac dysrhythmias, and left-sided heart failure
   d. Treatment is directed at cause: if obstructive, enlarged tonsils or adenoids may be removed
   e. Use of a CPAP device is often effective
3. Narcolepsy: overwhelming daytime sleepiness caused by lack of chemical (hypocretin) that regulates sleep; client may doze while involved in activities; treated with stimulants, such as amphetamines
4. Parasomnias: abnormal behavioral or physiologic events associated with stages of sleep and that interfere with sleep; treatment consists of relaxation technique and sleep hygiene practices
   a. Somnambulism: sleepwalking that occurs in stages III and IV NREM sleep; it is episodic and occurs 1–2 hours after falling asleep; sleepwalker does not notice dangers such as stairs and requires protection from injury
   b. Sleeptalking: talking occurs during NREM sleep, before REM sleep
   c. Nocturnal enuresis: bedwetting, more common in male children over 3 years old; often occurs 1–2 hours after falling asleep, when rousing from stage III and IV of NREM sleep
   d. Bruxism: clenching and grinding teeth during stage II NREM sleep
5. Sleep deprivation: syndrome in which client's prolonged disturbance results in a decrease in amount, quality, and consistency of sleep
   a. REM sleep deprivation can be caused by alcohol, shift work, jet lag, or extended ICU hospitalization and can result in excitability, confusion, and emotional lability; delay procedures or medications when possible to avoid waking a client during REM sleep
   b. NREM sleep deprivation can be caused by same factors as REM deprivation, as well as hypothyroidism, depression, sleep apnea, and age (common in older adults), and can result in withdrawal, excessive sleepiness, and hyporesponsiveness

NCLEX® c. A client with both REM and NREM sleep deprivation may have marked fatigue, perceptual distortions, and difficulty with concentration, judgment, and attention

E. Health promotion to improve sleep

1. Environmental controls: ensure appropriate lighting, ventilation, and temperature; keep noise level to a minimum
2. NCLEX® Promote bedtime routines: respect client's customary routines to promote relaxation; provide hygiene such as washing face, brushing teeth, and voiding; allow listening to music or praying, children's bedtime stories, or adults' conversations with caregivers or family members if possible
3. NCLEX® Promote comfort: provide backrubs, change of linen/clothing, position for comfort; administer analgesics to treat pain, which may promote and help maintain sleep; listen to client's concerns to alleviate emotional stress and promote relaxation; avoid heavy meal 3 hours before bedtime, decrease fluid intake 2 hours before sleep, and avoid alcohol, caffeine, and heavily spiced foods
4. Promote activity: encourage adequate exercise during day to reduce stress and a nonstrenuous activity prior to sleep
5. NCLEX® Pharmacologic aids (sedatives and hypnotics) should be used as a last resort and be taken prn (as necessary); teach desired and adverse effects of medications (they vary in onset and duration); regular use may lead to drug tolerance and possibly rebound insomnia

IV. URINARY ELIMINATION NEEDS

A. Healthy urinary function

1. Normal urine output (UO) is 60 mL/hr or 1500 mL/day; should remain 30 mL/hr (0.5 mL/kg/hr) or higher to ensure continued healthy kidney function
2. Urine usually consists of 96% water
3. Solutes found in urine may be organic (urea, ammonia, uric acid, and creatinine) or inorganic (sodium, chloride, potassium, sulfate, magnesium, and phosphorus)
4. Table 26–2 describes characteristics of healthy urine and possible abnormal findings

Table 26–2 Characteristics of Normal and Abnormal Urine

Characteristic	Normal	Abnormal	Nursing Considerations
Amount in 24 hours (adult)	1200–1500 mL	Under 1200 mL Over 1500 mL	Normal UO is approximately equal to fluid intake. Report UO less than 30 mL/hr, which may indicate decreased blood flow to kidneys.
Color, clarity	Straw, amber; transparent	Dark amber Cloudy Dark orange Red or dark brown Mucus plugs, viscid, thick	Concentrated urine is darker, while dilute urine is pale yellow to almost clear. Some foods and drugs discolor urine. White blood cells, bacteria, pus, prostatic fluid, sperm, or vaginal drainage may cause cloudy urine. Red blood cells in urine (hematuria) may be seen as pink, bright red, or rusty brown urine. Don't confuse menstrual blood in urine with hematuria.
Odor	Faint, aromatic	Offensive	Some foods (e.g., asparagus) cause a musty odor; infected urine can have a fetid odor; urine high in glucose has a sweet odor.
Sterility	No microorganisms present	Microorganisms present	Urine specimens may be contaminated by bacteria from perineum during collection.
pH	4.5–8	Under 4.5 Over 8	Freshly voided urine should be somewhat acidic. Alkaline urine (high pH) may indicate alkalosis, urinary tract infection, or a diet high in fruits and vegetables. More acidic urine (low pH) is found in acidosis, starvation, diarrhea, or with a diet high in proteins or cranberries.
Specific gravity (SG)	1.010–1.025	Under 1.010 Over 1.025	Concentrated urine has a higher SG; dilute urine has a lower SG.
Glucose	Not present	Present	Glucosuria indicates high blood glucose levels (>180 mg/dL) possibly associated with undiagnosed or uncontrolled diabetes mellitus (DM) or gestational DM.
Ketone bodies	Not present	Present	Ketones (end products of fatty acid breakdown) may be present in urine with uncontrolled DM, starvation, or excessive aspirin ingestion.
Blood	Not present	Occult (microscopic) Bright red	Hematuria may indicate urinary tract infection, kidney disease, or bleeding from urinary tract.
Protein	Not present	Present	Proteinuria can occur with damage to glomerular membrane of kidney.

Source: Adapted from Berman, A., Snyder, S., & Frandsen, G. (2016). *Kozier & Erb's fundamentals of nursing: Concepts, process, and practice* (10th ed.). New York, NY: Pearson Education, p. 1183.

B. Common abnormal assessment findings

1. Urgency: strong desire to void may be caused by inflammation or infection in bladder or urethra
2. Dysuria: painful or difficult voiding
3. Frequency: voiding that occurs more than usual when compared with client's regular pattern or generally accepted norm of voiding once every 3–6 hours
4. Hesitancy: undue delay and difficulty in initiating voiding
5. Polyuria: a large volume of urine voided at any given time
6. Oliguria: a small volume of urine or output between 100 and 500 mL/24 hr
7. Nocturia: excessive urination at night, interrupting sleep
8. Hematuria: RBCs in urine

C. Common urinary elimination problems

1. Urinary retention: bladder emptying is impaired, urine accumulates, and bladder becomes overdistended; causes include prostatic hyperplasia, surgery, medications such as anticholinergics, antidepressants, antipsychotics, antiparkinsonian agents, antihypertensives
2. Urinary tract infections (UTI): infectious process leads to inflammation (*-itis*) in any portion of urinary tract
   a. Lower UTI: urethritis affects urethra; cystitis affects urinary bladder (and is most common UTI); prostatitis affects prostate gland
   b. Upper UTI: pyelonephritis affects renal pelvis and parenchyma (functional portion of kidney tissue)
3. Incontinence: involuntary urination
   a. Stress incontinence: involuntary loss of urine of less than 50 mL occurring with increased abdominal pressure through coughing, laughing, or lifting
   b. Reflex incontinence: involuntary loss of urine at predictable intervals when bladder reaches a specific volume
   c. Urge incontinence: involuntary loss of urine soon after a strong urge to void
   d. Functional incontinence: involuntary, unpredictable passage of urine
   e. Total incontinence: continuous and unpredictable involuntary loss of urine

D. Urinary diversion devices: ureterostomy is a surgical rerouting of urine from kidneys to a site other than bladder, usually when bladder is removed or diseased

1. Cutaneous ureterostomy: ureter is brought directly to skin surface to form a small stoma; disadvantages include that stomas provide microorganisms with direct access to kidneys from skin, small stomas may present difficulty in fitting pouches, and stenosis of stomas may occur as a complication
2. Ileal conduit: a segment of ileum is separated from small intestine and formed into a pouch with open end brought out through abdominal wall to form a stoma; ureter is implanted into ileal pouch (see Figure 26–1)

E. Common urinary tests

NCLEX®

1. Urinalysis: macroscopic and microscopic analysis of urine to determine physical and chemical characteristics (see again Table 26–2)
2. Urine culture/sensitivity: a clean-catch specimen or catheterized specimen is needed to identify infecting organism and most effective antibiotic; culture requires 24–72 hours for organism growth and identification

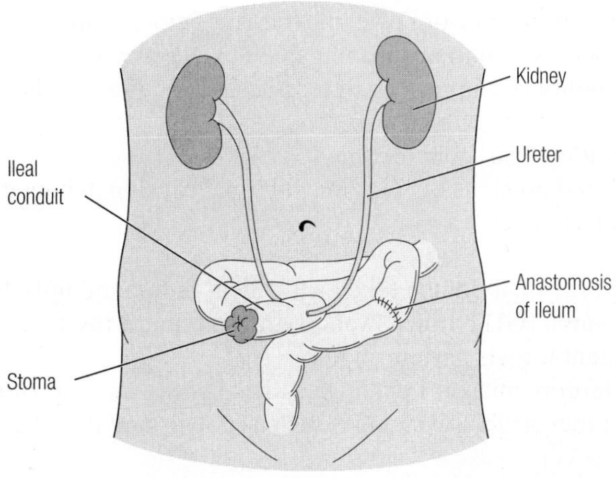

Figure 26–1

Ileal conduit as it is connected to abdominal organs.

3. Intravenous pyelogram (IVP) or intravenous urogram (IVU): IV injection of a radiopaque contrast medium concentrates in urine to aid visualization of kidneys, ureters, and bladder
4. Renal scan: IV injection of radiotraces or isotopes evaluates renal size, shape, position, function, or blood flow to kidneys; is recorded by a scintillation camera
5. Ultrasound: high-frequency sound waves are used to create images of urinary system
6. Cystoscopy: directly visualizes urethra and bladder with a cystoscope that is a self-contained optical lens system and provides a magnified illuminated view of bladder

NCLEX®

7. Bladder scan at bedside: detects amount of urine in bladder to help determine need for voiding or straight catheterization; may be done by nurses or other personnel trained to use portable device

F. Teaching and health promotion for urinary elimination

NCLEX®

1. Adequate hydration: daily intake of 1500 mL of measurable fluids recommended; if prone to development of stones or infections, increase to 2000–3000 mL per day; if experiencing abnormal fluid losses, additional fluids are necessary

NCLEX®

2. Personal hygiene: teach client to wash perineum with soap and water daily and wipe after defecation; instruct female clients to wipe from front to back (urinary meatus toward anus) after voiding and discard after each wipe; for recurrent infections, avoid tub baths
3. Empty bladder completely: regular exercise increases abdominal muscle tone that assists in bladder emptying; teach **Kegel exercises** to strengthen pelvic floor muscles—contract perineal muscles and hold for a count of 3–5 seconds and relax; do 10 contractions five times daily

NCLEX®

4. Infection prevention measures
   a. Drink eight 8-ounce glasses of water daily
   b. Empty bladder at least every 2–4 hours while awake, avoiding voluntary retention; if client is incontinent, instruct to void according to a timetable rather than urge to void (bladder training), void at regular intervals (habit training), or supplement habit training by reminding client to void (prompted voiding)
   c. For women: wear cotton briefs; cleanse perineum from front to back after elimination; void before and after sexual intercourse; avoid bubble baths, feminine hygiene sprays, and douches
   d. Explain that client can maintain urine acidity by taking vitamin C, drinking at least two glasses of cranberry juice per day or using cranberry supplements, and avoiding excess milk products and sodium bicarbonate
   e. Teach client symptoms and prevention measures of UTI and importance of reporting symptoms promptly

V. BOWEL ELIMINATION NEEDS

NCLEX®

A. Factors that influence bowel elimination (see Table 26–3)

B. Characteristics of normal stool

1. Color: varies from light to dark brown; foods and medications may affect color
2. Odor: aromatic, affected by ingested food and person's bacterial flora
3. Consistency: formed, soft, semisolid; moist
4. Frequency: varies with diet; once a day is a common pattern
5. Amount: varies with diet (about 100–400 grams/day)

NCLEX®

C. Common bowel elimination problems

1. Constipation: abnormal infrequency of defecation and abnormal hardening of stools
2. Impaction: accumulated mass of dry feces that cannot be expelled
3. Diarrhea: increased frequency of bowel movements (more than three times a day) as well as liquid consistency and increased amount; accompanied by urgency, discomfort, and possibly incontinence
4. Incontinence: involuntary elimination of feces, usually indicates a health problem at any age after toilet-training
5. Flatulence: expulsion of gas from rectum
6. Hemorrhoids: dilated portions of veins in anal canal causing itching and pain and possible bright red bleeding upon defecation

D. Diagnostic tests

1. Abdominal film: x-ray of abdomen taken with client in flat and upright positions
2. Upper gastrointestinal (GI) barium swallow: fluoroscopic x-ray exam of esophagus, stomach, and small intestines after client ingests barium sulfate
3. Barium enema: fluoroscopic x-ray exam visualizing entire large intestine after client is given a barium enema, which outlines structural changes such as polyps and diverticulitis

Table 26-3 Factors That Influence Bowel Elimination

Factor	Effect on Bowel Elimination
Age	Infants and toddlers: have immature control of bowel elimination; daytime control is achieved by age 2½ with toilet-training School-age and adolescents: have similar bowel habits as adults; however, school-age children involved in play may delay elimination Older adults: prone to constipation because of slowing of GI motility and decreased food intake and activity
Diet	Sufficient bulk is needed to provide fecal volume Low-residue or low-fiber diet may provide insufficient volume to stimulate reflex for defecation Irregular eating can interfere with regular elimination Diarrhea can be caused by spicy or overly sweet foods Gas-producing foods include cabbage, onions, beans, and cauliflower A laxative effect is exerted by bran, prunes, figs, and alcohol Constipating foods include cheese, eggs, pasta, and lean meat
Fluid intake	Healthy elimination requires an intake of 2000–3000 mL/day Inadequate fluid intake or excessive fluid loss may lead to hard feces
Activity	Stimulates peristalsis; immobility, weak muscles from lack of exercise, or impaired neurologic functioning can lead to constipation
Personal habits	Repeatedly ignoring urge to defecate allows continued water absorption from bowel and feces to harden; reflexes tend to be progressively weakened and may be lost
Positioning	Normal bowel elimination is facilitated by thigh flexion (increases intra-abdominal pressure) and a sitting position, which increases downward pressure on rectum Using a bedpan while in a supine position is uncomfortable and does not facilitate defecation, so place client in a semi-sitting position
Psychological	Anxiety or anger can increase peristalsis and lead to diarrhea Depression slows intestinal activity, resulting in constipation
Pain	Pain or discomfort during defecation may lead client to suppress urge to defecate, causing constipation
Medications	Many drugs have a constipating effect, including antidepressants, antipsychotic and antiparkinsonian agents, morphine, and codeine
Surgery	General anesthetics may cause a slowing of intestinal movement resulting in constipation Surgery in abdominal area that involves handling of intestines may cause cessation of intestinal movement (paralytic ileus) that lasts for 24–48 hours
Pregnancy	There is decreased intestinal secretion and colon is displaced upward, laterally, and posteriorly Peristaltic activity is decreased, causing constipation Venous pressure increases, causing hemorrhoids later in pregnancy

4. Endoscopy: use of a flexible tube (fiberoptic endoscope) to visualize GI tract; images produced are transmitted to a video screen
5. Upper endoscopy: a telescopic eyepiece is inserted through mouth; EGD—esophagogastroduodenoscopy
6. Lower endoscopy: a telescopic eyepiece is inserted through rectum—proctosigmoidoscopy

E. Health promotion for elimination problems

NCLEX® 1. Constipation: increase fluid intake; instruct client to drink liquids and fruit juices (especially prune juice) and to eat foods high in roughage or fiber, such as raw fruits and vegetables, bran products, whole-grain cereals, and bread

NCLEX® 2. Diarrhea: encourage oral intake of fluids and bland foods; avoid spicy and fatty foods, alcohol, beverages with caffeine, and high-fiber foods

3. Flatulence: limit chewing gum, carbonated drinks, use of drinking straws, and gas-producing foods such as cabbage, cauliflower, beans, and onions

F. Bowel diversion ostomies

1. An ostomy is a surgical opening in abdominal wall for elimination of feces or urine; bowel diversion ostomies are classified according to permanence, anatomic location, and construction of stoma
2. Permanence: colostomies can be temporary (for traumatic injuries or inflammatory conditions) or permanent (birth defect or disease such as cancer)

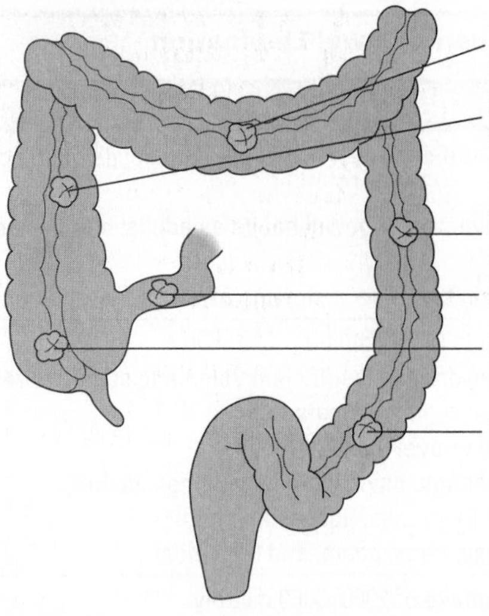

Figure 26–2

Locations of various bowel diversion ostomies.

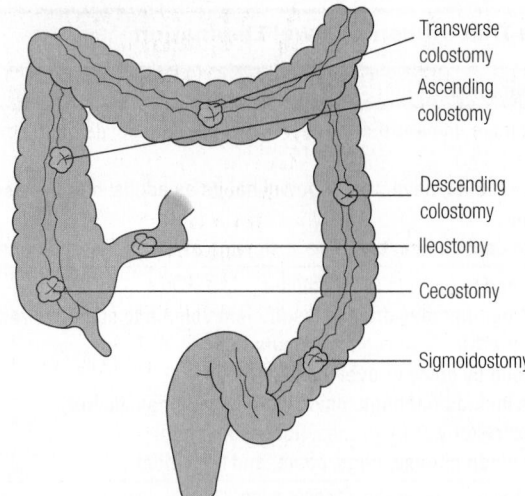

3. Anatomic location (see Figure 26–2): identifies site in small or large bowel from which ostomy empties
4. Construction of stoma
   a. Single: one end of bowel as opening
   b. Loop: a loop of bowel brought out into abdominal wall and supported by a rod or bridge; has two openings—proximal (active) and distal (inactive); usually performed as emergency surgery and situated often in right transverse colon
   c. Divided: two separated stomas; opening from digestive end is colostomy and distal end is mucus fistula (bowel continues to secrete mucus)
   d. Double-barreled: proximal and distal loops are sutured together and both ends are brought out through the abdominal wall

G. Health promotion for clients with ostomies

NCLEX®

1. For a client with a colostomy, dietary teaching needs to include information about:
   a. Foods that cause stool odor: asparagus, beans, eggs, fish, onions, garlic
   b. Foods that increase gas: cabbage, onions, beans, and cauliflower
   c. Foods that thicken stool: applesauce, bananas, rice, tapioca, cheese, yogurt
   d. Foods that loosen stool: chocolate, dried beans, fried foods, highly spiced foods, leafy green vegetables, raw fruits and vegetables

NCLEX®

2. For a client with ileostomy, teaching to relieve food blockage should include:
   a. Drink warm fluids or grape juice if not vomiting
   b. Take a warm shower
   c. Assume a knee-chest position
   d. Massage peristomal area
   e. Remove pouch if stoma is swollen and apply one with a larger opening
   f. Eat a low-residue diet initially; avoid foods that cause blockage such as popcorn, nuts, cucumbers, celery, fresh tomatoes, figs, blackberries, and caraway seeds
   g. Limit high-fiber foods and chew them well if eaten

   NCLEX®

   h. Know signs of blockage: abdominal cramping, swelling of stoma, and absence of ileostomy output for 4–6 hours

VI. SENSORY AND PERCEPTUAL NEEDS

A. Factors affecting sensation and perception

1. Illness may result in hospitalization; this change of environment may affect mentation, especially for older clients; in some cases, mental status changes result from an underlying disease process
2. Developmental stage affects sensory perception
   a. Infants have adequate sensory organs but have no mental concepts to understand sensory input
   b. As development occurs, person develops understanding of sensory input
   c. Adults have many learned responses to sensory cues; with aging, sensory input diminishes because of decreased sense organ functioning

NCLEX®

3. Medications can affect both sensory function and awareness; many drugs decrease level of consciousness (LOC); others contribute to mental confusion; in older adults, polypharmacy may lead to drug interactions that cause decreased sensory functioning

4. Stress can be described as eustress (optimal stress level that stimulates enhanced functioning) or distress (excessive stress that reduces ability to function and may limit amount of sensory input client can manage)
   a. Illness and hospitalization can both cause distress
   b. Hospitals and other in-patient facilities now try to create aesthetic environments conducive to healing (bright and cheerful walls, pictures, carpeted floors) to reduce stress
5. Personal lifestyle influences ability to manage amount of stimulation perceived by senses

B. Sensory and perceptual alterations

1. Three factors known to contribute to alterations in client behavior include (but are not limited to) sensory deprivation, sensory overload, and sensory deficits
2. **Sensory deprivation**: a lack of meaningful stimuli; reduced amount of incoming stimuli because of either decreased environmental stimuli or impairment in one or more of client's senses; can lead to disorientation over time
   NCLEX® a. Risk factors for sensory deprivation include dysfunction of senses (vision or hearing impairment, impaired sensation because of neurological problem), medications, immobility, isolation, and language barriers
   NCLEX® b. See Box 26–4 for clinical signs and symptoms of sensory deprivation
   c. Hospital rooms have clocks, calendars, and boards that identify work-shift caregivers to provide meaningful stimuli and promote orientation to surroundings
3. **Sensory overload**: an increase in intensity of stimuli to levels beyond normal; occurs when client is unable to process amount or intensity of stimuli or when exposed to numerous stimuli that are not meaningful
   a. Increased internal stimuli (such as anxiety) and increased unfamiliar external stimuli (noise, equipment, multiple healthcare personnel) can lead to sensory overload
   b. Sensory overload leads to sleep deprivation, which reduces individual coping abilities; when overloaded with sensory stimuli, client may feel out of control
   NCLEX® c. Contributing factors to overload could be pain, anxiety, and lack of sleep; incidence is increased in clients in intensive care units after 2–3 days
   d. Refer again to Box 26–4 for clinical signs and symptoms of sensory overload
4. **Sensory deficit**: impairment of both reception and perception of one or more senses; when loss is gradual, individual can compensate; for instance, clients with impaired vision may decrease area in which they travel alone

C. Common sensory deficits

1. Visual: vision is important in aiding clients to interact with environment
   a. Clients with visual impairment may wear glasses or contact lenses to correct refraction errors of lens
   b. Refraction errors include myopia (nearsightedness), hyperopia (farsightedness), and presbyopia (loss of lens elasticity that reduces ability to focus on close objects; occurs with aging, around age 45, and requires corrective lenses—"reading" glasses or bifocals)

Box 26–4

Signs of Sensory Deprivation and Sensory Overload

Sensory Deprivation

- Excessive yawning, drowsiness, sleeping
- Decreased attention span, difficulty concentrating, decreased problem solving
- Impaired memory
- Periodic disorientation, general or nocturnal confusion
- Preoccupation with somatic complaints, such as palpitations
- Hallucinations or delusions
- Crying, annoyance over small matters, depression
- Apathy, emotional liability

Sensory Overload

- Increased muscle tension
- Fatigue and inability to sleep
- Irritability and restlessness
- Inability to concentrate
- Decreased problem-solving performance

c. Cataracts: often seen after age 65; lens opacity blocks light rays and distorts and impairs visual field; surgical removal is often required as cataract progresses; see also Chapter 63
d. Glaucoma: a painless blockage in circulation of aqueous fluid in eye that leads to an increase in intraocular pressure and possibly blindness; see also Chapter 63
e. Diabetic retinopathy: leading cause of blindness among adults age 20–70; proliferative retinopathy or neurovascular disease occurs when ischemic retinal blood vessels (BVs) bleed, causing vitreous hemorrhage, which can be repetitive and may lead to permanent visual loss
f. Macular degeneration: degenerative changes in BVs in macular area of retina; macular BVs leak and damage macula; scarring occurs and visual loss results; symptoms are blurring and distortion of visual images; see also Chapter 63

2. Hearing: difficulty with hearing may make client feel isolated, interfere with health teaching, and even increase client's risk of injury
   a. Conductive hearing loss results from interrupted transmission of sound waves through outer and middle ear; possible causes are a tear in eardrum (tympanic membrane); obstruction in auditory canal caused by swelling or other factors; degeneration of hammer, anvil, and stirrup from infection; or continuous low-sensory input
   b. Sensorineural hearing loss results from damage to inner ear, auditory nerve, or hearing center in brain from viral infection or ototoxic medications (whose names often end with *mycin*)
   c. **Presbycusis** is age-related gradual loss of hearing ability; more common in men than in women
3. Balance: a gradual reduction of muscle power and contraction, which can also affect balance, occurs with aging, especially after age 50; degenerative joint changes may occur, making movement more restricted
4. Taste: decreased ability to taste can reduce appetite and contribute to poor nutrition; if a corresponding loss of smell occurs, client's appetite will fail to be stimulated by aroma of food
5. Smell: in addition to its effect on appetite, loss of smell can be a safety issue; with decrease in smell, client will not be aware of a gas leak, for example
6. Touch: tactile deprivation can occur from disease or an injury that causes destruction or damage to nerve cells
   a. Children born with myelomeningocele have damage to nerves below level of pathology; injuries that destroy nerves exert same effect; loss of tactile ability may contribute to safety issues, such as risk for burns if cannot feel heat
   b. Peripheral neuropathy interferes with innervation of peripheral nerves and can occur with aging, diabetes, or arteriosclerosis
   c. Multisensory deficit conditions: some conditions, such as stroke, cause damage to more than one sense depending on affected area(s) of brain; results may be decreased sensation and/or paresis or paralysis of extremities, as well as aphasia, blindness or other visual impairment, or impaired swallowing

NCLEX®

D. Promoting self-care

1. Screening and prevention: early detection of sensory deprivation is an important health-screening function
   a. Routine auditory testing is done at birth and during early school years
   b. Periodic vision screening of all school-age children is done
   c. Health fairs often provide a means to screen many healthy people
   d. Be aware of disease processes that can lead to sensory deprivation, and screen for symptoms to detect sensory problems early
   e. Teach measures to protect sensory organs; encourage protective eye and ear gear; emphasize, especially to teenagers, risk of ear damage from loud noise or music
   f. Teach clients general health measures such as regular eye and ear exams
   g. The Occupational Safety and Health Administration (OSHA) provides workplace regulations and guidelines to limit hazards affecting senses; OSHA guidelines are carefully followed in healthcare settings also
2. Assistive aids: encourage use of specific aids to support sensory function, promote use of other senses, communicate effectively, and work to ensure client's safety

NCLEX®

   a. Visual and hearing aids: give eyeglasses to clients upon awakening and assist in storage at bedtime; ensure that hearing aid is in place and functioning during daytime and prior to any explanations about care or treatment; see Box 26–5 for information on possible visual and auditory aids
   b. For clients with smell and taste deficits, supply diets that include a variety of flavors, temperatures, and textures to stimulate taste buds
   c. Evaluate each client who has a sensory deficit to determine appropriate assistive device

Box 26–5

Aids for Clients with Visual and Auditory Deficits

For Clients with Visual Deficits

- Prescription eyeglasses
- Proper lighting in rooms, including nightlights
- Shades on windows to reduce glare
- Large-print, recorded, or Braille books
- Magnifying glass
- Contrasting colors in environment
- Large numbers on clocks, watches, and phone
- Seeing-eye dog
- Red-tipped cane or laser cane

For Clients with Auditory Deficits

- Hearing aids
- Closed-caption service for television
- Telephone with amplifiers
- Flashing alarm clocks, smoke detectors, doorbells, and phone
- Cochlear implants
- Service dogs
- Telecommunication device for deaf (TDD phone)
- Wireless page, phone, and e-mail service

3. Communication
   a. Client with a sensory deficit is at risk for not accurately interpreting information shared during communication
   b. Convey respect to client and enhance his or her self-esteem
   c. A person with a hearing deficit needs to concentrate at all times during a conversation
   d. A client with visual deficits might misinterpret nonverbal clues during conversation
   e. See Box 26–6 for tips on communicating with clients who have visual or hearing deficits

VII. SKIN INTEGRITY AND WOUND CARE

A. Healthy skin integrity

1. Layers of skin
   a. Epidermis: outermost layer of stratified squamous epithelial cells
   b. Dermis: second layer composed of connective tissue that gives elasticity to skin; has BVs, nerve fibers, glands, and hair follicles
   c. Subcutaneous tissue: made of adipose tissue; provides support and blood flow to dermis
2. Skin glands: sebaceous glands, soporiferous glands, and cerumenous glands
   a. Sebaceous glands (within dermis) secrete an oily substance called sebum that protects hair from drying, prevents excessive water evaporation, and inhibits growth of certain bacteria on skin
   b. Soporiferous (sweat) glands produce a watery secretion and have two types: apocrine (primarily found in axilla and pubic areas; produce odor when decomposed by bacteria) and eccrine (chiefly found on palms of hands, soles of feet, and forehead; cools body through evaporation)
   c. Ceruminous glands secrete a thick, oily substance called cerumen, a waxy secretion of external ear (also known as earwax)
3. Skin alterations related to aging
   a. Epidermis thins and has a lower water content, leading to dry skin
   b. Elasticity and some fatty cushion are lost, resulting in wrinkles and fragile skin
   c. BVs in skin also become more fragile, leading to easy bruising

B. Classification of wounds

1. A wound is a physical break in skin or mucous membrane; may be superficial (affecting skin surface only) or deep (involving blood vessels, nerves, muscle, fascia, tendons, ligaments, and bones)

Box 26–6

Communicating with Clients Who Have a Visual or Hearing Deficit

Visual Deficit

- Always announce presence and identify self by name when entering room
- Stay in client's field of vision if vision loss is partial
- Speak in a warm and pleasant tone of voice, but not with excessive loudness
- Always explain what you will do before touching client
- Explain sounds in environment
- Indicate when conversation has ended and you are leaving the room

Hearing Deficit

- Before initiating a conversation, position yourself where client can see you or gently touch client
- Decrease background noises (e.g., radio) before speaking
- Talk at a moderate rate and in a normal tone of voice; do not shout (does not make voice more distinct)
- Address client directly; do not turn away while speaking; ensure client can see your face easily and that it is well lit
- Avoid talking with chewing gum or other items in mouth; avoid covering mouth with hand
- Keep voice at about same volume throughout each sentence; don't drop voice at end of each sentence
- Always speak as clearly and accurately as possible; articulate consonants with particular care
- Do not "overarticulate," which is just as troublesome as mumbling; pantomime or write ideas, or use sign language or finger spelling when appropriate
- Use longer phrases, which may be easier to understand than short ones; also, choose words carefully: "Fifteen cents" and "fifty cents" may be confused, but "half a dollar" is clear
- Pronounce names with care; add a reference to name for easier understanding—for example, "Joan, the girl from the office"
- Change to a new subject at a slower rate, ensuring that client follows the change; a key word or two at the beginning of a new topic is a good indicator

Source: Adapted from Berman, A., Snyder, S., & Frandsen, G. (2016). *Kozier & Erb's fundamentals of nursing: Concepts, process, and practice* (10th ed.). New York, NY: Pearson Education, p. 915.

2. Wounds are classified according to continuity of surface and type of damage
   a. Open wound: break in skin that can be superficial or deep; examples are an abrasion, laceration, or puncture
   b. Closed wound: injury with no break in skin; examples are contusion and ecchymosis; may be caused by a blow or other type of trauma
3. Superficial, partial, and full thickness refer to depth of injury and are used most often to describe burns
   a. Superficial thickness involves epidermal layer only, such as a mild sunburn or burn from contact with hot object
   b. Partial thickness involves entire epidermis, part of dermis; sweat glands and hair follicles are intact
   c. Full thickness involves epidermis and dermis, extending to subcutaneous tissue and possibly even to muscle and bone
4. Noninfected and infected wounds
   a. A noninfected or clean wound has no pathogenic microorganisms and heals without infection
   b. An infected wound or septic wound has pathogenic microorganisms; clinical signs and symptoms of infection develop
5. Surgical wound: an intentional wound made for therapeutic purposes using a sharp cutting instrument; it is a clean wound that heals without infection
6. Pressure injuries: lesions caused by unrelieved pressure, which also damages underlying tissues; see Table 26–4 for staging of pressure injuries

Table 26–4 Staging of Pressure Injuries

Stage	Description
I	Skin is intact, erythema noted but does not blanch (whiten when pressure applied) Client may report tingling or burning Darker-skinned clients may have skin discoloration, warmth, edema, and induration as indicators
II	Superficial partial-thickness skin loss that involves epidermis and possibly dermis Appears like a blister, abrasion, or a shallow crater
III	Full-thickness skin loss with necrotic tissue seen in subcutaneous layer that extends down to (but not through) underlying fascia Injury appears as a deeper crater with or without undermining of surrounding tissue
IV	Full-thickness skin loss with tissue necrosis or damage extending down to muscle, bone, and possibly other tissues such as tendons or joint capsule Undermining of tissue and sinus tracts may also be present

a. Contributing factors include immobility, fragile skin in older adults, moisture, malnutrition, shearing, and friction

NCLEX®

b. Assess client's relative risk using scales such as Braden scale or Norton scale; Braden scale rates six areas: sensory perception, moisture, activity mobility, nutrition, and friction and shear (total score ranges from low of 6 to high of 24; a lower score indicates a higher risk); Norton scale rates five areas: physical condition, mental condition, activity, mobility, and continence (total score ranges from 5 to 20; lower score indicates a higher risk)

c. Assess existing pressure injuries for healing using a tool such as Pressure Ulcer Scale for Healing (PUSH), which evaluates wound size, exudate amount, and type of tissue present in wound bed

C. Wound healing

1. Three phases

a. Inflammatory: fibrin network of protein fibers forms in wound; blood flow increases; damaged tissue then heals; drying fibrin and protein form a scab that seals skin in 3–4 days

b. Proliferative phase: fibroblasts grow to form granulation tissue (4–21 days), which is friable (easily damaged), soft, and pinkish red in color because of new capillaries; epithelial cells grow from edges; connective tissue fills area forming a scar that is stronger than granulation tissue; a large wound requiring excessive granulation tissue for closure can lead to formation of a **keloid**, a large, uneven scar

c. Maturation or remodeling phase (healing of scar): often occurs by weeks 3–4, but can extend for 2 years after injury; a fully healed wound has tensile strength of up to 80% of preinjury state (more susceptible to future injury)

2. Factors affecting wound healing

NCLEX®

a. Age: factors that inhibit healing in older adults include age-related vascular changes, cardiovascular disease or diabetes (which reduce blood flow to area), immune system changes, possible nutritional deficiencies, and slower rate of cell renewal

NCLEX®

b. Nutrition: protein helps build new tissue; vitamin C aids maturation of fibrous tissue and protein synthesis; undernutrition results in inadequate nutrient stores, while obesity tends to decrease blood flow to tissue and increase risk of infection

Memory Aid

Remember that foods containing protein or vitamin C are good choices for clients who have healing wounds.

c. Condition of tissues: wound contamination and infection slow healing process; organisms present in wound compete with cells for O_2 and nutrition

d. Efficiency of circulation: regular exercise promotes circulation and faster healing; factors that restrict local blood supply to a wound (damaged arteries, edema of tissues, and dehydration) interfere with healing; anemia and blood dyscrasias may interfere with O_2 delivery; conditions such as diabetes and liver dysfunction can delay healing; smoking may limit O_2 supply to tissues

e. Rest, anxiety, and stress: adequate rest of injured part aids wound closure; anxiety and stress can stimulate release of hormones that slow healing

NCLEX®

f. Medications: anti-inflammatory drugs such as steroids and hormones slow formation of fibrous tissue and therefore impair healing

3. Wound closures
   a. **Primary intention**: wound edges are well approximated and wound heals without infection; tissues return to a healthy state with minimal inflammation and little to no scarring
   b. **Secondary intention**: healing occurs by granulation when wound is extensive and edges cannot or should not be approximated; healing time is prolonged; carries greater risk for infection and results in deeper, more extensive scarring
   c. Surgical interventions: sutures, staples, and clips are devices used to approximate wound edges; some sutures absorb and others must be removed; staples and clips are alternatives to suturing and are usually made of silver; these require removal in about 7–10 days
4. Complications that affect wound healing
   a. Hemorrhage: assess internal hemorrhage by distention in area of wound; external hemorrhage is noted by blood on or leaking through dressing; if bleeding is severe, client may exhibit signs of shock; risk of hemorrhage is greater within first 48 hours; if pressure dressings do not successfully stop bleeding, surgical intervention may be needed
   b. Infection: noted by redness, swelling, heat, and pain at site; purulent exudate may be noted; client may be anorexic, nauseous, febrile, and have chills; wound culture and antibiotic therapy are warranted
   NCLEX® c. **Dehiscence**: accidental reopening of suture line (usually abdominal, but could occur with any wound) with tissue separation under wound; caused by infection or factors that impede wound healing; clients often "feel something giving way"; place client in bed with head of bed low to eliminate gravity and with knees bent to decrease pull on suture line; cover wound with large, sterile, wet saline dressings; notify surgeon immediately because repair of surgical site is necessary
   NCLEX® d. **Evisceration**: internal organs (viscera) protrude through incisional edges after dehiscence; contributing factors include infection, poor nutrition, failure of suture material, dehydration, and excessive coughing; repaired surgically

D. Wound assessment and management

1. Inspect wound and gently palpate surrounding area regularly
2. Note whether wound edges are approximated; a healing ridge may be noted during healing
3. *NCLEX®* Note presence and characteristics of wound drainage; outline drainage on dressing, noting date and time
4. *NCLEX®* Observe for signs of infection: redness, swelling, increased tenderness, or disruption of wound edges; note also body temperature and white blood cell count
5. Purposes for dressing a wound
   a. Absorb drainage
   b. Splint or immobilize wound to provide rest
   c. Protect wound from mechanical injury or contamination
   d. Promote hemostasis
   e. Provide mental and physical comfort for client
6. Purposes for maintaining a wound undressed
   a. Eliminate conditions that favor growth of microorganisms
   b. Allow for better wound observation and assessment
   c. Facilitate bathing and hygiene
   d. Avoid adhesive tape reaction
   e. Avoid friction and irritation that destroy new epithelial cells
7. Wound irrigation: may be needed to cleanse or flush wound to enhance healing; normal saline and antibiotic solutions are most commonly used

E. Wound management products

1. *NCLEX®* Wound cleansers: all wounds should be cleansed appropriately; in clean wounds where tissue is granulating, minimize disruption of wound bed; clean wound gently and rinse away debris with normal saline
2. Enzymatic debriding agent: an enzyme product such as collagenase may be applied to necrotic tissue to digest it
3. Dressings: a variety of dressing materials are available, each with different purposes; some provide barrier protection from contamination; some may be impregnated with antibiotics; others are moist and aid in liquefying necrotic tissue; see Table 26–5
4. Bandages are strips of cloth used to wrap a body part
   a. Made of gauze (light and porous) or an elasticized material (which provides pressure to area)
   b. Widths vary from 1 to 4 inches and are determined by body part to be wrapped
   c. Purposes are to anchor dressings, immobilize or provide support to a body part, or promote venous return

Table 26–5 Types of Dressings

Dressing Type	Description
Gauze	Plain or impregnated with an antimicrobial for use on full- and partial-thickness wounds Packs and fills wound; absorbs drainage May be applied dry, wet-to-moist, and wet-to-wet
Transparent film	Adhesive plastic semipermeable dressing that allows oxygen into wound but not liquids and bacteria Protects wound from contamination and friction, prevents fluid evaporation from wound, and aids wound assessment
Impregnated nonadherent	Cotton or synthetic material that is impregnated with saline, zinc-saline, antimicrobials, petrolatum, or others Protects partial- and full-thickness wounds that do not have exudate Requires secondary dressing to keep it in place, hold in moisture, and protect wound
Hydrocolloid	Contains adhesive wafer, paste, or powder; can be worn up to 7 days Inner layer absorbs exudates and forms hydrated gel over wound, while outer film provides occlusive seal Protects wound from contamination and eliminates risk of maceration of surrounding skin
Hydrogel	Water or glycerin is primary component of jelly-like sheet, granules, or gels; maintains moist wound bed and helps liquefy necrotic tissue or slough Permeable to oxygen and can fill dead spaces in a wound Secondary occlusive dressing is required
Alginate (exudate absorbers)	Nonadherent dressings of powder, beads, granules, ropes, sheets, or paste; requires secondary dressing Purpose is to absorb up tp 20 times their weight in drainage
Polyurethane foam	Nonadherent hydrocolloid dressing that absorbs large amounts of exudate while keeping wound moist Requires secondary dressing for an occlusive environment, or tape around edges to secure it Skin around area needs protection from maceration
Clear absorbent acrylic	Transparent absorbent wafer with an acrylic layer that absorbs exudates and allows moisture to evaporate Aids in wound assessment while protecting from bacteria and shearing forces; for 5- to 7-day use
Collagen	Derived from animal sources (often pig or cow); comes in a variety of forms Used to halt bleeding and stimulate cell proliferation in wound bed to help healing

d. Pad bony prominences and apply bandage with body part in normal position

e. Apply bandage from distal to proximal area to support blood return

NCLEX® **f.** Use even pressure while applying bandage, especially when using elastic bandages that could impair circulation

NCLEX® **g.** Inspect and palpate area regularly—more frequently on a fresher wound, less frequently on an older wound; note neurovascular status of extremity (temperature, blanching, and sensation) and pain (evaluate for its cause)

VIII. MOBILITY NEEDS

A. Common causes of immobility

1. Pain: reduces spontaneous movement and may inhibit client from participating in care activities, including coughing and deep breathing
2. Motor and nervous system impairment: disorders of musculoskeletal system (such as arthritis or amputation) and nervous system (such as multiple sclerosis or Parkinson's disease) can limit mobility; certain neurological diseases can cause muscles to become stiff or lose function (such as stroke)
3. Functional problems: some chronic conditions that limit supply of O_2 and nutrients or increase cardiac work affect activity tolerance, such as chronic obstructive lung disease, congestive heart failure, angina, and obesity
4. Generalized weakness: from age-related loss of muscle tone, flexibility and reaction time, decreased bone density, or chronic illness
5. Psychological problems: emotional disorders such as depression or stress can reduce motivation and energy to participate in activities
6. Medically induced immobility
   - **a.** Clients may be placed on bedrest or have activity restrictions to allow healing of body parts
   - **b.** Orthopedic devices (traction, casts, splints, braces) can also cause immobility

NCLEX®

B. Major complications of immobility

1. Psychological effects: powerlessness and possible reduced self-esteem
2. Muscle atrophy and joint contractures; disuse osteoporosis
3. Pressure injuries
4. Orthostatic intolerance (postural or orthostatic hypotension)
5. Deep vein thrombosis
6. Pneumonia
7. Decrease in peristalsis (paralytic ileus)
8. Kidney stones

C. Nursing interventions for impaired mobility

1. Explain benefits of exercise
   a. Improves tone and strength of muscles, joint flexibility and range of motion (ROM)
   b. Promotes pulmonary ventilation, which prevents pooling of secretions in lungs and reduces risk of pneumonia
   c. Improves GI motility and tone, improving digestion and elimination
   d. Decreases bone loss of calcium, which helps maintain acidic urine to decrease risk for renal calculi
2. Types of exercise
   a. Isometric: muscle tension or resistance is produced without a change in muscle length; strengthens muscle groups that will be used later in ambulation; teach client to push or pull against a stationary object; muscles exercised are abdominal, gluteus, and quadriceps
   b. Isotonic: exercises that shorten muscle to produce contraction and active movement with no significant change in resistance, so force of contraction stays stable; increase muscle tone and maintain joint flexibility; examples are using a trapeze to lift body or pushing body into a sitting position
   c. Passive ROM: accomplished with assistance of a caregiver who supports client's body part while moving it
   d. Active ROM: isotonic exercises of each joint in body that are performed by client; can maintain or improve muscle strength; prevent deterioration of joint movement and subsequent contractures

D. Assistive ambulation device: crutches

NCLEX®

1. Assist client in moving and ambulating; require rubber tips to prevent slipping on floors; various types of crutches are available (see Figure 26–3)
   a. An axillary crutch with hand bars (underarm crutch) is most frequently used crutch
   b. A Lofstrand or forearm crutch is used as a substitute for a cane; consists of a single metal tube with a handle and a cuff for forearm; allows user to release hand bar because metal cuff maintains crutch placement and prevents it from falling
   c. Canadian or elbow extensor crutch is used for client whose forearm extensor muscles are weak; it allows upper arm to provide stability to crutch

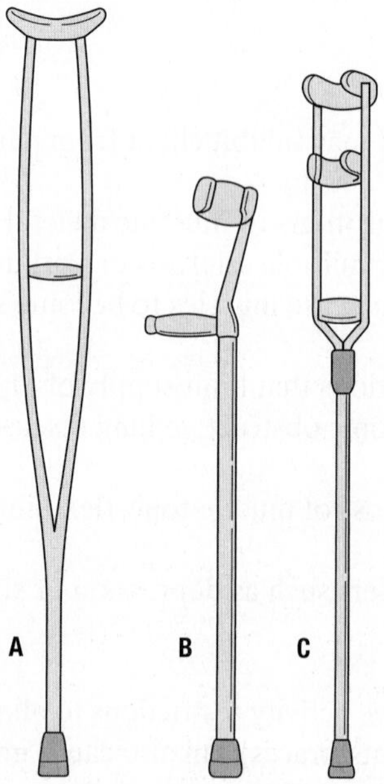

Figure 26–3

Three types of crutches: (A) axillary crutch; (B) Lofstrand crutch; (C) Canadian or elbow extension crutch.

NCLEX®

2. Measuring for crutches
   a. Measure client who is lying supine from anterior fold of axilla to heel of foot and add 2.5 cm (1 in.)
   b. Also measure placement of hand on crutch while client stands and adjust crutch so that it maintains elbow at a 30-degree angle
   c. With client standing erect, ensure that shoulder rest of crutch is 3 fingerwidths (2.5–5 cm, or 1–2 in.) below axilla

NCLEX®

3. Safety with crutches
   a. Place rubber tip on end of crutch
   b. Teach client appropriate gait
   c. Prior to gait training, encourage client to prepare for crutch walking by pushing body off the bed with hands and arms
   d. While using crutches, have client bear weight on arms, not axillae, to avoid nerve damage to axillae caused by continued pressure
4. Gait used for crutch walking depends on client's ability to bear weight and maintain balance; client alternates body weight between one or both legs and crutches; see Box 26–7
5. When going up stairs, client should first move unaffected (stronger) leg onto step while placing weight on crutches, then transfer weight to stronger leg on stairs and move crutches and affected leg up to same step; then repeat (affected leg is always supported by crutches)
6. When going down stairs, client should place weight on stronger leg and move crutches and affected leg down one step, transfer weight to crutches, and move stronger leg to same step; then repeat (affected leg is always supported by crutches)

E. Cane: assists a client to walk with greater balance and support

1. Three types of canes: quad cane (four feet), tripod cane (three feet) and straight cane
2. A rubber cap is fitted at tip of cane to prevent slipping
3. Canes are adjustable; length should allow elbow to bend 15–30 degrees (cane handle is at level of client's greater trochanter)
4. Client should hold cane on unaffected (stronger) side for best support and position tip of straight cane (or nearest tip of other canes) 15 cm (6 in.) to side and 15 cm (6 in.) in front of near foot

Box 26–7

Crutch Walking Gaits

Four-Point Gait: Partial Weight-Bearing

- Client must be able to bear weight on both legs.
- Safest gait, providing three points of support at all times.
- Requires constant shifting of weight and coordination of movement of legs and crutches.

Three-Point Gait: Requires One Leg to Be Able to Bear Weight of Entire Body

- Used for non-weight-bearing or partial weight-bearing on affected leg.
- Movements alternate between affected leg with both crutches, and then unaffected leg.

Two-Point Gait: Requires Partial Weight-Bearing on Both Legs

- Client can move at a faster gait than with four-point gait.
- Two points are used to support body at all times.
- Crutch movement is similar to swinging of arms while walking.
- May be used when client has bilateral prostheses on lower legs.

Swing-Through Gait: Weight-Bearing Gait That Requires Strength and Coordination

- Client moves both crutches forward together.
- Then the client lifts his or her body weight and swings through.

Swing-To Gait: Weight-Bearing on Both Legs

- Similar to swing-through gait except body motion is only to level of crutches.
- Useful for clients with paralysis of legs and hips.

NCLEX®

5. Client should move cane forward 30 cm (12 in.) or other comfortable distance while bearing weight on both legs; next client should move affected (weaker) leg forward while bearing weight on cane and stronger leg; finally, client moves unaffected (stronger) leg forward ahead of cane while weight is borne by cane and weaker leg

F. **Walker: provides more support than a cane**
1. Used for clients with poor balance, cardiac problems, or cannot use crutches
2. Standard walker has four legs with rubber tips on feet and plastic grips for hands
3. Client must be partial weight-bearing and have strength in wrists and arms
4. Client uses upper body to propel walker forward; sequence of movement is walker first, then affected (weaker) foot, and finally unaffected (stronger) foot
5. Two- or four-wheeled walker is useful if client is too weak or not stable enough to move walker by lifting it; some walkers have an attached seat to allow client to sit and rest as needed during walk
6. Walkers are height-adjustable

G. **Other assistive devices**
1. Should be used when weight to be lifted exceeds 16 kg (35 lb) or other conditions warrant use of device
2. Include floor-based and ceiling lifts, slings, sit-to-stand assist devices, friction-reducing devices, sliding boards, transfer sheets, and lateral transfer and transport chairs

Check Your NCLEX–RN® Exam I.Q.

You are ready for testing on this content if you can:

- Assist a client with personal hygiene needs.
- Evaluate a client's ability to perform activities of daily living.
- Plan nursing care to promote rest and sleep.
- Assess the elimination needs of a client.
- Provide care to a client to assist with urinary and bowel elimination.
- Take action to prevent complications of immobility.
- Assess a client's wound-healing status.
- Implement nursing measures to promote wound healing.
- Assess a client's need for assistive devices.
- Implement care for a client using an assistive device.

PRACTICE TEST

PRACTICE TEST

1 During a nursing assessment, the client states he is 70 years old and has a history of staphylococcus infections, increased intraocular pressure, and blurred vision. The nurse concludes that which item reported by the client is a risk factor for the development of cataracts?

1. History of staphylococcus infections
2. Increased intraocular pressure
3. Stated age of client
4. Long duration of blurred vision

2 A 92-year-old client who is very hard of hearing is hospitalized. Which action by the nurse is appropriate when conducting the admission interview and assessment of the client?

1. Use a cotton swab to clean cerumen in the client's ear before the interview.
2. Speak louder into the client's ear determined to have better hearing.
3. Maintain normal pitch of the voice and face the client during the interview.
4. Put new batteries in the hearing aid to ensure proper functioning.

3 A 72-year-old client has been in the ICU for the past 2 days. Which intervention would be the most appropriate in decreasing the risk for sensory deprivation? Select all that apply.

1. Remove equipment from the room.
2. Explain procedures and routines to the client upon admission.
3. Provide a clock and calendar in the client's room.
4. Maintain a balance of activity and rest periods.
5. Maintain constant conversation when in the client's room.

4 The nurse must apply an elastic bandage to support a client's sprained ankle. Which action should the nurse take during this procedure?

1. Moderately stretch the bandage and wrap it from distal extremity to proximal.
2. Wrap the extremity loosely enough to insert two fingers beneath the bandage.
3. Maintain a tight stretch with each wrap of the bandage.
4. Start proximal to the injury site and work distally.

5 All of the following clients visit the emergency room during one shift. For which clients should the nurse expect the healthcare provider to prescribe an antibiotic? Select all that apply.

1. Cat bite to the hand of an elderly client
2. Laceration from broken glass in a 6-year-old client
3. Stab wound in the arm of a 37-year-old client
4. Closed fracture to the ankle of a 40-year-old soccer player
5. A wrist sprain in a 17-year-old who was playing basketball

6 A client on complete bedrest is at risk for disuse syndrome. The nurse should consider which client goal as appropriate?

1. The client has shorter periods of immobility.
2. The client remains free of contractures in lower extremities.
3. The nurse turns the client every 2 hours.
4. The nurse performs passive range of motion to lower extremities every 4 hours.

7 An older adult client who was hospitalized 3 days ago is having trouble sleeping with some periods of confusion during waking hours. What is the best interpretation by the nurse regarding this client data?

1. The client is unable to manage health proactively.
2. The client is having difficulty coping with hospitalization.
3. The client may be experiencing hallucinations triggered by confusion.
4. The client is having a disrupted sleep cycle because of the environment.

8 An 80-year-old client has been admitted to the nursing unit with Parkinson's disease. Which action by the nurse would be most appropriate in preventing disuse syndrome?

1. Providing for the nutritional needs of the client
2. Promoting weight-bearing exercises
3. Encouraging 8 glasses of fluid in 24 hours
4. Turning and positioning every 2 hours

9 A client is admitted with a pressure injury on the left hip. The nurse has entered the following goal on the standardized care plan, "skin heals by June 12." Prior to this date, the nurse evaluates progress on reaching this goal. Which statement is the best notation of progress toward the goal?

1. Turned every 2 hours; avoided positioning on left side
2. Wet to moist dressing changed every 4 hours
3. No additional areas of skin breakdown noted
4. Wound less reddened; granulation tissue noted

10 In assessing a client who has been immobilized because of illness, the nurse would most likely document the state of the client's muscles as which of the following?

1. Hypertrophied
2. Atrophied
3. Flexible
4. Hardened

11 A female client can move her right arm and leg but has hemiplegia on the left side. What should the nurse instruct the unlicensed assistant to perform on the client's left side during care?

1. Active range of motion
2. Passive range of motion
3. Isotonic exercises
4. Isometric exercises

12 A client has weakness of the lower extremities and uses crutches for mobility. What client behavior should indicate to the nurse that the client needs further teaching about using crutches?

1. Uses the swing-to gait
2. Uses axillary crutches
3. Bears weight on the armpits
4. Replaces rubber tips on the crutches

13 A male client sustained numerous types of wounds when he lost control of his motorcycle and was thrown onto the pavement. The client asks the nurse which wounds will heal best. The nurse's reply is based on analysis that which type of wound would generally be least likely to scar?

1. A wound that heals by primary intention
2. A wound that heals by secondary intention
3. A wound that becomes infected
4. A wound to an extremity

14 A postoperative client tells the nurse that he developed dehiscence after his last surgery and wants to make sure it doesn't happen this time. Which nursing intervention should the nurse implement that would be most effective in preventing dehiscence in a postoperative client?

1. Helping the client lose weight
2. Preventing vomiting
3. Administering antibiotics
4. Keeping the wound dry

15 An older adult client's postoperative abdominal wound is still healing weeks after the surgery. The client asks the clinic nurse why the wound is healing so slowly. Which factors should the nurse identify that negatively affect healing in older adults? Select all that apply.

1. Vascular changes
2. Nutritional status
3. Decreased activity
4. Keloid formation
5. Nutrient absorption

16 A client admitted to the hospital for gallbladder surgery is diagnosed as having a vitamin C deficiency. The nurse places high priority on assessing this client for which development postoperatively?

1. Unusual muscle weakness
2. Mental confusion
3. Delayed wound healing
4. Ataxia upon ambulating

17 The nurse is assessing a client with a mobility problem to determine an appropriate assistance device. The client's lower extremities have no paralysis, but are very weak. Upper-body strength is also reduced. The nurse should suggest which device for this client?

1. Cane
2. Four-wheeled walker
3. Canadian or elbow extension crutch
4. Lofstrand crutch

18 The nurse is evaluating a client using a cane. Which assessment made by the nurse would indicate that the client is using the cane appropriately?

1. Client holds the cane with the hand on the stronger side.
2. Client holds the cane with the hand on the affected side.
3. Client moves the cane and the affected leg together.
4. The cane tip is made of aluminum to prevent slippage.

19 A client is at risk for developing a pressure injury and is placed on a repositioning regimen. The client does not like to lie on his side and complains about the need to turn. Which explanations by the nurse may enhance compliance? Select all that apply.

1. "Turning helps maintain skin integrity by alternating areas of pressure."
2. "Excess pressure interferes with skin absorption of vitamin D."
3. "Changing positions will promote circulation and prevent contractures."
4. "Changing position helps prevent skin breakdown that could ultimately lead to infection."
5. "A repositioning schedule is a standard part of hospital policy."

20 The nurse is changing the abdominal dressing of a client who is 4 days postoperative. The nurse notes a moderate amount of serosanguineous drainage, wound edges not approximated, and puffy tissue protruding through the wound. What condition should the nurse suspect from theses manifestations?

1. Hemorrhage
2. Normal healing by primary intention
3. Normal healing by secondary intention
4. Evisceration

21 The nurse needs to conduct an admission interview with a 74-year-old client who is hearing impaired. What should the nurse do to enhance the client's ability to hear? Select all that apply.

1. Position self to be within the client's line of vision
2. Dim the lights in the room
3. Overarticulate words
4. Turn down the television in the room
5. Use a moderate rate and the same tone for all words

ANSWERS & RATIONALES

1 **Answer: 3 Rationale:** Age above 65 is a risk factor for cataracts. Increased intraocular pressure and blurred vision are signs of glaucoma. History of staph infection is not a risk factor for cataracts. **Cognitive Level:** Applying **Client Need:** Basic Care and Comfort **Integrated Process:** Nursing Process: Assessment **Content Area:** Fundamentals **Strategy:** The core issue of the question is knowledge of factors that increase client risk for conditions affecting sensory perception. Use the process of elimination and nursing knowledge to make a selection.

2 **Answer: 3 Rationale:** Hearing loss, especially of upper-range tones, is common in older adults. Speaking to the client slowly and in a normal-pitched voice while facing the client is the best means of communication. Cleaning cerumen from the client's ears will not overcome age-related hearing loss. Depending on the level of hearing loss, speaking louder into the ear with the better hearing may still not be an effective action. The question states that the client is hard of hearing without reference to a hearing aid; if a hearing aid is used, changing the batteries may not be an effective action. **Cognitive Level:** Applying **Client Need:** Basic Care and Comfort **Integrated Process:** Communication and Documentation **Content Area:** Fundamentals **Strategy:** Apply knowledge related to communicating with a client who is hearing impaired. Remember that if the age of the client is included in the stem, it is important in determining the correct option. Consider the question as it is written and do not make assumptions.

3 **Answer: 3, 4 Rationale:** Providing the client with a clock and calendar helps the client to be oriented to time and date. These would be meaningful stimuli for the client and decrease the chance for sensory deprivation. Activities and rest periods should be spaced and planned to balance high and low levels of sensory stimuli. It may not be realistic in an ICU to remove equipment from the room. Explaining all procedures and routines would increase the risk of overload. Continuous conversation is not therapeutic and could place the client at risk for sensory overload as a different problem. **Cognitive Level:** Applying **Client Need:** Basic Care and Comfort **Integrated Process:** Nursing Process: Implementation **Content Area:** Fundamentals **Strategy:** The core issue of the question is nursing actions that can prevent the client from experiencing sensory deprivation. Use knowledge of basic nursing measures to help a client stay oriented to time, place, and person make appropriate selections.

4 **Answer: 1 Rationale:** To prevent vascular impairment, proper application of elastic bandages is required. Wrapping distal to proximal is compatible with the flow of venous return. Wrapping the bandage evenly while stretching it moderately ensures that there will be even tension applied to the extremity while not occluding circulation. Wrapping the bandage loosely enough to be able to insert two fingers will not secure the bandage in place or provide adequate support for the injury. Excessive tension when applying an elastic bandage would cause circulation to be compromised. Wrapping in a proximal to distal direction would inhibit venous return. **Cognitive Level:** Applying **Client Need:** Basic Care and Comfort **Integrated Process:** Nursing Process: Implementation **Content Area:** Fundamentals **Strategy:** The core issue of the question is knowledge of basic wound care procedures. Use nursing knowledge of these procedures and concepts related to blood flow to make your selection.

5 **Answer: 1, 2, 3 Rationale:** A cat bite, a laceration, and a stab wound all impair skin integrity, which could lead to infection, and thus may require prophylactic use of an antibiotic. A closed fracture or a sprain do not involve a break in the skin so there is no specific risk of infection. **Cognitive Level:** Analyzing **Client Need:** Basic Care and Comfort **Integrated Process:** Nursing Process: Implementation **Content Area:** Fundamentals **Strategy:** The core issue of the question is appropriate use of antibiotic therapy. Restate this question in the following way: "Which client is *not* at risk for infection?" Use the process of elimination and nursing knowledge to make selections that address the risk of infection.

6 **Answer: 2 Rationale:** Disuse syndrome is a result of prolonged immobility. Stating "the client remains free of contractures" describes in active terms the desired outcome for the client. Using "shorter periods of immobility" does not provide a specific expectation or outcome for the client. Stating that the nurse will turn the client every 2 hours is an intervention and not a goal. A goal needs to state a specific expectation or outcome for the client. Stating that the nurse will perform passive range of motion every 4 hours is an intervention and not a goal. A goal needs to state a specific expectation or outcome for the client. **Cognitive Level:** Applying **Client Need:** Basic Care and Comfort **Integrated Process:** Nursing Process: Planning **Content Area:** Fundamentals **Strategy:** Apply knowledge related to the nursing process, the pathophysiology of disuse syndrome, and appropriate client goals. Recall that goal statements are indicators of what the nurse wants to happen as a result of care. With these general principles in mind, eliminate each of the incorrect responses.

7 **Answer: 4 Rationale:** Changes in environment bring about uncertainty, and the client may be unable to sleep or may sleep less well than at home. Other than being hospitalized, there is no data to support that the client is unable to proactively manage health. It is more likely that the client's difficulty with sleep has a physiological basis rather than a psychological one (difficulty coping). Although the client has periods of confusion, there is no data presented that indicates the client is experiencing hallucinations. **Cognitive Level:** Analyzing **Client Need:** Basic Care and Comfort **Integrated Process:** Nursing Process: Diagnosis **Content Area:** Fundamentals **Strategy:** Exercise the ability to draw correct conclusions about client assessment data given specific client circumstances. In this case, the original problem is sleeping, and the correct answer is one that focuses on this problem.

8 **Answer: 2 Rationale:** Weight-bearing exercise is the best approach to preventing disuse syndrome. Disuse syndrome occurs because the stresses of weight-bearing are absent and the bone releases calcium. While nutritional needs of a client with Parkinson's is an appropriate nursing intervention, it does not address the prevention of disuse syndrome. Encouraging fluids is important for the elderly client because they become easily dehydrated due to a decreased sense of thirst; however, it does not address the prevention of disuse syndrome. Turning and repositioning every 2 hours is an important nursing intervention to prevent skin breakdown; this action does not specifically address the

prevention of disuse syndrome. **Cognitive Level:** Applying **Client Need:** Basic Care and Comfort **Integrated Process:** Nursing Process: Implementation **Content Area:** Fundamentals **Strategy:** Apply knowledge related to the cause of disuse syndrome and the nursing interventions that will minimize it. Use concepts of basic nursing care to answer the question.

9 **Answer: 4 Rationale:** The description refers to the wound itself and is the best indication of the wound's current status. A decrease in redness and the presence of granulation are indicators that there is progress toward the goal of injury healing. Turning the client every 2 hours evaluates whether the plan of care is carried out and does not focus on client goal achievement. Changing the dressing every 4 hours evaluates whether wound care was carried out according to the plan of care; it does not reflect client goal achievement. Noting that no additional areas of breakdown have occurred indicate that the client's condition has not worsened since admission, but does not indicate whether the pressure injury is actually healing. **Cognitive Level:** Applying **Client Need:** Basic Care and Comfort **Integrated Process:** Communication and Documentation **Content Area:** Fundamentals **Strategy:** Apply knowledge regarding the nursing process and the concepts of documentation. Distinguish which option most accurately answers the question.

10 **Answer: 2 Rationale:** After immobilization, unexercised muscles will atrophy. Hypertrophy is the opposite of atrophy. Flexibility is a term most frequently applied to joint movement. Hardened is a term that describes muscles that have been developed by exercise or activity. **Cognitive Level:** Knowledge **Client Need:** Basic Care and Comfort **Integrated Process:** Communication and Documentation **Content Area:** Fundamentals **Strategy:** This question requires application of basic nursing knowledge and terminology to a client situation. Select the term that is a common finding in clients who are immobilized.

11 **Answer: 2 Rationale:** Passive range of motion is most appropriate because the client is unable to move the left side of the body on her own because of hemiplegia. Active range of motion requires the client to move the body independently. Isotonic exercises require the ability to tighten the muscles on the left side. Isometric exercises require the ability to perform resistance with the muscles on the left side. **Cognitive Level:** Applying **Client Need:** Basic Care and Comfort **Integrated Process:** Nursing Process: Implementation **Content Area:** Fundamentals **Strategy:** The critical words in the question are *hemiplegia on the left side*. This indicates that the client cannot move the left side of the body and is unable to actively participate in exercising the joints. The wording of the question tells you that there is only one correct answer.

12 **Answer: 3 Rationale:** The weight of the body should be borne on the arms, not the axillae. When clients allow the axillae to bear the weight of the body, they are at risk of developing crutch palsy (nerve damage). This behavior would require additional client teaching. The ability to perform the swing-to gait represents correct use of crutches, and therefore no further teaching is needed on those points. Axillary crutches are crutches that are appropriately positioned beneath the axilla of the body. If a client is able to use axillary crutches without bearing weight on the armpits, no further teaching is needed. Placing new rubber tips on the crutches indicates an awareness of equipment safety that requires no further teaching. Worn crutch tips can cause a client to slip or fall. **Cognitive Level:** Analyzing **Client Need:** Reduction of Risk Potential **Integrated Process:** Nursing Process: Evaluation **Content Area:** Fundamentals **Strategy:** The core issue of the question is proper use of crutches. Keep in mind that this question has a negative stem and the correct answer is the option that reflects incorrect information.

13 **Answer: 1 Rationale:** Primary intention healing occurs when the wound edges are well approximated; wounds that heal by primary intention are least likely to scar. Wounds that heal by secondary intention have edges that cannot be approximated. The chance for scarring is greater for wounds that heal by secondary intention. Wounds that become infected are more likely to scar due to prolonged healing time, decreased probability of approximated wound edges, and increased chance of tissue loss. The further away from the heart, the longer the wound may take to heal. However, the location of a wound is not significant in regard to the likelihood of scarring. **Cognitive Level:** Applying **Client Need:** Basic Care and Comfort **Integrated Process:** Nursing Process: Diagnosis **Content Area:** Fundamentals **Strategy:** The core issue of this question is knowledge of physiological wound healing. The question should be read carefully because the client asks which wounds will heal best and the stem asks which wound is least likely to scar.

14 **Answer: 2 Rationale:** Activities that are likely to lead to dehiscence include vomiting and coughing because they increase intra-abdominal pressure. Clients who are obese and those with poor nutrition are candidates for dehiscence. Since the client is already postoperative, encouraging weight loss at this time would not affect risk for dehiscence, and there is no indication that the client is overweight. Administering antibiotics is effective in preventing or treating infection. Antibiotic therapy alone cannot prevent dehiscence. Keeping a wound dry will promote healing and prevent infection; however, this action alone will not prevent dehiscence. **Cognitive Level:** Analysis **Client Need:** Basic Care and Comfort **Integrated Process:** Nursing Process: Planning **Content Area:** Fundamentals **Strategy:** The core issue of the question is knowledge of risk factors for dehiscence. Recall that dehiscence is most likely to occur when there is some type of stress on the incision line. Consider that vomiting puts sudden tension on the suture line to select it as the option that is most likely to be harmful to the client.

15 **Answer: 1, 2, 5 Rationale:** Vascular changes in older adults, such as atherosclerosis and atrophy of capillaries, impair blood flow to the wound and negatively affect healing. Wound healing requires increased dietary intake of protein and vitamin C. The nutritional status of an older adult may be inadequate for a variety of reasons, such as difficulty with chewing or swallowing; lack of access to food sources; or food choices restricted by financial status. In older adults, deficient absorption of nutrients can occur because of chewing difficulties, decreased peristalsis, and/or reduced secretion of digestive enzymes—all of which can contribute to a delay in healing. A decreased activity level with aging does not diminish local blood supply to a healing wound. Keloid formation is an abnormal type of healing of a wound, which is not specific to the older adult client. **Cognitive Level:** Analysis **Client Need:** Basic Care and Comfort **Integrated Process:** Nursing Process: Evaluation **Content Area:** Fundamentals **Strategy:** The core issue of the question is age-related changes that have a negative impact on wound healing. This question has more than one correct answer and each option should be approached as a true/false statement before selecting the answer.

16 **Answer: 3 Rationale:** Protein and vitamin C are necessary for building and maintaining tissues. A deficiency of vitamin C would prolong wound healing. A vitamin C deficiency is not associated with unusual muscle weakness. Mental confusion is not a manifestation of vitamin C deficiency. Ataxia upon ambulating does not occur with vitamin C deficiency. **Cognitive Level:** Understanding **Client Need:** Basic Care and Comfort **Integrated Process:** Nursing Process: Diagnosis **Content Area:** Fundamentals **Strategy:** The core issue of this question is the role of vitamin C in wound healing. Use nursing knowledge and the process of elimination to make a selection.

17 **Answer: 2 Rationale:** The client has bilateral weakness of the lower extremities, and the proper assistive device is one that will provide bilateral support. In this case, a four-wheeled walker provides the most support and does not require the client to lift the walker as steps are taken. A cane would provide only limited support for a client with very weak lower extremities. A Canadian or elbow extension crutch requires adequate upper-body strength, which this client does not have. A Loftstand crutch extends only to the forearm and is not the best choice for a client with reduced upper-body strength. **Cognitive Level:** Analyzing **Client Need:** Safety and Infection Control **Integrated Process:** Nursing Process: Evaluation **Content Area:** Fundamentals **Strategy:** The core issue of the question is the assistive device that will provide the safest support to the client. The critical points of upper- and lower-extremity weakness in the stem of the question guide you to look for an option that provides bilateral support and minimal upper body strength.

18 **Answer: 1 Rationale:** To provide maximum support and appropriate body alignment while walking, the cane is held in the hand on the stronger side. The cane and the strongest leg should be advanced together in order to provide a stable stance when the weak leg is advanced. The tip of the cane should be rubber to prevent slipping. **Cognitive Level:** Applying **Client Need:** Safety and Infection Control **Integrated Process:** Nursing Process: Evaluation **Content Area:** Fundamentals **Strategy:** The core issue of the question is the proper use of a cane as an assistive aid. Use the process of elimination and basic nursing knowledge to make a selection.

19 **Answer: 1, 3, 4 Rationale:** Turning a client is one of the principal methods of preventing skin breakdown caused by pressure. When a client's position is changed, circulation to the previous areas of pressure is restored and the joints can be moved and aligned to prevent development of contractures. A loss of skin integrity places the client at risk for bacterial invasion and subsequent infection. Unless the skin loss is extensive, the skin will continue to absorb vitamin D. Making a reference to policy does not promote client understanding or compliance. **Cognitive Level:** Applying **Client Need:** Basic Care and Comfort **Integrated Process:** Teaching and Learning **Content Area:** Fundamentals **Strategy:** The core issue of the question is promoting compliance through client teaching about the benefits of turning and repositioning. Because there is more than one correct answer, look at each option as a true/false statement.

20 **Answer: 4 Rationale:** Evisceration occurs when internal viscera protrude from an incision that is dehiscing. In this situation, the nurse notes changes in wound appearance such as increased serosanguineous drainage, edges lacking approximation, and the protruding viscera. The nurse notes a moderate amount of serosanguineous drainage, which should be nearly diminished by the fourth day postoperative. However, this description does not fit hemorrhage. Healing by primary intention includes well-approximated incision edges and no signs of infection or complication. Secondary healing is when the wound is extensive and the edges cannot or should not be approximated; healing time is prolonged. **Cognitive Level:** Analyzing **Client Need:** Basic Care and Comfort **Integrated Process:** Nursing Process: Diagnosis **Content Area:** Fundamentals **Strategy:** The core issue of this question is the ability to draw accurate conclusions about the status of a surgical wound. Use the process of elimination and basic nursing knowledge to make a selection.

21 **Answer: 1, 4, 5 Rationale:** The nurse should select a position within the client's line of vision to enable the client to read lips during the conversation. It is good to decrease background noises that interfere with the client's ability to hear the nurse. It is also helpful to speak at a moderate rate and use the same voice tone throughout each sentence, not dropping the tone at the end of a sentence. The lighting should not be dimmed because doing so would interfere with the client's ability to see the nurse clearly in order to read lips. Words should not be overarticulated; exaggerated, unnatural movement of the lips can distort words for the client who relies on lip reading to compensate for hearing loss. **Cognitive Level:** Applying **Client Need:** Basic Care and Comfort **Integrated Process:** Communication and Documentation **Content Area:** Fundamentals **Strategy:** The core issue of the question is effective communication strategies with a client whose hearing is impaired. Remember to focus on enhancing the client's vision during communication and use a moderate overall approach (i.e., not excessive or insufficient). When there are multiple correct answers to a question, consider each option as a true/false statement.

Key Terms to Review

circadian synchronization p. 380
dehiscence p. 392
dyspnea p. 376
evisceration p. 392
hyperventilation p. 376
hypoventilation p. 376
Kegel exercises p. 384
keloid p. 391
orthopnea p. 377
presbycusis p. 388
pressure injury p. 375
primary intention p. 392
secondary intention p. 392
sensory deficit p. 387
sensory deprivation p. 387
sensory overload p. 387

References

Ball, J., & Bindler, R., & Cowen, K. (2015). *Principles of pediatric nursing: Caring for children* (6th ed.). Hoboken, NJ: Pearson Education.

Berman, A., Snyder, S., & Frandsen, G. (2016). *Kozier & Erb's fundamentals of nursing: Concepts, process, and practice* (10th ed.). New York, NY: Pearson Education.

Craven, R., & Hirnle, C., & Henshaw, C. (2017). *Fundamentals of nursing: Human health and function* (8th ed.). Philadelphia, PA: Wolters-Kluwer.

Potter, P., Perry, A., Stockert, P., Hall, A. (2017). *Fundamentals of nursing* (9th ed.). St. Louis, MO: Mosby.

Smith, S., Duell, D., Martin, B., Aebersold, M., & Gonzalez, L. (2017). *Clinical nursing skills: Basic to advanced skills* (10th ed.). New York, NY: Pearson Education.

Test Yourself

Are you ready for the NCLEX-RN® or course exams? Access the NEW web-based app that provides students with thousands of practice questions in preparation for the NCLEX experience.

Maintaining the Function of Tubes and Drains 27

In this chapter

Cross Reference

Other chapters relevant to this content area are

Meeting Nutritional Needs	Chapter 25
Meeting Basic Human Needs	Chapter 26
Perioperative Care	Chapter 48
Respiratory Disorders	Chapter 55
Renal and Genitourinary Disorders	Chapter 58
Gastrointestinal Disorders	Chapter 59

I. RESPIRATORY TUBES

A. Tracheostomy tube

1. Overview
   a. A **tracheostomy** is a surgically created opening into trachea into which a tracheostomy tube can be placed to establish a patent airway
   b. Tracheostomy tubes can be temporary or permanent, and may be attached to humidified air, oxygen, or to a mechanical ventilator as needed (see Figure 27–1A)
   NCLEX® c. Variations in tubes include double-lumen or single-lumen (inner cannula or no inner cannula), cuffed or cuffless, and fenestrated or nonfenestrated (see Table 27–1)
2. Therapeutic management
   a. Maintain head of bed elevated at least low Fowler's (30 degrees) and preferably semi-Fowler's or high Fowler's position
   NCLEX® b. Ensure that a manual resuscitation (Ambu) bag is at bedside at all times
   NCLEX® c. Keep spare tracheostomy (trach) set of same size, obturator, and clamps at bedside for use if trach is accidentally removed
   d. Ensure that air and oxygen (O_2) flowing into airway is humidified as prescribed because bypassing nose and mouth eliminates natural humidification process

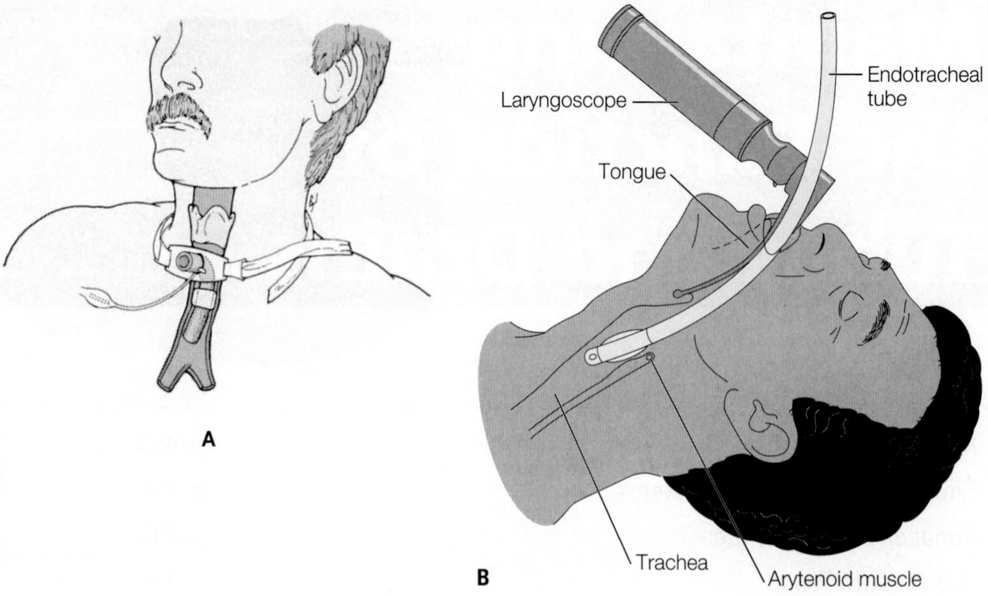

Figure 27–1

(A) Tracheostomy tube in place. (B) Endotracheal tube positioned in trachea.

Table 27–1 Comparison of Features of Tracheostomy Tubes

Feature	Present	Absent
Inner cannula (a removable inner tube within an outer tracheostomy tube)	Double-lumen tubes have both inner and outer cannulas; inner one can be removed for easy cleaning, especially with heavy secretions, and may be reusable or disposable.	Single-lumen tubes have no inner cannula and may be used short term or in clients not anticipated to have copious respiratory secretions.
Cuff (a balloon that seals airway)	Cuffed tube prevents air loss during mechanical ventilation and prevents aspiration of saliva, gastric contents, or tube feedings; inflated with air using syringe attached to pilot balloon.	Cuffless tube is often selected for long-term use in clients who do not need mechanical ventilation and are at low risk of aspiration.
Fenestration (holes to allow air flow between larynx and trachea)	Fenestrated trach is used frequently during weaning so client regains ability to breathe naturally; it allows client to speak.	Nonfenestrated tubes have no holes and are ideal for clients on mechanical ventilation or who cannot speak.

e. Encourage coughing and deep breathing to reduce risk of atelectasis and pneumonia

f. Assess respiratory status, including breath sounds, at regular intervals, minimally every 4 hours

g. Monitor and document O_2 saturation and/or arterial blood gas results and note trends

NCLEX® **h.** Suction client as indicated (cough, noisy respirations, or adventitious breath sounds); hyperoxygenate client before and after, suction for no more than 10 seconds at one time; assess secretions for blood or signs of infection (purulent secretions); see Chapter 26 for suctioning procedure

NCLEX® **i.** Assess stoma for redness or signs of infection; assess for and report subcutaneous emphysema (subcutaneous air, also called crepitus)

j. Perform trach care every 8 hours; use normal saline to cleanse site and inner cannula unless agency policy is different

k. Change trach ties daily or more often if soiled; have assistant hold trach in place so client cannot cough it out; if assistance is unavailable, place new ties before cutting and removing old ones to prevent tube dislodgement; a commercial tube holder that is soft and uses Velcro closure may be used instead of ties

l. Monitor cuff pressures (if inflated) at least every 8 hours per agency policy (should not exceed 20 mmHg); see endotracheal tube section that follows for cuff inflation techniques

NCLEX® **m.** Provide for alternate means of communication (word or picture board, writing pad) if client cannot talk because of cuff inflation

NCLEX® **n.** If client is prescribed oral intake while trach is in place, inflate cuff to reduce risk of aspiration and sit client upright during meals and for 1 hour afterward as ordered

NCLEX®
o. Before capping with Passey-Muir valve or plugging trach as final stage of weaning before trach removal, ensure that fenestrated trach is in use (necessary for plugging and is preferred for capping) and that cuff, if present, is deflated; note that cuff inflation during capping and plugging will occlude client's airway, leading to respiratory distress and arrest

NCLEX®
3. Complications (see Table 27–2)
4. Planned removal

NCLEX®
a. Suction trachea and oropharyngeal area to remove any secretions
b. Ensure that cuff is deflated
c. Healthcare provider cuts sutures that hold tracheostomy in place and withdraws tube during exhalation
d. Place dry sterile dressing over stoma and tape gently in place
e. Stoma closes over next few days and leaves small scar

Table 27–2 Complications of Tracheostomy

Complication	Prevention and Therapeutic Management
Short term	
Tube dislodgment (accidental removal)	Secure tube properly and do not allow client to pull at tube. Prevent traction on tube and avoid excessive tube movement. Keep spare tube of same size at bedside. Follow agency policy if tube displacement occurs. If dislodged in first 72 hours after placement, manually ventilate using resuscitation bag while an assistant gets emergency assistance. If dislodged more than 72 hours after placement, extend neck and separate tissues of stoma to restore airway; use retention sutures and/or tracheal dilator (curved clamp) to hold stoma open; insert obturator into trach tube, insert tube into trachea, remove obturator, ventilate with resuscitation bag, and assess air exchange and respiratory status; if unsuccessful or ineffective, get emergency assistance.
Tube obstruction	Assess client for respiratory difficulty, audible noisy respirations, thick and viscous tracheal secretions, and newly increased peak pressure on mechanical ventilator. Humidify oxygen, suction client as needed, and keep inner cannula clean. Encourage client to cough and deep breathe. Prepare for rapid tube replacement if obstruction is caused by cuff prolapse over distal end of tube.
Long term	
Tracheomalacia (tracheal dilation and erosion from high cuff pressures)	Assess for signs such as air leak around cuff, lost tidal volume (mechanical ventilation), or food particles or fluids in tracheal secretions (aspiration). Monitor cuff pressures and air volumes needed to keep cuff inflated per agency policy; identify and report increases. Monitor for and report onset of bleeding caused by pressure. Progress client to use of uncuffed tube at earliest opportunity.
Tracheoesophageal fistula (abnormal connection between posterior tracheal wall and esophagus from high cuff pressure)	Assess for signs similar to tracheomalacia above. Use soft feeding tube instead of nasogastric (NG) tube for feeding as possible prevention. Assess for client coughing, choking, or respiratory distress while taking food or fluids. Administer supplemental oxygen by mask to treat hypoxemia. Prepare for possible insertion of gastric or jejunostomy feeding tube if NGT pressure in esophagus is contributing factor.
Tracheal stenosis (narrowed tracheal lumen from scar formation caused by cuff irritation)	Observe for respiratory difficulty, increased coughing, inability to manage secretions, or difficulty in speaking after cuff deflation or trach tube removal. Prevent by avoiding high cuff pressures and avoiding traction or pulling on tube, keeping properly secured and using correct cuff pressures. Prepare client for surgical dilation of trachea for definitive treatment as needed.
Tracheal-innominate artery fistula (lateral tracheal wall erodes into artery because of pressure from distal tip of tube)	Prevent by keeping tube in midline position and avoiding traction on tube from any cause. Assess for pulsation of trach tube with each heartbeat and notify healthcare provider immediately if noted. Note fresh bleeding at or through stoma and report immediately. Remove tube immediately and apply direct pressure to blood vessel at stoma site. Prepare client for immediate life-saving surgical repair.

B. *Endotracheal tube* (ETT) (see Figure 27–1B, p. 404)

1. Overview
   a. An artificial airway that maintains airway patency and allows for mechanical ventilation; intended for short-term use, up to 10–14 days
   b. Consists of a long tube with a universal adapter at proximal end for attachment to oxygen source or ventilator, inflatable cuff at distal end (to prevent air leak, loss of tidal volume, or aspiration), and pilot balloon at proximal end for cuff inflation
2. Routes of insertion
   a. Orotracheal: allows for use of larger diameter tube and reduces respiratory effort; disadvantages are discomfort to client, possible displacement by tongue movement, and occlusion from biting on tube (oral airway may be used to prevent this)
   b. Nasotracheal: smaller diameter tube (more comfortable for client), prevents dislodgement by tongue, but increases respiratory effort; contraindicated with bleeding disorders, epistaxis, or nasal obstruction
3. Therapeutic management
   NCLEX® a. To assess placement after insertion, ventilate with manual resuscitation bag, and auscultate for bilateral breath sounds; if only right-sided breath sounds and chest expansion are noted, tube needs to be pulled back slightly (from right mainstem bronchus) until bilateral breath sounds and chest movements are present
   b. Auscultate over epigastric area to ensure esophageal intubation did not occur (ventilation sounds will be louder over stomach than chest; abdomen will rise and fall with ventilations); tube is removed immediately if this occurs
   c. A carbon dioxide (CO_2) analyzer is often used to check proper placement in trachea per agency protocol
   NCLEX® d. Confirm placement by portable chest x-ray; distal tip of tube should be 1–2 cm above carina (point of bifurcation of right and left mainstem bronchi)
   e. Tape tube in place or use other securing device; note position of tube (document centimeter marking at lip line) and monitor placement at least every 8 hours
   NCLEX® f. Ensure manual resuscitation bag is kept at bedside at all times
   NCLEX® g. Perform respiratory assessments every 4 hours and as needed; suction client as indicated by results of assessment as with tracheostomy
   h. Check cuff pressure every 8 hours or per agency policy; ensure it does not exceed 20 mmHg by anaeroid manometer using either minimal occluding volume or minimal leak technique
   i. Inflate cuff using minimal occluding volume technique by injecting air into pilot balloon just until no air leakage sounds can be heard during inspiration with stethoscope placed over trachea
   j. Inflate cuff using minimal leak technique by injecting air into pilot balloon until sealed and then deflating slightly so that no harsh sounds can be heard during inspiration but slight leak is heard at peak of inspiration
   k. Insert oral airway if orotracheal route is used to prevent client from biting tube or displacing tube with tongue movement
   l. Reposition orotracheal tube from one side of mouth to other daily with assistance of one other person; assess oral cavity for ulceration or necrosis
   m. Provide oral care every 2 hours to prevent drying and cracking of lips and mucous membranes
   NCLEX® n. Provide for alternative means of communication (word or picture board, writing pad)
4. Removal (extubation)
   a. Hyperoxygenate; suction endotracheal tube well; then suction oropharyngeal area
   b. Elevate head of bed to at least semi-Fowler's position
   c. Cuff is deflated and client is asked to inhale; at peak inspiration, tube is removed
   d. Encourage client to cough and deep breathe to clear residual secretions in throat
   e. Apply oxygen using delivery device and amount prescribed
   NCLEX® f. Monitor closely for first 30 minutes after extubation and frequently thereafter; notify healthcare provider if respiratory rate or effort show steady increase, oxygen saturation decreases, or respiratory distress occurs
   g. Explain that sore throat and hoarse voice are common and to limit talking; report hoarseness that doesn't improve over time (may indicate vocal cord damage)

II. CLOSED CHEST DRAINAGE SYSTEMS

A. Overview

1. A **chest tube** restores negative pressure to intrapleural space by draining air (pneumothorax), blood (hemothorax), or large amounts of fluid (pleural effusion) from pleural cavity
2. Closed chest drainage systems have three chambers: collection, water seal, and suction (Figure 27–2)

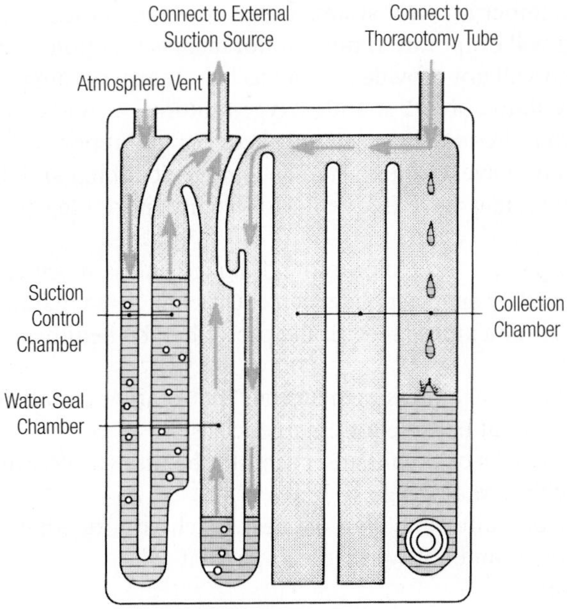

Figure 27–2

Disposable closed chest drainage system with three chambers: collection, water seal, and suction.

NCLEX® 3. Collection chamber connects chest tube to system; consists of marked columns (generally three) that indicate amount of drainage collected

NCLEX® 4. Water seal chamber (middle chamber) is filled to 2-cm marking; water allows air to escape system but not to reenter; during inhalation and exhalation, water moves up and down (oscillation; also called tidaling) in a tube in this chamber to indicate patency

NCLEX® 5. Suction control chamber allows use of suction to provide negative pressure to chest, which aids in reinflating lung more quickly by removing air, blood, pus, or effusion; suction level is determined by amount of water added to this chamber; when working properly, gentle, continuous bubbling occurs in this chamber

6. Some closed chest drainage systems use "dry" suction, controlled by adjusting suction knob to appropriate level; both types are connected to low wall suction using a connecting tube, but no bubbling in suction control chamber is present using "dry" system

7. Heimlich valve (one-way flutter valve): used instead of chest tube drainage system for selected ambulatory clients who have pneumothorax or to treat tension pneumothorax; valve allows air to escape chest cavity but not reenter; ensure arrow on valve housing points away from client

B. Therapeutic management

1. Maintain occlusive dressing (secured with large strips of wide tape or Elastoplast) at chest tube insertion site; reinforce as needed, but contact healthcare provider if dressings need to be changed

NCLEX® 2. Secure all chest tube and suction tubing connections with tape

NCLEX® 3. Keep collection apparatus 30.5 cm (12 in.) below chest level to allow gravity to promote chest drainage; keep tubing straight to prevent dependent loops or obstructions

NCLEX® 4. Monitor chest tube drainage at 1- to 4-hour intervals; report and document bright red blood, sudden increase in drainage, or consistent drainage greater than 100 mL/hour (provider may also specify volume to report)

5. Maintain 2-cm water level in water seal chamber; low water volume creates higher suction than may be desired, contributing to pleural tissue damage

NCLEX® 6. Assess for fluctuation in water seal chamber (tube is patent); absence of fluctuation may indicate tube obstruction, loop, or kink (requires correction) or full lung re-expansion (indicating tube is ready for removal); check client condition and time frame to aid in interpretation

NCLEX® 7. Assess for bubbling in water seal chamber

a. Continuous bubbling indicates an air leak in system and must be corrected; if leak is not found, notify surgeon

b. Intermittent bubbling that occurs with inspiration indicates drainage of air (pneumothorax) from pleural space and proper tube function; continue to monitor

8. Assess suction control chamber for correct amount of suction by either dial (dry system) or water level (fluid system); add sterile water if level is low (excessive wall suction speeds evaporation); remove excessive water by aspirating from rubber seal in chamber

9. Suction control chamber in "wet" system that uses water should have gentle, continuous bubbling; vigorous bubbling will evaporate water but not increase suction, and lack of continuous bubbling will not harm client but will not provide suction to help reexpand lung
10. Assess respiratory status, breath sounds, oxygen saturation, and comfort level every 4 hours or as indicated; assess that dressing is intact and check for and report subcutaneous emphysema
11. Change client position every 2 hours and encourage coughing and deep breathing
12. Anticipate that client may have frequent (up to daily) portable chest x-rays to monitor lung reexpansion
13. *NCLEX®* Do not milk or strip chest tube to promote drainage unless specifically prescribed by healthcare provider and allowed by agency policy (can cause changes in pleural pressure and/or tissue damage)
14. *NCLEX®* Do not clamp chest tube unless specifically prescribed by healthcare provider and allowed by agency policy
15. *NCLEX®* Keep a clamp and occlusive dressing materials (petrolatum gauze, dry sterile gauze, wide adhesive tape) and sterile water at bedside for emergency use
16. *NCLEX®* If drainage system cracks or breaks, insert chest tube into sterile water bottle to reestablish underwater seal and replace with new drainage system
17. *NCLEX®* If chest tube is accidentally pulled out of chest, pinch skin together, apply occlusive dressing using materials noted above, and notify surgeon immediately
18. Chest tube removal
    a. Indicated when fluctuation stops in water seal chamber, chest x-ray shows full lung expansion, and client has returned to normal or baseline respiratory status
    b. *NCLEX®* Obtain suture removal set, petrolatum gauze, dry sterile gauze or Telfa gauze, and wide adhesive tape; premedicate client with oral medication 30 minutes prior to removal if possible
    c. Instruct client to take deep breath, then hold breath (Valsalva) or exhale according to healthcare provider preference just prior to tube removal
    d. Open and prepare dressing materials just prior to tube removal; assist with application of dressing, and obtain follow-up chest x-ray if prescribed
    e. Assess and document respiratory status postremoval

III. RENAL AND URINARY TUBES

A. ***Nephrostomy tube***: drains urine from pelvis of kidney directly into urinary drainage bag, bypassing lower urinary system

1. Position tube (no kinks or compression) to maintain patency; do not clamp
2. Monitor and record urine output carefully; report output of less than 30 mL/hr or no drainage for 15 minutes or more
3. *NCLEX®* Irrigate tube only with a healthcare provider prescription; use a maximum of 5 mL sterile normal saline using strict surgical aseptic technique; inject slowly and gently
4. Report and document immediately if irrigation fails to restore tube patency

B. **Urinary catheters**

1. Types include straight catheter (for intermittent catheterization), indwelling urinary catheter (inflated balloon keeps catheter in bladder), and triple lumen or three-way catheter (allows for balloon inflation, urinary drainage, and inflow of bladder irrigation)
2. Insert using sterile technique; measure and record initial outflow amount and characteristics of urine
3. Properly position drainage bag below level of bladder (if indwelling) and secure catheter to thigh to prevent traction of balloon against urethra and bladder neck
4. Measure and record outputs accurately
5. Provide catheter care with soap and warm water using standard precautions
6. Wash front to back for females; in males retract foreskin if present, and return to original position after cleansing
7. Explain procedure to client just prior to removal; empty and record drainage, deflate balloon, and withdraw catheter while client exhales to reduce discomfort

C. ***Suprapubic catheter***

1. Inserted surgically through abdominal wall above symphysis pubis and into urinary bladder to drain urine
2. Attached to a closed urinary drainage system and uses principles of care associated with urinary drainage systems
3. Monitor catheter patency, urine output, client fluid intake, and client's general comfort
4. Change dressing around suprapubic catheter using sterile technique, tape in an occlusive fashion, and secure catheter to abdomen to prevent accidental dislodgement

5. If placement is temporary, catheter is allowed to drain for 48–72 hours, then a clamping schedule (3–4 hours at a time) may be prescribed until client can void satisfactory urine volume
6. If placement is permanent, client may not need to wear a dressing after insertion tract has healed (takes 6 weeks to 6 months); if catheter dislodges before full tract healing, catheter must be replaced within 30 min to avoid skin closure

IV. NASOGASTRIC TUBES

A. Overview

1. A **nasogastric tube** is inserted via naris to stomach to decompress stomach (remove food and fluids), reduce risk of aspiration, administer medications or enteral feedings, irrigate stomach (to remove toxins or poisons), or allow surgical anastomoses to heal (gastric surgery)
2. Commonly used is Salem sump, a double-lumen tube with air vent that allows for continuous (rather than intermittent) suction for gastric decompression; keep air vent above level of stomach and do not clamp; 30 mL air can be instilled through vent as needed to promote drainage through drainage lumen
3. Much less commonly used tube is Levin tube, a single-lumen tube that requires use of intermittent suction (lack of air vent causes tube to collapse if continuous suction is used)

NCLEX® **B. Insertion procedure (see Box 27–1)**

C. Therapeutic management

1. Assess placement
   - *NCLEX®* a. Chest x-ray is most reliable method of assessing tube placement
   - *NCLEX®* b. Aspirate gastric contents using piston syringe and apply to strip of pH test paper (pH of 4 or lower is consistent with gastric placement; pH of 6 or higher indicates intestinal placement); note that enteral feedings could alter pH and make this method less reliable
   - c. Inserting 5–10 mL air into tube while listening over epigastric area with stethoscope for "whooshing" or popping sound is a less reliable method than x-ray or gastric pH measurement
   - *NCLEX®* d. Check placement every 4 hours after insertion
2. Assess residual prior to and regularly during enteral feedings (see Chapter 25)
3. Irrigate tube with 30–50 mL water or saline as ordered to check tube patency; instill fluid using piston syringe and aspirate contents back; repeat if tube is difficult to irrigate or sluggish; document fluid instilled and aspirated back on intake and output record
4. Assess naris for ulceration from pressure when changing tape daily; provide nose care by removing any crusted areas with moist swabs
5. Provide mouth care every 2 hours; presence of tube in nose leads to mouth breathing and dryness

Box 27-1

Nasogastric Tube Insertion

1. Explain procedure, perform hand hygiene; sit client upright (high Fowler's position)
2. Place distal end of tube at tip of nose and measure to earlobe and then to xiphoid process to determine distance for tube insertion; mark tube to indicate point at which to stop insertion
3. Lubricate distal 5–7.6 cm (2–3 in.) of tube with lidocaine gel or water-soluble gel according to policy (not oil-based lubricant, which could cause pneumonia if tube enters trachea)
4. Ask client to tilt head downward (to close epiglottis so tube will enter esophagus)
5. Insert tube into naris and advance upward and backward until meeting resistance at back of nose; rotate catheter gently and advance into nasopharynx
6. Ask client to take sips of water if able while tube is advanced gently into stomach
7. Stop tube insertion and pull back on tube if client coughs or chokes during procedure; when client's respiratory status returns to normal, continue insertion
8. Stop advancing tube once tape reaches naris; check placement as outlined below
9. Tape tube in place
10. Place tube to low continuous (Salem sump) or intermittent (Levin) suction for gastric decompression
11. Do not begin enteral feedings by nasogastric tube (see Chapter 25) until placement confirmed by x-ray

6. Tube removal
    a. Check prescription, perform hand hygiene, apply gloves, and remove tape securing tube to nose
    b. Ask client to take a deep breath and hold it, then withdraw tube slowly and evenly over 3–6 seconds; coil tube around hand for control
    c. Provide comfort care and document procedure

V. NASOENTERIC (INTESTINAL) TUBES

A. Overview

1. A **nasoenteric (intestinal) tube** is used to treat intestinal obstruction; inserted nasally into stomach and passes into intestine via peristalsis assisted by balloon at lower end of tube filled with tungsten; common tubes are Andersen tube and Miller Abbott tube
2. Once tube has reached intestines it is secured to nose once final placement is verified by abdominal x-ray
3. Suction is applied once tube is in place for bowel decompression and removal of accumulated intestinal secretions

B. Therapeutic management

1. Check healthcare provider prescription and agency policy regarding tube advancement and removal
2. *NCLEX®* After tube insertion into stomach, maintain client position on right side initially to facilitate tube passage through pyloric sphincter of stomach into small intestine; then reposition client side to side every 2 hours to faciliate migration of tube to area of obstruction
3. *NCLEX®* Wait until tube has reached final placement, as verified by x-ray (may take several hours), before securing to nose with tape
4. *NCLEX®* Perform routine abdominal assessments and measure abdominal girth
5. Monitor and record amount and characteristics of tube drainage; if tube becomes blocked, notify physician; a small amount of air may be prescribed to help clear lumen
6. Remove tube according to institutional policy and procedure
    a. Aspirate tungsten and air using 5 mL syringe
    b. Withdraw tube approximately 15 cm (6 in.) each hour or as prescribed
    c. Dispose of tungsten as per agency policy

VI. COMBINED ESOPHAGEAL AND GASTRIC TUBES

A. Overview

1. Exert pressure against or provide tamponade to bleeding esophageal varices
2. Contraindicated with history of esophageal surgery or ulceration or necrosis of esophageal area
3. Airway management is an ongoing priority concern
4. *NCLEX®* **Sengstaken-Blakemore tube** has three lumens; one gastric lumen provides low intermittent gastric suction while round gastric balloon (in area of lower esophageal sphincter) and tubular esophageal balloon apply pressure against bleeding blood vessels
    a. Gastric balloon is inflated first, and then esophageal balloon is inflated (25–45 mmHg pressure) if gastric balloon is insufficient to stop bleeding
    b. Traction on tube is needed to maintain position of inflated balloons
    c. Check placement of tube by x-ray of chest and upper abdomen
    d. Prepare to insert NG tube in opposite naris to suction secretions that accumulate above esophageal balloon in esophagopharyngeal area to prevent aspiration
5. Minnesota tube is similar to Sengstaken-Blakemore tube but has additional (fourth) lumen to drain secretions from esophagopharyngeal area, eliminating need for separate NG tube placement in this area

B. Therapeutic management

1. Position client upright for insertion
2. Check all balloons prior to insertion and label each lumen
3. Double-clamp lumens to avoid air leaks
4. *NCLEX®* Keep head of bed raised after insertion
5. Obtain chest and upper abdominal x-ray to verify placement
6. Release esophageal balloon pressure intermittently per agency policy to prevent esophageal injury from ulceration or necrosis
7. *NCLEX®* Keep scissors at bedside to cut tube to rapidly deflate balloons if respiratory distress occurs

8. Monitor for complications
   a. Continued bleeding: steady or increased bloody drainage from gastric suction port; notify healthcare provider
   b. NCLEX® Esophageal rupture: upper abdominal and back pain, hypotension, tachycardia; report immediately: this is medical emergency

VII. TUBES FOR GASTRIC LAVAGE

A. Overview

1. NCLEX® Used to remove toxins from stomach due to drug or chemical poisoning or overdose
2. An **Ewald tube** is a large, reusable tube with a single lumen used for one-time rapid irrigation followed by aspiration of stomach contents
3. A Lavacuator tube has a lavage/vent lumen for irrigation and another lumen to provide continuous suction so that irrigation and suction can occur simultaneously

B. Therapeutic management

1. Determine that poison is appropriate for removal by lavage prior to procedure
2. Substances that have probably already been absorbed or substances that must be dialyzed out would contraindicate a need for irrigation
3. NCLEX® Airway management is a priority because of risk of aspiration, especially with possible decreased level of consciousness depending on poison or substance overdosed

VIII. WOUND AND MISCELLANEOUS DRAINS

A. Closed wound drainage systems

1. Consists of wound drain connected to electric suction apparatus or portable drainage suction (such as Jackson-Pratt drain or Hemovac drain)
2. Tube is sutured into place in surgery and attached to drainage reservoir
3. NCLEX® Measure and record drainage every shift; notify healthcare provider if drainage stops or increases suddenly or is brighter red in color; drainage should decrease over time
4. NCLEX® Wear gloves when emptying reservoir; avoid touching drainage port to prevent infection while uncapping port and draining fluid into collection device
5. NCLEX® Reestablish suction after emptying by compressing device with one hand while cleansing drainage port with alcohol swab and then closing cap or plug before releasing pressure; check device every 4 hours to be sure system is still compressed (which provides suction)
6. Often removed between 3 and 5 days postop, so prepare to teach some clients how to empty and maintain system at home

B. *Penrose drain*

1. A surgical drain less commonly used but may be optimal when excessive serosanguineous or purulent drainage is expected from wound
2. Usually inserted via a stab wound a few inches away from original incision to keep incision dry; drain is often 1.3–3.8 cm (0.5–1.5 in.) in diameter and up to 25–35 cm (10–14 in.) long
3. Advantage is preventing formation of abscesses because of excessive drainage
4. Drain may be drawn out or shortened by 2.5–5 (1–2 in.) each day as drainage lessens
5. NCLEX® Thick dressings, need for frequent dressing changes, and careful assessment of underlying skin are all priorities based on nature of drainage
6. Use of sterile technique is essential to prevent infection

C. *T-tube*

1. A T-shaped device inserted into common bile duct to maintain duct patency and allow drainage following cholecystectomy with bile duct exploration until surgical edema decreases
2. Keep T-tube below level of surgical wound and attached to sterile drainage device
3. Monitor drainage for color and consistency; up to 500 mL is expected in first 24 hours postop, decreasing to less than 200 mL in 2 or 3 days, and minimal after that; color is blood tinged at first and changes to brown-green
4. Assess for bile leakage during dressing changes and ensure tubing is properly secured after dressing change to prevent traction or pulling on tube
5. NCLEX® Assess for blockage of tube: absence of drainage, jaundice, and pale-colored stools
6. NCLEX® Follow clamping schedule before and after meals when prescribed
7. If client will be discharged with T-tube (may be left in for 7–10 days), teach client care of T-tube, how to clamp, and signs of infection to report

Check Your NCLEX–RN® Exam I.Q.

You are ready for testing on this content if you can:

- Use critical-thinking skills and scientific principles when caring for a client with a therapeutic tube or drain.
- Assess the client for patency and function of a therapeutic tube or drain.
- Monitor the progress of a client who has a therapeutic tube or drain.
- Teach the client and family pertinent information about a therapeutic tube or drain.
- Teach a client or family self-care of a therapeutic tube or drain as appropriate.

PRACTICE TEST

1 A client has returned to the nursing unit following a tracheostomy. In what order of importance would the nurse make the following assessments?

1. Respiratory rate and breath sounds
2. Amount of oxygen ordered to be delivered
3. Time when client last received pain medication
4. Status of tracheostomy dressing

Fill in your answer below:

Answer: 1 2 4 3

2 The nurse is providing care to a client who is 2 weeks postoperative for a tracheostomy. The nurse sees the tracheostomy tube come out when the client coughs. What should be the nurse's first action?

1. Call aloud for help.
2. Suction the stoma to remove residual secretions.
3. Grasp and spread the retention sutures to open the stoma.
4. Attempt to reinsert a new tracheostomy tube.

3 The client has just had emergency intubation for respiratory distress. Immediately following insertion of the endotracheal tube, what action by the nurse is most appropriate?

1. Tape the tube securely in place.
2. Assess for bilateral breath sounds.
3. Call for a chest x-ray to determine placement.
4. Provide the client an alternative method of communication.

4 Which respiratory assessment finding is of greatest concern to the nurse following endotracheal tube extubation?

1. Increased respiratory rate from 16 to 20 bpm
2. Scattered bilateral rhonchi
3. Expectoration of whitish yellow secretions
4. A harsh or crowing sound with inspiration

5 A client with a closed chest drainage system tries to get out of bed alone and disconnects the chest tube from the drainage system, which falls on the floor. In what order of importance should the nurse perform corrective actions after entering the client's room?

1. Submerge the tube in sterile water or saline.
2. Set up and attach a new closed chest drainage system.
3. Assess the client's respiratory status.
4. Check the client's pulse and blood pressure.

Fill in your answer below:

Answer: ________

6 Following chest tube insertion, the nurse notes continuous bubbling in the suction control chamber of the closed chest drainage system. What action should the nurse plan to take at this time?

1. Document and continue to monitor the bubbling.
2. Add water to the suction control chamber.
3. Remove water from the suction control chamber.
4. Turn up the suction on the wall suction unit.

7 During routine chest tube assessment, the nurse notes the presence of continuous bubbling in the water seal chamber of the closed chest drainage system. Which conclusion should the nurse draw from this data?

1. A new pneumothorax has developed.
2. There is an air leak in the system.
3. The wall suction unit is set on intermediate or high level.
4. The drainage tube connections are taped too tightly.

8 The client is scheduled for removal of a chest tube at 0900. At approximately 0830, what action should the nurse take?

1. Obtain a telephone report of the chest x-ray findings from radiology.
2. Administer a dose of a PRN analgesic to the client.
3. Ensure that a suture-removal set and dressing materials are available.
4. Explain to the client the upcoming removal procedure.

9 After a client's nephrostomy tube has stopped draining, the healthcare provider prescribes irrigation of the tube. How many milliliters (mL) is the maximum of fluid the nurse should use to carry out this procedure safely? Provide a numeric answer.

Fill in your answer below:

________ mL

10 A surgical client returns to the nursing unit with a nephrostomy tube in place. What is an appropriate action by the nurse when caring for this client?

1. Maintain patency with hourly irrigations.
2. Keep a clamp at the bedside.
3. Ensure the tubing is free of kinks.
4. Securely attach the drainage bag to the bedrail.

11 A nurse is assigned to a client with a nasogastric tube and is checking gastric pH to verify correct tube placement. Which pH reading should the nurse expect if the tube is properly positioned?

1. 4
2. 6
3. 7
4. 8

12 Which landmarks should the nurse use to correctly measure a client prior to nasogastric tube insertion? Select all that apply.

1. Tip of nose
2. Sternal notch
3. Mandibular joint
4. Tip of earlobe
5. Xiphoid process

13 A client with a partial bowel obstruction will undergo nasoenteric tube placement later in the day. The nurse should explain to the client that which position will be used after placement to promote tube migration to the intended area?

1. Flat and on the left side
2. Flat and on the right side
3. Head of bed elevated and on the left side
4. Head of bed elevated and on the right side

14 A client underwent insertion of a nasoenteric tube for partial bowel obstruction the previous evening. The nurse notes that the tube is not taped at the nose. Which action by the nurse is most appropriate at this time?

1. Call the healthcare provider immediately.
2. Securely tape the tube in place.
3. Note the finding on the client's flowsheet.
4. Call the radiology department to schedule an abdominal x-ray.

15 The nurse is receiving a report on a client who has a Sengstaken-Blakemore tube in place. The nurse expects that the client has which health problem as the primary reason for tube placement?

1. Cirrhosis of the liver
2. Esophageal varices
3. Portal hypertension
4. Abdominal ascites

16 The nurse has just assisted with insertion of a Sengstaken-Blakemore tube. The presence of what equipment is a priority at the bedside before the nurse leaves the client's room?

1. Suction
2. Oxygen
3. Scissors
4. Laryngoscope

PRACTICE TEST

17. The nurse working in the emergency department is awaiting arrival of a client who ingested half a bottle of acetaminophen a short while ago. The nurse should anticipate that which tube will be used to evacuate the client's stomach upon arrival?

1. Minnesota
2. Sengstaken-Blakemore
3. Ewald
4. Miller-Abbott

18. The nurse is aware that the client who underwent gastric lavage for overdose of a prescribed medication will need careful assessment for treatment complications. Which assessment should be the nurse's priority?

1. Respiratory rate and breath sounds
2. Heart rate and blood pressure
3. Skin color and body temperature
4. Urine output and peripheral edema

19. The nurse has emptied a Jackson Pratt wound drainage device and needs to reestablish suction to the tube. Which action should the nurse take to accomplish this objective?

1. Ensure the tubing has no kinks.
2. Squeeze the collection chamber.
3. Wipe the port with alcohol.
4. Close the cap on the device.

20. A client who underwent pelvic surgery the previous day has a Penrose drain placed in the lower abdomen. The nurse should take which action in the care of this wound drain?

1. Ensure that the drain stays in the original position placed by the surgeon.
2. Minimize number of gauze dressings around the tube for easier assessment.
3. Frequently assess the abdominal skin for irritation or breakdown.
4. Notify the surgeon if a large amount of drainage occurs.

21. The nurse has an order to insert a nasogastric tube into the stomach of an assigned client. In what order should the nurse perform the actions to complete the procedure? Place the options in the correct order. All options must be used.

1. Place distal end of tube at tip of nose and measure to earlobe and then to xiphoid process to determine distance for tube insertion
2. Insert tube into the nares and advance upward and backward until resistance is met; rotate catheter gently and advance into nasopharynx
3. Sit the client upright in a high Fowler's position
4. Ask client to take sips of water if able while tube is advanced gently into stomach
5. Tape tube to the client's nose to hold it securely in place

Fill in your answer below:

Answer: ____________________

ANSWERS & RATIONALES

ANSWERS & RATIONALES

1. **Answer: 1, 2, 4, 3 Rationale:** The status of the client's airway and breathing is the highest (first) priority assessment. Second, the delivery rate of oxygen is assessed to meet oxygenation needs and prevent hypoxia. Third, the dressing is assessed for signs of bleeding/hemorrhage. Fourth, the time lapse since any analgesic medication can be determined after the client is assessed for a patent airway, adequate oxygenation, and wound drainage/bleeding. **Cognitive Level:** Analyzing **Client Need:** Basic Care and Comfort **Integrated Process:** Nursing Process: Planning **Content Area:** Adult Health: Respiratory **Strategy:** Remember the ABCs—airway, breathing, and circulation—and Maslow's hierarchy of needs. In questions asking for priority setting, all options will be correct, and you need to select options in order of importance. Remembering the ABCs of *airway*, *breathing*, and *circulation* may help with questions that relate to respiratory or circulatory disorders or procedures, and note that these are physiological needs. The assessment of pain and the need for medication occurs after the ABCs, making it a lower priority.

2. **Answer: 3 Rationale:** The priority action of the nurse is to restore a patent airway. With this in mind, the nurse spreads the retention sutures to reopen the stomal opening of the tracheostomy. The nurse should call aloud for help so assistance will arrive to aid in tube reinsertion; however, establishing a patent airway is the first priority. The nurse cannot leave the client because a patent airway must be manually maintained. Suctioning the tracheostomy is not the priority action for the nurse to take. The nurse could reinsert a new tracheostomy tube if allowed by agency policy, since the tube has been in place for more than 72 hours; however, the stoma needs to be opened first. **Cognitive Level:** Analyzing **Client Need:** Basic Care and

Comfort **Integrated Process:** Nursing Process: Implementation **Content Area:** Adult Health: Respiratory **Strategy:** Remember the ABCs: *airway*, *breathing*, and *circulation*. The correct answer is one that directly affects the client's airway, which is opening the stoma. The other options are incorrect because they either are not the first action or may not be done at all.

3 **Answer: 2 Rationale:** The first action by the nurse is to assess for bilateral breath sounds as an initial indication of correct tube placement. After this is done, the tube should be securely taped in place to prevent dislodgement, a chest x-ray is needed to confirm tube placement, and then the nurse can assure the client about alternative communication means. **Cognitive Level:** Analyzing **Client Need:** Basic Care and Comfort **Integrated Process:** Nursing Process: Implementation **Content Area:** Adult Health: Respiratory **Strategy:** Remember the ABCs: *airway*, *breathing*, and *circulation*. The correct answer is one that directly affects the client's airway, which is assessing for bilateral breath sounds. Because the question asks for the priority action of the nurse, the other actions must be systematically eliminated.

4 **Answer: 4 Rationale:** A harsh or crowing sound with inspiration indicates stridor, which is consistent with airway narrowing and edema following endotracheal tube removal. This is of greatest concern because it could lead to upper respiratory obstruction. The nurse needs to notify the healthcare provider. An increase in respiratory rate from 16 to 20 bpm bears watching for trends; however, the respiratory rate is still within normal limits. The clients may be expected to have secretions that result in the development of rhonchi immediately after tube removal. The healthcare provider may order a culture of respiratory secretions to rule out the presence of an infection; however, this finding would not warrant the nurse's greatest concern. **Cognitive Level:** Analyzing **Client Need:** Basic Care and Comfort **Integrated Process:** Nursing Process: Assessment **Content Area:** Adult Health: Respiratory **Strategy:** Note the critical words *greatest concern*. This tells you that the correct option is the finding that is most abnormal. Use the process of elimination and knowledge of normal and abnormal physical assessment data to make a selection.

5 **Answer: 1, 3, 2, 4 Rationale:** The priority (first) action of the nurse is to submerge the tube in sterile water or saline to reestablish the underwater seal. This will prevent the client from sucking air through the chest tube into the pleural space during inspiration, thereby causing pneumothorax. Second, after the underwater seal is reestablished, the nurse would assess the client's respiratory status to try to detect new or enlarged pneumothorax, which is a medical emergency. Third, after reestablishing the underwater seal and assessing the client's respiratory status, a new closed chest drainage system is attached. Fourth (last), the nurse should obtain the client's full vital signs and then report the incident to the healthcare provider. **Cognitive Level:** Analyzing **Client Need:** Basic Care and Comfort **Integrated Process:** Nursing Process: Implementation **Content Area:** Adult Health: Respiratory **Strategy:** When prioritizing nursing actions, it can be helpful to visualize what should be done and the reason for the order of the actions. Recall that an underwater seal is critical to chest tube functioning to select the first action. Second, consider the ABCs and check for breathing. The client needs to be stabilized before vital signs are taken and the healthcare provider notified.

6 **Answer: 1 Rationale:** The nurse should document this normal finding and continue to monitor. Fluid addition and removal are based on fluid level, not on bubbling action of suction. The nurse should not turn up suction because the gentle bubbling indicates proper function. Increased suction could cause more rapid evaporation of water from chamber. **Cognitive Level:** Analyzing **Client Need:** Basic Care and Comfort **Integrated Process:** Nursing Process: Planning **Content Area:** Adult Health: Respiratory **Strategy:** The wording of the question indicates that there is a single correct answer. Recall that gentle bubbling is normal to guide your answer. Use nursing knowledge about closed chest drainage systems and the process of elimination to make a selection.

7 **Answer: 2 Rationale:** Continuous bubbling in the water seal chamber most often indicates a leak or loose connection in the system, and air is being sucked continuously into the closed chest drainage system. If the client experienced a new large pneumothorax, there could be rapid bubbling, but this is not the most likely explanation. Turning up the suction on the wall unit would increase the bubbling in the suction control chamber, not the water seal chamber. Taping the connections too tightly is not a concern. **Cognitive Level:** Analyzing **Client Need:** Basic Care and Comfort **Integrated Process:** Nursing Process: Diagnosis **Content Area:** Adult Health: Respiratory **Strategy:** The core issue of the question is the significance of finding continuous bubbling in the water seal chamber. Use the process of elimination and knowledge of closed chest drainage systems to make a selection.

8 **Answer: 2 Rationale:** The client should be premedicated approximately 30 minutes prior to chest tube removal if the client has an analgesic prescription and the medication can be given at this time. It is the healthcare provider's responsibility to determine the results of the daily chest x-ray. Obtaining equipment for removal of the chest tube is necessary; however, this action does not have to take place in the time indicated. Explaining the procedure to the client is important, but it can be done earlier or later than the time frame indicated. **Cognitive Level:** Analyzing **Client Need:** Basic Care and Comfort **Integrated Process:** Nursing Process: Planning **Content Area:** Adult Health: Respiratory **Strategy:** The core issue of the question is what action is timely *30 minutes* before chest tube removal. Analyze each option to determine whether each needs to occur at that time. Recall that analgesics are usually given about 30 minutes prior to a painful procedure to select the correct option.

9 **Answer: 5 Rationale:** The maximum amount of fluid that should be used to irrigate a nephrostomy tube is 5 mL. The nurse should also use strict aseptic technique to prevent infection of the renal pelvis as a result of the procedure. **Cognitive Level:** Applying **Client Need:** Basic Care and Comfort **Integrated Process:** Nursing Process: Planning **Content Area:** Adult Health: Renal and Genitourinary **Strategy:** The core issue of the question is knowledge of appropriate volumes of fluid that should be used to irrigate tubes such as a nephrostomy tube. Memorize this number if the question was difficult.

10 **Answer: 3 Rationale:** The nurse should ensure that the tubing is free of kinks or other obstructions to urine flow. The tube is irrigated only if prescribed. There is no situation that warrants clamping a nephrostomy tube; this action should be avoided. Securely attaching the drainage bag to the bedrail is dangerous because it could cause traction when the client moves in bed and cause the nephrostomy tube to become dislodged. **Cognitive Level:** Applying **Client Need:** Basic Care and

Comfort **Integrated Process:** Nursing Process: Implementation **Content Area:** Adult Health: Renal and Genitourinary **Strategy:** Use general principles of tube management to answer the question, and apply the basic concepts of safe nursing to find the correct answer. Remember that the tubing should be kept free of kinks and that nephrostomy tubes should not be clamped. Recognize the danger of securing a drainage bag in a manner that could cause dislodgement or injury.

11 **Answer: 1 Rationale:** Gastric pH is acidic and readings should be 4 or less if the tube is placed properly in the stomach. A pH reading of 6 or more is indicative of tube placement in the intestine. **Cognitive Level:** Analyzing **Client Need:** Basic Care and Comfort **Integrated Process:** Nursing Process: Diagnosis **Content Area:** Adult Health: Gastrointestinal **Strategy:** The core issue of the question is knowledge of pH readings that are consistent with placement of a nasogastric tube in the stomach. Knowledge about the pH readings in specific areas of the body and the ability to distinguish between acidic and alkaline pH readings is essential to answer the question.

12 **Answer: 1, 4, 5 Rationale:** The nurse correctly measures the length of an NG tube prior to insertion by first placing the tip of the tube at the tip of the nose. The second landmark that the nurse should use prior to placement of an NG tube is the tip of the earlobe; measure the distance from tip of the nose to the tip of the earlobe. The third landmark that the nurse should use is the xiphoid process; measure the distance from the tip of the nose to the tip of the earlobe to the xiphoid process and mark the tube at this length prior to insertion of an NG tube. The sternal notch and mandibular joint are not landmarks used for measuring the length of an NG tube prior to placement. **Cognitive Level:** Application **Client Need:** Basic Care and Comfort **Integrated Process:** Nursing Process: Planning **Content Area:** Adult Health: Gastrointestinal **Strategy:** The core issue of the question is knowledge of the process of obtaining the correct measurement of the tube length by properly measuring a client before nasogastric tube insertion. Use specific nursing knowledge and the process of elimination to make a selection.

13 **Answer: 4 Rationale:** For the tube to migrate to the area of intestinal blockage, the tube must pass through the pyloric sphincter of the stomach and into the intestines. Positioning the client with head elevated and on the right side will help the tube migrate into the intestines. Positioning the client on the left side will interfere with the passage of the weighted end of the tube through the pyloric sphincter. Positioning the client flat on the left side does not enlist the aid of gravity and does not aid peristalsis to move the tube past the pyloric sphincter. Positioning the client flat on the right side eliminates gravity as an aid to tube passage. **Cognitive Level:** Analyzing **Client Need:** Basic Care and Comfort **Integrated Process:** Teaching and Learning **Content Area:** Adult Health: Gastrointestinal **Strategy:** The core issue of the question is knowledge of proper client position following nasoenteric tube placement. Visualize the anatomy of the body and the laws of gravity when teaching the client about tube movement into the intestines. *Gravity* should be a prime consideration as a possible influence whenever answering questions related to tube placement.

14 **Answer: 3 Rationale:** Because the nasoenteric tube needs to migrate into the proper position, an action confirmed by x-ray, the nurse should note the finding on the medical record. The nurse should not call the healthcare provider based on this finding. The tube is not taped in place until it has reached proper position. The nurse is not responsible for scheduling an x-ray without a prescription, although the nurse could check to see if such a prescription exists and has been processed. **Cognitive Level:** Analyzing **Client Need:** Basic Care and Comfort **Integrated Process:** Nursing Process: Implementation **Content Area:** Adult Health: Gastrointestinal **Strategy:** The core issue of the question is knowledge that nasoenteric tubes are not taped until they have reached final position. Use specific nursing knowledge and the process of elimination to answer this question.

15 **Answer: 2 Rationale:** A Sengstaken-Blakemore tube is inserted to control bleeding from esophageal varices, which is the primary health problem of concern with use of this tube. The underlying health problem for this client may be portal hypertension, which is a complication of cirrhosis of the liver; however, the Sengstaken-Blakemore tube is not inserted to treat cirrhosis. The underlying health problem for this client may be portal hypertension; however, the Sengstaken-Blakemore tube is not inserted to treat portal hypertension. Abdominal ascites is a condition that may accompany cirrhosis; however, a Sengstaken-Blakemore tube is not inserted to treat abdominal ascites. **Cognitive Level:** Analyzing **Client Need:** Basic Care and Comfort **Integrated Process:** Nursing Process: Diagnosis **Content Area:** Adult Health: Gastrointestinal **Strategy:** The core issue of the question is knowledge of the rationale for placement of a Sengstaken-Blakemore tube. Use knowledge of pathophysiology and the process of elimination to make a selection.

16 **Answer: 3 Rationale:** Scissors need to be kept at the bedside of a client who has a Sengstaken-Blakemore tube. If the tube becomes dislodged and the client cannot breathe, the nurse cuts the tube to allow the balloons to deflate and restore a patent airway. A suction machine is generally helpful as an airway adjunct. Oxygen may be appropriate for a client with a Sengstaken-Blakemore tube, but it is not the priority bedside equipment needed in this situation. A laryngoscope is used to insert an endotracheal tube and it does not apply to this question. **Cognitive Level:** Analyzing **Client Need:** Basic Care and Comfort **Integrated Process:** Nursing Process: Planning **Content Area:** Adult Health: Gastrointestinal **Strategy:** The core issue of the question is knowledge that tube dislodgement can block the airway and that scissors are needed for rapid balloon deflation if this occurs. Use nursing knowledge and the process of elimination to make a selection.

17 **Answer: 3 Rationale:** An Ewald tube is a large-bore tube used to evacuate stomach contents rapidly following poisoning or overdose. A Minnesota tube and a Sengstaken-Blakemore tube are used for clients with bleeding esophageal varices. A Miller-Abbot tube is a nasoenteric tube used to decompress the bowel with small bowel obstruction. **Cognitive Level:** Applying **Client Need:** Basic Care and Comfort **Integrated Process:** Nursing Process: Planning **Content Area:** Adult Health: Gastrointestinal **Strategy:** The core issue of the question is knowledge of the use of various types of drainage tubes. Use nursing knowledge and the process of elimination to make a selection.

18 **Answer: 1 Rationale:** Because the risk of aspiration with gastric lavage is of concern to the nurse, assessment of respiratory status, including respiratory rate and breath sounds, is of priority. Other vital signs, such as heart rate and blood pressure, are important as a measure of general condition but are not focused on detection of complications of this procedure. Skin color and body temperature should be

assessed routinely, as a change can occur with hypoxia; however, respiratory assessment is a priority intervention aimed at preventing hypoxia. Urine output is of general concern, but peripheral edema is not a priority. **Cognitive Level:** Analyzing **Client Need:** Basic Care and Comfort **Integrated Process:** Nursing Process: Assessment **Content Area:** Adult Health: Gastrointestinal **Strategy:** The core issue of the question is knowledge that gastric lavage can lead to aspiration as a complication. Use nursing knowledge and the process of elimination to make a selection.

19 **Answer: 2 Rationale:** The nurse should squeeze the collecting chamber to reestablish negative pressure and suction to the device. The tubing should always be free of kinks to prevent obstruction. The nurse should wipe the port with alcohol before closing the collecting chamber to reduce the risk of infection; however, this action does not reestablish negative pressure and suction to the device. The cap of the wound drainage device is closed in order to maintain the negative pressure necessary to create suction; just closing the cap does not reestablish negative pressure and suction. **Cognitive Level:** Analyzing **Client Need:** Basic Care and Comfort **Integrated Process:** Nursing Process: Implementation **Content Area:** Adult Health: Integumentary **Strategy:** The core issue of the question is which action by the nurse will reestablish suction to a Jackson Pratt wound-drainage device. Use nursing knowledge and the process of elimination to make a selection.

20 **Answer: 3 Rationale:** The nurse should assess the skin for irritation and breakdown from contact between abdominal skin and wound drainage with dressing changes. The drain may be advanced over several days for gradual removal; a Penrose drain is not expected to remain in the original position. If an insufficient number of gauze dressings are used around drain, the likelihood of skin breakdown is increased. The surgeon does not need to be notified of large amounts of drainage because the finding is expected. **Cognitive Level:** Applying **Client Need:** Basic Care and Comfort **Integrated Process:** Nursing Process: Planning **Content Area:** Adult Health: Integumentary **Strategy:** The core issue of the question is knowledge that this type of drain can cause skin irritation by nature of the volume of drainage. Use nursing knowledge and the process of elimination to make a selection.

21 **Answer: 3, 1, 2, 4, 5 Rationale:** The head of client's bed is raised first because airway and breathing are the priority. The tube is measured for accurate length of insertion second, after the client is positioned for promotion of adequate respiration. The third step is to advance the tube past the nasopharynx. The fourth step requires the client to take sips of water to help with tube advancement into the stomach. Finally (fifth step), the tube is taped securely to the client's nose to maintain placement and prevent dislodgement. **Cognitive Level:** Applying **Client Need:** Basic Care and Comfort **Integrated Process:** Nursing Process: Planning **Content Area:** Adult Health: Gastrointestinal **Strategy:** The core issue of the question is knowledge of the insertion procedure for a nasogastric tube. Use nursing knowledge to sequence the steps that the nurse needs to take. Mentally visualize the procedure to aid in answering the question.

Key Terms to Review

chest tube p. 406
endotracheal tube p. 406
Ewald tube p. 411
nasoenteric (intestinal) tube p. 410
nasogastric tube p. 409
nephrostomy tube p. 408
penrose drain p. 411
Sengstaken-Blakemore tube p. 410
suprapubic catheter p. 408
tracheostomy p. 403
T-tube p. 411

References

Berman, A., Snyder, S., & Frandsen, G. (2016). *Kozier & Erb's fundamentals of nursing: Concepts, process, and practice* (10th ed.). New York, NY: Pearson Education.

Craven, R., & Hirnle, C., & Henshaw, C. (2017). *Fundamentals of nursing: Human health and function* (8th ed.). Philadelphia, PA: Wolters-Kluwer.

LeMone, P., Burke, K., Bauldoff, G., & Gubrud, P. (2015). *Medical surgical nursing: Clinical reasoning in patient care* (6th ed.). Hoboken, NJ: Pearson Education.

Lewis, S., Dirksen, S., Heitkemper, M., & Bucher, L. (2014). *Medical surgical nursing: Assessment and management of clinical problems* (9th ed.). St. Louis, MO: Elsevier Science.

Potter, P., Perry, A., Stockert, P., Hall, A. (2017). *Fundamentals of nursing* (9th ed.). St. Louis, MO: Mosby.

Smith, S., Duell, D., Martin, B., Aebersold, M., & Gonzalez, L. (2017). *Clinical nursing skills: Basic to advanced skills* (10th ed.). New York, NY: Pearson Education.

Test Yourself

Are you ready for the NCLEX-RN® or course exams? Access the NEW web-based app that provides students with thousands of practice questions in preparation for the NCLEX experience.

28 Integrative Therapies

In this chapter

Cross Reference

Other chapters relevant to this content area are

Promoting Healthy Lifestyle Choices	Chapter 16
Culturally Relevant Care	Chapter 19

I. NONPHARMACEUTICAL INTEGRATIVE THERAPIES

A. *Massage*

1. Relaxes muscles and leads to release of lactic acid that accumulates during exercise
2. Stretches joints and relieves pain; improves blood and lymph flow
3. Reduces anxiety and provides for relaxation and sense of well-being; enhances readiness for meditative state

Memory Aid

Massage is a basic touch therapy that many clients respond well to. Consider this therapy as an early choice for clients who are tense and cannot sleep.

4. When providing back massage, cover areas other than back to avoid chilling
   a. Warm lotion before applying to back
   NCLEX® b. Use combination of circular and long strokes; continue massage for 3–5 minutes in an unhurried manner
   NCLEX® c. Assess skin during back massage; document findings and client response to massage
5. *NCLEX®* Use caution, especially over bony prominences, in massaging clients at risk for skin breakdown, to prevent damage to skin and underlying tissue; do not massage nonblanching, reddened areas

B. *Progressive relaxation*

1. Reduces chronic pain and relieves stress by controlling bodily responses to anxiety and tension
2. Consists of tensing and then relaxing seven major muscle groups
3. *NCLEX®* Leads to decreased oxygen consumption, muscle tension, metabolism, and vital signs (heart rate, respiratory rate, and blood pressure)
4. Should be done for minimum of 10 minutes
5. Assist client to assume correct posture, such as sitting with feet flat on floor (body parts supported, joints slightly flexed, and arms and legs uncrossed)

Memory Aid

Position clients properly before engaging in progressive relaxation. The body must be fully supported to prevent risk of fall or other injury.

6. Tense and release muscles in specific sequence (more than one sequence available):
   a. Right fist, left fist, then both fists
   b. Both fists and both arms
   c. Toes, then ankles, then knees
   d. Buttocks and groin
   e. Stomach and lower back
   f. Chest and upper back, then shoulders
   g. Forehead, then jaw
7. Use with deep breathing and statements of positive affirmation (e.g., "Let go of the tension") to enhance relaxation

C. *Imagery*

1. Uses power of imagination to assist with physical, psychological, or spiritual healing
2. Often involves visualization but can also use other senses to create desired image
3. When imagery is assisted, it is called guided imagery
4. *NCLEX®* Consists of creating one or more of several types of images
   a. Healing a specific body part or increasing energy in a bodily area (body–mind)
   b. Destroying microorganisms or increasing local circulation (correct biologic)
   c. Being in a healed state (end state)
   d. Experiencing sense of unity, light, power, or spirituality (generalized healing)
   e. Connecting with higher levels of consciousness (transpersonal)

D. *Meditation*

1. Produces combined state of deep peace and rest along with mental alertness
2. May or may not be associated with religious practice or prayer
3. Includes relaxation and focused attention; may focus on an object (concentrative meditation) or remain open to all stimuli (mindfulness meditation)
4. General guidelines
   a. Choose specific time (early morning or evening, at least 2 hours after meal) and comfortable, distraction-free environment
   b. Keep spine straight and body relaxed; may sit cross-legged on floor or be upright in straight-backed chair
   c. Close eyes and place palms on thighs
   d. *NCLEX®* Use deep breathing or relaxation exercises; focus on either breathing or selected mental image; let distracting thoughts drift out of mind without focusing on them
   e. Perform daily for 10–20 minutes at a time

E. *Music therapy*

1. Often used in preoperative holding and cardiac units, birthing and counseling rooms, rehabilitation units, and for sleep induction
2. Used to alter ordinary level of consciousness, change mental focus, or change perception of time
3. Type of music chosen (classical, New Age, etc.) depends on client preferences and therapy goals
4. *NCLEX®* Choose music without words to enhance relaxation
5. Typical use is for approximately 20 minutes
6. Encourage client to let body respond to music spontaneously (such as relax muscles, lie down, hum, or clap)

F. Humor and laughter

1. Helps clients to establish relationships by decreasing social distance and placing people at ease
2. Helps to relieve anxiety and tension, anger or aggression
3. Helps to facilitate learning if carefully planned
4. Laughter raises heart and respiratory rates and increases oxygen exchange and muscle tension
5. A relaxation phase follows laughter, which reverses these changes
6. *NCLEX®* Humor can stimulate endorphin production, which reduces pain
7. Has healing properties because it fosters positive emotions

G. *Clinical aromatherapy*

1. Essential oils from plants can be used to either stimulate or calm client, improve sleep, change eating habits, or enhance immune system

NCLEX®
2. Essential oils stimulate sense of smell and may be inhaled, added to bath water, massaged into body, or applied as cold or warm compresses
3. Common essential oils used in home are chamomile, eucalyptus, ginger, jasmine, lavender, and tea tree
4. Oils vary in quality and are unregulated; caution clients to use carefully
5. Teach client to store and use only as directed
   - **a.** Dilute essentials oils with a carrier oil such as sunflower, grapeseed, or soy oil before applying to skin; oils (other than lavender or tea tree oil) are irritating to skin if undiluted
   - NCLEX® **b.** Before using topical application of oil, test skin for allergies with a small amount of diluted oil
   - **c.** Do not use near eyes or ingest internally (ingestion might be fatal)
   - **d.** Store in dark-covered bottles and keep away from light and heat according to product recommendation
   - NCLEX® **e.** Consult healthcare provider before using essential oils if pregnant or have respiratory problems such as asthma (some oils can cause bronchospasm)

Memory Aid

Essential oils are chemicals. As such, they can be toxic. Use them cautiously after consulting with healthcare provider.

H. Integrative therapies requiring specialized training

1. Acupuncture and acupressure are therapies that use fine needles or finger pressure, respectively, applied to specific points on body to relieve pain, treat selected illnesses, and promote general wellness
   - **a.** Qi (life energy, pronounced *chee*) flows along meridians (pathways) in body and can get blocked or congested near skin surface where qi forms tiny whirlpools; therapy seeks to release blockage of qi and relieve symptoms
   - **b.** Reflexology is a form of pressure used most commonly on feet but also on hands and ears
2. Hand-mediated biofield therapies include therapeutic touch, healing touch, and Reiki
   - **a.** These involve use of hands on or near body with intention to facilitate healing
   - **b.** They have no role in diagnosis of illness and are not intended to replace conventional therapy for organic disease

I. Nurses' role

1. Assess client's use of nonpharmaceutical integrative therapies
2. Communicate openly with client to build trust
3. Educate client about how to evaluate data sources, such as Internet or infomercials
4. Do not provide advice regarding use of integrative therapy regimens; instead, communicate data to healthcare provider, who will collaborate with client

II. USE OF HERBS AS DIETARY SUPPLEMENTS

A. General use

NCLEX®
1. Not intended for acute illness episodes or long-term therapy
2. Appropriate as adjunct to conventional Western therapies and should not replace a healthy diet

NCLEX®
3. Therapeutic effectiveness is slower than prescription medications; may take as long as several weeks, depending on herb
4. Many herbs are available in multiple forms, including teas, extracts, tinctures, and capsules or tablets containing powdered or freeze-dried forms of herb
5. Formulations vary in their potency and recommended dosage, with frequent lack of consensus on dosing
6. Most herbs are multipurpose, used, for example, as skin wash, gargle, compress, lotion, and eye bath

NCLEX®
7. Safe use in pregnancy and lactation is either contraindicated or unknown and may dry up breast milk during lactation; ginger may be an exception
8. Although they may be effective in children, herbs should be avoided in acute, sudden-onset illness

NCLEX®
9. Many herbs interact with other herbs, food, and prescription medications

B. Safety, labeling, and purity

1. Labels should contain specific directions for dosing and use
2. Only standardized extract, when available, should be used

3. Not all herbs have empirical support for their safety and efficacy
4. Much research and standardization originates in Europe, particularly in Germany
NCLEX® 5. Many herbs contain toxic substances (e.g., belladonna, hemlock, lily of the valley, and sassafras)
6. Healthcare providers should report all adverse effects of herbs to Food and Drug Administration (U.S.) or Health Canada (Canada)

C. Nurses' role and client education

1. Obtain a complete history and physical before starting any therapy with herbs
2. Herbs are not effective for and should not be used to treat acute illness
NCLEX® 3. Herbs take longer to work than do prescription medications, usually weeks
4. Report use of all herbs to healthcare provider
NCLEX® 5. Explain that client should start with one herb at a time, at lower than recommended doses, and closely monitor response
6. Teach client to know particular use, dosing, and safe administration of each herb and take only as directed
NCLEX® 7. Herbs may cause allergic reactions and adverse effects; if one occurs, discontinue herb and report symptoms to healthcare provider
8. Become familiar with specific herb–herb, herb–drug, and herb–food interactions
9. Teach client to purchase herbs from a reputable source, be aware of where and how herb was processed, and purchase standardized form of herbs if possible
10. Realize terms such as *natural* or *all natural* do not equate with safety or efficacy
11. Become familiar with various names by which particular herbs are identified
12. Teach client to avoid use of herbs in pregnancy, lactation, and in children
13. Teach client to accurately assess advertising claims; few definitive clinical trials have demonstrated safety and efficacy of selected agents
14. Continue to read new evidence that emerges from research as a professional obligation
15. Refrain from recommending or endorsing any particular product or agent

III. SPECIFIC HERBAL SUPPLEMENTS (SEE ALSO TABLE 28–1)

A. Bilberry (*Vaccinium myrtillus*, European blueberry, huckleberry, whortleberry)

1. Relative of blueberry and cranberry; shrub with small, sweet, black berries
2. Active ingredients: anthocyanoside (antioxidant bioflavonoid), pectin (soluble fiber)
3. Stabilizes collagen activity
4. Prevents production and release of compounds that promote inflammation, such as histamine and prostaglandins
5. Relaxes smooth muscle in vasculature; reduces permeability and strengthens capillary wall membrane
6. Inhibits platelet aggregation

B. Black cohosh (*Cimicifuga racemose*, black snakeroot, bugroot, rattleweed, rattleroot, squawroot, cimifuga)

1. Active ingredients: triperpenoid glycosides, isoflavones, aglycones
2. Binds to estrogen receptors
3. Inhibits luteinizing hormone
4. Apparent estrogen-like activity

C. Echinacea (*Echinacea purpurea*, snake root, purple or American cone flower, sampson root, black sampson, hedgehog, survey root)

1. Member of daisy family, with nine species
NCLEX® 2. Active ingredients: polysaccharides, alkylamides, flavonoids, caffeic acid derivatives (echinacosides), essential oils, and others
3. Available in capsule, tablet, candle, glycerite, hydroalcoholic extract, fresh-pressed juice, lollipop, lozenge, tea, and tincture forms
4. Activates T-lymphocytes and intensifies phagocytosis of macrophages
5. Stimulates tumor necrosis factor, interferon, and interleukin
6. Nonspecific stimulation of immune system

Memory Aid

Recall that Echinacea is an ingredient in some sore throat drops. This will aid in remembering that it is most effective if used early for colds and sore throats.

Table 28–1 Uses, Interactions, Contraindications/Side Effects of Common Herbs

Name	Uses	Interactions	Contraindications/Side Effects
Bilberry	Simple diarrhea Eye disorders: retinopathy, night blindness, glaucoma, cataracts Antioxidant	Use cautiously with aspirin, anticoagulants, vitamin E, fish oils, feverfew, garlic, ginger, ginkgo	May prolong coagulation time Iron absorption is ↓ when taken internally Contraindicated in lactation as well as pregnancy
Black cohosh	Menopause, dysmenorrhea, premenstrual syndrome	Potentiates hormone replacement medications (do not use together)	Dizziness, nausea, slowed pulse, increased sweating
Echinacea	Antimicrobial for colds and influenza Boosts immune system and ↑ resistance to infection (upper respiratory and urinary) Treat herpes simplex and Candida infection Topically: improves wound healing, provides antioxidant protection from UV A and B rays	May ↓ effectiveness of immunosuppressants (including corticosteroids) Use with antifungals (which ↑ liver enzymes) can cause liver damage Do not use with other hepatotoxicants (such as anabolic steroids, amiodarone, methotrexate, ketoconazole) Many tinctures contain large amounts of alcohol	Do not use in presence of autoimmune disease (e.g., HIV/AIDS, collagen disease, multiple sclerosis, tuberculosis), severe illness, or allergy to sunflower/daisy family Use longer than 8 weeks may cause hepatotoxicity and immunosuppression May influence fertility by spermatozoa enzyme interference Contraindicated in alcoholism, children, pregnancy, and lactation Risk of allergic reaction and anaphylaxis
Feverfew	Principle uses: prevention of recurrent migraine headaches, treatment of arthritis Relief of menstrual pain Asthma Dermatitis, psoriasis Antipyretic (promotes diaphoresis)	Do not use while taking prescription drugs for headache May interfere with blood clotting mechanism; do not use with aspirin or anticoagulants such as warfarin (Coumadin), or with bilberry, garlic, ginger, ginkgo	Cross-allergy to ragweed Adverse effects: lip and tongue swelling, mouth ulcers and ↓ taste from chewing leaves, abdominal colic, palpitations, ↑ menstrual flow, rebound headaches Sudden withdrawal may cause post-feverfew syndrome (muscle aches, pain, and stiffness); taper off to discontinue Avoid use in pregnancy, lactation, ↓ age 2
Garlic	Principle uses: ↓ cholesterol (triglycerides and low-density lipoproteins); ↑ high-density lipoproteins ↓ BP in mild hypertension (use should be monitored by health care provider [HCP]) Anticoagulant, antibacterial, antiviral, antifungal	↑ anticoagulant effect of anticoagulants, aspirin, and herbs that affect coagulation (bilberry, feverfew, ginger, ginkgo) Further ↓ blood glucose with hypoglycemic agents for diabetes May ↑ or ↓ effectiveness of drugs for HIV	Adverse effects: contact dermatitis, vertigo, garlic breath, hypothyroidism, GI irritation, nausea and vomiting (N/V) with large doses Enteric-coated tablets containing powdered form may reduce bad breath but are not as potent as raw garlic Contraindicated in pregnancy, GI (peptic ulcer and GERD) and bleeding disorders Chronic use may lower hemoglobin levels
Ginger	Principle use: antiemetic; ↑ appetite, digestion aid; alleviates dyspepsia Anti-inflammatory in treatment of rheumatoid arthritis and osteoarthritis Relieves muscle pain May ↓ motion sickness and relieve vertigo	May ↑ anticoagulant effects of bilberry, feverfew, garlic, ginkgo, or other anticoagulants such as aspirin or warfarin (Coumadin)	Adverse effects: headache, anxiety, insomnia, ↑ blood pressure, tachycardia, asthma attack, postmenopausal bleeding Contraindicated for postoperative nausea in clients with ↑ risk of bleeding and for treatment of hyperemesis gravidarum Severe overdose: possible CNS depression and dysrhythmias Conflicting data regarding safe use in pregnancy (FDA: relatively safe)
Ginkgo	Improves attention and memory, headaches Macular degeneration Intermittent claudication Erectile dysfunction Tinnitus	May ↑ anticoagulant effects of bilberry, feverfew, garlic, ginger, or aspirin or other anticoagulants such as warfarin (Coumadin)	Side effects: mild GI upset, ↑ risk bleeding Large doses my cause restlessness, headache, N/V, diarrhea, dizziness, or palpitations Avoid use of unprocessed leaves (contain allergens related to urushiol [chemical in poison ivy]) Avoid use in pregnancy, lactation, and children

Table 28–1 (Continued)

Name	Uses	Interactions	Contraindications/Side Effects
Ginseng	Counteracts physical and mental fatigue and ↑ stamina and concentration ↑ Body's ability to resist stress and disease; ↑ vitality Regulates blood pressure May ↓ mood swings Regulates blood glucose levels in type 2 diabetes mellitus	↑ Potency of estrogen in oral contraceptives leading to weight gain, breast pain, and vaginal bleeding May cause mania with MAOIs May cause irritability with caffeine May ↓ effectiveness of glaucoma medications	Most side effects reported are related to excessive or inappropriate use Avoid concurrent use with stimulants, such as coffee, tea, cola May potentiate MAOI actions Adverse effects: insomnia, palpitations, pruritus, nervousness, euphoria Do not use when acutely ill with cold or flu or if diagnosed with hypoglycemia
Hawthorn	Treats mild hypertension, athero- and arteriosclerosis, early heart failure Treats (prevents) chronic angina (not intended for acute angina)	May interfere with digoxin pharmacodynamics and monitoring Contraindicated with concomitant use of prescription antihypertensives or nitrates	Supervision of HCP needed for those with existing cardiac disease Adverse effects: nausea, fatigue, perspiration and cutaneous eruption of hands, increased CNS depression and sedation Contraindicated in pregnancy and lactation
Milk thistle	Adjunct antioxidant therapy in liver disease; close monitoring by HCP needed Treats overdose of death cap mushroom ↓ hepatotoxicity of psychoactive drugs such as phenothiazines	↓ Effectiveness of oral contraceptives	May trigger menstruation Insoluble in water, do not take in tea form Avoid alcohol-based extract in decompensated cirrhosis Cross-allergy to ragweed Adverse effects: loose stools, diarrhea in high doses Contraindicated in pregnancy and lactation
Saw palmetto	May treat symptoms of BPH with HCP supervision Helps initiate urine stream; ↓ urinary frequency, residual volumes, nocturia, dysuria	May potentiate finasteride (Proscar), resulting in overdose May interfere with iron absorption	Insoluble in water; do not take in tea form Adverse effects: nausea, abdominal pain, ↑ BP, headache, diarrhea with large doses Contraindicated in pregnancy and lactation
St. John's wort	Treats mild to moderate depression Not intended to treat suicidal ideation, psychotic behavior, or severe depression Possible antibacterial, antiviral, wound-healing properties	Do not use concurrently with prescription antidepressants, especially SSRIs or MAOIs Do not use concurrently with opioids, amphetamines, or OTC cold and flu preparations May inhibit absorption of iron May decrease digoxin levels	Avoid foods containing tyramine (aged cheese, smoked meats, liver, figs, dried or cured fish, yeast, beer, Chianti wine) Adverse effects (may last 2–4 weeks): GI distress, fatigue, pruritus, weight gain, headache, dizziness, restlessness May cause photosensitivity; avoid sun exposure, especially if fair-skinned Contraindicated in pregnancy, lactation, and in children
Valerian root	Sedative for insomnia, reduction of anxiety Muscle pain Menstrual and intestinal cramps Benzodiazepine withdrawal	Do not use concurrently with other sedatives, anxiolytics, or antidepressants Do not use with alcohol or disulfiram (Antabuse)	May be used safely while operating machinery or car, but monitor CNS effects Adverse effects: headache; upset stomach; others with long-term use or overdose (2.5 grams): excitability, insomnia, cardiac dysfunction, blurred vision, hepatotoxicity May cause hepatotoxicity; monitor liver function and avoid use in liver disease Extract contains 40–60% alcohol; avoid use in clients with alcoholism Contraindicated in pregnancy and lactation

7. Stabilizes hyaluronic acid (in connective tissue) to protect cells and connective tissue from microorganism invasion and attack from free radicals
8. Inhibits lipoxygenase to reduce inflammation

D. Feverfew (*Tanacetum parthenium*, bachelor's button, febrifuge plant, feather few, feather foil)

1. Short, bushy perennial of daisy family; has yellow flowers and yellow-green leaves resembling chamomile
2. Active ingredients: sesquiterpene lactones, especially parthenolide, essential oils
3. Suppresses secretion of granules in platelets and neutrophils to inhibit platelet aggregation
4. May suppress production of prostaglandins (thromboxane, leukotriene)
5. Inhibits release of serotonin

E. Garlic (*Allium sativum*, stinking root or rose, nectar of the gods, camphor of the poor, poor-man's treacle, rustic treacle)

1. Empirical support for effectiveness and use; most widely researched herb
2. Active ingredients (23 constituents): allicin (odorless, sulfur-containing amino acid), ajoene
3. Should be crushed or bruised to effectively convert various enzymes, protein, lipids, amino acids, and other ingredients to allicin
4. Allicin and ajoene not found in dried garlic but may be present if dried at low temperatures or taken in enteric-coated tablets
5. NCLEX® Inhibits platelet aggregation
6. Well-documented research shows that it reduces and inhibits metabolism of cholesterol
7. Increases bile acid secretion

F. Ginger (*Zingiber officinal*, Jamaica ginger, African ginger, Cochin ginger, black ginger, race ginger)

1. Green-purple flower resembling orchid
2. Active ingredient: sesquiterpenes, aromatic ketones (gingerols), and volatile oils
3. Inhibits thromboxane production to enhance effects of anticoagulation
4. Inhibits leukotrienes and prostaglandins to produce anti-inflammatory and analgesic effect

G. Ginkgo (*Ginkgo biloba*, GBE 761, GBE, GBX, Tebonin, Tebofortan, Ginkogink)

1. Active ingredients: flavone glycosides, flavonoids, terpene lactones (such as ginkgolides and bilobalide)
2. Ginkgo biloba extract referred to as GBE
3. Flavonoids act as antioxidants by destroying lipid layer of cell membrane
4. Flavone glycosides produce mild platelet aggregation
5. Ginkgolides antagonize platelet-activating factor to decrease coagulation
6. Bilobalide increases cerebral circulation to improve tissue perfusion and increase memory
7. Protects brain from effects of hypoxia

H. Ginseng, Korean (*Panax ginseng*, American ginseng, Panaschinseng)

1. Active ingredients: triterpenoid saponin glycosides (ginsenosides, panaxosides)
2. Possible effect on pituitary gland with action similar to corticosteroids
3. Improves serum glucose, glycosylated hemoglobin (HbA_{1c}), and amino-terminal propeptide concentrations
4. Hypertensive effect with low doses, hypotensive effect with higher doses

I. Hawthorn (*Crataegus oxyacantha*, Mayblossom, Maybush, whitehorn, LI 132)

1. Small to medium tree of several species; leaves, flowers, berries (fruit) are used in standardized extracts
2. Active ingredients: flavonoids, primarily procyanidins and proanthocyanidins
3. Acts as antioxidant that decreases damage by free radicals to cardiovascular system by increasing levels of vitamin C intracellularly
4. Increases coronary and myocardial circulation
5. Decreases peripheral vascular resistance to decrease blood pressure
6. Increases strength of myocardial contraction (positive inotropic effect) and decreases heart rate (negative chronotropic effect)
7. Angiotensin-converting enzyme (ACE) activity that prevents the conversion of angiotensin I to angiotensin II, a potent vasoconstrictor
8. Decreases total plasma cholesterol and low-density lipoprotein (LDL) levels

J. Milk thistle (*Silbyum marianum*, Mary thistle, Marian thistle, Lady's thistle, Holy thistle, silymarin, the "liver herb")

1. Tall plant, prickly leaves, milky sap, member of daisy family
2. Active ingredients: silymarin (and component silybinin) act as hepatoprotectant
3. Promotes glutathione production, a powerful endogenous antioxidant
4. Binds to hepatocyte membrane and blocks uptake of toxins into liver cell
5. Stimulates nucleolar polymerase A activity to promote new liver cell growth
6. Stimulates regeneration of liver by stimulating protein synthesis
7. Inhibits action of leukotriene by Kupffer cells
8. Stabilizes liver cell membrane by decreasing turnover rate of phospholipids

Memory Aid

Note that the words *milk* and *thistle* both contain the letters *l* and *i*, which may help you to associate this herb with the liver.

K. Saw palmetto (*Serenoa repens*, sabal, American dwarf palm tree, LSESR)

1. Shrublike palm tree with reddish-brown to black berries
2. Active ingredients: saturated and unsaturated fatty acids and sterols from berries (liposterolic acid)
3. Reduces action of 5-alpha-reductase enzyme that converts testosterone to dehydrotestosterone (DHT) in aging
4. No effect on prostate-specific antigen (PSA)
5. May reverse testicular and mammary gland atrophy
6. May increase sperm production and increase sexual vigor

L. St. John's wort (*Hypericum perforatum*, amber, goat weed, touch-and-heal, Johnswort, witch's herb, klamath weed, chassediable, devil's scourge)

1. Yellow perennial flower with red-pigmented leaves containing small black dots
2. Active ingredient: hypericin from red-pigmented leaves, pseudohypericin and flavonoids, tannin, and others
3. Inhibits reuptake of serotonin; actions not well determined or understood
4. Low monoamine oxidase inhibitor (MAOI) with effects comparable to imipramine, but produces fewer side effects than prescription antidepressants

M. Valerian root (*valerian officinalis*, wild valerian, garden heliotrope, setwall, capon's tail, all-heal, Amantilla, Baldrian wurzel, benedicta)

1. Tall perennial with hollow stem, leaves, and white or red flowers
2. Active ingredients: valepotriates and susquiterpine derivatives, valeric acid, valeranone, and others
3. Binds weakly to gamma-aminobutyric acid (GABA) receptor sites to decrease CNS activity, causing sedation with decreased side effects
4. Action similar to benzodiazepines but nonaddicting and produces no morning hangover

Memory Aid

Remember that valerian is an ingredient often found in teas that are recommended for sleep.

IV. NONHERBAL DIETARY SUPPLEMENTS

A. Overview

1. Nonherbal dietary supplements (also known as specialty supplements) are a diverse group of products derived from plant or animal sources
2. Generally more specific in action than herbal supplements and are targeted at one condition or a small range of related conditions
3. Some have legitimate health claims backed by research (such as amino acids, glucosamine and chondroitin, fish oils) while others do not
4. Caution clients to be skeptical about health claims of individual products until research results demonstrate advertised benefit

B. Claims of common nonherbal dietary supplements

1. Amino acids: to build protein, increase muscle strength and endurance
2. Carnitine: a variety of claims, including increased energy and better sports performance
3. Coenzyme Q10: antioxidant and prevention of heart disease
4. DHEA (dehydroepiandrosterone): enhance immune system and memory (made from wild yam and soy)
5. Fish oils: reduce cholesterol, enhance brain function and improve visual acuity
6. Glucosamine and chondroitin: alleviate osteoarthritis and other joint problems
7. *Lactobacillis acidophilus*: maintain intestinal health
8. Melatonin: aid in onset of sleep and reduce jet lag during travel
9. Methyl sulfonyl methane (MSM): reduce pollen and food allergy symptoms; relieve pain and inflammation caused by arthritis
10. Vitamin C: prevent or reduce severity of colds

PRACTICE TEST

Check Your NCLEX–RN® Exam I.Q.

You are ready for testing on this content if you can:

- Identify appropriate uses of integrative and complementary therapies.
- Assess a client regarding need for integrative and complementary therapies.
- Teach a client about integrative and complementary therapy choices.
- Participate in providing integrative and complementary therapies to a client.
- Evaluate the outcomes of integrative and complementary therapies for a client.

PRACTICE TEST

1 Which assessment data would prohibit the use of imagery with a client?

1. No previous history of using imagery techniques
2. States anxiety level of 6 on a 0–10 scale
3. Client feels reluctant to close eyes for the imagery session
4. Client has a history of psychosis

2 The nurse has determined that music therapy may be appropriate for use with a client. Which strategies should the nurse consider when choosing the music? Select all that apply.

1. Choose only music with words.
2. Choose music that is 5–7 minutes in duration.
3. Allow the client to choose music of his or her choice.
4. Encourage the client to respond to the music.
5. Ask the client not to analyze the music.

3 The nurse is using meditation with a client to help him decrease his pain. Which factor is important to consider when using this type of therapy?

1. The type of meditation is best determined by the nurse.
2. The client's condition will influence the use of meditation.
3. Meditation is best taught when the client is in an outpatient setting.
4. A certified professional should teach the client how to perform meditation.

4 The client asks the nurse how humor therapy affects the client physiologically. Which effects should the nurse explain are attributed to laughter? Select all that apply.

1. Decreases heart rate and blood pressure
2. Increases salivary immunoglobulin A (S-IgA)
3. Produces an antagonist response to stress hormones
4. Decreases the immune response by decreasing T-lymphocytes
5. Changes temperature set point in the brain

5 The nurse decides to teach a client with hypertension the progressive relaxation technique. Which instructions should the nurse give to the client when using this relaxation method?

1. Sit in an upright position with legs crossed.
2. Place sensors on the forehead to monitor physiological activity.
3. Contract and relax the body's muscles in groups from head to feet.
4. Monitor breathing pattern while repeating a word or phrase out loud.

6 The nurse teaches the client about massage therapy. Which statement by the client demonstrates a correct understanding of the benefits of massage? Select all that apply.

1. "Massage reduces blood clot formation."
2. "Massage impacts lymphatic drainage."
3. "Massage increases the lactic acid in muscle."
4. "Massage ultimately improves blood flow."
5. "Massage creates a sense of wakefulness."

7 A nurse is preparing to present information to a women's group about the cautions associated with aromatherapy. What information is appropriate to include for the audience? Select all that apply.

1. Aromatic oils are produced by a standard-quality formula.
2. The oils should be stored in dark glass containers.
3. Test for allergies by applying a small amount of oil to the skin before use.
4. Essential oils should not be used during pregnancy.
5. Production of essential oils is tightly controlled.

8 The nurse is preparing a presentation for staff about the effects of humor in nursing situations. What feedback would indicate to the nurse that the participants understand the role of humor in the healthcare setting?

1. Understanding that humor increases the social distance between people
2. Noting that humor promotes effective teaching and learning
3. Anticipating that humor fosters the expression of anger and aggression
4. Accepting that humor is ineffective as a coping mechanism

9 The nurse is evaluating the effectiveness of guided imagery for a client with preoperative anxiety. Which client statement should indicate to the nurse that the therapy has been successful?

1. "I hope that I don't have dreams about the images we used tonight."
2. "It is a real challenge to concentrate while I have so much on my mind."
3. "I will need to set up some practice time for next week."
4. "The images and exercises are selected to reduce anxiety about the surgery."

10 The nurse is using progressive relaxation on a client who is experiencing a great deal of stress. What nursing action is necessary in order to protect the client's safety prior to the start of the session?

1. Evaluate the client's muscle strength.
2. Determine if the client is taking sedatives.
3. Place the client in a totally supported position.
4. Obtain information regarding client allergies.

11 The nurse is teaching the client's partner how to perform a back massage on the client. Which observation by the nurse indicates that the partner understands how to perform the activity? Select all that apply.

1. The client is lying on the bed in his pajamas.
2. The client's back is being rubbed with large, circular motions.
3. The partner places the bottle of lotion in warm water prior to the massage.
4. The partner massages the client's back for 3–5 minutes.
5. The partner firmly massages reddened areas noted on the client.

12 The nurse taught the client about meditation. Which statement by the client demonstrates a correct understanding of this activity?

1. "Meditation is a technique used to quiet the mind and focus on the future."
2. "Meditation involves self-reflection on my religious convictions."
3. "Meditation is a pure concept with one clearly defined technique."
4. "Meditation involves both relaxation and focus of attention."

13 The nurse is performing an imagery session with a group of clients. What instruction should the nurse give the clients?

1. "Try to concentrate on your breathing, letting go of all your stress."
2. "Imagine that your body is using its energy to heal itself."
3. "Contract the muscles of your arm and then relax."
4. "Listen to music of your choice and let the music take you away."

PRACTICE TEST

14 A client is using aromatherapy to treat stress. Which assessment data indicates an allergic reaction in a client who has received an aromatherapy session?

1. Development of a rash
2. Increased skin turgor
3. Decreased pigmentation
4. Peripheral edema

15 The preoperative waiting area has soft instrumental music playing in the background. What purpose should the nurse recognize in regard to this utilization of music? Select all that apply.

1. Music produces a hypermetabolic state in the listener.
2. Music reduces the physiological stress, pain, and anxiety.
3. Music enhances the functions of the left hemisphere of the brain.
4. Music helps mask the normal noises found in the hospital setting.
5. Music without words more effectively enhances relaxation.

16 A client tells the nurse that walking causes right leg pain. The pain is described as muscle cramping or burning that subsides with rest. Based on the symptoms, the nurse supports the use of what herb?

1. Feverfew
2. Garlic
3. Ginkgo
4. Ginseng

17 A client is taking chlorpromazine. Based on the route of metabolism of this prescribed medication, the nurse is not surprised to learn the client uses which herb?

1. Valerian root
2. Ginger
3. Milk thistle
4. Hawthorn

18 Which therapeutic change in laboratory values would the nurse anticipate in the client taking garlic?

1. Increased platelet aggregation
2. Increased white blood cell count
3. Decreased serum cholesterol levels
4. Decreased serum glucose levels

19 The female client tells the nurse that she is planning a pregnancy soon. In providing client education about the use of herbs during pregnancy, which statement by the nurse is most appropriate?

1. "Most herbs are safe when taken as directed."
2. "Only herbs in the topical form are safe."
3. "Certain herbs are safe and effective when taken in lower doses."
4. "You should discuss the use of any herbs with your healthcare provider."

20 The client presents to the healthcare clinic with an abrasion to the left knee from a fall. After cleaning the abrasion, the nurse might support the use of which client-chosen herb as adjunct therapy to treat the abrasion?

1. Echinacea
2. Ginger
3. Valerian root
4. Feverfew

21 A client scheduled for arthroscopic knee surgery has been taking ginger for relief of arthritic pain. The client asks the nurse about postoperative use of ginger for continued relief of pain and postoperative nausea. What essential information should the nurse provide?

1. Ginger cannot be used safely postoperatively.
2. Ginger would not be effective for postsurgical pain and nausea.
3. Ginger may be repeated every 4 hours as needed.
4. Ginger may potentiate the effects of opioid medications.

22 The nurse would include which intervention when planning care for the client who is taking hawthorn?

1. Monitor blood glucose levels
2. Monitor blood pressure
3. Monitor white blood cell count
4. Monitor temperature

23 The client tells the nurse that a neighbor recommends the use of bilberry in treating simple diarrhea. The nurse supports the client's use based on knowledge of which action of bilberry?

1. Anthocynanosides in the berry decrease peristalsis.
2. The berry contains pectin, which acts as a soluble fiber.
3. Bilberry acts to counteract antimicrobial suppression of normal intestinal flora.
4. Action of the berry works to decrease bacterial or viral causes of diarrhea.

24 The nurse instructs the client taking St. John's wort that which food preferred by the client may be safely consumed while taking this herb?

1. Chocolate
2. Aged cheeses
3. Beer
4. Vanilla ice cream

25 Which client would benefit from the therapeutic effects of garlic? Select all that apply.

1. The client with decreased blood pressure
2. The client with liver disease
3. The client with coronary artery disease
4. The client with a bleeding disorder
5. The client with peripheral vascular disease

ANSWERS & RATIONALES

1 **Answer: 4 Rationale:** In clients with a history of organic brain syndrome or psychosis, deep relaxation may exacerbate symptoms of psychosis. Other relaxation methods should be instituted. The client does not need prior experience to gain the benefits of imagery. The client reporting an anxiety level of 6 on a 0–10 scale will benefit from the imagery session. Closing the eyes aids in establishing a state of internal awareness but is not necessary for an imagery session. The client could gaze at a fixed point 1–2 feet away instead of closing his or her eyes. When the client begins to trust the process, his or her eyes will get heavy and close. **Cognitive Level:** Applying **Client Need:** Basic Care and Comfort **Integrated Process:** Nursing Process: Assessment **Content Area:** Fundamentals **Strategy:** To answer this question, the nurse needs to know what clients will benefit from imagery and what contraindications may exist for use of this technique.

2 **Answer: 3, 4, 5 Rationale:** Music selections should be based on the type of music the client perceives as relaxing. The nurse should encourage the client to let the body respond to the music in any way it wishes, such as humming, relaxing muscles, or clapping. Analyzing the music will shift the client's focus from relaxing to thinking about the music. Any distracting thoughts should simply be let go, and the client should be instructed to concentrate on the music. Music without words is recommended so that the client does not concentrate on the words. Music therapy needs to be at least 20 minutes in length to be effective. **Cognitive Level:** Applying **Client Need:** Basic Care and Comfort **Integrated Process:** Teaching and Learning **Content Area:** Fundamentals **Strategy:** The answer to this question reflects the critical elements that should be considered when using music therapy with a client.

3 **Answer: 2 Rationale:** The client's condition is important when determining the appropriateness of this holistic therapy. The client needs to be involved in deciding which type of meditation to learn. Meditation can be used in any facility and is not restricted to outpatient settings. Anyone can learn how to meditate; it does not require a certified professional to learn this activity. **Cognitive Level:** Applying **Client Need:** Basic Care and Comfort **Integrated Process:** Nursing Process: Assessment **Content Area:** Fundamentals **Strategy:** This question requires knowledge about the process of meditation along with an understanding of when it is appropriate for the nurse to initiate meditation with a client.

4 **Answer: 2, 3 Rationale:** Research suggests that humor therapy increases IgA levels in the saliva, which helps prevent upper respiratory infections. Laughter decreases stress hormones such as cortisol. The sympathetic nervous system is stimulated with humor therapy, leading to an increase in heart rate, respiratory rate, blood pressure, and oxygen saturation. The arousal state is followed by a relaxation state in which vital signs return to or below pre-laughter baseline. Laughter increases T-lymphocyte cells, thereby increasing the immune response. Temperature is not affected by laughter. **Cognitive Level:** Analyzing **Client Need:** Basic Care and Comfort **Integrated Process:** Nursing Process: Implementation **Content Area:** Fundamentals **Strategy:** An understanding of the physiological effects of humor and laughter on the body is needed in order to answer this question correctly.

5 **Answer: 3 Rationale:** The progressive relaxation response requires the client to contract and relax muscles in groups from head to feet in order to gain a deeper state of relaxation. The client needs to be in a comfortable position for relaxation to occur; sitting upright with legs crossed is not essential. Electromyogram sensors are applied to the forehead when using biofeedback to assess the physiological response to relaxation technique. Repeating a phrase or word silently in rhythm with breathing helps the client turn off other thoughts and focus on a neutral, monotonous stimulus. **Cognitive Level:** Applying **Client Need:** Basic Care and Comfort **Integrated Process:** Nursing Process: Implementation

Content Area: Fundamentals **Strategy:** Knowledge of the process involved in performing progressive relaxation is necessary in order to answer this question.

6 **Answer: 1, 2, 4 Rationale:** Massage stimulates circulation, thereby helping to prevent the formation of blood clots. Massage also stimulates the lymphatic system, enhancing lymphatic drainage. Because massage stimulates circulation, it helps to improve blood flow. Massage causes the release of lactic acid that has accumulated during exercise. Massage creates a state of relaxation and can promote sleep. **Cognitive Level:** Applying **Client Need:** Basic Care and Comfort **Integrated Process:** Teaching and Learning **Content Area:** Fundamentals **Strategy:** Knowledge and an understanding of the physiological effects of massage on the body are needed to answer this question. With multiple correct answers, think of each option as a true or false statement.

7 **Answer: 2, 3 Rationale:** Many oils should be kept out of the sunlight and heat to prevent deterioration. Essential oils can be toxic and produce an allergic reaction in some individuals. Essential oils are distilled from flowers, roots, bark, leaves, wood, resins, citrus rinds, and more; the quality of essential oils varies. Some essential oils are unsafe during pregnancy, while others are considered safe, so it is critical to contact the primary care provider prior to trying aromatherapy during pregnancy. There is little government regulation over the production of essential oils. **Cognitive Level:** Analyzing **Client Need:** Basic Care and Comfort **Integrated Process:** Nursing Process: Implementation **Content Area:** Fundamentals **Strategy:** The core issues of the question are that essential oils can cause an allergic reaction and are affected by light. Note the wording of the question indicates that there is more than one correct answer.

8 **Answer: 2 Rationale:** Humor reduces the anxiety of the person teaching and gains the audience's attention, both of which facilitate learning. Humor decreases the social distance between people, putting them at ease. Humor helps individuals act out impulses in a safe, nonthreatening environment, thus dissipating anger and aggression. Humor diminishes anxiety and fear, reducing tension and enabling the client to confront and deal with the situation. **Cognitive Level:** Analyzing **Client Need:** Basic Care and Comfort **Integrated Process:** Teaching and Learning **Content Area:** Fundamentals **Strategy:** An understanding of the benefits of humor therapy is needed to answer the question correctly.

9 **Answer: 4 Rationale:** The statement about anxiety reduction indicates that the client understands the process and outcomes of guided imagery. The statement about dreams indicates the imagery session increased the client's anxiety level. The statement about difficulty concentrating indicates that the client did not focus well, which prevents total relaxation. The statement focused on the following week indicates the therapy was unsuccessful because guided imagery needs to be practiced daily to obtain the desired effect. **Cognitive Level:** Analyzing **Client Need:** Basic Care and Comfort **Integrated Process:** Nursing Process: Evaluation **Content Area:** Fundamentals **Strategy:** Understanding that the purpose of imagery is to help the client relax will help you choose the correct answer. Analyze and evaluate the client's comments carefully.

10 **Answer: 3 Rationale:** It is essential to have the body supported as the muscles begin to relax. The client could sustain injury if a fall occurs as muscle tension diminishes. It is not necessary to evaluate muscle strength prior to the relaxation therapy. It is not necessary to assess for the use of sedatives because this therapy will cause relaxation. It is not pertinent to know the client's allergies before performing progressive relaxation. **Cognitive Level:** Applying **Client Need:** Basic Care and Comfort **Integrated Process:** Nursing Process: Implementation **Content Area:** Fundamentals **Strategy:** The core issue of the question is the knowledge that a client can become so relaxed during the progressive relaxation session that falling is a risk if the body is not adequately supported.

11 **Answer: 3, 4 Rationale:** Warmed lotion helps enhance relaxation; this is accomplished by placing the bottle into warm water or rubbing the lotion briskly in the palms prior to touching the client. Massages should last 3–5 minutes and be given in an unhurried manner. In order to be effective, the skin being massaged needs to be exposed. Massaging the back requires long strokes along the spine with small, circular strokes peripherally. Reddened areas may indicate problems with pressure on areas over bony prominences; massage to the areas can result in additional damage to underlying tissue. **Cognitive Level:** Analyzing **Client Need:** Basic Care and Comfort **Integrated Process:** Nursing Process: Evaluation **Content Area:** Fundamentals **Strategy:** Knowledge about the steps in giving a back massage is important to answer this question. When multiple answers are correct, consider each option as a true/false statement.

12 **Answer: 4 Rationale:** All types of meditation involve relaxation and focused attention. Meditation involves focusing on the present moment and not on the future. Although meditation was at one time viewed as a religious practice, religious conviction is not required for meditation. Many types of meditation exist, and the techniques differ. **Cognitive Level:** Analyzing **Client Need:** Basic Care and Comfort **Integrated Process:** Nursing Process: Evaluation **Content Area:** Fundamentals **Strategy:** In order to answer this question correctly, you need to know the definition of meditation, the types of meditation, and how meditation is utilized.

13 **Answer: 2 Rationale:** Imagery involves visualization to assist in healing. An image often used in imagery is the healing of an ill area of the body. Others are destroying certain foreign substances (e.g., cancer cells) or connecting with a higher level of consciousness. Instructions to concentrate on breathing and consciously letting go of stress are appropriate for a client who wants to meditate. The instructions to systematically contract and relax specific muscles or areas are appropriate for progressive relaxation exercises. Listening to music can be an effective relaxation technique, but is not essential for the use of imagery. **Cognitive Level:** Applying **Client Need:** Basic Care and Comfort **Integrated Process:** Nursing Process: Implementation **Content Area:** Fundamentals **Strategy:** To answer this question, it is necessary to recall the difference between imagery and other nonpharmacological therapies such as meditation, progressive relaxation, and music therapy.

14 **Answer: 1 Rationale:** Dermatitis or eczema is a common allergic reaction to topical aromatherapy. A small area of skin should be tested before aromatherapy is administered to a large area. Skin turgor is not affected by aromatherapy. Aromatherapy is not known to change the pigmentation of the skin involved. Edema is not an expected side effect of aromatherapy. **Cognitive Level:** Analyzing **Client Need:** Basic Care and Comfort **Integrated Process:** Nursing Process: Evaluation **Content Area:** Fundamentals **Strategy:** The question requires that the nurse know what to look for when a

client has an allergic reaction to essential oils used in aromatherapy.

15 **Answer: 2, 4, 5 Rationale:** Music therapy helps reduce the stress and anxiety of the preoperative client. Soft instrumental music is effective in helping to mask normal noises found in the hospital setting, contributing to the reduction of anxiety and stress. The effects of music enhancing relaxation are more effective if the listener is not distracted by words. Music therapy causes a hypometabolic state that stimulates the parasympathetic system and causes relaxation as a response. Music therapy stimulates the right hemisphere of the brain where creativity resides. **Cognitive Level:** Analysis **Client Need:** Basic Care and Comfort **Integrated Process:** Nursing Process: Evaluation **Content Area:** Fundamentals **Strategy:** Knowledge regarding the physiological effects of music is needed to answer this question correctly. When a question has more than one correct answer, consider each option as a true/false statement.

16 **Answer: 3 Rationale:** All of the symptoms described suggest intermittent claudication. Ginkgo is the only herb effective for this condition because its anticoagulant properties will enhance blood flow to the extremities. Feverfew is noted to inhibit platelet aggregation, suppress the production of prostaglandins, and inhibit the release of serotonin. Garlic inhibits platelet aggregation, reduces and inhibits metabolism of cholesterol, and increases bile acid secretion. Ginseng may have an effect on the pituitary gland similar to corticosteroids, improves serum glucose, and can increase or decrease blood pressure depending on the dosage. **Cognitive Level:** Analyzing **Client Need:** Basic Care and Comfort **Integrated Process:** Nursing Process: Evaluation **Content Area:** Fundamentals **Strategy:** The core issue of the question is recognizing the effect of ginkgo in treating signs of intermittent claudication. Use this knowledge and the process of elimination to determine the correct option.

17 **Answer: 3 Rationale:** Chlorpromazine, a phenothiazine, is metabolized in the liver. Milk thistle, the liver herb, is known to reduce the risk of hepatotoxicity caused by phenothiazines. Valerian root decreases CNS activity and produces sedation without the side effects of some medications prescribed for sleep induction. Ginger can enhance the effects of anticoagulation and produce anti-inflammatory and analgesic effects. Hawthorn increases coronary and myocardial circulation, decreases blood pressure, increases strength of myocardial contraction, lowers heart rate, and decreases total cholesterol and LDL levels. **Cognitive Level:** Analyzing **Client Need:** Basic Care and Comfort **Integrated Process:** Nursing Process: Planning **Content Area:** Fundamentals **Strategy:** The core issue of this question is recognition that milk thistle has a beneficial effect on the liver. Use this knowledge and the process of elimination to determine the correct option.

18 **Answer: 3 Rationale:** Garlic is used most widely to reduce total serum cholesterol and triglyceride levels. Garlic would reduce, not increase, platelet aggregation, thus leading to bleeding tendencies. Although garlic has been shown to boost immunity, it has not demonstrated effects on the white blood cell count. There is no known relationship between garlic and serum glucose levels. **Cognitive Level:** Applying **Client Need:** Basic Care and Comfort **Integrated Process:** Nursing Process: Diagnosis **Content Area:** Fundamentals **Strategy:** The core issue of the question is the use of garlic as an aid in reducing cholesterol and triglyceride levels. Use this knowledge and the process of elimination to determine the correct option.

19 **Answer: 4 Rationale:** Although some sources recommend ginger for morning sickness, other sources claim safety during pregnancy is unknown. Black cohosh has been known to promote labor and should be avoided until birth is imminent. The use of any herb should be discussed with the healthcare provider, particularly in pregnancy and lactation. Most herbs are contraindicated at this time, regardless of the form and even when taken as directed or in lower doses. **Cognitive Level:** Analyzing **Client Need:** Basic Care and Comfort **Integrated Process:** Teaching and Learning **Content Area:** Fundamentals **Strategy:** The core issue of the question is that many herbs have unknown or adverse effects on the developing fetus and are therefore used cautiously or avoided during pregnancy. Use this knowledge and the process of elimination to determine the correct option.

20 **Answer: 1 Rationale:** Echinacea is effective when used topically to promote wound healing. It is also used internally to boost the immune system, particularly in the prevention and adjunct treatment of colds and influenza. Ginger enhances effects of anticoagulation and produces an anti-inflammatory and analgesic effect. Valerian root decreases CNS activity, causing sedation with decreased side effects, but nonaddicting, and produces no morning hangover. Feverfew inhibits platelet aggregation, may suppress production of prostaglandins, and inhibits the release of serotonin. **Cognitive Level:** Applying **Client Need:** Basic Care and Comfort **Integrated Process:** Nursing Process: Planning **Content Area:** Fundamentals **Strategy:** The core issue of the question is the use of echinacea in wound healing and immune system enhancement. Note the correlation between these properties and the skin injury of the client. Use this knowledge and the process of elimination to determine the correct option.

21 **Answer: 1 Rationale:** Ginger inhibits thromboxane production. The inhibition of this prostaglandin reduces platelet aggregation, increasing the risk of bleeding in the postoperative client. Ginger would be effective in controlling pain and nausea, however, postoperatively is unsafe due to the tendency to cause bleeding. Ginger can be repeated every 4 hours, but this true statement regarding dosing does not address the issue of safety when used postoperatively. There is no data to support ginger as potentiating the effects of opioid medications. **Cognitive Level:** Analyzing **Client Need:** Basic Care and Comfort **Integrated Process:** Teaching and Learning **Content Area:** Fundamentals **Strategy:** The core issue of the question is the risk of bleeding associated with the use of ginger. Note the association of that property of this herb and the word *postoperative* in the stem of the question. Use this knowledge and the process of elimination to determine the correct option.

22 **Answer: 2 Rationale:** The nurse should monitor blood pressure in the client taking hawthorn, which is known to decrease peripheral vascular resistance, thus decreasing blood pressure. There is no evidence that hawthorn has an effect on blood glucose, white blood cell count, or client temperature. **Cognitive Level:** Applying **Client Need:** Basic Care and Comfort **Integrated Process:** Nursing Process: Planning **Content Area:** Fundamentals **Strategy:** The core issue of the question is the effect of hawthorn on hemodynamics, such as lowering blood pressure and decreasing vascular resistance. Use this knowledge and the process of elimination to determine the correct option.

23 **Answer: 2 Rationale:** One of the principle active ingredients of bilberry is pectin, a soluble fiber that decreases diarrhea. Anthocyanosides do not decrease peristalsis. Bilberry does not counteract microbial suppression of normal intestinal flora. Bilberry does not have antibacterial or antiviral properties. **Cognitive Level:** Analyzing **Client Need:** Basic Care and Comfort **Integrated Process:** Nursing Process: Implementation **Content Area:** Fundamentals **Strategy:** The core issue of this question is recognition that bilberry contains pectin and that pectin is used to control diarrhea. Use this knowledge and the process of elimination to determine the correct option.

24 **Answer: 4 Rationale:** The psychotherapeutic effects of St. John's wort are not well understood. The herb is thought to work by inhibiting serotonin reuptake, but it may have a slight inhibition of monoamine oxidase (MAO). It is therefore correct for the nurse to instruct the client that it is safe to eat ice cream while taking St. John's wort. Chocolate, aged cheeses, and beer contain tyramine, which may lead to severe hypertension when consumed while taking MAO inhibitors (MAOIs). **Cognitive Level:** Analyzing **Client Need:** Pharmacological and Parenteral Therapies **Integrated Process:** Nursing Process: Implementation **Content Area:** Pharmacology **Strategy:** The core issue of the question is the risk of interactive effects of foods containing tyramine with the MAOI effect of St. John's wort. Use this knowledge and the process of elimination to determine the correct option.

25 **Answer: 3, 5 Rationale:** The client with coronary artery disease or peripheral vascular disease would benefit most from use of garlic because of its ability to lower cholesterol and triglyceride levels. Garlic is not helpful in treating low blood pressure or liver disease. Because it inhibits platelet aggregation, the use of garlic by clients with a bleeding disorder could be hazardous. **Cognitive Level:** Analyzing **Client Need:** Basic Care and Comfort **Integrated Process:** Nursing Process: Diagnosis **Content Area:** Fundamentals **Strategy:** The core issue of the question is the use of garlic as an aid in reducing cholesterol and triglycerides as serum lipids. Use this knowledge and the process of elimination to determine the correct option.

Key Terms to Review

clinical aromatherapy p. 420
imagery p. 419
massage p. 418
meditation p. 419
music therapy p. 419
progressive relaxation p. 418

References

Adams, M., & Urban, C. (2016). *Pharmacology: Connections to nursing practice* (3rd ed.). New York, NY: Pearson Education.

Berman, A., Snyder, S., & Frandsen, G. (2016). *Kozier & Erb's fundamentals of nursing: Concepts, process, and practice* (10th ed.). New York, NY: Pearson Education.

Craven, R., & Hirnle, C., & Henshaw, C. (2017). *Fundamentals of nursing: Human health and function* (8th ed.). Philadelphia, PA: Wolters-Kluwer.

Fontaine, K. L. (2014). *Complementary and alternative therapies for nursing practice* (4th ed.). Upper Saddle River, NJ: Pearson Education, Inc.

Potter, P., Perry, A., Stockert, P., Hall, A. (2017). *Fundamentals of nursing* (9th ed.). St. Louis, MO: Mosby.

Test Yourself

Are you ready for the NCLEX-RN® or course exams? Access the NEW web-based app that provides students with thousands of practice questions in preparation for the NCLEX experience.

Dosage Calculation and Medication Administration

29

In this chapter

Cross Reference

Other chapters relevant to this content area are

Pediatric Dosage Calculation and Medication Administration	Chapter 30
Intravenous Therapy	Chapter 31

I. GENERAL PRINCIPLES OF MEDICATION ADMINISTRATION

A. Medication names

1. **Generic name**: a name that reflects chemical family of a drug and does not change according to manufacturer; an example is hydromorphone
2. **Brand name** or **trade name**: a proprietary name given to a generic drug by its manufacturer, resulting in various names for same drug; for example, Dilaudid is trade name for generic drug hydromorphone

B. Medication prescription components

1. Include date and time of prescription, drug name, dose, route, frequency, any special parameters (such as blood pressure [BP] or pulse) for administering or withholding dose, and prescriber signature
2. Medication prescriptions must conform to agency policies and guidelines and use The Joint Commission–approved abbreviations and symbols (aimed at reducing medication errors)
3. *NCLEX®* Call prescriber immediately if prescription is difficult to read or for any questions; do not administer a medication that has an unclear prescription
4. *NCLEX®* Under law, nurses are responsible for their own actions (e.g., if a drug prescription is written incorrectly, nurse who administers it is also responsible for error)
5. Telephone prescriptions are recorded by nurses as agency policy allows, must include all elements noted above, and must be cosigned by prescriber as soon as possible and within time frame of agency policy (usually 24 hours)
6. Verbal prescriptions are generally discouraged and tend to be used during emergency or near emergency situations; these are recorded as soon as possible and appropriately signed

C. Essential concepts of pharmacology

1. **Pharmacokinetics**: study of how body absorbs, distributes, metabolizes or biotransforms, and excretes drugs (four processes)
2. **Absorption**: process by which a drug moves from administration site into bloodstream; drugs are absorbed through gastrointestinal (GI) tract, respiratory tract, or skin, and absorption depends on correct drug form being administered by correct route
3. **Distribution**: movement of drug from site of absorption to site of action; depends on vascularity for speed of onset and on chemical and physical drug properties to attract drug to a certain area of body where it will exert its effect
4. **Metabolism/biotransformation**: conversion of a drug by enzymatic action of liver into a less active substance that is easily excreted through renal or biliary systems; can be affected by a variety of factors, including disease states
5. **Excretion**: elimination of drug and metabolites from body, primarily through kidneys but also through feces, respiration, perspiration, saliva, and breast milk
6. Prescriber determines frequency of drug dosing according to drug's **half-life** (time it takes for total amount of drug to diminish by one-half); a drug's half-life provides information about its accumulation in body with repeated doses

D. Principles and process of medication administration

1. Determine completeness and accuracy of prescription
2. *NCLEX®* Check client allergies to prescribed medication and to any of its ingredients
3. Assess client condition related to why medication is being prescribed
4. *NCLEX®* Check prescribed medication against other prescribed medications for interactions; be aware of **side effects** (mild), **adverse effects** (more severe), and **toxic effects** (most harmful) associated with high doses
5. *NCLEX®* Calculate dose properly, using any conversions needed (see next section)
6. Check expiration date and do not use any medication for which expiration date has passed
7. Label all drawn-up or reconstituted medications with drug name, dose, date, time, and initials
8. Discard any partially used single-dose containers; label multiuse vials with date, time, and initials when opened or apply expiration date stickers used by some agencies (many expire 30 days after initial use; see product literature and agency policy)
9. *NCLEX®* Complete six rights when administering medications: right drug, dose, route, time, client, and documentation (date, time, initials and/or signature, site if parenteral, any parameters such as BP, pulse, or blood glucose)
10. *NCLEX®* Address any client concerns about medication; do not administer a medication that client questions until prescription is rechecked
11. Follow universal principles of medication administration and complete client teaching related to medication therapy (see Box 29–1)

II. MEASUREMENT AND CONVERSION SYSTEMS

A. Medication measurement systems

1. **Metric system**: a decimal system of measurement based on units of 10; gram is a unit of weight, and liter is a unit of liquid volume (see Table 29–1)
2. Apothecary system: oldest system of pharmacologic measurement, not used any longer for drug dosage calculation
3. Household: a less accurate system of measurement based on drops, teaspoons, tablespoons, cups, and glasses

B. Conversions

1. When a medication prescription is written in one system and medication label uses another system, one system must be converted to equivalent measure in other
2. See Table 29–2 for weight and volume equivalents between metric and household measurement systems
3. When converting within metric system, move decimal point three places to right to convert from a larger unit of measure to a smaller unit of measure (e.g., 2.5 grams converts to 2500 milligrams) and three places to left to convert from a smaller unit of measure to a larger unit of measure (e.g., 3000 milliliters converts to 3 liters)
4. Perform all conversions before calculating medication dosage

Box 29–1

Universal Principles for Medication Administration and Related Client Teaching

Administration Principles

- Assess current medications (including OTC drugs and herbal products) with previously prescribed medications (medication reconciliation) and client's history of allergies to identify any potential risks to client.
- Administer doses on time to maintain therapeutic blood levels.
- Do not break, crush, or allow client to chew sustained release or enteric-coated preparations.
- Be aware of side effects and adverse effects of medications and monitor client to maintain client safety.
- Provide both verbal and written instructions to client, and provide phone number to call if questions arise or problems occur.

Client Teaching

- Understand medication actions, side effects, signs of toxicity, how to self-administer, importance of follow-up with prescriber, and importance of adhering to plan for periodic laboratory testing if needed.
- Do not take any over-the-counter (OTC) drugs or herbal products without first consulting prescriber.
- Take exactly as prescribed and do not miss or double doses.
- Report adverse effects promptly.
- Do not discontinue drug without consulting prescriber.
- Do not drink alcohol while taking prescription medications.

Table 29–1 Metric System Abbreviations and Equivalents

Metric System Abbreviations	Metric System Equivalents
Volume: milliliter = mL liter = L	***Volume:*** 1 mL = 0.001 L 1 L = 1,000 mL
Weight: microgram = mcg milligram = mg gram = g kilogram = kg	***Weight:*** 1 mcg = 0.000001 g 1 mg = 0.001 g or 1,000 mcg 1 g = 1,000 mg or 1,000,000 mcg 1 kg = 1,000 g (or 2.2 lb [pounds])
Length: meter = m	

Table 29–2 Approximate Metric and Household System Equivalents

Metric	Household
1 mL	15 gtt (drop)
5 mL	60 gtt = 1 tsp (teaspoon)
15 mL	3 tsp = 1 tbsp (tablespoon)
30 mL	2 tbsp (1 ounce)
240 mL	1 cup (8 ounces)
500 mL	1 pint (16 ounces)
1000 mL	1 quart (2 pints)
4000 mL	1 gallon (4 quarts)

III. DOSAGE CALCULATIONS

A. **Medications are prescribed in a specific amount or weight per volume;** for instance, if a single tablet has 100 mg of medication, the volume of that tablet is 1; a medication that comes in 80 mg per 2 mL of liquid has a volume of 2

B. **A few liquid medications are prescribed by volume alone** because they are available in only one strength, such as a dose of 30 mL of a liquid antacid

C. **Common formulas for calculating medications** are ratio and proportion, "desired over have," and dimensional analysis (see Box 29–2)

Memory Aid

No single drug calculation formula is better than any other. Choose one that works for you and use it consistently.

D. **When giving liquid medications for injection,** round amounts greater than 1 mL to nearest tenth (0.1) to coincide with calibrations on syringe (see next section)

E. **When giving liquid medications for injection,** round amounts less than 1 mL to nearest hundredth (0.01) to coincide with calibrations on syringe (see next section)

F. **Rules for rounding generally require carrying out decimals to one place further than needed** and then rounding back only once at very end of calculation

IV. ORAL MEDICATIONS

A. **Tablets may be divided into partial dosages** (e.g., half) only when scored (marked in half with indented line)

B. **Extended-release and enteric-coated medications**

NCLEX®

1. Do not break or crush enteric-coated medications, which are designed for release and absorption in small intestine

Box 29–2

Calculating Medication Dosages

Formula 1 "Desired over Have"

$$\frac{\text{Dose ordered (desired)}}{\text{Dose on hand (have)}} \times \text{Amount available (quantity)} = \text{Amount to give}$$

Example: Lasix 60 mg IV is prescribed and medication is labeled as 80 mg per 2 mL.

$$\frac{60 \text{ mg}}{80 \text{ mg}} \times 2 \text{ mL} = 1.5 \text{ mL}$$

Formula 2 Ratio and Proportion

Dose prescribed is to (:) dose on hand as (::) *x* quantity is to (:) quantity available
Multiply the two outer values by the inner value and *x* to solve.
Example: Lasix 60 mg IV is prescribed and medication is labeled as 80 mg per 2 mL.

$60 \text{ mg} : 80 \text{ mg} :: x : 2$
$80x = 120; x = 1.5 \text{ mL}$

Formula 3 Dimensional Analysis

Uses a set of rules to set up problems for solving

Rule 1: Multiplying one side of an equation by a conversion factor will not change the value of the equation.

Rule 2: Set up the problem in fractions called factors so that all labels cancel from the numerator and denominator except the label desired in the answer.

Example: Lasix 60 mg IV is prescribed and medication is labeled as 80 mg per 2 mL.

$$\text{mL} = \frac{2 \text{ mL}}{80 \text{ mg}} \times 60 \text{ mg}$$

$$\text{mL} = \frac{120}{80} = 1.5$$

NCLEX® 2. As a rule, do not break or crush extended-release medications; some scored formulations can be broken without affecting release mechanism; some mixed-release capsules can be opened and contents sprinkled on food; read product literature carefully

3. Abbreviations used in brand names identifying drugs as extended-release include CR (controlled release), CRT (controlled-release tablet), LA (long acting), SA (sustained action), SR (sustained release), TR (time release), and XL or XR (extended length or release)

C. Liquid doses

1. Medicine cup holds a maximum volume of 30 mL and has calibrations in 5 mL increments, teaspoons, tablespoons, and ounces
2. Use medicine cup to pour liquid volumes of 5 mL or greater; hold cup in level position at eye level and measure to middle of meniscus
3. Use syringe with needle removed to draw up liquid volumes less than 5 mL
4. If a calibrated dropper is supplied with medication, it may be used (often used with children)

V. ENTERAL MEDICATIONS

A. Perform hand hygiene and place client in semi-Fowler's position

B. Determine correct tube placement

1. It may not be possible to reliably determine placement of small-bore enteral tubes by any technique other than radiography, which is most reliable
2. Nasogastric tube: aspirate stomach contents and check pH (should be 4 or less), or auscultate air insufflation (less reliable); drainage color should be greenish tan to clear
3. Nasointestinal tubes: aspirate stomach contents and check pH (should be higher than 6); color of duodenal fluid should be deep yellow
4. Percutaneous endoscopic gastrostomy (PEG) and percutaneous endoscopic jejunostomy (PEJ) tubes do not require placement verification prior to each dose administration

C. Enteral medication administration procedure

1. Flush enteral tube with approximately 30 mL water prior to administering medication
2. Administer medication in solution or elixir forms when available; crush tablets to a fine powder and mix in warm water to make a solution or suspension; do not mix medications—administer each medication separately; flush well between medications

NCLEX® 3. If client is receiving enteral feeding, ensure compatibility of medication and feeding; if they are not compatible, turn off tube feeding for 30–60 minutes before and after medication administration

4. Flush enteral tube with approximately 30 mL of water following each medication

NCLEX® 5. If enteral tube is connected to suction, disconnect from suction for at least 30 minutes after administering medication

NCLEX® 6. Maintain client in semi-Fowler's position for at least 30 minutes following administration of medication

VI. INJECTIONS

A. See Box 29–3 for withdrawing medications from a vial

B. See Box 29–4 for withdrawing medications from an ampule

C. Maintain sterility while assembling syringe and needle; select appropriate-size needle and syringe based on volume and type of medication, desired site, client's size, and viscosity of medication

Box 29–3

Withdrawing Medications from a Vial

1. Remove vial cap.
2. Cleanse rubber top of vial with alcohol.
3. Tighten needle on syringe or use needleless syringe.
4. Fill plunger with amount of air equal to amount of solution to be withdrawn.
5. Inject air into vacant area of vial, keeping needle above surface of medication.
6. Invert vial, touching only syringe barrel and plunger tip. Withdraw medication.
7. While syringe remains attached to vial, expel any air bubbles from syringe by tapping side of syringe sharply.
8. Recheck amount of medication in syringe.
9. Remove syringe from vial and recap needle, if appropriate, using scoop technique.

Box 29–4

Withdrawing Medications from an Ampule

1. Tap neck of ampule to move solution to body of ampule.
2. Using a pad to protect fingers, break ampule away from you.
3. Use a filter needle to withdraw solution. Solution can be withdrawn from either an upright or inverted position—insert needle, without touching sides of neck, with bevel down and touching bottom of ampule (it is not necessary to add air).
4. Return ampule to upright position.
5. Tap barrel below bubbles to dislodge air in syringe.
6. Eject air with syringe in upright position.
7. Recheck amount of medication in syringe.
8. Remove filter needle and replace with appropriate needle.

NCLEX®

D. **See Table 29–3 for a summary of syringes, needles, and uses;** see Figure 29–1 for examples of 3 mL, insulin, and tuberculin syringes, with illustration of various calibrations
E. **Some medications are supplied in single-use prefilled cartridges** and are placed in a cartridge holder for injection; these generally have sufficient volume to allow a second medication to be added, if prescribed

Table 29–3 Summary of Syringes, Needles, and Uses

Use/Purpose	Site	Maximum Volume	Syringe	Needle Size	Needle Angle
Insulin Slow absorption to produce a sustained effect	Abdomen, lateral and posterior areas of upper arm or thigh, scapular area, upper ventrodorsal gluteal areas	1 mL	Insulin—calibrated on 100-unit scale	Nonremovable 1 cm (⅜ in.) 29 gauge	45° or 90°
Intradermal or intracutaneous Antigens and skin testing, slow absorption	Inner lower arm or scapular area, upper chest	0.1 mL	1 mL tuberculin syringe	1 cm (⅜ in.) 25–27 gauge	10–15° just under epidermis; bevel of needle up
Subcutaneous Absorbed slowly for sustained effect	Abdomen, lateral and posterior aspects of upper arm or thigh, scapular area, upper ventro-and dorsogluteal areas	1 mL	0.5–3 mL syringe	1–1.5 cm (⅜ – ⅝ in.) 25 gauge	1.5 cm (⅝ in.) –45° when 1 in. of tissue can be grasped 1 cm (⅜ in.) –90° when 5 cm (2 in.) of tissue can be grasped
Intramuscular Rapid absorption *Ventrogluteal*—preferred for adults *Vastus lateralis*—-preferred for infant < 7 months of age	Ventrogluteal, dorsogluteal, vastus lateralis, deltoid	*Adult deltoid* 0.5–1 mL *Adult gluteus medius* 1–4 mL	1–5 mL syringe	*Deltoid* 1.5–2.5 cm (⅝ – 1 in.) 23–25 gauge *Vastus lateralis, ventrogluteal, and dorsogluteal* 3.8 cm (1.5 in.)	90°

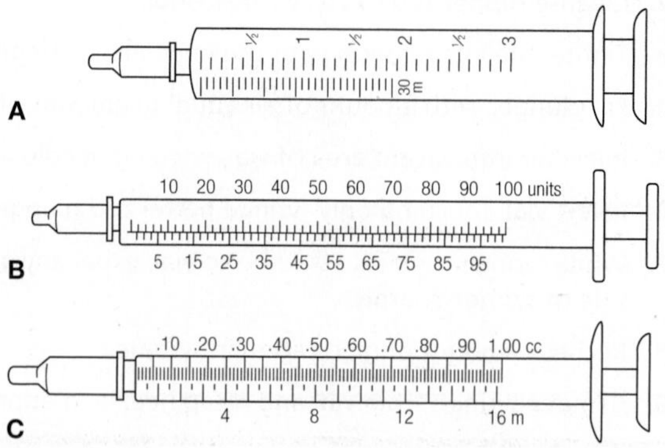

Figure 29–1

Three kinds of syringes for injection: (A) 3-milliliter (mL) hypodermic syringe is calibrated in tenths (0.1) mL and minims. (B) Insulin syringe is calibrated in 100 units for use with U100 insulin. (C) Tuberculin syringe is calibrated in tenths and hundredths (0.01) of an mL and in minims.

F. **If medication is supplied in powder form,** reconstitute (dissolve) dose using sterile water or normal saline in volume specified in drug insert; recognize that total volume of solution after reconstitution may be larger because powder adds volume

G. **Using anatomical landmarks,** select site of injection appropriate for type of injection and medication (e.g., intramuscular, intradermal, or subcutaneous); see Box 29–5 for a summary of injection sites

Box 29–5

Summary of Injection Sites

Intramuscular

Ventrogluteal

- Place client in side-lying position.
- Use right hand for left anterior hip and left hand for right anterior hip.
- Place palm over greater trochanter and point index finger toward client's anterior-superior iliac spine; spread out index finger from other three fingers to form a V area.
- Inject at a 90-degree angle within V area.

Dorsogluteal (less commonly used; not for use in infants and small children)

- Place client either in prone position with toes pointed inward or in side-lying position with upper knee flexed and in front of lower leg.
- Draw imaginary line between greater trochanter and postero-superior spine (prominence) of iliac crest.
- Inject at 90-degree angle lateral and superior to imaginary line.

Vastus Lateralis

- Place client in supine position.
- Inject at a 90-degree angle using anterior-lateral middle third of thigh between greater trochanter and lateral femoral condyle.

Deltoid

- Palpate lower edge of acromion and midpoint of lateral aspect of arm. Inject at 90-degree angle 5 cm (2 in.) below acromion process within triangle between boundaries.
- Alternate method—place four fingers across deltoid muscle with first finger on acromion process; site is three finger breadths below acromion process.

Z-Track Injection

- An alternative method of intramuscular injection designed to reduce seepage of medication into subcutaneous tissues.
- Prior to injection, displace skin, insert needle at 90-degree angle while skin remains displaced; remove needle and allow skin to return to neutral position, eliminating an intact needle tract.
- Use this method for medications that are irritating to subcutaneous tissues.

Subcutaneous

Most Common Sites

- Lateral-posterior aspect of upper arms
- Anterior thighs
- Lower quadrants of abdomen (outside 5-cm [2-in.] radius of umbilicus): preferred site for heparin

Other Sites

- Scapular areas
- Dorsogluteal

Intradermal

- Forearms
- Upper back beneath scapulae
- Upper chest

H. Use standard injection procedure to administer medication dose

1. Perform hand hygiene and put on gloves
2. Cleanse area with alcohol swab and wait for it to dry (usually 30 seconds)
3. Inject medication using procedure specific to route
4. Discard syringe and needle into a sharps container

I. Specific information appropriate to injection sites

1. **Intradermal (ID)**: gently pull skin taut; do not aspirate; inject medication slowly and observe for wheal formation and blanching at site
2. **Subcutaneous (subcut)**: grasp subcutaneous tissue; hold syringe like a dart (between thumb and forefinger) and insert needle; release tissue; aspirate (except with heparin or insulin) and inject medication slowly if no blood appears (if blood returns, withdraw needle, discard, and prepare a new injection); with insulin administration, rotate injection sites systematically to minimize tissue damage (**lipodystrophy**, atrophy, or hypertrophy of tissue), which affects absorption
3. **Intramuscular (IM)**: hold syringe like a dart; spread skin taught or grasp skin in geriatric client; use quick, darting motion to insert needle; aspirate and inject medication slowly unless blood returns (if blood returns, withdraw needle, discard, and prepare new injection); Z-track technique prevents "tracking" and is used to administer medications irritating to subcutaneous tissue (e.g., hydroxyzine)—pull skin approximately 2.5 cm (1 in.) laterally away from injection site, inject medication, withdraw needle, then release tissue

VII. INTRAVENOUS (IV) MEDICATIONS

A. Adding medications to *intravenous* (IV) fluids for infusion helps to maintain constant therapeutic blood levels; examples are potassium (e.g., 20 mEq added to 1 liter of IV solution) or heparin (25,000 units added to 250 mL solution)

1. To add medication to an IV solution, prepare medication from a vial or ampule and draw into syringe
2. Some medications supplied in powder form (such as antibiotics) may be reconstituted by attaching vial to IV solution injection port, squeezing IV fluid into vial, mixing, and squeezing liquid back into IV bag

B. To add medication to a new IV container

1. Clean injection port with alcohol swab and allow to dry for 30 seconds
2. Remove needle cap from syringe, insert needle through center of injection port, and inject medication
3. Mix medication and solution by gently rotating bag
4. Complete and attach medication label to IV solution; include name and dose of medication, date and time, and nurse's initials
5. Proceed with setting up IV for administration

C. To add medication to an existing infusion

1. Ensure there is sufficient IV solution in container to dilute medication properly
2. Proceed as with adding a medication to a new IV container

D. Injection by IV bolus or IV push

1. A **bolus**, or IV push, is a direct injection of a medication intravenously
2. Used to obtain rapid therapeutic serum concentrations when medications cannot be diluted, or to administer emergency drugs
3. Administration via heparin/saline lock device (no IV solutions running)
   a. Prepare syringe with medication and two syringes with flush solution, usually normal saline, according to agency policy, attach needleless device to syringes, and label all syringes
   b. Perform hand hygiene and put on gloves
   c. Cleanse infusion port with alcohol swab and let dry for 30 seconds
   d. Instill normal saline to flush IV access device according to agency policy
   e. Cleanse port again and attach syringe with medication to infusion port
   f. Inject medication at recommended IV push rate
   g. Flush IV access device again per agency policy

Memory Aid

Look up in a drug handbook or other standard reference the infusion rate of IV push medications. They vary in length, but most should be given over 1 minute or longer.

4. IV push medication through port of infusing IV line
   a. Draw up medication as prescribed
   b. Pinch off IV tubing or shut off IV pump before injecting medication

c. Cleanse IV tubing injection port and inject medication over appropriate time frame through port close to client and remove syringe
d. Resume IV infusion

5. Piggyback infusion without interrupting existing IV
NCLEX®
a. Ensure compatibility of piggyback medication with any other currently infusing IV solutions and any additives (such as potassium) or currently infusing medications; if incompatible, discontinue primary infusion temporarily if safe to do so or start a second IV line; set up secondary set following procedure for setting up an IV
b. Hang existing infusion set lower than piggyback secondary set
c. Cleanse uppermost infusion port with alcohol swab and let dry for 30 seconds
d. Connect secondary set to primary set using needleless access device above existing IV roller clamp
e. Maintain existing IV roller clamp position and regulate piggyback rate using roller clamp on secondary tubing or programming secondary rate and volume into infusion pump; piggyback solution will infuse first, and existing IV will resume at original rate when complete
f. When intermittent solution is in a syringe pump, connect syringe to secondary access port on pump; follow protocols for specific pump to administer intermittent medication as either a continuous infusion or an infusion that interrupts existing IV

VIII. TOPICAL MEDICATIONS

A. Medications applied to skin

NCLEX®
1. Perform hand hygiene and apply gloves to prevent **topical** drug absorption through fingertips
2. Remove prior applications remaining on client's skin unless otherwise specified
3. Remove ointments and creams from their containers and apply to skin with tongue depressors in thin layers unless otherwise specified
4. For transdermal patch or premeasured paper, read package insert for application directions
   a. Remove previously applied patch or paper and cleanse skin
   b. Record date and time of application and initials directly onto transdermal patch, and remove protective covering
   c. Place prescribed amount of medication directly on premeasured paper and apply immediately; secure paper with tape
   NCLEX®
   d. Alternate application areas to prevent skin irritation and apply to clean, dry, intact, and hairless skin

B. Nasal medications

1. Apply gloves after performing hand hygiene
2. Ask client to blow nose and tilt client's head back
3. Nasal spray: occlude one nostril with gloved finger and have client inhale through nose while squeezing medication bottle; client may self-medicate if able
4. Bottle with dropper: fill dropper with prescribed amount of medication, place dropper just inside nare, and instill correct number of drops
5. Wipe excess medication with tissue
6. Repeat with other nostril if appropriate
NCLEX®
7. Instruct client not to sneeze or blow nose and to keep head tilted back for 5 minutes until medication is absorbed

C. *Ophthalmic* (eye) medications

1. Ophthalmic drops
   a. Tilt client's head slightly backward and ask client to look up
   b. Supply tissue so that client can wipe off excess medication
   c. Hold eyedropper 1.3–1.9 cm (½–¾ in.) above eyeball
   d. Expose lower conjunctival sac by pulling down on cheek, creating a "cup"
   NCLEX®
   e. Drop prescribed number of drops into center of lower conjunctival sac while applying pressure to inner canthus to reduce systemic absorption of medication
   f. Instruct client to close eyelids and move eyes; gently massage closed lid
   g. Remove excess medication with tissue
2. Ophthalmic ointment
   a. Supply tissue so that client can wipe off excess medication
   b. Put on gloves
   c. Gently separate eyelids with two fingers, grasping lower lid immediately below lashes; exert pressure downward over bony prominence of cheek to form a trough
   d. Instruct client to look upward

NCLEX® e. Apply ointment along inside edge of entire lower eyelid, from inner canthus to outer canthus
f. Instruct client to close eyelids and move eyes to spread ointment under lids and over eye surface
g. Remove excess medication with tissue
h. Instruct client that vision may be blurred temporarily following administration of an ointment

D. Otic (ear) medications

1. Position client on side with ear to be treated facing up
2. Fill medication dropper with prescribed amount of medication
3. Put on gloves
4. NCLEX® Straighten ear canal; for an infant or young child, pull pinna of ear gently downward and backward; in an adult, pull pinna gently upward and backward
5. Instill medication drops, holding medication slightly above ear
6. Insert cotton loosely into ear canal, if prescribed
7. Instruct client to remain on side for 5–10 minutes

E. Vaginal medications

1. Position client in dorsal recumbent or Sims' position
2. Perform hand hygiene and put on gloves
3. Suppository: remove foil wrapper and insert suppository into applicator
4. Cream: attach medication tube to applicator and squeeze tube to fill applicator with prescribed dose; remove tube
5. Insert applicator into vaginal canal 7.5 to 10 cm (3–4 in.), push plunger until all medication is released, and remove applicator
6. Instruct client to lie quietly for 15 minutes until medication is absorbed; vaginal medications may be prescribed at bedtime to aid retention
7. Wash applicator and return to appropriate storage area

F. Rectal medications

1. Place client in Sims' (left lateral) position
2. Perform hand hygiene and put on gloves
3. Remove foil wrapper from suppository
4. Apply small amount of water-soluble lubricant to suppository
5. Use index finger to insert suppository flat end first so it is approximately 10 cm (4 in.) beyond external sphincter in adults to ensure retention (studies indicate that inserting flat end first promotes better retention than inserting tapered end first)
6. Instruct client to lie quietly for 15 minutes while medication is absorbed

IX. INHALATION MEDICATIONS

A. Metered-dose inhaled (MDI) medication

1. Shake canister before each puff to mix medication and propellant
2. Instruct client to:
   a. Hold inhaler 5 cm (2 in.) away from mouth
   b. Exhale through pursed lips
   c. Depress **inhalation** device, inhaling slowly and deeply through mouth
   d. Hold breath for 10 seconds and slowly exhale through pursed lips
   NCLEX® e. Wait 2–5 minutes (as drug literature recommends) between puffs
3. Clean device according to manufacturer's instructions

B. Spacer with MDI

1. Insert MDI mouthpiece into spacer
2. Remove mouthpiece cover from spacer
3. Shake MDI with spacer
4. Hold MDI and spacer with drug canister upright
5. Instruct client to inhale, exhale slowly through pursed lips, then close lips around spacer mouthpiece
6. Activate MDI canister by pushing it further down into plastic adapter while client inhales slowly and deeply
7. Instruct client to hold breath for 10 seconds, then exhale and relax
8. Wipe mouthpiece after use
9. Remove rubber end of spacer, rinse with warm water, and dry thoroughly

Check Your NCLEX–RN® Exam I.Q.

You are ready for testing on this content if you can:

- Assess the medication schedule of a client.
- Calculate medication dosages with accuracy.
- Reconstitute or mix medications appropriately.
- Verify dosage calculations before administering medications.
- Identify proper procedures for medication administration.
- Utilize the "six rights" of medication administration.
- Dispose of unused medications properly.

PRACTICE TEST

1 The nurse is administering an intradermal tuberculin skin test to a client. The nurse prepares to use which angle of needle entry for the injection?

1. 10–15 degrees
2. 30–40 degrees
3. 45 degrees
4. 90 degrees

2 The nurse is preparing to administer a watery medication via an intramuscular injection into the deltoid muscle of a 73-kg (160-lb) male. What is the preferred needle size for the medication, muscle, and weight of the client?

1. 3.8 cm (1.5 in.), 20 gauge
2. 2.5 cm (1 in.), 20 gauge
3. 3.8 cm (1.5 in.), 25 gauge
4. 2.5 cm (1 in.), 25 gauge

3 A nurse giving an intramuscular injection places the heel of the hand on the client's greater trochanter, with the fingers pointing toward the client's head. The nurse places the index finger on the client's anterior-superior iliac spine, while the middle finger is stretched dorsally, palpating the iliac crest. After giving the injection in the triangle formed, the nurse documents the injection as being given in which intramuscular injection site?

1. Vastus lateralis
2. Ventrogluteal
3. Dorsogluteal
4. Rectus femoris

4 A client is postoperative with an IV in place. During assessment, the client rates pain at being 6 on a 0–10 scale. The nurse notes a prescription in the client's chart for morphine sulfate 6–8 mg every 4 hours as needed for pain. Given the prescription and the client's condition, what action should the nurse take?

1. Administer 8 mg morphine sulfate intramuscularly (IM)
2. Administer 6 mg morphine sulfate through the IV
3. Withhold the pain medication and contact the prescriber
4. Give one 10 mg dose of morphine sulfate to regain pain control.

5 The healthcare provider gives the nurse a telephone prescription for acetaminophen 500 mg by mouth every 4 hours as needed for a temperature elevation higher than 37.8°C (100°F). What is the nurse's appropriate response?

1. Remind the provider that nurses are not permitted to write medication prescriptions over the telephone.
2. Write a "telephone order" and sign it, reminding the provider to cosign it within 24 hours.
3. Record the prescription and sign the provider's name first, followed by the nurse's signature.
4. Ask another nurse to listen to the telephone prescription and record the prescription with both nurse's names.

6 A client with a history of renal impairment is prescribed a medication known to be excreted through the kidneys. What parameters should the nurse monitor to detect adverse reactions to the medication?

1. Serum blood urea nitrogen (BUN) and creatinine
2. Color and odor of the urine
3. Urine sugar and acetone levels
4. Serum hemoglobin and hematocrit

PRACTICE TEST

7. A client has a continuously running peripheral intravenous (IV) infusion. The healthcare provider prescribes the addition of an antibiotic as a piggyback infusion four times a day. What should the nurse do in order to administer the antibiotic safely?

1. Start a new IV access to avoid compatibility issues with the antibiotic.
2. Start a new IV access to avoid too much volume at one IV site.
3. Increase the continuous infusion to facilitate administration of the antibiotic.
4. Check if the antibiotic is compatible with the continuous infusion solution.

8. The nurse is preparing to administer an oral medication to a client. Upon entering the client's room, the nurse finds that the client has developed vomiting and diarrhea, is confused, and has a fever. What should the nurse do next? Select all that apply.

1. Administer the medication IM.
2. Give the medication as prescribed.
3. Withhold the medication.
4. Omit this dose of medication.
5. Notify the healthcare provider.

9. After the nurse has prepared an IM injection for a preoperative client, another client becomes entangled in IV tubing and yells for help. As the nurse rushes to assist, the surgery orderly arrives for the preoperative client. The nurse asks a second nurse to give the injection to the preoperative client. What is the best response by the second nurse?

1. Offer to assist the second client.
2. Give the client the preoperative medication.
3. Prepare a new syringe for the preoperative client.
4. Explain that the nurse should give the prepared medication.

10. A client is in the bathroom. When the nurse enters the room to give medications, the client asks the nurse to leave the pills on the bedside table. What is the best nursing action?

1. Leave the medication on the bedside table.
2. Wait in the room until the client comes out of the bathroom.
3. Go into the bathroom and give the client the pills.
4. Return later with the medication and explain this to the client.

11. The client has a prescription for dexamethasone 6 mg IV push stat. Available is a vial of dexamethasone containing 4 mg/mL. The nurse should draw ______ milliliters into the syringe for the dose. Record your answer rounding to one decimal place.

Fill in your answer below:
Answer: ________ mL

12. The client has a prescription for cefotaxime 1 gram IV q6h. The reconstituted vial in the client's medication drawer is labeled with a concentration of 95 mg/mL. For the intermittent infusion, the nurse should add ______ milliliters of solution to the IV bag. Record your answer rounding to one decimal place.

Fill in your answer below:
Answer: ________ mL

13. The client has a prescription for glyburide 1.25 mg before breakfast and dinner. Available are 2.5 mg tablets. The nurse should plan to administer ______ tablet(s). Record your answer rounding to one decimal place.

Fill in your answer below:
Answer: ________ tablet(s)

14. The client has a prescription for lorazepam 0.5 mg IV q6h PRN for agitation. Available is a vial containing 2 mg/mL. The nurse should draw up ______ milliliters of solution for injection. Record your answer rounding to two decimal places.

Fill in your answer below:
Answer: ________ mL

15 A client has a temperature of 101.2°F (38.4°C). There is a prescription for acetaminophen 650 mg PO for fever, and 325 mg tablets are available. The nurse should give ______ tablets. Record your answer rounding to the nearest whole number.

Fill in your answer below:
Answer: ________ tablet(s)

16 A client has a prescription for cefazolin 2 grams IVPB. Available are vials filled with powder containing 1 gram of cefazolin. The instructions state to "dilute each 1 gram with 10 mL of sterile water." After reconstituting the medication, ______ total milliliters of solution should be drawn up to prepare the dose. Record your answer rounding to the nearest whole number.

Fill in your answer below:
Answer: ________ mL

17 A client has a prescription for a dose of digoxin 0.25 mg IV push. Available is a vial containing 0.125 mg/mL. The nurse should draw up ______ milliliters to administer the dose. Record your answer rounding to the nearest whole number.

Fill in your answer below:
Answer: ________ mL

18 The client has a prescription to receive methylprednisolone 120 mg IVPB q6h. Available is a solution containing 40 mg/mL. The nurse should add ______ milliliters of medication to the IV piggyback solution. Record your answer rounding to the nearest whole number.

Fill in your answer below:
Answer: ________ mL

19 The client has a prescription to receive 40 mg prednisone by mouth daily. Available are 10 mg tablets. The nurse should prepare to give ______ tablets. Record your answer rounding to the nearest whole number.

Fill in your answer below:
Answer: ________ tablet(s)

20 The nurse is to administer 600 mg of ibuprofen, which is available in a strength of 200 mg per tablet. The nurse would give ______ tablets to administer the dose. Record your answer rounding to the nearest whole number.

Fill in your answer below:
Answer: ________ tablet(s)

ANSWERS & RATIONALES

1 **Answer: 1 Rationale:** For an intradermal injection, the needle enters the skin at a 10- to 15-degree angle and the medication forms a bleb under the epidermis. The other options would permit the medication to be deposited too deeply into either subcutaneous or muscle tissue, depending on needle length and size of client. **Cognitive Level:** Applying **Client Need:** Pharmacological and Parenteral Therapies **Integrated Process:** Planning **Content Area:** Pharmacology **Strategy:** The core issue is knowledge of the correct needle angle to achieve the appropriate depth of penetration. The option that has the smallest angle, which will keep the injection from going too deeply, should be selected for an intradermal injection.

2 **Answer: 4 Rationale:** Several factors indicate the size and length of the needle to be used: the muscle, the type of solution, the amount of adipose tissue covering the muscle, and the age of the client. A smaller needle such as a 23- to 25-gauge needle that is 2.5 cm (1 in.) long is commonly used for the deltoid muscle. A 3.8-cm (1.5-in.), 20-gauge needle is appropriate for an injection of a viscous medication into a larger muscle, well-covered by adipose tissue. Commonly, a smaller 23- to 25-gauge needle that is 2.5 cm (1 in.) long is appropriate for an injection of watery medication into the deltoid muscle. A 2.5-cm (1-in.) long needle is usually appropriate for an injection into the deltoid muscle. More viscous solutions require a larger gauge (e.g., 20 gauge). A smaller 23- to 25-gauge needle is appropriate for an injection of watery medication into the deltoid muscle. However, a 3.8-cm

(1.5-in.) needle is appropriate for an injection into a larger muscle, well covered by adipose tissue. **Cognitive Level:** Analyzing **Client Need:** Pharmacological and Parenteral Therapies **Integrated Process:** Nursing Process: Implementation **Content Area:** Pharmacology **Strategy:** The critical concepts in the question are that the deltoid muscle commonly requires the use of a shorter needle and a watery solution allows the use of a smaller-gauge needle. Use the process of elimination to choose the option that combines these concepts.

3 **Answer: 2 Rationale:** The ventrogluteal site is in the gluteus medius muscle with the greater trochanter, the anterior-superior iliac spine, and the iliac crest as the landmarks. The vastus lateralis is located on the thigh. The dorsogluteal is located on the buttocks. The rectus femoris is located on the thigh. **Cognitive Level:** Analyzing **Client Need:** Pharmacological and Parenteral Therapies **Integrated Process:** Communication and Documentation **Content Area:** Pharmacology **Strategy:** Basic knowledge of injection sites and landmarks is necessary to answer this question. Utilize knowledge of anatomy and physiology to select the option that matches the description given in the question. Visualize the description.

4 **Answer: 3 Rationale:** The essential elements that must be present in order to implement a prescription are name of the drug, date and time the prescription was written, dosage, route, frequency, and signature of the prescriber. This client's prescription is missing a route so the prescriber must be contacted for clarification. Nurses may not independently administer a medication without all of the essential parts of the prescription. Administering medication in larger doses than prescribed constitutes practicing medicine without a license. **Cognitive Level:** Analyzing **Client Need:** Pharmacological and Parenteral Therapies **Integrated Process:** Nursing Process: Implementation **Content Area:** Pharmacology **Strategy:** The core issue of the question is recognizing and understanding that medication cannot be given with an incomplete prescription. Apply knowledge about medication administration to select the correct answer.

5 **Answer: 2 Rationale:** When the nurse documents a telephone prescription, the words "telephone order" and the prescriber's name must be recorded and the prescriber must cosign it, usually within 24 hours. A nurse can take a telephone prescription from a healthcare provider. The prescription needs to be designated as a "telephone order." It is unnecessary for a second nurse to listen to a telephone prescription. The nurse who takes the telephone prescription should read the prescription back to the healthcare provider for validation. **Cognitive Level:** Applying **Client Need:** Pharmacological and Parenteral Therapies **Integrated Process:** Communication and Documentation **Content Area:** Fundamentals **Strategy:** The core issue of the question is knowledge of how to properly record a *telephone order*. The wording of the question tells you that only one option is correct. Use the process of elimination and basic nursing knowledge to make a selection.

6 **Answer: 1 Rationale:** Blood levels of two metabolically produced substances, urea and creatinine, are routinely used to evaluate renal function. Both are normally eliminated by the kidneys and are measured as serum BUN and creatinine. The color and odor of the urine are general observations and are not specific to detect adverse renal reactions. Sugar and acetone in urine are found in diabetes mellitus with ketoacidosis and are not indicators of kidney function. Serum hemoglobin is a measure of the RBC count but does not reflect kidney function. **Cognitive Level:** Applying **Client Need:** Pharmacological and Parenteral Therapies **Integrated Process:** Nursing Process: Evaluation **Content Area:** Fundamentals **Strategy:** The core issue of the question is knowledge of what to assess to determine kidney function as an indicator for the clearance of medications. Use the process of elimination and basic nursing knowledge to make a selection.

7 **Answer: 4 Rationale:** Before making a decision about how to infuse the antibiotic, the nurse should check compatibility of the antibiotic with the continuous IV solution. If the drug and infusion were incompatible, the nurse would stop the infusion during the period of antibiotic administration and flush the line carefully before and after the antibiotic. It is always inadvisable to start a second IV site unless absolutely necessary. Increasing the IV flow rate constitutes changing a medical prescription, and does not address the issue of compatibility. **Cognitive Level:** Applying **Client Need:** Pharmacological and Parenteral Therapies **Integrated Process:** Nursing Process: Implementation **Content Area:** Pharmacology **Strategy:** The core issue of the question is the need to check compatibility of medications and IV solutions as a beginning point to decision making. Eliminate each of the incorrect options because they do not begin with compatibility checks or are incorrect nursing actions.

8 **Answer: 3, 5 Rationale:** The correct action should be to withhold the medication and call the prescriber. The prescriber should be called regarding the client's change of condition and the inability to administer the prescribed medication. The nurse cannot change the route that a medication is to be given without a prescription. Oral medications should not be administered to clients who are vomiting, which could interfere with the ability to absorb the medication and possibly initiate further vomiting. The nurse should not just omit the dose without notifying the prescriber of the client's change in condition. **Cognitive Level:** Applying **Client Need:** Pharmacological and Parenteral Therapies **Integrated Process:** Nursing Process: Implementation **Content Area:** Fundamentals **Strategy:** Use the process of elimination and general measures for administering medications safely to make a selection. When there is more than one correct answer for a question, consider each option as a true/false statement.

9 **Answer: 1 Rationale:** It would be prudent for the second nurse to assist the second client so that the first nurse may continue medication administration. The nurse who prepares the medication must be the nurse to give the medication. Preparation of a new syringe by the second nurse is acceptable but requires wasting of the original medication, additional time for the preparation, and unnecessary expense; therefore, this is not the best action. The explanation is appropriate, but does not resolve the issue of the preoperative client. **Cognitive Level:** Analyzing **Client Need:** Pharmacological and Parenteral Therapies **Integrated Process:** Nursing Process: Implementation **Content Area:** Fundamentals **Strategy:** The core issue of the question is the principle that nurses may not administer medications prepared by another nurse. Look at each option carefully with consideration given to client needs, time constraints, and expenses.

10 **Answer: 4 Rationale:** Informing the client that the nurse will return with the medication meets the principles of medication administration and the client's needs. Medications should not be left at the bedside, with certain exceptions that are ordered in advance (e.g., nitroglycerin and cough syrup). Waiting in the room for the client is an example of poor time management by the nurse. Going into the bathroom to give the client medication is an unnecessary invasion of the client's privacy. **Cognitive Level:** Applying **Client Need:** Pharmacological and Parenteral Therapies **Integrated Process:** Nursing Process: Implementation **Content Area:** Fundamentals **Strategy:** Use the process of elimination. There is one correct answer utilizing basic principles of medication administration.

11 **Answer: 1.5 Rationale:** Use the following formula to solve the problem:

$$\frac{\text{Amount desired}}{\text{Amount on hand}} \times \text{Quantity}$$

Thus,

$$\frac{6}{4} \times 1 = 1.5$$

Cognitive Level: Applying **Client Need:** Pharmacological and Parenteral Therapies **Integrated Process:** Nursing Process: Implementation **Content Area:** Fundamentals **Strategy:** Use knowledge of basic pharmacological math to set up the question. Carefully review your work and double-check placement of decimals for accuracy.

12 **Answer: 10.5 Rationale:** One gram is equal to 1000 mg. Use the following formula as one way to set up the problem:

Cross-multiply 95 by x and 1000 by 1 to yield $95x = 1000$. Divide 1000 by 95 to yield 10.52 or 10.5 mL.

Cognitive Level: Applying **Client Need:** Pharmacological and Parenteral Therapies **Integrated Process:** Nursing Process: Implementation **Content Area:** Fundamentals **Strategy:** Use knowledge of basic pharmacological math to set up the question. Carefully review your work and double-check placement of decimals for accuracy.

13 **Answer: 0.5 Rationale:** The following is one way to set up the calculation:

Cross-multiply 2.5 by x and 1.25 by 1 to yield $2.5x = 1.25$. Divide 1.25 by 2.5 to yield 0.5 tablet.

Cognitive Level: Applying **Client Need:** Pharmacological and Parenteral Therapies **Integrated Process:** Nursing Process: Implementation **Content Area:** Fundamentals **Strategy:** Use knowledge of basic pharmacological math procedures to set up the question. Check your work carefully and double-check placement of decimals for accuracy.

14 **Answer: 0.25 Rationale:** The following is one way to set up the calculation:

Cross-multiply 2.0 by x and 0.5 by 1 to yield $2x = 0.5$ Divide 0.5 by 2 to yield 0.25 mL.

Cognitive Level: Applying **Client Need:** Pharmacological and Parenteral Therapies **Integrated Process:** Nursing Process: Implementation **Content Area:** Fundamentals **Strategy:** Use knowledge of basic pharmacological math procedures to set up the question. Carefully review your work and double-check placement of decimals for accuracy.

15 **Answer: 2 Rationale:** The following is one way to set up the calculation:

Cross-multiply 325 by x and multiply 650 by 1 to yield $325x = 650$. Divide 650 by 325 to yield 2 tablets.

Cognitive Level: Applying **Client Need:** Pharmacological and Parenteral Therapies **Integrated Process:** Nursing Process: Implementation **Content Area:** Fundamentals **Strategy:** Use knowledge of basic pharmacological math procedures to set up the question. Check your work carefully.

16 **Answer: 20 Rationale:** Since the dose is 2 grams and each vial contains 1 gram, the nurse needs to use two vials. The nurse then adds 10 mL of sterile water to each vial of powder, based on the directions. Once both vials are reconstituted, the concentration of each solution is 1 gram/10 mL. The nurse then must draw up the contents of both vials, making the total volume 20 mL. **Cognitive Level:** Applying **Client Need:** Pharmacological and Parenteral Therapies **Integrated Process:** Nursing Process: Implementation **Content Area:** Fundamentals **Strategy:** Use knowledge of basic pharmacological math procedures to set up the question. Check your work carefully.

17 **Answer: 2 Rationale:** The following is one way to set up the calculation:

Cross-multiply 0.125 by x and 0.25 by 1 to yield $0.125x = 0.25$. Divide 0.25 by 0.125 to yield 2.0 mL.

Cognitive Level: Applying **Client Need:** Pharmacological and Parenteral Therapies **Integrated Process:** Nursing Process: Implementation **Content Area:** Fundamentals **Strategy:** Use knowledge of basic pharmacological math to set up the question. Carefully review your work and double-check placement of decimals for accuracy.

18 **Answer: 3 Rationale:** The following is one way to set up the calculation:

Cross-multiply 40 by x and 120 by 1 to yield $40x = 120$. Divide 120 by 40 to yield 3.0 mL.

Cognitive Level: Applying **Client Need:** Pharmacological and Parenteral Therapies **Integrated Process:** Nursing Process: Implementation **Content Area:** Fundamentals **Strategy:** Use knowledge of basic pharmacological math procedures to set up the question. Check your work carefully for accuracy.

19 **Answer: 4 Rationale:** The following is one way to set up the calculation:

Cross-multiply 10 by x and 40 by 1 to yield $10x = 40$. Divide 40 by 10 to yield 4 tablets.

Cognitive Level: Applying **Client Need:** Pharmacological and Parenteral Therapies **Integrated Process:** Nursing Process: Implementation **Content Area:** Fundamentals **Strategy:** Use knowledge of basic pharmacological math to set up the question. Check your work carefully for accuracy.

20 **Answer: 3 Rationale:** The following is one way to set up the calculation:

Cross-multiply 200 by x and 600 by 1 to yield $200x = 600$. Divide 600 by 200 to yield 3 tablets.

Cognitive Level: Applying **Client Need:** Pharmacological and Parenteral Therapies **Integrated Process:** Nursing Process: Implementation **Content Area:** Pharmacology **Strategy:** Use knowledge of the apothecary system and simple dosage calculation.

Key Terms to Review

absorption p. 434
adverse effects p. 434
biotransformation p. 434
bolus p. 440
brand name p. 433
distribution p. 434
excretion p. 434
generic name p. 433
half-life p. 434
inhalation p. 442
intradermal (ID) p. 440
intramuscular (IM) p. 440
intravenous (IV) p. 440
lipodystrophy p. 440
metabolism p. 434
metric system p. 434
ophthalmic p. 441
pharmacokinetics p. 434
side effects p. 434
subcutaneous (subcut) p. 440
topical p. 441
toxic effects p. 434
trade name p. 433

References

Berman, A., Snyder, S., & Frandsen, G. (2016). *Kozier & Erb's fundamentals of nursing: Concepts, process, and practice* (10th ed.). New York, NY: Pearson Education.

Giangrasso, A., & Shrimpton, D. (2014). *Ratio and proportion dosage calculations* (2nd ed.). Upper Saddle River, NJ: Pearson Education.

Olson, J., Giangrasso, A., & Shrimpton, D. (2013). *Medical dosage calculations: A Dimensional analysis approach* (10th ed.). Upper Saddle River, NJ: Pearson Education.

Smith, R., Duell, D., Martin, B., Gonzalez, L., & Aebersold, M. (2017). *Clinical nursing skills: Basic to advanced skills* (9th ed.). New York, NY: Pearson Education.

Test Yourself

Are you ready for the NCLEX-RN® or course exams? Access the NEW web-based app that provides students with thousands of practice questions in preparation for the NCLEX experience.

Pediatric Dosage Calculation and Medication Administration

30

In this chapter

Cross Reference

Other chapters relevant to this content area are

Dosage Calculation and Medication Administration	Chapter 29
Intravenous Therapy	Chapter 31

I. DOSAGE CALCULATION USING BODY WEIGHT

A. Consists of two steps:

1. Calculate body weight (often in kilograms)
2. Calculate actual drug dosage

B. Converting body weight between pounds (lb) and kilograms (kg): see Box 30–1

C. Calculating pediatric drug dosages: see Box 30–2

1. Drugs are often ordered in mg/kg/day (total daily dose) or mg/kg/dose (actual single dose or divided daily dose)
2. Occasionally a pediatric drug may be ordered in mg/lb/day
3. Most pediatric drugs are given in divided doses rather than a single daily dose
4. *NCLEX®* It is critical to check ordered dose against safe dosage range to ensure that dose is within recommended range
5. *NCLEX®* Question an order for a drug that does not fall within safe dosage range

Box 30–1

Converting Body Weight between Pounds and Kilograms

Recall that 2.2 pounds (lb) = 1 kilogram (kg).

To convert from pounds to kilograms, divide the pounds by 2.2.

To convert from kilograms to pounds, multiply the kilograms by 2.2.

Express either pounds or kilograms to the nearest tenth (e.g., 20.6 kg or 45.3 lb).

Box 30–2

Calculating Pediatric Drug Dosages Using Body Weight

Calculating a Single Pediatric Dose by Body Weight

1. Multiply child's weight in kilograms by dosage ordered per kilogram.
   Example: A pediatrician orders a dose of 15 mg of a drug per kilogram of body weight (15 mg/kg).

$$20 \text{ kg weight} \times \frac{15 \text{ mg of drug}}{1 \text{ kg}} = 300 \text{ mg of drug should be given as the dose}$$

2. Calculate volume (tablets, solution) using a standard pharmaceutical math calculation (such as "desired over have multiplied by quantity" or ratio and proportion; see Chapter 29).

Calculating a Single Pediatric Dose from a Total Daily Dose Using Body Weight

1. Multiply child's weight in kilograms by daily dosage ordered per kilogram.
   Example: A pediatrician orders a dose of 45 mg of a drug per kilogram of body weight per day (45 mg/kg/day).

$$20 \text{ kg weight} \times \frac{45 \text{ mg of drug per day}}{1 \text{ kg}} = 900 \text{ mg of drug should be given per day}$$

2. Divide total daily dose by number of doses per day to calculate amount of a single dose.
   Example (continued from above): 900 mg of drug per day divided by 3 doses per day = 300 mg per dose.

II. DOSAGE CALCULATION USING BODY SURFACE AREA (BSA)

A. ***Body surface area* is a measurement of total amount of skin surface of the body;** it is possibly a more important factor than weight for calculating precise medication dosages for infants and children in selected circumstances

B. **A pediatric client's BSA can be estimated using a *nomogram*** as shown in Figure 30–1; a nomogram is a chart that contains graphs for height, BSA, and weight; an online BSA calculator can also be used

C. **Use simple multiplication** when dose is ordered based on either milligrams or micrograms (mcg) of drug per meters squared (m^2) (see Box 30–3)

D. **Use a formula** to calculate a pediatric drug dose when dosage is specified only for adults (see Box 30–3)

III. ORAL MEDICATIONS

A. **Children under 5 years old** often have difficulty swallowing tablets and capsules

B. **Most medications for pediatric use** are available in both solid dose forms (pill, tablet) and liquid forms (suspension, elixir, syrup)

C. **If a child cannot swallow** a pill or tablet easily, dose may need to be crushed if drug formulation allows

NCLEX® 1. Do not crush enteric-coated, time-release, or extended-release medications

2. If oral medications are crushed, disguise taste by mixing with a small amount of flavored substance such as applesauce or juice

NCLEX® D. **Check child's mouth** to ensure that oral pills or tablets are swallowed if given whole

E. **When preparing liquid medications,** use standard medication preparation procedures

1. Use a syringe or calibrated medicine cup or dropper, especially if volumes are 5 mL or less

2. Measure medication dose accurately

NCLEX® 3. Mix suspensions well before pouring and administer immediately so dose does not precipitate out of suspension

4. If it is necessary to disguise taste of a liquid dose, mix in 30 mL or less of a flavored liquid such as juice

F. **Wear clean gloves when administering medications** to avoid coming in contact with child's saliva

NCLEX® G. **To administer dose to an infant,** place small amounts of liquid along inside of mouth slowly and allow time for infant to swallow before giving more (to prevent aspiration and reduce likelihood of spitting out dose)

H. **To administer dose to a small child,** sit child sideways in own lap or in parent/caregiver's lap; place child's closest arm under adult's arm and behind back; gently hold child's other arm near elbow, use dominant hand to give dose

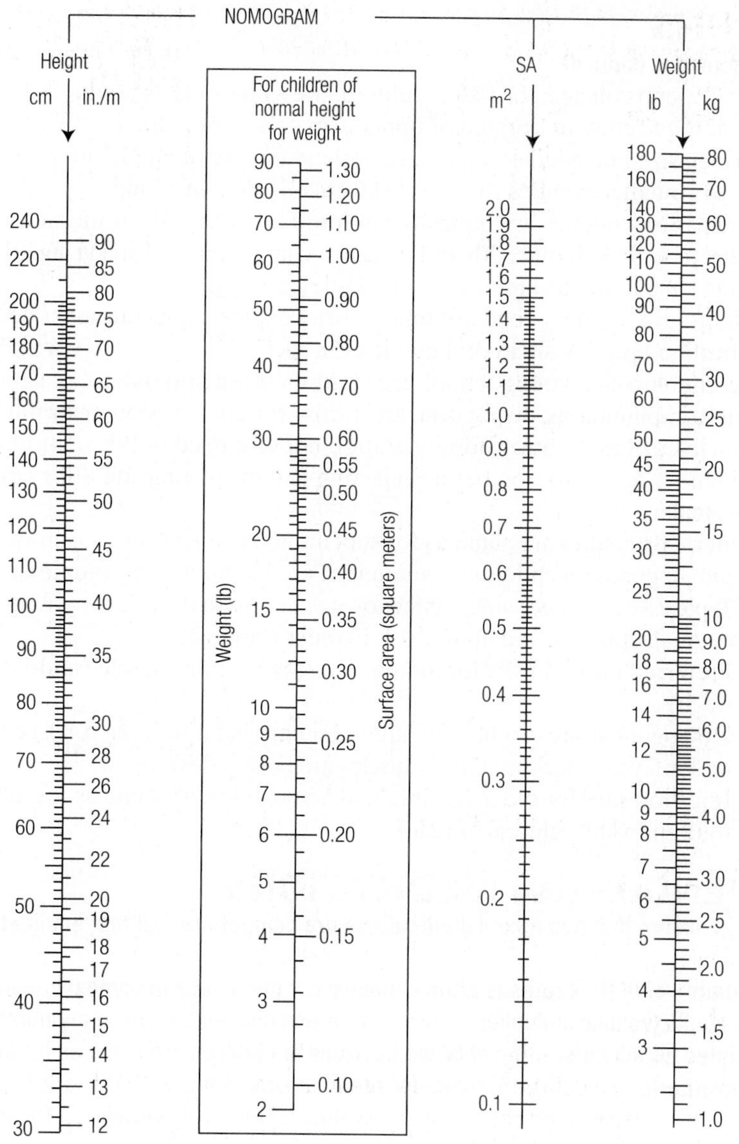

Figure 30–1

West nomogram for infants and children. Obtain child's height and weight and note those points on the nomogram. Draw a connecting line between these two points; the point where the line intersects the BSA column indicates the body surface area in square meters (m^2).

Box 30–3

Calculating Pediatric Drug Dosages Using Body Surface Area

Calculating a Single Pediatric Dose Ordered by Body Surface Area

1. Multiply recommended dosage (in milligrams or micrograms per m^2) by body surface area (m^2).
   Example:

   2.5 (mg per m^2) $\times$ 0.8 (m^2) $=$ 2 mg dose

2. Calculate dose volume (tablets, solution) using a standard pharmaceutical math calculation (such as "desired over have multiplied by quantity," ratio and proportion, or dimensional analysis; see Chapter 29).

Calculating a Single Pediatric Dose from an Adult Dose Using Body Surface Area

1. Divide child's body surface area (m^2) by 1.73 (m^2) and then multiply it by adult dose.
   Example:

   $$\frac{0.8\ m^2}{1.73\ m^2} \times 25\ \text{mg (adult dose)} = 11.56\ \text{mg (child's dose)}$$

2. Calculate volume (tablets, solution) using a standard pharmaceutical math calculation (such as "desired over have multiplied by quantity," ratio and proportion, or dimensional analysis; see Chapter 29).

IV. INJECTIONS

A. Subcutaneous (subcut)

1. Site depends on age; for older children, use same sites as adults, but newborns, infants, and toddlers often require use of dorsum of upper arm or anterior thigh
2. Syringe size and needle length also depend on size of child, but infants and children often require 25- to 26-gauge needles that are 1–1.6 cm (3/8- to 5/8-in.) long
3. *NCLEX®* Medication volumes are typically not more than 0.5 mL for infant and 2 mL for large child; calculate doses to nearest hundredth and measure using a tuberculin syringe if less than 1 mL
4. Inject subcutaneous medications at 45-degree angle
5. Infants and toddlers need minimal to brief explanations but must be held securely for dose injection, as outlined previously in oral medication section
6. Preschoolers and young school-age children often understand reason for injection and benefit from simple explanations, distraction, and praise for cooperation; restraint is on an as-needed basis
7. *NCLEX®* Principles of medication administration not discussed in this section are same as for adult, including guidelines for aspiration before injecting and massaging site after administration (see Chapter 29)

B. Intramuscular

1. General principles are same as for subcutaneous injections; variations are presented here
   a. Site depends on child's age, amount of muscle mass, and volume of medication to be injected
   b. *NCLEX®* Typical volumes per single injection site are up to 0.5 mL for young infant, up to 1 mL for older infant or small children, and up to 2 mL in older (large) child
   c. *NCLEX®* Preferred injection site for infants is vastus lateralis muscle (middle third of anterior-lateral aspect of thigh)
   d. Dorsogluteal site can be used after child has been walking for 1 year, but it is not ideal for children under 5 years because these muscles are poorly developed
   e. Injection sites for older children and adolescents are same as for adult and include vastus lateralis, deltoid, and ventrogluteal muscles

V. INTRAVENOUS (IV) MEDICATIONS

NCLEX® A. **Always ensure that two mixed medications are compatible** and that medications and IV solutions are compatible

B. **Calculation of IV flow rates is often unnecessary due to use of pumps;** however, formula for calculation is same as for adults (volume multiplied by drop factor and divided by time in minutes)

C. **Principles for administration of IV medications to children** are same as for adults but with special considerations

1. For infants and children, place IV medications along with diluent in an IV administration set with a volume control chamber (such as a Soluset, Buretrol, Metriset); these sets have a small drop factor (60 drops/mL)
2. Take special care to ensure that tubing contains no air to prevent air injection into child's vein and subsequent air embolus
3. *NCLEX®* Use an electronic controller or pump to regulate IV fluids and intermittent IV medications
4. When setting pump or controller, calculate volume of added medications into total volume (e.g., set 55 mL as volume to be infused if IV bag has 50 mL and 5 mL of medication has been added)
5. For intermittent medication infusions, select port close to child (ensures medication is delivered at proper time; with slowly running IVs, medication could take more time to travel from distal port to child's vein)
6. *NCLEX®* Check on IV medication and site several times during administration to ensure that site is patent without infiltration and to assess for medication side effects

VI. PEDIATRIC CONSIDERATIONS FOR OTHER ROUTES

A. Ophthalmic

1. Young children fear anything being placed in eyes; communicate in a manner to reduce anxiety and promote cooperation during procedure
2. Take care to maintain sterility in a child who is less than cooperative
3. Apply ointment or drops as for adults and close eyelids to prevent leakage
4. *NCLEX®* Encourage child not to squeeze eyes shut and have child lie quietly for 30 seconds

B. Otic

1. Use sterile technique if tympanic membrane is ruptured and draining
2. *NCLEX®* For children under 3 years of age, pull pinna straight back and slightly downward to straighten ear canal

NCLEX® 3. For older children, pull pinna back and upward as for an adult

C. Nasal

1. Saline drops are commonly given to infants with nasal congestion
2. Because nasal medications drain into back of throat, they may cause tickling, bad taste, and occasional difficulty breathing
3. *NCLEX®* Check child for choking or vomiting after instillation of drops
4. Keep child in same position for 5 minutes after administration to allow medication to contact nasal mucosa

D. Aerosol: as per adults

E. Rectal

1. If suppository needs to be cut in half, do so lengthwise
2. Obtain assistance if needed to keep child in side-lying position (or prone in parent's lap if small enough)
3. *NCLEX®* After lubricating, insert gently into rectum just beyond internal sphincter
4. Hold buttocks together until urge to expel medication has passed (may be 5–10 minutes)

Check Your NCLEX–RN® Exam I.Q.

You are ready for testing on this content if you can:

- Calculate pediatric medication dosages with accuracy.
- Verify dosage calculations before administering medications.
- Apply principles of medication administration by various routes to pediatric clients.

PRACTICE TEST

1 A 4-month-old client has D_5 ½ NS IV prescribed to run at a rate of 40 mL/hr. While the unlicensed assistant obtains an infusion pump, the nurse sets the drip rate at how many drops/minute, using a Soluset with microdrip tubing (drop factor of 60 gtt/mL)? Provide a numerical answer. Record your answer rounding to the nearest whole number.

Fill in your answer below:
Answer: ________ drops/min

2 A 3½-month-old infant has an order for acetaminophen suspension 45 mg by mouth q4h prn. The product label lists a concentration of 500 mg/5 mL. After determining that the dosage is safe, the nurse should administer how many mL? Record your answer, rounding to two decimal places.

Fill in your answer below:
Answer: ________ mL

3 A 4-year-old client's medication prescription reads cefotaxime 1380 mg IV every 8 hours. The client weighs 13.8 kg. Which nursing action is appropriate if the safe dosage range for a child from 1 month to 12 years of age is listed as 100–200 mg/kg/day given in divided doses?

1. Give the dose as scheduled and document it appropriately.
2. Question the order for the excessively high dose.
3. Administer the slightly high dose but give it at half the recommended rate.
4. Withhold the dose and question the prescriber, since it is below the recommended range.

4 A 6-year-old client who weighs 18 kg has a prescription for vancomycin 240 mg IV every 6 hours. The safe dose range for a child is listed as 40 mg/kg/day, with divided doses given every 6 hours. What is the best nursing action?

1. Question the dosage of the order.
2. Question the frequency of the order.
3. Administer the dose, being sure to use an infusion pump.
4. Give the dose over at least 60–90 minutes to avoid adverse effects.

5 A 5-year-old client has an order for baclofen one-half of a 10-mg tablet by mouth three times per day. The safe dose range for a 2- to 7-year-old child is 10–15 mg/day in divided doses. Which nursing action is most appropriate?

1. Question the total daily dose ordered.
2. Question the single dose ordered.
3. Refuse to give the dose because the child's weight is not factored into the dose.
4. Administer the dose as ordered.

6 A 3-year-old client has a prescription for 120 mg acetaminophen every 4–6 hours prn for pain. The maximum total dose is 2.6 grams/day for a child of 2–3 years. The nurse could legally administer how many doses per 24-hour period? Record your answer as a whole number.

Fill in your answer below:
Answer: ________ doses/24 hours

7 A client has a prescription for cefotaxime 1180 mg IV q6h. The reconstituted medication vial is labeled as having a concentration of 95 mg/mL. The nurse should draw up ____ milliliters of solution to add to the bag of IV solution for the intermittent infusion. Record your answer, rounding to one decimal place.

Fill in your answer below:
Answer: ________ mL

8 A 6-year-old client has a prescription for fexofenadine one-half of a 60 mg tab by mouth twice daily. The nurse calculates the child's total daily dose as ____ milligrams. Record your answer rounding to the nearest whole number.

Fill in your answer below:
Answer: ________ mg

9 A nurse is reviewing insulin administration techniques with a 13-year-old client who has uncontrolled diabetes. The nurse evaluates that the client is using proper procedure after noting that the client performs which action during self-injection?

1. Aspirates before injection but does not massage the site following injection
2. Uses a 45-degree injection angle and aspirates before injection
3. Uses a 90-degree angle and massages the site following injection
4. Uses a 90-degree injection angle and does not massage the site following injection

10 A 15-year-old client admitted with dehydration is prescribed a bolus infusion of 0.9% sodium chloride (normal saline, NS) 500 mL IV for 1 hour. An infusion device is available that counts the number of drops per minute delivered. The IV tubing has a drop factor of 10 drops/mL. If the bolus is to infuse on time, the nurse should set the drip rate to ____ drops per minute. Record your answer, rounding to the nearest whole number.

Fill in your answer below:
Answer: ________ drops/minute

11 A 6-year-old postoperative client who weighs 44 pounds has a medication order for cefazolin 500 mg IV every 6 hours. The safe dose range of cefazolin for a child is 25–100 mg/kg/day in three to four divided doses. To determine whether the child's dose is within the safe dose range, the nurse first calculates that this child's prescribed dose is ______ mg/kg/day? Record your answer, rounding to the nearest whole number.

Fill in your answer below:
Answer: ________ mg/kg/day

12 A child who sustained a head injury is prescribed mannitol 20 grams IV. Available is a bag of 20% solution that contains 20 grams mannitol in 100 mL volume. If infusing the dose over 90 minutes using an infusion pump that can be set to tenths of a milliliter, the nurse should set the infusion pump at how many mL/hour? Record your answer, rounding to one decimal place.

Fill in your answer below:
Answer: _________ mL/hr

13 A child who weighs 55 pounds is prescribed ceftazidime 250 mg IV every 8 hours. The safe dose range of ceftazidime for a child is 30–50 mg/kg/day in three divided doses. What is the total daily dose ordered for this client in mg/kg/day? Record your answer, rounding to the nearest whole number.

Fill in your answer below:
Answer: _________ mg/kg/day

14 A child is prescribed a bolus of 0.9% sodium chloride (normal saline, NS) 400 mL by the IV route. To infuse this volume over 90 minutes, the nurse should set the infusion pump at ____ mL/hour. Record your answer, rounding to the nearest whole number.

Fill in your answer below:
Answer: _________ mL/hr

15 A nurse is about to administer a dose of acetaminophen 200 mg via nasogastric tube to a child. Available is a suspension with a concentration of 80 mg per 5 mL. The nurse should administer how many mL to give the dose? Record your answer, rounding to one decimal place.

Fill in your answer below:
Answer: _________ mL

ANSWERS & RATIONALES

1 **Answer: 40 Rationale:** Use the following formula to calculate the rate of IV solutions:

$$\frac{\text{Volume} \times \text{drop factor}}{\text{Time (in minutes)}}$$

Set up the problem as follows:

$$\frac{40 \times 60}{60}$$

Multiply 40 by 60 to yield 2400 and divide 2400 by 60 (or cancel out the 60s) to yield 40 drops/minute. **Cognitive Level:** Applying **Client Need:** Pharmacological and Parenteral Therapies **Integrated Process:** Nursing Process: Implementation **Content Area:** Pharmacology **Strategy:** Use knowledge of basic IV calculation to set up the question. Calculate the problem carefully and double-check your answer for accuracy.

2 **Answer: 0.45 Rationale:** One way to set up the problem is to use the following formula:

$$\frac{\text{45 mg (dose desired)}}{\text{500 mg (available)}} \times \frac{\text{x (unknown)}}{\text{5 mL (quantity)}}$$

Cross-multiply 500 by x and cross-multiply 45 by 5 to yield $500x = 225$. Divide 225 by 500 to yield 0.45 mL. **Cognitive Level:** Applying **Client Need:** Pharmacological and Parenteral Therapies **Integrated Process:** Nursing Process: Implementation **Content Area:** Pharmacology **Strategy:** Use knowledge of basic dosage calculation to set up the question. Calculate the problem carefully and double-check your answer for accuracy.

3 **Answer: 2 Rationale:** To calculate the daily dose, first divide the number of mg (1380) by the client's weight in kg (13.8) to yield a single dose of 100 mg/kg. Because there are three doses ordered during a 24-hour period, multiply 100 by 3 to yield 300 mg/kg/day. Since the dose range is 100–200 mg/kg/day, the dosage is excessively high and the nurse should question the order as part of safe nursing practice. **Cognitive Level:** Analyzing **Client Need:** Pharmacological and Parenteral Therapies **Integrated Process:** Nursing Process: Implementation **Content Area:** Pharmacology **Strategy:** Use knowledge of basic pediatric dosage calculation to set up the question. Calculate the problem carefully and double-check your answer for accuracy. Remember that any dose that falls outside the safe dosage range needs to be questioned.

4 **Answer: 1 Rationale:** First calculate the total daily dose by dividing 240 mg by 18 kg to yield a single dose of 14.44 mg/kg. Multiply the single dose by 4 doses (every 6 hours) to yield a total daily dose of 57.76 mg/kg/day. Since this exceeds the safe total daily dose of 40 mg/kg/day, the nurse should question the dosage. Administering the dose with an infusion pump or over a longer time is still unsafe. The frequency of the order is not the problem. **Cognitive Level:** Analyzing **Client Need:** Pharmacological and Parenteral Therapies **Integrated Process:** Nursing Process: Implementation **Content Area:** Pharmacology **Strategy:** Use knowledge of basic pediatric dosage calculation to set up the question. Calculate the problem carefully and double-check your answer for accuracy. Remember that any dose

that falls outside the safe dosage range needs to be questioned.

5 **Answer: 4 Rationale:** The dose can be administered as prescribed. The order to give half of a 10-mg tab means that the dose is actually 5 mg. If there are three doses per day, the total daily dose is 15 mg, which is within the safe dosage range. The total daily dosage does not need to be questioned. The amount of the single dose is not an issue. The drug does not require weight to be factored when determining the safe dose range. **Cognitive Level:** Analyzing **Client Need:** Pharmacological and Parenteral Therapies **Integrated Process:** Nursing Process: Implementation **Content Area:** Pharmacology **Strategy:** Use knowledge of basic pediatric dosage calculation to set up the question. Calculate the problem carefully and double-check your answer for accuracy. Recall that any dose that falls within the safe dosage range may be administered.

6 **Answer: 6 Rationale:** Convert 2.6 grams to 2600 mg. Since a single dose is 120 mg, the client could receive this dose 21 times (2600 divided by 120 = 21.66) within a 24-hour period without exceeding the top of the dosage range. However, since the medication is prescribed every 4–6 hours, the nurse can legally administer the medication a maximum of six times (every 4 hours). **Cognitive Level:** Analyzing **Client Need:** Pharmacological and Parenteral Therapies **Integrated Process:** Nursing Process: Planning **Content Area:** Pharmacology **Strategy:** Use knowledge of basic math calculation to determine your answer. If the drug can be given no more frequently than every 4 hours, it cannot exceed six doses, since 24 divided by 4 is 6.

7 **Answer: 12.4 Rationale:** The following formula illustrates one way to set up the problem:

$$\frac{1180 \text{ mg (dose desired)}}{95 \text{ mg (available)}} = \frac{x\text{(unknown)}}{1 \text{ mL (quantity)}}$$

Multiply 95 by x and multiply 1180 by 1 to yield $95x = 1180$. Divide 1180 by 95 to yield 12.421 or 12.4 mL after rounding down to the nearest tenth. **Cognitive Level:** Analyzing **Client Need:** Pharmacological and Parenteral Therapies **Integrated Process:** Nursing Process: Implementation **Content Area:** Pharmacology **Strategy:** Use knowledge of basic dosage calculation procedures to set up the question. Calculate the problem carefully and double-check your answer for accuracy.

8 **Answer: 60 Rationale:** One-half of a 60-mg tablet is 30 mg. Because the dose is ordered twice a day, the total daily dose is 30 multiplied by 2 doses, yielding 60 mg. **Cognitive Level:** Analyzing **Client Need:** Pharmacological and Parenteral Therapies **Integrated Process:** Nursing Process: Implementation **Content Area:** Pharmacology **Strategy:** Use knowledge of basic math calculation to set up the problem. Calculate carefully and double-check your answer for accuracy.

9 **Answer: 4 Rationale:** Correct administration technique is to use a 90-degree angle (insulin syringes have a short, 1.3-cm (1/2-in.) needle), avoid aspiration before injection (e.g., to avoid tissue complications over time), and avoid massaging the area after injection (which would enhance quicker absorption of the dose). **Cognitive Level:** Analyzing **Client Need:** Pharmacological and Parenteral Therapies **Integrated Process:** Nursing Process: Evaluation **Content Area:** Pharmacology **Strategy:** The core issue of the question is knowledge of subcutaneous injection techniques. Use the process of elimination and nursing knowledge to answer the question. To help eliminate incorrect answers, recall that insulin and heparin should not be massaged and that a 90-degree angle is used for injection.

10 **Answer: 83 Rationale:** Since the infusion device delivers fluid in drops/min, the nurse must calculate the number at which to set the machine. The formula to use is

$$\frac{\text{Volume} \times \text{drop factor}}{\text{Time in minutes}}$$

Thus, set up the problem as follows:

$$\frac{500 \times 10}{60}$$

Multiply 500 by 10 to yield 5000 and divide it by 60 to obtain a flow rate of 83.33 gtt/min, which rounds down to 83 drops/minute. **Cognitive Level:** Analyzing **Client Need:** Pharmacological and Parenteral Therapies **Integrated Process:** Nursing Process: Implementation **Content Area:** Pharmacology **Strategy:** Use basic IV calculation procedures to set up the question. Calculate the problem carefully and double-check your answer for accuracy.

11 **Answer: 100 Rationale:** First convert the client's weight to kg by dividing 44 by 2.2 to yield a weight of 20 kg. Next, calculate the daily drug dose by dividing the number of mg (500) by the client's weight in kg (20) to yield a single dose of 25 mg/kg. Because there are four doses (every 6 hours) prescribed during a 24-hour period, multiply 25 by 4 to yield a total daily dose of 100 mg/kg/day. **Cognitive Level:** Analyzing **Client Need:** Pharmacological and Parenteral Therapies **Integrated Process:** Nursing Process: Implementation **Content Area:** Pharmacology **Strategy:** Use knowledge of basic dosage calculation to set up the question. Calculate the problem carefully and double-check your answer for accuracy.

12 **Answer: 66.7 Rationale:** Because the infusion pump delivers fluid in mL/hour, the nurse needs to calculate the equivalent hourly rate when infusing the 100 mL over 90 minutes. The problem can be set up to cancel out the labels and end up with mL/hour:

$$\frac{100 \text{ mL (volume)}}{90 \text{ minutes (time)}} \times \frac{60 \text{ minutes}}{1 \text{ hour}}$$

Multiply 100 by 60 to yield 6000 and divide it by 90 (90 × 1) to obtain an equivalent hourly flow rate of 66.66 or 66.7 mL/hr. This answer also makes common sense because if the medication were infusing over 90 minutes, then two-thirds of it would infuse in 1 hour; 66.7 mL is two-thirds of 100 mL. **Cognitive Level:** Analyzing **Client Need:** Pharmacological and Parenteral Therapies **Integrated Process:** Nursing Process: Implementation **Content Area:** Pharmacology **Strategy:** Use knowledge of basic math calculation to set up the question. Read the question carefully, noting that the time needs to convert from minutes to hours in order to have the correct labeling. Calculate the problem carefully and double-check your answer for accuracy.

13 **Answer: 30 Rationale:** First convert the child's weight to kg by dividing 55 by 2.2 to yield a weight of 25 kg. Then calculate the daily dose of the medication by dividing the mg (250) by the client's weight in kg (25) to yield a single dose of 10 mg/kg. Because there are three doses (every 8 hours) ordered during a 24-hour period, multiply 10 by 3 to yield a total daily dose of 30 mg/kg/day. **Cognitive Level:** Analyzing **Client Need:** Pharmacological and Parenteral Therapies **Integrated Process:** Nursing Process: Implementation **Content Area:** Pharmacology **Strategy:** Use knowledge of basic pediatric dosage calculation to set up the question. Calculate the problem carefully and double-check your answer for accuracy.

14 **Answer: 267 Rationale:** Since the infusion pump delivers fluid in mL/hour, the nurse must calculate the equivalent hourly rate when infusing the 400 mL over 90 minutes. The problem can be set up as follows to cancel out the labels and end up with mL/hour:

$$\frac{400\text{ mL (volume)}}{90\text{ minutes (time)}} \times \frac{60\text{ minutes}}{1\text{ hours}}$$

Multiply 400 by 60 to yield 24,000 and divide it by 90 (90 × 1) to obtain an equivalent hourly flow rate of 266.66 or 267 mL/hr. **Cognitive Level:** Analyzing **Client Need:** Pharmacological and Parenteral Therapies **Integrated Process:** Nursing Process: Implementation **Content Area:** Pharmacology **Strategy:** Use knowledge of basic math calculation to set up the question. Read the question carefully, noting that the time needs to convert from minutes to hours in order to have the correct labeling. Calculate the problem carefully and double-check your answer for accuracy.

15 **Answer: 12.5 Rationale:** The problem can be set up using ratio and proportion as follows:

$$\frac{200\text{ mg (dose desired)}}{80\text{ mg (available)}} = \frac{x\text{(unknown)}}{5\text{ mL (quantity)}}$$

Cross-multiply 80 by x and cross-multiply 200 by 5 to yield $80x = 1{,}000$. Divide 1,000 by 80 to yield 12.5 mL. **Cognitive Level:** Analyzing **Client Need:** Pharmacological and Parenteral Therapies **Integrated Process:** Nursing Process: Implementation **Content Area:** Pharmacology **Strategy:** Use knowledge of basic pediatric dosage calculation to set up the question. Calculate the problem carefully and double-check your answer for accuracy.

Key Terms to Review

body surface area (BSA) p. 450

nomogram p. 450

References

Giangrasso, A., & Shrimpton, D. (2014). *Ratio and proportion dosage calculations* (2nd ed.). Upper Saddle River, NJ: Pearson Education.

Olson, J., Giangrasso, A., & Shrimpton, D. (2013). *Medical dosage calculations: A dimensional analysis approach* (10th ed.). Upper Saddle River, NJ: Pearson Education.

Pickar, G. (2008). *Dosage calculations* (8th ed.). Clifton Park, NY: Delmar Learning.

Smith, R., Duell, D., Martin, B., Gonzalez, L., & Aebersold, M. (2017). *Clinical nursing skills: Basic to advanced skills* (9th ed.). New York, NY: Pearson Education.

31 Intravenous Therapy

In this chapter

Cross Reference

Other chapters relevant to this content area are

Blood and Blood Component Therapy Chapter 32
Total Parenteral Nutrition Chapter 33
Fluid and Electrolyte Imbalances Chapter 53

I. OVERVIEW OF INTRAVENOUS (IV) THERAPY

A. Indications

1. Replaces fluid and electrolytes for clients unable to have oral intake (such as NPO status, or problems related to swallowing or GI tract)
2. Provides a route for nutrients to be given via parenteral nutrition for clients with increased caloric needs beyond what can be ingested orally (such as with severe burns); see also Chapter 33
3. Provides vascular access to deliver medications that require a constant blood level, would be destroyed by GI tract, or would be too irritating if given by another route
4. Provides rapid vascular access for emergency medications, fluids, and blood products directly into bloodstream, ensuring prompt onset of action

B. Types of fluids provided by IV route

1. Hydrating solutions (see Table 31–1)
2. Total parenteral nutrition (TPN); see Chapter 33

C. Equipment needed for IV therapy

1. Catheters and needles
   a. Over-the-needle catheters: 16-gauge (large) to 26-gauge (small) plastic catheter fits over a needle that pierces skin and vein; once in vein, needle is withdrawn and discarded, leaving catheter in place; available in a variety of lengths and gauges (diameters); use smallest appropriate length and gauge of catheter (based on size of vein and solution prescribed); use 19-gauge or larger to infuse blood products
   b. Winged needle or butterfly: steel needle with plastic flaps (wings) attached to shaft to facilitate venipuncture; commonly used to obtain blood samples or for short-term therapy
   c. These devices come in needle styles designed to protect healthcare workers from accidental needlesticks
2. Infusion pumps and "smart" pumps
   a. Deliver fluids by exerting positive pressure on tubing or fluid to maintain fluid flow despite increased venous resistance

Table 31–1 Hydrating Solutions

Solution	Uses	Nursing Implications
Isotonic 0.9% sodium chloride (normal saline or NS) Lactated Ringer's (LR) 5% dextrose in water (D_5W)	Has same osmolality as plasma, so it remains in extracellular compartment, expanding vascular volume NS and LR are crystalloid solutions that ↑ fluid volume in both intravascular and interstitial spaces with minimal fluid volume expansion NS is the only solution to be administered with blood products D_5W is isotonic on initial administration but provides free water when metabolized (hypotonic), expanding intra- and extracellular fluid volumes	Assess for signs of hypervolemia • Bounding pulse • Shortness of breath • Distended neck veins Assess for signs of hypovolemia • Urine output < 30 mL/hr • Weak, thready pulse • Subnormal temperature • Flat neck veins
Hypotonic 0.45% sodium chloride (½ NS) 0.33% sodium chloride (⅓ NS) 0.225% sodium chloride (¼ NS)	Has lower osmolality than plasma; treats cellular dehydration through fluid shifting out of blood vessels into cells by osmosis; promotes elimination by kidneys	Do not administer if risk for third-space fluid shift or fluid sequestration in a body space (results in circulating volume loss and ↑ risk for organ failure or ↑ intracranial pressure) Administer slowly to prevent cellular edema
Hypertonic 5% dextrose in 0.9% sodium chloride (D_5NS) 5% dextrose in 0.45% sodium chloride (D_5 ½ NS) 5% dextrose in lactated Ringer's (D_5LR) 10% dextrose in water ($D_{10}W$) 50% dextrose in water ($D_{50}W$) 3% or 5% sodium chloride	Has higher osmolality than plasma, causing fluid to shift from cells into vascular compartment, expanding vascular volume 10% dextrose—stand-by solution for clients receiving TPN 50% dextrose—used for hypoglycemia Dextrose > D_5W	Do not administer to clients with kidney or heart disease or clients who are dehydrated; monitor for signs of hypervolemia ↓ Pull fluids out of something
Volume expanders (colloid solutions) Albumin 5% Albumin 25% Dextran 40 Hydroxyethyl starch (HES) products Plasma protein fraction	Colloid solutions contain substances that cannot diffuse through capillary walls, resulting in ↑ plasma volume and ↑ osmotic pressure, causing fluids to move into vascular compartment; used to treat hypovolemic shock	Establish baseline vital signs, lung and heart sounds, and central venous pressure; reassess per agency protocol Administer with a large-gauge (18–19 gauge) needle Monitor intake and output Monitor for resolving hypovolemia and signs of rebound hypervolemia
Nutrient 5% dextrose (D_5W) 5% dextrose in 0.45% sodium chloride (D_5 ½ NS)	Contain some form of carbohydrate (e.g., dextrose, glucose) and water D_5W provides 170 calories per liter	Useful in preventing dehydration but does not provide sufficient calories to promote wound healing, weight gain, or normal growth in children
Electrolyte 0.9% sodium chloride (NS) Ringer's solution (has sodium chloride, potassium, calcium) 5% dextrose in 0.45% sodium chloride (D_5 ½ NS)	Saline and electrolytes restore vascular volume and replace electrolytes LR is also an alkalinizing solution to treat metabolic acidosis D_5 ½ NS is an acidifying solution to treat metabolic alkalosis	Monitor fluid and electrolytes Monitor arterial blood gases Monitor intake and output

b. Regulate rate at preset limits; alarms are triggered when fluid level is low, air is in line, or an occlusion is present

c. Are used when volume needs to be carefully controlled, such as with central line infusions, solutions containing medication, and parenteral nutrition; commonly used by agencies for all IV infusions to promote safety

d. Smart pumps have a computer that is programmed with agency-specific drug library data sets and protocols; data is logged from pump to pharmacy computer about drug infusion, programmed rate and volume, and all alerts (alarms)

3. Syringe pumps
   a. Battery or electronic operated devices to control speed of medication infusion through an existing primary IV line
   b. Pharmacy dispenses new syringe for each dose, but microbore tubing may be reused for 48–72 hours per agency policy; a sterile cap is used each time primary tubing is accessed
4. Tubing: may be vented or nonvented
   a. Vented tubing is used with glass bottles to allow air to replace fluid as it infuses; nonvented tubing is used with plastic (nonrigid) bags
   b. If infusions flow by gravity, drip chamber of tubing determines size of drop
   c. Drip chambers are either macrodrip (drop factor of 10–20 drops [gtt] per mL) or microdrip (60 gtt/mL); microdrip chambers are used with pediatric or critically ill clients, or client receiving small fluid volumes (less than 50 mL/hr)
5. Filters: devices that may be part of infusion set or an addition to infusion line; filters remove contaminants (air, bacteria, or particulate matter); not all medications or solutions can or must be filtered
   NCLEX® a. TPN requires a filter change every 24 hours when tubing is changed; filters used for other purposes may be changed every 24 to 72 hours per agency policy
   NCLEX® b. Some medications, such as phenytoin and pantoprazole require a filter change with each dose
   NCLEX® c. Use a filter whenever blood is transfused; many blood administration sets have an in-line filter
   d. To prime a filter, point filter downward so proximal half fills with fluid first, then invert to complete priming

II. TYPES OF INTRAVENOUS INFUSIONS

A. Peripheral *intravenous* infusion
1. IV device with an internal tip that terminates in a peripheral vein
2. In adults, internal tip lies between fingertips and shoulder
3. Some fluids and medications cannot be administered by peripheral line because of fluid characteristics
4. Peripheral devices are usually rotated every 72 to 96 hours per agency policy and current evidence-based practice

B. Central intravenous infusion
1. IV device with an internal tip that lies in central venous system; these can include such catheters as central venous catheter (CVC) or peripherally inserted central catheter (PICC line)
2. Internal tip most commonly ends at superior vena cava
3. These devices can remain in place for long periods of time
4. Any fluid or medication that can be given IV can be given via a central line
5. NCLEX® Most central lines require sterile dressings to reduce risk of contamination; agency policy and type of dressing determine frequency of dressing changes

C. Continuous infusion: an uninterrupted infusion that runs 24 hours a day

D. Intermittent infusion
1. An infusion designed for clients who do not require IV fluid replacement therapy but require an IV access
2. An intermittent infusion device (saline lock or prn adapter) is fitted to end of IV catheter providing a connection for intermittent solution or medication administration
3. These devices require a saline flush at least once every 8 hours and before and after medication administration
4. Some central lines require saline flush be followed by a heparin flush (10 units/mL or 100 units/mL solutions) per agency policy to maintain patency

III. PROCEDURES AND SKILLS FOR INTRAVENOUS THERAPY

A. Preparing for IV therapy
1. NCLEX® Verify allergies, such as latex; use latex-free IV catheter, tubing, and injection ports for clients with latex allergy; also beware of rubber stoppers on vials
2. Gather equipment (IV catheter, tourniquet, antiseptic wipes, gauze or semipermeable transparent membrane dressing, tape, IV fluid and tubing, filter if indicated, pump and regulator device as appropriate, and gloves)
3. Verify healthcare provider prescription and perform hand hygiene
4. Prepare equipment
   a. Obtain needleless adapter to connect to venous access device if device does not include one
   b. Remove outer wrappers from tubing, connect tubing and filter device, and close tubing roller clamp
   NCLEX® c. Remove outer wrapper around IV bag; inspect bag for leaks (small amount of condensation is normal), tears, discoloration, cloudiness, or particulate matter; do not use bag if any of these conditions are present

d. Hang IV bag on pole
e. Using aseptic technique, remove port cap on IV bag and plastic protector from IV tubing spike (end with drip chamber) and insert spike into IV bag
f. Squeeze drip chamber until it is partially full
g. Remove protective cap on tubing if it is not an air-vented cap, open roller clamp to prime tubing and filter; invert and tap Y injection sites to remove air during priming, replace protective tubing cap
h. If prescribed solution is in a glass bottle (such as to administer medication that would absorb into plastic IV bag), use vented tubing, or solution will not infuse

B. Inserting an IV line

1. Follow agency policy when starting and maintaining an IV
2. *NCLEX®* Wear gloves for protection from bloodborne pathogens; insertion is a sterile procedure
3. Prepare client for infusion, explain procedure, and obtain client's permission for procedure; use client identification procedures
4. Identify appropriate vein for cannulation
   a. In adults, peripheral IVs are inserted in hand and forearm moving from proximal metacarpals to shoulder depending on age; use nondominant side if possible
   b. Peripheral IVs in children can also include scalp and leg or foot veins; do not use leg or foot veins in adults (risk of thrombus formation)
   c. *NCLEX®* Avoid sites where veins are sclerotic, inflamed, or have decreased blood flow (on side affected by stroke or mastectomy); also avoid skin areas that are infected or edematous
5. Use tourniquet to distend vessel
   a. *NCLEX®* Verify absence of latex allergy before applying
   b. In absence of a tourniquet, a blood pressure cuff may be used; some older adult clients may be accessed without a tourniquet
   c. Place tourniquet 10 to 15 cm (4–6 in.) above proposed site tightly enough to obstruct venous circulation but not arterial circulation (use light stroking, gravity, and/or topical heat application to aid vein distention)
6. Prepare skin; clean site with alcohol followed by cleansing agent such as chlorhexidine wipe; clean skin in a circular manner, starting at inside and moving outward; allow cleansing agent to dry on skin for up to 2 minutes
7. Introduce needle at a 10- to 30-degree angle with bevel up; once blood return occurs, hold needle still and advance catheter by pushing it forward off needle until hub is in contact with insertion site
8. Release tourniquet and remove needle from catheter
9. Connect catheter to IV tubing and apply sterile dressing to insertion site; apply label to dressing that identifies length and gauge of catheter, date and time of insertion, and nurse's initials
10. Complete and apply date sticker to IV tubing
11. Initiate prescribed flow rate: pumps are set to deliver fluid in mL/hr; if allowed to flow by gravity, calculate drip rate by multiplying volume by drop factor and dividing by time in minutes; for example, to administer 1000 mL in 8 hours with a drop factor of 15 drops/mL, set up problem as follows:

$$\frac{\text{Total infusion volume} \times \text{drop factor}}{\text{Total time of infusion in minutes}} = \text{drops/minute}$$

$$\frac{1000 \text{ mL} \times 15}{8 \times 60 \text{ min (480 min)}} = 31.25 \text{ drops/min (31 drops/minute)}$$

12. Dispose of sharps in rigid sharps disposal container
13. Document date, time, solution, amount, infusion device, rate, site location, and condition of site and dressing

C. Maintaining an IV infusion

1. Ensure that correct solution is infusing
2. Check rate of flow hourly or more often per policy for selected situations
3. Inspect patency of IV tubing and needle
4. Maintain solution container 3 feet above IV site for gravity infusion devices; keep bag higher than IV pump when using a pump
5. Inspect tubing for kinks or obstructions; ensure tubing is not hanging below IV site
6. Splint a joint per agency policy if IV is positional (movement of arm impedes flow of solution)
7. Ensure tight connections to prevent leakage
8. Discontinue solution and remove IV access device if there is no blood return and acceptable drip rate cannot be established

NCLEX®

9. Inspect insertion site for fluid infiltration (IV access device becomes dislodged from vessel, causing fluid to flow into interstitial tissues and other complications); see Table 31–2 for list of complications and associated nursing care

Table 31–2 Complications of IV Therapy

Complication	Nursing Implications
Infection (catheter-related) (sepsis)—common occurrence with TPN solutions that have high glucose concentration that invites bacteria; characterized by fever, chills, erythema, or drainage at insertion site, elevated white blood count, and possibly septic shock	Use strict aseptic technique when working with IVs. Change IV solutions at least every 24 hours. Change IV tubing and dressings every 72 to 96 hours per agency protocols (TPN tubing every day). When discontinuing central line, remove catheter and apply an occlusive dressing. Monitor site for 48 hours; catheter tip may be sent to lab for culture if sepsis is suspected.
Air embolism—air is introduced into IV line during catheter insertion, tubing change, or administration of solutions and medications; characterized by respiratory distress, chest pain, dyspnea, hypotension, and weak and rapid pulse	When changing tubing or reflux valves on CVADs without Groshong valves or catheters, instruct client to perform Valsalva maneuver (forcefully exhale with glottis, nose, and mouth closed). Ensure all catheter connections are tight. Ensure all connections on central lines are luer lock, not slip lock. During insertion of a percutaneous CVC, position client in head-down position with head turned in opposite direction of insertion site. If an air embolism is suspected, clamp the catheter, position the client in left Trendelenburg's position, administer oxygen, and contact healthcare provider.
Hypersensitivity reaction—sensitivity to medication; characterized by flushing, itching, and urticaria	Check client allergies prior to administering medications. Stop the infusion and check vital signs. Notify the healthcare provider and continue to monitor client.
Circulatory overload—also called speed shock; fluids are administered faster than circulation can accommodate; characterized by cough, dyspnea, crackles, distended neck veins, tachycardia, hypertension, S_3 heart sounds, and cardiac rhythm	Be watchful for this complication in very young and older adult clients, and clients with cardiac, renal, respiratory, and liver disorders. Use IV pumps or controllers to regulate infusion rate. Do not "catch up" with IV solutions that fall behind schedule. Carefully monitor fluid volumes when administering multiple concurrent IV solutions or medications. Check client's IV infusion rates at least hourly per agency protocols. Avoid selecting an IV container with a larger volume than needed over a 24-hour period. Monitor client's vital signs, intake and output, breath and heart sounds. For signs and symptoms of fluid volume overload: slow or stop infusion rate per order, place client in high Fowler's position, administer oxygen and diuretics per order, and notify healthcare provider.
Infiltration—localized swelling, coolness, pallor, and discomfort at IV site	Stop IV and remove venous access device. Apply a warm compress to infiltration site and elevate arm on a pillow. Restart infusion at another site.
Phlebitis—inflammation of a vein; characterized by warmth, swelling, red streak at vein site, pain along course of the vein, and localized warmth	Inspect and palpate IV site at least every 8 hours for redness; if phlebitis is detected, discontinue infusion and remove venous access device. A prescription is not required to remove and replace a peripheral catheter that shows symptoms of phlebitis. Apply warm compresses to venipuncture site. Select a large vein when administering irritating solutions or medications. Dilute irritating medications (e.g., promethazine) and administer over prescribed time via infusion pump; if client reports pain at site, further dilute medication and slow the flow rate.
Hypoglycemia—↓ blood glucose (BG) level related to TPN being abruptly discontinued or excessive insulin administration; characterized by BG less than 70 mg/dL, hunger, diaphoresis, weakness, anxiety	Monitor blood glucose per agency protocols (at least every day). Gradually decrease infusion when discontinuing TPN. Have 10% dextrose available as stand-by (medical prescription required for prn use).
Hyperglycemia—↑ BG related to TPN administration or use of excessive solutions in diabetic clients; characterized by BG greater than 200 mg/dL, excessive thirst, fatigue, restlessness, confusion, weakness, and diuresis	Monitor blood glucose per agency protocols (at least every day). Check medications affecting blood glucose levels (e.g., steroids). Begin infusion at a slow rate (40 mL/hr) and gradually increase. Do not "catch up" if infusion rate falls behind.

10. Instruct client to notify the nurse of these conditions:
    a. Flow rate changes or solution stops dripping
    b. Solution container is nearly empty
    c. There is blood in IV tubing or at insertion site
    d. There is discomfort or swelling at insertion site
11. At least every 8 hours, document solution, amount, infusion device, rate, site location, and condition of site and dressing

IV. CENTRAL VENOUS ACCESS DEVICES (CVADS)

A. **A CVAD enters a central vein that empties into superior vena cava;** placement can occur in numerous settings but all placements must be verified by x-ray
   1. Percutaneous (nontunneled) catheter: a single or multiple lumen catheter is inserted by healthcare provider
   2. Tunneled catheter (Hickman, Broviac, Groshong)
      a. Terminates in a central vein
      b. Remainder of catheter passes through a subcutaneous tract and exits on chest or abdominal wall
      c. Dacron cuff triggers scar formation that prevents ascending tract infection
      d. Does not require a sterile dressing once subcutaneous tract has healed
   3. PICC
      a. Inserted into basilic or cephalic vein just above or below antecubital space of right arm by healthcare provider or specially trained IV therapy nurse
      b. Used for longer-term inpatient or outpatient therapy
      c. Although insertion site is in periphery, catheter terminates in superior vena cava
   4. Implantable venous access ports (Port-a-Cath, Infusaport, Mediport)
      a. Surgically implanted into small subcutaneous pocket, usually on upper chest using local anesthesia
      b. Port is attached to catheter that terminates in a central vein
      c. Most subcutaneous ports are accessed with a Huber needle to prolong life of port's septum
   5. Midline venous access device
      a. Shorter version of a PICC, with catheter terminating in axilla
      b. Used for 2 weeks or less and cannot be used for medications or fluids that are irritants or vesicants
   6. Peripheral access system (PAS) ports are similar to a subcutaneous port except port itself is implanted in antecubital area

B. **Internal tips: internal tip of catheter comes in two versions**
   1. Open-tipped: end of catheter opens directly into bloodstream; if flushing techniques are not performed correctly, blood can back up into catheter causing occlusion; must be flushed with saline followed by heparin flush solution to maintain patency when not in use; two types are:
      a. Hickman: adult form of open-tipped catheter
      b. Broviac: pediatric version, which usually means smaller lumen size
   2. Closed-tip catheter or Groshong: has a valve on its internal tip that prevents backflow of blood; routinely flushed with double volumes of saline but do not require heparin flush solution; advantages are:
      a. Decreased risk of air emboli or bleeding
      b. Elimination of heparin flush
      c. Elimination of catheter clamping
      d. Reduced flushing protocols between use

C. **Lumens: central catheters may have a single, double, or triple lumen;** each lumen corresponds to a separate catheter and has a separate exit point
   1. Multiple lumens allow for administration of incompatible drugs
   2. Blood drawn from one lumen will not be contaminated by drugs administered through another lumen of catheter
   3. Each lumen is treated as a separate catheter and is flushed according to agency policy

D. **Indications for use of CVAD**
   1. Long-term IV therapy or IV medication administration
   2. Obtaining frequent blood specimens
   3. Central venous pressure (CVP) monitoring
   4. Administration of TPN and medications that are irritating to veins, thus requiring a high-flow vein for rapid dilution
   5. Sclerosed peripheral veins or limited peripheral venous access

E. Nursing care

NCLEX®
1. Take special precautions with all CVADs to ensure asepsis and catheter patency; refer again to Table 31–2 for complications
2. Site care: subclavian, jugular, and PICC sites
   a. Require air occlusive dressings: dressings should be changed when soiled or loose

NCLEX®
   b. Follow agency protocol for frequency of dressing changes—usually every 2–7 days; gauze dressings must be changed at least every 48 hours; semipermeable transparent membrane dressings may remain in place for up to 1 week
   c. Follow agency protocol for cleaning solution and types of dressing; isopropyl alcohol followed by an antiseptic are often used to clean insertion site
   d. Using surgical asepsis and wearing a surgical mask, clean area 5 cm (2 in.) in diameter around site using alcohol swab; use a circular motion starting at center and work outward; allow to dry, clean with approved antiseptic; allow to dry, then apply air occlusive dressing over entire insertion site

NCLEX®
   e. Assess site for redness, swelling, tenderness, or drainage, and compare length of external portion of catheter with its documented length to assess for displacement
   f. Document date, condition of site, and dressing
3. Site care: implantable devices
   a. Follow agency protocols for cleaning solutions and types of dressings; isopropyl alcohol and approved antiseptic are often used to clean insertion site
   b. Before accessing port, using aseptic technique, clean an area 5 cm (2 in.) in diameter around port with an alcohol swab, using a circular motion starting at center and working outward; allow alcohol to dry before cleaning with antiseptic; allow to dry before accessing

NCLEX®
   c. Assess site for redness, swelling, tenderness, or drainage
   d. Access site with an appropriate primed needle, usually a Huber needle; assess for patency by aspirating blood and then flushing according to policy
   e. Apply a sterile dressing
4. Catheter care and flushing
   a. Each lumen of catheter should be flushed according to agency policy; frequency of flush varies among catheters and may be as often as once a shift; subcutaneous ports that are not in use may not require flushing more often than once a month
   b. Volume of flush solution should be at least twice the internal volume of catheter; closed-tip catheters (Groshong) should have flushing volume doubled
   c. Flush solution is usually saline; some medications are incompatible with saline, and D_5W may be substituted
   d. For open-tip catheters, saline flush is followed by a heparin flush; volume should approximate internal volume of catheter

NCLEX®
   e. Syringes smaller than 10 mL should not be used for flushing because higher pressure exerted with injection may contribute to catheter rupture

NCLEX®
   f. Have client bear down (Valsalva maneuver) during tubing change and/or ensure catheter is clamped during tubing change; exception is Groshong catheter because of one-way valve
   g. Blood draws: use distal lumen if possible; discard appropriate amount of blood prior to obtaining sample; following blood aspiration, flush line with a double volume of saline prior to instillation of weak heparin solution (if appropriate); change injection cap following a blood draw
5. Client teaching: provide clients with these instructions:
   a. Do not allow anyone to measure BP on arm with a PICC or midline catheter or PAS port
   b. Wear a Medic-Alert bracelet if device will be implanted for a long time
   c. PICC, midline catheters, and nonimplanted CVADs: there is no activity restriction but do not immerse site in water
   d. Implanted CVADs: no restriction of activities is necessary; there are no restrictions regarding bathing or swimming when device is not accessed

V. INTRAVENOUS MEDICATION ADMINISTRATION

A. Mixtures of medications within large volumes of IV fluids provide and maintain a constant, well-diluted level of a medication in bloodstream

B. To add medication to an IV solution, prepare medication from a vial or ampule and draw into a syringe

C. To add medication to a new IV container

1. Clean injection port with an alcohol swab and let dry for 30 seconds

2. Remove needle cap from syringe, insert needle through center of injection port, and inject medication into IV solution
3. Mix medication in solution by gently rotating bag end over end several times
4. Complete and attach a medication label to IV solution, with drug name and dose, date and time, and nurse's initials
5. Proceed with setting up IV for administration

D. To add medication to an existing infusion

1. Ensure there is sufficient IV solution to properly dilute medication
2. Proceed as with adding a medication to a new IV container

E. Injection by *bolus* or push method

1. Direct injection of a medication by IV push is used to obtain rapid increase in serum concentration, when drug cannot be diluted, or to administer emergency drugs
2. With intermittent infusion device when no solutions are running
   a. Prepare medication, draw up into a syringe, and label syringe so that it will not be confused with syringe containing normal saline irrigating solution
   b. Wash hands and put on gloves
   c. Cleanse infusion port with alcohol swab and let dry for 30 seconds; flush IV access device per agency policy
   d. Cleanse infusion port again
   e. Remove needle from syringe, attach a needleless adaptor, and then attach syringe with medication to needleless port access device
   f. Administer medication following recommended IV push rate (*NCLEX®*)
   g. Flush IV access device per agency policy

F. Piggyback infusion

1. To administer intermittent infusion without disconnecting existing IV
   a. Set up secondary set following procedure for setting up an IV
   b. Hang existing infusion set lower than piggyback secondary set
   c. Cleanse upper infusion port with alcohol swab and let dry for 30 seconds
   d. Connect secondary set to primary set using a needleless adapter placed above existing IV roller clamp
   e. Maintain existing IV roller clamp position and regulate piggyback rate using roller clamp on secondary tubing; piggyback solution will infuse first and, when complete, existing IV will resume at original rate
2. To administer an intermittent infusion using an infusion pump that is regulating existing IV:
   a. When intermittent solution is in an IV bag, set up secondary administration set following procedure for setting up an IV; connect infusion tubing to secondary access port on pump; follow protocols for specific pump for administering intermittent medication as either a continuous infusion or an infusion interrupting existing IV
   b. When intermittent solution is in a syringe, connect syringe to secondary access port on pump; follow protocols for specific pump for administering intermittent medication as either a continuous infusion or an infusion interrupting existing IV

G. Tandem infusion (not often used)

1. An intermittent method of administering medications through an existing IV
2. Ensure that existing IV solution and intermittent infusion are compatible and client's condition, vein, and gauge of access device can tolerate volume of fluid
3. Medication will be administered in a second bag of fluid, usually 50–100 mL, by secondary line into Y port of a continuously running infusion
4. Use procedure similar to piggyback infusion but hang secondary infusion and existing infusion at same level
5. Maintain existing IV rate and regulate piggyback rate using roller clamp on secondary tubing; primary and secondary solutions will run concurrently at their respective rates

VI. SPECIAL CONSIDERATIONS IN IV THERAPY

A. IV lines increase risk of bacteremia and sepsis by breaking skin as a line of defense

B. Various preparations (such as EMLA cream or intradermal lidocaine) may be used to numb site before IV insertion, but these are considered to be drugs and must be prescribed by a healthcare provider

C. Solutions and medications administered by IV route act within seconds to minutes and cannot be retrieved once infused or injected

D. It is a critical nursing responsibility to ensure that medications and IV solutions are compatible before administration; this includes any additives (such as potassium) to an IV line, not only primary solution and intermittent medication

E. The young and old are at greater risk of circulatory overload as a speed-related complication of IV infusion

NCLEX® **F. Clients who have cardiac, renal, respiratory, or liver disease** may also be at greater risk of circulatory overload as a speed-related complication of IV infusion

NCLEX® **G. Certain IV additives should be avoided in specific disease states**

1. Clients with diabetes mellitus should not receive dextrose
2. Clients with heart failure or other conditions posing risk for excess fluid volume should not receive sodium in IV fluids; if sodium-containing solutions are necessary, they should be infused cautiously and with use of an IV pump
3. Clients with liver disease should not receive lactated Ringer's because of possible lack of ability to convert lactate to bicarbonate
4. Clients with renal failure should not receive potassium additives in IV solutions because they cannot excrete it

VII. DISCONTINUING AN IV

A. Indications

1. Client is able to take fluids orally
2. IV medication is no longer needed
3. Access route for emergency fluid and drug administration is no longer needed

B. Procedure

1. Gather equipment: (2 × 2 gauze, clean gloves, and tape)
2. Explain procedure to client
3. Turn off IV infusion
4. Apply gloves and loosen dressing and tape by peeling edges back; stabilize catheter to prevent vein injury
5. Fold sterile gauze in half or quarters and hold steadily over insertion site while withdrawing IV catheter flush to skin; apply pressure when catheter is completely removed from vein
6. NCLEX® Hold pressure for 2 minutes or until bleeding stops; assess site for bleeding, redness, or hematoma formation; apply fresh gauze and tape in place
7. Inspect catheter tip to be sure it is intact
8. NCLEX® Document procedure and volume of IV fluid infused
9. Recheck site in 15 minutes for redness, swelling, or hematoma formation

Check Your NCLEX–RN® Exam I.Q.

You are ready for testing on this content if you can:

- Use nursing knowledge and skills in caring for a client receiving IV therapy via peripheral or central vein.
- Assess and monitor a client receiving IV therapy, including an infusion pump.
- Initiate, maintain, and discontinue a client's IV using appropriate technique.
- Document a peripheral or central IV infusion accurately.
- Monitor a client for complications of IV therapy.
- Provide care to a client with a central venous access device.
- Provide client teaching about IV therapy.

PRACTICE TEST

1 A client has a continuously running peripheral infusion. The healthcare provider prescribes an antibiotic as a piggyback infusion four times per day. In order to administer the antibiotic, the nurse should do which of the following? Select all that apply.

1. Avoid compatibility issues by starting an additional IV access.
2. Start a new IV access to eliminate the problem of too much volume for one site.
3. Flush the IV line before and after infusion of an incompatible drug.
4. Check to see if the antibiotic is compatible with the continuous infusion.
5. Change the flow rate to facilitate the administration of the antibiotic.

2 The family of a home infusion client calls the home health nurse one night to report that the electronic infusion pump alarm is sounding. What should the nurse anticipate as the cause of the infusion pump alarming? Select all that apply.

1. The client's pulse and blood pressure are falling.
2. The client is experiencing a reaction to the medication.
3. The prescribed infusion is complete.
4. There is an incompatibility with the medications.
5. An occlusion has interrupted the infusion.

3 The home health nurse is monitoring a client who performs self-care of a central line. The nurse observes the client doing all of the following activities. Which activity indicates the need for further education?

1. Flushing the central line with a 3-mL syringe
2. Cleaning the needleless injection cap with alcohol before accessing
3. Using sterile gloves to change the central line dressing
4. Wearing a mask while changing the central line dressing

4 The client has a tunneled Groshong catheter for intermittent medication administration. After administering the medication, the nurse prepares to do which of the following?

1. Clamp the catheter after medication administration.
2. Flush the catheter with heparin at scheduled times.
3. Flush the catheter with saline after medication administration.
4. Initiate a Valsalva maneuver when disconnecting medication tubing.

5 The client has a percutaneous jugular central venous line that is capped and used for intermittent infusions. After administering the medication, the best method to maintain patency is to do which of the following?

1. Flush the line first with 3–5 mL of normal saline, then with 1–3 mL of heparinized normal saline.
2. Flush the line with 3–5 mL of normal saline.
3. Flush the line with 3–5 mL of heparinized normal saline.
4. Flush the line first with 3–5 mL of heparin, then with 1–3 mL of normal saline.

6 The nurse is caring for a client with a Hickman central line. While changing the central line dressing, the nurse notes that the injection cap (e.g., heplock adapter) is of the slip lock variety instead of a Luer-Lok device. The nurse recognizes that this adapter puts the client at risk for which complication?

1. Sepsis
2. Occlusion
3. Phlebitis
4. Air embolism — prevented w/ luer lock

7 The client is to receive the intravenous medication vancomycin. To prevent adverse reactions from rapid infusion, by what method should the nurse plan to administer this drug?

1. Using gravity
2. With a regulator
3. Electronic infusion pump
4. Elastomeric pump

8 The healthcare provider is going to prescribe a hypotonic intravenous solution for a client with cellular dehydration. The nurse would expect which fluid to be administered?

1. 0.9% normal saline
2. 5% dextrose in normal saline
3. Lactated Ringer's solution
4. 0.45% sodium chloride

9 The nurse is caring for several clients with central venous catheters. While changing the tubing on the central lines, the nurse would not need to instruct the client to perform Valsalva maneuver when the client has which catheter?

1. Groshong
2. Single-lumen
3. Percutaneous
4. Accessed subcutaneous venous port

10 A client who is receiving 5% dextrose in 0.45% sodium chloride has a prescription to receive one unit of packed red blood cells. Prior to hanging the blood, the nurse will prime the blood tubing with which solution?

1. 5% dextrose
2. Lactated Ringer's
3. 0.9% sodium chloride
4. 5% dextrose in 0.45% sodium chloride

11 While assessing a client's intravenous (IV) line, the nurse notes that the area is swollen, cool, pale, and causes the client discomfort. What complication should the nurse document?

1. Infiltration
2. Phlebitis
3. Infection
4. Air embolism

12 The client is receiving 5% dextrose and 0.45% sodium chloride intravenously and is complaining of pain at the IV site. The nurse assesses the site and notes erythema and edema. What is the appropriate action for the nurse to take? Select all that apply.

1. Slow the infusion to a keep-open rate.
2. Discontinue the IV and apply a warm compress to the IV site.
3. Apply antibiotic ointment to the IV site.
4. Gently pull back on the IV catheter to attempt repositioning.
5. Relocate the IV site and document the event.

13 The nurse is preparing to start a peripheral intravenous (IV) line in a client. The client's record indicates a latex allergy. What action should be taken by the nurse?

1. Utilize a new tourniquet for this client.
2. Use a blood pressure cuff to distend the vein.
3. Avoid putting povidone iodine on the skin.
4. Initiate a latex-free alternative therapy.

14 The nurse is inserting an intravenous (IV) line into a client. After piercing the skin and entering the vein, what manifestation should cause the nurse to refrain from advancing the catheter?

1. Blood backflow into the IV catheter
2. Mild resistance with advancement
3. No reports of client discomfort
4. IV catheter was inserted bevel side up

15 The nurse is inserting a peripheral intravenous (IV) line. Place the following steps in order to perform this procedure correctly.

1. Apply a tourniquet above insertion site.
2. Insert catheter at 5- to 15-degree angle through skin.
3. Select a vein and cleanse the skin.
4. Attach tubing primed with IV solution.
5. Gather the appropriate equipment.

Fill in your answer below:

Answer: ________

ANSWERS & RATIONALES

1 **Answer: 3, 4, 5 Rationale:** If the drug and infusion were incompatible, the nurse would stop the infusion during the period of antibiotic administration and flush the line carefully before and after the antibiotic. Before making a decision about how to infuse the antibiotic, the nurse should check compatibility of the antibiotic with the continuous IV solution. The flow rate of the IVPB antibiotic may need to be adjusted to accommodate the prescribed rate of delivery. A determination of drug compatibility with the IV solution needs to be made first. Starting a second IV site should be avoided if possible. The continuous IV fluid is paused while the antibiotic infusion is occurring. It is inadvisable to start a second IV site unless absolutely necessary. **Cognitive Level:** Analyzing **Client Need:** Pharmacological and Parenteral Therapies **Integrated Process:** Nursing Process: Implementation **Content Area:** Fundamentals **Strategy:** The core issue of the question is the knowledge regarding the administration of IVPB medications when a continuous IV infusion exists. It is critical to check for compatibilities when infusing IV solutions through the same line. With multiple correct answers, approach each option as a true/false statement.

2 **Answer: 3, 5 Rationale:** Alarms sound on electronic infusion devices when the infusion is interrupted by an occlusion or when it is complete. The alarm on an electronic infusion device would not be activated by a fall in the client's pulse and blood pressure, the client experiencing a medication reaction, nor incompatibility with the prescribed medications. **Cognitive Level:** Analyzing **Client Need:** Pharmacological and Parenteral Therapies **Integrated Process:** Nursing Process: Diagnosis **Content Area:** Fundamentals **Strategy:** The core issue of this question is the ability to interpret the significance of an alarm on an infusion pump. Use knowledge of pump function in general. When there is more than one correct answer, consider each option as a true/false statement.

3 **Answer: 1 Rationale:** All catheters should be flushed with syringes with barrels of 10 mL or larger. The smaller the barrel size, the greater the pressure that comes from the tip. Smaller syringes could damage the catheter. The needleless injection cap is cleansed with alcohol to prevent the introduction of microbes into the circulatory system. Care of a central line is a sterile process due to the possibility of infection. Wearing a mask is part of the sterile process required for central line care in order to prevent contamination of the site. **Cognitive Level:** Analyzing **Client Need:** Pharmacological and Parenteral Therapies **Integrated Process:** Nursing Process: Evaluation **Content Area:** Fundamentals **Strategy:** The wording of the question tells you the correct option is an incorrect statement. Use knowledge of IV catheter flush protocols and the process of elimination to make a selection.

4 **Answer: 3 Rationale:** The catheter is designed so that only saline is used as a flush. Groshong catheters have a three-way pressure-sensitive valve that restricts air from entering the venous system and prevents backflow of blood, so the catheter should not be clamped. The Groshong catheter does not require a heparin flush. Groshong catheters have a three-way pressure-sensitive valve that restricts air from entering the venous system and prevents backflow of blood; therefore, the client does not need to perform the Valsalva maneuver. **Cognitive Level:** Applying **Client Need:** Pharmacological and Parenteral Therapies **Integrated Process:** Nursing Process: Implementation **Content Area:** Fundamentals **Strategy:** The core issue of the question is knowledge of proper management and care of Groshong catheters. Use this knowledge and the process of elimination to make a selection.

5 **Answer: 1 Rationale:** Central venous access devices that are not Groshong catheters are flushed per agency protocols with heparinized normal saline (100 or 10 units per 1 mL of normal saline). When medications are administered, the access device is flushed first with normal saline, then with heparinized normal saline. Heparin is incompatible with many medications; for this reason, normal saline is used prior to the administration of heparinized saline that maintains patency of the catheter. **Cognitive Level:** Applying **Client Need:** Pharmacological and Parenteral Therapies **Integrated Process:** Nursing Process: Implementation **Content Area:** Fundamentals **Strategy:** The core issue of the question is knowledge of proper management and care of central venous catheters. Use this knowledge and the process of elimination to make a selection.

6 **Answer: 4 Rationale:** One of the complications of IV therapy is air embolism, which is the introduction of air into the vein. Air embolism can be prevented by using Luer-Lok devices on all attachments. The chances of sepsis, occlusion, or phlebitis are not increased by the use of a slip lock injection cap on a Hickman central line. **Cognitive Level:** Analyzing **Client Need:** Pharmacological and Parenteral Therapies **Integrated Process:** Nursing Process: Diagnosis **Content Area:** Fundamentals **Strategy:** The core issue of the question is the ability of the nurse to detect situations that could lead to complications of IV therapy. Use knowledge of these risks to aid in making a selection.

7 **Answer: 3 Rationale:** The device that provides the most accurate infusion rate is the electronic infusion pump. Gravity IV infusions can be difficult to control, even with a roller clamp, because the rate can be impacted by a change in height of the infusion, the position of the intravenous catheter, and the client's activities. The roller clamp is subject to tampering. A regulator is an in-line device where the flow rate is set by a dial rather than relying on gravity. An elastromeric device is a mechanical device used to control the rate of infusion by tubing size; it is used with home infusions to simplify medication administration. **Cognitive Level:** Analyzing **Client Need:** Pharmacological and Parenteral Therapies **Integrated Process:** Nursing Process: Planning **Content Area:** Fundamentals **Strategy:** The core issue of the question is the best method to prevent speed-related adverse reactions from a drug infused intravenously. Use knowledge of IV infusion devices and the process of elimination to make a selection.

8 **Answer: 4 Rationale:** 0.45% sodium chloride (one-half normal saline) is a hypotonic solution that draws fluid from the vascular compartment into the cells. Normal saline is an isotonic solution that remains in the vascular compartment and expands vascular volume. A solution of 5% dextrose in normal saline is hypertonic until the glucose is metabolized; then it is isotonic. Lactated Ringer's is an isotonic solution that would not be effective in treating cellular dehydration. **Cognitive Level:** Applying **Client Need:** Pharmacological and Parenteral Therapies **Integrated Process:** Nursing Process: Planning **Content Area:** Fundamentals **Strategy:** The core issue of the question is knowledge of the tonicity of various intravenous solutions. Use this knowledge and the process of elimination to make a selection.

9 **Answer: 1 Rationale:** The Groshong catheter is designed with a three-way pressure-sensitive valve that restricts air from entering the venous system and prevents backflow of blood. The single-lumen catheter does not have a pressure-sensitive valve to restrict air from entering the venous system; therefore, the Valsalva maneuver will be used to prevent the formation of an air embolus. A percutaneous catheter requires the client to perform the Valsalva maneuver during tubing change in order to prevent the formation of an air embolus. The Valsalva maneuver should be performed when changing the tubing on an accessed subcutaneous venous port in order to prevent the formation of an air embolus. **Cognitive Level:** Applying **Client Need:** Pharmacological and Parenteral Therapies **Integrated Process:** Nursing Process: Implementation **Content Area:** Fundamentals **Strategy:** The core issue of the question is knowledge of various central venous catheters and which ones pose the greatest risk of air embolism, requiring performance of the Valsalva maneuver.

10 **Answer: 3 Rationale:** 0.9% sodium chloride (normal saline) is the only solution that can be administered with blood or blood products. The 5% dextrose, lactated Ringer's, or 5% dextrose in 0.45% sodium chloride solutions may cause the blood cells to clump or cause clotting. **Cognitive Level:** Applying **Client Need:** Pharmacological and Parenteral Therapies **Integrated Process:** Nursing Process: Implementation **Content Area:** Fundamentals **Strategy:** The core issue of the question is the knowledge that only normal saline is compatible with any blood product. Use this knowledge and the process of elimination to make a selection.

11 **Answer: 1 Rationale:** Infiltration is leakage of fluids into the surrounding tissues, resulting in edema around the insertion site, blanching, and coolness of skin around the site. Phlebitis is inflammation to the lumen of a vein manifested by warmth, swelling, a red streak and pain along the course of the vein, and localized warmth. Infection is characterized by fever, chills, erythema, or drainage at the IV insertion site. An air embolism occurs when air is introduced into an IV line; characterized by respiratory distress, chest pain, dyspnea, hypotension, and a weak and rapid pulse. **Cognitive Level:** Analyzing **Client Need:** Pharmacological and Parenteral Therapies **Integrated Process:** Communication and Documentation **Content Area:** Fundamentals **Strategy:** The core issue of the question is the ability to accurately interpret an

IV complication. Use knowledge of various IV complications and the process of elimination to make a selection.

12 **Answer: 2, 5 Rationale:** The IV is discontinued and restarted at a new site. Applying a warm compress to an area of phlebitis dilates the vessel, improving circulation, and reduces the resistance to blood flow from within the vein reducing the pain. The site of the IV will need to be changed in order to prevent further damage of the current site. The event will need to be documented; however, the healthcare provider does not need to be contacted unless a change in the IV prescription is necessary. The client is exhibiting signs of phlebitis; continuing the infusion at that site and at any rate would only increase the phlebitis. The nurse cannot change the infusion rate without a healthcare provider's prescription. Applying antibiotic ointment to the IV site will not affect the development of phlebitis. Repositioning the IV catheter will not affect the development of phlebitis. **Cognitive Level:** Applying **Client Need:** Pharmacological and Parenteral Therapies **Integrated Process:** Nursing Process: Implementation **Content Area:** Fundamentals **Strategy:** The core issue of the question is the ability to accurately interpret an IV complication and initiate the correct nursing action. When there is more than one correct answer to a question, look at each option as a true/false statement.

13 **Answer: 2 Rationale:** A blood pressure cuff can be used as an alternative method of vein distention. Tourniquets are made of latex, so a new tourniquet would not resolve the latex issue. Avoiding providone iodine does not resolve the latex issue. The nurse cannot initiate an alternative therapy without a healthcare provider's prescription. **Cognitive Level:** Analyzing **Client Need:** Safety and Infection Control **Integrated Process:** Nursing Process: Planning **Content Area:** Fundamentals **Strategy:** The core issue of the question is providing for safety of the client who has a latex allergy. Use this knowledge and the process of elimination to make a selection.

14 **Answer: 2 Rationale:** The nurse would refrain from advancing the catheter if mild resistance is noted during the insertion process. A backflow is normal on insertion of an IV catheter, indicating that the vein has been pierced. Once the catheter is in the vein, the client should not experience pain. The IV should be inserted bevel side up in order for the skin to be more easily pierced. **Cognitive Level:** Applying **Client Need:** Pharmacological and Parenteral Therapies **Integrated Process:** Nursing Process: Implementation **Content Area:** Fundamentals **Strategy:** The core issue of the question is knowledge of normal IV insertion procedure. Use this knowledge and the process of elimination to make a selection.

15 **Answer: 5, 3, 1, 2, 4 Rationale:** The first step is to gather equipment. For the second step, the nurse selects a vein and cleanses the site. In the third step, the nurse applies a tourniquet and inserts the catheter. The fourth step is insertion of the catheter. Finally, the nurse attaches the primed tubing and regulates the drip rate. Additional steps are to release the tourniquet, continue to assess the site, apply a dressing, and document the procedure. **Cognitive Level:** Analyzing **Client Need:** Pharmacological and Parenteral Therapies **Integrated Process:** Nursing Process: Implementation **Content Area:** Fundamentals **Strategy:** Using nursing knowledge and mental visualization of the process, place the steps in the correct order.

Key Terms to Review

References

Ball, J., & Bindler, R., & Cowen, K. (2015). *Principles of pediatric nursing: Caring for children* (6th ed.). Hoboken, NJ: Pearson Education.

Berman, A., Snyder, S., & Frandsen, G. (2016). *Kozier & Erb's fundamentals of nursing: Concepts, process, and practice* (10th ed.). New York, NY: Pearson Education.

LeMone, P., Burke, K., Bauldoff, G., & Gubrud, P. (2015). *Medical surgical nursing: Clinical reasoning in patient care* (6th ed.). Hoboken, NJ: Pearson Education.

Lewis, S., Dirksen, S., Heitkemper, M., & Bucher, L. (2014). *Medical surgical nursing: Assessment and management of clinical problems* (9th ed.). St. Louis, MO: Elsevier Science.

Smith, S., Duell, D., Martin, B., Aebersold, M., & Gonzalez, L. (2017). *Clinical nursing skills: Basic to advanced skills* (9th ed.). New York, NY: Pearson Education.

Blood and Blood Component Therapy

32

In this chapter

Cross Reference

Other chapters relevant to this content area are

Intravenous Therapy	Chapter 31
Fluid and Electrolyte Imbalances	Chapter 53

I. SOURCES OF BLOOD FOR TRANSFUSION

A. Anonymous donor

1. An anonymous person (at least 17 years old) who donates blood to a blood bank
2. May donate one unit (pint) every 8 weeks (56 days)

B. *Designated donor*

1. A donor who has volunteered to donate for a client or has been selected by client; is often a relative who has compatible blood type
2. Does not reduce risk for transmission of bloodborne infections
3. Client often has less anxiety about receiving blood products from a known donor

C. *Autologous donor*

1. Client donates own blood for future transfusion
2. NCLEX® Process begins 4–6 weeks before scheduled surgery or procedure and ends at least 3 days before transfusion date
3. NCLEX® May donate every 3 days as long as hemoglobin (Hgb) level is satisfactory (no less than 11 grams/dL); iron supplements may be prescribed
4. Especially useful for clients who have a rare blood type, history of transfusion reactions, and to prevent transmission of bloodborne viral infections
5. NCLEX® Contraindicated in clients with acute infection (including bacteremia), leukemia, significant cardiovascular or cerebrovascular disease, Hgb less than 11 grams/dL, or hematocrit (Hct) less than 33%

D. *Blood salvage*

1. A type of autologous donation in which blood is suctioned (often during or after surgery) from body cavities, joint spaces, or other enclosed areas
2. Blood may be "washed" to remove cellular and tissue debris before reinfusion

II. COMPATIBILITY

A. *Compatibility* testing is completed to prevent a client who receives blood or a blood product from having a transfusion reaction

NCLEX® **B. Client's blood is typed to determine blood group (see Table 32–1) and Rh type (positive or negative)**

C. Antibody screening may also be done (e.g., prescription reads "type and screen") to detect antibodies other than anti-A and anti-B; this is often prescribed when client is likely to need blood in very near future but not immediately

Table 32–1 Blood Group Compatibility

Blood Group	Can Be Donor for	Can Be Recipient of
O (universal donor)	O, A, B, AB	O
A	A, AB	O, A
B	B, AB	O, B
AB (universal receiver)	AB	O, A, B, AB

D. ***Cross-match* is done (e.g., prescription reads "type and cross-match") when a unit of blood is to be transfused to client;** donor red blood cells (RBCs) are added to recipient's serum and Coomb's serum; if no RBCs agglutinate, the cross-match is compatible

NCLEX® E. **After a sample of client's blood is drawn for typing, a special identification (blood bank bracelet) is placed on client's wrist;** this bracelet has a unique blood donor number that must be matched to blood identification tag on any unit of blood client receives

III. BLOOD COMPONENTS

A. **Packed red blood cells (PRBCs)**
1. Used to replace RBCs lost because of anemia or actual blood loss; RBCs increase oxygen-carrying capacity of blood
2. The use of packed red blood cells has largely replaced the use of whole blood except in situations of trauma accompanied by severe blood loss
3. NCLEX® A unit of RBCs often contains a volume of 250 mL, although it can be supplied in bags containing up to 400 mL; check bag for actual volume
4. NCLEX® Each transfused unit should raise hemoglobin by 1 gram/dL and hematocrit by 2–3%; blood sample should be drawn at 4–6 hours posttransfusion (not earlier) to evaluate effectiveness
5. Washed RBCs are nearly free of residual plasma, WBCs, and platelets, and are used in clients who have severe reactions to components in plasma
6. Intended outcome is that client has increased RBC count and that symptoms of anemia (such as fatigue) resolve

B. **Fresh frozen plasma (FFP)**
1. Contains clotting factors and aids in volume expansion (though volume expansion is not primary purpose); RBCs and platelets have been removed
2. Used to correct bleeding due to multiple factor deficiencies, or for factor deficiency for which no specific replacement is available
3. Requires ABO and Rh compatibility testing prior to use
4. A unit of FFP is often 200–250 mL in volume; actual volume is labeled on bag
5. NCLEX® Infuse as rapidly as possible and within 6 hours of thawing to preserve viability of clotting factors and reduce risk of septicemia
6. Intended outcome is return to normal results of coagulation studies, such as partial thromboplastin time (PTT) and prothrombin time (PT)

C. **Cryoprecipitate**
1. Derivative of FFP that replaces various clotting factors found in blood, such as factor VIII, factor IX, fibronectin, and fibrinogen; concentrates of factor VIII and IX are also available
2. Originally used to treat hemophilia and von Willebrand's disease, but also treats disseminated intravascular coagulopathy (DIC) and other causes of acute bleeding (such as obstetric emergencies and cardiothoracic surgery)
3. NCLEX® Can be frozen for up to 1 year but must be used immediately upon thawing; infused over 15–30 minutes
4. Intended outcome is improvement in client's clinical picture, fibrinogen level, and results of coagulation studies

D. **Platelets**
1. Play an important role in blood coagulation and homeostasis; used to treat thrombocytopenia or dysfunctional platelets
2. A transfusion of platelets can range from a volume of 50–70 mL to 200–400 mL, depending on client need; actual volume is noted on bag
3. NCLEX® Infuse as rapidly as possible immediately after obtaining from blood bank
4. Intended outcome is improved platelet count (increase of 10,000/mcL per concentrate) at 1 hour and 24 hours posttranfusion

E. Granulocytes

1. Provides granulocytes to help fight an infection in a client with sepsis or who is neutropenic and not responding to antibiotic therapy
2. Intended outcome is improvement in client's clinical picture, negative culture results, and increase white blood cell (WBC) and granulocyte (WBC differential) counts

F. Albumin

1. Expands blood volume by providing plasma proteins that cannot diffuse through capillary walls; increased osmotic pressure in blood vessels causes interstitial fluids to move back into vascular compartment
2. Used to treat hypovolemic shock and restore blood proteins in hypoproteinemia
3. Available in concentrations of 5–25%; a bottle of albumin 25 grams/100 mL (25%) provides albumin content equal to that found in 500 mL of blood
4. *NCLEX®* Intended outcome is improved serum albumin level and resolution of hypovolemic shock, severe edema, or hyperproteinemia

IV. ADMINISTRATION OF BLOOD PRODUCTS

A. Safe administration of blood products is a vital concern to client and nurse

NCLEX® **B. For proper procedure for administering blood, see Box 32–1**

Box 32–1

Procedure for Blood Administration

- Verify client consent; obtain baseline vital signs 5 minutes prior to initiating transfusion (some agencies require specific healthcare provider approval to administer blood with client temperature elevation greater than 100°F [37.8°C])
- Ensure a suitable vein and appropriate-gauge needle (18- or 20-gauge preferred; must be large enough to allow blood to infuse without damaging cells)
- Set up blood infusion equipment:
  - Obtain a Y-set with blood filter; using aseptic technique, insert spike into a container of 0.9% sodium chloride (normal saline) and prime the tubing; ensure that solution covers filter and one-third of drip chamber above filter; back-prime other Y leg with saline; never use a solution containing dextrose because it will cause blood to clump
  - Start saline solution just prior to hanging unit of blood
- Obtain correct blood component from blood bank by checking requisition form against blood bag label with lab technician; verify client's name, identification (ID) number, blood type (A, B, AB, or O) and Rh group, blood donor number, and expiration date; note any abnormal color, RBC clumping, gas bubbles, and extraneous material; refuse to accept any blood product if date is expired or any abnormalities are noted
- With another nurse, compare client's ID bracelet against tag on unit of blood; ask client to state and spell name, ask date of birth, and compare name and identification number (located on client's blood bank ID band), number on blood bag label, and ABO group and Rh type on blood bag label; if information does not match exactly, notify blood bank and do not administer blood; sign appropriate form with second nurse according to agency protocol
- Immediately hang blood—it must be hung within 20–30 minutes of receipt from blood bank:
  - Wash hands and apply gloves
  - Invert blood bag gently several times to mix cells with plasma
  - Insert remaining Y-set spike into blood bag
  - Open upper clamp on Y-set arm to blood
  - Close upper clamp below IV saline solution and open upper clamp below blood bag to allow blood to run into saline-filled drip chamber
- Begin transfusion at a slow rate of about 2 mL per minute; stay with client for first 15 minutes; check vital signs at 5 minutes, 15 minutes, and every 30 minutes from time transfusion is started; monitor for reactions: bacterial, allergic, or hemolytic
- After first 15 minutes, increase rate of infusion; an entire unit of blood must be administered within 4 hours, but often infuses in approximately 1.5–2 hours if client can tolerate speed and volume in that time frame
- Monitor lung sounds every hour until 1 hour after transfusion is complete
- Measure posttransfusion vital signs and document procedure and client's reaction in health record

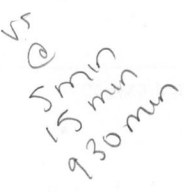

NCLEX®

C. Additional safety concerns

1. Blood products are released from blood bank only to personnel specified in agency policy
2. All agencies have very specific procedures related to blood product procurement and use
3. Store blood only in designated blood bank refrigerator
4. Do not add any medications or any solution other than normal saline to blood or blood products
5. Infuse blood product according to recommended time frame, which may vary with type of blood product being given
6. To reduce risk of septicemia, change blood administration set every 4 hours or with each unit of blood
7. A filter is used for every blood transfusion; this is typically built into blood administration tubing, but check to see that one is present

V. COMPLICATIONS

A. Transfusion reaction

1. Types of reaction are hypersensitivity, hemolytic, febrile, and bacterial reactions
2. Prescreen clients for risk by asking whether they have ever had a transfusion, a reaction to it, and any symptoms exhibited during reaction

NCLEX®

3. Assessment: see Table 32–2
4. Delayed reaction can occur days to months after a transfusion and manifests with increased temperature, decreased hematocrit, and mild jaundice

NCLEX®

5. Management
    a. Stop transfusion of blood or blood product
    b. Maintain IV access with infusion of normal saline (0.9% sodium chloride)
    c. Assess client and measure vital signs as often as every 5 minutes; do not leave client unattended
    d. Ensure that blood bank and healthcare provider are notified
    e. Provide supportive care and be ready to administer medications according to type of reaction; see Table 32–2 again
    f. Draw blood sample per policy for culture, retyping, and/or Hgb/Hct levels
    g. Obtain urine specimen for Hgb measurement; observe voidings for hemoglobinuria (hematuria)
    h. Return blood product bag, tubing, labels, and transfusion record to blood bank

B. Circulatory overload (formerly called speed shock)

1. Results from excessively rapid infusion of blood product beyond what client's circulatory system can tolerate

NCLEX®

2. Assessment: signs of fluid overload
    a. Tachycardia and bounding pulse
    b. Hypertension

Table 32–2 Blood Transfusion Reactions

Type and Cause	Assessment	Management
Hypersensitivity (antibodies in donor blood)	Fever Urticaria Anaphylactic shock	Airway management/oxygen Supportive care including treatment of shock state Diphenhydramine
Febrile (nonspecific and most common)	Fever	Premedication with acetaminophen or aspirin Airway management/oxygen Supportive care
Hemolytic (blood incompatibility)	Nausea and vomiting Lower back pain Tachycardia Hypotension Hemoglobinuria and ↓ urine output	Airway management/oxygen Supportive care Diphenhydramine
Bacterial (septicemia from contaminated blood product)	Fever and chills Tachycardia Hypotension/shock	Blood culture Antibiotic therapy Fluid resuscitation Vasopressors Corticosteroids

c. Distended neck veins
d. Crackles upon lung auscultation, dyspnea, and possibly cough

NCLEX®
3. Management
a. Slow infusion rate
b. Elevate head of bed to upright with feet dependent
c. Assess for cardiac dysrhythmias
d. Notify healthcare provider
e. Supportive care includes orders for oxygen and diuretics; morphine sulfate may be prescribed for vasodilating effect

C. Bloodborne infection (communicable disease)
1. Screening techniques and antibody testing of donor blood have greatly reduced this risk
2. Specific disease risks include hepatitis B and C, human immunodeficiency virus, Epstein-Barr virus, cytomegalovirus, human T-cell leukemia, and malaria

D. Electrolyte imbalances
1. Hyperkalemia
a. Occurs when potassium is released from hemolyzed cells in stored blood
b. Risk is greater to those with renal disease; these clients should receive fresh blood or blood that has not been stored very long
c. Monitor serum potassium level and signs of hyperkalemia (see Chapter 53)

NCLEX®
d. Slow tranfusion rate, notify healthcare provider, and carefully assess cardiac status if signs of hyperkalemia occur

2. Hypocalcemia
a. Occurs when calcium binds with citrate in banked blood and is excreted
b. Clients receiving multiple transfusions are at greater risk
c. Monitor serum calcium level and for signs of hypocalcemia (see Chapter 53)

NCLEX®
d. Slow tranfusion rate, notify healthcare provider, and assess client if signs of hypocalcemia occur (such as twitching of cheek, called Chvostek's sign)

E. Iron overload
1. Occurs only in those requiring repeated transfusions over time; delayed complication of transfusion
2. Assessment findings include nausea and vomiting, hypotension, and elevated iron level in blood

NCLEX®
3. Management: administer desferoxamine via subcutaneous or IV route to clear iron via kidneys; teach client that urine will appear red during exretion of iron; monitor serum iron levels

Check Your NCLEX–RN® Exam I.Q.

You are ready for testing on this content if you can:

- Safely administer blood and blood products.
- Monitor a client during administration of blood and blood products.
- Complete proper documentation of blood and blood product therapy.
- Monitor the client's response to therapy with blood and blood products.

PRACTICE TEST

1 A client is to receive a unit of packed red blood cells (PRBCs). The nurse and another nurse have confirmed that the correct blood for the client has been obtained from the blood bank. Immediately prior to starting the blood transfusion, what client assessment should the nurse make?

1. Vital signs
2. Skin color
3. Hemoglobin level
4. Urine output

2 The nurse is preparing to administer a unit of packed red blood cells (PRBCs). When obtaining the necessary supplies, the nurse should obtain which IV solution to hang with the unit of blood?

1. Ringer's lactate
2. 5% dextrose in 0.9% sodium chloride
3. 5% dextrose in 0.45% sodium chloride
4. 0.9% sodium chloride

PRACTICE TEST

3 The nurse returns to evaluate a client whose blood transfusion has been infusing for 30 minutes. Upon assessment, the nurse notes that the client is dyspneic and auscultates the presence of crackles in the lung bases with an apical heart rate of 110 beats per minute. What complication should the nurse suspect that the client is experiencing?

1. Immune response to transfusion
2. Hypovolemia
3. Fluid overload
4. Polycythemia vera

4 The nurse determines that a client receiving a unit of packed red blood cells (PRBCs) is experiencing a transfusion reaction. After stopping the blood transfusion, what actions should the nurse promptly take next? Select all that apply.

1. The healthcare provider should be notified.
2. Obtain a white blood cell count.
3. Run normal saline at keep vein open (KVO) rate.
4. Infuse a normal saline bolus.
5. Obtain vital signs every 5 minutes.

5 A client who takes warfarin arrives at the emergency department following a gunshot wound. The client's prothrombin time is twice the desired amount. The nurse expects the healthcare provider will order a transfusion of which blood product?

1. Fresh frozen plasma
2. Random donor platelets
3. Red blood cells
4. Crystalloids

6 An adult female client has a hemoglobin level of 9.2 grams/dL. The nurse interprets that this is most likely related to what condition?

1. Leukemia
2. Amenorrhea
3. Vitamin B_{12} deficiency anemia
4. Iron-deficiency anemia

7 The nurse has received an order to transfuse a client with one unit of packed red blood cells (PRBCs). In preparation for the infusion, the nurse selects the appropriate tubing for blood administration. The nurse is aware that the tubing is manufactured with which feature?

1. A macrodrip chamber
2. An air vent
3. An in-line filter
4. Tinting that protects blood from exposure to light

8 A postoperative client is to receive a transfusion of platelets because of a critically low platelet count. What knowledge should the nurse have related to the function of platelets?

1. Improves hemoglobin and hematocrit levels
2. Prevents formation of deep vein thrombosis
3. Decreases bleeding from a surgical site
4. Returns prothrombin time to expected range

9 The nurse has received an order to transfuse two units of PRBCs to a client. Each 350 mL unit is to infuse over a 2-hour period. The nurse would administer the infusion at an hourly rate of _____ mL/hour. Record your answer rounding to a whole number.

Fill in your answer below:
Answer: _________ mL/hour

700

10 A nurse has received a report on a client being admitted with anemia who requires a blood transfusion. The nurse will anticipate which assessment findings? Select all that apply.

1. Tachycardia
2. Hypertension
3. Headache
4. Diaphoresis
5. Bounding peripheral pulses

↓O_2

11 A client is scheduled for elective surgery in 4 weeks. When the nurse in the surgeon's office initiates preoperative education, the client expresses concern regarding the potential need for a blood transfusion. What is the nurse's best response to the client's concern?

1. "It is unlikely that you will lose that much blood during the surgery."
2. "Blood transfusions are safer now than in the past."
3. "Your family may be able to donate blood for you."
4. "You may want to consider an autologous blood transfusion."

12 A nurse is caring for an immunocompromised client with cancer who is a candidate for granulocyte transfusion. At what white blood cell count level should the nurse implement neutropenic precautions for this client?

1. 10,500/mm^3
2. 7650/mm^3
3. 6000/mm^3
4. 2000/mm^3

13 Shortly after a blood transfusion is initiated, a client experiences an adverse reaction. The nurse documents the event according to hospital policy. What should the nurse do with the remainder of the blood that has not been transfused?

1. Discard the blood in the appropriate biohazard bag.
2. Return the blood to the blood bank.
3. Send the blood to the chemistry laboratory for analysis.
4. Send the blood to the infection control department.

14 A client with a low hemoglobin and hematocrit is to receive a unit of packed red blood cells (PRBCs). Prior to initiating the transfusion, the nurse determines that the client's temperature is 100.8°F (38.2°C) orally. Based on this finding, what is the most appropriate action for the nurse to take?

1. Delay hanging the blood and notify the healthcare provider.
2. Begin the transfusion as prescribed.
3. Administer 650 mg of acetaminophen and begin the transfusion.
4. Administer an antihistamine and begin the transfusion.

15 A client presents to the emergency department following a motorcycle accident. The client is in hypovolemic shock. The healthcare provider has ordered plasma expansion. What blood product should the nurse anticipate that the client will receive?

1. Packed red blood cells
2. Cryoprecipitate
3. Platelets
4. Albumin

16 A client has received a granulocyte transfusion. What laboratory result should the nurse assess to determine if the client has benefited from the transfusion?

1. Hemoglobin and hematocrit levels
2. Erythrocyte count
3. White blood cell count
4. Platelet count

17 A client has experienced an adverse reaction to a blood transfusion manifested by the development of pruritic rash and urticaria. What treatment should the nurse anticipate will be ordered for the client?

1. Diphenhydramine
2. Acetaminophen
3. Hydrocortisone cream
4. Aspirin

ANSWERS & RATIONALES

1 **Answer: 1 Rationale:** Vital signs are taken immediately prior to beginning the transfusion. Because most blood transfusion reactions occur within 15 minutes of starting infusion, it is of great importance to establish the preinfusion baseline immediately prior to beginning the transfusion. Skin color, hemoglobin levels, and urine output would be important considerations; however, they would not be so essential that they should take place immediately prior to the start of the transfusion. **Cognitive Level:** Applying **Client Need:** Pharmacological and Parenteral Therapies **Integrated Process:** Nursing Process: Assessment **Content Area:** Fundamentals **Strategy:** The question focuses on the action that should be taken immediately prior to beginning a blood transfusion. Knowledge of the appropriate process is essential.

2 **Answer: 4 Rationale:** Normal saline is the solution of choice when used as an adjunct to a transfusion. Ringer's lactate, 5% dextrose in 0.9% sodium chloride, and 5% dextrose in 0.45% sodium chloride are contraindicated due to the potential for clotting and hemolysis. **Cognitive Level:** Applying **Client Need:** Pharmacological and Parenteral Therapies **Integrated Process:** Nursing Process: Implementation **Content Area:** Fundamentals **Strategy:** The focus of the question is compatibility of blood with intravenous solutions. Use nursing knowledge and the process of elimination to select the correct answer.

3 **Answer: 3 Rationale:** Circulatory overload is a complication associated with rapid transfusion administration. Symptoms include bounding pulse, dyspnea, and crackles in the lungs. Crackles in the lungs would not be associated with immune response to transfusion, hypovolemia, or polycythemia vera. **Cognitive Level:** Analyzing **Client Need:** Pharmacological and Parenteral Therapies **Integrated Process:** Nursing Process: Diagnosis **Content Area:** Fundamentals **Strategy:** The core issue of the question is the ability to recognize signs of circulatory overload. Use nursing knowledge and the process of elimination to make a selection.

4 **Answer: 1, 3, 5 Rationale:** The healthcare provider (HCP) should be notified, but the nurse is to stop the transfusion immediately and keep the IV line open with normal saline. The client should be closely monitored and not left alone. The nurse is to stop the transfusion immediately and keep the IV line open with normal saline. The client will need to be monitored closely. Vital signs should be obtained as frequently as every 5 minutes, and the client should not be left alone. A white blood cell count would be ordered by the HCP; however, this action would not be independently initiated by the nurse without contacting the HCP first. A saline bolus would be ordered by the HCP; however, this action would not be independently initiated by the nurse without contacting the HCP first. **Cognitive Level:** Analyzing **Client Need:** Pharmacological and Parenteral Therapies **Integrated Process:** Nursing Process: Implementation **Content Area:** Fundamentals **Strategy:** The core issue of the question is the ability to take proper action when a transfusion reaction is suspected. When there is more than one correct answer to a question, each option should be considered as a true/false statement.

5 **Answer: 1 Rationale:** A transfusion of FFP is indicated for clients who are actively bleeding with a prothrombin time greater than 1.5–2.0 times the control in seconds. Platelets would be indicated for the client with thrombocytopenia. Red blood cells would be appropriate for the client with anemia. Crystalloids are given to help establish or maintain an adequate fluid and electrolyte balance. **Cognitive Level:** Analysis **Client Need:** Pharmacological and Parenteral Therapies **Integrated Process:** Nursing Process: Planning **Content Area:** Fundamentals **Strategy:** The core issue of the question is the ability to anticipate the need for fresh frozen plasma. Use nursing knowledge and the process of elimination to make a selection.

6 **Answer: 4 Rationale:** Iron-deficiency anemia can result from blood loss and is common in menstruating women; this is the most likely source of anemia in an adult female client. Leukemia is reflected in the white blood cell count. Amenorrhea, the absence of menstruation, is unlikely to cause iron-deficiency anemia. Vitamin B_{12}–deficiency anemia is often associated with dietary deficiency, such as experienced by vegetarians or those who avoid dairy products. **Cognitive Level:** Analyzing **Client Need:** Pharmacological and Parenteral Therapies **Integrated Process:** Nursing Process: Diagnosis **Content Area:** Fundamentals **Strategy:** The core issue of the question is the ability to anticipate the needs of a client with iron-deficiency anemia. Use nursing knowledge related to growth and development to help answer this question.

7 **Answer: 3 Rationale:** An in-line filter is required for the administration of blood, and blood administration tubing comes from the manufacturer with the filter in place. Tubing for blood administration is not manufactured with a macrodrip chamber, an air vent, or tinting that protects the blood from light, a feature that is not necessary for blood administration. **Cognitive Level:** Understanding **Client Need:** Pharmacological and Parenteral Therapies **Integrated Process:** Nursing Process: Planning **Content Area:** Fundamentals **Strategy:** The core issue of the question is knowledge that an *in-line filter* is required for blood transfusion. Use nursing knowledge and the process of elimination to make a selection.

8 **Answer: 3 Rationale:** A transfusion of platelets is indicated for the client with active bleeding. A transfusion with PRBCs would result in increased hemoglobin and hematocrit levels. Platelet administration is not associated with the prevention of deep vein thrombosis. The administration of platelets is not associated with the return of the prothrombin time to normal. **Cognitive Level:** Understanding **Client Need:** Pharmacological and Parenteral Therapies **Integrated Process:** Teaching and Learning **Content Area:** Fundamentals **Strategy:** The core issue is knowledge related to *platelet transfusion therapy*. Recall that platelets are critical for proper blood clotting to select the correct answer.

9 **Answer: 175 Rationale:** To calculate, divide the total volume by the number of hours, and the dividend is the hourly rate. **Cognitive Level:** Applying **Client Need:** Pharmacological and Parenteral Therapies **Integrated Process:** Nursing Process: Implementation **Content Area:** Fundamentals **Strategy:** Use knowledge of pharmacological math to calculate the infusion rate.

10 **Answer: 1, 3 Rationale:** Key features of anemia include coolness to touch, intolerance to cold, tachycardia, orthostatic hypotension, and headaches. Hypertension, diaphoresis, and bounding peripheral pulses are not associated with anemia. **Cognitive Level:** Applying **Client Need:** Pharmacological and Parenteral Therapies **Integrated Process:** Nursing Process: Assessment **Content Area:** Fundamentals **Strategy:** The core issue of the question is the ability to anticipate the needs of a client with moderately severe anemia. When there is more than one correct answer to a question, consider each option as a true/false statement.

11 **Answer: 4 Rationale:** An autologous transfusion involves the collection of the client's blood prior to the anticipated need, thus compatibility is not problematic and the potential for contamination is eliminated. It would not be appropriate for the nurse to predict blood loss as a result of a surgical procedure. Stressing the safety of blood transfusions may elicit a false sense of comfort for the client. While the family may be able to donate blood, this would not be as potentially beneficial to the client as an autologous blood transfusion. Not all relatives share the same blood type. **Cognitive Level:** Applying **Client Need:** Pharmacological and Parenteral Therapies **Integrated Process:** Communication and Documentation **Content Area:** Fundamentals **Strategy:** The core issue of the question is knowledge of various types of transfusions. Use nursing knowledge, therapeutic communication skills, and the process of elimination to make a selection.

12 **Answer: 4 Rationale:** The nurse should consider implementing neutropenic precautions when the white blood cell count is at or below 2,000/mm^3. The normal white blood cell count is between 5000 and 10,000/mm^3; no neutropenic precautions are necessary as long as the WBC falls within the normal range (6000/mm^3 and 7650/mm^3) or above (10,500/mm^3). **Cognitive Level:** Applying **Client Need:** Reduction of Risk Potential **Integrated Process:** Nursing Process: Implementation **Content Area:** Fundamentals **Strategy:** The core issue of the question is knowledge of white blood cell counts. Use nursing knowledge to eliminate the WBC count that falls within the normal range.

13 **Answer: 2 Rationale:** When a transfusion reaction has occurred, the nurse must return any remaining blood to the blood bank. If a reaction had not occurred, the nurse would dispose of the blood in an appropriate biohazard bag. It would not be appropriate for the nurse to send the blood to the laboratory or to the infection control department. **Cognitive Level:** Applying **Client Need:** Pharmacological and Parenteral Therapies **Integrated Process:** Nursing Process: Implementation **Content Area:** Fundamentals **Strategy:** The core issue of the question is knowledge of critical actions to take when a transfusion reaction occurs. Use nursing knowledge and the process of elimination to make a selection.

14 **Answer: 1 Rationale:** Because the client is febrile, the nurse must notify the healthcare provider. The healthcare provider will determine if the client can tolerate the transfusion or if additional therapeutic intervention is warranted, which may include the administration of acetaminophen or an antihistamine. The nurse cannot administer medications without an order from the healthcare provider. **Cognitive Level:** Applying **Client Need:** Pharmacological and Parenteral Therapies **Integrated Process:** Nursing Process: Implementation **Content Area:** Fundamentals **Strategy:** The core issue of the question is knowledge of critical actions to take when a client requiring a blood transfusion has an elevated temperature. It is also essential that principles for drug administration are applied when making an answer selection.

15 **Answer: 4 Rationale:** Albumin is used as a plasma expander and is used in the treatment of hypovolemic shock. PRBCs are indicated in the treatment of anemia. Cryoprecipitate is administered to treat von Willebrand's disease and fibrinogen levels below 100 mg/dL. Platelets are indicated in the treatment of thrombocytopenia. **Cognitive Level:** Analyzing **Client Need:** Pharmacological and Parenteral Therapies **Integrated Process:** Nursing Process: Planning **Content Area:** Fundamentals **Strategy:** The core issue of the question is knowledge of the uses of various blood products. Use nursing knowledge and the process of elimination to make a selection.

16 **Answer: 3 Rationale:** Granulocyte transfusions are administered to neutropenic clients with infections for white blood cell replacement. Hemoglobin and hematocrit levels, erythrocyte count, and platelet count would not be appropriate for evaluating this therapy. **Cognitive Level:** Applying **Client Need:** Pharmacological and Parenteral Therapies **Integrated Process:** Nursing Process: Evaluation **Content Area:** Fundamentals **Strategy:** The core issue of the question is knowledge of appropriate outcomes of blood component therapy. Identification and understanding of the blood components are essential for answering the question correctly.

17 **Answer: 1 Rationale:** Diphenhydramine is administered for the treatment of allergic reaction. Diphenhydramine competes with H_1 receptors on effector cells, thus blocking effects of histamine. Acetaminophen would provide symptomatic relief from signs and symptoms of a transfusion reaction, but not be effective in stopping the reaction. Hydrocortisone would provide symptomatic relief from signs and symptoms of a transfusion reaction. Aspirin would not be indicated for treatment of a transfusion reaction. **Cognitive Level:** Applying **Client Need:** Pharmacological and Parenteral Therapies **Integrated Process:** Nursing Process: Planning **Content Area:** Fundamentals **Strategy:** The core issue of the question is knowledge of appropriate treatments for transfusion reactions. Use nursing knowledge and the process of elimination to make a selection.

Key Terms to Review

autologous donor p. 471	**compatibility** p. 471	**designated donor** p. 471
blood salvage p. 471	**cross-match** p. 472	**transfusion reaction** p. 474

References

Adams, M., & Urban, C. (2016). *Pharmacology: Connections to nursing practice.* New York, NY: Pearson Education.

Berman, A., Snyder, S., & Frandsen, G. (2016). *Kozier & Erb's fundamentals of nursing: Concepts, process, and practice* (10th ed.). New York, NY: Pearson Education.

LeMone, P., Burke, K., Bauldoff, G., & Gubrud, P. (2015). *Medical surgical nursing: Clinical reasoning in patient care* (6th ed.). Hoboken, NJ: Pearson Education.

Smith, S., Duell, D., Martin, B., Aebersold, M., & Gonzalez, L. (2017). *Clinical nursing skills: Basic to advanced skills* (10th ed.). New York, NY: Pearson Education.

Test Yourself

Are you ready for the NCLEX-RN® or course exams? Access the NEW web-based app that provides students with thousands of practice questions in preparation for the NCLEX experience.

33 Total Parenteral Nutrition

In this chapter

Cross Reference

Other chapters relevant to this content area are

Meeting Nutritional Needs	Chapter 25
Intravenous Therapy	Chapter 31

I. BASIC CONCEPTS OF PARENTERAL NUTRITION

A. Overview of two types

1. **Total parenteral nutrition (TPN)** is provided intravenously through a central venous line when a client cannot take or tolerate oral or enteral feedings (see Box 33–1); may be utilized in home setting as well as hospital; most common form of parenteral nutrition
2. **Peripheral parenteral nutrition (PPN)** is used to supplement a client's inadequate nutrient intake; administered using a peripheral IV line; solution has a maximum concentration of 10% dextrose to avoid irritation of peripheral blood vessel walls, phlebitis, and sclerosis
3. TPN meets client's need for energy and prevents catabolism of protein from muscle and fat from subcutaneous tissue
4. Composition of solution includes amino acids for protein (concentrations of 3.5–20%; should supply 15–20% of daily calories), dextrose for carbohydrate (typically 25% of final concentration of solution providing 60–70% of calories), vitamins, minerals, trace elements (often twice weekly), electrolytes (according to individual need), and water
5. Lipids may be added to primary bag or infused as separate emulsion; provide up to 30% of calories and prevent or treat deficiency of fatty acids
6. Occasionally, regular insulin may be added to minimize blood glucose elevations in clients with diabetes mellitus, and heparin can be added to prevent clotting at tip according to individual need and agency protocol
7. Types of solutions
   a. TPN: formulas with amino acids and dextrose in a volume of 2–3 liters infused over 24 hours
   b. Total nutrient admixture (TNA): also called 3-in-1 solution; contains amino acids, dextrose, and lipids; daily volume prescribed to be given over 24 hours

Box 33–1

Examples of Indications for TPN

Nonfunctional or poorly functioning GI tract (severe bowel inflammatory disease, malabsorption (several causes), severe GI side effects of chemo- or radiation therapy)

Conditions requiring bowel rest (extensive GI surgery, GI trauma, bowel obstruction)

High nutrient needs of client (burns, massive trauma, extensive wounds, malnutrition, cancer, acquired immunodeficiency syndrome)

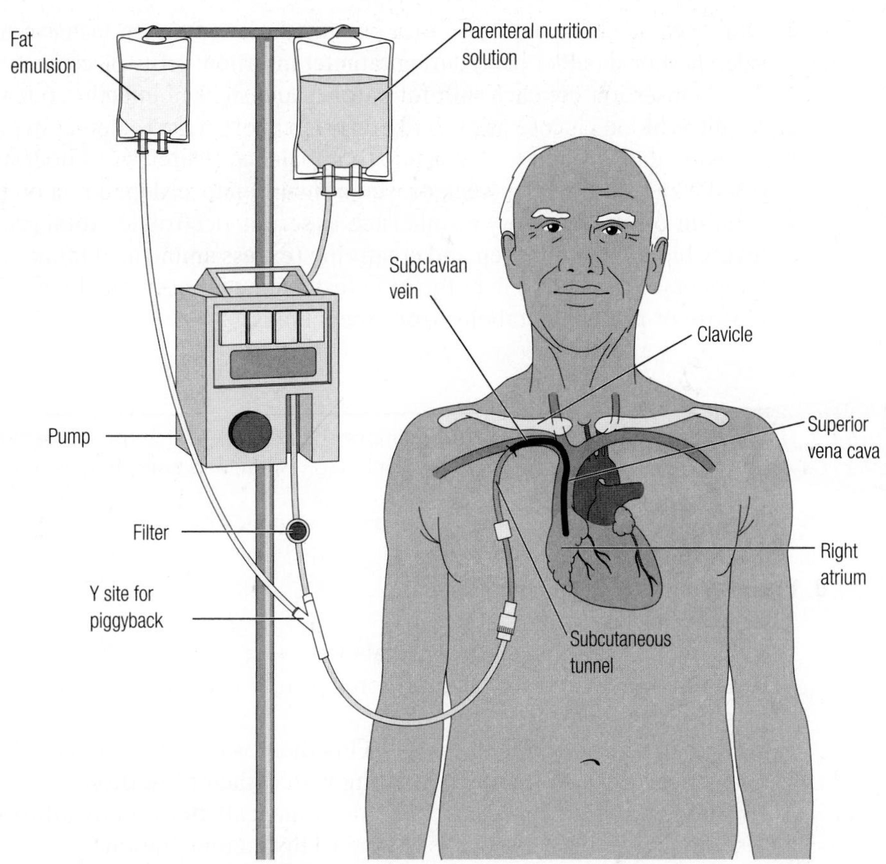

Figure 33–1

Total parenteral nutrition administered via right subclavian vein.

c. **Lipids** (fat emulsion): supplement TPN and provide fatty acids such as linoleic, linolenic, oleic, palmitic, and stearic acids; intermittent infusion of 10% fat emulsion (500 mL volume) may be given one to three times weekly

B. Access sites

1. Peripheral line (used for PPN)
   a. Peripheral veins are used for access to provide nutrient supplementation
   b. Peripheral route often used for up to 10 days
   NCLEX® c. Maximum dextrose concentration is 10% to avoid irritation of blood vessel walls, phlebitis, and sclerosis
2. Central line (typical TPN)
   a. Utilizes catheter inserted percutaneously into a central vein (see Figure 33–1); dextrose concentrations in solution are greater than 10% (often 25%)
   b. Triple-lumen catheter common; 18-gauge middle lumen used for TPN infusion (other ports used for medication administration or IV blood draws according to agency policy); TPN administration through line limited to 4 weeks or less
   c. Peripherally inserted central catheter (PICC) line is increasingly popular; catheter is inserted into basilic or cephalic vein and advanced to superior vena cava; used when TPN needed for more than 4 weeks
   d. Single-lumen catheters require secondary IV access site for other medications or IV fluids

Memory Aid

Do not administer or piggyback medications and blood into a line used for TPN. This will help to avoid incompatibilities and prevent infection.

II. NURSING MANAGEMENT

A. Assessment

NCLEX® 1. Obtain baseline assessment data, such as client weight, vital signs, breath sounds (risk for fluid overload), and any prescribed laboratory tests (such as blood glucose)
2. If a lipid solution is being used, assess for allergy to eggs since fat emulsions may use egg yolk phospholipids as an emulsifier

3. During catheter insertion, assess for pneumothorax (dyspnea, tachycardia, absent breath sounds on affected side, chest or shoulder pain) during catheter insertion; verify placement by x-ray following insertion

NCLEX® 4. Assess insertion site each shift for patency and signs of infection (clear transparent dressing often used)

NCLEX® 5. Monitor blood glucose as prescribed (often every 6 hr) to detect hyperglycemia

NCLEX® 6. Measure daily weight to determine fluid balance (1 liter = 1 kilogram) and nutritional weight gain 0.5–0.9 kg (1.1–2 lb) per week or weight maintenance, depending on individual client need

NCLEX® 7. Monitor other laboratory results, such as serum electrolytes, total protein, prealbumin and albumin levels, blood urea nitrogen and creatinine (excess amino acid intake will cause increased levels), total lymphocyte count, and liver function test results (abnormally high values may indicate problems with glucose or protein metabolism, or excess lipids)

Memory Aid

In severely malnourished clients, watch for "refeeding syndrome," a precipitous drop in serum potassium, magnesium, and phosphate levels.

B. Planning and implementation

1. Client goals
   a. Maintains fluid and electrolyte balance
   b. Gains weight according to nutritional plan or maintains current weight and avoids loss of essential nutritional elements
   c. Remains free of complications of TPN therapy (see section that follows)

NCLEX® 2. Use strict aseptic technique if assisting with catheter insertion

NCLEX® 3. Ensure that placement is correct before using catheter for any infusion

4. Use standard agency protocols to begin TPN administration
   a. Keep TPN solution in refrigerator until 30–60 minutes prior to use to retard bacterial growth; change TPN bag and tubing every 24 hours to prevent infection
   b. Administer TPN or PPN through IV tubing that has an inline filter to remove any crystals present in solution (0.22-micron filter without use of lipids; 1.2-micron filter or larger if lipids added)
   NCLEX® c. Check every ingredient in TPN solution against prescription; notify pharmacy and do not hang if any discrepancies are found; prescriptions should be renewed daily
   d. Do not add any other medication to solution once dispensed for use by pharmacy
   NCLEX® e. Do not hang a solution that is cloudy, dark in color, has visible fat globules (if lipids present); return to pharmacy for replacement
   f. Do not piggyback anything other than lipids into TPN line
5. Administer TPN using an electronic infusion device only
6. TPN rate is often started low (50 mL/hr) and gradually increased (often to 80–125 mL/hr) as client tolerates (based on fluid balance, blood glucose [BG], and electrolyte balance); ensure accuracy of flow rate
7. Use special tubing if lipid infusion is hung separately; use 1.2 micron filter or larger (not smaller filter in standard IV tubing) to allow lipids to pass through into vein; use an electronic infusion device and piggyback into TPN line below the level of the TPN inline filter to ensure free flow
8. Begin lipid infusion at rate of 1 mL/minute, titrate upward as prescribed according to client tolerance; monitor vital signs every 10 minutes for first half hour to detect adverse reactions (see section that follows); measure serum lipids if prescribed 4 hours postinfusion
9. Maintain steady prescribed rate of TPN infusion
   a. Maintain accurate intake and output records every shift
   b. Do not attempt to "catch up" a solution that has fallen behind schedule; with an appropriate prescription, it may be safe to restart the rate at 10% higher than the original rate to restore lost nutrients, but this is highly individualized and requires a prescription
   c. Do not discontinue TPN abruptly; taper rate down as prescribed to prevent hypoglycemia
   NCLEX® d. If a new TPN solution is not available when previous one has infused, hang 10% dextrose in water solution at prescribed rate to prevent hypoglycemia until TPN is available
   e. If central line is removed because of dislodgement, sepsis, or leakage, the central TPN solution cannot be infused peripherally; a peripheral solution with a maximum concentration of 10% dextrose must be used
10. Implement measures to prevent infection
   a. Change catheter dressing according to protocol using strict aseptic technique
   b. Monitor temperature every 4 hours

c. Assess insertion site each shift if clear dressing is used and with each dressing change if gauze dressing is used

11. Monitor fingerstick glucose levels as prescribed to detect hyperglycemia
12. Collaborate with healthcare provider and dietitian to evaluate whether goals of therapy are being met

Memory Aid

Change a transparent central line dressing every 72 to 96 hours as per agency policy; change gauze dressing more frequently according to policy; change any dressing that is loose, wet, or soiled to prevent infection from contamination.

C. Client/family teaching

1. Includes intended purpose and effects of therapy and adverse effects that must be self-monitored
2. Home care skills
   - a. How to self-administer TPN
   - b. Technique for changing sterile dressing
   - c. Clean hands before any contact with tubing or access area
   - d. Do not allow caregivers with an infectious disease to work with catheter
   - e. Monitor daily weight, and report more than 1.4 kg (3 lb) per week gain (fluid overload/retention)
   - f. Monitor BG and report elevations
   - g. Monitor catheter patency and report edema at catheter insertion site, jugular vein distention, and edema of affected arm (if applicable)
   - h. Monitor for catheter displacement (leakage at insertion site, pain/discomfort during infusion)

NCLEX® **D. Evaluation of outcomes**

1. Weight gain is satisfactory
2. Fluid and electrolytes are within normal limits
3. Client is free of complications of TPN therapy

III. COMPLICATIONS

NCLEX® **A. Complications of TPN (see Table 33–1)**

B. Adverse effects of lipids

1. See Box 33–2
2. If adverse reactions occur, discontinue lipid solution and notify prescriber; prepare to provide supportive measures according to symptoms

Table 33–1 Complications of Total Parenteral Nutrition

Complication	Client Manifestations	Nursing Management
Fluid overload (because of excess volume or hypertonicity)	Bounding pulse and increased BP, lung crackles, headache, jugular vein distention, excessive weight gain above goal	*Prevention:* always use electronic infusion device; do not "catch up" solutions that fall behind schedule; monitor weight daily and I&O every 8 hours *Intervention:* raise head of bed to alleviate respiratory symptoms; apply oxygen as prescribed; correctly carry out prescribed therapies, such as diuretics
Air embolism (potentially fatal entry of air into catheter during insertion or tubing changes)	Rapid-onset respiratory distress, dyspnea, apprehension, chest pain, rapid and weak pulse, low BP, churning heart murmur (hallmark sign)	*Prevention:* check catheter and tubing connections; have client use Valsalva maneuver during tubing and cap changes; place client in head-down position with head turned to opposite side (if tolerated) for cap and tubing changes to increase intrathoracic venous pressure *Intervention:* clamp catheter; place client in left Trendelenburg position (traps air in right ventricle away from pulmonic valve); notify healthcare provider; apply oxygen as prescribed
Infection/sepsis (catheter-related; high-dextrose solution excellent medium for bacterial growth)	Fever and chills; redness, swelling, tenderness, or drainage at insertion site; elevated WBC count; possible signs of septic shock	*Prevention:* use strict aseptic technique in all aspects of catheter and site care; change solution every 12–24 hours as prescribed and tubing every 24 hours per agency protocol; change dressing per protocol depending on dressing type (see text) *Intervention:* send tip of catheter for C&S upon catheter removal; arrange for blood cultures to be drawn if prescribed; administer antibiotics as prescribed

Table 33–1 *(continued)*

Complication	Client Manifestations	Nursing Management
Hyperglycemia (elevated BG level from dextrose load in solution, infusion rate, or diabetes)	Glucose levels greater than 200 mg/dL, thirst, fatigue, confusion, restlessness, weakness, and diuresis; coma when severe	*Prevention:* assess for history of glucose intolerance (e.g., diabetes); assess for use of medications that lead to hyperglycemia (e.g., corticosteroids); begin infusion at slow rate (often 40–60 mL/hr) and titrate ↑ over time as prescribed; use infusion pump *Intervention:* monitor BG levels q 6 hr or as prescribed; administer prescribed regular insulin to keep BG less than 200 mg/dL
Hypoglycemia (low BG level from abrupt termination of TPN or excess insulin)	Glucose level less than 70 mg/dL; weakness and shakiness, anxiety, diaphoresis, possible hunger	*Prevention:* use infusion pump for TPN; gradually ↓ rate of infusion when discontinuing therapy; hang 10% dextrose in water solution for 1–2 hr post-TPN as prescribed *Intervention:* monitor BG 1 hour after terminating TPN; administer glucose as needed

Box 33–2

Adverse Effects of Lipids

Chills	Dyspnea and cyanosis	Vertigo
Fever and flushing	Nausea and vomiting	Thrombophlebitis
Diaphoresis	Headache	Allergic reaction
Chest and back pain	Pressure over eyes	

Check Your NCLEX–RN® Exam I.Q.

You are ready for testing on this content if you can:

- Identify various types of access for TPN therapy.
- Begin, maintain, and discontinue TPN therapy.
- Appropriately monitor TPN flow rate.
- Provide nursing care to the client receiving TPN therapy.
- Monitor for adverse effects or complications of TPN.
- Provide client/family teaching related to TPN.

PRACTICE TEST

1 What nursing responsibilities will be included while caring for a client receiving total parenteral nutrition (TPN)? Select all that apply.

1. Covering blood glucose levels with a sliding scale of regular insulin
2. Inspecting solution to ensure "layering" of contents is absent
3. Adjusting rate of solution to the client's output every shift
4. Changing injection caps on the intravenous tubing every shift
5. Monitoring of liver function test results

2 Clients experiencing profound malnutrition may experience refeeding syndrome when first initiating total parenteral nutrition (TPN). What should the nurse do to determine if this occurs?

1. Monitor potassium, phosphorus, and magnesium levels closely.
2. Check blood glucose levels every 6 hours.
3. Assess client for hyperactive bowel sounds.
4. Assess client's level of consciousness every shift.

3 What condition should lead the nurse to conclude that a client's total parenteral nutrition (TPN) solution needs to be administered through a central venous catheter?

1. The client will be receiving fluids at a rate of 150–200 mL/hr.
2. The client will be receiving an infusion with a high caloric content.
3. The end concentration of dextrose in the solution will be 25%.
4. The use of a peripheral vein would require more frequent site changes.

4 A client recovering from multiple trauma is started on total parenteral nutrition (TPN) therapy. What should the nurse determine to be a major goal of this therapy?

1. Prevent a negative nitrogen balance in the client.
2. Maintain a high urine output.
3. Provide adequate hydration.
4. Ensure client receives needed trace minerals.

5 A client has had a central venous catheter inserted in the subclavian vein for initiation of total parenteral nutrition (TPN) therapy. What assessment finding best indicates to the nurse that the client may have a pneumothorax?

1. Client complains of sharp chest pain.
2. Pulse oximetry is 90% on room air.
3. Catheter insertion site is red and swollen.
4. Radial pulse is rapid.

6 A client, recovering from severe weight loss secondary to Crohn's disease, is being discharged and has received instructions on home parenteral nutrition. When the nurse instructs the client to obtain and monitor a weekly weight, what goal of therapy is being addressed?

1. To maintain current weight
2. A weight gain of 0.2 kg (0.5 lb) per week
3. A weight gain of 0.9 kg (2 lb) per week
4. A monthly weight gain of 1.8 kg (4 lb)

7 Total parenteral nutrition (TPN) is being initiated on a client with malabsorption syndrome. Prior to starting the infusion, what nursing responsibilities should the nurse complete? Select all that apply.

1. Calculating the nutrients for an individualized formula
2. Obtaining the client's baseline weight
3. Performing an EKG on client prior to starting infusion
4. Checking for allergies to wheat
5. Confirming the availability of an electronic delivery device

8 Prior to hanging a total parenteral nutrition (TPN) solution, the nurse checks the content of the solution. Which ingredients should the nurse expect to be included? Select all that apply.

1. Trace minerals
2. NPH insulin
3. Electrolytes
4. ~~Diuretic~~
5. Multivitamin

reg insulin can be added
only reg

9 A client is receiving an infusion of TPN at 83 mL/hr. The infusion is stopped for 4 hours while the client is off the nursing unit. When the client returns, the standing order indicates the infusion should be restarted at a rate of 10% greater than the baseline rate. The infusion should be run at ______ mL/hour. Record your answer as a whole number.

Fill in your answer below:
91.3 mL/hr

10 The nurse is careful to ensure that a client's total parenteral nutrition (TPN) infusion is discontinued gradually. What complication should the nurse be aware of that this measure will prevent?

1. Refeeding syndrome
2. Hypovolemia
3. Hyponatremia
4. Rebound hypoglycemia

11 The nurse is preparing to hang the next scheduled bag of total parenteral nutrition (TPN) solution. What actions should the nurse perform prior to hanging the bag? Select all that apply.

1. Irrigate the intravenous port with heparin.
2. Remove solution from refrigerator 1 hour prior to hanging it.
3. Infuse 100 mL of normal saline to clear the intravenous line.
4. Have sterile gloves available for changing bags of solution.
5. Compare every ingredient with healthcare provider's order.

12 A client who will be receiving total parenteral nutrition (TPN) has a subclavian catheter inserted. What is the most important action by the nurse before beginning the infusion?

1. Obtain the client's baseline weight.
2. Confirm x-ray report of correct catheter placement.
3. Determine if the client is afebrile.
4. Check intake and output for the past 24 hours.

PRACTICE TEST

13 A client recovering from a multiple trauma is receiving continuous total parenteral nutrition (TPN) therapy while remaining on a regular diet. Which nursing action is most important when caring for this client?

1. Monitor blood glucose levels closely.
2. Assess urine output.
3. Encourage intake of high-protein foods.
4. Offer nutritional supplements at bedtime.

14 A client admitted with malnutrition has received total parenteral nutrition (TPN) for 2 weeks. What is the nurse's best evaluation for the effectiveness of the treatment?

1. Monitor recent blood glucose levels.
2. Check for recent weight gain.
3. Check prealbumin levels.
4. Evaluate skin turgor.

15 The nurse is assisting a new graduate nurse in the preparation of a continuous infusion of total parenteral nutrition (TPN) solution. The nurse explains that which action by the new graduate nurse is unnecessary?

1. Donning sterile gloves when connecting tubing to the solution bag
2. Attaching tubing that contains a micron filter to the solution bag
3. Checking solution for evidence of layering and cracking
4. Reviewing accuracy of ingredients of TPN solution

ANSWERS & RATIONALES

1 **Answer: 1, 2, 5 Rationale:** TPN contains a 20–50% glucose solution, which often causes hyperglycemia and is routinely regulated by giving regular insulin. The solution should be clear and homogenous without layering or cracking. Abnormally high levels may indicate problems with glucose or protein metabolism or excess lipids. TPN solutions are infused at a steady rate; strict input and output are monitored, but infusion rate is regulated only by a healthcare provider order. Injection caps are changed per institution protocol, usually every 72 hours. More frequent changes increase risk for bacterial contamination. **Cognitive Level:** Analysis **Client Need:** Pharmacological and Parenteral Therapies **Integrated Process:** Nursing Process: Implementation **Content Area:** Fundamentals **Strategy:** The question asks for nursing responsibilities and the wording of the question indicates the correct options are true statements. Consider each option as a true/false statement. Recall both the effects of TPN solution on the body and the nursing responsibilities associated with TPN therapy in order to answer this question correctly.

2 **Answer: 1 Rationale:** Magnesium, potassium, and phosphate levels may drop because magnesium (needed for ATP synthesis) and phosphorus (a component of ATP) are utilized rapidly as the TPN solution is metabolized, and potassium is taken up intracellularly in energy metabolism. Blood glucose is checked frequently but is not related to refeeding syndrome. Bowel sounds and level of consciousness would be part of a routine assessment but do not reflect refeeding syndrome. A client's level of consciousness should be assessed every shift and more often when appropriate. This assessment is not reflective of refeeding syndrome. **Cognitive Level:** Applying **Client Need:** Pharmacological and Parenteral Therapies **Integrated Process:** Nursing Process: Assessment **Content Area:** Fundamentals **Strategy:** The question requires specific knowledge of refeeding syndrome. Use the process of elimination to determine the correct answer.

3 **Answer: 3 Rationale:** TPN solutions contain hypertonic glucose (20–50%), which would cause severe irritation and phlebitis to a peripheral vein. Central veins are much larger, and the solution becomes diluted quickly. A rate of 150–200 mL/hr would provide excessive fluid volume and calories; typically TPN is started at 50 mL/hr and may be gradually increased to a maximum rate of 80–125 mL/hr. The infusion is of a high caloric content, but this fact does not explain why it must be given centrally. Peripheral sites do require more frequent changes, but frequency of changes does not influence the decision to use a central vein. **Cognitive Level:** Analysis **Client Need:** Pharmacological and Parenteral Therapies **Integrated Process:** Nursing Process: Diagnosis **Content Area:** Fundamentals **Strategy:** Recalling the effect of osmolarity on blood vessels is essential in answering this question; use this knowledge to select the correct answer.

4 **Answer: 1 Rationale:** TPN provides a readily available source of carbohydrates, fats, and proteins in order to restore or maintain positive nitrogen balance. Recovery from multiple trauma utilizes protein and fat stores, leading to a negative nitrogen balance. TPN helps to maintain urine output, but the primary purpose is to spare the body's own energy stores. TPN provides some hydration, but the primary purpose is to spare the body's own energy stores. Trace minerals are added to TPN solutions but are not the primary reason TPN solutions are used. **Cognitive Level:** Applying **Client Need:** Pharmacological and Parenteral Therapies **Integrated Process:** Nursing Process: Planning **Content Area:** Fundamentals **Strategy:** A key word in the question is *major*, indicating some or all of the options may be correct, but one is considered more important. Recognize the *major* purpose of TPN is to provide calories and nutrition. The correct answer is more global and pertains to the nutritional needs.

5 **Answer: 1 Rationale:** Inspiration into a deflated lung produces sharp chest pain as resistance to airflow is met and is a sign of a pneumothorax. Oxygenation would decrease as ventilation capacity is decreased, but this effect could be attributed to many factors and is not the best indicator of a pneumothorax. A red and swollen insertion site is a sign of irritation or infection. A rapid pulse is not a specific indicator of pneumothorax. **Cognitive Level:** Analyzing **Client Need:** Pharmacological and Parenteral Therapies **Integrated**

Process: Nursing Process: Assessment **Content Area:** Fundamentals **Strategy:** Note the question asks for the best answer, indicating one option is a better choice. Omit the options that could be symptomatic of many respiratory and cardiovascular problems. Select the correct answer through elimination.

6 **Answer: 3 Rationale:** A 0.9-kg (2-lb) weekly gain is the ideal weight gain when TPN is given to restore nutritional balance and improve weight. It demonstrates the treatment is effective. Maintenance of weight would be a goal if weight gain were not desired. Weight gains of 0.5 kg (1.1 lb) or less per week are less than desirable. A monthly weight gain of 1.8 kg (4 lb) is an average weekly gain of 0.5 kg (1.1 lb); weight gains of 0.5 kg (1.1 lb) or less per week is less than desirable. **Cognitive Level:** Applying **Client Need:** Pharmacological and Parenteral Therapies **Integrated Process:** Teaching and Learning **Content Area:** Fundamentals **Strategy:** Key words in the question are *weekly* and *desired goal*. Also note the client is receiving the TPN to improve weight. Use this information to select the correct answer.

7 **Answer: 2, 5 Rationale:** A baseline weight is needed to provide a foundation for clinical therapy and to assess response to treatment. There is no need to assess for an allergy to wheat. TPN administration needs to be carefully monitored to prevent fluid and nutrient overload; an electronic delivery device is necessary. A dietitian calculates the nutrients for an individualized formula. It is not necessary to have a baseline EKG. **Cognitive Level:** Applying **Client Need:** Pharmacological and Parenteral Therapies **Integrated Process:** Nursing Process: Implementation **Content Area:** Fundamentals **Strategy:** Recall the nurse's role in the administration and monitoring of TPN therapy. Use this information to eliminate the incorrect options and correctly answer the question. Consider each option as a true/false statement.

8 **Answer: 1, 3, 5 Rationale:** In addition to the base solution, TPN contains trace minerals, electrolytes, and multivitamins. Regular insulin may be added, but NPH cannot. If a diuretic was needed because of an underlying client condition, it would not be added to the TPN solution. **Cognitive Level:** Applying **Client Need:** Pharmacological and Parenteral Therapies **Integrated Process:** Nursing Process: Planning **Content Area:** Fundamentals **Strategy:** Specific knowledge regarding the content of TPN is needed to answer this question correctly. Consider each option as a true/false statement and systematically eliminate ingredients that you recognize as inappropriate.

9 **Answer: 91 Rationale:** If TPN infusion is interrupted, the nurse should not play "catch-up," but TPN can be safely restarted at up to 10% of the baseline rate with an appropriate order to help replace nutrients missed. **Cognitive Level:** Applying **Client Need:** Pharmacological and Parenteral Therapies **Integrated Process:** Nursing Process: Implementation **Content Area:** Fundamentals **Strategy:** Correctly calculate by multiplying the baseline rate of 83 by 10% to yield 8.3 mL. Next, add the 8.3 mL to the baseline rate of 83 mL/hr to yield 91.3 mL/hr. Round the 0.3 down to the nearest whole number, making the correct answer 91 mL/hour.

$83 \text{ mL} \times 10\%$
$83 \text{ mL} \times .10 = 8.3 \text{ mL}$
$83 \text{ mL} + 8.3 \text{ mL} = 91.3 \text{ mL}$

Calculate carefully and recheck your answer.

10 **Answer: 4 Rationale:** TPN should be gradually discontinued over a 24- to 48-hour period to allow for adjustment in metabolic function and prevent a sudden drop in blood glucose. Refeeding syndrome occurs when TPN is first initiated, and not at the time of discontinuing the therapy. Some level of hypovolemia may occur, but it is not as significant a risk as hypoglycemia. Hyponatremia is not as significant a risk as hypoglycemia. **Cognitive Level:** Analyzing **Client Need:** Pharmacological and Parenteral Therapies **Integrated Process:** Nursing Process: Diagnosis **Content Area:** Fundamentals **Strategy:** The question indicates the action should be done gradually, implying that abrupt withdrawal would have consequences. Consider each option in terms of what would occur if the solution were stopped suddenly.

11 **Answer: 2, 5 Rationale:** It is recommended that TPN be brought to room temperature before infusing to prevent client discomfort and lowering of body temperature. Every ingredient in the TPN must be compared to and validated by the healthcare provider's order; the pharmacy should be notified of discrepancies. It is not necessary to irrigate the IV line with heparin. It is not necessary to irrigate the IV line with saline. Bags should be changed using aseptic technique, but sterile gloves are not needed. **Cognitive Level:** Applying **Client Need:** Pharmacological and Parenteral Therapies **Integrated Process:** Nursing Process: Implementation **Content Area:** Fundamentals **Strategy:** Knowledge of nursing responsibilities related to TPN is necessary. Although protocols differ among institutions, the options are general and apply to basic principles. When there is more than one correct answer, consider each option as a true/false statement.

12 **Answer: 2 Rationale:** Confirmation of correct catheter placement is essential before TPN is started to ensure infusion will enter the superior vena cava. Obtaining a baseline weight is important, as is determining if the client is afebrile, but not of highest priority. Intake and output should be monitored once TPN is started. **Cognitive Level:** Analyzing **Client Need:** Pharmacological and Parenteral Therapies **Integrated Process:** Nursing Process: Planning **Content Area:** Fundamentals **Strategy:** The core concept in the question is identifying the action that must be taken before TPN therapy can be started, and the key word is *most*, indicating all or some of the options are important, but one has a higher priority. Analyze each option and select the one that is most critical.

13 **Answer: 1 Rationale:** The client is at greater risk for hyperglycemia because he or she is both receiving TPN and taking in additional calories on a regular diet. The other options are appropriate, but not of highest priority. **Cognitive Level:** Analyzing **Client Need:** Pharmacological and Parenteral Therapies **Integrated Process:** Nursing Process: Implementation **Content Area:** Fundamentals **Strategy:** Recall TPN solutions contain a high caloric content and, combined with another source of calories, will increase risk of hyperglycemia for client. The key word in the stem is *most*, since all of the options are correct.

14 **Answer: 3 Rationale:** Prealbumin levels are the best indicators of protein stores and nitrogen balance, reflecting the client's nutritional status. Checking blood glucose levels assesses for hypoglycemia and hyperglycemia, but is not appropriate for effectiveness of treatment. Assessment of weight gain is indicated but is not the best indicator of nutritional status because fluid retention may influence the weight gain. Skin turgor is a measure of hydration status. **Cognitive Level:** Analyzing **Client Need:** Pharmacological and Parenteral Therapies **Integrated Process:** Nursing Process: Evaluation **Content Area:** Fundamentals **Strategy:** The question asks that

you evaluate effectiveness of treatment. A key word is *best*, indicating that some or all options are partially correct. Eliminate options that don't measure an outcome of treatment and then select the option that is a more specific measurement.

15 **Answer: 1** **Rationale:** Aseptic technique is used when changing solution bags. Sterile gloves are not needed and would be contaminated as soon as the outside of the bag is touched. TPN requires use of a special micron filter. Solutions that are layered or cracked should not be used. The primary provider must order the content of TPN, based on the nutritional needs of the client. The nurse checks for accuracy of the TPN solution by comparing the contents with the current order. **Cognitive Level:** Analyzing **Client Need:** Pharmacological and Parenteral Therapies **Integrated Process:** Nursing Process: Diagnosis **Content Area:** Fundamentals **Strategy:** The word *unnecessary* is significant and indicates that three of the options are important or required for the task. Look for the option that represents a wrong answer.

Key Terms to Review

lipids p. 481

peripheral parenteral nutrition (PPN) p. 480

total parenteral nutrition (TPN) p. 480

References

Adams, M., Holland, L., & Urban, C. (2017). *Pharmacology for nurses: A pathophysiologic approach* (5th ed.). New York, NY: Pearson Education.

Adams, M., & Urban, C. (2016). *Pharmacology: Connections to nursing practice* (3rd ed.). New York, NY: Pearson Education.

Berman, A., Snyder, S., & Frandsen, G. (2016). *Kozier & Erb's fundamentals of nursing: Concepts, process, and practice* (10th ed.). New York, NY: Pearson Education.

LeMone, P., Burke, K., Bauldoff, G., & Gubrud, P. (2015). *Medical surgical nursing: Clinical reasoning in patient care* (6th ed.). Hoboken, NJ: Pearson Education.

Lewis, S., Dirksen, S., Heitkemper, M., & Bucher, L. (2014). *Medical surgical nursing: Assessment and management of clinical problems* (9th ed.). St. Louis, MO: Elsevier Science.

Smith, S., Duell, D., Martin, B., Aebersold, M., & Gonzalez, L. (2017). *Clinical nursing skills: Basic to advanced skills* (10th ed.). New York, NY: Pearson Education.

Test Yourself

Are you ready for the NCLEX-RN® or course exams? Access the NEW web-based app that provides students with thousands of practice questions in preparation for the NCLEX experience.

Maternal and Newborn Medications 34

In this chapter

Cross Reference

Other chapters relevant to this content area are

Reproduction, Family Planning, and Infertility	Chapter 8
Uncomplicated Antenatal Assessment and Care	Chapter 9
Uncomplicated Labor and Delivery Care	Chapter 10
Uncomplicated Postpartum Assessment and Care	Chapter 11
Uncomplicated Newborn Care	Chapter 12
Complicated Antenatal Care	Chapter 49
Complicated Labor and Delivery Care	Chapter 50
Complicated Postpartum Care	Chapter 51
Complicated Newborn Care	Chapter 52

I. OXYTOCIN

A. Overview

1. A uterine stimulant that increases frequency and force of uterine contractions or stimulates contractions with uterine inertia
2. Helps to augment labor in clients who are at term and induce labor in clients with maternal diabetes, preeclampsia, eclampsia, and erythroblastosis fetalis
3. Cervical changes are observable once active phase of labor is attained
4. Stimulates letdown reflex in breastfeeding mother and relieves pain from breast engorgement
5. Controls postpartum hemorrhage and promotes postpartum uterine involution
6. May be used to manage an incomplete abortion

B. Administration considerations

1. Dilute as ordered in IV solution and hang as a titratable IV drip, using an IV pump
2. Use normal saline as a primary line, with medication piggybacked at secondary port or stopcock
3. Monitor effects on contractions (frequency, duration, force) while titrating dosage
4. Nasal spray may be used to promote milk ejection
5. *NCLEX®* Keep magnesium sulfate (antidote) on hand for use if needed to relax uterus
6. *NCLEX®* Safety point: Do not confuse brand names Pitocin (oxytocin) with Pitressin (vasopressin)

C. Side/adverse effects

1. Maternal: rare and with IV use, causes more rapid, painful contractions from effects on uterine smooth muscle; also hypersensitivity, cardiac dysrhythmias, hypotension, hypertension if given following use of vasopressors, water intoxication (hyponatremia and hypochloremia), nausea and vomiting (N/V); uterine atony can occur after oxytocin is discontinued
2. Fetal: tachycardia; rare adverse effects include dysrhythmias, intracranial hemorrhage, hypoxia

D. Nursing considerations

1. Use flowsheet to record baseline maternal BP and other vital signs, weight, input and output (I&O), contractions (frequency, duration, strength), and fetal heart rate (FHR) and tones
2. Continue to monitor maternal pulse and BP, FHR, contractions, and resting uterine tone at least every 15 minutes
3. Record time oxytocin was initiated and any changes in dosage
4. *NCLEX®* Monitor for hypertonic contractions (less than 2 minutes apart, greater than 90 seconds long, and about 50 mm Hg in strength), and shut off IV drip if uterine hyperstimulation or nonreassuring FHR occurs; turn client onto left side, increase rate of normal saline IV, and apply oxygen via facemask
5. Effects of drug will diminish 2–3 minutes after discontinuing oxytocin; assess for uterine atony and possible postpartum hemorrhage
6. Watch for hypertensive crisis in clients also receiving local or regional anesthesia (caudal, spinal); signs include sudden onset of intense occipital headache, palpitations, hypertension, stiff neck, N/V, fever and sweating, photophobia and dilated pupils, constricting chest pain, and bradycardia or tachycardia
7. *NCLEX®* Monitor I&O; report signs of water intoxication (drowsiness, headache, confusion, anuria, weight gain); report decreasing urine output with adequate intake
8. Keep emergency resuscitation equipment available

E. Client teaching

1. Purpose and effect of medication
2. Importance of reporting sudden, severe headache immediately

II. ERGOT ALKALOIDS

A. Overview

1. Used to control postpartum or postabortal hemorrhage; should not be used before delivery of placenta
2. Stimulates uterine muscle to produce firm tetanic contractions and increases frequency of contractions
3. *NCLEX®* Produce arterial vasoconstriction and possible vasospasm of coronary arteries
4. Common ergot alkaloid medications are listed in Box 34–1

B. Administration considerations: causes rebound uterine relaxation

C. Side/adverse effects

1. *NCLEX®* Contraindicated in pregnancy or hypersensitivity to ergot, hypertension
2. Should be used cautiously in unstable angina and recent myocardial infarction
3. Significant increase in systolic and diastolic BP, cardiac dysrhythmias
4. Uterine cramping
5. Decreased milk production
6. *NCLEX®* **Ergotism** or overdose: N/V, weakness, muscle pain, insensitivity to cold, paresthesia of extremities

Box 34–1	
Ergot Alkaloids	Ergonovine Methylergonovine

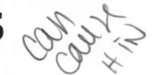

D. Nursing considerations

1. Closely monitor BP after administration; if hypertension noted, withhold dose and notify prescriber
2. Monitor lochia and uterine contractions (strength, duration, and frequency) after administration
3. *NCLEX®* Assess and report as indicated hypertension, chest pain, ergotism, or hypersensitivity (shortness of breath, itching)
4. Administer analgesics as needed to control pain of uterine contractions caused by ergot

E. Client teaching

1. Indication for administration
2. Route of administration (oral, IM, possible IV in emergency) and possible side effects, such as cramping
3. Report increased blood loss, increased temperature, or foul-smelling lochia
4. *NCLEX®* Perform pad count to monitor bleeding
5. Do not smoke because of increased/additive vasoconstriction with ergonovine use

III. PROSTAGLANDINS

terminate preg, promote delivery

A. Overview

1. **Prostaglandins** terminate pregnancy from 12th week through second trimester (Table 34–1); can also be used to stimulate myometrium and ripen cervix to promote delivery
2. Dinoprostone has FDA approval only for cervical ripening (softening, dilating, and effacing) prior to labor induction; available as a gel
3. Carboprost tromethamine has FDA approval for control of postpartum bleeding unresponsive to oxytocin and for inducing abortion at 13–20 weeks' gestation
4. Misoprostol (a synthetic analog of prostaglandin E1) is used off-label for pharmacological abortion, cervical ripening, and control of postpartum bleeding

B. Administration considerations

1. *NCLEX®* Client should remain supine for 20–30 minutes after receiving dinoprostone
2. Before dinoprostone, client should receive antiemetic and antidiarrheal medications

C. Side/adverse effects

1. *NCLEX®* Diarrhea, N/V, stomach cramping, possible increase in BP
2. Uterine cramping and possible uterine rupture
3. Tension headache, fever, chills, flushing, cardiac dysrhythmias, hypertension
4. Uterine tetany may develop with prelabor or intrapartum administration
5. Contraindicated with acute pelvic inflammatory disease, placenta previa or unexplained vaginal bleeding, fetal malpresentation or nonreassuring FHR pattern; use cautiously in hypertension and with history of asthma

D. Nursing considerations

1. *NCLEX®* Prenatal: obtain baseline maternal VS, FHR pattern, and Bishop score; have client void before drug administration
2. Have client lie supine with lateral tilting or lie on side for 30–60 minutes (gel) or 2 hours (vaginal insert) after administration
3. Prepare to discontinue treatment as prescribed for Bishop score of 8 (ripened cervix), presence of three or more contractions every 10 minutes (effective labor pattern), or occurrence of adverse effects
4. If labor augmentation is needed, oxytocin may be used 6–12 hours after termination of prostaglandin therapy
5. *NCLEX®* Postpartum: monitor lochia and BP, be prepared for client to develop diarrhea

E. Client teaching

1. Prenatal: report long or continuous contractions, as uterine tetany may develop; count fetal movement as an indicator of fetal well-being
2. Postpartum: prepare client for route of administration and possible side effects

Table 34–1 Common Prostaglandins

Category	Generic (Trade Name)	Route	Indications for Use
Prostaglandin E2	Dinoprostone	Intracervical gel or vaginal insert	Ripen cervix prior to induction of labor or abort fetus that has died
Prostaglandin F2	Carboprost tromethamine	IM	Postpartum hemorrhage

Table 34–2 Common Uterine Relaxant Medications

Generic Name	Notes
Terbutaline sulfate	Not FDA-approved for preterm labor but commonly used
Nifedipine	Not FDA-approved for preterm labor but commonly used
Magnesium sulfate	Not FDA-approved for preterm labor but commonly used

IV. TOCOLYTICS (UTERINE RELAXANTS)

A. Overview

1. Inhibit contractions and arrest preterm labor for 24–72 hours so that corticosteroids (betamethasone) can be given to facilitate fetal lung maturity
2. Used to stop contractions to allow intrauterine fetal resuscitation when uterine hyperstimulation is present
3. Common uterine relaxant medications (Table 34–2)

B. Administration considerations

1. Start at lowest possible dose and increase as indicated until contractions cease
2. If GI symptoms occur, advise client to take oral medication with food
3. Dilute IV terbutaline in prescribed IV solution and use an infusion pump for administration

C. Side/adverse effects

NCLEX®
1. Beta-adrenergics: maternal and fetal tachycardia, palpitations, tremors, jitteriness and anxiety, pulmonary edema
2. Nifedipine may cause or exacerbate constipation
3. Nausea and vomiting
4. Contraindicated with maternal eclampsia or severe preeclampsia, intrauterine infection, active vaginal bleeding, cardiac disease, or cervical dilation more than 4 cm; also contraindicated with fetal gestational age over 37 weeks, fetal demise or lethal anomalies, fetal distress, or chronic intrauterine growth restriction

D. Nursing considerations

1. Position client on left side (enhances placental perfusion, reduces pressure on cervix)
2. Assess vital signs, I&O, fetal status, and status of labor per agency protocols
3. If mother uses terbutaline during pregnancy, monitor neonate for hypoglycemia
4. Nifedipine: avoid grapefruit juice during administration (interferes with effect)

E. Client teaching

1. Possible side effects and coping strategies
2. Use and dose of oral medications and importance of taking them on time
3. NCLEX® Nifedipine: encourage client to change position slowly due to possible orthostatic hypotension
4. Teach how to self-monitor pulse
5. Importance of consulting healthcare provider prior to taking over-the-counter (OTC) medications

V. MAGNESIUM SULFATE

A. Overview

1. When given parenterally, acts as central nervous system (CNS) depressant and also depresses smooth, skeletal, and cardiac muscle function
2. Used to arrest preterm labor (common off-label use) and to prevent or to treat seizures with preeclampsia and eclampsia

B. Administration considerations

1. Use in conjunction with beta-adrenergics increases risk of pulmonary edema
2. Administer using an infusion pump; a loading dose may be given over 20–30 minutes
3. Continuous IV infusion should not be used for 2 hours prior to delivery; IV infusion increases risk of newborn magnesium toxicity
4. When used for preeclampsia, may be prescribed for 12–24 hours postpartum

C. Side/adverse effects

1. NCLEX® Respiratory depression leading to respiratory arrest
2. NCLEX® Decreased or absent deep tendon reflexes and muscle weakness
3. Decreased urine output, pulmonary edema, and hyponatremia

4. Nausea and vomiting
5. Contraindicated in pulmonary edema, heart block, heart failure, and renal failure; use cautiously with severe renal disease

D. **Nursing considerations**

NCLEX® 1. Check patellar reflex prior to initial dose and any subsequent doses; depressed reflex could indicate risk for respiratory arrest

NCLEX® 2. Monitor hand grasps and deep tendon reflexes hourly for signs of toxicity

3. Monitor vital signs every 30–60 minutes, especially respiratory rate (needs to be 16/min or greater for additional doses to be safe)

NCLEX® 4. Call prescriber for respiratory depression if respirations less than 12/minute

NCLEX® 5. Ensure that calcium gluconate (antidote) is available at bedside

NCLEX® 6. IV infusion flow rate is generally adjusted to maintain urine flow of at least 30–50 mL/hour, monitor I&O hourly; be certain to use infusion pump

7. Monitor IV site closely to avoid extravasation
8. Monitor serum magnesium levels for target range of 4–7.5 mEq/L and call prescriber if greater than 7 mEq
9. Measure daily weight accurately

E. **Client teaching**

1. Side effects of medication
2. Report signs of preeclampsia, including headache, epigastric pain, and visual disturbance
3. Report any signs of confusion

VI. ANALGESICS

A. **Overview (Box 34–2)**

1. Used to manage moderate to severe pain of labor
2. Common opioid agonist analgesic is fentanyl; less common is meperidine
3. Common opioid agonist-antagonists are butorphanol tartrate and nalbuphine
4. Epidural or intrathecal opioid agents commonly include fentanyl and sufentanil; sufentanil should be used in combination with low-dose bupivacaine if by epidural route

NCLEX® 5. Antidote to opioids is naloxone

B. **Administration considerations**

1. Do not administer in early labor because it could slow labor
2. Birth should occur more than 4 hours or less than 1 hour after dose of meperidine to minimize neonatal CNS depression
3. Agonist-antagonists provide adequate analgesia, less respiratory depression and N/V, but equal or greater sedation when compared to meperidine

NCLEX® 4. Do not use agonist-antagonists for women with opioid dependence because antagonist activity could precipitate withdrawal (abstinence) symptoms in mother and neonate (irritability, hyperactive reflexes, tremors, seizures, yawning, sneezing, vomiting, and diarrhea; excessive crying in neonate)

C. **Side/adverse effects**

1. Meperidine, hydromorphone, fentanyl, and sufentanil: N/V, sedation, drowsiness or confusion, tachycardia or bradycardia, hypotension, dry mouth, urinary retention, pruritis, respiratory depression
2. Butorphanol or nalbuphine: confusion, sedation, N/V, sweating; respiratory depression less likely to occur

D. **Nursing considerations**

1. Meperidine, hydromorphone, fentanyl, and sufentanil
   a. Monitor FHR and uterine contractions
   b. Assess for respiratory depression less than 12 breaths/minute

NCLEX® c. Assess newborn for respiratory depression if born within 1–4 hours of dose

Box 34–2

Analgesics during Labor

Opioid Agonists	Opioid Agonist-Antagonists
Meperidine	Butorphanol
Hydromorphone	Nalbuphine
Fentanyl and sufentanil	

d. Keep naloxone available as antidote; note, naloxone will also lead to withdrawal symptoms in an opioid-dependent client
e. Keep siderails raised per agency protocol for safety
f. Supplement pain relief using nonpharmacological methods, such as deep breathing and imagery
g. Monitor urine output (risk of urinary retention)

2. Butorphanol or nalbuphine
   a. Similar to opioid analgesics
   b. Watch for withdrawal symptoms if administered to opioid-dependent women and neonates
3. For all medications, monitor reduction in pain

E. Client teaching

1. Purpose and expected effects of medication
2. Use of nonpharmacological pain relief measures

VII. RH_0(D) IMMUNE GLOBULIN

A. Overview

1. Prevents anti-Rh_0(D) antibody formation (isoimmunization) in Rh-negative women
2. Used when there is potential or actual exposure to Rh-positive blood: pregnancy, labor and delivery, amniocentesis, chorionic villus sampling, termination of pregnancy, abdominal trauma, or transfusion

B. Administration considerations

1. *NCLEX®* Administer within 72 hours of potential or actual exposure to Rh-positive blood
2. *NCLEX®* Readminister with each subsequent possible or actual exposure
3. Do not administer if client has developed positive antibody titer to Rh antigen
4. *NCLEX®* In typical pregnancy, administer at 28 weeks' gestation and within 72 hours of delivery
5. Do not administer to newborn infant

C. Side/adverse effects

1. Tenderness at injection site and slight elevation in temperature
2. *NCLEX®* Contraindicated with hypersensitivity to human immunoglobulins and in Rh-positive women

D. Nursing considerations: administer as described previously

E. Client teaching: purpose and effects of medication and need for repeat injections with subsequent pregnancies

VIII. BETAMETHASONE

A. Overview

1. Synthetic glucocorticoid (corticosteroid) that increases surfactant production to accelerate maturation of fetal lungs
2. *NCLEX®* Prevention of neonatal respiratory distress syndrome (RDS) as an unlabeled use

B. Administration considerations

1. Administered to a client in preterm labor between 28 and 32 weeks' gestation
2. *NCLEX®* Used if client and fetus can safely tolerate inhibition of labor for 48 hours
3. Administer as once-daily dose IM

C. Side/adverse effects

1. Contraindicated during lactation
2. Similar to other corticosteroids, such as risk for infection, delayed wound healing, hyperglycemia in a mother with diabetes mellitus, and pulmonary edema because of sodium and water retention

D. Nursing considerations

1. Monitor maternal vital signs, lung sounds, I&O, and fetal well-being
2. Monitor for increased temperature and WBCs as general indicators of infection; monitor blood glucose levels to detect hyperglycemia

E. Client teaching: purpose and intended effects of medication to parents

IX. LUNG SURFACTANTS

A. Overview

1. **Surfactant** lowers surface tension on alveolar surfaces during respiration, which improves gas exchange
2. Stabilizes alveoli against collapse at resting pressures
3. *NCLEX®* Beractant and calfactant are common surfactants to prevent or treat RDS in premature infants

B. Administration considerations

1. Given by intratracheal route via endotracheal tube every 4–6 hours until condition improves
2. Do not suction within 2 hours after dose unless significant airway obstruction occurs

C. Side/adverse effects

1. Oxygen desaturation and transient bradycardia; possible mucus plug development or pulmonary hemorrhage
2. Crackles and moist breath sounds occur transiently after dose; does not necessarily indicate suctioning is needed

D. Nursing considerations

1. Ensure proper endotracheal tube placement prior to dosing
2. Monitor heart rate, lung sounds, chest expansion, facial expression during administration
3. Monitor oxygen saturation and periodically assess arterial or transcutaneous oxygen and CO_2 levels

E. Client teaching: purpose and intended effects of medication to parents

X. PHYTONADIONE OR VITAMIN K_1

A. Overview

1. Fat-soluble vitamin that aids synthesis of clotting factors II, VII, IX, and X in immature newborn liver
2. Prevents and treats hemorrhagic disease of newborn until neonate has intestinal flora to absorb vitamin K from GI tract

B. Administration considerations

NCLEX®
1. Administer IM in vastus lateralis thigh muscle (lateral aspect, middle third), often within 1 hour of birth but may be delayed until after first breastfeeding in birthing area
2. Protect from light
3. Be sure to give prior to circumcision procedure

C. Side/adverse effects: hyperbilirubinemia, bleeding on second or third day

D. Nursing considerations

1. Monitor for signs of bleeding, such as bruising at injection site, bleeding from umbilical cord, nose, or GI tract

NCLEX®
2. Assess for jaundice and monitor results of bilirubin levels to detect hyperbilirubinemia

E. Client teaching: purpose and intended effects of medication to parents

XI. NEONATAL EYE PROPHYLAXIS

A. Overview

1. Mandated by law for prophylaxis against ophthalmic neonatorum (caused by *Neisseria gonorrhoeae* and *Chlamydia trachomatis*), which could be transmitted to neonate during birth
2. Common agent is erythromycin ophthalmic ointment 0.5%

B. Administration considerations

NCLEX®
1. Apply up to but within 1 hour of delivery (allow time for eye contact that promotes parent–infant bonding)
2. Cleanse eyes before application of dose
3. Administer 1 cm ribbon of ointment along each lower conjunctival sac, from inner canthus to outer canthus
4. Gently close eye and manipulate to ensure spread of ointment
5. Do not rinse eyes following dose, but may wipe away excess after 1 minute with sterile cotton
6. Use a new tube of ointment for each neonate

C. Side/adverse effects: blurring of vision possible after application of ointment, sensitivity reaction may cause edema and inflammation of eyes, which subsides in 24–48 hours

D. Nursing considerations: as noted previously

E. Client teaching: purpose and effects of medication to parents

XII. SELECTED POSTPARTUM/NEWBORN VACCINES

A. Rubella vaccine (maternal)

1. Indicated for nonimmune postpartum clients who have a rubella titer less than 1:8
2. Should be administered before discharge by subcutaneous route
3. Side/adverse effects include hypersensitivity and transient rash
4. Contraindicated if client has an allergy to eggs

NCLEX®
5. Should not be administered if client or family members with whom client resides have an immunocompromised state

NCLEX®
6. Client should use contraception and avoid pregnancy for 1–3 months or as prescribed following rubella immunization

B. Hepatitis B vaccine

1. Recommended for all newborns, with first dose administered IM before newborn is discharged from birthing center
2. Obtain parental consent beforehand
3. Administer IM in vastus lateralis thigh muscle (lateral aspect, middle third)
4. If mother is positive for hepatitis B surface antigen, newborn should also received hepatitis B immune globulin within 12 hours of birth
5. Document administration on vaccination card provided to parents; this will be needed as hepatitis B series continues

Check Your NCLEX–RN® Exam I.Q.

You are ready for testing on this content if you can:

- Apply knowledge of expected actions and effects of maternal and newborn medications to client care.
- Correctly administer maternal and newborn medications to clients.
- Assess for side effects and adverse effects of maternal and newborn medications.
- Take appropriate action if a client has an unexpected response to a maternal or newborn medication.
- Monitor a client for expected outcomes or effects of treatment with maternal or newborn medications.

PRACTICE TEST

1 What should the nurse anticipate being included in the therapeutic plan of care for a postpartum client with subinvolution?

1. Oral methylergonovine maleate
2. Oxytocin IV infusion for 8 hours
3. Oral fluids to 3000 mL per day
4. Blood replacement

2 In which postpartum client should the nurse conclude that methylergonovine maleate is contraindicated?

1. A client with a blood pressure of 120/60
2. A client with a heart rate of 60
3. A client with a blood pressure of 140/100
4. A client with a respiratory rate of 12

3 A postpartum client has an epidural catheter in place following delivery of an infant via cesarean section. The nurse determines that which medication is a priority to have on hand for use if needed?

1. Meperidine hydrochloride
2. Betamethasone
3. Carboprost
4. Naloxone

4 The nurse is monitoring a client in labor who is receiving oxytocin as a continuous infusion to augment labor. What observations of the client would indicate to the nurse that the infusion needs to be stopped? Select all that apply.

1. Contractions lasting 120 seconds
2. Maternal blood pressure increase from 124/82 to 130/86
3. Early fetal heart rate decelerations on the fetal monitor
4. The mother squeezing her eyes shut during each contraction
5. Development of nausea and vomiting

5 The nurse is evaluating the status of a pregnant client receiving magnesium sulfate. What manifestation should indicate to the nurse that the medication is having the intended effect?

1. BP has stabilized at 128/76.
2. Serum magnesium level reaches 2.2 mEq/L.
3. Contractions are steady at a frequency of every 4 minutes.
4. There is an absence of seizure activity.

6 The nurse notes that the newly postpartum client is Rh-negative and her baby is Rh-positive. Which maternal laboratory result would be important to interpret next in determining if the client is a candidate for $Rh_0(D)$ immune globulin?

1. Hemoglobin level
2. Direct Coombs' test
3. Indirect Coombs' test
4. Bilirubin level

7 In addition to routine assessment and care, nursing care of the client who is receiving terbutaline to prevent premature labor should include assessing for what indicator of an adverse drug effect?

1. Oral temperature every 2 hours
2. Fetal heart tones every 30 minutes
3. Breath sounds every 4 hours
4. Deep tendon reflexes every 4 hours

8 A client in premature labor is scheduled to receive a dose of betamethasone. In teaching the client about this medication, how should the nurse explain the purpose and expected action of the medication?

1. Stops uterine contractions
2. Prevents infection
3. Hastens fetal lung maturity
4. Prevents cervical dilatation

9 The nurse is preparing to administer an intramuscular injection of phytonadione to a healthy newborn. What is the best explanation for the nurse to give the neonate's mother regarding the medication?

1. "This medication is specifically used to treat hemorrhagic disease of the newborn."
2. "This medication supplies vitamin K, which the newborn cannot produce in the first 5–8 days of life."
3. "This medication is a multivitamin that has many effects, including helping to produce prothrombin in the blood."
4. "This medication is also known as vitamin K, and it is a water-soluble vitamin that is deficient in newborns."

10 The nurse is caring for a newborn 30 minutes after birth. What should the nurse do when administering a prescribed dose of ophthalmic erythromycin? Select all that apply.

1. Withhold the dose for 2 hours to allow for parent–infant bonding.
2. Administer the dose across each lower conjunctival sac.
3. Irrigate the eyes after the dose to flush out microorganisms.
4. Use a new tube of ointment for the prescribed dose.
5. Explain to the mother that the medication will cause infant eye irritation.

11 The laboratory test results for a 24-week prenatal client indicate that the client does not have immunity to German measles. What notation should the nurse include in the plan of care?

1. $Rh_0(D)$ immune globulin will be given at the next visit.
2. $Rh_0(D)$ immune globulin will be administered within 2 days of delivery.
3. Rubella vaccine will be prescribed for the next visit.
4. Rubella vaccine will be provided after delivery on the day of discharge.

12 A breastfeeding mother and her newborn are to be discharged from the postpartum unit. The client has no immunity to rubella, and is prescribed to receive rubella vaccine on the day of discharge. What is the most important instruction for the nurse to include in the discharge plan? Select all that apply.

1. Utilize a reliable method of contraception.
2. Continue to breastfeed the newborn.
3. Avoid public outings for 2 weeks due to contagious period.
4. Have the infant screened for active rubella virus at the 2-month checkup.
5. Avoid becoming pregnant for at least 6 months.

13 A primigravida with blood type A-negative is at 28 weeks' gestation. Today, the client is to receive a prescribed $Rh_0(D)$ immune globulin injection. Which statement by the client demonstrates to the nurse that more teaching is needed related to this therapy?

1. "I'm getting this shot so that my baby won't develop antibodies against my blood, right?"
2. "I understand that if my baby is Rh-positive, I'll be getting another one of these injections."
3. "This shot will prevent me from becoming sensitized to Rh-positive blood."
4. "This shot should help to protect me in future pregnancies if this baby is Rh-positive like my husband."

PRACTICE TEST

14 A pregnant woman is having an exacerbation of asthma. What factor is most important for the nurse to consider in delivering aerosol medication?

1. Aerosol medication is used instead of postural drainage.
2. The droplets produced should be large enough to dilate the bronchioles.
3. The aerosol delivers medication to the lower respiratory tract.
4. Aerosol medications are contraindicated in pregnancy.

15 What explanation should the nurse give to a new nurse about the reason that phytonadione is administered to the neonate? Select all that apply.

1. It prevents the neonate from acquiring maternal gonorrhea.
2. It inhibits the production of prothrombin by the liver.
3. The neonate lacks the intestinal flora for vitamin K production.
4. The neonate cannot absorb vitamin K from the gastrointestinal tract.
5. Administration of phytonadione to a neonate is state law.

16 A pregnant client is receiving magnesium sulfate. What should the nurse evaluate as a sign of excessive blood levels of the drug?

1. Development of seizures
2. Disappearance of the knee-jerk reflex
3. Increase in respiratory rate
4. Increase in blood pressure

17 After receiving magnesium sulfate, a pregnant client develops signs of toxicity. What should the nurse be prepared to administer?

1. Oxygen
2. Epinephrine
3. Potassium chloride
4. Calcium gluconate

18 Before administering IV magnesium sulfate therapy to a client with preeclampsia, which set of parameters should the nurse consider as the highest priority?

1. Urinary glucose, acetone, and specific gravity
2. Temperature, blood pressure, and respirations
3. Urinary output, respirations, and patellar reflexes
4. Level of consciousness, funduscopic appearance, and knee reflex

19 A client with preeclampsia is receiving magnesium sulfate. For what effect should the nurse observe the client during administration of the drug?

1. Dry, pale skin
2. Hyporeflexia
3. Agitation
4. Increased respirations

20 A client in active labor is to have an epidural block. While this is being administered, what nursing action takes priority?

1. Checking the uterine contractions for an increase in strength
2. Positioning the mother flat in bed to avoid postspinal headache
3. Telling the mother she will feel the need to void more frequently
4. Monitoring maternal blood pressure for possible hypotension

21 A client is receiving magnesium sulfate for severe preeclampsia. What nursing actions are appropriate interventions? Select all that apply.

1. Limit fluid intake to 1000 mL/24 hours.
2. Prepare for the possibility of a precipitate delivery.
3. Restrict visitors and keep the room darkened and quiet.
4. Obtain calcium gluconate for use as an antagonist if necessary.
5. Assess for patellar reflexes.

ANSWERS & RATIONALES

1 **Answer: 1 Rationale:** Methylergonovine provides long-sustained uterine contraction. It is commonly used to treat late postpartum hemorrhage (subinvolution). Oxytocin and prostaglandin are more frequently used to treat early postpartum hemorrhage caused by uterine atony. Increased fluid intake is a general, helpful measure for any client who has lost body fluid volume, but it is not a specific therapy. When blood products are used, they are generally ordered for early postpartum hemorrhage. **Cognitive Level:** Applying **Client Need:** Pharmacological and Parenteral Therapies **Integrated Process:** Nursing Process: Planning **Content Area:** Maternal–Newborn **Strategy:** Specific knowledge of methylergonovine is needed to answer this question. Use medication knowledge and the process of elimination to make your selection.

2 **Answer: 3 Rationale:** Ergonovine has a side effect of raising blood pressure. A woman with hypertension or gestational hypertension would not be a good candidate for use of ergonovine. This client has a normal blood pressure, which is not a contraindication for prescribing ergonovine. A pulse of 60 is not a contraindication to use of ergonovine. A respiratory rate of 12 is not a contraindication to use of ergonovine. **Cognitive Level:** Analyzing **Client Need:** Pharmacological and Parenteral Therapies **Integrated Process:** Nursing Process: Planning **Content Area:** Pharmacology **Strategy:** Specific knowledge of ergonovine maleate is needed to answer this question. Use nursing knowledge and the process of elimination to make your selection.

3 **Answer: 4 Rationale:** Naloxone is the antidote to the opioid analgesics that are used with epidural analgesia. If respiratory depression occurs, this medication needs to be readily available for use. Meperidine is an opioid analgesic, but is not used for epidural analgesia. Betamethasone is a glucocorticoid used to enhance fetal lung maturity before premature delivery. Carboprost is a prostaglandin for cervical ripening. **Cognitive Level:** Analyzing **Client Need:** Pharmacological and Parenteral Therapies **Integrated Process:** Nursing Process: Planning **Content Area:** Pharmacology **Strategy:** The core issue of the question is a priority medication to have on hand during epidural analgesia. Use the process of elimination to select the antidote needed for respiratory depression, a priority adverse effect of epidural analgesia.

4 **Answer: 1, 5 Rationale:** Contractions lasting longer than 90 seconds indicate uterine hyperstimulation, which is a reason to stop the oxytocin infusion. Nausea and vomiting is an adverse effect related to the use of oxytocin, and a reason to stop the administration of the medication. The increase in blood pressure is not significant enough to be of concern. Early decelerations of fetal heart rate do not indicate fetal distress; rather, they are a reassuring sign. Squeezing the eyes shut during contractions could have variable meanings, including coping with the contraction, and needs to be correlated with other client data for proper interpretation. **Cognitive Level:** Analyzing **Client Need:** Pharmacological and Parenteral Therapies **Integrated Process:** Nursing Process: Assessment **Content Area:** Pharmacology **Strategy:** The core issues of the question are knowledge of adverse effects of oxytocin and how to recognize them in the woman in labor. When there is more than one correct answer to a question, consider each option as a true/false statement.

5 **Answer: 4 Rationale:** The danger of preeclampsia is that it can progress to eclampsia, characterized by seizure activity. Magnesium sulfate is given to prevent seizures. Magnesium sulfate would not be given when the BP has stabilized at 128/72, when serum magnesium level reaches 2.2 mEq/L, or when contractions are steady at every 4 minutes. **Cognitive Level:** Analyzing **Client Need:** Pharmacological and Parenteral Therapies **Integrated Process:** Nursing Process: Evaluation **Content Area:** Pharmacology **Strategy:** The core issue of the question is the action of magnesium sulfate in a client with preeclampsia. Use drug knowledge and the process of elimination to make a selection.

6 **Answer: 3 Rationale:** An indirect Coombs' test assesses for the presence of Rh antibodies in maternal blood, an indication that the mother is a candidate for Rh_0(D) immune globulin. Hemoglobin is not a determinant for the administration of Rh_0(D) immune globulin. Direct Coombs' test and bilirubin tests are conducted on the newborn. **Cognitive Level:** Analyzing **Client Need:** Pharmacological and Parenteral Therapies **Integrated Process:** Nursing Process: Diagnosis **Content Area:** Pharmacology **Strategy:** The core issue of the question is the laboratory indicator that signals the need for administration of Rh_0(D) immune globulin. Specific knowledge of this drug is needed to answer this question. Use the process of elimination.

7 **Answer: 3 Rationale:** Terbutaline, a beta-adrenergic agent, has many maternal and fetal side effects, including tachycardia, cardiac arryhthmias, and pulmonary edema. In addition to taking routine vital signs, the nurse should assess for pulmonary edema. The frequency of assessment of oral temperature depends on the intensity and length of the drug therapy, as well as surrounding circumstances. The frequency of assessment of fetal heart tones and oral temperature depends on the intensity and length of the drug therapy, as well as surrounding circumstances. Deep-tendon reflex assessment is not indicated. **Cognitive Level:** Analysis **Client Need:** Pharmacological and Parenteral Therapies **Integrated Process:** Nursing Process: Assessment **Content Area:** Pharmacology **Strategy:** The core issue of the question is knowledge that terbutaline is a beta-adrenergic drug that can lead to adverse effects, including pulmonary edema. Use the ABCs to help focus on breathing and respiratory assessment.

8 **Answer: 3 Rationale:** Corticosteroids such as betamethasone have been shown to enhance fetal lung maturity and prevent respiratory distress. Betamethasone does not stop labor. A side effect of betamethasone is an increased risk of infection. Betamethasone does not stop cervical changes. **Cognitive Level:** Applying **Client Need:** Pharmacological and Parenteral Therapies **Integrated Process:** Nursing Process: Implementation **Content Area:** Pharmacology **Strategy:** Specific medication knowledge is needed to answer the question. Recall that a drug ending in *-sone* is likely to be a steroid, and this hastens lung maturity in the fetus at risk for premature delivery.

9 **Answer: 2 Rationale:** Phytonadione is given to supply vitamin K, which the newborn cannot produce in the early days of life because of lack of the intestinal flora needed to

synthesize it. Although phytonadione does treat hemorrhagic disease of the newborn, its use in the healthy infant is prophylactic. Phytonadione is given to supply vitamin K; the medication is not a multivitamin. Phytonadione is not water-soluble, it is fat-soluble. **Cognitive Level:** Analyzing **Client Need:** Pharmacological and Parenteral Therapies **Integrated Process:** Communication and Documentation **Content Area:** Pharmacology **Strategy:** Note the critical word *best* in the stem of the question, which tells you that more than one or all answers might be factually correct. Note also the critical word *healthy*, which eliminates the option pertaining to disease.

10 **Answer: 2, 4 Rationale:** The nurse would give the ophthalmic dose by applying a 0.5–1 cm ribbon of ointment into each lower conjunctival sac. To prevent a possible contamination, a new tube is used for each newborn. The dose can be delayed up to an hour after birth, but not 2 hours. The eyes are not cleansed or irrigated after the dose. Ophthalmic erythromycin does not cause eye irritation; the previously used silver nitrate (1%) solution caused eye irritation in the neonate. **Cognitive Level:** Applying **Client Need:** Pharmacological and Parenteral Therapies **Integrated Process:** Nursing Process: Implementation **Content Area:** Pharmacology **Strategy:** Use the process of elimination, keeping in mind principles of aseptic technique and standard procedure for administration of eye medications. When more than one answer is correct, consider each option as a true/false statement.

11 **Answer: 4 Rationale:** German measles is also termed rubella. Pregnant women are tested at their first prenatal visit for immunity to rubella. If the client is found to be nonimmune, immunization will be given after delivery, before discharge. $Rh_0(D)$ immune globulin would not be given. **Cognitive Level:** Applying **Client Need:** Pharmacological and Parenteral Therapies **Integrated Process:** Communication and Documentation **Content Area:** Pharmacology **Strategy:** Look for key differences in the answers. Here we have rubella and Rh isoimmunization, both of which are tested during pregnancy. Rh isoimmunization is prevented by giving $Rh_0(D)$ immune globulin at 28 weeks and again after delivery if the baby is found to be Rh-positive, Coombs'-negative. Rubella vaccine is not given during pregnancy.

12 **Answer: 1, 2 Rationale:** The rubella vaccine is prepared with a live virus; therefore, it is not appropriate to administer during pregnancy. Clients are counseled to avoid pregnancy for 3 months after immunization. It is not necessary for the mother to stop breastfeeding the newborn after receiving a rubella vaccine. Rubella vaccine does not cause the recipient to become contagious; this is an unnecessary action. Rubella vaccine, given to the mother, does not place the infant at risk for acquiring the disease. After receiving a rubella vaccine, pregnancy should be avoided for 2–3 months. **Cognitive Level:** Analyzing **Client Need:** Pharmacological and Parenteral Therapies **Integrated Process:** Nursing Process: Planning **Content Area:** Pharmacology **Strategy:** Knowledge of immunizations is critical to planning care for clients. Rubella vaccine is a live-virus vaccine, and therefore pregnancy should be avoided while immunity is formed. When there is more than one correct answer, consider each option as a true/false statement.

13 **Answer: 1 Rationale:** This client statement indicates that she does not understand the fundamental indications for treatment of this potential blood incompatibility. If the infant is found to be Rh-positive, the client will be given $Rh_0(D)$ immune globulin within 72 hours of delivery to block any antigen–antibody formation. If an Rh-negative client is carrying an Rh-positive infant, the potential for mixing of fetal blood into the maternal system could occur at midpregnancy and at delivery of the placenta. This client statement indicates that she does understand the fundamental indications for treatment of this potential blood incompatibility and the need to block any antigen–antibody formation. **Cognitive Level:** Analyzing **Client Need:** Pharmacological and Parenteral Therapies **Integrated Process:** Nursing Process: Evaluation **Content Area:** Pharmacology **Strategy:** Mapping out the case management of a client with Rh-negative blood is helpful in choosing potential interventions throughout pregnancy.

14 **Answer: 3 Rationale:** Aerosol medications are delivered via a liquid mist, which delivers medication to the lower respiratory tract. Postural drainage would be done if indicated. The droplets of the aerosol medication need to be small, not large. Drugs are always administered during pregnancy after evaluating both the benefit to the mother and the risks to the fetus. **Cognitive Level:** Analysis **Client Need:** Pharmacological and Parenteral Therapies **Integrated Process:** Nursing Process: Planning **Content Area:** Pharmacology **Strategy:** Remember the underlying principle of respiratory care entails postural drainage, mist oxygen that delivers medication to the lower respiratory tract, and oral medications to decrease viscous secretions. The pregnant client actually breathes in more volume than the nonpregnant client. The nurse would be wise to monitor the fetal effects of the medications given to the mother; in this case, beta-adrenergic agents cause fetal tachycardia.

15 **Answer: 3, 4 Rationale:** The neonate intestinal tract is sterile at birth. Colonization of bacteria in the gut necessary for vitamin K synthesis takes approximately a week to occur. The neonate cannot absorb vitamin K from the gastrointestinal tract due to a lack of intestinal flora. Phytonadione is vitamin K and does not prevent neonate contamination from maternal gonorrhea. Vitamin K is a fat-soluble vitamin that aids the synthesis of clotting factors in the immature liver of the neonate. The administration of phytonadione to a neonate is not mandated by state law. **Cognitive Level:** Analysis **Client Need:** Pharmacological and Parenteral Therapies **Integrated Process:** Communication and Documentation **Content Area:** Pharmacology **Strategy:** Vitamin K is critical to normal clotting; careful attention to the subtle differences in the available answers will support better scores. When more than one answer is correct, consider each option as a true/false statement.

16 **Answer: 2 Rationale:** Magnesium sulfate is a CNS depressant; therefore, disappearance of the patellar or knee-jerk reflex would indicate serious CNS depression. It is given to prevent seizures, relax smooth muscles resulting in a decrease in blood pressure, and would not cause an increase in respiratory rate. **Cognitive Level:** Analyzing **Client Need:** Pharmacological and Parenteral Therapies **Integrated Process:** Nursing Process: Evaluation **Content Area:** Pharmacology **Strategy:** Remember your CNS assessments and that the patellar reflex is a specific indicator of CNS integrity. In a client receiving magnesium sulfate, you would expect the patellar reflex to be decreased or absent.

17 **Answer: 4 Rationale:** The antidote for magnesium sulfate is calcium gluconate. Oxygen, epinephrine, and potassium chloride will not reverse the effects of magnesium sulfate toxicity. **Cognitive Level:** Remembering **Client Need:** Pharmacological and Parenteral Therapies **Integrated**

Process: Nursing Process: Implementation **Content Area:** Pharmacology **Strategy:** Calcium gluconate is an antidote for excessive magnesium sulfate, and safe practice indicates that this drug should be available at the bedside.

18 **Answer: 3 Rationale:** Excretion of magnesium sulfate is primarily accomplished through the renal system. Critical assessments prior to administration of the drug would be focused on the body's ability to excrete the medication and the status of the CNS. Both assessments should be within normal limits, or the prescribing healthcare provider should be notified. Urinary glucose, acetone, and specific gravity may be important data but they are not of highest priority for this client. Vital signs are important data, but they are not a high priority specific to a client receiving magnesium sulfate therapy. A funduscopic assessment would not be performed prior to starting magnesium sulfate therapy. **Cognitive Level:** Analyzing **Client Need:** Pharmacological and Parenteral Therapies **Integrated Process:** Nursing Process: Assessment **Content Area:** Pharmacology **Strategy:** The key to answering this question correctly is to focus on indications for stopping the drug; if these signs are present prior to administration, they must be reported to the prescriber and recorded as baseline data.

19 **Answer: 2 Rationale:** Magnesium sulfate acts as an anticonvulsant medication when given to pregnant women with preeclampsia to diminish the risk of seizures. The drug is a CNS depressant and therefore acts to reduce CNS activity. Agitation, dry and pale skin, and increased respirations would not be expected effects. **Cognitive Level:** Understanding **Client Need:** Pharmacological and Parenteral Therapies **Integrated Process:** Nursing Process: Implementation **Content Area:** Pharmacology **Strategy:** Understanding the actions of CNS depressants is essential in finding the correct answer. Remember that CNS depressants should diminish reflex activity, not stop it altogether, or the client will cease respiratory and cardiac function.

20 **Answer: 4 Rationale:** Epidural medications cause vasodilatation, which can lead to hypotension. This is the primary risk factor the nurse needs to monitor after placement. Checking the uterine contractions is appropriate but not the priority nursing action during the administration of an epidural block. An epidural is a nerve block and is not a source of postspinal headaches. An epidural does not create a sensation of needing to void. **Cognitive Level:** Analyzing **Client Need:** Pharmacological and Parenteral Therapies **Integrated Process:** Nursing Process: Implementation **Content Area:** Pharmacology **Strategy:** Remember that many local anesthetics cause vasodilation and the effects should be a nursing priority.

21 **Answer: 3, 4, 5 Rationale:** It is important to keep the room quiet; too much stimulation may trigger seizures. The most critical incident that could occur in a client receiving magnesium sulfate is toxic CNS depression, which could affect respiratory and cardiac function. Therefore, the antidote should be available at the bedside. The nurse should assess for patellar reflexes to detect excessive dosing. It is not necessary to severely limit fluid intake. It is not necessary to prepare for precipitous birth. **Cognitive Level:** Analyzing **Client Need:** Pharmacological and Parenteral Therapies **Integrated Process:** Nursing Process: Implementation **Content Area:** Pharmacology **Strategy:** The critical word in the stem of the question is *appropriate*, which tells you that the correct options are also correct interventions. Use knowledge of magnesium sulfate and the process of elimination to make a selection.

Key Terms to Review

ergotism p. 490 **prostaglandins** p. 491 **surfactant** p. 494

References

Adams, M., Holland, L., & Urban, C. (2017). *Pharmacology for nurses: A pathophysiologic approach* (5th ed.). New York, NY: Pearson Education.

Adams, M., & Urban, C. (2016). *Pharmacology: Connections to nursing practice* (3rd ed.). New York, NY: Pearson Education.

Davidson, M., London, M., & Ladewig, P. (2016). *Olds' maternal newborn nursing and women's health across the lifespan* (10th ed.). New York, NY: Pearson Education.

London, M., & Davidson, M. (2014). *Contemporary maternal–newborn nursing care* (8th ed.). Upper Saddle River, NJ: Pearson Education.

London, M., Ladewig, P., Davidson, M., Ball, J., Bindler, R., & Cowen, K. (2014). *Maternal and child nursing care* (4th ed.). Upper Saddle River, NJ: Pearson Education.

Wilson, B., Shannon, M., & Shields, K. (2016). *Pearson nurse's drug guide 2016.* New York, NY: Pearson Education.

35 Psychiatric Medications

In this chapter

Cross Reference

Other chapters relevant to this content area are

Mental Health Disorders	Chapter 21
Substance Use and Addictive Disorders	Chapter 22
Crisis Intervention and Suicide	Chapter 23

I. GENERAL GUIDELINES FOR PSYCHIATRIC MEDICATIONS (SEE BOX 35–1)

II. ANTIPSYCHOTICS

A. Phenothiazines

1. Are **neuroleptics** (drugs used to treat psychosis); also called typical (traditional) antipsychotic agents (Box 35–2)
2. Assist in improving thought processes and positive symptoms in schizophrenia and other psychoses; are less effective in treating negative symptoms
3. Typical antipsychotics are predominantly dopamine **antagonists** (DA), which block postsynaptic D_2 receptors in several DA tracts in brain
4. Selected agents are also used as antiemetics and antihistamines; chlorpromazine is also used for intractable hiccups
5. **Tolerance** to antipsychotic medications is very uncommon; they are the most toxic drugs used in psychiatry
6. *NCLEX®* Medication effects can usually be seen in 1–2 days, but substantial improvement usually takes 2–4 weeks and full effects may not occur for several months
7. Initially, a thorough baseline evaluation is needed, including laboratory tests such as white blood cell (WBC) count and electrocardiogram (ECG)
8. Side/adverse effects
   a. Gynecomastia, galactorrhea, amenorrhea (occasionally), and weight gain
   b. Sedation and orthostatic hypotension
   c. *NCLEX®* **Anticholinergic effects** (dry mouth, blurred vision, urinary retention, photophobia, constipation, tachycardia)
   d. *NCLEX®* **Extrapyramidal symptoms (EPS)** include **akathisia** (an uncontrollable need to move), **parkinsonism** (a set of symptoms that resembles Parkinson's disease), **tardive dyskinesia** (presence of involuntary

BOX 35–1

General Guidelines for Psychiatric Medications

Administration Principles

- Perform medication reconciliation (including prescribed drugs, OTC drugs, and herbal products) and assess history of allergies to identify potential risks to client.
- Administer doses on time to maintain therapeutic blood levels.
- Do not break or allow client to chew sustained release or enteric-coated preparations.
- Many drugs cause CNS depression, so monitor for adverse effects and maintain a safe environment.
- Provide both verbal and written instructions to client, and provide phone number to call if questions arise or problems occur.
- When risk of suicide is of concern, do not allow access to large quantities of medication; ensure that doses are swallowed and not "cheeked."

Client Teaching

- Understand medication actions, side/adverse effects, signs of toxicity, importance of follow-up with prescriber and follow-up laboratory tests, and how to self-administer.
- Do not take any OTC or herbal preparations without first consulting prescriber.
- Take exactly as prescribed and do not miss or double doses.
- Report adverse or toxic effects promptly.
- Many psychiatric medications cause CNS depression; do not drive, use hazardous equipment, or engage in other activities requiring alertness until individual effects are known.
- Do not drink alcohol or take other OTC medications that cause drowsiness to avoid interactive effects.
- Do not discontinue without consulting with prescriber.

movements of body and extremities, chewing motions, and protruding tongue), and **dystonia (**facial grimacing, involuntary and/or abnormal eye movements)

e. Agranulocytosis is rare, marked by a severe deficit or lack of granulocytic WBCs (neutrophils, basophils, eosinophils)

NCLEX® **f. Neuroleptic malignant syndrome (NMS)**, characterized by catatonia, rigidity, stupor, unstable blood pressure (BP), hyperthermia, profuse sweating, dyspnea, and incontinence; treated with bromocriptine and dantrolene if usual treatment for hyperthermia is ineffective; drug must be changed

NCLEX® **g.** Overdoses are not usually fatal; treatment is supportive (e.g., gastric lavage to empty the stomach); can cause severe central nervous system (CNS) depression (somnolence to coma, hypotension), EPS (parkinsonism, dystonia, akathisia, tardive dyskinesia) and restlessness or agitation, seizures, hyperthermia, increased anticholinergic symptoms, and dysrhythmias

h. Low-potency drugs are more likely to cause sedation and hypotension, whereas high-potency drugs cause more EPS

Box 35–2

Typical and Atypical Antipsychotic Drugs

Typical Antipsychotics	Atypical Antipsychotics
Phenothiazine	Aripiprazole
Chlorpromazine	Clozapine
Fluphenazine	Olanzapine
Perphenazine	Paliperidone
Trifluoperazine	Quetiapine
Nonphenothiazine	Risperidone
Haloperidol	Ziprasidone
Loxapine	
Molindone	
Pimozide	
Thiothixene	

9. Nursing considerations

NCLEX®

a. Observe client taking medication in an inpatient setting to ensure medications are swallowed and not "cheeked"

b. Monitor vital signs and urine output

NCLEX®

c. Monitor and manage side effects, as appropriate (see Table 35–1)

Table 35–1 Interventions for Side Effects of Antipsychotic Drugs

Side Effects	Nursing Interventions
	Peripheral Nervous System Effects
Constipation	Increase fluid intake and dietary fiber intake; provide laxatives as needed
Dry mouth	Advise client to use sugarless hard candy or gum and take sips of water often
Nasal congestion	Suggest OTC nasal decongestants that are safe for use with antipsychotic agents
Blurred vision	Ask client to avoid dangerous tasks (symptom usually lasts only a short time at beginning of treatment; eye drops should be used for short-term need)
Mydriasis	Advise client to report any eye pain immediately
Photophobia	Advise client to wear sunglasses when in sunlight
Orthostatic hypotension	Advise client to get out of chair or bed slowly, to sit before standing, and to rise slowly; observe to see if change to another antipsychotic is advisable
Tachycardia	This is usually a reflex response to hypotension; with effective treatment of hypotension, reflex tachycardia usually decreases; with clozapine, withhold dose if pulse rate is over 140
Urinary retention	Encourage client to void when urge is present and to void frequently; catheterize for residual urine; client should closely monitor output; older men with benign prostatic hyperplasia are particularly susceptible
Urinary hesitation	Provide privacy; encourage client to take time to void, run water in sink, or pour warm water over perineum
Sedation	Help client to get up, get dressed, and begin the day early
Weight gain	Advise client to maintain appropriate diet
Agranulocytosis	Monitor WBC counts weekly; there is a high incidence of agranulocytosis for clients who are taking clozapine If WBC is less than 3500 cells/mm^3 prior to therapy, no treatment should begin After treatment has begun, a WBC count under 3000 cells/mm^3 (and granulocytes under 1500 cells/mm^3) warrant interruption of treatment to monitor for infection; if WBC count is under 2000 cells/mm^3 (granulocytes less than 1000 cells/mm^3), halt therapy with this particular drug; if infection develops, antibiotics should be prescribed
	Central Nervous System Effects
Akathisia	Usually develops within first 2 months of therapy Client experiences an uncontrollable need to move; occurs most often with high-potency antipsychotics Treatment is usually with beta-blockers, benzodiazepines, and anticholinergic drugs; antipsychotic should be changed to a lower potency agent Distinguish between akathisia and exacerbation of psychosis; if akathisia is confused with anxiety or psychotic agitation, antipsychotic dosage may be increased, making akathisia more intense
Dystonias	Acute: Often occur early in treatment and are dangerous and severe. Oculogyric crisis or torticollis are most common Immediate treatment includes antiparkinson drug or antihistamine; reassure client Obtain order for IM administration when client begins treatment with antipsychotics, or if in acute state of dystonia, call prescriber immediately For less acute dystonias, notify prescriber when an order for an antiparkinson drug is warranted
Drug-induced parkinsonism	A chronic disease characterized by a fine, slowly spreading tremor, muscular parkinsonism weakness and rigidity, and a peculiar gait induced by some antipsychotic drugs; asess for three major symptoms: tremors, rigidity, and bradykinesia; report to prescriber immediately; antiparkinson drugs will be indicated
Tardive dyskinesia (TD)	Develops in 15–20% of clients during long-term therapy; risk is related to duration of treatment and dose; often symptoms are irreversible; assess for signs using Abnormal Involuntary Movement Scale (AIMS); anticholinergic agents will worsen TD, so use is contraindicated
Neuroleptic malignant syndrome	This is a fatal side effect of antipsychotic drugs; routinely take client's temperature and encourage adequate water intake; assess for rigidity, tremor, and similar symptoms
Seizures	Occur in approximately 1% of clients taking antipsychotics; clozapine causes an even higher rate (up to 5% of clients taking 600–900 mg/day) For clozapine doses higher than 600 mg/day, an EEG should be performed; seizure activity may warrant discontinuing use of clozapine

NCLEX®
d. Consider long-acting depot injections such as haloperidol and fluphenazine for long-term therapy of schizophrenia; usually reduces rate of relapse

NCLEX®
e. Monitor results of periodic WBC counts and other laboratory studies

10. Client teaching
   a. Take medication as prescribed; discontinuing therapy is a major relapse factor for clients with schizophrenia
   b. Take oral doses with food, milk, or a full glass of water to decrease gastric irritation
   c. Dilute most concentrates in 120 mL of distilled or acidified tap water or fruit juice just before use; avoid skin contact with liquid to prevent contact dermatitis

NCLEX®
d. Use sunscreen and protective clothing such as long sleeves, pants, and hats when outdoors to prevent photosensitivity

Memory Aid

Many drugs cause photosensitivity as a side effect; when protection from the sun is an option, consider carefully whether this could be the correct answer.

e. Expect observable response after 7–10 days, but full effects take 3–6 weeks

NCLEX®
f. Expect urine color to change from yellow to pinkish or red-brown; this is an expected change and is not harmful

NCLEX®
g. Change position slowly to avoid orthostatic hypotension

NCLEX®
h. Report fever, malaise, and other signs of infection such as sore throat; these may indicate agranulocytosis

i. Follow-up WBC count and liver function studies are needed
j. Avoid sudden withdrawal of drug, which may lead to return of psychotic symptoms
k. Learn about other drugs that may be used to treat EPS (see Box 35–3)

B. Atypical antipsychotic drugs

1. Exert both dopamine receptor subtype 2 (D_2) and serotonin receptor subtype 2 ($5HT_2$) receptor-blocking action (DA and 5HT antagonists)
2. Blockage of serotonin receptors is thought to liberate dopamine in cortex and may explain some reduction in negative symptoms
3. Atypical agents cause few or no EPS

NCLEX®
4. Used to treat positive and negative symptoms of schizophrenia and other disorders with psychotic features and to treat mood symptoms, hostility, violence, suicidal behavior, and cognitive impairment seen in schizophrenia

Memory Aid

Remember that typical drugs are effective against positive symptoms of schizophrenia, while atypical antipsychotics are effective against both positive and negative symptoms.

5. Especially useful for clients experiencing first psychotic episode and are not responding well to typical antipsychotics or have had dose-limiting side effects from traditional neuroleptics
6. Refer back to Box 35–2 for listing of antipsychotic drugs
7. Side/adverse effects

NCLEX®
a. Clozapine: agranulocytosis, requiring weekly WBC count and a limit of not more than a 1-week supply of drug to enforce compliance with weekly labwork; NMS and seizures are also of concern

Memory Aid

Remember that clozapine begins with *c* and associate that with *CBC* to help you remember that white blood cell counts can drop with this medication, requiring close monitoring.

Box 35–3

Medications Used to Treat Extrapyramidal Symptoms

Anticholinergic: Benztropine

Antihistamine: Diphenhydramine

Dopamine agonist: Amantadine

   b. Risperidone: orthostatic hypotension, insomnia, agitation, headache, anxiety, rhinitis, NMS
   c. Olanzapine: few incidents of EPS, but NMS and seizures are possible
   d. Aripiprazole is similar to others but with increased risk of suicidal tendency
   e. *NCLEX®* In general, side effects of atypical antipsychotics include weight gain, anticholinergic effects, sedation and cardiac effects, with a low incidence of EPS
8. Nursing considerations
   a. Clozapine is usually given one to two times daily
   b. Risperidone is usually administered PO in one to two daily doses; for debilitated or elderly clients or for those with renal or hepatic impairment, dosage should be reduced
   c. *NCLEX®* Because of risk of fatal agranulocytosis, clozapine is reserved for clients with severe schizophrenia who have not responded to traditional antipsychotic drugs
9. Client teaching: as per Box 35–1

III. ANTIDEPRESSANTS

A. Tricyclic antidepressants (TCAs)

1. TCAs block monoamine reuptake, elevate mood, increase activity and alertness, decrease client's preoccupation with morbidity, improve appetite, and regulate sleep patterns
2. *NCLEX®* Therapeutic effect occurs in 1–3 weeks, with maximum effect in 6–8 weeks
3. Other uses include treatment of chronic insomnia, attention-deficit/hyperactivity disorder (ADHD), and panic disorder
4. Common medications are listed in Table 35–2

Table 35–2 Medications Commonly Used to Treat Depression

Drug Class and Generic Name	Nursing Responsibilities
Tricyclic Antidepressants (TCAs)	
Amitriptyline Clomipramine Desipramine Doxepin Imipramine Nortriptyline Protriptyline Trimipramine	• Educate client early about potential side effects • Inform client that side effects will diminish with time and, if needed, management alternatives can be implemented • Advise that response will take time and continued use is essential • Inform client that first-time treatment for major depression should continue for 6–12 months • Warn client of a possible significant weight gain • Monitor for improvement; if no change or minimum change after 2–4 weeks, it may be necessary to change medication
Second-Generation Tetracyclics	
Amoxapine Maprotiline	• General considerations are same as for tricyclics
Selective Serotonin Reuptake Inhibitors (SSRIs)	
Citalopram Escitalopram Fluoxetine Fluvoxamine Paroxetine Sertraline	• Inform client to take medication as prescribed; abrupt discontinuation of drug is contraindicated • Continuously monitor client for side/adverse effects, particularly in area of sexual dysfunction; client may be reluctant to discuss
Monoamine Oxidase Inhibitors (MAOIs)	
Isocarboxazid Phenelzine Selegiline Tranylcypromine	• Educate client concerning a tyramine-restricted diet • Caution client about side effects and adverse effects of MAOIs • Educate client about careful use of OTC or other prescription drug and be sure client understands seriousness of effects • Monitor efficacy of drugs and continuously re-educate client to avoid abruptly discontinuing medication or not taking it as prescribed

Table 35–2 *(continued)*

Drug Class and Generic Name	Nursing Responsibilities
	Atypical Antidepressants
Serotonin-norepinephrine reuptake inhibitors (SNRIs) Desvenlafaxine Duloxetine Venlafaxine *Norepinephrine and dopamine reuptake inhibitors* Bupropion *Norepinephrine reuptake inhibitor* Reboxetine *Combined reuptake inhibitor and receptor blocker* Mirtazapine Nefazodone Trazodone	• Instruct client about adverse/side effects of medication, especially seizure risks at higher drug doses • Instruct client about importance of taking this and all medication as prescribed • Use ordinary measures to manage mild side effects such as nausea, dry mouth, constipation, CNS sedation (somnolence) or agitation, changes in appetite, and sweating • Instruct client to report severe adverse effects and signs of sexual dysfunction, especially priapism, immediately

a. TCAs are equally effective; major differences are in side effects; for example, doxepin has sedative effects and is more useful in clients with insomnia

b. Older adults and those with glaucoma, constipation, or prostatic hyperplasia can be especially sensitive to anticholinergic effects of TCAs; therefore, a TCA such as desipramine with weak anticholinergic effects would be more appropriate with such clients

5. Administration considerations

a. Dosing with TCAs is individualized and based on clinical response or plasma drug levels (must be above 225 ng/mL for antidepressant effects to occur)

b. TCAs have long half-lives, so may be taken daily in a single dose

c. Once-a-day dosing at bedtime is more easily incorporated into daily routine, promotes sleep (sedative effect), and reduces intensity of daytime side effects

d. For clients at risk for suicide, do not allow access to large quantity of medication; keep hospitalized until risk of suicide has been ruled out

6. Significant drug interactions

NCLEX® **a.** TCAs taken with a monoamine oxidase inhibitor (MAOI) can lead to severe hypertension from excessive adrenergic stimulation of heart and blood vessels

b. TCAs potentiate responses to direct-acting sympathomimetics (e.g., epinephrine and norepinephrine) by blocking uptake of these drugs into adrenergic terminals, prolonging their presence in synaptic space

c. TCAs decrease responses to indirect-acting sympathomimetics (e.g., ephedrine and amphetamine) by blocking uptake of these drugs into adrenergic nerves, preventing them from reaching their site of action in nerve terminal

NCLEX® **d.** TCAs exert anticholinergic actions of their own; thus, they intensify effects of other medications with anticholinergic actions (antihistamines and OTC sleep aids); avoid these products while taking TCAs

e. CNS depression caused by TCAs adds to CNS depression caused by other drugs; avoid use of CNS depressants, including alcohol, antihistamines, opioids, and barbiturates

7. Side/adverse effects

NCLEX® **a.** Most common are orthostatic hypotension, sedation, and anticholinergic effects

b. Most serious is cardiac toxicity; clients over age 40 and those with heart disease should have baseline ECG and then every 6 months

NCLEX® **c.** Adverse effects of each drug are more fully described in Table 35–3

8. Nursing considerations

a. Advise clients of possible side effects and that therapeutic response takes some weeks to achieve; clients and families often become impatient when client is experiencing drug side effects while still having original symptoms

b. Refer back to Table 35–2 for nursing responsibilities with TCAs, and see Table 35–3 for manifestations of common adverse effects

Table 35–3 Most Common Adverse Effects from Antidepressant Medications

Effect	Manifestations
Orthostatic hypotension	Major decrease in BP with body position changes
Anticholinergic	Blockade of muscarinic cholinergic receptors, which produces dry mouth, blurred vision, photophobia, constipation, urinary hesitancy, tachycardia
Sedation	Sleepiness and difficulty maintaining arousal (caused by blockade of histamine receptors in CNS)
Cardiac toxicity	Decreased vagal influence (secondary to muscarinic blockade) and acting directly on bundle of His to slow conduction
Seizures	Lower seizure threshold
Hypomania	Mild mania can occur
Sexual dysfunction	Anorgasm, delayed ejaculation, decreased libido
Hypertensive crisis from dietary tyramine	Although MAOIs normally produce hypotension, can also cause severe hypertension if client eats tyramine-rich foods

9. Client teaching
   a. Side effects diminish with time and symptoms will lessen as medication regime is followed
   b. Encourage client and family to utilize other available therapies as well
   c. Refer back to Box 35–1 and Tables 35–1 and 35–2 for specific points to include in teaching

B. MAOIs

1. Because of potentially fatal food and drug interactions, MAOIs are not a first choice to treat depression unless client has atypical depression
2. Monoamine oxidase (MAO) is an enzyme present in liver, intestinal wall, and terminals of monoamine-containing neurons; it converts monoamine transmitters (norepinephrine, serotonin, and dopamine) into inactive products; in liver and intestine, MAO inactivates tyramine and other biogenic amines in food
3. MAOIs decrease amount of MAO in liver that breaks down amino acids tyramine and tryptophan
4. MAOIs have been used with some success to treat bulimia, obsessive–compulsive disorder, and panic disorder
5. Common antidepressant medications: refer again to Table 35–2
6. Contraindications: clients over age 60 or those with pheochromocytoma, heart failure, liver disease, severe renal impairment, cerebrovascular defect, cardiovascular disease, or hypertension
7. Significant drug interactions
   NCLEX® a. Taking SSRIs with MAOIs can cause **serotonin syndrome** (agitation, sweating, confusion, fever, hyperreflexia, tachycardia, hypotension, muscle rigidity, ataxia); avoid this combination
   NCLEX® b. Antihypertensive drugs potentiate hypotensive effects of MAOIs
   c. Meperidine can produce hyperthermia in clients taking MAOIs and should be avoided
8. NCLEX® Significant food interactions
   a. Dietary tyramine, some other dietary constituents, and indirect-acting sympathomimetics (e.g., amphetamine, methylphenidate, ephedrine, cocaine) can precipitate a hypertensive crisis in clients taking MAOIs
   NCLEX® b. See Box 35–4 for lists of foods to avoid or use cautiously while taking an MAOI
9. NCLEX® Side/adverse effects
   a. Orthostatic hypotension
   b. Edema, weight gain
   c. Reports of insomnia, anxiety, agitation, hypomania, and even mania
   d. Sexual dysfunction
10. Nursing considerations
    a. Assess client for ability to adhere to strict dietary regime
    NCLEX® b. Consult with prescriber about changes in vital signs to avoid potentially fatal hypertensive crisis
11. Client teaching
    a. Teach symptoms of orthostatic hypotension and to avoid injury by rising from bed or chair slowly
    NCLEX® b. Provide dietary teaching to avoid hypertensive crisis (include written list of foods to avoid)

C. SSRIs

1. Block reuptake of serotonin and intensify transmission at serotonergic synapses; effects are often seen after 1–3 weeks and similar to TCA effects

Box 35–4

Foods to Avoid or Limit When Taking Monoamine Oxidase Inhibitors

Foods to Avoid

- Dairy: aged cheeses such as Roquefort, blue, brie, and camembert; sour cream, yogurt, all cheeses except those noted below
- Meats and fish: aged/cured such as hot dogs, bologna, pepperoni, salami, sausage
- Fruits and vegetables: canned figs, papaya products (including meat tenderizers), raisins, broad bean pods, tofu, soybean extracts
- Alcohol: draft beer, Chianti red wine
- Other: sauerkraut, soy sauce, yeast extracts, soups (especially miso) that have protein extract, and Brewer's yeast or extracts
- Drugs: other antidepressant drugs, nasal and sinus decongestants, allergy, hay fever and asthma remedies, narcotics (especially meperidine), epinephrine, stimulants, cocaine, amphetamines

Consume with Caution

- Cheeses: mozzarella, cottage, ricotta, cream, processed
- Meats and fish: beef and chicken liver, meats, herring
- Fruits and vegetables: raspberries, bananas, small amounts only of avocado, spinach
- Alcohol: wine
- Other: monosodium glutamate, pizza, small amounts only of chocolate, caffeine, nuts, dairy products
- Drugs: insulin, oral antidiabetics, oral anticoagulants, thiazide diuretics, anticholinergic agents, muscle relaxants

2. SSRIs have the same efficacy as TCAs, exhibit fewer side effects than either TCAs or MAOIs, and have shorter time between initial dose and beginning of reduced signs and symptoms of depression
3. All SSRIs are effective in treatment of obsessive–compulsive disorder (OCD), panic disorder, and bulimia nervosa
4. Common antidepressant medications (refer again to Table 35–2)
5. Administration considerations
   a. Most SSRIs should not be prescribed for clients with a hypersensitivity to drug or severe hepatic or renal disease
   NCLEX® b. Lowered drug doses or longer dosing interval may be needed with impaired hepatic function, multiple drug therapy, or older adult clients
   NCLEX® c. To prevent serotonin syndrome, SSRIs should not be administered with MAOIs
   d. If a client is on an MAOI and is transferred to fluoxetine, at least 5 weeks should elapse before beginning the fluoxetine; to transfer from fluoxetine to MAOIs, at least 2 weeks should elapse before beginning MAOI
   e. In a client taking fluoxetine and warfarin, monitor coagulation closely because fluoxetine is highly bound to plasma proteins and may displace other highly bound drugs such as warfarin
   NCLEX® f. Monitor complete blood count (CBC) for decreased red blood cells (RBCs), WBCs, and platelets, and monitor bleeding time for increase
6. Side/adverse effects
   NCLEX® a. Common initial side effects include nausea, drowsiness, dizziness, headache, sweating, anxiety, insomnia, anorexia, and nervousness; generally milder and better tolerated than TCAs
   b. Sexual dysfunction is experienced by 20–40% of clients, and must be discussed with client
7. Nursing considerations
   a. Monitor mood changes; notify prescriber if client demonstrates an increase in anxiety, nervousness, or insomnia
   NCLEX® b. Assess for suicidal tendencies, especially during early drug therapy when client begins to have increased energy and can act on suicidal thoughts
   NCLEX® c. Restrict amount of drug available to client to prevent overdose
   d. Monitor appetite, nutritional intake, and weight
8. Client teaching: as per Box 35–1 and notify prescriber if a rash occurs, which may indicate hypersensitivity

D. Atypical antidepressants

1. Serotonin-norepinephrine reuptake inhibitors (SNRIs): desvenlafaxine, venlafaxine, and duloxetine
2. Norepinephrine and dopamine reuptake inhibitors (NDRIs): bupropion
3. Combined reuptake inhibitor and receptor blocker: trazodone, nefazodone, and mirtazapine
4. Administration considerations: bupropion can cause dose-related seizures, but does not have cardiotoxic, anticholinergic, and antiadrenergic side effects; dosage should be reduced in older adults or those with severe hepatic or renal disease
5. Side/adverse effects
   a. Most common side effects of bupropion are agitation and insomnia
   b. Common side effects of trazodone are sedation, orthostatic hypotension, nausea, and vomiting; in contrast to tricyclic agents, it lacks anticholinergic actions and is not cardiotoxic; it may cause priapism (sustained erection)
   c. Most common side effect of venlafaxine is nausea, but can also cause either CNS stimulation (nervousness, insomnia) or sedation
   d. Major adverse effect of bupropion is seizure activity
   e. Adverse effects of trazodone frequently include CNS changes
   f. Side effects among drugs may vary as they inhibit reuptake of different neurotransmitters (serotonin, norepinephrine, and dopamine) and may also act as a receptor blocker (trazodone, nefazodone, and mirtazapine)
   g. Some common side effects include insomnia, dry mouth, constipation, elevated BP and pulse, dizziness, sweating, blurred vision, headache, drowsiness, increased appetite, and increased blood glucose (duloxetine)
6. Nursing considerations
   a. Assess clients with a history of bipolar disorder taking bupropion for symptoms of mania
   b. Monitor BP and pulse rate before and during initial therapy; clients with preexisting cardiac disease should have ECG monitored before and periodically during therapy to detect dysrhythmias
   NCLEX® c. Assess mental status and mood changes frequently; assess for suicidal tendencies, especially during early therapy; restrict amount of drug available to client
7. Client teaching: as per Box 35–1

IV. MOOD STABILIZERS

A. Lithium

1. Used to control manic episodes in bipolar disorder and for long-term prophylaxis against recurrent mania and depression
2. Alters many neurotransmitter functions, possibly correcting an ion exchange abnormality or normalizing neurotransmission of norepinephrine, serotonin, dopamine, and acetylcholine
3. Common mood-stabilizing medications are listed in Box 35–5
4. Administration considerations
   a. Precise dosing is based on serum lithium levels
   NCLEX® b. Mood-stabilizing effects are usually seen in 5–7 days after initial doses, but full effect usually takes 2–3 weeks
   c. Adjunctive therapy with a benzodiazepine can provide the sedation clients need
   NCLEX® d. Contraindicated with sensitivity to drug; use cautiously in debilitated, dehydrated, or older adult clients; those with cardiac, renal, or thyroid disease or diabetes mellitus

Box 35–5

Commonly Used Mood-Stabilizing Drugs

Lithium-Based Drugs	**Atypical Antipsychotic Drugs**
Lithium carbonate	Aripiprazole
Lithium citrate	Asenapine
Antiseizure Drugs	Olanzapine
Carbamazepine	Quetiapine
Gabapentin	Risperidone
Lamotrigine	Valproate sodium
Valproic acid/divalproex	Ziprasidone

e. Should be used only where therapy (including blood levels) may be closely monitored (every 1–2 months and as needed based on client behaviors)

NCLEX® f. Large changes in sodium intake may alter renal elimination of lithium; increasing sodium intake will increase renal excretion; conditions leading to loss of sodium (such as dehydration, sweating, diuretics, diarrhea) may lead to toxicity

NCLEX® g. Therapeutic level and the toxic levels are very close; therapeutic range is 0.8–1.4 mEq/L, while the toxic dose is 1.5 mEq/L or greater

h. It is essential to monitor serum lithium levels frequently because of risk of toxicity

5. Side/adverse effects

a. Fatigue, headache, lethargy

b. Abdominal pain, anorexia, bloating, diarrhea, nausea, dry mouth, metallic taste in mouth

c. Polyuria, glycosuria, nephrogenic diabetes insipidus, and renal toxicity

d. Also reported are weight gain, muscle weakness, hyperirritability, rigidity, and tremors

e. Toxic effects classified as mild, moderate, or severe

NCLEX® f. Mild toxicity (1.5 mEq/L) leads to mild CNS changes: lethargy, decreased concentration, slight muscle weakness, coarse hand tremors, and mild ataxia

NCLEX® g. Moderate toxicity (1.5–2.5 mEq/L) leads to GI symptoms (nausea, vomiting [N/V], severe diarrhea), blurred vision, tinnitus, muscle tremors/twitching, slurred speech, worsening ataxia/incoordination

NCLEX® h. Severe toxicity (higher than 2.5 mEq/L) leads to nystagmus, hyperreflexia, impaired level of consciousness (LOC), hallucinations, muscle twitching/fasciculations, seizures, or renal shutdown; coma and death may result

6. Nursing considerations

a. Assess mood, ideation, and behaviors frequently; initiate suicide precautions if indicated

NCLEX® b. Monitor intake and output ratios; report significant changes in totals

NCLEX® c. Unless contraindicated, provide fluid intake of at least 2000–3000 mL/day

d. Monitor weight at least every 3 months

NCLEX® e. Assess client for signs of lithium toxicity (vomiting, diarrhea, slurred speech, decreased coordination, drowsiness, muscle weakness, or twitching); if these occur, report before administration of next dose

7. Client teaching

a. Take medication even if feeling well; take a missed dose as soon as remembered unless within 2 hours of next dose (6 hours if extended release)

NCLEX® b. May cause dizziness or drowsiness: avoid driving, operating heavy machinery, and other activities requiring alertness until response to medication is known

NCLEX® c. Low sodium levels may lead to toxicity: drink 2000 to 3000 mL fluid each day and eat a diet with consistent and moderate sodium intake

NCLEX® d. Avoid excessive amounts of coffee, tea, and cola (because of diuretic effect); avoid activities that cause excess sodium loss; notify prescriber of fever, vomiting, and diarrhea, which also cause sodium loss

e. Weight gain may occur: follow principles of a low-calorie diet

f. Consult with prescriber before taking any OTC medications, before use of contraception, or if pregnancy is suspected

g. For clients with cardiovascular disease or over 40 years of age: understand need for ECG evaluation before and periodically during therapy; report any irregular pulse, difficulty breathing, or fainting

B. Other mood stabilizer medications

1. A variety of antiepileptic and atypical antipsychotic drugs (see Box 35–5 again) also demonstrate beneficial effects in bipolar disorder when lithium is ineffective, although they may not be FDA approved for this use

2. Carbamazepine and valproate sodium have acute antimanic and long-term mood-stabilizing effects in bipolar disorder; are better than lithium in treating mixed or dysphoric bipolar states and in clients who are rapid cyclers

3. Lamotrigine is used for long-term maintenance therapy to prevent or delay relapses

4. Atypical antipsychotics help control symptoms of mania; may be used in combination with lithium to stabilize mood, although olanzapine may be used for long-term maintenance therapy

5. Contraindications

a. Carbamazepine: hypersensitivity or bone marrow depression; pregnancy unless potential benefits outweigh fetal risks; use cautiously in clients with cardiac or hepatic disease, prostatic hyperplasia, or increased intraocular pressure

b. Valproate: hypersensitivity or hepatic impairment; avoid use with products containing tartrazine; use cautiously with bleeding disorders, liver disease, organic brain disease, bone marrow depression, renal impairment, and in children (increased risk of hepatotoxicity); safe use in pregnancy not established

NCLEX®
6. Side/adverse effects
   a. Side effects generally include dizziness, ataxia, sedation, headache, N/V, double or blurred vision, prolonged bleeding time, transient leukopenia
   b. Adverse effects tend to include heart block, bone marrow depression, respiratory depression, exfoliative dermatitis, Stevens-Johnson syndrome, liver failure, pancreatitis
7. Nursing considerations
   a. Assess frequently for seizure activity when taking carbamazepine and assess for facial pain because of possibility of trigeminal neuralgia
   b. (NCLEX®) Measure WBC count weekly and provide weekly medication refill if client does not develop agranulocytosis; drug should be stopped if this sign of bone marrow depression occurs
   c. Check routine CBC and serum iron weekly during first 2 months and yearly thereafter to monitor for anemia caused by bone marrow depression
   d. (NCLEX®) Perform liver function tests, urinalysis, and BUN routinely; measure serum ionized calcium levels at least every 6 months
8. Client teaching
   a. Take around the clock, exactly as directed
   b. (NCLEX®) Immediately report fever, sore throat, mouth ulcers, easy bruising, petechiae, unusual bleeding, abdominal pain, chills, rash, pale stools, dark urine, or jaundice
   c. Use sunscreen and protective clothing to prevent photosensitivity reactions with carbamazepine
   d. For female clients: use a nonhormonal form of contraception while taking carbamazepine
   e. Carry information, such as a Medic-Alert tag/bracelet, describing disease and medication regimen at all times
   f. Understand importance of follow-up monitoring
   g. (NCLEX®) For divalproex, be sure to take medication exactly as directed; abrupt withdrawal may lead to seizures in a susceptible client

V. ANXIOLYTICS AND SEDATIVE-HYPNOTICS

A. Benzodiazepines (BZs)

1. BZ molecules and GABA bind to each other at GABA receptor sites, resulting in *inhibition* of neurotransmission that results in a clinical decrease in anxiety level
2. **Metabolites** (result of drug biotransformation) are pharmacologically active, so drug effects persist long after parent drug is gone from plasma
3. Major indications for use are anxiety, insomnia (sedative-hypnotic effect), and seizure disorders
4. Other uses include alcohol withdrawal, skeletal muscle relaxation, substance-induced (except for amphetamines) and psychotic agitation in crisis situations
5. Common anti-anxiety medications are listed in Box 35–6

Memory Aid Remember that a drug that ends with the suffix *-zepam* is a benzodiazepine.

6. Administration considerations
   a. (NCLEX®) BZs should be started at low doses and gradually increased to achieve desired clinical response
   b. For treatment of anxiety, BZs are usually dosed at bedtime or twice daily, only occasionally are three doses/day required
   c. Treatment for insomnia should be no longer than 7–10 days to avoid rebound insomnia; use sleep hygiene techniques also to establish regular sleep pattern
   d. (NCLEX®) BZs are contraindicated with drug sensitivity or during pregnancy or lactation (cross blood–brain barrier and enter breast milk with ease and develop quickly to toxic levels)
   e. BZs should not be used with clients who have preexisting CNS depression, severe uncontrolled pain, or narrow-angle glaucoma
   f. Because liver is site of drug biotransformation, drugs that interfere with liver metabolism (e.g., alcohol) dangerously compound BZ effects

Box 35–6

Anxiolytic and Sedative-Hypnotic Medications

Anxiolytics	**Benzodiazepine Antagonist**
Benzodiazepines	Flumazenil
Alprazolam	***Sedative-Hypnotics***
Chlordiazepoxide	**Barbiturates**
Clonazepam	Butabarbital
Clorazepate	Pentobarbital
Diazepam	Phenobarbital
Flurazepam*	Secobarbital
Lorazepam	**Other Sedative-Hypnotics**
Oxazepam	Chloral hydrate
Quazepam	Eszopiclone*
Temazepam*	Meprobamate
Triazolam*	Ramelteon*
Nondiazepine Anxiolytics	Zaleplon*
Buspirone	Zolpidem*

*Used to treat insomnia

NCLEX® **7.** Side/adverse effects
- **a.** Hypotension
- **b.** Dry mouth, ataxia, dizziness, drowsiness, nausea
- **c.** Withdrawal symptoms (increased anxiety, flulike symptoms, tremors)

8. Nursing considerations
- **a.** Assess degree and manifestation of anxiety before client begins therapy
- NCLEX® **b.** Assess client for drowsiness, light-headedness, and dizziness periodically during treatment; these usually disappear as therapy progresses
- **c.** Monitor BP, pulse, and respirations, and provide supportive care as needed
- NCLEX® **d.** Prolonged therapy may lead to psychological or physical dependence; risk is greater with larger drug doses; restrict amount of drug available to client

9. Client teaching
- **a.** As per Box 35–1
- **b.** If dose is missed, take within 1 hour or skip dose and return to regular schedule
- **c.** If medication is less effective after a few weeks, check with prescriber; do not increase dose
- NCLEX® **d.** Abrupt withdrawal of drug may cause sweating, vomiting, muscle cramps, tremors, and seizure

B. Benzodiazepine antagonist

NCLEX® **1.** Flumazenil is a BZ antagonist that selectively blocks BZ receptors but does not block adrenergic or cholinergic receptors

NCLEX® **2.** Can reverse *sedative* effects of BZs but may not reverse BZ-induced *respiratory depression*

3. Because it does not stimulate CNS or block other receptors, it can be given for suspected BZ overdose and to reverse effects of BZs following general anesthesia

4. Works within 30 to 60 seconds of IV administration

5. Contraindicated with hypersensitivity; if receiving BZs for life-threatening medical problems, including status epilepticus or increased intracranial pressure; and for clients with serious TCA overdose

NCLEX® **6.** Side effects: dizziness, agitation, confusion, N/V, hiccups, paresthesia, rigors, and shivering; principle adverse effect is seizures (occur most often with epilepsy or physical dependence on BZs)

7. Nursing considerations
- **a.** Assess LOC and respiratory status before and throughout therapy
- **b.** Establish that client has patent airway before administration
- NCLEX® **c.** Institute seizure precautions

NCLEX® d. For suspected BZ overdose: if no effects are seen after giving flumazenil, consider other causes of decreased LOC (alcohol, barbiturates, opioid analgesics)
e. Observe client for at least 2 hours after last dose for resedation; hypoventilation may occur
8. Client teaching
a. Client may appear alert at time of discharge but sedative effects of BZ may reoccur; avoid driving or other activities requiring alertness for at least 24 hours after discharge
NCLEX® b. Do not drink *any* alcohol or take nonprescription drugs for at least 18–24 hours after discharge
c. Resume usual activities only when no residual effects of BZs remain

C. Barbiturates
1. Cause relatively nonselective CNS depression and are prototypes of general CNS depressants; used for daytime sedation, induction of sleep, suppression of seizures, and general anesthesia
2. Can cause tolerance and dependence, have a high abuse potential, and are subject to multiple drug interactions; powerful respiratory depressants
3. Common sedative-hypnotic medications (see again Box 35–6)
4. Administration considerations
a. Avoid intramuscular (IM) route; barbiturate solutions are highly alkaline and can cause pain and necrosis when injected IM
NCLEX® b. As dosage is increased, response progresses from *sedation* to *sleep* to *general anesthesia*
NCLEX® c. At hypnotic doses, barbiturates may reduce BP and heart rate; in contrast, toxic doses can cause profound hypotension and shock (from direct depressant effects on both myocardium and vascular smooth muscle)
NCLEX® d. Tolerance to sedative and hypnotic effects and to other effects that underlie barbiturate abuse develops with repeated drug use
5. Side/adverse effects
a. Long half-lives can produce residual effects (hangover) when taken to treat insomnia; can manifest as sedation, impaired judgment, reduced motor skills
b. Paradoxical excitement (especially in older adult or debilitated clients)
c. Barbiturates can intensify sensitivity to pain and may cause pain directly; their use has produced muscle pain, joint pain, and pain along nerves
NCLEX® d. Acute barbiturate overdose produces a classic triad of symptoms: *respiratory depression*, *coma*, and *pinpoint pupils*, frequently accompanied by *hypotension* and *hypothermia*
6. Nursing considerations
NCLEX® a. Monitor respiratory status, pulse, and BP frequently
NCLEX® b. Prolonged therapy may lead to psychological or physical dependence; restrict amount of drug available, especially if client is depressed, suicidal, or has a history of addiction
c. Monitor client for safety, alertness, and assist as needed with ambulation or self-care
7. Client teaching
a. As per Box 35–1
b. For female using oral contraceptives: use additional nonhormonal contraceptive during therapy

D. Nonbenzodiazepine anxiolytics and miscellaneous agents
1. Buspirone: used to manage anxiety; binds to serotonin and dopamine receptors and increases norepinephrine metabolism in brain
2. Buspirone's major advantages are that it is nonsedative, has no abuse potential, and does not enhance CNS depression caused by BZs, alcohol, barbiturates, and related drugs; major disadvantage is delayed onset of anxiolytic effects
3. Zolpidem, eszopiclone, and zaleplon are used for short-term treatment of insomnia; produce CNS depression; have no analgesic properties but produce sedation and induction of sleep; ramelteon treats chronic insomnia in those who have difficulty falling asleep
4. Administration considerations
a. Giving buspirone with food delays absorption but enhances bioavailability (by reducing first-pass metabolism in liver)
b. Zolpidem, eszopiclone, ramelteon, and zaleplon are usually given just before bedtime because of rapid onset of action
5. Side effects
a. Most common reactions are dizziness, nausea, headache, daytime drowsiness, dream disturbances, and unpleasant taste (eszopiclone, ramelteon)
b. Adverse effects include paradoxical excitation, mood changes, tachycardia, blurred vision, confusion, myalgia

6. Nursing considerations
   - NCLEX® a. Assess degree and manifestations of anxiety before and periodically during therapy with buspirone
   - NCLEX® b. Clients changing from other antianxiety agents should receive gradually decreasing doses; buspirone will not prevent withdrawal symptoms
   - NCLEX® c. With zolpidem, there may be a potential for physical or psychological dependence if used longer than 7–10 days; limit the amount of drug available to client
   - d. With zolpidem, assess alertness at time of peak effect; notify prescriber if desired sedation doesn't occur
7. Client teaching
   - a. As per Box 35–1
   - NCLEX® b. With buspirone, report any chronic abnormal movements such as dystonia (muscle rigidity), motor restlessness, involuntary movements of facial or cervical muscles, or if pregnancy is suspected
   - NCLEX® c. With drugs used for insomnia, go to bed immediately after taking dose because of rapid onset of action

VI. DRUGS TO TREAT ALZHEIMER'S DISEASE

A. Alzheimer's disease (AD) is a degenerative neurological disease of uncertain etiology that leads to chronic, progressive loss of cognitive function; structural changes in brain include accumulation of beta-amyloid protein and neurofibrillatory tangles

B. Drug therapy for Alzheimer's disease (see Box 35–7)

1. Memantine reduces high levels of glutamate (major excitatory neurotransmitter of CNS) associated with progression of AD
2. Reversible cholinesterase inhibitors (donepezil, galantamine, rivastigmine) improve function in cognition, behavior, and activities of daily living
3. Side/adverse effects: GI (nausea, vomiting, diarrhea, abdominal cramps) and possibly headache, dizziness, muscle cramps; severe effects include renal failure (memantine), hallucinations, and depression
4. NCLEX® Nursing considerations
   - a. Monitor for intended effects on cognition, behavior, and ADLs and for side/adverse effects
   - b. Atropine IV is antidote for overdose (noted by signs of cholinergic crisis such as nausea, vomiting, bradycardia, hypotension, respiratory depression, and seizures)

VII. DRUGS TO TREAT ATTENTION-DEFICIT/HYPERACTIVITY DISORDER

A. Attention-deficit/hyperactivity disorder is characterized by unusually short attention span and hyperactive behavior; usually first diagnosed in childhood

B. Drug therapy for ADHD (see Box 35–8)

1. Consists of drugs that are CNS stimulants, which have a calming effect on children and increase their alertness and ability to attend to stimuli
2. In contrast to children, use of CNS stimulants by adults increases activity level and agitation
3. Side/adverse effects: anorexia and weight loss, tachycardia and increased blood pressure, agitation and dizziness

Box 35–7

Drugs to Treat Alzheimer's Disease

- Donepezil
- Galantamine
- Memantine
- Rivastigmine

Box 35–8

Drugs to Treat Attention-Deficit/Hyperactivity Disorder

Amphetamine	Dextroamphetamine and amphetamine
Atomoxetine	Lisdexamfetamine
Dexmethylphenidate	Methamphetamine
Dextroamphetamine	Methylphenidate

NCLEX®

4. Nursing considerations
   a. Obtain baseline electrocardiogram
   b. Monitor blood pressure, height, and weight during therapy

NCLEX®

5. Client and family teaching
   a. Avoid OTC and herbal medications; monitor for drug side effects
   b. Several weeks of therapy may be needed before there is noticeable therapeutic effect
   c. To prevent insomnia, last dose of day should be taken at least 6 hours before bedtime (14 hours for extended-release formulations)
   d. A drug-free period may be prescribed by healthcare provider if growth retardation occurs during therapy

VIII. SUBSTANCE MISUSE

A. Alcohol abuse and disulfiram (Antabuse) therapy

1. Alcohol is a CNS depressant that causes general (relatively nonselective) depression of CNS function, primarily by enhancing GABA
2. Effect of alcohol on CNS is dose-dependent; low dosage primarily affects cortical brain function (thought processes, self-restraint, motor function); as dosage increases, CNS depression deepens, reflexes diminish greatly, and level of consciousness (LOC) is impaired
3. Management of withdrawal (outpatient vs. inpatient) depends on degree of alcohol dependence
4. Most medical treatment for withdrawal includes use of BZs—chlordiazepoxide, diazepam, and lorazepam; a regime of atenolol (a beta-adrenergic blocking agent) used in conjunction with BZs decreases amount of BZs necessary for safe detoxification
5. Disulfiram inhibits enzyme *alcohol dehydrogenase*, which catalyzes a major step in breakdown of alcohol

NCLEX®

6. When enzyme is inhibited and an individual drinks alcohol, blood concentrations of toxic metabolite *acetaldehyde* increase significantly, producing unpleasant symptoms of flushing, tachycardia, nausea, vomiting, and hypotension
7. Administration considerations
   a. Disulfiram is used only with highly selected individuals in good physical health
   b. At least 12 hours should elapse from last alcohol intake and initial dose
   c. Relatively long half-life of disulfiram ensures that several days must elapse between stopping medication and safely drinking alcohol; this probably decreases impulsive relapse
8. Adverse effects/toxicity: acetaldehyde syndrome (from ingesting alcohol and disulfiram) is noted by marked respiratory depression, cardiovascular collapse, cardiac dysrhythmias, myocardial infarction, acute heart failure, seizures, and death
9. Nursing considerations
   a. Simultaneous use with alcohol can precipitate acetaldehyde syndrome
   b. Disulfiram effects may persist for about 2 weeks after last dose
10. Client teaching
    a. Avoid all forms of alcohol, including alcohol in sauces, cough and cold syrups, aftershave lotions, colognes, and liniments
    b. Adhere to all forms of self-help groups, both individual and group therapies, while using disulfiram therapy to establish a recovery program

B. Opioids

1. Opioids (e.g., morphine, heroin) are major drugs of abuse; usually Schedule II substances
2. Opioid toxicity produces a classic triad of symptoms: respiratory depression, coma, and pinpoint pupils
3. Naloxone, an opioid antagonist, rapidly reverses opioid poisoning
4. Naloxone dosage must be titrated carefully; too much naloxone reverses client from intoxicated state to withdrawal
5. Because of short half-life, naloxone must be given every few hours until opioid has dropped to a nontoxic level
6. Nalmefene, a long-acting opioid antagonist, is an alternative to naloxone; because of its long half-life, nalmefene does not require repeated dosing; however, if dose is excessive in an opioid-dependent person, it will lead to prolonged withdrawal
7. Methadone, a long-acting oral opioid, is commonly used to ease opioid withdrawal and prevent abstinence syndrome; once stabilized on methadone, withdrawal is accomplished by administering it in gradually smaller doses

8. With methadone withdrawal, abstinence syndrome is mild, with symptoms resembling those of moderate influenza; entire process of methadone substitution and withdrawal takes about 10 days
9. Objective of maintenance methadone therapy is to avoid withdrawal and need to procure illicit drugs; methadone maintenance is most effective in conjunction with nondrug measures directed at altering patterns of drug use

C. Cocaine

1. Is a fine, white, odorless powder extracted from coca plant; it passes blood–brain barrier readily and causes an instant high; when taken IV (mainlining), it is rapidly metabolized by liver, so "rush" does not last long
2. Exerts both CNS and peripheral nervous system (PNS) effects because it blocks norepinephrine and dopamine reuptake into presynaptic neurons; it depletes these neurotransmitters
3. Is highly addictive and produces mild physical withdrawal but severe psychological withdrawal
4. Treatment is aimed at restoring depleted neurotransmitters; three approaches include use of amino acid catecholamine precursors (such as tyrosine and phenylalanine), TCAs, and dopamine agonist bromocriptine

D. Cannabis (marijuana/hashish)

1. Marijuana is derived from the Indian hemp plant *Cannabis sativa*; major psychoactive substance is delta-9-tetrahydrocannabinol (THC), an oily chemical with high lipid solubility
2. Produces three main subjective effects: euphoria, sedation, and hallucinations
3. Common effects of low-dose THC include euphoria and relaxation; an increased sensitivity to visual and auditory stimuli; enhanced sense of touch, taste, and smell; increased appetite and more intense perceived flavor of food; distortion of time (seems to move more slowly)
4. Cannabinoids are sometimes used to treat N/V (in contrast to traditional antiemetics) caused by cancer chemotherapy; THC is approved for stimulating appetite in clients with AIDS

Check Your NCLEX–RN® Exam I.Q.

You are ready for testing on this content if you can:

- Apply knowledge of expected actions and effects of psychiatric medications to client care.
- Correctly administer psychiatric medications to clients.
- Assess for side effects and adverse effects of psychiatric medications.
- Take appropriate action if a client has an unexpected response to a psychiatric medication.
- Monitor a client for expected outcomes or effects of treatment with psychiatric medications.

PRACTICE TEST

1 The client is reporting vague dread; she is pacing and hyperventilating. Her jaw is clenched, and she is wringing her hands. What type of medication should the nurse conclude that this client needs?

1. A barbiturate
2. An anxiolytic
3. An antipsychotic
4. A CNS stimulant

2 What would be a priority clinical problem to address for a client taking zolpidem?

1. Reduced ability for self-care
2. Potential for violence
3. Sleep disturbance
4. Dehydration

3 A client has an order for 30 mg of flurazepam. The nurse determines that the client understands the effects of this medication by which client statement?

1. "After I take my medication at bedtime, I can watch the boxing match on TV and then go to sleep."
2. "Once I take my medicine, I should be able to go to bed and read for a short time."
3. "I will take my medicine, go straight to bed, and go to sleep."
4. "I will take my medicine before preparing for bed and the next day's work."

PRACTICE TEST

4. The nurse is conducting medication teaching with a client about clozapine. The nurse should include information about what weekly intervention?

1. Physical exam by a psychiatrist
2. Hematological monitoring
3. Follow-up visits with a prescriber
4. Urinalysis

5. A client is taking sertraline. The nurse explains to the client that how much time will pass before the onset of the medication occurs?

1. 5–7 days
2. 1–4 weeks
3. 4–6 weeks
4. 8–12 weeks

6. A client is taking phenelzine. The visiting nurse is evaluating for client safety. What should the nurse include as priority teaching?

1. Limiting daily intake of salt
2. Encouraging a fluid intake of at least 2000 mL
3. Encouraging the client to have scheduled blood tests on time
4. Restricting foods containing tyramine

7. The client is diaphoretic, disoriented, and has a temperature of 100°F (37.8°C). Additionally, the client complains of insomnia, anxiety, and an inability to sit still. What should the nurse suspect regarding this client? Select all that apply.

1. Withdrawing from alcohol use
2. Demonstrating flu symptoms
3. Withdrawing from an antipsychotic medication
4. Abruptly discontinuing lithium carbonate
5. Withdrawing from CNS depressants

8. Immediately after taking a dose of alprazolam, the client says, "I know I shouldn't feel this guilty, but I don't want to take medicine that makes me feel this way." What would be the most appropriate response by the nurse?

1. "You can't worry what people say about the medicine you take."
2. "Once the medication begins to work, you'll feel differently about taking it."
3. "Let's talk about how you're feeling about taking alprazolam."
4. "Your long-term mental health will benefit from taking this medication."

9. The client is taking carbamazepine for treatment of mania. The nurse should remind the client that laboratory testing will be needed to assess for which adverse effect?

1. Neuroleptic malignant syndrome
2. Agranulocytosis
3. Thrombocytopenia
4. Anemia

10. A client with schizophrenia has been taking haloperidol for 3 weeks with good effect. Today, he comes to group but is complaining of feeling like his legs are on fire. The nurse notes that he is moving continuously and leaves group early. The nurse should document and report that the client is experiencing which medication side effect?

1. Anticholinergic effects
2. Gustatory hallucinations
3. Akathisia
4. Oculogyric crisis

11. A client is taking trazodone. The nurse concludes the client understands the desired effects and major side effects of the drug by making which statement? Select all that apply.

1. "I can go downstairs to the bathroom during the night if I have a nightlight."
2. "I am drinking more fluids so the medication will work effectively."
3. "I should not worry about becoming addicted to this medication."
4. "I have been prescribed this medication to treat my insomnia."
5. "If I have a problem with priapism, I will notify my doctor immediately."

12 The client is hospitalized because of a suicide attempt while in a manic phase. The client has now been taking chlordiazepoxide for 2 days. What is the most important safety measure for the nurse to implement with this client?

1. Frequently remind the client to remain visible to the nurses at all times.
2. Elicit the client's promise to tell someone about any suicidal feelings.
3. Make a contract for safety.
4. Enforce the client's promise to eat all meals in the dining room.

13 If an overdose of benzodiazepines is suspected, the nurse should anticipate what medication order to reverse that drug's effects?

1. Diazepam
2. Triazolam
3. Fluvoxamine
4. Flumazenil

14 The nurse is making a plan of care for a client who is prescribed fluphenazine 1 mg daily at bedtime. The nurse will include which intervention for the side effects of the medication?

1. Remind the client to rise slowly when getting out of bed or a chair.
2. Assess for dizziness or lightheadedness frequently during the day.
3. Make sugarless hard candy, gum, and water available during the day.
4. Monitor the client frequently for manifestations of confusion.

15 A client, in an inpatient locked unit on suicide precautions, has been taking imipramine for 5 days. Currently, the client expresses an increase in appetite, a desire to participate in group therapy, and a request for her mother to visit later in the week. What consideration should the nurse make regarding changes to the nursing care plan at this time?

1. It is not safe after 5 days to address too many changes at once.
2. Positive changes in client behavior indicate a need to change the focus of care.
3. Behavior indicates a decreased possibility of another suicide attempt.
4. The client is less likely to attempt suicide if there is no change in the care plan.

16 A client who is receiving thioridazine 100 mg t.i.d. comes to the clinic with the chief complaint of a "dry mouth." To what should the nurse conclude this side effect is related?

1. High anticholinergic effects of thioridazine
2. Extrapyramidal side effects (EPS)
3. Weight loss effect from the medication
4. Neuroleptic malignant syndrome (NMS) side effect

17 A client asks the nurse if it is true that marijuana is not just a street drug but has legitimate uses. What therapeutic uses should the nurse relate to the client regarding marijuana? Select all that apply.

1. Stimulates appetite
2. Promotes organization and motivation
3. Heightens auditory sensitivity
4. Acts as an antibacterial agent
5. Promotes relaxation

18 The client who was recently attacked and robbed in her apartment has developed anxiety accompanied by immobilizing apprehension. A short-term anxiolytic has been prescribed. What is the primary nursing priority for this client?

1. Help client learn alternative responses to the anxiety.
2. Promote client's involvement in group or community support activities.
3. Provide for physical safety.
4. Assist with desensitization to phobic place (apartment).

19 A client admitted to the inpatient unit with a diagnosis of paranoid schizophrenia is prescribed risperidone. After 5 days of treatment, the client reports feeling dizzy. What should the nurse explain to the client is associated with this manifestation?

1. The desired effect of sedation
2. The side effect of loss of appetite
3. Anticholinergic side effect of this agent
4. The side effect of orthostatic hypotension

20 What should be the nurse's highest priority when caring for a client who, after withdrawing from alcohol, is beginning to use disulfiram?

1. Becoming socially reintegrated
2. Learning about the disease process
3. Remaining abstinent
4. Remaining in the rehabilitation unit

ANSWERS & RATIONALES

1 **Answer: 2 Rationale:** This client is suffering from anxiety and the appropriate type of medication is an anxiolytic. Barbiturates are sedative-hypnotics, which would not be prescribed. The client is not suffering from psychosis or hallucinations, so an antipsychotic is inappropriate. A CNS stimulant is inappropriate for the signs and symptoms described. **Cognitive Level:** Analyzing **Client Need:** Physiological Pharmacological and Parenteral Therapies **Integrated Process:** Nursing Process: Diagnosis **Content Area:** Pharmacology **Strategy:** This question requires you to interpret the client's symptoms as being representative of anxiety, and to choose the drug category that is effective against it. Focus on the client manifestations to eliminate each of the incorrect options.

2 **Answer: 3 Rationale:** Zolpidem is a sedative-hypnotic medication used to treat insomnia. Therefore, sleep disturbance is the appropriate priority clinical problem. There is not enough information in the question to determine whether reduced ability for self-care, potential for violence, or dehydration would be pertinent for the client. **Cognitive Level:** Analyzing **Client Need:** Pharmacological and Parenteral Therapies **Integrated Process:** Nursing Process: Diagnosis **Content Area:** Pharmacology **Strategy:** First, recall that zolpidem is a sedative-hypnotic medication. Next, consider its use as a bedtime sleep aid to make the appropriate selection.

3 **Answer: 2 Rationale:** The medication normally works within 30 minutes to 1 hour after administration. The medication will not work instantly. The client should not take a sedative and then stay active for an extended period of time. Watching stimulating shows on television at bedtime is not conducive to sleep. **Cognitive Level:** Analyzing **Client Need:** Pharmacological and Parenteral Therapies **Integrated Process:** Nursing Process: Evaluation **Content Area:** Pharmacology **Strategy:** The word *understands* in the stem of the question tells you the correct answer is also a true statement. Recall that the medication is used to enhance sleep, and utilize principles of good sleep hygiene to eliminate each of the incorrect options.

4 **Answer: 2 Rationale:** In order to safely monitor clozapine, a weekly blood test is mandatory. If the client does not have the hematologic exam, the medication is not given for the following week. This is to monitor for agranulocytosis, the drug's major adverse effect. A weekly physical exam is unnecessary. Follow-up visits are done periodically, but might not be needed weekly with the prescriber. Weekly urinalysis is unnecessary when taking clozapine. **Cognitive Level:** Applying **Client Need:** Pharmacological and Parenteral Therapies **Integrated Process:** Nursing Process: Assessment **Content Area:** Pharmacology **Strategy:** The core issue of the question is knowledge of possible adverse effects of clozapine. Recall that the drug can cause bone marrow depression and agranulocytosis to choose the correct monitoring technique.

5 **Answer: 2 Rationale:** Sertraline is an antidepressant of the SSRI type. These agents work within 1 to 4 weeks, not 5–7 days, 4–6 weeks, or 8–12 weeks. **Cognitive Level:** Remembering **Client Need:** Pharmacological and Parenteral Therapies **Integrated Process:** Nursing Process: Implementation **Content Area:** Pharmacology **Strategy:** Specific knowledge of the time frame in which SSRIs exert an effect is needed to answer this question. Use medication knowledge and the process of elimination to make a selection.

6 **Answer: 4 Rationale:** With an MAOI, such as phenelzine, the client must restrict foods that contain tyramine. Intake of tyramine-containing foods could lead to severe hypertension and other complications. Limiting salt, increasing fluid intake, and need for blood testing are not major teaching considerations for MAOIs. **Cognitive Level:** Applying **Client Need:** Pharmacological and Parenteral Therapies **Integrated Process:** Teaching and Learning **Content Area:** Pharmacology **Strategy:** The core issue of the question is knowledge regarding priority teaching for a client taking phenelzine, which is an MAOI. From there, recall that foods high in tyramine need to be avoided to make the correct selection.

7 **Answer: 1, 5 Rationale:** These symptoms are commonly seen in withdrawal from alcohol. The symptoms are commonly seen during withdrawal from CNS depressants. A client would usually not be complaining of disorientation or insomnia with flu-like symptoms. Individuals do not usually have withdrawal symptoms from antipsychotic medications. These are not signs of lithium carbonate being discontinued. **Cognitive Level:** Analyzing **Client Need:** Pharmacological and Parenteral Therapies **Integrated Process:** Nursing Process: Diagnosis **Content Area:** Pharmacology **Strategy:** Clients withdrawing from a substance are likely to experience the opposite effects of the original drug. With this in mind, review the client's symptoms, and note that they represent excitation of the CNS. You can deduce that the original substance was some type of CNS depressant, leading you to the correct answer. When there is more than one correct answer, consider each option as a true/false statement.

8 **Answer: 3 Rationale:** In the correct response, the nurse acknowledges the client's feelings, and asks the client to discuss his or her feelings and thoughts. An open and trusting nurse–client relationship helps support the client in decisions related to medication therapy. The nurse is not addressing the client's comment by talking about other people. The comment about when it starts to work dismisses the client's feelings; there is no way to determine how the client will feel over time. The statement about long-term mental health may or may not be a correct statement; however, it does not address the client's feelings or concern. **Cognitive Level:** Applying **Client Need:** Psychosocial Integrity **Integrated Process:** Communication and Documentation **Content Area:** Mental Health **Strategy:** The correct answer is one that is the most therapeutic response by the nurse. Use knowledge of communication techniques and the process of elimination to make a selection.

9 **Answer: 2 Rationale:** The most serious side effect of carbamazepine is agranulocytosis (low WBC count). Neuroleptic malignant syndrome is not common with carbamazepine. There is no need for routine monitoring for low platelet count while taking carbamazepine. There is no need for routine monitoring for anemia while taking carbamazepine. **Cognitive Level:** Applying **Client Need:** Pharmacological and Parenteral Therapies **Integrated Process:** Nursing Process: Implementation **Content Area:** Pharmacology **Strategy:** The core issue of the question is that an adverse effect of carbamazepine is agranulocytosis. With this in mind, eliminate each of the incorrect responses that do not address this concern.

10 **Answer: 3 Rationale:** Akathisia is an uncontrollable need to move; a common extrapyramidal side effect after long-term use of haloperidol. Anticholinergic effects would include dry mouth, urinary hesitance, constipation, mydriasis, tachycardia, and diminished lacrimation. Gustatory hallucination is tasting something that is not present. Oculogyric crisis involves painful twisting and turning of the head and neck. **Cognitive Level:** Analyzing **Client Need:** Pharmacological and Parenteral Therapies **Integrated Process:** Nursing Process: Assessment **Content Area:** Pharmacology **Strategy:** The core issue of the question is correct identification of side effects of haloperidol. Knowledge of terminology will help identify the connection between *gustatory* referring to taste and *oculo-* referrring to eyes; also, the word *akathisia* is consistent with the client's presentation, while the word *anticholinergic* is not.

11 **Answer: 3, 4, 5 Rationale:** The abuse potential for trazodone is minimal. Trazadone is an atypical antidepressant that is used more for insomnia than for depression. Priapism is a penile erection that occurs without stimulation and is an adverse side effect to trazadone; the doctor should be notified. For safety reasons, it is not a good practice when taking trazodone as a sleep aid to ambulate in low lighting because the drug produces a profound sedative effect. Taking more fluids will not increase the effectiveness of the medication. **Cognitive Level:** Analyzing **Client Need:** Pharmacological and Parenteral Therapies **Integrated Process:** Nursing Process: Evaluation **Content Area:** Pharmacology **Strategy:** First, recall that trazodone is often used as a sleep aid. Knowledge regarding the adverse effects of this drug will be helpful in finding the correct answer. When there is more than one correct answer to a question, consider each option as a true/false statement.

12 **Answer: 3 Rationale:** The client needs to make an agreement with the nurse to remain safe, or to report to the nurse if not feeling safe. The agreement to remain visible to the nurses at all times is too vague, and does not give specific responsibility to the nurse or the client. The promise to tell is vague, and does not make the client specifically accountable to the healthcare professionals. Eating all meals in the dining room does not keep the client safe for 24 hours, only during meals. **Cognitive Level:** Applying **Client Need:** Pharmacological and Parenteral Therapies **Integrated Process:** Nursing Process: Implementation **Content Area:** Pharmacology **Strategy:** Note that the question contains a key phrase: *most important safety measure*. This tells you that more than one option might be partially or totally correct. Keep in mind that medication therapy alone is not sufficient in treating this client and select another appropriate intervention.

13 **Answer: 4 Rationale:** Flumazenil is the only drug available that acts as an antagonist to the benzodiazepines. Diazepam and triazolam are benzodiazepines and would not be prescribed to counteract the overdose of a drug from the same classification. Fluvoxamine is a selective serotonin reuptake inhibitor (SSRI) type of antidepressant. **Cognitive Level:** Applying **Client Need:** Pharmacological and Parenteral Therapies **Integrated Process:** Nursing Process: Planning **Content Area:** Pharmacology **Strategy:** Specific knowledge of the antidote to benzodiazepines is needed to answer this question. It might help to remember that the antidote to benzodiazepines is a generic drug name that contains the letters *ze*, and is not a benzodiazepene itself.

14 **Answer: 3 Rationale:** Dry mouth occurs from the anticholinergic effects seen with fluphenazine. Orthostatic hypotension is not a major side effect of fluphenazine. Dizziness or lightheadedness is a sign of orthostatic hypotension, which is not a major side effect of fluphenazine. Confusion is not a side effect of fluphenazine. **Cognitive Level:** Applying **Client Need:** Pharmacological and Parenteral Therapies **Integrated Process:** Nursing Process: Planning **Content Area:** Pharmacology **Strategy:** First, eliminate options that are similar in referring to orthostatic hypotension. Select between the remaining options by choosing the anticholinergic effects, which are of concern.

15 **Answer: 1 Rationale:** Imipramine is very slow to become effective, taking 2–6 weeks, not 5 days. It is better to make gradual changes once the medication is more effective. It is not appropriate to change the care plan after such a short time of therapy; this client needs additional observation and evaluation of behavioral changes. The likelihood of another suicide attempt is high; gradual change and monitoring for changes in mood and behavior are still very critical for this client after only 5 days. The decision to not change the care plan should not influence the client's likelihood of attempting suicide; gradual change and monitoring for changes in mood and behavior are still very critical for this client. **Cognitive Level:** Analyzing **Client Need:** Pharmacological and Parenteral Therapies **Integrated Process:** Nursing Process: Planning **Content Area:** Pharmacology **Strategy:** To answer this question correctly, recall that antidepressants generally take more than 5 days for full effect. With this in mind, realize that the client is still a safety risk, and choose the option that keeps the client safest while medication therapy is progressing.

16 **Answer: 1 Rationale:** With thioridazine, the anticholinergic side effects of dry mouth, constipation, urinary retention, and blurred vision are usually severe. Dry mouth is not associated with extrapyramidal side effects or neuroleptic malignant syndrome. There is usually not a weight loss as a side effect of thioridazine; there is usually a weight gain. **Cognitive Level:** Analyzing **Client Need:** Pharmacological and Parenteral Therapies **Integrated Process:** Nursing Process: Diagnosis **Content Area:** Pharmacology **Strategy:** Specific knowledge of the intended effects and side effects of thioridozine is needed to answer the question. Use the process of elimination to make your selection.

17 **Answer: 1, 3, 5 Rationale:** Marijuana has been used for individuals with AIDS and on chemotherapy for cancer by enhancing the client's sense of taste and smell, which increases their appetite. Common effect of low doses of marijuana is an increased sensitivity to auditory stimuli. Low doses of marijuana do produce a state of relaxation. Marijuana does not promote organization and motivation. Marijuana does not have antibacterial properties. **Cognitive Level:** Applying **Client Need:** Pharmacological and Parenteral Therapies **Integrated Process:** Nursing Process: Implementation **Content Area:**

ANSWERS & RATIONALES

Pharmacology **Strategy:** The core issue of the question is legitimate uses for marijuana. To aid in making the correct selection, keep in mind that an effect of the drug is to stimulate appetite and the senses and promote relaxation. When there is more than one correct answer to a question, consider each option as a true/false statement.

18 **Answer: 3 Rationale:** The need for physical safety is the primary nursing priority for the client at this time. Teaching alternative responses to anxiety is an appropriate nursing intervention, but should be addressed once physical safety is established. Involvement in group or community support activities is appropriate; however, the need for physical safety is the primary nursing priority for the client at this time. Helping to desensitize the client to phobic reaction related to place is an appropriate nursing intervention. This need should be addressed once physical safety is established. **Cognitive Level:** Analyzing **Client Need:** Pharmacological and Parenteral Therapies **Integrated Process:** Nursing Process: Planning **Content Area:** Pharmacology **Strategy:** Note that the drug prescribed is an anxiolytic. Next, relate the cause of the anxiety to the need for the medication. Choose the option that targets the best concern of the client and is congruent with the need for the medication.

19 **Answer: 4 Rationale:** Risperidone has very few side effects; they include orthostatic hypotension and insomnia, agitation, headache, anxiety, and rhinitis. The effect of dizziness is not a desired effect of risperidone. There is no information in the question that indicates that the client has a loss of appetite. Risperidone does not cause sedation. **Cognitive Level:** Analyzing **Client Need:** Pharmacological and Parenteral Therapies **Integrated Process:** Nursing Process: Evaluation **Content Area:** Pharmacology **Strategy:** The core issue of this question is recognition of dizziness as a sign of orthostatic hypotension. With this concept in mind, eliminate each of the other options because they do not relate to this concern.

20 **Answer: 3 Rationale:** The principle of remaining abstinent is one of the three most important goals of treatment for alcoholism. It is also critical when taking disulfiram, in order to avoid adverse effects from the interaction of the medication and alcohol. The other goals of becoming socially reintegrated, learning about the disease process, and remaining in the rehab unit are important but not the priority. They may help concurrent psychiatric conditions and long-term prevention of relapse. **Cognitive Level:** Applying **Client Need:** Pharmacological and Parenteral Therapies **Integrated Process:** Nursing Process: Planning **Content Area:** Pharmacology **Strategy:** The core issue of the question is the interactive effect of disulfiram and alcohol. With this in mind, eliminate each of the incorrect options because they do not address this critical concern.

Key Terms to Review

agranulocytosis p. 503
akathisia p. 502
antagonists p. 502
anticholinergic effects p. 502
dystonia p. 503
extrapyramidal symptoms (EPS) p. 502
metabolite p. 512
neuroleptic malignant syndrome (NMS) p. 503
neuroleptics p. 502
parkinsonism p. 502
serotonin syndrome p. 508
tardive dyskinesia (TD) p. 502
tolerance p. 502

References

Adams, M., Holland, L., & Urban, C. (2017). *Pharmacology for nurses: A pathophysiologic approach* (5th ed.). New York, NY: Pearson Education.

Adams, M., & Urban, C. (2016). *Pharmacology: Connections to nursing practice* (3rd ed.). New York, NY: Pearson Education.

American Psychiatric Association. (2013). *Diagnostic and statistical manual of mental disorders.* (5th ed.). Arlington, VA: Author.

Kniesl, C., & Trigoboff, E. (2013). *Contemporary psychiatric-mental health nursing* (3rd ed.). Upper Saddle River, NJ: Pearson Education.

Lehne, R. (2016). *Pharmacology for nursing care* (9th ed.). St. Louis, MO: Saunders.

Wilson, B., Shannon, M., & Shields, K. (2016). *Pearson nurse's drug guide 2016.* New York, NY: Pearson Education.

Respiratory Medications 36

In this chapter

Cross Reference

Other chapters relevant to this content area are

Dosage Calculation and Medication Administration	Chapter 29
Immunological and Anti-Infective Medications	Chapter 45
Respiratory Disorders	Chapter 55

I. BRONCHODILATORS

A. Beta-agonists (sympathomimetics)

1. Sympathetic nervous system (SNS) **adrenergic agonists** raise intracellular levels of cAMP (cyclic adenosine monophosphate) to dilate constricted bronchi and bronchioles by relaxing smooth muscle
2. Used during an **acute asthma attack**, characterized by bronchospasm with shortness of breath and wheezing, for quick airway dilation and relief of bronchospasm; used also for emphysema and acute and chronic bronchitis
3. **Sympathomimetics** can have $beta_1$ or $beta_2$ activity; $beta_1$ adrenergic receptors increase heart rate and force of myocardial contraction
4. Beta-adrenergic agents can be classified as **catecholamines** released from adrenal medulla in response to SNS stimulation or **noncatecholamines**, which are not released by SNS; all beta-adrenergic agents stimulate $beta_2$ receptors; catecholamines affect both alpha and beta receptors and cause cardiovascular effects
5. Selective $beta_2$ agonists are preferred for bronchial smooth muscle dilation because they produce fewer cardiac side effects
6. Common bronchodilator medications are listed in Box 36–1

Memory Aid

If a medication ends in *-terol* or *-terenol*, it is a sympathomimetic type of bronchodilator.

7. Administration considerations

NCLEX®

   a. Adverse effects may occur with albuterol, levalbuterol, and pirbuterol if used too frequently because they lose $beta_2$-specific actions at larger doses ($beta_1$ receptors are stimulated, leading to elevated heart rate [HR], nausea, anxiety, palpitations, and tremors)

Box 36–1

Common Bronchodilators

Beta Agonists/Sympathomimetics	**Methylxanthine**
Albuterol	Theophylline
Arformoterol	**Anticholinergics**
Formoterol fumarate	Ipratropium
Levalbuterol hydrochloride	Tiotropium
Metaproterenol sulfate	
Pirbuterol acetate	
Salmeterol	
Terbutaline sulfate	

NCLEX® **b.** Use with caution in young children and monitor for tremors, restlessness, hallucinations, dizziness, palpitations, tachycardia, and gastrointestinal (GI) difficulties

c. Salmeterol is not used in an acute asthma attack because of slow onset of action (20 minutes); do not dose more often than every 12 hours because of the 12-hour duration of action

NCLEX® **d.** Contraindicated with hypersensitivity to sympathomimetics or with tachydysrhythmias

e. Use with caution in clients with cardiovascular disease because of potential for increasing myocardial oxygen demand

f. Use with caution in clients with hypertension, diabetes mellitus, seizures, and hypothyroidism

NCLEX® **g.** Children under 12 should not use inhalations of albuterol and terbutaline

NCLEX® **h.** Concurrent use of monoamine oxidase inhibitors (MAOIs) may lead to hypertensive crisis

8. Side/adverse effects

NCLEX® **a.** May cause nervousness, tremors, increased HR, and increased blood pressure (BP) when $beta_1$ receptors are stimulated

b. With alpha- and beta-adrenergic stimulation, may lead to insomnia, restlessness, anorexia, tremors, cardiac stimulation, anginal pain, and vascular headache

c. Additional side effects may include hypokalemia, hyperglycemia, nausea and vomiting (N/V), chest pain, and dysrhythmias

NCLEX® **d.** Paradoxic bronchospasm and urinary retention may also occur

9. Nursing considerations

a. Monitor older adults carefully

NCLEX® **b.** Monitor vital signs, especially HR and BP, when administering beta-agonists (because of cardiovascular effects)

NCLEX® **c.** Proper use of metered-dose inhaler (MDI) is essential for maximum benefit (see Box 36–2 for client teaching about use and care of inhalers)

d. At times, use of multiple drugs is effective and dosages of each can be reduced

NCLEX® **e.** Note amount, color, and character of sputum

f. Monitor baseline and periodic pulmonary function tests during therapy

g. Administer oral medications with meals to decrease GI irritation

h. Solutions may remain diluted for 24–48 hours

NCLEX® **i.** Monitor blood glucose (BG) levels closely in diabetic clients because some medications may elevate BG; an adjustment in maintenance doses of antidiabetic drugs may be indicated

10. Client teaching

a. If diabetic, monitor BG level closely

NCLEX® **b.** Report chest pain, palpitations, seizures, headaches, hallucinations, or blurred vision to prescriber

c. Do not take more than prescribed dose because of risk for hypertension, tachycardia, dysrhythmias, and angina

d. Record prn use of these drugs, noting date, time, symptoms, and effectiveness

NCLEX® **e.** Wait 1–3 minutes (some references suggest 3–5 minutes) between inhalations of aerosol medications

f. Avoid eye contact with inhaler spray

g. Avoid contact with allergens and avoid contact with smoke and other irritants, such as aerosol hairspray, perfumes, and cleaning products

h. Increase fluid intake if not contraindicated by other diseases

Box 36–2

Client Education about the Use and Care of Metered-Dose Inhalers

- ➤ Insert medication firmly into inhaler.
- ➤ Remove cap and hold inhaler upright.
- ➤ Shake inhaler for 3–5 seconds to ensure even mixing of medication in propellant.
- ➤ Tilt head back slightly and hold inhaler upright.
- ➤ Position inhaler 2.5–5 cm (1-2 in.) away from open mouth or attach it to spacer/holding chamber (preferred for best effectiveness); if a medicine chamber is used, seal lips around mouthpiece.
- ➤ Press on inhaler while beginning to breathe in slowly through mouth.
- ➤ Breathe in slowly and deeply for 3–5 seconds.
- ➤ Hold breath for 8–10 seconds as able to allow medication to move down into airways.
- ➤ Wait 1–3 minutes per product directions before next inhalation if another is prescribed.
- ➤ Rinse mouth with water and blow nose.
- ➤ Use mild soap and water to clean mouthpiece; allow to air dry.
- ➤ Store inhaler at room temperature.

Note: In addition to metered-dose inhalers, medication inhalation devices include dry powder inhalers and nebulizers.

i. Teach clients early symptoms of respiratory difficulty (activity intolerance and waking at night with asthma symptoms) for early intervention

NCLEX® **j.** Avoid caffeine, which may increase nervousness and insomnia from bronchodilating drugs

NCLEX® **k.** An inhaled bronchodilator is treatment of choice in an acute asthma attack

l. Nervousness and tremors may occur when a medication is newly administered, but they frequently decrease over time

m. Use inhaled preparations properly (have client demonstrate proper use)

NCLEX® **n.** Understand care of nebulizer and/or inhaler: wash daily in warm water and dry; use white vinegar to rinse the nebulizer tubing; read and follow manufacturer's instructions about use, storage, and cleaning of equipment

o. Anticipated response to use of nebulizer or inhaler is absence of wheezing and dyspnea

B. *Xanthine*-type bronchodilator: theophylline

1. Inhibits phosphodiesterase (PDE), which leads to increased levels of cAMP and bronchial dilation due to smooth muscle relaxation
2. Can also increase catecholamine levels, inhibit calcium ion movement into smooth muscle, inhibit prostaglandin synthesis, and inhibit release of bronchoconstrictive substances from leukocytes and **mast cells** (which contain histamine, prostaglandins, and thromboxanes)
3. By bronchodilation, increases ability of cilia to clear mucus from airways
4. Used to treat bronchoconstriction associated with chronic obstructive pulmonary disease (COPD, including chronic bronchitis, asthma, and emphysema) and other chronic respiratory disorders
5. Has a slow onset of action, so is used to prevent rather than treat asthma attacks; can be used during an asthma attack if it is mild to moderate

NCLEX® 6. Used IV to treat **status asthmaticus** (a bout of severe asthma that cannot be controlled with typical medications) if no response to faster-acting beta agonist)

Memory Aid

If the medication ends in *-phylline*, it is a xanthine type of bronchodilator and has a therapeutic range of 10–20 mcg/mL.

7. Administration considerations

a. Use cautiously in older adults because of risk for increased sensitivity

NCLEX® **b.** Carefully monitor serum drug levels and therapeutic response to avoid potential toxicity; therapeutic range of theophylline is 10–20 mcg/mL

c. Xanthines have a stimulating effect on CNS, which may be enhanced in children
NCLEX® d. Use cautiously in clients with cardiovascular disorders
e. Theophylline doses should be based on lean body weight because it does not enter adipose tissue
f. Theophylline can enter breast milk and cross placenta
NCLEX® g. Dosages are often started low and titrated up as needed for relief of symptoms
h. Those who smoke cigarettes metabolize these drugs more quickly and thus may need higher doses for therapeutic effects
i. Theophylline levels may be increased in liver disease, congestive heart failure (CHF), and acute viral infections because of impaired biotransformation
j. Avoid with known hypersensitivity to xanthines; tachydysrhythmias; hyperthyroidism (exacerbates disease); history of seizure disorders unless unresponsive to other drugs (can cause seizures); peptic ulcer disease, acute gastritis, or other GI disorders because of increased gastric acid secretion
NCLEX® k. Avoid caffeinated drinks and foods, which have additive effects with xanthines
NCLEX® 8. Side/adverse effects
a. N/V, anorexia, and gastroesophageal reflux during sleep
b. Sinus tachycardia, chest pain, palpitations, and ventricular dysrhythmias
c. Hyperglycemia and transient increased urination
NCLEX® d. Tremors, dizziness, hallucinations, restlessness, agitation, headache, and insomnia
9. Nursing considerations
NCLEX® a. Assess for toxicity (restlessness, insomnia, irritability, tremors, N/V); tends to occur when theophylline level exceeds 20 mcg/mL
NCLEX® b. Assess client for hypoxia if restlessness occurs to differentiate cause
c. Refrigerate suppository forms
NCLEX® d. Children may exhibit hyperactive behavior while taking theophylline because of CNS stimulation
10. Client teaching
a. Refrigerate suppository forms
b. Notify prescriber if suppositories cause rectal burning, itching, or irritation
NCLEX® c. Notify prescriber if palpitations, N/V, weakness, dizziness, chest pain, or seizure occur
d. Comply with monitoring blood levels periodically
NCLEX® e. Avoid use of caffeine-containing products (tea, coffee, cola, chocolate), which could lead to an additive effect with xanthines
NCLEX® f. Avoid contact with allergens if possible; avoid contact with smoke and other respiratory irritants such as aerosol hairspray, perfumes, and cleaning products
g. Increase fluid intake if no contraindication because of other disease process
h. Take medications even when there are no symptoms of asthma
i. Take medications with food if GI symptoms develop

II. INHALED CORTICOSTEROIDS

A. Overview

1. Decrease airway inflammation by inhibiting inflammatory mediators, such as **histamine**, leukotriene, cytokines, and prostaglandins
2. Decreased inflammation also reduces mucosal edema, secretions, and bronchoconstriction
3. May aid in increasing responsiveness of bronchial smooth muscle to beta-agonists
4. Appear to help inhibit movement of fluid and protein into tissues as well as inhibit production of prostaglandins, **leukotrienes** (substances released after exposure to an allergen), and **interleukins** (plasma proteins that increase during inflammatory process)
5. Promote mobilization of mucus by increasing mucociliary action
6. Used in chronic asthma to decrease inflammation and therefore decrease airway obstruction, and are used prophylactically, not during acute attack
7. Treats bronchospastic disorders when bronchodilators are not completely effective
8. Used to treat chronic bronchitis, COPD, and cystic fibrosis
9. Common inhaled drugs are listed in Box 36–3; oral corticosteroids such as prednisone and methylprednisolone may also be used

Memory Aid Many corticosteroids contain *-cort* or *-sone* in either the generic or trade name.

Box 36–3

Inhaled Corticosteroid Medications

Beclomethasone dipropionate	Fluticasone propionate
Budesonide	Mometasone furoate
Ciclesonide	Triamcinolone acetonide
Flunisolide	

B. Administration considerations

NCLEX® 1. Proper technique is essential when administering medications via inhalation
2. Beclomethasone has greater anti-inflammatory action and causes fewer side effects than dexamethasone
NCLEX® 3. If client is also taking a systemic corticosteroid, that dose may need to be decreased with addition of inhaled corticosteroids
4. Beclomethasone, flunisolide, and fluticasone are available as nasal solutions for treatment of allergic rhinitis
5. Monitor for impaired bone growth in children receiving inhaled corticosteroids
NCLEX® 6. Contraindicated with known allergy, psychosis, fungal infection, acquired immunodeficiency syndrome (AIDS), tuberculosis, idiopathic thrombocytopenia, and in children under age 2 years
7. Use cautiously in clients with diabetes, glaucoma, osteoporosis, ulcers, renal disease, CHF, myasthenia gravis, seizure disorders, inflammatory bowel disease, hypertension, thromboembolic disorders, esophagitis, and infections (due to risk for suppressed immune system)
NCLEX® 8. Because of possible decreased response to skin test antigens, postpone skin testing if possible until after corticosteroid therapy

C. Side/adverse effects

1. Pharyngeal irritation, sore throat, and **rhinitis** (inflamed nasal mucous membranes)
2. Coughing or dry mouth; oral fungal infections
3. Increased susceptibility to infection, dermatologic effects, and osteoporosis
4. Diarrhea, N/V, and stomach upset
5. Headache, fever, dizziness, angioedema, rash, urticaria, and paradoxical bronchospasm
6. Menstrual disturbances
7. Palpitations
8. Adrenocortical insufficiency, fluid and electrolyte disturbances, nervous system effects, and endocrine effects if absorbed systemically

D. Nursing considerations

1. Assess sputum color and viscosity for signs of infection
2. Children may need prescriber's order to keep an inhaler with them at school

E. Client teaching

1. Keep equipment clean and in working order per manufacturer's guidelines
NCLEX® 2. Rinse mouth after use of inhalation devices such as **inhaler** or **nebulizer**
NCLEX® 3. Do not abruptly stop taking this medication; taper dose slowly over a 2-week period under direction of prescriber
4. Wear a bracelet or necklace to identify self as a steroid user
NCLEX® 5. Learn symptoms of steroid use, including moon face, acne, increased fat pads, increased edema; notify prescriber if these symptoms arise
6. Report signs of decreased steroid levels, including nausea, dyspnea, joint pain, weakness, and fatigue
NCLEX® 7. Report weight gain of more than 5 pounds per week
8. Avoid contact with allergen responsible for producing allergic response if possible
9. Take drug at approximately same time each day for maximal effectiveness
NCLEX® 10. If taking two inhaled medications at same time, use corticosteroid last after bronchodilator to ensure best penetration into lung tissue
NCLEX® 11. Use inhaled corticosteroids as maintenance drugs; they are ineffective in acute bronchospasm

III. INHALED MAST CELL STABILIZERS

A. Overview

1. Stabilize mast cells to prevent release of bronchoconstrictive and inflammatory substances when stimulated by allergen; therefore, inflammation is limited
2. Used to prevent and treat inflammation of airways and decrease mucosal edema, mucous secretions, and bronchoconstriction

3. Used for prophylaxis of acute asthma attacks and to prevent and treat allergic rhinitis
4. Common medication: cromolyn; available as oral spray or nebulizer solution for oral inhalation

B. Administration considerations

NCLEX® 1. Bronchodilator and corticosteroid doses may be decreased with use of this drug
NCLEX® 2. Use cautiously with impaired hepatic or renal function; lower doses may be needed
3. Administer using proper inhalation technique
4. It may take 3 weeks of daily dosing to see therapeutic effects
NCLEX® 5. Do not use in clients with acute bronchospasm, status asthmaticus, or hypersensitivity to drug

C. Side/adverse effects

1. Headache
2. Dry mouth and unpleasant taste
NCLEX® 3. Cough and irritation of throat and trachea, bronchospasm
NCLEX® 4. Erythema, rash, urticaria

D. Nursing considerations

NCLEX® 1. Use cautiously in clients with coronary heart disease and/or cardiac dysrhythmias
2. Pulmonary function testing may be prescribed prior to therapy

E. Client teaching

1. Use inhaler properly to ensure maximal drug effectiveness; use spacer as appropriate
2. Record frequency and severity of asthma attacks
NCLEX® 3. Allow 2–4 weeks for full medication effectiveness
NCLEX® 4. Rinse mouth after taking medication to avoid dry mouth
5. Do not take during an acute attack because symptoms may be aggravated
NCLEX® 6. Optimally, take bronchodilator 20–30 minutes prior to taking cromolyn or according to product literature; wait a minimum of 3–5 minutes between inhalations

IV. LEUKOTRIENE MODIFIERS

A. Overview

1. Leukotrienes are substances released during an allergic response; they cause inflammation, bronchoconstriction, and mucus production that leads to coughing, sneezing, and shortness of breath
2. Leukotriene modifiers reduce airway inflammation by either blocking leukotriene receptors or blocking an enzyme that controls leukotriene synthesis
3. Provide relief of inflammatory symptoms of asthma
4. Used for prophylaxis and chronic treatment of asthma in adults and children over age 12; they are not used in managing an acute asthma attack
5. Common leukotriene modifiers are listed in Box 36–4

Memory Aid

If a medication ends in *-lukast*, it is a leukotriene modifier.

B. Administration considerations

1. Leukotriene modifiers are oral drugs used in adults and children age 12 and older
NCLEX® 2. They exert localized effects in lungs and therapeutic effects may take up to a week
NCLEX® 3. They are used alone or in combination with corticosteroids

C. Side/adverse effects

1. Headaches may occur with all drugs
2. Zileuton may also cause dyspepsia, nausea, dizziness, insomnia, and hepatotoxicity
3. Zafirlukast may cause nausea and diarrhea
4. Monitor clients over age 55 for infection

Box 36–4
Leukotriene Modifiers

Montelukast	Zafirlukast
Zileuton	

D. Nursing considerations

1. Be sure drug is prescribed for chronic, not acute, treatment of asthma
2. NCLEX® Monitor liver enzymes during zileuton therapy and discontinue drug if elevated to five times normal value or if liver dysfunction develops

E. Client teaching

1. NCLEX® Expect drugs to take a week before therapeutic effects are seen
2. NCLEX® Follow-up liver function studies may be needed
3. NCLEX® Drugs prevent some asthma symptoms but are not to be used for acute attacks
4. Avoid contact with specific allergen if possible
5. Increase fluid intake if not contraindicated because of other disease processes
6. Take zafirlukast 1 hour before or 2 hours after meals
7. Montelukast and zileuton may be taken with or without food

V. ANTIHISTAMINES

A. Overview

1. **Antihistamines** (histamine antagonists) are used to treat allergies, allergic rhinitis (hay fever), allergic conjunctivitis, allergic contact dermatitis, vertigo, motion sickness, insomnia, allergic reactions, cough, and sneezing and runny nose from common cold
2. Compete with histamine for H_1 receptor sites and thereby block action of histamine following its release; work best early in response because they do not displace histamine from H_1 receptors
3. Cause bronchial smooth muscle relaxation and reduce bronchial, salivary, gastric, nasal, and **lacrimal** (tear) secretions
4. Reduce itching (urticaria) and are used to treat anaphylactic shock
5. Can be used to prevent or treat allergic reactions to medications
6. Common antihistamines are listed in Box 36–5

B. Administration considerations

1. NCLEX® Treat symptoms but not the cause of a problem
2. Should not be used to treat acute asthma attack or lower respiratory disorder
3. Most antihistamines are tolerated better when taken with meals
4. Hydroxyzine is effective with pruritis
5. Azelastine is topically applied to nasal mucosa and action peaks in 2–3 hours; it does not tend to cause drowsiness but does leave an unpleasant taste in mouth
6. NCLEX® Antihistamines may be used as premedication before administering blood products to decrease risk of allergic reactions
7. Oral antihistamines act in 15–60 minutes and last 4–6 hours; sustained-release medications last 8–12 hours
8. Use a rapid-acting agent with an acute allergic reaction
9. Longer-acting agents give more consistent relief with chronic allergic conditions
10. Should be used cautiously with history of increased intraocular pressure, cardiac or renal disease, hypertension, bronchial asthma, stenosing peptic ulcer disease, prostatic hyperplasia, convulsive disorders, or during pregnancy
11. NCLEX® Can mask positive skin test results; discontinue use for 3 days (72 hours) before allergy skin testing

Box 36–5 Antihistamines

Second-Generation or Less Sedating Antihistamines	First-Generation or Traditional Antihistamines
Acrivastine with pseudoephedrine	Brompheniramine
Azelastine	Chlorpheniramine
Cetirizine	Clemastine
Desloratadine	Cyproheptadine
Fexofenadine	Dexchlorpheniramine
Levocetirizine	Dimenhydrinate
Loratidine	Diphenhydramine
Olapatadine	Promethazine
	Triprolidine

C. Side/adverse effects

NCLEX® 1. Drowsiness is main side effect; children can experience paradoxical excitement

NCLEX® 2. **Anticholinergic** side effects include dry mouth and nose, changes in vision, difficulty urinating, and constipation

3. Sedation from drowsiness to deep sleep, dizziness, syncope, muscular weakness, unsteady gait, paradoxical excitement (especially in older adults), restlessness, insomnia, and nervousness

4. Anorexia, N/V, diarrhea, constipation, and jaundice

NCLEX® 5. Urinary retention, impotence, vertigo, visual disturbances, blurred vision, tinnitus, hypotension, syncope, and headache

6. Hemolytic anemia, leukopenia, thrombocytopenia, and pancytopenia

D. Nursing considerations

1. Cetirizine, loratadine, and fexofenadine may be used in children over age 6

2. Help client determine precipitating factors and symptoms of allergic reactions

NCLEX® 3. Assess for drowsiness and dizziness, especially during first few days of therapy

4. Encourage fluid intake of 2000–3000 mL/day to loosen secretions unless contraindicated by another condition

NCLEX® 5. Administer at bedtime to reduce side effect of drowsiness

6. Administer intramuscular antihistamines deep into large muscles

7. Intravenous injection should be over a few minutes; see product literature

E. Client teaching

1. Take with meals to decrease stomach upset

2. Avoid contact with allergen if possible; if unable, take medication prior to exposure

3. Do not take more than one medication at a time

NCLEX® 4. Contact prescriber if excessive sedation, confusion, or hypotension occur

5. Use hard, sugarless candy to relieve dry mouth

6. Increase fluid intake; antihistamines may dry and thicken respiratory tract secretions and make them difficult to expectorate

7. Take loratadine on an empty stomach to increase absorption

8. Avoid prolonged exposure to sunlight because of potential for sunburn

9. Take medication at bedtime to reduce drowsiness, which should become less significant after repeated doses

NCLEX® 10. Do not take antihistamines for 72 hours prior to allergen skin testing to reduce likelihood of false-negative results

VI. MEDICATIONS TO CONTROL AIRWAY SECRETIONS

A. Nasal *decongestants*

1. Relieve nasal stuffiness by shrinking swollen nasal mucous membranes

2. Adrenergic agents (sympathomimetics) cause vasoconstriction, decreasing blood flow to nasal mucosa and thereby reducing swelling

3. Corticosteroids can also be administered by nasal route to suppress inflammatory response

4. Used to relieve nasal congestion and nasal discharge caused by acute or chronic rhinitis (common cold), sinusitis, hay fever, and other allergies

5. May be used to decrease local blood flow prior to nasal surgery or as an aid to visualizing nasal mucosa during diagnostic exams

6. Common medications to control bronchial secretions are listed in Box 36–6

Memory Aid

A medication that ends in *-zoline* is a nasal decongestant, although not all nasal decongestants end in *-zoline*.

7. Administration considerations

a. Can be used topically (with sprays or drops) or orally

NCLEX® b. Sustained use of topical drugs (longer than 3 days or in excessive amounts) can cause rebound congestion; therefore, oral agents should be used if needed for longer than 3 days

c. Topical drugs are potent decongestants with prompt onset of action

d. Topical drugs are preferred if client has cardiovascular disease because of decreased risk of cardiovascular side effects

Box 36–6

Medications That Control Bronchial Secretions

Nasal Decongestants

Naphazoline

Oxymetazoline

Phenylephrine hydrochloride

Pseudoephedrine hydrochloride

Tetrahydrozoline

Xylometazoline

Expectorant

Guaifenesin

Antitussives

Nonopioid type

Benzonatate

Dextromethorphan

Opioid type

Codeine phosphate or sulfate

Hydrocodone with homatropine

Mucolytics

Sodium chloride solution by nebulization

Acetylcysteine (nebulizer)

Dornase alfa (a proteolytic enzyme for clients with cystic fibrosis only)

8. Side/adverse effects
   a. Local nasal mucosal irritation and dryness
   b. Rebound congestion is common
   c. Nervousness, insomnia, palpitations, and tremor (with systemic absorption) are rare
9. Nursing considerations
   NCLEX® a. Assess client's medical history to determine risk for side effects; older adults with significant cardiac disease should avoid nasal decongestants (high risk for hypertension, dysrhythmias, nervousness, and insomnia)
   b. To administer nose drops, have client lie down or sit with neck hyperextended
   c. Wash medication droppers after each use to prevent contamination
   d. Client should squeeze nasal spray container once, avoid touching nares with spray dispenser, and rinse tip of dispenser after each use
   e. Observe client for intended decrease in nasal congestion
   NCLEX® f. Assess for tachycardia, hypertension, and cardiac dysrhythmias; also observe for rebound nasal congestion, chronic rhinitis, and ulceration of the nasal mucosa
10. Client teaching
   NCLEX® a. Avoid concurrent use of caffeine, which can cause nervousness, tremors, and insomnia
   b. Avoid smoking because it increases secretions and decreases ciliary action
   c. Avoid exposure to crowds to minimize spread of disease
   NCLEX® d. Increase fluid intake to 2000–3000 mL/day unless contraindicated by another medical condition
   NCLEX® e. Nasal congestion in infants can decrease ability to suck effectively; apply nasal solution prior to feeding to increase infant's ability to feed
   f. Avoid eating or drinking for 30 minutes after medication administration
   g. Practice good hand hygiene
   NCLEX® h. Rinse droppers and spray bottles after each use to avoid contamination

B. *Expectorant*

1. Expectorants reduce viscosity of secretions and increase mucus flow in respiratory tract to aid removal by cough reflex and ciliary action
2. Used to relieve nonproductive cough associated with common cold, bronchitis, laryngitis, and influenza
3. Common expectorant is guaifenesin (see Box 36–6); found in many OTC cough and cold products
4. NCLEX® Administration considerations: use with caution in older adults or debilitated clients, or those with asthma and respiratory insufficiency
5. Side/adverse effects: N/V, gastric irritation, rash, dizziness, and headache
6. Nursing considerations: none specific to this group
7. Client teaching
   NCLEX® a. Report a fever or cough to prescriber if it lasts longer than a week
   NCLEX® b. Increase fluid intake if not contraindicated by other disease processes

c. Avoid smoking because it increases secretions and decreases ciliary action
d. Avoid drinking fluids for 30 minutes after use

C. *Antitussives*

1. **Opioid** (narcotic) and nonopioid antitussives suppress cough reflex by directly affecting cough center; nonopioid antitussives do so without CNS suppression
2. Peripherally acting agents (glycerin, ammonium chloride) have local anesthetic effects to decrease irritation of pharyngeal mucosa; available in gargles, lozenges, and syrups; lozenges increase saliva flow to suppress cough
3. Used to stop a nonproductive cough or a dry, hacking, nonproductive cough that interferes with rest and sleep
4. Common antitussive medications are listed in Box 36–6
5. Administration considerations
   NCLEX® a. There is risk for addiction and CNS and respiratory depression with opioids
   b. Most are given as liquid or as oral tablets; syrup form may soothe irritated mucosa in pharynx
   c. Dextromethorphan is preferred over codeine because it provides desired effect without use of opioids; available in many OTC products and does not require a prescription
   d. Dextromethorphan is contraindicated with asthma, emphysema, chronic headaches, or hypersensitivity
   NCLEX® e. Codeine preparations are contraindicated with respiratory depression, increased intracranial pressure, severe liver or renal disease, hypothyroidism, adrenal insufficiency, or seizure disorders
6. Side/adverse effects
   a. Dizziness, headache, drowsiness or sedation, N/V, constipation, pruritus, nasal congestion, dry mouth, blurred vision, and sweating
   NCLEX® b. Dependence and respiratory depression with codeine
   c. Dry mouth, palpitations, thickened respiratory mucus, anorexia, urinary retention or frequency, diarrhea, photosensitivity, and dysuria with nonopioids
   d. Nasal congestion and burning of the eyes with benzonatate
7. Nursing considerations
   a. Assess for inability to cough effectively from excessive cough suppression
   b. Observe for listed side effects and potential drug dependence
   NCLEX® c. Cough may be a useful diagnostic tool and protective measure for client; use antitussives cautiously for irritating, nonproductive, ineffective cough
8. Client teaching
   NCLEX® a. Notify prescriber if cough lasts longer than a week or if persistent headache, fever, or rash occurs
   b. Do not drink liquids for 30–35 minutes after taking a chewable tablet or a lozenge
   c. Avoid smoking because it increases secretions and decreases ciliary action
   d. For excessive respiratory secretions, understand benefits of coughing, deep breathing, and ambulation
   NCLEX® e. Liquefy secretions with increased oral intake up to 2000–3000 mL/day unless contraindicated

D. *Mucolytics*

1. Administered by inhalation to liquefy (thin) mucus in respiratory tract and aid in removal of viscous secretions
2. Used with sinusitis and common cold
3. An oral form of acetylcysteine can be used to treat acetaminophen overdose
4. Common mucolytic medications are listed in Box 36–6
5. Administration considerations
   a. Used less often because of questionable effectiveness
   NCLEX® b. These drugs are nebulized using a face mask or a mouthpiece; can be instilled into a tracheostomy
   c. Acetylcysteine is effective 1 minute after inhalation or immediately after direct instillation; maximal effect is in 5–10 minutes
   NCLEX® d. Activated charcoal limits effectiveness of acetylcysteine when used as antidote to acetaminophen overdose
6. Side/adverse effects: oral irritation, sore throat, cough and bronchospasm, N/V, headaches
7. Nursing considerations
   NCLEX® a. May cause bronchospasm and are usually given with bronchodilators
   b. Suction client if cough is ineffective
   c. Rinse mouth after therapy to decrease oropharyngeal irritation
   NCLEX® d. Discard unused medication after 4 days
8. Client teaching
   NCLEX® a. Increase fluid intake unless contraindicated by other disease processes
   b. Avoid smoking because it increases secretions and decreases ciliary action

VII. OXYGEN

A. Indications

1. **Hypoxia**, deficiency of oxygen (O_2) in cells and tissues, and **hypoxemia**, deficiency of O_2 in arterial blood
2. Conditions associated with decreased arterial oxygen (PaO_2) levels (pulmonary edema), decreased cardiac output (myocardial infarction), decreased blood O_2-carrying capacity (anemia), increased O_2 demand (sepsis, sustained fever), and others

B. Types of delivery systems

1. Nasal cannula (nasal prongs): most common form of O_2 delivery
   a. Prongs insert into nostrils and tubing attaches to oxygen source and flowmeter
   b. Client can eat and talk with a nasal cannula
   c. *NCLEX®* Oxygen can be administered at a rate ranging from 1 L/min to 6 L/min
   d. Dryness of mucous membranes can occur
2. Nasal catheter: inserted into throat through a nostril, change to other nostril every 8 hours; not used frequently because of client discomfort; gastric distention sometimes occurs
3. Oxymizer: a nasal cannula with a reservoir that can deliver approximately twice the concentration of O_2 than a regular cannula without use of a mask
4. *NCLEX®* Face mask: a mask that fits over client's mouth and nose
   a. Simple face mask: flow rate is 5–10 L/min with O_2 delivery capabilities of 40–60%
   b. Partial rebreather mask: consists of a face mask with a reservoir bag; some exhaled air goes into reservoir bag and is mixed with 100% O_2 for next inhalation; permits conservation of O_2 and can deliver 70–90% O_2 at rates of 6–15 L/min
   c. Nonrebreather mask: delivers highest concentration of O_2 by mask (60–100% O_2 at flow rates of 6–15 L/min); no exhaled air goes into reservoir bag; reservoir bag contains O_2, which client breathes in with inspiration; exhaled air passes through side vents
   d. Venturi mask: percentage of O_2 is adjusted by a dial at end of mask; amount of air pulled into system varies with needed amount of O_2 and gives precise O_2 concentrations

C. Oxygen toxicity

1. *NCLEX®* Prolonged exposure to high O_2 concentrations can damage lung tissue
2. Exact amount of O_2 and length of time required to cause O_2 toxicity depends on degree of underlying lung disease; some sources say lung damage can occur with O_2 delivery of greater than 50% for more than 24–48 hours
3. *NCLEX®* **Atelectasis**, or alveolar collapse, can result with O_2 administration at rates of 60% for more than 36 hours or 90% for more than 6 hours
4. Adult respiratory distress syndrome (ARDS) can result from breathing 80–100% oxygen for more than 24 hours
5. Symptoms of O_2 toxicity begin as a nonproductive cough, substernal chest pain, GI upset, and dyspnea; as it worsens, client develops decreased vital capacity, lung compliance, and hypoxemia; atelectasis, pulmonary edema, and pulmonary hemorrhage can result if not reversed
6. *NCLEX®* Oxygen should be weaned as soon as possible according to O_2 saturation (SaO_2) level

D. Nursing considerations (see also Chapter 26)

1. Oxygen therapy can be anxiety-provoking; provide sufficient explanation and allow client to express anxieties
2. Flow rate is measured in liters per minute (L/min); it is a measure of O_2 delivered but is not completely accurate because there is loss of O_2 content with leaking and mixing with room air
3. Oxygen analyzers are available to measure percentage of O_2 client inhales; this is recommended every 4 hours
4. *NCLEX®* Clients with COPD should not receive O_2 at more than 2 L/min by nasal cannula because higher levels of O_2 in bloodstream can cause hypoventilation; a COPD client's drive to breathe is from low levels of O_2 tension
5. *NCLEX®* Check O_2 delivery system frequently to ensure proper functioning
6. Oxygen should be humidified when client is receiving rates higher than 2 L/min
7. A face mask should fit client's face to avoid unnecessary leakage; if mask is too snug, skin irritation can occur
8. Masks can be changed to a nasal cannula during meals with prescriber order
9. *NCLEX®* The reservoir bag on a partial rebreather should deflate slightly with inspiration
10. Provide reassurance if client becomes claustrophobic
11. *NCLEX®* Flaps on side of nonrebreather mask should open during exhalation and close during inhalation
12. *NCLEX®* Monitor SaO_2 with pulse oximeter during O_2 therapy; with prescriber order, O_2 may be titrated to achieve desired SaO_2 level

13. Assess for signs of hypoxia and respiratory distress, changes in vital signs and color changes (pallor, dusky, cyanosis)
14. Monitor arterial blood gases (ABGs) per healthcare provider
15. Normal arterial O_2 levels decrease with age
16. NCLEX® Provide oral care for comfort because of potential drying of mucous membranes
17. Identify clients at high risk for developing O_2 toxicity

E. Client teaching

1. Expect noise with flow of O_2
2. NCLEX® Avoid open flames with O_2 administration because it is flammable
3. NCLEX® Ensure there are no frayed electrical cords near O_2 so there are no sparks causing combustion
4. NCLEX® Do not smoke when O_2 therapy is being utilized
5. Expect delivery to cause dryness of mouth and nasal mucosa
6. NCLEX® Remove O_2 when using an electric razor
7. Continue O_2 therapy at home as prescribed
8. NCLEX® Keep O_2 tank in holder and away from direct sunlight to reduce effects of heat
9. Understand signs of hypoxia and report them to prescriber

Check Your NCLEX–RN® Exam I.Q.

You are ready for testing on this content if you can:

- Apply knowledge of expected actions and effects of respiratory medications to client care.
- Correctly administer respiratory medications to clients.
- Assess for side effects and adverse effects of respiratory medications.
- Take appropriate action if a client has an unexpected response to a respiratory medication.
- Monitor a client for expected outcomes or effects of treatment with respiratory medications.

PRACTICE TEST

1 A client with heart failure is taking digoxin and furosemide. A new diagnosis of acute bronchitis is made, and albuterol via inhalation is started. The nurse should anticipate that this client is at risk for what complication?

1. Hyperkalemia
2. Hypernatremia
3. Hypocalcemia
4. Hypokalemia

2 A client with asthma has begun drug therapy with formoterol fumarate. The client also takes a monoamine oxidase inhibitor (MAOI). For what complication should the nurse assess the client?

1. Hypotension
2. Hypertension
3. Tachycardia
4. Bradycardia

3 A client who has diabetes mellitus begins drug therapy with albuterol for exercise-induced asthma. Which follow-up finding should indicate to the nurse that the client is experiencing a side effect of this medication?

1. Blood glucose level 152 mg/dL
2. Blood glucose level 57 mg/dL
3. Potassium level 5.4 mEq/L
4. Potassium level 3.1 mEq/L

4 The nurse is teaching a client with chronic obstructive pulmonary disease (COPD) how to administer multiple medications by inhalation. Which statement by the client indicates an understanding of the instruction? Select all that apply.

1. "If my symptoms get worse, I can double my dosage."
2. "I will wait at least 1 minute between use of my different inhalers."
3. "I should consult my prescriber before using over-the-counter medications."
4. "I cannot rinse my inhaler equipment because it is not supposed to get wet."
5. "I should store my inhaler in the refrigerator door between uses."

5 A client reports nervousness and tremors after beginning drug therapy with salmeterol. Which statement by the nurse is most appropriate?

1. "The symptoms are common at first, but decrease over time."
2. "Stop taking the medicine because the symptoms will only get worse."
3. "Drinking coffee or tea will help decrease the symptoms."
4. "Those symptoms indicate a worsening of the disease process."

6 The nurse is teaching the client about home administration of theophylline. Which statement by the client reflects an understanding of the instruction?

1. "I can crush the sustained-release forms so they are easier to swallow."
2. "If a dose is omitted, I can take a double dose the next time."
3. "I should take the medication as soon as symptoms occur."
4. "Taking the medication with food will prevent stomach upset."

7 A client who takes theophylline complains of restlessness. Which is the most appropriate action for the nurse to take first?

1. Assess the client for hypoxia.
2. Explain that this is a toxic reaction, and call the prescriber.
3. Assess the client for other signs and symptoms of theophylline toxicity.
4. Call the prescriber to obtain an order for a theophylline level.

8 A client asks the nurse why beclomethasone was prescribed for his chronic obstructive pulmonary disease (COPD). Which statement by the nurse is most appropriate?

1. "Beclomethasone prevents airway dilation."
2. "Beclomethasone decreases inflammation, and makes it easier to breathe."
3. "Beclomethasone suppresses the immune response."
4. "Beclomethasone decreases responsiveness to medications that dilate the airway."

9 The nurse is teaching a client about cromolyn. Which statement should the nurse make about the mechanism of action for cromolyn?

1. Relaxes bronchial smooth muscle to assist with bronchodilation
2. Limits inflammation and bronchoconstriction with exposure to allergens
3. Helps to liquefy respiratory secretions to promote expectoration
4. Promotes bronchoconstriction of overly dilated airways

10 The nurse is assessing the client who takes cromolyn. Which symptom indicates to the nurse that the client is experiencing a potential side effect? Select all that apply.

1. Vomiting
2. Dry mouth
3. Tachycardia
4. Headache
5. Throat irritation

11 A client beginning medication therapy with montelukast asks the nurse how the medication is helping the symptoms. Which is the nurse's best response?

1. "Montelukast decreases inflammation and mucus secretion."
2. "Montelukast increases mucus secretion and bronchodilation."
3. "Montelukast prevents smooth muscle contraction by nervous system stimulation."
4. "Montelukast protects the airway from the effects of allergen exposure."

12 The client asks the nurse about self-care related to newly prescribed zafirlukast. What is an appropriate response by the nurse?

1. Renal function tests should be monitored.
2. Liver function tests should be monitored.
3. Fluid intake should be decreased.
4. The medication should be taken with meals.

13. A client asks the nurse if there is a benefit to taking second-generation antihistamines instead of first-generation antihistamines. What is the nurse's best response in identifying the fewer side effects of second-generation antihistamines?

1. Nausea
2. Anxiety
3. Drowsiness
4. Euphoria

14. A client asks the nurse about drug interactions with diphenhydramine. The nurse informs the client that which substances will increase the effects of diphenhydramine? Select all that apply.

1. Alcohol
2. Opiates
3. Caffeine
4. Antianxiety agents
5. Tricyclic antidepressants

15. The nurse is teaching a client proper technique for self-administration of nasal sprays. Which explanation should the nurse use in order to provide accurate information?

1. "Squeeze the bottle twice in each nostril for an adequate dose."
2. "Inhale while holding your finger over the other nostril."
3. "Rinsing the tip of the spray bottle can contaminate the medication."
4. "Lying down for administration ensures the medication is instilled."

16. The nurse is developing a teaching plan for a client using a nasal decongestant. What instruction should the nurse include in the teaching plan?

1. "Be sure to stay on the medication for at least 7 days."
2. "Decrease fluid intake to 1L/day to decrease nasal secretions."
3. "Avoid eating or drinking for 30 minutes after medication administration."
4. "Decrease smoking activity while using this medication."

17. The nurse is preparing to teach the client important information related to self-administration of guaifenesin. What information should the nurse include in the teaching plan?

1. Side effects include nausea, vomiting, and rash.
2. Report a cough to the prescriber if it lasts longer than 2 weeks.
3. Take the medication with meals.
4. If the medication is not effective, double the dose.

18. The nurse is assessing a client for side effects of an opioid antitussive. Which side effect is the most significant if noted during assessment?

1. Dry, cracked lips
2. Report of blurred vision
3. Inability to stay awake
4. Respirations of 10/min

19. Which statement by the client taking a mucolytic indicates a need for further teaching?

1. "I will drink at least 2–3 liters of fluid each day."
2. "I will avoid smoking."
3. "I will rinse my mouth after I take my medicine."
4. "I should discard what I do not use of the medicine after a week."

20. The nurse has an order to administer 50% oxygen to a client with pulmonary edema. Which oxygen administration system should the nurse select that allows that percentage of oxygen to be delivered?

1. Nasal cannula
2. Nonrebreather mask
3. Partial rebreather mask
4. Venturi mask

ANSWERS & RATIONALES

1 **Answer: 4 Rationale:** Risk of hypokalemia is worsened by the concurrent use of a potassium-wasting diuretic and a beta-agonist (albuterol) medication. Furthermore, the risk of cardiac glycoside toxicity is worse in the presence of hypokalemia. Hyperkalemia, hypernatremia, and hypocalcemia are not of concern with this drug regimen. **Cognitive Level:** Analyzing **Client Need:** Pharmacological and Parenteral Therapies **Integrated Process:** Nursing Process: Diagnosis **Content Area:** Pharmacology **Strategy:** The core issue of this question is the effect of taking a potassium-losing diuretic with other cardiac or respiratory medications, which helps you to focus on hypokalemia. Note also that two options are opposites, so there is a greater chance that one of these is the correct answer.

2 **Answer: 2 Rationale:** Concurrent use of an MAOI and a beta-agonist such as formoterol can lead to hypertensive crisis. Hypotension is not of concern with this combination of medications; the client is at risk for a hypertensive crisis. The beta-agonist could lead to tachycardia, but since no specific agent is listed, the nurse should consider the potential interaction of the MAOI and the beta-agonist first. Bradycardia is not of concern with this combination of medications; it is more likely that the client will experience tachycardia. **Cognitive Level:** Analyzing **Client Need:** Pharmacological and Parenteral Therapies **Integrated Process:** Nursing Process: Assessment **Content Area:** Pharmacology **Strategy:** The core issue of the question is interactive effects of beta-agonists and MAOIs. Use the process of elimination, and recall that an agonist type of drug enhances the action of a system, in this case the beta-adrenergic system. Then recall that these effects include increased pulse and blood pressure. Note also that two of these options are opposites, making it more likely that one of them is the correct answer.

3 **Answer: 1 Rationale:** Albuterol is a beta-adrenergic agent used to dilate bronchial airways. It can cause an increased blood glucose level, which is especially an issue for a client with diabetes mellitus. These clients should be instructed to monitor blood glucose levels because an adjustment in maintenance doses of hypoglycemic agents could be indicated. Hypoglycemia, hyperkalemia, and hypokalemia are not expected effects of the medication. **Cognitive Level:** Analyzing **Client Need:** Pharmacological and Parenteral Therapies **Integrated Process:** Nursing Process: Assessment **Content Area:** Pharmacology **Strategy:** The core issue of the question is knowledge that beta-adrenergic medications stimulate the sympathetic nervous system, and that one of the end effects of the stimulation is increased blood glucose. Correlate this knowledge with the client in the question, who has diabetes, to make a correct selection relative to hyperglycemia.

4 **Answer: 2, 3 Rationale:** The client should wait at least 1 minute between inhalations. OTC products should not be added without consulting the prescriber. Dosages should be taken exactly as prescribed. Inhaler equipment should be cleaned with mild soap, rinsed, and dried daily. The inhaler should be stored at room temperature. **Cognitive Level:** Applying **Client Need:** Pharmacological and Parenteral Therapies **Integrated Process:** Nursing Process: Evaluation **Content Area:** Pharmacology **Strategy:** The core issue of the question is correct administration procedure for inhaled medications. The wording of the question tells you the correct answers are options phrased as true statements. When more than one answer is correct, consider each option as a true/false statement.

5 **Answer: 1 Rationale:** Nervousness and tremors might be experienced when salmeterol (a beta-agonist) is newly administered, but they frequently decrease over time. Clients should not terminate medication use without consulting the prescriber. Caffeine would exacerbate the problem. The symptoms are likely related to the medication, and not to the disease process. **Cognitive Level:** Analyzing **Client Need:** Pharmacological and Parenteral Therapies **Integrated Process:** Communication and Documentation **Content Area:** Pharmacology **Strategy:** Knowledge of the side effects with a beta-adrenergic agent will be helpful in answering the question. Combine information about the drug with the principles of therapeutic communication to select the correct answer.

6 **Answer: 4 Rationale:** Taking the medication with food can decrease GI symptoms. Sustained-release forms should not be crushed or chewed because doing so irritates the gastric mucosa and changes the absorption of the medication. Medications should be taken as prescribed, without omissions or doubled doses. Theophylline should be taken at all times and as prescribed, not just when the client is symptomatic. **Cognitive Level:** Applying **Client Need:** Pharmacological and Parenteral Therapies **Integrated Process:** Teaching and Learning **Content Area:** Pharmacology **Strategy:** The core issues of the question are general medication knowledge and instructions for use of theophylline. Eliminate the options that are not consistent with the general principles for self-administration of medication.

7 **Answer: 1 Rationale:** Because restlessness is often an early indicator of hypoxia, the first action is to assess for hypoxia. The nurse should perform additional assessment before calling the prescriber to report a toxic reaction. After ruling out hypoxia as a cause of restlessness, the nurse should assess the client for other possible signs and symptoms of toxicity (insomnia, irritability, nausea/vomiting, tremors). Requesting an order for a theophylline level may be appropriate after performing all assessments. **Cognitive Level:** Analyzing **Client Need:** Pharmacological and Parenteral Therapies **Integrated Process:** Nursing Process: Planning **Content Area:** Pharmacology **Strategy:** The question contains the word *first*, which indicates that more than one option might be technically correct, but one is best. All the incorrect options refer to the theme of toxicity. If options are very similar, none of them can be correct. Use the integrated principles of nursing process: assessment and ABCs to help determine the correct answer.

8 **Answer: 2 Rationale:** Beclomethasone is an inhaled corticosteroid that is thought to decrease inflammation and dilate the airway. Preventing airway dilation is undesirable for this client, and the exact opposite action of beclomethasone. The exact mechanism of action is unknown. Beclomethasone, like any other corticosteroid, does suppress the immune response, but this is not the rationale for administration of the medication. Inhaled corticosteroids are thought to increase responsiveness of bronchial smooth

muscle to beta-agonist drugs. **Cognitive Level:** Applying **Client Need:** Pharmacological and Parenteral Therapies **Integrated Process:** Teaching and Learning **Content Area:** Pharmacology **Strategy:** Use medication knowledge and the process of elimination to make a selection. Knowledge about the pathology of COPD will be helpful in identifying the correct answer.

9 **Answer: 2 Rationale:** Cromolyn is a nonsteroidal agent that stabilizes mast cells so bronchoconstrictive and inflammatory substances are not released when stimulated with an allergen. It is used to treat inflammation of the airway. Cromolyn is a nonsteroidal agent; not a bronchodilator. Cromolyn is a nonsteroidal agent; not an expectorant. Cromolyn is used to treat inflammation of the airway. It does not cause bronchoconstriction. **Cognitive Level:** Applying **Client Need:** Pharmacological and Parenteral Therapies **Integrated Process:** Teaching and Learning **Content Area:** Pharmacology **Strategy:** Use medication knowledge in conjunction with knowledge of the pathophysiology of COPD to select the correct answer.

10 **Answer: 2, 4, 5 Rationale:** Side effects of cromolyn include dry mouth, headaches, and throat irritation. Vomiting and tachycardia are not side effects of cromolyn. **Cognitive Level:** Applying **Client Need:** Pharmacological and Parenteral Therapies **Integrated Process:** Nursing Process: Assessment **Content Area:** Pharmacology **Strategy:** Specific medication knowledge is needed to answer this question. Use the process of elimination to make a selection.

11 **Answer: 1 Rationale:** Leukotriene modifiers such as montelukast block the action of leukotrienes, and therefore decrease mucous secretion and reduce inflammation, preventing bronchoconstriction. Montelukast blocks the action of leukotrienes and decreases mucous secretion. Leukotriene modifiers such as montelukast do not prevent smooth muscle contraction; they decrease mucous secretion and reduce inflammation. Leukotrienes are released when a client is exposed to an allergen. Leukotriene modifiers such as montelukast do not protect the airway from the effects of allergen exposure. **Cognitive Level:** Applying **Client Need:** Pharmacological and Parenteral Therapies **Integrated Process:** Teaching and Learning **Content Area:** Pharmacology **Strategy:** Specific medication knowledge is needed to answer this question. Use the process of elimination to make a selection.

12 **Answer: 2 Rationale:** Liver function tests should be monitored with leukotriene modifiers because of the potential for liver dysfunction with this type of medication. Renal studies are unnecessary in relation to this medication. Fluid intake should be increased unless contraindicated by another condition, in order to thin secretions and assist in their mobilization. The medication should be taken 1 hour before or 2 hours after meals. **Cognitive Level:** Applying **Client Need:** Pharmacological and Parenteral Therapies **Integrated Process:** Teaching and Learning **Content Area:** Pharmacology **Strategy:** Recall that metabolism and excretion of many drugs occurs in either the hepatic or renal systems. This provides a clue that two of the options may be correct. Associate the letter *l* in *leukotrienes* with the letter *l* for *liver*.

13 **Answer: 3 Rationale:** Second-generation antihistamines cause less sedation than do first-generation medications, so the client experiences less drowsiness. They are selective for peripheral H1 histamine receptors, and do not cross the blood–brain barrier. Nausea, anxiety, and euphoria are unrelated as comparison points between first- and second-generation antihistamines. **Cognitive Level:** Applying **Client Need:** Pharmacological and Parenteral Therapies **Integrated Process:** Teaching and Learning **Content Area:** Pharmacology **Strategy:** Recall that second-generation drugs generally have some type of improvement over first-generation drugs. In this case, since antihistamines often cause drowsiness, it is easy to reason that this side effect would be decreased in second-generation medications in this category.

14 **Answer: 1, 2, 4, 5 Rationale:** The effects of first-generation antihistamines, such as diphenhydramine, are increased with alcohol, opioid analgesics, antianxiety agents, and tricyclic antidepressants. The consumption of caffeine, a stimulant, would not have an additive effect when taking diphenhydramine. **Cognitive Level:** Analyzing **Client Need:** Pharmacological and Parenteral Therapies **Integrated Process:** Teaching and Learning **Content Area:** Pharmacology **Strategy:** Recall first that first-generation antihistamines cause drowsiness, and look for an option that would have an additive effect. Eliminate any choice that acts as a stimulant. When there is more than one correct answer, consider each option as a true/false statement.

15 **Answer: 2 Rationale:** The proper application of nasal spray decongestants is with the client sitting and squeezing the bottle once, holding a finger over the other nostril, and inhaling. Unless otherwise specified, administering more than a one-squeeze application would increase the dose. The applicator should be rinsed after each use to prevent contamination. The proper application of nasal spray decongestants is with the client in a sitting position. **Cognitive Level:** Applying **Client Need:** Pharmacological and Parenteral Therapies **Integrated Process:** Teaching and Learning **Content Area:** Pharmacology **Strategy:** A key word in the question is *accurate*. The core issue of the question is the instruction that is a true statement. Use the process of elimination and knowledge of basic medication administration procedures to make a selection.

16 **Answer: 3 Rationale:** Avoidance of eating or drinking for 30 minutes after medication administration allows the medication time to work. Nasal spray decongestants should not be taken for more than 3 days because they can cause rebound congestion. Fluid intake should be increased to 2–3 L/day, not decreased, to liquefy secretions. Smoking should be avoided because it increases secretions and decreases ciliary action. **Cognitive Level:** Applying **Client Need:** Pharmacological and Parenteral Therapies **Integrated Process:** Teaching and Learning **Content Area:** Pharmacology **Strategy:** The wording of the question tells you the correct answer is also a true statement. Eliminate the options that are least likely to be true. Choose the correct option using knowledge about the side effects of decongestants.

17 **Answer: 1 Rationale:** It is important to teach clients side effects of medications. The side effects of expectorants include nausea, vomiting, gastric irritation, and rash. If a cough lasts longer than 1 week (not 2), it should be reported to the prescriber. The client should avoid eating or drinking for 30 minutes after medication administration to allow the medication to work. The medication should be taken as directed, and doses should not be doubled. **Cognitive Level:** Applying **Client Need:** Pharmacological and Parenteral Therapies **Integrated Process:** Nursing Process: Planning **Content Area:** Pharmacology **Strategy:** Use the process of elimination and general medication knowledge to answer the question. Eliminate options with excessive time frames, those that

hinder medication absorption, and any option that does not support standard medication teaching.

18 **Answer: 4 Rationale:** The most significant side effect of an opioid antitussive is respiratory depression, evidenced by a respiratory rate of 10, when normal is 12–20 breaths/minute. Dry, cracked lips, blurred vision, and inability to stay awake are potential side effects of opioid antitussives; however, the most significant side effect is respiratory depression. **Cognitive Level:** Analyzing **Client Need:** Pharmacological and Parenteral Therapies **Integrated Process:** Nursing Process: Assessment **Content Area:** Pharmacology **Strategy:** The key words *most significant* tell you that more than one option might be technically correct, and that you must select the most important option. Use the ABCs (airway, breathing, and circulation) to make your selection.

19 **Answer: 4 Rationale:** Unused medication should be discarded after 4 days, not 7. This statement indicates that the client needs additional teaching. Increasing fluids assists with thinning secretions; this statement does not indicate a need for additional teaching. The client does not need further teaching if there is an understanding that avoidance of smoking is necessary; smoking increases secretions and decreases ciliary action. Rinsing the mouth after administration is an appropriate action because this action decreases oropharyngeal irritation. **Cognitive Level:** Applying **Client Need:** Pharmacological and Parenteral Therapies **Integrated Process:** Nursing Process: Evaluation **Content Area:** Pharmacology **Strategy:** The phrase *further teaching* tells you the correct answer is an incorrect or false statement. Eliminate options that indicate that the client is expressing an understanding of appropriate actions.

20 **Answer: 4 Rationale:** The Venturi mask has a dial to set the percentage of oxygen, and can administer 50% oxygen. The nasal cannula can administer up to 6 L/min, which is approximately 44% oxygen. The nonrebreather mask administers 60–100% oxygen. The partial rebreather mask administers 70–90% oxygen. **Cognitive Level:** Applying **Client Need:** Pharmacological and Parenteral Therapies **Integrated Process:** Nursing Process: Implementation **Content Area:** Pharmacology **Strategy:** Specific knowledge of the various concepts related to oxygen therapy is needed to answer this question. Use the process of elimination to make a selection, and remember that Venturi masks deliver precise oxygen concentrations.

Key Terms to Review

acute asthma attack p. 523
adrenergic agonists p. 523
anticholinergic p. 530
antihistamines p. 529
antitussives p. 532
atelectasis p. 533
catecholamines p. 523
decongestants p. 530
expectorant p. 531
histamine p. 526
hypoxemia p. 533
hypoxia p. 533
inhaler p. 527
interleukins p. 526
lacrimal p. 529
leukotrienes p. 526
mast cells p. 525
mucolytics p. 532
nebulizer p. 527
noncatecholamines p. 523
opioid p. 532
rhinitis p. 527
status asthmaticus p. 525
sympathomimetics p. 523
xanthines p. 526

References

Adams, M., Holland, L., & Urban, C. (2017). *Pharmacology for nurses: A pathophysiologic approach* (5th ed.). New York, NY: Pearson Education.

Adams, M., & Urban, C. (2016). *Pharmacology: Connections to nursing practice* (3rd ed.). New York, NY: Pearson Education.

Berman, A., Snyder, S., & Frandsen, G. (2016). *Kozier & Erb's fundamentals of nursing: Concepts, process, and practice* (10th ed.). New York, NY: Pearson Education.

Lehne, R. (2016). *Pharmacology for nursing care* (9th ed.). St. Louis, MO: Saunders.

LeMone, P., Burke, K., Bauldoff, G., & Gubrud, P. (2015). *Medical surgical nursing: Clinical reasoning in patient care* (6th ed.). Hoboken, NJ: Pearson Education.

Lewis, S., Dirksen, S., Heitkemper, M., & Bucher, L. (2014). *Medical surgical nursing: Assessment and management of clinical problems* (9th ed.). St. Louis, MO: Elsevier Science.

Smith, S., Duell, D., Martin, B., Aebersold, M., & Gonzalez, L. (2017). *Clinical nursing skills: Basic to advanced skills* (10th ed.). New York, NY: Pearson Education.

Wilson, B., Shannon, M., & Shields, K. (2016). *Pearson nurse's drug guide 2016.* New York, NY: Pearson Education.

Test Yourself

Are you ready for the NCLEX-RN® or course exams? Access the NEW web-based app that provides students with thousands of practice questions in preparation for the NCLEX experience.

37 Cardiovascular Medications

In this chapter

Cross Reference

Other chapters relevant to this content area are

Dosage Calculation and Medication Administration	**Chapter 29**
Cardiovascular Disorders	**Chapter 56**

I. NITRATES

A. **Increase flow of oxygenated blood to myocardium** by dilating coronary and systemic blood vessels (BVs)
B. **Dilation of systemic vascular bed** leads to pooling of blood in peripheral BVs and reduced **preload** (volume in left ventricle just prior to contraction) and **afterload** (resistance to blood being ejected by left ventricle) and myocardial oxygen (O_2) demand
C. **Common nitrate medications are listed in Box 37–1**

Memory Aid

Remember that drugs that are nitrates have the letters *nitro-* or *nitr-* in them.

Box 37–1	
Nitrates	Nitroglycerin Isosorbide mononitrate Isosorbide dinitrate

D. Administration considerations

1. Ensure oral mucous membranes are moist when giving sublingual (SL) nitroglycerin (NTG) tablets
2. For a hospitalized client, keep NTG tablets at bedside with a healthcare provider (HCP) prescription if policy allows; instruct client to report all chest pain episodes; count tablets daily if kept at bedside
3. Administer intravenous (IV) NTG as a continuous or intermittent infusion (not IV push) using an infusion pump; dose is often **titrated** (adjusted according to a predetermined parameter, such as chest pain)

NCLEX®
4. IV NTG is available in glass bottles and must be infused only through manufacturer-supplied IV tubing; regular polyvinylchloride IV tubing can absorb 40–80% of NTG

NCLEX®
5. Monitor blood pressure (BP) and heart rate (HR) every 15 minutes when using IV form of NTG and titrating medication; be prepared to treat hypotension by decreasing or stopping NTG infusion

NCLEX®
6. Use gloves or an applicator to spread NTG paste or ointment evenly and avoid absorption of medication into nurse's skin

NCLEX®
7. Rotate location of NTG paste or patch to reduce skin irritation and enhance absorption; place on hairless areas and avoid scar tissue or lesions; appropriate areas include chest, upper abdomen, anterior thigh, or upper arm
8. NTG dosing regimen should allow for an 8- to 10-hour nitrate-free period to prevent development of tolerance; apply NTG patch in morning and remove at bedtime

NCLEX®
9. Do not administer any nitrate to a client who has hypersensitivity to nitrates, is hypotensive, has severe bradycardia or tachycardia, or has used erectile dysfunction medications such as sildenafil within 24 hours (causes profound hypotension)

E. Side/adverse effects

NCLEX®
1. Headache (50%), mild or severe orthostatic hypotension, flushing, blurred vision, dry mouth
2. Weakness, dizziness, vertigo, and faintness
3. Nausea and vomiting (N/V), fecal and urinary incontinence, abdominal pain

F. Nursing considerations

NCLEX®
1. Ensure client sits or lies down before taking NTG dose to prevent dizziness or fainting
2. Allow SL tablet to dissolve naturally under tongue; if mouth is dry, instruct client to take a sip of water before placing tablet under tongue

NCLEX®
3. Give no more than three tablets total, one every 5 minutes; monitor BP after each dose; notify HCP if client becomes hypotensive or if pain is unrelieved after third dose

NCLEX®
4. Remove paste or patch each day at designated time before applying next dose
5. Store ointment in a cool, dry place with cap attached tightly
6. Check IV infusion concentration carefully because different dilutions are possible

NCLEX®
7. During IV NTG use, monitor BP and HR frequently (as often as every 5–15 minutes)

G. Client teaching

1. All forms of NTG may cause dizziness and headache; rest for at least 15 minutes after taking SL medication to avoid dizziness
2. Report to HCP if symptoms become worse or increase in frequency
3. Sit down near phone when taking sublingual (SL) NTG tablets in case it becomes necessary to call for help

NCLEX®
4. If pain persists after three NTG tablets (or sprays) at 5-minute intervals, notify HCP or emergency medical services because persistent pain could indicate an impending myocardial infarction (MI)

NCLEX®
5. NTG degrades in heat, light, or moisture; store medication in original container in a cool, dry place

NCLEX®
6. Replace NTG tablets every 3–6 months after opening; each tablet should cause a slight stinging or tingling sensation when placed under tongue if fresh
7. Write down emergency numbers and place them next to phone with home address and exact directions
8. Take a SL or spray NTG before an event that might cause angina, such as stair climbing, exercise, or sexual intercourse; shake spray prior to use
9. Keep a written record for prescriber of times, dates, amount of medication required for relief of each attack, and possible precipitating factors

10. If wearing an NTG patch or paste and experiencing an anginal attack, an NTG tablet may be taken SL following safety measures outlined above
11. Swimming or bathing with an NTG patch in place is acceptable
12. Frequent and prolonged use of NTG may reduce efficacy, requiring a medication adjustment

II. BETA-ADRENERGIC BLOCKERS

A. **Block $beta_1$ adrenergic receptors found chiefly in cardiac muscle**; at higher doses, may also block $beta_2$ adrenergic receptors in airways, leading to increased airway resistance, especially in clients with asthma or chronic obstructive pulmonary disease (COPD)

Memory Aid

Use the number to remember the organs affected by beta-adrenergic receptors. Remember β_1—you have one heart, and β_2—you have two lungs.

B. **Used therapeutically to manage hypertension, angina pectoris, acute MI, and supraventricular tachycardia**

NCLEX® C. **Block cardiac effects of beta-adrenergic stimulation, resulting in:**
1. Reductions in HR, myocardial **irritability** (cardiac muscle response to a variety of external stimuli such as hypoxia), and force of contraction
2. A negative **inotropic** (force of contraction) and **chronotropic** (heart rate) effect
3. Depression of **automaticity** (heart's ability to initiate impulses on its own without external stimulation) of sinus node
4. Reduction in atrioventricular (AV) node and intraventricular **dromotropic** (conduction velocity) effect

D. **Also useful in controlling panic attacks and stage fright** in some clients

E. **Common medications are listed in Box 37–2**

Memory Aid

Recognize beta-adrenergic blockers because they end in *-olol* or *-lol*.

F. **Administration considerations**
1. Assess client before, during, and after initial dose
2. NCLEX® Monitor BP, apical pulse, and cardiac rhythm frequently during initial administration; if given orally, assess client 30 minutes before and 60 minutes after initial dose
3. Prior to next dose, reassess BP, HR, and cardiac rhythm
4. Give drug at consistent times with or without meals; recommended before meals and at bedtime
5. NCLEX® Use of beta-adrenergic blockers with calcium channel blockers (see section to follow) may increase adverse response, including bradycardia and hypotension
6. Tablets may be crushed as needed (prn) before administration and taken with fluid of choice
7. NCLEX® Do not discontinue therapy abruptly; dosage is reduced gradually over 1–2 weeks, observe client for paradoxical reactions such as hypertension and tachycardia
8. NCLEX® Contraindicated with first-degree heart block (PR interval greater than 0.2 second), heart failure, bradycardia, shock, significant aortic or mitral valve disease, hyperactive airway syndrome (asthma or bronchospasm), severe seasonal allergies (allergic rhinitis during pollen season), concurrent use of psychotropic that augments adrenergic system or within 2 weeks of a monoamine oxidase inhibitor (MAOI)

Box 37–2

Common Beta-Adrenergic Blockers

Acebutolol	Nadolol
Atenolol	Nebivolol
Betaxolol	Penbutolol
Bisoprolol	Pindolol
Labelalol	Propranolol
Metoprolol	Timolol

9. Use cautiously before and after major surgery, with renal or hepatic impairment, diabetes mellitus, myasthenia gravis, or Wolff-Parkinson-White (WPW) syndrome, and systemic allergies to insect stings

G. Side/adverse effects

1. Dizziness, sleep disturbances, depression, confusion, agitation, or psychosis
2. *NCLEX®* Hypotension, bradycardia, heart block, acute heart failure, and peripheral paresthesias resembling Raynaud's phenomenon
3. Laryngospasm or bronchospasm
4. Dry eyes with a gritty sensation, blurred vision, tinnitus, or hearing loss
5. Dry mouth, N/V, heartburn, diarrhea, constipation, abdominal cramps, and flatulence
6. Agranulocytosis, hypo- or hyperglycemia, and hypocalcemia in clients with hyperthyroidism

H. Nursing considerations

1. *NCLEX®* Take apical pulse and BP before administering; evaluate for fluid volume overload as sign of heart failure
2. Monitor intake and output (I&O) and daily weight
3. *NCLEX®* Withhold dose if HR is less than 60 beats per minute (bpm) or if systolic BP is less than 90 mmHg

Memory Aid

Many cardiovascular drugs that have antihypertensive and vasodilating effects cause orthostatic hypotension and dizziness, so assist client to arise slowly from lying to sitting, and from sitting to standing positions; provide a safe environment to decrease injury in case of falls.

4. *NCLEX®* Assess for history of asthma, allergies, or COPD; realize beta-blockers may lead to bronchospasm in clients with no previously documented history of pulmonary disease
5. Assess HR, BP, and respiratory status carefully during periods of dosage adjustment; maintain effective communication with prescriber
6. Restrict dietary sodium as prescribed to prevent fluid volume overload; check with prescriber regarding sodium restriction or concurrent use of a diuretic
7. Fasting longer than 12 hours may induce hypoglycemia, which is worsened by beta-blocker therapy because signs are masked
8. Review results of periodic renal, hepatic, cardiac, and hematologic studies
9. *NCLEX®* Beta-blockers may induce false-negative exercise tolerance electrocardiogram (ECG) results

I. Client teaching

1. How to check pulse and BP and their desired ranges, how to record daily measurements, and when to call prescriber
2. *NCLEX®* Abrupt withdrawal can lead to severe paradoxical or rebound reactions, including sweating, tremulousness, severe headache, malaise, palpitations, hypertension, MI, and life-threatening heart rhythm disturbances
3. Establish a routine for taking medication and strive to comply with plan for results; write out a daily schedule for medication
4. *NCLEX®* Notify prescriber if any dizziness or lightheadedness occurs; avoid driving or operating machinery until these symptoms are relieved

Memory Aid

Teach clients taking antihypertensive or vasodilating drugs to take measures to reduce risk of orthostatic hypotension; avoid use of hot baths and hot tubs and limit amount of time spent out of doors in hot weather to minimize risk of orthostatic BP changes.

5. *NCLEX®* Stop smoking (may offset desired outcomes of controlled HR, BP, and prevention of angina); smoking also increases hepatic metabolism of beta-blockers, leading to unpredictable or reduced drug effects
6. Avoid OTC medications and herbal supplements without consulting prescriber
7. Inform all HCPs, including ophthalmologist or optometrist, of medication use; beta-blockers may lower intraocular pressure
8. Reduce salt intake while taking medication

III. CALCIUM CHANNEL BLOCKERS

A. **Are class IV antidysrhythmic drugs that inhibit calcium ion influx** through slow channels into cells of myocardial and arterial smooth muscle (cardiac and peripheral BV)
   1. Intracellular calcium remains below levels needed to stimulate cell
   2. Dilate coronary arteries and arterioles and prevent coronary artery spasm
   3. Increase myocardial O_2 delivery to prevent angina
   4. Slow conduction through sinoatrial (SA) node and AV node, lowering HR and decreasing strength of cardiac contraction (negative inotropic effect)
   5. Decrease automaticity and **conductivity** (amount of force and pressure to pump blood out of ventricles) by blocking flow of calcium into cell
   6. Decrease systemic vascular resistance (SVR) and thus afterload by dilating peripheral arterioles
   7. Reduce arterial BP (antihypertensive effect) and HR

B. **Used for vasospastic angina** (Prinzmetal's variant or angina at rest), chronic stable (classic and activity-induced) angina, and essential hypertension; IV form is useful in atrial fibrillation, atrial flutter, and supraventricular tachycardia

C. **Common medications are listed in Box 37–3**

Memory Aid

Recognize many calcium channel blockers by noting the suffix *-dipine*. This is not true for all, however; exceptions are verapamil and diltiazem.

D. **Administration considerations**
   1. Administer oral diltiazem before meals and at bedtime and oral verapamil with food to reduce gastric irritation
   2. Evaluate BP and ECG before initiation of therapy
   3. Monitor for headache; an analgesic may be required
   4. Use infusion pump to administer IV forms of verapamil and diltiazem and carefully follow package directions
   5. *NCLEX®* Withhold dose if BP is less than 90/60
   6. Contraindicated with known hypersensitivity to drug, sick sinus syndrome (without artificial pacemaker), second- or third-degree heart blocks
   7. Does not alter serum calcium levels

E. **Adverse effects and toxicity**
   1. Headache, dizziness, nervousness, insomnia, confusion, tremor, and gait disturbance
   2. *NCLEX®* Postural hypotension, heart block and profound bradycardia, heart failure, possible syncope, palpitations, and fluid volume overload
   3. N/V, constipation, and impaired taste
   4. Skin rash

F. **Nursing considerations**
   1. Obtain baseline BP and ECG; monitor closely during dose adjustment (including orthostatic changes)
   2. Monitor hepatic and renal lab test results
   3. May induce hyperglycemia; monitor diabetic clients closely

Box 37–3

Common Calcium Channel Blockers

Selective for Blood Vessels	Nonselective: Heart and Blood Vessels
Amlodipine	Diltiazem
Clevidipine	Verapamil
Felodipine	
Isradipine	
Nicardipine	
Nifedipine	
Nisoldipine	

4. Can cause constipation; increase fiber and fluids as tolerated
5. Monitor for signs of CHF (dyspnea, crackles, frothy pink-tinged sputum)

G. Client teaching

NCLEX® 1. Take radial pulse before each dose (especially verapamil); report an irregular pulse or if slower than identified parameter (such as 50 or 60)
NCLEX® 2. Change position slowly to prevent orthostatic (postural) hypotension
3. Avoid driving if dizziness or faintness is noted; report these symptoms immediately
NCLEX® 4. Report gradual weight gain and evidence of edema; may indicate onset of CHF
NCLEX® 5. Avoid grapefruit and grapefruit juice when taking verapamil
6. Use typical measures to prevent constipation (fluids, fiber, activity)

IV. ANGIOTENSIN-CONVERTING ENZYME (ACE) INHIBITORS

A. Block conversion of angiotensin I to angiotensin II, which prevents peripheral vasoconstriction and reduces blood volume by inhibiting secretion of aldosterone

NCLEX® **B. Used to treat hypertension;** preferred for hypertensive clients with diabetic nephropathy; useful in myocardial infarction and in clients with heart failure

C. Common ACE inhibitors are listed in Box 37–4

Memory Aid

Generic names of ACE inhibitors can be recognized because they end in *-pril.*

D. Administration considerations

1. Discontinue with prescriber supervision if pregnancy is detected
2. Give moexipril and captopril 20–60 minutes before meals (decreased absorption with food)
3. When initiating therapy, watch for first dose effect (profound hypotension with syncope); prevent by giving while sitting or lying down

E. Side/adverse effects

1. Headache, dizziness, anxiety, fatigue, insomnia, nervousness
NCLEX® 2. Hypotension and palpitations
3. N/V, abdominal pain, constipation
NCLEX® 4. Persistent dry nonproductive cough, dyspnea
5. Rash, arthralgia, impotence, and dysgeusia (altered taste)
NCLEX® 6. Angioedema, leukopenia, agranulocytosis, pancytopenia, thrombocytopenia
7. Cerebrovascular accident (CVA), MI, and hypertensive crisis

F. Nursing considerations

1. Do not administer to pregnant or lactating women
NCLEX® 2. Monitor labs for increased potassium, liver enzymes, bilirubin, BUN and creatinine, and decreased sodium levels and WBC count
NCLEX® 3. Take BP before giving dose and monitor regularly
NCLEX® 4. Monitor for rashes or hives and for peripheral edema
5. Discontinue diuretics 2–3 days before ACE inhibitor therapy

G. Client teaching

1. Report peripheral edema, signs of infection, facial swelling, loss of taste, or difficulty breathing
2. Do not skip doses or stop taking drug (may cause serious rebound increase in BP)
NCLEX® 3. Persistent, dry cough is a side effect and does not indicate respiratory disease or infection
NCLEX® 4. Avoid potassium-containing salt substitutes to prevent hyperkalemia

Box 37–4

Common ACE Inhibitors

Benazepril	Moexipril
Captopril	Perindopril
Enalapril	Quinapril
Fosinopril	Ramipril
Lisinopril	Trandolapril

5. Monitor for petechiae, bruising, or bleeding with captopril
6. Taste of food may be diminished during the first month of therapy
7. Take captopril 20 minutes to 1 hour before a meal

V. ANGIOTENSIN II RECEPTOR BLOCKERS (ARBs)

A. **Act as antagonists at angiotensin II receptor of vascular smooth muscle,** blocking vasoconstriction and aldosterone-secreting effects and lowering BP
B. **Common ARB medications are listed in Box 37–5**

Memory Aid

ARBs are easily recognized because they end in the suffix *-sartan*.

C. **Administration considerations**
1. Discontinue immediately if pregnancy is detected
2. NCLEX® Use cautiously in clients with renal or hepatic disease

D. **Side/adverse effects**
1. Hypotension and dizziness, tachycardia or bradycardia
2. Cough, GI upset, insomnia, nasal congestion, and myalgia
3. NCLEX® Neutropenia and hyperkalemia

E. **Nursing considerations**
1. NCLEX® Monitor client taking diuretics for additive hypotension
2. NCLEX® Regularly assess renal function, potassium level, and WBC with differential
3. Do not administer to pregnant or lactating women
4. NCLEX® Monitor BP and apical pulse regularly

F. **Client teaching**
1. Do not discontinue medication abruptly
2. NCLEX® Avoid salt substitutes because of potassium content
3. Notify HCP immediately if pregnancy is suspected
4. If using oral contraceptives, use alternate birth control methods
5. Maintain adequate hydration

Box 37–5

Common Angiotensin II Receptor Blockers (ARBs)

Candesartan	Olmesartan
Eprosartan	Telmisartan
Irbesartan	Valsartan
Losartan	

VI. DIRECT-ACTING VASODILATORS

A. **Potent antihypertensive agents that act directly on arterial smooth muscles**
B. **Produce peripheral vasodilation,** resulting in lowered arterial BP, increased HR, and increased cardiac output (CO)
C. **Some may also be used as an adjunct** in treating heart failure or to treat Raynaud's disease by increasing blood flow to extremities
D. **Common direct-acting vasodilators are listed in Box 37–6**
E. **Administration considerations**
1. Take oral forms with food to increase bioavailability
2. NCLEX® May give IV hydralazine undiluted by IV push at a rate of 10 mg/min
3. NCLEX® Infuse sodium nitroprusside cautiously using an IV pump; when mixed, it appears orange; must be covered in a foil pouch to avoid exposure to light to prevent decomposition during infusion

Box 37–6

Direct-Acting Vasodilators

Diazoxide	Minoxidil
Hydralazine	Nitroprusside

4. Do not mix with other IV solutions
5. Discontinue all vasodilators slowly to avoid paradoxical hypertensive effects
6. Monitor HR and BP closely during administration to prevent sudden hypotension
7. Contraindicated in compensatory hypertension (arteriovenous shunt, coarctation of aorta), inadequate cerebral perfusion leading to a decreased cerebral perfusion pressure (CPP), or hypovolemia

NCLEX®
8. Monitor cyanide and serum thiocyanate levels after 48–72 hours of nitroprusside therapy, especially in clients with impaired renal function

F. Side/adverse effects

1. Headache, dizziness, tremors, apprehension, and muscle twitching

NCLEX®
2. Angina, palpitations, tachycardia or bradycardia, flushing, paradoxical rise in BP, ECG changes, profound hypotension, shock, and dysrhythmias
3. Systemic lupus erythematosus (SLE)–like syndrome (with hydralazine), edema
4. Anorexia, N/V, constipation or diarrhea, abdominal pain, and paralytic ileus
5. Difficulty urinating and glomerulonephritis
6. Decreased hematocrit and hemoglobin, anemia, agranulocytosis (rare)
7. Rash, irritation at IV site, urticaria, pruritus, fever, chills, arthralgia, eosinophilia, and cholangitis; excessive hair growth with minoxidil
8. With sodium nitroprusside, thiocyanate toxicity (profound hypotension, tinnitus, fatigue, pink skin color, metabolic acidosis, and loss of consciousness)

G. Nursing considerations

1. Assess carefully baseline HR, BP, cardiac rhythm, ECG, and neurological status

NCLEX®
2. When administering IV vasodilators:
   a. Establish a large, stable IV site because infusions are irritating to tissue; administer with an IV infusion pump
   b. Monitor BP every 5–15 minutes during initial infusion and medication adjustment
   c. Monitor input and output (I&O)
   d. If hypotension occurs, decrease infusion and monitor client closely; if sudden, severe hypotension occurs, discontinue medication; maintain airway, breathing, and circulation (ABCs); establish IV site; contact HCP, and initiate emergency protocols as needed
3. Check BP, heart rate, and cardiac rhythm before each oral dose

H. Client teaching

1. How to self-monitor pulse and BP

NCLEX®
2. Possibility of headache and palpitations within 2 to 4 hours after first oral dose
3. Stop smoking as this negates positive effects of medication
4. Monitor weight daily and report edema

NCLEX®
5. Avoid hot tubs and baths that might induce profound vasodilation and hypotension

VII. ALPHA ADRENERGIC ANTAGONISTS (CENTRAL AND PERIPHERAL)

A. Centrally acting sympatholytics

1. Stimulate $alpha_2$ receptors in CNS to inhibit sympathetic cardio-accelerator and vasoconstrictor centers
2. Decrease sympathetic outflow from CNS, resulting in decreased arterial pressure

B. Peripheral anti-adrenergics

1. Deplete catecholamine stores in peripheral nervous system (PNS) and some act in CNS
2. Decrease total peripheral resistance, HR, and CO

C. Common alpha adrenergic antagonists are listed in Box 37–7

D. Administration considerations

NCLEX®
1. Do not discontinue abruptly; may result in rebound hypertension
2. Guanabenz: allow 1–2 weeks before adjusting dose
3. Guanfacine: give at bedtime to decrease daytime sleepiness; allow 3–4 weeks before adjusting dose
4. Methyldopa: allow 2 days for maximum response before adjusting dose
5. Contraindicated in hypersensitivity, active hepatitis or cirrhosis, co-administration with MAOIs (methyldopa), heart failure (methyldopa), history of mental depression, active peptic ulcer disease, ulcerative colitis, asthma, and bronchitis (reserpine)

E. Side/adverse effects

1. Sedation, headache, weakness, dizziness, and decreased mental acuity
2. Involuntary choreoathetoid movements, parkinsonism, depression, nightmares

Box 37–7

Alpha$_1$ and Alpha$_2$ Blockers

Alpha$_1$ Blockers	**Adrenergic Neuron Blockers (Peripherally Acting)**
Doxazosin	Reserpine
Prazosin	Guanabenz acetate
Terazosin	Guanfacine
Alpha$_2$ Blockers	
Clonidine	
Methyldopa	
Alpha and Beta Blockers (Centrally Acting)	
Carvedilol	
Labetalol	

3. Bradycardia, orthostatic hypotension, aggravation of angina, edema
4. GI disturbance, rash, gynecomastia, galactorrhea, amenorrhea, impotence, dry mouth, weight gain
5. Myocarditis, hemolytic anemia, thrombocytopenia
6. Hepatic necrosis
7. Severe rebound hypertension

F. Nursing considerations

1. Administer orally; tablets may be crushed and do not need to be given with food unless GI upset occurs
2. IV methyldopa should be given over 30–60 minutes; do not give subcutaneously or IM
3. *NCLEX®* Apply transdermal systems (clonidine) to dry, hairless skin of chest or upper arm; assess areas for rash
4. *NCLEX®* Monitor labs for elevated liver enzymes, alkaline phosphatase, bilirubin, BUN, creatinine, potassium, sodium, and uric acid
5. May prolong prothrombin times
6. *NCLEX®* Obtain baseline BP and apical pulse, and monitor weight regularly
7. *NCLEX®* Assess client for peripheral edema
8. Dry mouth may contribute to development of dental caries, periodontal disease, oral candidiasis, and discomfort

G. Client teaching

1. *NCLEX®* Possible need for sodium restriction and weight reduction; report weight gain of more than 2.3 kg (5 lb) per week
2. Relieve dry mouth by sipping water or chewing sugarless gum
3. Treat nausea by eating unsalted crackers, noncola beverages, or dry toast
4. Report mental acuity changes to HCP
5. Some drugs cause urine to become darker
6. *NCLEX®* Do not drive a car or perform hazardous activities if drowsiness occurs
7. *NCLEX®* Take medication as prescribed; do not stop abruptly to avoid rebound hypertension

VIII. CARDIAC GLYCOSIDES

A. Used primarily to treat heart failure but also used to treat atrial **dysrhythmias** such as atrial tachycardia, atrial flutter, and atrial fibrillation

B. Increases *contractility* (force of contraction) and efficiency of myocardial contraction

C. Positive inotrope that increases force of myocardial contraction

D. Negative chronotrope and dromotrope (decreases heart rate and conduction velocity through AV node, respectively)

E. Common medication: digoxin

F. Administration considerations

1. May be given with or without food
2. Tablet may be crushed and mixed with fluid or food; pediatric elixir is available
3. *NCLEX®* IV push digoxin may be administered undiluted or diluted per package insert over 5 minutes; client may receive a loading dose (digitalization) to achieve adequate serum drug levels
4. Do not administer digoxin IM; causes tissue irritation and great variation in bioavailability
5. Infiltration into subcutaneous tissue can cause local irritation and tissue sloughing

6. Contraindicated in clients with known hypersensitivity or digoxin toxicity or those with ventricular dysrhythmias or second- or third-degree heart block
7. Full digitalizing dose should not be given if client has received digoxin during previous week
NCLEX® 8. Use cautiously with following conditions: renal insufficiency, hypokalemia, advanced heart disease, acute MI, mild heart block, cor pulmonale, hypothyroidism, and lung disease
9. Use cautiously in pregnant or nursing mothers, children, premature infants, and older adults

NCLEX® **G. Side/adverse effects**

1. Fatigue, muscle weakness, headache, confusion, drowsiness, dizziness, and malaise
2. Bradycardia, dysrhythmias, hypotension, A-V heart block, and diaphoresis
3. Anorexia, N/V, or diarrhea
4. Visual disturbances (blurred vision, green or yellow vision, photophobia, or halo effect)
5. Digoxin toxicity may be unrecognized because it may present same early manifestations as a flu, such as anorexia, N/V, diarrhea, visual disturbances

H. Nursing considerations

1. Obtain baseline data and perform ongoing physical assessments, including neurological status, HR, BP, and cardiac rhythm
2. Check baseline serum digoxin level prior to initiating digoxin therapy
   a. Blood level is 0 if client has not taken digoxin before
   NCLEX® b. Therapeutic levels are 0.5–2.0 ng/mL (ranges vary slightly among texts)
   NCLEX® c. Toxic levels are greater than 2 ng/mL
3. Assess baseline and ongoing serum electrolytes, creatinine clearance, magnesium, and calcium
4. Monitor older clients taking digoxin and a diuretic to treat CHF or atrial fibrillation for digoxin toxicity
NCLEX® 5. Take apical pulse for 1 full minute prior to dose, noting rate, rhythm, and quality; if changes are noted, withhold dose and notify prescriber; an ECG will likely be ordered
NCLEX® 6. Withhold dose if client has symptoms of digoxin toxicity (anorexia, N/V, diarrhea, or visual disturbances)
7. In children, early signs of toxicity include cardiac dysrhythmias; children rarely demonstrate anorexia, N/V, diarrhea, or visual disturbances
NCLEX® 8. Provide foods high in potassium, such as oranges, bananas, fruit juices, dried fruits, vegetables, and potatoes if client is taking loop (potassium-wasting) diuretics
NCLEX® 9. Monitor I&O and daily weight, especially with impaired renal failure; auscultate breath sounds for crackles
NCLEX® 10. Antidote: digoxin immune Fab used in extreme toxicity
NCLEX® 11. Assess extremities for edema as indicator of fluid volume overload

I. Client teaching

NCLEX® 1. Measure pulse rate for 1 full minute prior to taking dose; contact prescriber before taking dose if pulse is below 60 beats/min or above 110 or if skipped beats are present
2. Suspect toxicity with N/V, anorexia, diarrhea, or visual disturbances such as halos or green or yellow vision; withhold dose and notify prescriber
NCLEX® 3. Weigh self daily with same clothes and at same time; report weight gain greater than 0.9 kg (2 lb) per day
4. Take as prescribed; do not skip or add additional dose

IX. ANTIDYSRHYTHMICS

A. Class IA (note all Class I drugs are fast sodium channel blockers)

1. Used to treat both atrial and ventricular dysrhythmias; prevent recurrence of premature ventricular contractions (PVCs) and ventricular tachycardia (VT) that are not severe enough to require cardioversion
2. Depress myocardial contractility and excitability and prolong **refractory period** (making cells able to respond only to strong stimulus)
3. Reduce rate of spontaneous diastolic depolarization in pacemaker cells, thereby suppressing ectopic focal activity
4. Disopyramide shortens sinus node recovery time and increases atrial and ventricular effective refractory period
5. Quinidine is classified as a chemical cardioversion agent used to convert atrial fibrillation to normal sinus rhythm
6. Common antidysrhythmics are listed in Box 37–8

Box 37–8

Common Antidysrhythmic Drugs

Class I: Sodium Channel Blockers	Class II: Beta-Adrenergic Blockers
Class IA Drugs	Acebutolol
Disopyramide	Esmolol
Procainamide	Propranolol
Quinidine gluconate	**Class III: Potassium Channel Blockers**
Quinidine sulfate	Amiodarone
Class IB Drugs	Dofetilide
Lidocaine	Dronedarone
Mexiletine	Ibutilide
Phenytoin	Sotalol
Class IC Drugs	**Class IV: Calcium Channel Blockers**
Flecainide	Diltiazem
Propafenone	Verapamil

7. Administration considerations
  a. Give first dose of disopyramide 6–12 hours after last quinidine dose and 3–6 hours after last procainamide dose
  b. Do not administer controlled-release capsules as loading dose when a rapid control is required or when creatinine clearance is less than 40 mL/min
  c. Do not crush or open controlled-release capsules (may deliver potentially toxic dose of medication)
  d. Start controlled-release form of capsule 6 hours after last dose of conventional capsule when switching between these forms
  e. Contraindicated in cardiogenic shock, second- or third-degree heart block, severe heart failure, and hypotension
  f. Assess blood glucose levels and serum potassium levels because hyperkalemia worsens toxic effects; correct hypokalemia and other electrolyte imbalances before initiating therapy
  g. Follow ECG results closely; notify HCP of conduction delays (prolonged QT interval, widening of QRS greater than 25%), HR less than 60 or greater than 120, unusual change in pulse rate, rhythm, or quality

8. Adverse effects/toxicity
  a. Blurred vision, dizziness, headache, fatigue, muscle weakness, seizures, paresthesias, nervousness, acute psychosis, and peripheral neuropathy
  NCLEX® **b.** Hypotension, chest pain, edema, dyspnea, syncope, bradycardia, tachycardia, increased dysrhythmias, CHF, cardiogenic shock, and heart block
  c. N/V, epigastric and abdominal pain, jaundice, dry mouth, constipation
  d. Urinary retention, frequency, urgency, and renal insufficiency
  e. Pruritis, urticaria, rash, photosensitivity, and laryngospasm
  f. Drying of nose, throat, and bronchial secretions
  g. Uterine contraction during pregnancy, precipitation of myasthenia gravis, agranulocytosis (decreased granulocytes), and thrombocytopenia

9. Nursing considerations
  NCLEX® **a.** Check apical pulse before administering the medication
  NCLEX® **b.** Monitor ECG and report any changes to HCP immediately
  c. Monitor BP, especially during dosage adjustment and with high doses
  d. Monitor I&O, especially in older adults and those with impaired renal function, prostatic hyperplasia, and urinary retention/hesitancy
  e. Monitor lab results as appropriate
  f. Assess for peripheral neuritis

10. Client teaching
  a. Weigh self daily and report gain of more than 0.9–1.8 kg (2–4 lb) per week
  b. Assess ankles and tibia daily for edema

NCLEX®
c. Avoid prolonged standing, and lie down if feeling lightheaded; avoid driving and other hazardous activities if dizzy or lightheaded
d. Be sure to avoid use of nasal decongestants without contacting prescriber
e. Avoid exposure to sunlight or ultraviolet radiation
f. Notify all other HCPs of medication and have regular eye exams for glaucoma

B. Class IB

1. Decrease refractory period and raise electrical stimulation threshold of ventricle during diastole
2. Suppress automaticity in the bundle of His–Purkinje system
3. Treat or prevent ventricular dysrhythmias
4. Common antidysrhythmic medications are listed in Box 37–8
5. Administration considerations
   a. Bolus dose of lidocaine may be given undiluted IVP at a rate of 25–50 mg/min; be sure to use lidocaine manufactured specifically for IV use
   b. Add 1 gram lidocaine to 250–500 mL of D_5W for infusion; flow rate should not be more than 4 mg/mL
   NCLEX® c. Use microdrip tubing and infusion pump for an infusion
   d. Discontinue IV infusion as soon as client's basic cardiac rhythm stabilizes
   e. Contraindicated in hypersenstivity to amide-type anesthetics, Stokes-Adams syndrome, untreated sinus bradycardia, and severe SA, AV, and intraventricular heart block
   NCLEX® f. Use cautiously with hepatic or renal disease, heart failure, hypovolemia or shock, myasthenia gravis, debilitated clients or older adults, and family history of malignant hyperthermia
6. Side/adverse effects
   a. Drowsiness or restlessness; confusion; disorientation; irritability; apprehension; euphoria; wild excitement; numbness of lips, tongue, and other paresthesias; chest heaviness; and difficulty speaking
   b. Dyspnea and difficulty swallowing, muscular twitching, tremors, psychosis, convulsions and respiratory depression with high doses
   NCLEX® c. Hypotension, lightheadedness, bradycardia, heart block, cardiovascular collapse, and cardiac arrest
   d. Tinnitus and decreased hearing; blurred vision, double vision, and impaired color perception
   e. Anorexia, N/V, and excessive perspiration
   f. Urticaria, rash, edema, and anaphylactoid reactions
7. Nursing considerations
   a. Assess ECG for prolonged PR interval, widened QRS, aggravation of dysrhythmias, and heart block
   b. Monitor BP frequently
   c. Assess CNS status at baseline and frequently during infusions
   NCLEX® d. Auscultate breath sounds for crackles and monitor respiratory rate
   NCLEX® e. Assess results of serum drug levels and creatinine levels
8. Notify prescriber if adverse effects occur; see previous section

C. Class IC

1. Decrease automaticity and conductivity through AV node and ventricles
2. Used to treat life-threatening ventricular dysrhythmias
3. Common antidysrhythmic medications are listed in Box 37–8
4. Administration considerations
   a. Medications are available in oral forms
   b. Do not increase dosages more frequently than every 4 days, especially with older adults or those with previous extensive myocardial damage
   c. Dosage reduction should be considered in severe liver dysfunction and with significant QRS widening
   d. Contraindicated with drug hypersensitivity, severe degrees of heart block or intraventricular block, cardiogenic shock, or hepatic failure
5. Side/adverse effects
   a. Headache, dizziness, prolonged lightheadedness, unsteadiness, paresthesias, fatigue, and fever
   NCLEX® b. Worsening dysrhythmias, chest pain, CHF, edema, and dyspnea
   c. Prolonged blurred vision and spots before eyes
   d. Nausea, constipation, and changes in taste perception
6. Nursing considerations
   NCLEX® a. Assess laboratory data and treat hypokalemia/hyperkalemia before initiating therapy
   NCLEX® b. Monitor ECG rhythm for adverse changes; client may need Holter monitoring for ambulatory assessment
   c. Determine threshold levels of pacemaker before initiating medication and at regular intervals thereafter
7. Client teaching: report any visual changes

D. Class II (beta-blockers): acebutolol, esmolol, propranolol; see previous section

E. Class III (potassium channel blockers)

1. Small but diverse class of drugs that prolong repolarization and refractory period and reduce automaticity
2. Decrease intraventricular conduction (thus prolonging QT interval)
3. Used to treat ventricular tachycardia (VT) and ventricular fibrillation (VF)
4. May also be used to treat supraventricular tachycardias
5. Common antidysrhythmic medications are listed in Box 37–8
6. Administration considerations
   a. Contraindicated with hypersensitivity to drug, cardiogenic shock, severe sinus bradycardia or heart block, and hepatic disease
   b. Use cautiously in hyper- or hypothyroidism, heart failure, electrolyte imbalance, preexisting pulmonary disease, cardiac surgery, and sensitivity to iodine
7. Side/adverse effects
   a. Vary depending on specific drug used; most have prodysrhythmic effects (ability to cause additional cardiac dysrhythmias)
   NCLEX® b. Bradycardia, hypotension, sinus arrest, cardiogenic shock, CHF, worsening dysrhythmias, and heart block
   NCLEX® c. Amiodarone: visual disturbances (corneal deposits, blurred vision, photophobia, xerostomia, macular degeneration, and cataracts), pneumonia-like syndrome (pulmonary toxicity may be fatal)
   d. Anorexia, N/V, and constipation
   e. Angioedema, hyperthyroidism or hypothyroidism, and hepatotoxicity
8. Nursing considerations
   NCLEX® a. Monitor BP during therapy to prevent hypotension, bradycardia
   b. Check laboratory and other reports for liver, lung, thyroid, GI, and neurological dysfunction
   NCLEX® c. Baseline and regular ophthalmic examinations with a slit-lamp are recommended throughout therapy with amiodarone
   d. Be alert to signs of pulmonary toxicity (amiodarone): dyspnea, fatigue, cough, pleuritic pain, or fever; auscultate breath sounds for adventitious sounds
   NCLEX® e. Report adverse reactions promptly
   f. Observe client already receiving other antiarrhythmic therapy for adverse effects, especially heart block and worsening dysrhythmias
9. Client teaching
   NCLEX® a. Monitor pulse daily and report HR less than 60 bpm
   b. Have regular ophthalmic examinations every 6 months to 1 year
   NCLEX® c. Photophobia may be eased by wearing darkened glasses, but some clients should avoid daylight entirely
   d. Skin reactions can occur with amiodarone (10–15% of clients); avoid sunlight, tanning beds, and sunlamps; wear protective clothing and a barrier-type sunblock to avoid exposure to sun (zinc-oxide or titanium-oxide preparations)

F. Class IV (calcium channel blockers): see previous section

G. Miscellaneous antidysrhythmic: Adenosine

1. Slows conduction through SA and AV nodes; interrupts reentry pathways through AV node
2. Depresses left-ventricular function (very temporary)
3. NCLEX® Treats supraventricular dysrhythmias
4. Administration considerations
   NCLEX® a. Rapid IV bolus: administer IV push over 1–2 seconds and follow with a rapid normal saline flush
   b. Expect sudden slowing of HR or even asystole for a brief period of time; do not repeat dose if high-grade AV heart block develops after first dose
   c. Store at room temperature to avoid crystallization; if crystals appear, dissolve by warming to room temperature
   d. Contraindicated in severe heart block, sick sinus syndrome (without a pacemaker), atrial fibrillation or atrial flutter, VT
   e. Use cautiously with asthma, pregnancy, hepatic failure, and renal failure
5. Side/adverse effects
   a. During conversion to sinus rhythm, many dysrhythmias can occur
   b. Facial flushing, transient dyspnea, or headache

NCLEX®
6. Nursing considerations
   a. Monitor ECG continuously and HR and BP every 15 minutes until stable
   b. Monitor carefully for bronchospasm, especially in clients with asthma
7. Client teaching: monitoring will be done during drug administration, and transient facial flushing may occur

X. ADRENERGIC AGONISTS (SYMPATHOMIMETICS)

A. **Mimic fight-or-flight response of sympathetic nervous system (SNS),** selectively stimulating alpha-adrenergic and beta-adrenergic receptors
B. **Stimulation of alpha-adrenergic receptors** results in vasoconstriction and increased systemic BP
C. **Stimulation of beta-adrenergic receptors** increases force and rate of myocardial contraction
D. **Used to treat shock**
E. **Common adrenergic agonists are listed in Box 37–9**
F. **Administration considerations**
   1. Drug must be diluted before administration; use infusion pump to control dose
   2. Client should be attended constantly during drug administration
   3. Contraindicated in uncorrected dysrhythmias, mesenteric or vascular thrombosis, profound hypoxia, hypercapnia, hypotension due to hypovolemia
   4. Use with caution in those receiving MAOIs or imipramine-type antidepressants
G. **Side/adverse effects**
   1. Anxiety, weakness, dizziness, tremor, restlessness
   2. Bradycardia, tachycardia, palpitations
   3. N/V, flushing, diaphoresis, sloughing upon extravasation
   4. Azotemia, shortness of breath, lung crackles, wheezing, bronchospasm
   NCLEX® 5. Severe hypertension, anaphylaxis
   NCLEX® 6. Arrhythmias, cardiac arrest, ventricular tachycardia
   7. Seizures, asthmatic episodes
H. **Nursing considerations**
   NCLEX® 1. Carefully monitor vital signs, ECG, and I&O
   2. Monitor for rebound hypertension
   3. Correct blood volume depletion first
   4. Monitor infusion site frequently; stay with client constantly during administration
   NCLEX® 5. Antidote for extravasation of dopamine: phentolamine mesylate diluted in normal saline injected at site of IV infiltration
I. **Client teaching**
   1. Report adverse reactions and side effects immediately
   2. Vital signs will be monitored frequently
   3. Report anginal pain while on dobutamine

Box 37–9

Adrenergic Agonists (Sympathomimetics)

Dopamine	Isoproterenol
Dobutamine	Norepinephrine
Epinephrine	

XI. ANTICOAGULANTS (SEE BOX 37–10)

A. **Oral medication; warfarin sodium**
   1. Oral **anticoagulants** prevent or delay blood coagulation and are used to treat and prevent thromboembolic disorders in clients at risk
   2. Warfarin prevents conversion of vitamin K, thereby decreasing its production in liver and subsequently reducing several clotting factors (II, VII, IX, and X)
   3. Vitamin K plays an active role in **extrinsic pathway** (forms fibrin and acts within seconds) in **clotting cascade** (a coagulation pathway)
   4. Warfarin is bound to plasma proteins (especially albumin), metabolized in liver
   5. Used to treat deep vein thrombosis (DVT), pulmonary embolism (PE), acute MI, heart valve replacement (bioprosthetic and mechanical), atrial fibrillation, and antiphospholipid syndrome

Box 37–10

Anticoagulants

Oral Anticoagulant	Direct Thrombin Inhibitors
Warfarin sodium	Argatroban
Heparin	Bivalirudan
Heparin sodium	Dabigatran
Low-Molecular-Weight Heparins	Desirudin
Dalteparin	Lepirudin
Enoxaparin	**Factor Xa Inhibitors**
Tinzaparin	Apixaban
Fondaparinux	Rivaroxaban

6. Administration considerations
   a. Warfarin is given orally at a usual dose of 1–15 mg daily
   b. Requires close monitoring because of a narrow therapeutic range, frequent need for dose adjustments, and high risk for food and drug interactions that can lead to either ineffective therapy or toxicity

   NCLEX®
   c. Full anticoagulant effect is seen at approximately 1 week; thus drug may be started during heparin therapy and overlap while heparin is tapered

   NCLEX®
   d. **Prothrombin time (PT)**, a laboratory test that measures extrinsic clotting response, and **international normalized ratio (INR)**, a standard reference range for reporting PT levels, are both used to monitor client response and determine ongoing dose
   e. Desired range of PT and INR vary based on indication for use; PT levels are usually maintained at 1.5–2.5 times control value; INR levels range from a usual 2.0 to 3.0 range to a higher level of 3.0 to 4.5 for specific prosthetics
   f. Warfarin is usually given in evening based on laboratory test results from earlier in day
   g. Therapy can last from several months to lifelong depending on specific need
   h. Refer to specific hospital protocol and prescriber's order for dose adjustments and monitoring of PT and INR levels
   i. Vitamin K is antidote for warfarin
   j. Contraindicated in pregnancy (may be given if needed during lactation), hemorrhage or bleeding tendencies, clients with malignant hypertension, and those with history of allergic reaction
7. Side/adverse effects

   NCLEX®
   a. Bleeding is the major adverse effect and is usually seen at higher dosage levels; also thrombocytopenia may occur
   b. Nausea, diarrhea, intestinal obstruction, anorexia, abdominal cramping
   c. Rash, urticaria, and purple toe syndrome (due to decreased perfusion from release of microemboli)
   d. Increased serum transaminase levels, hepatitis, jaundice
   e. Burning sensation in feet
   f. Transient hair loss

NCLEX®
8. Nursing considerations
   a. Monitor baseline and ongoing PT and INR; report high or low abnormal values (ineffective therapy vs. toxicity)
   b. Review drug and dietary history for potential drug and food interactions; be sure to include nutritional and herbal supplements; monitor to ensure steady intake of vitamin K in diet

   NCLEX®
   c. Institute bleeding precautions (see Box 37–11)
   d. If client experiences adverse effects or toxicity, withhold warfarin dose; depending on INR or client manifestations, administration of phytonadione (vitamin K) may be indicated
   e. For significant bleeding, prescriber may order transfusion of fresh frozen plasma (FFP) or prothrombin concentrate

NCLEX®
9. Client education
   a. Bleeding precautions (see Box 37–11)
   b. Stress need for frequent (weekly to monthly) follow-up blood tests to ensure safe therapy
   c. Point-of-care (POC) testing is available for self-monitoring PT and INR; prescriber may establish a home protocol to help manage care and necessary dose adjustments
   d. Take dose daily; do not stop therapy unless prescriber orders a dose to be withheld (pending PT and INR results) or client experiences a bleeding episode

Box 37–11

Bleeding Precautions for Clients Taking Anticoagulant and Fibrinolytic (Thrombolytic) Drugs

- Use a soft toothbrush and ensure gentle mouth care to minimize even mild trauma that could lead to bleeding.
- Use an electric razor rather than a straight razor for shaving.
- Use work gloves, do not go barefoot, and take other ordinary precautions as appropriate to avoid minor trauma to skin.
- Observe for and report to prescriber evidence of bleeding, including bleeding gums, epistaxis (nosebleed), ecchymosis (bruising), petechiae, tarry stools, hematuria, hematemesis.
- Notify healthcare providers, including dentists, about use of medications that cause bleeding, especially prior to any procedures or surgery.
- Avoid use of OTC drugs that could increase risk of bleeding, such as aspirin or nonsteroidal anti-inflammatory drugs (NSAIDs).

NCLEX®
e. Maintain steady daily intake of dietary vitamin K; foods high in vitamin K such as liver, cheese, egg yolk, leafy vegetables (broccoli, cabbage, spinach, and kale), and oils (peanut, corn, olive, or soybean) might be limited during therapy according to HCP directions

B. Heparin and related medications

1. Heparin plays an active role in the **intrinsic pathway** (where fibrin formation occurs) of clotting cascade; inhibits conversion of fibrinogen to fibrin, prevents formation of a fibrin clot, and inhibits thrombin
2. Molecular weight of heparin varies depending on whether drug is unfractionated heparin (UFH) or **low-molecular-weight heparin (LMWH)**
3. Has immediate effect and is treatment of choice for DVT, PE, and embolism resulting from atrial fibrillation
4. Also used as a prophylaxis for clients at risk for thrombi following surgery
5. Also used in a weak concentration as a flush solution to maintain access and prevent thrombus formation in vascular access devices
6. LMWH is a class of heparin molecule consisting of heparin fragments, with enoxaprin being most commonly used
7. Heparin sodium is most commonly used anticoagulant for treatment and prevention of recurrent thromboembolic episodes
8. Refer to Box 37–10 for a list of heparin anticoagulants
9. Administration considerations
   a. Heparin can be administered IV or subcutaneously
   b. LMWH has a higher bioavailability when compared to standard UFH
   NCLEX®
   c. **Activated partial thromboplastin time (APTT)** is used to monitor heparin therapy; results are trended over time to determine client response
   d. Low-dose UFH therapy: used as a prophylactic treatment for DVT; dosage ranges from 5,000 units subcutaneously every 8 to 12 hours or three doses in the immediate postoperative period depending on protocol; enoxaparin or Lovenox (an LMWH) comes in prefilled syringes ready for individual use
   e. High-dose UFH therapy achieves a therapeutic APTT; normal APTT value is 25–40 seconds, and therapeutic values are often 1.5–2.0 times control
   NCLEX®
   f. Use an infusion pump for IV administration; use a dedicated infusion line because of its incompatibility profile
   g. Be sure to carefully identify strength on product label; several concentrations of IV heparin are available; some are used only as flushes for IV lines
   NCLEX®
   h. **Protamine sulfate** is antidote that reverses action of heparin; dose depends on amount of heparin given and time period following its administration; however, do not give more than 50 mg IVP in a 10-minute period
   i. Hypersensitivity reaction can be seen in clients receiving heparin, so epinephrine 1:1000 should be readily available if a reaction develops
   j. Contraindicated with uncontrolled bleeding, known hypersensitivity, and thrombocytopenia
   NCLEX®
   k. Should not be given with aspirin or nonsteroidal anti-inflammatory drugs (NSAIDs), which increase risk of bleeding

NCLEX® **10.** Side/adverse effects
- **a.** Hemorrhage, hematuria, epistaxis, bleeding gums
- **b.** Thrombocytopenia **heparin-induced platelet aggregation (HIPA)**, a more serious form of thrombocytopenia with platelet count less than 100,000/mm^3; also called white clot syndrome; can be fatal if not treated aggressively; begins 3–12 days following start of heparin therapy
- **c.** Clients who are on heparin therapy longer than 6 months are prone to develop osteoporosis

11. Nursing considerations
- **a.** Monitor client's baseline labs according to heparin protocol (specifically APTT); commonly measured q 6 hours; when level is critically high, infusion may be stopped for 1 or more hours and APTT measured in 2–3 hours
- **b.** Obtain daily weight for client on weight-based heparin protocol
- NCLEX® **c.** Institute bleeding precautions, hemocult all stools, and evaluate pertinent labs
- **d.** Verify with pharmacy or another RN the correct dosage of heparin before administering or adjusting heparin infusion
- NCLEX® **e.** Evaluate dosage for safety and therapeutic range (normal adult dosage range of 20,000–40,000 units/24 hr); heparin is usually infused in units per hour
- NCLEX® **f.** Have antidote available (protamine sulfate)
- NCLEX® **g.** Subcutaneous administration of heparin requires rotation of sites; *do not aspirate or rub injection site*
- NCLEX® **h.** When administering heparin by subcutaneous route, inject into abdomen using a small (1.6-cm [5/8-in.], 25- to 27-gauge) needle at a *90-degree angle*

12. Client teaching
- **a.** Heparin administration if used after discharge
- **b.** Frequent bloodwork monitoring is required to ensure effective anticoagulation
- **c.** As per Box 37–11

C. Direct thrombin inhibitors
1. Bind reversibly to thrombin to prevent fibrin formation
2. Exhibit same anticoagulant actions and have same indications as heparin and LMWHs
3. Are given by IV route except for desirudin, which is given by subcutaneous route
4. A common adverse effect is bleeding and less common adverse effect is allergic reaction
5. Nursing considerations and client teaching is similar to other anticoagulants

XII. ANTIPLATELET AGENTS

A. Prevent or disrupt aggregation of platelets needed to form a clot by blocking certain enzyme pathways

B. Often used as adjuncts to other anticoagulants such as warfarin

C. Used often for clients with history of MI, stroke, and cardiac surgery

D. Common medications
1. Aspirin: most common antiplatelet agent; other therapeutic properties include analgesic, anti-inflammatory, and antipyretic actions
2. Ticlopidine: can be used by clients who cannot take aspirin
3. Dipyridamole: used for antiplatelet effect and in cardiac stress testing
4. Clopidrogrel: used as a form of secondary prevention for clients who have had MI, stroke, and peripheral arterial disease
5. Glycoprotein inhibitors prevent platelet activation and thrombus formation with recent MI, CVA, and percutaneous coronary intervention; a disadvantage is that they are expensive
6. Antiplatelet medications are listed in Box 37–12

E. Administration considerations
1. Aspirin is administered in dosages ranging from 81 to 325 mg/day (baby ASA to adult strength); it can also be given as an enteric-coated preparation to minimize GI upset
2. Dipyridamole has a better profile when used with clients who have prosthetic mechanical heart valves; contraindicated in pregnant or lactating clients
3. Ticlopidine has been used effectively as a preventive measure in clients at risk for MI
4. Glycoprotein inhibitors are administered by continuous IV infusion
5. NCLEX® Aspirin is contraindicated with known hypersensitivity to salicylates, bleeding disorders, asthma, or GI bleeding; do not give to children because of risk for developing Reye syndrome
6. Antiplatelet agents are generally contraindicated with conditions that increase risk of bleeding

F. Side/adverse effects
1. NCLEX® Aspirin: blood dyscrasias, hemorrhage, GI symptoms, increased bleeding tendencies, hemorrhage, N/V, dizziness, confusion, tinnitus, and ototoxicity

Box 37–12

Antiplatelet Drugs

Anagrelide	Ticagrelor
Aspirin	*Glycoprotein IIb/IIIa Receptor Antagonists*
Dipyridamole	Abciximab
Vorapaxar	Eptifibatide
Adenosine Diphosphate (ADP) Receptor Blockers	Tirofiban
Clopidogrel	*Drugs for Intermittent Claudication*
Prasugrel	Cilostazol
Ticlopidine	Pentoxyphylline

2. Dipyridamole: GI symptoms such as N/V, CNS alterations, headache, and dizziness
3. Ticlopidine: serious blood dyscrasias such as agranulocytosis and neutropenia; GI symptoms such as N/V and jaundice
4. Clopidrogrel: flulike symptoms, chest pain, edema, and hypertension
5. Glycoprotein receptor antagonists: dyspepsia, dizziness, pain at injection site, hypotension, bradycardia
6. NCLEX® In general: bruising, hematuria, tarry stools, other signs of bleeding

G. Nursing considerations
1. Perform baseline hematological labs on admission; monitor coagulation studies
2. Monitor vital signs and for bleeding
3. Antiplatelet drugs should be stopped at least 7 days prior to a planned surgery
4. NCLEX® Older adult clients may require closer monitoring to avoid toxicity because tinnitus and ototoxicity may be harder to assess if baseline hearing is already diminished
5. NCLEX® Lifespan concerns: children, pregnant women, and lactating women should not take antiplatelet medications

H. Client teaching
1. Carry a Medic-Alert bracelet
2. NCLEX® Monitor for and report side effects related to bleeding; may use bleeding precautions (see Box 37–11) on advice of prescriber
3. Adults should not self-treat pain with aspirin for more than 5 days without consulting prescriber
4. Maintain adequate fluid intake to prevent salicylate crystalluria
5. Prolonged use of aspirin can lead to iron-deficiency anemia (especially important for females of childbearing age)

XIII. THROMBOLYTICS

A. *Thrombolytics* activate *fibrinolytic system* to dissolve or break down a thrombus or blood clot, which reestablishes blood flow and increases perfusion to an ischemic area

B. Conversion of plasminogen to plasmin helps break down clot by digesting fibrin and degrading fibrinogen and other procoagulant proteins into soluble fragments

C. Indicated for clients at risk for developing thrombus with resultant ischemia, such as acute MI, arterial thrombosis, DVT, pulmonary embolism, and occlusion of catheters or shunts, with primary use in emergency and critical care settings

D. Common thrombolytic medications are listed in Box 37–13

Memory Aid

Remember that the suffix *-ase* often indicates a fibrinolytic/thrombolytic drug if it is given IV.

Box 37–13

Thrombolytics

Alteplase	Streptokinase
Reteplase	Tenecteplase

E. Administration considerations

1. Record baseline vital signs and obtain baseline coagulation studies
2. Give IV according to specific protocols; monitor IV sites for signs of infiltration and/or phlebitis; change IV site to opposite extremity if any problems are noted with IV
3. NCLEX® Place client on cardiac monitor during administration
4. NCLEX® Antidote to streptokinase is aminocaproic acid
5. Contraindicated in clients with active bleeding, clients who are pregnant, or clients who have a recent history of CVA, severe uncontrolled hypertension, recent trauma, or neoplasm

F. Side/adverse effects (dose-related)

1. NCLEX® Hemorrhage
2. NCLEX® Hypersensitivity reactions
3. N/V and hypotension
4. Cardiac dysrhythmias; reperfusion dysrhythmias may pose further problems for acutely ill client

G. Nursing considerations

1. Monitor coagulation studies and continue to assess client during therapy
2. NCLEX® Monitor for vital sign changes because drug may cause variations in pulse, BP, and temperature
3. Maintain adequate IV site for administration; observe closely for infiltration
4. NCLEX® Institute bleeding precautions and limit invasive procedures and injections to reduce risk of bleeding
5. NCLEX® If bleeding occurs, medication should be stopped; fresh frozen plasma (FFP) and packed red blood cells (PRBCs) may be ordered
6. Monitor client closely for development of dysrhythmias
7. Maintain aseptic technique to prevent infection
8. Provide adequate nutrition and rest to support client

H. Client teaching

1. Treatment methods and medication administration; measurable signs of clinical response may not occur for 6–8 hours after therapy is started
2. NCLEX® Bleeding precautions as per Box 37–11
3. Lifestyle changes may be needed to prevent further abnormal clotting
4. Discontinue medication if bleeding occurs and notify HCP

XIV. ANTIHYPERLIPIDEMICS

A. HMG-coenzyme A reductase inhibitors

1. Also called *statins*; reduce LDL cholesterol levels when diet therapy has not been effective
2. Have a dose-dependent effect on HDL cholesterol; lipoprotein levels are not affected by statins
3. Common antihyperlipidemic medications are listed in Box 37–14
4. Usually administered at night to increase effectiveness because cholesterol synthesis normally occurs during evening hours

Memory Aid

The suffix *-statin* indicates the cholesterol-lowering drugs known as HMG-coenzyme A reductase inhibitors.

Box 37–14

Antihyperlipidemic Drugs

HMG-Coenzyme A Reductase Inhibitors ("Statins")

Atorvastatin
Fluvastatin
Lovastatin
Pitavastatin
Pravastatin
Rosuvastatin
Simvastatin

Bile Acid Sequestrants

Cholestyramine
Colesevelam
Colestipol

Fibric Acid Derivatives

Fenofibrate
Fenofibric acid
Gemfibrozil

5. Contraindicated with active liver disease, abnormal serum transaminase levels, and during pregnancy and lactation
6. Monitor for elevation of liver function tests
7. Side/adverse effects
   NCLEX® a. GI upset, dyspepsia, flatulence, pain, and myalgias
   b. Headache, rash, dizziness, sinusitis
8. Nursing considerations
   NCLEX® a. Monitor lipid levels within 2–4 weeks after initiation of therapy
   b. May be given without regard to food
9. Client education
   NCLEX® a. Take dose with evening meal to coincide with body's timing of cholesterol production
   b. Required lab monitoring for compliance and client response
   NCLEX® c. Report immediately any unexplained muscle pain, tenderness, yellowing of skin or eyes, or loss of appetite (liver toxicity)
   d. Avoid or minimize alcohol intake

B. Bile acid sequestrants

1. Work in GI tract to bind with bile acids; liver cells respond by sending cholesterol to maintain bile acid synthesis, lowering plasma levels of LDL cholesterol
2. Indicated for use with elevated cholesterol levels with or without high triglyceride levels
3. Common medications: cholestyramine, colesevelam, and colestipol
   a. Colestipol and colesevelam are available as a tablet or powder, given in two to four doses before meals and at bedtime
   b. Cholestyramine is available as a powder, given two to four times daily before meals and at bedtime
4. Administration considerations
   NCLEX® a. Do not crush, chew, or cut colestipol tablets; they should be given with adequate fluids
   NCLEX® b. Mix powdered drug forms at bedside to prevent overthickening and esophageal obstruction; they may be plain or have flavoring; cholestyramine powder contains phenylalanine and should not be used in clients with phenylketonuria (PKU)
   c. Administer bile acids alone to avoid binding with other medications; give other drugs 1–2 hours before or 4–6 hours after bile acid administration
   d. Mix contents of one packet with at least 120–180 mL of water or other preferred liquid; dissolve before administration because drug is irritating to mucous membranes
5. Side/adverse effects
   NCLEX® a. Abdominal pain, dyspepsia, bloating, reflux, and constipation
   NCLEX® b. Associated fat-soluble vitamin deficiencies (A, D, K) and decreased erythrocyte folate levels
6. Nursing considerations
   a. Not often used as first-line therapy because of poor compliance
   b. Vitamin deficiencies may require supplementation, if not discontinuation of bile acids, to restore normal levels
   c. Increase fluids and fiber to counteract constipation as tolerated
   d. If client develops GI symptoms, dosage reduction may be needed to maintain adherence to therapy
   e. Serum cholesterol levels are reduced within 24–48 hours after starting therapy
   NCLEX® f. Assess baseline cholesterol and triglyceride levels; trend results to determine client response
   g. Decreased levels of LDL cholesterol should be seen within 1 month of therapy
   h. Long-term use of cholestyramine can increase bleeding tendency
7. NCLEX® Client teaching
   a. Proper administration and scheduling of medication to maximize effect
   b. Be alert for signs and symptoms indicating side effects of these agents
   c. Follow-up serum cholesterol levels are necessary
   d. Increase high-bulk diet with adequate fluid intake; report constipation immediately

C. Fibric acid agents

1. Act on very low lipid–density lipoproteins (VLDL) and chylomicrons to reduce triglyceride levels
2. HDL cholesterol levels are increased but this is not primary effect; also has variable effect on LDL
3. Indicated for use with elevated triglyceride and cholesterol levels resistant to dietary management
4. Common antihyperlipidemic medications are listed in Box 37–14
5. Administration considerations
   a. Usually given in divided doses, 30 minutes prior to morning and evening meals
   b. Contraindicated in clients with gallbladder disease, renal problems, liver or biliary cirrhosis, and in pregnant or lactating women

6. Side/adverse effects
   NCLEX® a. Abdominal or epigastric pain, jaundice
   b. Blurred vision, headache, and depression
   c. Rash, dermatitis, pruritus with gemfibrozil
   d. Back pain, muscle cramps, myalgia, and swollen joints
   NCLEX® e. Client may develop gallbladder disease and acute appendicitis
   f. Hypokalemia; eosinophilia in white blood cell count
7. Nursing considerations
   NCLEX® a. Obtain baseline lipid levels, monitor periodically
   b. If there is no response to therapy or if liver function tests are persistently abnormal after 3 months, then therapy should be discontinued
   c. Decreased hemoglobin, hematocrit, and WBC count may be seen with the use of gemfibrozil
   d. Monitor client for potential side effects and adverse effects
   NCLEX® e. Monitor closely for right upper quadrant (RUQ) abdominal pain or vomiting
NCLEX® 8. Client teaching
   a. Need for periodic labwork to evaluate response
   b. Immediately report unexplained bleeding or any serious side effects such as acute appendicitis or gallbladder disease
   c. Restrict fat and alcohol intake

D. Nicotinic acid (niacin, vitamin B_3)

1. Water-soluble vitamin that lowers most lipoprotein levels (total cholesterol, LDL, triglycerides, and lipoproteins) and increases HDL levels
2. Indications for use are high cholesterol levels and as adjunctive therapy when dietary management is ineffective
3. Causes peripheral vasodilation and can be used for clients with peripheral vascular disease
4. Pellagra (dermatitis, diarrhea, and dementia) is a clinical deficiency state associated with niacin deficiency
NCLEX® 5. Dosage to lower cholesterol is high (greater than 3 grams/day) in contrast to normal vitamin dose (500 mg/day in adults)
6. Administration considerations
   a. Tablets should be taken whole; do not crush or divide the pill
   b. Can be taken with meals to prevent GI upset
   NCLEX® c. Flushing is a common side effect caused by niacin's vasodilator properties; usually subsides after an hour
   d. Oral nicotinic acid should be taken with cold water
   e. Contraindicated with liver disease and/or unexplained elevated serum transaminases and with active peptic ulcer disease
   f. Contraindicated in clients with severe hypotension because of vasodilation
   g. Leads to increases in blood glucose, uric acid, and serum transaminase levels
7. Side/adverse effects
   NCLEX® a. Flushing, postural hypotension, vasovagal attacks
   b. Pruritus, increased sebaceous gland activity
   c. Dyspepsia, epigastric pain, and nausea
   d. Dark-colored urine
   e. Megadose therapy has been associated with liver damage, hyperglycemia, hyperuricemia, and cardiac dysrhythmias
NCLEX® 8. Nursing considerations
   a. Dosing of nicotinic acid varies depending on whether prescribed to reduce cholesterol levels or merely as a vitamin supplement; be aware of specific dosing levels
   b. Expect side effect of flushing when administering medication
   c. Evaluate client for food sources high in niacin (dairy, meats, tuna, and egg) and assess dietary intake
9. Client teaching
   NCLEX® a. Change position slowly to avoid sudden BP drop
   b. Avoid direct exposure to sunlight
   NCLEX® c. Flushing in face, neck, and ears may occur within 2 hours after oral ingestion and immediately after IV administration and may last several hours; alcohol and niacin cause increased flushing
   d. Periodic follow-up labwork will be done to determine response to therapy
   e. Do not self-medicate with additional sources of niacin, which can lead to overdose

XV. HEMOSTATICS

A. Systemic hemostatics

1. Systemic **hemostatics** are substances that inhibit bleeding after an injury
2. Common medications
   a. Aminocaproic acid and tranexamic acid impede **fibrinolysis**

   NCLEX® b. Aminocaproic acid is used to treat hyperfibrinolysis-induced hemorrhage after surgery, aplastic anemia, hepatic cirrhosis, and some neoplastic disease states; it is also an antidote to thrombolytic drugs

   c. Tranexamic acid is used 1 day before and 2–8 days after dental or other surgery in clients with hemophilia

   NCLEX® d. Phytonadione (vitamin K_1) is antidote to warfarin and is fat-soluble; used to reverse excess effects of oral anticoagulants

   e. Menadiol sodium diphosphate (vitamin K_4), is a water-soluble compound

   f. Vitamin K is also used as mandatory treatment to prevent hemorrhagic disease of newborn
3. Nursing considerations
   a. Assess client's baseline labs for renal and liver function

   NCLEX® b. Monitor PT levels and response to therapy for vitamin K administration

   NCLEX® c. Monitor client's coagulation profile as antifibrinolytics can cause **hypercoagulation**, or rapid coagulation of blood

   d. Rotate injection sites for vitamin K; assess for signs of local irritation

   e. Monitor client closely for signs of hypersensitivity and allergic reaction

   f. Monitor client closely during parenteral infusion because of risk for volume overload and adverse reactions

   g. Use an infusion pump for IV administration
4. Client teaching
   a. Dietary sources of vitamin K

   b. Periodic PT levels will be drawn to monitor response to therapy

   c. Monitor for signs and symptoms of bleeding

   d. Use of yogurt and buttermilk products in diet can help restore normal intestinal flora that aid in synthesis of vitamin K; clients receiving antibiotic therapy or who have intestinal problems may benefit from this supportive therapy

   e. Report difficulty urinating or reddish-brown urine (caused by myoglobinuria) while taking aminocaproic acid

   f. Report chest pain, arm or leg pain, or difficulty breathing

B. Topical thrombin

1. Used to stop oozing of blood or minor bleeding from capillaries
2. Administration considerations
   a. Available as a spray or gelatin sponge

   b. Irrigation with normal saline may be needed to prevent further tissue destruction with removal
3. Nursing considerations
   a. Assess local site for signs of hypersensitivity, and document findings; antihistamine such as diphenhydramine may be prescribed to prevent or treat allergic reaction

   NCLEX® b. Remove topical hemostatics per product guidelines; irrigate site with normal saline if necessary to prevent further tissue destruction with removal; document site assessment

XVI. ANTIANEMIC AGENTS

A. Iron salts

1. Iron is an essential trace element that aids oxygen transport, tissue respiration, and enzyme reactions
2. Iron is stored as ferritin; ferritin levels reflect visceral iron stores that are available to body; transferrin levels reflect how iron is transported in body
3. Common antianemic medications are listed in Box 37–15

Box 37–15 Iron Salts

Ferrous fumarate	Ferymoxytol
Ferrous gluconate	Iron dextran injection
Ferrous sulfate	Iron sucrose

4. Administration considerations
   a. NCLEX® Oral iron is given with meals to decrease gastric upset
   b. NCLEX® Iron dextran is administered by Z-track technique to minimize discomfort, prevent tissue discoloration, and ensure absorption
   c. There is risk of anaphylaxis following iron dextran administration; a test dose may be prescribed to determine client response
   d. Monitor client for intake of dietary sources of iron to avoid potential overdosing and toxicity
   e. NCLEX® Liquid (elixir) iron is administered by straw to avoid discoloration of tooth enamel
   f. Contraindicated in clients with ulcerative colitis, peptic ulcer disease, cirrhosis, hemolytic anemia, and iron overload syndromes (hemosiderosis and hemochromatosis)
   g. NCLEX® Vitamin C can increase absorption of oral iron
5. Side/adverse effects
   a. Upset stomach, N/V, diarrhea, and constipation
   b. NCLEX® Dark and tarry stools
   c. Discoloration of skin and pain upon injection
   d. **Pica** (ingestion of nonfood items) can interfere with iron levels and cause anemia; pregnant women are most likely to be affected
   e. Iron can accumulate in body, leading to potentially toxic levels
   f. Chelation therapy removes iron from body; additional supportive measures include airway maintenance, correction of acidosis, and administration of IV fluids
6. Nursing considerations
   a. Monitor client for expected side effects, such as tarry stools
   b. Since anemia is often a symptom of a disease, assess for underlying cause
   c. If client does not show a clinical response to iron therapy, notify prescriber
   d. Refer to dietitian as needed for instruction on foods rich in iron
   e. Evaluate client for pica if there is a high index of suspicion
   f. NCLEX® Monitor reticulocyte count, which will increase if RBC production is increasing
   g. If hemoglobin and hematocrit levels do not rise following iron therapy, additional testing may be required to determine type of anemia
7. NCLEX® Client education
   a. Proper self-administration of oral iron medications
   b. NCLEX® Importance of adequate food sources to maintain iron levels; these include lean meats, liver, egg yolks, dried beans, green vegetables (e.g., spinach)
   c. NCLEX® Expected changes in characteristics of stool (black, tarry)

B. Vitamin B_{12} (cyanocobalamin)

1. Water-soluble vitamin used in many coenzyme reactions during metabolism of carbohydrate, protein, and fat
2. NCLEX® Found primarily in foods of animal origin (liver, meat, shellfish, and dairy food items)
3. Deficiency of vitamin B_{12} affects neurological, hematological, and GI systems
4. Vitamin B_{12} is considered an extrinsic factor, whereas intrinsic factor is released by parietal cells in stomach
5. NCLEX® Clients with GI surgeries with partial or complete removal and/or anastomosis of stomach cannot produce intrinsic factor and will require weekly and then monthly vitamin B_{12} injections for life; a nasal form is now available as well
6. **Pernicious anemia** is name of anemia that results from vitamin B_{12} deficiency; classified as a megaloblastic macrocytic anemia
7. Atrophic gastritis is associated with vitamin B_{12} deficiency
8. Because B-complex vitamins work together, it is likely that more than one deficiency exists, making assessment and treatment of other anemias (such as folic acid deficiency) necessary
9. Adverse effects are rare but include diarrhea, hypokalemia, flushing, itching, rash, peripheral vascular thrombosis, pulmonary edema, and heart failure

C. Folic acid (folate)

1. Is a water-soluble B-complex vitamin that is essential for normal DNA and RNA synthesis
2. NCLEX® Found primarily in fresh green vegetables, dried beans, and wheat products
3. Deficiency of folic acid is seen in megaloblastic anemia and often accompanies vitamin B_{12} deficiency
4. NCLEX® Deficiency of folic acid during pregnancy is linked to neural birth defects such as spina bifida
5. Perform baseline and periodic assessments to evaluate effects of therapy, including follow-up labwork; client may note brighter yellow urine
6. Adverse effects are rare but include warmth or flushing during IV use, irritability, depression, loss of appetite, nausea, dyspnea, itching, or rash

Check Your NCLEX–RN® Exam I.Q.

You are ready for testing on this content if you can:

- Apply knowledge of expected actions and effects of cardiovascular medications to client care.
- Correctly administer cardiovascular medications to clients.
- Assess for side effects and adverse effects of cardiovascular medications.
- Take appropriate action if a client has an unexpected response to a cardiovascular medication.
- Monitor a client for expected outcomes or effects of treatment with cardiovascular medications.

PRACTICE TEST

1 A client is prescribed to receive a continuous infusion of IV nitroglycerin. What consideration should the nurse make in preparing to administer this medication?

1. Cover the solution with a plastic bag.
2. Maintain the solution in a glass bottle.
3. Replace the solution every 2 hours due to instability.
4. Prepare the solution under a laminar flow hood.

2 A client with angina pectoris received nitroglycerin tablets sublingually for chest pain. The client reports a severe headache shortly after the medication is administered. What interpretation should the nurse make based on the client's statement?

1. This is a common but unhealthy response to the medication.
2. This common response will diminish as tolerance to the medication develops.
3. This is a response caused by cerebral hypoxia induced by the medication.
4. This is an adverse reaction that should be reported to the prescriber immediately.

3 Diltiazem is prescribed for a client with chronic, stable angina. Which statement by the client indicates to the clinic nurse that the client needs additional medication information?

1. "I will call the prescriber if shortness of breath occurs."
2. "I will rise slowly when getting out of bed."
3. "I will take the medication after meals."
4. "I may notice changes in mental alertness until my dose is regulated."

4 A client with diabetes mellitus is newly diagnosed with hypertension. After learning that the client has a 15-year history of smoking one pack of cigarettes daily, the nurse would consult with the prescriber regarding which antihypertensive medication?

1. Diltiazem
2. Propranolol
3. Prazosin
4. Furosemide

5 The nurse has given medication instructions to the client receiving nicardipine for angina. What client statement should indicate to the nurse that further client teaching is needed?

1. "I will keep track of angina episodes, and report them if they increase."
2. "Edema and weight gain are expected side effects of the medication."
3. "I will report a pulse rate of fewer than 50 beats per minute."
4. "I will take any missed dose as soon as remembered, unless it is almost time for the next dose."

6 A client with hypertension has been given a prescription to treat the disorder. The nurse should explain that cough and loss of taste are side effects if which antihypertensive agent has been prescribed?

1. Lisinopril
2. Propranolol
3. Diltiazem
4. Furosemide

7 The healthcare provider prescribes losartan for a client with hypertension. When the client questions how this medication works, the nurse explains that it promotes vasodilation by which action?

1. Preventing calcium from going into the cells
2. Promoting epinephrine and norepinephrine
3. Promoting release of aldosterone
4. Inhibiting conversion of a substance that would cause vasoconstriction

8 A client with hypertension monitors his blood pressure daily and is prescribed verapamil sustained release 240 mg daily and hydrochlorothiazide 12.5 mg daily. The client states that if his systolic BP reading is lower than 140, he skips his medication for the day. What would be the most appropriate response by the nurse? Select all that apply.

1. "As long as the systolic is lower than 140, it is OK to skip the dose."
2. "You should not skip doses unless instructed by the prescriber."
3. "Maybe you won't even need your BP medications in a few more months."
4. "Your prescriber may want to stop the hydrochlorothiazide and have you take only the verapamil."
5. "Your lower systolic blood pressure is a response to the medication."

9 Adenosine is to be administered to a client in the emergency department. Before preparing the medication, the nurse ensures that which priority piece of equipment is operational?

1. A pulse oximetry machine
2. An IV infusion pump
3. A cardiac monitor
4. An endotracheal tube

10 The home health nurse would be most concerned that a client is experiencing digoxin toxicity after noting which manifestations during a routine visit? Select all that apply.

1. Palpitations
2. Anorexia
3. Fatigue
4. Taste alterations
5. Visual disturbances

11 A client is experiencing multiform, premature ventricular contractions (PVCs) that are resistant to amiodarone therapy. The nurse checks the medication cart to ensure that which alternate medication is available for immediate use?

1. Digoxin
2. Metoprolol
3. Verapamil
4. Lidocaine

12 The nurse is preparing to administer amiodarone IV. Which item should the nurse assure is in use at this time?

1. Oxygen therapy
2. Noninvasive blood pressure monitoring
3. Continuous cardiac monitoring
4. Oxygen saturation monitoring

13 Which medication does the nurse anticipate will be used for a pregnant client who requires anticoagulation therapy?

1. Low-molecular-weight heparin
2. Epoetin alfa
3. Heparin
4. Enoxaparin

14 A client is taking warfarin for atrial fibrillation. The nurse would include in a teaching plan that the client will need to remain on drug therapy for what period of time?

1. 6 months
2. 2–3 months
3. Indefinite, or long-term
4. 1 year

15 A client is placed on ticlopidine following a stroke. What follow-up bloodwork is indicated in managing the client?

1. Frequent CBC monitoring to evaluate for blood dyscrasias
2. Monthly PT and INR levels to evaluate for clotting problems
3. ABGs to evaluate respiratory status
4. Serum chemistries to monitor for potential electrolyte imbalances

16 A client is undergoing percutaneous transluminal coronary angioplasty (PTCA) and requires an antiplatelet agent. What drug should the nurse anticipate administering to this client immediately following the procedure?

1. Heparin
2. Abciximab
3. Clopidogrel
4. Aspirin

17 A client is receiving thrombolytic therapy. The nurse monitors the client for which potential problems? Select all that apply.

1. Headache
2. Bruising
3. Hematuria
4. Bone pain
5. Hypotension

18 The nurse would assess a client who is receiving anistreplase for which manifestation?

1. Dry mouth
2. Decreased urine output
3. Decreased clotting times
4. Cardiac dysrhythmias

19 For what manifestation should the nurse monitor a client taking folic acid to treat megaloblastic anemia?

1. Brighter-yellow urine
2. Dark-green or black stools
3. Temperature elevations
4. Increased pulse rate

20 Which measures should the nurse utilize when administering ferrous sulfate elixir? Select all that apply.

1. Mix the medication with milk to decrease GI effects.
2. Administer the oral form of the medication with food.
3. Administer the medication through a straw.
4. Mix the medication with carbonated beverages to minimize gastric upset.
5. Increase dietary intake of vitamin C to promote absorption.

21 A client has an order to receive 5,000 units of heparin subcutaneously. Available is a vial labeled "Heparin 10,000 units per mL." The nurse should administer ______ mL of heparin solution. Record your answer rounding to one decimal place.

Fill in your answer below:
Answer: ______ mL

ANSWERS & RATIONALES

1 **Answer: 2 Rationale:** Intravenous nitroglycerin (NTG) must be prepared only in glass bottles and infused via the manufacturer-provided tubing. There is no indication that the solution needs to be covered by a plastic bag. NTG is stable in a glass bottle for 24 hours. The preparation of NTG solution does not require laminar flow ventilation. **Cognitive Level:** Applying **Client Need:** Pharmacological and Parenteral Therapies **Integrated Process:** Nursing Process: Implementation **Content Area:** Pharmacology **Strategy:** The core issue of the question is knowledge that nitroglycerin adsorbs into plastic, making it necessary to use a glass bottle and special IV tubing from the manufacturer. Use nursing knowledge related to pharmacology and the process of elimination to make a selection.

2 **Answer: 2 Rationale:** The incidence of headache decreases over time as the client develops tolerance to the medication. Headache is a common side effect (not adverse reaction) related to the vasodilation properties of nitroglycerin. Headache is not an indication of cerebral hypoxia induced by nitroglycerine; the medication has vasodilation properties. The client should be encouraged to continue to use nitroglycerine as needed; acetaminophen or aspirin can be taken for the headache, according to the preference of the prescriber. **Cognitive Level:** Analyzing **Client Need:** Pharmacological and Parenteral Therapies **Integrated Process:** Nursing Process: Diagnosis **Content Area:** Pharmacology **Strategy:** The core issue of the question is knowledge of common adverse effects of nitroglycerin therapy. Use nursing knowledge related to pharmacology and the process of elimination to make a selection.

3 **Answer: 3 Rationale:** Diltiazem is usually administered before meals and at bedtime to increase the absorption of medication. The client should notify the prescriber if shortness of breath, irregular heartbeat, pronounced dizziness, nausea, or constipation develops. Postural hypotension can occur, so the client must be instructed to rise slowly to avoid

dizziness and falling. The medication can cause a decrease in mental alertness until the body adjusts and the proper dosage is established. **Cognitive Level:** Analyzing **Client Need:** Pharmacological and Parenteral Therapies **Integrated Process:** Nursing Process: Evaluation **Content Area:** Pharmacology **Strategy:** The wording of the question tells you that the correct answer is an incorrect statement. Recall information about calcium channel blockers and use the process of elimination to make a selection.

4 **Answer: 2 Rationale:** Adverse effects of beta-adrenergic blockers such as propranolol include their potential to cause bronchospasm and to mask hypoglycemia attacks. Therefore, the clients who are at risk for these conditions should not utilize beta-blockers as antihypertensive medications. Diltiazem is a calcium channel blocker, which would not directly affect the client's conditions. Alpha blockers such as prazosin do not directly affect the client's conditions. Furosemide is a diuretic, which will not directly affect the client's conditions. **Cognitive Level:** Applying **Client Need:** Pharmacological and Parenteral Therapies **Integrated Process:** Nursing Process: Implementation **Content Area:** Pharmacology **Strategy:** The core issue of the question is knowledge of contraindications for beta-adrenergic blockers, such as propranolol. Use nursing knowledge related to pharmacology and the process of elimination to make a selection.

5 **Answer: 2 Rationale:** Nicardipine is a calcium channel blocker. Weight gain and edema are potential signs of heart failure, and must be reported to the prescriber. The client taking this medication should keep track of angina episodes and report any increase in the episodes or change in the pattern. The client should be taught to check his pulse, note the rate, and report if the heart rate is lower than 50 beats per minute. The client may take a missed dose of medication if not too close to the next dose; otherwise, the dose should be omitted. **Cognitive Level:** Analyzing **Client Need:** Pharmacological and Parenteral Therapies **Integrated Process:** Nursing Process: Evaluation **Content Area:** Pharmacology **Strategy:** The core issue of the question is knowledge of teaching points regarding calcium channel blockers, such as nicardipine. The wording of the question tells you that the correct answer is an incorrect statement. Use nursing knowledge related to pharmacology and the process of elimination to make a selection.

6 **Answer: 1 Rationale:** Cough and loss of taste are common side effects of angiotensin-converting enzyme (ACE) inhibitors such as lisinopril. They disappear with discontinuation of the medication. Cough and loss of taste are not common side effects of propranolol, which is a beta-adrenergic blocker. Diltiazem, a calcium channel blocker, does not cause the side effects of cough and loss of taste. Furosemide, a diuretic, will not cause the client to develop a cough or loss of taste as side effects. **Cognitive Level:** Analyzing **Client Need:** Pharmacological and Parenteral Therapies **Integrated Process:** Teaching and Learning **Content Area:** Pharmacology **Strategy:** The core issue of the question is knowledge that ACE inhibitors lead to cough and loss of taste perception. From there, you must be able to identify which drug is an ACE inhibitor. Recall that these drugs end in *-pril* to help make a selection.

7 **Answer: 4 Rationale:** Losartan is an angiotensin II antagonist that inhibits the conversion of angiotensin I to angiotensin II. Because angiotensin II is a powerful vasoconstrictor, this inhibition results in vasodilation and normalizing blood pressure. The client should be assessed for dizziness, cough, and diarrhea while taking this medication. Calcium channel blockers prevent calcium from entering cells, but don't promote vasodilation. Epinephrine and norepinephrine are sympathomimetic antihypotensives, which promote vasoconstriction. The primary effect of aldosterone is sodium reabsorption, which would cause an elevation in blood pressure and not be prescribed for a client with hypertension. **Cognitive Level:** Applying **Client Need:** Pharmacological and Parenteral Therapies **Integrated Process:** Teaching and Learning **Content Area:** Pharmacology **Strategy:** The core issue of the question is knowledge of the mechanism of action of angiotensin-receptor blockers. To reach the correct answer, it is necessary to recognize that the drug is in this class. Use nursing knowledge related to pharmacology and the process of elimination to make a selection.

8 **Answer: 2, 5 Rationale:** Lack of adherence to pharmacologic treatment strategies prevents the client from establishing good control of the disease, and ultimately places him at risk for developing long-term complications of hypertension. Noncompliance with the therapeutic program is a significant problem in people with hypertension. It is an important nursing activity to reinforce the need for the client to adhere to the medication as prescribed. The client should not skip doses of medications without consulting the prescriber. The comment about not needing medications is inappropriate; the client may require long-term treatment for hypertension. The prescriber is responsible for adjusting the client's medication regimen; to state HCTZ may be stopped is not an appropriate comment. **Cognitive Level:** Applying **Client Need:** Pharmacological and Parenteral Therapies **Integrated Process:** Communication and Documentation **Content Area:** Pharmacology **Strategy:** The core issue of the question is knowledge that antihypertensive medications need to be taken as scheduled without missing or skipping doses. Use nursing knowledge related to pharmacology and the process of elimination to make a selection. When more than one answer is correct, consider each option as a true/false statement.

9 **Answer: 3 Rationale:** Adenosine is an antidysrhythmic used in the treatment of paroxysmal supraventricular tachycardia (SVT). Cardiac performance must be assessed before and throughout treatment by cardiac monitoring. A pulse oximetry machine and IV infusion pump might be helpful in assessing oxygenation, but are not priority items. An endotracheal tube may be used if an emergency necessitates mechanical ventilation, but the tube itself is a rather isolated item. **Cognitive Level:** Analyzing **Client Need:** Pharmacological and Parenteral Therapies **Integrated Process:** Nursing Process: Planning **Content Area:** Pharmacology **Strategy:** The core issue of the question is the most important piece of equipment needed to monitor a client receiving adenosine. Recall that this drug is an antidysrhythmic to help select the cardiac monitor as the appropriate answer.

10 **Answer: 2, 5 Rationale:** Anorexia, nausea, and visual disturbances are signs of digoxin toxicity. Palpitations, fatigue, and taste alterations are not signs of digoxin toxicity. **Cognitive Level:** Analyzing **Client Need:** Pharmacological and Parenteral Therapies **Integrated Process:** Nursing Process: Assessment **Content Area:** Pharmacology **Strategy:** The core issue of the question is knowledge of the signs of digoxin toxicity. Recall that early signs are usually more subtle than are later signs. Use nursing knowledge related to pharmacology and the process of elimination to make a selection. When more than one answer is correct, consider each option as a true/false statement.

11 **Answer: 4 Rationale:** Amiodarone is a class III antidysrhythmic used to treat ventricular dysrhythmias. Other medications that might be prescribed include procainamide, lidocaine, or magnesium sulfate. Digoxin would not be used as a primary treatment of ventricular dysrhythmias because it is a cardiac glycoside. Metoprolol would not be used as a primary treatment of PVCs because it is a beta blocker. Verapamil would not be used as a primary treatment of ventricular dysrhythmias because it is a calcium channel blocker. **Cognitive Level:** Analysis **Client Need:** Pharmacological and Parenteral Therapies **Integrated Process:** Nursing Process: Planning **Content Area:** Pharmacology **Strategy:** The core issue of the question is knowledge of first-line treatment for PVCs. Use nursing knowledge related to pharmacology and the process of elimination to make a selection.

12 **Answer: 3 Rationale:** Amiodarone is a class III antiarrhythmic that is often used as first-line treatment for life-threatening ventricular dysrhythmias. The client should have continuous EKG monitoring, and the medication should be infused through an IV pump. Oxygen therapy might be needed, but its use is unrelated specifically to this medication. Noninvasive blood pressure monitoring is not critical during administration of this medication, although it may generally be a useful adjunct. Oxygen saturation monitoring is not critical during administration of this medication. **Cognitive Level:** Analysis **Client Need:** Pharmacological and Parenteral Therapies **Integrated Process:** Nursing Process: Implementation **Content Area:** Pharmacology **Strategy:** The core issue of the question is knowledge of what parameter needs to be monitored carefully during amiodarone therapy. Recall that the drug is an antidysrhythmic agent to make the final selection.

13 **Answer: 3 Rationale:** Heparin is the drug of choice in pregnancy. Low-molecular-weight heparins are not recommended for use during pregnancy. Epoetin alfa is a colony-stimulating growth factor, and is not used for anticoagulation. Low-molecular-weight heparins, of which enoxaparin is an example, are not recommended for use during pregnancy. **Cognitive Level:** Applying **Client Need:** Pharmacological and Parenteral Therapies **Integrated Process:** Nursing Process: Planning **Content Area:** Pharmacology **Strategy:** The core issue of the question is knowledge of the anticoagulant that is safe to use during pregnancy. Use nursing knowledge related to pharmacology and the process of elimination to make a selection.

14 **Answer: 3 Rationale:** Clients who have atrial fibrillation are at risk to develop emboli. Therapy with warfarin is considered to be ongoing in nature, in order to prevent such an occurrence. Clients who have atrial fibrillation are at risk to develop emboli; six months is too short to achieve a preventative goal. In addition, the likelihood of emboli formation does not significantly diminish unless the client is anticoagulated on a long-term basis. **Cognitive Level:** Applying **Client Need:** Pharmacological and Parenteral Therapies **Integrated Process:** Nursing Process: Planning **Content Area:** Pharmacology **Strategy:** The core issue of the question is knowledge that treatment for prevention of blood clot formation from atrial fibrillation is indefinite. Use nursing knowledge related to pharmacology and the process of elimination to make a selection.

15 **Answer: 1 Rationale:** A client taking ticlopidine should be monitored for potential blood dyscrasias that can occur with this drug. Monthly PT and INR levels are not indicated as follow-up for ticlopidine, but are used in conjunction with warfarin therapy. ABGs are not indicated in the management of clients who are taking ticlopidine. There are no reported electrolyte imbalances with the use of ticlopidine. **Cognitive Level:** Applying **Client Need:** Pharmacological and Parenteral Therapies **Integrated Process:** Nursing Process: Planning **Content Area:** Pharmacology **Strategy:** The core issue of the question is knowledge of adverse effects of ticlopidine that can be detected using laboratory monitoring. Use nursing knowledge related to pharmacology and the process of elimination to make a selection.

16 **Answer: 2 Rationale:** Abciximab is often given IV following this type of procedure, to help prevent possible reocclusion of the coronary artery that has been treated. Abciximab is often given IV following this type of procedure, it can be administered in conjunction with weight-based heparin therapy, but heparin alone is an anticoagulant agent. Clopidogrel is an example of an antiplatelet agent that is given orally and is not utilized in this particular acute-care setting. Aspirin is an example of an antiplatelet agent that is given orally and is not utilized in this particular acute-care setting. However, aspirin can be given later as follow-up to the procedure, to prevent possible complications related to vessel occlusion. **Cognitive Level:** Analyzing **Client Need:** Pharmacological and Parenteral Therapies **Integrated Process:** Nursing Process: Planning **Content Area:** Pharmacology **Strategy:** The core issue of the question is knowledge of drugs that have antiplatelet properties and that can be used following interventional cardiology procedures such as PTCA, and which would have an immediate effect. Use nursing knowledge related to pharmacology and the process of elimination to make a selection.

17 **Answer: 2, 3, 5 Rationale:** The client receiving thrombolytic therapy should be monitored closely for skin bruising, which can be an indication of bleeding. Urine should be monitored for the presence of occult or obvious blood, indications of hemorrhage or bleeding. When on thrombolytic therapy, the client's blood pressure should be monitored for dose-related or hemorrhage-related hypotension. Headache is not directly related to thrombolytic therapy. Bone pain is not directly related to thrombolytic therapy. **Cognitive Level:** Analyzing **Client Need:** Pharmacological and Parenteral Therapies **Integrated Process:** Nursing Process: Assessment **Content Area:** Pharmacology **Strategy:** The core issue of the question is knowledge that thrombolytics can lead to bleeding. With this in mind, recall the various ways that bleeding can manifest in a client taking drugs that interfere with clotting. Use nursing knowledge related to pharmacology and the process of elimination to make a selection. When there is more than one correct answer, consider each option as a true/false statement.

18 **Answer: 4 Rationale:** The use of thrombolytic agents can cause cardiac irritation and lead to reperfusion dysrhythmias that can be life-threatening. The nurse must be aware of the serious likelihood that treatment can cause further cardiac compromise. Dry mouth, decreased urine output, and decreased clotting times are not seen with thrombolytic therapy. **Cognitive Level:** Applying **Client Need:** Pharmacological and Parenteral Therapies **Integrated Process:** Nursing Process: Assessment **Content Area:** Pharmacology **Strategy:** The core issue of the question is knowledge that thrombolytic drugs can cause reperfusion dysrhythmias as a result of clot lysis. Use nursing knowledge related to pharmacology and the process of elimination to make a selection.

19 **Answer: 1 Rationale:** Folic acid (in large doses) can cause the urine to become discolored and turn to a brighter-yellow color. Dark-green or black stools are more commonly associated with iron therapy. Temperature elevations and increased pulse rate are not associated with folic acid. **Cognitive Level:** Applying **Client Need:** Pharmacological and Parenteral Therapies **Integrated Process:** Nursing Process: Evaluation **Content Area:** Pharmacology **Strategy:** The core issue of the question is knowledge of expected side effects of folic acid. Recall that B-complex vitamins can turn the urine a brighter or darker yellow as an aid to answering the question. Use nursing knowledge related to pharmacology and the process of elimination to make a selection.

20 **Answer: 2, 3, 5 Rationale:** The oral form of ferrous sulfate is usually taken with food to minimize GI upset. Liquid iron preparations can cause staining of teeth. It is important for the nurse to be aware of proper administration methods, which include drinking the mixture through a straw. Vitamin C promotes the absorption of ferrous sulfate when the medication is taken orally. Mixing ferrous sulfate with milk will decrease its absorption. Mixing medication with carbonated beverages will decrease its absorption. **Cognitive Level:** Analyzing **Client Need:** Pharmacological and Parenteral Therapies **Integrated Process:** Nursing Process: Implementation **Content Area:** Pharmacology **Strategy:** The core issue of the question is knowledge of the administration considerations that should be made when giving ferrous sulfate. Keeping other administration principles in mind helps you to eliminate the incorrect options. When more than one answer is correct, consider each option as a true/false statement.

21 **Answer: 0.5 Rationale:** To calculate the dose, divide the desired dose (5,000 units) by the dose on hand (10,000 units) and multiply that by the quantity (1 mL). The result is 0.5 mL. **Cognitive Level:** Applying **Client Need:** Pharmacological and Parenteral Therapies **Integrated Process:** Nursing Process: Implementation **Content Area:** Pharmacology **Strategy:** The core issue of the question is the ability to calculate a drug dose. If necessary, memorize this basic formula for use in solving many medication questions.

Key Terms to Review

activated partial thromboplastin time (APTT) p. 555
afterload p. 540
anticoagulants p. 553
automaticity p. 542
chronotropic p. 542
clotting cascade p. 553
conductivity p. 544
contractility p. 548
dromotropic p. 542
dysrhythmias p. 548
extrinsic pathway p. 553
fibrinolysis p. 561
fibrinolytic system p. 557
hemostatics p. 561
heparin-induced platelet aggregation (HIPA) p. 556
hypercoagulation p. 561
inotropic p. 542
international normalized ratio (INR) p. 554
intrinsic pathway p. 555
irritability p. 542
low molecular weight heparin (LMWH) p. 555
pernicious anemia p. 562
pica p. 562
preload p. 540
protamine sulfate p. 555
prothrombin time (PT) p. 554
refractory period p. 549
thrombolytics p. 557
titrated p. 541

References

Adams, M., Holland, L., & Urban, C. (2017). *Pharmacology for nurses: A pathophysiologic approach* (5th ed.). New York, NY: Pearson Education.

Adams, M., & Urban, C. (2016). *Pharmacology: Connections to nursing practice* (3rd ed.). New York, NY: Pearson Education.

Berman, A., Snyder, S., & Frandsen, G. (2016). *Kozier & Erb's fundamentals of nursing: Concepts, process, and practice* (10th ed.). New York, NY: Pearson Education.

Lehne, R. (2016). *Pharmacology for nursing care* (9th ed.). St. Louis, MO: Saunders.

Wilson, B., Shannon, M., & Shields, K. (2016). *Pearson nurse's drug guide 2016.* New York, NY: Pearson Education.

Neurologic and Musculoskeletal Medications

38

In this chapter

Cross Reference

Other chapters relevant to this content area are

Dosage Calculation and Medication Administration	Chapter 29
Psychiatric Medications	Chapter 35
Neurologic Disorders	Chapter 57
Musculoskeletal Disorders	Chapter 61

I. ANALGESICS

A. Opioids

1. Used to relieve severe acute and chronic pain
2. Produce effects by binding to opioid receptors in CNS and peripheral tissues
3. Labeled controlled substances by Food and Drug Administration (FDA)
4. Cross blood–brain and placental barriers and also into breast milk
5. Common opioid medications are listed in Box 38–1
6. Administration considerations
   - *NCLEX®* **a.** Use caution because of possibility of dependence
   - **b.** Determine client's pattern of use if long term; be aware that some opioids are used as street drugs
   - **c.** May increase intracranial pressure (ICP)
   - **d.** Closely monitor clients with severe heart, liver, or kidney disease or respiratory or seizure disorders
   - **e.** Decrease dosages for older adults or debilitated clients
   - *NCLEX®* **f.** Additional CNS depression can occur if used with barbiturates, other narcotics, hypnotics, antipsychotics, or alcohol
7. Side/adverse effects
   - **a.** Nausea and vomiting (N/V), anorexia
   - *NCLEX®* **b.** Sedation, respiratory or circulatory depression

Box 38–1

Common Opioid Analgesics

Pure Agonists	Mixed Agonists-Antagonists
Codeine	Buprenorphine
Fentanyl	Butorphanol tartrate
Hydrocodone	Nalbuphine
Hydromorphone	Pentazocine
Oxycodone	
Levorphanol	
Meperidine	
Methadone	
Morphine sulfate	
Oxymorphone	
Sufentanyl	
Tramadol	

Memory Aid

Remember that opioid analgesics are CNS depressants; watch for sedation as an early sign and respiratory rate decrease as a later sign of CNS depression.

   c. Constipation, gastrointestinal (GI) cramps, urinary retention, oliguria
   d. Pruritis, light-headedness, dizziness, increased ICP
8. Nursing considerations
   NCLEX® a. Assess pain type, intensity (pain scale), and location prior to administration
   NCLEX® b. Assess respiratory rate, depth, and rhythm; if less than 12, withhold medication
   c. Assess for CNS changes, including changes in level of consciousness (LOC); monitor vital signs (VS) regularly
   NCLEX® d. Assess for allergic reaction such as rash or urticaria
   e. Administer opioids for pain and antiemetics for N/V
   f. Evaluate therapeutic response and maintain comfort
9. NCLEX® Client teaching
   a. Avoid other CNS depressants while using opioids
   b. Use caution in ambulation, and avoid smoking, driving, and strenuous activities without assistance until drug response is known
   c. Report any CNS changes, allergic reactions, or shortness of breath
   d. If using medication on a long-term basis, be aware of withdrawal symptoms, including N/V, cramps, fever, faintness, and anorexia

B. Opioid antagonists

1. Include naloxone, naltrexone for reversal of CNS depression, and alvimopan and methylnatrexone for treatment of opioid-induced bowel constipation
2. Compete with opioids at opiate receptor sites, blocking opioid effects
3. NCLEX® Reverse respiratory depression induced by overdose of opioids, pentazocine, and propoxyphene (naloxone and naltrexone)
4. Onset of effect is 1–2 minutes, duration is 45 minutes; remain with client because CNS depression could recur when drug wears off
5. Side/adverse effects
   NCLEX® a. Reversal of analgesia
   b. Increased or decreased blood pressure (BP), tachycardia, hyperpnea, N/V
   c. Tremors, drowsiness, nervousness, convulsions
   d. Ventricular tachycardia and fibrillation, pulmonary edema

6. Nursing considerations

NCLEX®
   a. Assess VS every 3 to 5 minutes initially (tachycardia, hypertension); taper to every 15 minutes, then every 30 minutes as client stabilizes, and then routine
   b. Assess arterial blood gases (ABGs) and respiratory function (rate, rhythm, lung sounds)
   c. Initiate cardiac monitoring and assess cardiac rhythm

NCLEX®
   d. Administer only with resuscitative equipment nearby
   e. Do not leave client alone; evaluate therapeutic response, LOC, and need to reverse respiratory depression

C. Nonopioids

1. Acetylsalicylic acid (aspirin)
   a. Inhibits prostaglandins involved in producing inflammation, pain, and fever
   b. Blocks pain impulses in CNS and provides relief of mild to moderate pain
   c. Antipyretic action results from vasodilation of peripheral vessels
   d. Powerfully inhibits platelet aggregation

NCLEX®
   e. Assess for allergy to salicylates prior to administration
   f. Decrease gastric irritation by administering with full glass of water, milk, food, or antacid, or by using an enteric-coated preparation

NCLEX®
   g. Side/adverse effects include visual changes, tinnitus, hepatotoxicity, allergic reactions and bleeding; instruct client to report these
   h. Instruct client not to combine with other OTC medications that also contain aspirin and avoid alcohol ingestion to decrease risk of GI bleeding

NCLEX®
   i. Warn client that aspirin should not be given to children or teens with flulike or chickenpox symptoms (can lead to Reye syndrome, characterized by encephalopathy and fatty liver degeneration)

2. Acetaminophen
   a. Used for mild to moderate pain or fever, especially when aspirin or nonsteroidal anti-inflammatory drugs (NSAIDs) are not tolerated; blocks pain impulses peripherally
   b. Antipyretic action occurs by inhibiting prostaglandins in CNS, resulting in peripheral vasodilation, sweating, and dissipation of heat

NCLEX®
   c. Do not use if allergic to acetaminophen or phenacetin
   d. Avoid use in anemia or hepatic diseases, including alcoholism, malnutrition, or thrombocytopenia

NCLEX®
   e. May cause **hepatotoxicity** at doses greater than 4 grams/day with chronic use; assess for dark urine, clay-colored stools, yellowing of skin or sclera, itching, abdominal pain, fever, and diarrhea, especially if on long-term therapy

NCLEX®
   f. Prepare to administer acetylcysteine as antidote for acetaminophen poisoning
   g. Evaluate client for therapeutic response, such as decreased pain or fever

3. NSAIDs
   a. Decrease prostaglandin synthesis by inhibiting an enzyme needed for biosynthesis
   b. Used for mild to moderate pain, osteo- or rheumatoid arthritis, and dysmenorrhea
   c. Common NSAID medications are listed in Box 38–2
   d. Decrease gastric irritation by administering with full glass of water or milk or with food
   e. Give dose at least 30 minutes prior to planned activity to minimize discomfort

NCLEX®
   f. Contraindicated with asthma, severe renal or hepatic disease, GI bleeding, bleeding disorders, peptic ulcer disease, anemia, or anticoagulant therapy

Box 38–2

Common Nonsteroidal Anti-Inflammatory Drugs

Celecoxib	Ketorolac
Diclofenac	Meclofenate
Diflunisal	Mefenemic acid
Etodolac	Meloxicam
Fenoprofen	Naproxen
Flurbiprofen	Oxaprozin
Ibuprofen	Piroxicam
Indomethacin	Sulindac
Ketoprofen	Tolmetin

NCLEX® **g.** Instruct client to report blurred vision, ringing or roaring in ears; may indicate toxicity

h. Evaluate for therapeutic response, including decreased pain, stiffness in joints, decreased swelling in joints, ability to move more easily; may take up to 1 month

D. Medications to treat headaches

1. Aimed at prevention with prophylactic therapy and acute symptomatic treatment during attack
   - **a.** Ergot alkaloids and triptans are serotonin receptor agonists; triptans are thought to act by constricting certain intracranial blood vessels and are used first; ergot alkaloids are used for migraine headaches unresponsive to triptans; ergot dose should be separated from triptan dose by at least 24 hours
   - **b.** Prophylaxis for migraine headaches includes beta-adrenergic blockers and antiepileptics
   - **c.** Mild analgesics and muscle relaxants are first-line medications for tension-type headaches; antidepressants may be used with counseling; ASA, acetaminophen, and ibuprofen are used for pain; amitriptyline is helpful for muscle contraction pain
   - **d.** Preventative therapies for cluster headaches may include high-dose calcium channel blockers, lithium, methysergide, or corticosteroids
2. Common medications for headaches are listed in Box 38–3
3. NCLEX® Administration considerations
   - **a.** For abortive treatment medications, take early in headache to be effective
   - **b.** Start with dose that was effective on last headache at start of this headache
   - **c.** Contraindicated with hypersensitivity to ergot alkaloids, pregnancy, cardiovascular disease, coronary artery disease, hypertension, sepsis, or severe pruritus
4. Nursing considerations
   - **a.** Carefully assess history, including past treatments that were effective
   - NCLEX® **b.** Assess for medication-specific side effects as well as efficacy of treatment
   - **c.** Provide a quiet and low-light environment
   - **d.** Obtain accurate dietary history to determine if onset of headache is associated with certain foods
   - **e.** Avoid prolonged medication use
   - NCLEX® **f.** Beware of ergotamine rebound or an increase in frequency and duration of headache
5. Client teaching
   - NCLEX® **a.** Identify triggers for headaches and how to ameliorate them
   - **b.** Keep a headache diary
   - **c.** Use stress reduction, stress management, lifestyle changes (including diet), to minimize headaches
   - **d.** Do not eat, drink, or smoke while tablet is dissolving (if using sublingual tablet)
   - **e.** Avoid prolonged exposure to cold weather (may increase adverse reactions to medication)
   - **f.** Do not increase dose without consulting prescriber
   - NCLEX® **g.** Use comfort measures during attack, such as lying in darkened, quiet room with cold compresses applied to head

Box 38–3

Medications Used to Treat Headaches

Ergot Alkaloids	Frovatriptan
Dihydroergotamine	Naratriptan
Ergotamine	Rizatriptan
Triptans	Sumatriptan
Almotriptan	Zolmitriptan
Eletriptan	

II. ANTIEPILEPTICS

A. Hydantoins

1. Inhibit spread of seizure activity in motor cortex
2. Used in general **tonic-clonic seizures** (grand mal seizures), **status epilepticus seizures** (seizures that last longer than 4 minutes), and **psychomotor seizures** (complex focal seizures)
3. Common antiepileptic medications are listed in Table 38–1
4. Administration considerations
   - **a.** Fosphenytoin should only be given IV for status epilepticus in emergency department or critical care area; monitor respiratory rate, BP, and ECG
   - **b.** Do not interchange chewable phenytoin products with capsules

Table 38–1 Antiepileptics

Type	Generic Names
Hydantoins	Fosphenytoin, phenytoin
Dicarbazepines	Carbamazepine, eslicarbazepine, oxcarbazepine
Succinimides	Ethosuximide, methsuximide
Benzodiazepines	Clobazam, clonazepam, clorazepate, diazepam, lorazepam
Barbiturates	Mephobarbital, phenobarbital, primidone
Miscellaneous	Ezogabine, felbamate, gabapentin, lacosamide, lamotrigine, levetiracetam, pregabalin, rufinamide, tiagabine, topiramate, valproic acid, vigabatrin, zonisamide

NCLEX® c. Phenytoin readily binds with protein, so do not give with gastric feedings, which inhibit uptake

d. Do not crush tablets or capsules of valproate sodium; take whole

e. Contraindicated with hypersensitivity, pregnancy, bradycardia, SA and AV node block, Stokes-Adams syndrome, hepatic failure

5. Side/adverse effects

NCLEX® a. Drowsiness, dizziness, insomnia, **paresthesias** (abnormal sensations), depression, suicidal tendencies, aggression, headache, confusion, slurred speech

NCLEX® b. **Nystagmus** (involuntary oscillation of eye), **diplopia** (double vision), blurred vision

NCLEX® c. Constipation, anorexia, N/V, weight loss, hepatitis, jaundice, **gingival hyperplasia** (increased growth of gum tissue)

d. Urine discoloration

e. Rash, hirsutism, lupus erythematosus, **Stevens-Johnson syndrome** (an acute inflammatory skin disorder)

f. Toxicity: bone marrow suppression (agranulocytosis, leukopenia, aplastic anemia, thrombocytopenia), N/V, ataxia, diplopia, cardiovascular collapse, slurred speech, confusion

6. Nursing considerations

NCLEX® a. Assess for seizure activity, including type, location, duration, and character; provide seizure precautions

b. Monitor cardiovascular status; monitor CBC with differential, platelet count, liver function tests, and calcium and magnesium levels

c. Assess respiratory status for depression, rate, depth, and character of respirations

NCLEX® d. Assess complete blood count (CBC) for blood dyscrasias; also assess for fever, sore throat, bruising, rash, and jaundice

e. Evaluate client for therapeutic responses such as decreases in severity and number of seizures or decreased ventricular dysrhythmias

f. Monitor blood glucose (BG) with diabetes; phenytoin can cause loss of glycemic control

NCLEX® g. Monitor results of serum drug levels to ensure they are in therapeutic range

Memory Aid

Therapeutic serum phenytoin level is 10–20 mg/dL. Memorize this value because it is an important one to know in practice and in test situations.

7. Client teaching

a. Carry Medic-Alert bracelet stating medication use

b. Urine may turn pink or red-brown but this is expected

NCLEX® c. Perform proper brushing of teeth with soft toothbrush and proper flossing to prevent gingival hyperplasia; maintain routine or more frequent dental exams

d. Do not change brands of medication once seizure activity has stabilized; bioavailability differs among formulations

B. Barbiturates

1. Decrease impulse transmission to cerebral cortex
2. Can be used in all forms of **epilepsy**, a chronic disorder characterized by recurring seizures; however, they have been largely replaced by newer drugs as first-line agents because of CNS depressant effects
3. Common medications are listed in Table 38–1

4. Administration considerations
   a. If prescribed by intramuscular (IM) route, inject into large muscle mass to prevent tissue sloughing; use less than 5 mL/site
   b. When prescribed IV, give slowly (after dilution) per product literature
5. Contraindicated with hypersensitivity, pregnancy, porphyria, and liver disease
6. Side/adverse effects
   NCLEX® a. Paradoxical excitement (older adults), drowsiness, lethargy, hangover headache, flushing, hallucinations
   b. Diarrhea, constipation, N/V
   c. Rash, urticaria, local pain or swelling or necrosis, Stevens-Johnson syndrome, angioedema, thrombophlebitis
7. Nursing considerations
   NCLEX® a. Assess mental status for changes in mood, sensorium, affect, and memory (long and short term)
   b. Assess for respiratory depression
   c. Assess for blood dyscrasias, fever, sore throat, bruising, rash, and jaundice
   NCLEX® d. Assess for seizure activity, including type, duration, and precipitating factors
   e. Obtain routine blood studies and liver function tests during long-term treatment
   f. Evaluate for therapeutic responses such as decreased seizures or increased sedation
8. Client teaching
   NCLEX® a. Avoid use of other CNS depressants; carry Medic-Alert bracelet stating medication use
   NCLEX® b. Avoid hazardous activities until stabilized on drug; drowsiness may occur
   c. Therapeutic effects may not be seen for 2–3 weeks

C. Succinimides

1. Inhibit spike and wave formation in absence seizures (petit mal), although recent research questions actual mechanism of action; may be used as one element of drug therapy for other types of seizures
2. Common medications are listed in Table 38–1
3. Administration considerations: give with food or milk to decrease GI symptoms; contraindicated with hypersensitivity
4. Side/adverse effects
   NCLEX® a. Drowsiness, dizziness, fatigue, euphoria, lethargy
   b. Anorexia, N/V, diarrhea, and abdominal pain
   NCLEX® c. Pink urine
   d. Urticaria, pruritic erythema, Stevens-Johnson syndrome
   e. Myopia, blurred vision
   NCLEX® f. Toxicity: bone marrow depression, ataxia, diplopia, and cardiovascular collapse
5. Nursing considerations
   a. Assess mental status for changes in mood, sensorium, affect, and behavior
   NCLEX® b. Monitor periodically renal studies (urinalysis, blood urea nitrogen [BUN], creatinine), CBC, and liver function test
   c. Assess for eye problems; may need regular ophthalmic exams
   d. Assess for allergic reactions such as red, raised rash or exfoliative dermatitis
   NCLEX® e. Assess for fever, sore throat, bruising, rash, or jaundice
6. Client teaching
   a. Carry ID card or Medic-Alert bracelet with medication, client's name, healthcare provider's name, and phone number
   NCLEX® b. Avoid driving and other activities that require alertness; avoid alcohol ingestion and other CNS depressants because they may increase sedation

D. Benzodiazepines

1. Enhance inhibitory neurotransmitter gamma-aminobutyric acid (GABA) to decrease anxiety and only as an adjunct for seizure activity
2. Used to treat delirium tremens; diazepam and lorazepam are used to treat status epilepticus; clonazepam and clorazepate are used for specific types of seizures when other drugs are not effective
3. Common medications are listed in Table 38–1
4. Administration considerations
   a. Give with food or milk to reduce GI symptoms; give IV injection into large vein
   NCLEX® b. Can lead to dependency; monitor client's use
5. Contraindicated with hypersensitivity, acute narrow-angle glaucoma or psychosis, children younger than 6 months, liver disease (clonazepam), or during lactation (diazepam)

6. Side/adverse effects
   NCLEX® a. Dizziness, drowsiness, confusion, headache, fatigue, blurred vision
   NCLEX® b. Orthostatic hypotension, ECG changes, tachycardia, respiratory depression
   c. Constipation, dry mouth, rash, itching, neutropenia
7. Nursing considerations
   NCLEX® a. Assess BP (lying, standing), pulse; if systolic BP drops 20 mmHg, withhold drug, notify healthcare provider because of orthostatic hypotension
   b. Assess hepatic and renal function (AST, ALT, bilirubin, creatinine, high-density lipoprotein), alkaline phosphatase
   c. Assess mental status for changes in mood, sensorium, affect, memory (long and short term)
   d. Assess respiratory status for depression, rate, rhythm, depth
   e. Assess for seizure activity, including type, duration, and precipitating factors
   f. Evaluate client for therapeutic responses such as reduced or absent seizure activity, anxiety

NCLEX® 8. Client teaching: avoid other CNS depressants, including alcohol; avoid hazardous activities until stabilized on drug; drowsiness may occur

E. Dicarbazepines and miscellaneous drugs

1. Dicarbazepines consist of carbamazepine, eslicarbazepine, and oxcarbamazepine (see Table 38–1)
   a. Inhibit nerve impulses by limiting influx of sodium ions across cell membrane in motor cortex; have other actions not explained by this mechamism, including analgesic, anticholinergic, antidysrhythmic, antidepressant, and sedative effects
   b. Used in tonic-clonic, complex-partial, and mixed seizures
   NCLEX® c. Give oral forms with food or milk to reduce GI symptoms
   d. When administered via NG tube, must be mixed with D_5W or NS and flushed with at least 100 mL solution afterward
   e. Contraindicated with hypersensitivity to carbamazepine or tricyclic antidepressants (TCAs), bone marrow depression, and concurrent use of MAOIs
   NCLEX® f. Side/adverse effects are many and include drowsiness, dizziness, confusion, N/V, constipation, diarrhea, tinnitis, dry mouth, blurred vision, nystagmus, thrombocytopenia, agranulocytosis, neutropenia, paralysis, worsening of seizures, Stevens-Johnson syndrome, and possible fatal reaction with MAOIs
   g. Assess for seizure activity, including type, duration, and precipitating factors
   h. Monitor blood, hepatic, and renal studies
   i. Assess mental status for changes in mood, sensorium, affect, and memory (long and short term)
   NCLEX® j. Assess for eye problems; may need regular ophthalmic exams
   NCLEX® k. Assess for blood dyscrasias, fever, sore throat, bruising, rash, or jaundice
   l. Evaluate client for therapeutic response such as decreased or absent seizure activity
   NCLEX® m. Instruct client to avoid other CNS depressants and activities that cause additive drowsiness
   n. Inform client that urine may turn pink to brown
2. Miscellaneous drugs
   a. Act in a variety of ways but all reduce or eliminate seizure activity
   b. Side/adverse effects depend on specific drug but may include dizziness, drowsiness, lightheadedness, confusion, agitation, tachycardia or palpitations, blurred vision, dry mouth, difficulty concentrating, memory impairment, and possible suicidal ideation
   c. Assess for seizure activity, including type, duration, and precipitating factors
   d. Monitor complete blood count and liver and renal function studies
   e. Monitor VS, mental status, coordination, and balance periodically; older adults are at increased risk for falls because of drug side effects
   NCLEX® f. Teach client to avoid use of alcohol and other CNS depressants while taking antiepileptic drugs
   NCLEX® g. Teach client to avoid abrupt discontinuation of antiepileptic drugs, which would lead to return of seizure activity and possible status epilepticus

III. CENTRAL NERVOUS SYSTEM (CNS) STIMULANTS

A. Anorexiants

1. Most act similarly to amphetamines, as indirect sympathomimetic amines with alpha- and beta-adrenergic activity
2. Used for **narcolepsy** (inability to stay awake during day), **attention-deficit disorder** (ADD), **attention-deficit/hyperactivity disorder** (ADHD), and as short-term adjunct for weight loss to control obesity
3. Common CNS stimulant medications are listed in Table 38–2

Table 38–2 CNS Stimulants and Other Drugs for Narcolepsy and Attention-Deficit/Hyperactivity Disorder (ADHD)

Type	Generic (Trade) Names	Use
Amphetamines and amphetamine-like drugs	Diethylpropion	Weight loss
	Amphetamine/dextro-amphetamine	Narcolepsy, weight loss
	Methylphenidate	Narcolepsy, ADHD
	Dexmethylphenidate	ADHD
	Dextroamphetamine	Narcolepsy, ADHD
	Lisdexamphetamine	ADHD
Nonstimulants	Atomoxetine	ADHD
	Clonidine	ADHD
	Guanfacine	ADHD
Other drugs for narcolepsy	Armadafinil	Narcolepsy
	Modafinil	Narcolepsy
	Sodium oxybate	Narcolepsy

4. Administration considerations
   NCLEX®
   a. Anorexiant effects are temporary
   b. To avoid insomnia, take 6 hours prior to bedtime
   c. Do not abruptly discontinue medication

NCLEX®
5. Contraindicated with hypersensitivity, angle-closure glaucoma, advanced cardiac disease, hyperthyroidism, agitated states, history of drug abuse, and children under 12 years
6. Side/adverse effects
   a. Restlessness, insomnia, decrease in seizure threshold in epilepsy
   b. Palpitations and tachycardia
   c. Dysmenorrhea

NCLEX®
7. Nursing considerations
   a. Assess BP and pulse during treatment
   b. Current dosage of antihypertensive and antidiabetic agents may need to be adjusted
   c. Evaluate client for therapeutic response such as decrease in weight over time
8. Client teaching
   a. Discuss all current medications (including OTC) with prescriber; serious or fatal interactions can occur
   b. Avoid driving or other hazardous activities until drug effect is determined

B. Amphetamines

1. Increase release of norepinephrine and dopamine in cerebral cortex to reticular activating system
2. Used in treating narcolepsy, exogenous obesity, ADD
3. Common medications are listed in Table 38–2
4. Administration considerations
   NCLEX®
   a. Give first dose on awakening and last dose no closer than 6 hours before bedtime
   b. Administer on empty stomach 30–60 minutes before meal
5. Contraindicated with hypersensitivity, hyperthyroidism, hypertension, glaucoma, severe arteriosclerosis, drug abuse, cardiovascular disease, anxiety, and lactation

NCLEX®
6. Side/adverse effects
   a. Hyperactivity, insomnia, restlessness, talkativeness
   b. Dry mouth, N/V, impotence, change in libido, palpitations, tachycardia
7. Nursing considerations
   NCLEX®
   a. Assess VS, especially BP, since anorexiants may reverse antihypertensive medication action
   b. Monitor CBC, urinalysis, and in diabetics, BG; changes in insulin may be required
   c. Assess mental status for mood, sensorium, and affect; stimulation, insomnia, or aggressiveness may occur
   d. Assess for withdrawal symptoms: headache, N/V, muscle pain, weakness
   NCLEX®
   e. Evaluate client for therapeutic responses such as decreased activity in ADHD, absence of sleeping during day in narcolepsy, decrease in weight
8. Client teaching
   a. Understand the importance of rest
   NCLEX®
   b. Avoid or decrease caffeine intake (coffee, tea, cola, chocolate); these substances may increase irritability or stimulation

C. Medications to treat narcolepsy and ADHD

1. Affect norepinephrine and dopamine have varying mechanisms of action to exert intended effects
NCLEX® 2. Administer medication at least 6 hours before bedtime
3. Common medications are listed in Table 38–2
4. Many are contraindicated with hypersensitivity, anxiety, history of Tourette's syndrome, children under 6 years, and glaucoma
5. Increased stimulation and increased amine effect occurs with caffeine
NCLEX® 6. Side/adverse effects vary but commonly include irritability, headache, dizziness, drowsiness, insomnia, nausea
7. Nursing considerations
    a. Assess VS, especially BP, since reversal of antihypertensive drug effects may occur
    b. Monitor CBC, urinalysis, and in diabetics, monitor BG closely; changes in insulin may be required
    c. Assess mental status for changes in mood, sensorium, and affect; stimulation, insomnia, and aggressiveness may occur
    d. Assess for withdrawal symptoms: headache, N/V, muscle pain, weakness
    NCLEX® e. Assess client for changes in appetite, sleep, speech patterns
    NCLEX® f. Assess client for increased attention span and decreased hyperactivity
    g. Evaluate client for therapeutic responses such as decreased activity in ADHD, absence of sleeping during day in narcolepsy, or decrease in weight
NCLEX® 8. Client education
    a. Avoid or decrease caffeine intake (coffee, tea, cola, chocolate); may increase irritability or stimulation

Memory Aid

Foods or beverages containing caffeine or theobromine (coffee, tea, cola, chocolate), which are CNS stimulants, are often contraindicated with medications that affect the CNS.

    b. Avoid hazardous activities until stabilized on drug; drowsiness may occur
    c. Seizure threshold is decreased in clients with seizure disorders

IV. ANTIPARKINSONIAN MEDICATIONS

A. Anticholinergics

1. Block or compete at central acetylcholine receptor sites in autonomic nervous system (ANS)
2. Used to decrease involuntary movements in parkinsonism
3. Common medications for Parkinson's are listed in Table 38–3
4. Administration considerations
    a. Parenteral dose of benztropine is given slowly; keep client at rest at least 1 hour after administering medication and monitor VS
    NCLEX® b. Monitor drug dosage carefully; even slight overdose can lead to toxicity
5. Contraindicated for clients with narrow-angle glaucoma, myasthenia gravis, or GI obstruction
6. Side/adverse effects: dry mouth, constipation, paralytic ileus, urinary retention or hesitancy, headache, or dizziness
NCLEX® 7. Nursing considerations
    a. Monitor intake and output (I&O); retention may cause decreased urine output; assess for urinary hesitancy and retention; palpate bladder if retention occurs
    b. Assess for constipation; increase fluids, bulk, and exercise to counteract this

Table 38–3 Medications Used to Treat Parkinson's Disease

Type	Generic (Trade) Names
Anticholinergics	Benztropine mesylate, biperiden hydrochloride, trihexyphenidyl hydrochloride
Dopamine replacement drugs	Levodopa/carbidopa, levodopa
Dopamine agonists	Apomorphine, bromocriptine, pramipexole, ropinirole, rotigotine
COMT inhibitors	Entacapone, tolcapone
Monoamine oxidase-B inhibitors	Rasagiline, seligeline
Miscellaneous drugs	Amantadine

c. If tolerance occurs during long-term therapy, dose may need to be increased or changed
d. Assess mental status for affect, mood, CNS depression, worsening of mental symptoms during early therapy
e. Evaluate client for therapeutic responses such as decreased tremors, secretions, absence of N/V

NCLEX® 8. Client education: avoid driving, other hazardous activities, or use of OTC cough and preparations with alcohol or antihistamines; drowsiness may occur

B. Medications affecting amount of dopamine in brain

1. Include levodopa, dopamine agonists, amantadine, and MAO type B inhibitors (see Table 38–3)
   a. L-dopa is the immediate, natural precursor of dopamine; replacement therapy with levodopa is most effective therapy for treating Parkinson's disease
   b. Catecholamine O-methyl transferase (COMT) inhibitors prevent destruction of levodopa in peripheral tissues, with same side effects as levodopa
   c. Amantadine (an antiviral) promotes the synthesis and release of dopamine
   d. Dopamine agonists (DA) directly stimulate specific subclasses of dopamine receptors
   e. MAO type B inhibitors (MAOBIs) increase dopamine activity by an incompletely understood mechanism
   NCLEX® f. DAs and MAOBIs are used to enhance the effects of L-dopa
   g. All increase availability of dopamine, which reduces symptoms of Parkinson's disease
2. NCLEX® Administration considerations
   a. Administer dose after meals for better absorption and to decrease GI symptoms
   b. Give levodopa and selegiline with a low-protein snack or meal
3. Contraindicated with hypersensitivity, narrow-angle glaucoma, and undiagnosed skin lesions
4. Significant food interactions
   a. Decreased levodopa and selegiline absorption with high-protein foods
   NCLEX® b. With selegiline, tyramine-containing foods may increase hypertensive reactions
5. Side/adverse effects
   a. Dry mouth, N/V, and constipation
   b. Dizziness, headache, depression, and cough
   c. Cardiac dysrhythmias and orthostatic hypotension
   NCLEX® d. Sleep disturbance, "on–off" phenomenon
   NCLEX® e. Amantadine: seizures, congestive heart failure (CHF), leukopenia
   f. Levodopa: hemolytic anemia, leukopenia, agranulocytosis
   g. DAs: seizures, shock
   h. MAOBIs: tachycardia or sinus bradycardia
   NCLEX® i. Levodopa toxicity: mental or personality changes, increased twitching, grimacing, tongue protrusion
6. Nursing considerations
   a. Assess BP and respirations
   b. Assess mental status for affect, mood, behavioral changes, depression; complete a suicide assessment
   NCLEX® c. Monitor for involuntary movement, akinesia, tremors, staggering gait, muscle rigidity, and drooling
   NCLEX® d. Evaluate for therapeutic responses such as decreased akathisia and increased mood
7. Client education
   NCLEX® a. Change positions slowly to prevent orthostatic hypotension
   b. Report side effects such as twitching and eye spasm; may indicate overdose
   NCLEX® c. Never discontinue drugs abruptly because this may precipitate parkinsonian crisis
   NCLEX® d. Do not take medication with foods high in protein

V. MEDICATIONS TO TREAT ALZHEIMER'S DISEASE

A. Action and use: reversible cholinesterase inhibitors raise acetylcholine level in cerebral cortex by slowing degradation of acetylcholine released in cholinergic neurons; memantine is an N-methyl-O-aspartate receptor antagonist

B. Common medications for Alzheimer's are listed in Box 38–4

Box 38–4

Medications Used to Treat Alzheimer's Disease

- Donepezil
- Galantamine
- Memantine
- Rivastigmine

C. Administration considerations

NCLEX® 1. Administer dose between meals; may give with meal to reduce GI symptoms
2. Adjust dosage to response no more frequently than every 6 weeks

D. Contraindications: hypersensitivity to drug or development of jaundice when taking drug

E. Side/adverse effects

NCLEX® 1. Insomnia, headache, dizziness, confusion, ataxia, anxiety, depression, hostility, and abnormal thinking
2. Constipation, diarrhea, N/V, and abdominal pain
3. Urinary frequency and incontinence
4. Rhinitis or cough; rash; seizures or hepatotoxicity

F. Nursing considerations

NCLEX® 1. Assess BP for hypotension or hypertension
2. Assess mental status for affect, mood, behavioral changes, depression, hallucinations, confusion; complete a suicide assessment
3. Assess GI status for side effects; monitor liver function test results
4. Assess client for urinary frequency and incontinence
5. Evaluate for therapeutic responses such as decreased confusion, improved mood

G. Client teaching

NCLEX® 1. Report side effects such as twitching, nausea, vomiting, sweating; they might indicate overdose
2. Dose may be taken with food to decrease GI upset
NCLEX® 3. Medication is not a cure; it only relieves symptoms

VI. MEDICATIONS TO TREAT MYASTHENIA GRAVIS (MG)

A. Actions and use

1. Inhibit breakdown of acetylcholine (Ach) at myoneural junction via acetylcholinesterase (AchE); used to treat muscle weakness associated with MG
NCLEX® 2. Edrophonium is used to diagnose MG
3. As symptoms worsen over time, AchE inhibitors alone may not be effective and corticosteroids may be added (for immunosuppressant effect)

B. Common medications for myasthenia gravis are listed in Box 38–5

C. Administration considerations

1. Administer prior to mealtimes for optimal absorption
NCLEX® 2. Administer doses on time to prevent muscle weakness from impairing ability to chew food and swallow medications

NCLEX® **D. Use of edrophonium (Tensilon) as diagnostic aid**

1. Aids in diagnosis of MG in an undiagnosed client or myasthenic crisis (undermedication) in a diagnosed client; positive findings noted when muscle tone improves within 30–60 seconds following IV dose, and improved muscle strength lasts 4–5 minutes (positive Tensilon test)
2. Diagnosis of cholinergic crisis (often caused by overmedication) in a diagnosed client is made when muscle strength does not improve after edrophonium injection, and symptoms may worsen (negative Tensilon test)

E. Contraindications: bowel obstruction or other conditions with GI motility, or urinary tract obstruction

NCLEX® **F. Side/adverse effects**

1. Increased bronchial secretions, sweating, drooling, and urge to urinate
2. Pinpoint pupils and eye watering, N/V, diarrhea

G. Nursing considerations

NCLEX® 1. Keep atropine sulfate available as antidote
NCLEX® 2. Keep equipment for respiratory support on hand; muscles of head, neck, and respiratory system are affected before muscles in the lower body
3. Observe client for weakness; if it begins 1 hour after drug dose, overdose or cholinergic crisis may be occurring; if it begins 3 or more hours after dose, myasthenic crisis (undermedication) may be occurring

Box 38–5

Medications Used to Treat Myasthenia Gravis

- Edrophonium
- Neostigmine
- Pyridostigmine
- Ambenonium

NCLEX® 4. Observe for subtle changes in speech and facial expression, ptosis, and decreased ability to swallow as indicators that additional medication is needed
5. Assess general neuromuscular strength, including gait and reflexes
6. Monitor VS, especially respirations, pulse, and BP

H. Client teaching

1. Report side effects such as twitching, N/V, sweating; they might indicate overdose
2. Do not increase or abruptly decrease dose; serious consequences may result
3. NCLEX® Medication is not a cure; it only relieves symptoms

VII. SKELETAL MUSCLE RELAXANTS

A. Direct-acting skeletal muscle relaxants are often used to treat *spasticity* in conjunction with physical therapy; dantrolene is only drug in its class used for this purpose; others are botulinum type A and B for cervical dystonia and type A only for wrinkles

1. Decrease synaptic responses at neurotransmitters to decrease frequency, severity of **spasms** (involuntary contractions of large muscles) and pain in musculoskeletal conditions
2. Reduce spasticity after spinal cord injury, stroke, and in cerebral palsy, multiple sclerosis; dantrolene is also used to treat malignant hyperthermia
3. Commonly used direct-acting drug is dantrolene, although centrally acting drugs are also effective in treating spasticity (see Box 38–6)
4. Contraindicated in hypersensitivity and active hepatic disease, and should be used cautiously with impaired respiratory and cardiac function
5. Side/adverse effects
   a. Dizziness, weakness, fatigue, drowsiness
   b. Photosensitivity, tachycardia and erratic BP, urinary retention
   c. Hepatotoxicity
6. Nursing considerations
   a. NCLEX® Monitor BP, weight, and hepatic function
   b. Monitor I&O; check for urinary retention or hesitancy
   c. Monitor for severe weakness or numbness in extremities
   d. NCLEX® Monitor for CNS depression, dizziness, drowsiness, or psychiatric symptoms
   e. Monitor results of liver and renal function studies
   f. NCLEX® Evaluate for therapeutic responses such as decreased pain or spasticity
7. NCLEX® Client teaching
   a. Do not discontinue medication quickly; spasticity, tachycardia will occur; it should be tapered off gradually by prescriber
   b. Notify prescriber of abdominal pain, jaundiced sclera, clay-colored stools, or change in color of urine
   c. Do not break, crush, or chew capsules

B. Centrally acting skeletal muscle relaxants are often used to treat muscle spasms associated with inflammation and injury

1. Depress multisynaptic pathways in spinal cord, causing skeletal muscle relaxation and/or sedation; have no effect on neuromuscular junction or muscle tissue
2. Used for adjunct relief of spasms in acute musculoskeletal conditions not associated with CNS disease
3. Common medications are listed in Box 38–6
4. NCLEX® Contraindicated in hypersensitivity, children under age 12, intermittent porphyria, and use cautiously in thyroid disease and cardiac disease including myocardial infarction (MI), heart block, and CHF
5. Side/adverse effects
   a. NCLEX® Dizziness, weakness, drowsiness, xerostomia

Box 38–6

Skeletal Muscle Relaxants

Direct-Acting Skeletal Muscle Relaxant

Dantrolene sodium

Centrally Acting Skeletal Muscle Relaxants

Baclofen
Carisoprodol
Chlorzoxazone
Cyclobenzaprine
Metaxalone
Methocarbamol
Orphenadrine
Tizanidine

b. Edema of tongue and face with sweating, myalgia
c. Unpleasant taste, coated tongue with discoloration, vomiting, anorexia, diarrhea with flatulence
d. Angioedema, anaphylaxis
e. Orthostatic hypotension, tachycardia, syncope, palpitations, vasodilation

6. Nursing considerations
a. Periodically monitor results of blood studies (including CBC, WBC with differentials) and liver studies (including AST, ALT, alkaline phosphatase)
b. Monitor results of EEG in clients with seizures
NCLEX® **c.** Assess for allergic reactions, including idiosyncratic reaction, anaphylaxis, rash, fever, and respiratory distress
d. Assess for severe weakness or numbness in extremities
NCLEX® **e.** Assess for CNS depression, dizziness, drowsiness, and psychiatric symptoms
f. Evaluate for therapeutic responses such as decreased pain, spasm, and spasticity

NCLEX® **7.** Client teaching
a. Do not discontinue medication abruptly; insomnia, nausea, headache, spasticity, tachycardia will occur
b. Avoid hazardous activities if drowsiness or dizziness occurs

Check Your NCLEX–RN® Exam I.Q.

You are ready for testing on this content if you can:

- Apply knowledge of expected actions and effects of neurologic and musculoskeletal medications to client care.
- Correctly administer neurologic and musculoskeletal medications to clients.
- Assess for side effects and adverse effects of neurologic and musculoskeletal medications.
- Take appropriate action if a client has an unexpected response to a neurologic or musculoskeletal medication.
- Monitor a client for expected outcomes or effects of treatment with neurologic and musculoskeletal medications.

PRACTICE TEST

1 A client is receiving oxcarbazepine to control seizures. What statement by the client to the nurse indicates an understanding regarding administration of this medication?

1. "I need to take an additional dose when I am having a stressful day."
2. "I will be able to stop taking this medicine in about a year."
3. "I will probably need to take this medicine all my life."
4. "I will never have another seizure if I take this medicine."

2 A client with a history of seizures is admitted with a partial occlusion of the left common carotid artery. The client has taken carbamazepine for 10 years. What is the most important nursing consideration when planning care for this client?

1. Obtain a history of seizure incidence.
2. Place an airway, suction, and restraints at the bedside.
3. Ask the client to remove any dentures.
4. Observe the client for increased restlessness and agitation.

3 A client with a history of seizures is scheduled for an arteriogram at 10:00 A.M. and is to have nothing by mouth before the test. The client is scheduled to receive a daily prescribed dose of phenytoin at 9:00 A.M. What action should the nurse take regarding this situation?

1. Omit the 9:00 A.M. dose.
2. Give the same dosage of the drug rectally.
3. Ask the prescriber if the drug can be given IV.
4. Administer the drug with 30 mL of water at 9:00 A.M.

4 The nurse is assessing a client with Parkinson's disease to determine effectiveness of medication therapy. The nurse would determine that the medication is not working optimally if the client is demonstrating which characteristic?

1. A flattened affect
2. Tonic-clonic seizures
3. Decreased intelligence
4. Changes in pain tolerance

5 The client with Parkinson's disease asks the nurse, "How will levodopa treat this disease?" What action of levodopa should the nurse incorporate into a response?

1. Improves myelination of neurons
2. Increases acetylcholine production
3. Replaces dopamine in the brain cells
4. Causes regeneration of injured thalamic cells

6 A female client who takes medications for seizures has been placed on warfarin for thrombophlebitis. After the weekly prothrombin time, the client mentions that she is out of her barbiturate sleeping pill and needs a refill. What is the most important reason that the nurse should instruct the client to obtain the refill immediately?

1. The client is at risk of developing withdrawal symptoms.
2. The absence of sleep could precipitate seizures.
3. Discontinuation of the drug can affect the prothrombin level.
4. Seizure control depends on the combined action of the medications.

7 A client is brought to the emergency department in the midst of a persistent tonic-clonic seizure. Diazepam is administered intravenously. The nurse anticipates that in addition to decreasing central neuronal activity, what other effect of diazepam will occur?

1. Slowing of cardiac contractions
2. Relaxation of peripheral muscles
3. Dilation of tracheobronchial structures
4. Promoting amnesia of the seizure episode

8 The nurse would assess for which symptoms of morphine overdose in a client receiving patient-controlled analgesia? Select all that apply.

1. A decrease in blood pressure and respiration rate
2. Dilated pupils and restlessness
3. Profuse sweating and a state of deep sleep
4. Constricted pupils and sedation
5. Lethargy and depressed reflexes

9 Levodopa is prescribed for a client with Parkinson's disease. What information should the nurse include in the teaching plan for the client about levodopa?

1. It is poorly absorbed if given with meals.
2. It must be monitored by weekly laboratory tests.
3. It causes an initial euphoria, followed by depression.
4. It can cause a side effect of orthostatic hypotension.

10 When caring for the client who is receiving phenytoin, the nurse emphasizes meticulous oral hygiene to the client. This nursing intervention is based on the nurse's knowledge that phenytoin has what effect on oral tissue?

1. It causes hyperplasia of the gums.
2. It increases alkalinity of the oral secretions.
3. It erodes and destroys tooth enamel.
4. It promotes bacterial growth at the gum lines.

11 The healthcare provider prescribes phenobarbital sodium for a client who has had a tonic-clonic seizure. What statement indicates to the nurse that the client understands the side effects of phenobarbital? Select all that apply.

1. "I can expect a loss of appetite or persistent fatigue."
2. "I might feel lightheaded or off balance."
3. "Diarrhea accompanied by an anal itch is common."
4. "Decreased tolerance to common foods can occur."
5. "I should be aware of becoming depressed."

12 The nurse administering methylphenidate is monitoring the client for side effects associated with this medication. Which assessment finding would the nurse disregard as unrelated to this medication?

1. Insomnia
2. Fever
3. Rash
4. Palpitations

13 The healthcare provider prescribes fosphenytoin for a client to control tonic-clonic seizures. The nurse explains in simple terms to the client that which expected effect may occur with use of the drug?

1. An antispasmodic action on the muscles
2. Prevention of central nervous system depression
3. Control of nerve impulses originating in motor cortex
4. Altered permeability of cell membranes to potassium

14 The nurse is providing medication information to a client taking benztropine for Parkinson's disease. Which subsequent client statement indicates the need for additional instruction?

1. "I may crush the tablets to make them easier to take."
2. "I should not drive until I know how this medication will affect me."
3. "I can take OTC medications for a cough or cold."
4. "I should never discontinue the medication abruptly."

15 The nurse is providing discharge instructions to a client with Alzheimer's disease and his family. Based on the knowledge that the prescribed medication therapy will not reverse Alzheimer symptoms, what should be included in this discussion?

1. Keep the client in his own home, regardless of circumstances.
2. Provide supervision to protect client from being injured or lost.
3. Encourage the client to interview potential homecare agencies.
4. Postpone the use of adaptive-assistive equipment as long as possible.

16 The nurse prioritizes which problem to be of greatest concern for the client newly diagnosed with Alzheimer's disease who is just beginning medication therapy?

1. Possible altered fluid and electrolyte balance
2. Generalized discomfort
3. Interruption in normal sleep patterns
4. Disturbances in thought processes

17 The nurse should include which items in an assessment of the client with Alzheimer's disease who is receiving rivastigmine?

1. Blood pressure (BP), mental status, and gastrointestinal (GI) status
2. Hemoglobin (Hgb), white blood cells (WBCs), and liver function tests
3. Hgb, red blood cells (RBCs), and mental status
4. BP, electrolytes, and edema in legs

18 A client's healthcare provider has prescribed amitriptyline as prophylaxis for migraine headaches. The nurse should warn the client about which over-the-counter (OTC) medication that might intensify the actions of amitriptyline?

1. Acetaminophen
2. Aspirin
3. Naproxen
4. Cimetidine

19 When administering anticholinergic medications for Parkinson's disease, what assessment finding should be of least concern to the nurse in regard to the medication?

1. Dry mouth
2. Constipation
3. Fever
4. Urinary retention or hesitancy

20 The client receiving phenytoin asks the nurse why the healthcare provider has prescribed folic acid with this medication. The nurse's response would be based on which item of information?

1. Phenytoin improves absorption of iron from foods.
2. Folic acid content in common foods is inadequate.
3. Folic acid prevents the neuropathy caused by phenytoin.
4. Phenytoin inhibits the absorption of folic acid from foods.

ANSWERS & RATIONALES

1 **Answer: 3 Rationale:** Clients with seizure disorders are rarely able to stop taking the anticonvulsants. Extra doses of oxcarbazepine are not taken in response to real or anticipated stress. There is no indication in this question whether medication therapy could be terminated near the 1-year mark. The goal of taking oxcarbazepine is to eliminate and/or control seizure activity; the use of the word never indicates a lack of understanding. **Cognitive Level:** Analyzing **Client Need:** Pharmacological and Parenteral Therapies **Integrated Process:** Nursing Process: Evaluation **Content Area:** Pharmacology **Strategy:** The wording of the question tells you that the correct answer is also a true statement. Use the process of elimination and medication knowledge to make a selection. Avoid selecting options that contain definitive terms such as *never*.

2 **Answer: 1 Rationale:** Carbamazepine is an antiepileptic drug that is effective in controlling seizures. Data collection before planning nursing care for a client with a seizure disorder should always include a history of seizure incidence. Putting an airway in place or restraining a client during a seizure could cause physical harm. Removal of dentures might be indicated during a seizure, but not at this time. Restlessness and agitation might be a prodromal phase in some clients, but a history of incidence is more important data. **Cognitive Level:** Analyzing **Client Need:** Pharmacological and Parenteral Therapies **Integrated Process:** Nursing Process: Planning **Content Area:** Pharmacology **Strategy:** The words *most important* in the stem of the question tell you that more than one or perhaps all options might be correct and that you must choose the best option. Use medication knowledge as well as knowledge of how to manage a client during a seizure to eliminate any of the incorrect options.

3 **Answer: 3 Rationale:** The therapeutic blood levels of the antiepileptic need to be maintained. The nurse should question the prescriber about alternate routes of administration. Omission of a dose is not prudent; the nurse should contact the prescriber. Changing the route of medication is not appropriate without a prescription. Administering the drug is a violation of the prescription related to the client's test; the prescriber should be contacted for alternative orders. **Cognitive Level:** Applying **Client Need:** Pharmacological and Parenteral Therapies **Integrated Process:** Nursing Process: Implementation **Content Area:** Pharmacology **Strategy:** The core issue of the question is how to maintain the client in a seizure-free state while NPO. Analyze each of the options to determine the method that will best protect the client from seizure activity and not violate the principles of medication administration.

4 **Answer: 1 Rationale:** Destruction of the neurons of the basal ganglia in Parkinson's disease results in decreased muscle tone. This gives the face a mask-like appearance, and causes a monotone speech pattern that can be interpreted as flat. If medication therapy was ineffective, the client would still exhibit symptoms of the disorder, such as flattened affect. Tonic-clonic seizures and decreased intelligence are not a common manifestation of Parkinson's disease. Clients with Parkinson's do not experience changes in their ability to tolerate pain. **Cognitive Level:** Applying **Client Need:** Pharmacological and Parenteral Therapies **Integrated Process:** Nursing Process: Assessment **Content Area:** Pharmacology **Strategy:** The core issue of the question is the symptom that should be abolished by medication therapy. Use medication knowledge and the process of elimination to make a selection.

5 **Answer: 3 Rationale:** Levodopa is the precursor of dopamine. It is converted to dopamine in the brain cells until needed as a neurotransmitter. Improvement in myelination of the neurons, increase in acetylcholine production, and regeneration of injured thalamic cells cannot be attributed to levodopa. **Cognitive Level:** Applying **Client Need:** Pharmacological and Parenteral Therapies **Integrated Process:** Communication and Documentation **Content Area:** Pharmacology **Strategy:** The wording of the question tells you that the correct option is also a true statement. Use medication knowledge and the process of elimination to make a selection.

6 **Answer: 3 Rationale:** Barbiturates decrease the body's response to warfarin. As a result, there is less suppression of prothrombin; when inhibition caused by barbiturates disappears, hemorrhage could result. Withdrawal symptoms are not a priority concern if the client just takes the barbiturate for sleep. Absence of sleep is not likely to result in seizure activity. Control of seizure activity is not dependent on combined use of phenytoin and the barbiturate sleep aid. **Cognitive Level:** Analyzing **Client Need:** Pharmacological and Parenteral Therapies **Integrated Process:** Nursing Process: Implementation **Content Area:** Pharmacology **Strategy:** The words *most important* in the stem of the question tell you that more than one or perhaps all options might be partially or totally correct, and that you must choose the most important option. The core issue of the question is knowledge of the interactive effects of barbiturates and warfarin.

7 **Answer: 2 Rationale:** Diazepam is a benzodiazepene tranquilizer and an anticonvulsant used to relax smooth muscles during seizures. Diazepam does not slow cardiac contractions. Diazepam does not dilate tracheobronchial structures. Diazepam does not promote amnesia of seizure activity. **Cognitive Level:** Applying **Client Need:** Pharmacological and Parenteral Therapies **Integrated Process:** Nursing Process: Diagnosis **Content Area:** Pharmacology **Strategy:** The wording of the question tells you that the correct option is also a true effect of the medication. Use medication knowledge and the process of elimination to make a selection.

8 **Answer: 1, 4, 5 Rationale:** Morphine could lower blood pressure; its major adverse effect is respiratory depression. Morphine can cause pupillary constriction and sedation. Morphine can lead to lethargy and depressed reflexes. Morphine can lead to lethargy and pupillary constriction. Morphine does not produce profuse sweating; the state of sedation caused by morphine should not be confused with deep sleep. **Cognitive Level:** Analyzing **Client Need:** Pharmacological and Parenteral Therapies **Integrated Process:** Nursing Process: Evaluation **Content Area:** Pharmacology **Strategy:** Use specific medication knowledge and the process of elimination to make a selection. When there is more than one correct answer, consider each option as a true/false statement.

9 **Answer: 4 Rationale:** Levodopa is the precursor of dopamine. It reduces sympathetic outflow by limiting vasoconstriction, which can result in orthostatic hypotension. Levodopa should be administered with food to minimize gastric irritation. Levodopa is not monitored by weekly laboratory tests. Levodopa does not cause initial euphoria followed by depression. **Cognitive Level:** Applying **Client Need:** Pharmacological and Parenteral Therapies **Integrated Process:** Nursing Process: Planning **Content Area:** Pharmacology **Strategy:** The wording of the question tells you that the correct option is also a true statement that would be included in client teaching. Use medication knowledge and the process of elimination to make a selection.

10 **Answer: 1 Rationale:** Gingival hyperplasia (overgrowth of gum tissue) is an adverse effect of long-term phenytoin therapy. Phenytoin does not increase alkalinity of oral secretions, erode or destroy tooth enamel, or promote bacterial growth at the gum line. **Cognitive Level:** Applying **Client Need:** Pharmacological and Parenteral Therapies **Integrated Process:** Nursing Process: Implementation **Content Area:** Pharmacology **Strategy:** The wording of the question tells you that the correct option is also a true statement that would be included in client teaching. Use medication knowledge and the process of elimination to make a selection.

11 **Answer: 1, 2, 5 Rationale:** Phenobarbital depresses the CNS, particularly the motor cortex, producing side effects such as lethargy, loss of appetite, and vertigo. It also depresses the CNS, particularly the motor cortex, producing side effects such as depression. Phenobarbital does not cause diarrhea or anal itching, nor does it cause a decreased tolerance to common foods or constipation. **Cognitive Level:** Applying **Client Need:** Pharmacological and Parenteral Therapies **Integrated Process:** Nursing Process: Evaluation **Content Area:** Pharmacology **Strategy:** Use medication knowledge and the process of elimination to make a selection. When there is more than one correct answer, consider each option as a true/false statement.

12 **Answer: 2 Rationale:** Fever is not a side effect of methylphenidate. Insomnia, rash, and palpitations are possible side effects of methylphenidate. **Cognitive Level:** Applying **Client Need:** Pharmacological and Parenteral Therapies **Integrated Process:** Nursing Process: Assessment **Content Area:** Pharmacology **Strategy:** Note that the stem of the question contains the word *not*, which indicates that the correct option is not an actual manifestation of the drug. Use knowledge of side/adverse medication effects to make a selection.

13 **Answer: 3 Rationale:** The primary action of fosphenytoin is to reduce voltage, frequency, and spread of electrical discharges within the motor cortex, resulting in inhibition of seizure activity. Fosphenytoin does not prevent central nervous system depression, control nerve impulses originating in the motor cortex, or cause altered permeability of cell membranes to potassium. **Cognitive Level:** Applying **Client Need:** Pharmacological and Parenteral Therapies **Integrated Process:** Teaching and Learning **Content Area:** Pharmacology **Strategy:** Use medication knowledge and the process of elimination to make a selection.

14 **Answer: 3 Rationale:** Many OTC cough and cold medications contain alcohol; medications with alcohol (another CNS depressant) should be avoided unless specifically directed by the provider. Benztropine may be crushed before administering the medication. Benztropine is a CNS depressant and the client should avoid activities such as driving until the effects of the medication are known. Benztropine should not be discontinued abruptly; it may precipitate a parkinsonian crisis. **Cognitive Level:** Analyzing **Client Need:** Pharmacological and Parenteral Therapies **Integrated Process:** Teaching and Learning **Content Area:** Pharmacology **Strategy:** Note that the question contains the words *more instruction*, which indicates that the correct answer option contains incorrect information. Use medication knowledge and the process of elimination to make a selection.

15 **Answer: 2 Rationale:** The client with Alzheimer's disease and his or her family will need much support. Medication therapy will delay progression of symptoms, but will not affect a cure. The primary concern is for the safety of the client, so constant supervision is necessary. The primary concern is for the safety of the client, so the family should be aware of behaviors that indicate the client cannot remain in his own home. Medication therapy will delay progression of symptoms, but will not affect a cure. The client may not have the cognitive ability to perform the interview process for hiring a homecare agency. The primary concern is for the safety of the client; the use of appropriate assistive devices can prevent client injuries. **Cognitive Level:** Applying **Client Need:** Pharmacological and Parenteral Therapies **Integrated Process:** Teaching and Learning **Content Area:** Pharmacology **Strategy:** The wording of the question tells you that the correct answer is an option that is a priority teaching measure. To make your selection, recall the nature of the disorder and that medication therapy will not reverse symptoms.

16 **Answer: 4 Rationale:** The disturbance in thought processes is the primary concern related to the client's status. Effective medication therapy will reduce the progression of symptoms of the dementia. Altered fluid and electrolyte status is not of concern. Generalized discomfort is not applicable given the information in the question. A disturbance in sleep pattern could become important later, but initially, the alteration in thought process is most significant. **Cognitive Level:** Analyzing **Client Need:** Pharmacological and Parenteral Therapies **Integrated Process:** Nursing Process: Diagnosis **Content Area:** Pharmacology **Strategy:** Note the key words *most important* in the stem of the question, which tells you that you need to prioritize your answer. Use knowledge of the key effects of medication therapy and the process of elimination to make a selection.

17 **Answer: 1 Rationale:** Rivastigmine increases the available acetylcholine in the brain; therefore, the parasympathetic system is stimulated. Blood pressure, mental status, and GI status would be affected. Hemoglobin, white blood cell count, and liver function do not relate to rivastigmine. Hemoglobin and red blood cell count do not relate to rivastigmine; however, mental status should be assessed. Blood pressure is an appropriate assessment, but electrolyte balance and edema in legs do not occur with use of rivastigmine. **Cognitive Level:** Applying **Client Need:** Pharmacological and Parenteral Therapies **Integrated Process:** Nursing Process: Assessment **Content Area:** Pharmacology **Strategy:** The wording of the question tells you that the correct option is also a true statement that would be included in client teaching. Use medication knowledge and the process of elimination to make a selection.

18 **Answer: 4 Rationale:** Cimetidine can increase the levels of amitriptyline in the blood, causing seizures, tachycardia, hypertension, or toxicity. Aspirin, acetaminophen, and naproxen do not intensify the effect of amitriptyline. **Cognitive Level:** Applying **Client Need:** Pharmacological and Parenteral Therapies **Integrated Process:** Teaching and Learning **Content Area:** Pharmacology **Strategy:** Options that are similar are not likely to be correct. All of the incorrect options relate to analgesia, and so must be eliminated.

19 **Answer: 3 Rationale:** Fever is not a side effect of anticholinergic medications; the presence of fever should be a concern, but it is not connected to the medication. Dry mouth, constipation, and urinary retention or hesitancy are possible side effects and should be noted by the nurse. **Cognitive Level:** Analyzing **Client Need:** Pharmacological and Parenteral Therapies **Integrated Process:** Nursing Process: Assessment **Content Area:** Pharmacology **Strategy:** The key words in the stem of the question are *least concerned*. This tells you that the correct answer is an option that is not characteristic of this medication. Use medication knowledge and the process of elimination to make a selection.

20 **Answer: 4 Rationale:** Phenytoin inhibits folic acid absorption and potentiates effects of folic acid antagonists. Folic acid is helpful in correcting some anemias that can result from phenytoin administration. Phenytoin inhibits iron absorption and causes the development of some anemias. Folic acid is adequate in a

well-balanced diet; however, phenytoin inhibits folic acid absorption and potentiates effects of folic acid antagonists. Folic acid does not prevent the neuropathy caused by phenytoin. **Cognitive Level:** Applying **Client Need:** Pharmacological and Parenteral Therapies **Integrated Process:** Nursing Process: Diagnosis **Content Area:** Pharmacology **Strategy:** Use knowledge of the key side effects of medication therapy and the process of elimination to make a selection.

Key Terms to Review

attention-deficit disorder p. 575
attention-deficit/hyperactivity disorder p. 575
diplopia p. 573
epilepsy p. 573
gingival hyperplasia p. 573
hepatotoxicity p. 571
narcolepsy p. 575
nystagmus p. 573
paresthesias p. 573
psychomotor seizures p. 572
spasms p. 580
spasticity p. 580
status epilepticus seizures p. 572
Stevens-Johnson syndrome p. 573
tonic-clonic seizures p. 572

References

Adams, M., Holland, L., & Urban, C. (2017). *Pharmacology for nurses: A pathophysiologic approach* (5th ed.). New York, NY: Pearson Education.

Adams, M., & Urban, C. (2016). *Pharmacology: Connections to nursing practice* (3rd ed.). New York, NY: Pearson Education.

Berman, A., Snyder, S., & Frandsen, G. (2016). *Kozier & Erb's fundamentals of nursing: Concepts, process, and practice* (10th ed.). New York, NY: Pearson Education.

Lehne, R. (2016). *Pharmacology for nursing care* (9th ed.). St. Louis, MO: Saunders.

Wilson, B., Shannon, M., & Shields, K. (2016). *Pearson nurse's drug guide 2016.* New York, NY: Pearson Education.

Test Yourself

Are you ready for the NCLEX-RN® or course exams? Access the NEW web-based app that provides students with thousands of practice questions in preparation for the NCLEX experience.

39 Renal Medications

In this chapter

Cross Reference

Other chapters relevant to this content area are

Age-Related Care of Older Adults	Chapter 17
Dosage Calculation and Medication Administration	Chapter 29
Renal and Genitourinary Disorders	Chapter 58

I. DIURETICS

A. Loop diuretics

1. **Diuretics** (agents that increase amount of urine excreted) inhibit electrolyte reabsorption in thick ascending loop of Henle, promoting excretion of sodium, water, chloride, and potassium
2. Mechanism of action involves renal vasodilation, to provide a temporary increase in glomerular filtration rate (GFR) and decrease in peripheral vascular resistance
3. Loop diuretics are more potent than thiazide diuretics, causing rapid diuresis and reducing vascular fluid volume, cardiac output, and blood pressure (BP)
4. Used in clients with low GFR and hypertensive emergencies
5. Also used in clients with edema, pulmonary edema, congestive heart failure (CHF), chronic renal failure (CRF), and hepatic cirrhosis
6. May be used as treatment in drug overdose to increase renal elimination
7. Common loop diuretics are listed in Box 39–1
8. Administration considerations

NCLEX®

   a. Take early in day to avoid nocturia
   b. Give IV doses slowly per drug literature; rapid injection may cause hypotension
   c. For IV infusion, dilute in 5% dextrose in water, 0.9% NaCl, or lactated Ringer's; use infusion fluids within 24 hours
   d. Administer IV furosemide slowly (20 mg/minute or less); hearing loss can occur if injected rapidly

Box 39–1 Common Loop Diuretics

Bumetanide	Ethacrynic acid
Furosemide	Torsemide

Memory Aid

Remember that loop diuretics can cause ototoxicity, so be sure to assess hearing and avoid exceeding recommended injection rates.

9. Side/adverse effects
    - NCLEX® **a.** Contraindicated with **anuria** (urine output less than 400 mL daily), electrolyte depletion
    - **b.** CNS: dizziness, headache, orthostatic hypotension, weakness
    - **c.** GI: nausea or vomiting (N/V), abdominal pain, elevated lipids with decreased high-density lipoprotein (HDL), pancreatitis, anorexia, constipation
    - **d.** GU: excessive urination, nocturia, urinary bladder spasms
    - NCLEX® **e.** Photosensitivity, sulfonamide allergy, and ototoxicity (tinnitus, hearing impairment, deafness, vertigo, and sense of fullness in ears)
    - **f.** Skin: dermatitis, urticaria, pruritis, and muscle spasm
    - **g.** Severe watery diarrhea is a side effect of ethacrynic acid
    - **h.** Electrolyte imbalances: hyponatremia, hypochloremia, hypokalemia, hypomagnesemia, hypocalcemia, and hypouricemia
    - **i.** Thrombocytopenia, systemic vasculitis, interstitial nephritis, thrombophlebitis, agranulocytosis, and aplastic anemia

NCLEX® 10. Nursing considerations and client teaching (see Box 39–2)

Box 39–2

Nursing Care and Client Education Related to Diuretic Therapy

Nursing Care

- Obtain baseline weight, VS (especially BP and pulse), breath sounds, edema, and hearing status when initiating diuretic therapy.
- Ensure that baseline and periodic laboratory studies (such as electrolytes, glucose, blood counts, uric acid, and liver and renal function studies) are completed as scheduled.
- Monitor for intended effects of therapy, such as increased urine output, reduced edema, and reduced blood pressure if prescribed as treatment for hypertension.
- Measure BP in lying, sitting, and standing positions to detect **orthostatic hypotension** (a fall of more than 10–15 mmHg of systolic blood pressure [SBP] or more than 10 mmHg of diastolic blood pressure [DBP] and a 10–20% increase in heart rate).
- Initiate fall prevention measures if dizziness or orthostatic hypotension occurs as a result of decreased circulating blood volume.
- Measure intake and output in hospitalized clients and record. Track 24-hour fluid volume status as a measure of fluid balance over days of time.
- Monitor serum electrolytes (especially potassium, as well as sodium and calcium) and uric acid levels; monitor hemoglobin and hematocrit (may increase due to hemoconcentration).
- Measure body weight daily at same time of day, in same amount of clothing, and with same scale. Report weight change of 1 kg (2.2 lb) in a 24-hour period.
- Assess for indicators of dehydration if excess drug effect: thirst, poor skin turgor, coated tongue.
- Encourage or limit dietary potassium depending on type of diuretic prescribed.

Client Education

- When taking potassium-wasting diuretics, eat foods high in potassium to prevent hypokalemia (such as bananas, cantaloupe).
- When taking potassium-sparing diuretics, limit foods high in potassium and avoid use of salt substitutes (often have potassium as ingredient).
- Restrict sodium intake generally to prevent fluid retention.
- Weigh self daily and report weight change of 1 kg (2.2 lb) in a 24-hour period.
- Avoid dehydration by avoiding beverages with alcohol or caffeine and replacing fluids during exercise or hot weather.

- Avoid exposure to intense heat as with baths, showers, and electric blankets.
- Take small, frequent amounts of ice chips or clear liquids if vomiting.
- During episodes of diarrhea, replace fluids in small amounts frequently.
- Because diuretics increase amount and frequency of urination, take dose in morning (daily) and afternoon (twice-daily dosing) to avoid nighttime urination (nocturia).
- Change position slowly to avoid dizziness and orthostatic hypotension.
- With loop diuretic use, report ringing in ears or hearing loss immediately; this indicates ototoxicity and may not be reversible. Photosensitivity can also occur while taking a loop diuretic.

B. Thiazide and thiazide-like diuretics

1. Increase urinary excretion of sodium and water by inhibiting sodium reabsorption in cortical diluting tubule of kidney
2. Hypotensive effect may be caused by direct arteriolar vasodilation and decreased total peripheral resistance
3. Used for edema and hypertension (SBP above 140 mmHg and DBP above 90 mmHg)
4. Not effective for immediate diuresis
5. Common thiazide diuretics are listed in Box 39–3
6. Administration considerations
   - *NCLEX®* **a.** Give medication early in the day to avoid nocturia
   - **b.** Thiazide diuretics are ineffective if creatinine clearance level is less than 30 mL/min
   - **c.** Allow 2–4 weeks for maximum antihypertensive effect
   - **d.** Metolazone is not recommended in children because safety has not been established
7. Side/adverse effects
   - *NCLEX®* **a.** Dizziness, vertigo, headache, and weakness
   - *NCLEX®* **b.** Fatigue, dehydration, orthostatic hypotension, hyperglycemia, and frequent urination
   - *NCLEX®* **c.** Electrolyte imbalance (hyponatremia, hypokalemia, hypomagnesemia, hypochloremia), jaundice, muscle cramps, photosensitivity, impotence, and hyperuricemia
   - *NCLEX®* **d.** Contraindicated with hypersensitivity to thiazide diuretics or sulfonamide derivatives, anuria, severely impaired renal or hepatic function, pregnancy or lactation
   - **e.** Renal failure, aplastic anemia, agranulocytosis, thrombocytopenia, and anaphylactic reaction
8. Nursing considerations
   - *NCLEX®* **a.** See Box 39–2
   - **b.** Clients with diabetes mellitus should check blood glucose as recommended because of risk of hyperglycemia

C. Potassium-sparing diuretics

1. Act in distal convoluted tubule to increase sodium excretion and decrease potassium secretion
2. Used for hypertension and edema associated with heart failure
3. Spironolactone is also used for cirrhosis of liver, primary hyperaldosteronism, hirsutism, and premenstrual syndrome
4. Common potassium-sparing diuretics are listed in Box 39–4
5. Administration considerations
   - **a.** Take with food or milk
   - *NCLEX®* **b.** Avoid salt substitutes, which are high in potassium

Box 39–3

Common Thiazide Diuretics

Short Acting	**Long Acting**
Chlorothiazide	Chlorthalidone
Hydrochlorothiazide	Indapamide
Intermediate Acting	Methyclothiazide
Bendroflumethiazide and nadolol	
Metolazone	

Box 39–4

Potassium-Sparing Diuretics

Sodium Channel Inhibitors	**Aldosterone Antagonists**
Amiloride	Eplerenone
Triamterene	Spironolactone

NCLEX® c. Avoid excessive ingestion of foods high in potassium
d. When administering spironolactone to children, crush tablet and mix in flavored syrup as oral suspension

6. Side/adverse effects
   a. CNS: headache, weakness, dizziness, and orthostatic hypotension
   b. GI: N/V, diarrhea, and constipation
   c. Impotence, muscle cramps, urticaria, gynecomastia, and breast soreness
   d. Dry mouth, photosensitivity, transient elevated blood urea nitrogen (BUN) and creatinine
   e. NCLEX® Aplastic anemia and thrombocytopenia
   f. NCLEX® Hyperkalemia (potassium greater than 5.1 mEq/L)
   g. Contraindicated with serum potassium levels greater than 5.5 mEq/mL, concurrent use with other potassium-sparing diuretics, fluid and electrolyte imbalances, anuria, acute and chronic renal insufficiency, diabetic nephropathy, hypersensitivity, and impaired hepatic function
7. NCLEX® Nursing considerations and client teaching
   a. See Box 39–2
   b. Discontinue potassium supplements and teach client to avoid eating large quantities of foods high in potassium
   c. NCLEX® Monitor for symptoms of hyperkalemia such as nausea, diarrhea, abdominal cramps, and tachycardia followed by bradycardia
   d. Side effects usually disappear after drug is stopped, but gynecomastia may persist
   e. With spironolactone, maximal diuresis may not occur until day 3 of therapy and diuresis may continue 2–3 days after the drug is stopped
   f. Triamterene may turn urine blue
   g. NCLEX® Avoid exposure to direct sunlight to prevent photosensitivity reaction

D. Carbonic anhydrase inhibitors

1. Achieve noncompetitive reversible inhibition of enzyme carbonic anhydrase, which promotes excretion of bicarbonate, sodium, potassium, and water
2. Used to treat edema caused by CHF, decrease intraocular pressure in open-angle glaucoma, and treat epilepsy and metabolic alkalosis
3. Common carbonic anhydrase inhibitors are listed in Box 39–5
4. Administration considerations
   a. Increasing dose does not appear to increase diuresis
   b. Do not administer with high-dose aspirin
   c. Intramuscular administration is not recommended
5. Side/adverse effects
   a. Confusion, drowsiness, and paresthesias
   b. Hearing dysfunction, GI upset, polyuria, and transient myopia
   c. Electrolyte imbalance, fever, rash, renal calculus, and photosensitivity
   d. Metabolic acidosis
   e. Anaphylaxis
   f. Bone marrow depression (thrombocytopenia purpura, hemolytic anemia, leukopenia, pancytopenia, and agranulocytosis)
   g. Severe reactions to sulfonamides, including Stevens-Johnson syndrome, toxic epidermal necrolysis, fulminant hepatic necrosis, coma, and death
   h. NCLEX® Contraindicated in narrow-angle or acute glaucoma, any situation with decreased sodium and/or potassium levels, marked kidney or liver dysfunction; use cautiously with chronic obstructive pulmonary disease (COPD)

Box 39–5

Carbonic Anhydrase Inhibitors

Acetazolamide
Methazolamide

6. Nursing considerations
   a. Monitor for signs and symptoms of dehydration
   b. Assess for alterations in skin integrity and for edema
   NCLEX® c. Assess VS, daily weight, and I&O
   d. Assess cardiovascular and respiratory status
   e. Assess changes in level of consciousness and activity level
   f. Assess dietary intake for foods high in salt
   g. Maintain fluid restriction as prescribed
7. Client education
   NCLEX® a. Do not take aspirin or aspirin-containing medications
   b. Report symptoms of anorexia, lethargy, or tachypnea
   NCLEX® c. Use caution while driving or performing tasks that require alertness, coordination, or physical dexterity because these drugs can cause drowsiness
   d. Monitor for signs of renal calculi
   e. Follow-up with scheduled lab tests is important
   NCLEX® f. Weigh self daily at same time of day and report acute weight gain or loss (more than 0.9–1.4 kg [2–3 lb] per day)
   g. Avoid foods and beverages containing high amounts of sodium

E. Osmotic diuretics

1. Increase osmotic pressure of glomerular filtrate in proximal tubule and loop of Henle inhibiting reabsorption of water and electrolytes, thus promoting diuresis
2. Used to prevent and manage acute renal failure (ARF) and oliguria
3. NCLEX® Used to decrease intracranial or intraocular pressure
4. Mannitol is used with chemotherapy to induce diuresis
5. Common osmotic diuretics are listed in Box 39–6
6. Administration considerations
   a. Medications are administered IV by slow infusion
   b. Urea turns to ammonia if left standing
   c. Do not infuse with blood or blood products
   NCLEX® d. Mannitol crystallizes at low temperatures
7. Side/adverse effects
   a. Headache, syncope, and hypotension
   b. Dry mouth, N/V, urine retention, electrolyte imbalance, and urticaria
   c. Seizures
   d. Thrombophlebitis, CHF, cardiovascular collapse
   e. Contraindicated with severely impaired renal function, marked dehydration, breastfeeding, hepatic failure, active intracranial bleed, anuria, severe pulmonary congestion, and severe CHF
8. Nursing considerations
   NCLEX® a. Maintain adequate hydration
   NCLEX® b. Monitor fluid and electrolyte balance, daily weight
   c. Indwelling catheter should be used in comatose clients for accurate I&O
   NCLEX® d. Monitor I&O and VS hourly while receiving mannitol
   e. Monitor renal function (BUN, creatinine), fluid balance, serum and urinary sodium and potassium levels
   NCLEX® f. Assess for signs of decreasing intracranial pressure if appropriate
   g. Monitor lung and heart sounds for signs of pulmonary edema
9. Client education
   a. Monitor weight
   b. Report immediately pain in chest or legs, shortness of breath, or apnea
   c. Change position slowly to prevent dizziness or orthostatic hypotension
   d. Drink only fluids prescribed if also on a fluid restriction
   e. Use sugarless hard candies to reduce dry mouth

Box 39–6

Common Osmotic Diuretics

Glycerin
Mannitol
Urea

Box 39–7

Common Urinary Tract Anti-Infectives

Sulfonamides	Urinary Antiseptics and Other Drugs for UTI
Sulfadiazine	Fosfomycin
Sulfadoxine-pyrimethamine	Methenamine
Sulfisoxazole	Nalidixic acid
Trimethoprim-sulfamethoxazole	Nitrofurantoin

II. URINARY ANTI-INFECTIVES

A. Overview

1. Act as **bacteriostatic** (inhibit growth of bacteria without destruction) and **bactericidal** (destroy bacteria) agents
2. Act as disinfectants within urinary tract and are used to treat urinary tract infections
3. Common urinary tract anti-infectives are listed in Box 39–7
4. Urinary anti-infectives may be combined with a urinary analgesic (such as phenazopyridine or pentosan polysulfate sodium) for relief of pain associated with urinary tract infections (dysuria)

B. Administration considerations

1. May take with food or milk to decrease GI upset
2. Check renal and hepatic function before administering
3. NCLEX® Oral suspension of nitrofurantoin may stain teeth; instruct client to rinse mouth following dose
4. NCLEX® Complete full course of therapy to prevent reinfection or overgrowth of resistant organisms

C. Side/adverse effects

1. Drowsiness, weakness, headache, dizziness
2. NCLEX® Sensitivity to light, blurred vision
3. GI distress, pruritis, rash, arthralgia
4. Seizures, increased intracranial pressure
5. Leukopenia, thrombocytopenia, angioedema
6. NCLEX® Contraindicated with hypersensitivity, megaloblastic anemia and folate deficiency, renal insufficiency, severe hepatic insufficiency, severe dehydration, anuria, oliguria, and seizure disorder

D. Nursing considerations

1. Drugs work best if client is well (but not overly) hydrated
2. Administer with meals to decrease GI distress
3. Monitor renal and liver function
4. Check urine pH before administration because some drugs work best in acidic urine
5. Cranberry juice or vitamin C may be added to acidify urine
6. Monitor CNS side effects
7. Large fluid intake while taking methenamine will reduce antibacterial effects by diluting drug and raising urinary pH

E. Client education

1. Long-term therapy is common even if feeling fine
2. NCLEX® Drink at least eight glasses of water daily
3. Take doses with meals to decrease GI distress
4. NCLEX® Avoid alkalizing fluids such as milk, fruit juices, or sodium bicarbonate
5. Notify prescriber of any new medications
6. NCLEX® Use sunscreen and avoid excessive exposure to sunlight
7. Notify prescriber of any CNS side effects
8. NCLEX® Nitrofurantoin may discolor urine brown; this is not harmful and will disappear after drug is discontinued
9. Phenazopyridine (urinary analgesic) causes orange or reddish discoloration to urine and will stain clothing

III. URINARY ANTISPASMODICS

A. Overview

1. Muscarinic antagonists (anticholinergics) that relax smooth muscles of the urinary tract to decrease bladder and detrusor muscle spasms
2. Used to manage lower urinary tract symptoms associated with hypermotility: dysuria, urgency, nocturia, suprapubic pain, frequency, and incontinence
3. Common antispasmodics are listed in Box 39–8

Box 39–8

Common Antispasmodic Medications

Darifenacin	Oxybutynin chloride
Dicyclomine	Propanetheline
Flavoxate	Tolterodine tartrate
Hyoscyamine	Trospium

B. Administration considerations: administer 1 hour before antacids or antidiarrheals

C. Side/adverse effects

1. Headache, insomnia, drowsiness, dizziness, confusion, excitement, palpitations
2. Blurred vision, dry mouth, GI distress, urinary hesitancy, urine retention, urticaria, leukopenia
3. NCLEX® Contraindicated in glaucoma, obstructive breathing, obstructive GI disease, severe ulcerative colitis, and myasthenia gravis; hypersensitivity to anticholinergics; paralytic ileus; unstable cardiovascular status; urinary tract obstruction

D. Nursing considerations

1. NCLEX® Monitor effect of medication and any CNS manifestations
2. Monitor I&O

E. Client education

1. NCLEX® Drowsiness and blurred vision may occur; use caution with driving or operating machinery; avoid alcohol, which increases drowsiness
2. NCLEX® Use hard, sugarless candy for dry mouth
3. Swallow pill whole and do not chew or crush; medication shell may appear in stool
4. Inform client of side effects and to report them to prescriber

IV. CHOLINERGIC AGENT

A. Overview

1. Direct-acting cholinergic agent is indicated for use with neurogenic bladder and urinary retention from nonobstructive causes
2. NCLEX® Contracts detrusor muscle of urinary bladder, which increases bladder tone and ability to initiate micturition (voiding)
3. Common medication: bethanechol chloride

B. Administration considerations

1. Give oral dose on empty stomach to reduce N/V (1 hour before or 2 hours after meals)
2. Alternate route is subcutaneous; do not give by IM or IV route to avoid life-threatening symptoms of cholinergic stimulation
3. NCLEX® Keep atropine sulfate available as an antidote

NCLEX® **C. Side/adverse effects**

1. Headache and malaise, flushing and increased sweating
2. Hypotension with dizziness and faintness; dyspnea or acute asthmatic attack
3. Blurred vision and lacrimation; urgency with urination or defecation
4. N/V, diarrhea, and abdominal cramps
5. Contraindications of cholinergic drugs include mechanical obstruction of GI or urinary tracts, peptic ulcer disease, COPD, bradycardia, parkinsonism, hypotension, and AV blocks

D. Nursing considerations

1. NCLEX® Monitor for 1 hour after subcutaneous dose for early signs of overdose: salivation, sweating, flushing, abdominal cramps, and nausea
2. NCLEX® Use atropine as prescribed for antidote
3. Monitor I&O to determine effectiveness
4. Monitor client's ambulation as needed according to response to drug

E. Client education

1. NCLEX® Change positions slowly, especially from lying to standing
2. Do not stand in place for long periods, and lie down at first sign of faintness
3. Use caution in activities to maintain safety because of risk of blurred vision

V. ERYTHROPOIETIC GROWTH FACTORS

A. Action and use

NCLEX® 1. Used to stimulate red blood cell (RBC) production to raise hematocrit (Hct)

2. Reverses anemia associated with chronic renal failure (CRF), HIV infection, and chemotherapy used to treat nonmyeloid malignancies

B. Common erythropoietic growth factors are listed in Box 39–9

C. Administration considerations

NCLEX® 1. Do not shake solution

NCLEX® 2. Use only one dose per vial, and do not reenter vial

3. Inspect solution for particulate matter prior to use

4. IV administration: may be given undiluted by direct IV as a bolus dose or during hemodialysis

5. Rotate injection sites if given subcutaneously to minimize irritation

D. Side/adverse effects

NCLEX® 1. Hypertension, headache, seizure

2. Iron deficiency, sweating, bone pain, arthralgias

3. Thrombocytosis, clotting of AV fistula

4. Contraindicated in uncontrolled hypertension, known hypersensitivity to mammalian cell-derived products and albumin

E. Nursing considerations

1. Evaluate serum ferritin and transferrin levels prior to beginning therapy

NCLEX® 2. BP may rise during early therapy as Hct increases; notify prescriber of a rapid rise in Hct greater than 4 points in 2 weeks

3. Do not give with any other drug solution

4. Initial effects can be seen within 1 to 2 weeks

NCLEX® 5. Hct reaches satisfactory levels (30–36%) in 2–3 months

6. Monitor for hypertensive encephalopathy in clients with CRF during period of increasing Hct

7. Client may require additional heparin during dialysis to prevent clotting of vascular access

F. Client education

NCLEX® 1. Self-monitor VS, especially BP

2. Headache is a common adverse effect; it should be reported if severe

NCLEX® 3. Avoid driving and other hazardous activity because of possible seizure, especially during first 90 days of therapy

4. Keep all follow-up appointments

Box 39–9

Erythropoietic Growth Factors

- Epoetin alfa
- Darbepoietin
- Peginesatide

Check Your NCLEX–RN® Exam I.Q.

You are ready for testing on this content if you can:

- Apply knowledge of expected actions and effects of renal medications to client care.
- Correctly administer renal medications to clients.
- Assess for side effects and adverse effects of renal medications.
- Take appropriate action if a client has an unexpected response to a renal medication.
- Monitor a client for expected outcomes or effects of treatment with renal medications.

PRACTICE TEST

1 A client is taking nalidixic acid for treatment of a urinary problem. The nurse explains to the client that the medication is best described as what type of drug?

1. An antispasmodic
2. A uricosuric
3. An anti-infective
4. An analgesic

2 The client with congestive heart failure (CHF) is eating a 1-gram-sodium diet, and will be having a potassium-sparing diuretic added to the medication regimen. The nurse prepares to conduct teaching about which medication that is likely to be prescribed?

1. Hydrochlorothiazide
2. Spironolactone
3. Furosemide
4. Methazolamide

3 The home healthcare nurse is visiting an older adult client who is taking torsemide twice daily. Which statements made by the client indicate the need for further teaching? Select all that apply.

1. "I will take my medication in the morning and before bedtime."
2. "I will change my position slowly, so that I don't fall."
3. "I will notify my physician if my ankles swell."
4. "I can drink coffee and tea in an effort to get enough fluid."
5. "I should expect to experience some ringing in my ears."

4 A client is receiving mannitol. The nurse assesses the client for evidence of which clinical problem, for which the client is at risk?

1. Dehydration
2. Somnolence
3. Tinnitus
4. Fatigue

5 The nurse is reviewing the medication administration record for a client newly admitted for congestive heart failure. The client is receiving hydrochlorothiazide. Which conditions should concern the nurse in relation to administration of this medication? Select all that apply.

1. Hyponatremia
2. Hypokalemia
3. Hypouricemia
4. Hyperchloremia
5. Hyperglycemia

6 The nurse is planning to administer furosemide 40 mg by the IV push route. What technique should the nurse use when administering this medication?

1. Push the medication steadily over 1 minute.
2. Give the medication slowly, diluted in 50 mL of NS.
3. Inject the medication over 2–3 minutes.
4. Dilute the medication with sterile water, and inject over 5 minutes.

7 A client is being prescribed oxybutynin for a neurogenic bladder. The nurse determines that the client is possibly experiencing toxic effects of this medication after noting which manifestation?

1. Restlessness
2. Drowsiness
3. Pallor
4. Bradycardia

8 The nurse is admitting a client with a hypertensive emergency and a history of renal insufficiency. The nurse should ensure that which diuretic is readily available for use if prescribed?

1. Furosemide
2. Hydrochlorothiazide
3. Chlorthalidone
4. Spironolactone

9 A client being discharged from the hospital is beginning medication therapy with bumetanide. The nurse instructs the client to contact the prescriber if which contraindication for use develops?

1. Increase in peripheral edema
2. Absence of urine output
3. Shortness of breath
4. Increase in blood pressure

PRACTICE TEST

10 The nurse notes while taking an admission history that a client is taking acetazolamide. The nurse next questions the client about a history of which medical condition?

1. Hypertensive crisis
2. Congestive heart failure (CHF)
3. Open-angle glaucoma
4. Peripheral vascular disease

11 A client is in the intensive care unit following a serious closed head injury. Mannitol is administered to decrease developing intracranial pressure. What is the priority manifestation the nurse should assess for after the drug is given?

1. Hypotension
2. Cardiovascular collapse
3. Seizures
4. Electrolyte imbalance

12 A client who has been taking bethanechol chloride for 3 days begins to complain of abdominal pain and difficulty breathing. After assigning another staff member to remain with the client, the nurse checks to see that which medication is available on the nursing unit?

1. Phytonadione
2. Atropine sulfate
3. Oxybutynin
4. Epinephrine

13 A client who requires diuretic therapy has a creatinine clearance less than 30 mL/min. The nurse checks the medication administration record, expecting to find a prescription for which diuretic?

1. Mannitol
2. Spironolactone
3. Chlorothiazide
4. Furosemide

14 The healthcare provider has prescribed oxybutynin for a 65-year-old female with urinary frequency and urgency. The nurse teaching the client about drug side effects should explain that which manifestations are associated with this medication? Select all that apply.

1. Dizziness
2. Increased bruising
3. Diarrhea
4. Dry mouth
5. Blurred vision

15 Phenazopyridine is prescribed to a client for relief of dysuria associated with urinary tract infection. The nurse explains that the client should expect which urine characteristic while taking phenazopyridine?

1. Decrease in volume
2. Odor that is foul
3. Increase in volume
4. Color that is orange or red

16 A client who has been prescribed nitrofurantoin reports a concern about onset of brown-colored urine to the home care nurse. Which is the best response by the nurse?

1. "The brown discoloration indicates you are not drinking enough fluids."
2. "If your urine is discolored then the medication may be past the expiration date."
3. "A brown color to the urine is consistent with drug toxicity; call the prescriber."
4. "This is an expected effect of the medication so there is no cause for concern."

17 A client who is taking spironolactone arrives in the emergency department reporting unrelieved edema in the legs. Which data shared by the nurse with the healthcare provider indicates a need to withhold the medication?

1. Blood glucose level of 170
2. Blood pressure of 110/70
3. Sodium level of 146 mEq/L
4. Potassium of 5.9 mEq/L

18 A client is admitted to an acute care facility due to anemia related to renal failure. Based on the nurse's knowledge about administration of hematopoietic growth factor, which action is not appropriate?

1. Gently shaking the medication for adequate mixing
2. Discarding the medication vial after the first dose
3. Giving undiluted medication as an IV bolus dose
4. Closely inspecting solution for particulate matter

19 The client beginning medication therapy with sulfisoxazole needs instructions for its use. What client teaching should the nurse include about the medication?

1. Call the prescriber if the urine turns dark brown.
2. Maintain a high fluid intake.
3. Restrict salt intake.
4. Decrease the dosage when symptoms are improving.

20 The nurse has an order to administer a first dose of epoetin to a client with chronic renal failure. The nurse would make note of which laboratory test results to establish a baseline? Select all that apply.

1. Hemoglobin of 9%
2. Hematocrit of 26%
3. White blood cell count 3,000/mm^3
4. Creatinine 3.2 mEq/L
5. Blood urea nitrogen 56 mg/dL

ANSWERS & RATIONALES

1 **Answer: 3 Rationale:** Nalidixic acid is an anti-infective agent. It is bactericidal, and inhibits microbial synthesis of DNA. The spectrum of microorganisms for which nalidixic acid is effective includes most Gram-negative organisms except *Pseudomonas*. Nalidixic acid is not an antispasmodic, uricosuric, or analgesic agent. **Cognitive Level:** Knowing **Client Need:** Pharmacological and Parenteral Therapies **Integrated Process:** Nursing Process: Planning **Content Area:** Pharmacology **Strategy:** The core issue of the question is knowledge of basic information about nalidixic acid and its uses. Use the process of elimination and nursing knowledge to make a selection.

2 **Answer: 2 Rationale:** Spironolactone is a potassium-sparing diuretic that promotes sodium excretion while conserving potassium. Hydrochlorothiazide and furosemide are diuretics, but are not potassium-sparing. Methazolamide is a carbonic anhydrase inhibitor. **Cognitive Level:** Applying **Client Need:** Pharmacological and Parenteral Therapies **Integrated Process:** Nursing Process: Planning **Content Area:** Pharmacology **Strategy:** The core issue of the question is knowledge of drugs that are potassium-sparing diuretics. Use the process of elimination and nursing knowledge to make a selection.

3 **Answer: 1, 4, 5 Rationale:** Taking medication at the same time each day improves compliance. In addition, morning and *early* evening are the best times to take torsemide, so as not to interrupt sleep. Tea and coffee are poor choices for hydration. They are mild diuretics, and can cause severe dehydration if used concurrently with diuretics. Tinnitus is an indication of ototoxicity when taking furosemide; this is an adverse effect and should be reported to the physician; the client needs additional teaching. A common side effect of torsemide is orthostatic hypotension; the client should be advised to rise slowly to prevent falls. Notifying the prescriber when edema is noticed is important, and should be emphasized by the nurse. **Cognitive Level:** Analyzing **Client Need:** Pharmacological and Parenteral Therapies **Integrated Process:** Nursing Process: Evaluation **Content Area:** Pharmacology **Strategy:** The critical words in the stem of the question are *need for further teaching*. This tells you that the correct answers are incorrect statements on the part of the client. Use the process of elimination and knowledge of diuretic therapy to narrow the selection to the one that utilizes additional diuretic substances. When more than one answer is correct, consider each option as a true/false statement.

4 **Answer: 1 Rationale:** The client receiving mannitol should be assessed for dehydration because the medication is an osmotic diuretic. Mannitol does not cause somnolence; clients receiving mannitol often exhibit improved neurological status after its use to treat increased intracranial pressure. Tinnitus would be of concern with loop diuretics. Fatigue is unrelated to drug therapy with mannitol. **Cognitive Level:** Analyzing **Client Need:** Pharmacological and Parenteral Therapies **Integrated Process:** Nursing Process: Diagnosis **Content Area:** Pharmacology **Strategy:** The core issue of the question is knowledge of unintended effects associated with the use of mannitol. Use the process of elimination and knowledge of drug side effects to make a selection.

5 **Answer: 1, 2, 5 Rationale:** The side effects of hydrochlorothiazide include electrolyte disturbances such as hyponatremia, hypokalemia, hypomagnesemia, and hypochloremia (not hyperchloremia). Hyperuricemia (not hypouricemia) would be of concern. Hyperglycemia is a concern especially in clients with diabetes mellitus. **Cognitive Level:** Analysis **Client Need:** Pharmacological and Parenteral Therapies **Integrated Process:** Nursing Process: Diagnosis **Content Area:** Pharmacology **Strategy:** To aid in correct selection of options, recall that diuretics can generally cause electrolyte disturbances as adverse effects. When there is more than one correct answer, consider each option as a true/false statement.

6 **Answer: 3 Rationale:** Furosemide should be given at a rate of 20 mg/minute or less; 40 mg should be pushed over a period of 2 minutes or more. Infusing the dose over 1 minute is too rapid and can cause hearing loss as a result of ototoxicity. Furosemide does not need to be further diluted before injection, and 50 mL of NS is too much for an IV push. Furosemide does not need to be further diluted before injection, and it is not typical to dilute drugs in sterile water. **Cognitive Level:** Applying **Client Need:** Pharmacological and Parenteral Therapies **Integrated Process:** Nursing Process: Implementation **Content Area:** Pharmacology **Strategy:** It is not typical to dilute IV push medications in sterile water or in a volume of 50 mL, which is usually given as an IV piggyback. Use knowledge of drug administration and adverse effects to select the correct answer.

7 **Answer: 1 Rationale:** Excessive dosing of oxybutynin produces nervousness, hallucinations, restlessness, tachycardia, confusion, flushed or red face, and signs of respiratory depression. Drowsiness, pallor, and bradycardia are the opposite of what

the nurse should expect. **Cognitive Level:** Analyzing **Client Need:** Pharmacological and Parenteral Therapies **Integrated Process:** Nursing Process: Assessment **Content Area:** Pharmacology **Strategy:** Note that when two options are opposite, one of them is likely correct. Use this strategy to eliminate two of the options first. Use the process of elimination and medication knowledge to choose the correct answer.

8 **Answer: 1 Rationale:** Furosemide is a loop diuretic. The antihypertensive action involves renal and peripheral vasodilation, a temporary increase in glomerular filtration rate (GFR), and decreased peripheral vascular resistance. For this reason, it is the drug of choice for clients with low GFR as a result of renal insufficiency. Hydrochlorothiazide, chlorthalidone, and spironolactone are not associated with use in clients with low GFR. **Cognitive Level:** Applying **Client Need:** Pharmacological and Parenteral Therapies **Integrated Process:** Nursing Process: Planning **Content Area:** Pharmacology **Strategy:** Specific knowledge of the benefits of furosemide as a loop diuretic and as the diuretic of choice with renal insufficiency is needed to answer this question. Take time to learn about this common medication if you had difficulty with this question.

9 **Answer: 2 Rationale:** Anuria is the absence of urine formation, and is a contraindication for using this medication. An increase in peripheral edema is not a contraindication for the use of bumetanide. Diuretics such as bumetanide are used to increase the amount of urine excreted in clients with pulmonary edema, which should relieve shortness of breath. An increase in blood pressure is not a contraindication to use of bumetanide. **Cognitive Level:** Applying **Client Need:** Pharmacological and Parenteral Therapies **Integrated Process:** Nursing Process: Implementation **Content Area:** Pharmacology **Strategy:** The core issue of the question is knowledge of expected effects and adverse effects of loop diuretics such as bumetanide. Knowing that diuretics help to relieve the symptoms in three of the options will help you to eliminate each of them.

10 **Answer: 3 Rationale:** Acetazolamide is a carbonic anhydrase inhibitor. Inhibition of carbonic anhydrase decreases the rate of formation of aqueous humor, and thereby reduces intraocular pressure. Acetazolamide may be used for treatment of edema caused by CHF, but it is not a first-line therapy. Acetazolamide does not have a therapeutic effect on hypertensive crisis or peripheral vascular disease. **Cognitive Level:** Analyzing **Client Need:** Pharmacological and Parenteral Therapies **Integrated Process:** Nursing Process: Assessment **Content Area:** Pharmacology **Strategy:** The critical word in the stem of the question is *next*, which tells you that more than one follow-up question might be appropriate, but you must select the most important one. Eliminate the options that are not targeted by this type of therapy. Use knowledge regarding the uses of the drug to select the correct answer.

11 **Answer: 2 Rationale:** Mannitol is an osmotic diuretic and cardiovascular collapse can occur because of the amount of fluid that can be lost. This life-threatening adverse effect should be the nurse's priority concern. Hypotension is an expected side effect. Seizure activity and electrolyte imbalance is possible so the client should be monitored; however, either of these is not the priority concern. **Cognitive Level:** Analyzing **Client Need:** Pharmacological and Parenteral Therapies **Integrated Process:** Nursing Process: Assessment **Content Area:** Pharmacology **Strategy:** The core issue in this question is being able to identify the effects of mannitol for treatment of increasing intracranial pressure. Knowledge regarding which manifestation is the highest priority will assist in selecting the correct answer.

12 **Answer: 2 Rationale:** The client is exhibiting signs of cholinergic toxicity, and atropine is the antidote. Phytonadione or vitamin K is the antidote to warfarin. Oxybutinin is indicated for use as a urinary antispasmodic. Epinephrine is used to treat severe hypersensitivity reactions (anaphylaxis). **Cognitive Level:** Analyzing **Client Need:** Pharmacological and Parenteral Therapies **Integrated Process:** Nursing Process: Assessment **Content Area:** Pharmacology **Strategy:** Use the process of elimination, focusing on the critical words *abdominal pain* and *difficulty breathing*. After determining that the client is experiencing adverse or toxic effects of the medication, choose the option that is an anticholinergic drug, which will treat the cholinergic symptoms.

13 **Answer: 4 Rationale:** Loop diuretics such as furosemide have the disadvantage of requiring more frequent dosing, but are advantageous in clients with creatinine clearance less than 30 mL/min. Mannitol, spironolactone, and chlorothiazide are not as helpful as diuretic agents when the client has a decreased creatinine clearance. **Cognitive Level:** Analyzing **Client Need:** Pharmacological and Parenteral Therapies **Integrated Process:** Nursing Process: Diagnosis **Content Area:** Pharmacology **Strategy:** The core issue of the question is knowledge that loop diuretics are the most beneficial type of diuretic for clients with low creatinine clearance levels. Specific knowledge of this drug category and the ability to recognize drugs from each diuretic class are needed to answer this question.

14 **Answer: 1, 4, 5 Rationale:** Oxybutynin is an antispasmodic medication used to restore normal voiding patterns in clients with spasms of smooth muscle of the urinary bladder. It produces anticholinergic side effects such as dizziness, dry mouth, and blurred vision. Periodic interruptions in therapy are recommended to assess continued need for this medication. It does not cause increased bruising or diarrhea. **Cognitive Level:** Applying **Client Need:** Pharmacological and Parenteral Therapies **Integrated Process:** Teaching and Learning **Content Area:** Pharmacology **Strategy:** Use the process of elimination. The core issue of this question is knowledge of side and adverse effects of this medication. Choose the options that indicate anticholinergic effects. When there is more than one correct answer, consider each option as a true/false statement.

15 **Answer: 4 Rationale:** Phenazopyridine is a urinary analgesic with a local anesthetic effect on the urinary tract mucosa, and relieves pain and dysuria associated with urinary tract infection. It causes the urine to have an orange-to-red color. Phenazopyridine has no effect on volume of urine. Foul odor to the urine can be caused by urinary tract infection. Phenazopyridine is a urinary analgesic with a local anesthetic effect; it has no effect on volume of urine. **Cognitive Level:** Applying **Client Need:** Pharmacological and Parenteral Therapies **Integrated Process:** Teaching and Learning **Content Area:** Pharmacology **Strategy:** The core issue of the question is knowledge of the effects of phenazopyridine on the urine. A critical word in the stem of the question is *dysuria*, which should remind you that the medication is a urinary analgesic, and as the only drug of its type, it causes orange-to-red discoloration in body fluids, including urine.

16 **Answer: 4 Rationale:** A brown discoloration of the urine is an expected effect of therapy with nitrofurantoin (a urinary antiseptic). It does not indicate insufficient fluid intake.

Brown-colored urine is unrelated to the expiration date of the medication. A brown color to the urine does not indicate drug toxicity. **Cognitive Level:** Applying **Client Need:** Pharmacological and Parenteral Therapies **Integrated Process:** Communication and Documentation **Content Area:** Pharmacology **Strategy:** The core issue of the question is knowledge of expected side effects of nitrofurantoin therapy. Recall drugs that commonly discolor urine to make the correct selection.

17 **Answer: 4 Rationale:** Spironolactone is a potassium-sparing diuretic that increases sodium excretion and decreases potassium secretion in the distal convoluted tubule. Potassium levels higher than 5.5 mEq/L are contraindicated with spironolactone, due to additive risk of hyperkalemia. Elevated blood glucose is not a priority issue related to this medication. A blood pressure of 110/70 is within normal limits, and does not warrant withholding the medication. An elevated sodium level could be alleviated by the medication, and thus it is not a reason to withhold the dose of medication. **Cognitive Level:** Analyzing **Client Need:** Pharmacological and Parenteral Therapies **Integrated Process:** Nursing Process: Assessment **Content Area:** Pharmacology **Strategy:** The core issue of the question is the need to monitor potassium levels in a client taking potassium-sparing diuretics. Use knowledge of expected effects of diuretics to eliminate the incorrect options.

18 **Answer: 1 Rationale:** The nurse should not shake hematopoietic growth factor medications. After the first dose of a hematopoietic growth factor is drawn from the vial, the vial should not be reentered; the vial should be discarded. Hematopoietic growth factor can be given undiluted as a direct IV bolus. Hematopoietic growth factor should be inspected for particulate matter before administration and discarded if it is present. **Cognitive Level:** Applying **Client Need:** Pharmacological and Parenteral Therapies **Integrated Process:** Nursing Process: Implementation **Content Area:** Pharmacology **Strategy:** The core issue of the question is knowledge related to the administration of hematopoietic growth factor. The stem of the question is worded so that an incorrect option is the correct answer. Knowledge related to this medication is necessary to answer correctly.

19 **Answer: 2 Rationale:** Each dose of this medication should be administered with a full glass of water, and the client should be encouraged to maintain a high fluid intake. Sulfisoxazole does not discolor urine brown (although nitrofurantoin does), and it is not harmful. It is not necessary to restrict salt intake when taking sulfisoxazole. Prescribed medication should be taken as directed and until complete; the dose should not be decreased even if symptoms improve. **Cognitive Level:** Applying **Client Need:** Pharmacological and Parenteral Therapies **Integrated Process:** Teaching and Learning **Content Area:** Pharmacology **Strategy:** Specific drug knowledge is needed to answer the question; however, recalling that fluid intake should be increased with urinary infections should help to eliminate the other incorrect options.

20 **Answer: 1, 2 Rationale:** Epoetin is given to stimulate red blood cell production in the client with chronic renal failure. For this reason, the nurse should look at the hemoglobin and hematocrit as baseline measurements. A white blood cell stimulant such as filgrastim would be given to raise white blood cell counts; a baseline for white blood cells is not necessary. Epoetin alfa will not treat creatinine or BUN levels; the client would be receiving dialysis to control these values. **Cognitive Level:** Analyzing **Client Need:** Pharmacological and Parenteral Therapies **Integrated Process:** Nursing Process: Assessment **Content Area:** Pharmacology **Strategy:** Use the process of elimination and knowledge of drug therapy. Recall that dialysis is needed to treat renal failure, and options that require dialysis can be eliminated first. Recall that clients in renal failure are anemic because of impaired ability to produce erythropoietin to eliminate the white blood cell count. When there is more than one correct answer; consider each option as a true/false statement.

Key Words to Review

anuria p. 588
bactericidal p. 592
bacteriostatic p. 592
diuretic p. 587
orthostatic hypotension p. 588

References

Adams, M., Holland, L., & Urban, C. (2017). *Pharmacology for nurses: A pathophysiologic approach* (5th ed.). New York, NY: Pearson Education.

Adams, M., & Urban, C. (2016). *Pharmacology: Connections to nursing practice* (3rd ed.). New York, NY: Pearson Education.

Berman, A., Snyder, S., & Frandsen, G. (2016). *Kozier & Erb's fundamentals of nursing: Concepts, process, and practice* (10th ed.). New York, NY: Pearson Education.

Lehne, R. (2016). *Pharmacology for nursing care* (9th ed.). St. Louis, MO: Saunders.

Wilson, B., Shannon, M., & Shields, K. (2016). *Pearson nurse's drug guide 2016*. New York, NY: Pearson Education.

40 Gastrointestinal Medications

In this chapter

Cross Reference

Other chapters relevant to this content area are

Dosage Calculation and Medication Administration	**Chapter 29**
Immunologic and Anti-Infective Medications	**Chapter 45**
Gastrointestinal Disorders	**Chapter 59**

I. GASTROINTESTINAL ANTISPASMODIC AND ANTI-INFLAMMATORY DRUGS

A. Overview

1. **Antispasmodics** are muscarinic antagonists (**anticholinergics**) that antagonize action of acetylcholine (Ach) at cholinergic receptor sites and slow intestinal motility
2. Antispasmodics are used to treat spasms of the gastrointestinal (GI) tract such as pylorospasm, ileitis, and reduce cramping and diarrhea with irritable bowel syndrome (IBS)
3. GI anti-inflammatory drugs (5-aminosalicylic acid agents) are useful for induction therapy for inflammatory bowel disease (IBD), although immunosuppressive agents (azathioprine, mercaptopurine, and methotrexate; see also Chapter 45) are better for maintenance therapy
4. Anti-inflammatories exert their action by inhibiting prostaglandins and leukotrienes (mediators of inflammation)

B. Common medications are listed in Box 40–1

NCLEX® **C. Administration considerations**: give antispasmodics 30–60 minutes before meals and at bedtime; anti-inflammatories may be given with or after meals to slow GI transit time, but timing should be consistent

Box 40–1

GI Antispasmodic and Anti-Inflammatory Drugs

Antispasmodic	Anti-inflammatory
Dicyclomine	Balsalizide
Hyoscyamine	Mesalamine
	Olsalazine
	Sulfasalazine

D. Contraindications

1. Antispasmodics
   a. Narrow-angle glaucoma, obstructive GI disease, paralytic ileus, obstructive uropathy
   b. Excreted in breast milk; may cause infant toxicity and decreased milk production
   c. Use with caution with renal dysfunction
2. Anti-inflammatories
   a. Hypersensitivity to aspirin for all in this class or sulfonamides for sulfasalazine
   b. Urinary obstruction
   c. Cautious use in hemotological disorders (risk of blood dyscrasias), liver disease (hepatotoxicity), dehydration (crystalluria), hyper- or hypoglycemia (increases insulin secretion)

E. Side/adverse effects

NCLEX® 1. Antispasmodics
   a. Common: dry mouth, blurred vision, drowsiness, constipation, urinary hesitancy, tachycardia
   b. Less common: confusion, paralytic ileus
2. Salicylate anti-inflammatories
   a. Common: headache, abdominal pain, nausea and vomiting (N/V), rash, allergic reactions
   b. Less common: hepatotoxicity, blood dyscrasias, salicylate hypersensitivity, crystalluria (sulfasalazine)

F. Nursing considerations

NCLEX® 1. Determine factors contributing to diarrhea to determine effective treatment
2. Clients who lose significant potassium with diarrhea are at risk for paralytic ileus and cardiac dysrhythmias; monitor serum electrolytes
NCLEX® 3. Monitor for metabolic acidosis (loss of bicarbonate and impaired renal excretion of acids)
NCLEX® 4. Monitor vital signs (VS), intake and output (I&O), and visual changes

G. Client teaching

NCLEX® 1. Avoid exposure to high temperatures (risk of hyperthermia if fluid losses occur)
NCLEX® 2. Follow recommended dietary/fluid interventions to decrease constipation
3. Report any additional medications prescribed
4. Monitor own I&O for adequacy

II. ANTIDIARRHEALS

A. Overview

1. Slow and/or inhibit GI motility by acting on intestinal wall nerve endings to reduce stool volume, increase viscosity, and decrease fluid and electrolyte loss
2. Used for symptomatic relief of acute, nonspecific diarrhea and diarrhea of inflammatory disease

B. Common antidiarrheals are listed in Box 40–2

C. Administration considerations

1. Shake suspensions well; chew tablets thoroughly; do not give at same time as other medications
NCLEX® 2. Stool may appear gray-black (may mask GI bleeding)
NCLEX® 3. Seek medical care if diarrhea persists for more than 2 days in an adult
4. Do not use to treat diarrhea in children; seek medical attention

Box 40–2

Antidiarrheals

Loperamide	Bismuth subsalicylate
Diphenoxylate with atropine	Octreotide
Difenoxin with atropine	

D. Contraindications

NCLEX® 1. Bloody diarrhea, diarrhea associated with pathogens such as *E. coli*, salmonella, shigella or pseudomembranous colitis, or other bacterial toxins
2. Avoid use if obstructive bowel disease is suspected

NCLEX® 3. Avoid bismuth subsalicylate if allergic to aspirin or other salicylates; avoid concurrent use of aspirin with bismuth subsalicylate to prevent additive effects
4. Difenoxin/atropine sulfate should not be used in children under age 2
5. Octreotide is used in severe diarrhea associated with cancer, ileostomy, and acquired immunodeficiency syndrome (AIDS)
6. Avoid concurrent use with monoamine oxidase inhibitors (MAOIs), which may increase risk of hypertensive crisis

E. Side/adverse effects

NCLEX® 1. Dry mouth, dizziness, drowsiness, constipation, N/V
2. Temporary darkening of stools and tongue may occur with bismuth salicylate
3. Central nervous system (CNS) and respiratory depression, hypotonic reflexes, angioedema, anaphylaxis, and paralytic ileus
4. Signs and symptoms of overdose include drowsiness, decreased blood pressure (BP), seizures, apnea, blurred vision, dry mouth, and psychosis

F. Nursing considerations

1. Note allergies
2. Document onset, duration, and frequency of symptoms, any previous therapies and current medications
3. Identify any causative factors and presence of comorbid conditions; perform stool analysis as prescribed

NCLEX® 4. Assess for evidence of dehydration or electrolyte imbalance; monitor vital signs and I&O

NCLEX® 5. Assess abdomen for tenderness, distention, bowel sounds, or masses

G. Client teaching

1. Drink fluids to avoid dehydration and alleviate dry mouth
2. Follow BRAT diet—bananas, rice, applesauce, tea/toast—to reduce episodes of diarrhea if recommended by healthcare provider

NCLEX® 3. Do not exceed prescribed dose; consult prescriber if diarrhea persists more than 2 days

NCLEX® 4. Use caution in activities requiring alertness if dizziness/drowsiness is present (possible side effects)
5. Report occurrence of fever, N/V, abdominal pain or distention

NCLEX® 6. Avoid dairy products, which could aggravate diarrhea
7. Use hygiene measures to avoid skin irritation or breakdown due to diarrhea

III. LAXATIVES

A. Bulk-forming laxatives

1. Overview
   a. Include nonabsorbable polysaccharide and cellulose derivatives
   b. **Laxatives** swell in water, forming an emollient gel that increases bulk in intestines, which stimulates peristalsis and decreases bowel transit time
   c. Generally produce laxative effect within 12–14 hours but may require 2–3 days for full effect
2. Common laxatives are listed in Box 40–3

Box 40–3

Laxatives

Bulk-Forming Laxatives	**Osmotic Laxatives**
Calcium polycarbophil	Polyethylene glycol
Methylcellulose	Glycerin
Psyllium	**Stool Softener (Surfactant)**
Stimulant Laxatives	Docusate sodium
Bisacodyl	**Saline Laxatives**
Castor oil	Magnesium citrate
Lubricant Laxative	Magnesium hydroxide
Mineral oil	Sodium biphosphate

NCLEX® 3. Administration considerations: since water increases bulk, give each dose with a full glass of liquid (240 mL); may cause intestinal and esophageal obstruction if insufficient liquid is given with dose

4. Contraindications
   a. Not recommended for clients with intestinal stenosis, ulceration, adhesions, or fecal impaction
   b. Use cautiously in clients with swallowing difficulties to prevent aspiration
5. Side/adverse effects
   a. Abdominal discomfort and/or bloating, flatulence, N/V, diarrhea
   NCLEX® b. Esophageal obstruction, swelling, or blockage may occur if insufficient fluid used in mixing a bulk-forming laxative
6. Nursing considerations
   a. Assess swallowing ability (monitor for aspiration), adequately mix agents in liquid, and encourage additional fluid intake
   NCLEX® b. If administered via feeding tube, use large-bore tube; give rapidly with adequate flushing
   c. Separate psyllium administration from digoxin, salicylates, and anticoagulants by 2 hours
7. Client teaching
   NCLEX® a. Take in additional fluids, engage in exercise, and increase dietary fiber
   b. Bulk-forming laxatives may decrease appetite if taken before meals
   c. Take medication 2 hours after meals and any oral medications
   d. Use sodium- and sugar-free preparations if appropriate for diet restrictions
   e. Full effect of medication may not occur for 2–3 days

NCLEX® **B. Stimulant cathartics**

1. Overview
   a. Stimulate peristalsis and may modify permeability of colonic mucosal cells, which results in intraluminal fluid and electrolyte secretion
   NCLEX® b. **Cathartics** are agents with purgative actions
   c. Defecation occurs 6–12 hours after oral administration; rectal dose of bisacodyl produces catharsis within 15 minutes to 2 hours
2. NCLEX® Common laxatives were listed in Box 40–3
3. NCLEX® Administration considerations: follow product directions; bedtime administration of dose promotes a morning bowel movement
4. NCLEX® Contraindications
   NCLEX® a. Abdominal pain, N/V, symptoms of appendicitis, rectal bleeding, gastroenteritis, intestinal obstruction, fecal impaction
   b. Castor oil may induce premature labor
5. Side/adverse effects
   a. Abdominal cramps, diarrhea, N/V, rectal burning/itching (suppository), laxative dependence
   b. Muscle weakness, hypokalemia, hypocalcemia, metabolic acidosis or alkalosis
6. Nursing considerations
   NCLEX® a. Evaluate for N/V, abdominal pain, diarrhea, fluid or electrolyte imbalances; evaluate for laxative dependence and offer counseling
   NCLEX® b. Encourage increased fluids and increased amounts of high-fiber foods in diet
7. Client teaching
   NCLEX® a. Avoid chronic use of laxatives (beyond 1 week)
   NCLEX® b. Increase fluid intake and diet high in fiber; report side effects to prescriber

C. Hyperosmotic cathartics

1. Overview: increase osmotic pressure in intestinal lumen, resulting in retention of water and softening of stool
2. Common laxatives were listed in Box 40–3
3. Administration considerations: follow product directions; glycerin is available only for rectal administration (suppository or enema) to treat acute constipation; laxative effect occurs within 15 to 30 minutes
4. Contraindications: bowel obstruction
5. Side/adverse effects
   a. Glycerin: rectal irritation and burning, hyperemia of rectal mucosa
   b. Polyethylene glycol: flatulence, abdominal cramps/bloating, diarrhea
   c. Fluid and electrolyte imbalances
6. NCLEX® Nursing considerations: monitor frequency and consistency of stools and for electrolyte imbalances, especially in older adults

7. Client teaching
   a. Medication may take 2–4 days for effect
   b. Contact prescriber if unusual bloating, cramping, or diarrhea occurs
   c. Prolonged use may result in electrolyte imbalance and laxative dependence

D. Stool softeners (*surfactants*)

1. Overview
   a. Used for clients at risk for constipation, such as during hospitalization and bedrest, after surgery, or when receiving opioid analgesics
   b. Stool softeners are often called emollient laxatives; anionic surfactants that lower fecal surface tension by allowing water and lipid penetration
   c. Some preparations combine a stool softener (docusate sodium) with a stimulant (casanthrol) to make a single combination product (e.g., Pericolace)
   NCLEX® d. Used for constipation associated with dry, hard stools and to decrease strain of defecation; fecal softening generally occurs in 1–3 days
2. Common medication: docusate sodium
3. Administration considerations: do not give with mineral oil; offer fluids after each oral dose
4. Contraindications
   a. Hypersensitivity to drug; heart failure (sodium content)
   NCLEX® b. Intestinal obstruction, undiagnosed abdominal pain, vomiting or other signs of appendicitis, fecal impaction, or acute abdomen
5. Side/adverse effects: bitter taste; mild abdominal cramping, diarrhea; dependence with long-term or excessive use
6. NCLEX® Nursing considerations: monitor frequency and consistency of stools and electrolyte balance, especially in older adults
7. NCLEX® Client teaching
   a. Take medication with milk or juice to decrease bitter taste
   b. Increase high-fiber foods in diet and fluid intake
   c. May require 1–3 days to soften fecal matter; avoid prolonged use

E. Lubricant laxative

1. Overview: lubricates feces and hinders water reabsorption into colon; not commonly used today because of unintended effects
2. Common medication: mineral oil
3. Administration considerations: may take 24–48 hours to work; do not give with food (may delay gastric emptying; separate by 2 hours); may interfere with absorption of some drugs, so alter administration times as needed
4. NCLEX® Contraindications: abdominal pain, N/V; symptoms of appendicitis or acute abdomen; fecal impaction or bowel obstruction
5. Side/adverse effects
   a. N/V, diarrhea, abdominal cramps; aspiration may cause lipoid pneumonia
   b. Laxative dependence may occur with excessive or long-term use
   c. Nutritional deficiencies and impaired absorption of fat-soluble vitamins (A, D, E, K)
6. Nursing considerations
   NCLEX® a. Because of possible aspiration and diminished vitamin absorption, do not give to children under age 6, pregnant women, older adults, or debilitated clients; do not administer to client lying flat in bed
   b. Do not administer medication at bedtime or within 2 hours of food because of possible decrease in gastric emptying
7. Client teaching
   NCLEX® a. Avoid chronic use; mineral oil may leak through anal sphincter; report side effects to prescriber
   b. Do not take medication when lying flat or at bedtime (risk of aspiration)

F. Saline laxatives

1. Overview
   a. Magnesium, sulfate, phosphate, and citrate salts used for rapid bowel evacuation, such as in preparation for procedures or surgery
   b. Mechanism of action is unclear, but may produce an osmotic effect that increases intraluminal volume and stimulates peristalsis
2. Common laxatives were listed in Box 40–3

NCLEX®

3. Administration considerations
   a. Use magnesium salts cautiously in renal impairment because absorption may cause hypermagnesemia
   b. Use sodium phosphate salts cautiously in clients with sodium restriction
   c. Concurrent use with antacids may inactivate both
4. Contraindications
   a. Not recommended for children under age 2 because of risk for hypocalcemia
   b. Contraindicated in presence of abdominal pain, N/V, signs of appendicitis or acute abdomen, intestinal obstruction, edema, CHF, megacolon, or impaired renal function
5. Side/adverse effects
   a. Cramping and urgency to defecate
   b. NCLEX® Safe when administered for short-term management; may cause significant fluid and electrolyte imbalances with prolonged use or in certain clients
6. Nursing considerations: encourage increased fluid intake to avoid dehydration since these drugs are salts; monitor drug effectiveness
7. Client teaching
   a. Avoid frequent or prolonged use to avoid laxative dependence; report side effects or lack of effectiveness to prescriber
   b. Increase fluid intake and dietary fiber as additional measures

IV. ANTIEMETICS

A. Overview

1. **Emesis** is a complex reflex brought about by activation of vomiting center in medulla oblongata
2. Certain stimuli activate vomiting center directly (e.g., GI irritation), while others (e.g., drugs, toxins, radiation) stimulate chemoreceptor trigger zone (CTZ) in medulla
3. Emetogenic compounds and antiemetic drugs produce their effects by affecting neuroreceptors (which are influenced by acetylcholine, histamine, serotonin, dopamine, benzodiazepines, and cannabinoids)
4. Phenothiazines suppress emesis by blocking dopamine receptors in CTZ
5. Cannabinoids are approved to treat N/V associated with cancer chemotherapy; mechanism of action is unknown; dronabinol also approved as appetite stimulant in AIDS

Memory Aid Cannabinoids can be recognized on sight because they end with the suffix *-abinol.*

6. Benzodiazepines: primary effect is suppression of anxiety; most effective for management of N/V associated with cancer chemotherapy when combined with metoclopramide and dexamethasone
7. Glucocorticoids: mechanism for suppressing chemotherapy-associated emesis is unknown; effective alone and in combination with other antiemetics
8. Antihistamines: anticholinergic effect reduces motion sickness and vomiting
9. Serotonin receptor antagonists: block serotonin receptors to reduce nausea

B. Common antiemetics are listed in Box 40–4

Memory Aid Serotonin antagonists can be recognized on sight because they end with the suffix *-setron.*

C. Administration considerations

1. Often antiemetic combinations work better than single-drug treatment, particularly for cancer chemotherapy induced emesis, suggesting more than one mechanism may trigger emesis
2. Prophylactic drugs are often given by mouth; however, active emesis is usually managed with parenteral or rectal dosing
3. NCLEX® Anticipatory N/V should be treated 1 hour before meals or therapy
4. Parenteral doses should be given deep IM to avoid drug leakage into subcutaneous tissues

Box 40–4

Antiemetics

Anticholinergics–Antihistamines	**Phenothiazine and Phenothiazine-like**
Cyclizine	Metoclopramide
Dimenhydrinate	Perphenazine
Diphenhydramine	Prochlorperazine
Doxylamine and pyridoxine	Promethazine
Hydroxyzine	**Serotonin (5-HT_3) Receptor Antagonists**
Meclizine	Dolasetron
Scopolamine	Granisetron
Benzodiazepines	Ondansetron
Lorazepam	Palonosetron
Cannabinoids	**Neurokinin (NK) Receptor Antagonists**
Dronabinol	Aprepitant
Nabilone	Fosaprepitant
Glucocorticoids	
Dexamethasone	
Methylprednisolone	

D. Contraindications

1. CNS depression and coma
2. Use cautiously in clients with glaucoma, seizures, intestinal obstruction, prostatic hyperplasia, asthma, cardiac, pulmonary, or hepatic disease

E. Side/adverse effects

NCLEX® 1. Phenothiazines: extrapyramidal reactions, anticholinergic effects, hypotension, and sedation
2. Cannabinoids: temporal disintegration, dissociation, depersonalization, and dysphoria
NCLEX® 3. Phenothiazines: agranulocytosis, thrombocytopenia

F. Nursing considerations

1. Dronabinol and nabilone have a high potential for abuse
2. Check VS regularly for hypotension or tachycardia
3. Observe for side effects and adverse reactions
4. Monitor I&O for urine retention
5. Observe for mood changes or involuntary movements
NCLEX® 6. Monitor lab values: liver function tests, electrolytes, blood urea nitrogen (BUN), and creatinine
NCLEX® 7. May mask response of skin testing; discontinue 4 days prior to testing
NCLEX® 8. Monitor for anticholinergic effects: dry mouth, constipation, visual changes

G. Client teaching

1. Avoid activities that require alertness; avoid alcohol and CNS depressants
2. Monitor blood glucose if diabetic
NCLEX® 3. Avoid excessive sunlight/ultraviolet light because of potential photosensitivity
NCLEX® 4. Use sugarless hard candy or ice chips to avoid dry mouth
5. Increase fluids and dietary fiber to decrease risk of constipation
6. Take medication 30–60 minutes before any activity that causes nausea

V. HISTAMINE H_2 ANTAGONISTS

A. Overview

1. Reduce gastric acid secretion by blocking histamine$_2$ in gastric parietal cells
2. Histamine **H_2 antagonists** (agents that decrease gastric secretion) are used to treat duodenal ulcer, gastric ulcer, hypersecretory conditions such as Zollinger-Ellison syndrome, reflux esophagitis

3. Used to prevent stress ulcers in critically ill clients; used in combination therapy to treat ***Helicobacter pylori*** (bacteria found in gastric mucosa) infection
4. Prototype agent, cimetidine, has highest rate of side effects

B. Common H_2 antagonists are listed in Box 40–5

Memory Aid

H_2 antagonists can be recognized on sight because they end with the suffix *-tidine*.

Box 40–5

Histamine 2 (H_2) Antagonists

Cimetidine	Famotidine
Ranitidine	Nizatidine

C. Administration considerations: drugs administered intravenously (IV) should not be mixed with other medications; avoid antacid use within 1 hour of administration

NCLEX® **D. Contraindications**: hypersensitivity to drug; use caution in clients with impaired renal or hepatic function

E. Side/adverse effects

1. Cimetidine: constipation, diarrhea, nausea, headache, fatigue, gynecomastia; rarely hepatitis, blood dyscrasias, dysrhythmias, skin reactions, confusion, anaphylaxis, galactorrhea
2. Others: headache, nausea, and dry mouth; rarely musculoskeletal pain, tachycardia, blood dyscrasias, blurred vision

F. Nursing considerations

1. NCLEX® Dosages are usually reduced with hepatic or renal impairment
2. Assess medications for possible interactions
3. Evaluate nutritional status and dietary interventions
4. Evaluate need for smoking cessation and alcohol abuse programs

G. Client teaching

1. Avoid smoking, which causes gastric stimulation
2. NCLEX® Avoid **antacid** (agent reducing acidity) use within 1 hour of dose
3. Take once-a-day dose at bedtime; otherwise take before meals
4. Avoid gastric irritants such as alcohol, aspirin, and nonsteroidal anti-inflammatory drugs (NSAIDs)
5. Report side effects to prescriber

VI. PROTON PUMP INHIBITORS (PPIs)

A. Overview

1. Block acid secretion by inhibiting H^+-K^+ ATPase at secretory surface of gastric parietal cells
2. Used to treat gastroesophageal reflux disease (GERD) or duodenal ulcers, active benign gastric ulcers, NSAID-associated gastric ulcers, pathological hypersecretory conditions such as Zollinger-Ellison syndrome

B. Common proton pump inhibitors are listed in Box 40–6

Memory Aid

A **proton pump inhibitor** can be recognized on sight because it ends with the suffix *-prazole*.

Box 40–6

Proton Pump Inhibitors

Esomeprazole	Pantoprazole
Lansoprazole	Rabeprazole sodium
Omeprazole	

C. Administration considerations
1. May give with antacids
2. If unable to swallow capsules, lansoprazole and esomeprazole capsules may be opened and sprinkled on applesauce before taking
3. Omeprazole, pantoprazole, and rabeprazole must be swallowed whole
4. To give per nasogastric (NG) tube, dilute capsule contents in 40 mL juice

D. Contraindications: not recommended in children or nursing mothers

E. Side/adverse effects
1. More common are headache, diarrhea, nausea, rash, dizziness, and abdominal pain
2. Rarely agranuloxytosis or other blood disorder can occur

F. Nursing considerations

NCLEX® 1. Document reason for therapy, duration of symptoms, drug efficacy, and any side effects
2. Monitor liver function tests, CBC, BUN, and creatinine; dose may be reduced in liver disease

G. Client teaching
1. Follow product directions and prescribed diet and activities to decrease symptoms
2. Medication is often for short-term therapy; keep healthcare appointments for continued signs and symptoms
3. Take early in morning 30–60 minutes before breakfast

VII. MUCOSAL PROTECTIVE AGENTS

A. Overview
1. Misoprostol is a synthetic prostaglandin E2 that stimulates production of protective mucus and inhibits gastric secretion; prevents gastric ulcers with high-dose NSAID or corticosteroid therapy
2. Sucralfate enhances mucosal defenses and produces a thick protective coating over ulcer, which protects against further erosion and aids healing

B. Common medications: misoprostol, sucralfate

C. Administration considerations

NCLEX® 1. Sucralfate should be taken 1 hour before meals and bedtime or 2 hours after meals or medications and not within 2 hours of antacids
2. Misoprostol should be taken with food

D. Contraindications

NCLEX® 1. Misoprostol is contraindicated in clients who are allergic to prostaglandins or who are pregnant or lactating; pregancy category is X; safety not established for those under age 18; use cautiously with clients with renal impairment and/or older than 64 years
2. Sucralfate has no known contraindications but safety in children and during lactation is not fully established

E. Side/adverse effects
1. Misoprostol: diarrhea, abdominal cramping, dysmenorrhea, menstrual disorders, and postmenopausal bleeding
2. Sucralfate: constipation; minimal adverse effects because little drug absorbed from GI tract

NCLEX® **F. Nursing considerations**: assess for pregnancy (misoprostol); assess effect of medication on GI symptoms and any side effects; monitor concurrent medications

G. Client teaching

NCLEX® 1. Avoid gastric irritants such as caffeine, alcohol, smoking, and spicy foods
2. Report side effects to prescriber for possible dosage change

NCLEX® 3. Follow contraceptive practices while on misoprostol
4. Do not take misoprostol if pregnant; discontinue use if pregnancy occurs or is suspected; report any abnormal vaginal bleeding; avoid pregnancy at least 1 month or one menstrual cycle after stopping medication
5. Increase fluids and fiber to decrease constipation

VIII. ANTACIDS

A. Overview
1. Gastric acid–neutralizing agent used for relief of hyperacidity associated with GI disorders
2. Used as antiflatulent (with simethicone) to alleviate symptoms of gas and bloating

B. Common antacids are listed in Box 40–7

NCLEX® **C. Administration considerations**: take at least 2 hours apart from other drugs where a drug interaction may occur

Box 40–7

Antacids

Aluminum hydroxide	Magnesium hydroxide and aluminum hydroxide
Calcium carbonate	Magnesium hydroxide, aluminum hydroxide, and simethicone
Calcium carbonate with magnesium hydroxide	Sodium bicarbonate
Magaldrate	
Magnesium hydroxide	
Magnesium trisilicate and aluminum hydroxide	

D. Contraindications

1. Safety has not been established for use of antacids by lactating women
2. Magnesium hydroxide: abdominal pain, N/V, diarrhea, severe renal dysfunction, fecal impaction, rectal bleeding, colostomy, ileostomy
3. Aluminum carbonate antacids: low serum phosphate level (causes additive hypophosphatemia); hypertension and heart failure (aluminum-based products contain sodium)
4. Calcium carbonate antacids: hypercalcemia and hypercalciuria, severe renal disease, renal calculi, GI hemorrhage or obstruction, dehydration

E. Side/adverse effects

1. Antacids increase gastric pH and may bind with other drugs, decreasing their absorption and effectiveness; separate their administration from other drugs by 1–2 hours or as recommended by drug literature
2. Prolonged use may alter aluminum, calcium, sodium, and phosphate levels
3. Belching, constipation, flatulence, diarrhea, and gastric distention
4. *NCLEX®* Aluminum-based products: constipation (most frequent), hypophosphatemia (anorexia, malaise, tremors, muscle weakness), aluminum toxicity (dementia) with prolonged use
5. *NCLEX®* Magnesium-based products: diarrhea (most frequent) unless combined with aluminum-based product
6. Calcium-based products: hypercalcemia and metabolic alkalosis
7. Sodium bicarbonate: may worsen hypertension and risk for heart failure (sodium content)

NCLEX® **F. Nursing considerations**

1. Shake suspension well; flush NG tube with water after administration
2. Liquid preparations act more quickly than tablets; follow liquid dose with 4 ounces of water to speed effectiveness

NCLEX® **G. Client teaching**

1. Take as directed; do not exceed maximum dose
2. Keep out of reach of children
3. May interact with certain medications; consult with healthcare provider before use
4. Do not use without medical advice if diagnosed with kidney disease

IX. TREATMENT REGIMENS FOR *HELICOBACTER PYLORI*

A. Overview

1. Antisecretory and antimicrobial action against most strains of *Helicobacter pylori* (*H. pylori*)
2. Used to eradicate *H. pylori* infection and to reduce risk of duodenal ulcer recurrence

B. Common medication combinations for *H. pylori* are listed in Box 40–8

C. Administration considerations

1. Swallow all pills whole except bismuth, which should be chewed
2. If dose is missed, continue with normal dosage regimen; do not double-dose
3. *NCLEX®* Do not administer if client has allergy to any component of therapy
4. Pregnant women should not take regimens containing clarithromycin

D. Side/adverse effects

1. Rash, N/V, diarrhea, abnormal taste, abdominal pain, dyspepsia
2. Transient CNS reactions (anxiety, behavior changes, tinnitus, vertigo), headache, photosensitivity, ventricular dysrhythmias

Box 40–8

Treatment Regimens for *Helicobacter pylori*

Omeprazole (or other PPI), clarithromycin, and amoxicillin

Ranitidine, bismuth subsalicylate, metronidazole, and tetracycline

Omeprazole (or other PPI), bismuth subsalicylate, metronidazole, and tetracycline

E. Nursing considerations

1. Note signs and symptoms, onset, and duration; document allergy status

NCLEX®
2. Determine pregnancy status; do not adminster bismuth subsalicylate to children because of risk of Reye syndrome
3. Document previous therapies used; document confirmation of infection

F. Client teaching

1. Understand importance of compliance; review drug packaging (some combinations are prepackaged)

NCLEX®
2. Avoid gastric irritants such as smoking, alcohol, and caffeine
3. Practice stress reduction techniques; avoid prolonged exposure to sun
4. Bismuth-containing preparations may cause darkening of tongue and stool
5. Report side effects or continued symptoms to prescriber
6. Do not double-dose if dose is missed; therapy usually lasts 7–14 days
7. Use additional contraception (antibiotics can decrease oral contraceptive effectiveness)

X. GALLSTONE-DISSOLVING AGENT

A. Ursodiol

1. Natural occurring bile acid that inhibits hepatic synthesis and secretion of cholesterol; used to dissolve gallbladder stones smaller than 20 mm
2. Absorbed in small bowel, secreted into hepatic bile ducts, and expelled into duodenum in response to eating

B. Administration considerations: use beyond 24 months has not been established

C. Contraindications: clients who have calcified cholesterol stones, radiopaque stones, or radiolucent bile pigment stones; acute cholecystitis, biliary obstruction, pancreatitis, allergy to bile acids, and chronic liver disease

D. Side/adverse effects

NCLEX®
1. Abdominal pain, N/V, constipation, diarrhea, rash
2. Headache, fatigue, anxiety, sweating, thinning of hair, arthralgia

E. Nursing considerations

NCLEX®
1. Document indications and length of therapy; if no dissolving of partial stone is noted in 12 months, drug will probably not be effective
2. Determine pregnancy status

F. Client teaching

1. Avoid antacid use with drug unless prescribed; report side effects to prescriber
2. Therapy may take up to 24 months and stones may recur; comply with follow-up visits
3. Be aware that birth control pills may decrease drug effect

XI. PANCREATIC ENZYME REPLACEMENT

A. Pancrelipase: enzyme (lipase, amylase, and protease) replacement therapy for cystic fibrosis, chronic pancreatitis, ductal obstructions, or pancreatic insufficiency

B. Administration considerations

1. Swallow tablets/capsules whole; do not crush or chew; if swallowing is difficult, open capsules and put contents in applesauce or pudding to swallow without chewing
2. Give medications before or with meals; do not give with antacids or iron

NCLEX® **C. Contraindications**: hypersensitivity to pork protein or enzymes, or with acute pancreatitis

NCLEX® **D. Side/adverse effects**: nausea, diarrhea, abdominal cramps, hyperuricemia

E. Nursing considerations

NCLEX®
1. Assess swallowing ability or difficulty
2. Monitor for side effects and monitor steatorrhea (should diminish with appropriate drug dose)
3. Assess and monitor to maintain good nutritional status; monitor uric acid levels

F. **Client teaching**
1. Follow dietary interventions; consult with dietitian for meal planning
2. Take before or with meals with plenty of water; report side effects to prescriber

XII. HEPATIC ENCEPHALOPATHY TREATMENT

NCLEX® A. **Lactulose:** promotes peristalsis and bowel elimination of ammonia from GI tract, leading to lower serum ammonia levels; used to prevent and treat portal systemic encephalopathy leading to hepatic coma

B. **Administration considerations:** give dose orally as a syrup or by rectal route

C. **Contraindications:** use in clients who require a low galactose diet; cautious use in clients with diabetes mellitus because of lactose and galactose content

NCLEX® D. **Side/adverse effects:** transient flatulence and intestinal cramps with initial dosing; diarrhea, dehydration, hypokalemia, and hypernatremia

NCLEX® E. **Nursing considerations:** monitor neurological status, serum ammonia levels, and fluid and electrolyte balance

F. **Client teaching:** intended effects and side effects of therapy

Check Your NCLEX–RN® Exam I.Q.

You are ready for testing on this content if you can:

- Apply knowledge of expected actions and effects of gastrointestinal medications to client care.
- Correctly administer gastrointestinal medications to clients.
- Assess for side effects and adverse effects of gastrointestinal medications.
- Take appropriate action if a client has an unexpected response to a gastrointestinal medication.
- Monitor a client for expected outcomes or effects of treatment with gastrointestinal medications.

PRACTICE TEST

1 A client who has been prescribed rabeprazole for symptoms of gastroesophageal reflux disease (GERD) has trouble swallowing pills. What alternate medication should the nurse expect to be prescribed for this client?

1. Omeprazole
2. Pantoprazole
3. Lansoprazole
4. IV esomeprazole

2 A nurse is teaching a female client newly diagnosed with *Helicobacter pylori* infection. The nurse expects that which medication will not be used after learning the client is pregnant?

1. Metronidazole
2. Amoxicillin
3. Clarithromycin
4. Calcium carbonate

3 A client is taking bismuth for diarrhea. For which side effect, unique to this medication, would a nurse monitor?

1. Darkening of the tongue
2. Dyspepsia
3. Abdominal pain
4. Diarrhea

4 A client's breath urease test is positive for *Helicobacter pylori* organisms. The nurse anticipates that which set of medications will be prescribed to eradicate this infection?

1. Antacids and amoxicillin
2. Omeprazole, ranitidine, and amoxicillin
3. Proton pump inhibitor, amoxicillin, and clarithromycin
4. Clarithromycin and bismuth salicylate

5 The nurse should interpret that which medication is prescribed at a safe and effective dosage range for an adult client who is experiencing nausea and vomiting?

1. Promethazine 25 mg every 4–6 hours prn
2. Prochlorperazine 200 mg every 6 hours
3. Metoclopramide 30 mg ac and HS
4. Trimethobenzamide hydrochloride 20 mg t.i.d. prn

PRACTICE TEST

6. A client is receiving omeprazole for esophageal reflux. The nurse should monitor the results of which laboratory studies? Select all that apply.

   1. Urinalysis
   2. Uric acid
   3. Liver enzymes
   4. Serum glucose
   5. Complete blood count (CBC)

7. When caring for a client with onset of severe nausea, the nurse telephones the healthcare provider for a prescription for which emetic that has the fastest onset of action?

   1. Oral promethazine
   2. Scopolamine transdermal
   3. Oral metoclopramide
   4. Haloperidol

8. A client has been diagnosed with severe erosive esophagitis. The nurse who is developing a medication teaching plan should anticipate that which medication is most appropriate to treat the disorder?

   1. Sucralfate
   2. Omeprazole
   3. Nizatidine
   4. Amoxicillin

9. A client has been advised to take an antacid to neutralize gastric acid and decrease pain from gastric irritation. What administration issues related to antacids should the nurse discuss with the client? Select all that apply.

   1. Chew the tablets and follow with 4 ounces of water.
   2. Take the antacid 2 hours after other prescribed oral medication.
   3. Take prescribed antacids on a regular basis for up to 6 weeks.
   4. Take antacids regularly after meals to prevent gastric irritation.
   5. Breastfeeding mothers can safely be prescribed the use of antacids.

10. A client who has a history of glaucoma is diagnosed with a gastrointestinal disorder. The nurse should consult with the healthcare provider if which medication is prescribed?

    1. Dicyclomine
    2. Omeprazole
    3. Metoclopramide
    4. Magnesium hydroxide

11. A client who needs to take a histamine H_2 antagonist has a history of multiple health problems. The nurse should explain that which drug should be avoided because it has the greatest number of drug interactions?

    1. Famotidine
    2. Ranitidine
    3. Nizatidine
    4. Cimetidine

12. A client newly diagnosed with a gastric ulcer has been prescribed sucralfate. Which beneficial effect related to this medication should the nurse explain to the client?

    1. It will reduce GI spasms.
    2. It will protect the eroded ulcer surface from stomach acid.
    3. It will help relieve nausea and vomiting.
    4. It will act as an anticholinergic.

13. A client with chronic pancreatitis has been prescribed pancrelipase. The nurse who is teaching the client about this medication should include that pancrelipase increases digestion of what types of nutrients?

    1. Proteins and starches
    2. Proteins and fats
    3. Starches and fats
    4. Vitamins and starches

14. A client with diarrhea for the past 24 hours reports taking loperamide the previous day per dosage instructions without relief. Currently, the client has a temperature of 102°F (38.9°C), excessive thirst, and severe abdominal cramping. What is the highest-priority action for the nurse at this time?

    1. Obtain a further history of digestive disorders.
    2. Discuss dietary factors that might be causing the diarrhea.
    3. Suggest acetaminophen for fever and pain.
    4. Notify the healthcare provider.

15 A parent of a 2-year-old child asks the nurse why bismuth subsalicylate should not be used to treat diarrhea in young children. The nurse should include which rationale in a response?

1. The taste is offensive to children.
2. It could lead to development of Reye syndrome.
3. It has a higher-than-recommended lead content.
4. The side effect of a darkened tongue frightens children.

16 The nurse is giving follow-up instructions to a client with irritable bowel syndrome (IBS). The nurse provides information about which medication that would be beneficial to treat both the diarrhea and constipation associated with IBS?

1. Methylcellulose
2. Docusate sodium
3. Dicyclomine
4. Bisacodyl

17 A 26-year-old female client who comes to the clinic for an annual health examination tells the nurse she will be getting married next month. The client has been taking misoprostol for several years following diagnosis of a gastric ulcer. What is the priority nursing intervention at this time?

1. Discuss whether to continue taking her oral contraceptive.
2. Discuss family planning.
3. Provide sexually transmitted infection (STI) counseling.
4. Explain the risks of using misoprostol during pregnancy.

18 A client with compensated congestive heart failure comes to the ambulatory care center reporting increased fatigue, weakness, and dizziness. Laboratory results indicate a low sodium level. Current medications include daily doses of furosemide, potassium, digoxin, and a prn bisacodyl suppository. What information would help determine the cause of the client's hyponatremia?

1. How frequently a bisacodyl suppository is used
2. Whether digoxin doses were skipped in the last week
3. Validation of compliance with prescribed amount of potassium
4. Frequency of dietary intake of salty foods in restaurants

19 A client with constipation has history of coronary artery disease and congestive heart failure. Which type of laxative is most appropriate for the nurse to recommend?

1. A bulk-forming laxative
2. A saline laxative
3. A stimulant laxative
4. PRN enemas

20 A client who comes to the clinic to get a prescription refill for dicyclomine hydrochloride tells the nurse she is leaving the next day for a vacation to Florida. What education should the nurse provide this client?

1. "Don't be so concerned about taking the medication on vacation."
2. "This medication makes you more sensitive to high temperatures."
3. "If you anticipate drinking alcohol, discontinue the medication."
4. "Take antacids with this medication to decrease any symptoms of GERD."

ANSWERS & RATIONALES

1 **Answer: 3 Rationale:** Lansoprazole capsules may be opened and sprinkled on applesauce or dissolved in 40 mL of juice; this is an appropriate substitution for the client who cannot swallow capsules or pills. Omeprazole and pantoprazole must be swallowed whole. Esomeprazole does not come in IV form; pantoprazole can be given IV over 15 minutes at a rate not more than 3 mg/min. **Cognitive Level:** Analyzing **Client Need:** Pharmacological and Parenteral Therapies **Integrated Process:** Nursing Process: Planning **Content Area:** Pharmacology **Strategy:** The core issue of the question is knowledge of the formulations of various proton pump inhibitors. Use medication knowledge and the process of elimination to make a selection. Eliminate the drug with the most invasive route of administration first.

2 **Answer: 3 Rationale:** Clarithromycin is not recommended for *Helicobacter pylori* infection during pregnancy. Metronidazole, amoxicillin, and calcium carbonate (an antacid) may be used by a pregnant client after consulting with the healthcare provider. **Cognitive Level:** Applying **Client Need:** Pharmacological and Parenteral Therapies **Integrated Process:** Nursing Process: Assessment **Content Area:** Pharmacology **Strategy:** The core issue of the question is knowledge of what medications are safe for use in pregnancy for a client with *Helicobacter pylori* infection. Use medication knowledge and the process of elimination to make a selection.

3 **Answer: 1 Rationale:** Bismuth-containing preparations can cause all the listed side effects, but transient darkening of the tongue and stool is a side effect specific to bismuth.

Dyspepsia, abdominal pain, and diarrhea can be caused by, but are not unique to, this medication. **Cognitive Level:** Applying **Client Need:** Pharmacological and Parenteral Therapies **Integrated Process:** Nursing Process: Assessment **Content Area:** Pharmacology **Strategy:** The critical word in the stem of this question is *unique*. This means that the answer is a side effect that does not occur with other drugs that are antidiarrheals. Use specific medication knowledge and the process of elimination to make a selection.

4 **Answer: 3 Rationale:** The highest rate of eradication of *Helicobacter pylori* infection is achieved by using a proton pump inhibitor and two antibiotics (usually clarithromycin and amoxicillin or metronidazole). Antacids/amoxicillin, omeprazole/ranitidine/amoxicillin, and clarithromycin/bismuth salicylate do not provide a level of effectiveness for eradication of *Helicobacter pylori*. **Cognitive Level:** Applying **Client Need:** Pharmacological and Parenteral Therapies **Integrated Process:** Nursing Process: Diagnosis **Content Area:** Pharmacology **Strategy:** The core issue of the question is knowledge of what medications are commonly used in treating *Helicobacter pylori* infection. Use medication knowledge and the process of elimination to make a selection.

5 **Answer: 1 Rationale:** Promethazine is usually given 25 mg every 4–6 hours prn. Dosing may start at 12.5 mg every 4–6 hours prn depending on client status; however, 25 mg is the usual dose. The normal dose of prochlorperazine is 5–10 mg t.i.d.–q.i.d; 200 mg is too high. The normal dose of metoclopramide is 10 mg, 30 minutes AC and HS; 30 mg is too high. The normal dose of trimethobenzamide hydrochloride is 250 mg t.i.d.–q.i.d. prn; 20 mg is too low. **Cognitive Level:** Applying **Client Need:** Pharmacological and Parenteral Therapies **Integrated Process:** Nursing Process: Diagnosis **Content Area:** Pharmacology **Strategy:** The core issue of the question is knowledge of the dosage range for various antiemetics. Use medication knowledge and the process of elimination to make a selection.

6 **Answer: 1, 3, 5 Rationale:** Urinalysis results should be monitored for hematuria and proteinuria. Omeprazole can cause an increase in liver enzyme levels (AST, ALT, alkaline phosphatase, and bilirubin), leading to adverse reactions of liver necrosis and hepatic failure. The nurse should monitor these lab values as they become available. It is rare, but agranulocytosis can occur; therefore, the CBC should be monitored to identify development of any hematological disorders. Uric acid should be monitored only as indicated based on an individual client's identified health need; there is no health need that indicates a need for this test. Omeprazole does not affect the serum glucose levels; monitoring is not necessary in relation to this drug administration. **Cognitive Level:** Analyzing **Client Need:** Pharmacological and Parenteral Therapies **Integrated Process:** Nursing Process: Planning **Content Area:** Pharmacology **Strategy:** The core issue of the question is knowledge of the laboratory values that could be affected by administration of omeprazole. With this group of medications, it is necessary to remember the liver and kidneys. Use medication knowledge and the process of elimination to make a selection. When more than one answer is correct, consider each option as a true/false statement.

7 **Answer: 2 Rationale:** All medications listed (promethazine, scopolamine, metoclopramide, and haloperidol) have antiemetic effects, but transdermal scopolamine has the fastest onset of action. For this reason, it is most effective in providing relief from nausea for a prolonged period of time. **Cognitive Level:** Applying **Client Need:** Pharmacological and Parenteral Therapies **Integrated Process:** Nursing Process: Implementation **Content Area:** Pharmacology **Strategy:** The core issue of the question is knowledge of onset of action of various antiemetics. Recall that transdermal systems begin to absorb into the skin immediately after application, while oral doses take various amounts of time to absorb through the GI tract. Use medication knowledge and the process of elimination to make a selection.

8 **Answer: 2 Rationale:** Because of their antisecretory effect, proton pump inhibitors such as omeprazole are the drugs of choice for moderate-to-severe erosive esophagitis. The course of therapy is usually 4–8 weeks. Sucralfate, nizatidine, and amoxicillin might be helpful for clients with *Helicobactor pylori*; however, proton pump inhibitors are the medication classification of choice for erosive esophagitis. **Cognitive Level:** Analyzing **Client Need:** Pharmacological and Parenteral Therapies **Integrated Process:** Nursing Process: Planning **Content Area:** Pharmacology **Strategy:** The core issue of the question is knowledge of the various GI medications that are useful in treating digestive system health problems. Recall that disorders that end in *-itis* involve inflammation, so the correct answer is one that reduces inflammation either by its own action or by inhibiting other irritants, such as gastric acid. Use medication knowledge of omeprazole as a proton pump inhibitor to make a selection.

9 **Answer: 1, 2, 4 Rationale:** Antacids should be chewed well and followed with 4 ounces of water for optimal effect. The client should allow at least 2 hours between taking the antacid and any other oral medication to avoid any issues related to absorption. Antacids should be taken regularly after meals in order to prevent gastric upset and provide better symptom control. Antacids should not be taken for longer than 2 weeks without further evaluation. Safety has not been established for the use of antacids by lactating women. **Cognitive Level:** Analyzing **Client Need:** Pharmacological and Parenteral Therapies **Integrated Process:** Nursing Process: Planning **Content Area:** Pharmacology **Strategy:** The core issue of the question is knowledge of medication administration procedures for antacids. Recall that antacids are more effective when given with fluid to help disperse medication in the stomach. Use medication knowledge and the process of elimination to make a selection. When more than one answer is correct, consider each option as a true/false statement.

10 **Answer: 1 Rationale:** Clients with glaucoma should not take anticholinergic agents such as dicyclomine because the medication affects pupillary dilatation, and therefore indirectly affects the outflow of aqueous humor. Prescribing omeprazole should not pose a problem for a client with glaucoma. It is safe to prescribe metoclopramide for gastric issues in a client with glaucoma. There are no contraindications regarding a client with glaucoma taking magnesium hydroxide. **Cognitive Level:** Analyzing **Client Need:** Pharmacological and Parenteral Therapies **Integrated Process:** Nursing Process: Intervention **Content Area:** Pharmacology **Strategy:** The core issue of the question is knowledge of medications that are contraindicated with glaucoma. Specific medication knowledge is needed to answer the question. Use medication knowledge and the process of elimination to make a selection.

11 **Answer: 4 Rationale:** Cimetidine decreases metabolism of beta-blockers, phenytoin, procainamide, quinidine, benzodiazepines, metronidazole, tricyclic antidepressants, and warfarin,

leading to increased risk of drug toxicity. Famotidine, ranitidine, and nizatidine are histamine-2 blockers that are newer than cimetidine, and have fewer side effects. **Cognitive Level:** Applying **Client Need:** Pharmacological and Parenteral Therapies **Integrated Process:** Nursing Process: Implementation **Content Area:** Pharmacology **Strategy:** The core issue of the question is knowledge of histamine antagonists that are highest in side or adverse effects. Specific medication knowledge is needed to answer the question. Use medication knowledge and the process of elimination to make a selection.

12 **Answer: 2 Rationale:** Sucralfate forms an adhesive barrier on the surface of the gastric mucosa, protecting it from gastric acid. Sucralfate does not help to reduce GI spasms. Sucralfate does not relieve nausea and vomiting. Sucralfate does not act as an anticholinergic. **Cognitive Level:** Applying **Client Need:** Pharmacological and Parenteral Therapies **Integrated Process:** Nursing Process: Implementation **Content Area:** Pharmacology **Strategy:** The core issue of the question is knowledge of the mechanism of action of sucralfate. Specific medication knowledge is needed to answer the question. Use this knowledge and the process of elimination to make a selection.

13 **Answer: 3 Rationale:** Pancrelipase, a pancreatic enzyme replacement, increases digestion of starches and fats, and thereby decreases the incidence of steatorrhea (fatty, frothy, foul-smelling stools). It does not increase the digestion of proteins and vitamins. **Cognitive Level:** Applying **Client Need:** Pharmacological and Parenteral Therapies **Integrated Process:** Teaching and Learning **Content Area:** Pharmacology **Strategy:** The core issue of the question is knowledge of the mechanism of action of pancrelipase. Specific medication and physiology knowledge is needed to answer the question. Use this knowledge and the process of elimination to make a selection.

14 **Answer: 4 Rationale:** Associated symptoms of fever, abdominal pain, and dehydration might suggest pathological diarrhea. The healthcare provider should be contacted for further evaluation. Obtaining a history of digestive disorders is appropriate but it is not the highest nursing priority. Identifying dietary factors that might be the cause of the diarrhea is not the highest nursing priority. Suggesting acetaminophen for fever and pain is an inappropriate nursing action. **Cognitive Level:** Analyzing **Client Need:** Pharmacological and Parenteral Therapies **Integrated Process:** Nursing Process: Implementation **Content Area:** Pharmacology **Strategy:** The stem of the question contains the critical words *highest priority*. This tells you that more than one of the options could be partially or totally correct. Use general nursing knowledge about diarrhea associated with fever, and the process of elimination, to make a selection.

15 **Answer: 2 Rationale:** Reye syndrome is a theorized complication of salicylate use in young children. Taste is not the primary or most important reason for not giving a child bismuth subsalicylate. Bismuth subsalicylate contains small amounts of naturally occurring lead, but it is not the most important reason for not giving the medication to a child. Darkening of the tongue may be frightening to a child, but it is not the primary issue for not giving a child bismuth subsalicylate. **Cognitive Level:** Analyzing **Client Need:** Pharmacological and Parenteral Therapies **Integrated Process:** Teaching and Learning **Content Area:** Pharmacology **Strategy:** Note the critical word *salicylate* in the stem of the question. Immediately associate this word with aspirin, which is contraindicated for use in children because of the risk of developing Reye syndrome.

16 **Answer: 1 Rationale:** Methylcellulose is a bulk-forming cellulose that absorbs intestinal fluids. This action helps prevent constipation and reduce or eliminate diarrhea. Docusate sodium is a laxative, which would not be effective in eliminating diarrhea. Dicyclomine is an antispasmodic medication, and not prescribed for constipation or diarrhea. Bisacodyl is a laxative and would not be prescribed for diarrhea. **Cognitive Level:** Applying **Client Need:** Pharmacological and Parenteral Therapies **Integrated Process:** Nursing Process: Diagnosis **Content Area:** Pharmacology **Strategy:** The core issue of the question is knowledge of a medication that relieves both constipation and diarrhea. With this in mind, you need to select a medication that regulates the bowel. Use medication knowledge and the process of elimination to make a selection.

17 **Answer: 4 Rationale:** A serious adverse effect of misoprostol is that a pregnant woman who takes the medication could experience a miscarriage. Misoprostol should be discontinued at least 1 month before pregnancy occurs. A discussion related to the client's use of oral contraceptives may be appropriate, but it has a lower priority than the discussion regarding adverse effects of misoprostol. A discussion related to family planning may be appropriate, but it has a lower priority than the discussion regarding adverse effects of misoprostol. Providing STI counseling is not supported by information in this question. **Cognitive Level:** Applying **Client Need:** Pharmacological and Parenteral Therapies **Integrated Process:** Nursing Process: Implementation **Content Area:** Pharmacology **Strategy:** The core issue of the question is associated risks of taking misoprostol during pregnancy. Eliminate the options that do not relate to misoprostol. Then choose the option that is more specific to the medication.

18 **Answer: 1 Rationale:** Bisacodyl is a stimulant laxative that can cause fluid and electrolyte imbalance. This can have additive effects because the diuretic use would also contribute to this finding. For this reason, the nurse should assess the use of the laxative. Determining whether digoxin doses were skipped in the last week, validating compliance with prescribed potassium, and determining frequency of dietary intake of salty foods in restaurants would not help determine the cause of the client's current symptoms. **Cognitive Level:** Analyzing **Client Need:** Pharmacological and Parenteral Therapies **Integrated Process:** Nursing Process: Diagnosis **Content Area:** Pharmacology **Strategy:** Note that the question contains the critical word *hyponatremia*. With this in mind, evaluate each option in terms of its relevance to the low sodium value. Eliminate each of the incorrect options because they would not cause the electrolyte imbalance stated in the question.

19 **Answer: 1 Rationale:** Bulk-forming laxatives, such as methylcellulose, absorb intestinal fluid, increasing stool volume, stimulating peristalsis, and decreasing straining on defecation. This type of laxative is the best choice for a client with a history of heart disease complicated by heart failure. A saline laxative is more likely to cause straining at stool for the client and therefore is less helpful for the client's overall status. A stimulant laxative is more likely to cause straining at stool for the client, and would not be recommended for a client with a history of heart disease and heart failure. PRN enemas are more likely to cause straining at stool for the client,

and therefore are less helpful for the client's overall status. **Cognitive Level:** Applying **Client Need:** Pharmacological and Parenteral Therapies **Integrated Process:** Nursing Process: Assessment **Content Area:** Pharmacology **Strategy:** The critical words in the stem of the question are *best choice*. This tells you that more than one option might be partially or totally correct, but one option is best. Keeping in mind that the client has heart disease, use the process of elimination to choose the bulk-forming laxative as least likely to cause strain on the heart.

20 **Answer: 2 Rationale:** Dicyclomine is an antispasmodic drug. Peripheral side effects include hot, flushed, dry skin; hyperthermia; and intolerance to high temperatures, manifested by dizziness. The client should not be advised to change the medication regimen because of vacation; this is an inappropriate comment by the nurse. The client should be reminded that any CNS effects of the medication will be enhanced by an intake of alcohol; but the nurse should not advise the client to discontinue the medication. There is nothing to indicate that the client has GERD. **Cognitive Level:** Analyzing **Client Need:** Pharmacological and Parenteral Therapies **Integrated Process:** Nursing Process: Planning **Content Area:** Pharmacology **Strategy:** The core issue of the question is adverse effects of dicyclomine. A clue in the question is the reference to Florida, which suggests that the option about effects of high temperature is the correct option.

Key Terms to Review

antacid p. 607
anticholinergics p. 600
antispasmodics p. 600
cathartic p. 603
emesis p. 605
H_2 antagonist p. 606
Helicobacter pylori p. 607
laxative p. 602
proton pump inhibitor p. 607
surfactant p. 604

References

Adams, M., Holland, L., & Urban, C. (2017). *Pharmacology for nurses: A pathophysiologic approach* (5th ed.). New York, NY: Pearson Education.

Adams, M., & Urban, C. (2016). *Pharmacology: Connections to nursing practice* (3rd ed.). New York, NY: Pearson Education.

Lehne, R. (2016). *Pharmacology for nursing care* (9th ed.). St. Louis, MO: Saunders.

Wilson, B., Shannon, M., & Shields, K. (2016). *Pearson nurse's drug guide 2016*. New York, NY: Pearson Education.

ANSWERS & RATIONALES

Endocrine Medications

41

In this chapter

Cross Reference

Other chapters relevant to this content area are

Dosage Calculation and Medication Administration	Chapter 29
Endocrine Disorders	Chapter 60

I. MEDICATIONS AFFECTING THE PITUITARY GLAND

A. Growth hormone (GH)

1. Regulates growth of organs and tissues, specifically length of long bones; replacement therapy is approved for use in children to treat growth hormone deficiency; GH suppressants are used to treat GH excess in children (gigantism) and adults (acromegaly)
2. Common medications that affect GH are listed in Table 41–1
3. Administration considerations
   a. Most are only given by subcutaneous (subcut) route; oral dose is inactivated by digestive enzymes; exception is bromocriptine, which is given orally

   NCLEX®

   b. Contraindicated for growth stimulation in children who are short unrelated to GH deficiency, during or after closure of epiphyseal plates in long bones, or with secondary intracranial tumors

Table 41–1 Drugs That Affect Growth Hormone (GH)

Generic Name	Actions/Uses
Bromocriptine	Suppresses GH level in children with GH excess in combination with octreotide
Lanreotide	Suppresses GH level in clients with acromegaly who have not responded to radiation therapy or are unable to tolerate surgery
Mecasermin	Recombinant DNA insulinlike growth factor (IGF) with same actions as GH; used for growth failure in children only (before bone epiphyses close)
Ocreotide	Suppresses intestinal peptide hormones, insulin, glucagons, and growth hormone
Pegvisomant	GH receptor antagonist
Somatropin	Used as GH replacement therapy

4. Side/adverse effects of GH replacement
   a. Metabolic: glucose intolerance, adrenocorticotropic hormone (ACTH) deficiency, or hypothyroidism

NCLEX®

   b. Renal: **hypercalciuria** (excess calcium excretion in urine) during first 2–3 months of treatment; risk of renal calculi with flank pain, colic, gastrointestinal (GI) upset, urinary frequency, chills, fever, and hematuria
   c. Local allergic reaction: pain and edema at injection site

NCLEX®

   d. Systemic allergic reaction: peripheral edema, headache, myalgia, and weakness
   e. Excess dosage: diabetes mellitus, atherosclerosis, enlarged organs, hypertension, and features related to acromegaly
5. Side/adverse effects of GH suppressants
   a. Most common are nausea and vomiting (N/V), diarrhea, headache, flushing, and injection site pain
   b. More serious effects are dysrhythmias (octreotide), elevated liver enzymes (pegvisomant), or hyper- or hypoglycemia (lanreotide)
6. Nursing considerations; ensure that growth rate is documented for at least 6–12 months prior to initiating treatment; ensure annual bone age assessments are performed
7. Client teaching for GH replacement
   a. Advise parents or caregivers about need for regular bone age assessments

NCLEX®

   b. An 8- to 13-cm (3- to 5-in.) growth rate is expected in first year and less in second year, with normal growth rate in subsequent years; subcutaneous fat diminishes during treatment but will return later
   c. Teach client/caregiver to document monthly height and weight measurements and to report any less-than-expected growth to prescriber

NCLEX®

   d. Teach signs and symptoms of slipped femoral epiphysis (hip or knee pain and limp) and to notify prescriber of same
8. Client teaching for GH suppressants
   a. Reconstitute gently (avoid shaking); inject solution at room temperature; rotate injection sites among abdomen, thighs, and buttocks
   b. Report jaundice, N/V, or right upper pain to prescriber (possible liver or gallbladder disease)
   c. Treatment is discontinued when adequate adult height is reached, epiphyseal plates fuse, or client fails to respond to GH

B. Antidiuretic hormone (ADH)

1. Promotes reabsorption of water; exerts vasopressor effect by constricting smooth muscle; increases aggregation of platelets

NCLEX®

2. Pituitary hormone replacement therapy for clients with diabetes insipidus (DI); also for use in hemophilia A, von Willebrand's disease type 1
3. Common medications for diabetes insipidus: see Box 41–1

Memory Aid

Medications that are pituitary hormone replacements usually end with the suffix *-pressin*.

4. Administration considerations
   a. Given by intranasal, subcut, IV, IM, or intra-arterial route as directed

NCLEX®

   b. Contraindicated with heart or vascular disease; vasoconstriction leads to elevated blood pressure (BP)
   c. Monitor serum and urine osmolality if given to treat diabetes insipidus
   d. Monitor Factor VIII coagulation level if given to promote hemostasis
5. Side/adverse effects
   a. Excess dosing can cause water intoxication; early signs are drowsiness, headache, and lethargy; later signs are seizures and coma
   b. Nasal congestion and irritation, rhinitis, abdominal cramps, nausea, heartburn, elevated BP, pain or swelling at injection site

NCLEX®

   c. IV route may cause anaphylaxis

Box 41–1

Drugs to Treat Diabetes Insipidus

Desmopressin

Vasopressin

6. Nursing considerations
   a. Give initial dose in evening to aid in uninterrupted sleep
   NCLEX® b. Check vital signs (VS), especially BP and pulse, before giving by IV and subcut routes
   c. Assess for mental status changes such as disorientation, lethargy, and behavioral changes related to fluid overload
   NCLEX® d. Measure daily intake and output (I&O) and daily weight to monitor water retention and sodium depletion; assess edema in extremities
   NCLEX® e. For nasal spray, inspect nares for intact nasal mucosa prior to dose
   f. Store nasal spray at room temperature; all other solutions need refrigeration
7. Client teaching
   a. Follow proper technique for nasal instillation (tube inserted into nostril to instill)
   b. May take missed dose up to 1 hour before next dose
   NCLEX® c. Report nasal congestion or upper respiratory tract infection to prescriber; also report signs of water retention such as shortness of breath and increases in weight, pulse, and BP

II. MEDICATIONS AFFECTING THE ADRENAL GLANDS

A. Mineralocorticoids

1. A **mineralocorticoid** is a steroid hormone that acts on kidneys to retain sodium and water and release potassium; synthesis is regulated by renin-angiotensin system
NCLEX® 2. Replacement therapy is required with adrenal gland failure or hypofunction (hypoaldosteronism)
3. Common medication: fludrocortisone

Memory Aid

Medications that replace hormones from the adrenal cortex (either glucocorticoid or mineralocorticoid) often have the syllable *cort* somewhere in the name.

4. Administration considerations
   a. Use with caution in disorders where fluid accumulation could be harmful, such as heart failure, hypertension, renal and possibly liver disease
   b. Monitor serum electrolyte levels because drug's hypokalemic effect may potentiate action of other drugs and hypernatremia can result if given with high-sodium drugs
5. Side/adverse effects
   a. Sodium and fluid retention, nausea, acne, thromboembolism
   b. Impaired wound healing, aggravation or masking of infection
   c. Anaphylactoid reactions are rare; may occur with hypersensitivity to glucocorticoids (fludrocortisone also has glucocorticoid properties)
6. Nursing considerations
   NCLEX® a. Used with glucocorticoids for replacement therapy
   b. Monitor serum electrolyte levels, weight, and I&O; report weight gain of 2.3 kg (5 lb) per week
   c. Monitor BP daily and more frequently during periods of dosage adjustment
   NCLEX® d. Check for signs of overdosage related to hypercorticism (psychosis, excess weight gain, edema, congestive heart failure [CHF], increased appetite, severe insomnia, and elevated BP)
   e. Check for signs of underdosage: weight loss, poor appetite, N/V, diarrhea, muscular weakness, increased fatigue, and low BP
7. Client teaching
   NCLEX® a. Report signs of low potassium associated with high sodium (muscle weakness, paresthesias, circumoral numbness, fatigue, anorexia, nausea, depression, delirium, diminished reflexes, polyuria, irregular heart rate, CHF, ileus)
   NCLEX® b. Eat foods high in potassium if so advised
   c. Salt intake regulates drug's effect: report signs of edema
   NCLEX® d. Weigh daily and report weight gain of 2.3 kg (5 lb) per week
   NCLEX® e. Report any infections, trauma, or unexpected stress, which may require increased dosage

B. *Glucocorticoids*

1. A glucocorticoid is a steroid hormone with metabolic effects on carbohydrate, protein, and fat metabolism, as well as anti-inflammatory and immunosuppressive activity
2. Synthesis is regulated by pituitary gland via negative feedback effect; may regulate metabolism of skeletal and connective tissues

3. Used in acute **adrenal insufficiency** (inability of adrenal glands to produce sufficient adrenocortical hormones) caused by trauma or thrombosis; chronic primary adrenal insufficiency (**Addison's disease**); and secondary adrenal insufficiency (diseased or destroyed adenohypophysis with inadequate production of ACTH)

NCLEX®
4. Many miscellaneous uses
   a. Allergic conditions (asthma, angioedema, transfusion reactions, and serum sickness)
   b. Dermatological conditions, such as dermatitis and pemphigus
   c. Inflammatory GI disorders, such as Crohn's disease and ulcerative proctitis
   d. Severe joint inflammation, bursitis, acute inflammatory states of arthritis, and systemic lupus erythematosus
   e. With antineoplastic agents to treat leukemias and lymphomas
   f. Transplant rejection prophylaxis
5. Common glucocorticoid medications are listed in Table 41–2
6. Administration considerations
   NCLEX® a. Routes of administration for systemic use to treat inflammatory conditions are IV, IM, and PO; routes for nonsystemic use are inhalation, nasal, ophthalmic, otic, and topical
   b. Contraindicated with systemic fungal infections and known hypersensitivity
   NCLEX® c. Monitor CBC and differential, serum electrolytes, and blood glucose (BG)
   d. With long-term therapy, monitor hypothalamic–pituitary–adrenal (HPA) axis function to check adrenal function

NCLEX®
7. Side/adverse effects
   a. Few side effects if high doses are given for only a few days
   b. Higher doses and prolonged therapy may alter tissue and organ metabolism, leading to muscle wasting and increased fat tissue deposits in trunk and face; changes in behavior and personality may also occur
   c. Prolonged therapy may suppress growth in children and lead to osteoporosis in adults; impaired glucose tolerance and diabetes mellitus may occur
   d. Prolonged therapy can suppress the HPA axis; **adrenal crisis** (acute, life-threatening state of profound adrenocortical insufficiency) may result if drug is abruptly withdrawn; taper dose slowly as ordered
   e. Toxicity may include anaphylactoid reactions, hypertriglyceridemia, peptic ulcers, acute pancreatitis, aseptic necrosis of bone, cataracts, glaucoma, hypertension, and opportunistic infections
   f. **Osteoporosis** (abnormal loss of bone density), decreased muscle mass, **cushingoid state** (having the appearance and facies characteristic of Cushing's disease), activation of latent tuberculosis or diabetes mellitus, vertebral compression fractures
8. Nursing considerations
   NCLEX® a. Check VS, BP, lung sounds, weight (including any history of gain or loss), N/V, and dependent edema
   b. Conduct mental status exam and assess for signs of depression, withdrawal, insomnia, and anorexia
   NCLEX® c. Check skin for striae, thinning, bruising, change in color, change in hair growth, and acne; with prolonged therapy, reposition immobilized clients carefully and limit use of adhesive tape on skin
   d. In children on prolonged therapy, monitor height and growth pattern
   e. Advise regular ophthalmic examinations with long-term therapy
   NCLEX® f. Check stool for occult blood periodically; GI bleeding could result
9. Client teaching
   NCLEX® a. Take oral doses with meals

Table 41–2 Drugs for Adrenal Replacement Therapy (Glucocorticoids)

Generic Name	Notes
Betamethasone	Little or no mineralocorticoid action
Cortisone acetate	Both mineralocorticoid and glucocorticoid action
Dexamethasone	Little or no mineralocorticoid action
Hydrocortisone	Both mineralocorticoid and glucocorticoid action
Methylprednisolone	Little mineralocorticoid action
Prednisolone	Both mineralocorticoid and glucocorticoid action
Prednisone	Little mineralocorticoid action
Triamcinolone	Little or no mineralocorticoid action

Box 41–2	
Drugs Used to Diagnose Adrenal Gland Insufficiency	Corticotropin HP Cosyntropin Metyrapone

b. If ordered every other day, take any missed dose immediately if remembered on same day; if remembered next day, take dose and readjust schedule to be every other day; do not double up missed doses

NCLEX® c. It may be advisable to lose weight, limit sodium intake, and increase potassium intake if excessive weight gain occurs

NCLEX® d. If diabetic, carefully monitor for increased BG levels

NCLEX® e. Report any blood in stool or black tarry stools, mood changes or insomnia, vision changes or headache, weight gain of more than 2.3 kg (5 lb) per week, irregular menses or pregnancy, irregular heart rate, excessive fatigue, severe abdominal pain, serious injury, or infection

f. Avoid strenuous activities if skin is fragile and bruises easily

g. Do not discontinue medication without notifying prescriber; do not increase or decrease dose on own; tapering of dose is necessary

h. Avoid immunizations during therapy and for 3 months after; avoid contact with anyone with measles or chickenpox or anyone receiving oral polio vaccine

i. Avoid skin testing during therapy

NCLEX® j. With long-term therapy, report any fever, cough, sore throat, malaise, and unhealed injuries; avoid contact with anyone with active infection

C. Adrenocorticotropic hormone (ACTH)

1. Directly stimulates adrenal cortex to synthesize adrenal steroids

NCLEX® 2. Used primarily to diagnose adrenal disorders such as Addison's disease and secondary adrenal insufficiency caused by pituitary dysfunction

3. Plasma cortisol levels are measured before and 1 hour after test dose; if no rise in cortisol then problem is in adrenal gland (Addison's disease; primary adrenocortical insufficiency); if cortisol level rises then problem is in hypothalamus or pituitary gland (secondary adrenocortical insufficiency)

NCLEX® 4. Limited use in treatment of adrenal insufficiency; corticosteroids used instead

5. Common medications for adrenal gland insufficiency are listed in Box 41–2; corticotropin and cosyntropin are used to diagnose etiology of insufficiency (Addison's disease versus CNS); metapyrone has an inhibiting action and is used to diagnose excess (Cushing's disease versus CNS)

6. Administration considerations: contraindicated with ocular herpes simplex, recent surgery, disorders such as CHF, scleroderma, osteoporosis, systemic fungoid infections, hypertension, sensitivity to porcine proteins, or conditions related to adrenocortical insufficiency or hyperfunction

7. Side/adverse effects

a. N/V, dizziness, drowsiness, or light-headedness

NCLEX® b. Hypersensitivity including urticaria, pruritus, and anaphylactic shock

8. Nursing considerations

NCLEX® a. Monitor VS and BP; observe closely for 15 minutes after dose for hypersensitivity reactions; assess for dizziness, fever, flushing, rash, and urticaria

b. Monitor plasma or urinary cortisol levels and serum electrolytes

9. Client teaching: drug action and possible results

III. MEDICATIONS AFFECTING THE THYROID GLAND

A. Thyroid hormones

1. Replacement therapy for **hypothyroidism** (decreased activity of thyroid gland with a variety of specific causes); have same action as naturally produced thyroid hormones in body

2. Used to diagnose and treat thyroid deficiency and **myxedema** (most severe form of hypothyroidism characterized by swelling of face, feet, and around eyes; may lead to coma and death), and to control goiter or thyroid carcinoma

3. Common medications for hypothyroid disorders are listed in Table 41–3

4. Administration considerations

NCLEX® a. Contraindicated in thyrotoxicosis, acute myocardial infarction (MI) and cardiovascular disease, morphologic hypogonadism, nephrosis, and uncorrected hypoadrenalism

Table 41–3 Drugs for Diagnosing and Treating Hypothyroid Disorders

Generic Name	Notes
Levothyroxine	Chemically pure form of T_4; preferred therapy for hypothythroidism Given IV for myxedema coma
Liothyronine	Chemically pure form of T_3; for adult hypothyroidism; not used for cretinism (T_3 does not cross blood–brain barrier as well as T_4).
Liotrix	Chemically pure T_4 and T_3 in 4:1 ratio; used for hypothyroidism
Dessicated thyroid	Older porcine formulation with less reliable concentrations than synthetic forms; used only by clients who have taken it for years

b. Use cautiously with cardiac disease; hypertension; renal insufficiency; pregnancy; concurrent use of **catecholamines** (drugs that mimic sympathetic nervous system effects); diabetes mellitus; **hyperthyroidism** (hyperfunction of thyroid gland), and malabsorption states

5. Side/adverse effects
   - *NCLEX®* a. Weight gain, vomiting, and tachycardia
   - *NCLEX®* b. Angina pectoris, coronary occlusion, or stroke in older adult or predisposed clients
   - c. Relative adrenal insufficiency in clients with inadequate pituitary function related to secondary hypothyroidism and secondary adrenal insufficiency; adrenal crisis
   - d. Overdosage causing signs of hyperthyroidism related to thyroid storm with shock and coma; thyrotoxicosis with CHF, angina, cardiac dysrhythmias, and shock
6. Nursing considerations
   - *NCLEX®* a. Assess VS, BP, weight and history of weight change, normal diet, energy level, mood, subjective feeling, and response to temperature
   - b. In children, check height
   - *NCLEX®* c. Monitor BG levels and results of thyroid function test results (serum T_4, free thyroxine, T_3 uptake, serum T_3, serum thyroid-stimulating hormone (TSH), protirelin test, thyroid uptake of radioiodine, TSH test, and thyroid suppression test)
   - d. Start older adults on lower dose and increase dose by small increments; assess for symptoms of stress that could lead to angina or stroke
7. Client teaching
   - a. Self-monitor pulse, weight, and height; wear medical alert identification
   - *NCLEX®* b. Adhere to dosage schedule and intervals; therapy is life-long; do not change brand without prescriber approval because of differences in bioavailability
   - *NCLEX®* c. Immediately report chest pain or other signs of aggravated cardiovascular disease
   - d. With juvenile hypothyroidism therapy, dramatic weight loss and catch-up growth can occur

B. Antithyroid medications

1. Used to treat hyperthyroidism and **Graves' disease** (pronounced hyperthyroidism often associated with enlarged thyroid gland and exophthalmos; also called thyrotoxicosis)
2. Common antithyroid medications are listed in Table 41–4
3. Administration considerations
   - a. Contraindicated with previous allergic or other severe reactions to thioamides
   - b. Impaired hepatic function may require reduced doses
   - *NCLEX®* c. Monitor results of laboratory studies: serum T_4, serum T_3, free T_4, free T_3, T_3 resin uptake, serum thyroid uptake of radioiodine, and thyroid suppression test

Table 41–4 Antithyroid Drugs

Generic Name	Notes
Methimazole	Inhibits thyroid hormone synthesis but not release.
Propylthiouracil	Inhibits thyroid hormone synthesis but not release; in peripheral tissues inhibits conversion of T_4 to T_3.
Potassium iodide (pima)	Has direct action on thyroid and used for short-term inhibition of thyroid hormone synthesis.
Radioactive iodide (^{131}I)	Radioisotope concentrates in thyroid and destroys tissue.

4. Side/adverse effects
   a. Fever, itching, skin rash, blood dyscrasias, peripheral neuropathy, joint pain and swelling, lupus-like syndrome
   NCLEX® b. Dizziness and alteration in taste
   c. Overdosage results in hypothyroidism
   d. Rare instances of agranulocytosis
5. Nursing considerations
   a. Assess for tingling of fingers and toes
   NCLEX® b. Monitor weight and check for hair loss and skin changes
   c. Check CBC, differential count, and thyroid and liver function tests
   NCLEX® d. Dilute oral iodine solutions well in milk, juice, or other beverage
   NCLEX® e. Assess for metallic taste in mouth, sneezing, edematous thyroid, vomiting, and bloody diarrhea
6. Client teaching
   a. Side effects may not appear for days or weeks after treatment begins
   NCLEX® b. Report fever, chills, sore throat, and unusual bleeding/bruising
   NCLEX® c. Take dose at same time of day and with meals or snack; space additional daily doses throughout day
   d. With radioactive iodine, clients may become hypothyroid and require thyroid hormone replacement; periodic thyroid evaluation is needed

IV. MEDICATIONS AFFECTING THE PARATHYROID GLANDS

A. Medications to treat hypocalcemia

NCLEX® 1. Calcium supplements replace calcium to supply body's metabolic needs, help maintain bone strength, and prevent calcium loss from bones
2. Used to treat mild hypocalcemia and to supplement dietary calcium; has additional use as antacid
3. Common medications for calcium deficiency are listed in Box 41–3
4. Administration considerations
   a. Given orally, dosage differs among different oral calcium salts
   NCLEX® b. Give with large glass of water and with meals or 1–1.5 hours after meals for better absorption

Memory Aid

Most drugs that directly or indirectly affect calcium levels will have *calci-* or *calc-* somewhere in the generic name.

   NCLEX® c. When used as antacid, should be given 1 hour after meals and at bedtime
   d. Contraindications: hypercalcemia, renal calculi, and hypophosphatemia
   NCLEX® e. Absorption may be reduced by foods such as spinach, Swiss chard, beets, bran, and whole grains
   f. Monitor results of periodic calcium levels for effectiveness
5. Side/adverse effects: constipation, flatulence, hypercalcemia (with frequent or high doses)
6. Nursing considerations
   NCLEX® a. Note number and consistency of stools; for constipation, a laxative or stool softener may be ordered
   b. With prolonged therapy, monitor weekly serum and urine calcium levels
   c. Observe for signs of hypercalcemia with frequent or high dosage
   d. Monitor for acid rebound if used as an antacid for more than 1–2 weeks
7. Client teaching
   NCLEX® a. Understand signs of hypercalcemia and report any N/V, constipation, frequent urination, lethargy, or depression

Box 41–3

Calcium Salts Used to Treat Mild Calcium Deficiency

Calcium acetate	Calcium gluconate
Calcium chloride	Calcium lactate
Calcium carbonate	Calcium phosphate tribasic
Calcium citrate	

NCLEX® b. Do not take with cereals or other foods high in oxalates that form insoluble, nonabsorbable compounds with calcium

c. If used as antacid, understand risk of acid rebound if used for more than 2 weeks

B. Vitamin D

1. Fat-soluble vitamin (can accumulate in body) needed for proper calcium absorption
2. Used to control hypocalcemia or vitamin D deficiency
3. NCLEX® Used in treatment of rickets, **osteomalacia** (abnormal loss of calcification of lamellar bone matrix, resulting in bone softening and fracture), and **hypoparathyroidism** (insufficient secretion by parathyroid glands caused by primary parathyroid dysfunction or abnormal serum calcium level)
4. Common medications for vitamin D deficiency are listed in Box 41–4
5. Administration considerations
   a. NCLEX® Adequate calcium is needed for optimal response to treatment
   b. Contraindications: hypercalcemia, vitamin D toxicity, malabsorption syndrome
6. Side/adverse effects
   a. Hypercalcemia from overuse (ataxia, fatigue, irritability, seizures, somnolence, tinnitus, hypertension, GI tract distress or constipation, and hypotonia in infants)
   b. NCLEX® Vitamin D hypercalcemia may lead to dysrhythmias in clients taking digoxin
   c. Hypervitaminosis D caused by large therapeutic doses may lead to hypercalcemia, hypercalciuria, bone pain, and calcium deposits in soft tissues
7. Nursing considerations
   a. NCLEX® Assess for any CNS problems; monitor BP, pulse, and I&O
   b. NCLEX® Monitor BUN, serum creatinine levels, serum calcium and phosphorus levels, serum alkaline phosphatase, and urinalysis
   c. If vitamin D toxicity occurs, make sure client stops drug immediately, drinks large amounts of fluid, and eats a low-calcium diet
8. Client teaching
   a. Make sure oral dose is swallowed intact without crushing or chewing tablet
   b. NCLEX® Consult prescriber before taking any OTC medications containing calcium, phosphorus, vitamin D, or substances high in vitamin D
   c. NCLEX® Do not drive or use heavy equipment if fatigue, vertigo, or weakness develop
   d. Avoid magnesium-containing antacids

C. Medications to treat hypercalcemia, osteoporosis, and *Paget's disease*

1. Reduce calcium release from bone, slow bone resorption and remodeling, and prevent high serum calcium concentrations
2. Specific drugs are used to treat hypercalcemia, Paget's disease (a nonmetabolic disease of bone), postmenopausal osteoporosis (abnormal loss of bone density), and heterotropic ossification after spinal cord injury and hip replacement
3. Common medications for calcium imbalances are listed in Box 41–5

Box 41–4

Drugs Used to Treat Vitamin D Deficiency

Calcitriol	Doxercalciferol
Cholecalciferol	Ergocalciferol
Dihydrotachysterol	Paricalcitol

Box 41–5

Drugs to Treat Hypercalcemia, Osteoporosis, and Paget's Disease

Bisphosphonates	*Miscellaneous Agents*
Alendronate	Calcitonin salmon
Etidronate	Cinacalcet
Ibandronate	Denosumab
Pamidronate	Raloxifene
Risedronate	Teriparatide
Tiludronate	
Zoledronate	

4. Administration considerations
   a. Given PO, IV, subcutaneously, or by intranasal spray (once daily in alternate nostrils)
   b. Contraindicated with known hypersensitivity or esophageal disorders
   c. Interacts with antacids, mineral supplements, calcium salts, vitamin D, and calcium-rich dairy products
   d. Decreased effects of digoxin occur when serum calcium is reduced
5. Side/adverse effects
   a. N/V, diarrhea, and dyspepsia with oral route
   b. Facial flushing and occasional inflammatory reaction at injection site
   c. Transient influenza-like symptoms with IV route
   d. Muscle spasms; leukopenia with chills, fever, or sore throat
   e. Nasal dryness and irritation with intranasal spray
   f. Allergic reactions with calcitonin salmon
   g. IV route may cause venous irritation, thrombophlebitis, nephrotoxicity (NCLEX®)
   h. Varying effects of hypocalcemia
   i. Toxicity with higher doses causes more severe hypocalcemia, GI distress such as severe esophagitis with ulceration, and severe nephrotoxicity
6. Nursing considerations
   a. Assess for signs of hypercalcemia (such as renal calculi) and hypocalcemia (tetany)
   b. Monitor weight and I&O if vomiting and diarrhea occur
   c. Monitor serum electrolytes, alkaline phosphatase, calcium and phosphorus, serum creatinine, BUN, liver function tests, CBC with differential, and urinalysis
   d. Monitor bone pain in clients with Paget's disease (NCLEX®)
   e. Check results of baseline values of bone mineral density (BMD) in hip, vertebrae, and forearm, and obtain periodic BMD values (NCLEX®)
7. Client teaching
   a. Depending on drug, teach how to self-administer subcut injection and to rotate sites
   b. Do not discontinue therapy without notifying MD
   c. Take PO doses of calcium regulators on empty stomach and remain upright for 30–60 minutes after taking (NCLEX®)
   d. Recognize signs of esophagitis; withhold drug and notify prescriber if difficulty swallowing or worsening heartburn occur (NCLEX®)
   e. Consume a diet sufficient in calcium and vitamin D; take in sufficient fluid (at least 6–8 glasses of water daily and possibly more if not contraindicated by other health problems) (NCLEX®)
   f. Understand use of metered-dose pump for nasal spray use; alternate nares

V. MEDICATIONS USED TO TREAT DIABETES MELLITUS

A. Insulin

1. Attaches to receptors on cell membranes to facilitate passage of glucose into cell; promotes conversion of glucose to glycogen; corrects **hyperglycemia** (higher than normal BG levels; normal BG is 70–110 mg/dL)
2. Treats type 1 diabetes mellitus (T1DM) and diabetic ketoacidosis (DKA); treats type 2 DM if oral antidiabetic agents are insufficient (NCLEX®)
3. Also lowers plasma potassium and magnesium levels (carried into cell with glucose); regular insulin IV and dextrose IV are used as emergency treatment of severe hyperkalemia
4. Types of insulin are listed in Table 41–5; premixed combinations of isophane and regular insulin are also available, see product literature (Humulin 70/30, Novolin 70/30, Humulin 50/50, Novolog Mix 70/30, and Humalog Mix 75/25) (NCLEX®)
5. Administration considerations
   a. Given only by injection (subcut, IM, IV); only regular insulin may be given IV; inactivated by digestive enzymes if given orally
   b. Injection sites include upper arms, thighs, abdomen, and infrascapular area (NCLEX®)
   c. One anatomical area is used at one time to maintain consistent absorption rates and prevent **lipodystrophy** (abnormal deposition of subcut fat at injection sites); sites within each area are used only once every 2–3 weeks and are 1.5 in. from previous site (NCLEX®)
   d. Only mix insulins that are compatible with one another and use according to manufacturer's guidelines (NCLEX®)
   e. Store unopened vials in refrigerator; opened vials can remain at room temperature for up to 1 month; do not freeze or place in warm areas (such as direct sunlight or hot car) (NCLEX®)
   f. Label vial with date and time opened and/or due to expire according to agency policy

Table 41–5 Types of Insulin Preparations

Action	Generic Name	Onset	Peak	Duration	Administration Notes
Rapid	Insulin lispro	5–15 min	0.5–1 hr	3–4 hr	Give subcut 5–10 min before meal; can give with isophane insulin (draw up lispro, aspart, or glulisine first) and give immediately
	Insulin aspart	10–20 min	1–3 hr	3–5 hr	
	Insulin glulisine	15–30 min	1 hr	3–4 hr	
Short	Insulin regular	30–60 min	2–4 hr	5–7 hr	Give subcut 30–60 min before meal; can give with isophane insulin (draw up regular first), but not glargine; can give IV if not mixed with isophane
Intermediate	Isophane insulin suspension	1–2 hr	4–12 hr	18–24 hr	Give subcut; cloudy in appearance; can mix with aspart, lispro, and regular, but not glargine
Long	Insulin detemir	Gradual	6–8 hr	Up to 24 hr	Give subcut 1–2 times daily; do not mix with any other insulins
	Insulin glargine	Gradual	None	Up to 24 hr	Give subcut once daily at same time of day; do not mix with any other insulins

Source: Adapted from Adams, M., & Urban, C. (2016). *Pharmacology: Connections to nursing practice* (3rd ed.). New York, NY: Pearson Education, Table 66.2, p. 1118.

g. Alternate methods of delivery include jet injectors, pen injectors, and portable and implantable insulin pumps

h. Insulin selection, doses, and timing are individualized to achieve glucose regulation in each client

NCLEX® i. Concurrent use of beta-adrenergic blocking agents could mask signs of hypoglycemia normally triggered by sympathetic nervous system (tachycardia and palpitations)

NCLEX® 6. Side/adverse effects

a. **Hypoglycemia** when BG level drops below 50 mg/dL (headache, confusion, drowsiness, fatigue, tachycardia, anxiety, sweating, and cool, clammy skin)

b. Coma related to inadequate insulin dosage as seen in uncontrolled diabetes with high BG levels and ketoacidosis or hyperosmolar coma

c. Coma related to insulin overdose caused by inadequate food intake, excessive exercise, or excessive insulin administration

7. Complications: lipodystrophy and local allergic reaction related to a contaminant in insulin preparation

8. Nursing considerations

a. Assess VS, weight, condition of skin and nails, and wound healing

NCLEX® b. Assess for long-term complications related to acceleration of atherosclerosis (hypertension, heart disease, stroke); retinopathy leading to possible blindness; nephropathy leading to possible renal failure; neuropathy leading to lower limb ulcerations and amputation, impotence, and gastroparesis

c. Consult with prescriber regarding insulin management when there is insufficient food intake or when client is NPO for surgery

d. Adhere to agency policy regarding insulin administration

NCLEX® e. Monitor results of random BG, fasting BG, glucose tolerance test, **glycosylated hemoglobin** A1C (represents average BG over past several weeks), serum electrolytes

f. Increase frequency of BG monitoring with fever, N/V, diarrhea, or other illness, to detect rises requiring adjustment of insulin dose

g. Check urine ketones if BG exceeds 250–300 mg/dL to detect early DKA

h. Be alert for signs of hypoglycemia and treat as indicated (15-gram carbohydrate snack or simple sugar if necessary)

9. Client teaching

NCLEX® a. Understand all aspects of insulin therapy, including syringe use, mixing of insulins, stability of mixture, injection technique and sites, and storage

NCLEX® b. Do not switch type or source of insulin or brand of syringe and avoid taking any new drug before notifying prescriber

NCLEX® c. Understand (and ensure family understands) signs of hyper- and hypoglycemia and self-treatment measures

d. Learn how to test BG levels

e. Follow dietary restrictions and weight control measures; consult dietitian

f. Engage in regular aerobic exercise appropriate to health and abilities

g. Understand foot care and related aspects of personal hygiene

NCLEX® h. Learn sick-day management of DM and insulin administration (continue to eat and take liquids as able, check BG, maintain insulin schedule, and call prescriber if BG is higher than 250 mg/dL)

i. Avoid smoking; avoid drinking alcoholic beverages unless approved by prescriber, since this can lead to hypoglycemia without proper food intake

j. Consult with prescriber before conceiving (if female)

k. Contact local home care agency and American Diabetes Association for additional follow-up and access to community-based resources

B. Oral antidiabetic (hypoglycemic) agents—sulfonylureas

1. Stimulate release of insulin from pancreatic islets
2. Used along with diet and exercise to reduce BG levels in type 2 DM
3. Common sulfonylurea medications are listed in Box 41–6
4. Administration considerations

a. Dose is given orally one to three times a day

b. Different agents possess different durations of action

NCLEX® c. May be used alone or prescribed with insulin

NCLEX® d. Contraindicated during pregnancy, in women who are nursing/lactating, or in clients allergic to sulfa or urea

Memory Aid

The classification name *sulfonylurea* provides the clue as to what allergies to look for as contraindications for use. Break the word into component parts. The syllable *sulf* can trigger an assessment of sulfa allergy, while *urea* should trigger an assessment of allergy to urea.

NCLEX® e. Beta-adrenergic blocking agents can suppress insulin release and delay response to hypoglycemia

5. Side/adverse effects

a. GI tract distress (nausea, heartburn)

b. Neurologic symptoms such as dizziness, drowsiness, or headache

NCLEX® c. Alcohol may cause a disulfiram-like reaction: flushing, palpitations, and nausea

d. Allergy noted by skin reaction

e. Blood dyscrasias and cholestatic jaundice

f. Hypoglycemia related to excess dosage, drug interactions, altered drug metabolism, or inadequate food intake, or because of renal or hepatic dysfunction

6. Nursing considerations

NCLEX® a. Assess VS, weight, condition of skin and nails, BG levels, glycosylated hemoglobin, and electrolyte and arterial blood gas levels as appropriate

b. Assess for long-term complications of diabetes as noted in previous section regarding nursing considerations with insulin

NCLEX® c. Consult with prescriber regarding management when client has insufficient food intake or is NPO for surgery

7. Client teaching

NCLEX® a. Principles are similar to those discussed in previous section for insulin therapy

b. Participate in individualized teaching plan based on previous knowledge, educational level, motivation to learn, and cultural considerations

c. Understand all aspects of drug therapy; take with food if GI upset

d. Take medication even if not feeling well

e. Take dose with first daily meal and take any missed dose as soon as remembered unless time for next dose; do not double up doses

NCLEX® f. Understand sick-day management of diabetes and PRN insulin administration

Box 41–6

Oral Antidiabetic Agents (Sulfonylureas)

First-Generation Agents	Second-Generation Agents
Chlorpropamide	Glimepiride
Tolbutamide	Glipizide
Tolazamide	Glyburide

g. Consult with prescriber before conceiving (females); discontinue drug during pregnancy and lactation (may need insulin)

C. Oral antidiabetic (hypoglycemic) agents—nonsulfonylureas

1. Act in a variety of ways; combination drugs are also available
   a. Biguanides decrease production and release of glucose by liver, increase glucose uptake by cells, and lower lipid levels
   b. Alpha-glucosidase inhibitors delay absorption of digested carbohydrates, which reduces BG elevation after meals
   c. Thiazolidinediones or "glitazones" inhibit glucose production in liver and increase cellular sensitivity to insulin
   d. Metiglinides stimulate insulin release from pancreas
   e. Incretin enhancers act as either DPP-4 inhibitors (prevent breakdown of incretins, which are hormones released by small intestine in response to meals) or GLP-1 agonists (which increase insulin secretion, decrease glucagon secretion, delay gastric emptying, and increase satiety)

NCLEX®

2. All decrease BG levels after meals in clients with type 2 DM not controlled by diet and exercise
3. Common nonsulfonylurea medications are listed in Box 41–7; note that several combinations of oral antidiabetic agents are available; read drug inserts carefully for administration and client teaching purposes
4. Administration considerations
   a. Given orally one to three times a day
   b. Alpha-glucose inhibitors are contraindicated with GI disorders such as bowel inflammatory disease, and bowel obstruction, and should be used cautiously in clients with GI distress or liver disease
   c. NCLEX® Thiazolidinediones should be used cautiously in clients with liver disease; may cause liver damage
   d. Biguanides and alpha-glucosidase inhibitors should not be taken together because of significant GI distress
   e. NCLEX® Alcohol may increase risk of hypoglycemia or lactic acidosis
5. Side/adverse effects
   a. All groups except biguanides have risk of hypoglycemia (tremors, palpitations, sweating)
   b. Other common side effects include GI symptoms such as anorexia, N/V, diarrhea, abdominal discomfort or flatulence
   c. Decreased vitamin B_{12} levels can occur with biguanides and incretin enhancers
   d. Lactic acidosis can occur with biguanides
   e. Symptoms of upper respiratory infection can occur with metiglinides, thiazolidinediones, and incretin enhancers
   f. Miscellaneous adverse effects: anaphylaxis and pancreatitis (metiglinides); hepatotoxicity, bone fractures, heart failure and myocardial infarction (thiazolidinediones); and angioedema, Stevens-Johnson syndrome (sitagliptin)
6. NCLEX® Nursing considerations
   a. Assess VS, weight, condition of skin and nails, serum BG levels, glycosylated hemoglobin, and electrolyte and arterial blood gas levels as appropriate
   b. NCLEX® Assess renal function and liver function studies

Box 41–7

Oral Antidiabetics/ Hypoglycemics (Nonsulfonylureas)

Alpha-Glucosidase Inhibitors	**Incretin Enhancers (DPP-4 Inhibitors)**
Acarbose	Alogliptin
Miglitol	Linagliptin
Biguanide	Saxagliptin
Metformin	Sitagliptin
Incretin Enhancers (GLP-1 Agonists)	**Meglitinides**
Albiglutide	Nateglinide
Exenatide	Repaglinide
Dulaglutide	**Thiazolidinediones**
Liraglutide	Pioglitazone
	Rosaglitazone

c. Assess for early signs of lactic acidosis (biguanide: metformin)
d. Assess for long-term complications of diabetes mellitus
e. Consult with prescriber regarding management when client has insufficient food intake or is NPO for surgery

NCLEX®

7. Client teaching
   a. Understand all aspects of diabetic management as outlined in previous client education section for sulfonylureas
   b. Understand early signs of hypoglycemia and lactic acidosis (hyperventilation, myalgia, malaise, unusual somnolence) and notify prescriber immediately if symptoms occur

D. Glucose-elevating medication—glucagon

1. Promotes breakdown of glycogen in liver (glycogenolysis) and converts amino acids to glucose (gluconeogenesis)

NCLEX®

2. Used for emergency treatment of severe hypoglycemia in clients who are unconscious or unable to swallow
3. Administration considerations
   a. Reconstitute according to manufacturer's directions

   NCLEX®

   b. Give IM, subcut, or by direct IV push; flush IV line with 5% dextrose instead of sodium chloride (NaCl) solution; incompatible with NaCl solutions or additives
   c. Incompatible in syringe with any other medication
   d. Contraindicated with hypersensitivity to glucagon or protein compounds
   e. Use cautiously in insulinoma and pheochromocytoma
4. Side/adverse effects: N/V, hypersensitivity, hyperglycemia, hypokalemia

NCLEX®

5. Nursing considerations

   NCLEX®

   a. Client usually responds/awakens within 5 to 20 minutes after administration, which is slower than response time to IV glucose

   NCLEX®

   b. After client awakens and is able to swallow, give oral carbohydrate
   c. After recovery, assess for persistent headache, nausea, and weakness

NCLEX®

6. Client teaching
   a. Proper testing of BG levels
   b. Be sure responsible family member knows how to administer subcut or IM dose to treat hypoglycemic reactions
   c. Notify prescriber immediately after reaction to determine cause

Check Your NCLEX–RN® Exam I.Q.

You are ready for testing on this content if you can:

- Apply knowledge of expected actions and effects of endocrine medications to client care.
- Correctly administer endocrine medications to clients.
- Assess for side effects and adverse effects of endocrine medications.
- Take appropriate action if a client has an unexpected response to an endocrine medication.
- Monitor a client for expected outcomes or effects of treatment with endocrine medications.

PRACTICE TEST

1 A young child who has been taking growth hormone for 1 month is complaining of flank pain, colic, and GI symptoms. The nurse concludes that this client is at increased risk for which adverse effect that is more likely to occur during the first few months of treatment?

1. Acute glomerulonephritis
2. Renal calculi
3. Bowel obstruction
4. Duodenal ulcer

2 A client with coronary artery disease and hypertension was recently diagnosed with diabetes insipidus. For what reason should the nurse conclude that treatment with antidiuretic hormone (ADH) is contraindicated for this client?

1. Fluid overload and elevated BP could occur.
2. Volume depletion and decreased BP could occur.
3. Overstimulation and agitation could occur.
4. Hypercalciuria and renal calculi could occur.

3 A client with cardiovascular disease has been recently diagnosed with hypothyroidism, and levothyroxine has been prescribed. Which manifestation related to this medication is most important for the client to report to the prescriber?

1. Increased urine output
2. Chest pain
3. Increase in appetite
4. Loose stools

4 A client with a history of cardiac disease is exhibiting severe symptoms of hypothyroidism, and is started on medication therapy with levothyroxine. The nurse anticipates that which principle will be followed for initiation of drug therapy?

1. Start with the highest dose, and titrate according to the client's response.
2. Start with the highest dose and give a beta blocker to prevent tachycardia.
3. Start with a low dose and gradually increase the dose over a period of weeks.
4. Administer a fixed dose calculated by client's weight; adjust as necessary.

5 A client with acute adrenal insufficiency (adrenal crisis) is admitted to the hospital. The nurse monitors for resolution of which manifestation to determine that drug therapy with cortisone has been effective? Select all that apply.

1. Restlessness
2. Weight loss
3. Vitiligo
4. Hypertension
5. Cardiac angina episodes

6 The nurse is assessing the laboratory data of a client diagnosed with Cushing's syndrome. The nurse would expect to note which laboratory values prior to initiation of drug therapy? Select all that apply.

1. Elevated plasma cortisol level
2. Decreased blood glucose level
3. Increased white blood cell count
4. Increased sodium level
5. Increased potassium level

7 The nurse is caring for a client who has just been diagnosed with Graves' disease. During client education, the nurse should include what information?

1. Atropine-like medications are safe to use.
2. Thyroid hormone replacement therapy is necessary.
3. A low-calorie diet will be ordered.
4. Propylthiouracil (PTU) will be prescribed.

8 A client with Graves' disease has been taking medication therapy as prescribed. Which finding, noted on cardiac assessment, indicates to the nurse that the client has not had a sufficient response to medication therapy?

1. Decreased systolic blood pressure
2. Narrowed pulse pressure
3. Bradycardia
4. Tachycardia

9 The nurse is caring for a client who recently was diagnosed with hypoparathyroidism. To determine the effectiveness of medication therapy with calcitrol, the nurse should assess laboratory findings to see if what change has occurred?

1. Hypercalcemia is resolving.
2. Hypocalcemia is resolving.
3. Hypermagnesemia is resolving.
4. Vitamin D levels are decreasing.

10 A client with type 2 diabetes mellitus has been prescribed pioglitazone. Which test does the nurse anticipate will be done before drug therapy is initiated with this medication?

1. Liver function tests
2. Thyroid function tests
3. Respiratory function tests
4. Pituitary function tests

11. A client newly diagnosed with adrenal insufficiency is to begin therapy with fludrocortisone. What therapeutic effect of this medication should the nurse explain to the client?

1. Decreases resorption of sodium by decreasing hydrogen and potassium excretion in the distal tubule
2. Increases resorption of sodium by increasing hydrogen and potassium excretion in the distal tubule
3. Decreases inflammation by suppressing migration of leukocytes and eliminating the body's immune response to certain stimuli
4. Increases inflammation by stimulating the production of leukocytes and enhancing the body's immune response to many stimuli

12. A homebound client with type 2 diabetes mellitus calls the nurse to report nausea and flulike symptoms for 2 days. What advice should the nurse give the client?

1. "Be sure to check your blood glucose level in the morning on a daily basis."
2. "Take half of your regular dose of insulin and oral hypoglycemic agent."
3. "Limit fluid intake, and eat only when you feel hungry."
4. "Test your urine for ketones if your blood glucose is higher than 240 mg/dL."

13. A client, just diagnosed with hypothyroidism, also takes sodium warfarin. Before giving any thyroid replacement hormone, the nurse should check the results of what laboratory value?

1. Complete blood count (CBC)
2. Prothrombin time (PT) or international normalized ratio (INR)
3. Activated partial thromboplastin time (APTT)
4. Warfarin level

14. A client who has been receiving calcium supplements for osteoporosis on a long-term basis is beginning drug therapy with digoxin. For what type of drug interaction would the home care nurse assess during future visits?

1. Hypocalcemia
2. Hyperkalemia
3. Digoxin toxicity
4. Hypermagnesemia

15. The nurse who is working in a women's health clinic has several clients to see during the day. Which client does the nurse anticipate will need medication teaching for calcium supplementation to treat primary osteoporosis?

1. A premenopausal client
2. An overweight client
3. An African American client
4. A Caucasian client

16. A client with osteoporosis has been prescribed hormone replacement therapy (HRT) in addition to calcium supplements. The nurse teaches the client that progesterone is given along with estrogen in this therapy to decrease occurrence of what condition?

1. Vaginitis
2. Endometrial or breast cancer
3. Benign breast tumors
4. Ovarian cysts

17. A client newly diagnosed with diabetes mellitus (DM) has begun taking insulin. The client asks the nurse about alcohol consumption. What information should the nurse provide to the client?

1. "Moderate-to-high alcohol consumption without food can cause your blood glucose level to go down too low."
2. "Moderate-to-high alcohol consumption without food can cause your blood glucose level to rise too high."
3. "Consumption of alcohol has no effect on your blood glucose, as long as you don't eat while drinking."
4. "As long as you only drink beer and wine, and not hard liquor, there should be no effect from the alcohol."

PRACTICE TEST

18 The nurse is instructing the newly diagnosed diabetic client how to mix regular insulin and isophane insulin. What should the nurse tell the client?

1. Shake the bottle of isophane insulin before withdrawing the amount.
2. Withdraw the isophane insulin first.
3. Withdraw the regular insulin first.
4. Inject air into the bottle of regular insulin first.

19 Metformin has been prescribed for a client newly diagnosed with type 2 diabetes mellitus. Which client statement about this medication validates to the nurse that the client understood the teaching?

1. Decreases sensitivity of peripheral tissue to insulin
2. Stimulates glucose production in the liver
3. Treats unstable type 2 diabetes mellitus
4. Decreases production of glucose by the liver

20 The healthcare provider has prescribed vitamin D for a client. The client asks the nurse about the purpose of the medication. What is the best response by the nurse?

1. "Vitamin D decreases intestinal absorption of calcium and phosphorus."
2. "Vitamin D helps regulate calcium and phosphorus balance."
3. "Vitamin D helps the kidneys rid the body of excess calcium and phosphorus."
4. "Vitamin D decreases blood levels of calcium and phosphorus."

ANSWERS & RATIONALES

1 **Answer: 2 Rationale:** Adverse/side effects during the first 2–3 months of treatment with growth hormone include hypercalciuria, with resultant renal calculi. The client taking growth hormone is not at increased risk for acute glomerulonephritis, bowel obstruction, or duodenal ulcer. **Cognitive Level:** Analyzing **Client Need:** Pharmacological and Parenteral Therapies **Integrated Process:** Nursing Process: Diagnosis **Content Area:** Pharmacology **Strategy:** Note the critical words in the question are *first few months*. This tells you that the adverse effect occurs soon after the start of medication therapy. Use medication knowledge and the process of elimination to make a selection.

2 **Answer: 1 Rationale:** Clients with coronary artery insufficiency and hypertensive cardiovascular disease who take ADH are at increased risk for developing fluid overload and edema. Volume depletion and decreased BP are the opposite of what can occur with this client. Overstimulation and agitation are not related to this client's situation. Hypercalciuria and renal calculi are not related to this client's situation. **Cognitive Level:** Analyzing **Client Need:** Pharmacological and Parenteral Therapies **Integrated Process:** Nursing Process: Diagnosis **Content Area:** Pharmacology **Strategy:** Note that two of the options are opposite, which could be a clue that one of them is correct. Recall that ADH causes fluid retention to link this information with the associated risks for a client with cardiac disease.

3 **Answer: 2 Rationale:** Clients with known cardiovascular disease who are prescribed thyroid hormone replacement therapy can develop chest pain that could lead to myocardial infarction. For this reason, it is the most important manifestation for the client to report. Increased urine output, increased appetite, and loose stools should be reported, but are of lesser priority. **Cognitive Level:** Analyzing **Client Need:** Pharmacological and Parenteral Therapies **Integrated Process:** Nursing Process: Planning **Content Area:** Pharmacology **Strategy:** The critical words in the stem of the question are *most important*, which tell you that more than one answer might be correct, and that you must prioritize your answer. Use the ABCs (airway, breathing, and circulation) to select the answer most important to a client with cardiac disease (which affects circulation).

4 **Answer: 3 Rationale:** Clients with severe symptoms of hypothyroidism and a history of cardiac disease must be started on the lowest dose possible of hormone therapy and have the dose gradually increased in order to prevent onset of severe hypertension, heart failure, and myocardial infarction (MI). Weight would not be an appropriate calculation factor. The highest possible starting dose, with or without a beta blocker, puts the client at risk for chest pain and subsequent MI. **Cognitive Level:** Analyzing **Client Need:** Pharmacological and Parenteral Therapies **Integrated Process:** Nursing Process: Planning **Content Area:** Pharmacology **Strategy:** The core issue of the question is knowledge of the principles of beginning a medication that stimulates metabolism in a client with heart disease. Use knowledge of pathophysiology to select the option that causes the least stress on the heart during initiation of therapy.

5 **Answer: 2, 3, 5 Rationale:** Clients with acute adrenal insufficiency will report anorexia, which generally leads to weight loss. Clients with acute adrenal insufficiency will exhibit integumentary symptoms such as vitiligo. Clients with acute adrenal insufficiency will exhibit cardiovascular symptoms related to anemia, such as angina. Lethargy, not restlessness, is seen with adrenal insufficiency. Hypotension, not hypertension, is seen with adrenal insufficiency. **Cognitive Level:** Analyzing **Client Need:** Pharmacological and Parenteral Therapies **Integrated Process:** Nursing Process: Evaluation **Content Area:** Pharmacology **Strategy:** The wording of the question tells you that the core issue is knowledge of signs and symptoms of adrenal insufficiency that should respond to drug therapy. Use nursing knowledge and the process of elimination to make a selection. When more than one answer is correct, consider each option as a true/false statement.

6 **Answer: 1, 3, 4 Rationale:** Clients with Cushing's syndrome or hypercortisolism have elevated levels of cortisol; drug therapy will reduce serum cortisol levels when given as directed. Clients with Cushing's syndrome or hypercortisolism have elevated white blood cell counts. Clients with Cushing's syndrome or hypercortisolism have increased sodium levels. Decreased blood glucose levels are opposite of what would be expected in Cushing's syndrome. An increased serum potassium level is opposite of what would be expected in Cushing's syndrome. **Cognitive Level:** Analyzing **Client Need:** Pharmacological and Parenteral Therapies **Integrated Process:** Nursing Process: Assessment **Content Area:** Pharmacology **Strategy:** The core issue of the question is knowledge of laboratory values that are expected to change once drug therapy is initiated for Cushing's syndrome. Use nursing knowledge and the process of elimination to make a selection. When more than one answer is correct, consider each option as a true/false statement.

7 **Answer: 4 Rationale:** Graves' disease is caused by elevated levels of thyroid hormone. Clients experience tachycardia, nervousness, insomnia, increased heat production, and weight loss. Medication therapy with an agent such as propylthiouracil will help control the disorder. Atropine-like drugs are contraindicated for clients with hyperthyroidism. Initiation of thyroid hormone replacement therapy would be indicated for hypothyroidism. A client with Graves' disease needs a high-calorie diet, not a low-calorie one; behavioral and metabolic activity increases, which results in weight loss. **Cognitive Level:** Analyzing **Client Need:** Pharmacological and Parenteral Therapies **Integrated Process:** Nursing Process: Planning **Content Area:** Pharmacology **Strategy:** The core issue of the question is the type of medication therapy that will be effective in treating hyperthyroidism or Graves' disease. Use nursing knowledge and the process of elimination to make a selection.

8 **Answer: 4 Rationale:** Cardiac problems related to Graves' disease and hyperthyroidism include increased systolic blood pressure, a widened pulse pressure, tachycardia, and other dysrhythmias. Appropriate control of the disorder with medication therapy would prevent these manifestations from occurring. **Cognitive Level:** Applying **Client Need:** Pharmacological and Parenteral Therapies **Integrated Process:** Nursing Process: Assessment **Content Area:** Pharmacology **Strategy:** The core issue of the question is knowledge of which symptoms should resolve once medication therapy for Graves' disease has begun. Recall that Graves' disease represents a hypermetabolic state, and then eliminate each option that does not correlate with excessive metabolic activity.

9 **Answer: 2 Rationale:** Management of hypoparathyroidism is aimed at correcting hypocalcemia, vitamin D deficiency, and hypomagnesemia. Hypercalcemia is an opposite manifestation and not appropriate to hypoparathyroidism. Hypermagnesemia is an opposite manifestation and not appropriate to hypoparathyroidism. A decreasing vitamin D level is the opposite of effective treatment of hypoparathyroidism. **Cognitive Level:** Applying **Client Need:** Pharmacological and Parenteral Therapies **Integrated Process:** Nursing Process: Diagnosis **Content Area:** Pharmacology **Strategy:** The core issue of the question is knowledge of abnormal laboratory values that should resolve with effective medication therapy for hypoparathyroidism. Use knowledge of medication actions to eliminate each of the incorrect options. Two options are opposite, which is a clue that one of them is likely to be the correct answer.

10 **Answer: 1 Rationale:** Pioglitazone is a thiazolidinedione type of oral antidiabetic agent; its action enhances insulin action and promotes glucose utilization in peripheral tissues. This drug improves sensitivity to insulin in muscle and fat tissue, and inhibits glucogenesis. Because of the potential for liver damage, clients taking drugs in this class must have liver function studies done before therapy is begun, and periodically thereafter. Thyroid, respiratory, and pituitary function tests are not necessary before beginning therapy with pioglitazone. **Cognitive Level:** Applying **Client Need:** Pharmacological and Parenteral Therapies **Integrated Process:** Nursing Process: Planning **Content Area:** Pharmacology **Strategy:** The core issue of this question is knowledge of the adverse effects of thiazolidinedione antidiabetic agents. Recall as a general strategy that many drug classes have adverse effects on the liver. Use medication knowledge and the process of elimination to make a selection.

11 **Answer: 2 Rationale:** Adrenocortical replacement therapy medications are divided into mineralocorticoids and glucocorticoids. Mineralocorticoids such as fludrocortisone increase resorption of sodium by increasing hydrogen and potassium excretion in the distal tubule. Glucocorticoids decrease inflammation by suppressing leukocyte migration, but they do not eliminate the body's immune response. Glucocorticoids decrease inflammation by suppressing leukocyte migration and modifying the body's immune response. **Cognitive Level:** Applying **Client Need:** Pharmacological and Parenteral Therapies **Integrated Process:** Teaching and Learning **Content Area:** Pharmacology **Strategy:** Specific medication knowledge about the effects of mineralocorticoid drug therapy is needed to answer this question. Use medication knowledge and the process of elimination to make a selection.

12 **Answer: 4 Rationale:** To prevent diabetic ketoacidosis, this client must regularly check urine ketone levels if the blood glucose level is higher than 240 mg/dL. If anorexia, nausea, or vomiting is present, sick-day diabetic management care requires clients to check their blood glucose level every 4–6 hours. Clients should not eliminate or adjust their doses of insulin or oral hypoglycemics. Meals should be eaten at regular times, and clients should consume foods and liquids that are more easily tolerated. **Cognitive Level:** Applying **Client Need:** Pharmacological and Parenteral Therapies **Integrated Process:** Teaching and Learning **Content Area:** Pharmacology **Strategy:** The core issue of the question is knowledge of how to manage medication therapy for a diabetic client during illness. With this in mind, choose the option that does not decrease the drug dose (since blood glucose rises during illness), and that provides for safe and effective treatment (contacting the prescriber when the level is excessive).

13 **Answer: 2 Rationale:** Thyroid hormones increase the effects of anticoagulants. Assessment of PT or INR will determine if the anticoagulant dosage must be decreased. The nurse also assesses the client for evidence of bruising or bleeding. A CBC could detect anemia caused by bleeding as a complication of excessive warfarin therapy, which should be monitored on a regular basis; however, it is not an essential test prior to thyroid replacement hormone therapy. APTT measures the effectiveness of heparin, and would not be appropriate for a client on Coumadin therapy. Thyroid hormones increase the effects of anticoagulants. Assessment of PT or INR will determine if the anticoagulant dosage must be decreased. Warfarin levels are not drawn. **Cognitive Level:** Analyzing **Client Need:** Pharmacological and Parenteral Therapies **Integrated Process:** Nursing Process: Assessment

Content Area: Pharmacology **Strategy:** The core issue of the question is an understanding of interactive effects of thyroid hormones and anticoagulants such as warfarin. Use knowledge of both medications and associated laboratory values to make a selection.

14 **Answer: 3 Rationale:** Digitalis toxicity could result when calcium supplements interact with digoxin. Clients must be instructed to take these two drugs at separate times of the day. Hypercalcemia could result when calcium supplements interact with digoxin. Clients must be instructed to take these two drugs at separate times of the day. Also, antacids must not be taken with digoxin. Hyperkalemia is not a concern with calcium supplementation. Hypomagnesemia could result when calcium supplements interact with digoxin. **Cognitive Level:** Analyzing **Client Need:** Pharmacological and Parenteral Therapies **Integrated Process:** Nursing Process: Assessment **Content Area:** Pharmacology **Strategy:** The core issue of the question is knowledge of the effects of calcium supplements in a client who also takes digoxin. Use knowledge of medication interactions and the process of elimination to make a selection.

15 **Answer: 4 Rationale:** Primary osteoporosis is more prevalent in Caucasian and Asian women. Primary osteoporosis most often occurs in postmenopausal women. Primary osteoporosis most often occurs in women who are thin and lean-built. Primary osteoporosis is not as prevalent in African American women. **Cognitive Level:** Analyzing **Client Need:** Pharmacological and Parenteral Therapies **Integrated Process:** Nursing Process: Diagnosis **Content Area:** Pharmacology **Strategy:** The core issue of the question is knowledge of the clients at risk for osteoporosis and amenable to therapy with calcium supplementation. Use general nursing knowledge and the process of elimination to make a selection.

16 **Answer: 2 Rationale:** Progesterone frequently is given along with estrogen as part of HRT to minimize the occurrence of endometrial or breast cancer. This regimen does not decrease the incidence of vaginitis, benign breast tumors, or ovarian cysts. **Cognitive Level:** Applying **Client Need:** Pharmacological and Parenteral Therapies **Integrated Process:** Teaching and Learning **Content Area:** Pharmacology **Strategy:** The core issue of the question is knowledge of the adverse effects of HRT given in addition to calcium supplementation for prevention or treatment of osteoporosis. Use knowledge of adverse drug effects and the process of elimination to make a selection.

17 **Answer: 1 Rationale:** Because of the risk of alcohol-induced hypoglycemia, clients must ingest alcohol only with or shortly after meals. If diabetes is well controlled, blood glucose levels are not affected by mild consumption of alcohol; however, food should be ingested shortly before, after, or during alcohol intake. The client should confer with the prescriber and dietitian to determine whether alcohol may be utilized as part of the overall caloric intake. The effects of alcohol on a diabetic client do not change in regard to the source of the alcohol. Male clients taking insulin may ingest two alcoholic beverages daily, and female clients may ingest one alcoholic beverage with, or in addition to, the regular meal plan. **Cognitive Level:** Applying **Client Need:** Pharmacological and Parenteral Therapies **Integrated Process:** Communication and Documentation **Content Area:** Pharmacology **Strategy:** The core issue of the question is knowledge of how alcohol can affect blood glucose levels in a client taking insulin. Use knowledge of interactive effects of medications and alcohol to make a selection.

18 **Answer: 3 Rationale:** The regular insulin should be withdrawn first to prevent the isophane insulin from mixing in the bottle with the regular insulin. Gently roll the bottle of isophane insulin to mix because vigorous shaking creates bubbles, leading to an inaccurate dose. Air must be injected into each bottle before withdrawing; first into the bottle of isophane insulin, and then into the bottle of regular insulin. **Cognitive Level:** Applying **Client Need:** Pharmacological and Parenteral Therapies **Integrated Process:** Teaching and Learning **Content Area:** Pharmacology **Strategy:** The core issue of the question is proper technique for drawing up mixed insulins. Choose the option that does not contaminate the regular insulin with the isophane insulin, which would necessitate discarding the contaminated vial.

19 **Answer: 4 Rationale:** Metformin is given to clients with stable type 2 diabetes mellitus to inhibit glucose production by the liver and increase sensitivity of peripheral tissue to insulin. Metformin does not stimulate glucose production in the liver. Metformin is not the drug of choice to treat unstable type 2 diabetes mellitus. Metformin does not decrease sensitivity of peripheral tissue to insulin. **Cognitive Level:** Analyzing **Client Need:** Pharmacological and Parenteral Therapies **Integrated Process:** Nursing Process: Evaluation **Content Area:** Pharmacology **Strategy:** The core issue of the question is knowledge of the actions of metformin on reducing blood glucose. Use medication knowledge and the process of elimination to make a selection.

20 **Answer: 2 Rationale:** Vitamin D regulates calcium and phosphorus levels by increasing blood levels, increasing intestinal absorption and mobilization from bone, and reducing renal excretion of both elements. Vitamin D does not decrease intestinal absorption of calcium and phosphorus. Vitamin D does not help the kidneys excrete excess calcium and phosphorus. Vitamin D does not decrease blood levels of calcium and phosphorus. **Cognitive Level:** Applying **Client Need:** Pharmacological and Parenteral Therapies **Integrated Process:** Teaching and Learning **Content Area:** Pharmacology **Strategy:** The core issue of the question is knowledge of the effects of vitamin D. Use medication knowledge and the process of elimination to make a selection.

Key Terms to Review

Addison's disease p. 620
adrenal crisis p. 620
adrenal insufficiency p. 620
catecholamine p. 622
cushingoid state p. 620
glucocorticoids p. 619
glycosylated hemoglobin p. 626
Graves' disease p. 622
hypercalciuria p. 618
hyperglycemia p. 625
hyperthyroidism p. 622
hypoglycemia p. 626
hypoparathyroidism p. 624
hypothyroidism p. 621
lipodystrophy p. 625
mineralocorticoid p. 619
myxedema p. 621
osteomalacia p. 624
osteoporosis p. 620
Paget's disease p. 624

References

Adams, M., Holland, L., & Urban, C. (2017). *Pharmacology for nurses: A pathophysiologic approach* (5th ed.). New York, NY: Pearson Education.

Adams, M., & Urban, C. (2016). *Pharmacology: Connections to nursing practice* (3rd ed.). New York, NY: Pearson Education.

Lehne, R. (2016). *Pharmacology for nursing care* (9th ed.). St. Louis, MO: Saunders.

Wilson, B., Shannon, M., & Shields, K. (2016). *Pearson nurse's drug guide 2016.* New York, NY: Pearson Education.

Test Yourself

Are you ready for the NCLEX-RN® or course exams? Access the NEW web-based app that provides students with thousands of practice questions in preparation for the NCLEX experience.

42 Integumentary Medications

In this chapter

Cross Reference

Other chapters relevant to this content area are

Dosage Calculation and Medication Administration	Chapter 29
Integumentary Disorders	Chapter 62

I. GENERAL AND PROTECTIVE AGENTS

A. Lotions, emollients, protectants, and cleansers

1. Lotions are either a liquid emulsion or a suspension of a powder in water; may have a drying effect on skin as water evaporates; shake any lotion before applying to skin; common preparations include calamine lotion, zinc stearate, and others
2. *NCLEX®* Some preparations of calamine lotion also contain diphenhydramine, which can cause drowsiness; use cautiously until effect is known
3. Emollients are occlusive agents that make skin soft by hydrating and filling gaps in stratum corneum created by dry, contracted skin cells
4. Emollients include silicone oils, propylene glycol, isopropyl palmitate, and octyl stearate; ingredients such as petrolatum, lanolin, cocoa butter, or mineral oil prevent evaporation of water from skin
5. *NCLEX®* Emollients can also function as skin protectants if they soothe **pruritus** (intense itching) due to exposed, traumatized nerve endings
6. Protectants are designed to protect skin from wetness or prevent and treat diaper rash, prickly heat, and/or chafing; they may be packaged as medicated ointments or powders, and often contain zinc oxide or petrolatum
7. Excessive flaking of skin on scalp that occurs with dandruff can be treated by use of 1% lotion of selenium sulfide or a shampoo that contains selenium
8. Specific cleansing agents may be used for clients who have specific needs; chlorhexidine cleanses and reduces microbe counts on skin; hydrogen peroxide is an antiseptic solution that may damage healing skin but is useful for cleansing debris from wound tubes such as tracheostomy tubes; povidone-iodine is used as a scrub on intact skin before surgery or other invasive procedures but can impair healing of skin wounds

NCLEX® 9. Nursing considerations: assess any skin symptom; apply to skin after bathing while skin is slightly moist unless otherwise directed; monitor for desired effect

NCLEX® 10. Client teaching
   a. Keep powders away from face to avoid inhalation
   b. Some preparations should not be used on broken skin
   c. If skin irritation or diaper rash worsens or does not improve within 7 days of treatment, consult healthcare provider

B. Soaks and wet dressings

NCLEX® 1. Soaks and wet dressings are useful in treating acute lesions that are oozing, weeping, and crusting, while scaling chronic lesions tend to respond best to moisturizing, lubricating preparations

NCLEX® 2. Open soaks are applied for 20 minutes, three times a day

3. Closed soaks use a water-impermeable substance (occlusion) over a wet soak to cause heat retention, which is excellent for debridement but may lead to skin maceration; are applied for 1–2 hours two to three times a day
4. Continuous closed soaks are left in place for 24 hours to treat thick crusts; it is important to rewet dressing four to five times a day
5. Common preparations include Burow's solution, acetic acid 0.1–1% solution, or a salt solution
6. Nursing considerations: assess any skin symptom and monitor for achievement of intended effects
7. Client teaching: proper procedure for type of soak recommended or prescribed

C. Rubs and liniments

1. Over-the-counter (OTC) preparations for temporary relief of minor aches and pains of muscles and joints associated with strains, bruises, sprains, sports injuries, simple backache, and arthritis
2. Contain various antiseptics, analgesics, local anesthetics; some contain salicylates that could lead to salicylate side effects (nausea and vomiting [N/V] or tinnitus) if used extensively
3. Common preparations often include salicylate or capsaicin (from cayenne pepper) as active ingredient
4. Nursing considerations: assess causative symptom, assess for allergy to ingredient (salicylates or cayenne) and monitor for effects of treatment

NCLEX® 5. Client teaching
   a. Remove other ointments (water in oil emulsions), creams, sprays, or liniments before applying product
   b. Apply to affected areas not more than three to four times daily
   c. Some products have specific directions (e.g., not to use with heating pad or tight bandage because skin irritation or burning could occur)

D. Sunscreen preparations

1. Help to prevent sunburn and later skin cancer by absorbing rays of ultraviolet (UV) light
2. Chemical absorbers formulated against UVB rays include cinnamates, p-aminobenzoic acid (PABA) and PABA esters, or salicylates; those formulated against UVA rays include benzophenones
3. Physical sunscreens reflect or scatter light to prevent skin penetration and contain ingredients such as titanium dioxide, zinc oxide, talc

NCLEX® 4. Effectiveness is indicated by sun protection factor (SPF); a SPF of 15 means product offers 15 times greater protection than no sunscreen; SPFs range from 4 to 70+

5. Sunscreens should be applied 30–60 minutes before sun exposure and should be reapplied after swimming, sweating, and every 2–3 hours; a minimum SPF of 15 is recommended

II. ANTIPRURITICS

A. Overview

1. Antipruritics stop intense itching of pruritis
2. Pruritus has a multitude of causes, and treatment must be tailored to specific cause
3. Types include winter pruritus, senior pruritus, lichen simplex chronicus, external otitis, pruritus ani (e.g., pinworm infestation in children), and genital pruritus
4. Antipruritic therapy for some types of pruritis might include topical corticosteroids to decrease inflammation and/or methods to promote skin hydration
5. Antipruritic therapy may also require use of a systemic antihistamine, such as hydroxyzine, chlorpheniramine, or cyproheptadine hydrochloride

B. Common topical preparations often contain ingredients such as colloidal oatmeal, mineral oil, glyceryl stearate, camphor, menthol, and phenol

C. Nursing considerations

1. Topical medications are often available OTC but oral medications may be prescribed if relief is insufficient
2. Take a history of systemic symptoms and any associated skin symptoms
3. *NCLEX®* Monitor for intended effects and any local or systemic adverse effects of any topical preparation
4. *NCLEX®* Monitor for drowsiness or other anticholinergic side effects if systemic antihistamines are used

NCLEX® **D. Client teaching**

1. Bathe less frequently, use mild soaps only, and use soap sparingly
2. Understand need to interrupt itch-and-scratch cycle because of negative effect of scratching
3. Maintain cool environment, especially in bedroom for sleep
4. Try to eliminate environmental source of trigger if possible

III. ANTI-INFECTIVES

A. Antibacterials

1. Topical antibiotics inhibit growth of *Staphylococcus* and *Streptococcus* on skin
2. Topical antibacterial therapy may be used prophylactically to prevent infections in wounds and injuries and to treat mild skin infections; oral antibiotic therapy may be needed for more serious infections
3. Common topical anti-infectives are bacitracin, erythromycin, gentamicin, metronidazole, mupirocin, neomycin, and tetracycline
4. *NCLEX®* Nursing considerations
   a. Assess skin lesion carefully and assess for hypersensitivity to antibacterial agent
   b. Monitor for healing or development of skin irritation or superinfection
5. *NCLEX®* Client teaching
   a. Wash hands before using any topical antibacterial agent; may wear gloves
   b. Generally, apply products sparingly and gently to affected area
   c. With some, a dressing should be applied; with others, it should not: follow product instructions
   d. Report lack of healing or worsening of condition

B. Antivirals

1. Used to treat cutaneous **herpes simplex** (an acute viral disease marked by groups of skin vesicles, often on borders of lips, nares, or genitals) or herpes zoster
2. With some infections an oral agent instead of a topical agent may be needed
3. Common medication: acyclovir 5% ointment

Memory Aid

Antiviral agents often can be recognized on sight because they contain *vir* in the beginning, middle, or end of the name.

4. *NCLEX®* Nursing considerations: assess skin symptoms and monitor for local adverse effects of topical product, such as mild pain, burning, stinging
5. *NCLEX®* Client teaching
   a. Wash hands before use and apply gloves or finger cot when applying product to avoid autoinnoculation of other body sites
   b. Apply as soon as symptoms of herpes lesions begin
   c. Apply sparingly and gently to affected area
   d. Wear loose clothing and keep area clean and dry
   e. Avoid sexual activity when skin lesions are present

C. Antifungals

1. Fungal infections of the skin, such as **tinea pedis** (athlete's foot) and tinea cruris (jock itch), tend to occur in warm, moist areas of body that are covered by clothing
2. Topical antifungals can be used if infection is mild and limited to glabrous (smooth, hairless) skin; clients with extensive disease or infection of hair and nails are best treated with systemic therapy
3. *NCLEX®* Advantages of topical use over systemic use: absence of serious adverse reactions or drug interactions, OTC availability of some preparations, ability to localize treatment to affected sites, no need to monitor laboratory tests

4. Common medications
   a. Topical agents are listed in Box 42–1
   b. Oral agents include fluconazole, griseofulvin, itraconazole, ketoconazole, and terbinafine

Memory Aid

Antifungal agents are easy to recognize on sight because they generally end with the suffix *-azole*.

5. Nursing considerations
   a. Assess skin symptom and predisposing factors, such as trauma, general health, suppressed immune status, hygiene practices, and exposure to infectious agent
   NCLEX® b. Monitor for intended effects and for local adverse effects (irritation, burning, or stinging)
   NCLEX® c. Monitor for skin sensitization, noted by increased redness, swelling, weeping, or any burning or itching not present before treatment began
   d. Systemic effects of topical products are negligible, since absorption rates are low

NCLEX® 6. Client teaching
   a. Use products as directed for full course of therapy (may be prolonged); apply liberally to clean and dry skin
   b. Leave exposed to air; do not apply protective dressing unless specifically prescribed
   c. Wear shower shoes or foot thongs in public or communal showers and locker rooms (tinea pedis)
   d. Avoid going barefoot, and wear footwear of natural fibers (leather shoes, cotton or wool socks) to prevent tinea pedis; change socks daily
   e. To avoid other fungal infections such as tinea cruris, keep affected areas clean, dry, and well ventilated (loose clothing), and use powders (with or without antifungal ingredients) to keep skin dry and prevent maceration

D. Antiparasitics

1. Used to treat infestations such as **scabies** (infestation caused by mites) or **pediculosis** (infestation caused by lice); may involve hair (tinea capitus), body (tinea corporis), or pubic area (tinea pubis)
2. Recurrence of scabies is generally related to reinfection from incomplete treatment but mite resistance may occur
3. Crotamiton can be used in clients with scabies and pediculosis capitis who are ragweed-sensitive
4. Common antiparasitics are listed in Table 42–1; oral ivermectin may be used for hard-to-treat head lice
5. Nursing considerations
   a. Assess skin symptom at baseline and during treatment
   NCLEX® b. Monitor for local adverse effects (irritation, pruritis, burning, stinging)
   c. Monitor for systemic effect of dizziness with lindane because it affects nervous system; avoid use in infants, children, and clients with known seizure disorders because of risk of seizures

Box 42–1

Topical Antifungals

Allylamines

Naftifine hydrochloride: cream gel

Terbinafine: cream

Imidazoles

Clotrimazole: cream, solution, lotion, vaginal tablets, cream

Betamethasone dipropionate with clotrimazole: cream, lotion

Econazole: cream

Ketoconazole: cream, shampoo

Miconazole: cream, powder, spray, vaginal suppository or cream

Oxiconazole: cream, lotion

Sulconazole nitrate: cream, solution

Miscellaneous

Ciclopirox: cream, lotion

Undecylenic acid: cream, powder

Nystatin: cream, ointment, powder, vaginal tablet

Tolnaftate: cream, solution, spray, liquid, powder, gel

Table 42–1 Antiparasitics

Agent	Uses
Crotamiton	Scabies
Malathion	Pediculosis capitis and their ova
Permethrin	Pediculosis capitis, scabies
Pyrethrin	Pediculosis capitis, pediculosis corporis, pediculosis pubis
Lindane	Pediculosis capitis, pediculosis pubis, scabies

NCLEX®

6. Client teaching: scabies
   a. Apply thin layer to dry skin from neck down over body; rub in thoroughly
   b. Permethrin and lindane: leave on 8–12 hours, remove thoroughly with washing
   c. Crotamiton: apply again after 24 hours, wash to remove it 48 hours after initial application

NCLEX®

7. Client teaching: pediculosis capitis
   a. Lindane lotion: apply lotion to dry hair, rub in thoroughly, leave on 12 hours, remove thoroughly
   b. Lindane shampoo: apply shampoo to dry hair, lather with small amount of water, work into hair for 4 minutes, rinse thoroughly
   c. Second treatment in 7–10 days may be needed with malathion

IV. CORTICOSTEROIDS

A. Overview

1. Topical corticosteroids are typically used to treat dermatitis, including atopic dermatitis (eczema), seborrheic dermatitis (a type of eczema), contact dermatitis (hypersensitivity response), psoriasis, and intertrigo
2. Responsiveness to topical corticosteroids varies: highly responsive diseases include psoriasis, atopic dermatitis in children, seborrheic dermatitis, intertrigo
3. Penetration of preparation varies according to skin site
4. Increased incidence of adverse reactions can occur when used on thin skin or under occlusive dressing, or in older adult or pediatric clients
5. Adverse effects more common in higher potency preparations
6. Local adverse reactions include atrophy, hypopigmentation, striae (NCLEX®)
7. Topical corticosteroids can cause systemic adverse reactions, including suppression of adrenal function (NCLEX®)
8. Low-potency agents are best used for diffuse eruptions, those involving face or occluded areas such as axilla or groin, and chronic dermatoses
9. Medium-potency agents are appropriate for acute flare-up of chronic dermatoses and acute self-limited eruptions with treatment periods of 14–21 days
10. High-potency agents are best for acute localized eruptions for only 7–14 days, but should be avoided on face, intertriginous areas, and perineum (areas susceptible to increased penetration and adverse reactions)
11. A twice-a-day application is usually sufficient; more frequent application does not appear to improve response
12. Mid- or high-potency corticosteroids should not be discontinued abruptly; may result in rebound flare-up of disorder (NCLEX®)

Memory Aid

A corticosteroid drug can often be recognized because it ends in the suffix *-sone* or *-one*. As an alternative, it may contain *cort* in the beginning, middle, or end of the drug name.

B. Common medications are listed in Box 42–2

C. Nursing considerations

1. Assess skin symptom at baseline and during therapy
2. Generally, corticosteroids are applied sparingly and gently in a thin film to affected area (NCLEX®)
3. Monitor for local adverse effects (acneiform skin eruptions, dryness, itching, burning, allergic contact dermatitis, hypopigmentation, overgrowth of bacteria/fungi/viruses)

Box 42-2

Topical Corticosteroids

Low Potency	Mometasone furoate 0.1%
Alclometasone 0.05%	Prednicarbate 0.1%
Desonide 0.05%	Triamcinolone acetonide 0.025–0.1%
Dexamethasone 0.1%	**High Potency**
Hydrocortisone 0.25–1%	Amcinonide 0.1%
Medium Potency	Fluocinonide 0.025%
Betamethasone benzoate 0.025%	Halcinonide 0.025%
Betamethasone valerate 0.1%	**Very High Potency**
Clocortolone 0.1%	Augmented betamethasone dipropionate 0.05%
Desoximetasone 0.025%	Clobetasol propionate 0.05%
Fluocinolone acetonide 0.025%	Diflorasone diacetate 0.05%
Flurandrenolide 0.025%	Halobetasol propionate 0.05%
Fluticasone propionate 0.05%	
Hydrocortisone valerate 0.2%	

NCLEX® 4. Monitor for systemic adverse effects, which are more likely to include hirsutism (usually of face), moon facies, alopecia (scalp area), and immunosuppression

NCLEX® **D. Client teaching**

1. Before using, wash and dry area gently; use exactly as directed; do not overuse
2. Do not apply to open wounds or weeping areas
3. Report worsening of condition, signs of infection, or lack of healing

V. KERATOLYTICS

A. Overview

1. Reduce thickness of hyperkeratotic stratum corneum (remove or soften this layer of skin)
2. Used to treat disorders such as actinic keratosis (rough, red or brown skin lesions on arms, back of hands, face, and scalp) caused by prolonged exposure to sun

B. Common keratinolytic medications are listed in Box 42–3; alpha-hydroxy acid and sulfur are ingredients with keratolytic action that may be found in some skincare products

NCLEX® **C. Nursing considerations**

1. Assess any skin symptom initially and during treatment as needed
2. Monitor for local adverse effects of topical preparations

NCLEX® **D. Client teaching**

1. Understand purpose, use, side effects, and anticipated length of treatment
2. Apply as directed; method will vary somewhat depending on use

VI. MEDICATIONS TO TREAT PSORIASIS

A. Overview

1. Reduce symptoms of **psoriasis**, a chronic inflammatory skin disorder characterized by red raised patches of skin with flaky thickened scales called plaques
2. Suppress rapid turnover of cells that give skin lesions their typical appearance

B. Common medications for psoriasis are listed in Box 42–4; consist of topical and systemic agents and systemic biologic drugs that interfere with immune component of psoriasis

Box 42–3

Keratinolytic Medications

Aminolevulinic acid

Diclofenac sodium 3%

Fluorouracil

Imiquimod 5% cream

Box 42-4

Medications to Treat Psoriasis

Topical Agents	Systemic Agents Including Biologicals
Anthralin	Acetretin
Calcipotriene	Alefacept
Coal tar	Cyclosporine
Corticosteroids	Methotrexate
Keratolytics	Ustekinumab
Tazarotene	

NCLEX®

C. Nursing considerations

1. Assess skin lesions initially and during treatment to determine effectiveness of therapy
2. Phototherapy may be used in addition to drug therapy to improve results
3. Anthralin: can cause skin redness or local irritation and may stain clothing, hair, and skin; apply at bedtime to remain on skin overnight
4. Calcipotriene: may take up to 1–3 weeks to achieve desired results; may cause local irritation; hypercalcemia could result from high-dose applications (vitamin D analogue)
5. Tazarotene: vitamin A derivative applied in evening (once daily) to affected skin; instruct client to use sunscreen and protective clothing (drug causes sensitization to light); assess for mild skin reactions (redness, itching, burning, dryness of skin) and more serious skin reactions (rash, desquamation, bleeding, development of inflammation or fissures)
6. Acetretin: derivative of vitamin A; teratogenic and embryotoxic; hepatotoxic effects include elevated triglyceride level and reduced HDL cholesterol level
7. Cyclosporine: immunosuppressant that inhibits both B and T cells; used for severe cases not responding to first-line agents; assess renal function (nephrotoxic)
8. Methotrexate: reduces epidermal cell proliferation; assess for GI side effects (such as diarrhea), signs of bone marrow depression (blood dyscrasias), and hepatotoxicity
9. Alefacept: reduces $CD4^+$ T lymphocytes; monitor $CD4^+$ T-cell count during therapy; contraindicated for clients with HIV infection or who have a history of malignancy (drug increases risk of developing cancer)
10. Ustekinumab: monoclonal antibody that reduces immune system activity but increases risk of some cancers; do not administer live virus vaccine during treatment and assess household members' need for vaccine; do not administer bacille Calmette-Guerin (BCG) vaccine from 1 year prior to drug treatment until 1 year after treatment is completed

NCLEX®

D. Client teaching

1. Monitor skin lesions regularly to determine effectiveness of therapy
2. Monitor for local adverse effects of topical preparations and systemic adverse effects of systemic medications and report them as directed to prescriber
3. See preceding nursing considerations section for relevant teaching points for individual medications
4. Acitretin: use two reliable forms of contraception beginning 1 month prior to treatment and continuing until at least 3 years after termination of treatment; if pregnancy occurs, notify prescriber and discuss options regarding pregnancy; take dose with meals and avoid alcohol and concurrent vitamin A supplements

VII. MEDICATIONS TO TREAT ACNE

A. Overview

1. Generally, a staged approach is used
2. Mild **acne** (noninflammatory and inflammatory lesions often on face, chest, back) with some comedones or few inflammatory lesions is treated with topical agents such as benzoyl peroxide (an OTC keratinolytic), salicylic acid, and topical antibiotics
3. Moderate acne consisting of *comedones* (blackheads) and **papules** (small, circumscribed, superficial, solid elevations of skin) can be managed by gradually increasing strength of topical tretinoin
4. Severe acne consisting of inflammatory papules and nodulocystic disease requires systemic antibiotics and isotretinoin
5. Choice of vehicle for topical preparation depends on whether client has dry or oily skin

Box 42–5

Medications to Treat Acne

Topical Retinoids	Oral Drug Therapy
Adapalene	Doxycycline
Azelaic acid	Erythromycin
Tazarotene	Isotretinoin
Tretinoin	Minocycline
Topical Antibiotics	Tetracycline
Clindamycin*	**Hormonal Therapy**
Erythromycin*	Oral contraceptives
Clindamycin and tretinoin gel	
Dapsone	
Sulfacetamide sodium	

*May be combined with benzoyl peroxide

NCLEX® 6. Local adverse reactions to some topical preparations include erythema, burning or stinging, excessive dryness, hypersensitivity, and susceptibility to sunburn

7. Most clients develop tolerance to local side effects within 3–4 weeks

B. Common acne medications are listed in Box 42–5

1. Retinoids are closely related to vitamin A and break up formation of clogged pores (may be called comedolytics); isotretinoin reduces size of sebaceous glands to decrease oil production
2. Antibiotics reduce redness and inflammation associated with moderate to severe acne, which reduces formation of cysts and pustules
3. Hormonal therapy (oral contraceptives) suppress sebum production and skin oiliness in pubertal females whose acne does not flare up at certain times during menstrual cycle

C. Nursing considerations

1. Assess skin lesions as baseline and periodically to evaluate effectiveness of therapy
2. Monitor for local adverse effects of topical preparations

NCLEX® 3. Monitor for systemic adverse effects as particular to individual medication

D. Client teaching

1. Understand purpose, use, side effects, and anticipated length of treatment
2. Treatment is designed to control, not cure; therefore, periodic breakouts (especially premenstrual flare-ups) may still occur

NCLEX® 3. With topical preparation, wash and dry skin; massage thin film gently into affected areas as ordered

NCLEX® 4. Avoid getting product into eyes, mouth, and mucous membranes; wash hands after use

NCLEX® 5. With certain preparations, minimize exposure to sun and UV light

NCLEX® 6. Isotretinoin is a teratogen; females of childbearing age must strictly avoid becoming pregnant; they should have negative pregnancy test within 2 weeks before starting therapy and monthly during therapy

NCLEX® 7. To prevent toxicity, avoid excess vitamin A intake with isotretinoin, which is a vitamin A metabolite, and comply with monthly triglyceride-level measurements (may be elevated as adverse effect)

VIII. BURN MEDICATIONS

A. Overview

1. Goals of therapy are to decrease inflammation, prevent infection, relieve pain, and promote healing
2. Topical agents are used to prevent infection in burn wounds, which could rapidly lead to sepsis

B. Common topical burn medications are listed in Table 42–2

C. Nursing considerations

NCLEX® 1. Apply thin layer of agent under sterile conditions once or twice daily to clean and debrided wound (ensure all areas of wound are fully covered continuously)

2. If hospitalized, client may undergo hydrotherapy (bathing in whirlpool) to aid debridement prior to reapplication

NCLEX® 3. Premedicate client with analgesic whenever possible 30 minutes prior to burn wound cleansing

4. Wound may be covered or left open

Table 42–2 Topical Burn Medications

Medication	Use	Notes
Mafenide	Bacteriostatic against *Pseudomonas aeruginosa* and *Clostridia*	Adverse reactions include pain, burning, or stinging at application site for first 20–30 minutes after application With impaired renal function, high blood levels of mafenide may lead to metabolic acidosis; watch for compensatory respiratory alkalosis, evidenced by hyperventilation
Silver sulfadiazine	Silver is toxic to bacteria; prevents replication of several organisms	Application is generally painless Watch for adverse reactions, including leukopenia, skin necrosis, erythema multiforme, skin discoloration, rashes Up to 10% may be absorbed; hazardous to use in clients with G6PD deficiency

NCLEX® 5. Monitor for adverse effects as outlined in Table 42–2

NCLEX® 6. Watch for signs of infection and monitor WBC count in clients receiving silver sulfadiazine because of leukopenic effect

D. Client teaching

1. Understand purpose, use, side effects, and anticipated length of treatment
2. Use as directed if using preparation as an outpatient

IX. DEBRIDING AGENTS

A. Overview

1. Debriding agents remove dirt, damaged tissue, and cellular debris from wound to prevent infection and promote healing
2. Effectiveness in removing necrotic tissue, clotted blood, purulent exudates, or fibrinous accumulations has been questioned
   a. Appear most effective when wound base has collagen that must be removed before epithelialization can proceed
   b. Specific indications may vary (e.g., collagenase is indicated for stage 3 and 4 pressure ulcers)

B. Common topical debriding agents are listed in Table 42–3

C. Nursing considerations: assess skin problem before use and monitor progress in wound healing

D. Client teaching: understand purpose, use, and side effects of medications and anticipated length of treatment

Memory Aid

Some enzymes that are used to debride wounds end in the suffix *-ase*. This may help you to choose an appropriate product at least some of the time.

Table 42–3 Topical Debriding Agents

Agent	Action	Notes
Collagenase	Digests collagen; active at pH 6–8, takes 10–14 days	Inactivated by extremes of pH, hydrogen peroxide, heavy metals like silver, detergents, iodine, nitrofurazone, and hexachlorophene
Sutilains	Digests necrotic soft tissues by proteolytic action	Same as for collagenase
Trypsin, Balsam Peru, castor oil (as combination product Granulex)	Source of trypsin is bovine pancreas	Balsam Peru is capillary bed stimulant used to improve circulation; castor oil used to reduce premature epithelial cornification

Check Your NCLEX–RN® Exam I.Q.

You are ready for testing on this content if you can:

- Apply knowledge of expected actions and effects of integumentary medications to client care.
- Correctly administer integumentary medications to clients.
- Assess for side effects and adverse effects of integumentary medications.
- Take appropriate action if a client has an unexpected response to an integumentary medication.
- Monitor a client for expected outcomes or effects of treatment with integumentary medications.

PRACTICE TEST

1 The nurse explains to a client that a product containing what ingredient would be the most useful agent to treat photoaging of the skin?

1. Propylene glycol
2. Salicylic acid
3. Alpha-hydroxy acids
4. Resorcinol

2 The nurse would include what information when explaining the use of a skin emollient to a client?

1. It requires shaking before each use.
2. It has a drying effect on the skin when the water evaporates.
3. It includes a corticosteroid component.
4. It fills the gaps in the stratum corneum.

3 What instructions should the nurse give the client who is receiving topical tretinoin for treatment of acne?

1. Apply tretinoin to affected areas each morning.
2. Use gloves to apply tretinoin to skin.
3. Avoid products containing vitamin C.
4. Apply to dry skin 30 minutes after washing.

4 A client's burn wound is infected and mafenide is prescribed. The nurse should conclude that the client is experiencing a systemic side effect from the medication after noting which assessment data?

1. An increase in respiratory rate from 16 to 24 breaths/min
2. A drop in systolic blood pressure by 10 mmHg
3. Increase in pain at the site of the burn wound
4. Development of a rash at the site of the burn wound

5 A female client who is using salicylic acid to treat psoriasis asks how long she will have to use this drug. What would be the best response by the nurse?

1. "The drug should not be needed after 3 months of therapy."
2. "Prolonged remission is uncommon, and maintenance therapy is needed."
3. "Each situation is so unique that the question cannot be answered accurately."
4. "The dermatologist caring for you is the best resource for your question."

6 The nurse would recommend that a client with excessive dandruff use a medicated shampoo that contains which active ingredient?

1. Silver sulfadiazine
2. Selenium sulfide
3. Corticosteroid
4. Lindane

7 It is winter and the client has extremely dry skin. Which type of preparation should the nurse recommend first?

1. Cleansing soap
2. Shake lotion
3. Emollient or emollient-containing lotion
4. Antipruritic lotion

8 A client with which integumentary disorder may benefit from a prescription for acyclovir?

1. Herpes simplex virus infection
2. Chronic dermatitis
3. Pseudofolliculitis
4. Candidiasis

9 A child has scraped his finger on a sharp spot on a shower door edge. The mother would like to use a topical antibiotic to prevent infection. Which agent would the pediatric telephone consultation nurse recommend?

1. Bacitracin
2. Malathion
3. Ketoconazole
4. Mafenide

PRACTICE TEST

10. An older adult client is being treated for a pressure ulcer. The nurse would anticipate using what type of agent to topically debride this ulcer?

1. Betamethasone
2. Ketoconazole
3. Tazarotene
4. Collagenase

11. The nurse is preparing to do tracheostomy care, and notes that the client's tracheostomy has encrusted debris around the tube. The nurse should dilute which antiseptic solution to half strength to most effectively clean the skin around the tracheostomy?

1. Povidone-iodine
2. Hydrogen peroxide
3. Chlorhexidine
4. Isopropyl alcohol

12. A client is prescribed to have topical application of sutilains. The nurse anticipates that this client has which type of integumentary problem?

1. Inflammation of external ear canal
2. Redness and itching of perirectal area
3. Dry skin on lower legs and feet
4. Pressure ulcer in coccyx area

13. A client is seeking treatment for a wart. What type of product should the nurse recommend to effectively remove this growth?

1. Astringent
2. Antiseptic
3. Keratinolytic
4. Proteolytic

14. The nurse would be most careful when using a topical drug for a client in which age group because of increased risk of toxicity?

1. Middle-aged adult
2. Older adult
3. Child
4. Adolescent

15. Which dermatologic medication would the nurse anticipate being prescribed for a client who has severe facial acne?

1. Doxycycline
2. Itraconazole
3. Benzoyl peroxide
4. Salicylic acid

16. A client has been using hydrocortisone 1% cream as a topical agent. For what medication actions should the nurse evaluate the client? Select all that apply.

1. Moisturizing
2. Drying
3. Antimicrobial
4. Anti-inflammatory
5. Vasoconstriction

17. A client with psoriasis needs to apply a lubricating lotion to a psoriatic plaque. The nurse plans to teach the client to use what type of substance?

1. Emollient
2. Antiseptic
3. Alcohol-based
4. Astringent

18. The nurse should plan to apply which prescribed agent to a burn wound that has been cleansed with sterile saline?

1. Adapalene
2. Silver sulfadiazine
3. Hydrocortisone
4. Acetic acid

19. A client has a wound infection that is resistant to treatment with several antiseptics. The nurse expects that the wound infection will most likely respond to treatment with which antiseptic?

1. Hydrogen peroxide
2. Phenol derivative
3. Isopropyl alcohol
4. Dakin's solution

20 The nurse is teaching a client about the use of sunscreen as a skin protective agent. What information should the nurse share with the client?

1. "Apply sunscreen 30–60 minutes before exposing skin to sunshine."
2. "Reapply sunscreen to skin every 4–6 hours when exposure to the sun continues."
3. "Reapply sunscreen immediately before going into the water to swim."
4. "Choose a sunscreen that has a minimum SPF factor of 8 for adequate skin protection."

ANSWERS & RATIONALES

1 **Answer: 3 Rationale:** Alpha-hydroxy acids are useful keratinolytics that help reduce the effects of photoaging. Propylene glycol is used to treat ichthyosis. Salicylic acid is a keratinolytic that is used to treat a variety of other skin disorders. Resorcinol is a keratinolytic that is used to treat a variety of other skin disorders. **Cognitive Level:** Applying **Client Need:** Pharmacological and Parenteral Therapies **Integrated Process:** Nursing Process: Implementation **Content Area:** Pharmacology **Strategy:** The core issue of the question is knowledge of products that assist the skin to appear younger and resist the aging effects of light. Use knowledge of these ordinary products and the process of elimination to make a selection.

2 **Answer: 4 Rationale:** Emollients contain petrolatum, oils, propylene glycol, or other substances, and make the skin soft and pliable by filling the gaps and increasing hydration of the dry stratum corneum. Shaking an emollient prior to application is not always needed. Emollients contain petrolatum, oils, propylene glycol, or other substances; they do not dry the skin. Dermasil does not contain corticosteroids. **Cognitive Level:** Applying **Client Need:** Pharmacological and Parenteral Therapies **Integrated Process:** Nursing Process: Implementation **Content Area:** Pharmacology **Strategy:** The core issue of the question is general knowledge of integumentary products that are emollients. Use knowledge regarding these ordinary products and the process of elimination to make a selection.

3 **Answer: 4 Rationale:** The area to be treated with tretinoin should be washed at least 30 minutes before applying. Tretinoin is a retinoic acid derivative that needs to be applied once daily in a thin layer before bedtime. It is not necessary to use gloves when applying tretinoin to affected skin. Increased intake of vitamin A, not vitamin C, needs to be avoided. **Cognitive Level:** Applying **Client Need:** Pharmacological and Parenteral Therapies **Integrated Process:** Nursing Process: Implementation **Content Area:** Pharmacology **Strategy:** The core issue of the question is knowledge of proper use of tretinoin. Use medication knowledge and the process of elimination to make a selection.

4 **Answer: 1 Rationale:** Mafenide can lead to metabolic acidosis, especially in clients who have impaired renal function. The client's system would attempt to compensate by inducing respiratory alkalosis, which the nurse would detect as an increase in respiratory rate. A drop in systolic blood pressure by 10 mmHg is unrelated to systemic effects of mafenide. Increased pain at the site of the burn may be a local effect of mafenide within 20 to 30 minutes after application, butit could also reflect inadequate pain management. Development of a rash at the site of the burn wound would be a local side effect of the medication. **Cognitive Level:** Analyzing **Client Need:** Pharmacological and Parenteral Therapies **Integrated Process:** Nursing Process: Assessment **Content Area:** Pharmacology **Strategy:** The core issue of the question is the ability to discriminate between local and systemic side effects of mafenide in a client with burn injury. Use medication knowledge and the process of elimination to make a selection.

5 **Answer: 2 Rationale:** There is no cure for psoriasis. Psoriasis is notoriously chronic and recurrent. The cause is unknown. For most clients the disease is recurrent, and therapy will need to be continued. **Cognitive Level:** Applying **Client Need:** Pharmacological and Parenteral Therapies **Integrated Process:** Teaching and Learning **Content Area:** Pharmacology **Strategy:** The core issue of the question is general knowledge about medications used to treat psoriasis. Use medication knowledge and the process of elimination to make a selection.

6 **Answer: 2 Rationale:** A 1% lotion of selenium sulfide or shampoo is used to relieve the itching and flaking of the scalp associated with dandruff. Silver sulfadiazine is a cream used in the prevention and treatment of infection in partial- and full-thickness burns. Corticosteroids can be used for many things, but dandruff is not one of them. A shampoo with lindane 1% would be used for pediculosis capitis. **Cognitive Level:** Analyzing **Client Need:** Pharmacological and Parenteral Therapies **Integrated Process:** Teaching and Learning **Content Area:** Pharmacology **Strategy:** The core issue of the question is general knowledge about medications used to treat dandruff. Use medication knowledge and the process of elimination to make a selection.

7 **Answer: 3 Rationale:** Emollient lotions are dilute dispersions of emulsified lipids in water. These provide smooth application and the most rapid hydration if applied to dry skin. Emollients (e.g., petrolatum) are occlusive agents that make the skin soft and pliable by increasing hydration of the stratum corneum. Excessive washing with harsh soaps strips stratum corneum of its natural lipids and exacerbates dry skin. No-shake lotion is made specifically for management of dry skin. Itching can occur with dry skin, but before an antipruritic lotion is used, an emollient lotion or emollient should be tried. **Cognitive Level:** Analyzing **Client Need:** Pharmacological and Parenteral Therapies **Integrated Process:** Nursing Process: Planning **Content Area:** Pharmacology **Strategy:** The core issue of the question is general knowledge about products used to treat dry skin. Use product knowledge and the process of elimination to make a selection.

8 **Answer: 1 Rationale:** Acyclovir is an antiviral agent that is useful in the treatment of herpes simplex viruses. Chronic dermatitis, pseudofolliculitis, and candidiasis may require therapy with an anti-infective, but not of the antiviral type. **Cognitive Level:** Applying **Client Need:** Pharmacological and Parenteral Therapies **Integrated Process:** Nursing Process: Implementation **Content Area:** Pharmacology **Strategy:** The core

issue of the question is knowledge of the uses of acyclovir in a client with herpes infection. Use medication knowledge and the process of elimination to make a selection. Remember that an antiviral medication often contains *vir* somewhere in its name.

9 **Answer:** 1 **Rationale:** Bacitracin is a topical antibiotic that is bactericidal against Gram-positive cocci and bacilli, including staphylococci and streptococci. These organisms might cause infection in a skin wound. Malathion is an antiparasitic agent for pediculosis. Ketoconazole is an antifungal agent. Mafenide is an agent used for burns. **Cognitive Level:** Applying **Client Need:** Pharmacological and Parenteral Therapies **Integrated Process:** Nursing Process: Implementation **Content Area:** Pharmacology **Strategy:** The core issue of the question is knowledge of the types of medications used for various skin conditions. Use medication knowledge and the process of elimination to make a selection. Remember that cuts or open wounds often heal effectively when topical antibiotics are used to prevent infection at the site.

10 **Answer:** 4 **Rationale:** An agent that would be useful for chemically debriding a pressure ulcer would be collagenase, which has enzymatic action. Betamethasone is a corticosteroid. Ketoconazole is an antifungal drug. Tazarotene is a vitamin A derivative that is used to treat psoriasis. **Cognitive Level:** Analyzing **Client Need:** Pharmacological and Parenteral Therapies **Integrated Process:** Nursing Process: Planning **Content Area:** Pharmacology **Strategy:** The core issue of the question is the type of topical agent to use when debridement is needed. Use medication knowledge and the process of elimination to make a selection. Enzymes often end in *-ase*, which makes them easy to recognize on sight.

11 **Answer:** 2 **Rationale:** Hydrogen peroxide is an oxidizing antiseptic that can be used to clean tracheostomy tubes and selected client wounds. Products containing povidone-iodine have cleansing action but may impair healing and are no longer commonly used. Chlorhexidine can be used as a cleaning agent, but it does not have the bubbling action of hydrogen peroxide. Isopropyl alcohol would be irritating or drying to the skin and should not be used. **Cognitive Level:** Applying **Client Need:** Pharmacological and Parenteral Therapies **Integrated Process:** Nursing Process: Implementation **Content Area:** Pharmacology **Strategy:** The core issue of the question is knowledge of the type of skin cleansing agent used for tracheostomy. Use knowledge of these agents and the process of elimination to make a selection.

12 **Answer:** 4 **Rationale:** Proteolytic enzymes such as sutilains can be used to chemically debride tissue in venous stasis ulcers, burn wounds, and pressure ulcers. Proteolytic enzymes would not be used to treat inflammation of external ear canal, redness and itching of perirectal area, or dry skin on lower legs and feet. **Cognitive Level:** Applying **Client Need:** Pharmacological and Parenteral Therapies **Integrated Process:** Nursing Process: Implementation **Content Area:** Pharmacology **Strategy:** The core issue of the question is knowledge of the debriding agents appropriate for use at various skin sites. Use knowledge of these agents and the process of elimination to make a selection.

13 **Answer:** 3 **Rationale:** A keratinolytic agent such as salicyclic acid is used to treat warts, as well as corns, calluses, and other keratin-containing skin lesions. Astringents cause topical vasoconstriction, and would not be effective to remove a wart. Antiseptics inhibit bacterial growth. Proteolytic enzymes are used to debride tissue, but not warts. **Cognitive Level:** Applying **Client Need:** Pharmacological and Parenteral Therapies **Integrated Process:** Teaching and Learning **Content Area:** Pharmacology **Strategy:** The core issue of the question is what type of medication is effective in treating warts. Begin to answer by reasoning that treatment of a wart includes breaking it down for removal. Next note the suffix *-lytic* in the correct option, which means "to break down."

14 **Answer:** 3 **Rationale:** Children have an increased risk of systemic toxicity from topically applied drugs because of the greater ratio of surface area to weight. Middle-age adults, older adults, and adolescents have a greater body surface area-to-weight ratio than a child; age is not a factor. **Cognitive Level:** Applying **Client Need:** Pharmacological and Parenteral Therapies **Integrated Process:** Nursing Process: Evaluation **Content Area:** Pharmacology **Strategy:** The core issue of this question is the age group that is at greatest risk because of its skin characteristics when topical drugs are used. Recall that the greater the area involved, the greater the risk of absorption and toxic effects. Finally, recall that infants and children have a greater skin surface-to-weight ratio than an adult of any age.

15 **Answer:** 1 **Rationale:** Severe acne is treated with doxycycline, a systemic antibiotic, or isotretinoin. Itraconazole is an antifungal agent. Benzoyl peroxide is a topical keratinolytic found in many OTC products that are used to treat mild acne. Salicylic acid is an exfoliative ingredient in many OTC products that are used to treat mild acne. **Cognitive Level:** Applying **Client Need:** Pharmacological and Parenteral Therapies **Integrated Process:** Nursing Process: Planning **Content Area:** Pharmacology **Strategy:** The core issue of the question is what type of medication is effective in treating acne. Since this condition is characterized by inflammation and drainage, consider that an agent that has a drying effect would be opposite to the characteristics of the condition, and would help reduce symptoms.

16 **Answer:** 4, 5 **Rationale:** Corticosteroids such as hydrocortisone are anti-inflammatory drugs. Corticosteroids such as hydrocortisone decrease erythema through vasoconstriction. Corticosteroids are not moisturizing agents. Corticosteroids are not drying agents. Corticosteroids do not exert antimicrobial action, and, in fact, they can increase risk of infection by suppressing the inflammatory response. **Cognitive Level:** Analyzing **Client Need:** Pharmacological and Parenteral Therapies **Integrated Process:** Nursing Process: Evaluation **Content Area:** Pharmacology **Strategy:** The core issue of the question is knowledge of the intended effects of corticosteroids as anti-inflammatory agents. Use this information and the process of elimination to make a selection. When there is more than one correct answer, consider each option as a true/false statement.

17 **Answer:** 1 **Rationale:** Psoriatic plaques need to be lubricated so that they are easier to loosen and remove. Emollients and lubricants are fatty or oily substances that can be used for this purpose because they keep skin soft and prevent water evaporation. Antiseptics, alcohol-based liquids, and astringents are harsher substances and might have a drying effect. **Cognitive Level:** Applying **Client Need:** Pharmacological and Parenteral Therapies **Integrated Process:** Teaching and Learning **Content Area:** Pharmacology **Strategy:** Note the word *lubricating* in the stem of the question. This tells you that regardless of the client's health problem, the agent is one that has a moisturizing effect on the skin. Use the process of

elimination and knowledge of the categories of skin products to make a selection.

18 **Answer: 2 Rationale:** Silver sulfadiazine is a metallic type of antiseptic that is widely used on burns. The silver in the solution is toxic to bacteria and prevents them from reproducing. Adapalene is a topical retinoid that is used to treat acne. Hydrocortisone is a topical corticosteroid that has a variety of uses, but is not for care of burn wounds. Acetic acid is an ingredient in a solution used when wet soak is prescribed. **Cognitive Level:** Applying **Client Need:** Pharmacological and Parenteral Therapies **Integrated Process:** Nursing Process: Planning **Content Area:** Pharmacology **Strategy:** The core issue of the question is the type of agent that would be effective in preventing microbial growth in a client with a burn injury. Use knowledge of topical antimicrobial agents and the process of elimination to make a selection.

19 **Answer: 4 Rationale:** A chlorine preparation such as Dakin's solution is used for infected wounds when other treatments are ineffective. They are useful because they also dissolve necrotic materials and blood clots; however, a disadvantage is that they delay blood clotting, which later could interfere with wound healing. Hydrogen peroxide, phenol derivatives, or isopropyl alcohol are not helpful in treating infections resistant to several antiseptics. **Cognitive Level:** Applying **Client Need:** Pharmacological and Parenteral Therapies **Integrated Process:** Nursing Process: Diagnosis **Content Area:** Pharmacology **Strategy:** The core issue of the question is knowledge of antiseptics that are useful in treating problems involving the skin. Use this knowledge and the process of elimination to make a selection.

20 **Answer: 1 Rationale:** Sunscreen should be applied 30–60 minutes before sun exposure to allow sufficient time for it to penetrate the skin. Sunscreen should be reapplied every 2 to 3 hours of continuous sun exposure. Sunscreen should be reapplied after swimming or sweating to maintain continuous skin protection. Sunscreen should have a minimum SPF factor of 15 for adequate skin protection. **Cognitive Level:** Applying **Client Need:** Pharmacological and Parenteral Therapies **Integrated Process:** Teaching and Learning **Content Area:** Pharmacology **Strategy:** The core issue of the question is knowledge of proper selection and application of sunscreen for skin protection. Use the process of elimination and knowledge of principles of sunscreen use to make a selection.

Key Terms to Review

acne p. 642
herpes simplex p. 638
papules p. 642
pediculosis p. 639
pruritus p. 636
psoriasis p. 641
scabies p. 639
tinea pedis p. 638

References

Adams, M., Holland, L., & Urban, C. (2017). *Pharmacology for nurses: A pathophysiologic approach* (5th ed.). New York, NY: Pearson Education, Inc.

Adams, M., & Urban, C. (2016). *Pharmacology: Connections to nursing practice* (3rd ed.). New York, NY: Pearson Education, Inc.

Lehne, R. (2016). *Pharmacology for nursing care* (9th ed.). St. Louis, MO: Saunders.

Wilson, B., Shannon, M., & Shields, K. (2016). *Pearson nurse's drug guide 2016.* New York, NY: Pearson Education, Inc.

43 Eye and Ear Medications

In this chapter

Cross Reference

Other chapters relevant to this content area are

Dosage Calculation and Medication Administration	Chapter 29
Respiratory Medications	Chapter 36
Eye and Ear Disorders	Chapter 63

I. MEDICATIONS TO TREAT GLAUCOMA

A. Beta-adrenergic blockers (antagonists)

1. Decrease production of **aqueous humor** (fluid formed by ciliary body in eye)
2. Reduce **intraocular pressure** (IOP; pressure within eye) in **open-angle glaucoma** (a change in appearance of optic disk resulting in visual loss)
3. Commonly used to manage chronic, primary open-angle glaucoma
4. Common glaucoma medications are listed in Box 43–1

Memory Aid

Remember that a beta-blocking drug can be recognized easily because it ends with the suffix *-olol* or *-lol*.

5. Administration considerations
   - NCLEX® a. Use nasolacrimal occlusion (press on inner canthus of eye) to minimize **systemic absorption** (entry of drug into body and circulating fluids)
   - NCLEX® b. Use cautiously in clients with renal failure, diabetes, asthma, and chronic obstructive pulmonary disease (COPD)
   - c. May mask symptoms of hyperthyroidism
   - d. Drug may be $beta_1$ selective (cardiac), $beta_2$ selective (pulmonary), or both $beta_1$ and $beta_2$ selective
   - e. Because it is $beta_1$ selective, betaxolol is usually preferred for clients with pulmonary disease
6. Contraindicated in hypersensitivity, sinus bradycardia, second- or third-degree heart block, cardiogenic shock, or congestive heart failure (CHF)
7. NCLEX® Adverse cardiovascular effects may occur when beta-adrenergic blockers are used in combination with other cardiovascular agents such as antihypertensives and antidysrhythmics
8. Side/adverse effects
   - NCLEX® a. Primarily local reactions: eye irritation, burning, stinging
   - NCLEX® b. Systemic adverse cardiorespiratory effects: bradycardia or tachycardia, CHF, dysrhythmias, hypotension, edema of lower extremities, wheezing, cough, exacerbation of asthma, and bronchospasm

Box 43–1

Medications to Treat Glaucoma

Beta-Adrenergic Blockers (Antagonists)

Betaxolol

Carteolol

Levobunolol

Metipranolol

Timolol

Alpha$_2$-Adrenergic Agonists

Apraclonidine

Brimonidine

Cholinergic Agonists

Carbachol

Echothiophate iodide

Pilocarpine

Carbonic Anhydrase Inhibitors

Acetazolamide

Brinzolamide

Dorzolamide

Methazolamide

Sympathomimetic

Dipivefrin

Osmotic Diuretics

Mannitol

Prostaglandin Agonists

Bimatoprost

Latanoprost

Tafluprost

Travoprost

c. Miscellaneous systemic adverse effects: nausea and vomiting (N/V) and neurologic effects such as weakness, ataxia, confusion, and depression

9. Nursing considerations

NCLEX® a. Obtain baseline data for vital signs (VS), neurologic status, vision, and IOP

b. Assess for cardiovascular disease, renal failure, diabetes, lactation, or thyrotoxicosis

c. Assess for local signs of hypersensitivity such as ocular burning, itching, redness, and swelling

NCLEX® d. Refer to Box 43–2 for administration of ophthalmic medications

10. Client teaching

NCLEX® a. Beta-blocking agents may mask symptoms of hypoglycemia

b. Inform prescriber if surgery is being considered; gradual withdrawal of beta-blocking agent 48 hours before surgery may be required (withdrawal is controversial)

Box 43–2

Administration of Ophthalmic Medications

Instillation of Eyedrops

- Perform hand hygiene.
- Cleanse exudates from eye(s) if necessary
- Tilt client's head toward side of affected eye
- Gently pull lower eyelid down and have client look up (this forms a "sac")
- Instill drops in conjunctival sac formed by lower lid, *not* onto eye
- Unless specifically indicated otherwise, apply gentle pressure for 30 seconds to 1 minute over inner canthus next to nose (prevents absorption through lacrimal duct and drainage of medication)
- Unless specifically indicated otherwise, client should close eye(s) gently. Avoid squeezing eye(s) tightly as this forces medication out

Instillation of Eye Ointment

- Follow same procedure for instillation of eyedrops except that ointment is expressed directly into lower conjunctival sac from inner canthus to outer canthus
- Unless specifically indicated otherwise, client should close eye(s) and gently massage eye(s) to distribute medication

Note: To avoid contamination and risk of infection, do not touch dropper or tube to eye, eyelashes, or any other surface. Remove contact lenses before instilling ophthalmic medications.

c. Have routine eye examinations and measurement of IOP
d. Do not stop medication unless instructed to do so by prescriber
NCLEX® e. Report symptoms of breathing difficulty, swelling of extremities, slow heart rate
NCLEX® f. Wear dark glasses and avoid bright light if photophobia is present

B. Adrenergic medications (alpha$_2$-adrenergic agonists)

1. Decrease production of aqueous humor and decrease IOP
2. Used to manage open-angle glaucoma (often in combination with other drugs), glaucoma secondary to **uveitis** (intraocular inflammatory disorder), to produce **mydriasis** (pupil dilation) for ocular examination, and to produce local hemostasis during eye surgery to control bleeding
3. Common medications for glaucoma: see again Box 43–1
4. Administration considerations: do not administer ophthalmic solution that contains precipitates or has turned brown
5. NCLEX® Contraindicated in treatment of narrow-angle (angle-closure) glaucoma or abraded cornea because pupil dilation further restricts ocular fluid outflow, precipitating an acute attack of glaucoma
6. Side/adverse effects
   a. NCLEX® Local reactions include eye pain and stinging on initial instillation
   b. CNS side effects include headache, blurred vision, brow ache, photophobia, and difficulty with night vision
   c. Systemic adverse effects are unusual but may include hypertension in clients with cardiovascular disease
7. Nursing considerations
   a. Obtain history of allergies or hypersensitivity to specific agents
   b. NCLEX® Obtain baseline VS, vision status, and IOP measurement
   c. Assess cardiac, respiratory, and renal function routinely
8. NCLEX® Client teaching
   a. Drugs may discolor contact lenses
   b. Do not blink for at least 30 seconds after instilling medication
   c. Report a decrease in visual acuity, floating spots, sensitivity to light, eye redness, or headache to healthcare provider

C. Cholinergic agonists (miotics, cholinesterase inhibitors)

1. Increase outflow of aqueous humor, decrease resistance to aqueous flow in open-angle and angle-closure glaucoma
2. Produce miosis before ophthalmic examination or after ophthalmic surgery
3. Often used for clients who fail to respond to first-line agents (beta-blockers)
4. Common medications: see again Box 43–1
5. Administration considerations
   a. NCLEX® Do not administer ophthalmic solution that contains precipitates or has turned brown
   b. Pilocarpine can be stored at room temperature
   c. Contraindicated in acute iritis or conditions in which pupillary constriction is not desirable
6. Side/adverse effects
   a. Visual blurring, myopia, irritation, reduced visual acuity in low light, and headache
   b. Systemic reactions include abdominal pain with diarrhea, bronchoconstriction, hypotension, N/V diuresis, diaphoresis, exacerbation of asthma
   c. NCLEX® Toxic effects produce ataxia, confusion, seizures, coma, respiratory failure, hypotension, and death
   d. Prolonged use of cholinergics may lead to retinal detachment, obstruction of tear drainage, and cataracts
   e. NCLEX® Acute toxicity is reversible by IV atropine, an anticholinergic agent that acts as antidote
7. Nursing considerations
   a. Obtain baseline VS, neurologic status, vision, and IOP data
   b. Assess for cardiovascular disease, renal failure, diabetes, lactation, or thyrotoxicosis
   c. NCLEX® Concurrent use with beta-adrenergic blocking agents may increase risk of cardiovascular reactions
   d. Assess for local signs of hypersensitivity such as burning, itching, redness, and swelling
8. Client teaching: miosis may cause difficulty adjusting quickly to changes in lighting; use proper administration technique

D. Carbonic anhydrase inhibitors (CAIs)

1. Nonbacteriostatic sulfonamides that lower IOP by decreasing aqueous humor production
2. Oral CAIs are used to treat open-angle, secondary, and angle-closure glaucoma
3. Ophthalmic CAIs are used to treat open-angle glaucoma and ocular hypertension

NCLEX® 4. Commonly used preoperatively in intraocular surgery
5. Common medications: see again Box 43–1

Memory Aid

Carbonic anhydrase inhibitors can often be recognized because many of them end with the suffix *-zolamide*.

6. Administration considerations
   - NCLEX® a. Oral acetazolamide is administered for maintenance
   - NCLEX® b. IV route is used preoperatively or to rapidly reduce increased IOP
   - c. To minimize nocturia, schedule doses early in day
   - d. Administer with caution to clients with adrenocortical insufficiency
   - NCLEX® e. Contraindicated with hypersensitivity to antibacterial sulfonamides, chronic noncongestive angle-closure glaucoma, hyponatremia, hypokalemia, or other electrolyte imbalances, or hepatic or renal dysfunction
7. Side/adverse effects
   - a. Oral agents: anorexia, diarrhea, diuresis, N/V, lethargy, weakness, weight loss, metallic bitter taste, and paresthesia of fingers, hands, and toes
   - NCLEX® b. Topical agents: topical allergic reaction, photosensitivity, superficial **keratitis** (inflammation of cornea)
   - NCLEX® c. Stevens-Johnson syndrome and bone marrow depression with acetazolamide
   - d. Acidosis, blood dyscrasias, hypokalemia
8. Nursing considerations
   - a. Potential exacerbation of renal stones; monitor renal function
   - NCLEX® b. Monitor for fluid volume depletion related to diuresis; monitor intake and output (I&O), skin turgor, mucous membranes, and weight
   - NCLEX® c. Monitor urinalysis, complete blood cell count (CBC), electrolytes
9. NCLEX® Client teaching
   - a. Unless contraindicated, eat diet high in potassium and low in sodium
   - b. Unless contraindicated, increase fluid intake to at least 2 liters per day to decrease risk of renal stones
   - c. Report changes in urine color, rashes, fever

E. Sympathomimetic agents

1. Lower IOP by decreasing aqueous humor production and increasing its outflow; used to manage open-angle glaucoma
2. Common medication (ophthalmic): dipivefrin
3. Administration considerations
   - a. Administer with caution to clients with cardiovascular disease, hypertension, asthma, diabetes mellitus, hyperthyroidism, and parkinsonism
   - NCLEX® b. Assess for sensitivity to sulfites
   - NCLEX® c. Avoid concurrent use with monoamine oxidase inhibitors (MAOIs)
   - NCLEX® d. Contraindicated with **narrow-angle glaucoma** (increased IOP from impaired rate of aqueous humor flow) or predisposition to narrow-angle glaucoma
4. Side/adverse effects
   - a. Local: brow pain, burning, eye irritation, headache, watering eyes, stinging, **photophobia** (sensitivity to light)
   - NCLEX® b. Systemic: hypertension, diaphoresis, tachycardia, palpitation, tremors, light-headedness
5. Nursing considerations
   - NCLEX® a. Obtain baseline IOP and vision data; measure baseline and periodic heart rate and BP to detect systemic effects
   - NCLEX® b. Maintain pressure on lacrimal sac for 1–2 minutes after instillation of drug to minimize systemic absorption
6. Client teaching
   - a. Discuss use of contact lenses with prescriber; use may or may not be permitted
   - b. Report increased heart rate, heart palpitations, or elevated BP to prescriber

F. Prostaglandin agonists

1. Increases aqueous humor outflow
2. Used to manage open-angle glaucoma and ocular hypertension
3. Common medications: see again Box 43–1

Memory Aid

Prostaglandin agonists can often be recognized because many of them end with the suffix *-prost*.

4. Administration considerations
   NCLEX® a. Administer 5 minutes apart from other prescribed antiglaucoma ophthalmic medications
   b. If pilocarpine is included in drug regimen, it should be administered 1 hour after prostaglandin agonist
5. Contraindications: hypersensitivity to latanoprost or benzalkonium chloride
6. NCLEX® Side/adverse effects
   a. Blurred vision, photophobia, burning, stinging, and itching
   b. Longer, thicker, darker eyelashes; increasing iris pigmentation
   c. Conjunctival hyperemia
7. Nursing considerations
   a. Assess for hypersensitivity to latanoprost or benzalkonium chloride
   b. Assess for burning, itching, stinging after initial administration of medication
8. NCLEX® Client teaching
   a. Drug may cause an increase in iris pigmentation
   b. Do not exceed once-a-day dose
   c. Remove contact lenses before dose and leave out for 15 minutes after
   d. Report burning, itching, stinging after administration to prescriber

II. MYDRIATICS AND CYCLOPLEGICS

A. Anticholinergic cycloplegics

1. Produce mydriasis (pupil dilation) and/or **cycloplegia** (paralysis of ciliary muscle)
2. Used to treat ocular pain secondary to inflammatory disorders such as uveitis and keratitis or for relaxation of ciliary muscle to improve measurement of refractive errors
3. NCLEX® Used preoperatively and postoperatively for intraocular surgery
4. Common mydriatic and cycloplegic ophthalmic medications: see Box 43–3
5. Administration considerations
   NCLEX® a. Use cautiously with primary glaucoma or predisposition to angle-closure glaucoma
   b. Apply ointment several hours before vision examination
   NCLEX® c. Compress lacrimal duct during administration and for 2–3 minutes after dose
   d. Contraindicated with severe systemic reactions to atropine or hypersensitivity to anticholinergic drugs
6. Side/adverse effects
   a. Local: blurred vision, photophobia, allergic lid reactions
   NCLEX® b. Systemic: confusion, delirium, drowsiness, dry mouth, flushing, and tachycardia
   NCLEX® c. Acute glaucoma can be precipitated by pupillary dilation; if not recognized and treated, acute glaucoma can result in blindness
   d. Dry mouth and tachycardia may be symptoms of scopolamine toxicity
7. Nursing considerations
   a. Obtain baseline IOP and vision status data
   b. Combination drugs produce greater mydriasis
   c. Systemic side effects are more pronounced in infants and children with blond hair and blue eyes
   NCLEX® d. Monitor for tachycardia, confusion, slurred speech, dry mouth, dry skin, weakness, drowsiness

Box 43–3

Mydriatic and Cycloplegic Ophthalmic Medications

Anticholinergics: Cycloplegics	Sympathomimetics: Mydriatics
Atropine sulfate	Phenylephrine
Cyclopentolate	
Homatropine	
Scopolamine hydrobromide	
Tropicamide	

8. Client teaching
   a. Mydriasis may last from 3 days (scopolamine) to 12 days (atropine)
   b. Blurred vision may occur
   NCLEX® c. Wear dark sunglasses and avoid bright light for photophobia
   d. Use sugarless hard candy to relieve dry mouth
   NCLEX® e. IOP and vision should be monitored over course of therapy
   NCLEX® f. Withhold dose if experiencing tachycardia and dry mouth (symptoms of toxicity) and contact prescriber

B. Sympathomimetics

1. Usually used to treat minor eye injuries and before eye examination
2. Common medication: phenylephrine
3. Administration and nursing considerations and client teaching: same as discussed in previous adrenergic section of chapter
4. Side/adverse effects
   a. Rebound **miosis** (constriction of pupils) may occur with phenylephrine
   b. Older adults with cardiac disease may experience BP elevations with phenylephrine

III. MEDICATIONS FOR EYE INFLAMMATION, INFECTION, AND ALLERGIC CONJUNCTIVITIS

A. Nonsteroidal anti-inflammatory drugs (NSAIDs)

1. Flurbiprofen is used to inhibit intraoperative miosis
2. Diclofenac is used to treat postoperative inflammation after cataract extraction
3. Ketorolac is used to treat conjunctivitis and seasonal allergic ophthalmic pruritis
4. Common anti-inflammatory ophthalmic medications: see Box 43–4
5. Administration considerations
   a. Systemic effects may be produced if absorbed
   NCLEX® b. NSAIDs may cause increased bleeding; closely monitor clients who have bleeding tendencies and have periodic CBC and coagulation studies done
   NCLEX® c. Contraindicated with sensitivity to aspirin or phenylacetic acid derivatives or to systemic NSAIDs
6. Side/adverse effects
   a. Local: transient burning or stinging on application, itching, allergic reaction, pain, and redness
   b. Systemic toxicity: bleeding

NCLEX® 7. Nursing considerations: assess for bleeding and local hypersensitivity symptoms (burning, itching, redness, and swelling)

8. Client teaching: NSAIDs may potentiate bleeding in clients with known bleeding tendencies

B. Corticosteroids

1. Indicated for allergic and inflammatory ophthalmic disorders of conjunctiva, cornea, and anterior segment of eye
2. Common anti-inflammatory ophthalmic medications: see again Box 43–4
3. Administration considerations
   NCLEX® a. Corticosteroids should be used for short-term treatment only
   b. Use with caution in clients with cataracts and chronic open-angle glaucoma

NCLEX® 4. Contraindicated with hypersensitivity and corneal abrasion; may mask hypersensitivity reactions to other drugs

Box 43–4

Anti-Inflammatory Drugs for Ophthalmic Use

Anti-Inflammatory Drugs (Nonsteroidal)

Diclofenac

Flurbiprofen

Ketorolac

Corticosteroids: Steroidal Anti-Inflammatory Drugs

Dexamethasone

Fluorometholone

Loteprednol etabonate

Prednisolone, gentamicin

Rimexolone

Ophthalmic Immunosuppressant and Anti-Inflammatory Drug

Cyclosporine

5. Side/adverse effects
   a. Local: stinging after application
NCLEX® b. Toxicity: visual disturbances, headache, and eye pain
NCLEX® 6. Nursing considerations: may mask symptoms of infection and hypersensitivity reactions; may increase susceptibility to infection
NCLEX® 7. Client teaching: avoid use of contact lenses during and for prescribed time after corticosteroid therapy; have eye(s) examined for progress

C. Antibacterial, antifungal, and antiviral agents

1. Antibacterial agents treat conjunctivitis, blepharitis, keratitis, uveitis, and hordeolum (external stye) or chalazion (internal stye)
2. Antifungal agents treat fungal blepharitis, conjunctivitis, and keratitis
3. Antiviral agents treat herpes simplex virus keratitis and herpes simplex virus keratoconjunctivitis
4. Common anti-infective ophthalmic medications are listed in Box 43–5
5. Administration considerations
NCLEX® a. If indicated, obtain culture from eye(s) before administering first dose
   b. Remove exudates from eyes before administering medication
   c. Do not administer ophthalmic anesthetics within 30 minutes of sulfonamides (sulfacetamide sodium); sulfonamides are incompatible with thimerosol and silver preparations
6. Side/adverse effects
   a. Local: dermatitis, itching, stinging, swelling
   b. Stevens-Johnson syndrome, systemic lupus erythematosus (SLE) with sulfacetamide sodium
NCLEX® 7. Nursing considerations
   a. Monitor infected eye(s) for pain, drainage, redness, swelling
   b. Store idoxuridine and trifluridine in cool place or refrigerator
NCLEX® 8. Client teaching: inform prescriber of photosensitivity, redness, swelling, increased drainage, pain, or if no improvement seen within a few days; ganciclovir may cause temporary blurred vision after each application

D. Medications to treat allergic conjunctivitis

1. Antihistamines and mast cell stabilizers decrease redness and itching associated with allergic conjunctivitis
2. Common medications for allergic conjunctivitis: see Box 43–6

Box 43–5

Anti-Infective Agents for Ophthalmic Use

Antibacterial	Sulfacetamide
Bacitracin	Tobramycin
Ciprofloxacin	**Antiviral**
Erythromycin	Ganciclovir
Gentamicin sulfate	Trifluridine
Ofloxacin	**Antifungal**
Polymyxin B sulfate	Natamycin

Box 43-6

Drugs to Treat Allergic Conjunctivitis

Antihistamines	**Mast Cell Stabilizer Drugs**
Azelastine	Azelastine
Bepotastine	Cromolyn sodium
Emedastine	Epinastine
Epinastine	Ketotifen fumarate
Ketotifen	Lodoxamide
Olopatadine	Nedocromil
	Olopatadine
	Pemirolast potassium

3. Administration considerations: these medications are supplied as ophthalmic solutions
4. Contraindications: hypersensitivity
5. Side/adverse effects of antihistamines: fatigue, dizziness, dry mouth, sore throat, cough, bitter taste, rhinitis
6. Side/adverse effects of mast cell stabilizers: dry mouth, headache, nausea, sneezing, transient eye stinging, nasal symptoms, bronchospasm, angioedema, and anaphylaxis
7. For further information, see Chapter 36 for antihistamines and mast cell stabilizers

E. Eye lubricants

1. Eye lubricants add moisture to eyes or replace tears, moisten contact lenses or artificial eyes, treat keratitis, and protect eyes when blink reflex is impaired (such as during surgery or certain neurologic disorders)
2. Common lubricants include carboxymethylcellulose, hydroxypropyl methylcellulose, polyvinyl alcohol, and petroleum-based ointments
3. Teach client that burning or discomfort can occur on instillation of drops and that allergic reaction is possible to preservative ingredients

IV. ANESTHETIC EYE MEDICATIONS

A. Action and use

1. Prevent initiation and transmission of nerve impulses
2. Prevent pain during diagnostic procedures such as **tonometry** (measurement of IOP, used to detect glaucoma), subconjunctival injections, removal of foreign bodies, surgical procedures, and removal of sutures

B. Common medications: lidocaine, proparacaine hydrochloride, tetracaine hydrochloride

C. Administration considerations: rapid onset within 20 seconds, and duration is 15–20 minutes; tetracaine can cause systemic toxicity

D. Contraindications: hypersensitivity

E. Side/adverse effects

1. Proparacaine causes allergic contact dermatitis, cycloplegia, conjunctival congestion, delayed corneal healing
2. Signs of CNS excitation (rare systemic effect): blurred vision, dizziness, nervousness, restlessness, and trembling, followed by CNS depression (dyspnea, drowsiness, dysrhythmias)

NCLEX® **F. Nursing considerations**

1. Protect eye from injury while anesthetized to avoid corneal damage (apply eye patch until blink reflex has returned)
2. Assess for hypersensitivity symptoms such as burning, itching, stinging

NCLEX® **G. Client teaching:** do not touch or rub the eye until anesthesia has worn off

V. AUDITORY MEDICATIONS

A. Antibiotics for ear

1. Topical otic antibiotics such as neomycin, gentamicin, and ciprofloxacin are used to manage external ear infections of external ear (external otitis)
2. A variety of oral systemic antibiotics may be prescribed to treat middle ear infections (otitis media)
3. Administration considerations
   a. Unless contraindicated, warm ear drops by holding medication bottle under warm running water, immersing bottle in a cup of warm water, or holding bottle in hand or pocket for 30 minutes prior to administration
   b. Assess client's baseline hearing status and presence of ear drainage, earache, erythema, pain, and **vertigo** (dizziness)
   c. Assess first that ear canal is clear and not impacted with *cerumen* (earwax)
   d. Assess for intact tympanic membrane
   NCLEX® e. Contraindicated in hypersensitivity and perforation of tympanic membrane
4. Side/adverse effects
   a. Local: burning, rash, redness, swelling, blurred vision
   b. Systemic: hypersensitivity reaction
5. Nursing considerations
   NCLEX® a. Assess for local adverse effects; discontinue use if hypersensitivity reaction occurs
   b. Monitor auditory canal for drainage and pain and monitor for hearing

6. Client teaching
   a. Inform prescriber of increased pain, drainage, or no improvement in symptoms within a few days of treatment
   NCLEX® b. Refer to Box 43–7 for instillation of otic medications

B. Corticosteroids

1. Used for anti-inflammatory, antipruritic, or antiallergenic effects; may be given with antibacterial or antifungal agents
2. Common corticosteroid medications for otic use are listed in Box 43–8
3. Administration considerations
   a. Assess client's hearing status and presence of ear drainage, earache, erythema, pain, and vertigo
   b. Assess first that ear canal is clear and not impacted with cerumen before medication administration and that tympanic membrane is intact
   c. May be given in combination with antibiotics to treat infections of external ear canal or mastoid cavity
4. NCLEX® Side/adverse effects: corticosteroids may mask infection or exacerbate an existing infection
5. NCLEX® Nursing considerations: assess for hypersensitivity and for symptom relief
6. Client teaching
   a. Hearing should be monitored during course of treatment
   b. Inform prescriber of new onset of ear drainage, heat, fever, odor, or pain, or if no improvement is seen within a few days of treatment

C. Other medications (over-the-counter medications)

1. Acetic acid (alcohol, glycerin, or propylene glycol) is used after swimming or bathing to restore normal acid pH to ear canal
2. Glycerin, mineral oil, and olive oil are emollients to relieve itching and burning in ear
3. Propylene glycol enhances antibacterial effects and acidity of acetic acid
4. Carbamide peroxide is an antibacterial agent that helps remove accumulated cerumen
5. Common OTC medications for otic use are listed in Box 43–9

Box 43–7

Administration of Otic Medications

For instillation of eardrops in older children and adults:

➤ Assess ear canal for cerumen or edema
➤ Tilt client's head toward unaffected side
➤ Gently pull pinna of ear up and back
➤ Instill eardrops—*do not* insert dropper into ear canal
➤ Gently massage area anterior to ear to facilitate entry of drops into ear canal

For instillation of eardrops in children 3 years and younger:

➤ Assess ear canal for cerumen or edema
➤ Tilt client's head toward unaffected side
➤ Gently pull pinna of ear slightly down and back
➤ Instill eardrops—*do not* insert dropper into ear canal
➤ Gently massage area anterior to ear to facilitate entry of drops into ear canal

Box 43–8

Corticosteroid Agents for Otic Use

Betamethasone	Dexamethasone
Hydrocortisone	Hydrocortisone with acetic acid

Box 43–9

Common OTC Agents for Otic Use

Acetic acid; aluminum acetate	Hydrocortisone, propylene glycol, alcohol, benzyl benzoate
Boric acid and isopropyl alcohol	Isopropyl alcohol
Carbamide peroxide	Isopropyl alcohol in glycerin
Carbamide peroxide and glycerin	

6. General considerations: generally considered safe and effective; contraindicated with hypersensitivity
7. Client teaching
   a. Seek evaluation by prescriber if symptoms do not improve within several days
   b. Inform prescriber if adverse reactions occur or if symptoms worsen

D. Medications that cause ototoxicity

1. Analgesics: aspirin and other salicylates, NSAIDs
2. Antibiotics: aminoglycosides (clarithromycin, tobramycin), erythromycin, streptomycin, vancomycin, chloramphenicol
3. Antineoplastic agents: cisplatin, nitrogen mustard
4. Loop diuretics (bumetanide, ethacrynic acid, furosemide, torsemide) and carbonic anhydrase inhibitor diuretic acetazolamide
5. Miscellaneous: quinine, quinidine

Check Your NCLEX–RN® Exam I.Q.

You are ready for testing on this content if you can:

- Apply knowledge of expected actions and effects of eye and ear medications to client care.
- Correctly administer eye and ear medications to clients.
- Assess for side effects and adverse effects of eye and ear medications.
- Take appropriate action if a client has an unexpected response to an eye or ear medication.
- Monitor a client for expected outcomes or effects of treatment with eye and ear medications.

PRACTICE TEST

1 A client being treated for glaucoma reports photophobia. What instructions should the nurse include in the client teaching?

1. Discontinue use of ophthalmic antiglaucoma medications.
2. Wipe eyes with tissue immediately after instilling eyedrops.
3. Wear dark glasses when outside, or when around bright lights.
4. Special glasses are necessary while being treated for glaucoma.

2 Which statement by the client indicates to the nurse that the client has an understanding regarding pilocarpine?

1. "I will see better at night."
2. "I may have trouble adjusting to darkness."
3. "It should not be difficult adjusting to changes from light to dark."
4. "I will not use the medication if I plan to drive."

3 The nurse is providing care to a client with glaucoma who is receiving methazolamide. The nurse should monitor for which electrolyte imbalances as part of the plan of care? Select all that apply.

1. Hyperkalemia
2. Hypokalemia
3. Hypocalcemia
4. Hypercalcemia
5. Hypernatremia

4 A client has a prescription for otic chloramphenicol. Which statement by the client should indicate a need for further instruction by the nurse?

1. "I will inform my doctor of increased ear pain."
2. "I will inform my doctor if my ear infection has not improved in 7 days."
3. "I will inform my doctor if I have an increase in drainage from my ear."
4. "I will inform my doctor if I experience any hearing disturbances."

5 A client is receiving pilocarpine for the treatment of glaucoma. Which symptom, if experienced by the client, does the nurse attribute to systemic absorption?

1. Diaphoresis
2. Constipation
3. Tachycardia
4. Hypertension

6 A client is receiving cyclopentolate and phenylphrine before an ocular examination. How should the nurse explain the purpose of the medication?

1. To constrict the pupil
2. To dilate the pupil
3. To provide anesthesia
4. To provide a prophylactic antibiotic

7 Which symptom, if described by a client, would lead the nurse to suspect a systemic side effect of atropine ophthalmic solution? Select all that apply.

1. Tachycardia
2. Slurred speech
3. Salivation
4. Diaphoresis
5. Confusion

8 Which statement demonstrates the client's understanding of proper administration of ophthalmic solutions?

1. "I will discard a medication if it has turned brown."
2. "I will discontinue medication that causes eye burning."
3. "I will use a cotton swab to apply my medication."
4. "I will not use any medication that is more than 1 month old."

9 In teaching a client about side effects of medications, for which over-the-counter medications would the nurse discuss ototoxicity? Select all that apply.

1. Aspirin
2. Vitamin C
3. Diphenhydramine
4. Vitamin A
5. Ibuprofen

10 During a follow-up visit at the clinician's office, a client states, "I insert the ear dropper deep into my ear so the medication doesn't run back out." What should be the nurse's response and priority teaching to the client?

1. The client's ear canal is likely obstructed with cerumen.
2. The client is using the appropriate technique for administering an otic solution.
3. The client should lie on the affected side for 5 minutes to promote absorption.
4. The medication dropper should not be inserted into the ear canal.

11 Which action, if observed by the nurse, demonstrates appropriate client technique for self-administering an ophthalmic medication?

1. Administers two different ophthalmic solutions 5 minutes apart.
2. Administers ophthalmic solution 5 minutes after ophthalmic ointment.
3. Administers two different ophthalmic solutions 2 minutes apart.
4. Administers ophthalmic ointment 2 minutes after ophthalmic solution.

12 The nurse is observing a client give a return demonstration of the administration of eyedrops. Which actions, if taken by the client, indicate an understanding of this procedure? Select all that apply.

1. The client pulls the lower lid of the eye down, forming a sac.
2. The client instills the medication into the conjunctival sac.
3. The client cleanses the eyelid with cotton balls moistened with warm tap water.
4. The client cleanses the eye from inner canthus to outer canthus.
5. The client promotes drainage of the medication toward the inner canthus.

13 The nurse is assessing a client with open-angle glaucoma who is receiving timolol for treatment. The nurse should expect what action of the timolol to promote the client's therapeutic response?

1. A decrease in the outflow of aqueous humor
2. An increase in the outflow of aqueous humor
3. A decrease in aqueous humor production
4. An increase in aqueous humor production

14 The nurse is providing information on safety measures to the family of an older adult client being treated with carbachol, an ophthalmic cholinesterase inhibitor. For what side effect are the safety measures implemented?

1. Difficulty in adjusting to quick changes in lighting due to miosis
2. Difficulty in adjusting to quick changes in lighting due to mydriasis
3. Medication side effect of constipation
4. Medication side effect of hypertension

15 The nurse is developing a plan of care for a client receiving acetazolamide for treatment of glaucoma. The nurse identifies that the client is at risk for developing which fluid and electrolyte imbalance?

1. Fluid overload
2. Dehydration
3. Hyperkalemia
4. Hypocalcemia

16 A client who just self-administered the first dose of ganciclovir calls the clinic and reports eye redness and swelling not present before treatment began. The nurse should instruct the client to take which action?

1. No action is necessary because these are normal manifestations of the medication.
2. Discontinue the medication and return to clinic immediately for evaluation.
3. If redness continues after 3 days, return to the clinic for evaluation.
4. Discontinue the medication until the next scheduled clinic appointment.

17 Which statement, if made by a client being treated with ophthalmic trifluridine, indicates an understanding of the medication instructions?

1. "I will stop the medication once healing has occurred."
2. "I will administer the treatment for 7 days."
3. "I will keep the medication in my pocket to avoid missing a dose."
4. "I will continue the medication for 5–7 days after healing has occurred."

18 The parent of a 2-year-old child exhibits correct administration technique for otic solutions by which action in a return demonstration?

1. The child's pinna is pulled down and back before administering the medication.
2. The child's pinna is pulled up and back before administering the medication.
3. The dropper is placed into the child's ear canal for instilling the medication.
4. The child's head is tilted toward the affected side for medication instillation.

19 A client who takes oral acetazolamide reports frequent urination during the night. Upon evaluation, what should the clinic nurse suspect is likely the cause of the nocturia?

1. The client takes oral acetazolamide on an empty stomach.
2. The client consumes 2,000 mL of fluid per day.
3. The client takes oral acetazolamide before supper.
4. The client takes oral acetazolamide with juice.

20 The nurse is orienting a newly hired nurse to the outpatient ophthalmic clinic. The nurse concludes that the new nurse understands the time frame for administering proparacaine hydrochloride for tonometry after observing which action?

1. Proparacaine is administered 15 minutes before the scheduled tonometry.
2. Proparacaine is administered immediately before the scheduled tonometry.
3. Proparacaine is administered 5 minutes before the scheduled tonometry.
4. Proparacaine is administered after the tonometry is completed.

ANSWERS & RATIONALES

1. **Answer: 3 Rationale:** Clients experiencing photophobia are instructed to wear dark sunglasses and to avoid bright lights. Not enough information is provided to warrant discontinuing the medication. Eyes should not be wiped with tissue immediately after instillation of drops. No special glasses are required. **Cognitive Level:** Applying **Client Need:** Pharmacological and Parenteral Therapies **Integrated Process:** Teaching and Learning **Content Area:** Pharmacology **Strategy:** Focus on the word *photophobia* and use the process of elimination to choose the answer that shields the eyes from light.

2. **Answer: 2 Rationale:** Difficulty in adjusting quickly to changes in illumination occurs as a result of miosis, an effect of pilocarpine. The client will experience more difficulty seeing at night. Driving is not contraindicated; however, nighttime driving might not be possible because of the miosis. **Cognitive Level:** Analyzing **Client Need:** Pharmacological and Parenteral Therapies **Integrated Process:** Nursing Process: Evaluation **Content Area:** Pharmacology **Strategy:** Specific knowledge of the important teaching points related to pilocarpine is needed to answer the question. Use this knowledge and the process of elimination to make a selection.

3. **Answer: 2, 5 Rationale:** The diuretic effects of methazolamide could lead to hypokalemia. The diuretic effects of methazolamide could lead to hypernatremia. Methazolamide will not cause hyperkalemia. Methazolamide will not cause hypocalcemia. Methazolamide will not cause hypercalcemia. **Cognitive Level:** Analyzing **Client Need:** Pharmacological and Parenteral Therapies **Integrated Process:** Nursing Process: Planning **Content Area:** Pharmacology **Strategy:** The core issue of the question is knowledge of electrolyte disturbances for which the client is at risk during therapy with methozolamide. Recall that the medication has a diuretic effect, and reason that potassium might be lost while sodium is retained. Use this knowledge and the process of elimination to make a selection. When there is more than one correct answer, consider each option as a true/false statement.

4. **Answer: 2 Rationale:** Superinfections are known to occur with this medication; therefore, 7 days is too long to seek further evaluation and treatment; this statement indicates a need for additional instruction. Informing the doctor of increased ear pain, increased ear drainage, and hearing disturbances are correct actions by the client. **Cognitive Level:** Analyzing **Client Need:** Pharmacological and Parenteral Therapies **Integrated Process:** Nursing Process: Evaluation **Content Area:** Pharmacology **Strategy:** The wording of the question tells you that the correct answer is an inaccurate statement. Use the process of elimination, and select the option that represents incorrect information.

5. **Answer: 1 Rationale:** Symptoms of systemic absorption of pilocarpine include diaphoresis, diarrhea, bradycardia, and hypotension. Constipation, tachycardia, and hypertension are not symptoms of systematic absorption of pilocarpine. **Cognitive Level:** Applying **Client Need:** Pharmacological and Parenteral Therapies **Integrated Process:** Nursing Process: Diagnosis **Content Area:** Pharmacology **Strategy:** The core issue of the question is recognition of signs of systemic absorption of pilocarpine. Specific knowledge of systemic effects of this medication is needed to answer the question. Use this knowledge and the process of elimination to make a selection.

6. **Answer: 2 Rationale:** Cyclomydril and other mydriatics are applied topically to produce mydriasis (dilated pupil) to facilitate ocular examination. Cyclomydril and other mydriatics do not provide anesthesia, nor do they prevent infection. **Cognitive Level:** Applying **Client Need:** Pharmacological and Parenteral Therapies **Integrated Process:** Teaching and Learning **Content Area:** Pharmacology **Strategy:** The core issue of the question is knowledge of the intended effects of cyclomydril. Note that the name of the drug contains the letters *myd*, which is also the beginning of the word *mydriasis* (meaning to dilate the pupils). Using simple word association will sometimes assist in making the correct selection.

7. **Answer: 1, 2, 5 Rationale:** Systemic side effects of ophthalmic atropine include tachycardia, slurred speech, and confusion. Salivation, which is the opposite of dry mouth, may be a side effect. Diaphoresis is unrelated to the use of ophthalmic atropine. **Cognitive Level:** Analyzing **Client Need:** Pharmacological and Parenteral Therapies **Integrated Process:** Nursing Process: Diagnosis **Content Area:** Pharmacology **Strategy:** The core issue of the question is knowledge of side/adverse effects of atropine. Recall that when used for cardiac reasons and as a pre-op medication, the medication speeds up heart rate. With this in mind, eliminate each of the incorrect responses. When there is more than one correct answer, consider each option as a true/false statement.

8. **Answer: 1 Rationale:** Ophthalmic solution that has darkened or become cloudy should be discarded. Many eye medications can cause the sensation of eye burning; medications should not be discontinued without first consulting the healthcare provider. Swabs should not be used to apply ophthalmic medication. Ophthalmic medications generally have a shelf-life of 3 months. **Cognitive Level:** Analyzing **Client Need:** Pharmacological and Parenteral Therapies **Integrated Process:** Nursing Process: Evaluation **Content Area:** Pharmacology **Strategy:** The core issue of the question is safe self-administration of ophthalmic medications. Use nursing knowledge and the process of elimination to answer the question.

9. **Answer: 1, 5 Rationale:** Aspirin can cause tinnitus, vertigo, and hearing loss, if ingested in high doses. Over-the-counter ibuprofen, if ingested in high doses, can cause ototoxicity. Vitamin C, dihyphenhydramine, and vitamin A do not present concerns about ototoxicity. **Cognitive Level:** Applying **Client Need:** Pharmacological and Parenteral Therapies **Integrated Process:** Nursing Process: Implementation **Content Area:** Pharmacology **Strategy:** The core issue of the question is an understanding of the types of drugs that can cause ototoxicity. Use nursing knowledge and the process of elimination to make a selection. When there is more than one correct answer, consider each option as a true/false statement.

10. **Answer: 4 Rationale:** Inserting objects, including medication droppers, into the ear canal can perforate the tympanic membrane; this is the priority teaching need. The ear canal may or may not be obstructed with cerumen, and the client needs teaching about the appropriate instillation technique; addressing the issue of cerumen is not the priority. The client is not demonstrating the proper technique for instilling ear medication. The client is instructed to lie on the unaffected side, not the affected side, to allow flow of medication into

the ear. While important, this is not the priority teaching need. **Cognitive Level:** Analyzing **Client Need:** Pharmacological and Parenteral Therapies **Integrated Process:** Nursing Process: Planning **Content Area:** Pharmacology **Strategy:** The core issue of the question is an understanding of the procedure for safe self-administration of an otic medication. Use nursing knowledge and the process of elimination to make a selection.

11 **Answer: 1 Rationale:** The recommended wait time between administrations of two ophthalmic solutions is 5 minutes. If an ophthalmic ointment is instilled, the waiting time is 10 minutes between the ointment and the next medication. **Cognitive Level:** Applying **Client Need:** Pharmacological and Parenteral Therapies **Integrated Process:** Nursing Process: Evaluation **Content Area:** Pharmacology **Strategy:** The core issue of the question is an understanding of the procedure for safe self-administration of an ophthalmic medication. Use nursing knowledge and the process of elimination to make a selection.

12 **Answer: 1, 2, 4 Rationale:** The client should pull the lower lid of the eye down, forming a sac. The client should instill the medication into the conjunctival sac. The client should cleanse the eye from inner canthus to outer canthus. The eye should be cleansed with sterile irrigating solution or sterile normal saline, not tap water, to decrease risk of contamination. Drainage of the medication should be directed toward the outer canthus and gentle pressure should be applied to the inner canthus to prevent systemic absorption of the medication. **Cognitive Level:** Analyzing **Client Need:** Pharmacological and Parenteral Therapies **Integrated Process:** Nursing Process: Evaluation **Content Area:** Pharmacology **Strategy:** The wording of the question tells you that the correct options are appropriate actions. Analyze each option to decide if it is a true or false statement, and select those that represent correct information.

13 **Answer: 3 Rationale:** Timolol is a beta-adrenergic blocker that decreases the production of aqueous humor, thereby decreasing intraocular pressure. Sympathomimetics also decrease aqueous humor production. A decrease in the outflow of aqueous humor is contraindicated for a client with glaucoma. Prostaglandins increase the outflow of aqueous humor to decrease intraocular pressure. An increase in aqueous humor production is contraindicated for a client with glaucoma. **Cognitive Level:** Analyzing **Client Need:** Pharmacological and Parenteral Therapies **Integrated Process:** Nursing Process: Evaluation **Content Area:** Pharmacology **Strategy:** Note that the drug name ends in *-olol*, and reason that the medication is a beta-blocking agent. With this in mind, recall the actions of beta-blocker medications in the eye. Use nursing knowledge and the process of elimination to make a selection.

14 **Answer: 1 Rationale:** Carbachol causes miosis (pupil constriction), making quick changes in illumination difficult. Nighttime is particularly hazardous for the elderly client. The client and family are instructed on methods such as lighting hallways and bathrooms at night to reduce the potential for injury. Mydriasis, pupil dilation, is not a concern when taking carbachol. Systemic side effects of carbachol include diarrhea. Systemic side effects of carbachol include hypotension. **Cognitive Level:** Applying **Client Need:** Pharmacological and Parenteral Therapies **Integrated Process:** Teaching and Learning **Content Area:** Pharmacology **Strategy:** Note that two options are opposites and when two options are opposite, consider the possibility that one of them is the correct answer. In this case, note that the client is elderly and is not in a situation (such as an eye exam) when the pupils would be dilated. With this in mind, eliminate the option that represents pupil dilation.

15 **Answer: 2 Rationale:** Carbonic anhydrase inhibitors produce increased urinary elimination and subsequent increased excretion of potassium. Clients are monitored for fluid volume deficit. Clients are monitored for fluid volume deficit, not excess. Clients are monitored for hypokalemia. The client should not experience hypocalcemia; however, the nurse should assess electrolytes, I&O, daily weights, mucous membranes, and skin turgor. **Cognitive Level:** Analyzing **Client Need:** Pharmacological and Parenteral Therapies **Integrated Process:** Nursing Process: Planning **Content Area:** Pharmacology **Strategy:** The core issue of the question is knowledge of what to monitor regarding side effects of carbonic anhydrase inhibitors. Use medication knowledge and the process of elimination to make a selection. Note also that two options are opposites, which suggests that one of them might be correct.

16 **Answer: 2 Rationale:** Redness and swelling are signs of hypersensitivity to ganciclovir. The medication should be discontinued, and the client should return to the clinic immediately for evaluation. **Cognitive Level:** Analyzing **Client Need:** Pharmacological and Parenteral Therapies **Integrated Process:** Nursing Process: Implementation **Content Area:** Pharmacology **Strategy:** Note that the question contains key information about adverse effects that began after the first dose of the medication. When symptoms suddenly appear, as in this question, consider the possibility of a hypersensitivity reaction and choose an option accordingly.

17 **Answer: 4 Rationale:** Trifluridine is used to treat viral infections such as herpes. It is administered for an additional 5–7 days after healing has occurred. Immediately discontinuing the medication is contraindicated. Stopping at 7 days is too limited of a time frame. Ophthalmic medications are stored in a cool, dry place, and some are recommended for refrigeration; a pocket is too warm. **Cognitive Level:** Analyzing **Client Need:** Pharmacological and Parenteral Therapies **Integrated Process:** Nursing Process: Evaluation **Content Area:** Pharmacology **Strategy:** The core issue of the question is knowledge of appropriate information about Viroptic as an ophthalmic medication. Use nursing knowledge and the process of elimination to make a selection.

18 **Answer: 1 Rationale:** The child's pinna is pulled down and back for administration of otic solutions. The pinna in the adult is pulled up and back. Droppers should never be inserted into the ear canal. The head is tilted toward the unaffected side so that medication will run into the ear canal. **Cognitive Level:** Analyzing **Client Need:** Pharmacological and Parenteral Therapies **Integrated Process:** Nursing Process: Evaluation **Content Area:** Pharmacology **Strategy:** One quick way to remember the direction for pulling the pinna is to associate the direction with the height of the person. Since an adult is taller, pull the pinna up and back, while for a child, who is shorter, pull the pinna down and back.

19 **Answer: 3 Rationale:** Acetazolamide, a carbonic anhydrase inhibitor, causes diuresis. The nurse should instruct the client to take the medication early in the day, to avoid nocturia. Acetazolamide may be taken with food to minimize gastrointestinal irritation. Clients receiving acetazolamide

are encouraged to consume at least 2000 mL of fluid per day to avoid fluid volume depletion. Acetazolamide may be taken with juice to minimize gastrointestinal irritation. **Cognitive Level:** Analyzing **Client Need:** Pharmacological and Parenteral Therapies **Integrated Process:** Nursing Process: Evaluation **Content Area:** Pharmacology **Strategy:** The core issue of the question is recognition of and client teaching to prevent nocturia, a side effect of carbonic anhydrase inhibitors. Use medication knowledge and general principles for timing the administration of diuretics to answer the question.

20 **Answer: 2** **Rationale:** The medication has a rapid onset, within 20 seconds, and a duration of 15–20 minutes. Proparacaine is administered beforehand to prevent pain during procedures such as tonometry and removal of foreign bodies. **Cognitive Level:** Analyzing **Client Need:** Pharmacological and Parenteral Therapies **Integrated Process:** Nursing Process: Evaluation **Content Area:** Pharmacology **Strategy:** Note that the name of the drug ends in *-caine* to help remember that this drug has an anesthetic action. With this in mind, choose the option that best protects an eye that has no sensation, which in this case is the option that utilizes the medication just prior to the exam.

Key Terms to Review

aqueous humor p. 650
cycloplegia p. 654
intraocular pressure p. 650
keratitis p. 653
miosis p. 655
mydriasis p. 652
narrow-angle glaucoma p. 653
open-angle glaucoma p. 650
photophobia p. 653
systemic absorption p. 650
tonometry p. 657
uveitis p. 652
vertigo p. 657

References

Adams, M., Holland, L., & Urban, C. (2017). *Pharmacology for nurses: A pathophysiologic approach* (5th ed.). New York, NY: Pearson Education.

Adams, M., & Urban, C. (2016). *Pharmacology: Connections to nursing practice* (3rd ed.). New York, NY: Pearson Education.

Lehne, R. (2016). *Pharmacology for nursing care* (9th ed.). St. Louis, MO: Saunders.

Wilson, B., Shannon, M., & Shields, K. (2016). *Pearson nurse's drug guide 2016.* New York, NY: Pearson Education.

Antineoplastic Medications

44

In this chapter

Cross Reference

Other chapters relevant to this content area are

Dosage Calculation and Medication Administration	Chapter 29
Cardiovascular Medications	Chapter 37
Gastrointestinal Medications	Chapter 40
Immunologic and Anti-Infective Medications	Chapter 45
Oncologic Disorders	Chapter 65

I. ALKYLATING AGENTS

A. Overview

1. Interfere with DNA replication by cross-linking or breaking DNA strands and through abnormal base pairing proteins
2. Most agents are **cell cycle–nonspecific**, which means that they exhibit a cytotoxic effect regardless of cell cycle stage; alkylating effect can occur anytime during cell life cycle, but cell death occurs when the cell attempts to duplicate the defective DNA strands
3. Chemical classes of alkylating agents are nitrogen mustards, nitrosureas, platinum compounds, and miscellaneous alkylating agents
4. Major toxicities occur in hematopoietic, gastrointestinal (GI), and reproductive systems

B. Common alkylating medications are listed in Box 44–1

C. Administration considerations

NCLEX® 1. Cyclophosphamide: oral doses may be given on an empty stomach; if nausea and vomiting (N/V) are severe, it may be taken with food; antiemetic agent should be given before administering drug

2. Mechlorethamine
   - *NCLEX®* a. Potent **vesicant** (causes severe skin and tissue necrosis if drug extravasates from vein)
   - b. Should be administered through side-arm portal of a freely running IV to avoid **extravasation** (infiltration of a drug that causes tissue damage); see signs and symptoms of extravasation in Table 44–1 and antidotes for vesicant drugs in Table 44–2
   - *NCLEX®* c. If drug should extravasate, subcutaneous (subcut) and intradermal injection with isotonic sodium thiosulfate and application of ice compresses may reduce local irritation
   - d. Short **nadir** period (6–8 days), which is lowest point to which blood counts will drop after chemotherapy administration

Box 44–1

Common Alkylating Agents

Nitrogen Mustards
Bendamustine
Chlorambucil
Cyclophosphamide
Estramustine
Ifosfamide
Mechlorethamine
Melphalan

Nitrosureas
Carmustine
Lomustine
Streptozocin

Platinum Compounds
Carboplatin
Cisplatin
Oxaliplatin

Miscellaneous Alkyating Agents
Busulfan
Dacarbazine
Procarbazine
Temozolamide
Thiotepa

Table 44–1 Signs and Symptoms of Extravasation

Assessment Parameter	Immediate Manifestations	Delayed Manifestations
Pain	Severe pain or burning that lasts minutes to hours and eventually subsides; usually occurs around needle site while drug is being given	Up to 48 hours
Redness	Blotchy redness around needle site; not always present at time of extravasation	Later occurrence
Ulceration	Develops insidiously; usually occurs 48–96 hours later	Later occurrence
Swelling	Severe swelling or puffiness; usually occurs immediately	Up to 48 hours
Blood return	Inability to obtain a blood return in IV line when drawing back gently with a syringe	Good blood return during administration
Other	Change in quality of infusion	Local tingling and sensory deficits

Table 44–2 Antidotes for Vesicant Therapy

Chemotherapeutic Drug	Antidote
Mechlorethamine Cisplatin	Thiosulfate
Dactinomycin	Apply ice and elevate; heat may enhance tissue damage
Doxorubicin	Cold pack with circulating ice water first 24–48 hours
Vinblastine Vincristine Vinorelbine	Hyaluronidase; apply warm pack for first 24–48 hours
Paclitaxel	Hyaluronidase; apply ice for first 24 hours

3. Carmustine: administer over 1–2 hours by slow IV infusion with constant monitoring if given peripherally; a vesicant—if possible, avoid starting IV in dorsum of hand, wrist, or antecubital veins
4. Lomustine: should be taken on an empty stomach to avoid nausea
5. Streptozocin: a vesicant—infuse via side arm portal of a freely flowing IV; administer antiemetic routinely before dose and every 4–6 hours after for first 24 hours
6. Carboplatin
   a. Do not use needles or IV sets containing aluminum
   b. Premedication with an antiemetic 30 minutes before and on a scheduled basis thereafter is generally recommended
   c. Dosage should not be repeated until neutrophil count is at least 2,000/mm^3

NCLEX® 7. Cisplatin

NCLEX® a. Provide hydration with 1–2 liters of IV fluid before and after administration

b. Administer parenteral antiemetic agent 30 minutes before therapy is started and give it on a scheduled basis throughout day and night as long as necessary

8. Busulfan: should be taken at same time every day; taking drug on an empty stomach may minimize N/V

D. Contraindications

1. Cyclophosphamide: childbearing age, serious infections including chickenpox and herpes zoster, immunosuppression, pregnancy (category C), and nursing mothers
2. Ifosfamide: **myelosuppression** (a decrease in red blood cell, white blood cell, and platelet counts usually related to chemotherapy), or known hypersensitivity to drug; use cautiously in clients with impaired renal function, prior radiation therapy, prior cytotoxic agents, pregnancy (category D drug), and nursing mothers
3. Mechlorethamine: myelosuppression, infectious granuloma, known infectious diseases (including herpes zoster), pregnancy (category D), and lactation
4. Carmustine: history of pulmonary function impairment, decreased platelets, leukocytes, or erythrocytes; safe use during pregnancy (category D) not established
5. Lomustine: decreased platelets, leukocytes, or erythrocytes; safe use during pregnancy (category D) not established
6. Streptozocin: hepatic and renal dysfunction; safe use during pregnancy (category C) not established
7. Carboplatin: history of severe reactions to carboplatin or cisplatin, severe bone marrow depression, impaired renal function, pregnancy (category D), and with other nephrotoxic drugs
8. Cisplatin: history of sensitivity to cisplatin or other platinum-containing compounds, impaired renal function and/or hearing, history of gout or urate renal stones; safe use in pregnancy (category D) and nursing women not established
9. Busulfan: therapy-resistant chronic lymphocytic leukemia, blast crisis of chronic myelogenous leukemia, bone marrow depression, pregnancy (category D), and nursing mothers

E. Significant assessment parameters

1. General
   a. Because bone marrow suppession (myelosuppression) is primary dose-limiting toxicity of this drug group, measure complete blood count (RBC, WBC with differential, and platelet count) before and during therapy, and for up to 6 weeks after last dose as appropriate to specific drug
   b. Withhold dose and notify provider if WBC is below 2000/mm^3 or platelet count is below 50,000/mm^3 (or other specified levels)
2. Cyclophosphamide: obtain baseline and periodic liver and renal function studies and serum electrolytes; microscopic urine examinations are recommended after large doses

NCLEX® 3. Busulfan: hematological toxicity may have abrupt onset; recovery from busulfan-induced **pancytopenia** (decrease in all blood cell components) may take from 1 month to 2 years; ovarian suppression, amenorrhea, and menopausal symptoms are common

NCLEX® 4. Ifosfamide: monitor urine before and during each dose for microscopic hematuria; hydrate with at least 3000 mL of fluid daily to reduce risk of **hemorrhagic cystitis** (excessive bleeding from bladder due to chemical irritation)

5. Carmustine
   a. Persistent N/V may occur 2 hours after drug administration and persist up to 6 hours; prior administration of an antiemetic will help
   b. Assess results of pulmonary function studies prior to and during therapy; report symptoms of lung toxicity to provider: cough, dyspnea, fever
   c. Assess for hepatic and renal insufficiency
6. Lomustine: monitor liver and kidney function tests
7. Streptozocin: assess for early evidence of renal dysfunction with hypophosphatemia, mild proteinuria, and changes in intake and output (I&O) pattern; perform liver function studies prior to each dose
8. Carboplatin

NCLEX® a. Monitor closely for signs of anaphylaxis caused by allergic reaction during first 15 minutes of infusion

b. Periodically monitor kidney function and creatinine clearance, although it has less renal toxicity than cisplatin

c. Monitor for peripheral neuropathy, ototoxicity, and visual disturbances, although they occur less frequently than with cisplatin

d. Monitor clients on diuretic therapy closely because carboplatin may also decrease serum sodium, potassium, calcium, and magnesium levels

9. Cisplatin
   a. Pretreatment electrocardiogram (ECG) is indicated because of possible myocarditis or focal irritation

   NCLEX®

   b. Monitor urine output (UO) and specific gravity for 4 consecutive hours before therapy and for 24 hours after therapy; report less than 100 mL/hr UO or specific gravity greater than 1.030; a UO of less than 75 mL/hr requires medical intervention
   c. Audiometric testing should be performed before initial dose
   d. Anaphylactic reactions may occur within minutes of drug administration
   e. Blood urea nitrogen (BUN), serum uric acid, serum creatinine, and urinary creatinine clearance should be assessed before initiating each course of therapy; nephrotoxicity usually occurs within 2 weeks and becomes more severe and prolonged with repeated rounds of therapy

   NCLEX®

   f. Suspect ototoxicity if client manifests tinnitus or difficulty hearing in high-frequency range
   g. Assess BP, mental status, pupils, and optic fundi every hour during therapy because hydration increases danger of elevated intracranial pressure
   h. Monitor and report abnormal bowel patterns because constipation may be an early sign of neurotoxicity

F. Adverse effects/toxicity

1. Common adverse effects with alkylating agents are headache, N/V, stomatitis, anorexia, and **alopecia** (partial or complete hair loss usually on scalp)
2. Common severe adverse effects with alkylating agents are bone marrow suppression, severe N/V, diarrhea, and possible hypersensitivity reactions
3. Cyclophosphamide
   a. Cardiotoxicity, acute cardiomegaly with high dose; prior radiation therapy and prior anthracycline therapy increases risk

   NCLEX®

   b. Hemorrhagic cystitis (occasionally chronic and severe)
   c. Metallic taste on administration

Memory Aid

Notice that the words *cyclophosphamide* and *cystitis* begin with *cy*. Use these letters to associate this drug with hemorrhagic cystitis of the bladder.

   d. **Acral erythema** (palmar redness) and sloughing of skin on palms of hands and soles of feet
   e. Diffuse hyperpigmentation
   f. Gonadal dysfunction
4. Ifosfamide

   NCLEX®

   a. Hemorrhagic cystitis, occasionally chronic and severe
   b. Hepatic dysfunction and nephrotoxicity
   c. Somnolence, confusion, and hallucinations
5. Carmustine
   a. Ocular infarctions, retinal hemorrhage, suffusion of the conjunctiva
   b. Delayed myelosuppression
   c. Pulmonary infiltration or fibrosis
6. Streptozocin: nephrotoxicity; insulin shock due to effect on pancreatic beta cells
7. Carboplatin

   NCLEX®

   a. Myelosuppression with pronounced thrombocytopenia
   b. Hepatotoxicity and ototoxicity, mild nephrotoxicity
8. Cisplatin
   a. Renal and hepatic toxicity; peripheral neuropathy; neurotoxicity

   NCLEX®

   b. Eighth cranial nerve damage because of ototoxicity
   c. Metallic taste on administration
9. Busulfan
   a. Pulmonary fibrosis, sometimes called *busulfan lung*
   b. Hepatic dysfunction leading to veno-occlusive disease
   c. Diffuse hyperpigmentation; development of bullae

Memory Aid

Notice that the word *busulfan* begins with *b*, which can help you to think of blue and pulmonary complications of therapy with busulfan.

G. Client and family education

1. Myelosuppression is severe and may be cumulative
   a. Teach that susceptibility to infection will increase; teach symptoms of sepsis
   b. Teach specific ways to avoid infection, such as avoiding large crowds and being near people with infections
   c. Teach neutropenic precautions for low WBCs
   d. Teach bleeding precautions for low platelet counts, such as preventing injury, avoiding over-the-counter (OTC) aspirin-containing medications (same precautions as used with anticoagulant therapy)
2. Cyclophosphamide
   a. Because of mutagenic potential, use adequate contraception during and for at least 4 months after termination of drug therapy
   NCLEX® b. Void frequently and maintain hydration with oral fluids to at least 3000 mL/24 hours
3. *NCLEX®* Ifosfamide: void frequently and maintain hydration; report any unusual bleeding or bruising
4. Carmustine: teach signs and symptoms of pulmonary toxicity
5. Streptozocin: teach signs and symptoms of hypoglycemia
6. Carboplatin
   NCLEX® a. Give special attention to strategies to prevent nausea
   b. Report paresthesias, visual disturbances, or symptoms of ototoxicity (hearing loss/tinnitis)
7. Cisplatin
   NCLEX® a. Continue maintenance of adequate hydration with oral fluids to at least 3000 mL/24 hours; report reduced UO, anorexia, N/V uncontrolled by antiemetics, fluid retention, and weight gain
   b. Keep vestibular stimulation to a minimum to avoid dizziness or falling
   NCLEX® c. Tingling, numbness, tremors of extremities, loss of position sense and taste, and constipation are early warning signs of neurotoxicity
8. Procarbazine
   NCLEX® a. Avoid foods high in tyramine (e.g., beer, wine, cheese, brewer's yeast, chicken livers, and bananas); may lead to hypertension and possible intracranial hemorrhage
   b. Disulfiram-like reaction can occur if client consumes alcohol and procarbazine

II. ANTIMETABOLITES

A. Overview

1. Inhibit protein synthesis, substitute erroneous metabolites or structural analogues during DNA synthesis, and inhibit DNA synthesis; have three subgroups
2. Folic acid analogs are structurally similar to folic acid and disrupt DNA replication
3. Pyrimidine analogs are structurally similar to pyrimidines (bases used in biosynthesis of DNA and RNA) and can act in a variety of specific ways
4. Purine analogs are bases (similar to pyrimidines) used in biosynthesis of nucleic acids
5. Most agents are **cell cycle–specific**, exhibiting cytotoxic effect during a specific phase of cell cycle, such as S phase
6. *NCLEX®* Most toxicity occurs in hematopoietic (myelosuppression) and GI systems
7. Used to treat leukemia, solid tumors, and lymphoma

B. Common antimetabolites are listed in Box 44–2

C. Administration considerations

1. Rotate IV sites every 48 hours to decrease hyperpigmentation
2. Determine whether prescribed dosage is standard or high and obtain prescription for appropriate rescue therapy before administration (i.e., leucovorin rescue therapy at specific times following methotrexate dose)

D. Contraindications

1. *NCLEX®* Myelosuppression
2. Pregnancy (category D) and nursing women
3. Concurrent administration of hepatotoxic drugs and hematopoietic depressants
4. Cautious use in following situations
   a. Clients with major surgery during previous month
   b. Previous use of alkylating agents
   c. History of high-dose pelvic irradiation
   d. Preexisting bone marrow impairment
   e. Men and women during childbearing years
   f. Hepatic or renal impairment

Box 44–2
Common Antimetabolites

Folic Acid Analogs	Purine Analogs
Methotrexate	Cladribine
Pemetrexed	Clofarabine
Pralatrexate	Fludarabine
Pyrimidine Analogs	Mercaptopurine
Capecitabine	Nelarabine
Cytarabine	Pentostatin
Floxuridine	Thioguanine
Fluorouracil	
Gemcitabine	

NCLEX® **E. Significant assessment parameters**
1. Assess baseline CBC, WBC differential, and platelet count prior to administration
2. Assess for signs and symptoms of infection or bleeding

F. Adverse effects/toxicity

NCLEX® 1. General adverse effects for this drug group include myelosuppression, N/V, mucosal inflammation or stomatitis, alopecia, photosensitivity with or without hyperpigmentation, and diarrhea (most commonly associated with antimetabolites)
2. Fluorouracil: cerebellar toxicity; cardiotoxicity resembling acute myocardial infarction (MI), angina, cardiogenic shock
3. Cytarabine
   a. Maculopapular rash, with or without fever; acryl erythema
   b. Cytarabine syndrome (rash with or without fever, myalgia, bone pain, malaise)
   c. Chemical conjunctivitis
   d. Acute neurotoxicity: cerebellar toxicity; clients over age 50 at highest risk
   e. Hepatotoxicity

G. Client and family education

NCLEX® 1. Teach importance of self-care measures to avoid infection and bleeding
NCLEX® 2. Assess condition of oral cavity, maintain scheduled mouth care, and report development of stomatitis to provider
NCLEX® 3. Maintain a low-residue diet after discharge and report excessive diarrhea (more than three loose stools in 24 hours) to healthcare provider
4. Darkening of veins, mucous membranes, and fingernails may occur
NCLEX® 5. Photosensitivity precautions should be followed year round: use sunscreen with a sun protection factor (SPF) of at least 15; avoid sun exposure between 10:00 a.m. and 2:00 p.m.; wear long sleeves and a large-brimmed hat

III. ANTITUMOR ANTIBIOTICS

A. Overview
1. Contain substances from bacteria that are able to kill cancer cells; were originally intended to be antibiotics, but were too cytotoxic for this use
2. Are divided into two groups: anthracyclines and nonanthracyclines
3. Anthracyclines tend to cause more cardiotoxicity than nonanthracyclines
4. Interfere with nucleic acid synthesis and function, inhibit ribonucleic acid (RNA) synthesis, and inhibit DNA synthesis
5. Most agents are cell cycle–nonspecific

NCLEX® 6. Major toxicities occur in hematopoietic, GI, reproductive, and cardiac systems (cumulative doses)

B. Common antitumor antibiotics are listed in Box 44–3

C. Administration considerations

NCLEX® 1. Most antitumor antibiotics are severe vesicants except for bleomycin (see again signs of extravasation in Table 44–1 and antidotes for vesicants in Table 44–2)

Box 44–3

Antitumor Antibiotics

Anthracyclines	Nonanthracyclines
Doxorubicin	Bleomycin
Doxorubicin liposomal	Dactinomycin
Daunorubicin	Mitomycin
Daunorubicin liposomal	Mitoxantrone
Epirubicin	
Idarubicin	

2. Administer slowly by IV push (IVP) via side-arm portal of a freely flowing IV
3. Maintain clear visualization of injection site during administration
4. IV catheter should have an excellent blood return, be recently placed, and not more than 48 hours old before administering vesicant therapy
5. *NCLEX®* Avoid use of antecubital veins, in dorsum of hand, or in wrist, where extravasation could damage underlying tendons and nerves
6. Avoid venous access in extremity with compromised venous or lymphatic drainage

D. Contraindications

1. Doxorubicin: myelosuppression, impaired cardiac function, obstructive jaundice, impaired hepatic or renal function, safe use in pregnancy not established
2. Bleomycin: history of hypersensitivity or idiosyncrasy to bleomycin; pregnancy (category D) and women of childbearing age; cautious use with compromised hepatic, renal, or pulmonary function; previous cytotoxic drug or radiation therapy
3. Mitoxantrone: hypersensitivity, myelosuppression, pregnancy (category D) and lactation, cautious use in impaired cardiac, renal, or hepatic function
4. Mitomycin: hypersensitivity, pregnancy (category D) and lactation, thrombocytopenia, and coagulation disorders

E. Significant assessment parameters

1. Doxorubicin
   a. Assess hepatic, renal, hematopoietic, and cardiac function prior to administration and at regular intervals thereafter
   b. Establish baseline data, including temperature, pulse, respirations, BP, body weight, laboratory values, I&O ratio and pattern, and cardiac ejection fraction; continue to track these
   c. *NCLEX®* Give prompt attention to report of stinging or burning at injection site
   d. *NCLEX®* Be alert to and report early signs of cardiotoxicity and hepatic dysfunction

Memory Aid

Notice that the word *doxorubicin* contains the letters *rub*. Think of ruby and red when you see this name to help you think of the heart and cardiotoxicity.

   e. Stomatitis is greatest at 2 weeks following therapy (coincides with nadir of drug), begins with burning sensation
   f. *NCLEX®* **Radiation recall**, erythema that develops in previously irradiated field, is common
2. Bleomycin
   a. *NCLEX®* Assess vital signs (VS); a febrile reaction is relatively common
   b. Bone marrow toxicity is rare
   c. *NCLEX®* Pulmonary toxicity occurs in about 10% of clients, usually in clients over 70 years of age and when cumulative dose reaches 400 units
   d. *NCLEX®* Radiation recall is common

Memory Aid

Notice that the word *bleomycin* begins with *bl*, which can help you to think of blue and pulmonary toxicity from chemotherapy with this agent.

3. Mitoxantrone
    a. Assess IV insertion site; transient blue discoloration may occur
NCLEX® b. Assess cardiac function throughout therapy; report signs of heart failure
NCLEX® c. Assess uric acid levels and initiate hypo-uricemic therapy before antileukemia therapy
4. Mitomycin
    a. Assess serum creatinine (drug is rarely given if greater than 1.7 mg/dL); assess platelet count, PT, and bleeding times
NCLEX® b. Assess I&O ratio and pattern, dysuria, hematuria, and oliguria; maintain hydration because drug is nephrotoxic

F. Adverse effects/toxicity

1. Common adverse effects for antitumor antibiotics are N/V, stomatitis, anorexia, and alopecia
2. More severe adverse effects of this drug class are myelosuppression, severe N/V, diarrhea, stomatitis, or mucositis
3. Anthracycline(s), which end in *-rubicin*
    a. Vesicant: flare-up reaction is common and may be difficult to distinguish from an extravasation
NCLEX® b. Cardiotoxicity leading to degenerative cardiomyopathy occurs over time
    c. Lifetime dosage is 450–550 mg/m^2
    d. Prior radiation therapy to chest wall may enhance risk of cardiotoxicity
    e. Hyperpigmentation of nail beds and dermal creases
4. Bleomycin
NCLEX® a. Anaphylactic reactions and pulmonary toxicity that is dose- and age-related can occur
    b. Mild febrile reaction commonly occurs
    c. Diffuse alopecia, hyperpigmentation of skin, vesiculation, acne, thickening of skin and nailbeds
5. Mitoxantrone
    a. An **irritant**: a drug capable of causing pain and inflammation at administration site if extravasation occurs
NCLEX® b. Sclera and urine may turn blue to blue-green
    c. Increased cardiotoxicity with cumulative dose higher than 180 mg/m^2
6. Mitomycin
NCLEX® a. Vesicant; has unique ability to produce ulceration at distal sites
    b. Myelosuppression is delayed and cumulative initial nadir is 4–6 weeks
NCLEX® c. Nephrotoxic; can cause hemolytic uremia syndrome

G. Client and family education

1. General strategies to treat common adverse effects as detailed in previous sections
2. Anthracycline
NCLEX® a. Alopecia, which may also involve eyelashes, eyebrows, beard/mustache, and pubic and axillary hair; regrowth of hair usually begins 2–3 months after completion of administration
NCLEX® b. Urine may turn red
3. Mitoxantrone
NCLEX® a. Blue-green urine is common for 24 hours after drug therapy and sclera may also take on a bluish color
    b. Stomatitis and mucositis may occur within 1 week of therapy

IV. PLANT EXTRACTS

A. Overview

1. Are derived from plants and include vinca alkaloids, taxanes, and topoisomerase inhibitors
2. Arrest or inhibit mitosis (mitotic inhibitors); most agents are cell cycle–specific, M-phase
3. Major toxicities occur in hematopoietic, integumentary, neurologic, and reproductive systems; also, hypersensitivity reactions may occur

B. Common plant extract medications are listed in Box 44–4

C. Administration considerations

1. Etoposide: administer by slow IVPB over 60–90 minutes to avoid hypotension
2. Paclitaxel
    a. Do not use equipment or devices containing polyvinyl chloride (PVC); administer via non-PVC tubing with an in-line filter of 0.22 micron or less
    b. Tissue necrosis occurs with extravasation
NCLEX® c. Requires strict premedication (preferably with dexamethasone, diphenhydramine, and either cimetidine or ranitidine) per protocol order set before administration to prevent anaphylaxis

Box 44–4

Plant Extracts

Vinca Alkaloids	Topoisomerase Inhibitors
Vinblastine	Etoposide
Vincristine	Irinotecan
Vinorelbine	Teniposide
Taxanes	Topotecan
Cabazitaxel	**Miscellaneous Natural Products**
Docetaxel	Eribulin
Paclitaxel	Omacetaxine

3. Vincristine and other vinca alkaloids
   a. Vesicant: administer into side-arm portal of freely flowing IV
   NCLEX® b. Hyaluronidase is antidote if extravasation occurs; also apply moderate heat to disperse drug and minimize sloughing

D. Contraindications

1. Etoposide: severe bone marrow depression, severe hepatic or renal impairment, existing or recent viral infection or bacterial infection, safe use in pregnancy (category D) and nursing mothers not established
2. Paclitaxel: hypersensitivity to paclitaxel, baseline neutropenia of less than 1500 cells/mm^3, cautious use in presence of cardiac arrhythmias and impaired liver function, pregnancy (category X)
3. Vincristine: obstructive jaundice, demyelinating neurologic diseases; preexisting neuromuscular disease, pregnancy (category D)

E. Significant assessment parameters

1. Etoposide
   a. Assess IV site before and after infusion; extravasation can cause thrombophlebitis and necrosis
   b. Be prepared to treat an anaphylactic reaction
   c. Monitor VS during and after infusion; if hypotension occurs, stop infusion
   NCLEX® d. Assess CBC, WBC, and differential, and hepatic and renal function before administration and periodically during treatment
2. Paclitaxel
   NCLEX® a. Monitor for hypersensitivity during first two administrations; immediately discontinue if angioedema and generalized urticaria develop
   NCLEX® b. Monitor VS frequently; bradycardia occurs in 12% of clients
   c. Assess for peripheral neuropathy
3. Vincristine
   a. Assess for leukopenia, which occurs in a significant number of clients
   NCLEX® b. Assess hand grasps and deep tendon reflexes; depression of Achilles reflex is earliest sign of neuropathy

F. Adverse effects/toxicity

1. Common adverse effects are N/V, anorexia, stomatitis, alopecia, and loss of energy and strength
2. More serious adverse effects are myelosuppression, severe N/V, diarrhea, mucositis, and hypersensitivity
3. Etoposide
   a. Acral erythema and sloughing of the skin on palms and soles
   b. Severe blood count fluctuations
   c. Fever and chills during infusion
4. Paclitaxel
   a. Transient bradycardia
   b. Peripheral neuropathy
   c. Hypersensitivity reaction including hypotension, bronchospasm, urticaria, and angioedema
   d. Alopecia
5. Docetaxel: neurotoxicity and severe fluid retention
6. Vincristine: neurotoxicity; loss of sensation on fingertips and soles of feet, paralytic ileus; depression of Achilles reflex is earliest sign

G. Client and family education

1. Etoposide

NCLEX®

   a. Inform about possible adverse effects (blood dyscrasias, alopecia, and carcinogenesis)
   b. Make position changes slowly, particularly from a recumbent position to avoid hypotension
   c. Inspect mouth daily for ulcerations and bleeding and avoid obvious irritants

2. Paclitaxel

NCLEX®

   a. Report dyspnea, chest pain, palpitations, or angioedema
   b. Stress need for periodic laboratory testing
   c. There is high probability of developing alopecia

3. Vincristine

NCLEX®

   a. Prevent constipation and report a change in bowel habits or paralytic ileus
   b. Alopecia is most common side effect; reversible after treatment is complete

V. HORMONES AND HORMONE MODULATORS

A. Overview

1. Corticosteroids: lyse lymphoid malignancies and have indirect effect on malignant cells
2. Estrogens: suppress testosterone production in males and alter response of breast cancers to prolactin
3. Antiestrogens: compete with estrogens for binding with estrogen receptor sites on malignant cells
4. Progestins: promote palliation and tumor cell regression; exact mechanism of action unknown
5. Gonadotropin-releasing hormone (Gn-RH) analogs: provide feedback to pituitary gland to increase production of interstitial cell–stimulating hormone (ICSH), which initially increases testosterone and then causes it to dramatically fall as pituitary becomes insensitive to Gn-RH
6. Antiandrogens: inhibit binding of androgens at androgen receptor sites in target tissues; indicated for use in metastatic/advanced prostate cancer
7. Androgens: hormone therapy with palliative use in metastatic/advanced carcinoma of breast; used if surgery and irradiation inappropriate; otherwise, tamoxifen is drug of choice for this purpose

B. Common hormones and hormone modulators are listed in Box 44–5

Box 44–5

Hormones and Hormone Modulators

Corticosteroids

Prednisone

Dexamethasone

Estrogens

Diethylstilbestrol

Ethinyl estradiol

Antiestrogens

Tamoxifen

Toremifene

Anastrozole

Exemestane

Fulvestrant

Letrozole

Raloxifene

Progestins

Medroxyprogesterone

Megestrol

Gonadotropin-Releasing Hormone (Gn-RH) Analogs

Degarelix

Leuprolide

Goserelin

Histrelin

Triptorelin

Antiandrogens (Androgen Receptor Blockers)

Abiraterone

Bicalutamide

Enzalutamide

Flutamide

Nilutamide

Androgens

Fluoxymesterone

Testosterone

Testolactone

Fluoxymesterone

C. Administration considerations

NCLEX® **1.** Corticosteroids: administer oral forms with meals; they may be crushed; give IV dose slowly by IVPB to prevent vaginal and anal burning

2. Estrogens

a. Give orally immediately after solid food

b. An exception is estramustine (combination of festrogen and nitrogen mustard); this must be taken with water an hour before meals; also requires no concurrent use of milk, dairy products, or calcium-containing products

3. Progestins: give orally without regard to meals

4. Estrogen antagonists: give orally; dosage may be decreased if side effects are severe

5. Androgens and antiandrogens: give orally

6. Gn-RH Analogs: give by IM, subcut, or subcut implant routes per drug literature

D. Contraindications

1. Corticosteroids: systemic infections, ulcerative colitis, diverticulitis, active or latent peptic ulcer disease; safe use in pregnancy (category C) and nursing mothers not established

NCLEX® **2.** Estrogens: known or suspected pregnancy, estrogen-dependent neoplasms, history of thromboembolic disorders

3. Progestins: severe arrhythmias if taking a calcium-channel blocker; psychiatric depression, pregnancy (category C); cautious use in lactation

4. Antiestrogens: first trimester of pregnancy (category C)

5. Gn-RH analogs: pregnancy (category X)

E. Significant assessment parameters

NCLEX® **1.** Corticosteroids

a. Establish baseline and trend data on BP, I&O, weight, and sleep patterns

b. Measure 2-hour postprandial blood glucose, serum potassium, and serum calcium prior to therapy and at regular intervals thereafter

c. Watch for changes in mood, emotional stability, and sleep patterns

2. Estrogens

NCLEX® **a.** Spotting or breakthrough bleeding may occur

b. Severe hypercalcemia may occur

3. Progestin

a. Assess weight periodically

b. Assess for allergic reactions, rash, urticaria, anaphylaxis, tachypnea

4. Antiestrogens: assess CBC, including platelet count, periodically

NCLEX® **5.** Androgens: monitor serum calcium levels; hypercalcemia can result, requiring temporary termination of therapy and treatment with large volumes of IV fluid

6. Antiandrogens: monitor liver function studies periodically to detect rare complication of hepatitis

F. Adverse effects/toxicity

1. Corticosteroids

a. Euphoria, headache, insomnia, psychosis

NCLEX® **b.** Edema

c. Muscle weakness, delayed wound healing, osteoporosis, spontaneous fractures

NCLEX® **d.** Hyperglycemia

NCLEX® **2.** Estrogens: thromboembolic disorders, nausea

3. Progestins: vaginal bleeding and breast tenderness; abdominal pain, N/V; increased appetite and weight gain

NCLEX® **4.** Antiestrogens: thrombosis; N/V (25% of clients); hot flashes, weight gain, changes in menstrual cycle, leaking from breasts

5. Gn-RH analogs

a. Hot flashes and decreased bone density in both men and women

b. Testicular atrophy and gynecomastia in men

c. Amenorrhea in women

NCLEX® **6.** Androgens: hypercalcemia; virilization (including clitoral enlargement, increased facial and body hair, deepened voice, increased libido, and male-pattern baldness)

NCLEX® **7.** Antiandrogens: gynecomastia, GI disturbances (N/V, constipation, diarrhea), and hepatitis

G. Client and family teaching: for all drug groups, teach about adverse effects and when to report them

VI. OTHER ANTINEOPLASTICS

A. Biological response modifiers (BRMs) and monoclonal antibodies (MABs); see Box 44–6

1. Kill tumor cells using body's immune system
2. BRMs consist of interferons and interleukins that alter bodily defenses to neutralize or aid removal of foreign cells; they have limited applications in chemotherapy but are also used to treat other immune system disorders (see also Chapter 45)
   a. Interferons are natural proteins produced by T cells in response to antigens and viral infections; they bind to specific receptors on cancer cell membranes to suppress cell division, enhance phagocytosis by macrophages, and aid cytotoxic actions of T lymphocytes
   b. Interferons used for hairy cell and chronic myelogenous leukemia include interferon alfa-2b and peginterferon alfa-2a; those used to treat other diseases are discussed in Chapter 45
   c. Common adverse effects of interferons are flulike symptoms (fever, chills, malaise), N/V, diarrhea, anemia, confusion and dyspnea; more serious adverse effects include tachycardia, hypotension, oliguria or anuria, pulmonary edema, and capillary leak syndrome
   d. Interleukin-2 activates cytotoxic T lymphocytes and promotes other areas of immune response; prototype drug aldesleukin is used to treat metastatic renal cell carcinoma
   e. Common adverse effects of aldesleukin are flulike symptoms, headache, fatigue, myalgia, anorexia, and diarrhea; more serious adverse effects are myelosuppression, anaphylaxis, hepatotoxicity, and suicide ideation
3. MABs attack antigens on surfaces of specific tumor cells; because of this specificity, they are also referred to as *molecularly targeted agents*; other MABs subdue overactive inflammatory cells, which aids in treatment of severe psoriasis and rheumatoid arthritis; such MABs are further discussed in Chapter 45
   a. Common adverse effects of MABs used to treat cancer include N/V, anorexia, stomatitis, rash, alopecia, fever and chills

Box 44–6

Biological Response Modifiers and Monoclonal Antibodies (Molecularly Targeted Agents)

Biological Response Modifiers

Aldesleukin
Interferon alfa-2

Monoclonal Antibodies and Molecularly Targeted Agents

Alemtuzumab
Axtinib
Bevacizumab
Bortezomib
Bosutinib
Brentuximab
Carfilzomib
Cabozantinib
Ceritinib
Cetuximab
Crizotinib
Dasatanib
Erlotinib
Gefitinib
Gemtuzumab
Ibritumomab
Imatinib
Ipilimumab
Lapatinib
Nilotinib
Obinutuzumab
Ofatumumab
Panitumumab
Pazopanib
Pertuzumab
Plerixafor
Ramucirumab
Regorafenib
Rituximab
Sorafenib
Sunitinib
Tositumomab
Trastuzumab
Vandetanib
Vemurafenib
Vismodegib
Ziv-aflibercept

b. More severe adverse effects are myelosuppression, severe N/V, diarrhea, severe hypersensitivity reactions, and pulmonary toxicity; each drug may additionally have unique adverse effects, see specific drug literature

B. Miscellaneous antineoplastics (act by unique mechanisms)

1. Drugs in this group are structurally dissimilar to groups already discussed and have unique actions and adverse effects; see Box 44–7
2. Angiogenesis inhibitors include thalidomide, enalidomide, and pomalidomide
   a. Prevent formation of new blood vessels needed by tumors for growth; do not kill cancer cells but inhibit their growth
   b. Have teratogenic properties and a limited distribution program
   c. Bevacizumab, a MAB, also inhibits angiogenesis by targeting vascular endothelial growth factor
3. Altretamine
   a. Is similar to alkylating agents; forms toxic metabolites that bind to macromolecules and have cytotoxic effect
   b. Adverse effects are mild N/V, mild neurotoxicity (ataxia, dizziness, vertigo, peripheral neuropathy), and severe myelosuppression (15% of clients)
4. Arsenic trioxide
   a. Toxic metal used for acute promyelocytic leukemia; action not fully understood but seems to cause DNA fragmentation with apoptosis
   b. GI side effects and neurotoxicity are common; skin reactions can occur (dermatitis, pruritus, and injection site inflammation); can cause QT prolongation and complete AV block, so drugs that prolong QT interval should be discontinued during therapy
5. Asparaginase and pegaspargase
   a. Deprive cancer cells of asparagine, an essential amino acid, which greatly reduces protein, RNA and DNA synthesis; pegaspargase has PEEG molecule bonded to prolong half-life and require fewer injections (3 doses vs. 21)
   b. Adverse reactions include hypersensitivity reactions (urticaria to anaphylaxis), hepatotoxicity (impaired synthesis of protein and clotting factors), neurotoxicity, and pancreatitis (possibly fatal)
6. Bexarotene
   a. A retinoid (an agent related to vitamin A); used for refractory T-cell lymphomas; used off-label for lung cancer, Kaposi's sarcoma, and metastatic breast cancer; pregnancy category X
   b. Adverse effects of oral route are hyperlipidemia, hypothyroidism, acute pancreatitis, anemia, anorexia, and photosensitivity
   c. Adverse effects of topical route are rash, erythema, and pruritus
7. Hydroxyurea
   a. Blocks incorporation of thymidine into DNA and may damage already formed DNA molecules
   b. Adverse effects include myelosuppression (especially neutropenia), GI side effects, and possible skin ulcers and gangrene
8. Ixabepilone
   a. Has same mechanisms of action as taxanes but different pharmacokinetics; used in combination with capecitabine to treat metastatic or advanced breast cancer resistant to first-line treatments such as taxanes

Box 44–7

Miscellaneous Antineoplastics

Angiogenesis Inhibitors	Bexarotene
Lenalidomide	Hydroxyurea
Pomalidomide	Ixabepilone
Thalidomide	Mitotane
Unique Drugs	Pegaspargase
Altretamine	Romidepsin
Arsenic trioxide	Vorinostat
Asparaginase	Zoledronic acid
Belinostat	

b. Adverse effects include GI effects, alopecia, fatigue, musculoskeletal pain, peripheral neuropathy, myelosuppression

9. Mitotane
   a. Similar to insectide DDT and forms links to proteins to poison cancer cells; used for advanced, inoperable adrenocorticoid cancer
   b. Adverse effects include GI symptoms, CNS effects (lethargy, drowsiness, vertigo), adrenal insufficiency, rash, and possible hemorrhagic cystitis
10. Vorinostat
   a. Arrests cell cycle and induces apoptosis; used for progressive or persistent cutaneous T-cell lymphoma
   b. Adverse effects include GI effects, altered taste, fatigue, chills, blood dyscrasias, and possible pulmonary embolism
11. Zoledronic acid
   a. Bisphosphonate used in multiple myeloma with osteolytic metastases; inhibits bone resorption by osteoclasts; also used to treat osteoporosis
   b. Adverse effects include flulike symptoms, bone and muscle pain, dysrhythmias, electrolyte imbalances, osteonecrosis of jaw

C. Drugs to reduce antineoplastic drug adverse effects

1. Do not have any antineoplastic drug actions; instead, they prevent adverse effects from occurring or treat/limit them once they occur
2. Antiemetics such as dronabinol, prochlorperazine, and ondansetron are used to treat N/V; see Chapter 40
3. Constipation is treated by laxatives and stool softeners, while diarrhea is treated by antidiarrheals; see Chapter 40
4. Myelosuppression is treated with drugs to increase red blood cell count (epoetin alfa), white blood cell count (filgrastim), or platelets (oprelvekin); see Chapter 45

VII. SAFE HANDLING OF CHEMOTHERAPEUTIC AGENTS

A. Drug preparation and administration

NCLEX® 1. All individuals preparing and administering cytotoxic drugs should be specially trained in safe handling procedures and comply with agency, government, and professional practice standards
2. Chemotherapy doses are generally individualized according to body weight (in kg) or body surface area (in m^2)
3. Most chemotherapy protocol order sets consist of short, intermittent, high-dose courses of medications (often in combination) to maximize cancer-cell kill while allowing healthy cells time to heal and recover
4. Chemotherapy drugs should be prepared for use in an air-vented space, such as a clean-air workstation or biohazard cabinet; access to this area should be limited

NCLEX® 5. Wear a disposable, leak-proof gown, surgical latex gloves, a mask, and eye protection when preparing chemotherapeutic agents

NCLEX® 6. Do not prepare or administer IV chemotherapy if pregnant because of possible risk to fetus

B. Safe handling of antineoplastic agents and spill management

NCLEX® 1. Use leak-proof, puncture-resistant containers to dispose of all antineoplastic drug preparation equipment; double-bag and identify container with a biohazard label
2. To avoid leaking medication from them, do not separate needle from syringe or break needles

NCLEX® 3. If drug accidentally touches nurse or client, wash area well with soap and water; immediately remove contaminated clothing; copiously flush eyes if involved while keeping eyelids open
4. Double-glove to clean a drug spill, washing hands before and after
5. For powdered medications, wear a mask and eye protection as well
6. Place spilled substance in a plastic bag; wipe remaining area with a damp cloth and place cloth in same bag; place this bag into another plastic bag (double-bag) and label it as biohazardous
7. All materials used for drug preparation and administration must be disposed of by incineration

NCLEX® **C. Disposal of client's body fluids**

1. Handle cautiously all body substances, such as blood, urine, vomitus, stool, and others; carefully follow standard precautions and other procedures as designated by agency policy
2. Wear gloves when in contact with all body substances; carefully dispose of them in toilet; clean containers carefully and thoroughly

VIII. NURSING MANAGEMENT OF TREATMENT SIDE EFFECTS

A. Neutropenia

NCLEX® 1. Neutropenia is an absolute neutrophil count (ANC) of 1,500/mm^3 or less
2. Lowest point (nadir) in WBC count after chemotherapy most commonly occurs 7–14 days following chemotherapy administration
3. Fever of more than 100.4°F (38°C) is most reliable and often only sign of infection in neutropenic clients

NCLEX® 4. Management
   - a. Avoid exposure to fresh fruits, vegetables, flowers, and live plants; people recently vaccinated with live organisms or viruses; or pet excreta including fish tanks and aquariums
   - b. Teach people who come in contact with client to wash hands prior to touching client
   - c. Encourage client to practice good personal hygiene
   - d. Prevent trauma to skin and mucous membranes
   - e. Culture urine, peripheral blood, all lumens of central venous catheters (CVCs) and suspected sources of infection; obtain chest x-ray (CXR); administer antibiotics as prescribed for empiric therapy
   - f. Institute neutropenic precautions for hospitalized clients whose ANC drops as described, using previously described measures
   - g. Administer filgrastim, a granulocyte colony-stimulating factor that increases production of neutrophils, either IV or subcut as prescribed; client may report bone pain 1–3 days before blood count increases, which may be controlled with nonopioid analgesics

NCLEX® 5. Client and family education
   - a. Report temperature greater than 100.4°F (38°C), shaking chills, dysuria, dyspnea, sputum production, or pain
   - b. Use meticulous hygiene to prevent infection
   - c. Avoid contact with people who have contagious illness
   - d. Teach self-administration of granulocyte colony-stimulating factor (G-CSF) for neutropenia or granulocyte/macrophage colony-stimulating factor (GM-CSF) for treatment of blood-forming organ cancers as prescribed

B. Thrombocytopenia

1. Bone marrow suppression decreases platelet production; circulating platelets diminish gradually because platelet lifespan is only 10 days
2. Assessment
   - a. Platelet count below 50,000/mm^3; risk significantly increases when platelet count falls below 20,000/mm^3
   - b. Petechiae, bruising, and hemorrhage (tachycardia, hypotension)
   - c. Neurologic changes, which may indicate intracranial bleeding

NCLEX® 3. Management
   - a. Institute bleeding precautions (refer to Chapter 37)
   - b. Decrease activity to prevent falls and maintain a safe environment
   - c. Discourage heavy lifting and Valsalva maneuver, which may increase risk of intracranial bleeding
   - d. Encourage client to eat a high-fiber diet and drink adequate liquids
   - e. Avoid using nail clippers; use a nail file instead
   - f. Avoid using vaginal douches, rectal suppositories, or enemas
   - g. Use water-soluble lubricant for sexual intercourse
   - h. Avoid intercourse when platelet count is below 50,000/mm^3
   - i. Instruct menstruating women to monitor pad count and amount of saturation; tampon use should be avoided
   - j. Encourage client to blow nose gently or wipe nose instead
   - k. Avoid administering aspirin or aspirin-containing products and NSAIDs
   - l. Apply pressure for 5–10 minutes following venipuncture, bone marrow biopsy, or other invasive procedures; platelet transfusion prior to procedure may be indicated

NCLEX® 4. Client and family education
   - a. Notify provider of symptoms of bleeding
   - b. Test urine and stool for occult blood
   - c. Implement other safety recommendations for daily management as above

C. Nausea and vomiting

1. **Anticipatory nausea**: a conditioned response resulting from repeated association of chemotherapy-induced N/V and stimulus from environment

2. Acute nausea: occurs 0–24 hours after chemotherapy administration
3. Delayed nausea: persistent vomiting lasting 1–4 days after chemotherapy administration
4. Assessment parameters
   a. Women have higher incidence than men
   b. Younger clients experience more nausea than older clients
   c. A history of motion sickness can predispose some to experience chemotherapy-induced nausea
   d. Dehydration may accelerate N/V

NCLEX® 5. Administer prescribed antiemetics as previously described; may also give metoclopramide, a prokinetic GI stimulant
6. Provide additional antiemetics to manage breakthrough nausea
7. Dexamethasone may be most effective agent in preventing anticipatory N/V
8. Client and family education
   NCLEX® a. Eat small, frequent meals and avoid fatty or spicy foods
   b. Notify prescriber if vomiting persists for 24 or more hours and client is unable to take oral hydration
   c. Maintain antiemetic schedule for 48–72 hours to avoid delayed nausea

D. Diarrhea

1. Chemotherapy affects rapidly dividing cells in GI mucosa; combined chemotherapy and radiation therapy to pelvis can have additive effect
2. Monitor number of stools, amount, and consistency

NCLEX® 3. Replace fluid and electrolytes, including potassium
4. Administer antidiarrheal(s) to reduce peristalsis, stool frequency, and volume

NCLEX® 5. Client and family education
   a. Eat a low-residue, high-protein, high-calorie diet to promote bowel rest
   b. Eliminate irritating foods, such as alcohol, coffee, cold liquids, popcorn, and raw fruits and vegetables
   c. Drink 6–8 glasses of water per 24-hour period
   d. Implement liquid diet if diarrhea is severe
   e. Avoid milk products and chocolate
   f. Decrease activity with severe diarrhea to provide rest, reduce peristalsis
   g. Clean rectal area with mild soap and water after each stool and apply moisture barrier
   h. Take warm sitz baths for comfort

E. Stomatitis

1. Epithelial cells of oral mucosa are destroyed, causing inflammatory response and denudation of oral mucosa
2. Initial presentation: burning sensation with no physical changes in oral mucosa, sensitivity to heat and cold, and salty and spicy foods

NCLEX® 3. Promote well-balanced intake, including protein intake of greater than 1 gram/kg of body weight

NCLEX® 4. Promote consistent, thorough oral hygiene after each meal and before sleep
5. Administer antifungal/antiviral medication for prophylaxis as directed

NCLEX® 6. Client and family education
   a. Use consistent oral hygiene and topical anesthetics per healthcare provider
   b. Avoid using hydrogen peroxide and products containing alcohol, which promote dryness and irritation

F. Constipation

1. Neurotoxic effects of chemotherapy can decrease peristalsis or cause paralytic ileus
2. Assess patterns of elimination including amount and frequency
3. Assess usual fiber and fluid intake
4. Determine laxative and cathartic use, including frequency and amounts taken

NCLEX® 5. Initiate bowel maintenance program for clients receiving neurotoxic chemotherapeutic agents or those at high risk for constipation
6. Recognize complications associated with constipation, such as fecal impaction
7. Client and family education
   a. Drink warm liquids to stimulate bowel movement
   NCLEX® b. Increase fiber intake to increase peristalsis and stool bulk
   NCLEX® c. Drink at least 8 glasses of water per day
   d. Exercise regularly
   e. Develop a regular bowel program, avoiding use of laxatives if possible

G. Alopecia

1. Cells responsible for hair growth have a high mitotic rate and are affected to some degree by many chemotherapeutic agents
2. Hair loss begins approximately 2 weeks after drug administration and continues until 3–5 months after last chemotherapy treatment is completed

NCLEX® 3. Devices to decrease circulation to scalp are contraindicated because they can also promote micrometastasis
4. Provide emotional support to client who is experiencing body image change
5. Client and family education
   a. Rationale and expected time frame of hair loss and regrowth
   NCLEX® b. Provide gentle hair care, avoiding permanent waves, coloring, peroxide, electric rollers, and curling irons until regrowth has been reestablished long enough for two haircuts
   c. Hair prosthesis (wig)
   d. Emotional support strategies to cope with changing body image

H. Cardiotoxicity

1. May occur within 24 hours to up to 4–5 weeks after therapy; self-limiting; warrants immediate drug discontinuation
2. Higher doses over a shorter period of time increase its incidence
3. Baseline ejection fraction should be assessed before administering cardiotoxic agents
4. Signs of cardiotoxicity include a variety of EKG changes (including premature ventricular contractions, ventricular tachycardia, bradycardia), angina, hypotension, atypical chest pain, cardiomegaly, and pulmonary congestion
5. Cardiotoxicity may manifest more commonly as cardiomyopathy leading to heart failure and less commonly as hemorrhagic myocardial necrosis
6. Maintain ongoing documentation of client's cumulative dose
7. Cardioprotective iron-chelating agents (e.g., dexrazoxane) may be prescribed to prevent cardiotoxicity in clients who have received 75% of their lifetime dose
8. Client and family education
   NCLEX® a. Recognize signs of heart failure and report them to prescriber as directed
   NCLEX® b. Chronic cardiotoxicity is dose-related and possibly irreversible

I. Pulmonary toxicity

1. Lung tissue is sensitive to toxic effects of chemotherapy, causing direct damage to alveoli and capillary endothelium; risk increases significantly after age 70
NCLEX® 2. Dyspnea is cardinal symptom
3. Deteriorating creatinine clearance (renal dysfunction) is an important predictor for pulmonary pneumonitis
4. High oxygen concentrations can enhance pulmonary toxicity of bleomycin
5. Monitor pulmonary function studies as indicated
6. Client education
   NCLEX® a. Recognize and report signs of pulmonary toxicity (e.g., dyspnea, chest pain, shallow breathing, chest wall discomfort)
   NCLEX® b. Use pursed-lipped breathing and use a small fan to decrease symptoms of dyspnea
   c. Use opioid analgesic as prescribed to decrease fear of air hunger
   NCLEX® d. Be aware of safety issues related to oxygen administration
   e. Explore with client and family their wishes for intubation and resuscitation; breastfeeding should be discontinued

J. Hemorrhagic cystitis

1. Bladder mucosal irritation and inflammation results from contact with acrolein, a metabolic by-product of cyclophosphamide and ifosfamide
2. Prior radiation therapy to pelvis or bladder increases risk
NCLEX® 3. Presents with dysuria, frequency, burning upon urination, and hematuria
NCLEX® 4. A chemoprotectant agent (mesna) may be given to bind to acrolein in bladder, inactivating it and allowing excretion from bladder; mesna may be part of combination product with ifosfamide (ifosfamide/mesna kit)
5. Client education
   a. Hemorrhagic cystitis is possible side effect of cyclophosphamide and ifosfamide; report signs to prescriber
   NCLEX® b. Void frequently and take medication early in day
   NCLEX® c. Drink at least 6–8 glasses of fluid daily and empty bladder at least every 4–6 hours

K. Hepatotoxicity

1. Caused by direct toxic effect on liver when drugs are metabolized
2. Prior liver infection, tumor involvement in liver, advanced age, total bilirubin higher than 2 mg/dL, or cirrhosis increase incidence
NCLEX® 3. Clinical manifestations include jaundice, ascities, fatigue, anorexia, nausea, hyperpigmentation, upper right quadrant pain, hepatomegaly, and changes in urine and stool

4. Avoid hepatotoxic drugs if liver function tests are abnormal
5. Client and family education
   a. Avoid alcohol-containing beverages
   b. Instruct client about signs of liver failure

L. Nephrotoxicity

1. Caused by direct damage to glomeruli, renal blood vessels, different parts of nephron, and/or precipitation of metabolites in acid environment of urine; leads to obstructive nephropathy
2. Advancing age, preexisting renal disease, poor nutritional status, and administration of other nephrotoxic agents predispose client to nephrotoxicity
3. *NCLEX®* Manifested by increasing serum creatinine, declining creatinine clearance, hypomagnesemia, proteinuria, and hematuria
4. Continuation of nephrotoxic agents should be reviewed if BUN is higher than 22 mg/dL and/or creatinine is higher than 2 mg/dL
5. *NCLEX®* Institute hydration of 3000 mL/day to prevent or minimize renal damage
6. *NCLEX®* Induce diuresis with mannitol or furosemide when administering cisplatin
7. *NCLEX®* Administer allopurinol to decrease uric acid level from high tumor-cell kill (e.g., leukemia, lymphoma, small-cell lung cancer)
8. Maintain alkaline urine with sodium bicarbonate to a pH level greater than 8 to prevent renal damage when giving high-dose methotrexate
9. Avoid administration of aspirin and NSAIDs
10. *NCLEX®* Client and family education: it is important to comply with measures to prevent nephrotoxicity, such as collecting 12- or 24-hour urine for creatinine clearance, increasing fluid intake, using measures to alkalinize urine, and completing leucovorin rescue and/or allopurinol therapy

M. Neurotoxicity

1. Caused by direct toxicity on nervous system, metabolic encephalopathy, or intracranial hemorrhage related to chemotherapy-induced coagulopathy
2. Risk factors
   a. Administration of agents that cross blood–brain barrier
   b. Specified chemotherapeutic agents, especially cumulative doses of vinca alkaloids
   c. Concurrent radiation therapy to brain
   d. Increased age
   e. Impaired renal function
3. *NCLEX®* Assess for fine motor losses, numbness, tingling, gait disturbance, constipation, and change in mentation, which are early warning signs
4. *NCLEX®* Use measures outlined in Table 44–3 for collaborative management of neurotoxicity
5. Client and family education: recognize and report to prescriber early warning signs

Table 44–3 Neurotoxicity

Area Affected	Assessment	Collaborative Management
Cerebrum	Confusion, memory loss, and level of consciousness	1. Use positive support and encouragement 2. Maintain a consistent schedule
Sensory	Decreased reflexes, numbness, decreased sensation, jaw pain, paresthesia of hands or feet	1. Avoid extreme temperatures 2. Use assistive devices as required 3. Use opioids, antidepressants, and antiepileptics for neuropathic pain
Autonomic	Abdominal pain, constipation, ileus, bladder atony	1. Recommend a high-fiber diet 2. Increase fluid intake 3. Administer stool softeners and laxatives as required 4. Start bowel management program 30 min after meals 5. Monitor for bladder infection with urinary retention
Auditory	Tinnitis, hearing loss	1. Report auditory changes 2. Reduce or discontinue chemotherapy agent

N. Sexual and reproductive dysfunction

1. Infertility occurs in men primarily through depletion of germinal epithelium that lines seminiferous tubules
2. Women experience reproductive dysfunction primarily because of hormonal alterations or direct effects that cause ovarian fibrosis and follicular destruction
3. Chemotherapy compromises fertility by exerting cytotoxic effects on gametogenesis; degree is related to therapeutic agent and duration of treatment
4. Approximately 40–100% of clients experience some sexual dysfunction after treatment; it is frequently underreported because it often is not assessed by healthcare personnel
5. *NCLEX®* Males should be encouraged to bank sperm before starting treatment
6. Although expensive (and not always successful), females should be informed of opportunities to bank oocytes or cryopreserve embryos
7. Water-based lubricants or estrogen supplements may help to decrease vaginal dryness
8. Client education and counseling
   a. Provide unbiased, sexually neutral environment to promote open discussion
   b. Identify whether sexual issues pose a problem for client and/or partner
   c. Explain implications of treatments on sexuality
   d. *NCLEX®* Provide information related to contraception; discourage pregnancy during treatment
   e. Advise client of possible long-term side effects on reproductive function
   f. *NCLEX®* Encourage communication between client and partner

Check Your NCLEX–RN® Exam I.Q.

You are ready for testing on this content if you can:

- Apply knowledge of expected actions and effects of antineoplastic medications to client care.
- Correctly describe administration of antineoplastic medications to clients.
- Assess for side effects and adverse effects of antineoplastic medications.
- Take appropriate action if a client has an unexpected response to an antineoplastic medication.
- Monitor a client for expected outcomes or effects of treatment with antineoplastic medications.

PRACTICE TEST

1 A client is receiving chemotherapy. The nurse determines that the client needs additional education about this therapy after observing which client behaviors? Select all that apply.

1. Is near individuals with upper respiratory infection
2. Keeps fresh flowers and plants in the home
3. Shaves with an electric razor
4. Trims nails with a nail clipper
5. Increases intake of fresh fruits and vegetables

2 A newly licensed registered nurse asks the nurse preceptor what qualifications are needed in order to administer chemotherapy agents. What is an accurate reply by the nurse preceptor?

1. "You have to hold a bachelor's degree in nursing."
2. "You must have special training in safe handling and administration procedures."
3. "You must have a specialty certification in oncology nursing."
4. "You need at least 1 year of clinical experience after graduation."

3 During an intravenous (IV) push administration of doxorubicin peripherally into client's left forearm, the nurse becomes unable to obtain a blood return. The client reports no discomfort at the site and no swelling is noted. What is the appropriate action by the nurse?

1. Remove the IV catheter and restart it at another site.
2. Flush the IV with saline to ensure no extravasation has occurred.
3. Reposition the needle in hopes of obtaining a blood return.
4. Since the client has no complaint of pain, continue the administration.

4 A client who is receiving chemotherapy reports having prolonged diarrhea at home without adequate management. The nurse should become concerned about which risk to this client regarding chemotherapy?

1. Malnutrition
2. Increased gastric motility
3. Insidious weight gain and jaundice
4. Renal failure

5 The nurse would apply which clinical label to nausea and vomiting experienced by a client 24 hours after administration of the chemotherapeutic drug cisplatin?

1. Delayed nausea and vomiting
2. Retching
3. Acute nausea and vomiting
4. Anticipatory nausea and vomiting

6 The client is receiving chemotherapy with fluorouracil and concurrent radiation therapy to the abdomen for colon cancer. The client is at greatest risk for developing which adverse effect?

1. Peripheral neuropathy
2. Alopecia
3. Thrombocytopenia
4. Diarrhea

7 The nurse would assess for pulmonary toxicity in a client receiving which chemotherapeutic agent?

1. Doxorubicin
2. Vincristine
3. Cyclophosphamide
4. Bleomycin

8 A client receiving cyclophosphamide as treatment for cancer experiences painful urination, dysuria, suprapubic pain, and blood in the urine. The nurse determines that these classic signs are compatible with what problem?

1. Thrombocytopenia
2. Hemorrhagic cystitis
3. Renal dysfunction
4. Urinary tract infection

9 For what major risk factors influencing gonadal toxicity would a nurse assess in a client who is receiving chemotherapy drugs?

1. Renal function, specific agents, and blood levels of chemotherapeutic drugs
2. Gender, age, and specific agents
3. Renal function, blood levels of drugs, and age
4. Age, blood levels of drugs, and gender

10 The nurse suspects that which class of chemotherapy drug is most likely to put a client at risk for developing a second malignancy?

1. Antimetabolite
2. Taxanes
3. Alkylating agent
4. Vinca alkaloid

11 The nurse caring for a client receiving chemotherapy incorporates which practices into the routine for the day's work shift? Select all the apply.

1. Anticipate dosage changes by the healthcare provider based on the client's lab values.
2. Administer oral drugs that are part of the treatment regimen for the client.
3. Encourage the client to consider alternative nonpharmaceutical treatment options.
4. Maintain dose intensity through management of treatment side effects.
5. Prevent exhaustion by assigning total care and assistance for the client.

12 What is the priority nursing assessment for a client who has experienced ototoxicity as a result of chemotherapy administration?

1. Chronic pain
2. Vertigo
3. Confusion
4. Visual changes

13 A 90-year-old client is exhibiting altered mental status after chemotherapy with a neurotoxic agent. Which statement provides appropriate reality orientation when the client first awakens in the morning? Select all that apply.

1. "I am going to write down my name, the date, and where you are on this wall board to help you remember."
2. "Did you sleep well? Which gown would you prefer to wear today, the pink or the blue?"
3. "Today is Tuesday, and we will be having pancakes and sausage for breakfast."
4. "This is your second day in St. Elizabeth's Hospital. My name is Susan, and I will be your nurse for today."
5. "Don't worry about your confusion, it is a common side effect when receiving chemotherapy and it should go away."

14 A client is receiving a continuous fluorouracil infusion. What statements should the nurse include when teaching the client about the importance of oral care during treatment? Select all that apply.

1. "Assess the inside of your mouth daily."
2. "Gently remove white patches in your mouth with your toothbrush."
3. "Eat a nonspicy, low-acid diet to prevent stomatitis pain."
4. "Call your healthcare provider if white patches appear on your tongue or mouth."
5. "Apply a lanolin-based gel with a cotton swab to oral sores."

15 The nurse is developing a plan of care for a client who will receive chemotherapy with a neurotoxic agent. At what appropriate time should the nurse plan to implement client and family education regarding these side effects?

1. When the client requests it
2. Before the treatment begins
3. When the symptoms occur
4. When the healthcare provider requests client education

16 What is an important intervention for a client receiving chemotherapy who has an absolute granulocyte count (AGC) of less than $500/mm^3$?

1. Assess the client's rectal temperature every 4 hours.
2. Administer broad-spectrum antibiotics as prescribed.
3. Encourage intake of fresh fruits to increase potassium level.
4. Bathe every other day to reduce risk of skin irritation.

17 The oncology nurse is providing care for a client receiving chemotherapy. What should be the highest-priority nursing intervention to decrease nausea in this client?

1. Avoid oral nutrition 24 hours before chemotherapy administration.
2. Encourage the client to eat salty snacks, such as potato chips.
3. Encourage the client to avoid fatty or spicy foods.
4. Administer an antiemetic each time vomiting is experienced.

18 The nurse would explain to a client receiving which chemotherapeutic agents that the drug could cause a metallic taste during administration and lead to taste changes? Select all that apply.

1. Etoposide
2. Cyclophosphamide
3. Doxorubicin
4. Prednisone
5. Mechlorethamine

19 A client is receiving bleomycin as treatment for cancer. For which of the following cardinal symptoms of pulmonary toxicity should the nurse assess?

1. Absent breath sounds in upper lobes
2. Generalized fatigue
3. Dyspnea on exertion and at rest
4. Respiratory acidosis on arterial blood gases

20 A client is receiving anthracycline chemotherapy agents. The oncology nurse should assess this client for what most well-known and common manifestation of chronic cardiac toxicity?

1. Cardiomyopathy
2. Asymptomatic bradycardia
3. Hemorrhagic myocardial necrosis
4. Coronary artery spasm

ANSWERS & RATIONALES

1 **Answer: 1, 2, 4, 5 Rationale:** Not all clients receiving chemotherapy experience concurrent leukopenia. However, these clients should avoid individuals with an upper respiratory infection to minimize the risk of developing an illness. Keeping fresh flowers and plants in the home provides a source of microbes, and they should be avoided to minimize risk of infection. A client on chemotherapy can develop thrombocytopenia and so should avoid activities that could result in injury and bleeding. For this reason, the client should use a nail file instead of a nail clipper when trimming the nails and should use an electric razor as a safe method for shaving. Fresh fruits and vegetables can be a source of microbes for the client on chemotherapy; all fruits and vegetables should be cooked or prepared in a manner that destroys any microbes. **Cognitive Level:** Analyzing **Client Need:** Pharmacological and Parenteral Therapies **Integrated Process:** Nursing Process: Evaluation **Content Area:** Pharmacology **Strategy:** The core issue of the question is safety measures for the client receiving chemotherapy. Apply knowledge regarding the effects of immunosupression that occur with this drug regimen to make a selection. When more than one answer is correct, consider each option as a true/false statement.

2 **Answer: 2 Rationale:** Before accepting an assignment to administer chemotherapy, the nurse should receive additional education on the management of treatment side effects, pharmacology, administration principles, and safe handling. A bachelor's degree might be helpful but is not a requirement to safely administer chemotherapy. Certification in oncology nursing is not required in order to administer chemotherapy safely. Upon graduation, the registered nurse has attained adequate knowledge to manage standard clinical problems; 1 year of clinical experience might be helpful but is not required to safely administer chemotherapy. **Cognitive Level:** Applying **Client Need:** Pharmacological and Parenteral Therapies **Integrated Process:** Communication and Documentation **Content Area:** Pharmacology **Strategy:** The core issue of the question is prerequisite qualifications to administering chemotherapy. Make your selection based on knowledge that this is a specialized skill requiring additional specialized training.

3 **Answer: 2 Rationale:** Clients can experience extravasation without pain, but not without swelling. With no evidence of swelling or pain, it is safe to flush with 20–30 mL of saline to ensure an extravasation has not occurred. It is not uncommon to lose a blood return during IV administration of a vesicant. Restarting the IV gives no assurance that the blood return will not be lost again. Repositioning the IV may increase the likelihood of infiltration due to manipulation. **Cognitive Level:** Analyzing **Client Need:** Pharmacological and Parenteral Therapies **Integrated Process:** Nursing Process: Implementation **Content Area:** Pharmacology **Strategy:** The core issue of the question is safe nursing practice relative to administration of IV medications that are chemotherapeutic agents. Choose the option that is safest in avoiding harm to the client if the line is infiltrated after losing a blood return. Eliminate options that are potentially dangerous, and then further eliminate the option that might be unnecessary and excessive at this point.

4 **Answer: 1 Rationale:** Prolonged diarrhea without adequate management will cause dehydration, nutritional malabsorption, and circulatory collapse. Increased gastric motility can accompany diarrhea; in itself, increased motility is not a resulting clinical problem. Weight loss rather than weight gain could result from uncontrolled diarrhea. Jaundice reflects a problem with the liver or gallbladder. Renal failure does not result from uncontrolled diarrhea. **Cognitive Level:** Analyzing **Client Need:** Pharmacological and Parenteral Therapies **Integrated Process:** Nursing Process: Diagnosis **Content Area:** Pharmacology **Strategy:** The core issue of the question is knowledge of complications of side effects from chemotherapeutic agents. Recall that nausea and vomiting deplete both fluid volume and nutrients and make the selection that is consistent with one of these.

5 **Answer: 1 Rationale:** Delayed nausea and vomiting may occur 24–48 hours after chemotherapy administration, primarily due to the ongoing effect that drug metabolites exert on CNS or GI tracts. Despite effective antiemetic regimens, 93% of clients receiving cisplatin experience delayed nausea. Retching is not a term used to label delayed nausea and vomiting. Acute nausea occurs 1–2 hours after chemotherapy administration. Anticipatory nausea occurs in approximately 25% of clients due to the classic conditioning response from prior therapy. **Cognitive Level:** Analyzing **Client Need:** Pharmacological and Parenteral Therapies **Integrated Process:** Nursing Process: Diagnosis **Content Area:** Pharmacology **Strategy:** The critical words in the stem of the question are *24 hours after*. From there, evaluate each option in terms of time frame; eliminate options that are focused on the present, or are future-oriented related to the chemotherapy administration.

6 **Answer: 4 Rationale:** Both fluorouracil and radiation therapy to the abdomen can cause diarrhea, making this the greatest adverse effect related to both therapies. Peripheral neuropathy is not related to either therapy. Alopecia is uncommon with fluorouracil and occurs with irradiation to the skull, and not the abdomen. Some myelosuppression could result from simultaneous fluorouracil and radiation therapy, but is not the greatest risk. **Cognitive Level:** Analyzing **Client Need:** Pharmacological and Parenteral Therapies **Integrated Process:** Nursing Process: Diagnosis **Content Area:** Pharmacology **Strategy:** Note that the stem of the question contains the critical words *greatest risk*. This tells you that multiple options are correct, and that you must prioritize your answer. Choose the option that is a lower GI symptom, which is the area that both chemotherapy and radiation therapy will target.

7 **Answer: 4 Rationale:** Pulmonary toxicity is a dose- and age-related toxic effect of bleomycin. Cardiotoxicity is a toxic effect of doxorubicin. Vincristine causes neurotoxicity. Cyclophosphamide can cause hemorrhagic cystitis. **Cognitive Level:** Analyzing **Client Need:** Pharmacological and Parenteral Therapies **Integrated Process:** Nursing Process: Assessment **Content Area:** Pharmacology **Strategy:** The core issue of the question is knowledge of toxicity caused by bleomycin. If you associate the *bl* in *bleomycin* with the color blue for cyanosis, this might help you to recall that this drug causes pulmonary toxicity.

8 **Answer: 2 Rationale:** Painful urination, dysuria, suprapubic pain, and blood-tinged urine can indicate drug-related hemorrhagic cystitis in a client receiving cyclophosphamide. A decreased platelet count might cause blood in the urine, but rarely causes the other symptoms. Renal dysfunction usually does not cause painful urination and dysuria. Although the client's signs and symptoms are compatible with urinary tract infection, the nurse should first expect drug toxicity as the cause of the problem. **Cognitive Level:** Analyzing **Client Need:** Pharmacological and Parenteral Therapies **Integrated Process:** Nursing Process: Diagnosis **Content Area:** Pharmacology **Strategy:** The core issue of the question is knowledge of toxicity caused by cyclophosphamide. If you associate the *cy* in *cyclophosphamide* with the beginning of the word *cystitis*, this might help you to recall that this drug can lead to hemorrhagic cystitis.

9 **Answer: 2 Rationale:** The likelihood that chemotherapy will affect a client's fertility depends in part on the client's gender and age and on the specific agent. Since chemotherapy affects rapidly dividing cells, men are more affected than women. Women over age 30 are less likely to regain ovarian function because they have fewer oocytes. Renal function and blood levels of chemotherapy drugs are not related to gonadal toxicity. **Cognitive Level:** Analyzing **Client Need:** Pharmacological and Parenteral Therapies **Integrated Process:** Nursing Process: Assessment **Content Area:** Pharmacology **Strategy:** The critical word in the stem of the question is *gonad*. From there, eliminate the options that refer to renal function. Eliminate the option regarding blood level of the drug and select the option addressing specific agents; not all agents have the same degree of gonadal toxicity.

10 **Answer: 3 Rationale:** A serious consequence of cancer chemotherapy is that the treatment that is intended to cure the client can contribute to development of a second malignancy. Alkylating agents such as procarbazine are the agents most likely to cause chemotherapy-related malignancies. Antimetabolites, taxanes, and vinca alkaloids do not tend to cause secondary malignancies. **Cognitive Level:** Analyzing **Client Need:** Pharmacological and Parenteral Therapies **Integrated Process:** Nursing Process: Diagnosis **Content Area:** Pharmacology **Strategy:** The core issue of the question is knowledge of chemotherapeutic agents that cause added risk for future malignancy. Specific knowledge of the drug classes is needed to answer the question. Use this knowledge and the process of elimination to make a selection.

11 **Answer: 1, 2, 4 Rationale:** The nurse should review laboratory values before administering chemotherapy and report alterations to the healthcare provider for possible dosage changes. Nurses administer oral medications to clients. Management of treatment side effects is important, so that the client's treatment program can remain on course; this is an essential function of nursing. It is inappropriate to influence the client's decision making related to alternative treatment options. The client may neither want nor need total care; during severe illnesses and treatment, the client's need or desire to maintain some level of independence should be respected. **Cognitive Level:** Analyzing **Client Need:** Pharmacological and Parenteral Therapies **Integrated Process:** Nursing Process: Planning **Content Area:** Pharmacology **Strategy:** The core issue of the question is knowledge of the nurse's role related to chemotherapy that is prescribed for a client. Use general nursing knowledge and the process of elimination to make a selection. When more than one answer is correct, consider each option as a true/false statement.

12 **Answer: 2 Rationale:** Since many chemotherapeutic agents can cause ototoxicity, continued administration could cause irreparable hearing loss and/or vestibular issues such as vertigo. Chronic pain would not be a consequence of ototoxicity. There are many causes of confusion, but ototoxicity is not among them. Visual changes are unrelated to ototoxicity. **Cognitive Level:** Applying **Client Need:** Pharmacological and Parenteral Therapies **Integrated Process:** Nursing Process: Diagnosis **Content Area:** Pharmacology **Strategy:** The core issue of the question is the ability to translate the label *ototoxicity* into data that the nurse needs to assess for while implementing nursing care. Use general nursing knowledge and the process of elimination to make a selection.

13 **Answer: 1, 4 Rationale:** Providing the client with visual reminders can help prevent anxiety in a client with altered mental status. The nurse should be specific when addressing a confused/disoriented client. The questions about the environment and the need to make choices might be too challenging, and could decrease the client's self-esteem. The statement about Tuesday and pancakes and sausage for breakfast does little to orient the client and provides irrelevant information. The nurse should not offer false hope, call attention to the client's mental status, or diminish the client's concerns. **Cognitive Level:** Analyzing **Client Need:** Pharmacological and Parenteral Therapies **Integrated Process:** Communication and Documentation **Content Area:** Pharmacology **Strategy:** The core issue of the question is communication techniques that will be most effective in a client who has experienced confusion secondary to neurotoxicity. Use knowledge of general communication techniques and the process of elimination to make a selection. When more than one answer is correct, consider each option as a true/false statement.

14 **Answer: 1, 3, 4 Rationale:** The client should assess the oral cavity daily when receiving chemotherapy. Inflammation of the mouth, stomatitis, is aggravated by spicy or acidic foods. White patches on the mouth or tongue should be reported to the healthcare provider so that an antifungal agent can be prescribed. The patches should not be manually removed because doing so will cause bleeding of the mucous membranes. A lanolin-based gel is not recommended treatment; the healthcare provider will prescribe topical anesthetic agents if necessary to help control pain and discomfort. **Cognitive Level:** Analyzing **Client Need:** Pharmacological and Parenteral Therapies **Integrated Process:** Teaching and Learning **Content Area:** Pharmacology **Strategy:** The core issue of the question is knowledge of oral assessment protocols for a client receiving chemotherapy. Use knowledge of the signs and symptoms of stomatitis and fungal infection to choose the correct options. When more than one answer is correct, consider each option as a true/false statement.

15 **Answer: 2 Rationale:** Education related to chemotherapeutic agents should occur before the treatment is administered. Although the nurse should assess client readiness, if the client does not want to receive education, then the nurse should educate the caregiver. Education related to chemotherapeutic agents should occur before the treatment is administered, rather than when the symptoms develop. Client education is a nursing intervention and does not require a prescription. **Cognitive Level:** Applying **Client Need:** Pharmacological and Parenteral Therapies **Integrated Process:** Teaching and Learning **Content Area:** Pharmacology **Strategy:** The core issue of the

question is appropriate timing of client and family teaching related to adverse effects of chemotherapy. Recall that a principle of client education is to conduct teaching about a problem beforehand whenever possible. This will easily help you to choose the correct option.

16 **Answer: 2 Rationale:** Broad-spectrum antibiotics may be prescribed for a client according to individual client circumstances when the client is notably neutropenic, and at great risk of infection. A rectal temperature should not be performed on a neutropenic client. The neutropenic client should avoid fresh fruits and vegetables, which can be a source of microbes. A daily bath will remove pathogens from the skin and decrease their potential for causing infection. **Cognitive Level:** Analyzing **Client Need:** Pharmacological and Parenteral Therapies **Integrated Process:** Nursing Process: Implementation **Content Area:** Pharmacology **Strategy:** The core issues of the question are recognition that the client is neutropenic and selection of an appropriate action. Eliminate options that increase the risk of infection. Then choose the option that focuses on infection instead of the possible risk of bleeding.

17 **Answer: 3 Rationale:** Avoiding fatty, spicy foods will often decrease nausea related to chemotherapy. Avoiding nutrition before treatments should be discouraged, and has little to no benefit. Salty foods might help, but potato chips are also high in fat. Antiemetics should be administered on a scheduled basis, not after vomiting has already occurred. **Cognitive Level:** Applying **Client Need:** Pharmacological and Parenteral Therapies **Integrated Process:** Nursing Process: Implementation **Content Area:** Pharmacology **Strategy:** The core issue of the question is knowledge of methods to reduce nausea and vomiting in a client receiving chemotherapy. Recall that fatty and spicy foods can aggravate nausea to help you make the appropriate selection. Note also that two options are opposite in terms of dietary fat, which is a clue that one of them might be the correct answer.

18 **Answer: 2, 5 Rationale:** Clients receiving cyclophosphamide commonly report a metallic taste in the mouth. Some clients become so sensitized to this taste that they become nauseated in anticipation of drug administration. Mechlorethamine can cause taste changes such as a metallic taste in the mouth. Unique side effects of etoposide are acral erythema and sloughing of the skin on palms and soles. Doxorubicin is associated with adverse cardiac effects but not taste changes. Prednisone is a corticosteroid that does not alter taste. **Cognitive Level:** Analyzing **Client Need:** Pharmacological and Parenteral Therapies **Integrated Process:** Nursing Process: Diagnosis **Content Area:** Pharmacology **Strategy:** The core issue of this question is knowledge of chemotherapeutic agents that cause metallic taste as a side effect of therapy. Specific medication knowledge is needed to answer this question. When there is more than one correct answer, consider each option as a true/false statement.

19 **Answer: 3 Rationale:** The cardinal sign of pulmonary toxicity is dyspnea, which can be present both on exertion and at rest. A client does not have absence of breath sounds in upper lobes with pulmonary toxicity. The client might have generalized fatigue, but this is not a cardinal sign. The client might have respiratory acidosis, but this is not a cardinal sign. **Cognitive Level:** Analyzing **Client Need:** Pharmacological and Parenteral Therapies **Integrated Process:** Nursing Process: Assessment **Content Area:** Pharmacology **Strategy:** The core issue of the question is recognition of manifestations of pulmonary toxicity in a client receiving chemotherapy for cancer. The critical word *cardinal* tells you that multiple options might be partially or totally correct, and you must prioritize your answer. Recall that a classic sign of respiratory distress or pulmonary toxicity is dyspnea to help you to prioritize this answer over the others.

20 **Answer: 1 Rationale:** Cardiomyopathy leading to heart failure is caused by cardiac toxicity and occurs in 40% of clients receiving anthracycline chemotherapy agents. Bradycardia may be a less common sign of cardiotoxicity, but the client is more likely to be symptomatic if caused by cardiotoxicity. Hemorrhagic myocardial necrosis is a less common presentation of cardiotoxicity. Coronary artery spasm is associated with Prinzmetal angina, but not cardiotoxicity due to chemotherapy. **Cognitive Level:** Analyzing **Client Need:** Pharmacological and Parenteral Therapies **Integrated Process:** Nursing Process: Assessment **Content Area:** Pharmacology **Strategy:** The critical words in the stem of the question are *most . . . common*. This tells you that more than one option might be partially or totally correct, and that you must prioritize your answer. Use medication knowledge and the process of elimination to make a selection.

Key Terms to Review

acral erythema p. 668
alopecia p. 668
anticipatory nausea p. 679
cell cycle–nonspecific p. 665
cell cycle–specific p. 669
extravasation p. 665
hemorrhagic cystitis p. 667
irritant p. 672
myelosuppression p. 667
nadir p. 665
pancytopenia p. 667
radiation recall p. 671
vesicant p. 665

References

Adams, M., Holland, L., & Urban, C. (2017). *Pharmacology for nurses: A pathophysiologic approach* (5th ed.). New York, NY: Pearson Education.

Adams, M., & Urban, C. (2016). *Pharmacology: Connections to nursing practice* (3rd ed.). New York, NY: Pearson Education.

Lehne, R. (2016). *Pharmacology for nursing care* (9th ed.). St. Louis, MO: Saunders.

Wilson, B., Shannon, M., & Shields, K. (2016). *Pearson nurse's drug guide 2016.* New York, NY: Pearson Education.

Immunologic and Anti-Infective Medications

45

In this chapter

Cross Reference

Other chapters relevant to this content area are

Dosage Calculation and Medication Administration	**Chapter 29**
Immunologic Disorders	**Chapter 66**
Communicable or Infectious Diseases	**Chapter 67**

I. IMMUNOMODULATORS

A. Description

1. Immunomodulators can either suppress or enhance immune response
2. An **immunosuppressant** interferes with body's response to an **antigen**, a substance that stimulates production of antibodies
3. An immunostimulant (either colony stimulant or cell stimulant) enhances body's ability to fight infection and disease and is often used as an aid in treating cancer

B. *Colony-stimulating factors*

1. Action and use
   a. Glycoproteins that increase WBC production to enhance cellular immunity, counteract **neutropenia** (abnormally low neutrophil count), and assist in mobilizing stem cells, allowing for stem cell collection
   b. Described as granulocyte colony-stimulating factors (G-CSF) or granulocyte and macrophage colony-stimulating factors (GM-CSF)
2. Common CSF medications are described in Table 45–1

Table 45–1 Common Colony- or Cell-Stimulating Medications

Generic Name	Actions
Colony-Stimulating Filgrastim Pegfilgrastim	Increases neutrophil (granulocyte) production in clients with cancer to prevent infection, so labeled as a G-CSF
Sargramostim	Increases production of granulocytes and macrophages before and after bone marrow transplantation, so labeled as a GM-CSF
Cell-Stimulating Aldesleukin	Increases lymphocytes, platelets, and tumor necrosis factor
Oprelvekin	Increases thrombocyte and megakaryocyte production, thus preventing thrombocytopenia

3. Administration considerations: read product directions carefully about reconstitution for intravenous (IV) or subcutaneous (subcut) use; monitor neutrophil counts as directed because they may influence therapy

NCLEX®

4. Contraindications: pregnancy, hypersensitivity to yeast or *E. coli* products
5. Side/adverse effects
   a. Nausea and vomiting (N/V), anorexia, constipation, diarrhea
   b. Headache, stomatitis, edema, rash, mucositis, generalized pain, bone pain
   c. Supraventricular dysrhythmias, tachycardia
   d. Renal or hepatic dysfunction, dyspnea, seizures, porphyria
   e. Adult respiratory distress syndrome (ARDS), pleural effusion
   f. Myocardial infarction (MI), gastrointestinal (GI) hemorrhage, thrombus formation
6. Nursing considerations for sargramostim
   a. Assess baseline CBC and platelet count and two times per week during therapy; assess for excessive myeloid blasts in bone marrow
   b. Assess renal and hepatic function
   c. Do not administer during pregnancy; use cautiously during lactation

NCLEX®

7. Nursing considerations for filgrastim
   a. Assess CBC, differential, and platelet count at baseline and two times per week during therapy
   b. Do not administer 24 hours before or after chemotherapy
   c. Assess for hypersensitivity to *E. coli* products
   d. Filgrastim is pregnancy category C; use cautiously with lactation
8. Client education for sargramostim or filgrastim
   a. Avoid exposure to infection because client's lowered WBC count increases risk of infection; be aware of signs and symptoms of infection and report immediately to healthcare provider
   b. Report difficulty breathing and fever
   c. CBC and platelet counts must be done periodically
   d. Report pain in joints and bones (filgrastim)

C. Cell-stimulating medications

1. Action and use
   a. Interleukins (ILs) are biological response modifiers that promote proliferation of T cells and activated B cells (IL-2) or stimulate platelet production to prevent thrombocytopenia (IL-1)
   b. Aldesleukin is used to treat renal carcinoma and metastatic malignant melanoma
   c. Oprelvekin is used following chemotherapy that causes **myelosuppression** (depressed bone marrow function in manufacture of blood cells); it increases thrombocyte and megakaryocyte production to prevent and treat thrombocytopenia in clients receiving chemotherapy
2. Common cell-stimulating medications are listed in Table 45–1
3. Administration considerations
   a. Aldesleukin: because of risk of serious side effects, should only be administered by healthcare providers familiar with its use
   b. Oprelvekin: can be given for 21 days or until platelet count is greater than 100,000 cells/mm^3
4. Side/adverse effects
   a. Aldesleukin: flulike symptoms, fatigue, myalgia, capillary leak syndrome, cardiac dysrhythmias, hypotension
   b. Oprelvekin: flulike symptoms, cardiac dysrhythmias, fluid retention

Table 45–2 Common Immunosuppressant Medications

Generic Name	Actions
Azathioprine	Prevents renal transplant rejection; administered for life
Basiliximab	Prevents acute renal transplant rejection in combination with cyclosporine and a glucocorticoid
Cyclosporine	Prevents rejection in solid organ transplant
Muromonab CD3	Suppresses T cells to prevent renal transplant rejection
Mycophenolate	Prevents rejection in renal, liver, and cardiac transplants
Sirolimus	Prevents renal transplant rejection in combination with cyclosporine and a glucocorticoid
Everolimus	Prevents renal transplant rejection
Tacrolimus	Prevents rejection in solid organ transplant, primarily liver transplant

5. Nursing considerations
   a. Assess CBC, with WBC differential, and platelet count
   b. Assess heart rate, BP, respirations, and lung sounds
   c. Maintain fluid and electrolyte balance
6. Client and family education
   a. Home medication administration
   b. Assessment of fluid retention and irregular heart rate
   c. Measures to assist in preventing infection
   d. Care and management of flulike symptoms

D. Immunosuppressants

1. Action and use
   a. Inhibit inflammatory response and block immune response to an antigen; inhibit T cells and block production of antibodies by B cells
   b. Prevent rejection of organs that have been transplanted

NCLEX®

2. Common immunosuppressant medications are listed in Table 45–2
3. Administration considerations: time frames for administration of individual drugs should be noted carefully to best prevent organ rejection
4. Side/adverse effects
   a. Increased risk for infection, hypertension, acne
   b. Hepatotoxicity and/or renal toxicity
   c. Flulike symptoms and/or headache, diarrhea, nausea and/or vomiting
   d. Contraindicated with allergy to drug or during pregnancy or lactation
5. Nursing considerations
   a. Assess for signs and symptoms of infection; provide supportive care for flulike symptoms
   b. Monitor results of CBC, platelet count, BUN, creatinine, and liver enzymes
   c. Assess nutritional status; encourage nutritious meals with small, frequent feedings
6. Client education: need for lab studies, prevention of infection, and all aspects of medication administration, including action, side effects, and nursing implications

II. MEDICATIONS TO TREAT MULTIPLE SCLEROSIS (MS)

A. Action and use

1. Goal is to decrease inflammation and suppress immune system to prevent nerve tissue destruction and decrease fatigue and ataxia
2. A wide variety of medications are used, including beta-adrenergic blockers, corticosteroids, anti-inflammatory agents, and interferon

NCLEX®

B. Common medications for multiple sclerosis are listed in Table 45–3

C. Administration considerations: read product literature carefully

D. Side/adverse effects

1. Interferons: muscle aches, flulike symptoms, local reactions, headache, anemia, myelosuppression, hepatotoxicity
2. Dimethyl fumarate: flushing, abdominal pain, nausea, diarrhea, lymphopenia
3. Glatiramer acetate: anxiety, arthralgia, back pain, malaise, flulike symptoms, lymphadenopathy, pain at injection site

Table 45–3 Common Medications to Treat Multiple Sclerosis

Generic Name	Actions
Dalfampridine	Potassium channel blocker that improves walking speed in MS
Dimethyl fumarate	Mechanism unknown in treating relapsing forms of MS
Fingolimod	Blocks capacity of lymphocytes to leave lymph nodes, reducing numbers of peripherally circulating lymphocytes to reduce relapse rate in MS
Glatiramer acetate	Immunomodulator that prevents destruction of brain and nerve tissue; used for long-term treatment
Interferon beta 1a Interferon beta 1b	Interferon that reduces severity of acute exacerbations; decreases demyelination in brain tissue; can be used for long-term treatment of relapsing forms
Mitoxantrone	An antineoplastic that suppresses activity of T and B cells and macrophages to slow disease process; approved for use in MS
Natalizumab	Monoclonal antibody that may inhibit movement of damaging immune cells across blood–brain barrier
Teriflunomide	A metabolite of leflunomide (drug that treats rheumatoid arthritis); suppresses division of B and T cells to reduce relapse rates and development of MS lesions in brain

4. Mitoxantrone: myelosuppression, cardiotoxicity, stomatitis, N/V, pain at injection site; also potentially fatal opportunistic viral brain infection (progressive multifocal leukoencephalopathy)
5. Natalizumab: headache, depression, fatigue, menstrual dysfunction, infections, and rarely anaphylaxis
6. Teriflunomide: alopecia, diarrhea, influenza, nausea, paresthesia, hepatotoxicity, leukopenia, severe skin reactions

E. Nursing considerations

1. Assess for signs of adverse effects and results of prescribed laboratory tests
2. Assess injection sites for inflammation and pain
3. Monitor for effects of treatment and exacerbations of disease

F. Client education

1. Side effects of medication and need for periodic laboratory studies
2. Report any side effects to prescriber
3. Supportive care of flulike symptoms, including adequate fluid intake, rest, and use of acetaminophen for relief of pain and fever
4. Signs and symptoms of cardiotoxicity for mitoxantrone

III. MEDICATIONS TO TREAT MYASTHENIA GRAVIS

A. Action and use

1. Acetylcholinesterase (Ach) inhibitors treat symptoms of myasthenia gravis (MG) by increasing concentration of acetylcholine at neuromuscular junction
2. Increase nerve impulse conduction and muscle strength

NCLEX® **B. Common medications for myasthenia gravis are listed in Table 45–4**

NCLEX® **C. Administration considerations**

1. Edrophonium: single dose is for diagnostic purposes only; may be repeated once to aid in uncertain diagnosis
2. Neostigmine: can be administered subcutaneously (subcut) during an acute exacerbation
3. Pyridostigmine: a timed-release preparation can be administered at bedtime; can also be administered IM during acute exacerbation
4. Contraindicated in pregnancy and lactation, bradycardia, intestinal or urinary obstruction
5. Use cautiously in clients with asthma, heart disease, Parkinson's disease, and seizure disorders

Table 45–4 Common Medications to Treat Myasthenia Gravis

Generic Name	Actions
Ambenonium	Long-acting medication to treat MG
Edrophonium	Used for diagnostic purposes; clients who exhibit temporary improvement in muscle strength, posture, and respiratory function with injected dose have MG
Neostigmine	Increases acetylcholine concentration, facilitating neuromuscular function; 2- to 4-hour duration of action
Pyridostigmine	Increases acetylcholine concentration facilitating neuromuscular function; taken every 3–6 hours

D. Side/adverse effects

1. Bradycardia, hypotension, or cardiac arrest
2. Increased gastric secretions, N/V, diarrhea
3. Increased urinary urgency and involuntary incontinence of stool
4. NCLEX® Severe cholinergic reactions: excessive salivation, sphincter relaxation, diarrhea, and vomiting

E. Nursing considerations

1. NCLEX® Assess respirations, heart rate, and general muscle strength, including swallowing, before dose
2. Administer with meals to enhance absorption and decrease GI irritation
3. NCLEX® Administer on time to prevent difficulty with respirations and swallowing caused by undermedication or late medication administration
4. Administer IV preparations slowly to prevent cholinergic reaction
5. NCLEX® Have atropine available as antidote to counteract cholinergic reaction
6. Assess response to medication and ability to perform activities of daily living

F. Client education

1. All aspects of drug administration, side effects; take with food to decrease GI irritation
2. Coordination of medication administration with activities of daily living
3. Overmedication will result in cholinergic reaction
4. How to assess apical pulse

IV. MEDICATIONS TO TREAT RHEUMATOID ARTHRITIS

A. Action and use

1. Early-stage rheumatoid arthritis (RA) is managed with NSAIDs, which have anti-inflammatory and analgesic action
2. Often disease-modifying antirheumatic drugs (DMARDs), which are a diverse group of drugs that modify immune or inflammatory response, are added to the drug regimen early in disease process
3. DMARDs used early in treatment of RA tend to include hydrochloroquine, methotrexate, or sulfasalazine
4. Biologic therapies are newest type of DMARD used to block inflammatory response, reduce joint inflammation, and slow joint damage
5. Multiple drugs may be used at one time to adequately control symptoms and delay disease progression
6. Older drugs are gold salts, D-penicillamine, cyclophosphamide, and cyclosporine, but they are more toxic than other DMARDs and are used rarely
7. Corticosteroids are used to relieve symptoms of flare-ups in moderate to severe RA, but are used in smallest possible doses and are not used long term because of their adverse effects

B. Common medications for rheumatoid arthritis are listed in Table 45–5

C. Administration considerations: check product literature for specific information

Table 45–5 Common Medications to Treat Rheumatoid Arthritis

Generic Name	Actions
Biological Therapies Adalimumab, certolizumab pegol, etanercept, golimumab, infliximab	Tumor necrosis factor (TNF) inhibitors that block steps in TNF-mediated cellular response to reduce inflammation and slow progression of joint damage; biologic therapies
Abatacept, anakinra	Block actions of interleukins in inflammatory pathways
Rituximab	Monoclonal antibody that inhibits B lymphocytes that play a role in inflammation in RA; used with methotrexate
Tocilizumab	Inhibits actions of interleukin-6 (IL-6) to inhibit inflammation and activation of immune response
Tofacitinib	Janus kinase inhibitor that blocks inflammatory mediators in moderate to severe RA
Nonbiologic Therapies Azathioprine, cyclosporine	Immunosuppressants that inhibit lymphocyte replication or disrupt T helper cells
Hydroxychloroquine	Not completely understood; reduces migration of eosinophils and neutrophils and probably inhibits synthesis of histamine and prostaglandins
Leflunomide	Inhibits inflammatory process by blocking enzyme DHODH
Methotrexate	Inhibits DNA synthesis and folic acid reductase to reduce inflammation; cytotoxic drug
Sulfasalazine	Anti-inflammatory drug that is also a sulfonamide and a salicylate

D. Side/adverse effects

1. Biologic therapies: local reactions at injection site, headache, nasopharyngitis, infections, lupus-like syndrome, heart failure exacerbations, Stevens-Johnson syndrome
2. Azathioprine: chills, fever, malaise, myalgia, myelosuppression, hepatotoxicity
3. Hydroxychloroquine: anorexia, N/V, headache, personality changes, retinopathy, agranulocytosis, aplastic anemia, seizures
4. Methotrexate: headache, glossitis, gingivitis, nausea, myelosuppression, hepatic cirrhosis, nephrotoxicity, pulmonary fibrosis, and teratogenicity
5. Sulfasalazine: headache, anorexia, N/V, leukopenia, Stevens-Johnson syndrome, reversible oligospermia

E. Nursing considerations

1. Avoid antacid use for at least 2 hours following medication administration
2. Assess for drug adverse effects
3. Assess for signs of infection (NCLEX®)
4. Monitor effects of medication therapy on RA symptoms and joint function

F. Client education

1. Protect self from infection
2. Comply with periodic laboratory studies
3. All aspects of medication administration, including side effects, action, use, and contraindications

V. MEDICATIONS TO TREAT SYSTEMIC LUPUS ERYTHEMATOSUS

A. Action and use

1. Aspirin, acetaminophen, NSAIDs, and corticosteroids are used to treat pain and inflammation associated with systemic lupus erythematosus (SLE)
2. Drugs with immunosuppressive action are helpful in treating autoimmune diseases

B. Common medications (NCLEX®)

1. NSAIDS (off-label use), sometimes in combination with an antimalarial drug such as hydroxychloroquine
2. Immunosuppressants such as belimumab, cyclophosphamide, methotrexate, and azathioprine are useful in severe cases
3. See previous section on RA and immunosuppressants for discussion of these drugs

VI. ANTIBIOTICS

A. Aminoglycosides

1. Action and use
   a. **Bactericidal**: aminoglycosides kill bacteria cells by affecting bacterial protein synthesis
   b. Used to treat a variety of serious systemic bacterial infections, sterilize bowel prior to surgery, or kill gut bacteria that produce ammonia (useful in treating hepatic encephalopathy)
2. Common aminoglycosides are listed in Box 45–1 (NCLEX®)

Memory Aid

Recognize an aminoglycoside by the suffix *-micin* or *-mycin*. Not all drugs that end in *-mycin* are aminoglycosides, but all aminoglycosides end in either *-mycin* or *-micin*.

3. Administration considerations
   a. IV route preferred but can be administered intramuscularly (IM)
   b. Oral route: poorly absorbed, so used orally to decrease bacteria in bowel before surgery or prevent absorption of ammonia (hepatic encephalopathy)

Box 45–1

Aminoglycosides

Amikacin	Paromomycin
Gentamicin	Streptomycin
Kanamycin	Tobramicin
Neomycin	

c. Contraindicated with allergy to aminoglycosides, preexisting renal disease, or if client is receiving other agents toxic to kidneys

4. Significant laboratory studies

NCLEX® a. **Peak drug level**: blood specimen drawn 30 minutes after completion of IV dose to determine that toxic levels do not occur; dose may need to be decreased if peak too high

NCLEX® b. **Trough drug level**: blood specimen drawn immediately prior to starting next IV dose to ensure that therapeutic drug levels are maintained between administrations; if drug level is too low, an increase in dose and/or dosing frequency may be indicated

c. WBC count to monitor effectiveness of drug in resolving infection

d. Serum creatinine and blood urea nitrogen (BUN) to monitor renal function; if creatinine level rises 3–4 days into treatment, renal damage has occurred

5. Side/adverse effects

a. Headache, paresthesias, skin rash, fever

b. Nephrotoxicity: increased with risk factors such as advancing age, hypotension, dehydration, preexisting renal disease, coadministration of other nephrotoxic drugs

c. Ototoxicity: may be irreversible; auditory impairment and vestibular damage; possible damage to 8th cranial nerve; risk is increased with impaired renal function and concurrent use of other ototoxic drugs, such as furosemide, vancomycin, amphotericin B, and certain antineoplastic agents

d. Neuromuscular blockade (inhibiting acetylcholine release): may be seen in clients with MG or those receiving neuromuscular blockers such as pancuronium bromide or succinylcholine; use calcium salts to reverse blockade

NCLEX® e. **Candidiasis**: secondary infection (usually of skin and mucous membranes) caused by *Candida albicans*; appears as discrete white plaques that are not easily removed

NCLEX® f. **Pseudomembranous colitis**: secondary infection of bowel (usually caused by *Clostridium difficile*) manifested by four to six watery stools per day with blood and/or mucus, abdominal pain, and fever; antibiotic is discontinued and vancomycin PO or metronidazole IV or PO is prescribed

6. Nursing considerations

a. See Box 45–2 for general nursing considerations with antibiotic therapy

Box 45–2

General Nursing Considerations for Antibiotic Therapy and Other Anti-Infectives

- Collect appropriate specimen for culture and sensitivity (C&S), whenever possible, before starting antibiotic therapy to ensure proper drug selection; empiric therapy may be started so that infection can be treated promptly
- Assess client's medication profile (including OTC and herbal products) for agents that may cause drug interactions
- Assess for allergy before administration and withhold dose and notify prescriber for documented hypersensitivity reaction (such as hives, urticaria, stridor, dyspnea, and anaphylaxis)
- Administer doses on time to maintain therapeutic blood levels; when IV antibiotic is scheduled at same time as another IV medication (e.g., famotidine), give IV antibiotic first to maintain standardized times and keep drug level within therapeutic range
- Assess for, document, and report adverse effects of prescribed antibiotic
- Monitor for superinfection:
  - Candidiasis: vaginal yeast infection or oral thrush; treated with appropriate anti-infective
  - Pseudomembranous colitis: four to six or more watery stools per day, accompanied by blood and mucus in stools, abdominal cramps, and fever; place client on contact precautions; original antibiotic is discontinued and another is selected
- Maintain adequate fluid hydration and increase fluids if indicated (up to 3 liters daily) depending on antibiotic class
- Ensure that client takes full course of therapy for full beneficial effects, even if signs of infection resolve; otherwise, microorganism regrowth and drug resistance can occur
- Observe for evidence that infection is resolving with symptom improvement within 48–72 hours of beginning therapy (decreased temperature, WBC count, and local signs of infection); report to prescriber if infection is not resolving and prepare to do additional cultures as prescribed

b. **Empiric therapy** (based on probable offending organism) is usually begun before test results available because of seriousness of infection
c. Monitor peak and trough aminoglycoside levels
d. Monitor for nephrotoxicity: monitor serum creatinine, BUN, urine creatinine clearance, urinalysis (urinary casts and proteinuria), and intake and output (I&O)
e. Monitor for ototoxicity: assess for dizziness, lightheadedness, tinnitus, fullness in ears, and hearing loss; monitor vestibular integrity with Romberg's test

NCLEX®
f. Maintain fluid hydration to protect kidneys; intake should be 2500–3000 mL/day unless contraindicated by other conditions

7. Client education

NCLEX®
a. See general teaching points for antibiotic therapy (Box 45–3)
b. Take oral drug with food if not contraindicated to reduce risk of GI upset

B. Cephalosporins

1. Action and use
a. Related to penicillins; **cross-sensitivity** may occur between penicillins and cephalosporins, meaning that hypersensitivity to one class may indicate hypersensitivity to the other occasionally
b. Usually bactericidal and inhibit bacterial cell wall synthesis
c. Used to treat a wide variety of infections
d. Most cephalosporins are excreted through urine; exceptions are cefoperazone and ceftriaxone, which are excreted in bile
2. Common cephalosporins are listed in Box 45–4

Memory Aid

Recognize a cephalosporin by the prefix or root *cef-* or *ceph-*.

3. Administration consideration
a. Check renal function before and during therapy; renal impairment significantly extends drug half-life; use extreme caution if creatine clearance is less than 50 mL/min
b. Separate oral administration of antacids, H_2-receptor antagonists, iron supplements, and foods fortified with iron by 2 hours before and after oral doses

Box 45–3

General Client Teaching Points for Antibiotic Therapy

- Know drug, dose, purpose, route, and schedule of drug regimen
- Take at evenly spaced intervals around the clock without disrupting sleep to maintain serum levels
- Take with food, if not contraindicated, to minimize GI upset
- If medication must be taken on empty stomach, take 1 hour before or 2 hours after a meal
- Ensure adequate fluid intake of 2000–3000 mL fluid intake daily if not contraindicated by heart failure, kidney disease, or other condition
- If using liquid preparation, use calibrated measuring device rather than household measurement (kitchen teaspoons can vary by 2–10 mL)
- Know side and adverse effects of drug and which ones require notification of prescriber
- Report signs of possible superinfection: sore throat or white patches in mouth (candida) or watery stools more often than four to six times per day (pseudomembranous colitis)
- Before taking any over-the-counter (OTC) drugs, check efficacy and possible adverse reactions with prescriber
- Take full course of therapy as ordered; do not discontinue drug on own even if feeling better and symptoms have resolved; do not "save" medication for future illnesses
- Do not take drugs with expired date; discard any drug that is not used (full course of therapy should be taken)
- Report to prescriber if symptoms aren't resolving or not feeling better after 48–72 hours

Box 45–4

Cephalosporins

First Generation	Cefditoren
Cefadroxil	Cefixime
Cefazolin	Cefotaxime
Cephalexin	Cefpodoxime
Second Generation	Ceftazidime
Cefaclor	Ceftibuten
Cefotetan	Ceftizoxime
Cefoxitin	Ceftriaxone
Cefprozil	**Fourth Generation**
Cefuroxime	Cefepime
Third Generation	**Fifth Generation**
Cefdinir	Ceftaroline

4. Side/adverse effects
   a. GI: N/V, mild diarrhea, abdominal cramps or distress, elevated liver enzymes, abdominal pain, colitis; pseudomembranous colitis

   NCLEX® b. Hypersensitivity occurs in 5–16% of clients; cross-sensitivity with penicillins can occur

   c. Other: fatigue, rash, pruritis, pain at injection site, oral or vaginal candidiasis, nephrotoxicity, pseudomembranous colitis
5. Nursing considerations as per Box 45–2
   a. Monitor injection site for induration and tenderness; provide warm compresses and gentle massage to site if painful or swollen; if phlebitis or redness at IV site develops, remove IV device and restart IV

   b. Monitor for renal toxicity: check serum creatinine, BUN, urine creatinine
6. Client education as per Box 45–3

   NCLEX® a. Drink fluids and maintain nutrition, especially protein, to ensure adequate protein for drug binding and efficacy of action

   b. Shake suspensions well immediately before administration; use a measuring device for liquid/suspension and not a kitchen teaspoon (may vary from 2–10 mL/teaspoon)

   NCLEX® c. Report manifestations of hypersensitivity to healthcare provider: difficulty breathing, severe rash, hives, severe headache, dizziness or weakness, aching joints

C. Fluoroquinolones

1. Action and use
   a. Newer class of broad-spectrum bactericidal antibiotics

   b. Inhibit nucleic acid synthesis needed by bacterial DNA; used in various bacterial infections of respiratory and GI tracts, bone and joint infections, UTIs, skin and soft tissue infections, and STIs
2. Common fluoroquinolones are listed in Box 45–5

Memory Aid

Recognize a fluoroquinolone by the suffix *-oxacin*.

3. Administration considerations
   a. Administer around the clock, evenly spaced, to maintain therapeutic blood level; avoid interrupting sleep if possible

   b. Oral drug is tolerated better with food

   c. Elimination of caffeine is decreased with ciprofloxacin, enoxacin, and norfloxacin
4. Side/adverse effects
   a. Common: N/V, diarrhea, headache, rash, insomnia, local inflammation and pain at injection site; corneal stinging and burning (ophthalmic use)

Box 45–5

Fluoroquinolones

First Generation	**Fourth Generation**
Nalidixic acid	Besifloxacin
Second Generation	Gemifloxacin
Ciprofloxacin	Moxifloxacin
Norfloxacin	
Ofloxacin	
Third Generation	
Gatifloxacin	
Levofloxacin	

b. Serious: anaphylaxis, **superinfections** (oral thrush from candida or diarrhea from alteration in normal bowel flora), photosensitivity, tendonitis and tendon rupture, seizures, peripheral neuropathy, hepatotoxicity, pseudomembranous colitis

5. Nursing considerations as per Box 45–2
   a. Separate drug from oral antacids, iron and zinc salts, or sucralfate by 2 hours
   b. Monitor renal function
   c. Provide more frequent meals with complete or complementary proteins to better ensure adequate albumin levels for drug efficacy
   d. Monitor for increased CNS irritability if client has history of epilepsy, alcohol abuse, or is concurrently taking theophylline
   e. Maintain hydration with 3 L fluid/day, if not contraindicated
6. Client education as per Box 45–3
   a. Take safety precautions including changing position slowly and avoiding driving and hazardous tasks if CNS effects occur
   b. Drink fluids and maintain nutrition, especially protein, to provide adequate protein for drug-binding and drug efficacy

   NCLEX®

   c. Wear sunglasses, long sleeved and long-legged garments, and hat to protect from direct sunlight; sunscreen or sunblock may not prevent photosensitivity reaction; avoid ultraviolet light, tanning beds, and direct sunlight

D. Macrolides and lincosamides

1. Action and use
   a. **Bacteriostatic** (inhibiting bacterial growth) but can be bactericidal in high doses with some bacteria; inhibit bacterial protein synthesis
   b. Highly protein-bound
   c. Used in upper and lower respiratory tract infections, whooping cough, diphtheria, Legionnaire's disease, chlamydial infections, skin and soft tissue infections caused by *Streptococcus* or *Haemophilus* organisms, and prophylaxis for recurring rheumatic fever if allergic to penicillin
   d. Clarithromycin is used with omeprazole to treat *Helicobacter pylori* associated with peptic ulcers
   e. Fidamoxicin is used to treat *C. difficile*-associated diarrhea
2. Common macrolides and lincosamides are listed in Box 45–6
3. Administration considerations
   a. If erythromycin form has bitter taste, give with juice or applesauce; give with food to reduce GI irritating effects
   b. Give clindamycin and lincomycin with at least 8 ounces of fluid or on an empty stomach

Box 45–6

Macrolides and Lincosamides

Azithromycin	Clindamycin
Clarithromycin	Lincomycin
Erythromycin	Telithromycin
Fidamoxicin	

4. Side/adverse effects
   a. Common: N/V, diarrhea, abdominal cramping, dry skin or burning with topical route
   b. Serious: anaphylaxis, ototoxicity, hepatotoxicity, superinfections, dysrhythmias, pseudomembranous colitis; with fidaxomicin GI bleeding, anemia and neutropenia can occur
5. Nursing considerations as per Box 45–2
   a. Assess GI function and elimination pattern; monitor for superinfections
   b. Observe for bleeding if taking oral anticoagulants
   c. Monitor liver enzymes, serum creatinine, BUN, creatinine clearance, and I&O
   d. Assess baseline hearing and monitor for hearing loss; consult prescriber for alternative drug if hearing loss occurs
   e. Hydrate with at least 2000–2400 mL/day if not contraindicated
6. Client education as per Box 45–3; include protein in diet because these drugs are highly protein bound and require protein for therapeutic efficacy

E. Penicillins (beta-lactams) and penicillinase-resistants

1. Action and use
   a. Most effective against infections caused by Gram-positive organisms; inhibit bacterial cell wall synthesis
   b. Extended spectrum penicillins are effective against infections caused by *Pseudomonas*; penicillinase-resistant penicillins are effective against *Staphylococcus*
   c. Increasing resistance developing, especially in facility-acquired infections
2. Common penicillins are listed in Box 45–7

Memory Aid

Recognize a penicillin by the suffix *-cillin*.

3. Administration considerations
   a. Oral dosing needs to be three to four times greater than parenteral dose because of hepatic first-pass effect and instability of penicillin in acid environment of stomach
   b. For serious systemic infections, parenteral route is recommended
   c. Penicillin G procaine or benzathine not to be given IV: lethal
   d. Most likely drug category to cause allergic reactions
   e. Use caution in anemia, thrombocytopenia, bone marrow depression, and concurrently with anticoagulants because some penicillins cause increased bleeding
4. Side/adverse effects
   a. *NCLEX®* Common: nausea, diarrhea, fever; a maculopapular, pruritic measles-like rash with ampicillin or amoxocillin is not a true allergic reaction but develops after 7–10 days of therapy and may last several days after discontinuing penicillin; not a contraindication to give drug in future
   b. *NCLEX®* Serious: nephrotoxicity and anaphylaxis (noted by urticaria, pruritis, severe dyspnea, stridor, tachycardia, hypotension, dizziness, loss of consciousness, and circulatory collapse)

Box 45–7

Penicillins

Natural Penicillins	Extended-Spectrum Penicillins
Penicillin G benzathine	Piperacillin
Penicillin G potassium	Piperacillin-tazobactam
Penicillin G procaine	Ticarcillin-clavulanate
Broad-Spectrum Penicillins	**Penicillinase-Resistant Penicillins**
Amoxicillin	Dicloxacillin
Amoxicillin-clavulanate	Nafcillin
Ampicillin	Oxacillin
Ampicillin-sulbactam	

NCLEX®

5. Nursing considerations as per Box 45–2
   a. Monitor renal studies, liver enzymes, and electrolytes; some penicillins contain sodium salts that can result in hypokalemia
   b. If mild diarrhea develops, give yogurt, buttermilk, or probiotics as per prescriber to restore normal flora; use absorbent antidiarrheal agents (kaolin and pectin); avoid antiperistaltic agents that delay or prevent elimination of intestinal toxins
6. Client education as per Box 45–3
   a. Take oral drug on empty stomach, 1 hour before meals or 2 hours after meals, except amoxicillin (not affected by food)
   b. NCLEX® Shake suspensions to disperse particles before measuring; use a calibrated device; most suspensions maintain potency for 14 days if refrigerated
   c. Take missed doses as soon as possible; do not double-dose if one missed
   d. NCLEX® Report rash, urticaria, pruritis, difficulty breathing
   e. Eat small, frequent meals with high-quality protein and drink six to eight glasses or more of water per day if not contraindicated by other conditions

F. Sulfonamides

1. Action and use
   a. First effective group of antibiotics; are bacteriostatic; inhibit metabolic pathways of bacteria
   b. Used to treat UTIs (especially caused by *E. coli*, most common cause), *chlamydia* infections, mild-to-moderate ulcerative colitis, active Crohn's disease, nocardiosis
   c. Silver sulfadiazine and mafenide prevent bacterial growth in burns and wounds
   d. Cross-sensitivity possible with penicillins and cephalosporins
2. Common sulfonamides are listed in Box 45–8

Memory Aid

Recognize a sulfonamide by the root *sulf* in the drug name.

3. Administration considerations: provide fluid intake of 2500–3000 mL/day to promote urine output of at least 1,500 mL/day to prevent crystalluria/stone formation; alkaline ash diet may help, which includes fruit (except plums, prunes, and cranberries), vegetables, and milk
4. Side/adverse effects
   a. Common: N/V, anorexia, rash, crystalluria
   b. NCLEX® Serious: anaphylaxis, blood dyscrasias, fulminant hepatic necrosis, hyperkalemia, Stevens-Johnson syndrome (an adverse reaction of skin that resembles appearance of partial-thickness burns), hyperkalemia
5. Nursing considerations as per Box 45–2
   a. Assess baseline and periodic laboratory tests for liver and renal function
   b. NCLEX® Hydration to assure daily urine output of 1500 mL or more to prevent crystalluria; alkalinize urine as indicated; keep accurate I&O record
   c. Provide small, frequent, nutritious meals with high-quality proteins; drugs that may be taken with food may decrease GI upset
6. Client education as per Box 45–3
   a. Take with food, if not contraindicated, to minimize GI upset
   b. Eat small, frequent meals with at least 2500–3000 mL fluid intake a day
   c. Empty bladder frequently, such as every 2 hours while awake
   d. NCLEX® Report flank or suprapubic pain, increased dysuria, disruption of skin integrity to healthcare provider

Box 45–8

Sulfonamides

Systemic	Topicals
Sulfadiazine	Silver sulfadiazine
Sulfadoxine-pyrimethamine	Mafenide
Sulfisoxazole	
Trimethoprim-sulfamethoxazole	
Sulfasalazine	

G. Tetracyclines

1. Action and use
   a. Broad spectrum; bacteriostatic; inhibit bacterial protein synthesis
   b. Used to treat acne vulgaris, Rocky Mountain spotted fever, **amebiasis** (a protozoan infection), typhus, cholera, syphilis (if allergic to penicillin), Lyme disease, *H. pylori* peptic ulcer disease
   c. Used as a sclerosing agent for pleural and pericardial effusion, such as in cancer metastasis; causes inflammation resulting in fibrosis, leaving scar tissue that does not allow fluid to accumulate
   d. Inhibits antidiuretic hormone (ADH) in treating syndrome of inappropriate antidiuretic hormone (SIADH)
2. Common tetracyclines (generic name ends in *-cycline*); see Box 45–9

Memory Aid

Recognize a tetracycline by the suffix *-cycline* in the drug name.

3. Administration considerations
   a. Oral: give with full glass of water on empty stomach at least 1 hour before or 2 hours after meals; food and milk products decrease absorption by half
   b. If topical, clean area with soap and water, rinse and dry well prior to application
   NCLEX® c. Tetracyclines bind to calcium, slowing rate of bone growth and causing yellow-brown tooth discoloration; usually contraindicated in children under age 8 and pregnant or lactating women
4. Side/adverse effects
   a. Common: N/V, diarrhea, abdominal cramping, flatulence, mild phototoxicity, rash, dizziness, local burning and stinging (topical route), dry mouth, bulky or loose stools
   b. Serious: anaphylaxis, superinfections, hepatotoxicity, exfoliative dermatitis, permanent tooth discoloration in children
   NCLEX® c. Hepatotoxicity; nephrotoxicity in clients with preexisting renal disease
5. Nursing considerations as per Box 45–2
   a. Assess for history of renal or liver problems and related laboratory results
   b. Monitor I&O
6. Client education as per Box 45–3
   NCLEX® a. Report side effects, particularly severe diarrhea
   NCLEX® b. Avoid exposure to direct sunlight or ultraviolet light or tanning beds; wear hat, long-sleeved and long-legged clothing, and sunglasses outside during and for a few days after treatment; sunscreen or sunblock may not prevent erythema
   c. Take oral doses with full glass of water on empty stomach (1 hour before or 2 hours after meal or dairy product) to promote absorption and decrease risk of esophagitis; report sudden dysphagia to prescriber
   d. Topical form may stain clothing or cause affected skin to reflect yellow or green fluorescence under an ultraviolet or "black" light

H. Urinary tract antiseptics

1. Action and use: drugs that act against bacteria in urine (UTIs) but have little or no systemic antibacterial effects
2. Common urinary tract antiseptics are listed in Box 45–10

Box 45–9
Tetracyclines

Demeclocycline	Tetracycline
Doxycycline	Tigecycline
Minocycline	

Box 45–10
Urinary Tract Antiseptics

Fosfomycin	Nalidixic acid
Methenamine mandelate	Nitrofurantoin
Methenamine hippurate	

3. Administration considerations

NCLEX®

a. Acidic urine inhibits bacteria from adhering to bladder wall, so acid ash diet may be recommended (meat, cheese, eggs, whole grains, as well as cranberries, prunes, and plums)
b. Alkaline ash diet may interfere with the required acidity of urine for antiseptic action; alkaline ash foods to avoid include fruits (except cranberries, prunes, plums), milk, vegetables

4. Side/adverse effects
a. Common: N/V, anorexia, diarrhea, epigastric distress, headache, back pain, blurred vision, fatigue, photophobia (nalidixic acid), brown urine (nitrofurantoin)
b. Serious: crystalluria, anaphylaxis, superinfections, and hemolytic anemia; with nitrofurantoin also Stevens-Johnson syndrome, hepatic necrosis, interstitial pneumonitis

5. Nursing considerations as per Box 45–2
a. Assess for previous renal or liver dysfunction
b. Encourage at least 3000 mL/day fluids, including cranberry juice, if not contraindicated by fluid restriction or other conditions
c. Give medication with or after food to limit GI adverse effects

6. Client education as per Box 45–3
a. Take with or after food to minimize GI distress

NCLEX®

b. Drink at least 3 liters of fluid a day unless contraindicated by other conditions
c. Include acid ash foods in diet (cranberries, prunes, plums, cheese, eggs, meat, whole grains); limit alkaline ash foods (citrus fruits and juices, vegetables)
d. Avoid drugs that may alkalinize urine, such as antacids, sodium bicarbonate
e. Nalidixic acid can cause photophobia; avoid bright sunlight, wear sunglasses, and report visual disturbances; photosensitivity can also occur several weeks after drug is discontinued so avoid direct sunlight or ultraviolet light
f. Nitrofurantoin may cause urine to be brown; may stain clothing
g. Do not drive or perform hazardous tasks if drowsiness or dizziness occurs

I. Miscellaneous antibiotics are listed in Box 45–11

1. Quinupristin/dalfopristin: used to treat bacteremia and life-threatening infections caused by vancomycin-resistant *Enterococcus faecium* (VREF); also complicated skin and skin structure infections
a. Administration considerations: IV use only, preferably via central line
b. Side/adverse effects: arthralgias, myalgias (possibly severe); with peripheral IV administration, frequently pain, inflammation, edema, and thrombophlebitis
c. Nursing considerations and client education: same as for other antibiotics

2. Vancomycin: bactericidal; parenteral antibiotic of choice for methicillin-resistant *Staphylococcus aureus* (MRSA) and other Gram-positive microorganisms; antibiotic-induced pseudomembranous colitis caused by *Clostridium difficile* and staphylococcal enterocolitis (oral drug form)

NCLEX®

a. Administration considerations: poorly absorbed from GI tract so indicated for local surface-infected areas of GI tract; IV dose should be through a central venous access device (CVAD) because of high risk for phlebitis; can cause necrosis if it extravasates
b. Side/adverse effects: nausea, hypotension, flushing; pain and thrombophlebitis at injection site; ototoxicity, nephrotoxicity, temporary leukopenia; "red neck (or man) syndrome": too rapid IV infusion results in profound hypotension, erythematous rash on face, neck, upper chest, and arms
c. Nursing considerations: as for other antibiotics; give IV dose over 60–90 minutes to avoid hypotension and red neck syndrome
d. Client education: as for other antibiotics; also, if client is receiving IV therapy in home, ensure appropriate knowledge and ability to perform procedures correctly, including monitoring BP and heart rate

Box 45–11

Miscellaneous Antibiotics

Monobactam	**Streptogramin**
Aztreonam	Quinupristin/dalfopristin
Carbapenems	**Other**
Doripenem	Daptomycin
Ertapenem	Metronidazole
Imipenem/cilastatin	Vancomycin
Meropenem	

3. Carbapenems
   a. May be used in serious infections of urinary tract, lower respiratory tract, bones, joints, skin and skin structures; intra-abdominal, gynecologic, and mixed infections
   b. Meropenem is used in bacterial meningitis because of its ability to enter CSF, especially if inflammation is present
   c. Administration considerations: preparations are specific for IM or for IV use; do not interchange; give IM deep into gluteal muscle
   d. Side/adverse effects: nausea, diarrhea, headache, confusion, seizures, superinfections, anaphylaxis
   e. Nursing considerations and client education: same as for other antibiotics; eat meals with high-quality protein; drink at least six to eight glasses of fluids a day
4. Aztreonam: a cell wall inhibitor with a beta lactam ring but does not have cross-sensitivity to penicillins or cephalosporins; given by parenteral route; adverse effects include N/V, diarrhea, candidiasis, pain at injection site; anaphylaxis and pseudomembranous colitis are rare
5. Metronidazole: active against bacteria and multicellular parasites; antibacterial uses include anaerobic infections and peptic ulcer disease; resistance is rare; adverse effects include nausea, dry mouth, headache; neurotoxicity can occur in high doses

VII. ANTIMYCOBACTERIALS

A. Antituberculins

1. Action and use
   a. Inhibit cell wall synthesis, protein synthesis, RNA synthesis
   b. Used as prophylaxis or treatment of pulmonary tuberculosis and extrapulmonary tuberculosis from *Mycobacterium tuberculosis*, to prevent or delay onset of *Mycobacterium avium* bacteremia in clients with acquired immunodeficiency syndrome (AIDS)
   c. Rifampin also eradicates *Neisseria meningitides* from nasopharynx of asymptomatic carriers, and is used prophylactically with exposure to *Haemophilus influenzae* type B (HIB) infection
2. Common antituberculin medications are listed in Box 45–12
3. Administration considerations
   a. Effectiveness depends on correct drug, correct combination therapy, adequate dosing and duration of therapy, and client adherence to therapy (directly observed therapy [DOT] may be needed)
   b. Multicombination drug therapy decreases risk or rate of developing resistance to any single drug; treatment protocols last 6 months (typical) to 9 months depending on specific client circumstances
   c. Use caution in renal or liver dysfunction, history of seizures, alcohol abuse
4. Side/adverse effects
   a. Common: N/V, anorexia, constipation, diarrhea, dyspepsia
   b. Serious: vary by drug, but tend to include hepatotoxicity, anaphylaxis, blood dyscrasias, optic neuritis (ethambutol and isoniazid)
   c. Others include headache, dizziness, malaise, fever, chills, arthralgia, flulike symptoms, weakness, skin rash, dry skin, photophobia, photosensitivity, vision changes
   NCLEX® d. Change in color to orange-red of excretions/secretions such as urine, tears, feces, perspiration (rifampin and rifabutin)

Box 45–12

Antituberculin Drugs

First-Line Agents	Bedaquiline
Ethambutol	Capreomycin
Isoniazid	Ciprofloxacin
Pyrazinamide	Cycloserine
Rifabutin	Ethionamide
Rifampin	Kanamycin
Rifapentine	Ofloxacin
Second-Line Agents	Streptomycin
Amikacin	
Aminosalicylic acid	

Memory Aid

Remember the *r* in rifampin can indicate a reddish-orange discoloration to body fluids.

5. Nursing considerations as per Box 45–2
   a. Assess baseline and periodic liver and renal function studies, C&S results, CBC with WBC differential, RBC indices, and platelet count
   b. Coadminister pyridoxine (vitamin B_6) and/or cyanocobalamin (vitamin B_{12})

   NCLEX®

   c. Encourage foods high in B-complex vitamin (especially pyridoxine), such as meat (chicken, beef, and pork), liver, soybeans, baked potato with skin, raw avocado to help reduce paresthesias
   d. Evaluate adherence to therapy to lessen risk of reinfection or drug resistance
6. Client education as per Box 45–3
   a. Take isoniazid 1 hour before meals
   b. Rifampin: may discolor urine, tears, saliva; may stain contact lens and undergarments
   c. Keep follow-up appointments and testing with healthcare provider
   d. Use infection control measures to protect self and others
   e. Avoid alcohol because of increased risk for hepatitis or disulfiram-like effect
   f. Use alternative contraception during therapy and for at least 1 month after therapy is discontinued if using oral contraceptives

B. Leprostatics

1. Action and use: treat leprosy and some AIDS-related opportunistic infections
2. Common medications: dapsone and clofazimine
   a. Dapsone is bacteriostatic against *Mycobacterium leprae* and *tuberculosis*, *Pneumocystis jerovici*, *Plasmodium*; inhibits folic acid synthesis
   b. Clofazimine is bactericidal against *Mycobacterium leprae* and *avium*
3. Administration considerations: give clofazimine with food
4. Side/adverse effects
   a. Common: skin pigmentation changes (reddish-brown); may resolve in weeks to months, dry skin, N/V, diarrhea, abdominal pain, headache, insomnia, malaise, paresthesias, nervousness, tinnitus, vertigo, vision changes
   b. Serious: dose-related hemolysis and methemoglobinemia (rhinitis, fatigue, difficulty breathing, cyanosis), toxic hepatitis, agranulocytosis (rare), male infertility (dapsone)
5. Nursing considerations as per Box 45–2; monitor WBC count with differential, serum electrolytes, albumin, and liver enzymes
6. Client education as per Box 45–3
   a. Reddish-brown skin discoloration may occur; resolves in months to years after drug is discontinued
   b. Ensure infection control measures are used
   c. Encourage hydration and good nutrition with complete or complementary proteins for tissue healing

VIII. ANTIVIRALS

A. Medications to treat herpesviruses

1. Action and use
   a. Virustatic; drugs convert to compound that is a counterfeit nucleotide, which terminate developing viral DNA chain; has little effect on host cells; effective during acute (not latent) phase of infection
   b. Used to treat broad spectrum of diseases, including cold sores, viral encephalitis, shingles, and genital infection
   c. Viruses include herpes simplex virus–1 (HSV-1) in oral herpes or herpes labialis, HSV-2 in genital herpes, herpes zoster virus (HZV) in shingles, herpes varicella zoster virus (VZV) in chickenpox, cytomegalovirus (CMV), some Epstein-Barr viruses (infectious mononucleosis), and herpesvirus–type 6 (roseola)
   d. Most frequently prescribed drugs for HSV and VZV include acyclovir, famciclovir, and valacyclovir
2. Common medications for herpesvirus infections are listed in Box 45–13

Memory Aid

Recognize an antiviral drug by the root *vir* in the drug name.

Box 45–13

Antivirals to Treat Herpesvirus Infections

Systemic Agents	**Topical Agents**
Acyclovir	Docusanol
Cidofovir	Idoxuridine
Famciclovir	Penciclovir
Foscarnet	Trifluridine
Ganciclovir	
Valacyclovir	
Valganciclovir	

3. Administration considerations
   a. Hydrate client to decrease risk or extent of nephrotoxicity
   b. Wear gloves for topical application to limit exposure to drug or lesions
   c. Preferred central venous access for IV administrations
4. Side/adverse effects
   a. Common: N/V, diarrhea, headache, pain, local inflammation at IV injection sites
   b. Serious: nephrotoxicity, thrombocytopenic purpura or hemolytic uremia syndrome, seizures and electrolyte imbalances (foscarnet), neutropenia (cidofovir), hematologic toxicity or bone marrow suppression (ganciclovir, valganciclovir)
   c. Topical: burning or stinging at application site, headache, photophobia, keratopathy, eyelid edema (ophthalmic use)

NCLEX®
5. Nursing considerations
   a. Assess baseline and periodic clinical data to monitor effectiveness of drug and side effects
   b. Assess renal function (creatinine, BUN, creatinine clearance, I&O), hepatic function (liver enzymes, bilirubin)
   c. Assess skin and lesions regularly; monitor for pain relief and resolution of infection
   d. Hydrate to decrease risk of nephrotoxicity (e.g., 2000–3000 mL/fluids per day) if not contraindicated by other conditions
6. Client education
   a. Similar principles as in antibiotic therapy (see Box 45–3); importance of completing full course of therapy with evenly distributed dosing that does not interrupt sleep (to improve effectiveness and prevent drug resistance)
   b. *NCLEX®* Avoid sexual intercourse if genital herpes being treated
   c. *NCLEX®* Avoid touching lesions to avoid spreading infection to new sites (autoinoculation)
   d. Avoid hazardous tasks and driving if drowsiness, dizziness, seizure activity occurs
   e. Follow up with labs and appointments with prescriber
   f. Eat frequent, small, high-protein meals and drink 2000–3000 mL/day in fluids
   g. *NCLEX®* Female clients should have annual Pap smear since there is increased risk of cervical cancer with genital herpes infection
   h. Antiviral agents treat but do not cure viral infections
   i. Notify prescriber for adverse drug effects or if lesions recur or do not heal

B. **Antiretroviral drugs** to treat human immunodeficiency virus (HIV) infection and acquired immunodeficiency syndrome (AIDS) include nucleoside and nucleotide reverse transcriptase inhibitors (NRTIs, NtRTIs), non-nucleoside reverse transcriptase inhibitors (NNRTIs), protease inhibitors, entry inhibitors, and integrase inhibitors (see Figure 45–1)

C. **Reverse transcriptase inhibitors (nucleoside, nucleotide, and non-nucleoside)**
1. Block viral reverse transcriptase; stops replication/growth; effectiveness diminishes over time; used in combination because resistant strains rapidly evolve if used alone
2. Used for all symptomatic HIV clients with a CD4 count less than $500/mm^3$ and some with higher counts; possible prophylaxis for known occupational HIV exposure
3. Common reverse transcriptase inhibitors are listed in Box 45–14
4. Administration considerations
   a. Food may slow absorption but does not affect total absorption
   b. May administer at bedtime for better tolerance of CNS adverse effects
   c. Contraindicated with concurrent use of drugs that cause peripheral neuropathy

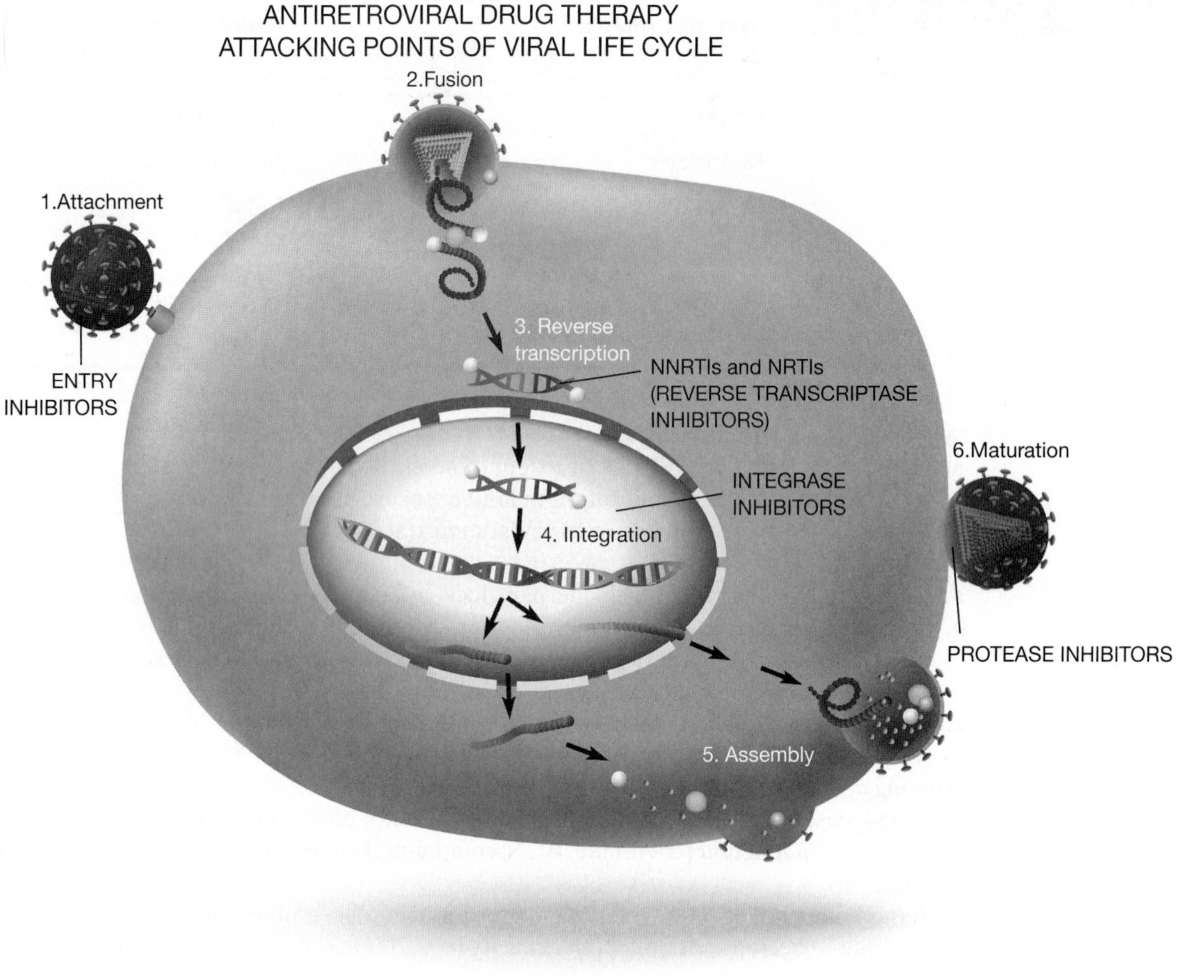

Figure 45–1 Antiretroviral drug therapy in HIV infection.

Box 45–14

Antiretrovirals for HIV and AIDS

Non-nucleoside Reverse Transcriptase Inhibitors

Delavirdine

Efavirenz

Etravirine

Nevirapine

Rilpivirine

Nucleoside and Nucleotide Reverse Transcriptase Inhibitors

Abacavir sulfate

Didanosine

Emtricitabine

Lamivudine

Stavudine

Tenofovir

Zidovudine

Protease Inhibitors

Atazanavir

Darunavir

Fosamprenavir

Indinavir

Lopinavir/ritonavir

Nelfinavir

Ritonavir

Saquinavir

Tipranavir

Entry Inhibitors

Enfuvirtide

Maraviroc

Integrase Inhibitors

Raltegravir

Dolutegravir

5. Side/adverse effects
   a. Non-nucleoside-type drugs: rash, fever, nausea, diarrhea, headache, stomatitis, paresthesias, Stevens-Johnson syndrome, hepatotoxicity (nevirapine), CNS toxicity (efavirenz), and severe depression (rilpiravine)
   b. Nucleoside- and nucleotide-type drugs: weakness, fatigue, myalgia, N/V, abdominal pain, anorexia, headache, rash, sleep disorders, bone marrow suppression with neutropenia and anemia, neurotoxicity, lactic acidosis with steatorrhea, pancreatitis (lamivudine), peripheral neuropathy (stavudine)
6. Nursing considerations
   a. Similar principles as for other anti-infective drugs (Box 45–2)
   b. Monitor renal and liver function (liver enzymes) and renal function (BUN, creatinine, I&O, daily weight) at baseline and periodically during therapy; monitor for reduced symptoms of AIDS or ARC and for increase in CD4 count
   c. Ensure client takes complete course and all drugs included in regimen to improve effectiveness and retard risk for emergence of resistant strains
   d. Assess client for complications of HIV infection (e.g., opportunistic infections, cancer, neurologic disease)
   e. Assess for and report adverse drug effects
   f. Provide safety measures to protect from injury if CNS adverse effects occur
   g. Assess nutritional intake and tolerance
   h. Monitor skin and mucous membranes frequently
7. Client education
   a. Similar principles as for other anti-infective therapy (Box 45–3)
   b. Caution about risks of dizziness or altered mentation; do not drive or perform hazardous tasks
   c. Avoid crowds and persons with infections
   d. Hair loss possible with zidovudine (AZT)
   e. Drugs do not cure but help manage infection; they reduce viral load, decrease risk for complications, and extend survival
   f. Practice good personal hygiene and safe-sex practices

D. Protease inhibitors

1. Inhibit cell protein synthesis to interfere with viral replication
2. Used in AIDS and AIDS-related complex (ARC) to decrease viral load and opportunistic infections, and in combination with other drugs to increase CD4 counts and decrease incidence or rate of development of drug resistance
3. Common protease inhibitors are listed in Box 45–14
4. Administration considerations
   a. Give saquinavir with high-fat meals or within 2 hours of full meal
   b. Give ritonavir with chocolate milk, nutritional supplement, or food (unpleasant taste)
   c. Indinavir requires an acidic gastric environment for absorption, so give dose 1 hour before or 2 hours after a light, low-fat snack; client should drink 1.5 liters or more of fluid daily
5. Side/adverse effects
   a. Common: N/V, diarrhea, abdominal discomfort, headache
   b. Serious: anemia, leukopenia, lymphadenopathy, pancreatitis, deep vein thrombosis, hemorrhagic colitis, nephrolithiasis (indinavir), thrombocytopenia and pancytopenia (saquinavir), cardiac arrest (atazanavir)
6. Nursing considerations
   a. Similar principles as for antibiotic therapy (Box 45–2)
   b. Monitor for hepatotoxicity (elevated liver enzymes, N/V, jaundice, enlarged or tender liver) and nephrotoxicity (elevated creatinine, BUN, creatinine clearance); keep accurate I&O
   c. Monitor CBC for blood dyscrasias such as neutropenia, thrombocytopenia, or anemia, and for improvement as evidenced by increased T cell count
   d. Monitor for side effects; if neutropenic, observe for occult signs of infection (e.g., lower back, flank, or suprapubic pain), normal temperature or low-grade fever related to UTI
   e. Provide neutropenic precautions as appropriate
7. Client education
   a. Similar principles as for antibiotic therapy (Box 45–3)
   b. Ensure fluid intake of at least 1500 mL/day
   c. Be aware of drug-specific self-administration instructions and follow them

d. Eat small, frequent meals with complete or complementary proteins
e. Use measures to protect self against infection

E. Entry inhibitors and integrase inhibitors (see again Box 45–14)

1. Enfuvirtide
   a. Entry inhibitor that interferes with fusion of viral and cell membranes, blocking entry of HIV into host cell
   b. Given by subcutaneous injection twice daily; injection site reaction is almost certain in first week, with severe pain, pruritus, erythema, cysts, abscesses, and cellulitis at injection site
   c. Other common adverse effects are nausea, diarrhea, fatigue, and increased risk for pneumonia
2. Maraviroc
   a. Entry inhibitor that blocks CCR5 coreceptor needed for viral entry into human cell; significantly reduces viral load and increases T cell production
   b. Dosed orally and may be given with or without food
   c. Adverse effects are upper respiratory infection, cough, fever, rash, and dizziness, risk for hepatotoxicity (may be preceded by systemic allergic reaction), increased risk for myocardial ischemia or infarction in clients with cardiac disease
3. Raltegravir
   a. Integrase inhibitor that inhibits viral integrase enzyme needed to insert viral DNA into human chromosome
   b. Given orally; headache and GI symptoms are most common adverse effects
4. Dolutegravir: approved in 2014 as an oral integrase inhibitor that can be given as a three-drug combination with abacavir and lamudivine

F. Medications for influenza and respiratory viruses

1. Have both prophylactic applications (amantadine and rimantadine) and treatment applications (oseltamivir and zanamivir); see Box 45–15
2. Virustatic; most viral replication occurs before symptoms appear; bacterial replication occurs as signs of infection emerge
3. Administration considerations: administer before flu season for prophylaxis and as soon as symptoms emerge when used for treatment
4. Side/adverse effects
   a. Amantadine and rimantadine (prophylaxis): nausea, dizziness, insomnia, difficulty concentrating, nervousness; orthostatic hypotension, urinary retention, leukopenia, seizures, and hallucinations; most are transient and resolve quickly after drug discontinued
   b. Oseltamivir and zanamivir (treatment): N/V, diarrhea, dizziness, bronchitis, bronchospasm, serious skin hypersensitivity reactions
5. Nursing considerations
   a. Similar principles as for other anti-infectives (Box 45–2)
   b. Assess hepatic and renal dysfunction and baseline neurologic status (orientation, affect, coordination, reflexes)
   c. Provide safety precautions if CNS adverse effects develop
   d. Keep accurate I&O; monitor for urinary retention
6. Client education
   a. As per other types of anti-infectives (Box 45–3)
   b. Change position slowly to minimize risk of orthostatic hypotension
   c. Report increased respiratory distress or severe adverse effects to prescriber
   d. If drowsiness, dizziness, lightheadedness, confusion, ataxia, or blurred vision occur, do not drive or perform hazardous tasks
   e. Drink at least six to eight glasses of fluids a day

Box 45–15

Medications for Influenza and Respiratory Viruses

Amantadine
Rimantadine
Oseltamivir
Zanamivir

IX. ANTIFUNGALS

A. Systemic antifungals

1. Fungistatic or fungicidal depending on therapeutic serum levels and sensitivity to fungi
2. Treat candida infections, cryptococcus, blastomycosis, histoplasmosis, aspergillus fumigates, and **tinea** infections (a fungal infection caused by ringworm)
3. Increased cell membrane permeability allows other drugs to enter fungus cell
4. Common systemic antifungal medications are listed in Box 45–16
5. Administration considerations
   a. Administer carefully as prescribed, especially IV dosages; nonliposomal form of drug should be used only for progressive and potentially life-threatening fungal infection
   b. May premedicate amphotericin with an antipyretic such as acetaminophen, an antihistamine such as diphenhydramine, an antiemetic, to reduce severity of fever/chills response; heparin or hydrocortisone added to IV solution may reduce risk for thrombophlebitis at IV site
   c. Administer over 2–6 hours to avert cardiovascular collapse (hypotension, shock) from too rapid infusion (amphotericin B)
   NCLEX® d. Hydrate with IV fluids usually 2 hours before and 2 hours after amphotericin B administration to decrease risk for nephrotoxicity
6. Side/adverse effects
   a. Common: vary by drug but tend to include fever, chills, N/V, diarrhea, headache, hypokalemia, hypomagnesemia, dizziness, and drowsiness
   b. Serious: anaphylaxis, anemia, leukopenia, agranulocytosis, thrombocytopenia, hepatic failure, nephrotoxicity, visual disturbances (voriconazole), cardiac dysrhythmias (posaconazole, voriconazole)
7. Nursing considerations
   a. Similar principles as for other anti-infectives (Box 45–2); check for incompatibility of solutions as there are many
   b. Monitor liver and renal laboratory studies throughout therapy
   c. Monitor WBC for improvement and for early detection of developing neutropenia, platelet count (thrombocytopenia), red blood cell count (anemia)
   d. Give potassium supplements if hypokalemia occurs
   e. Protect amphotericin B from light, and monitor client's I&O
8. Client education
   a. Similar principles as for other anti-infectives (Box 45–3); know length of therapy (e.g., amphotericin B may be given over weeks or months)
   b. Take oral agents with food to minimize GI distress
   c. Report adverse effects such as burning at IV site, increased bleeding or bruising, evidence of superinfection
   d. Febrile reaction may decrease over time
   e. Fluid intake of 2000–3000 mL/day if not contraindicated by other conditions

B. Topical antifungals

1. Action and use
   a. Local infections of skin and mucous membranes of oropharynx, vagina, or intestines caused by *Candida* species; infections of tinea pedis (athlete's foot), tinea cruris (in scrotal, crural, anal, and genital areas, called "jock itch"), tinea corporis (skin), tinea unguium or onychomycosis (nail fungus), tinea manus, tinea versicolor (infection of skin with yellow or beige brawny patches)
   b. Use vaginal tablets up to 6 weeks prior to delivery to prevent newborn thrush
2. Common topical antifungal medications are listed in Box 45–17; see product literature because individual drugs may be available as a cream, gel, ointment, powder, shampoo, troche, vaginal suppository, or oral dose

Box 45–16

Systemic Antifungal Medications

Amphotericin B	Fluconazole
Anidulafungin	Itraconazole
Caspofungin	Ketoconazole
Flucytosine	Posaconazole
Micafungin	Voriconazole

Box 45–17

Topical Antifungal Medications

General	Econazole
Butenafine	Fluconazole
Ciclopirox	Itraconazole
Griseofulvin	Ketoconazole
Naftifine	Luconazole
Nystatin	Miconazole
Tavaborole	Oxiconazole
Terbinafine	Sulconazole
Tolnaftate	Terconazole
Undecylenic acid	Tioconazole
Azoles	
Butoconazole	
Clotrimazole	

3. Administration considerations
   a. Oral tablets or lozenges/troches are not to be chewed or swallowed whole; swallow saliva as lozenge/troche dissolves slowly over 5–30 minutes; avoid food or drink during and for 30 minutes after dose
   b. For oral infections in client with dentures, remove dentures at bedtime; with oral suspension, remove dentures before each rinse or before each oral lozenge/troche

   NCLEX®
   c. For application to skin: wear latex gloves, cleanse area with tepid water (soap if prescribed), dry thoroughly (without application of heat), and apply antifungal to infected area sparingly; do not cover with an occlusive dressing or tight clothing; wash hands well after removing gloves
   d. For treatment of tinea pedis (athlete's foot), apply antifungal powder such as nystatin to inside of shoes and stockings
   e. For vulvovaginal use: insert one full applicator or one vaginal tablet at bedtime as instructed; continue therapy during menstruation
   f. Avoid contact of antifungal with eyes; with certain agents, avoid contact with mucous membranes

   NCLEX®
   g. Do not apply occlusive dressing unless prescribed; client should avoid restrictive clothing in areas of infection
4. Side/adverse effects
   a. Common: dry skin, stinging at application site, pruritus, urticaria, contact dermatitis
   b. Serious: hypersensitivity (-azoles), granulocytopenia (griseofulvin), cholestatic hepatitis and neutropenia (oral terbinafine)
5. Nursing considerations
   a. Ensure complete course of therapy taken and observe for clinical signs of improvement
   b. Observe for clinical evidence of liver dysfunction, such as upper right quadrant tenderness, abdominal discomfort or bloating, lethargy, mentation changes, icterus, enlarged liver, elevated liver enzymes
   c. Withhold application and collaborate with prescriber if severe burning or exacerbation of lesions occurs
6. Client education
   a. Know drug name, purpose, dose, strength, how to apply, schedule of administration, length of therapy
   b. Observe site for improvement within first week of therapy; some infections require 2–4 weeks of treatment; notify prescriber if condition worsens or no improvement is noted in 1–2 weeks
   c. Store in tightly covered container at room temperature; if vaginal tablet or suppository, store as recommended, usually in refrigerator or above 59°F (15°C); avoid freezing or excess heat with all products
   d. If taken vaginally, refrain from sexual intercourse or have partner wear condom to avoid burning or irritation of penis or urethra

   NCLEX®
   e. Wash clothing and linens in contact with infectious sites with soap and water after each treatment; ointments may be removed from fabric with commercial cleaning products
   f. If severe burning, stinging, or eruptions occur, discontinue use and notify prescriber

X. ANTIPROTOZOALS

A. Antimalarials

1. Action and use: treatment or prophylaxis of malarial infection; chloroquine is used as treatment for **giardiasis** (protozoan intestinal infection) and amebiasis outside GI tract
2. Common antiprotozoal medications are listed in Box 45–18
3. Administration considerations
   a. Separate drug from antacid administration by 4 hours before or after antacids
   b. Administer with food to decrease GI distress: chloroquine, hydroxychloroquine, and pyrimethamine; administer quinine with food to decrease GI distress and mask bitter taste; do not crush capsule
   NCLEX® c. For prophylaxis, take as prescribed, such as same day every week when entering high-risk area and for 10 weeks after departing
4. Side/adverse effects
   a. Common: N/V, diarrhea, headache, anorexia, abdominal cramping, visual changes (blurred vision, photophobia, difficulty focusing), myalgias
   b. Serious: vary by drug but may include hemolytic anemia in clients with G6PD deficiency, cardiac rhythm disturbances (bradycardia, tachycardia, atrioventricular block, QT prolongation), hypotension, neutropenia, agranulocytosis, psychosis, cinchonism (tinnitus, ototoxicity, vertigo, fever, vision disturbances) with quinine
   c. Other: with chloroquine and hydroxychloroquine there may be alopecia, bleaching of scalp or hair (including eyebrows, body hair), and freckles; bluish-black hue of skin or mucous membranes, rash, pruritis
5. Nursing considerations
   a. Similar principles as for other anti-infectives (Box 45–2)
   b. Assess for and report adverse effects
   c. If client is taking antiepileptics, monitor drug levels of these agents
   d. Ensure regular ophthalmic exams, ECGs, and lab tests as prescribed
6. Client education
   a. Similar principles as for other anti-infectives (Box 45–3)
   b. If weekly dosing, take on same day every week
   c. Do not drive or perform hazardous tasks if drowsiness, dizziness, vertigo, visual disturbances occur; report adverse effects to prescriber
   NCLEX® d. Chloroquine: sunglasses may reduce photophobia; urine may become rusty yellow or brown

B. Other antiprotozoals

1. Action and use
   a. Treat diarrhea caused by amebiasis, giardiasis, cryptosporidiosis, or other infections common in areas with poor sanitation (water, sewer)
   b. Some are bacteriocidal as well as amebicidal, especially in GI tract
2. Common antiprotozoal medications are listed in Box 45–18
3. Administration considerations: see specific product literature

Box 45–18

Antiprotozoal Medications

Antimalarials	Melarsoprol
Artemether/lumefantrine	Metronidazole
Atovaquone/proguanil	Miltefosine
Chloroquine	Nifurtimox
Hydroxychloroquine	Nitazoxanide
Mefloquine	Paromomycin
Primaquine	Pentamidine
Quinine	Pyrimethamine
Other Antiprotozoal Medications	Sodium stibogluconate
Eflornithine	Suramin
Iodoquinol	Tinidazole

4. Side/adverse effects
   a. Common: N/V, diarrhea, headache, anorexia, abdominal cramping
   b. Serious: vary by drug but may include blood dyscrasias, nephrotoxicity, hepatotoxicity, CNS disturbances such as seizures, confusion, paresthesias or peripheral neuropathy, visual problems (blurring, unable to focus, seeing halos), ototoxicity with tinnitus and hearing loss (eflornithine), substernal pain and electrocardiogram (ECG) changes (sodium stibugluconate), cough and pneumonia (sodium stibugluconate)

NCLEX® 5. Nursing considerations: ensure complete course of therapy is taken for full benefit

NCLEX® 6. Client education
   a. Know drug, dose, purpose, schedule, proper administration technique
   b. Take full course of therapy for best effect
   c. Know clinical manifestations of infections and drug side effects to report

XI. ANTIHELMINTHICS

A. Action and use: treatment for intestinal round worms, pinworm, and hook worms

B. Common antihelminthic medications are listed in Box 45–19

C. Administration considerations
1. Mebendazole: may be chewed, swallowed whole, crushed, mixed with food
2. Pyrantel: may take with food
3. Thiabendazole: take after meals

D. Side/adverse effects
1. Common: N/V, diarrhea, abdominal cramps, anorexia, pruritus, fever, headache, dizziness, malaise, arthralgia and lymphadenopathy (ivermectin), urinary odor (thiabendazole)
2. Serious: leukopenia, acute inflammatory or allergic response (ivermectin), nephrotoxity or jaundice (thiabendazole), cerebrospinal reaction syndrome (praziquantel)

E. Nursing considerations
1. Similar principles as for other anti-infectives (Box 45–2)
2. Monitor hepatic, renal, or hematological laboratory results
3. Collect stool specimen for ova and parasites (O&P) for baseline and follow-up to verify eradication of infectious agents

F. Client education
1. Similar principles as for other anti-infectives (Box 45–3)
2. Do not repeat drug therapy for continued infection until 1 week after initial treatment
3. Practice personal hygiene to prevent transmission
4. Urine odor may occur with thiabendazole

Box 45–19

Antihelminthics

Albendazole	Praziquantel
Ivermectin	Pyrantel
Mebendazole	Thiabendazole

Check Your NCLEX–RN® Exam I.Q.

You are ready for testing on this content if you can:

- Apply knowledge of expected actions and effects of anti-infective and immunologic medications to client care.
- Correctly describe administration of anti-infective and immunologic medications to clients.
- Assess for side effects and adverse effects of anti-infective and immunologic medications.
- Take appropriate action if a client has an unexpected response to an anti-infective or immunologic medication.
- Monitor a client for expected outcomes or effects of treatment with anti-infective and immunologic medications.

PRACTICE TEST

1 A client has a new order to receive vancomycin to treat a systemic infection. The nurse anticipates the prescription would indicate which route for optimal administration?

1. Peripheral venous access
2. Central venous access
3. Intramuscular
4. Oral

2 Gentamicin therapy is to be initiated. Which laboratory test result would indicate to the nurse that the client is manifesting a common adverse effect?

1. Elevated urine creatinine clearance
2. Increased prothrombin time (PT)
3. Increased serum creatinine
4. Hypokalemia

3 A client who is taking isoniazid is experiencing paresthesia as a common side effect. The nurse should teach the client to include what foods in the diet? Select all that apply.

1. Liver
2. Peanuts
3. Raw avocados
4. Raw apples
5. Baked potato with skin

4 A client who takes digoxin is to begin drug therapy with amphotericin B. The nurse anticipates that the client could experience digitalis toxicity for which reason?

1. Hypokalemia
2. Antifungal attaching to receptors before digoxin
3. Increased plasma concentration of amphotericin B
4. Increased gastrointestinal absorption of digoxin and amphotericin B

5 A client is receiving levofloxacin in addition to an oral anticoagulant. What treatment should the nurse anticipate administering if the client experiences an adverse drug effect as a result of this combination?

1. Albumin
2. Platelets
3. Protamine sulfate
4. Phytonadione (vitamin K)

6 The nurse assesses a client taking doxycycline as being jaundiced and lethargic. What laboratory study would be most specific for the nurse to assess?

1. Bilirubin
2. Alkaline phosphatase (ALP)
3. Alanine aminotransferase (ALT)
4. Aspartate aminotransferase (AST)

7 A client taking ampicillin develops a macular rash on the chest. What conclusion should the nurse draw about this assessment finding?

1. This reaction is Stevens-Johnson syndrome.
2. A minor rash usually precipitates the development of more severe reactions.
3. A minor rash requires notification of the prescriber, but might be well tolerated and might fade with continued treatment.
4. Hypersensitivity reactions requiring discontinuation of the antibiotic occur to some extent with many clients taking a penicillin agent.

8 A client is started on erythromycin as treatment for pneumonia. The nurse should teach the client to contact the healthcare provider for which reasons? Select all that apply.

1. Improvement of fever, cough, or respiratory effort is not observed in 48–72 hours.
2. Fluids can be taken orally, but still cannot eat after 24 hours.
3. Anorexia and nausea develop within 24 hours.
4. Fever fluctuates.
5. Changes in response to verbal stimuli are noted.

PRACTICE TEST

9 A child with otitis media is taking trimethoprim-sulfamethoxazole as a suspension. What instructions should the nurse provide to the mother?

1. Do not allow the child to drink water immediately after taking the medication.
2. The medication is to be taken on an empty stomach.
3. The medication must be kept refrigerated.
4. Use a calibrated measuring device.

10 A client receiving an anti-infective drug begins to wheeze. The nurse anticipates initial administration of what drug?

1. Epinephrine
2. Methylprednisolone
3. Atropine sulfate
4. Dopamine

11 An adult client is prescribed to take metronidazole 250 mg by mouth three times a day for confirmed trichomoniasis. After taking the drug for 24 hours, the client reports flushing, dizziness, pounding headache, sweating, abdominal cramps, nausea, and irritability. What important data should the nurse assess at this time? Select all that apply.

1. History of alcohol abuse
2. Current over-the-counter medications
3. History of liver disease
4. Whether tablets were crushed before administration
5. Whether food was given with the medication

12 The nurse assesses the client receiving cefotazime and notes three diarrhea stools in the past 24 hours, rectal itching, glossitis, and fever. What adverse effect should the nurse conclude the client is exhibiting?

1. Leukocytosis
2. Opportunistic infection
3. Bone marrow depression
4. Drug failure against original infective organism

13 What teaching or intervention is appropriate for a client taking an antibiotic that causes diarrhea secondary to elimination of normal intestinal flora?

1. Test stool for occult blood daily.
2. Include yogurt or buttermilk products in the diet.
3. Arrange for IV administration instead of oral route.
4. Take antacids with antibiotic to reduce diarrhea.

14 A disulfiram-like reaction occurs in a client taking cefoperazone sodium. The nurse suspects this reaction is a drug interaction resulting from the client's ingestion of which substance within the last few hours?

1. Caffeine in tea or coffee
2. Sulfamethoxazole for a chronic urinary tract infection
3. Over-the-counter cough suppressant
4. Ampicillin, which has a cross-sensitivity to cephalosporins

15 The nurse evaluates for an adverse reaction to tobramycin by conducting what assessment?

1. Capillary refill
2. Romberg test
3. Chvostek sign
4. Babinski reflex

16 What should the nurse teach an adult premenopausal client receiving griseofulvin for a systemic antifungal condition?

1. If taking oral contraceptives, use an alternative form of contraception during and for 1 month after use of griseofulvin.
2. Record number of absorbent products used daily to monitor for increased menstrual flow while taking griseofulvin.
3. Check blood pressure (BP) daily if taking an oral contraceptive and griseofulvin, as both can increase BP.
4. Avoid taking calcium supplements concurrently with griseofulvin.

17 Due to the mechanisms of action with tetracycline, what does the nurse anticipate that the client will need for the drug to be effective?

1. A competent immune system
2. Concurrent administration of iron
3. Supplemental pyridoxine HCl (vitamin B_6)
4. Weekly evaluation of complete blood count

18 A client is receiving long-term oral anticoagulation therapy and is also taking a beta-lactam penicillin. What lab result should the nurse assess for during this therapy?

1. Decreased bleeding time
2. Increased thrombin time (TT)
3. Increased prothrombin time (PT)
4. Increased activated partial thromboplastin time (aPPT)

19 Appropriate teaching for a young adult female related to a new prescription for ampicillin orally would include which of the following? Select all that apply.

1. Client may notice development of red, scaly skin.
2. Observe for clinical extrapyramidal tract manifestations.
3. Change positions slowly to avoid orthostatic hypotension.
4. Oral contraceptives may lose effectiveness.
5. Vaginal itching and discharge can occur.

20 A female client is taking sargramostim following a bone marrow transplant. During an assessment, the client voices concern about her hair falling out. Based on this assessment, what should be the nurse's priority concern?

1. General skin integrity
2. Alopecia
3. Client's body image
4. Client's anxiety level

21 A client receiving aldesleukin reports new-onset fever and pain. What should be the priority concern for this client?

1. Risk for dehydration because of flulike symptoms
2. Possible issues with airway in response to fever
3. Excess fluid intake in response to flulike symptoms
4. Weak cough related to increased pulmonary secretions

22 The nurse should assess a client receiving oprelvekin frequently for which manifestations? Select all that apply.

1. Dehydration
2. Congestive heart failure (CHF)
3. Anxiety
4. Hyperuricemia
5. Irregular apical pulse

23 For what condition would the nurse expect to administer a medication that would increase the concentration of acetylcholine at neuromuscular junctions?

1. Multiple sclerosis
2. Parkinson's disease
3. Myasthenia gravis
4. Lupus erythematosus

24 A client is admitted to the emergency department with a 7.6-cm (3-in.) laceration over the left eye. The nurse should assess for which priority factor related to risk of infection before beginning drug therapy to prevent infection?

1. The client's temperature
2. The date of the client's last tetanus vaccine
3. If the client's blood pressure is decreased
4. Whether the client is taking corticosteroid medication

25 A client is preparing to travel to the rainforest region of South America. What is the most common medication that the nurse should expect to be prescribed for this client?

1. Zidovudine
2. Mefloquine
3. Rimantadine
4. Filgrastim

26 In conducting client teaching about interferon beta 1b, what should the nurse explain as the goal for administering this medication?

1. Cure the client of multiple sclerosis.
2. Prevent signs and symptoms of anaphylaxis.
3. Destroy nerve tissue that is laden with plaque.
4. Decrease demyelination in brain tissue.

27 What should the nurse instruct the client to do to decrease renal insufficiency side effects in clients receiving cyclophosphamide?

1. Consume a diet high in fiber.
2. Have creatinine level assessed weekly.
3. Drink 3000 mL of fluid per day.
4. Take hydrochlorothiazide (HCTZ).

28 To assess a client's baseline before administering azathioprine, the nurse should put highest priority on evaluating which laboratory test result?

1. Creatinine
2. Uric acid
3. PT and PTT
4. Red blood cell count

29 Azathioprine and allopurinol are administered to a client diagnosed with multiple sclerosis and gout. It is important for the nurse to assess the results of which laboratory test in this client?

1. Creatinine
2. Uric acid
3. Blood glucose
4. Blood urea nitrogen (BUN)

30 A client is scheduled for diagnostic testing for myasthenia gravis. What medication is necessary for the nurse to prepare for this testing?

1. Ambenonium
2. Edrophonium
3. Neostigmine
4. Physostigmine

31 What points should the nurse include in a teaching plan for a client receiving medications to treat multiple sclerosis? Select all that apply.

1. Indications of pulmonary edema
2. Restriction of oral fluids
3. Requirement to avoid crowds
4. Enhancement of muscle strength
5. Chest pain

32 A client has been exposed to hepatitis A. Which client factor would be an indication for withholding administration of immune serum globulin to the client?

1. The client has received a hepatitis B vaccine.
2. The client has recently fallen and suffered a hip fracture.
3. The client has a history of a coagulation disorder.
4. The client is scheduled for foreign travel.

ANSWERS & RATIONALES

1 **Answer: 2 Rationale:** Vancomycin can cause thrombophlebitis; the best route of administration is with central IV where the drug will be diluted enough to lessen irritation to the vein. Peripheral IV administration increases the risk of thrombophlebitis from irritating effects of the drug. Intramuscular administration of vancomycin is contraindicated. Vancomycin is not absorbed in the GI tract, so the oral route is used only to treat *Clostridium difficile* associated with antibiotic-induced pseudomembranous colitis. **Cognitive Level:** Applying **Client Need:** Pharmacological and Parenteral Therapies **Integrated Process:** Nursing Process: Planning **Content Area:** Pharmacology **Strategy:** Focus on the critical word *systemic* in the stem of the question. Use this word and knowledge of safe administration of this drug to eliminate the incorrect options regarding best route.

2 **Answer: 3 Rationale:** Increased serum creatinine indicates renal dysfunction. Nephrotoxicity is a common adverse effect of aminoglycosides such as gentamicin. The urine creatinine clearance would be decreased in renal impairment. Coagulation disturbances are not attributed to this class of antibiotic as a direct adverse reaction. Hypokalemia is not attributed to this class of antibiotic as a direct adverse reaction. **Cognitive Level:** Applying **Client Need:** Pharmacological and Parenteral Therapies **Integrated Process:** Nursing Process: Diagnosis **Content Area:** Pharmacology **Strategy:** Note the critical words *common adverse effect* in the stem. Recall that aminoglycosides often adversely affect the kidneys. Identify the option that indicates renal impairment as the correct answer.

3 **Answer: 1, 3, 5 Rationale:** Peripheral neuritis is the most common side effect of isoniazid. Adding vitamin B_6 (pyridoxine) to the client's intake is the therapy to correct this side effect. The diet may be supplemented with vitamin B_6. Foods highest in vitamin B_6 include beef liver and chicken liver. A food other than meat that could be included is raw avocados, as well as baked potato with skin, raw banana, figs, and soybeans. Peanuts are not a food source high in vitamin B_6. Raw apples are not high in pyridoxine. **Cognitive Level:** Applying **Client Need:** Pharmacological and Parenteral Therapies **Integrated Process:** Nursing Process: Implementation **Content Area:** Pharmacology **Strategy:** The core issue of the question is knowledge of what nutrient will reduce adverse drug effects of INH. Recall that vitamin B_6 will assist in this action, and then choose the food that is highest in this vitamin. When more than one answer is correct, consider each option as a true/false statement.

4 **Answer: 1 Rationale:** Amphotericin-induced hypokalemia might potentiate toxicity of digoxin because hypokalemia is a primary cause for digitalis toxicity. Antifungal agents and cardiac glycosides do not compete for the same receptor sites. Amphotericin B is available for only IV and topical routes; gastrointestinal absorption is not a concern. **Cognitive Level:** Understanding **Client Need:** Pharmacological and Parenteral Therapies **Integrated Process:** Nursing Process:

Diagnosis **Content Area:** Pharmacology **Strategy:** The core issue of the question is knowledge of drug interaction of digoxin and amphoteracin B. Use specific nursing knowledge and the process of elimination to make a selection.

5 **Answer: 4 Rationale:** Absorption of vitamin K from the intestines can be interrupted, and prolonged bleeding can result due to inadequate serum level of prothrombin (hypoprothrombinemia). Appropriate therapy is to administer phytonadione or menadiol sodium diphosphate. Since intestinal absorption might not be optimal, the parenteral route is preferred. Eradication of the intestinal flora can occur during antibiotic therapy. Prolonged bleeding can occur with levofloxacin; however, albumin, a plasma expander, is not indicated unless there is notable blood loss. The nurse must assess for and protect against increased bleeding because levofloxacin can cause prolonged bleeding; however, there is no indication that the client has notable blood loss requiring platelets. Protamine sulfate is an antidote to heparin and is not appropriate or effective if bleeding should occur from the administration of levofloxacin. **Cognitive Level:** Analyzing **Client Need:** Pharmacological and Parenteral Therapies **Integrated Process:** Nursing Process: Planning **Content Area:** Pharmacology **Strategy:** The core issue of the question is knowledge of drug interaction between levofloxacin and oral anticoagulants. Recall that vitamin K reverses bleeding to help identify the drug that reverses the effect of oral anticoagulant drugs.

6 **Answer: 3 Rationale:** ALT is specific for diagnosing and monitoring liver disease or impairment. Differential diagnosis of etiology of jaundice between hepatic dysfunction and hemolysis of red blood cells is indicated by the bilirubin. ALP is a protein found in all body tissues, and while liver tissue has a high amount of ALP, this test is not as liver-specific as the ALT results. AST can help to diagnose or monitor heart disease or disease of the liver. **Cognitive Level:** Analyzing **Client Need:** Pharmacological and Parenteral Therapies **Integrated Process:** Nursing Process: Diagnosis **Content Area:** Pharmacology **Strategy:** The core issue of the question is the laboratory test that will help evaluate the presence of jaundice as an adverse effect of doxycycline. Use specific nursing knowledge and the process of elimination to make a selection.

7 **Answer: 3 Rationale:** A minor rash is the most common side effect of the penicillins and might be relatively insignificant. Its presence does not signify an allergic reaction and does not prohibit future administration of penicillin. However, the nurse closely monitors for further hypersensitivity reaction because other clinical manifestations could develop, such as fever, urticaria, chills, erythema, Stevens-Johnson syndrome, respiratory distress, and anaphylaxis. Stevens-Johnson syndrome is a more serious aberration of the skin associated with antimicrobial adverse reactions; it resembles a second-degree burn in that necrolysis separates the epidermis from the dermis, causing blisters. If itching occurs, an antihistamine such as diphenhydramine may be prescribed. All available antimicrobials are capable of stimulating an exaggerated immune response, but not all clients experience allergy with antibiotic therapy. **Cognitive Level:** Analyzing **Client Need:** Pharmacological and Parenteral Therapies **Integrated Process:** Nursing Process: Diagnosis **Content Area:** Pharmacology **Strategy:** The core issue of the question is the significance of a rash that develops in a client taking ampicillin. Use specific nursing knowledge and the process of elimination to make a selection. Recall that not all drug rashes indicate hypersensitivity to aid in choosing the correct option.

8 **Answer: 1, 5 Rationale:** Improvement in clinical manifestations of the infection should be noted within 48–72 hours. Otherwise, compliance with prescribed drug therapy should be assessed, and adjustment of drug, dose, and/or administration frequency might be needed. A side effect of erythromycin is ototoxicity, resulting in hearing loss preceded by tinnitus. A baseline hearing assessment should be made prior to administering the drug. The client's ability to take in fluids can temporarily sustain his nutritional status for a few days, particularly if dietary supplements are also included, which is appropriate for client education. Anorexia and nausea can be common sequelae in systemic infections, and would not warrant contacting the healthcare provider unless the manifestations became increasingly worse. A fluctuating febrile state can be a common sequela in systemic infection; in itself, it would not be considered a reason to contact the healthcare provider. **Cognitive Level:** Analyzing **Client Need:** Pharmacological and Parenteral Therapies **Integrated Process:** Teaching and Learning **Content Area:** Pharmacology **Strategy:** The core issues of the question are unsatisfactory progress or adverse side effects after beginning erythromycin and indicators that need to be reported to the prescriber. Use specific nursing knowledge and the process of elimination to make a selection. When there is more than one correct answer, consider each option as a true/false statement.

9 **Answer: 4 Rationale:** The volume of a household teaspoon can vary by 2–10 mL, so a calibrated device is necessary for accurate dosing. The suspension is to be shaken to disperse the particles just prior to measurement. It is recommended that a glass of water be given with the medication, and that adequate urinary output be maintained. Food does not interfere with absorption of the medication and could help to minimize gastrointestinal side effects. The medication is stable at room temperature (although the taste might be more palatable if cold). **Cognitive Level:** Applying **Client Need:** Pharmacological and Parenteral Therapies **Integrated Process:** Teaching and Learning **Content Area:** Pharmacology **Strategy:** The core issue of the question is the proper method of administration of trimethoprim-sulfamethoxazole to a child. Use specific nursing knowledge and the process of elimination to make a selection.

10 **Answer: 1 Rationale:** Epinephrine is the primary drug used when bronchoconstriction causes inadequate respiratory exchange, as in anaphylactic shock. Marked improvement in respiration occurs within a few minutes after subcutaneous administration of 0.1–0.5 mL of 1:1000 strength epinephrine. Corticosteroids may be given to minimize the inflammation and edema but are not the initial agent given. Atropine might minimize secretions but would not be given unless vagal-induced bradycardia or asystole occurred; then atropine could be given as an IV bolus rapidly before, during, or after cardiopulmonary arrest. Dopamine, a catecholamine (as is epinephrine), may be given to increase blood pressure if shock develops. **Cognitive Level:** Analyzing **Client Need:** Pharmacological and Parenteral Therapies **Integrated Process:** Nursing Process: Implementation **Content Area:** Pharmacology **Strategy:** The core issue of the question is knowledge of drugs that are used to treat hypersensitivity or anaphylactic reactions. Think of the necessity to preserve the airway first. Use specific nursing knowledge and the process of elimination to make a selection.

11 **Answer: 1, 2 Rationale:** A disulfiram-like effect is associated with certain drugs, including metronidazole. Onset is usually within 15 to 30 minutes of ingestion of alcohol, but can occur up to 72 hours after metronidazole has been discontinued. The reaction lasts approximately 20–30 minutes but can remain up to 24 hours. This is an important assessment for the nurse to make. Over-the-counter drugs, such as cold and cough preparations, may contain alcohol. This is an important factor for the nurse to assess. Metronidazole, if prescribed for clients with liver disease, should be given in smaller doses; however, this information should be noted prior to this medication being prescribed. Metronidazole tablets can be crushed for the client who cannot swallow the medication whole. However, metronidazole ER (extended-release form) cannot be chewed or crushed and must be swallowed whole. There is no indication that the medication is the extended-release form. Metronidazole tablets can be taken safely before, with, or after meals or with food or milk to decrease GI distress. This is not important for the nurse to assess in regard to the presenting manifestations. **Cognitive Level:** Analyzing **Client Need:** Pharmacological and Parenteral Therapies **Integrated Process:** Nursing Process: Implementation **Content Area:** Pharmacology **Strategy:** The core issue of the question is to determine the connection between Flagyl and the presenting manifestations. Use specific nursing knowledge and the process of elimination to make selections. When more than one answer is correct, consider each option as a true/false statement.

12 **Answer: 2 Rationale:** Opportunistic infections or superinfections are manifested by these signs and symptoms. Common ones are vaginal and GI tract infections, including candidiasis and diarrhea. They often result from broad-spectrum antibiotic use that destroys bacteria in the normal flora, allowing the resistant pathogens to proliferate. Early recognition and intervention with administration of sensitive anti-infectives is important in controlling discomfort and the severity of the reaction. The manifestations exhibited by the client do not represent leukocytosis, bone marrow depression, or drug failure against the original infective organism. **Level:** Analyzing **Client Need:** Pharmacological and Parenteral Therapies **Integrated Process:** Nursing Process: Diagnosis **Content Area:** Pharmacology **Strategy:** The core issue of the question is knowledge of adverse drug effects of cefotazime and their significance. Use specific nursing knowledge and the process of elimination to make a selection.

13 **Answer: 2 Rationale:** Yogurt and buttermilk products can decrease the diarrhea as well as add protein to the diet to provide albumin for drug binding. Clients are not usually taught to test their stool for occult blood. Visible blood or mucus in the stool with increased number of stools indicates the possibility of pseudomembranous colitis, which should be reported to the healthcare provider. The route of administration of antibiotics is not the cause of destruction of normal flora. Antacids would interfere with the effectiveness of the antibiotic and should not be taken; yogurt or buttermilk products are a more beneficial treatment for diarrhea. **Cognitive Level:** Applying **Client Need:** Pharmacological and Parenteral Therapies **Integrated Process:** Nursing Process: Implementation **Content Area:** Pharmacology **Strategy:** The core issue of the question is knowledge of client teaching points related to antibiotic therapy that has diarrhea as a side effect. Use specific nursing knowledge and the process of elimination to make a selection.

14 **Answer: 3 Rationale:** Disulfiram- or antabuse-like reactions can occur when cephalosporins are taken with ingestion of alcohol (as in a cough suppressant) during and up to 72 hours after discontinuation of the cephalosporin. Caffeine would not cause this reaction. Sulfamethoxazole prescribed for a chronic urinary tract infection or ampicillin, which has a cross-sensitivity to cephalosporins, would not cause this reaction. **Cognitive Level:** Analyzing **Client Need:** Pharmacological and Parenteral Therapies **Integrated Process:** Nursing Process: Diagnosis **Content Area:** Pharmacology **Strategy:** The core issue of the question is knowledge of the causes of disulfiram-like drug reactions. Use specific nursing knowledge and the process of elimination to make a selection.

15 **Answer: 2 Rationale:** Vestibular ototoxicity as well as cochlear ototoxicity can occur with administration of an aminoglycoside such as tobramycin. A positive Romberg test indicates vertigo or loss of balance, and can suggest a vestibular problem. Assessing capillary refill is one method of assessing peripheral circulation; it is not an appropriate assessment for adverse reactions to tobramycin sulfate. Chvostek sign is seen in tetany and hypocalcemia; it is not an appropriate assessment for adverse reactions to tobramycin sulfate. Babinski reflex, if present in the adult, reflects a possible lesion in the corticospinal tract of the spinal cord; it is not an appropriate assessment for adverse reactions to tobramycin sulfate. **Cognitive Level:** Analyzing **Client Need:** Pharmacological and Parenteral Therapies **Integrated Process:** Nursing Process: Assessment **Content Area:** Pharmacology **Strategy:** The core issue of the question is knowledge of assessment techniques that will help determine whether ototoxicity is occurring in a client taking tobramycin. Use specific nursing knowledge and the process of elimination to make a selection.

16 **Answer: 1 Rationale:** Griseofulvin can interfere with the effectiveness of estrogen-containing oral contraceptives. Griseofulvin does not cause increased bleeding unless the client is also on anticoagulant therapy. Griseofulvin has no known effect on blood pressure. Griseofulvin has no known interaction with calcium supplement intake. **Cognitive Level:** Applying **Client Need:** Pharmacological and Parenteral Therapies **Integrated Process:** Teaching and Learning **Content Area:** Pharmacology **Strategy:** The core issue of the question is knowledge of key teaching points regarding systemic griseofulvin. Use specific nursing knowledge and the process of elimination to make a selection.

17 **Answer: 1 Rationale:** Bacteriostatic agents inhibit or retard bacterial growth and replication, but they do not kill all the bacteria. These agents depend on the host's defense mechanisms to finish eliminating the bacteria. Tetracyclines are bacteriostatic. Iron, as well as antacids, laxatives, food, and dairy products, should be given 1 hour before or 2 hours after administration of a tetracycline. These substances interfere with the absorption of tetracyclines. Supplemental vitamin B_6 is indicated with isoniazid administration. Weekly evaluation of the complete blood count is unnecessary. **Cognitive Level:** Understanding **Client Need:** Pharmacological and Parenteral Therapies **Integrated Process:** Nursing Process: Diagnosis **Content Area:** Pharmacology **Strategy:** The core issue of the question is the mechanism of action of tetracycline, and how it leads to eradication of infection. Use specific nursing knowledge and the process of elimination to make a selection.

18 **Answer: 3 Rationale:** The prothrombin time (PT) and the international normalization ratio (INR) values are standard tests

to monitor warfarin levels. Beta-lactam antibiotics can cause increased PT and INR. The bleeding time evaluates the integrity of the vascular and platelet factors associated with stagnated blood. Thrombin time evaluates the fibrinogen-to-fibrin conversion factor that can be used to gauge heparin effectiveness; if the client is receiving oral anticoagulant therapy, it is with warfarin. The APPT is currently used most often in regulating heparin therapy; the client is receiving oral anticoagulant therapy. **Cognitive Level:** Analyzing **Client Need:** Pharmacological and Parenteral Therapies **Integrated Process:** Nursing Process: Diagnosis **Content Area:** Pharmacology **Strategy:** The core issue of the question is the expected change in laboratory results for a client taking a beta-lactam penicillin and an oral anticoagulant. Use specific nursing knowledge and the process of elimination to make a selection.

19 **Answer: 1, 4, 5 Rationale:** The development of exfoliative dermatitis, which presents as red, scaly skin, is possible with ampicillin therapy. All skin changes should be reported to the healthcare provider for evaluation; they may be nonallergenic and not an absolute contraindication to future therapy. Extrapyramidal tract manifestations are not noted with ampicillin therapy. Orthostatic hypotension does not occur with ampicillin therapy. Antibiotics, especially aminopenicillins such as ampicillin, can decrease the effectiveness of oral contraceptives; therefore, alternative contraceptive methods should be used during and for 1 month following ampicillin therapy. Ampicillin can cause superinfections, which may be manifested by the presence of vaginal itching and vaginal discharge. **Cognitive Level:** Analyzing **Client Need:** Pharmacological and Parenteral Therapies **Integrated Process:** Teaching and Learning **Content Area:** Pharmacology **Strategy:** The core issue of the question is client teaching that is needed for a client beginning drug therapy with ampicillin. Use specific nursing knowledge and the process of elimination to make a selection. When there is more than one correct answer, consider each option as a true/false statement.

20 **Answer: 3 Rationale:** It is the responsibility of the nurse to address the client's body image related to alopecia, which is a side effect of the medication. Noting general skin integrity does not address the client's concern. Alopecia is not the primary concern; rather, it is how the client reacts to the alopecia. Anxiety may or may not be applicable but there is insufficient information to make that determination. **Cognitive Level:** Analyzing **Client Need:** Pharmacological and Parenteral Therapies **Integrated Process:** Nursing Process: Diagnosis **Content Area:** Pharmacology **Strategy:** The core issue of the question is knowledge of how adverse drug effects of sargramostim can affect a client, necessitating formulation of a nursing diagnosis. Use specific nursing knowledge and the process of elimination to make a selection.

21 **Answer: 1 Rationale:** Potential flulike symptoms can occur with aldesleukin. For this reason, the nurse must provide for adequate fluid and electrolyte balance to prevent dehydration. A possible issue with airway is not a priority because airway concerns are not a side effect of aldesleukin. Excess fluid intake is not anticipated to be a typical overreaction to flulike symptoms associated with aldesleukin therapy. Weak cough may often be a priority concern; however, increased pulmonary secretions are not expected with aldesleukin therapy. **Cognitive Level:** Analyzing **Client Need:** Pharmacological and Parenteral Therapies **Integrated Process:** Nursing Process: Diagnosis **Content Area:** Pharmacology **Strategy:** The core issue of the question is knowledge of how adverse drug effects of aldesleukin can affect a client, necessitating formulation of a nursing diagnosis. Take care to discriminate when airway clearance is not the priority concern. Use specific nursing knowledge and the process of elimination to make a selection.

22 **Answer: 2, 5 Rationale:** Oprelvekin can cause cardiopulmonary insufficiency with irregular heart rate and fluid retention. Thus, it is a nursing priority to assess the client frequently for signs and symptoms of congestive heart failure. Dehydration is not a probable or priority concern with oprelvekin therapy. While anxiety can occur with the development of CHF, as a result of oprelvekin therapy, it is not the priority concern. Hyperuricemia is not a priority concern with oprelvekin therapy. **Cognitive Level:** Analyzing **Client Need:** Pharmacological and Parenteral Therapies **Integrated Process:** Nursing Process: Assessment **Content Area:** Pharmacology **Strategy:** The core issue of the question is knowledge of adverse drug effects of oprelvekin. Use specific nursing knowledge and the process of elimination to make a selection. When there is more than one correct answer, consider each option as a true/false statement.

23 **Answer: 3 Rationale:** Myasthenia gravis is treated by the administration of medications that would increase the concentration of acetylcholine at neuromuscular junctions, such as pyridostygmine. The drugs of choice to treat multiple sclerosis are beta-adrenergic blockers, corticosteroids, anti-inflammatory agents, and interferon, none of which increases the concentration of acetylcholine at neuromuscular junctions. Parkinson's disease does result from decreased concentration of acetylcholine at neuromuscular junctions. Cytoxic drugs along with NSAIDs and corticosteroids are used to treat lupus erythematosus; they do not increase the concentration of acetylcholine at neuromuscular junctions. **Cognitive Level:** Understanding **Client Need:** Pharmacological and Parenteral Therapies **Integrated Process:** Nursing Process: Planning **Content Area:** Pharmacology **Strategy:** Knowledge related to the pathophysiological cause of myasthenia gravis is useful when selecting the correct answer. Use specific nursing knowledge and the process of elimination to make a selection.

24 **Answer: 2 Rationale:** It is recommended that every client have a tetanus vaccine every 10 years to prevent infection caused by tetanus. The primary opportunity for this assessment is following a laceration. Temperature and decreased blood pressure do not address the risk of infection caused by trauma while the client is in the emergency department. Delayed wound healing is a possibility with corticosteroid therapy, but assessment of tetanus immunization status takes priority. **Cognitive Level:** Understanding **Client Need:** Pharmacological and Parenteral Therapies **Integrated Process:** Nursing Process: Assessment **Content Area:** Pharmacology **Strategy:** The critical words in the question are *laceration* and *emergency department*, which indicates that the injury is the result of trauma and is subject to contamination. Recall that the skin is the first line of defense against infection, and the client will need to be assessed for the need for a tetanus vaccine.

25 **Answer: 2 Rationale:** Mefloquine is frequently prescribed as a prophylaxis for malarial infection when traveling into regions where there is a high population of mosquitoes and increased risk of contracting malaria. Zidovudine is an antiviral medication prescribed for treatment of AIDS and

ANSWERS & RATIONALES

HIV. Rimantadine is a medication prescribed for influenza or respiratory infections; while this may be a recommended medication, it is not the most common. Filgrastim is a colony-stimulating factor prescribed for neutropenia, low white blood cell count; it would not be prescribed prophylactically. **Cognitive Level:** Applying **Client Need:** Pharmacological and Parenteral Therapies **Integrated Process:** Nursing Process: Planning **Content Area:** Pharmacology **Strategy:** Knowledge about malaria will be helpful in selecting the correct answer. Dissect each drug name to look for a hint regarding its use; *flu* for respiratory infection, *vir* for virus, *neu* for neutrophils, and *quine* for quinine (used to treat malaria).

26 **Answer: 4 Rationale:** Interferon beta 1b reduces the severity of acute exacerbations of multiple sclerosis by decreasing demyelination in brain tissue. There is no cure for multiple sclerosis; the manifestations can only be managed through the use of medications. Preventing signs and symptoms of anaphylaxis does not accurately reflect the action of interferon beta 1b. The destruction of nerve tissue that is laden with plaque is not a desirable or effective goal in treating multiple sclerosis. **Cognitive Level:** Applying **Client Need:** Pharmacological and Parenteral Therapies **Integrated Process:** Nursing Process: Implementation **Content Area:** Pharmacology **Strategy:** The core issue of the question is knowledge of goals of drug therapy with interferon beta 1b. Use specific nursing knowledge and the process of elimination to make a selection.

27 **Answer: 3 Rationale:** Adequate fluid intake greater than 2000–3000 mL per day allows the kidneys to flush renal toxins and prevents renal insufficiency. Consuming a diet high in fiber is a general measure to prevent constipation. Having a weekly assessment of creatinine level would be a monitoring function but would not prevent renal insufficiency. The nurse would not instruct the client to take additional medication that is not specifically part of the plan of care. **Cognitive Level:** Applying **Client Need:** Pharmacological and Parenteral Therapies **Integrated Process:** Teaching and Learning **Content Area:** Pharmacology **Strategy:** The core issue of the question is knowledge of measures to prevent the development of renal side effects with use of cyclophosphamide. Use specific nursing knowledge and the process of elimination to make a selection.

28 **Answer: 1 Rationale:** The most significant laboratory test to utilize prior to medication therapy with azathioprine is creatinine level because renal and hepatic function should be assessed for baseline parameters. Monitoring uric acid levels is irrelevant for the administration of azathioprine. A decreased platelet count can occur with the administration of azathioprine, but laboratory values for PT and PTT provide information related to blood clotting. An RBC evaluates an important component of the blood; however, a risk related to the administration of azathioprine would be increased white cell count (infection). **Cognitive Level:** Applying **Client Need:** Pharmacological and Parenteral Therapies **Integrated Process:** Nursing Process: Evaluation **Content Area:** Pharmacology **Strategy:** The core issue of the question is knowledge of adverse drug effects of azathioprine and of which laboratory test to use as a baseline measure. Use specific nursing knowledge and the process of elimination to make a selection.

29 **Answer: 2 Rationale:** Azathioprine is administered to treat multiple sclerosis, and allopurinol is administered to treat symptoms of gout. When these two medications are administered together, the dose of azathioprine should be reduced. The uric acid level and client symptoms should be assessed to determine the control of gout. The creatinine level indicates kidney function. Blood glucose levels are not important during the administration of azathioprine and allopurinol. BUN is a laboratory indicator related to renal function. **Cognitive Level:** Applying **Client Need:** Pharmacological and Parenteral Therapies **Integrated Process:** Nursing Process: Assessment **Content Area:** Pharmacology **Strategy:** The core issue of the question is knowledge of drug interactive effects of azathioprine and allopurinol. Use specific nursing knowledge and the process of elimination to make a selection.

30 **Answer: 2 Rationale:** Edrophonium is used for diagnostic purposes. Clients who receive an injection of edrophonium and exhibit a temporary relief of symptoms are diagnosed with myasthenia gravis, which is characterized by a decrease in the concentration of acetylcholine in the neuromuscular junction. Ambenonium, neostigmine, and physostigmine are not used to diagnose myasthenia gravis. **Cognitive Level:** Applying **Client Need:** Pharmacological and Parenteral Therapies **Integrated Process:** Nursing Process: Planning **Content Area:** Pharmacology **Strategy:** The core issue of the question is knowledge of medications used for diagnosis of myasthenia gravis. Use specific nursing knowledge and the process of elimination to make a selection.

31 **Answer: 1, 5 Rationale:** Medications used to treat symptoms of multiple sclerosis have been noted to increase pulmonary edema. The restriction of oral fluids could increase risk of urinary tract infection. Avoiding crowds is useful to avoid infection, but does not specifically relate to medication teaching. Activities that could effectively enhance muscle strength could increase fatigue; if done to excess, it could lead to exacerbation of symptoms. Medications used to treat symptoms of multiple sclerosis have been noted to increase pulmonary edema, leading to chest pain and shortness of breath. **Cognitive Level:** Applying **Client Need:** Pharmacological and Parenteral Therapies **Integrated Process:** Teaching and Learning **Content Area:** Pharmacology **Strategy:** The core issue of the question is knowledge of essential teaching points for a client being treated with drug therapy for multiple sclerosis. Use specific nursing knowledge and the process of elimination to make a selection. When more than one answer is correct, consider each option as a true/false statement.

32 **Answer: 3 Rationale:** Immune serum globulin should not be administered to clients with a history of coagulation disorders. Having received a hepatitis B vaccine does not represent contraindication to immune serum globulin. Immune serum globulin is safe to administer to a client who recently experienced a traumatic hip fracture. There is no reason to withhold immune serum globulin because of upcoming foreign travel. **Cognitive Level:** Analyzing **Client Need:** Pharmacological and Parenteral Therapies **Integrated Process:** Nursing Process: Assessment **Content Area:** Pharmacology **Strategy:** The core issue of the question is knowledge of safe administration of serum immune globulin. Use specific nursing knowledge and the process of elimination to make a selection.

Key Terms to Review

amebiasis p. 701
antigen p. 689
bactericidal p. 694
bacteriostatic p. 698
candidiasis p. 695
colony-stimulating factors p. 689
cross-sensitivity p. 696
empiric therapy p. 696
giardiasis p. 711
immunosuppressant p. 689
myelosuppression p. 690
neutropenia p. 689
peak drug level p. 695
pseudomembranous colitis p. 695
superinfection p. 698
tinea p. 709
trough drug level p. 695

References

Adams, M., Holland, L., & Urban, C. (2017). *Pharmacology for nurses: A pathophysiologic approach* (5th ed.). New York, NY: Pearson Education.

Adams, M., & Urban, C. (2016). *Pharmacology: Connections to nursing practice* (3rd ed.). New York, NY: Pearson Education.

Lehne, R. (2016). *Pharmacology for nursing care* (9th ed.). St. Louis, MO: Saunders.

Wilson, B., Shannon, M., & Shields, K. (2016). *Pearson nurse's drug guide 2016.* New York, NY: Pearson Education.

Test Yourself

Are you ready for the NCLEX-RN® or course exams? Access the NEW web-based app that provides students with thousands of practice questions in preparation for the NCLEX experience.

46 Common Laboratory Tests

In this chapter

Cross Reference

Other chapters relevant to this content area are

Common Diagnostic Tests and Procedures	Chapter 47
Fluid and Electrolyte Imbalances	Chapter 53
Acid–Base Imbalances	Chapter 54

I. GENERAL PRINCIPLES OF SPECIMEN COLLECTION

A. Routine specimens

NCLEX® 1. Usually collected in early morning before intake of food and fluids; if done in fasting state, withhold food and fluids for 8–12 hours prior to test

2. Collect using standard precautions to protect against exposure to blood or other body fluids; use strict aseptic technique to protect client from infection

NCLEX® 3. Label specimens with client name, date, exact time of collection, and type of specimen

NCLEX® 4. On laboratory requisition slip, note client identifying information as per agency policy, possible diagnosis, and test (or tests) being requested; record any factors that could interfere with results, such as foods or prescribed drugs

NCLEX® 5. Avoid shaking blood specimens to avoid hemolysis and send promptly to lab

6. Values that fall within laboratory reference range are considered normal

NCLEX® 7. Critical (panic) values are abnormal results that could increase risk of harm to client; these are sent immediately to nursing unit and must be reported to charge nurse and/or healthcare provider

NCLEX® **B. Twenty-four-hour urine specimens**

1. Obtain a 24-hour specimen collection container (with preservative if indicated) from lab
2. Label container with client's name, date, test, and time started and time completed (e.g., 12/29/17 08:00 to 12/30/17 08:00); place container on ice if indicated
3. Place 24-hour specimen collection sign above client bed, in bathroom, and on chart or electronic health record as a reminder to save all urine collected during specified time period
4. At beginning of collection period, have client void and discard this urine; save all urine for next 24 hours
5. Instruct client to void each time into container, such as a specimen hat, and avoid contaminating specimen with feces or bathroom tissue
6. Transfer voided specimen into collection device using standard precautions
7. At end of collection time, have client void and save this specimen
8. Complete laboratory requisition and send urine collection to lab; document specimen completion and pertinent observations of urine in client record

II. ARTERIAL BLOOD GASES

A. Consist of *serum* (blood) pH, partial pressure of arterial oxygen (PaO_2), partial pressure of carbon dioxide ($PaCO_2$), bicarbonate (HCO_3^-), and base excess

B. See Table 46–1 for normal reference ranges

C. See Chapter 54 for further discussion of arterial blood gases (ABGs)

III. SERUM ELECTROLYTES

A. Consist of cations and anions: sodium, potassium, calcium, and magnesium are cations; chloride and phosphorus are anions

B. Standard reported values include sodium, potassium, chloride, bicarbonate; others are prescribed as needed; see Table 46–2 for normal reference ranges

C. See Chapter 53 for further discussion of full range of electrolytes

Table 46–1 Normal Arterial Blood Gases

Test	Normal Adult Reference Ranges	
	U.S.	Canada
Serum pH	7.35–7.45	7.35–7.45
Oxygen (PaO_2)	80–100 mmHg	80–100 mmHg
Carbon dioxide ($PaCO_2$)	35–45 mmHg	35–45 mmHg
Bicarbonate (HCO_3^-)	22–26 mEq/L	22–26 mmol/L
Oxygen saturation (SaO_2)	95–100%	95–100%
Base excess	+3 to −3	+3 to −3

Table 46–2 Normal Serum Electrolytes

Test	Normal Reference Ranges	
	U.S.	Canada
Sodium (Na^+)	135–145 mEq/L	135–145 mmol/L
Potassium (K^+)	3.5–5.1 mEq/L	3.5-5.0 mmol/L
Chloride (Cl^-)	95–105 mEq/L	95–105 mmol/L
Bicarbonate (venous)	23–29 mEq/L	23-29 mmol/L
Calcium (Ca^{++})	Total: 8.5–10.5 mg/dL or 4.5–5.5 mEq/L Ionized 4.0–5.0 mg/dL or 2.5 mEq/L	Total: 2.2–2.58 mmol/L Ionized 1.0–1.15 mmol/L
Magnesium (Mg^{++})	1.6–2.5 mg/dL or 1.5-2.5 mEq/L	0.65–1.05 mmol/L
Phosphate ($PO4^-$)	3–4.5 mg/dL	3–4.5 mg/dL

Note: Normal laboratory values vary from agency to agency.

IV. GLUCOSE STUDIES

A. Fasting blood glucose (FBG)

1. Glucose is an end product of carbohydrate digestion, glycogenolysis, and gluconeogenesis
2. Primary fuel source for cellular energy, especially for brain and red blood cell function

NCLEX®
3. Used to diagnose diabetes mellitus and hypoglycemia; see Table 46–3 for normal adult reference range

NCLEX®
4. Client must fast for 8–12 hours prior to drawing lab sample, with no ingestion of foods, beverages, or medications (oral antidiabetics or insulin)

B. Random blood glucose

1. Measures blood glucose as above but in nonfasting state
2. May be checked using capillary blood obtained via fingerstick

NCLEX®
3. See Table 46–3 for normal reference range

C. Two-hour postprandial blood glucose: measures serum glucose 2 hours after eating

D. Glucose tolerance test (GTT)

1. Used as a screening test for clients at risk of DM and as diagnostic aid
2. Glucose levels should rise and fall in predictable amounts following ingestion of a specific glucose load (see Table 46–3); with DM, glucose levels peak at higher levels and fall more slowly than normal

NCLEX®
3. Client teaching
   a. Eat high-carbohydrate (CHO) diet (200–300 grams daily) for 3 days prior to test (give client list of high-CHO foods as needed)
   b. Do not drink alcohol or coffee or smoke for 36 hours before test (eliminates alcohol, caffeine, and nicotine as interfering factors with test results)
   c. Fast for 10–16 hours before test as instructed by healthcare provider
   d. Do not take any oral antidiabetic medications or insulin prior to test
   e. Do not exercise vigorously for 8 hours before or after test; sit quietly during test
   f. Test consists of baseline glucose level, ingestion of oral or IV glucose load, and series of blood glucose samples
   g. Two-hour GTT takes about 3 hours to complete; abnormal results may require a longer (3- to 5-hour) GTT

E. Glycosylated hemoglobin A_{1c}

1. Measures glucose that binds irreversibly to hemoglobin for life of red blood cell (RBC lifespan is 120 days)

NCLEX®
2. Indicates glycemic control over 3–5 weeks (takes into account continuous production and destruction of RBCs); some sources report 3- to 4-month time frame
3. See Table 46–3 for interpretation of results; no fasting is required before test

F. Diabetes mellitus autoantibody panel

1. Used to identify type 1 DM, evaluate insulin resistance, and determine insulin allergy
2. Does not require fasting; normal value is a titer less than 1:4 with no antibody detected

Table 46–3 Normal Adult Glucose Levels

Test	Normal Adult Reference Ranges	
	U.S.	Canada
Fasting blood glucose	70–110 mg/dL	4–6 mmol/L
Random (capillary) glucose	60–110 mg/dL	3.6–5.6 mmol/L
2-hour postprandial blood glucose	<140 mg/dL	<7.8 mmol/L
Oral glucose tolerance test (OGTT), nonpregnant		
Fasting baseline	70–110 mg/dL	4-6 mmol/L
60-minute sample	<200 mg/dL	<11.1 mmol/L
120-minute sample	70–120 mg/dL	<7.8 mmol/L
Glycosylated hemoglobin A_{1c}		
Normal	3.5–6%	4-6%
Good diabetic control	7% or lower	7% or lower
Fair diabetic control	7–8%	7–8%
Poor diabetic control	>8%	>8%

V. COADULATION STUDIES

A. Prothrombin time (PT) and international normalized ratio (INR)

1. Measures time needed for prothrombin (a vitamin K–dependent glycoprotein produced in liver) to form a fibrin clot via extrinsic clotting pathway
2. Commonly used to assess effectiveness of oral anticoagulant warfarin or to diagnose disseminated intravascular coagulopathy (DIC), vitamin K deficiency, or liver dysfunction

NCLEX®
3. Normal reference ranges for PT may vary slightly by lab but are generally 11–13 seconds (U.S. and Canada); normal level is control value plus or minus 2 seconds; therapeutic range for warfarin is 1.5–2 times the control value

NCLEX®
4. INR is similar to PT but standardizes normal values across all lab systems; therapeutic range for warfarin is 2.0–3.0 for standard therapy and 3.0–4.5 for high-dose therapy; baseline normal reference range is 0.8–1.2 (U.S. and Canada)
5. Draw baseline PT before beginning oral anticoagulation and repeat at specified intervals to monitor progress of therapy; apply pressure to venipuncture site for 3–5 mins

NCLEX®
6. Report abnormals or any values outside therapeutic ranges; low values indicate ineffective therapy and high values indicate risk for bleeding or hemorrhage

NCLEX®
7. Teach client to maintain steady but moderate intake of green leafy vegetables (they are rich in vitamin K and will decrease PT/INR)

B. Activated partial thromboplastin time (aPTT)

1. Measures time needed for recalcified, citrated plasma to clot after adding activated thromboplastin reagent; reflects intrinsic clotting pathway
2. Commonly used to assess heparin therapy; can screen for all clotting factor deficiencies except VII and XIII
3. Elevated in liver disease and DIC

NCLEX®
4. Normal reference range is 20–35 seconds (24–36 seconds in Canada); therapeutic range for heparin therapy is 1.5–2.5 times the control in seconds (often 60–80 secs)
5. Draw baseline aPTT before beginning heparin therapy and repeat at specified intervals to monitor progress of therapy

NCLEX®
6. Do not draw lab sample from vein in same arm in which heparin is infusing

NCLEX®
7. Report abnormals or any values outside therapeutic ranges; low values indicate ineffective therapy and high values indicate risk for bleeding or hemorrhage

C. Bleeding time

1. Evaluates overall functioning of platelets in achieving hemostasis
2. Normal adult reference range is 1–3 minutes (Duke method), 3–6 minutes (Ivy method), 180–570 seconds (Canada)
3. Skin puncture is done to determine time needed for bleeding to stop
4. Ensure that client has not received drugs that interfere with test (aspirin, aspirin-containing products, anticoagulants) for 3 days prior to test, and apply pressure dressing after procedure if needed

D. D-dimer

1. Evaluates for hypercoagulability state by assessing secondary fibrinolysis that yields fibrin degradation fragments
2. Normal value is 0.5 mcg/mL FEU (fibrinogen equivalent units) or 0–3 nmol/L; results are prolonged in conditions such as DIC, deep vein thrombosis, pulmonary embolism, and other arterial or venous thromboses

VI. COMPLETE BLOOD COUNT

A. Hematocrit (Hct)

1. Is the proportion of RBCs to **plasma** (liquid portion of blood), reported as a percentage
2. Can be falsely elevated when white blood cell (WBC) counts are markedly elevated (referred to as "buffy coat")
3. Can be falsely lowered with hemodilution (increased water component of blood)

NCLEX®
4. Normal reference range is 40–50% for males and 38–47% for females (U.S.); range in Canada is 0.37–0.49 for males and 0.36–0.46 for females

B. Hemoglobin (Hgb)

1. Hemoglobin is a major component of erythrocytes that combines loosely with oxygen (O_2) and carbon dioxide (CO_2) for transport in circulation
2. Abnormal hemoglobinopathies include sickle cell disease and thallasemias; decreased Hgb commonly indicates anemia

3. Normally, Hgb and Hct levels parallel each other; Hct is usually three times higher than Hgb level

NCLEX® 4. Normal reference range is 13.5–18 grams/dL for males and 12–16 grams/dL for females in U.S.; range in Canada is 138–180 grams/L for males and 120–160 grams/L in females

C. Red blood cell (RBC) count (erythrocyte count)

1. RBCs are formed in bone marrow and removed by liver, spleen, and bone marrow
2. Lifespan of RBC is approximately 120 days
3. Carry hemoglobin molecules responsible for O_2 transport to tissues
4. Normal reference range: 4.0–5.5 million cells/microliter for adult females and 4.5–6.2 million cells/microliter for adult males in U.S.; range in Canada is 4.1×10^{12}/L to 5.1×10^{12}/L for females and 4.5×10^{12}/L to 5.3×10^{12}/L for males

NCLEX® 5. Abnormal values indicate anemia or blood dyscrasias; further evaluation of anemia can be done by evaluating RBC indices (mean corpuscular volume [MCV], mean corpuscular hemoglobin [MCH], and mean corpuscular hemoglobin concentration [MCHC])

D. Platelet count

NCLEX® 1. Normal reference range: 150,000–450,000 per cubic mm (mm^3) in U.S.; Canadian range is 150×10^9/L to 350×10^9/L

2. Platelets are produced in bone marrow and have a lifespan of about 10 days
3. When microtrauma occurs and damages blood vessels, platelets aggregate to form hemostatic plug to initiate clot formation
4. Platelet aggregation is inhibited by drugs such as aspirin
5. Decreased platelet levels (thrombocytopenia) occur with cancer chemotherapy from bone marrow suppression, idiopathic thrombocytopenic purpura (ITP), most leukemias, uremia, and some infections such as infectious mononucleosis

NCLEX® 6. An insufficient number of platelets leads to increased risk of bleeding; bleeding precautions should be instituted if platelet count drops below 50,000 cells/mm^3 or 50×10^9/L

E. WBC

1. Consist of agranulocytes (monocytes and lymphocytes; no stainable granules in nucleus) and granulocytes (neutrophils, eosinophils, and basophils)

NCLEX® 2. Normal total WBC reference range: 5000–10,000 cells/mm^3 (U.S.) and 4.5×10^9/L to 11×10^9/L (Canada); see Table 46–4 for normal WBC differential reference ranges

3. Neutrophils defend against inflammation, tissue injury, and infection

NCLEX® a. A "shift to the left" indicates a greater number of neutrophils are immature (bands) because of need for more rapid production to combat inflammation or infection

   b. A "shift to the right" indicates cells with excessive nuclear segments, seen with liver disease, megaloblastic and pernicious anemias, and Down syndrome

4. Eosinophils increase during allergic and parasitic conditions and decrease with higher levels of steroids
5. Basophils increase during healing process and decrease when steroid levels rise
6. Monocytes ("monos") are second line of defense against bacterial infection and foreign substances; these macrophages ingest larger particles and debris from cellular destruction; may also kill tumor cells—mechanism unclear
7. Lymphocytes ("lymphs") elevate during chronic and viral infections and lymphocytic leukemia; consist of B lymphocytes and T lymphocytes

Table 46–4 White Blood Cell Differential Counts

Cells	Normal Adult Reference Ranges	
	U.S.	Canada
Neutrophils (total)	50–70% or 2500–7000 cells/microliter	55–70%
Segments (mature)	50–65% or 2500–6500 cells/microliter	50–65% or 2500–6500 cells/microliter
Bands (immature)	0–5% or 0–500 cells/microliter	0–5% or 0–500 cells/microliter
Eosinophils	1–3% or 100–300 cells/microliter	1–4%
Basophils	0.4–1.0% or 40–100 cells/microliter	0–2%
Lymphocytes	25–35% or 1700–3500 cells/microliter	20–40%
Monocytes	4–6% or 200–600 cells/microliter	2–8%

VII. CARDIOVASCULAR FUNCTION STUDIES

A. Serum lipids

1. Primary measurements include total cholesterol, low-density lipoproteins (LDLs), high-density lipoproteins (HDLs), and triglycerides
2. Normal reference ranges: see Table 46–5
3. *NCLEX®* Elevated levels (except for HDLs) increase risk of heart disease, stroke, and peripheral vascular disease; high HDL levels seem to be cardioprotective; elevated triglycerides indicate hyperlipidemia (possibly familial)
4. *NCLEX®* Teach client to avoid alcohol intake for 24 hours before test and avoid high-cholesterol foods the evening before blood is drawn
5. Client must fast (except water) for 12–14 hours prior to test

B. Creatine kinase (CK) or creatinine phosphokinase (CPK)

1. *NCLEX®* An enzyme found in large amounts in cardiac and skeletal muscle and in low amounts in brain tissue; enzyme is released from cells upon cell death
2. Enzyme can be fractionated into isoenzymes to identify tissue of origin; CK-MB is cardiac band; CK-MM is skeletal muscle band; CK-BB is brain tissue band
3. *NCLEX®* Normal reference range and pattern of elevation: see Table 46–6
4. Avoid intake of alcohol 24 hours prior to test
5. Avoid injections, which could lead to falsely elevated value
6. Instruct client to avoid excessive physical exertion if monitoring skeletal muscle band; make note of soft tissue injury or falls that could cause false elevations
7. *NCLEX®* Monitor results serially over 3 days if monitoring myocardial infarction (MI) and correlate with clinical picture

C. Troponins

1. Regulatory proteins found in skeletal and cardiac muscle (striated muscle cells)
2. Released into bloodstream with myocardial cell death; early indicator of cardiac damage; myoglobin also rises (12–90 mcg/L normal); peaks in 8–12 hrs
3. *NCLEX®* Normal reference range and pattern of elevation: see Table 46–6
4. *NCLEX®* Monitor results serially over 3 days and correlate with clinical picture

Table 46–5 Serum Lipid Levels

Type of Lipid	Normal Adult Reference Ranges	
	U.S.	Canada
Cholesterol (total)	<200 mg/dL	<5.2 mmol/L
LDL	<130 mg/dL	<3.5 mmol/L ideal; <2.0 target if moderate to high risk of heart disease
HDL	60 mg/dL and above	>1.5 mmol/L
Triglycerides	<200 mg/dL	0.45–1.69 mmol/L

Table 46–6 Cardiac Enzymes

Enzyme/Isoenzyme	Normal Adult Reference Range		Pattern of Elevation and Decline
	U.S.	Canada	
Creatine kinase (CK)	Males 55–170 units/L Females 30–135 units/L	Males 38–174 U/L Females 26–140 U/L	Begins to rise 4–6 hours after myocardial or skeletal muscle damage
CK-MM	94–100%	96–100%	Peaks at 18–24 hours
CK-MB	0–6%	0–6%	Returns to normal within 3–4 days
CK-BB	0%	0%	
Cardiac troponins			Rise within 3 hours of myocardial infarction
Troponin I	<0.05 ng/mL	<0.05 mcg/L	Returns to normal in 5–9 days (I) or 10–14 days (T)
Troponin T	<0.3 ng/mL	<0.3 mcg/L	

D. Natriuretic peptides

1. Neuroendocrine peptides useful in identifying and monitoring heart failure
2. There are three major types secreted in response to increased hemodynamic load
   a. Atrial natriuretic peptide (ANP): secreted in response to atrial stretch or endocrine stimulation (renin-aldosterone system)
   b. Brain natriuretic peptide (BNP): secreted in response to ventricular stretch or endocrine stimulation (renin-aldosterone system); there is a positive correlation between dyspnea as a sign of heart failure and rising BNP levels
   c. C-type natriuretic peptide (CNP): produced by vascular endothelial cells and has vasodilative properties

VIII. THYROID FUNCTION STUDIES

A. Thyroxine (T_4)

1. Major hormone secreted by thyroid gland
2. Aids in diagnosis of hypo- or hyperthyroidism with low or high levels, respectively
3. Normal reference range: 4.6–12 mcg/mL (59–155 pmol/L) T_4 or 0.8–1.5 ng/dL (10–19 pmol/L) free T_4

B. Triiodothyronine (T_3)

1. A short-acting but potent thyroid hormone; present only in small amounts in blood
2. More useful for diagnosing hyperthyroidism than hypothyroidism
3. Normal reference range: 70–204 ng/dL (1.08–3.14 nmol/L) T_3 or 2.6–4.8 pg/mL (0.04–0.07 pmol/L) free T_3

C. Thyroid-stimulating hormone (TSH)

1. A hormone secreted via negative feedback loop by anterior pituitary gland in response to decreased T_4
2. Used with results of T_4 level to differentiate between pituitary and thyroid dysfunction
   a. Decreased T_4 and normal or elevated TSH is consistent with thyroid disorder
   b. Decreased T_4 and decreased TSH is consistent with pituitary disorder
3. Normal reference range: 0.4–4.2 microinternational units/mL (U.S. and Canda)

D. No special preparation is needed for any thyroid test, but results can be affected by antithyroid drugs or radionuclide scan within 7 days prior to test

IX. RENAL FUNCTION STUDIES

A. Blood urea nitrogen (BUN)

1. Formed in liver as end product of protein metabolism; consists of nitrogen portion of urea
2. Excreted via kidneys with only small amounts reabsorbed in renal tubules
3. NCLEX® Normal reference range: see Table 46–7
4. NCLEX® Rises with reduced glomerular filtration rate (GFR), increased dietary protein, increased catabolism (such as starvation), crush injuries, febrile illness, and with hemoconcentration from dehydration
5. Decreases with overhydration, inadequate protein intake, or severe liver disease (inadequate conversion of ammonia to urea)
6. NCLEX® Assess concurrently with serum creatinine for true indication of renal status; if BUN and creatinine rise together, indicates renal insufficiency or failure

B. Serum creatinine

1. End product of muscle creatine metabolism; specific indicator of GFR and renal status
2. NCLEX® Elevated levels commonly indicate renal insufficiency or failure
3. Teach client to avoid eating red meat for 24 hours prior to test and heavy exercise 8 hours prior in order to avoid falsely high values
4. Normal reference range: see Table 46–7

Table 46–7 Renal Function Tests

Renal Function Test	Normal Adult Reference Ranges	
	U.S.	Canada
Blood urea nitrogen (BUN)	8–22 mg/dL	3.6–7.1 mmol/L
Serum creatinine	0.6–1.3 mg/dL	44–133 micromol/L
Creatinine clearance	85–125 mL/min men 75–115 mL/min women	1.42–2.08 mL/s men 1.25–1.92 mL/s women
Serum osmolality	280–300 mOsm/kg water	280–300 mmol/kg water
Urine osmolality	250–900 mOsm/kg water	250–900 mmol/kg water

Box 46–1

Estimating Serum Osmolality Using Laboratory Values

Formula:	**2(Na+) + BUN/2.8 + Blood glucose/18**
Example:	2(137) + 10/2.8 + 110/18
	276 + 3.57 + 6.11 = 286

Note: Na+ = serum sodium, BUN = blood urea nitrogen

C. Creatinine clearance
1. Compares serum creatinine with creatinine excreted in a volume of urine over a period of hours (2, 12, 24)
2. Collection procedure is same as for a 24-hour urine; no preservative is needed in collection device
3. Normal reference range: see Table 46–7
4. Decreases progressively with renal insufficiency and failure as GFR declines

D. Serum osmolality
1. Reflects concentration of serum (number of osmotically active particles in solution)
2. Can be calculated using serum Na^+, BUN, and BG levels (see Box 46–1) but calculated value can be up to 9 mOsm less than drawn value
3. Normal reference range: see Table 46–7
4. Values rise with dehydration (more particles per volume of solution) and decrease with fluid overload (fewer particles per volume of solution)
5. Often used to detect risk of increased intracranial pressure

E. Urine osmolality
1. Measures concentration of urine; see Table 46–7 for normal reference range
2. High values indicate kidneys are conserving water, while low values may reflect increased fluid intake, effect of diuretics, diabetes insipidus, or renal damage; clinical correlation is needed

X. URINALYSIS

A. Normal results: see Table 46–8

B. Possible causes of abnormal results: see Table 46–9

C. Nitrites
1. If present, nitrites suggest urinary tract infection (UTI) with Gram-negative bacteria
2. Mechanism: when Gram-negative bacteria (such as common *E. coli*) are present in urine, dietary nitrates in urine are converted to nitrites
3. False-negatives can result if urine does not sit in bladder long enough (≥4 hours) for reaction to take place, if infection is not caused by Gram-negative organism, or if dietary nitrate is absent

D. Leukocyte esterase

NCLEX®

1. Simple test that may be done on a voided urine sample; positive result suggests UTI
2. Mechanism: WBCs contain esterases that react with substances in urine if sufficient bacterial colonies present

Table 46–8 Normal Urinalysis Findings

Component	Normal Findings (U.S. and Canada)
Color	Ranges from pale yellow to amber
Clarity	Clear when first excreted
Odor	Faint aromatic
Specific gravity	1.010–1.025
pH	4.5–8
Protein	None
Glucose	None
Ketones	None
Sediment	0–3 RBCs, 0–4 WBCs; occasional cast; occasional renal epithelial cell

Table 46–9 Possible Causes of Abnormal Urinalysis Findings

Urinalysis	Significance of Abnormal Findings
Color	Pale: diabetes insipidus, drinking of excess free water
	Reddish: RBCs
	Burgundy: porphyria
	Orange: phenazopyridine or rifampin
	Green: bile
	Black-brown: mercury poisoning
	Milky: pus, fat globules
Clarity	Cloudy: infection, phosphate precipitation from standing
	Turbid: spermatozoa, prostatic fluid
Odor	Sweet: acetonuria
	Strong: drugs, asparagus
	Ammonia: after standing for a time
Specific gravity	Decreased: diabetes insipidus, diuretics, excessive intake of free water
	Increased: diabetes mellitus, hypovolemia, liver disease, heart failure, SIADH, IV contrast medium
pH	Acid: acidosis, diabetes mellitus, fever, starvation, dehydration
	Alkaline: citrus, salicylate poisoning, sodium bicarbonate, urinary tract infection; urine becomes alkaline after standing because urea-splitting bacteria result in ammonia production
Protein	Transient: fever, stress
	0.5 gram/day: chronic pyelonephritis
	0.5–4 grams/day: multiple myeloma, diabetic nephropathy
	5 grams/day: nephrotic syndrome, glomerulonephritis
Glucose	Present: diabetes mellitus
Ketones	Present: acidosis, diabetic ketoacidosis, starvation, dieting (fat breakdown)
Sediments	Casts: clumps of material or cells that form in renal collecting tubule, assuming shape of tubule; are seen in various renal disease states
	Granular casts: acute tubular necrosis, glomerulonephritis, UTI, stress, renal transplant rejection
	Pus: glomerulonephritis
	RBC casts: glomerulonephritis
	WBCs: UTI
	RBCs: bleeding within glomeruli, transfusion reaction, malaria, hemolytic anemia

XI. LIVER FUNCTION STUDIES

A. Alanine aminotransferase (ALT)

1. Enzyme found primarily in liver cells but also found in small amounts in heart, kidney, and skeletal muscle
2. Normal reference range: see Table 46–10
3. Rises as high as 200–400 units with hepatitis or liver damage from drugs and chemicals
4. *NCLEX®* Used to differentiate between jaundice caused by liver disease (often >300 units/L) and causes outside liver (often <300 units/L)
5. There is no food or fluid restriction before test

B. Aspartate aminotransferase (AST)

1. An enzyme found mainly in heart muscle and liver, with moderate amounts also found in skeletal muscle, kidneys, and pancreas
2. Normal reference range: see Table 46–10
3. *NCLEX®* Rises with cellular injury and release of enzyme into circulation, such as with liver disease or injury, myocardial infarction, pancreatitis, and musculoskeletal trauma
4. False elevations can be caused by intramuscular injections

Table 46–10 Liver Function Tests

Liver Function Test	Normal Reference Ranges	
	U.S.	Canada
Alanine aminotransferase (ALT)	10–25 units/L	10–55 U/L men, 7–30 U/L women
Aspartate aminotransferase (AST)	8–38 units/L	10–40 U/L men, 9–25 U/L women
Bilirubin	Total: 0.1–1.2 mg/dL adults and 1–11.7 mg/dL neonate	$<$21 micromol/L adult and $<$200 micromol/L neonate
	Direct: 0.1–0.3 mg/dL adults and $<$0.6 mg/dL neonate	Direct: $<$5 micromol/L adults and $<$10 micromol//L neonate
	Indirect: calculate by subtracting direct from total	Indirect: calculate by subtracting direct from total
Ammonia	35–65 micrograms/dL	25–46 micromol/L

C. Bilirubin

1. A by-product of hemoglobin breakdown; produced also by liver, spleen, and bone marrow
2. Consists of total bilirubin, direct or conjugated bilirubin (excreted by GI tract), and indirect or unconjugated bilirubin (circulates protein-bound in blood)
3. Normal reference ranges: see Table 46–10
4. *NCLEX®* Levels are elevated with jaundice and liver disease, alcohol and many drugs (note those administered on lab requisition)
5. Draw infant blood sample from heel of foot
6. *NCLEX®* Protect specimen from sunlight and artificial light and avoid hemolysis
7. Teach client to reduce intake of yellow vegetables (beans, carrots, sweet potatoes, squash) for 3–4 days before test and to fast for 4 hours prior to test

D. Ammonia

1. End product of nitrogen breakdown during protein metabolism
2. Metabolized by liver and excreted via kidneys
3. Normal reference range: see Table 46–10
4. *NCLEX®* Elevated results indicate liver disease and possibly encephalopathy (degree of elevation does not correlate directly with risk for hepatic coma)
5. Teach client not to smoke for 24 hours prior to test and to fast (except for water) for 8–10 hours before test

XII. PANCREATIC ENZYMES

A. Amylase

1. Produced by pancreas and salivary glands for CHO digestion and excreted via kidneys
2. Normal reference range: 25–151 units/L
3. *NCLEX®* Increased with pancreatitis; elevation begins 3–6 hours after pain begins, peaks in 24 hours, and returns to normal in 2–3 days
4. Many drugs affect results, so list them on lab requisition; false results can occur if measured within 72 hours of cholecystography with radiopaque dyes

B. Lipase

1. Produced by pancreas to break down fats and triglycerides into fatty acids and glycerol
2. Normal reference range: 10–140 units/L
3. *NCLEX®* Increased with pancreatic disorders; may rise as late as 24–36 hours after onset of disorder and return to normal as much as 14 days later

XIII. METABOLIC FUNCTION STUDIES

A. Albumin

1. A plasma protein that maintains oncotic pressure (to prevent edema) and transports water-insoluble substances (fatty acids, hormones, bilirubin, drugs)
2. *NCLEX®* Normal reference range: see Table 46–11
3. *NCLEX®* May be decreased in malnourished states and monitored as an indicator of nutritional status

B. Total protein

1. Consists of circulating albumin and globulins in serum; serve many functions, including tissue growth and repair, pH buffering, enzymes, hormones, and coagulation factors

Table 46–11 Tests Reflecting Metabolic Function

Test	Normal Adult Reference Ranges	
	U.S.	Canada
Prealbumin	12–50 mg/dL adults	120–150 mg/L
Albumin	3.4–5.0 grams/dL	34–50 grams/L
Total protein	6.0–8.0 grams/dL	60–80 grams/L
Alkaline phosphatase	4.5–1.3 King-Armstrong units/dL	4.5–1.3 King-Armstrong units/dL
Uric acid	4.0–8.0 mg/dL adult males, 3.5–7.3 mg/dL females	0.24–0.47 mmol/L adult males, 0.21–0.43 mmol/L females

NCLEX® 2. Normal reference range: see Table 46–11
NCLEX® 3. May be decreased with malnutrition, low-protein diet, GI disorders, severe liver disease, chronic renal failure, severe burns, or water intoxication
4. May be increased with dehydration (hemoconcentration), vomiting, diarrhea, and myeloma
5. Teach clients to avoid high-fat foods for 24 hours prior to test

C. Prealbumin

1. Also known as thyroxin-binding prealbumin or transthyretin
2. Sensitive indicator of recent changes in catabolism because half-life is less than 2 days
3. Used to screen for nutritional problems and gauge effectiveness of nutrition therapy
4. Normal reference range: see Table 46–11
5. Low values indicate need for comprehensive nutritional evaluation (history, weight, anthropometric measurements, calorie count)
6. High values are found in renal failure because of poor renal excretion

D. Alkaline phosphatase

1. Enzyme present in intestines, liver, bone, and placenta
2. Normal reference range: see Table 46–11
NCLEX® 3. Rises with periods of bone growth and with liver disease or bile duct obstruction
4. Results may be affected by hepatotoxic drugs administered during 12 hours prior to test
5. Fasting may be required for 12 hours prior to test

E. Uric acid

NCLEX® 1. By-product of purine metabolism; elevated in gout; affected by diet and renal function
2. Normal reference range: see Table 46–11
3. Excessive uric acid can lead to kidney stone formation as renal clearance occurs
NCLEX® 4. Teach client to avoid high-purine foods (liver, kidney, brain, heart, sweetbreads, scallops, sardines) for 24 hours prior to test; otherwise, no food or drink restriction
5. Write medications taken on lab requisition, since many drugs affect results

XIV. IMMUNE FUNCTION STUDIES

A. Human immunodeficiency virus (HIV) tests

1. Consist of enzyme-linked immunosorbent assay (ELISA), Western blot, immunofluorescence assay (IFA), and HIV Type 1 and Type 2 Antibodies Immunoassay
NCLEX® 2. ELISA is tested first and repeated in duplicate (if positive) with same blood sample; if one test is negative, client should be retested in 3–6 months
NCLEX® 3. A positive Western blot or (IFA) confirms diagnosis of HIV; if ELISA is positive and Western blot of IFA is negative, repeat testing should be done in 3–6 months
4. Most recent approved tests are HIV Type 1 and Type 2 Antibodies Immunoassay and HIV1/2 antigen/antibody combination immunoassay; these test for specific antibodies and follow algorithmic guidelines to determine test results

B. CD4 T cell counts

1. Function of T helper cells is primarily to help B cells and increase immunoglobulin production
2. Normal reference range: 500–1600 cells/microliter (mcL)
NCLEX® 3. CD4 counts decrease with HIV, causing increased risk of infection at levels of 200–499 cells/mcL and severe risk when count is less than 200 cells/mcL

C. CD4 to CD8 ratio

1. CD8 or T suppressor cells are responsible for down-regulation of immune response or once an infection has been eradicated

2. Normal ratio of CD4 to CD8 cells is 2:1
3. With decrease in CD4 counts as HIV progresses to acquired immunodeficiency syndrome (AIDS) and client condition worsens, this ratio decreases

D. Viral load testing

1. Measures amounts of HIV viral RNA or other viral protein in blood

NCLEX® 2. Values increase or decrease according to current level of infection

XV. THERAPEUTIC DRUG LEVELS

A. Overview

1. Measure amount of drug circulating in bloodstream; see Table 46–12

NCLEX® 2. Measurements required before and after drug administration (such as aminoglycoside antibiotics) are referred to as peak and trough drug levels
   a. Trough level is drawn when circulating dose is lowest (just prior to next dose)
   b. Peak level is drawn when circulating dose is highest (approximately 30 minutes after drug has finished infusing and dose has equilibrated in bloodstream)
3. Drug levels need to remain within therapeutic range at all times

NCLEX® 4. High drug levels could cause signs of toxicity; low levels could result in symptoms of original health problem (ineffective dose)

NCLEX® **B. Nursing considerations**

1. Teach client not to take daily dose before routine drug level is drawn
2. Alert prescriber immediately of abnormal levels so dosage adjustment can be made

Table 46–12 Common Therapeutic Drug Levels

Drug	Therapeutic Range	Drug	Therapeutic Range
Acetaminophen	10–20 mcg/mL	Magnesium	4.0–7.0 mg/dL
Amitriptyline	120–150 ng/mL	Phenytoin	10–20 mcg/mL
Carbamazepine	5–12 mcg/mL	Procainamide	4–10 mcg/mL
Clozapine	1000–2000 nmol/L	Salicylate	100–250 mcg/mL
Digoxin	0.5–2.0 ng/mL	Theophylline	10–20 mcg/mL
Gentamicin	5–10 mcg/mL	Tobramycin	5–10 mcg/mL
Lidocaine	1.5–5.0 mcg/mL	Valproic acid	50–100 mcg/mL
Lithium	0.5–1.3 mEq/L	Vancomycin	15–20 mg/L

Check Your NCLEX–RN® Exam I.Q.

You are ready for testing on this content if you can:

- Collect blood and body fluid specimens correctly for laboratory analysis.
- Perform client teaching about specimen collection for laboratory analysis.
- Identify normal and abnormal values for common laboratory tests.
- Correlate pathophysiology with results of laboratory tests.
- Make appropriate clinical decisions after reviewing laboratory test results, including notification of primary care provider.

PRACTICE TEST

1 Eighteen hours after surgery, the urine output of a client who underwent removal of a pituitary tumor is markedly increased, and the urine specific gravity is 1.002. The nurse expects to note which corresponding findings when reviewing results of laboratory tests? Select all that apply.

1. Serum sodium 148 mEq/L
2. Serum potassium 3.4 mEq/L
3. Serum osmolality 263 mOsm/L
4. Blood urea nitrogen 7 mg/dL
5. Hematocrit 51%

PRACTICE TEST

2 The nurse would be most concerned about which laboratory value obtained for a client receiving furosemide therapy?

1. Blood urea nitrogen 20 mg/dL
2. Hematocrit 46%
3. Creatinine 1.1 mg/dL
4. Potassium 3.2 mEq/L

3 The nurse inserts a nasogastric tube, and it immediately drains 1000 mL of fluid. Which electrolyte assessment is of greatest concern to the nurse at this time?

1. Sodium
2. Potassium
3. Chloride
4. CO_2 content

4 A client who was just admitted to the nursing unit has a uric acid level of 9.5 mg/dL. Which question would the nurse ask initially?

1. "Do you have a history of gallbladder disease?"
2. "Do you drink large amounts of green tea?"
3. "Do you have a history of gout?"
4. "Do you have any pains in the flank area?"

5 The nurse is caring for a client who received a renal transplant 24 hours previously. Which trend in laboratory studies indicates to the nurse that the new kidney is functioning? Select all that apply.

1. Hemoglobin 12%, increased from 11.8%
2. Serum creatinine 1.6 mg/dL, decreased from 1.9 mg/dL
3. Serum sodium 140 mEq/L, increased from 136 mEq/L
4. Serum phosphate 4.4 mg/dL, decreased from 4.8 mg/dL
5. Blood urea nitrogen level 29 mg/dL, decreased from 35 mg/dL

6 The nurse is caring for a client who has just returned from the operating room. Blood loss was minimal, but the client was given large volumes of crystalloid fluid during the procedure. Which laboratory test results suggest overhydration? Select all that apply.

1. Sodium 147 mEq/L
2. Hemoglobin 14%
3. Hematocrit 33%
4. Calcium level 8.8 mg/dL
5. Blood urea nitrogen 8 mg/dL

7 A client is being evaluated for possible appendicitis. An elevation of which laboratory test result suggests most strongly to the nurse the presence of an acute bacterial infection?

1. Neutrophils
2. Erythrocytes
3. Lymphocytes
4. Platelets

8 The nurse is assigned to care for a client admitted with meningitis who has had a spinal tap performed. Which cells in the cerebrospinal fluid (CSF) suggest that the client has a viral meningitis infection?

1. Platelets
2. Neutrophils
3. Red blood cells
4. Lymphocytes

9 In caring for a female client who has a urinary tract infection (UTI) with more than 100,000 colonies of *Escherichia coli* bacteria, what corresponding findings would the nurse expect to see on the client's urinalysis report? Select all that apply.

1. Positive nitrites
2. Positive leukocyte esterase
3. Negative red blood cells (RBCs)
4. Negative white blood cells (WBCs)
5. Positive glucose

10 The nurse is reviewing the results of follow-up laboratory studies on a client diagnosed with hyperlipidemia. The nurse concludes that the client has been compliant with diet and medication therapy if the total cholesterol level is less than how many mg/dL? Provide a numeric answer.

Fill in your answer below:

Answer: _____ mg/dL

11 A nurse notes the client's albumin level is 2.4 grams/dL. The nurse should plan to assess the client for which of the following at this time? Select all that apply.

1. Peripheral edema
2. Inelastic skin turgor
3. Hypoactive bowel sounds
4. Dry mucous membranes
5. Lung crackles

12 A client is admitted with complaints of severe nausea and vomiting for several days. The nurse expects the client is at risk for experiencing which acid–base imbalance?

1. Metabolic acidosis
2. Metabolic alkalosis
3. Respiratory acidosis
4. Respiratory alkalosis

13 Troponin levels are ordered on a client to confirm a myocardial infarction. When should the nurse plan to have blood drawn for this test?

1. Within 1–2 hours of onset of chest pain
2. Within the first 24 hours of onset of chest pain
3. Between 6 and 24 hours of onset of chest pain
4. Between 24 and 48 hours of onset of chest pain

14 The nurse would anticipate that a client with cirrhosis of the liver would have increased levels of which laboratory values? Select all that apply.

1. Albumin
2. Bilirubin
3. Ammonia
4. Prothrombin time
5. Calcium

15 The nurse notes that the international normalized ratio (INR) of a client with aortic valve replacement taking sodium warfarin is 2.6. What action should the nurse take at this time?

1. Encourage the client to eat additional foods high in vitamin K.
2. Administer the daily dose of warfarin as prescribed.
3. Monitor the client closely for signs of a deep vein thrombosis.
4. Withhold the next scheduled dose of warfarin and notify the prescriber.

16 A client is being evaluated for primary hypothyroidism, and has had blood drawn to determine thyroid-stimulating hormone (TSH) and T_4 levels. The nurse concludes that which test results pattern would support this diagnosis?

1. Elevated TSH and elevated T_4 levels
2. Elevated TSH and decreased T_4 level
3. Decreased TSH and elevated T_4 level
4. Decreased TSH and decreased T_4 level

17 A client is admitted with dehydration secondary to prolonged nausea and vomiting. Which serum laboratory test results would the nurse expect to note as a result of the dehydration? Select all that apply.

1. Sodium 138 mEq/dL
2. Potassium 4.2 mEq/dL
3. Blood urea nitrogen (BUN) 30 mg/dL
4. Hematocrit 49%
5. Total protein 6.8 mg/dL

18 The nurse is establishing a plan of care for a client who has a hemoglobin level of 7.6 grams/dL. What should the nurse identify as a priority physiological area of concern for the client?

1. Ability to tolerate activity
2. Constipation
3. Risk for dehydration
4. Insufficient caloric intake

19 The nurse should assess for Trousseau's sign in a client after noting which electrolyte abnormality?

1. Potassium 3.3 mEq/L
2. Sodium 131 mEq/L
3. Chloride 94 mEq/L
4. Calcium 7.7 mEq/L

20 The white blood cell (WBC) count of a client is 18,000 cells/microliter. The nurse attributes this value to which health problem?

1. Rheumatoid arthritis
2. History of alcoholism
3. Viral infection
4. Wound dehiscence

21 The nurse would assess the client for fever and other signs of infection if the client's white blood cell (WBC) count was noted to be greater than _____ cells/mm^3 on the laboratory report. Provide a numerical response that is a whole number.

Fill in your answer below:
_____ cells/mm^3

ANSWERS & RATIONALES

1 **Answer: 1, 5 Rationale:** Diabetes insipidus is a potential complication following surgery on the pituitary gland. Edema of the remaining pituitary gland can inhibit release of antidiuretic hormone (ADH), resulting in loss of water from glomeruli into collecting tubules of the nephrons. The client excretes large volumes of urine with a low urine specific gravity. As water is removed from the vascular compartment, the serum sodium and hematocrit become concentrated. The blood urea nitrogen and serum osmolality would be expected to be elevated rather than low as the client loses body water. The serum potassium would not be low. **Cognitive Level:** Analyzing **Client Need:** Reduction of Risk Potential **Integrated Process:** Nursing Process: Assessment **Content Area:** Adult Health: Endocrine and Metabolic **Strategy:** This question calls for specific knowledge of altered ADH secretion that can occur after pituitary surgery. Remember that ADH results in movement of free water (i.e., water without sodium) into collecting tubules of the nephron, which results in large volumes of water being removed from the blood. The specific gravity (concentration) of the urine decreases. In addition, removal of water from the serum concentrates (and thereby elevates) the serum sodium and hematocrit. Recall also that hemoconcentration could also raise, not lower, other lab values.

2 **Answer: 4 Rationale:** Furosemide inhibits reabsorption of sodium, water, and potassium from the distal renal tubules and the loop of Henle, leading to diuresis. The most common electrolyte disturbance associated with furosemide administration is hypokalemia. The creatinine value is within normal limits. The BUN and hematocrit could rise or fall, depending on the amount of fluid retained in the vascular compartment. **Cognitive Level:** Analyzing **Client Need:** Reduction of Risk Potential **Integrated Process:** Nursing Process: Assessment **Content Area:** Adult Health: Renal and Genitourinary **Strategy:** This question calls for specific knowledge of the action of furosemide, and knowledge that hypokalemia is a common side effect. Use nursing knowledge and the process of elimination to make a selection.

3 **Answer: 2 Rationale:** Hypokalemia is an almost universal complication of loss of gastric hydrochloric acid. In this scenario, loss of the hydrogen ions results in a metabolic alkalosis. In turn, compensation for this loss takes place in the nephron, where hydrogen ions are retained. The nephron is obligated to excrete potassium, which could result in profound hypokalemia and require vigilant IV replacement. Sodium, chloride, and other electrolytes might be affected, but not to the degree that potassium homeostasis is altered. The CO_2 content might be affected, but this is of less concern than potassium depletion, which could lead to cardiac dysrhythmias. **Cognitive Level:** Applying **Client Need:** Reduction of Risk Potential **Integrated Process:** Nursing Process: Diagnosis **Content Area:** Adult Health: Gastrointestinal **Strategy:** This question calls for specific knowledge that loss of hydrochloric acid triggers the mechanism whereby the kidneys lose potassium. Use nursing knowledge and the process of elimination to make a selection.

4 **Answer: 3 Rationale:** Elevated uric acid levels are commonly seen with gout, which is a disorder of purine metabolism, and this is the initial question to ask the client. Uric acid does not rise with gallbladder disease. The uric acid level is not affected by green tea. Although the client could experience renal stones from precipitation of uric acid crystals (causing flank pain), this is not the initial question to ask, since renal stones are a complication of gout. **Cognitive Level:** Analyzing **Client Need:** Reduction of Risk Potential **Integrated Process:** Nursing Process: Assessment **Content Area:** Adult Health: Endocrine and Metabolic **Strategy:** Note the stem of the question has the critical word *initially*, which indicates more than one option might be technically correct but one is best. Use nursing knowledge related to uric acid level and gout, and the process of elimination, to make a selection.

5 **Answer: 2, 5 Rationale:** Serum creatinine and blood urea nitrogen (BUN) are often associated with renal function, although serum creatinine is the most reliable indicator of kidney function. Decreases in serum creatinine and BUN are often dramatic following renal transplantation. Regular monitoring of these levels is imperative in assessing the function of the transplanted kidney. Hemoglobin levels can increase postoperatively due to blood transfusions. Serum sodium levels might fluctuate according to an individual client's sodium–water balance. Serum phosphate might decrease long term as the kidney increases excretion of phosphates; however, this is not a reliable indicator of renal function. **Cognitive Level:** Analyzing **Client Need:** Reduction of Risk Potential **Integrated Process:** Nursing Process: Assessment **Content Area:** Adult Health: Renal and Genitourinary **Strategy:** This question calls for the specific knowledge that creatinine is the best indicator of renal function and that BUN is another key indicator. Note the wording of the question indicates that more than one option may be correct.

6 **Answer: 3, 5 Rationale:** The hematocrit is an indicator of the proportion of red blood cells in a given volume of blood.

The hematocrit might decrease when cell volume of the blood is decreased because of blood loss or when the liquid portion of the blood volume increases, such as when large volumes of intravenous (IV) fluid are administered. The blood urea nitrogen varies according to hydration status; it rises with dehydration and falls with fluid overload, such as when large volumes of IV fluid are administered. Hemoglobin, sodium, and calcium levels would not be altered. **Cognitive Level:** Analyzing **Client Need:** Reduction of Risk Potential **Integrated Process:** Nursing Process: Assessment **Content Area:** Adult Health: Endocrine and Metabolic **Strategy:** This question requires understanding of how fluid overload affects laboratory values. Specifically, it requires knowledge that the BUN can decrease and that hematocrit can be reduced even if there is no blood loss. Note that the wording of the question suggests that more than one option is likely to be correct.

7 **Answer: 1 Rationale:** Neutrophils are responsible for destruction of bacterial invaders. In acute bacterial infections, such as appendicitis, the percentage of neutrophils (especially immature bands) in the complete blood count will increase. This presence of an increased number of bands is known as a "shift to the left." Lymphocytes are responsible for destruction of viruses. Erythrocytes and platelets are not affected by infections. **Cognitive Level:** Analyzing **Client Need:** Reduction of Risk Potential **Integrated Process:** Nursing Process: Assessment **Content Area:** Adult Health: Gastrointestinal **Strategy:** This question calls for specific knowledge that neutrophils are responsible for destroying bacteria, and will be elevated in acute bacterial infections. Use nursing knowledge and the process of elimination to make a selection.

8 **Answer: 4 Rationale:** Lymphocytes are responsible for the destruction of viruses. Thus, the presence of lymphocytes in the CSF suggests that the meningitis is viral in etiology. This is significant because the infection is most commonly self-limiting, and will not respond to antibiotic therapy (as would bacterial meningitis). The presence of neutrophils would suggest bacterial meningitis. Normally, CSF is free of all cell types, including platelets and red blood cells. **Cognitive Level:** Applying **Client Need:** Reduction of Risk Potential **Integrated Process:** Nursing Process: Diagnosis **Content Area:** Adult Health: Neurological **Strategy:** This question calls for the specific knowledge that lymphocytes are responsible for destruction of viruses. Use nursing knowledge and the process of elimination to make a selection.

9 **Answer: 1, 2 Rationale:** Nitrites are likely to be positive with UTI. A positive leukocyte esterase suggests a UTI. Leukocytes (white blood cells) contain esterases that react with substances contained in urine. More than 100,000 colonies of bacteria (per high-powered field) are needed before the client can be diagnosed with a UTI. RBCs are also usually positive because of the effect of infection on tissue. WBCs are present in the urine to fight infection. Glucose in the urine should be negative and a positive finding would indicate glucose intolerance rather than UTI. **Cognitive Level:** Applying **Client Need:** Reduction of Risk Potential **Integrated Process:** Nursing Process: Diagnosis **Content Area:** Adult Health: Renal and Genitourinary **Strategy:** This question calls for specific knowledge that leukocyte esterase will be positive urine infected with bacteria. Use nursing knowledge and the process of elimination to make a selection.

10 **Answer: 200 Rationale:** To maintain health, the goal for total serum cholesterol is to keep the value below 200 mg/dL. **Cognitive Level:** Analyzing **Client Need:** Reduction of Risk Potential **Integrated Process:** Nursing Process: Assessment **Content Area:** Adult Health: Cardiovascular **Strategy:** The core issue of the question is knowledge of normal serum cholesterol levels. Use nursing knowledge and the process of elimination to make a selection.

11 **Answer: 1, 5 Rationale:** Albumin is a protein responsible for increasing osmotic pressure and maintaining intravascular fluid volume. Low albumin levels reduce intravascular colloid osmotic pressure, which allows fluid to move out of blood vessels and into interstitial tissues. This fluid retention will be assessed as peripheral edema, lung crackles, and fluid weight gain. Skin turgor will be elastic when fluid shifts into the interstitial spaces. Bowel sounds and mucous membranes would not be affected. **Cognitive Level:** Analyzing **Client Need:** Reduction of Risk Potential **Integrated Process:** Nursing Process: Planning **Content Area:** Adult Health: Endocrine and Metabolic **Strategy:** Determine that this test result is an abnormally low albumin level. Recall that albumin is necessary for maintenance of fluid balance between body compartments and then select all options that indicate fluid retention.

12 **Answer: 2 Rationale:** The loss of gastric acids is a metabolic problem that leads to an excess of alkaline fluids in the body. Metabolic acidosis does not occur when acids are being lost from the body. Respiratory acidosis occurs when the body retains carbon dioxide. Respiratory alkalosis occurs when the client exhales excess carbon dioxide. **Cognitive Level:** Applying **Client Need:** Reduction of Risk Potential **Integrated Process:** Nursing Process: Diagnosis **Content Area:** Adult Health: Endocrine and Metabolic **Strategy:** First, determine if the imbalance is metabolic or respiratory. Loss of GI fluids is a metabolic function, so options indicating a respiratory problem can be eliminated. Next, determine if the imbalance is acid or base. Loss of body acids will lead to an excess of bicarbonate in the body and an alkaline state.

13 **Answer: 3 Rationale:** Troponin is a specific marker for cardiac injury. Elevations in serum levels usually begin 4–6 hours after onset of symptoms. The elevation peaks in 12–24 hours. Drawing the blood in the first 2 hours would be too soon. "Within the first 24 hours of onset" is too vague because this could include the first few hours when levels would be falsely low. Waiting longer than 24 hours would miss the times for peak levels. **Cognitive Level:** Applying **Client Need:** Reduction of Risk Potential **Integrated Process:** Nursing Process: Planning **Content Area:** Adult Health: Cardiovascular **Strategy:** The question calls for specific knowledge of troponin release times following myocardial infarction. Recall the times for elevation and return to normal and choose the option that is closest and most specific to this pattern.

14 **Answer: 2, 3, 4 Rationale:** The cirrhotic liver is unable to completely break down bilirubin, and serum levels are elevated. Ammonia is normally converted to urea in the liver; serum levels are increased with liver damage. Prothrombin times are increased when the liver is unable to synthesize clotting factors. In cirrhosis, the damaged liver is unable to properly metabolize amino acids and synthesize albumin, resulting in decreased serum concentrations. Calcium levels should be unaffected by cirrhosis. **Cognitive Level:** Applying **Client Need:** Reduction of Risk Potential **Integrated Process:** Nursing Process: Assessment **Content Area:** Adult

Health: Gastrointestinal **Strategy:** This question tests knowledge of liver functions and cirrhosis. Recall the liver's function as related to each of the laboratory values, and systematically eliminate incorrect options.

15 **Answer: 2 Rationale:** The usual therapeutic INR level during medication therapy with sodium warfarin is 2–3. The next dose should be given as scheduled. Encouraging the client to eat more foods high in vitamin K would reduce effectiveness of the drug. The client would be at risk for deep vein thrombosis when blood clotting is accelerated, not slowed. The dose would be withheld only if the client's level is above the therapeutic range; there is no need to notify the prescriber. **Cognitive Level:** Analyzing **Client Need:** Reduction of Risk Potential **Integrated Process:** Nursing Process: Implementation **Content Area:** Adult Health: Cardiovascular **Strategy:** First, determine if the level is expected. Recall that in order to be therapeutic, the INR usually needs to fall within the 2–3 range. With this in mind, select the option that is consistent with routine nursing care.

16 **Answer: 2 Rationale:** In primary hypothyroidism, the thyroid gland does not produce thyroxine (T_4), despite being stimulated by the pituitary gland (with elevated TSH) to do so. Elevated TSH and T_4 levels are seen with secondary hyperthyroidism caused by excessive TSH production by the pituitary. A decreased TSH and elevated T_4 are seen with primary hyperthyroidism, not hypothyroidism. Decreased TSH and T_4 levels are seen in secondary hypothyroidism due to insufficient pituitary secretions. **Cognitive Level:** Applying **Client Need:** Reduction of Risk Potential **Integrated Process:** Nursing Process: Assessment **Content Area:** Adult Health: Endocrine and Metabolic **Strategy:** The question requires knowledge of pituitary and thyroid hormone functions. First eliminate options with an increased T_4 level, which would not be seen with hypothyroidism. Next, recall the negative endocrine feedback loop to differentiate between test results expected with primary and secondary hypothyroidism.

17 **Answer: 3, 4 Rationale:** Dehydration results in loss of fluids, causing a hemoconcentration of BUN, which is elevated. The hematocrit would be elevated secondary to hemoconcentration from dehydration. The sodium is normal and would be more likely to be elevated from hemoconcentration with dehydration. The potassium level is normal, and would most likely be lower because of losses from the vomiting. The total protein level is normal, and would not likely be influenced by dehydration. **Cognitive Level:** Analyzing **Client Need:** Reduction of Risk Potential **Integrated Process:** Nursing Process: Assessment **Content Area:** Adult Health: Gastrointestinal **Strategy:** The question requires analysis of fluid losses on common lab values. Recall that vomiting leads to loss of sodium, potassium, and water. Eliminate values that are normal; look for abnormal values.

18 **Answer: 1 Rationale:** Hemoglobin is the oxygen-carrying component of red blood cells. When levels are decreased, the client will be fatigued with possible decompensation during activity (which could lead to safety concerns). Although of general concern if it occurred, constipation would not be as high in priority when the client has a low hemoglobin level. Risk for dehydration would not be as high in priority when the client has a low hemoglobin level because low hemoglobin is an indicator of anemia. Insufficient calories might be the cause of the low hemoglobin, but only if the proper nutrients are deficient and the anemia is not caused by blood loss. **Level:** Analyzing **Client Need:** Reduction of Risk Potential **Integrated Process:** Nursing Process: Diagnosis **Content Area:** Adult Health: Hematological **Strategy:** The question asks to choose a priority, indicating all options may be partially or totally correct. Eliminate options that do not directly relate to risks of low hemoglobin (which include reduced oxygenation and activity intolerance).

19 **Answer: 4 Rationale:** Hypocalcemia causes excitability of skeletal, cardiac, and smooth muscle tissues. Evidence of this is seen in Trousseau's sign, a carpopedal spasm. Hypokalemia, hyponatremia, and hypochloremia would not cause this sign. **Cognitive Level:** Applying **Client Need:** Reduction of Risk Potential **Integrated Process:** Nursing Process: Assessment **Content Area:** Adult Health: Endocrine and Metabolic **Strategy:** Specific knowledge of Trousseau's sign is needed to answer this question. Recall this carpopedal spasm is seen with low calcium and magnesium levels. Eliminate the other options because low levels of the other electrolytes would lead to muscle weakness, not neuromuscular excitability.

20 **Answer: 4 Rationale:** Tissue injury, such as with wound dehiscence, can cause a significant increase in WBCs. The WBC count may not increase with rheumatoid arthritis. The WBC count does not increase with alcoholism. Viral infection could lead to an increase in lymphocytes, but the overall WBC count does not rise to such high levels overall with viral infections. **Cognitive Level:** Analyzing **Client Need:** Reduction of Risk Potential **Integrated Process:** Nursing Process: Assessment **Content Area:** Adult Health: Gastrointestinal **Strategy:** First, determine that the WBC is abnormally high. Recall conditions that elevate the WBC, such as bacterial infections, stress, and tissue injury. Evaluate each option to eliminate conditions in which the WBC is decreased or unaffected.

21 **Answer: 10,000 Rationale:** The normal range for the WBC count is 5000–10,000/mm^3. For this reason, the nurse would be concerned about the risk of infection if the exceeded 10,000. **Cognitive Level:** Analyzing **Client Need:** Reduction of Risk Potential **Integrated Process:** Nursing Process: Assessment **Content Area:** Adult Health: Hematological **Strategy:** The core issue of the question is knowledge of normal laboratory values. Use this knowledge to choose an answer. Since specific knowledge is needed to answer correctly, memorize this value if you found the question difficult.

Key Terms to Review

plasma p. 725

serum p. 723

References

Centers for Disease Control (2014, June 27). Quick reference guide. Laboratory techniques for the diagnosis of HIV infection. Updated recommendations. Available at www.cdc.gov/hiv/pdf/guidelines_testing_recommendedlabtestingalgorithm.pdf.

Corbett, J. (2013). *Laboratory tests and diagnostic procedures with nursing diagnoses* (8th ed.). Upper Saddle River, NJ: Pearson Education.

Fischbach, F., & Dunning, M. (2014). A *manual of laboratory and diagnostic tests* (9th ed.). Philadelphia: Lippincott Williams & Wilkins.

Kee, J. (2017). *Pearson's handbook of laboratory and diagnostic tests* (8th ed.). New York, NY: Pearson Education.

Kozier, B., Erb, G., Berman, A., Snyder, S., Buck, M., Yiu, L., et al. (2014). *Fundamentals of Canadian nursing* (3rd ed.). Toronto, ON, Canada: Pearson Canada.

Leeuwen, A., & Bladh, M. (2015). *Davis's comprehensive handbook of laboratory and diagnostic tests with nursing implications* (6th ed.). Philadelphia: F. A. Davis.

Smith, S., Duell, D., Martin, B., Aebersold, M., & Gonzalez, L. (2017). *Clinical nursing skills: Basic to advanced skills* (10th ed.). New York, NY: Pearson Education.

Test Yourself

Are you ready for the NCLEX-RN® or course exams? Access the NEW web-based app that provides students with thousands of practice questions in preparation for the NCLEX experience.

47 Common Diagnostic Tests and Procedures

In this chapter

Cross Reference

Other chapters relevant to this content area are

Common Laboratory Tests **Chapter 46**

I. GENERAL DIAGNOSTIC TESTS

A. Client safety in diagnostic testing

1. Client safety for any diagnostic test implies knowledge of procedure, risks and benefits, and pre- and postcare

NCLEX® 2. Ensure that informed consent form is signed and witnessed, especially for invasive diagnostic tests involving penetration of tissues or blood vessels (contrast dye, radioisotopes)

NCLEX® 3. Before beginning a diagnostic test, a *time-out* or pause is called to double-check that right procedure is being carried out on right client at right site

B. *Biopsy*

1. Overview
   - **a.** Removes and examines body tissue to detect malignancy or other disease process
   - **b.** Methods include aspiration by suction, brush method (scrapes cells using stiff bristles), excision by surgical cutting, needle aspiration, or punch biopsy (using punch-type instrument)
   - **c.** Common sites: breast, uterine endometrium, thyroid, kidney, colon, liver, bone marrow (often sternum, iliac crest); see Figure 47–1A
2. Preprocedure care
   - **a.** Take baseline vital signs (VS)
   - **b.** Client teaching: biopsy site will be anesthetized just prior to procedure; with needle biopsy client may be asked to take a breath and hold it
   - **c.** Keep client NPO for 6 hours prior to liver biopsy to decrease liver congestion
3. Postprocedure care
   - **a.** Monitor VS as prescribed
   - *NCLEX®* **b.** Apply pressure to site for 20 minutes (kidney); place client on right side (liver) to reduce risk of bleeding (see Figure 47–1B); apply pressure dressing to any site
   - **c.** Observe for bleeding at site and instruct client to report bleeding
   - *NCLEX®* **d.** Instruct client to rest and avoid heavy lifting for 24 hours or longer if indicated (liver, kidney)

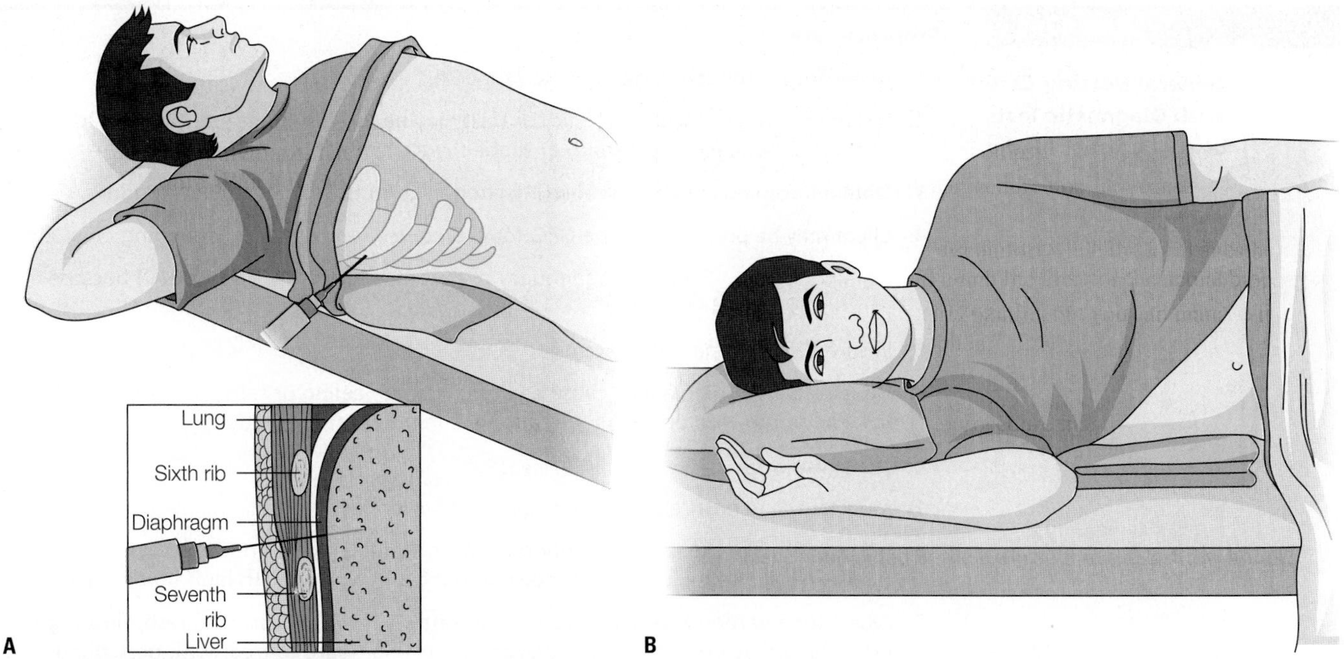

Figure 47–1 Liver biopsy. (**A**) Common liver biopsy site; (**B**) right-sided positioning after liver biopsy.

e. Increase fluid intake and teach client to report decreased urine output or burning on urination (kidney)
f. Do not administer aspirin, anticoagulants (heparin or warfarin), or nonsteroidal anti-inflammatory drugs (NSAIDs) from immediately after biopsy until 2 weeks post-biopsy to prevent bleeding

C. *Computed tomography (CT) scan*

1. Overview
   a. A radiological procedure that uses x-ray images taken at multiple angles to create a composite three-dimensional image that distinguishes minor differences in tissue density
   b. Common areas for scanning are head and brain, chest (thoracic), abdomen, spine, long bones, joints, and pelvis; may be done with or without contrast dye (most are without contrast)
   c. Protective shields must be worn by personnel and over client's reproductive area to prevent adverse effects of x-ray exposures (clients of child-bearing age should have urine pregnancy test done before CT scan)
2. Preprocedure care
   a. Ensure informed consent when contrast is used
   NCLEX® b. See Box 47–1 for general nursing care of clients having diagnostic tests using contrast media
   c. No food or fluid restriction if contrast medium is not used
   d. Ensure client has patent IV access if contrast medium to be used
   e. Remove metal objects prior to scanning
   f. Explain that machine is circular and makes series of "clicking" sounds, test is not painful, and usually takes about 15 minutes

NCLEX® 3. Postprocedure care: see Box 47–1 for postprocedure care of clients receiving contrast media; client can resume usual diet and activity unless otherwise prescribed

D. Fluoroscopy

1. Overview
   a. Views organs in motion on fluorescent screen (commonly thorax, heart, abdomen, brain)
   b. Often used with many diagnostic tests for visualization and guidance
   c. Room is darkened for visualization and those remaining in room should wear protective aprons to prevent exposure
2. Preprocedure care
   a. Explain that there is no discomfort with procedure
   b. Ask if client is pregnant or suspects pregnancy (contraindication to procedure); complete a pregnancy test if indicated

Box 47–1

General Nursing Care with Diagnostic Tests Using Contrast Media

Preprocedure

1. Assess for allergy to iodine or contrast media.
2. If client is allergic, hypoallergenic contrast may be used or client may be premedicated with prednisone (corticosteroid) or diphenhydramine (antihistamine).
3. Obtain informed consent because injection of contrast is an invasive procedure.
4. Client may be prescribed to be NPO for 4–8 hours preprocedure, depending on study.
5. Obtain baseline VS and note adequacy of preprocedure urine output (UO) because contrast is cleared by kidneys.
6. Ensure client has patent IV access.
7. Explain contrast media may cause a warm, flushed feeling or salty, fishy, or metallic taste in mouth, and possibly nausea for 1–2 minutes after injection.

Postprocedure

1. Monitor UO to ensure clearance of contrast via kidneys.
2. Increase fluid intake to aid excretion of contrast unless contraindicated by heart failure, renal disease, or other condition that could worsen with high fluid intake.
3. Assess for and report delayed reaction to contrast medium (dyspnea, rash, flushing, urticaria, tachycardia, decreased UO, and others); prepare to treat with prescribed antihistamines or corticosteroids.

c. Barium sulfate is given to clients undergoing abdominal procedures
d. Advise that x-ray personnel may give specific instructions during test

3. Postprocedure care
a. Food and fluids permitted after abdominal and thorax fluoroscopy, but cardiac catheterization aftercare is performed following fluoroscopy of heart (see section later in chapter)
b. Laxative is usually ordered postfluoroscopy of abdomen

E. ***Magnetic resonance imaging (MRI)***

1. Overview
a. Produces images similar to CT scanning but does not use ionizing radiation, so client is free of hazards caused by exposure to x-rays
b. Consists of magnet enclosed in large, doughnut-shaped cylinder; client is guided into cylinder until area being diagnosed is within magnetic field
NCLEX® c. Contraindications to MRI are implanted metal devices (pacemakers or wires, aneurysm or surgical clips, metal rods or screws in bones, some hearing aids, nerve stimulators)

2. Preprocedure care
a. Screen for implanted metal objects, which are contraindications for test
NCLEX® b. Remove all jewelry and other metal objects (eyeglasses, hearing aids, hair pins, cosmetics that may have metallic fragments)
c. Food and fluids are not restricted for adults; children may be NPO for 4 hours
NCLEX® d. IV access may be inserted for contrast (usually gadolinium is used—nonallergenic, but may affect calcium absorption for next 24 hours)
e. Explain that procedure involves lying on narrow table that will slide into machine; clients with claustrophobia may need sedation or use of open machine if available; test is painless
NCLEX® f. Advise that machine makes loud noises (clicks and thumps) but earplugs are available and client can communicate with personnel via intercom; family member or friend may remain in room with client (no radiation)
g. MRI machines have weight limits; obese and claustrophobic clients may need to use open scanner if available

3. Postprocedure care: none specific

F. ***Nuclear imaging study*** **(also called radionuclide imaging or radioisotope scan)**

1. Overview
a. Scintillation camera records distribution of radioisotope in specific organ(s) after inhalation, oral, or IV administration

b. Common radioisotopes: technetium-99m, thallium-201, iodine-131, gallium citrate, and indium 111 (to label white blood cells)

2. Preprocedure care

a. Keep NPO if prescribed depending on area being scanned

NCLEX® b. Administer prescribed blocking agent (Lugol's solution, potassium perchlorate) prior to radioiodine study except for thyroid scan

c. Adhere to protocols for administering radioisotopes and waiting periods before scanning; ensure client arrives on time for scan

d. Instruct to avoid high-iodine foods and iodized salt for 3 days prior to thyroid scan

NCLEX® e. Explain that radionuclide leaves body in 6–24 hours and should not affect other people

f. Explain that scans cause no discomfort, to lie still during procedure unless asked to change position, and more than one imaging session may be needed (client may need to return at specified times)

NCLEX® g. Remove jewelry and other metal objects in area under study

3. Postprocedure care: none specific

G. Positron emission tomography (PET) scan

1. Overview

a. Detects blood flow (often to brain or heart) to diagnose disease

b. Measures concentrations of positron-emitting isotope after receiving a substance tagged with a radionuclide (radioactive glucose, rubidium 82, oxygen 15, nitrogen 13)

2. Preprocedure care

a. Ensure that client has patent IV access and measure VS

b. Teach client to follow instructions given during test, Velcro straps may be used to limit movement during test, and radiation from test is short-lived

3. Postprocedure care

a. Monitor VS; avoid postural hypotension by moving client slowly to upright position

b. Increase fluid intake to aid in clearing radioisotope via kidneys

H. *Ultrasonography* (sonogram)

1. Overview

a. Uses a probe (transducer) over skin surface or in body cavity to produce ultrasound beam that is reflected or echoed from tissues and can be captured by computer into scans, graphs, or audible sounds (Doppler)

b. Can be used for many body tissues to detect abnormalities such as masses, cysts, edema, fluid, and stones; evaluates blood flow in arteries and veins

2. Preprocedure care

a. Restrict food and fluids for 4–8 hours prior to tests of abdomen, abdominal aorta, gallbladder, liver, spleen, and pancreas

NCLEX® b. Have client eat fat-free meal on evening prior to abdominal, gallbladder, liver, pancreas, kidney, or liver sonogram

NCLEX® c. For pelvic and renal ultrasound (including obstetrics), client should drink 720 mL (24 oz) water 1 hour prior to exam or three to four 240-mL (8-oz) glasses of clear fluid 90 minutes prior to exam; teach client not to void until after test is completed

d. Explain that ultrasound gel is applied to skin surface of site being examined; probe is moved smoothly with light pressure over area

e. Advise that test is usually painless and no radiation is involved

3. Postprocedure care: none specific

I. *X-rays*

1. Overview

a. Uses radiation (x-ray beams) to detect abnormal size, structure, and shape of bone or tissues, such as chest, heart, abdomen (flat plate), KUB (kidneys, ureter, bladder), skull, and skeletal

NCLEX® b. Client and personnel wear protective garb over reproductive organs; pregnant clients should avoid x-rays, especially during first trimester (perform urine pregnancy test prior to x-rays)

2. Preprocedure care

a. Food and fluids are generally not restricted unless client may go to surgery following tests (such as to repair bone fractures)

NCLEX® b. Remove hairpins, glasses, jewelry, and other metallic objects prior to test

c. Explain that more than one x-ray film may be needed and that client may need to wait while staff ensures that films are of good quality

3. Postprocedure care: none specific

II. RESPIRATORY DIAGNOSTIC TESTS

A. Bronchoscopy

1. Overview
   a. Allows for direct inspection or visualization of larynx, trachea, and bronchi using a metal or flexible fiberoptic bronchoscope
   b. Indicated to diagnose tracheobronchial tumor or bleeding site, remove foreign body or mucus plugs, or obtain samples for cytologic examination or culture
   c. Client generally receives premedication and local anesthetic sprayed in throat and sometimes nose (if fiberoptic instrument used) before insertion of bronchoscope
2. Preprocedure care
   a. Ensure that informed consent form is completed and preprocedure or preoperative checklist is completed
   NCLEX® b. Assess for allergies to drugs (especially analgesics, anesthetics, and antibiotics), food, and latex
   NCLEX® c. Have client void before giving premedication
   d. Remove dentures, contact lenses, and jewelry
   e. Obtain baseline VS; ensure admission VS also available for comparison
   f. Instruct client to relax during test if using local anesthesia (general anesthesia could be used); throat may be sore after procedure but will resolve
3. Postprocedure care
   a. Monitor VS every 15 minutes for first hour, every 30 minutes for second hour, and then hourly until stable
   NCLEX® b. Keep head of bed (HOB) elevated in semi-Fowler's position; if unconscious, position client on side with head slightly elevated to prevent aspiration
   c. Assess for and notify healthcare provider of respiratory distress (dyspnea, wheezing, apprehension, decreased breath sounds)
   NCLEX® d. Explain that coughing with minimal blood-tinged mucus may be expected; assess for and immediately report hemoptysis (coughing up excessively bloody secretions)
   NCLEX® e. Do not give food or fluids until cough, gag, and swallow reflexes have returned (usually 2–8 hours postprocedure); offer ice chips and sips of water before giving food
   f. Offer throat lozenges to relieve sore throat once client is taking food and fluids
   g. Assess and report complications, including laryngeal edema, bronchospasm, pneumothorax, cardiac dysrhythmias, and bleeding from biopsy site

B. *Pulmonary function tests*

1. Overview
   a. Detect pulmonary dysfunction, differentiate obstructive and restrictive lung disease, evaluate response to drug therapy (e.g., bronchodilators or steroids), and obtain baseline parameters for pulmonary rehabilitation
   b. Common pulmonary tests include vital capacity tests, lung volume studies, flow volume loop, diffusion capacity test, bronchial provocation studies, exercise studies, pulse oximetry, nutritional studies (indirect calorimetry), and body plethysmography
2. Preprocedure care
   a. Contact laboratory for specific restrictions, which can vary among labs
   NCLEX® b. Instruct client to avoid eating heavy meal prior to test and to avoid smoking for 4–6 hours before test
   c. Record age, height, and weight for predicting normal range of results
   d. Tell client to wear nonrestrictive clothing
   e. Cancel test if client has active cold, fever, or is under influence of alcohol
   NCLEX® f. Withhold medications that affect results, including sedatives and narcotics; check whether bronchodilators are allowed (may be withheld prior and given during test)
   g. Help client practice breathing patterns for test, such as normal breathing, rapid breathing, forced deep inspiration, and forced deep expiration
3. Postprocedure care: none specific

C. Ventilation scan (pulmonary ventilation scan)

1. Overview
   a. A nuclear lung scan performed after client inhales a mixture of air, oxygen, and radioactive gas
   b. Often performed with pulmonary perfusion scan to differentiate between respiratory disease (ventilatory problem) and vascular abnormality in lungs

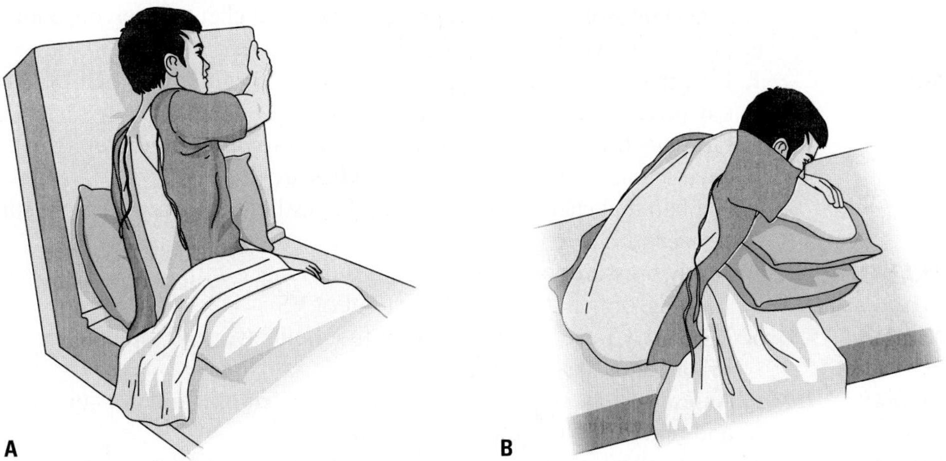

Figure 47–2

Common positions for thoracentesis. (**A**) Sitting to one side, holding arm upward and to front; (**B**) sitting and leaning forward over pillow on bed or table. **A** **B**

2. Preprocedure care
   a. There is no food or fluid restriction
   b. Remove all jewelry and other metal objects from neck and chest area
   NCLEX® c. Explain that client will inhale radioactive gas and will be asked to take deep breath and hold it while single image of lung is taken; other images will be recorded during three phases of test: wash-in (gas builds up in lungs), equilibrium (steady state), and wash-out (gas is expelled while breathing room air)
3. Postprocedure care
   NCLEX® a. Assess respiratory status and breath sounds; report changes in rate and difficulty breathing
   b. Assess for and report chest pain, especially if pulmonary embolism is suspected as underlying problem

D. *Thoracentesis*

1. Overview
   a. An invasive procedure that uses a needle inserted through chest wall to remove fluid or air in pleural space to ease breathing, or to inject chemotherapeutic agents into pleural space
   b. Often done at bedside after chest x-ray is done to pinpoint best insertion site
   c. Aspirating needle is attached to syringe and stopcock (turned to off position to ensure no air enters pleural space during insertion); fluid is aspirated into syringe or drained into tubing and container attached to stopcock
2. Preprocedure care
   a. Record baseline VS and ensure informed consent is signed
   b. Position client sitting to one side or sitting and leaning over a pillow (see Figure 47–2)
   c. Explain that local anesthetic will be administered
   NCLEX® d. Ensure that strict aseptic technique is maintained while handling equipment and supplies for procedure
3. Postprocedure care
   a. Assess respiratory status and breath sounds; report changes in rate and difficulty breathing
   b. Apply pressure dressing over site and monitor client for pain as anesthetic wears off; a mild analgesic may be prescribed
   c. Monitor site for bleeding or signs of infection

III. CARDIOVASCULAR DIAGNOSTIC TESTS

A. *Angiography* (angiogram)

1. Overview
   a. Injection of contrast dye via catheter into femoral, brachial, subclavian, carotid, or other arteries to visualize blood vessels; also called arteriography
   b. Used to detect aneurysms, thrombosis, emboli, space-occupying lesions, stenosis, and plaques, and to evaluate cerebral, pulmonary, and renal blood flow
   c. Type of study is specified by prefacing *angiography* or *angiogram* with name of area being studied, such as cerebral angiography or pulmonary angiogram
2. Preprocedure care
   NCLEX® a. Keep client NPO for 8–12 hours prior to test
   NCLEX® b. Cleanse skin and clip hair at access site per agency policy
   c. Discontinue anticoagulants, such as heparin, for specified time prior to test (e.g., 6 hours)

d. See again Box 47–1 for preprocedure care of clients receiving contrast medium
e. Have client void before procedure
NCLEX® f. Ensure that client has patent IV access and begin prescribed IV fluids at time specified; administer any prescribed premedication
g. Give cleansing enema as prescribed prior to renal angiography to enhance visualization; perform vascular studies before any barium studies are done
h. Explain that client will receive local anesthetic and must remain still during procedure

3. Postprocedure care
NCLEX® a. Apply pressure for up to 30 minutes or longer until bleeding has stopped; check site for bleeding, swelling, or hematoma with each set of VS
NCLEX® b. Monitor VS every 15 minutes for first hour, every 30 minutes for 2 hours, every hour for next 4 hours, or longer until stable, then routine
NCLEX® c. Assess peripheral pulses in affected area (femoral and dorsalis pedis or radial) with VS and document and report diminished or absent pulses
NCLEX® d. Note neurovascular status of affected extremity (color, temperature, motion, sensitivity) when assessing pulses and report abnormal findings (pale, cool, numbness, weakness)
e. Monitor body temperature every 4 hours for 24–48 hours per protocol
f. Maintain bedrest for 6–8 hours; restrict activities until following day
NCLEX® g. Apply sandbag, pressure device, cold compress, or ice bag to site as prescribed to relieve edema or discomfort
NCLEX® h. See Box 47–1 for postprocedure care of clients receiving contrast medium
i. Explain that coughing may be expected following pulmonary angiography
NCLEX® j. Assess for and report dysphagia and respiratory distress after cerebral angiography, and also for weakness or numbness in an extremity, confusion, slurred speech, visual changes (possible transient ischemic attack)

B. *Cardiac catheterization*

1. Overview
a. Also known as cardiac angiography, angiocardiography, and coronary arteriography
b. Right-heart catheterization uses femoral vein access to diagnose tricuspid or pulmonic valve stenosis or regurgitation, pulmonary hypertension, and septal defects
c. Left-heart catheterization uses brachial or femoral artery access up through aorta to diagnose mitral or aortic valve stenosis or regurgitation, coronary artery disease, left ventricular hypertrophy, and ventricular aneurysm
d. Left-sided catheterization is more commonly performed and uses principles of angiography outlined in previous section

NCLEX® 2. Preprocedure care
a. Ensure that informed consent is signed and that provider has discussed possible risks with client and family
b. Restrict food and fluids for 8 hours before test or as per agency policy
c. Provide preprocedure care to clients receiving contrast medium (see again Box 47–1); administer any prescribed antihistamines and corticosteroids on evening before or on day of test
d. Withhold medications, including anticoagulants such as heparin, for 6–8 hours as prescribed
e. Cleanse and clip/prep insertion site on morning of procedure
f. Measure and record client's height and weight to calculate amount of contrast needed (1 mL/kg body weight), and record baseline VS and peripheral pulses
g. Ensure client voids before receiving premedication (given 30 minutes to 1 hour prior)
NCLEX® h. Explain that cardiac cath room has a padded table; IV fluids will be given; cardiac rhythm will be monitored; skin anesthetic will be applied to injection site; client may feel flushed or warm during or after injection of contrast and this will pass; client may be asked to cough or deep-breathe during procedure; coughing can reduce nausea from contrast and possible cardiac dysrhythmias

NCLEX® 3. Postprocedure care
a. Monitor VS (BP, pulse, respirations) every 15 minutes for an hour, every 30 minutes until stable, then every hour as prescribed, and then every 4 hours; monitor temperature every 4 hours
b. Assess catheter insertion site for bleeding or hematoma; change dressing as needed
c. Assess peripheral pulses, neurovascular status of affected extremity, pain or discomfort
d. Assess cardiac rhythm and report rate or rhythm abnormalities
e. Assess for and report chest pain, chest heaviness, shortness of breath, and abdominal or groin pain
f. Administer prescribed analgesics for comfort and antibiotics if prescribed

g. Instruct client to remain on bedrest for 8–12 hours or per agency policy
h. Client may turn from side to side and HOB may be elevated to no more than 30 degrees (some agencies have head flat or only 15-degree elevation); affected leg must be kept straight for 8–12 hours; if arm used for access, it must be immobilized for 3 hours (smaller blood vessel)
i. Provide postprocedure care to clients receiving contrast medium (see again Box 47–1)
j. Assess for and report signs of complications, including myocardial infarction, dysrhythmias, cardiac tamponade, and pulmonary or cerebral embolism

C. *Echocardiography*

1. Overview
a. A noninvasive ultrasound test to identify abnormalities in heart size, structure, and function, and to diagnose valvular disease
b. Handheld transducer is moved over chest in area of heart and other identified areas; sound waves are emitted and reflected back to produce images that appear on a video screen and are recorded on videotape and paper
c. Several specific types of studies are available, including M-mode, two-dimensional, spectral Doppler, color Doppler, transesophageal, contrast, and stress echocardiography
2. Preprocedure care
a. Measure and record baseline VS
b. There is no food or fluid restriction and no medications need to be withheld unless instructed by provider; exceptions are transesophageal and stress echocardiography, which require NPO status 4 hours prior to test
NCLEX® c. For transesophageal test, client will be given IV sedation
NCLEX® d. For contrast test, an IV access line must be inserted
e. Have client undress from waist up and wear hospital gown
f. Explain procedure to client (outlined earlier in general ultrasound section)
g. Explain that client will lie supine or on left side
3. Postprocedure care: none for most tests; client is monitored during recovery for 1–2 hours after transesophageal test

D. *Electrocardiography* (electrocardiogram or ECG, EKG)

1. Overview
NCLEX® a. Measures electrical activity of heart; detects cardiac dysrhythmias and electrolyte imbalance (hyperkalemia—tall peaked T wave)
NCLEX® b. Electrodes are placed on extremities and chest (excess hair may be shaved in small spots) and electrical activity is recorded with each heartbeat
c. Records cardiac waveforms or complexes in 12 leads: six limb leads (three bipolar: leads I, II, and III; three unipolar: leads aVR, aVL, and aVF); and six chest or precordial leads (V1 through V6); see Figure 47–3
NCLEX® 2. Preprocedure care
a. No food or fluid restriction is needed; no consent form is required
b. Position client supine and expose arms and legs for limb lead placement
c. Clothing should be removed to waist, with females given a gown to wear
d. Note medications client is receiving, since some drugs (e.g., antidysrhythmics and beta-blockers) may alter readings

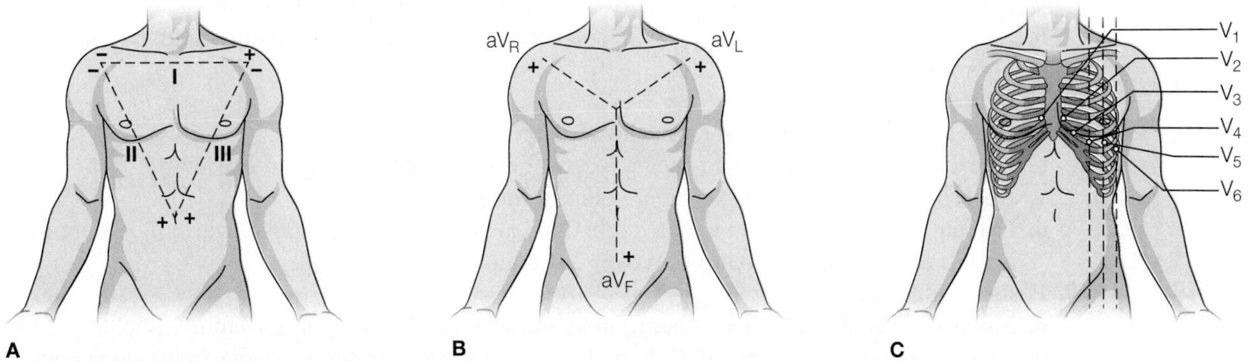

Figure 47–3 12 leads of ECG: (**A**) bipolar limb leads (I, II, III); (**B**) unipolar limb leads (aVR, aVL, aVF); (**C**) unipolar precordial leads (V1–V6).

   e. Instruct client to relax muscles and breathe normally during ECG, and that procedure does not cause pain or electric shock
   f. Instruct client to state if chest pain is experienced during ECG
3. Postprocedure care: remove electrode paste or jelly if used and assist client to dress if needed

E. Holter monitoring

1. Overview
   a. Evaluates heart rate and rhythm during normal activities over a 24-hour period; identifies cardiac dysrhythmias
   b. Consists of a recording device and clock inside a 1-pound monitor that is worn by client
   NCLEX® c. Client keeps a diary to record timing of symptoms such as palpitations, chest pain, shortness of breath, syncope, vertigo, and usual daily activities (eating, exercise, sleep) for correlation with ECG readings
2. Preprocedure care
   a. No food or fluid restriction is necessary
   b. Clean and shave as necessary skin areas needed for electrode placement
   c. Place five to seven electrodes on chest as per particular monitor
   NCLEX® d. Instruct client to avoid vigorous exercise or sweating, and not to shower, take a bath, or swim until electrodes are removed
   e. Postprocedure care: none specific except to review items in diary with client for clarification if necessary

F. Stress/exercise tests

1. Overview
   a. Include a variety of specific tests, such as treadmill exercise electrocardiography, exercise myocardial perfusion imaging test (thallium or technetium stress test), nuclear dipyridamole or dobutamine stress test
   b. Used to screen for coronary artery disease, evaluate myocardial perfusion, differentiate between cardiac ischemia and infarct, develop cardiac rehabilitation program, evaluate cardiac status for work capability, and evaluate effectiveness of cardiac drug therapy
   c. Electrodes are applied to chest; baseline VS are recorded and monitored periodically during test, and client exercises per age-based protocol on treadmill or bicycle (except persantine test, prescribed for those who cannot tolerate exercise)
2. Preprocedure care
   a. Maintain NPO status after midnight (dipyridamole, dobutamine) or for 2–3 hours prior to test (others)
   NCLEX® b. Avoid alcohol, caffeine, and nicotine during NPO status
   NCLEX® c. Instruct client to wear comfortable clothes (shorts or slacks with belt, sneakers or tennis shoes with socks, shirt with buttons in front for ECG electrodes)
   NCLEX® d. Test can be stopped if client has dyspnea, severe fatigue, or chest pain (client should report these), rapid increase in pulse rate or BP, life-threatening dysrhythmias, or palpitations
   e. Make note of any medications, such as beta-blockers, that could interfere with test results
3. Postprocedure care
   a. Return client to department for any follow-up testing
   b. Record VS and ECG tracings at end of test and 5–10 minutes later
   NCLEX® c. Explain client can resume usual activity but may need to avoid strenuous activity or taking hot baths or showers posttest depending on procedure

G. Venography (venogram), also called phlebography

1. Overview
   a. A fluoroscopic or x-ray exam of deep leg veins after contrast dye injection
   b. Detects deep vein thrombosis (DVT) and congenital venous abnormalities and aids in selecting vein for arterial bypass grafting
2. Preprocedure care
   a. NPO for 4 hours before test (some hospitals permit clear liquids)
   b. Provide preprocedure care to clients receiving contrast dye (see again Box 47–1)
   c. Record baseline VS and have client void prior to procedure
   d. Explain that client will lie on x-ray table tilted at 40- to 60-degree angle, tourniquet is applied above ankle, and dye is injected into vein over 2–4 minutes
3. Postprocedure care
   a. Monitor VS until stable, then as per routine, and assess peripheral pulses (femoral, popliteal, dorsalis pedis)
   NCLEX® b. Assess injection site for bleeding, hematoma, or infection (redness, edema, pain); document and report if any of these are found
   NCLEX® c. Elevate extremity as prescribed; if DVT is found, expect prescriptions for bedrest, heparin, leg elevation, and warm, moist compresses

IV. RENAL OR URINARY DIAGNOSTIC TESTS

A. Cystoscopy and cystography (cystogram)

1. Overview
   a. *Cystoscopy* is direct visualization of bladder wall and urethra using a cystoscope (tubular lighted telescopic lens), usually by urologist
   b. *Cystography* is instillation of contrast dye into bladder using a catheter
   c. Purposes are to detect and remove urinary calculi, determine cause of hematuria or urinary tract infection (UTI), and detect tumors or prostatic hyperplasia
2. Preprocedure care
   NCLEX® a. Ensure informed consent is signed before giving premedication (usually 1 hour before test)
   NCLEX® b. Record baseline VS and urine characteristics (amount, color, odor, specific gravity)
   c. Assess for allergy to medications, food, and latex
   NCLEX® d. Explain that procedure will be done under local or general anesthesia; local anesthesia will be injected into urethra several minutes before cystoscope is inserted
   e. Complete preoperative or preprocedure checklist as per agency policy
3. Postprocedure care
   NCLEX® a. Monitor VS every 15 minutes for an hour, then possibly every half-hour until stable
   NCLEX® b. Monitor UO for 48 hours after cystoscopy; increase fluid intake if less than 240 mL in 8 hours; report low UO to provider
   c. Apply heat to lower abdomen to relieve pain and muscle spasm as ordered; explain that some pressure or burning may be present after test
   NCLEX® d. Assess for and report gross hematuria; blood-tinged urine may be expected
   e. Monitor for complications: hemorrhage, bladder perforation, urinary retention, and infection
   NCLEX® f. Explain that slight burning on urination is expected for 1–2 days after procedure; use analgesic if prescribed and avoid alcoholic beverages for 2 days after test (bladder irritant)

B. Intravenous pyelography (IVP)

1. Overview
   a. Also called excretory urography because test visualizes entire urinary tract (not just pelvis of kidney)
   b. Consists of injecting IV radiopaque contrast and taking series of x-rays at specified times (3, 5, 10, 15, and 20 minutes postinjection), and a final x-ray after client voids to visualize residual dye in bladder
   c. Used to identify abnormal kidney size, shape, or function and renal calculi, tumors, and cysts
2. Preprocedure care
   a. Keep client NPO for 8–12 hours prior to test
   NCLEX® b. Administer laxative on evening before test and enema on morning of test as prescribed
   c. Provide preprocedure care to clients receiving contrast dye (see again Box 47–1)
   NCLEX® d. Check blood urea nitrogen (BUN) lab result (test might be canceled if greater than 40 mg/dL [normal 8–22 mg/dL])
NCLEX® 3. Postprocedure care: monitor VS and UO; provide care to client receiving contrast medium (see again Box 47–1)

C. Retrograde pyelography (retrograde pyelogram)

1. Overview
   a. May be performed after or in place of IVP and is usually done in conjunction with cystoscopy
   b. Consists of injecting contrast dye via catheter into ureters and renal pelvis to diagnose suspected nonfunctioning kidney, unlocated calculus, tumor, or renal stricture
2. Preprocedure care
   NCLEX® a. NPO for 8 hours prior to test; some clients may be allowed water to avoid dehydration unless undergoing general anesthesia
   b. Administer laxative and/or cleansing enema as prescribed
   NCLEX® c. Provide preprocedure care to clients receiving contrast medium (see again Box 47–1)
   d. Explain that legs are placed in stirrups; pressure and urge to void (but not pain) may occur when cystoscope is inserted
3. Postprocedure care
   a. Monitor VS and provide postprocedure care to clients receiving contrast medium (see again Box 47–1)
   NCLEX® b. Monitor UO and report if less than 240 mL in 8 hours or if client does not void in 8 hours
   c. Assess for and report hematuria; explain to client that blood-tinged urine is common
   d. Provide prescribed analgesics for pain or discomfort and report severe pain
   NCLEX® e. Observe for and report signs of infection (fever, chills, abdominal pain, tachycardia, and later hypotension)

V. NEUROLOGIC DIAGNOSTIC TESTS

A. *Electroencephalography* (EEG)

1. Overview
   a. Measures electrical impulses produced by brain cells to detect seizure disorder, brain tumor, abscess, and intracranial hemorrhage, and to assist in determinating brain death
   b. Electrodes are applied to scalp and brain activity is recorded on moving paper
   c. Procedure may be performed while client is awake, drowsy, asleep, undergoing stimuli (hyperventilation, flashes of bright light), or combinations of these
2. Preprocedure care
   NCLEX® a. Shampoo hair night before test and instruct client not to use oil or hair spray on hair
   NCLEX® b. Food and fluids are permitted and encouraged (hypoglycemia could affect results) but client may not have alcohol (CNS depressant) or coffee, tea, cola (CNS stimulants) before test
   c. Do not administer sleep aids or other sedatives on night before test because they affect readings; check with provider whether other medications should be given or withheld (such as antiepileptics)
   d. Explain that procedure is painless and may be done with client lying down or seated in reclining chair
   e. Explain electrode placement and that electric shock will not occur; alleviate any client fears including that machine cannot determine intelligence and cannot read client's mind
   NCLEX® f. Observe for and report seizure activity; note whether client is extremely anxious, restless, or upset
3. Postprocedure care
   NCLEX® a. Shampoo client's hair to remove paste or collodion; acetone may be used to remove paste
   b. Allow client to resume normal activity unless client was sedated

B. Myelography (myelogram)

1. Overview
   a. Fluoroscopic and radiologic exam of spinal subarachnoid space (spinal canal) using contrast agent (oil- or water-based)
   b. Detects spinal lesions (herniated intervertebral disks, spinal cysts or tumor, or spinal nerve root injury)
2. Preprocedure care
   NCLEX® a. NPO for 4–8 hours prior to test; client may have light breakfast or clear liquids in morning if test is scheduled for afternoon
   b. Administer cleansing enema if prescribed to remove feces and gas to improve visualization
   c. Administer prescribed premedications such as sedative or narcotic analgesic and atropine
   d. Provide preprocedure care to clients receiving contrast medium (see again Box 47–1)
   NCLEX® e. Explain that spinal puncture will be performed and contrast will be injected; table may be tilted as contrast enters spinal column to enhance visualization of structures
   f. Instruct client to tell healthcare provider of any discomfort (such as pain going down legs)
3. Postprocedure care
   NCLEX® a. Monitor VS until stable per protocol; monitor UO and notify provider if client does not void in 8 hours
   NCLEX® b. Position client properly: keep head of bed flat if oil-based contrast used and elevated to 60 degrees for 8 hours or longer if water-based contrast was used (to prevent irritation from residual dye; oil-based dye is aspirated out but some microdroplets could remain)
   NCLEX® c. Increase fluid intake to excrete contrast via kidneys and to replace lost spinal fluid
   d. Provide postprocedure care to clients receiving contrast media (see again Box 47–1)
   e. Assess for signs of chemical or bacterial meningitis (severe headache, fever, chills, stiff neck, irritability, photophobia, and seizures)
   f. Encourage use of good body mechanics

C. Lumbar puncture (LP or spinal tap)

1. Overview
   a. A procedure in which cerebrospinal fluid is withdrawn through a needle inserted into subarachnoid space of spinal canal at level of L_3–L_4 or L_4–L_5 disk interspace (see Figure 47–4A)
   b. Used to help diagnose multiple sclerosis, subarachnoid hemorrhage, brain tumor or abscess, encephalitis, viral infections, and assess intraspinal pressure
2. Preprocedure care
   a. Assess and document baseline VS; ensure client consent and obtain sterile LP tray
   b. Have client void prior to procedure

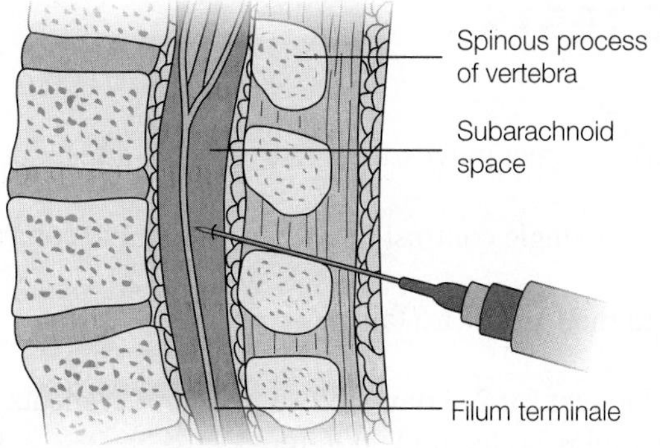

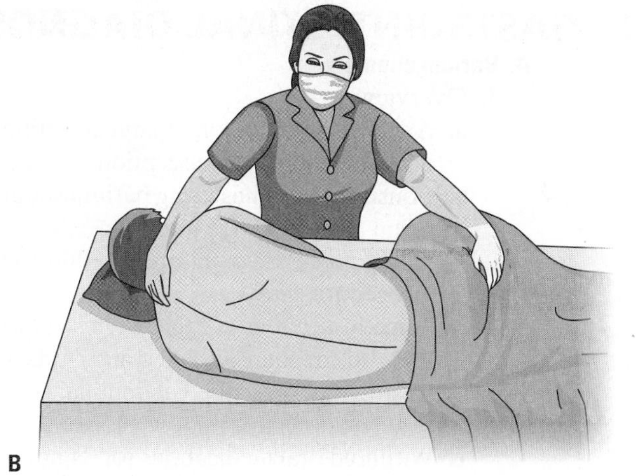

Figure 47–4

Lumbar puncture. (**A**) Needle insertion into spinal subarachnoid space; (**B**) positioning client for lumbar puncture.

NCLEX® c. Assist client to lie on one side in fetal position with head flexed on chest, back bowed, and knees drawn up to abdomen (see Figure 47–4B)
   d. Assist healthcare provider and provide reassurance to client during procedure
3. Postprocedure care
   a. Monitor VS per protocol; apply dressing to site

NCLEX® b. Monitor for and report neurologic changes (irritability, fever, hypertension, nonreactive pupils, numbness or tingling in lower extremities)
   c. Administer prescribed analgesic for headache
   d. Maintain client on bedrest for 4–8 hours with head flat in bed in either a supine or prone position
   e. Monitor puncture site for bleeding, hematoma, or CSF leakage
   f. Encourage increased fluid intake up to 3000 mL/24 hr to replace lost CSF, if not contraindicated by another condition

VI. MUSCULOSKELETAL DIAGNOSTIC TESTS

A. *Arthroscopy*

1. Overview
   a. An endoscopic examination of interior joint (usually knee) using fiberoptic endoscope; usually preceded by arthrography (x-ray exam of joint using air, contrast media, or both)
   b. Used to diagnose and/or surgically treat meniscal, patellar, extrasynovial, and synovial problems
2. Preprocedure care
   a. No food or fluid restriction if done using local anesthetic; NPO after midnight for spinal and general anesthesia
   b. Assess involved skin area for lesion or infection; document and report if found
3. Postprocedure care
   a. Assess VS and local bleeding or swelling; report abnormal findings
   b. Apply covered ice bag to area if prescribed and analgesics for pain or discomfort
   c. Instruct client to rest joint for specified amount of time and avoid excessive use of joint for 2–3 days after procedure; minimize walking

B. Bone densitometry (bone mineral density or BMD)

1. Overview
   a. Detects early osteoporosis by determining density of bone mineral content by dual-energy x-ray absorptiometry (DEXA)
   b. Normal result is determined according to client age, sex, and height
   c. Most frequent population is postmenopausal women, who are at risk for greatest annual bone loss
2. Preprocedure care
   a. Food and fluids do not need to be restricted

NCLEX® b. Teach client to remove all metal objects in area of scan; test takes 30–60 minutes and is not painful
3. Postprocedure care: none

VII. GASTROINTESTINAL DIAGNOSTIC TESTS

A. Barium enema

1. Overview
   a. An x-ray examination of large intestine (colon) to detect polyps, tumor, diverticuli, intestinal stricture or obstruction, intussusception, or ulceration
   b. Consists of administering barium sulfate (alone as single contrast or with air as double contrast) via rectal tube into large intestine
   c. Filling process is monitored by fluoroscopy, and then x-rays are taken

NCLEX®
2. Preprocedure care
   a. Some institutions ask that clients eat low-residue diet for 2–3 days before test (tender meats, eggs, bread, clear soup, pureed bland fruits and vegetables, boiled milk, potatoes)
   b. Ensure that prescribed abdominal x-rays, ultrasound and radionuclide studies, and proctosigmoidoscopy are done prior to this test
   c. Withhold oral medications for 24 hours prior to test unless prescribed by provider
   d. Provide, or instruct client to take, clear liquid diet for 18–24 hours before test and maintain water and clear liquid intake 24 hours prior to maintain hydration
   e. Administer laxatives (such as magnesium citrate) in late afternoon or early evening (4:00–8:00 p.m.) of day before test
   f. Administer cleansing enema or laxative suppository such as bisacodyl on evening before test as ordered
   g. Administer saline enemas in early morning of day of procedure until clear (maximum of three) if prescribed
   h. Black coffee or tea is permitted up to 1 hour prior to test
3. Postprocedure care
   a. Instruct client to try to expel barium in bathroom or on bedpan immediately after test

NCLEX®
   b. Increase fluid intake for hydration and to prevent constipation from retained barium

NCLEX®
   c. Administer ordered laxative or oil retention enema to expel barium; laxative may need to be repeated on day following test

B. Cholangiography

1. Overview
   a. May be done as IV, percutaneous, or T-tube cholangiography
   b. IV test examines biliary ducts to detect strictures, stones, or tumor, but gallbladder may not be well visualized
   c. Percutaneous test is indicated when biliary obstruction is indicated because contrast is injected directly into biliary tree
   d. T-tube test may be done 7–8 hours after cholecystectomy to explore common bile duct for patency and determine if any gallstones are blocking duct after gallbladder removal; dye is injected into T-shaped tube, which is placed into common bile duct during surgery to promote drainage
2. Preprocedure care
   a. NPO for 8 hours prior to test
   b. Take usual precautions regarding allergy to contrast media
   c. Provide laxative (evening before test) and cleansing enema (morning of test) as prescribed; for T-tube test, only cleansing enema may be prescribed
3. Postprocedure care
   a. Monitor VS per protocol and instruct client to remain in bed for 6 hours after percutaneous test
   b. T-tube may or may not be taken out after procedure
   c. Provide postprocedure care to clients receiving contrast medium (see again Box 47–1); otherwise, no specific aftercare is indicated

C. Cholecystography (oral)

1. Overview
   a. An x-ray test to visualize stones in gallbladder or determine obstruction in cystic duct
   b. Oral contrast medium is administered, which concentrates in gallbladder in 12–14 hours
   c. Specific sequence of dietary instructions must be followed for best results
   d. Liver disease, inadequate client preparation, obstruction of cystic duct, and diarrhea (eliminates contrast agent) can interfere with results
2. Preprocedure care

NCLEX®
   a. Assess allergy history; assess for signs of jaundice (yellow sclera, skin or serum bilirubin greater than 3 mg/dL); notify provider if found

b. Provide fat-free diet for 24 hours before test (some agencies suggest high-fat meal at noon to empty gallbladder and low-fat meal in evening)

NCLEX®

c. Begin NPO status with sips of water after dinner the evening before test

d. Administer radiopaque tablets 2 hours after dinner according to package directions with total of 240 mL (8 oz) of water

e. Saline enema may be prescribed on morning of test in some agencies to clear GI tract

f. Explain to client that fasting x-rays will be taken and then high-fat meal or fat-containing substances will be given in x-ray department; follow-up x-rays will be done over next 1–2 hours to monitor gallbladder emptying

g. Explain that test does not cause discomfort

h. Explain that client should not become alarmed if test needs to be repeated but should remain on low-fat diet until repeat test is completed

3. Postprocedure care: none specific

D. *Colonoscopy*

1. Overview

a. A procedure to view colon using long, flexible fiberoptic endoscope to detect tumors, polyps, diverticulitis, inflammatory bowel disease, and lower GI bleeding

b. Tube is inserted anally and advanced through rectum, sigmoid colon, and large intestine to cecum, and air is used to insufflate area for better visualization

2. Preprocedure care

a. Withhold medications that interfere with coagulation (aspirin, NSAIDs) and alcohol 1 week prior to test

b. Explain that another person must be available to drive client home if performed on outpatient basis

c. Follow preprocedure preparation: clear liquid diet for 24 hours before test; bowel preparation (using citrate of magnesia, laxatives, or polyethylene glycol) on day before test to clear bowel of feces; and NPO after midnight

d. Avoid soap solution enemas, which could irritate wall of colon

e. Record baseline VS

NCLEX®

f. Explain that client will lie in Sims or left lateral position, will receive IV moderate sedation immediately before test

3. Postprocedure care

a. Monitor VS and report abnormal changes

b. Do not administer anything by mouth following IV moderate sedation until cough, gag, and swallow reflexes have returned

c. Assess for and report anal bleeding, abdominal distention, severe pain or abdominal cramps, or fever; increased flatus is expected

NCLEX®

d. Maintain client safety postsedation

e. If polyps were removed during procedure, instruct client to avoid high-fiber foods for 1–2 days and avoid heavy lifting for 7 days

E. Endoscopic retrograde cholangiopancreatography (ERCP)

1. Overview

a. Examines biliary and pancreatic ducts endoscopically after injection of contrast medium into duodenal papilla

b. Identifies causes of biliary obstruction (jaundice usually present), such as stricture, cyst, stones, tumor

c. May be done as follow-up to ultrasound, CT scan, liver scan, or biliary tract x-rays

2. Preprocedure care

a. Maintain NPO status for 8 hours prior to test

b. Obtain baseline VS and assess for allergies to contrast media

c. Ensure that informed consent is obtained and that client voids before premedication (mild sedative or narcotic and atropine, usually)

NCLEX®

d. Explain that local anesthetic is sprayed in throat to decrease gag reflex prior to insertion of endoscope

3. Postprocedure care

a. Monitor VS including temperature (fever could indicate infection) and respiratory rate (respiratory status could be compromised from anesthetic spray in throat and/or endoscope)

NCLEX®

b. Ensure cough, gag, and swallow reflexes are present before offering food and fluids

c. Provide warm saline gargles or lozenges to reduce sore throat caused by endoscope; may be needed for a few days

NCLEX®

d. Note and report presence of persistent abdominal pain, discomfort, or fullness

F. Esophagogastroduodenoscopy

1. Overview
   a. Also includes or is known as gastroscopy, esophagoscopy, esophagogastroscopy, duodenoscopy, endoscopy
   b. Directly visualizes esophagus, stomach, and duodenum with flexible fiberoptic endoscope
   c. Used to diagnose esophageal, gastric, or duodenal disease; diverticulosis or *H. pylori* infection; to obtain cytologic specimens; or to remove foreign bodies
2. Preprocedure care
   NCLEX® a. NPO status for 8–12 hours before test; if done as emergency and NPO status not possible, perform stomach lavage/suction to prevent aspiration
   b. Record baseline VS and have client void
   c. Administer any prescribed premedication; client's usual prescribed medications may often be taken at 6:00 a.m. on day of test; check with provider
   NCLEX® d. Give client hospital gown to wear and remove dentures, eyeglasses, and jewelry; note any loose teeth
   e. Explain that client may feel some pressure with insertion of scope, but that IV sedation and local anesthetic to throat will be used
3. Postprocedure care
   NCLEX® a. NPO for 2–4 hours after test as prescribed; ensure that gag and swallow reflexes have returned before offering fluids or food
   b. Monitor VS
   c. Explain that "burping up air" or passing gas is expected because air is instilled during procedure to visualize area
   d. Provide gargles, lozenges, or analgesics for throat discomfort, which is expected and caused by endoscope
   e. Observe for possible complications, such as perforated GI tract; assess for and report epigastric, abdominal, or back pain; dyspnea; fever; tachycardia; and subcutaneous emphysema in neck

G. Gastric analysis

1. Overview
   a. Examines acidity of gastric secretions via nasogastric (NG) tube during basal state (without stimulation) and at peak secretion (with drug stimulation)
   b. Decreased levels indicate pernicious anemia, gastric malignancy, and atrophic gastritis
   c. Increased levels indicate peptic ulcer (duodenal) or Zollinger-Ellison syndrome
2. Basal gastric analysis
   NCLEX® a. NPO for 8–12 hours prior to test and restrict smoking for 8 hours
   b. Restrict selected drugs (antacids, steroids, cholinergics, and anticholinergics) and coffee and alcohol for at least 24 hours prior; note on test request form if not complied with
   c. Record baseline VS and remove loose dentures
   d. Insert NG tube; obtain residual gastric specimen and four additional specimens 15 minutes apart
   e. Label first set of specimens as basal specimens with client name, date, time, and specimen number
3. Stimulation test (a continuation of basal gastric analysis test)
   a. Administer gastric stimulant such as histamine or pentagastrin
   b. Obtain four to eight specimens 15 minutes apart depending on agent used
   c. Label peak specimens obtained after stimulation with client name, date, time, and specimen number
   d. Monitor VS postprocedure; remove NG tube if inserted only for test

H. Gastrointestinal (GI) series

1. Overview
   a. Also known as upper GI series, barium swallow, or small bowel series
   b. Consists of fluoroscopic and x-ray exams of esophagus, stomach, and small intestine after ingestion of oral barium sulfate or water-soluble contrast such as gastrografin
   c. Used to detect ulcers, polyps, tumors, strictures, hiatal hernia, foreign bodies, or esophageal varices
2. Preprocedure care
   NCLEX® a. Low-residue diet may be prescribed for 2–3 days prior to test
   NCLEX® b. Maintain NPO status with no smoking for 8–12 hours before test
   c. Withhold medications for 8 hours before test unless otherwise prescribed; withhold narcotics and anticholinergics for 24 hours (reduce gastric motility)
   d. Administer laxatives as prescribed on evening before test
   e. Explain that client swallows a chalk-flavored (chocolate or strawberry) barium meal or gastrografin and x-rays are taken periodically over 1–2 or 4–6 hours depending on length of area to be visualized; follow-up film (post–GI series) at 24 hours may be prescribed as well

3. Postprocedure care
   a. Check with radiology department that studies are completed before giving late breakfast or late lunch
   NCLEX® b. Administer prescribed laxative following test to excrete barium
   NCLEX® c. Explain to client that stool will be light in color for some days after test and to notify provider if no bowel movement within 2–3 days

VIII. REPRODUCTIVE DIAGNOSTIC TESTS

A. Fetal nonstress test (NST)

1. Overview
   a. Evaluates fetal functioning and well-being in response to fetal movement
   b. Inexpensive, rapidly accomplished, lacks side effects, and helps identify at-risk fetuses for mothers with high-risk pregnancy conditions (such as diabetes and gestational hypertension)
   c. Monitors fetal heart rate (FHR) with fetal movement (should accelerate 15 beats/min for 15 seconds)
   d. If FHR does not increase within 20 minutes, can rub mother's abdomen or make loud noise nearby to stimulate fetal movement
   e. If no increase in FHR after 40 minutes, test indicates a nonreactive fetus; normal is a reactive fetus
2. Preprocedure care
   a. Obtain informed consent and measure baseline VS and FHR
   b. Position mother in semi-Fowler or lateral position with roll or wedge under right hip to displace uterus to left slightly
   NCLEX® c. Instruct client to press pressure transducer when she feels fetus move so FHR acceleration can be monitored
3. Postprocedure care: encourage client to rest; provide general instruction to report bleeding, continuous contractions, or lack of fetal movement
4. Nonreactive test may be followed up with contraction stress test
   a. Evaluates fetal functioning during spontaneous or induced uterine contractions
   b. May also be performed as routine test for selected high-risk mothers
   c. Uses nipple stimulation or oxytocin to stimulate uterine contraction
   NCLEX® d. Normal result is absence of late decelerations in FHR during three contractions; presence of late decelerations indicates condition that leads to placental dysfunction or insufficient blood supply

B. Hysteroscopy

1. Overview
   a. Visualizes uterine cavity; allows for endometrial biopsy or polyp removal
   b. Contraindicated with cervical or vaginal infection, pelvic inflammatory disease, purulent vaginal discharge, or if cervical surgery performed previously
   c. Risks to procedure include perforation of uterus and infection
2. Preprocedure care
   a. Obtain menstrual history because test should be done after menses but before ovulation
   b. Restrict food and fluids for 8 hours before test
   c. Have client void before test
   d. Explain that client will be in lithotomy position; hysteroscope will be inserted and carbon dioxide will be instilled to distend uterus for visualization
3. Postprocedure care
   a. Monitor VS and assess for excessive bleeding or discharge
   b. Explain that cramping may occur following test and mild analgesic will reduce discomfort; report severe discomfort or shortness of breath immediately
   c. Advise to avoid sexual intercourse or douching for 2 weeks or as instructed by provider

C. Mammography

1. Overview
   a. X-ray examination of breasts to detect cysts or tumors
   b. Detects approximately 90% of breast malignancies
   NCLEX® c. Frequency is determined by current evidence and client's individual history
2. Preprocedure care
   a. Food and fluids are not restricted prior to test
   NCLEX® b. Instruct client not to use ointment, powder, or deodorant on breasts or underarms on day of test; client will need to remove clothes to waist and wear a paper gown that opens in front
   c. Explain that procedure will not cause pain but some discomfort may occur during breast compression

- **d.** Explain that client will need to wait while films are developed, and reassure client that additional films are sometimes needed and not to be alarmed

3. Postprocedure care: none specific

D. Papanicolaou (Pap) smear

1. Overview
- **a.** A cytologic test to detect precancerous lesions or cancerous cells of cervix
- **b.** Also identifies viral, fungal, and parasitic conditions and evaluates response to chemotherapy or radiation therapy

2. Preprocedure care
- **a.** Food and fluids are not restricted
- *NCLEX®* **b.** Client should not douche, insert vaginal medications, or have sexual intercourse for 24 hours before test
- **c.** Obtain menstrual history, including any problems, and document whether or not client is taking any hormones or oral contraceptives
- **d.** Ask client to remove all clothes; provide paper gown; breast examination is done after Pap smear is taken
- **e.** Explain that client will lie on examining table in lithotomy position and speculum will be inserted into vagina to aid in specimen collection

3. Postprocedure care: none specific; provide tissues so client can remove lubricant before dressing

IX. INTEGUMENTARY DIAGNOSTIC TESTS

A. Tuberculin skin test

1. Overview
- **a.** Screens for tuberculosis
- **b.** Tine test or Mono-Vacc test is multipuncture test that uses tines impregnated with purified protein derivative (PPD); used for mass screening and is read in 48–72 hours
- *NCLEX®* **c.** Mantoux test involves injection of PPD intradermally using a tuberculin (1 mL) syringe with a 25- to 27-gauge needle; read in 48–72 hours

2. Preprocedure care
- **a.** Food and fluids are not restricted
- *NCLEX®* **b.** Assess whether client has tested positive to test before; test should only be performed if previous results were negative
- **c.** Cleanse inner aspect of forearm with alcohol and let dry before injecting 0.1 mL of antigen intradermally

3. Postprocedure care
- *NCLEX®* **a.** Explain that client needs to return to have results read in 48–72 hours; a 72-hour reading is more accurate; client may be asked to return for reading at 72 hours if 48-hour result is questionable
- *NCLEX®* **b.** Explain that positive test does not always indicate active infectious disease but that organism is present in body in either an active or dormant state; follow-up x-ray and sputum cultures are indicated

B. Other skin tests

1. Include tests for blastomycosis, coccidioidomycosis, histoplasmosis, trichinosis, and toxoplasmosis

2. Procedures are similar to that described above for tuberculosis

NCLEX® **3.** For allergy skin tests, injected area may be outlined with a marker and a diagram made of injection sites, especially if more than one antigen is planted concurrently; antihistamines are withheld 3–4 days prior to avoid false negatives

Check Your NCLEX–RN® Exam I.Q.

You are ready for testing on this content if you can:

- Apply knowledge from foundational sciences to the care of clients undergoing diagnostic testing.
- Correlate client pathophysiology with specific nursing interventions needed before and after diagnostic testing.
- Assess a client appropriately before and after diagnostic testing.
- Compare the results of client assessments before and after diagnostic testing.
- Monitor the results of serial or periodic diagnostic tests.
- Reinforce client teaching about diagnostic tests.

PRACTICE TEST

1 A client is about to undergo skin biopsy to determine if a skin lesion is malignant. The client asks how much the biopsy will hurt. Which response by the nurse is best?

1. "We will give you a pain pill in just a moment that will minimize any pain during the biopsy."
2. "Luckily, this type of procedure does not cause any pain for most people."
3. "You may feel some discomfort while the local anesthetic is injected, but this will numb the area for the actual biopsy."
4. "The procedure is fairly painful, but you can manage it afterward with acetaminophen."

2 The client is about to undergo a computed tomography (CT) scan of the head with contrast. Which question by the nurse is most important to ask while preparing the client for the test?

1. "Have you ever had a procedure like this before?"
2. "Do you have an allergy to iodine?"
3. "Would you like something to drink before you leave the unit?"
4. "Have you voided in the bathroom in the last few hours?"

3 The client is scheduled for a magnetic resonance imaging (MRI) study of the spine. The outpatient nurse gives the client which instructions as part of preprocedure care? Select all that apply.

1. "Do not eat anything after midnight the day before the test."
2. "You will be able to drive yourself home after the test."
3. "Expect to stay in the MRI department for an hour afterward for observation."
4. "Do not wear any metal, such as jewelry or hairclips."
5. "Do not drink any liquids for 6 hours before the test."

4 A client will undergo a radionuclide scan of the thyroid. A nursing assistant asks what needs to be done to protect staff from any residual radiation after the scan. What is an appropriate response by the nurse? Select all that apply.

1. "Everyone must stand 6 feet away from the client for 24 hours. I should put a sign above the bed."
2. "Using standard precautions for handling body fluids will be sufficient to protect staff."
3. "I have arranged for the client to be moved to a private room for 48 hours after the test."
4. "The client will need to be on contact precautions. Can you call the central processing department for a cart with gowns and gloves?"
5. "The amount of residual radiation is quite small."

5 A 17-year-old girl is brought to the emergency department for x-rays after twisting her ankle. Which question is most important for the nurse to ask the client before sending her to the radiology department?

1. "Do you experience claustrophobia when in small spaces?"
2. "Are you wearing any necklaces or other metal objects?"
3. "When was your last monthly period?"
4. "Have you ever had an x-ray before?"

6 A female client is returning to the nursing unit following a pelvic ultrasound. What should the nurse plan to do for the client at this time? Select all that apply.

1. Make the client comfortable.
2. Instruct the client to drink at least one quart of water over the next hour.
3. Explain that analgesic medication is available to relieve the expected cramping pain.
4. Tell the client that she will be able to eat in 1 hour.
5. Ask the client if she needs anything.

7 A client who underwent bronchoscopy 4 hours ago is asking for something to drink to ease a sore throat. The nurse obtains some juice for the client after noting which assessment data?

1. Respiratory rate has ranged from 16 to 18.
2. Breath sounds are clear bilaterally.
3. The client has had no hemoptysis.
4. Gag and swallow reflexes have returned.

8 A client underwent angiography of the left leg. Which data obtained during the current assessment is of concern to the nurse? Select all that apply.

1. Skin paler on left foot than right.
2. Skin temperature cooler on left foot than right.
3. Left dorsalis pedis pulse audible by Doppler, previously 2.
4. Dressing at femoral access site has trace amount of dark red blood.
5. Client reports slight numbness and tingling in the left leg.

9 The client who will undergo a cardiac catheterization says to the nurse: "I am nervous about having a cardiac catheterization. Can you tell me what to expect?" Which response by the nurse is appropriate? Select all that apply.

1. "The procedure will be done in the operating room to help ensure sterile conditions."
2. "The room will be brightly lit at all times."
3. "The insertion of the catheter in the femoral area will be one of the few painful moments of the procedure."
4. "The provider will ask you to lie still except to do specific things, such as cough or take a deep breath."
5. "There will be a fluoroscopy screen in the room, which the staff may look at during the procedure."

10 A client scheduled for a cardiac echocardiogram at 9:00 a.m. the next day asks whether eating breakfast before the test is allowed. What response by the nurse is appropriate?

1. "Yes, we can arrange for your breakfast tray to arrive a half-hour early so that you have time to eat before the test."
2. "Yes, but you will need to get up at 5:00 a.m. so that you will be without food or fluids for 4 hours before the test."
3. "Yes, but you can only drink clear liquids, such as apple juice, and you cannot eat solid food until after the test."
4. "No, you cannot eat or drink before the test, but you can have a full breakfast after the test."

11 A client has just received a Holter cardiac monitor to wear for the next 24 hours. The nurse determines that the client understands its use when the client makes which statement?

1. "I should write in the diary what I am doing every half-hour."
2. "I should only take a bath, not a shower, for the next 24 hours."
3. "I can continue with my usual activity and exercise pattern while wearing the monitor."
4. "I need to try to walk a total of 3 miles over the next 24 hours while wearing the monitor."

12 A client who underwent cystography 16 hours ago has a urinary output of 180 mL in the previous 8 hours. Which actions should the nurse take at this time? Select all that apply.

1. Measure the specific gravity of the urine.
2. Document the volume on the client's flowsheet.
3. Encourage the client to drink more fluids.
4. Notify the healthcare provider.
5. Compare the output to the client's intake during the previous shift.

13 The nurse has assigned an unlicensed assistant to work with a client who just returned to the nursing unit at 0945 after electroencephalography. What direction should the nurse give the assistant regarding care to the client?

1. "Do not give any food or fluids until lunchtime."
2. "Wash the client's hair at your earliest opportunity."
3. "Keep the client on bedrest for the remainder of the shift."
4. "Encourage the client to drink fluids to flush dye through the kidneys."

14 A client has just returned to the nursing unit after a myelogram using water-based contrast to diagnose a herniated intervertebral disk. The nurse should assist the client to which position in bed after transferring from the stretcher?

1. Supine, with the head of the bed elevated 60 degrees
2. Supine, with the head of the bed elevated 15 degrees
3. Left side-lying, with the head of the bed flat
4. Any position of the client's choice, with the head of the bed elevated 30 degrees

15 A client has received discharge instructions after undergoing arthroscopy of the knee earlier in the day. The nurse concludes that the client understands self-care after discharge when the client makes which statement?

1. "I should not expect to need pain medication following this procedure."
2. "I should apply warm, moist heat to my knee to maintain comfort."
3. "I should limit my activities, including walking, for 2–3 days."
4. "I should expect increased swelling and perhaps some bleeding in the knee area after going home."

16 A client with gastroesophageal reflux disease has just undergone esophagogastroscopy. The nurse places highest priority on continuing to monitor which client data?

1. Inability to swallow saliva
2. Temperature of 99.4°F (37.4°C) oral
3. Client report of heartburn
4. Client report of sore throat

17 The nurse has given instructions to a client who will have a barium swallow in 3 days. The nurse determines that the client understands how to properly prepare for the test after the client makes which statement?

1. "I should eat a low-fat meal for 2 days, and then have clear liquids the day before the test."
2. "I should stop taking all medication except antacids the day before the test."
3. "I should not eat or drink anything after midnight just prior to the test."
4. "I should eat a high-carbohydrate diet for 3 days before the test."

18 The nurse is providing instructions to a client who is returning home following a colonoscopy. Which statement would be appropriate for the nurse to include? Select all that apply.

1. "You may drive in about 6 hours, after the medication given during the procedure has fully worn off."
2. "It is all right to eat and drink, but it is helpful to resume the diet gradually."
3. "You should call the healthcare provider if you feel distended or begin passing gas."
4. "Bleeding from the rectum is expected after this procedure, but call the healthcare provider if it gets severe."
5. "Avoid activities requiring mental alertness for 24 hours after the test."

19 The nurse would give which instruction regarding preprocedure care to a woman who is scheduled for a mammogram?

1. "Drink liquids, but don't eat breakfast on the morning of the mammogram."
2. "Do not use any lotions or deodorant on the chest or underarms before the mammogram."
3. "Take a mild analgesic such as acetaminophen before coming in for the mammogram."
4. "Plan a light schedule for the day of the mammogram, so you can rest after the procedure."

20 The nurse has given an intradermal injection of purified protein derivative (PPD) to a client to screen for tuberculosis. After noting that the current day is Monday, when should the nurse instruct the client to return to have the result read?

1. Tuesday or Wednesday
2. Wednesday or Thursday
3. Thursday or Friday
4. Friday or the following Monday

21 A client will undergo basal gastric acid secretion analysis. The client is taking several medications. Which types of drugs should the nurse withhold prior to the test? Select all that apply.

1. Anticholinergic
2. Cardiac glycoside
3. Antacid
4. Diuretic
5. Corticosteroid

ANSWERS & RATIONALES

1 **Answer: 3 Rationale:** The area is anesthetized using a local anesthetic before skin biopsy, so the client should only feel discomfort while the anesthetic is administered. Analgesics are not given before the procedure. The procedure is not pain-free. The client may take medication such as acetaminophen following the procedure, but this does not address the client's question about pain during the procedure. **Cognitive Level:** Analyzing **Client Need:** Reduction of Risk Potential **Integrated Process:** Communication and Documentation **Content Area:** Adult Health: Integumentary **Strategy:** The core issue of the question is pain during skin biopsy. Use knowledge that local anesthesia is used during the procedure to make your selection.

2 **Answer: 2 Rationale:** Because a contrast agent will be used for the test, it is most important for the nurse to ask about an allergy to iodine. While it is good to know if the client has had a similar test to determine possible anxiety, it is not the priority. The client should not have anything to eat or drink for 4 hours prior to the test. It is generally helpful for the client to void before leaving the unit to avoid having to do so during the test, but this is a lower-priority item than assessing for allergy. **Cognitive Level:** Analyzing **Client Need:** Reduction of Risk Potential **Integrated Process:** Nursing Process: Assessment **Content Area:** Adult Health: Neurologic **Strategy:** The core issue of the question is knowledge that a client who is allergic to iodine may have an allergic reaction to iodinated contrast media. Memorize this important point if this question was difficult.

3 **Answer: 2, 4 Rationale:** The client can drive home after the test. Because the MRI scanner uses magnets, the client cannot wear any metal, and clients who have implanted metal might be ineligible for this study. The client does not need to withhold food after midnight on the evening before the test. The client does not need to remain in the department for additional observation after the test. The client does not need to withhold fluids before the test. **Cognitive Level:** Applying **Client Need:** Reduction of Risk Potential **Integrated Process:** Communication and Documentation **Content Area:** Adult Health: Musculoskeletal **Strategy:** The core issues of the question are that the client does not need to withhold food or fluids before the test, and also that metal cannot be worn in the vicinity of an MRI scanner because of the magnetic field. Note the wording of the question suggests more than one option is likely to be correct.

4 **Answer: 2, 5 Rationale:** The amount of residual radioactivity following radionuclide scanning is very small, and poses no risk to visitors or staff. Using standard precautions in handling blood or body fluids is sufficient for protection. It is unnecessary to stand 6 feet away from the client, use a private room, or place the client on contact precautions. **Cognitive Level:** Applying **Client Need:** Reduction of Risk Potential **Integrated Process:** Communication and Documentation **Content Area:** Adult Health: Endocrine and Metabolic **Strategy:** The core issue of the question is knowledge that the amount of radioactivity following radionuclide imaging is very small. With this in mind, eliminate each of the incorrect options, which contain excessive and unnecessary steps for protection of staff.

5 **Answer: 3 Rationale:** The most important question is to determine whether the client could be pregnant, since x-rays are contraindicated during pregnancy, especially during the first trimester. Asking about fear of small or enclosed spaces would be important for MRI machines and possibly for CT scanning machines. The question second in importance would be whether the client is wearing any metal, but possible pregnancy is a priority. It is helpful, but not of highest priority, to know if the client has had an x-ray before, to alleviate concerns. **Cognitive Level:** Analyzing **Client Need:** Reduction of Risk Potential **Integrated Process:** Nursing Process: Assessment **Content Area:** Adult Health: Musculoskeletal **Strategy:** The core issue of the question is knowledge that x-rays are contraindicated during pregnancy. Note the critical words *most important* in the question, which indicates more than one option could be correct, and you must prioritize your answer. Use knowledge of x-rays and the process of elimination to make a selection.

6 **Answer: 1, 5 Rationale:** There is no special aftercare following pelvic ultrasound. For this reason, the nurse should make the client comfortable and ask if she needs anything before leaving the room. The client does not need to drink fluids, should not have cramping pains, and does not need to wait an hour before eating. **Cognitive Level:** Applying **Client Need:** Reduction of Risk Potential **Integrated Process:** Nursing Process: Planning **Content Area:** Adult Health: Renal or Genitourinary **Strategy:** The core issue of the question is knowledge that there is no special aftercare following ultrasound. Use nursing knowledge and the process of elimination to answer. Note the wording of the question suggests that more than one option is likely to be correct.

7 **Answer: 4 Rationale:** Before offering food or fluids to a client following bronchoscopy, it is essential to ensure that gag and swallow reflexes have returned. A local anesthetic is used to numb the throat to ease passage of the bronchoscope, and if protective reflexes have not returned, the client could aspirate. A normal respiratory rate is unrelated to whether the client can eat or drink after the procedure. Clear breath sounds are normal and are assessed during routine monitoring of the client. Absence of hemoptysis is a favorable sign that the client may be free of complications from the procedure, but is not related to resuming oral intake. **Cognitive Level:** Analyzing **Client Need:** Reduction of Risk Potential **Integrated Process:** Nursing Process: Assessment **Content Area:** Adult Health: Respiratory **Strategy:** The core issue of the question is knowledge that gag and swallow reflexes need to be present before offering clients food or beverages to prevent aspiration. Think of gag and swallow reflexes as a possible priority concern whenever a client has had a procedure ending in *-oscopy*.

8 **Answer: 1, 2, 3, 5 Rationale:** Paler skin on the affected extremity is an adverse neurovascular change and should be of concern to the nurse. Cooler skin temperature can occur with decreased peripheral perfusion and should be investigated further. A diminishing strength of the dorsalis pedis pulse indicates that blood flow to the affected leg is decreased. Slight numbness and tingling in the affected leg is an adverse neurovascular change that may be the result of diminished local blood flow after the procedure. A bandage that has a small amount of old blood is expected and is not of concern at this time. **Cognitive Level:** Analyzing **Client Need:** Reduction of Risk Potential **Integrated Process:** Nursing Process:

Diagnosis **Content Area:** Adult Health: Cardiovascular **Strategy:** The core issue of the question is adverse change in the neurovascular status of a client who underwent angiography. The critical words in the stem of the question are *of concern*, which guides you to look for data that is abnormal. Note that the wording of the question indicates that more than one option is likely to be correct.

9 **Answer: 4, 5 Rationale:** The client is asked to lie still except for specific requests, such as to cough or deep-breathe to aid in catheter movement, or to terminate cardiac dysrhythmias caused by irritation of the catheter. The fluoroscopy screen may be used to view catheter movement and also the flow of dye after injection. The procedure is done in a special cardiac catheterization room in the radiology department, not in the operating room. The lights in the room may be dimmed at times so catheter movement can be visualized on a fluoroscopy screen. The catheter insertion site is anesthetized with a local anesthetic, so the client should feel pressure but not pain. **Cognitive Level:** Applying **Client Need:** Reduction of Risk Potential **Integrated Process:** Teaching and Learning **Content Area:** Adult Health: Cardiovascular **Strategy:** The core issue of the question is knowledge of typical events during a cardiac catheterization. Knowledge of these factors helps alleviate client fears. Use nursing knowledge and the process of elimination to make a selection.

10 **Answer: 1 Rationale:** There is no restriction of food or fluids prior to a cardiac (or any) echocardiogram. This test uses sound waves emitted from and reflected back to a transducer, and it is noninvasive. The client does not need to be NPO for 4 hours before the test. There is no need for a clear liquid restriction in the diet. The client does not have to wait until after the test to eat or drink. **Cognitive Level:** Analyzing **Client Need:** Reduction of Risk Potential **Integrated Process:** Teaching and Learning **Content Area:** Adult Health: Cardiovascular **Strategy:** The core issue of the question is knowledge of client preparation for echocardiography. Recall that this is a noninvasive test and uses only ultrasound waves (and thus has no special restrictions) to eliminate each of the incorrect options.

11 **Answer: 3 Rationale:** The client should go about his usual daily activities and exercise pattern while wearing the monitor, and should record activities and any symptoms experienced in the diary. The client does not need to make diary entries every 30 minutes, but as needed to provide an overview of activity so that it can be correlated with any cardiac abnormalities on the time-stamped electrocardiogram being recorded. The client should not take a bath or a shower while wearing the device, which has electrical circuitry. The client does not need to walk a total of 3 miles during the 24-hour period. **Cognitive Level:** Analyzing **Client Need:** Reduction of Risk Potential **Integrated Process:** Nursing Process: Evaluation **Content Area:** Adult Health: Cardiovascular **Strategy:** The core issue of the question is knowledge of proper use of a Holter monitor. The wording of the question indicates only one option is a correct statement. Use nursing knowledge and the process of elimination to make a selection.

12 **Answer: 2, 3, 4, 5 Rationale:** The urine output should be documented on the flowsheet as a routine nursing action. Because the urine output is 60 mL less than the expected minimum urine output of 240 mL in 8 hours, the nurse should encourage the client to drink additional fluids. The nurse should notify the healthcare provider because the urine output is only 75% of the minimum volume (240 mL) that is acceptable in an 8-hour period. It is appropriate to compare the client's fluid intake to the urine output to determine if insufficient intake is a contributing cause. Measuring the urine specific gravity is not a routine nursing action at this time. **Cognitive Level:** Analyzing **Client Need:** Reduction of Risk Potential **Integrated Process:** Nursing Process: Implementation **Content Area:** Adult Health: Renal and Genitourinary **Strategy:** The critical words in the question are *at this time*. The wording of the question also suggests that more than one answer is likely to be correct. Use this nursing knowledge of routine actions for decreased urine output to make a selection.

13 **Answer: 2 Rationale:** The unlicensed assistant should wash the client's hair to remove the paste or colloidon that was used to secure the electrodes to the head for the diagnostic test. The client should be able to eat and drink as usual. The client can resume usual activity unless otherwise prescribed. There is no dye used in this diagnostic test. **Cognitive Level:** Applying **Client Need:** Reduction of Risk Potential **Integrated Process:** Nursing Process: Implementation **Content Area:** Adult Health: Neurologic **Strategy:** Recall that electroencephalography requires no special aftercare except to cleanse the client's scalp because of the electrode paste. Use this knowledge and the process of elimination to make a selection.

14 **Answer: 1 Rationale:** Following myelogram with water-based contrast, the client lies supine and the head of the bed needs to be elevated to 60 degrees to reduce the risk of meningeal irritation from any residual contrast in the spinal fluid. A head of the bed raised to 15 degrees is an insufficient amount of head elevation to prevent headache from meningeal irritation as a complication of the procedure. If an oil-based contrast was used, the head of the bed would need to remain flat. Using any position of the client's choice, even with head elevated to 30 degrees, might not prevent meningeal irritation. **Cognitive Level:** Applying **Client Need:** Reduction of Risk Potential **Integrated Process:** Nursing Process: Implementation **Content Area:** Adult Health: Neurological **Strategy:** The core issue of the question is knowledge of correct head position following myelogram using water-based contrast. Use nursing knowledge and the process of elimination to make a selection.

15 **Answer: 3 Rationale:** The client should limit joint movement, including walking, for 2–3 days after arthroscopy. Analgesics are often needed to manage pain, and the client should be instructed about what to use and how often to take it. The healthcare provider may prescribe ice to control swelling, but not heat, which would aggravate swelling. Increased swelling and bleeding after discharge should be reported, because these are abnormal findings and could indicate a complication of the procedure. **Cognitive Level:** Analyzing **Client Need:** Reduction of Risk Potential **Integrated Process:** Nursing Process: Evaluation **Content Area:** Adult Health: Musculoskeletal **Strategy:** The core issue of the question is knowledge of measures to prevent complications and aid healing after arthroscopy. Use nursing knowledge about postarthroscopy care and the process of elimination to make a selection.

16 **Answer: 1 Rationale:** Because the throat is anesthetized so the client can tolerate the endoscope, the client's gag and swallow reflexes are temporarily lost during any upper endoscopy procedure, such as esophagogastroscopy. The nurse's priority is to monitor for return of these protective airway reflexes. While mildly elevated temperature and reports of heartburn also warrant continued monitoring, they are of lesser priority than concerns related to the client's airway. A temporary sore throat is expected and warrants routine

follow-up assessment. **Cognitive Level:** Analyzing **Client Need:** Reduction of Risk Potential **Integrated Process:** Nursing Process: Assessment **Content Area:** Adult Health: Gastrointestinal **Strategy:** Use the ABCs (airway, breathing, and circulation) to answer the question. Options that involve the airway are frequently the highest priority items. Use nursing knowledge and the process of elimination to make a selection.

17 **Answer: 3 Rationale:** The client should not eat or drink anything for 8–12 hours before the test, so the client should not eat or drink anything after midnight. A low-fat diet is unnecessary before this test. Oral medications including antacids are usually withheld before the procedure. A high-carbohydrate diet does not provide any benefit in preparation for this test. **Cognitive Level:** Analyzing **Client Need:** Reduction of Risk Potential **Integrated Process:** Nursing Process: Evaluation **Content Area:** Adult Health: Gastrointestinal **Strategy:** The core issue of the question is knowledge of dietary preparation before a barium swallow or upper GI series. Use ordinary logic to determine that the GI organs would be difficult to visualize if they contained food or fluid. Use nursing knowledge and the process of elimination to make a selection.

18 **Answer: 2, 5 Rationale:** The diet may be resumed after colonoscopy, but the client usually tolerates it better if it is resumed gradually. The client should not drive or perform other activities requiring mental alertness for about 24 hours, until all medications have fully worn off. It is normal to pass gas and feel bloated because of the carbon dioxide used to insufflate the colon to visualize the area. It is abnormal for bleeding to be present, and the client should notify the healthcare provider if it occurs. **Cognitive Level:** Analyzing **Client Need:** Reduction of Risk Potential **Integrated Process:** Teaching and Learning **Content Area:** Adult Health: Gastrointestinal **Strategy:** The core issue of the question is knowledge of self-care following colonoscopy. Use nursing knowledge and the process of elimination to make a selection.

19 **Answer: 2 Rationale:** The client should avoid using any skin products, such as lotions or deodorant, on the skin of the breast or underarm prior to mammogram. The client may eat and drink as usual. Although the procedure might cause some women discomfort with compression of the breast, it is not necessary to premedicate with analgesics. There is no activity restriction following the test. **Cognitive Level:** Applying **Client Need:** Reduction of Risk Potential **Integrated Process:** Teaching and Learning **Content Area:** Adult Health: Reproductive **Strategy:** The core issue of the question is knowing to avoid skin products to prevent possible skin damage before a radiographic procedure such as a mammogram. The wording of the question tells you that only one option is correct. Use nursing knowledge and the process of elimination to make a selection.

20 **Answer: 2 Rationale:** A Mantoux test (or PPD test) to screen for tuberculosis should be read in 48–72 hours. If the test was planted on Monday, the result must be read in 2–3 days, which is Wednesday or Thursday. The options of reading the test on Tuesday or Wednesday, reading it on Thursday or Friday, and reading it on Friday or the following Monday are either partially or completely incorrect. **Cognitive Level:** Applying **Client Need:** Reduction of Risk Potential **Integrated Process:** Nursing Process: Implementation **Content Area:** Adult Health: Respiratory **Strategy:** The core issue of the question is knowledge of specific time frames for reading a PPD test. Remember when there is more than one part to an option, the entire option must be correct for that option to be the correct answer. Use nursing knowledge and the process of elimination to make a selection.

21 **Answer: 1, 3, 5 Rationale:** Selected drugs (anticholinergics, cholinergics, antacids, and corticosteroids) and coffee and alcohol should be restricted for at least 24 hours prior to test; note on the test request form if the client has not complied with the restrictions. There is no reason to withhold a cardiac glycoside or a diuretic because these medications would not affect the test results. **Cognitive Level:** Applying **Client Need:** Reduction of Risk Potential **Integrated Process:** Nursing Process: Implementation **Content Area:** Adult Health: Gastrointestinal **Strategy:** The core issue of the question is knowledge of drugs that could interfere with basal gastric acid testing and analysis. The wording of the question tells you that more than one option might be correct. Use nursing knowledge and the process of elimination.

Key Terms to Review

angiography p. 745
arthroscopy p. 751
biopsy p. 740
cardiac catheterization p. 746
colonoscopy p. 753
computed tomography (CT) scan p. 741
echocardiography p. 747
electrocardiography p. 747
electroencephalography p. 750
magnetic resonance imaging (MRI) p. 742
nuclear imaging study p. 742
pulmonary function tests p. 744
thoracentesis p. 745
ultrasonography p. 743
x-ray p. 743

References

Berman, A., Snyder, S., & Frandsen, G. (2016). *Kozier & Erb's fundamentals of nursing: Concepts, process, and practice* (10th ed.). New York, NY: Pearson Education.

Corbett, J. (2013). *Laboratory tests and diagnostic procedures with nursing diagnoses* (8th ed.). Upper Saddle River, NJ: Pearson Education.

Fischbach, F., & Dunning, M. (2014). A *manual of laboratory and diagnostic tests* (9th ed.). Philadelphia: Lippincott Williams & Wilkins.

Kee, J. (2017). *Pearson's Handbook of laboratory and diagnostic tests* (8th ed.). New York, NY: Pearson Education.

Leeuwen, A., & Bladh, M. (2015). *Davis's comprehensive handbook of laboratory and diagnostic tests with nursing implications* (6th ed.). Philadelphia: F. A. Davis.

Smith, S., Duell, D., Martin, B., Aebersold, M., & Gonzalez, L. (2017). *Clinical nursing skills: Basic to advanced skills* (10th ed.). New York, NY: Pearson Education.

Perioperative Care

48

In this chapter

Cross Reference

Other chapters relevant to this content area are

Preventing and Controlling Infection	Chapter 7
Maintaining the Function of Tubes and Drains	Chapter 27
Blood and Blood Component Therapy	Chapter 32

I. OVERVIEW OF PERIOPERATIVE NURSING

NCLEX®

A. Perioperative phases

1. **Preoperative phase** begins with decision to have surgery and ends with transport of client to operating room (OR); general nursing activities include client identification, client assessment, identifying potential or actual health problems, and beginning teaching about postoperative self-care
2. **Intraoperative phase** (surgical period) begins when client is transferred to operating table and ends with admission to postanesthesia care unit (PACU); general nursing activities include:
   a. Preparing client for induction of anesthesia
   b. Maintaining homeostasis and asepsis throughout procedure
   c. Assisting surgeon and team as needed by providing an aseptic, hazard-free environment and necessary supplies in a timely manner
3. **Postoperative phase** begins with client's admission to PACU and ends with a follow-up evaluation in either a clinical setting or home; general nursing activities include:
   a. Assessing for physical adaptation following anesthesia and surgical intervention
   b. Assisting in orienting client who is regaining consciousness
   c. Providing continuity of information between nursing units about client progress after surgery

B. Summary of nursing responsibilities during preoperative period

1. Interview: current health status, allergies, medication currently taking, previous surgical experiences, mental status, understanding of surgical procedure and anesthesia, smoking habit, alcohol and drug use, coping strategies, social resources, and cultural considerations
2. Arranging for preadmission testing, consultations, and education about postsurgical recovery
   a. Scheduling appropriate prescribed laboratory tests, electrocardiogram, x-rays

b. Ensuring reports are available on chart
c. Reporting to surgeon or anesthesiologist any pertinent abnormalities
d. Asking client if arrangements for autologous or directed blood donation (family/friends) have been made; if so, attach pertinent lab requisitions

NCLEX®

3. Day of surgery: after appropriate identification of client, verify completion of paperwork and secure valuables; if procedure is being performed on an outpatient basis, verify transportation home; then complete these activities:
   a. Determine client's cognitive understanding of procedure and obtain signed **informed consent** form; ensure consent is obtained before administering premedication with sedative effects; some agencies have client mark limb that will be operated on, if appropriate
   b. Perform a physical assessment and record vital signs (VS)
   c. Implement preoperative teaching for postoperative care
   d. Physical preparation: may include skin preparation, antiembolism stockings, catheterization, and starting an intravenous (IV) infusion
   e. Complete preoperative checklist: client wears identification and allergy bracelets; consents are signed for anesthesia, surgical procedure, and for blood transfusion; limb disposal or sterilization procedure, if appropriate; history and physical exam, consultations, lab and diagnostic test results are in record; assist client to remove clothing, jewelry, dentures, and other articles and to don hospital gown
   f. If client refuses to remove wedding band, tape in place and notify operating room personnel; leave eyeglasses in place if consistent with hospital policy; keep hearing aid(s) in place
   g. Have client void before administering any preoperative medications that affect level of consciousness (narcotics, sedatives); after medicating client, raise side rails as per agency policy and ensure call bell is in reach

C. Summary of nursing responsibilities during intraoperative period

1. Participate with rest of surgical team in protocol to prevent "wrong site, wrong procedure, wrong patient" surgery; includes verification of correct client, marking of operative site, and a final "time-out" before procedure begins to perform final verification of correct client, procedure, and site
2. Administer IV infusions and medications as needed

NCLEX®

3. Provide safe, effective care
   a. Position client to ensure functional alignment and exposure of surgical site
   b. Apply grounding device
   c. Provide emotional and physical support if awake
   d. Account for all equipment and supplies
   e. Maintain aseptic environment
   f. Perform physiological monitoring
   g. Assess fluid loss or gain
   h. Monitor cardiac, respiratory, and neurologic status
   i. Monitor client response to preoperative medications
4. Nursing roles during surgery
   a. Circulating nurse assists scrub nurses and surgeons; sterile scrubbing and gloving not necessary
   b. Scrub nurses assist surgeons; maintain sterile gowns, gloves, shoe covers; wear eye protection and caps
   c. Circulating nurse and scrub nurse account for used sponges, needles, and instruments during case

D. Summary of nursing responsibilities during postoperative period

1. Immediate care
   a. Assess effects of anesthetic agents and surgical procedure
   b. Monitor vital functions
   c. Provide comfort and pain relief

NCLEX®

2. Ongoing care
   a. Assess for client adaptation to effects of surgery
   b. Provide pain management
   c. Position client appropriately
   d. Promote use of incentive spirometry
   e. Assist with postoperative exercises
   f. Maintain hydration
   g. Promote urinary elimination
   h. Maintain suction to devices as needed
   i. Provide wound care
   j. Continue client teaching and discharge planning

II. PURPOSES AND TYPES OF SURGERY AND ANESTHESIA

NCLEX® **A. Purposes**

1. Diagnostic or exploratory: establishes a diagnosis, such as a breast biopsy
2. Curative: removes pathological cause, such as removal of cancer
3. Ablative: removes a diseased body part, such as tonsils for tonsillitis
4. Reconstructive: restores function or appearance, such as cleft lip repair
5. **Palliative**: relieves or reduces pain or symptoms, such as resecting sensory nerves for intractable pain

B. General classification of surgery

1. Major (higher risk) versus minor (lower risk)
   a. Major: may include prolonged intraoperative period, a large loss of blood, involvement of a vital organ, or postoperative complications; examples are lung surgery, colectomy
   b. Minor: usually associated with few complications, may be described as "one-day surgery" or outpatient surgery; examples are cyst removal, ingrown toenails

NCLEX® 2. Urgency classification (see Table 48–1)

C. Administration of *anesthesia* (partial or complete loss of sensation)

1. Anesthetic agents are drugs used to achieve a partial or complete loss of pain sensation; client may be conscious or unconscious

NCLEX® 2. **Moderate sedation** (formerly conscious sedation)
   a. An anesthesia state involving minimal depression of level of consciousness (LOC), allowing client to respond to verbal and physical stimuli; client maintains a patent airway while pain threshold is raised; an example is during balloon angioplasty
   b. Uses IV narcotics and anti-anxiety agents

NCLEX® 3. **Regional anesthesia**: loss of sensation in one part of body; see Table 48–2

NCLEX® 4. General anesthesia
   a. Anesthesia that involves loss of all sensation and consciousness
   b. Usually administered by IV infusion or by inhalation of gases
   c. Examples of use: major surgery, exploratory laparotomy

D. Stages of general anesthesia (see Table 48–3)

E. Preanesthesia classification of client's physical condition

1. Anesthesiologist reviews client's medical history as well as current data related to diagnosis, medication use, allergies, and drug reactions
2. Client is then assigned a risk category for surgery, from I (healthiest) to VI (brain death; organs being donated) or E for emergency surgery

Table 48–1 Urgency Classification of Surgery

Classification	Description	Example
Emergent	Performed immediately to save client's life, limb, or organ	Testicular torsion
Urgent	Requires prompt attention, usually within 24 hrs	Fracture reduction
Required	Needed for client's well-being, often within weeks to months	Cholecystectomy, if not acute
Elective	Needed but condition is not imminently life-threatening; surgery will improve client's life	Plastic surgery
Optional	Based on client preference	Gastric stapling

Table 48–2 Types of Regional Anesthesia

Type	Description
Local	Injected in a specific area for minor surgical procedures, such as lidocaine for suturing a small wound.
Nerve block	Anesthetic agent is injected into and around a nerve or group of nerves, such as a pudendal block used to numb perineum for an episiotomy.
Epidural block	Anesthetic agent injected into epidural space to anesthetize larger areas, such as in vaginal childbirth; client is awake and aware of surroundings but feels no pain.
Spinal anesthesia	Anesthesia is injected through a lumbar puncture into subarachnoid space, such as for hernia repairs or cesarean-section deliveries; client is conscious but has no sensation or movement of lower extremities up to a specific area.

Table 48–3 Stages of Anesthesia

Stage	Characteristics
Stage I	Beginning of anesthesia; client is drowsy and dizzy; pain sensation is depressed
Stage II	Excitement stage; client has irregular breathing, involuntary motor movements; avoid stimulating client, which can trigger vomiting, holding the breath, and increased activity; ensure client safety by proper use of safety straps
Stage III	Stage of anesthesia appropriate for surgical procedures; client has skeletal muscle relaxation, constricted pupils, absence of eyelid reflex
Stage IV	Medullary depression; client is near death; pupils are fixed and dilated, respirations are weak, pulse is rapid and thready

NCLEX® 3. General health problems that increase overall surgical risk are malnutrition (delayed wound healing and infection), obesity (impaired respiratory and cardiac function, impaired wound healing), cardiac conditions, blood coagulation disorders (bleeding), lung disease (reduced pulmonary function), renal disease (impaired regulation of fluids, electrolytes, and drug excretion), diabetes mellitus (delayed healing, wound infection), and liver disease (impaired drug detoxification, prothrombin production for clotting, and nutrient metabolism for healing)

F. Anesthetic agents may be administered by either inhalation or IV routes

1. Inhalation anesthetic agents are inhaled in gaseous forms
   - a. Administered by mask or by endotracheal tube; induction is usually rapid
   - b. Drugs are eliminated by respiratory system
   - c. With normal lung function, recovery rate is predictable
2. IV anesthesia
   - a. Administered alone or combined with inhalation anesthetic; rapid onset of unconsciousness
   - b. Metabolized primarily by liver and excreted by kidneys
   - c. Reversal agents may be required to stop drug effects

III. COMPONENTS OF PREOPERATIVE ASSESSMENT

A. Client's history

1. Medical history: current and past
   - NCLEX® a. Family history of malignant hyperthermia
   - b. Current health status including any chronic disease that might affect response to surgery and anesthesia
   - c. Past medical illnesses and treatments; previous surgical experiences including complications that occurred with previous surgical or anesthesia experience (such as malignant hyperthermia)
   - d. Report of severe anxiety associated with surgery
2. NCLEX® Medication use: all current medications, including prescription, over-the-counter, and herbal or other agents
3. NCLEX® Allergies
   - a. Food or medication
   - b. Environmental: latex allergies, tape, soap, and antiseptic agents
4. Tobacco use: may indicate potential problems of respiratory tract; identify type of product and amount and frequency of use; when possible, urge client to stop smoking 6–8 weeks before major surgery
5. Alcohol and controlled substance use: assess type of product, amount and frequency, and potential for problems with withdrawal
6. Psychosocial and economic factors: occupation and financial concerns, support systems, spiritual needs and cultural beliefs, coping mechanisms used in the past, and fear and anxiety about procedure (e.g., changes in body image, pain, grieving loss of a body part)

B. Physical assessment

1. Assessment of factors that will affect response to surgery or anesthesia
2. NCLEX® See Table 48–4 for summary of important preoperative physical assessments

C. Diagnostic screening

1. Laboratory tests are done before surgery to screen for existing abnormalities and to use as a baseline for future assessments
2. Additional tests may be prescribed related to specific condition
3. NCLEX® Verify that test results are available; abnormal findings may need to be corrected prior to surgery
4. See Table 48–5 for routine preoperative screening tests

Table 48–4 Components of Preoperative Physical Assessment

Focus	Specific Assessments
General	Overall appearance, gestures, facial expression Height and weight (obesity increases risk) Vital signs (hypertension increases risk)
Head and neck	Oral mucous membranes (hydration status) Loose teeth, dentures, and orthodontia work Soft palate, nasal sinuses, cervical lymph nodes Presence of jugular venous distention
Integumentary	Skin over entire body noting areas where skin is thin, dry, has poor turgor or breakdown
Chest and lungs	Adventitious breath sounds Degree of chest expansion, presence of cough, upper airway congestion, and/or obstructed nasal passages
Cardiovascular	Apical rate and rhythm Color and temperature of extremities Presence of pacemaker, A-V fistula or graft
Gastrointestinal	Determination of distention of abdomen versus obesity Baseline bowel sounds and elimination patterns Gag reflex and history of nausea/vomiting postoperatively Validation of NPO (nothing by mouth) status when applicable; anesthetics depress GI functioning; clients are usually NPO for 6–8 hours before surgery to reduce risk of vomiting and aspiration
Genitourinary and reproductive	Alterations in urinary elimination, color, appearance, and usual amount of urine output Presence of abnormal vaginal discharge, uterine bleeding in women Pregnancy status
Neurologic and mobility status	Baseline level of consciousness Presence of sensory or perceptual deficits Range of motion and ability to perform activities of daily living

Table 48–5 Routine Preoperative Screening Tests

Test	Purpose for Assessment
Urinalysis	Urine composition and possible abnormal components
Chest x-ray	Respiratory status and heart size
Electrocardiogram	Preexisting cardiac disease or rhythm abnormalities
Complete blood count (CBC)	RBCs, hemoglobin, and hematocrit for O_2-carrying capacity; WBCs as indicator of immune function (infection)
Blood typing and cross-matching	Blood transfusion, ABO and Rh matching
Serum electrolytes	Electrolyte balance (Na^+, K^+, Ca^{++}, Mg^{++}, Cl^-, HCO_3^-)
Fasting blood glucose	Detection or control of diabetes mellitus
BUN and creatinine	Renal function
ALT, AST, LDH, bilirubin	Liver function
Serum albumin and total protein	Nutritional status

IV. INFORMED CONSENT

A. Description

1. Written permission obtained from client prior to any invasive procedure or one that has potentially serious side effects or complications
2. Client has right to accept or reject procedure after receiving explanation

NCLEX®

3. Informed consent includes providing client with information about the following:
   a. Nature and purpose of a treatment or procedure
   b. Expected outcomes and probabilities of success, material risks, benefits, and consequences of treatment

c. Alternatives to procedure and supporting information
d. Effect of not having procedure or treatment, including effect on prognosis

B. Three elements of informed consent

1. Given voluntarily

NCLEX® 2. Given by an individual with capacity and competence to understand what procedure involves:
a. Adults have legal authority to make decisions for themselves
b. If client is a minor, parent or legal guardian has right to provide consent
c. Many states recognize emancipated minors who can provide consent for themselves
d. Many states allow minors to provide consent for treatment in cases related to sexually transmitted infections, pregnancy, abortion, and contraception
e. Legal power of attorney for health care allows another person to make decisions if client becomes incapacitated

3. Sufficient information must be provided to client to allow for an informed decision
a. Healthcare workers must communicate in a way client can understand
b. An interpreter may be needed to ensure adequate communication

4. In emergencies, when informed consent cannot be obtained from client or next of kin, consent is implied by law; specific information about emergency situation and reason informed consent was not obtained must be documented in medical record

C. Nurse's role with informed consent

1. Informed consent is part of healthcare provider–client relationship

NCLEX® 2. Healthcare provider has obligation to obtain consent

3. Because nurse does not perform surgery or procedures, obtaining informed consent is not a nursing responsibility; nurses can reinforce healthcare provider's explanations

NCLEX® 4. Nurse can serve as witness to the following:
a. Authority on consent form is authentic
b. Client has capacity to make informed consent
c. Client has authority to consent
d. Consent is being given voluntarily

V. DEVELOPMENTAL CONSIDERATIONS OF CLIENTS HAVING SURGERY

NCLEX® **A. Children and adolescents**

1. Take care with all children and adolescents while explaining procedures because they may misinterpret meaning
2. Infancy: surgery and separation from parents may interfere with bonding; infants have no understanding of events but are aware of adult emotions; no explanations about procedures are required for infant, but parents will need complete preparation
3. Toddler: may experience separation anxiety; their security lies in presence of their caregivers; when caregivers are not present, child may suffer; immediately prior to a procedure, give toddler a brief, simple explanation
4. Preschoolers: often view illness as punishment for bad behavior; have an inadequate understanding of cause–effect and thus misinterpret relationships; continue to give simple explanations in close proximity to time of procedure; play therapy may help preschooler to express feelings
5. School-age children: better able to withstand separation from parents and are accustomed to dealing with adults other than family; they fear pain and mutilation and require more complete, yet age-appropriate instructions; they may benefit from pictures, dolls, and videos as teaching aids
6. Adolescents: concerns are separation from peers and body image/physical attractiveness; protect child's privacy

B. Adults

1. Fear of unknown and separation from support systems
2. Dependence and loss of control
3. Disruption in career goals, family living patterns, and financial worries
4. Concern over disability and/or death

VI. PHYSICAL PREPARATION OF CLIENTS HAVING SURGERY

A. Preparing for anesthesia

1. Anesthetic needs and risks are assessed by anesthesiologist
2. Type of anesthetic along with method of administration, risks, and recovery is explained

Table 48–6 Classifications of Possible Preoperative Medications

Drug Class	Preoperative Use	Major Side Effects
Anti-infectives	Reduce risk of infection prophylactically	Antibiotic resistance; first dose hypersensitivity
Anticholinergics	Reduce body fluid secretion (e.g., saliva)	GI system depression
Antiemetics	Reduce risk of emesis and aspiration	Respiratory depression
H_2-receptor blockers	Reduce gastric acidity and reflux	Rebound acidity
Opioid analgesics	Reduce dosages needed of anesthetics	CNS depression
Benzodiazepines	Reduce anxiety and as a medication enhancer	CNS depression
Barbiturates	Sedation and as narcotic enhancer; not often used	CNS, respiratory depression

B. Preparing skin
1. Purpose: cleansing and removing transient microbes from skin
2. Cleansing begins with morning shower or bath; surgical site is then cleansed with an antimicrobial agent immediately prior to surgical procedure
3. Hair removal from surgical site may be prescribed to further reduce microbial growth; take care to maintain intact skin (clip but don't shave)

C. Preparing GI tract

NCLEX®
1. Client is placed on NPO status prior to OR to reduce risk of vomiting or aspiration, prevent contamination of operative site from fecal material, and reduce postoperative nausea, vomiting, gastric distention, or bowel obstruction
2. Colon cleansing may be prescribed for surgical procedures involving GI tract to reduce contamination of surgical field; postoperative constipation may be prevented; cleansing may occur using enemas, laxatives, and oral antibiotics (such as neomycin)

D. Preparation on day of surgery

NCLEX®
1. Routine care for most outpatient as well as hospitalized clients
   a. Consent form is signed
   b. Preoperative medications are given
   c. Emotional support to client and family is provided
   d. Preoperative teaching is completed, including postoperative routine
2. General care
   a. Record VS for baseline information
   b. Remove dentures, bridgework (or both); note on chart presence of loose teeth
   c. Have client put on hospital gown without undergarments in many cases (for children and minor procedures, there may be exceptions)
   d. Have client void to empty bladder
   e. Remove cosmetics and nail polish
   f. Remove jewelry per agency policy and place in secure area for safekeeping; if client does not want to remove wedding band, it can be taped in place; in certain situations, removal of wedding band may be required because of risk of postoperative edema
   g. Leave hearing aids in place and note on preoperative checklist
   h. Remove eyeglasses, contact lenses, and other prostheses
   i. Antiembolism stockings may be prescribed to promote venous return from legs

E. Preoperative medications
1. May be prescribed at a scheduled time or "on call" to OR
2. Purposes include to sedate or tranquilize, decrease respiratory tract secretions, provide analgesia, reduce gastric acid, reduce nausea, and prevent vomiting
3. Classifications of preoperative medication: see Table 48–6

VII. INTRAOPERATIVE FACTORS AFFECTING POSTOPERATIVE PHASE

A. Principles of perioperative asepsis
1. General
   a. Keep sterile supplies dry and unopened
   b. Check package sterilization expiration date to verify sterility
   c. Maintain general cleanliness in surgical suite

NCLEX®
   d. Maintain **surgical asepsis** (techniques to keep sites free of microorganisms) throughout procedure (refer back to Chapter 7, Table 7–1, p. 67)

2. Personnel with signs of illness should not report to work
3. **Surgical scrub**, a specific handwashing technique used by OR personnel to reduce microorganisms on hands and arms; is done for length of time designated by hospital policy
   a. A sensor-controlled or knee- or foot-operated faucet allows water to be turned on and off without use of hands
   b. Remove all rings and watches
   c. Use liquid soaps to prevent spread of microorganisms
   d. Keep fingernails short and well trimmed; clean fingernails with a nail stick under running water; artificial nails pose risk of infection and are prohibited
   e. Hold hands higher than elbows throughout procedure so run-off goes to elbows; this allows hands to be cleanest area
   f. A scrub brush facilitates removal of microorganisms; clean all areas of skin on hands and arms in sequence, starting at hands and ending at elbows
   g. After rinsing, dry hands with sterile towels, drying first one arm from hand to elbow, then using a second towel to dry second hand

NCLEX®

4. Maintaining a **sterile field** (a microoganism-free area)
   a. Create a sterile field using sterile drapes
   b. Use sterile field to place sterile supplies to be available during procedure
   c. Drape equipment prior to use
   d. Keep drapes dry and out of contact with nonsterile objects
   e. Utilize sterile technique while adding or removing supplies from sterile fields

NCLEX®

5. Sterile supplies and solutions
   a. Check expiration dates for sterility
   b. Don't use solutions that were opened prior to current use
   c. "Lip" solutions after initial use by pouring a small amount of liquid out of bottle into a waste container to cleanse bottle lip

B. Potential environmental health hazards during intraoperative period

1. Injuries caused by equipment
   a. Laser tools used for a surgical procedure can cause burns
   b. Improperly grounded cautery devices can cause burns
   c. Ensure proper grounding for electrical equipment and check equipment prior to beginning surgical procedure

NCLEX®

2. Latex allergy affects many people, both clients and hospital personnel
   a. Clients with spina bifida and those who have had multiple surgical procedures are at greatest risk
   b. Exposure can occur percutaneously, mucosally, parenterally, and via inhalation
   c. Symptoms can vary from contact dermatitis to anaphylaxis
   d. Symptoms in an anesthetized client would include flushing, facial swelling, urticaria, bronchospasm, hypotension, and cardiac arrest
   e. Be aware of equipment that contains latex, including tourniquets, manual resuscitation (Ambu) bags, balloon catheters, surgical gowns, boots, and drapes

NCLEX®

3. Exposure to blood and body fluids
   a. Concern for client and staff alike
   b. Use goggles and fluid-protectant shields; gloves worn for extended period can leak and should be changed periodically
   c. Use caution with sharps

C. Potential intraoperative complications

1. Nausea and vomiting: ensure that client is NPO for prescribed time period
2. Hypoxia and respiratory complications
   a. Loss of pharyngeal and cough reflexes may lead to aspiration of secretions or vomitus
   b. Respiratory depression can occur from anesthetic agents
   c. Respiratory muscles become weakened or paralyzed by neuromuscular agents
   d. Positioning can negatively affect lung expansion
   e. Tissue perfusion is monitored by anesthesiologist
   f. Use of a pulse oximeter assists with monitoring oxygenation
3. Hypothermia
   a. Related to OR temperature and exposure of internal organs
   b. Minimized by preventing exposure of nonsurgical body parts, use of head covering and blankets, warmed IV fluids and anesthetic agents

NCLEX®

4. Malignant hyperthermia
   a. Excessive heat production related to stress, trauma, infection; may be attributed to anesthetic agent; seen more commonly in males; there is a tendency toward development if inherited as an autosomal-dominant trait
   b. Symptoms include rapid rise in body temperature, tachycardia, tachypnea, and respiratory and metabolic acidosis
   c. Skin initially appears flushed, then becomes mottled and cyanotic
   d. Treatment includes use of 100% oxygen, cooling blankets and ice packs, cool IV fluids, and stomach irrigation
   e. Can be fatal
5. Paresthesia and impaired skin integrity related to positioning
6. Excessive fluid and blood loss

VIII. POSTOPERATIVE NURSING CARE

A. Assessments in immediate period following surgery in PACU (see Box 48–1)

1. Confirm client's identity
2. Receive report from surgical nurse: surgical procedure, anesthesia, drugs, and IV fluids administered and estimated blood loss
3. Note location, types, and conditions of catheters, **drains**, or packs; drains are tubes inserted into wounds to allow removal of excessive **serosanguineous** (fluid composed of serum and blood) or **purulent** (containing pus) material from wound

B. Nursing management in PACU

NCLEX®

1. Maintain a patent airway and adequate respirations: priority nursing concern
   a. May be impaired by continued effects of anesthetic drugs, relaxation of tongue, oropharyngeal secretions, or vomitus
   b. Position client on side unless contraindicated (helps prevent aspiration if vomiting occurs)
   c. Monitor respiratory rate (should be 10–30 breaths/minute)
   d. Assess breath sounds for crackles (fluid) or rhonchi (secretions) and suction as necessary
   e. Wheezing or stridor may signal broncho- or laryngospasm; assess carefully and maintain airway; notify surgeon or anesthesiologist immediately
   f. Assess for return of cough, gag, and swallow reflexes
   g. If client had spinal anesthesia, do not elevate legs on pillow because diaphragm muscles could become impaired

Box 48–1

Clinical Assessment in the Postanesthetic Phase

- Airway patency including presence of protective airway reflexes (e.g., gag, cough, swallow)
- Respirations: adequacy of respiratory rate, rhythm, and depth; use of accessory muscles; oxygen saturation; breath sounds
- Circulation: heart rate and rhythm, BP, peripheral pulse volume and equality, capillary refill, skin color (pale, pink, dusky, cyanotic)
- Neurologic and musculoskeletal: level of consciousness, mobility and sensation in extremities
- Fluid balance: intake and output, minimum urine output of 30 mL/hr, IV infusions (type, rate, amount remaining in bag), other losses (amount of volume of blood, gastric or other tube drainage; if amount is appropriate), signs of fluid overload or dehydration
- Status of surgical drains and/or dressings at operative site: dressing dry and intact or presence and type of drainage; type and patency of surgical drain and amount, type, and color of drainage (example: T-tube)
- Pain or discomfort: pain location and characteristics, presence of nausea and vomiting
- Protective environment: correct postoperative positioning if applicable, call bell within reach (and client understands use), appropriate use of bed rails

NCLEX®

2. Maintain cardiovascular stability
   a. Client is typically on a cardiac and respiratory monitor
   b. Monitor vital signs (VS) according to hospital policy (often every 15 minutes) until stable and then every 30 minutes until PACU discharge
   c. Report changes in VS immediately; small but persistent trends are early signs that client's condition is deteriorating
   d. Apply sequential compression devices (SCDs) or antiembolism stockings as prescribed to promote circulation in lower extremities
3. Assess for hypotension or shock
   a. May be related to fluid or blood loss or as a reaction to drugs
   b. Symptoms: restlessness, decreased urine output (UO), cool, moist skin, pallor followed by cyanosis, and dropping BP with increasing pulse
   c. Monitor and maintain IV infusion flow rates to prevent hypovolemia as a cause of shock

NCLEX®

4. Assess for hemorrhage
   a. Monitor dressings and drains for amount of discharge; observe appearance and amount of urine (concentrated and decreased volume with hypovolemia); observe for distention of body tissues
   b. A client with excessive blood loss may require a transfusion; ensure blood product and type are correct (see Chapter 32)
5. Assess for hypertension and dysrhythmias
6. Relieve pain and anxiety
   a. Pain can negatively affect VS and recovery
   b. Assess location, intensity, characteristics, and cause of pain
   c. Administer analgesics (often opioids by IV) as prescribed
   d. Observe effectiveness of analgesics
7. Neurologic status
   a. Assess LOC with vital signs and prn
   b. Frequently attempt to arouse client until fully awake
   c. Orient to environment when awake
   d. Maintain quiet environment during recovery period from anesthesia
8. Temperature
   a. Measure temperature
   b. Apply warm blankets or postoperative warming device such as Bair hugger to keep client warm if hypothermic from surgery

NCLEX®

9. Integumentary
   a. Monitor status of incision if visible; otherwise, monitor status of incisional dressing
   b. Assess for skin redness or breakdown because of surgical positioning or burns from cautery or grounding pad; report and complete incident report if found

NCLEX®

C. Discharge criteria from PACU

1. Aldrete postanesthesia recovery score
   a. Used to monitor recovery of client from anesthesia to determine readiness for PACU discharge
   b. Consists of five areas that are each scored from 0 to 2: activity, respiration, circulation, consciousness, and oxygen saturation
   c. Maximum score is 10 and many PACUs require a score of 9 for discharge
2. A more comprehensive set of discharge criteria from PACU include the following:
   a. Conscious and oriented
   b. Can maintain a clear airway, deep-breathe and cough freely, and has no respiratory distress
   c. Has stable VS that are consistent with preoperative measurements for at least 30 minutes
   d. Has demonstrated return of cough, swallow, and gag reflexes
   e. Able to move all extremities (assumes no impairment before surgery)
   f. Has adequate intake and urine output
   g. Afebrile or febrile state has been managed
   h. Has dressings that are dry and intact with no overt drainage

D. Nursing management on clinical unit

1. Review postoperative prescriptions for fluids and diet allowed, IV solutions and medications, other medications, positioning in bed, activity permitted (including ambulation), intake and output measurement (may be automatic in some agencies), and laboratory tests

2. Review PACU record for surgical procedure performed, type of anesthesia used, postoperative diagnosis, estimated blood loss, medications administered in PACU, and presence and location of any drains

NCLEX®

3. Immediate nursing interventions upon arrival to nursing unit
   a. Assess breathing and apply oxygen if prescribed
   b. Check VS and skin warmth, moisture, color
   c. Assess surgical site (approximation of wound edges, edema or bleeding, or status of dressing) and wound drains
   d. Note and document wound **exudate** (fluid and cells that accumulate in a wound); exudate varies in appearance: **serous** (like serum—watery and clear), purulent (thick and contains pus; may be blue, green, or yellow tinged), **sanguineous** (bloody and may be dark red or bright red depending on freshness of blood)
   e. Connect tubes to drain devices or suction
   f. Perform pain assessment and utilize appropriate pain relief interventions
   g. Position client properly using support devices as necessary
   h. Monitor IV fluids and infusion pumps
   i. Monitor UO hourly or less frequently as prescribed; hourly UO should be 30 mL or more
   j. Bladder distention is possible for up to 24 hours following spinal anesthesia; client should void spontaneously within 6–8 hours postoperatively; if unable to void, catheterization may be prescribed and repeated as necessary
4. Ongoing nursing interventions on surgical unit

NCLEX®

   a. Encourage incentive spirometer, deep-breathing and coughing exercises every 2 hours while awake to prevent atelectasis and pneumonia; encourage client to sit up in bed and place hands one on top of the other directly on wound (splint incision) to reduce discomfort of coughing; monitor oxygen saturation with VS
   b. Teach and encourage leg exercises (such as foot circles, ankle pumps), use of support stockings or SCDs; assess for Homans sign or calf pain with client foot dorsiflexion during routine assessments
   c. Keep call light, emesis basin, ice chips, bedpan, urinal within reach
   d. Communicate with family and significant others

NCLEX®

   e. Monitor for infection by noting wound characteristics (*REEDA*: *r*edness, *e*rythema, *e*cchymosis, *d*rainage, *a*pproximation of wound edges), temperature, and WBC test results; administer prophylactic or other antibiotics on time to maintain therapeutic blood levels
   f. Teach self-care according to surgical procedure and client and family needs
   g. Encourage activity as tolerated

NCLEX®

   h. Promote GI status: perform abdominal assessment including bowel sounds each shift; provide diet and fluids once bowel sounds return; begin with clear liquids and advance to full liquids, soft and regular as prescribed and tolerated (no N/V, abdominal distention); encourage early ambulation to promote bowel function

NCLEX®

   i. Continue to monitor UO and compare to intake; diuresis from mobilization of fluids given during surgery can occur by second postoperative day

NCLEX®

   j. Provide for adequate pain management using patient-controlled analgesia or other opioids; assess pain at least every 4 hours; document pain rating, location, quality, and other characteristics; consider cultural beliefs and practices regarding pain management; assess effectiveness of pharmacologic and nonpharmacologic (e.g., music, distraction, massage) measures
   k. Provide wound care as prescribed (monitor incision, change dressing as prescribed); document findings; one complication of surgery is **dehiscence** (partial or total rupture of a sutured wound), which may be preceded by sudden straining as occurs during coughing (see also section on complications that follows)

NCLEX®

   l. Provide emergency care if client experiences evisceration after dehiscence of an abdominal incision: remain with client and call for help; assist client to a low Fowler's position with knees bent (prevents added tension on incision line); cover bowel loops and other abdominal contents with sterile normal saline dressings that are kept moist; monitor vital signs for possible impending shock; prepare client for surgery as needed, and document in client record (observations, actions taken, client outcomes)

NCLEX®

   m. Participate in discharge planning according to client needs: include in discharge teaching diet, activity, medications, and when to call surgeon for complications; schedule follow-up care; ensure that home care or other support services are in place (see Box 48–2)

Box 48–2

Common Postsurgical Discharge Instructions

Diet

- Drink at least six to eight glasses of fluid daily unless otherwise prescribed (water is beneficial)
- Adhere to any diet restrictions (provide individualized instruction according to diet)
- Eat well-balanced meals that are high in vitamin C and protein to aid wound healing

Activity

- Maintain activity restriction if prescribed by surgeon
- Resume activities gradually (all clients)
- Avoid heavy lifting for 6 weeks after major surgery
- Avoid lifting more than 4.5 kg (10 lb) or performing activities involving pushing or pulling with an abdominal incision
- Often may return to work in 6–8 weeks (depending on surgery and client status preoperatively)

Medications

- Continue to take pain medication as needed; follow directions on prescription bottle
- Take other medications as prescribed (teach specifics about medication action, dose, how to take, and side/adverse effects to watch for and report)

Wound Care

- Take care of incision and/or change dressing as taught (specific information is individualized to client and surgery; provide 1–2 days of dressing materials or according to hospital policy)
- Cover incision with plastic wrap before showering (if allowed)
- Sutures or staples are often removed in surgeon's office 7–14 days postoperatively
- Steri-Strips will fall off by themselves (if used instead of sutures or if applied for support when sutures are removed before discharge)

Follow-up Care

- Contact surgeon if signs of complications occur (fever, signs of wound infection, increased pain, other signs specific to surgery)
- Keep follow-up appointments to aid in continued recovery from surgery

IX. POSTOPERATIVE COMPLICATIONS (SEE TABLE 48–7)

Table 48–7 Potential Postoperative Problems

Problem	Description	Cause	Clinical Signs	Preventive Interventions
Respiratory Pneumonia	Inflammation of alveoli	Infection, toxins, or irritants causing inflammatory process; immobility and impaired ventilation result in atelectasis and promote growth of pathogens	Elevated temperature, cough, expectoration of blood-tinged or purulent sputum, dyspnea, chest pain	Deep-breathing exercises and coughing, moving in bed, early ambulation
Atelectasis	Condition in which alveoli collapse and are not ventilated	Mucous plugs blocking bronchial passageways, inadequate lung expansion, analgesics, immobility	Dyspnea, tachypnea, tachycardia; diaphoresis, anxiety; pleural pain, decreased chest wall movement; dull or absent breath sounds; decreased oxygen saturation (SpO_2)	Deep-breathing exercises and coughing, moving in bed, early ambulation

Table 48–7 Potential Postoperative Problems (*continued*)

Problem	Description	Cause	Clinical Signs	Preventive Interventions
Pulmonary embolism	Blood clot that has moved to lungs and blocks a pulmonary artery, thus obstructing blood flow to a portion of lung	Stasis of venous blood from immobility, venous injury from fractures or during surgery, use of oral contraceptives high in estrogen, preexisting coagulation or circulatory disorder	Sudden chest pain, shortness of breath, cyanosis, shock (tachycardia, low BP)	Turning, ambulation, antiemboli stockings, sequential compression devices (SCDs)
Circulatory				
Hypovolemia	Inadequate circulating blood volume	Fluid deficit, hemorrhage	Tachycardia, decreased UO, decreased BP	Early detection of signs; fluid and/or blood replacement
Hemorrhage	Internal or external bleeding	Disruption of sutures, insecure ligation of blood vessels	Overt bleeding (dressings saturated with bright blood; bright, free-flowing blood in drains or chest tubes), increased pain, increasing abdominal girth, swelling or bruising around incision	Early detection of signs
Hypovolemic shock	Inadequate tissue perfusion resulting from markedly reduced circulating blood volume	Severe hypovolemia from fluid deficit or hemorrhage	Rapid weak pulse, dyspnea, tachypnea; restlessness and anxiety; UO less than 30 mL/hr; decreased BP; cool, clammy skin, thirst, pallor	Maintain blood volume through adequate fluid replacement, prevent hemorrhage; early detection of signs
Thrombophlebitis	Inflammation of veins, usually of legs and associated with a blood clot	Slowed venous blood flow due to immobility or prolonged sitting; trauma to vein, resulting in inflammation and increased blood coagulability	Aching, cramping pain; affected area is swollen, red, and hot to touch; vein feels hard; discomfort in calf when foot is dorsiflexed or when client walks (Homans sign)	Early ambulation, leg exercises, antiemboli stockings, SCDs, adequate fluid intake
Thrombus	Blood clot attached to wall of vein or artery (most commonly leg veins)	Thrombophlebitis for venous thrombi; disruption or inflammation of arterial wall for arterial thrombi	*Venous:* same as thrombophlebitis *Arterial:* pain and pallor of affected extremity; decreased or absent peripheral pulses	*Venous:* same as thrombophlebitis *Arterial:* maintain prescribed position; early detection of signs
Embolus	Foreign body or clot that has moved from its site of formation to another area of body (e.g., lungs, heart, or brain)	Venous or arterial thrombus; broken IV catheter, fat, or amniotic fluid	In venous system, usually becomes a pulmonary embolus (see pulmonary embolism); signs of arterial emboli may depend on location	Turning, ambulation, leg exercises, SCDs; careful maintenance of IV catheters
Urinary				
Urinary retention	Inability to empty bladder, with excessive accumulation of urine in bladder	Depressed bladder muscle tone from narcotics and anesthetics; handling of tissues during surgery on adjacent organs (rectum, vagina)	Fluid intake larger than output; inability to void or frequent voiding of small amounts, bladder distention, suprapubic discomfort, restlessness	Monitoring of fluid intake and output, interventions to facilitate voiding, urinary catheterization as needed
Urinary tract infection	Inflammation of bladder, ureters, or urethra	Immobilization and limited fluid intake, instrumentation of urinary tract	Burning sensation when voiding, urgency, cloudy urine, lower abdominal pain	Adequate fluid intake, early ambulation, aseptic straight catheterization only as necessary, good perineal hygiene

(*continued*)

Table 48–7 Potential Postoperative Problems (*continued*)

Problem	Description	Cause	Clinical Signs	Preventive Interventions
Gastrointestinal				
Nausea and vomiting		Pain, abdominal distention, ingesting food or fluids before return of peristalsis, certain medications, anxiety	Complaints of feeling sick to stomach, retching or gagging	IV fluids until peristalsis returns; then clear fluids, full fluids, and regular diet; antiemetic drugs if prescribed; analgesics for pain
Constipation	Infrequent or no stool passage for abnormal length of time (e.g., within 48 hours after solid diet started)	Lack of dietary roughage, analgesics (decreased intestinal motility), immobility	Absence of stool elimination, abdominal distention, and discomfort	Adequate fluid intake, high-fiber diet, early ambulation
Tympanites	Retention of gases within intestines	Slowed motility of intestines due to handling of bowel during surgery and effects of anesthesia	Obvious abdominal distention, abdominal discomfort (gas pains), absence of bowel sounds	Early ambulation; avoid using a straw, provide ice chips or water at room temperature
Postoperative ileus	Intestinal obstruction characterized by lack of peristaltic activity	Handling bowel during surgery, anesthesia, electrolyte imbalance, wound infection	Abdominal pain and distention; constipation; absent bowel sounds; vomiting	Early ambulation; chewing gum; early oral intake and feeding
Wound				
Wound infection	Inflammation and infection of incision or drain site	Poor aseptic technique; laboratory analysis of wound swab identifies causative microorganism	Purulent exudate, redness, tenderness, elevated body temperature, wound odor	Keep wound clean and dry, use surgical aseptic technique when changing dressings
Wound dehiscence	Separation of a suture line before incision heals	Malnutrition (emaciation, obesity), poor circulation, excessive strain on suture line	Increased incision drainage, tissues underlying skin become visible along parts of incision, possible report of "popping" sensation after coughing or moving	Adequate nutrition, appropriate incisional support, and avoidance of strain
Wound evisceration	Extrusion of internal organs and tissues through incision	Same as for wound dehiscence	Opening of incision and visible protrusion of organs; sudden leakage of serosanguineous fluid from previously dry wound	Same as for wound dehiscence
Psychological				
Postoperative depression	Mental disorder characterized by altered mood	Weakness, surprise nature of emergency surgery, news of malignancy, severely altered body image, other personal matter; may be a physiologic response to some surgeries	Anorexia, tearfulness, loss of ambition, withdrawal, rejection of others, feelings of dejection, sleep disturbances (insomnia or excessive sleeping)	Adequate rest, physical activity, opportunity to express anger and other negative feelings

Source: Berman, A. Snyder, S., & Frandsen, G. (2016). *Kozier & Erb's fundamentals of Nursing: Concepts, Process, and Practice* (10th ed.). New York, NY: Pearson Education, pp. 884–885.

Check Your NCLEX–RN® Exam I.Q.

You are ready for testing on this content if you can:

- Determine a client's readiness for surgery.
- Prepare a client for surgery.
- Monitor a client before, during, and after surgery.
- Provide preoperative, intraoperative, and postoperative care to a client.
- Assess a client's response to recovery from various types of anesthesia.
- Provide client education about preoperative and postoperative care.
- Assess a client's response to a surgical procedure.
- Evaluate effectiveness of interventions designed to prevent postoperative complications.

PRACTICE TEST

1 The nurse has taught the client to perform deep-breathing and coughing exercises. The nurse determines that the client needs additional teaching when the client is observed doing which activities? Select all that apply.

1. Sitting upright before deep breathing and coughing
2. Taking deep breaths before attempting to cough
3. Placing both hands vertically and slightly on either side of the incision
4. Using a pillow for splinting during coughing
5. Use gentle coughing efforts that sound like clearing the throat

2 A toddler who has not had surgery before is being prepared for a surgical procedure. The child's mother expresses concern about the child's psychological adaptation to surgery. While planning for postoperative care, the nurse recognizes that the child is likely to have which greatest concern based on age?

1. Anticipated pain
2. Body image changes
3. Communication difficulties
4. Separation from parents

3 A client is being prepared for surgery. When the nurse asks that the client remove a wedding ring, the client refuses. What would be an appropriate response by the nurse? Select all that apply.

1. Encourage the client to use soapy water to remove the ring if it is tight.
2. Explain that the hospital cannot be responsible for jewelry worn during surgery.
3. Notify the surgeon's office that the surgeon must see the client in the preoperative holding area.
4. Tape the ring in place before the client is transported to the preoperative holding area.
5. Make a notation on the preoperative checklist that the ring is in place.

4 The nurse is caring for clients in the preoperative holding area. The nurse notes that one client, who is an older adult, has an increased surgical risk based on which factor?

1. Decreased kidney function, leading to potential fluid and electrolyte imbalances
2. Increased hunger sensations, leading to postoperative complications from hyperacidity
3. Inability to comprehend the seriousness of surgical interventions, leading to noncompliance
4. Poor cardiovascular status, leading to decreased pain sensation

5 A client who takes numerous medications is being prepared for surgery. The nurse reviewing the client medication list is most concerned about which medication that increases surgical risk?

1. An antidysrhythmic
2. A sedative-hypnotic
3. A corticosteroid
4. An oral hypoglycemic

6 The following clients are in the preoperative holding area. The nurse determines that the client undergoing which procedure is having the most serious or major surgery?

1. Tonsillectomy
2. Biopsy of the breast
3. Arthroscopy
4. Nephrectomy

7 Each of the following clients will be having surgery this morning. The nurse concludes that which client is most likely to be at higher overall surgical risk?

1. A client who has dementia
2. A client who is culturally different than the medical personnel
3. A client who has mild anxiety
4. A client who has had previous surgeries

PRACTICE TEST

8 The nurse is preparing a client for surgery. Prior to completing the skin preparation, the nurse assesses the surgical site for which finding?

1. Presence of pustules or abrasions
2. Absence of hair growth
3. Presence of lanugo
4. Absence of pulsation

9 When the nurse asks the client about previous surgeries, the client asks why this information is important. The nurse responds that previous surgeries can have which effect on the client?

1. Interfere with the absorption of anesthetic agents.
2. Affect the ability of the client to comprehend the instructions prior to surgery.
3. Affect the central nervous system.
4. Alter the client's responses to surgery.

10 A client who arrives for an outpatient surgical procedure has the odor of alcohol on the breath. Before completing the preoperative assessment, the nurse reports this finding to the surgeon, after drawing which conclusion about the significance of this finding?

1. Alcohol can affect the client's response to anesthesia and surgery.
2. Alcohol can increase the risk for respiratory complications.
3. Alcohol can decrease the effectiveness of preoperative sedatives or hypnotics.
4. Physiological and psychological responses are slowed down by recent alcohol intake.

11 When the staff nurse asks questions about the preoperative client's vision and hearing, a family member asks why these questions are important. What reply by the nurse provides the primary reason for seeking this information?

1. "This will help us determine the need for additional resources after discharge."
2. "This will help assess the risk of accidents in the home after surgery, which could affect the surgical outcome."
3. "This helps identify any unanticipated needs prior to beginning the surgery."
4. "This will help us to individualize how we provide preoperative and postoperative teaching."

12 A client is admitted for surgery. During the preoperative assessment, the nurse learns the client was taking warfarin but stopped it a few days ago per surgeon instructions. The nurse should include assessing for which specific problem when developing the postoperative plan of care?

1. Delirium tremens
2. Respiratory depression
3. Bleeding or oozing at the surgical wound site
4. Hypovolemia

13 While planning postoperative care for an obese client prior to surgery, the nurse should be most concerned about which risk that is increased by obesity during the postsurgical recovery period?

1. Impaired wound healing
2. Fluid overload
3. Pressure ulcer development
4. Inability to regulate body temperature

14 The postsurgical unit nurse is implementing measures to prevent thrombophlebitis. Which measure should be the priority action by the nurse?

1. Apply prescribed sequential compression devices.
2. Reinforce importance of smoking cessation.
3. Assess the legs with each set of vital signs.
4. Teach the client to report Homans sign.

15 A client has been admitted for surgery for resection of nerve roots. The client, observing the written comment that the surgery is palliative, asks what this means. The nurse should offer which explanation?

1. The surgery schedule is overbooked, so the client's surgery could be delayed.
2. The surgeon is against performing the surgery.
3. The exact surgical procedure has not been decided.
4. The procedure will be done to relieve pain, but it will not cure the problem.

16 The progress note in the health record indicates a plan to let a client's wound heal by tertiary intention. The nurse concludes that healing has occurred after making which observation of the wound?

1. The wound is smaller but irregular.
2. Very little scarring has occurred.
3. Tissue loss prevents the edges from approximating.
4. A wide scar is present over the area of wound closure.

17 The nurse assesses the wound of a postoperative client to have moderate drainage with a greenish tinge. The nurse should take which priority action next?

1. Document the expected findings.
2. Check for bleeding at the base of the wound.
3. Take the pulse and blood pressure, and compare with previous readings.
4. Note the latest temperature and white blood cell (WBC) count.

18 A client is scheduled for surgery and has been placed on NPO status. The client reports thirst and hunger and asks for breakfast. The nurse should explain that NPO status has which purpose?

1. To make anesthesia induction easier
2. To avoid the risk of aspiration
3. To prevent excessive bleeding
4. To allow for more rapid wound healing

19 The nurse is teaching a client about wound care in preparation for discharge. How should the nurse evaluate the effectiveness of home care teaching on wound care? Select all that apply.

1. Give a paper-and-pencil quiz.
2. Have the caregiver or client demonstrate the procedure.
3. Have the client or caregiver explain the procedure.
4. Have the client or caregiver critique a video on the procedure.
5. Ask the client detailed questions while demonstrating the procedure.

20 A 78-year-old client with chronic obstructive pulmonary disease (COPD) has had abdominal surgery and suddenly feels something "let go" in the incision underneath the dressing when coughing. What should be the nurse's immediate actions? Select all that apply.

1. Have someone notify the healthcare provider.
2. Open the dressing and view the problem.
3. Apply pressure over the site.
4. Use a sterile dressing and sterile saline to keep the open incision moist.
5. Sit the client upright in bed.

ANSWERS & RATIONALES

1 **Answer: 3, 5 Rationale:** Placing the hands directly on the incision during coughing (instead of slightly to each side) will diminish the discomfort associated with coughing. The client should cough forcefully (instead of weakly, as in clearing the throat) to eliminate secretions effectively. Sitting up before coughing, taking deep breaths before coughing, and using a pillow to splint incision are correct and do not require further teaching by the nurse. **Cognitive Level:** Applying **Client Need:** Reduction of Risk Potential **Integrated Process:** Nursing Process: Evaluation **Content Area:** Fundamentals **Strategy:** The words *needs more teaching* in the stem of the question indicates the incorrect client statement is the correct option. Note the wording of the question indicates more than one option is likely to be correct. Use knowledge of nursing fundamentals to answer the question.

2 **Answer: 4 Rationale:** The child fears separation from her parents during the toddler years. The child has no previous experiences to compare to this experience, so she will not anticipate pain before the surgery. A toddler cannot anticipate any changes in her body. A toddler does not worry about communication. **Cognitive Level:** Applying **Client Need:** Reduction of Risk Potential **Integrated Process:** Nursing Process: Planning **Content Area:** Fundamentals **Strategy:** The critical word *greatest* in the stem of the question provides a clue that more than one option could be partially true. Use knowledge of growth and development to make a selection, recalling that toddlers fear separation from their parents.

3 **Answer: 4, 5 Rationale:** Taping a wedding band in place is acceptable for the client who does not wish to remove it, unless there is danger the finger might swell during or after surgery. Documenting the presence of the ring on the

preoperative checklist alerts staff in the surgical suite of its presence. Encouraging the client to use soapy water assumes the ring is tight, and that the client wishes to remove it. Explaining that the hospital cannot be liable creates unnecessary anxiety at a time when it already is likely to be increased. The surgeon does not need to see the client in the preoperative holding area. **Cognitive Level:** Applying **Client Need:** Reduction of Risk Potential **Integrated Process:** Nursing Process: Implementation **Content Area:** Fundamentals **Strategy:** Identify the core issue of the question, which is the method of safeguarding client property during surgery. Choose options that meet the needs of the client and protect both the hospital and the client's property.

4 **Answer: 1 Rationale:** With increased age, there is a greater likelihood that the kidneys start to degenerate. This can lead to reduced glomerular filtration rate and makes the client generally more at risk for fluid and electrolyte imbalances. Hunger does not necessarily lead to complications from hyperacidity. Other factors (when diet is resumed, whether a nasogastric tube is in place, and whether drugs are prescribed to decrease stomach acidity) will all affect stomach acidity. Comprehension is not altered in older adults unless the client has a form of dementia, which is a clinical diagnosis and not an age-related change. Cardiovascular problems do not necessarily diminish pain sensations. **Cognitive Level:** Analyzing **Client Need:** Reduction of Risk Potential **Integrated Process:** Nursing Process: Diagnosis **Content Area:** Fundamentals **Strategy:** For questions that ask you to choose one client over others, determine which client description indicates the worst client status or greatest risk for complications. In this case, note that fluid and electrolyte balance poses the greatest risk in the intraoperative period, which is the core issue of the question.

5 **Answer: 3 Rationale:** Corticosteroids can lead to salt and water retention, and can also delay wound healing. An antidysrhythmic helps to regulate the cardiac rhythm. A sedative-hypnotic can interfere with uptake of the anesthetics, but does not affect healing. An oral hypoglycemic agent is used for diabetes, but the medication itself does not pose added risk to the client during surgery. **Cognitive Level:** Analyzing **Client Need:** Reduction of Risk Potential **Integrated Process:** Nursing Process: Assessment **Content Area:** Fundamentals **Strategy:** To answer this question, recall the actions and adverse effects of each drug class listed. Use the process of elimination, focusing on the risk to the client during an actual surgical procedure, to make your selection.

6 **Answer: 4 Rationale:** A nephrectomy is a major type of surgery because the kidney is a major vital organ, loss of blood is likely to be greater than with the other mentioned surgeries, and there is greater likelihood of complications. A tonsillectomy, biopsy, and arthroscopy are all examples of minor surgery because they do not involve a high degree of risk. **Cognitive Level:** Analyzing **Client Need:** Reduction of Risk Potential **Integrated Process:** Nursing Process: Diagnosis **Content Area:** Fundamentals **Strategy:** The core issue of the question is the degree of surgical risk associated with each procedure. Use the process of elimination, focusing on the nature of each surgical procedure and the seriousness of each one.

7 **Answer: 1 Rationale:** Dementia affects the person's understanding of the proposed surgery and ability to cooperate with the perioperative care; it also affects the medications given. Cultural differences should not pose a risk unless the client's beliefs are contrary to the proposed measures. Mild anxiety will not create a risk. Previous surgeries do not increase risk and could possibly be helpful for the client, who can then draw on previous experiences. **Cognitive Level:** Analyzing **Client Need:** Reduction of Risk Potential **Integrated Process:** Nursing Process: Assessment **Content Area:** Fundamentals **Strategy:** The core issue of the question is the degree of surgical risk associated with each client circumstance. Use the process of elimination, recalling that physiological issues take precedence over psychosocial ones, and that previous surgery might or might not be relevant to the current surgery.

8 **Answer: 1 Rationale:** Abrasions, pustules, or other skin conditions have to be assessed and documented because they can interfere with wound healing or increase the risk of infection. Lack of hair growth or presence of lanugo or fine hair will not interfere with the skin preparation. Pulsation is not always visible or available to assess, depending on the part of the body being operated on. **Cognitive Level:** Applying **Client Need:** Reduction of Risk Potential **Integrated Process:** Nursing Process: Assessment **Content Area:** Fundamentals **Strategy:** The core issue of the question is knowledge of integumentary risks to a surgical procedure. Use the process of elimination, focusing on skin breaks or alterations as the option that interferes with the protective function of the skin.

9 **Answer: 4 Rationale:** Previous surgeries can affect the physiological or psychological responses of the client to the planned surgery. Previous surgeries can reveal possible difficulties or problems with certain anesthetic agents, but do not interfere with absorption of anesthetics, hinder comprehension of instructions, or affect the central nervous system. **Cognitive Level:** Applying **Client Need:** Reduction of Risk Potential **Integrated Process:** Nursing Process: Implementation **Content Area:** Fundamentals **Strategy:** Focus on the issue of the question, which is the need to gather assessment data that could put the client at risk during the surgical procedure. With this concept in mind, eliminate each of the other options that are false statements.

10 **Answer: 1 Rationale:** Alcohol affects the central nervous system, and therefore the client's response to surgery and the anesthetic itself. Smoking, not alcohol (in small amounts), poses respiratory risks. Alcohol could have an additive or synergistic effect with any preoperative sedatives or hypnotics because both depress the central nervous system. Past and recent intake of alcohol can impact responses, which can be either slowed down or escalated. **Cognitive Level:** Applying **Client Need:** Reduction of Risk Potential **Integrated Process:** Nursing Process: Diagnosis **Content Area:** Fundamentals **Strategy:** The core issue of the question is knowledge that alcohol has an interactive effect with anesthesia and possibly other medications used during surgery. Focus on the option that safeguards the client's physical status as the reason for notifying the surgeon.

11 **Answer: 4 Rationale:** The ability of the client to see and hear could affect the preoperative and postoperative teaching methods used. The need for referrals for postdischarge resources depends not only on the client's vision and hearing, but also on family supports and the client's physical and mental status. Vision and hearing impairments could interfere with safety postdischarge, but this is not a primary reason for the assessment at this time. *Unanticipated needs* is a very general term that can be applied not just to vision and hearing but also to any area of client functioning. **Cognitive Level:** Applying **Client Need:** Reduction of Risk Potential **Integrated Process:** Teaching and Learning

ANSWERS & RATIONALES

Content Area: Fundamentals **Strategy:** Focus on the critical word *preoperative*, which should help you select an option that is linked in time with the reason for the assessment.

12 **Answer: 3 Rationale:** Anticoagulants inhibit clotting of the blood, putting the client at increased risk for bleeding postoperatively. If the client was abusing alcohol, the nurse would need to assess for onset of delirium tremens caused by alcohol withdrawal. Respiratory compromise might occur if the client takes sedatives or hypnotics. Hypovolemia is a general risk in the intraoperative and postoperative period, but this risk would be heightened if the client is taking diuretics. **Cognitive Level:** Applying **Client Need:** Reduction of Risk Potential **Integrated Process:** Nursing Process: Planning **Content Area:** Fundamentals **Strategy:** The core issue of the question is knowledge that warfarin sodium is an anticoagulant, and that this medication increases risk of bleeding unless stopped for a sufficient amount of time before surgery (approximately 7 days, depending on client and surgery). Of the two options that relate to bleeding, choose *bleeding or oozing at the surgical wound site* over *hypovolemia* because of the critical word *specific* in the stem of the question.

13 **Answer: 1 Rationale:** Wound and cardiovascular complications are more common among clients who are obese. The client has no risk for fluid overload. Pressure ulcers occur more frequently in clients who are thin rather than obese because of pressure over bony prominences. The client who is obese does not have a problem with the temperature regulating center in the hypothalamus, although adipose tissue can insulate and prevent heat loss. **Cognitive Level:** Applying **Client Need:** Reduction of Risk Potential **Integrated Process:** Nursing Process: Planning **Content Area:** Fundamentals **Strategy:** Recall that obesity leads to increased cardiovascular risks in general, and that it can also be a risk factor for poor wound healing after surgery. Eliminate fluid overload and body temperature regulation first, as being least related to the core issue of the question, and choose impaired wound healing over pressure ulcer development as the priority risk.

14 **Answer: 1 Rationale:** Sequential compression devices facilitate venous return from the lower extremities by alternately inflating and deflating. Smoking can contribute to cardiovascular events, but cessation will not necessarily lessen the chance of thrombophlebitis in the immediate postsurgical period. Assessment of the leg will help with detection but not prevention of thrombophlebitis. Homans sign is pain on dorsiflexion of the leg, and this assessment is a means of detection but not prevention. **Cognitive Level:** Applying **Client Need:** Reduction of Risk Potential **Integrated Process:** Teaching and Learning **Content Area:** Fundamentals **Strategy:** Focus on the critical word in the stem, *prevent*. Discriminate between those options that address assessment and those that address prevention.

15 **Answer: 4 Rationale:** A surgical procedure that relieves symptoms of disease or pain but does not cure is described as palliative. The scheduling of the surgery would not have anything to do with the name or category of surgery. There is no term to describe a surgery that the surgeon does not want to perform. A surgical procedure that has not been decided would not be named or documented. **Cognitive Level:** Applying **Client Need:** Reduction of Risk Potential **Integrated Process:** Teaching and Learning **Content Area:** Fundamentals **Strategy:** Use the process of elimination, selecting the answer that is an accurate description of the meaning of the term *palliative*. Recall that the word *palliate* means "to lessen or reduce," which may help in selecting the correct option.

16 **Answer: 4 Rationale:** A wide scar occurs in tertiary intention because the edges are not approximated, and they regenerate via granulation. A wound that is smaller but irregular is consistent with a wound that has healed by secondary intention. Very little scarring is expected in a wound that heals by primary intention. Tissue loss that prevents edges from approximating is consistent with a wound that is healing by secondary intention. **Cognitive Level:** Analyzing **Client Need:** Reduction of Risk Potential **Integrated Process:** Nursing Process: Evaluation **Content Area:** Fundamentals **Strategy:** First, recall the definition of *tertiary intention*. Then, visualize the appearance of the wound to make your selection.

17 **Answer: 4 Rationale:** Purulent drainage, which often indicates wound infection, is made up of tissue debris, WBCs, and bacteria, and can have different colors, depending on the type of bacteria. The next action by the nurse would be to gather additional data that could indicate infection, such as elevated temperature and WBC count. The nurse would document the findings at some point, but this is not the priority action because green drainage is not an expected finding. It is not a priority to assess for bleeding within the wound at this time. There is no specific reason to measure pulse and BP at this time, since these vital signs are not precise indicators of infection. **Cognitive Level:** Analyzing **Client Need:** Reduction of Risk Potential **Integrated Process:** Nursing Process: Assessment **Content Area:** Fundamentals **Strategy:** The critical words in the stem of the question are *priority action*. This means that the correct option is one that contains a critical-thinking sequence based on the information presented. Correlate the word *greenish* with infection, and then choose the option that assesses for signs of infection.

18 **Answer: 2 Rationale:** By keeping the stomach empty during surgery, the risk of vomiting and aspiration is decreased. NPO status does not make anesthesia induction easier, prevent excessive bleeding, or allow for more rapid wound healing. **Cognitive Level:** Applying **Client Need:** Reduction of Risk Potential **Integrated Process:** Nursing Process: Implementation **Content Area:** Fundamentals **Strategy:** Use knowledge of basic principles of preoperative care to make a selection. The wording of the question tells you that there is only one correct choice.

19 **Answer: 2, 3 Rationale:** Return demonstration is the best way to evaluate teaching of a procedure. Ideally, the teaching is done over a few days and is then evaluated. Having the client explain the procedure is also appropriate because it indicates that the client has the necessary knowledge to perform the procedure. Giving a paper-and-pencil quiz and having the client critique a video would measure cognitive aspects of learning but are not realistic measures. Asking the client detailed questions during the procedure is not helpful because it detracts from learning. **Cognitive Level:** Analyzing **Client Need:** Reduction of Risk Potential **Integrated Process:** Teaching and Learning **Content Area:** Fundamentals **Strategy:** Use fundamental principles of teaching and learning to answer the question, recalling that the best methods of evaluation involve knowledge and action on the part of the client, which can be determined by verbal explanation and return demonstration.

20 **Answer: 1, 2, 4 Rationale:** The nurse should have someone else notify the healthcare provider so the nurse can stay with the client. The symptoms are of possible dehiscence and evisceration; the nurse needs to assess the problem before

taking quick follow-up action. A sterile dressing and sterile normal saline are used to maintain a moist environment until the client goes back to surgery. Applying pressure over the wound will not return the contents into the abdominal cavity if they have eviscerated, and pressure could decrease blood flow, causing tissue hypoxia or necrosis. The client should be placed in a low Fowler position with the knees slightly elevated to reduce tension on the abdomen. **Cognitive Level:** Analyzing **Client Need:** Reduction of Risk Potential **Integrated Process:** Nursing Process: Implementation **Content Area:** Fundamentals **Strategy:** Note that the wording of the question indicates that more than one option is likely to be correct. Select options that protect the wound and reduce the client's anxiety.

Key Terms to Review

anesthesia p. 765
dehiscence p. 773
drains p. 771
exudate p. 773
informed consent p. 764
intraoperative phase p. 763
moderate sedation p. 765
palliative p. 765
postoperative phase p. 763
preoperative phase p. 763
purulent p. 771
regional anesthesia p. 765
sanguineous p. 773
serosanguineous p. 771
serous p. 773
sterile field p. 770
surgical asepsis p. 769
surgical scrub p. 770

References

Ball, J., & Bindler, R., & Cowen, K. (2015). *Principles of pediatric nursing; Caring for children* (6th ed.). Hoboken, NJ: Pearson Education.

Berman, A., Snyder, S., & Frandsen, G. (2016). *Kozier & Erb's fundamentals of nursing: Concepts, process, and practice* (10th ed.). New York, NY: Pearson Education.

LeMone, P., Burke, K., Bauldoff, G., & Gubrud, P. (2015). *Medical surgical nursing: Clinical reasoning in patient care* (6th ed.). Hoboken, NJ: Pearson Education.

Smith, S., Duell, D., Martin, B., Aebersold, M., & Gonzalez, L. (2017). *Clinical nursing skills: Basic to advanced skills* (10th ed.). New York, NY: Pearson Education.

Complicated Antenatal Care 49

In this chapter

Cross Reference

Other chapters relevant to this content area are

Reproduction, Family Planning, and Infertility **Chapter 8**
Uncomplicated Antenatal Assessment and Care **Chapter 9**
Uncomplicated Labor and Delivery Care **Chapter 10**
Uncomplicated Postpartum Assessment and Care **Chapter 11**
Uncomplicated Newborn Care **Chapter 12**
Immunologic and Anti-Infective Medications **Chapter 45**
Common Laboratory Tests **Chapter 46**
Common Diagnostic Tests and Procedures **Chapter 47**
Complicated Labor and Delivery Care **Chapter 50**
Complicated Postpartum Care **Chapter 51**
Complicated Newborn Care **Chapter 52**

I. ASSESSMENT AND DIAGNOSTIC TESTING FOR HIGH-RISK PRENATAL CLIENT

A. ***Biophysical profile (BPP)***
   1. A method of assessing fetal well-being by determining scores on five criteria: fetal breathing, fetal movements, muscle tone, fetal heart rate (FHR) acceleration, and amniotic fluid volume
   2. Total score ranges from 0 to 10; criterion scores are 2 (normal) or 0 (abnormal)
   3. A total score of 8–10 is normal, and the risk of fetal asphyxia increases as scores decline from 6 downward

B. ***Doppler blood flow analysis***
   1. A noninvasive study of fetal blood flow across placenta; can be done as early as 15 weeks
   2. Velocity waveforms from umbilical artery are reported as systolic/diastolic (S/D) ratios
   3. Abnormal ratios (above 95th percentile or reversing after 18–20 weeks' gestation) have been associated with intrauterine growth restriction (IUGR)

C. ***Nonstress test (NST)***
   1. A screening test that assesses fetal well-being; analyzes response of FHR to fetal movement
   2. Advantages: noninvasive, easily interpreted, and can be done in outpatient setting at low cost; good indicator of fetal well-being
   3. Disadvantages: high number of false-positive results caused by fetal sleep cycles, medications, fetal immaturity; not a good predictor of fetal compromise

   NCLEX®
   4. Test procedure: place client in semi-Fowler position; an ultrasound transducer and tocodynamometer record contractions and FHR; client is asked to press a hand-held marker when fetal movement is felt
   5. Episodes of fetal movement are compared to changes in FHR; acoustical stimulation can be done if absence of fetal movement

NCLEX® 6. Findings: normal (reactive) if there are two or more accelerations during a 20-minute period that are at least 15 beats above baseline and last for 15 seconds each

NCLEX® 7. If these criteria are not met within 40 minutes, test is considered nonreactive (nonreassuring) and further testing is indicated

D. ***Contraction stress test (CST)***

1. Assesses fetal ability to withstand stress of uterine contractions and evaluates placental capacity for O_2/CO_2 exchange; since contractions reduce blood flow to fetus, can predict a fetus that may not tolerate stress of labor
2. Indications: factors that place fetus at risk for asphyxia such as IUGR, diabetes, postdate, nonreactive NST, and BPP score less than 6
3. Contraindications: third-trimester bleeding, previous cesarean birth with classical uterine incision; premature rupture of membranes, cervical insufficiency, cerclage in place, multiple gestation, and history of preterm labor (if being done before term)

NCLEX® 4. Test procedure: explain procedure and verify informed consent; have client void and lie in semi-Fowler or side-lying position; begin electronic monitoring of contractions and FHR; after obtaining baseline fetal heart tracing, contractions (if not spontaneous) are initiated with nipple self-stimulation or IV oxytocin

NCLEX® 5. Findings: when at least three contractions of 40- to 60-second duration occur in a 10-minute time period, the FHR pattern is assessed; result is reassuring (negative) if no late decelerations occur; not reassuring (positive) if late decelerations occur with more than 50% of contractions; suspicious or equivocal if there are nonpersistent late decelerations or decelerations associated with hyperstimulation

E. ***Amniocentesis***

1. Overview: an invasive procedure performed on outpatient basis but near a birthing center; a sterile needle is inserted through abdominal wall to uterine cavity (see Figure 49–1) to collect sample of amniotic fluid; often done at 15–20 weeks' gestation
2. Purpose: prenatal diagnosis of genetic disorders, metabolic defects, congenital anomalies, assess fetal lung maturity, and follow-up on abnormalities found on ultrasound

NCLEX® 3. Complications: infrequent but may include vaginal spotting, cramping or amniotic fluid leakage, chorioamnionitis, Rh isoimmunization, needle injury to fetus, or fetal loss (rare)

4. Test procedure: explain procedure and verify informed consent; if client is more than 20 weeks' gestation, she should empty bladder (minimize risk of puncture) and assume supine position with possibly a wedge under left hip to avoid pressure of uterus on vena cava; abdomen is cleansed; using sterile technique, healthcare provider inserts a needle using ultrasound guidance and withdraws 15–20 mL of fluid

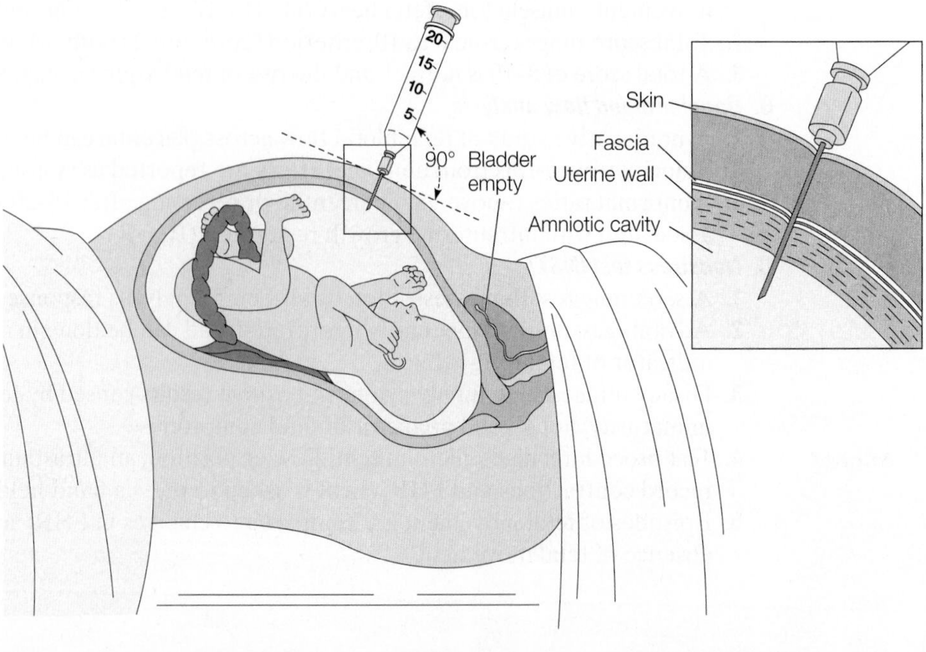

Figure 49–1

Amniocentesis.

NCLEX® 5. Obtain baseline vital signs (VS) and FHR; monitor every 15 minutes during procedure and for 30 minutes after

NCLEX® 6. Rh-negative clients should receive Rh_0(D) immune globulin after procedure because of risk of isoimmunization from fetal blood

7. Follow-up: instruct client to contact healthcare provider for lack of fetal movement or unusual fetal hyperactivity, clear or bloody vaginal drainage, abdominal pain, uterine contractions, fever, chills
8. Inform client to increase fluid intake and engage in only light activities for 24 hours

F. Tests to evaluate fetal lung maturity

1. **Lecithin to sphingomyelin (L/S) ratio**
   a. Obtained via amniocentesis to assess fetal lung maturity
   b. Ratio of 2:1 or higher indicates probable lung maturity and low risk of fetal respiratory distress syndrome (RDS); contamination with meconium or blood may alter results
2. **Phosphatidylglycerol (PG)**
   a. Obtained via amniocentesis; phospholipid found in pulmonary surfactant
   NCLEX® b. Presence in amniotic fluid indicates fetal lung maturity and low risk of RDS

G. *Nitrazine test*

1. Uses a nitrazine test strip to determine presence of amniotic fluid in vaginal secretions
2. Amniotic fluid is slightly alkaline (pH 7.0–7.5) and turns strip blue
3. Vaginal secretions are acidic ((pH 4.5–5.5) and does not cause color change in test strip (beige)

H. *Fetal fibronectin (fFN) test*

1. Glycoprotein produced by fetal tissues and found in cervicovaginal secretions before 16–20 weeks' gestation and again near term
2. Absence of fFN between 20 and 34 weeks' gestation is a positive indicator that client has low risk for premature rupture of membranes or premature birth
3. NCLEX® A positive finding (presence of fFN) indicates a high risk for labor within 2 weeks and warrants further evaluation by sterile speculum exam, nitrazine test, and assessment of cervicovaginal secretions for ferning (presence of amniotic fluid)

I. *Chorionic villus sampling (CVS)*

1. Involves collection of a small specimen of tissue from edge of developing placenta to detect genetic, metabolic, and DNA abnormalities
2. Advantages: earlier diagnosis and rapid return of results compared to amniocentesis; can be performed at 10–12 weeks' gestation with results returned in 1 day (direct preparation method) or 7–10 days (tissue culture)
3. Test preparation: instruct client to come for procedure with full bladder; explain procedure and obtain informed consent; use lithotomy position
4. Test procedure: using sterile technique, healthcare provider visualizes cervix using ultrasound guidance, a suction cannula is used to collect specimen transvaginally or transabdominally (if necessary)
5. Rh-negative clients should receive Rh_0(D) immune globulin postprocedure
6. Complications (rare): vaginal spotting or bleeding, miscarriage, rupture of membranes, and chorioamnionitis; limb anomalies if procedure done before 10 weeks' gestation
7. Follow-up includes teaching client signs of complications to report, when results will be available, that test does not detect neural tube defects, and arranging genetic counseling as needed

II. PREGESTATIONAL CONDITIONS

A. Cardiac disease

1. Pregnancy increases workload on heart; cardiac output increases 30–50% by mid-pregnancy (cardiac workload greatest at 28–30 weeks' gestation when blood volume peaks)
2. A compromised heart with inadequate cardiac capacity and decreased reserves may be unable to adapt to added requirements of pregnancy
3. Treatment options and outcome depend on degree of cardiac compromise
4. Clients with class I and II cardiac disease have potential for good pregnancy outcome, while class III or IV clients may have serious maternal or fetal compromise (Table 49–1)
5. NCLEX® Nursing assessment: most common complication of heart disease during pregnancy is heart failure (HF)
   a. Edema of varying degree from pedal edema, pitting edema, generalized edema (anasarca), and pulmonary edema
   b. Dyspnea on exertion, increasing fatigue, dyspnea at rest, moist cough, basilar crackles, pallor then cyanosis of nail beds, circumoral cyanosis
   c. Tachycardia, irregular pulse, murmurs, chest pain

Table 49–1 New York Heart Association Classification of Functional Capacity for Clients with Cardiac Disease

Classification	Functional Capacity
I	Uncompromised: No limitation on physical activity and no symptoms during ordinary activity
II	Slightly compromised: Normal activity causes fatigue, palpitation, dyspnea, or angina; asymptomatic at rest
III	Markedly compromised: May be comfortable at rest but less than usual activity causes fatigue, dyspnea, palpitations, or angina
IV	Severely compromised: Cannot perform any activity without increasing discomfort; may experience angina and cardiac insufficiency while at rest

6. Collaborative management
   a. Monitor client and fetal well-being more frequently during pregnancy; changes in maternal VS or signs of fetal compromise may indicate inability to handle increasing demands on heart

   NCLEX®
   b. Teach adequate nutrition for pregnancy and provide prenatal vitamins and iron to prevent anemia; some clients may be prescribed a low-sodium diet to prevent fluid retention

   NCLEX®
   c. Instruct client to avoid excessive weight gain and emotional stress, which place added stress on cardiac reserves
   d. Teach client to report signs of infection so treatment may begin early
   e. Diagnostic procedures may include cardiac auscultation, electrocardiogram, echocardiogram, and possible cardiac catheterization
   f. Medications may include digoxin (a cardiac glycoside), antidysrhythmics (control cardiac dysrhythmias), and diuretics (reduce fluid retention)

   NCLEX®
   g. Heparin is considered safe for use in pregnancy if an anticoagulant is indicated (pregnancy category C); warfarin is a pregnancy category X drug (Table 49–2) and must be avoided

   NCLEX®
   h. Teach client to avoid exertion and to plan frequent rest periods
   i. During labor, monitor VS frequently, apply cardiac monitor and external fetal monitor, apply oxygen as needed, maintain bedrest with client lying either in semi-Fowler position with lateral tilt or on side with head and shoulders elevated
   j. Remain with client during labor for support, keep her informed of labor progress, encourage sleep or relaxation between contractions, and use shorter and moderate pushing efforts with complete relaxation between contractions

   NCLEX®
   k. Observe client carefully for complications from hemodynamic changes immediately after delivery; extravascular fluid returns to bloodstream causing risk for decompensation during first 48 hours postpartum

B. Diabetes mellitus

1. A pancreatic endocrine disorder affecting carbohydrate (CHO) metabolism resulting from inadequate production or use of insulin (see also Chapter 60)
2. Affects pregnancy by decreasing need for insulin during first trimester because of hPL (human placental lactogen), then increasing insulin demand toward end of first trimester through end of pregnancy

Table 49–2 FDA Pregnancy Categories for Prescription Drugs

Category	Risk to Fetus	Examples of Drugs
A	Controlled studies in women do not demonstrate risk to fetus in first trimester, and possibility of fetal harm appears remote.	RDA dose of Vitamin C
B	Animal studies have not demonstrated fetal risk but there are no controlled studies in women, or animal studies show an adverse effect not confirmed in controlled studies in women in first trimester.	Acetaminophen Penicillins
C	Animal studies show adverse effects and there are no controlled studies in women, or studies in women and animals are not available. Drug should be given only if potential benefit justifies potential risk to fetus.	Zidovudine Heparin
D	Positive evidence of fetal risk in humans, but benefits to mother may be acceptable despite risk in certain situations.	Phenobarbitol
X	Risks to fetus clearly outweigh any possible benefit to mother. Drug is contraindicated in women who may become pregnant.	Warfarin Diethylstilbestrol

NCLEX®
3. Maternal risks during pregnancy are decreased by tight control of blood glucose (70–110 mg/dL), but include hydramnios (excess amniotic fluid from excess fetal urination due to hyperglycemia), ketoacidosis, preeclampsia and eclampsia, dystocia (difficult labor because of large fetus), and worsening retinopathy

NCLEX®
4. Fetal risks result from high maternal blood glucose levels and include congenital anomalies, **macrosomia** (excessive growth leading to large infant size from persistent hyperglycemia and fetal hyperinsulinism), and post-birth hypoglycemia, polycythemia, hyperbilirubinemia, hypocalcemia, and respiratory distress syndrome

5. **Gestational diabetes** occurs in a previously nondiabetic client when pancreas is unable to meet increased demands for insulin production during pregnancy
   a. Risk factors: family history of diabetes, maternal obesity (BMI greater than 30), polycystic ovarian syndrome, previous large-for-gestational-age (LGA) infants, previous unexplained stillbirth
   b. Classic symptoms of diabetes mellitus: thirst (polydipsia), hunger (polyphagia), frequent urination (polydipsia), glycosuria

NCLEX®
   c. Other symptoms include blurred vision, recurrent urinary tract infections and vaginal candidiasis (yeast) infections caused by altered pH in reproductive tract, ketonuria, polyhydramnios, and LGA fetal size
   d. Detection includes diabetes screening at 24–28 weeks' gestation with a 50-gram oral glucose tolerance test (GTT); if BG equals or is greater than 140 mg/dL at 1 hour, a 3-hour 100-gram oral GTT is performed

6. Antepartum management of diabetes
   a. Teach prescribed ADA diet with no concentrated sweets

NCLEX®
   b. Monitor glucose levels with capillary glucose self-testing, fasting blood glucose, and glycosylated hemoglobin (HbA_{1c}) (see Chapter 46)

NCLEX®
   c. Medications: insulin (human) of the intermediate, regular, and/or analog (lispro and aspart) types should be carefully regulated and adjusted as pregnancy progresses with up to a fourfold dose increase needed at term; recent evidence suggests that oral hypoglycemics glyburide (a second-generation sulfonylurea) and metformin (a biguanide) may be safe for use in gestational diabetes

NCLEX®
   d. Instruct client in frequent BG and urine ketone testing and to keep a diary of test results and activity levels

NCLEX®
   e. Encourage regular nonstrenuous exercise such as walking for weight and BG control
   f. Monitor fetal well-being: quadruple screening at 15–20 weeks, ultrasound for anomalies, amniotic fluid volume, and fetal size; fetal movement counts, weekly NST from 28–32 weeks, possible oxytocin challenge test (OCT), BPP, and amniocentesis for lung maturity; L/S ratio needs to be 1:3 (normal is 1:2); PG should be present
   g. Monitor client for development of complications: infection, preeclampsia, and diabetic ketoacidosis

7. Intrapartum management of diabetes
   a. Many pregnancies go to full term, but some clinicians prefer to induce labor at 38–39 weeks for clients with type 1 diabetes mellitus to reduce problems caused by decreased perfusion as placenta ages; cesarean birth may be needed if fetus has nonreassuring status; preterm birth should be preceded by testing of fetal lung maturity
   b. During labor, maternal glucose levels are measured hourly (maternal need for insulin decreases significantly during labor), longer-acting insulins replaced with regular insulin, and client should have two IV lines (one with 5% dextrose solution and second with saline in case IV insulin is needed)

NCLEX®
8. Postpartum management of diabetes: insulin requirements drop dramatically after delivery of placenta and removal of hormonal influences; client may need no insulin or a very decreased dose; those with gestational diabetes generally require no insulin but an oral hypoglycemic may be used if glucose is elevated

C. Substance abuse

1. Description and etiology
   a. Pregnant women may be reluctant to disclose substance use but may also recognize a need for care and be responsive to caring interventions; some clients may delay seeking care or present in labor with no prenatal care; all pregnant women should be screened for substance abuse including assessment of physical signs
   b. Substances frequently used are nicotine, alcohol, heroin, methadone, diazepam, amphetamines, marijuana, cocaine/crack, and MDMA (Ecstasy); effects on pregnancy include spontaneous abortion, IUGR, preterm labor, placental abruption, stillbirth, neonatal addiction, and fetal alcohol syndrome (FAS)

2. Nursing assessment

NCLEX®
   a. Establish trusting relationship with client by remaining open, matter-of-fact, and nonjudgmental; women seeking prenatal care want to improve and safeguard their health and that of fetus
   b. Encourage client to describe all substances used, amounts, times and triggers to use, and any previous attempts to discontinue use
   c. Evaluate client's motivation, support systems, and personal strengths that may be elicited to change behaviors

3. Collaborative management

NCLEX®
   a. Monitor client for complications: anemia, inadequate nutrition and weight gain, hypertension, preterm labor; random urine toxicology screens may be prescribed

NCLEX®
   b. Monitor fetal growth and well-being: fundal height, ultrasound, NST, BPP

NCLEX®
   c. Teach client about potential negative effects of substances used on pregnancy and fetus/neonate

NCLEX®
   d. Assist with referrals for client as indicated: smoking cessation classes, Alcoholics Anonymous, addiction counseling, psychological counseling, and possible hospitalization
   e. Reinforce teaching about nutrition and effects on fetal development; teach client danger signs of pregnancy including signs of preterm labor and abruption of placenta

NCLEX®
   f. Support client's efforts to change negative behaviors
   g. Client may need to be followed by a perinatologist during pregnancy; an addicted neonate will require intensive care at birth
   h. "Cold turkey" drug withdrawal is not advised because of risk to fetus; clients with heroin addiction may receive methadone hydrochloride—a narcotic agonist analgesic that blocks severe symptoms of heroin withdrawal
   i. Preferred methods for pain management during labor include psychoprophylaxis, regional or local anesthetics (such as pudendal block local infiltration), but pain medication should not be withheld because of fear of contributing to further addiction

D. HIV/AIDS

1. Overview: human immunodeficiency virus (HIV) is transmitted through contact with infected blood and body secretions, is characterized by decreased immunity and increased susceptibility to opportunistic infections, and over years of time may lead to acquired immunodeficiency syndrome (AIDS); see also Chapter 66

NCLEX®
2. Maternal and fetal risks: priority focus is on maintaining health of mother, preventing transmission to a possibly seronegative father, and preventing mother-to-child transmission (repeated exposure to virus through unsafe sex practices or IV drug use with contaminated needles, vaginal birth, and breastfeeding)

NCLEX®
3. Current maternal treatment with antiretroviral therapy (ART) is recommended to all infected women to reduce risk of perinatal transmission; drugs include a nucleoside reverse transcriptase inhibitor (NRTI) backbone including one or more drugs with high level of placental passage (zidovudine, lamivudine, tenofovir, or abacavir); see Chapter 45 for additional drug information

NCLEX®
4. Maternal HIV antibodies cross placenta so all infants of HIV-positive mothers will test positive at birth and until maternal antibodies are depleted at between 15 and 18 months of age

5. Collaborative management
   a. Antibodies to HIV are detected with ELISA test and results confirmed by Western blot test or immunofluorescence assay (IFA); see also Chapter 47
   b. Provide emotional support and reproductive counseling to client and family
   c. Evaluate client for other sexually transmitted infections and hepatitis B
   d. Review lab results for signs of anemia, thrombocytopenia, leukopenia, and decreased CD-4 T-lymphocyte counts

NCLEX®
   e. Monitor client for signs of opportunistic infection: fever, weight loss, fatigue, candidiasis, cough, skin lesions
   f. Monitor fetal growth and well-being
   g. Protect uninfected fetus from HIV during labor and birth by avoiding invasive procedures such as vaginal exam after rupture of membranes, fetal scalp electrode monitoring, fetal scalp sampling, and vacuum extraction when possible
   h. Avoid episiotomy to decrease amount of maternal blood in vaginal canal
   i. Avoid or limit oxytocin use when possible to reduce incidence of vaginal tears or need for episiotomy
   j. Place highly absorbent pads under mother's hips during delivery to absorb maternal blood and amniotic fluid

NCLEX®
   k. Suction fluids from neonate immediately after delivery

NCLEX® l. Provide zidovidine as prescribed during labor and delivery to reduce risk of neonatal transmission

m. Remove neonate from maternal blood after delivery and bathe newborn as soon as possible to remove all maternal secretions; delay any newborn injections or heelsticks until after bath

NCLEX® n. Encourage mother to formula-feed infant to avoid transmission by breast milk

E. Rh-sensitization

1. Overview
   a. Rh-negative women who have Rh-positive embryo/fetus (from an Rh-positive father) may become sensitized to Rh antigen with contact between maternal and fetal blood; other causes are blood transfusion of Rh-positive blood to an Rh-negative woman or fetomaternal blood contact during amniocentesis or other invasive procedure
   b. Sensitized Rh-negative women develop anti-Rh antibodies, which may cross placenta in subsequent Rh-positive pregnancies and attack and destroy fetal RBCs
   c. Sensitized effects of Rh incompatibility and sensitization are progressively severe

NCLEX® 2. Hemolysis of fetal erythrocytes leads to greatly increased immature RBC production, termed **erythroblastosis fetalis**; continued RBC destruction and resulting anemia leads to jaundice and marked fetal edema known as **hydrops fetalis**, which may lead to fetal heart failure, hepatosplenomegaly, severe generalized edema (anasarca), multiple organ system failure, and possible fetal death

NCLEX® 3. Breakdown of RBCs releases bilirubin, causing jaundice; high levels of circulating bilirubin can cause **kernicterus**, a yellow staining of basal ganglia and brain, and may result in permanent neurologic damage

NCLEX® 4. Nursing assessment
   a. All pregnant women should be tested for blood group and Rh factor, and have routine antibody screening; note history of previous miscarriage, blood transfusions, or infants experiencing jaundice
   NCLEX® b. If client is Rh-negative, infant's father is tested for Rh status; an Rh-negative father and mother will only produce Rh-negative offspring who will not be affected by Rh-incompatibility
   NCLEX® c. An indirect **Coombs' test** on maternal blood determines whether Rh-negative client has developed antibodies to Rh antigen; serial antibody screening should continue throughout pregnancy; a direct Coombs' test on infant's blood after birth identifies maternal antibodies attached to fetal RBCs

5. Collaborative management
   a. Provide support and education to client and family; client should wear or carry Rh-negative identification and recognize that she may need $Rh_0(D)$ immune globulin with future pregnancies
   b. Unsensitized Rh-negative clients should receive 300 mcg of $Rh_0(D)$ immune globulin IM at 28 weeks and also within 72 hours of delivery
   c. Antibodies in immune globulin bind with Rh antigens in maternal circulation to provide passive immunity (mother will not become sensitized to Rh antigens and will not produce antibodies)
   NCLEX® d. $Rh_0(D)$ immune globulin is not given to mothers who are already sensitized and have antibodies (positive indirect Coombs' test)
   NCLEX® e. $Rh_0(D)$ globulin is also given after abortion, ectopic pregnancy, amniocentesis, and any other situation that might result in maternal exposure to fetal Rh antigen
   NCLEX® f. Evaluate fetus for onset of complications by serial ultrasound for amniotic fluid volume, fetal size, and development of edema or enlarged heart
   g. A sinusoidal electronic fetal monitoring pattern indicates severe fetal anemia; BPP may be used to identify a compromised fetus
   h. Amniocentesis or percutaneous umbilical cord blood sampling (PUBS) may be used to determine fetal Rh; both procedures carry risk of causing maternal exposure and sensitization, so $Rh_0(D)$ immune globulin should be given
   i. Intrauterine exchange transfusion (replacement with Rh-negative blood to stop destruction of fetal RBCs) may be performed for severely affected fetus until viability is reached
   NCLEX® j. An early delivery with phototherapy and exchange transfusions may be planned if fetus is developing anemia close to term

III. GESTATIONAL AND PRELABOR CONDITIONS

A. Hyperemesis gravidarum

1. Overview
   a. Extreme nausea and vomiting (N/V) during first half of pregnancy associated with dehydration, weight loss, and electrolyte imbalances; emesis is much more severe than in common "morning sickness" of early pregnancy

b. Cause remains unclear but may be related to high hcG level, higher estradiol level, lower prolactin level, hypofunction of anterior pituitary gland and adrenal cortex, corpus luteum abnormalities, and psychological factors
c. High level of hCG, also found in gestational trophoblastic disease (hydatidiform mole, molar pregnancy), is associated with severe N/V
d. Fetus is at risk for abnormal development, IUGR, or death from lack of nutrition, hypoxia, and maternal ketoacidosis

2. Nursing assessment
a. Intractable vomiting during first 20 weeks of pregnancy but especially during first trimester
NCLEX® b. Dehydration: poor skin turgor, dry mucous membranes, possible hypotension, tachycardia, and increased hematocrit and urine specific gravity
c. Manifestations of electrolyte or acid–base imbalance (acidosis): ketosis, confusion, drowsiness, muscle weakness, cramps, clumsiness, tremors, irregular heartbeat, decreased level of consciousness (LOC)
d. Manifestations of starvation: muscle wasting, ketonuria, jaundice, bleeding gums (vitamin deficiency), weight loss

3. Collaborative management
NCLEX® a. If severe, client may need IV fluid therapy with glucose, electrolytes, and vitamins or parenteral nutrition therapy
NCLEX® b. Monitor VS, daily weight, intake and output (I&O), and calorie count
c. Monitor serum laboratory results for electrolyte imbalances and urine for ketones
d. Administer prescribed antiemetic medications such as phenothiazines or antihistamines as prescribed to control N/V
NCLEX® e. Encourage six small feedings/day after acute N/V pass; foods that are low fat, easily digested carbohydrates, and salty foods may be better tolerated at first; encourage having liquids between meals rather than with meals; clear liquids may be better tolerated at first
f. Monitor fetal growth with serial ultrasounds and ongoing monitoring of fetal heart rate and activity level
g. Refer for additional counseling and support as indicated

B. *Ectopic* pregnancy

1. Overview
a. Implantation of fertilized ovum outside uterus; most commonly a fallopian tube narrowed by scarring or adhesions; other sites are ovary or elsewhere in abdominal cavity
b. Risk factors for tubal damage that can lead to ectopic pregnancy include ascending infections, pelvic inflammatory disease (PID), use of IUD contraception, or tubal surgery

2. Nursing assessment
a. Last normal menstrual period (LNMP) is consistent with possible pregnancy; possible subjective symptoms of pregnancy, such as breast tenderness and nausea, are present
NCLEX® b. Possible irregular vaginal bleeding and unilateral lower abdominal pain
NCLEX® c. With rupture with subsequent bleeding into abdominal cavity, client may have increased and severe pain with abdominal rigidity, referred right shoulder pain, and signs of shock

3. Implementation and collaborative care
NCLEX® a. Monitor BP, pulse, and respirations every 15 minutes or more often if indicated
NCLEX® b. Treat shock with oxygen and IV fluids with at least an 18-gauge needle in case blood products need to be given; obtain type and cross-match if hemorrhage is suspected; medicate for pain as prescribed
c. Medical treatment is methotrexate as a single or two-dose approach; this is an option for stable healthy client with unruptured ectopic pregnancy of 4 cm or less and no fetal heart movement
d. Surgical treatment is salpingostomy via laparoscope if future pregnancy is desired
NCLEX® e. Provide standard preoperative and postoperative care and teaching; offer emotional support to client and family; facilitate grieving; provide Rh_0(D) immune globulin for Rh-negative mothers with an Rh-positive partner

C. *Gestational trophoblastic disease (GTD)*

1. Overview
a. Pathological proliferation of trophoblastic cells (outermost layer of embryonic cells) that includes hydatiform mole (molar pregnancy), invasive mole (chorioadenoma destruens), and choriocarcinoma (a form of cancer)
b. **Hydatiform mole** is characterized by trophoblastic cells that grow rapidly into fluid-filled, grapelike clusters; a complete mole develops from an empty ovum that contains no genetic material; a partial mole may have an abnormal embryo that usually spontaneously aborts in first trimester

c. A complete mole may lead to development of choriocarcinoma, a rapidly growing malignant neoplasm
d. An invasive mole (chorioadenoma destruens) is similar to a complete mole but involves uterine myometrium

2. Nursing assessment
a. Variable vaginal bleeding usually occurs during first trimester; may be brown, like prune juice, and may contain some grapelike vesicles
NCLEX® b. Unusual uterine enlargement measured by fundal height; no fetal parts can be palpated and no FHR heard; "snowstorm" pattern seen on ultrasound
c. Abnormal labs include very high hCG levels and very low maternal AFP levels
NCLEX® d. Complications: anemia, hyperemesis gravidarum (probably associated with high hCG levels), infection (often with late diagnosis and spontaneous abortion of mole), disseminated intravascular coagulopathy, ovarian cysts, hyperthyroidism, and possible trophoblastic pulmonary embolism

3. Collaborative management
NCLEX® a. Monitor client for signs of hemorrhage, hypertension, or other complications
b. Prepare client and assist with suction uterine evacuation of molar pregnancy (may be followed by oxytocin to contract uterus); hysterectomy may be chosen by clients who do not want to preserve fertility to reduce risk of choriocarcinoma
c. Monitor for postsurgical hemorrhage and infection as with any surgery
NCLEX® d. Weekly hCG levels are done initially until three negative results are obtained, then monthly for 6 to 12 months to rule out choriocarcinoma; reinforce need for diligent follow-up care
NCLEX® e. Client should avoid pregnancy for 1 year after molar pregnancy to avoid confusion between new pregnancy or development of cancer
f. Provide emotional support for client and family who are grieving pregnancy loss and living with fear of developing a malignancy

D. *Cervical insufficiency*

NCLEX® 1. Overview: a painless cervical effacement and dilatation without contractions or pain because of structural or functional defect of cervix
2. Risk factors can be congenital (bicornuate uterus or exposure to DES [diethylstilbestrol]), acquired (inflammation and infection, cervical trauma, cone biopsy, subclinical uterine activity, increased uterine volume/multiple gestation), and hormone relaxin
3. Nursing assessment
a. Previous unexplained second-trimester pregnancy losses may indicate undiagnosed cervical insufficiency
NCLEX® b. Client may present for care completely dilated with bulging membranes
4. Collaborative management
a. Provide emotional support and grief support group referral for client with pregnancy loss from cervical insufficiency
NCLEX® b. Provide client teaching if client is managed on bedrest at home for a cervix just beginning to efface (shorten)
NCLEX® c. Provide teaching about cervical **cerclage** (placement of a surgical stitch in cervix to prevent spontaneous abortion or preterm birth
d. Monitor for signs of preterm labor or infection; client may receive progesterone supplementation or a tocolytic (drug to stop labor) and an antibiotic and anti-inflammatory drugs as indicated
NCLEX® e. Instruct client to contact provider if contractions begin because cesarean delivery is performed or suture must be removed before vaginal birth can be accomplished

E. Spontaneous *abortion*

1. Overview
a. An unintended pregnancy loss related to chromosomal abnormalities (often in first trimester), teratogenic drugs, faulty implantation, weakened cervix, placental abnormalities, and maternal disease, infection, or endocrine imbalance
b. Classification of spontaneous abortion is presented in Box 49–1
2. Nursing assessment
NCLEX® a. Vaginal spotting or bleeding is common; client may pass clots and tissue
b. Pelvic cramping or dull backache is usually present
c. Falling hCG levels indicate death of embryo; ultrasound is used to identify gestational sac and note whether there is current cardiac movement
3. Collaborative management
NCLEX® a. Instruct client that typical management of threatened abortion is with bedrest at home and abstinence from coitus; client should notify healthcare provider if bleeding or cramping worsens

Box 49–1

Classification of Spontaneous Abortion

Terminology associated with spontaneous abortion helps to classify the clinical condition.

- Threatened abortion: Presence of vaginal bleeding, cramping, or backache but cervix remains closed. May resolve without threatening fetus or leading to expulsion.
- Imminent (inevitable) abortion: Presence of increased cramping and bleeding; cervix dilates, and membranes may rupture.
- Incomplete abortion: Expulsion of some products of conception; some tissue is retained (most often placenta); internal cervical os is dilated.
- Complete abortion: Expulsion of all products of conception; uterus is contracted and cervix is closed.
- Missed abortion: Fetus has died in utero but is not expelled; signs of pregnancy reverse (no uterine growth, breast changes resolve); client may be at risk for DIC if products of conception are retained after 4 weeks.
- Recurrent pregnancy loss: Abortion occurs in three or more consecutive pregnancies.
- Septic abortion: Infection is present; can occur with unrecognized rupture of membranes, pregnancy with IUD in place, or attempt to end pregnancy by unqualified person.

NCLEX® **b.** Assess current amount of bleeding; instruct client to save all clots and tissue that may be passed for further examination

c. Monitor BP, pulse, and respirations frequently if bleeding is heavy; evaluate client for signs of impending shock

d. Initiate IV therapy with at least an 18-gauge needle as prescribed

e. Assist with dilatation and curettage (D&C) as indicated for an incomplete abortion

NCLEX® **f.** Provide emotional support, but not false hope, to client and family; never discount importance of even a very early pregnancy

g. Engage in reflective listening; explore client's feelings and explain grief cycle; provide resources, such as referral to pregnancy loss support groups

NCLEX® **h.** Give $Rh_0(D)$ immune globulin to Rh-negative clients with Rh-positive partners within 72 hours of abortion

F. *Placenta previa*

1. Overview

a. Placenta is abnormally implanted in lower uterine segment or over internal cervical os; with contraction and dilation of lower uterine segment in later pregnancy, placental villi are torn from uterine wall, causing bleeding

b. May be a low implantation near cervix, marginal previa at edge of internal cervical os, partial previa covering part of os, or complete placenta previa covering entire os

c. A client with complete previa undergoes cesarean delivery, usually with a classical uterine incision to avoid placenta; decisions about vaginal versus cesarean delivery for other types of previa depend on proximity of os to placenta's lower edge

2. Nursing assessment

NCLEX® **a.** Episodic painless bright red vaginal bleeding; uterus is soft without contractions; each successive bleeding episode is usually heavier than previous one; profuse hemorrhage can occur as cervix dilates under placenta

b. Maternal VS, FHR with external fetal monitor, onset of pain, and uterine contractility

3. Collaborative management

NCLEX® **a.** To avoid profuse hemorrhage, never perform vaginal exam or other actions that stimulate uterine activity on pregnant client with painless vaginal bleeding

NCLEX® **b.** Maintain preterm clients on bedrest (side-lying preferred), possibly with bathroom privileges as long as there is no active bleeding, until fetal maturity is reached or until hemorrhage warrants immediate cesarean delivery

NCLEX® **c.** Monitor maternal VS to rule out ascending infection or shock

NCLEX® **d.** Assess blood loss by weighing peripads and bed pads that are bloody (1 gram = 1 mL); report blood loss during a specified period as prescribed (e.g., 50 mL blood loss in 20 minutes)

e. Monitor serial hemoglobin and hematocrit levels; obtain blood group and type; have two units of cross-matched blood available

Memory Aid

Remember when weighing small amounts of blood or other fluids that one gram equals one milliliter (1 g = 1 mL); weigh the dry object (such as peripad) and subtract weight from that of wet object to obtain weight of blood or other fluids.

f. Perform continuous external fetal monitoring and other testing as indicated

g. Maintain IV access with at least an 18-gauge needle, if indicated, and provide replacement fluids (lactated Ringer's) as prescribed

NCLEX® h. Provide emotional support to client on bedrest; facilitate family visits

NCLEX® i. Promote adequate nutrition with prenatal vitamins and iron to prevent maternal anemia

j. Assist with double setup procedure if indicated: healthcare provider performs a careful vaginal exam in OR with equipment and staff ready to perform either cesarean or vaginal delivery depending on whether bleeding is caused by placenta previa or is increased bloody show of advanced labor

k. Provide routine preoperative and postoperative cesarean care if indicated; instruct client about location of uterine incision as it relates to future desire for a vaginal birth after cesarean (VBAC)

G. ***Abruptio placentae***

1. Premature separation of normally implanted placenta from uterine wall
2. Three types: marginal abruption (at periphery of placenta; may cause bleeding), central (placenta separates centrally, trapping blood; no external bleeding), and complete (almost total separation; massive bleeding (see Figure 49–2)
3. Risk factors include maternal hypertension, abdominal trauma, domestic violence, uterine fibroids, multiple gestation, smoking, alcohol and cocaine use
4. Maternal risks are hemorrhagic shock and renal failure as a consequence of shock; fetal risks are death or consequences of premature labor, anemia, and hypoxia (such as neurologic defects or brain damage if severe)
5. Nursing assessment

NCLEX® a. Presence of dark red vaginal bleeding depending on type; abdomen may increase in size as bleeding continues

b. A central abruption causes severe pain from distention of uterine muscle from trapped blood; uterus is irritable and fetus shows consistent late decelerations

NCLEX® c. Bleeding behind placenta is forced into myometrium and may result in a Couvelaire uterus, which becomes bluish-purple, extremely irritable, distended, and rigid; uterus does not contract efficiently after delivery, leading to postpartum hemorrhage

d. Marginal placental abruption may present with more vaginal bleeding but less pain than a concealed abruption

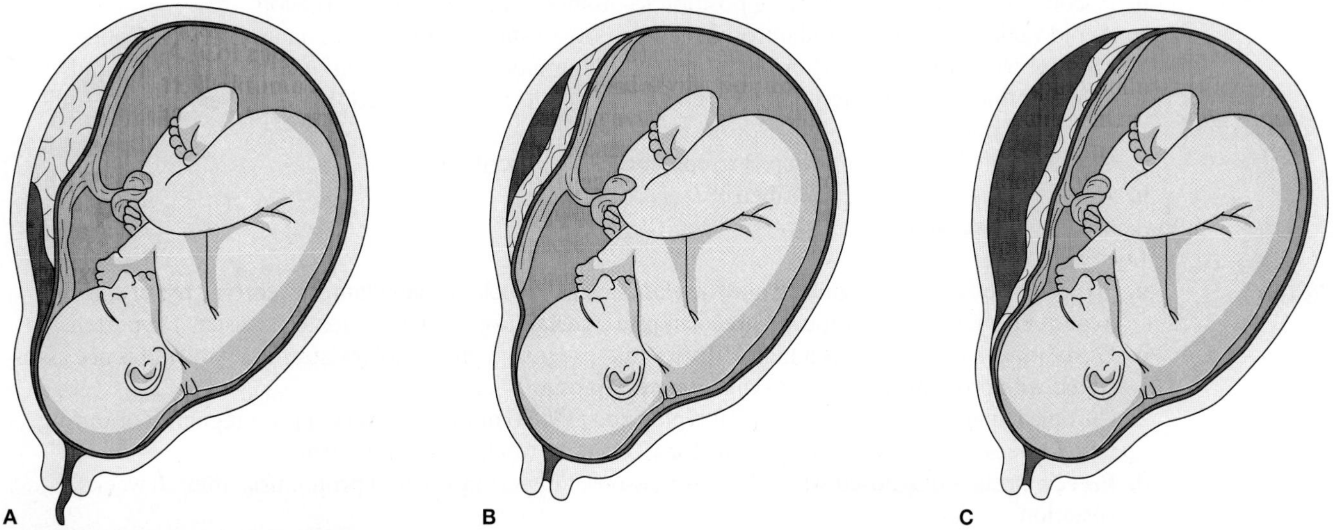

Figure 49–2 Abruptio placentae. (**A**) Marginal—external bleeding, (**B**) central-concealed bleeding, (**C**) complete.

Memory Aid

Differentiate between abruptio placentae and placenta previa by characteristic of bleeding and uterine status. Bleeding is dark red (if present) in abruptio placentae and bright red with placenta previa. Uterus is tender/painful/rigid in abruptio placentae and soft/nontender in placenta previa.

6. Collaborative management
   a. Monitor maternal VS for impending shock (increasing pulse and respirations, decreasing BP)

   NCLEX® b. Monitor fetus continuously for signs of distress: increased fetal movement, changes in baseline FHR, late decelerations

   NCLEX® c. Assess client for bleeding, uterine activity, and abdominal pain; place on external fetal monitor to evaluate uterine irritability and fetal well-being; palpate uterine tone

   d. Measure client's abdominal girth at umbilicus for baseline size and repeat hourly to evaluate occult bleeding; an alternative method is to measure distance from symphysis pubis to top of uterine fundus

   e. Review lab values to estimate blood loss (hemoglobin and hematocrit) and monitor for DIC (decreased platelets and fibrinogen; increased fibrin degradation products, prolonged PT and PTT)

   f. Monitor client for signs of developing coagulation defects: unusual bleeding from injection sites, gums, development of petechiae

   NCLEX® g. Administer IV fluids, oxygen, and blood products as prescribed; monitor I&O; a urinary catheter may be inserted with expected urine output of 30 mL/hour or greater

   h. Carefully monitor client and fetus if vaginal delivery is attempted; prepare for emergency cesarean delivery if fetus develops distress

   i. Provide ongoing information and emotional support for client and family

H. Premature rupture of membranes (PROM)

1. Spontaneous rupture of amniotic membrane before labor begins
2. Preterm PROM (PPROM) involves membrane rupture prior to 37 weeks' gestation; risk factors include infection, cervical insufficiency, and trauma
3. Prolonged rupture of membranes refers to membranes ruptured more than 24 hours before birth; healthcare providers may induce labor rather than risk possible ascending infection

NCLEX® 4. Nursing assessment: gush of fluid from vagina with continued leakage and pooling in vaginal vault; positive nitrazine test (alkaline pH indicating amniotic fluid)

5. Collaborative management

   NCLEX® a. Note time, color, consistency, and amount of fluid at time of rupture; obtain a baseline maternal temperature

   b. Evaluate client's temperature every 2 hours; other VS may be routine; if temperature elevates, assess hydration status

   c. Assess fetal heart tracings for adverse signs (tachycardia, loss of variability, late decelerations); an unengaged fetus is at risk for prolapsed cord when membranes rupture

   NCLEX® d. Encourage client to use side-lying position to promote uteroplacental perfusion

   e. Avoid vaginal exams to avoid introducing microorganisms that may cause an ascending infection

   f. Monitor client for signs of **chorioamnionitis** (inflammation and infection of fetal membranes and amniotic fluid): elevated temperature, abdominal tenderness, increased WBCs and erythrocyte sedimentation rate

   g. Obtain vaginal culture for group B streptococcus as prescribed

   h. Administer antibiotics if prescribed

I. Preeclampsia and eclampsia

1. Overview

   NCLEX® a. Hypertension during pregnancy may be classified as preeclampsia-eclampsia, chronic hypertension, hypertension with superimposed preeclampsia or eclampsia, and gestational (transient) hypertension

   b. Gestational hypertension is a high BP after mid-pregnancy that resolves after delivery and is not associated with proteinuria or other signs of preeclampsia

   c. Chronic hypertension exists when BP is elevated (140/90 mmHg or higher) pre-pregnancy or during first 20 weeks of pregnancy, or persists for 12 or more weeks after childbirth

   d. **Preeclampsia** is diagnosed when there is new-onset hypertension and proteinuria after 20 weeks' gestation

NCLEX®

e. Mild preeclampsia is characterized by BP higher than 140/90 after 20 weeks' gestation and proteinuria of 1–2+ by dipstick or less than 2 grams protein in a 24-hour urine

f. Severe preeclampsia is characterized by a BP of 160/110 or higher and proteinuria 3+ or greater or more than 500 mg protein in a 24-hour urine

g. Sudden onset of severe edema indicates a need for evaluation for preeclampsia or renal disease

NCLEX®

h. **Eclampsia** is the term for preeclampsia that has progressed to include maternal generalized seizures or coma

NCLEX®

i. HELLP (hemolysis, elevated liver enzymes, and low platelet count) syndrome may be associated with severe preeclampsia; the client is at risk for hemorrhage, pulmonary edema, and hepatic rupture

j. Fetal complications include IUGR, fetal distress from hypoxia, and death

Memory Aid

Remember HELLP to recall a syndrome that is a complication of preeclampsia: **H**emolysis, **E**levated **L**iver enzymes, and **L**ow **P**latelet count

2. Nursing assessment

NCLEX®

a. Symptoms usually develop during third trimester (most frequently in last 10 weeks of gestation) except in cases of GTD; client is at risk for seizures and other complications up to 48 hours after delivery; see Table 49–3

b. Although no longer considered diagnostic, client may develop generalized edema (puffy hands, face, and dependent areas such as ankles/lower legs)

c. Weight gain may be used as a proxy for edema: assess for weight gain of more than 1.5 kg/month (3.3 pounds) in second trimester or more than 0.5 kg/week (1.1 pounds) in third trimester

d. Systemic responses with severe preeclampsia: CNS irritability or cerebral edema cause severe or continuous headache, hyperreflexia (greater than +2, baseline, or clonus), or visual disturbances (blurred vision, seeing spots or flashing lights); renal damage is indicated by oliguria (less than 30 mL/hr); portal hypertension may result in epigastric pain and may precede hepatic rupture

3. Collaborative management: the only cure for preeclampsia is delivery of placenta; goal is to deliver healthy, viable infant while safeguarding mother's health

NCLEX®

a. Bedrest at home is indicated if preeclampsia is mild; hospitalization if severe until fetus is mature enough for delivery; bedrest on lateral side-lying position (often left) to facilitate uteroplacental perfusion

b. Maintain quiet, calm environment to decrease CNS stimulation; use seizure precautions for clients with severe preeclampsia who are at risk of progressing to seizures

NCLEX®

c. Provide a diet high in protein and carbohydrates with no added salt

NCLEX®

d. Implement frequent assessments (every 15 minutes to 1–4 hours as indicated by client condition) to include BP, pulse and respirations, deep tendon reflexes, and clonus checks; assess client for headache, visual disturbances, and epigastric pain

e. Monitor fluid balance: record strict I&O; evaluate urine for protein; assess daily weight

Table 49–3 Comparison of Mild and Severe Preeclampsia

	Mild Preeclampsia	Severe Preeclampsia
Blood pressure	140/90 or higher on two occasions 6 hours apart	160/110 or higher on two occasions 6 hours apart while on bedrest
Proteinuria	Trace to +1 dipstick or less than 2 grams in 24-hour urine	3+ to 4+ dipstick or more than 5 grams in 24-hour urine
Urine output	Normal	Oliguria; often less than 500 mL/day
Laboratory results	Normal creatinine and platelets, and normal to minimal increase in liver enzymes	Elevated creatinine, decreased platelets, elevated liver enzymes
Visual disturbances	Absent to minimal spots or "sparkles," blurred vision, or photophobia	Common spots or "sparkles," blurred vision, photophobia, or temporary blindness
Fetal growth	Normal	Restricted; reduced amniotic fluid volume

f. Monitor fetal well-being by continuous electronic fetal monitoring, serial NSTs, BPP, or others as indicated

NCLEX®

g. For severe preeclampsia, administer magnesium sulfate as prescribed for seizure prevention; monitor client for signs of magnesium toxicity (CNS depression of deep tendon reflexes and respirations, sweating, flushing; see also Chapter 34); keep calcium gluconate available as antidote

h. Institute standard care of client with seizures if seizure activity occurs (see also Chapter 57)

i. Prepare for induction or cesarean birth when fetus is mature or if maternal condition worsens

j. Evaluate newborn for signs of depression related to magnesium sulfate

k. Continue to monitor client for complications; seizures may occur for 48 hours after delivery

Check Your NCLEX–RN® Exam I.Q.

You are ready for testing on this content if you can:

- Implement nursing care for pregnant clients undergoing diagnostic testing.
- Determine whether the condition of a pregnant client undergoing diagnostic testing has changed from preprocedure to postprocedure.
- Position clients appropriately for diagnostic testing.
- Take action to prevent complications of diagnostic procedures.
- Implement nursing care for clients experiencing complications of pregnancy.
- Instruct clients who have a complication of pregnancy about ongoing care.

PRACTICE TEST

1 A client at 24 weeks' gestation has been scheduled for an amniocentesis. Which actions should the nurse plan to take in the care of this client? Select all that apply.

1. Monitor maternal vital signs and fetal heart rate during procedure.
2. Instruct that an ultrasound machine will be used during the procedure.
3. Assist the woman in assuming a supine position with a wedge under left hip.
4. Have a consent form signed for epidural analgesia.
5. Explain that 60 mL of amniotic fluid will be withdrawn.

2 The client is scheduled to have an amniocentesis for assessment of lung maturity. She seems upset and says that she doesn't understand how this test could tell if a baby's lungs are mature. What is the best response by the nurse?

1. "Please try not to worry about that. Your healthcare provider knows the procedure well."
2. "The fluid changes color as the fetal lungs mature. We look at the color to determine lung maturity."
3. "A chemical called lecithin is made by the fetal lungs and increases as pregnancy continues. It flows into amniotic fluid, where we can measure it."
4. "The amount of bilirubin in amniotic fluid increases as the lungs mature. We check for yellow-colored fluid to assess lung maturity."

3 The nurse determines that which potential problem should be a focus of care for a client undergoing an amniocentesis?

1. Dehydration because of NPO status
2. Aspiration because of anesthesia
3. Anxiety about well-being of fetus
4. Inadequate amniotic fluid volume

4 The nurse assesses that which maternal conditions in the third trimester would be a contraindication for conducting a contraction stress test? Select all that apply.

1. Intrauterine growth restriction
2. Diabetes mellitus
3. Pregnancy at 42 weeks' gestation
4. Marginal abruptio placentae
5. Third-trimester bleeding

5 A primigravida is hospitalized at 32 weeks' gestation after a second hemorrhage from a complete placenta previa. The client appears subdued and sad after learning she will remain hospitalized until delivery. She says she is worried about her husband, who will be at home alone much of the time. The nurse interprets the client's response as indicating which psychological state?

1. Anxiety
2. Denial
3. Immaturity
4. Ineffective coping

6 The nurse reviews the client's chart for results of which diagnostic test that will best indicate a diagnosis of erythroblastosis fetalis?

1. Amniocentesis
2. Biophysical profile
3. Indirect Coombs' test
4. Percutaneous umbilical blood sampling

7 The nurse caring for a client with a concealed abruptio placentae should prepare to assess the client for which complication as a priority after delivery?

1. Retained placental fragments
2. Urinary tract infection
3. Uterine atony
4. Vaginal hematoma

8 A pregnant client with class II heart disease progressed through pregnancy without complications and is admitted to the hospital in active labor. Soon after admission, the client reports shortness of breath and the nurse auscultates lung crackles. The nurse anticipates administering which medications based on the client's history? Select all that apply.

1. Penicillin
2. Metoprolol
3. Furosemide
4. Digoxin
5. Procainamide

9 The nurse conducts client teaching with a pregnant client who has placenta previa and who states her religious beliefs prohibit receiving blood or blood products. The nurse evaluates that the teaching has been effective if the client makes which statement?

1. "A judge will force me to accept a transfusion if I really need it."
2. "I might have to sign out of the hospital against medical advice (AMA)."
3. "I will meet with the dietician to increase the amount of iron in my diet."
4. "There is little chance that I will bleed heavily during this pregnancy."

10 The nurse would assess the pregnant client with a history of multiple sexual partners for which complication of pregnancy of greatest concern in this situation?

1. Ectopic pregnancy
2. Premature rupture of membranes
3. Preeclampsia
4. Rh-incompatibility

11 The nurse anticipates that a pregnant client with a history of which health problems might benefit from a scheduled cesarean birth to have an improved outcome for the infant? Select all that apply.

1. Diabetes mellitus
2. Active genital herpes lesions
3. Human immunodeficiency virus
4. Systemic lupus erythematosus
5. Class I heart disease

12 Which short-term client outcome would be most appropriate for a client admitted to the hospital with hyperemesis gravidarum and unable to tolerate regular food and fluid intake?

1. Measures own hourly intake and output (I&O)
2. Maintains present weight
3. Identifies favorite foods in the diet
4. Verbalizes risks to the fetus

13 A prenatal client with type 1 diabetes mellitus asks the clinic nurse whether she will be able to breastfeed her baby. Which response by the nurse is most accurate?

1. "Breastfeeding is contraindicated for insulin-dependent moms."
2. "Certainly, breastfeeding will be beneficial for both of you."
3. "I think this is a good idea because it also prevents pregnancy."
4. "You will have a lot of difficulty maintaining a stable blood sugar."

14 A full-term pregnant client is admitted with membranes that ruptured 4 hours ago and occasional mild contractions. The fetus has healthy indicators on external monitoring. What is the priority intervention in the nursing plan of care for this client?

1. Encourage ambulation
2. Monitor vital signs
3. Promote rest
4. Provide clear liquids

15 A prenatal client at 14 weeks' gestation reports continuous nausea and vomiting and a severe headache. The blood pressure is elevated and fundal height is 21 centimeters. Which diagnostic test does the nurse anticipate will be prescribed to confirm a hydatidiform mole?

1. Biophysical profile
2. Human chorionic gonadotropin
3. Maternal serum alpha-fetoprotein
4. Sonography

16 An HIV-positive client in active labor with newly ruptured membranes is being transported to the hospital via ambulance. The nurse anticipates priority administration of which medication to this client?

1. Antibiotics
2. Immune globulin
3. Oxytocin
4. Zidovudine

17 A pregnant client who acknowledges use of crack cocaine during pregnancy asks the nurse not to inform the baby's father about the substance use. Which responses by the nurse would be appropriate? Select all that apply.

1. "You must be worried about how he will react to that information."
2. "This is your pregnancy and your body, so I'll keep your information private."
3. "Your baby will probably not survive, so there is no need for him to know."
4. "Have you considered that he deserves to know that the baby may be at risk?"
5. "What reaction do you think the baby's father will have?"

18 A client experiencing profuse hemorrhage from placenta previa is being prepared for an emergency cesarean birth. The client exhibits signs of hypovolemia. The nurse makes it a priority to place the client in which position?

1. Knee-chest
2. Left lateral
3. Semi-Fowler
4. Trendelenburg

19 Which clinical focus is of highest priority for a client with a missed abortion who has developed disseminated intravascular coagulopathy (DIC)?

1. Grief regarding loss of fetus
2. Risk for infection
3. Risk for bleeding
4. Anxiety about possible death

20 A client with premature rupture of membranes (PROM) at 33 weeks' gestation is to be given betamethasone to increase fetal lung maturity. The nurse checks the client's record to ensure that the client does not have what disorder that could be affected by this drug?

1. Diabetes mellitus
2. History of alcohol abuse
3. Incompetent cervix
4. Intrauterine growth restriction (IUGR)

21 The nurse concludes that a client is at risk for preeclampsia when the vital signs taken today show that the blood pressure has shown which pattern of elevation since the previous prenatal visit?

1. 90/56 to 110/70
2. 130/60 to 146/92
3. 122/70 to 138/82
4. 134/74 to 138/88

22 A client who has experienced a spontaneous abortion at 8 weeks asks why this happened. What would the nurse include in a response to address the most common cause of "miscarriage"?

1. Chromosome abnormalities
2. Environmental teratogens
3. Excessive activity
4. Substance abuse

23 The nurse explains to a client who had a cervical cone biopsy several years ago that she is now at increased risk for which complication of pregnancy?

1. Ectopic pregnancy
2. Cervical insufficiency
3. Gestational trophoblastic disease
4. Placenta previa

24 A pregnant client visits the prenatal clinic for a routine visit during the second trimester of pregnancy. Which assessment findings should lead the nurse to suspect development of a central abruptio placentae?

1. Painless vaginal bleeding
2. Abdominal pain
3. Leakage of amniotic fluid
4. New onset hypertension

ANSWERS & RATIONALES

1 **Answer: 1, 2, 3 Rationale:** Maternal vital signs and FHR are monitored during procedure. The test is completed on an outpatient basis under guidance of ultrasound visualization. The client is positioned on her back with a wedge under her left hip to avoid hypotension from pressure of the uterus on the vena cava. Epidural analgesia is not used for the procedure. Approximately 15–20 mL of amniotic fluid is aspirated for the procedure. **Cognitive Level:** Applying **Client Need:** Reduction of Risk Potential **Integrated Process:** Nursing Process: Planning **Content Area:** Maternal–Newborn **Strategy:** The wording of the questions tells you that more than one option is likely to be correct. Visualize the procedure and choose standard safe actions for a pregnant client (positioning, monitoring vital signs). Recall that the procedure uses ultrasound to choose that option. Recall that a local skin anesthetic may be used, but not epidural analgesia, to eliminate that option. Finally, realize that 60 mL is a large amount of fluid to consider that option incorrect.

2 **Answer: 3 Rationale:** The amount of lecithin increases as the fetal lungs mature. The ratio of lecithin to sphingomyelin is used to assess lung maturity. To ask a client not to worry or state the healthcare provider knows the procedure well does not provide information to the client. The color of the amniotic fluid is not useful in determining lung maturity. Bilirubin levels in amniotic fluid do not determine lung maturity. **Cognitive Level:** Applying **Client Need:** Reduction of Risk Potential **Integrated Process:** Communication and Documentation **Content Area:** Maternal–Newborn **Strategy:** Recall that amniotic fluid is clear to eliminate options referring to color change of amniotic fluid. Next, eliminate the response that is not therapeutic.

3 **Answer: 3 Rationale:** Most women view invasive antenatal testing with anxiety because of the reason for the test, the impending results, and concern about maternal and fetus complications. A client does not have to be NPO prior to amniocentesis. Amniocentesis does not require anesthesia, although a local anesthetic may be used to numb the skin before needle insertion. Because only 15–20 mL of fluid is removed, the client is not at risk for having inadequate amniotic fluid volume. **Cognitive Level:** Analyzing **Client Need:** Reduction of Risk Potential **Integrated Process:** Nursing Process: Diagnosis **Content Area:** Maternal–Newborn **Strategy:** Use knowledge of the procedure to assist in eliminating incorrect options. First, recall there is no need for NPO status or anesthesia. Next, choose anxiety as a psychosocial issue because the amount of fluid loss is so small as to not present a physiological issue.

4 **Answer: 4, 5 Rationale:** Contractions elicited during the test could cause increased bleeding if an abruption is present or if there is already bleeding in the third trimester. Intrauterine growth restriction, diabetes mellitus, and postterm (42 weeks) pregnancy are all indications for completing a contraction stress test. **Cognitive Level:** Analyzing **Client Need:** Reduction of Risk Potential **Integrated Process:** Nursing Process: Assessment **Content Area:** Maternal–Newborn **Strategy:** Note the critical word *contraindication* in the stem of the question. This tells you that the correct answer is likely an item that could pose risk of harm to the fetus. From there, recall that abruptio placentae can lead to bleeding to help you choose correctly.

5 **Answer: 1 Rationale:** The client has stated that she is worried, which creates anxiety. The information presented does not represent denial or immaturity. There is not enough data to determine whether the client's coping is effective at this time. **Cognitive Level:** Analyzing **Client Need:** Physiological Adaptation **Integrated Process:** Communication and

Documentation **Content Area:** Maternal–Newborn **Strategy:** Note that the client exhibits appropriate nonverbal behavior (subdued and sad), and is able to articulate a concern (worried about husband). Consider that all of these are expected reactions to choose anxiety over the other options.

6 **Answer: 4 Rationale:** Percutaneous umbilical blood sampling (PUBS) obtains an actual sample of fetal blood for analysis. Amniocentesis, biophysical profile, and indirect Coombs' test provide information about fetal well-being, but do not directly sample the fetal erythrocytes. **Cognitive Level:** Analyzing **Client Need:** Reduction of Risk Potential **Integrated Process:** Nursing Process: Diagnosis **Content Area:** Maternal–Newborn **Strategy:** Note the word *erythroblastosis* in the question, and correlate that with erythrocytes or red blood cells. Eliminate amniocentesis and biophysical profile first because they are not related to red blood cells. Then choose option PUBS over indirect Coombs' test because it allows access to fetal cells, not to maternal cells.

7 **Answer: 3 Rationale:** A concealed abruption could result in a Couvelaire uterus, which doesn't contract effectively after delivery, leading to uterine atony. Retained placental fragments, urinary tract infection, or vaginal hematoma could occur in any client. **Cognitive Level:** Analyzing **Client Need:** Physiological Adaptation **Integrated Process:** Nursing Process: Assessment **Content Area:** Maternal–Newborn **Strategy:** Specific knowledge of the risks of concealed abruptio placentae is needed to answer the question. Use nursing knowledge and the process of elimination to make your selection.

8 **Answer: 1, 3, 4 Rationale:** Prophylactic antibiotics such as penicillin are given during labor to prevent bacterial endocarditis. A diuretic such as furosemide and a cardiac glycoside such as digoxin may help counteract the new signs of decreased cardiac output (crackles and shortness of breath). An antihypertensive such as metoprolol or an antidysrhythmic such as procainamide would be used only as needed. **Cognitive Level:** Analyzing **Client Need:** Physiological Adaptation **Integrated Process:** Nursing Process: Planning **Content Area:** Maternal–Newborn **Strategy:** The core issue of the question is the significance of adverse cardiopulmonary assessment findings with class II heart disease during labor. Use nursing knowledge and the process of elimination to make your selection. Consider that an antibiotic is the only drug listed that could prevent a new problem (infection), while a cardiac glycoside and diuretic will manage symptoms of decreased cardiac output because of increased cardiac demand during labor.

9 **Answer: 3 Rationale:** The client is likely to lose some blood with a placenta previa. Increasing iron in her diet is a positive response that does not interfere with her religious beliefs. A judge will not force a transfusion. The client will not need to sign out AMA to avoid receiving a transfusion, even if one is indicated. It is not possible to predict that amount of bleeding that could be experienced by a specific client with placenta previa. **Cognitive Level:** Analyzing **Client Need:** Physiological Adaptation **Integrated Process:** Nursing Process: Evaluation **Content Area:** Maternal–Newborn **Strategy:** The core issue of this question is culturally competent care to reduce risk of complications. First, eliminate options that fail to provide care or that go against the client's wishes. Next, choose the option about iron because it is a positive behavior and avoids having to guess about the unknown (amount of bleeding to expect during pregnancy).

10 **Answer: 1 Rationale:** The client with multiple partners is at high risk for sexually transmitted infection and ascending infection that can lead to blockage in the fallopian tubes. Ultimately, this process could lead to ectopic pregnancy. Premature rupture of membranes is not associated with multiple partners. The number of sexual partners does not influence development of preeclampsia. Rh-incompatibility has to do with Rh blood type of the father. **Cognitive Level:** Analyzing **Client Need:** Physiological Adaptation **Integrated Process:** Nursing Process: Assessment **Content Area:** Maternal–Newborn **Strategy:** Note the critical words *multiple sexual partners* and *greatest concern* in the question. This tells you that the correct answer has a connection to risks associated with multiple sex partners. Use knowledge of complications of sexually transmitted infections to choose correctly.

11 **Answer: 2, 3 Rationale:** A client with active herpes lesions should undergo cesarean delivery to prevent transmission of the virus during vaginal birth. The chance of transmission of HIV is less than 1% if the infant is delivered by cesarean prior to membrane rupture. A client with diabetes mellitus does not require cesarean delivery based on this diagnosis alone. A client with systemic lupus erythematosus does not require cesarean delivery based on this diagnosis alone. A client with class I heart disease does not require cesarean delivery based on this diagnosis alone. **Cognitive Level:** Applying **Client Need:** Physiological Adaptation **Integrated Process:** Nursing Process: Planning **Content Area:** Maternal–Newborn **Strategy:** The core issue of the question is knowledge of methods of transmitting infection from mother to newborn during the delivery process. Choose the options that represent risk of neonatal infection and eliminate all of the remaining options.

12 **Answer: 2 Rationale:** A short-term outcome of maintaining present weight is appropriate while the client is being stabilized in the hospital. While I&O are important measurements, they do not need to be done hourly, and this intervention would help evaluate whether a goal of fluid balance is maintained. Being able to identify favorite foods is not sufficient to ensure adequate nutritional intake. Verbalizing risks of malnutrition to the fetus does nothing to alter the condition. **Cognitive Level:** Analyzing **Client Need:** Physiological Adaptation **Integrated Process:** Nursing Process: Planning **Content Area:** Maternal–Newborn **Strategy:** The critical words in the question are *client outcomes*. With this in mind, eliminate options that do not represent the outcome or end result of appropriate care.

13 **Answer: 2 Rationale:** Breastfeeding should be encouraged because it benefits both the mother and her infant. Breastfeeding is not contraindicated for diabetic mothers. Breastfeeding might or might not help prevent future pregnancy during lactation. Breastfeeding does not necessarily lead to loss of blood glucose control with careful management. **Cognitive Level:** Applying **Client Need:** Physiological Adaptation **Integrated Process:** Nursing Process: Implementation **Content Area:** Maternal–Newborn **Strategy:** Note the critical words *most accurate*, which indicates the correct answer is one that is a true statement, while the others are false to a greater or lesser degree. First eliminate the options that contain the words *contraindicated* and *a lot of difficulty*. Then choose the option that is most true.

14 **Answer: 2 Rationale:** The client with premature ruptured membranes is at risk for developing an infection and should have vital signs, specifically temperature, monitored every

2 hours. The client may be on bedrest, not ambulating, following rupture of the membranes. Promoting rest and providing clear liquids are slightly lower priorities for this client. **Cognitive Level:** Analyzing **Client Need:** Physiological Adaptation **Integrated Process:** Nursing Process: Planning **Content Area:** Maternal–Newborn **Strategy:** The core issue of the question is knowledge of infection as the key risk following rupture of the membranes. Eliminate options that do not address this risk.

15 **Answer: 4 Rationale:** Ultrasound confirms the diagnosis of molar pregnancy that is indicated by the client's symptoms. Biophysical profile is inappropriate before the third trimester because that test evaluates the fetus. The client will have high hCG levels and low maternal serum alpha-fetoprotein levels, but these are not conclusive for hydatidiform mole. **Cognitive Level:** Applying **Client Need:** Reduction of Risk Potential **Integrated Process:** Nursing Process: Assessment **Content Area:** Maternal–Newborn **Strategy:** The core issue of the question is the best method to determine hydatidiform mole. Choose sonography over the others because it is the only one that allows direct visualization of the reproductive structures and differentiates true pregnancy from hydatidiform mole.

16 **Answer: 4 Rationale:** The rate of transmission of HIV to the newborn decreases sharply if the mother is given prophylactic zidovudine orally during pregnancy and by IV during labor. An antibiotic could be administered if the membranes were ruptured for an extended time before delivery. There is no indication in the question for immune globulin, which would provide passive immunity against a specific type of infection. There is no indication in the question for oxytocin, which would induce labor. **Cognitive Level:** Analyzing **Client Need:** Physiological Adaptation **Integrated Process:** Nursing Process: Planning **Content Area:** Maternal–Newborn **Strategy:** The core issue of the question is management of the HIV client in active labor to prevent HIV transmission to the newborn. Eliminate oxytocin first because it stimulates labor. Choose zidovudine over the others listed that related to infection because it is antiviral rather than antibacterial and the immunity is needed by the neonate rather than the mother.

17 **Answer: 1, 5 Rationale:** Addressing the client's worry is a therapeutic response to the client's concerns. Asking about the father's reaction gathers more data and also provides an opportunity to assess possible client safety concerns. Stating to keep the information private is nontherapeutic because it does not explore the client's concern. Stating the baby is not likely to survive is inaccurate. Asking whether the father deserves to know is judgmental. **Cognitive Level:** Applying **Client Need:** Psychosocial Integrity **Integrated Process:** Communication and Documentation **Content Area:** Maternal–Newborn **Strategy:** The core issue of the question is a therapeutic response to a concern shared by the client. Eliminate each of the incorrect options systematically because they do not invite further sharing of information between client and nurse.

18 **Answer: 2 Rationale:** The left lateral position facilitates uteroplacental perfusion. Knee-chest position will not aid circulation and is unlikely to be maintained by a client in shock. Semi-Fowler position would decrease maternal cerebral perfusion. Trendelenburg puts the weight of the gravid uterus against the maternal lungs. **Cognitive Level:** Analyzing **Client Need:** Physiological Adaptation **Integrated Process:** Nursing Process: Implementation **Content Area:** Maternal–Newborn **Strategy:** The core issue of the question is how to maintain uteroplacental perfusion for the client in shock. Choose the position that turns the client to the left side and takes pressure of the gravid uterus off the great vessels in the abdomen.

19 **Answer: 3 Rationale:** The client with DIC is at risk for bleeding or hemorrhage, which takes priority because of associated physiological consequences such as hypovolemia or shock. The client is likely to be experiencing grief related to fetal loss but this is a psychosocial concern that can be addressed once the client is physiologically stable. The client could experience infection, but this risk is no greater than for other clients. The client may or may not be concerned about death, but physiological interventions to stabilize the client would take priority. **Cognitive Level:** Analyzing **Client Need:** Physiological Adaptation **Integrated Process:** Nursing Process: Diagnosis **Content Area:** Maternal–Newborn **Strategy:** The issue of the question is knowledge of complications of DIC, specifically hemorrhage and loss of circulating volume. With this in mind, focus on physiologically based nursing diagnoses and choose risk for bleeding and hemorrhage because it is a more specific diagnosis.

20 **Answer: 1 Rationale:** Glucocorticoids raise the blood glucose, and this has implications for diabetic control in a client with diabetes mellitus. A history of alcohol abuse, incompetent cervix, and IUGR are not contraindications for giving betamethasone. **Cognitive Level:** Applying **Client Need:** Physiological Adaptation **Integrated Process:** Nursing Process: Assessment **Content Area:** Maternal–Newborn **Strategy:** The core issue of the question is knowledge of key side effects of betamethasone, which helps to select the client for whom it has implications. Recall that the glucocorticoids often end in *-sone* to help you recognize the drug as a glucocorticoid. Recall next the risk of elevating blood glucose levels to choose diabetes mellitus over the others.

21 **Answer: 2 Rationale:** A systolic blood pressure of 140 mmHg and a diastolic blood pressure of 90 mmHg are diagnostic for preeclampsia. The other blood pressure changes (90/56 to 110/70, 120/70 to 138/82, and 134/74 to 138/88) do not meet the criteria for either the systolic or the diastolic blood pressure reading. **Cognitive Level:** Analyzing **Client Need:** Physiological Adaptation **Integrated Process:** Nursing Process: Assessment **Content Area:** Maternal–Newborn **Strategy:** Specific knowledge of the criteria for preeclampsia is needed to answer this question. Choose the option that has the greatest degree of change in both systolic and diastolic measurements.

22 **Answer: 1 Rationale:** The majority of early abortions are related to abnormal chromosomes. The client might fear that she has caused the loss; she should be provided with accurate information. The majority of early abortions are not related to environmental teratogens, excessive activity, or substance abuse. **Cognitive Level:** Applying **Client Need:** Physiological Adaptation **Integrated Process:** Communication and Documentation **Content Area:** Maternal–Newborn **Strategy:** Specific knowledge of the etiologies of spontaneous abortion is needed to answer the question. Use nursing knowledge and the process of elimination to make your selection.

23 **Answer: 2 Rationale:** Cervical trauma and scarring, such as from cervical cone biopsy, can result in cervical incompetence during pregnancy. The client who had a cervical cone

biopsy is not at greater risk for ectopic pregnancy, gestational trophoblastic disease, or placenta previa. **Cognitive Level:** Analyzing **Client Need:** Physiological Adaptation **Integrated Process:** Teaching and Learning **Content Area:** Maternal–Newborn **Strategy:** Note the critical word *cervical* in the stem of the question, and choose the option that also refers to the cervix.

24 **Answer: 2 Rationale:** Abdominal pain or uterine tenderness is a classic sign of a central placental abruption, which is characterized by separation of placenta from the uterine wall. Painless vaginal bleeding would occur with placenta previa; there is no bleeding in a central abruption, in which blood is trapped between the placenta and uterine wall. Premature rupture of membranes is associated with leakage of amniotic fluid. New onset of hypertension should be further assessed to determine development of preeclampsia. **Cognitive Level:** Analyzing **Client Need:** Physiological Adaptation **Integrated Process:** Nursing Process: Assessment **Content Area:** Maternal–Newborn **Strategy:** Visualize the pathophysiology of abruptio placentae and associate it with the various signs and symptoms that may be associated with it.

Key Terms to Review

abortion p. 791
abruptio placentae p. 793
amniocentesis p. 784
biophysical profile (BPP) p. 783
cervical insufficiency p. 791
cerclage p. 791
chorioamnionitis p. 794
chorionic villus sampling (CVS) p. 785
contraction stress test (CST) p. 784
Coombs' test p. 789
Doppler blood flow analysis p. 783
eclampsia p. 795
ectopic p. 790
erythroblastosis fetalis p. 789
fetal fibronectin test (fFN) p. 785
gestational diabetes p. 787
gestational trophoblastic disease (GTD) p. 790
hydatiform mole p. 790
hydrops fetalis p. 789
kernicterus p. 789
lecithin to sphingomyelin (L/S) ratio p. 785
macrosomia p. 787
nitrazine test p. 785
nonstress test (NST) p. 783
preeclampsia p. 794
placenta previa p. 792
phosphatidylglycerol (PG) p. 785

References

Davidson, M., London, M., & Ladewig, P. (2016). *Olds' maternal newborn nursing and women's health across the lifespan* (10th ed.). New York, NY: Pearson Education.

Kee, J. (2017). *Pearson's handbook of laboratory and diagnostic tests* (8th ed.). New York, NY: Pearson Education.

Ladewig, P., London, M., & Davidson, M. (2014). *Contemporary maternal–newborn nursing care* (8th ed.). Upper Saddle River, NJ: Pearson Education.

London, M., Ladewig, P., Davidson, M., Ball, J., Bindler, R., & Cowen, K. (2014). *Maternal and child nursing care* (4th ed.). Upper Saddle River, NJ: Pearson Education.

Lowdermilk, D., Perry, S., Cashion, M., & Alden, K. (2016). *Maternity and women's health care* (11th ed.). St. Louis, MO: Elsevier.

Complicated Labor and Delivery Care

50

In this chapter

Cross Reference

Other chapters relevant to this content area are

Reproduction, Family Planning, and Infertility	Chapter 8
Uncomplicated Antenatal Assessment and Care	Chapter 9
Uncomplicated Labor and Delivery Care	Chapter 10
Uncomplicated Postpartum Assessment and Care	Chapter 11
Uncomplicated Newborn Care	Chapter 12
Maternal and Newborn Medications	Chapter 34
Complicated Antenatal Care	Chapter 49
Complicated Postpartum Care	Chapter 51
Complicated Newborn Care	Chapter 52

I. GENERAL NURSING CARE OF CLIENT

A. High-risk factors

1. May develop at any time during labor in client who was healthy throughout pregnancy
2. Etiology may be related to fetus, birth passage, relationship between birth passage and fetus, and psychosocial considerations

B. Client response to onset of high-risk factors in labor

1. Stress, fear, and anxiety brought about by unexpected complications during labor may have profound effects on maternal and fetal outcomes
2. Maternal anxiety can increase tension, produce higher pain perception, and may make labor contractions less effective
3. Catecholamines released during stress produce vasoconstriction that may negatively affect uterine blood flow

C. Nursing care

1. Basic intrapartal care is still important
2. Nursing care during complicated labor requires additional special knowledge and skill in assessment and care of mother and fetus
3. Be aware that family may be overwhelmed with concerns and less capable of providing needed emotional support

II. PROBLEMS WITH THE FETUS

A. Fetal *malpositions*

1. Ideal fetal position is flexed with cephalic occiput in right or left anterior quadrant of maternal pelvis
2. Various types of malpositions are possible
3. Occiput posterior (OP) position
   a. Right or left OP position usually rotates to occiput anterior (OA) as labor progresses
   b. Failure to rotate may be related to small maternal pelvis, poor contractions, inadequate pushing effort (often from epidural anesthesia), abnormal flexion of head, or large fetus
   NCLEX® c. Maternal risks include prolonged labor, higher rate of cesarean birth, extension of midline episiotomy, perineal lacerations, and anal sphincter injury
   NCLEX® d. Maternal symptoms include intense back pain in labor, dysfunctional labor pattern, prolonged active phase, hypotonic labor (not enough pressure of head on cervix), arrest of dilatation and/or descent
4. Occiput transverse (OT) position
   a. Incomplete rotation of OP position to OA results in fetal head being in horizontal or transverse position
   b. If pelvic structure is adequate, vaginal delivery can be accomplished by stimulating contractions with oxytocin and use of forceps
5. Collaborative management of fetal malpositions
   a. Key maternal assessments are pain and coping skills
   NCLEX® b. Knee-chest position used twice daily may provide a downward slant to vaginal canal, and pelvic rocking may facilitate rotation
   NCLEX® c. Apply sacral counterpressure with heel of hand to reduce back pain
   d. If rotation accomplished, encourage client to lie in Sims position on side opposite from fetal back
   e. Provide support and encouragement by keeping client and family informed of progress, praising efforts to maintain control, and encouraging relaxation with contractions
   f. Anticipate rotation with forceps (instruments applied to fetal head) and forceps-assisted birth or vacuum extraction (suction cup applied to fetal head) if rotation not accomplished
   NCLEX® g. Risks of forceps use are fetal ecchymosis or edema of face, transient facial paralysis, maternal lacerations, or episiotomy extensions
   NCLEX® h. Risks of vacuum extraction are newborn cephalohematoma, retinal hemorrhage, and intracranial hemorrhage

B. Fetal *malpresentations*

1. Include cephalic malpresentations (sinciput or military, brow and face), shoulder (transverse lie), breech, and compound presentation
2. A sinciput (military) presentation has head that is neither flexed nor extended and usually self-corrects by flexion when head reaches pelvic floor
3. Brow presentation is least common; fetal forehead is presenting part and head is slightly extended instead of flexed; because of this, widest diameter of fetal head enters birth canal (called occipitomental)
   a. Causes may include high parity, placenta previa, uterine or fetal anomaly, cephalopelvic disproportion (CPD), or multiparity
   b. Maternal risks include longer labor and possible cesarean birth
   c. Neonatal risks include facial edema, bruising, exaggerated molding of head, damage to trachea and larynx, and cerebral and neck compression
4. With face presentation, fetal head is hyperextended more than in brow presentation; occurs more often with maternal contracted pelvis or multiparity; there is increased risk of CPD, prolonged labor, and cesarean birth
   a. Anticipate vaginal delivery if mother's pelvis is adequate and infant's chin (mentum) is in anterior position
   NCLEX® b. Anticipate cesarean birth if mentum is posterior and does not rotate to anterior in late stages of labor, or if signs of fetal distress occur
   NCLEX® c. Do not place fetal monitor electrode on presenting part (infant's face); requires external fetal heart rate (FHR) monitoring
   NCLEX® d. Edema and bruising of face, eyes, and lips are common; prepare clients for this before seeing infant for first time
5. Breech presentations
   a. Three types (see Figure 50–1)

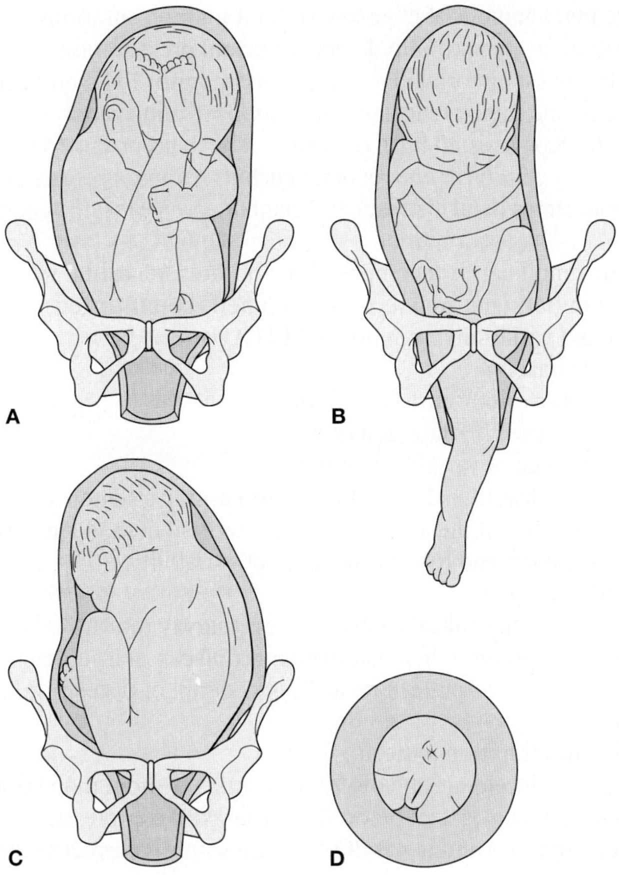

Figure 50–1

Breech presentation. (**A**) Frank breech: sacrum is presenting part, knees extended. (**B**) Incomplete (footling) breech: one or both feet presenting, increasing risk of umbilical cord prolapse. (**C**) Complete breech: sacrum is presenting part, knees flexed, left sacral anterior position shown. (**D**) On vaginal exam, nurse may feel anal sphincter; tissue of fetal buttocks feels soft.

b. Incidence increased with earlier gestational age, placenta previa, hydramnios, high parity, multiple gestation, oligohydramnios, uterine anomalies, and fetal anomalies such as anencephaly and hydrocephaly

NCLEX® **c.** Maternal concern is increased likelihood of cesarean birth, while fetal risks include compressed or prolapsed umbilical cord, entrapment of fetal head, injury to fetal head, meconium aspiration, and asphyxia at birth

NCLEX® **d.** Current therapy includes maternal positioning exercises with hips higher than torso two to three times daily to provide room for fetus to change position and **external cephalic version** (ECV) at 36–38 weeks, which involves manipulating fetus through abdominal wall using a forward or backward rolling motion to convert from breech (or shoulder) to cephalic presentation before onset of labor

e. Collaborative management during ECV includes applying external fetal monitor, starting IV fluids, administering a beta-mimetic drug (terbutaline subcutaneously or, if contraindicated, intravenous infusion of magnesium sulfate) to relax uterine muscle, closely monitoring FHR during version attempt, and discontinuing version if undue maternal or fetal distress occurs

f. **Cesarean birth**: most breech presentations are delivered by planned cesarean (operative abdominal) delivery to reduce risk of complications

6. Shoulder presentation (transverse lie): acromium process is presenting part

a. Occurs more often with grand multiparity with relaxed uterine muscles, preterm fetus, placenta previa, hydramnios, and bony dystocia

b. ECV is attempted at 39 weeks (may convert spontaneously in earlier weeks); labor may or may not be induced if version is successful and cervix is favorable

NCLEX® **c.** Vaginal delivery is not possible with shoulder presentation; cesarean birth is indicated

7. Compound presentations: more than one part of fetus presents

a. Most common type is a hand or arm prolapsing beside head

NCLEX® **b.** Risk of cord compression and prolapse is increased

c. Vaginal versus cesarean birth depends on size of fetus, presence of fetal distress, and progress in labor

8. Collaborative management of clients with fetal malpresentations
    - NCLEX® **a.** Leopold's maneuvers may help detect abnormal presentation
    - NCLEX® **b.** Observe closely for abnormal labor patterns; monitor FHR and contractions continuously
    - **c.** Provide client and family teaching, client support, and encouragement
    - **d.** Anticipate forceps-assisted birth or cesarean birth according to presentation
    - **e.** Be prepared for childbirth emergencies such as neonatal resuscitation

C. Nonreassuring fetal status (fetal distress): transient or chronic insufficient oxygen supply to meet demands of fetus

1. Causes include umbilical cord compression and uteroplacental insufficiency
2. Most common initial signs are meconium-stained (green-tinged) amniotic fluid (in vertex presentation) and variations from normal FHR pattern
3. Changes in FHR baseline
    - NCLEX® **a.** Tachycardia (above 160): early sign of distress
    - **b.** Bradycardia (below 110): late sign of distress
4. Decreased or absence of variability of heart rate
    - **a.** Heart rate varies less than 2–5 beats/minute, causing a flattened appearance to heart rate
    - **b.** Indicates depression of the autonomic nervous system that controls heart rate
    - **c.** Fetal sleep, sedation, and hypoxia may affect variability
5. Late deceleration pattern
    - NCLEX® **a.** FHR slows following peak of contraction and slowly returns to baseline rate during resting phase
    - **b.** Indicates fetal response to hypoxia from uteroplacental insufficiency
    - **c.** Considered an ominous pattern regardless of depth of deceleration of FHR and requires immediate intervention
6. Severe variable deceleration pattern
    - NCLEX® **a.** FHR repeatedly decelerates below 90 beats/min for more than 60 seconds before returning to baseline
    - **b.** Indicates interference of fetal blood flow from cord compression
    - **c.** Leads to fetal hypoxia and low APGAR scores unless corrective steps taken
7. Collaborative management
    - **a.** Assess FHR baseline, variability, and pattern of periodic changes
    - **b.** Assess contraction pattern and maternal response to labor
    - NCLEX® **c.** Change maternal position, increase rate of IV fluids, and administer oxygen at 6–10 L/min as prescribed
    - NCLEX® **d.** Institute **intrauterine resuscitation** (corrective measures to improve oxygen exchange within maternal–fetal circulation) based on FHR pattern (see Box 50–1); for late deceleration, take steps to improve uteroplacental blood flow and for severe variable deceleration, take steps to relieve cord compression
    - **e.** Provide appropriate information and emotional support to client and family
    - **f.** Maintain continuous monitoring of FHR, uterine activity, and labor progress
    - NCLEX® **g.** Prevent meconium aspiration with possible suction of neonate's nasopharynx prior to delivery of chest and abdomen; visualize larynx and vocal cords with deep suction immediately after delivery and before first breath is taken

Memory Aid

To correctly perform nasotracheal suction on an infant, slightly hyperextend head to a "sniffing" position with chin up and head tilted back slightly.

- **h.** **Amnioinfusion**: warmed sterile saline is instilled through an intrauterine pressure catheter when signs of cord compression are present; increases volume of liquid to relieve pressure on cord and increase perfusion to fetus; monitor FHR monitor continuously and discontinue infusion when signs of cord compression disappear

D. Prolapsed umbilical cord

1. Cause: fetus is not firmly engaged, allowing room for umbilical cord to move beyond (prolapse) or alongside presenting part (occult prolapse), causing cord compression that can lead to decreased oxygen transport and nonreassuring fetal status
2. Contributing factors include rupture of membranes before engagement of presenting part, small fetus, breech presentation, multifetal pregnancy, and transverse lie (shoulder presentation)

Box 50–1

Nursing Management of Nonreassuring Fetal Status

Late decelerations (uteroplacental insufficiency)
Goal is to improve maternal blood flow to placenta

- Reposition mother on her left side
- Administer O_2 by face mask at 6–10 L/min
- Maintain continuous electronic fetal monitoring
- Increase IV fluids
- Discontinue oxytocin infusion if labor is being induced
- Notify healthcare provider immediately

Severe variable decelerations or prolonged bradycardia (cord compression)
Goal is to relieve pressure on umbilical cord

- Reposition mother on either side; if no improvement, reposition to opposite side
- Administer O_2 by face mask at 6–10 L/min
- Trendelenburg or knee-chest position if not corrected
- Perform vaginal examination and apply upward digital pressure on presenting part to relieve pressure on umbilical cord

3. Collaborative management
   a. Identify client at risk for prolapsed umbilical cord; keep laboring client with ruptured membranes in horizontal position until fetal head is well engaged as preventive measure
   b. *NCLEX®* Place mother's hips higher than head using either knee-chest or Trendelenburg position
   c. Administer O_2 by face mask at 6–10 L/min
   d. Maintain continuous electronic fetal monitoring
   e. *NCLEX®* Perform sterile vaginal exam as indicated, and if loop of cord is discovered, push fetal presenting part upward with fingers to relieve pressure on cord until healthcare provider arrives
   f. *NCLEX®* If cord protrudes through vagina, determine that pulsation is present and wrap cord loosely with warm sterile saline–soaked towel or dressing to prevent drying; do not allow dressing or towel to cool, which could cause spasms of umbilical cord vessels and decrease fetal oxygenation
   g. Prepare for rapid delivery, often by cesarean birth

E. Macrosomia

1. A fetal weight of more than 4000 grams at birth
2. More common with pre-pregnancy maternal obesity, excessive maternal weight gain, multiparity, maternal diabetes mellitus and gestational diabetes, postterm pregnancy, and maternal birth weight
3. Maternal risks include CPD, dysfunctional or prolonged labor, soft-tissue lacerations during vaginal birth, postpartum hemorrhage, and puerperal infection
4. Fetal risks include asphyxia, meconium aspiration, shoulder dystocia, upper brachial plexus injury and fractured clavicles, hypoglycemia, polycythemia, and hyperbilirubinemia
5. Cesarean birth is planned for fetus weighing 4500 grams or more, with mixed views about vaginal versus cesarean birth if weight is 4000–4500 grams

III. PROBLEMS WITH PELVIC STRUCTURES

A. *Cephalopelvic disproportion (CPD)*

1. Occurs when fetal head is larger than bony maternal pelvis (at inlet, outlet, or between these) and cannot pass through birth canal
2. Android and platypelloid pelvic types predispose to CPD
3. Contracted pelvic inlet: anterior–posterior diameter less than 10 cm; transverse diameter less than 12 cm
   a. Makes engagement difficult
   b. Influences fetal position and presentation
4. Contracted pelvic outlet: interischial tuberous diameter less than 8 cm; often occurs with a midpelvic contracture (interspinous diameter less than 9.5 cm)
5. *NCLEX®* Signs and symptoms: fetal head does not descend despite strong contractions
6. Maternal risks include prolonged labor, exhaustion, premature rupture of membranes, necrosis of maternal soft tissues with delay or descent, hemorrhage, and uterine rupture
7. Fetal risks include hypoxia and birth trauma

8. **Trial of labor (TOL)**: labor is allowed to continue or may even be stimulated with oxytocin when pelvic measurements are borderline to see if fetal head will descend, making vaginal delivery possible; if progressive changes in dilatation and station do not occur, or if obvious CPD is present, a cesarean birth is performed

B. **Shoulder dystocia:** an obstetric emergency resulting from difficulty or inability to deliver shoulders

1. Inability to deliver shoulders leads to fetal hypoxia and death; fetal macrosomia increases risk
2. NCLEX® Maternal risks: lacerations and tears of birth canal and postpartum hemorrhage
3. NCLEX® Neonatal risks: hypoxia, fractures of clavicle, and injury to neck and head
4. Collaborative management
   a. Identify client at risk for shoulder dystocia: obesity, increased fundal height, history of macrosomia, maternal diabetes or gestational diabetes, prolonged second-stage labor
   b. NCLEX® Assist with positioning during delivery: use McRoberts maneuver, flexing thighs up onto abdomen to change angle of pelvis, increase pelvic diameters, and facilitate delivery of shoulders
   c. Assess for maternal and newborn injury following delivery

IV. PROBLEMS WITH UTERINE CONTRACTIONS

A. ***Induction of labor***

1. Is defined as stimulation of uterine contractions before spontaneous onset of labor; **labor augmentation** is artificial stimulation of uterine contractions when spontaneous contractions do not lead to progressive cervical dilation or fetal descent
2. Cervical ripening (softening and effacement of cervix) may be done before labor induction using misoprostol (synthetic PGE_1 analog) or prostaglandins (PGE_2) gel (see also Chapter 34); monitor FHR, uterine activity, and maternal vital signs (VS)
3. **Amniotomy** or artificial rupture of membranes (AROM): use of an amniohook instrument to create a tear in amniotic membrane during sterile vaginal exam if cervix is at least 2 cm dilated
   a. NCLEX® Assess fetus for presentation, position, station (head should be engaged to reduce risk of cord prolapse); assess FHR prior to and immediately after AROM to detect umbilical cord prolapse or fetal distress
   b. Assist client to semi-reclining position and place disposable pads or towels under buttocks to absorb amniotic fluid
   c. Assess color, odor, and amount of fluid, and note meconium-stained fluid or blood; change pads as needed to promote comfort
   d. NCLEX® Take maternal temperature every 1–2 hours after AROM to detect infection; vaginal exams should use sterile technique and should be kept to a minimum

Memory Aid

Remember that *-otomy* means "cutting into"; amniotomy is thus artificial rupture of amniotic membranes.

4. Oxytocin administration (see also Chapter 34)
   a. Use **Bishop score** to assess maternal readiness for induction by determining dilatation, effacement, station, cervical consistency, and position of cervix
   b. NCLEX® Begin external fetal monitoring and monitor FHR closely throughout induction
   c. NCLEX® Assess and record maternal VS, intake and output (I&O), and contraction frequency and intensity
   d. NCLEX® Always administer using IV infusion pump for safety; stop infusion immediately for contractions closer than 2 minutes apart or lasting longer than 60 seconds, insufficient uterine relaxation between contractions, or for any indication of fetal distress
5. Contraindications to induction or augmentation of labor are any contraindications to spontaneous labor and vaginal birth

B. ***Dystocia* or difficult labor:** abnormal labor pattern with cervical dilatation of less than 0.5 cm per hour over 4 hours during active labor stage, or less than 1 cm per hour of fetal descent during second labor stage

1. **Tachysystole labor pattern**: more than five contractions in a 10-minute period with less than 60 seconds of relaxation between contractions, or uterine contractions lasting longer than 2 minutes
   a. Risk factors include high oxytocin dose or incremental intervals less than 30 minutes, cocaine use, placental abruption, and uterine rupture
   b. Fetal risks include hypoxia caused by decreased uteroplacental blood flow and possible prolonged pressure on fetal head (leading to cephalohematoma, caput succedaneum, excessive molding)

c. Ensure use of continuous fetal monitoring and stop oxytocin infusion if in use; tocolytic agents may be prescribed if needed

NCLEX®
d. Provide comfort and support, such as changing position to left lateral side-lying, high Fowler, or rocking in a rocking chair; maintain quiet environment; assist with back massage, effleurage, guided imagery, and relaxation exercises

e. Provide hydration and monitor I&O

f. Be prepared to institute intrauterine resuscitation measures for nonreassuring fetal status: position client on left side, apply oxygen by face mask, increase IV fluids by at least a 500 mL bolus

2. **Hypotonic labor pattern**: infrequent contractions with low amplitude; cervical dilatation may be less than 1 cm/hour (*prolonged labor*) or no change in dilatation (if this lasts longer than 2 hours is considered *arrest of progress*)

a. More commonly occurs in first stage of labor in nulliparous client

b. Maternal risks are maternal exhaustion, stress on coping ability, intrauterine infection if prolonged labor after membranes rupture, and postpartum hemorrhage from insufficient uterine contractions after birth

c. Fetal risks are nonreassuring fetal status from prolonged labor and fetal sepsis from pathogens ascending birth canal

NCLEX®
d. Medical treatment includes ruling out CPD (which would require cesarean birth) and initiating active management of labor, which includes amniotomy, timed cervical exams, and labor augmentation with oxytocin

e. Nursing management includes monitoring fetal status, assessing maternal stress and coping, and maintaining adequate fluid intake (oral or IV) and nourishment (light snacks in early labor)

3. Deviations from normal progress in labor can be documented using a **labor graph (Friedman curve),** which plots cervical dilatation and descent of fetal head over time

C. ***Preterm labor:*** labor occurring between 20 and 37 weeks' gestation

NCLEX®
1. May be difficult to diagnose because many symptoms similar to normal pregnancy: abdominal, back and pelvic pain, menstrual-like cramps, vaginal discharge (pinkish or mucus-like), pelvic pressure, urinary frequency, or diarrhea

2. Criteria for diagnosis of preterm labor: uterine contractions every 5 minutes for 20 minutes (or 8 contractions in 60 minutes), and documented cervical change or cervical effacement of 80% or more (or cervical dilation greater than 1 cm)

NCLEX®
3. Immediate actions to be taken by clients experiencing premature labor symptoms for more than 15 minutes while physically active

a. Empty bladder

b. Lie down in a side-lying position, left side preferred

c. Drink three to four (8-ounce) cups (0.7–0.9 L) of water

d. Palpate abdomen for uterine contractions; if 10 minutes apart or closer for 1 hour, contact healthcare provider

e. Soak in warm tub bath with uterus completely submerged under water

f. Rest for 30 minutes after symptoms subside and slowly resume activity

g. If symptoms do not subside, contact healthcare provider

4. Collaborative management (in-hospital)

NCLEX®
a. Promote bedrest with client in left side-lying position

b. Monitor maternal VS and I&O

NCLEX®
c. Continuously monitor uterine contractions and FHR

NCLEX®
d. Administer prescribed **tocolytic agents** (drugs to stop contractions) if labor continues, including magnesium sulfate, nifedipine (calcium channel blocker), terbutaline (beta adrenergic), prostaglandin synthetase inhibitors (indomethacin, sulindac, and celecoxib); see also Chapter 34

NCLEX®
e. Administer betamethasone or dexamethasone to stimulate fetal lung maturation

f. Provide client and family teaching regarding signs and management of preterm labor at home

g. Provide emotional support encouraging client and family to express feelings and concerns

D. ***Precipitous labor and delivery:*** labor lasting less than 3 hours and resulting in rapid birth

1. Contributing factors include multiparity, large pelvis, previous precipitous labor, small fetus in favorable position, and recent maternal cocaine use

NCLEX®
2. Maternal risks: cervical, vaginal, or rectal lacerations and postpartum hemorrhage from undetected lacerations or inadequate uterine contractions after birth

NCLEX®
3. Fetal risks: hypoxia (decreased perfusion to intervillous spaces), cerebral trauma and brachial plexus injuries from rapid descent through birth canal

4. Collaborative management
   a. Identify client at risk for precipitous labor and birth
   NCLEX® b. Have precipitous delivery tray available with cord clamp, scissors, and hemostat
   c. Do not leave client; send someone else to call for healthcare provider assistance; do not try to prevent delivery
   d. Instruct client to pant or blow to decrease urge to push
   NCLEX® e. Have amniohook available to rupture membranes when head crowns if needed
   f. Support perineum with a sterile towel as crowning occurs
   NCLEX® g. Apply gentle pressure on fetal head to prevent rapid delivery; lacerations of maternal perineum and damage to fetal head can occur with sudden expulsion of infant's head

Memory Aid

Remember to "protect the head" during a precipitous birth. Apply enough pressure to guide the descent and prevent rapid intracranial pressure changes within the infant's molded skull.

   NCLEX® h. After delivery of head, suction infant's mouth, then each naris, with bulb syringe
   NCLEX® i. Check around infant's neck for possible tight umbilical cord; if present, cord must be clamped and cut before delivery

Memory Aid

Remember that umbilical cord could choke fetus and is dangerous. If, during delivery, it can't be loosened and slipped away from infant's neck, two clamps should be applied to cord and cord should be cut between these clamps.

   j. Place hands on each side of infant's head and instruct client to push gently
   k. Deliver posterior shoulder and apply gentle downward pressure to move anterior shoulder under symphysis pubis (facilitates birth of anterior shoulder)
   l. Support infant's body with a sterile towel during expulsion from birth canal
   m. Dry infant and cover to keep warm; place infant on mother's abdomen or breast for skin contact and to aid uterine contractions as soon as stable
   n. Clamp and cut umbilical cord
   o. Observe for signs of placental separation: gush of bright blood; lengthening of the cord
   p. Gently pull cord while massaging fundus to deliver placenta
   NCLEX® q. Continue to massage fundus to prevent hemorrhage or put infant to breast
   r. Inspect perineum for lacerations or tears

E. Postterm pregnancy

1. Extends more than 294 days or 42 weeks past first day of last menstrual period (2 weeks past estimated date of birth at 40 weeks)
2. Maternal risks include probable labor induction, increased risk for large-for-gestational-age (LGA) infant and subsequent perineal trauma, increased risk of infection, and increased risk of forceps-assisted, vacuum-assisted, or cesarean birth
3. Fetal risks include decreased placental perfusion (oxygenation, nutrient supply), oligohydramnios (less amniotic fluid), macrosomia, nonreassuring fetal status with possible meconium or meconium aspiration, and low 5-minute Apgar score
4. Treatment includes assessment using nonstress test (NST) and biophysical profile (BPP) 2–3 times weekly to evaluate fetal well-being, and induction of labor (some prefer this at 41 weeks) or cesarean birth

F. Uterine prolapse

1. Vigorous massage of fundus and pulling on umbilical cord to speed placental separation may cause prolapse of cervix and lower uterine segment through introitus
2. **Uterine inversion**: turning inside out of uterus; may be complete (visible outside introitus) or incomplete (partially inverted and not visible): either can result in hemorrhage and shock and requires correction manually by healthcare provider, or by laparotomy if unsuccessful

G. ***Uterine rupture***: tearing open or separation of uterine wall

NCLEX®
1. Rare but serious complication, caused by separation of scar from previous classical cesarean, uterine trauma, intense uterine contractions, overstimulation of labor with oxytocin, difficult forceps-assisted birth, and external cephalic or internal version
2. Risk factors: overdistension of uterus with multifetal pregnancy or hydramnios, labor after previous cesarean birth, previous uterine surgery, and abdominal trauma
3. Types
   a. Complete: extends through uterine wall into peritoneal cavity
   b. Incomplete: extends into peritoneum covering uterus but not into peritoneal cavity
4. Collaborative management
   a. Attempt to prevent by identifying clients at risk and avoiding hyperstimulation of uterus during induction
   b. (NCLEX®) May be silent or have dramatic signs and symptoms: sudden, sharp lower abdominal pain, tearing sensation, signs of shock, cessation of contractions, cessation of FHR, and if complete, palpation of fetal parts through abdominal wall
   c. (NCLEX®) Monitor for and treat shock with oxygen, intravenous fluids, and blood products
   d. Prepare client for immediate cesarean birth
   e. Complete rupture may require hysterectomy if unable to repair, while incomplete rupture may require laparotomy and repair

V. PROBLEMS WITH MATERNAL PSYCHOLOGICAL STATUS

A. Factors influencing psyche of client in labor
1. Fear, anxiety, and perception of situation
2. Self-image
3. Preparation for childbirth
4. Support systems and coping ability
5. Underlying psychological disorder, most frequently depression or anxiety

B. Effects of fear and anxiety on labor progress
1. Epinephrine is secreted in response to stress, leading to vascular changes that divert blood from uterus to skeletal muscles
2. Oxygen and glucose supplies decrease, and lactic acid accumulates in uterine muscle, resulting in increased (worsened) experience of pain
3. With a decrease in available energy supply to support effective contractions, labor progress is slowed

C. Collaborative management
1. Assess client's past experiences with, preparation for, and expectations of labor and birth
2. (NCLEX®) Assess client's current coping behaviors and their effectiveness with current situation; encourage client to use coping behaviors that work well
3. Establish trusting relationship with client and family using a calm, caring, and nonjudgmental approach to therapeutic interactions
4. (NCLEX®) Provide frequent attention and remain at bedside with client and family as able during labor
5. Identify sources of distress and and work to reduce them
6. Offer methods to promote comfort and relaxation
7. Acknowledge client's pain, fears, and any other symptoms expressed
8. Keep client and family informed; provide clear but succinct information about environment, labor process and progress, breathing and relaxation techniques, and any medical procedures planned
9. Keep client's external environment free from excessive stimuli
10. Promote self-image by praising efforts to manage labor

VI. CESAREAN BIRTH

A. Overview
1. Delivery of infant by an abdominal and uterine incision
2. Purpose is to facilitate delivery to preserve health of mother and fetus
3. Major indications for cesarean birth include complete placenta previa, CPD, placental abruption, active genital herpes, umbilical cord prolapse, failure to progress in labor, nonreassuring fetal status, and benign and malignant tumors that obstruct birth canal

NCLEX® **B. Maternal risks**
1. Cesarean births carry a higher mortality rate than vaginal births
2. Postoperative complications include infection, reactions to anesthetic agents, blood clots, and bleeding
3. Less frequent problems include ureteral injury, bladder laceration, and wound infection

C. Surgical techniques
1. Skin incisions
   a. Vertical (infraumbilical midline) between navel and symphysis pubis
   b. Transverse (Pfannenstiel) across lowest part of abdomen just below pubic hair line
2. Uterine incisions
   a. Classical: through upper uterine segment
   b. Low transverse cervical: in lower uterine segment (Kerr incision)
   c. Lower uterine segment vertical (Selheim incision)

D. Collaborative management
1. Determine indication for cesarean birth
2. Assess client's understanding of indication, procedure, and implications for recovery from cesarean birth
3. Assess whether cesarean birth was discussed in childbirth preparation classes
   a. Clients and families cope better if they have time to learn about cesarean birth
   b. Emergency cesarean birth increases anxiety and alters couple's expectations about childbirth

NCLEX®

4. Preoperative care
   a. Assess NPO status (being NPO decreases risk of aspiration)
   b. Explain procedure so that client and family know what to expect
   c. Obtain client signature on consent form
   d. Perform abdominal and perineal prep
   e. Insert indwelling urinary catheter to prevent bladder distention during surgery
   f. Start IV fluids using an IV catheter adequate in gauge for blood product administration if needed
   g. Administer an antacid PO or agent to lower gastric acidity IV to decrease risk of lung damage if acidic gastric contents are aspirated during surgery
   h. Assist with positioning on operating table (often slanted to one side or with wedge placed under right hip to displace uterus about 15 degrees from midline); reduces vena cava compression and supine maternal hypotension; apply straps to prevent falls or injury during surgery
   i. Continue to monitor FHR until immediately before surgery and then ensure any internal fetal scalp monitor is removed
   j. Perform instrument count and record (this is repeated three times during procedure to ensure no instruments are left in abdomen); may be checked with portable x-ray if needed

NCLEX®

5. Intraoperative care
   a. Assist father, partner, or support person who is attending cesarean birth with donning surgical attire and positioning near client's head; include support person in surgical experience
   b. Provide heated crib and supplies to receive newborn
   c. Provide immediate care to newborn or assist nursery personnel as needed; assess Apgar score, complete initial assessment, and complete identification procedures just as with vaginal birth
   d. Provide assistance to surgical team and provide immediate care for mother
   e. Assist with measures to promote bonding with infant after delivery

NCLEX®

6. Postoperative care
   a. Begin postanesthesia care unit (PACU) monitoring of VS, oxygen saturation, and cardiac monitoring; monitor VS every 15 minutes for first hour and longer if needed until stable, then every 30 minutes until PACU discharge
   b. Assess abdominal dressing and perineal pad every 15 minutes for first hour; gently palpate fundus to determine whether firm or boggy (if boggy, massage until firm while supporting incision)
   c. Assess urinary catheter and urine output; assess for blood tinge to detect surgical trauma to bladder
   d. Apply and maintain sequential devices (SCDs) to prevent deep vein thrombosis
   e. With general anesthesia, position client on side to facilitate drainage of secretions and turn, cough, and deep-breathe hourly
   f. With spinal or epidural anesthetic, assess every 15 minutes for return of sensation
   g. Administer medications for pain as needed
   h. Facilitate parent–infant contact and bonding

E. Trial of labor after cesarean (TOLAC)
1. Labor and vaginal birth after a previous cesarean is considered a safe option if indication for cesarean birth is not likely to be repeated
2. Contraindications
   a. Previous classical incision into uterus
   b. Large infant (over 4000 grams)

c. Malpresentation
d. Pelvic measurements inadequate
e. Any fetal or placental problem that may require cesarean birth
f. Delivery in an alternative birth setting: it is necessary to have access to a facility where emergency cesarean birth could be performed

NCLEX®
3. Risks of TOLAC
   a. Possible uterine rupture and hemorrhage: less likely to occur if previous uterine incision was in the lower uterine segment
   b. Failure of trial of labor, requiring a repeat cesarean
4. Benefits of TOLAC
   a. Ability to experience labor and vaginal delivery (desired by some clients)
   b. Vaginal delivery is less costly than cesarean birth with faster, easier recovery period and less risk of complications
   c. Does not preclude induction or augmentation of labor
5. Collaborative management
   a. NCLEX® Monitor uterine activity and progress in labor; identify deviations from normal progress in labor and report to healthcare provider (essential)
   b. NCLEX® Monitor FHR and response to contractions, identify and report indications of fetal distress quickly
   c. NCLEX® Observe for indications of uterine rupture, including signs of shock or hemorrhage, report of "ripping or tearing" sensation or sharp uterine pain, abrupt cessation of contractions, abrupt onset of fetal distress, and more easily palpable fetus (lying outside uterus)
   d. Be alert and prepared for possible emergency cesarean birth
   e. Provide support and encouragement for client attempting TOLAC

Check Your NCLEX–RN® Exam I.Q.

You are ready for testing on this content if you can:

- Assess the client experiencing complications of labor and delivery.
- Provide care to the client experiencing complications of labor and delivery.
- Take action to prevent fetal distress during complications of labor and delivery.
- Evaluate client's response to interventions to treat complications of labor and delivery.
- Communicate effectively to increase client and family understanding of complications of labor and delivery.

PRACTICE TEST

1 The nurse caring for a high-risk client in labor observes the presence of variability of the fetal heart rate (FHR) of 10–12 beats per minute as recorded by the internal fetal monitor. What interpretation should the nurse make about the fetal condition or state?

1. Fetal hypoxia
2. Fetal well-being
3. Umbilical cord compression
4. Uteroplacental insufficiency

2 The nurse locates fetal heart tones in the right upper quadrant of the abdomen. This finding should cause suspicion that the fetus is in what presentation?

1. Occiput posterior
2. Occiput transverse
3. Breech
4. Shoulder

3 A client's contractions have become less frequent and less intense in the past hour. Vaginal examination reveals 6-cm dilatation and 0 station, which is unchanged since the last examination over 2 hours ago. The nurse should take which action at this time?

1. Notify the healthcare provider of the last exam.
2. Continue to observe for 1 hour for further progress.
3. Encourage the client to turn on her side and rest.
4. Prepare for cesarean birth.

PRACTICE TEST

4. The nurse is assisting in the delivery of a client whose infant has shoulder dystocia. How should the nurse have the client move to perform McRoberts maneuver to assist with delivery?

1. Flex the thighs against the abdomen
2. Place legs in stirrups
3. Assume a side-lying position for delivery
4. Sit upright for delivery

5. The nurse explains to a client with premature labor that betamethasone will be administered for which purpose?

1. Stop uterine contractions
2. Prevent infection
3. Hasten fetal lung maturity
4. Prevent cervical dilatation

6. After teaching the pregnant client and her husband about premature labor, the nurse evaluates the instruction was effective when the client makes which statement? Select all that apply.

1. "I will call the office if I notice excessive fetal movement."
2. "I will call the office if I have back pain that does not go away."
3. "I will lie down and rest awhile if I notice watery vaginal discharge."
4. "I will call the office for abdominal cramps or pressure that don't stop after I drink three to four cups of liquid and rest for an hour."
5. "I don't need to worry about occasional irregular contractions."

7. The client is admitted in active labor with a breech presentation. Which sign would indicate to the nurse that there is fetal distress?

1. Meconium-stained amniotic fluid
2. Fetal heart rate (FHR) of 180 beats/minute
3. Mild variable decelerations
4. Increased FHR variability

8. The labor graph (Friedman curve) shows that a nulliparous client has not made any progress in cervical dilatation or station since she was 7 cm and 0 station over 2 hours ago. What interpretation should the nurse make from this information?

1. A prolonged deceleration phase
2. Protracted active phase
3. Arrest of descent
4. Secondary arrest of dilatation

9. The nurse is admitting to the maternity unit a client who is at risk for precipitous birth. Once the admission procedures have been completed, which action by the nurse should take priority?

1. Instruct the client to pant or blow during contractions
2. Avoid rupturing the amniotic membrane at all times
3. Remove a towel from the shelf to support perineum when crowning occurs
4. Leave the client's room to get extra assistance in case of rapid delivery

10. The client in labor says she was told she is having hypertonic uterine contractions but does not understand how these could harm the baby. How would the nurse explain the relationship between hypertonic contractions and risk of fetal distress?

1. Maternal exhaustion occurs, producing a buildup of lactic acid.
2. Umbilical cord compression occurs, decreasing oxygen supply to the fetus.
3. Increased uterine tone and frequent contractions interfere with blood flow to fetus through the uterine arteries.
4. Placental separation can occur, which can be harmful to both mother and fetus.

11. After the initial care following amniotomy, the nurse should include which assessment every 2 hours?

1. Maternal blood pressure and pulse
2. Fetal movement
3. Color and consistency of amniotic fluid
4. Oral temperature

12 Which condition of the pregnant client places her at increased risk for uterine inversion during the current labor and delivery?

1. Forceps delivery of a previous infant
2. Fundal pressure during delivery of the head and body
3. Precipitous birth of less than 3 hours' duration
4. Traction on the umbilical cord and vigorous fundal massage in the third stage

13 What is the priority nursing goal in helping a client during a complicated labor?

1. Establish a trusting relationship.
2. Ensure that the client knows what to expect.
3. Prevent invasion of privacy.
4. Prevent fear and anxiety.

14 The onset of late decelerations on the fetal monitor should lead the nurse to suspect which condition?

1. Head compression
2. Cord compression
3. Decreased uteroplacental blood flow
4. Close uterine contractions

15 A client asks what *trial of labor* means. What is the best response by the nurse?

1. "The healthcare provider is giving you more time to make progress in labor before considering cesarean birth."
2. "You will need to make progress in the next hour, or a cesarean birth will be planned."
3. "Even though your pelvis is small, sometimes it is possible to deliver your baby vaginally."
4. "A cesarean birth will be done because you already went into labor and have not made much progress."

16 The nurse should suspect cephalopelvic disproportion (CPD) after noting documentation of which data for a laboring client?

1. Pelvic outlet is less than 9 cm.
2. Midpelvis is contracted.
3. Fetal shoulders are too large to pass through the bony pelvis.
4. Fetal head is too large to pass through the bony pelvis.

17 The nurse explains to a pregnant client at 37 weeks' gestation that a Bishop score is being completed to determine which of the following?

1. The client's readiness for labor
2. The fetus's readiness for labor
3. Progress during induction
4. Cervical changes in labor

18 Which of the following priority items should the nurse assess because of the potential impact on the laboring client's psychological status?

1. Attitude about parenting
2. Relationship with the client's own mother
3. Self-image
4. Beliefs about health

19 A pregnant client in the active phase of labor has contractions that occur every 3–4 minutes, are 35 seconds in duration and have mild intensity. What conclusion about the client's status does the nurse draw from this data?

1. Tachysystolic uterine dysfunction
2. Hypotonic uterine dysfunction
3. Normal uterine activity
4. Progressive labor pattern

20 In preparing the client in labor for vacuum extraction, it is important to explain that the infant might initially have which appearance after delivery? Select all that apply.

1. Edema of the caput
2. Red marks on the face
3. Edema of the face
4. Swelling of the eyes
5. Bruising of the scalp

ANSWERS & RATIONALES

1 **Answer: 2 Rationale:** Variability of FHR indicates fetal well-being. The presence of variability is assessed by internal fetal monitoring, since there is less artifact that could be mistaken for variability of heart rate. Hypoxia can cause loss of variability of the FHR. Umbilical cord compression can cause severe variable decelerations or prolonged bradycardia of FHR. Uteroplacental insufficiency can cause late decelerations of FHR. **Cognitive Level:** Analyzing **Client Need:** Physiological Adaptation **Integrated Process:** Nursing Process: Assessment **Content Area:** Maternal–Newborn **Strategy:** The core issue of the question is knowledge of the significance of variability in FHR. Recall that less or loss of variability may be a cause for concern, depending on the circumstances leading to it. Use nursing knowledge and the process of elimination to make a selection.

2 **Answer: 3 Rationale:** Fetal heart tones are heard loudest over the fetal back. In breech presentation, this tends to be above the umbilicus. Fetal heart tones are heard just below the midline of the umbilicus in shoulder presentation or transverse lie. The terms occiput posterior and occiput transverse refer to head positions (fetal malpositions) rather than fetal malpresentations. **Cognitive Level:** Analyzing **Client Need:** Physiological Adaptation **Integrated Process:** Nursing Process: Diagnosis **Content Area:** Maternal–Newborn **Strategy:** Specific knowledge related to fetal position and associated location of fetal heart sounds is needed to answer the question. Use nursing knowledge and the process of elimination to make your selection.

3 **Answer: 1 Rationale:** The nurse should suspect cephalopelvic disproportion (CPD) because of the lack of progress since the last exam. The healthcare provider might assess the maternal pelvis by CT, MRI, or other means, or could stimulate contractions with oxytocin, opting for a trial of labor (TOL). Lack of progress could be caused by inadequate contractions, and a vaginal delivery could be possible, so it is too early to anticipate cesarean birth. Encouraging rest and continued observation will do nothing to resolve the problem. **Cognitive Level:** Analyzing **Client Need:** Physiological Adaptation **Integrated Process:** Nursing Process: Implementation **Content Area:** Maternal–Newborn **Strategy:** The core issues of the question are recognition of lack of progress in labor and the nurse's decision-making ability once this is detected. Eliminate options that do nothing to help labor progress again, and choose notifying the healthcare provider over preparing for cesarean birth because there is not enough information yet to indicate that cesarean birth is needed.

4 **Answer: 1 Rationale:** Flexing the thighs against the abdomen (McRoberts maneuver) increases the pelvic angle from symphysis pubis to sacrum, and facilitates delivery by making the bony pelvis less restrictive. Placing the legs in stirrups is not sufficient to make the bony pelvis less restrictive. Assuming a side-lying position or sitting upright for delivery will not make the bony pelvis less restrictive. **Cognitive Level:** Applying **Client Need:** Physiological Adaptation **Integrated Process:** Nursing Process: Implementation **Content Area:** Maternal–Newborn **Strategy:** Specific knowledge of the McRoberts maneuver is needed to answer this question. Use nursing knowledge and the process of elimination to make your selection.

5 **Answer: 3 Rationale:** Corticosteroids such as betamethasone have been shown to enhance fetal lung maturity and prevent respiratory distress. Betamethasone does not stop labor or cervical changes. A side effect of betamethasone is increased risk of infection. **Cognitive Level:** Applying **Client Need:** Pharmacological and Parenteral Therapies **Integrated Process:** Nursing Process: Implementation **Content Area:** Maternal–Newborn **Strategy:** Specific knowledge of the purpose of betamethasone late in pregnancy is needed to answer this question. Use nursing knowledge and the process of elimination to make your selection.

6 **Answer: 2, 4, 5 Rationale:** Signs of premature labor can include persistent back pain. The client should be instructed to empty her bladder, lie down on her side, and drink three to four cups of water. If symptoms do not disappear within an hour, the healthcare provider should be notified. Excessive fetal movement can sometimes indicate fetal distress, but is not a sign of premature labor. Watery vaginal discharge should be reported sooner rather than later after lying down and resting because the fluid could be amniotic fluid. Occasional irregular contractions are called Braxton Hicks contractions and are normal during pregnancy. **Cognitive Level:** Analyzing **Client Need:** Physiological Adaptation **Integrated Process:** Teaching and Learning **Content Area:** Maternal–Newborn **Strategy:** The wording of the question tells you that correct answers are options that contains a true statement. Eliminate the option with watery discharge because this symptom should not be ignored and would not be relieved by rest. Eliminate the option about excessive movement because this is not of concern.

7 **Answer: 2 Rationale:** An FHR greater than 160 beats per minute is considered fetal tachycardia, an early sign of distress. Meconium passage often occurs in breech presentation because of pressure on the presenting part, and is not an indication of fetal distress in this situation. Mild variable decelerations and increased FHR variability are not indications of fetal distress and occur more frequently in breech presentations. **Cognitive Level:** Analyzing **Client Need:** Physiological Adaptation **Integrated Process:** Nursing Process: Assessment **Content Area:** Maternal–Newborn **Strategy:** The core issue of this question is the ability to correlate knowledge of breech presentation with knowledge of fetal distress. Choose correctly by recalling that the normal fetal heart rate (FHR) is 120–160 beats per minute. An FHR outside this range is generally a cause for concern regardless of the specific situation.

8 **Answer: 4 Rationale:** Dilatation has stopped (arrested) after considerable progress. The cause could be hypotonic uterine contractions, malposition, or cephalopelvic disproportion. The terms *prolonged* and *protracted* when describing labor indicates that progress occurs at a very slow rate. Arrest of descent occurs when the station, rather than cervical dilatation, does not change. **Cognitive Level:** Analyzing **Client Need:** Physiological Adaptation **Integrated Process:** Nursing Process: Assessment **Content Area:** Maternal–Newborn **Strategy:** Note the critical phrases *not made any progress* and *over 2 hours ago*. Correlate these phrases with the word *arrest* to eliminate options using the term *prolonged* or *protracted*. Choose *secondary arrest of dilatation* because dilatation has not

changed and because the word *secondary* implies that labor was active at one time, which is true in this case.

9 **Answer: 1 Rationale:** When a client is at risk for precipitous (rapid) birth, the nurse should instruct the client to pant or blow to decrease the urge to push during the contractions, which may slow down the speed of delivery. The nurse should be prepared to rupture the amniotic membrane with an amniohook if crowning occurs before the amniotic membrane has ruptured. A sterile towel (not a clean towel) should be used to support the perineum when crowning occurs. The nurse should not leave the client alone; the nurse should call for someone else to request assistance from healthcare providers. **Cognitive Level:** Application **Client Need:** Physiological Adaptation **Integrated Process:** Nursing Process: Implementation **Content Area:** Maternal–Newborn **Strategy:** Specific knowledge of nursing interventions during precipitous labor is needed to answer the question. Visualize the process and choose the option that protects the safety of the mother and fetus.

10 **Answer: 3 Rationale:** Frequent contractions and increased uterine muscle tone impede the blood flow through uterine arteries to the placenta. While maternal exhaustion and lactic acid accumulation can occur over time, they do not immediately threaten fetal well-being. The incidence of umbilical cord compression is not increased. Hypertonic contractions are not necessarily associated with placental separation. **Cognitive Level:** Applying **Client Need:** Physiological Adaptation **Integrated Process:** Communication and Documentation **Content Area:** Maternal–Newborn **Strategy:** The core issue of the question is how hypertonic uterine contractions affect fetal well-being. Eliminate maternal exhaustion and placental separation as least likely to happen, then eliminate umbilical cord compression because this may or may not occur, depending on the position of the fetus.

11 **Answer: 4 Rationale:** The risk of infection is increased after amniotomy (rupture of membranes). The nurse should assess temperature every 2 hours. Blood pressure, pulse, and fetal movement are checked more often during active labor. Color and consistency of amniotic fluid are assessed immediately after rupture, and each time the underpad is changed. **Cognitive Level:** Applying **Client Need:** Physiological Adaptation **Integrated Process:** Nursing Process: Assessment **Content Area:** Maternal–Newborn **Strategy:** Recognize that the term *amniotomy* (*-otomy* means "cutting into") refers to artificial rupture of the membranes. Correlate this with increased risk for infection as a complication to choose temperature as the answer.

12 **Answer: 4 Rationale:** Although not always preventable, uterine inversion can occur because of excessive traction on the umbilical cord during the third stage of labor with or without vigorous fundal massage to remove the placenta, especially if the placenta is implanted in the fundus. Previous forceps delivery, fundal pressure during delivery of head and body, and precipitous birth are not associated with inversion. **Cognitive Level:** Analyzing **Client Need:** Physiological Adaptation **Integrated Process:** Nursing Process: Diagnosis **Content Area:** Maternal–Newborn **Strategy:** Specific knowledge of the etiology and risks of uterine inversion is needed to answer this question. Use nursing knowledge and the process of elimination to make your selection.

13 **Answer: 1 Rationale:** Establishing a trusting relationship with the client and her family is a priority. A trusting relationship increases the likelihood of cooperation and compliance during a crisis. In an emergency situation such as a complicated labor, the nurse might have little time to ensure that the client knows what to expect or to protect her privacy. It is not always possible to prevent fear and anxiety. **Cognitive Level:** Applying **Client Need:** Psychosocial Integrity **Integrated Process:** Nursing Process: Planning **Content Area:** Maternal–Newborn **Strategy:** Note the critical word *priority* in the question, which tells you all options might be partially or totally correct, and you must choose the most important one. A client experiencing a complicated labor is likely to experience both fear and lack of knowledge. Choose a trusting relationship over the others as it is the foundation for assisting the client through the labor process and reducing fear and lack of knowledge.

14 **Answer: 3 Rationale:** Uteroplacental insufficiency (UPI) is believed to be the cause of late decelerations. The insufficiency or decreased uteroplacental blood flow leads to fetal hypoxia. Several factors including maternal hypotension, anemia, vasoconstriction, uterine tetany, and dehydration can be primary causes of UPI. Head compression causes early decelerations. Cord compression causes variable decelerations. Close uterine contractions is incorrect because it might not lead to UPI and eventual late deceleration. **Cognitive Level:** Analyzing **Client Need:** Physiological Adaptation **Integrated Process:** Nursing Process: Diagnosis **Content Area:** Maternal–Newborn **Strategy:** Specific knowledge of the significance of late decelerations is needed to answer this question. Use nursing knowledge and the process of elimination to make your selection.

15 **Answer: 1 Rationale:** A trial of labor means that the client will be followed closely and given more time to show progress before considering a cesarean birth. Placing a time limit of 1 hour or stating that vaginal delivery is sometimes possible makes cesarean birth seem inevitable and can increase the client's anxiety. Cesarean birth is incorrect because the client will be allowed to continue laboring as long as some progress is made. **Cognitive Level:** Applying **Client Need:** Physiological Adaptation **Integrated Process:** Communication and Documentation **Content Area:** Maternal–Newborn **Strategy:** Recall the definition of the term *trial of labor*. Eliminate systematically those options that are not consistent with its meaning. The wording of the question indicates only one option is correct.

16 **Answer: 4 Rationale:** CPD means that the fetal head is too large to pass through the bony pelvis. A pelvic outlet of less than 9 cm and a contracted midpelvis refer to a smaller-than-normal pelvis, but do not take into account the fetal head size. Fetal shoulders that are too large to pass through the bony pelvis refers to shoulder dystocia. **Cognitive Level:** Analyzing **Client Need:** Physiological Adaptation **Integrated Process:** Nursing Process: Diagnosis **Content Area:** Maternal–Newborn **Strategy:** Specific knowledge of CPD is needed to answer this question. Consider the word *disproportion* in the question to determine the correct answer must have two elements that are compared. Use nursing knowledge and the process of elimination to make your selection.

17 **Answer: 1 Rationale:** The Bishop score, an assessment of the mother's physical readiness for labor, takes into account cervical dilatation, effacement, consistency, cervical position, and station before contractions begin. The higher the score, the more likely a client can be successfully induced. The Bishop score does not evaluate the condition of the fetus, progress during labor, or cervical changes during

labor. **Cognitive Level:** Analyzing **Client Need:** Physiological Adaptation **Integrated Process:** Nursing Process: Implementation **Content Area:** Maternal–Newborn **Strategy:** Recall that a Bishop score focuses primarily on the mother rather than the fetus and on readiness for labor (rather than progress during labor) to choose correctly. Note also that the client in the question is at 37 weeks' gestation, which suggests that the client is not in labor.

18 **Answer: 3 Rationale:** Self-image refers to how a client feels about herself. A positive self-image enables a client to deal with labor and delivery realistically, even in the event of complications. Research has shown that self-image impacts the laboring client's psyche. Attitude about parenting, relationship with own mother, and health beliefs have not been identified as having a significant impact during labor. **Cognitive Level:** Analyzing **Client Need:** Psychosocial Integrity **Integrated Process:** Nursing Process: Assessment **Content Area:** Maternal–Newborn **Strategy:** Note that the focus of the question is on the client in active labor. With this in mind, choose the self-image option because it is the only one that specifically relates to the client's current status.

19 **Answer: 2 Rationale:** Hypotonic uterine dysfunction occurs most often during the active phase. It is characterized by contractions that have become further apart, less intense, and of shorter duration. Normal uterine contractions are typically 2–3 minutes apart, strong, and last 45–60 seconds in the active phase of labor. Tachysystolic uterine dysfunction would be characterized by long, strong contractions with little resting time between contractions. A progressive labor pattern would show contractions that get longer, stronger, and closer together. **Cognitive Level:** Analyzing **Client Need:** Physiological Adaptation **Integrated Process:** Nursing Process: Assessment **Content Area:** Maternal–Newborn **Strategy:** Note that the question contains the critical words *mild intensity* and *active phase*. Reasoning that active labor should be characterized by strong contractions, you would select hypotonic uterine contractions because it contains the word *hypotonic*. Alternatively, eliminate normal uterine activity and progressive labor pattern because they are similar, and eliminate hypertonic uterine dysfunction because the word *hypertonic* conveys the opposite of what the client in the question is experiencing.

20 **Answer: 1, 5 Rationale:** Suction applied over the occiput commonly causes edema and bruising of the scalp. Although it might appear to be a deformity of the fetal head, the edema disappears in 2–3 days and the bruising resolves more gradually. Suction is not applied to the face and thus would not cause facial red marks, facial edema, or swelling of the eyes. **Cognitive Level:** Applying **Client Need:** Physiological Adaptation **Integrated Process:** Nursing Process: Planning **Content Area:** Maternal–Newborn **Strategy:** Note the critical word *vacuum* in the stem of the question, and eliminate as incorrect any options that refer to a part of the face, rather than to the head itself.

ANSWERS & RATIONALES

Key Terms to Review

amnioinfusion p. 806
amniotomy p. 808
Bishop score p. 808
cephalopelvic disproportion (CPD) p. 807
cesarean birth p. 805
dystocia p. 808
external cephalic version p. 805
hypotonic labor pattern p. 809
induction of labor p. 808
intrauterine resuscitation p. 806
labor augmentation p. 808
labor graph (Friedman curve) p. 809
malpresentations p. 804
malpositions p. 804
precipitous labor and delivery p. 809
preterm labor p. 809
tachysystole labor pattern p. 808
tocolytic agents p. 809
trial of labor after cesarean (TOLAC) p. 812
trial of labor (TOL) p. 808
uterine inversion p. 810
uterine rupture p. 811

References

Davidson, M., London, M., & Ladewig, P. (2016). *Olds' maternal newborn nursing and women's health across the lifespan* (10th ed.). New York, NY: Pearson Education.

Kee, J. (2017). *Pearson's handbook of laboratory and diagnostic tests* (8th ed.). New York, NY: Pearson Education.

Ladewig, P., London, M., & Davidson, M. (2014). *Contemporary maternal–newborn nursing care* (8th ed.). Upper Saddle River, NJ: Pearson Education.

London, M., Ladewig, P., Davidson, M., Ball, J., Bindler, R., & Cowen, K. (2014). *Maternal and child nursing care* (4th ed.). Upper Saddle River, NJ: Pearson Education.

Lowdermilk, D., Perry, S., Cashion, M., & Alden, K. (2016). *Maternity and women's health care* (11th ed.). St. Louis, MO: Elsevier.

Complicated Postpartum Care 51

In this chapter

Cross Reference

Other chapters relevant to this content area are

Reproduction, Family Planning, and Infertility	Chapter 8
Uncomplicated Antenatal Assessment and Care	Chapter 9
Uncomplicated Labor and Delivery Care	Chapter 10
Uncomplicated Postpartum Assessment and Care	Chapter 11
Uncomplicated Newborn Care	Chapter 12
Maternal and Newborn Medications	Chapter 34
Complicated Antenatal Care	Chapter 49
Complicated Labor and Delivery Care	Chapter 50
Complicated Newborn Care	Chapter 52

I. NURSING CARE OF THE HIGH-RISK POSTPARTUM CLIENT

NCLEX®

A. Assessment

1. Degree of homeostasis, amount of intrapartum blood loss, hematocrit, hemoglobin, and complete blood cell (CBC) count results
2. Vital signs: elevated temperature, blood pressure (BP), heart rate; low BP, symptoms of shock
3. Fundus: height, tone, and position
4. Lochia: amount, color, consistency, odor, and presence/size of clots (larger than quarter-size of concern)
5. Perineum: edema, ecchymosis, pain, hemorrhoids
6. Bladder: distension and displacement, ability to void
7. Bowel: constipation, distended abdomen, decreased or absent bowel sounds (risk of ileus)
8. Breasts: cracked, bleeding, or blistered nipples; engorgement, red streaks, lumps, clogged milk ducts
9. Homans sign (nonspecific), redness, tenderness, areas of heat in calves, severe abdominal or flank pain
10. Rest, activity tolerance
11. Bonding or attachment behaviors, maternal–infant interaction

B. Implementation

1. Teach client normal adaptation
2. Observe for actual or potential problems in immediate postpartum period (first 2 hours after delivery) and continue into later postpartum period
3. Administer treatment or medication as prescribed

4. Educate client about signs of complications prior to discharge
5. Reinforce importance of keeping appointment for postpartum checkup
6. Provide client with telephone numbers to call if questions arise

II. POSTPARTUM HEMORRHAGE

A. *Early-postpartum hemorrhage*

NCLEX® 1. A blood loss greater than 500 mL in first 24 hours after vaginal delivery or 1000 mL after cesarean delivery; clinical definition is decrease in hematocrit of 10% from prebirth level or excessive bleeding that leads to hemodynamic instability or need for blood transfusion
2. Most common cause is uterine atony (over 50%)
3. Other causes include genital tract lacerations, episiotomy, retained placental fragments, hematomas (vulvar, vaginal, or subperitoneal), uterine inversion, uterine rupture, problems of placental implantation, and coagulation disorders
4. **Uterine atony**
   NCLEX® a. Description: relaxation of uterus; after birth, contraction of interlacing uterine muscles occludes open areas at site of placental attachment; absent or ineffective uterine contractions can cause significant blood loss
   NCLEX® b. Predisposing factors that overdistend uterus: delivery of a large infant (macrosomia), multiple gestation, hydramnios/polyhydramnios
   NCLEX® c. Predisposing factors that affect uterine contractility: multiparity, precipitous labor, dysfunctional or prolonged labor, prolonged third stage of labor, retained placental fragments
   d. Predisposing medications: general anesthesia (halothane), magnesium sulfate, nifedipine, terbutaline
   e. Predisposing maternal condition: preeclampsia or placenta previa, coagulation disorders
5. Lacerations
   a. Description: tears of perineum, vagina, or cervix associated with a firm uterus and bright red bleeding or a steady stream or trickle of unclotted blood
   NCLEX® b. Predisposing factors: nulliparity, epidural anesthesia, precipitous childbirth (less than 3 hrs), macrosomia, forceps or vacuum-assisted birth, use of oxytocin
6. Retained placental fragments
   a. Description: retention in uterus of pieces of placenta, generally caused by partial separation of placenta during fundal massage before spontaneous placental separation; may lead to early or late postpartum hemorrhage
   b. Preventive measures include avoiding uterine massage before placental separation and inspection of placenta for intactness or evidence of missing cotyledons on maternal side or presence of vessels that cross to edge of placenta outward along membranes on fetal side
7. **Hematoma**
   a. Description: a collection of blood, often vulvar or vaginal, resulting from birth trauma or inadequate hemostasis at site of repair of laceration or incision; a subperitoneal hematoma (involving uterine artery branches or broad ligament blood vessels) is rare but most dangerous because significant blood loss can occur without signs until client becomes hemodynamically unstable
   NCLEX® b. Predisposing factors: episiotomy, forceps or vacuum-assisted births, genital tract lacerations, preeclampsia, primiparity, prolonged second stage of labor, macrosomia, clotting disorder, or history of vulvar varicosities
8. **Disseminated intravascular coagulopathy (DIC)**
   a. Overview: complex disorder of blood-clotting mechanisms; consumption of clotting factors because of widespread clotting in microcirculation leads to general diffuse hemorrhage; oozing from puncture sites or development of petechiae may be initial clues of coagulopathy
   NCLEX® b. Predisposing factors: preeclampsia, amniotic fluid embolism, sepsis, abruptio placentae, prolonged intrauterine fetal demise syndrome
9. Other causes of early postpartum hemorrhage: uterine rupture or uterine inversion

B. *Late-postpartum hemorrhage*

NCLEX® 1. Description: occurs most often 24 hours to 6 weeks after childbirth because of **subinvolution** (failure of uterus to return to normal size) or retained placental tissue; blood loss may be excessive but usually poses less risk than immediate postpartum hemorrhage
2. Lochia often fails to progress from rubra to serosa to alba normally; lochia rubra that exists longer than 2 weeks is suggestive of subinvolution
3. Subinvolution as causative factor is most commonly diagnosed at 4- to 6-week postpartum exam with bimanual palpation of an enlarged, softer than usual uterus

C. Nursing assessment

NCLEX® 1. Assess client's history and labor and delivery record for predisposing factors to various causes of postpartum hemorrhage

NCLEX® 2. Assess vaginal bleeding after delivery every 10–15 minutes for 1 hour, then every 30 minutes for 1 hour until stable; more frequent assessments may be needed depending on condition

a. Bleeding may be slow and continuous or rapid and profuse

b. Blood may escape from vagina or pool in uterus and vagina, becoming evident as clots

NCLEX® c. Bleeding from a laceration occurs in presence of a firm uterus and may be noted as a slow, steady trickle

d. Assess bleeding visually, through pad count, or weighing material used to absorb blood

NCLEX® e. Assist client to a side-lying position to check pad underneath client; blood may accumulate unseen

f. Weigh peri-pads or other absorbent materials to estimate blood loss if careful measurement is needed

NCLEX® 3. Palpate fundus for firmness, assess for height in relation to umbilicus and position

4. Assess bladder for fullness and distension, which can displace uterus, making it more difficult to contract

5. Assess VS, oxygen saturation, skin color and temp, level of consciousness (LOC), UO, and other indicators for typical signs of hypovolemic shock

6. Assess carefully any complaint of pain such as pelvic pain or backache; if perineal pain is reported, examine for signs of hematoma: edema, ecchymosis, fluctuant mass, tense overlying skin, and extreme tenderness at site

D. Implementation

1. Remain with client

NCLEX® 2. Massage boggy uterus gently but firmly, cupping uterus between two hands and avoiding overly aggressive massage (to avoid injury and reactive relaxation of musculature)

3. If bleeding is excessive, healthcare provider may perform bimanual massage

NCLEX® 4. Monitor vital signs up to every 15 minutes as indicated, intake and output (I&O), LOC, fundal tone and placement, and amount of bleeding during episode of acute hemorrhage

5. Initiate perineal pad counts if steady free flow of blood and possible pad weighing (1 mL = 1 gram); also have client turn to side in bed to assess for pooling of blood underneath client

NCLEX® 6. Encourage frequent voiding to prevent bladder distension that contributes to uterine atony; a urinary catheter may be inserted during postpartum hemorrhage if unable to void

7. Monitor hematocrit values if available and notify provider if a decrease of 10% or more occurs

8. Replace fluids by IV and administer blood products as prescribed (usually 3 mL normal saline or lactated Ringer's to 1 mL blood loss)

9. Elevate legs 30 degrees as blood volume becomes depleted (modified Trendelenburg or shock position)

10. Assist with preoperative preparation if necessary for surgical removal of placental fragments (dilatation and curettage), ligation of bleeding vessel, suturing of laceration, or to correct more serious causes of bleeding, such as uterine rupture (see also Chapter 50)

11. Provide adequate rest and assistance with self-care once stabilized because of fatigue associated with anemia from blood loss; assist also with infant care or encourage partner to assist in client and infant care as appropriate

NCLEX® 12. Uterine stimulants may be prescribed to prevent or manage uterine atony and hemorrhage, depending on whether it is early or late; these often include oxytocin, methylergonovine maleate (commonly used for subinvolution), or prostaglandin; hypertension is a common adverse effect; see Chapter 34 for additional information

III. POSTPARTUM INFECTIONS

A. Reproductive tract infections

1. Any infection in reproductive system within 6 weeks of delivery

2. Predisposing factors: prolonged rupture of amniotic membranes, obstetric trauma (episiotomy and lacerations of perineum, vagina, or cervix), invasive procedures (internal fetal monitoring, multiple vaginal exams), retained placental fragments, chorioamnionitis, preexisting bacterial vaginosis, manual removal of placenta, use of forceps or vacuum extraction, compromised health status (nutrition, anemia, obesity, smoking, alcohol or drug use), lapses in aseptic technique by staff

NCLEX® 3. Cesarean birth is single most significant risk (as high as 35% without antibiotic prophylaxis)

4. Localized infections of perineum, vulva, and vagina

a. Local infection may extend through venous circulation, resulting in infectious thrombophlebitis or septicemia

b. Local infection may extend through lymphatic vessels, resulting in **pelvic cellulitis/parametritis**, an infection involving connective tissue of broad ligament or connective tissue of all pelvic structures
c. Can lead to **peritonitis**, an infection involving peritoneal cavity

5. **Endometritis or endomyometritis**: localized infection of uterine lining, usually beginning at placental site; more common after cesarean birth; antibiotic prophylaxis at time of cord-clamping reduces incidence of postpartum endometritis in both elective and emergent cesarean births
6. Nursing assessment (see Table 51–1)
   - NCLEX® a. Temperature higher than 100.4°F (38°C) on any 2 of first 10 days postpartum excluding first 24 hours, when taken orally at least four times daily
   - NCLEX® b. Endometritis: foul-smelling lochia, fever, uterine tenderness on palpation, lower abdominal pain, tachycardia, and chills
   - c. Pelvic cellulitis: fever, chills, malaise, abdominal pain, subinvolution of uterus (larger and softer), tachycardia, local and referred rebound tenderness
   - NCLEX® d. Abnormal laboratory results: positive culture, postpartum leukocytosis—white blood cell (WBC) level of 14,000–16,000/mm^3 is not unusual; an increase in WBC level greater than 30% in 6 hours indicates infection
7. Implementation
   - a. Administer prescribed antibiotics, analgesics, and antipyretics
   - b. Promote comfort; change linen frequently
   - NCLEX® c. Promote adequate nutrition and hydration (3000–4000 mL/day); monitor and record I&O
   - NCLEX® d. Use aseptic technique and good hand hygiene; provide frequent perineal care and educate client in correct technique
   - NCLEX® e. Assess VS, especially temperature; monitor laboratory results
   - f. Assess fundus for involution and lochia; encourage semi-Fowler position to facilitate drainage
   - g. Promote adequate rest and sleep; allow family and friends to visit per client's wishes
   - h. Encourage client to care for self first before caring for infant; allow client to care for and feed infant per client's condition; provide positive reinforcement

B. Wound infections

1. Infections of abdominal incision (cesarean birth), episiotomy, or repaired laceration
2. NCLEX® Predisposing factors: obesity, diabetes mellitus, prolonged postpartum hospitalization, premature rupture of membranes (PROM), metritis, prolonged labor, anemia, steroid therapy, immunosuppression
3. Nursing assessment
   - NCLEX® a. REEDA assessment; see Box 51–1
   - b. Generalized fever and/or induration (hardening) of site, localized tissue warmth
   - c. Tenderness

Table 51–1 Summary of Specific Reproductive System Infections and Assessment Findings

Type of Infection	Assessment Findings
Endometritis (metritis)	Fever initially 101–102°F (38.3–38.9°C); then sawtooth temperature elevations between 101 and 104°F (38.3–40°C) Uterine tenderness on palpation of fundus or on bimanual exam Grimacing, guarding, reports of pain; prolonged or bothersome afterpains Subinvolution of uterus Positive bacteria culture of lochia
Pelvic cellulitis (parametritis)	Prolonged elevation of temperature to 102–104°F (38.9-40°C) with fluctuations Abdominal pain extending laterally; possible rebound tenderness Hypotension, subinvolution, chills, decreased bowel sounds, nausea, and vomiting
Peritonitis	Elevated temperature up to 105°F (40.5°C) and severe pain Paralytic ileus and abdominal rigidity; frequent vomiting with dehydration Possibly weak and thready pulse; rapid, shallow respirations Excessive thirst and marked anxiety
Septic pelvic thrombophlebitis	Elevation of temperature to 105°F (40.5°C); dramatic fluctuations possible Pain in flank or lower abdomen
Bacteremia and septic shock	Rapid elevation of temperature to 103–104°F (39.4–40°C) Profuse, foul-smelling lochia Symptoms of shock, including urine output less than 30 mL/hr, tachycardia, hypotension

Box 51–1

REEDA Assessment

Redness: erythema around wound
Edema: swelling of tissues
Ecchymosis: skin discoloration
Discharge: purulent drainage from incision site
Approximation of skin edges: gaping of the wound edges

4. Implementation

NCLEX®
   a. Assess incision or episiotomy site every 8–12 hours for signs of infection; document and report adverse REEDA signs and induration

Memory Aid

Use the mnemonic **REEDA**. See Box 51–1 to remember to assess episiotomies and wounds for **r**edness, **e**dema, **e**cchymosis, **d**ischarge, and **a**pproximation of wound edges.

   b. Assess vital signs; monitor laboratory results

NCLEX®
   c. Use aseptic technique and appropriate hand hygiene; provide frequent wound or perineal care; educate client in correct technique
   d. Administer antibiotics, analgesics, and antipyretics as prescribed

NCLEX®
   e. Promote adequate nutrition and hydration (3000–4000 mL/day); monitor and record I&O
   f. Promote comfort, change linens frequently
   g. Promote adequate rest and sleep; allow family and friends to visit per client's wishes
   h. Encourage client to care for self first before taking care of baby; allow client to care for and feed infant per client's condition; provide client positive reinforcement

C. Breast infection (*mastitis*)

1. An infection of breast interlobular connective tissue, primarily in lactating women; onset is usually at 2–8 weeks' postpartum or any other time that breastfeeding frequency decreases
2. Predisposing factors
   a. Traumatized tissue, fissured or cracked nipples
   b. Engorgement, milk stasis or failure to empty breasts, missed feedings
   c. Lowered maternal defenses caused by fatigue, stress, or poor diet
   d. Poor hand hygiene practices or breasts not air-dried after feeding
   e. Restrictive clothing, plastic lined breast pads (trap moisture), and constricting or underwire bra

NCLEX®
3. Nursing assessment
   a. Routine daily assessment of breast consistency, skin color, surface temperature, nipple condition, and presence of pain
   b. Warm, reddened, painful area on breast, often wedge-shaped
   c. Axillary lymph nodes enlarged or tender
   d. Flu-like symptoms (fever, chills, headache, muscle aches, and malaise)
   e. Diagnosis by healthcare provider is usually on basis of clinical signs and symptoms
4. Implementation
   a. Administer prescribed antibiotics (or antifungal if candida is responsible), analgesics compatible with breastfeeding, such as nonsteroidal anti-inflammatory drugs (NSAIDs), and antipyretics
   b. Culture and sensitivity of breast milk may be prescribed if case is severe or nonresponsive to antibiotics (after washing breast, first 3 mL expressed and discarded before midstream sample obtained); note that infection is usually not transmitted to breast milk

NCLEX®
   c. Promote comfort: a well-fitting, supportive bra is needed 24 hours a day
   d. Promote adequate nutrition, hydration, rest, and sleep; increase fluid intake to 2–2.5 L/daily
   e. Provide local application of warm, moist heated compresses for comfort

NCLEX®
   f. Remind mother and staff to use meticulous handwashing technique before handling breasts or assisting with breastfeeding; continue and increase breastfeeding as advised by healthcare provider

NCLEX®
   g. Educate client regarding breast care, proper positioning of infant on breast and latch on, let-down reflex, necessity for frequent breastfeeding, signs of complications, and telephone numbers client can call with questions; provide client positive reinforcement

NCLEX®
   h. Change position of infant for feeding to relieve pressure on same area of nipple; breastfeed frequently to prevent stasis of milk

D. *Urinary tract infections* (UTI)

1. Can occur as **cystitis** (lower urinary tract infection) and often appears 2–3 days after birth, or as **pyelonephritis** (upper urinary tract infection); postdelivery urinary tract infections are usually caused by *E. coli* bacteria and generally occur soon after vaginal delivery

NCLEX® 2. Predisposing factors: retention of residual urine, bacteria introduced during catheterization, and bladder traumatized by childbirth

NCLEX® 3. Nursing assessment
   a. Overdistension of bladder in early postpartum period
   b. Urinary frequency with small volume voided, urgency, burning, dysuria, hesitancy and dribbling, nocturia, and possible hematuria
   c. Elevated temperature; low-grade temperature occurs with cystitis, higher fever occurs with pyelonephritis
   d. Flank pain, costovertebral angle tenderness, chills, nausea and vomiting (N/V) with pyelonephritis

4. Implementation
   NCLEX® a. Monitor bladder frequently during recovery period to institute preventative measures
   b. Obtain prescribed culture and sensitivity of urine prior to giving antibiotics
   c. Administer prescribed antibiotics; commonly sulfamethoxazole/trimethoprim, nitrofurantoin, or, in case of sulfa allergy, amoxicillin or axoxicillin-clavulanate
   d. Promote comfort; administer analgesic, antispasmodic, antipyretic medications
   NCLEX® e. Promote nutrition and hydration; increase oral fluids to at least 8–10 8-ounce glasses daily, especially water
   f. Acidify urine with low-sugar juices (such as cranberry, plum, apricot, and prune) and vitamin C; avoid foods and beverages that alkalinize urine, such as carbonated beverages, coffee, citrus fruits, tomatoes, and chocolate
   g. Encourage voiding at first urge and at least every 2–4 hours while awake; wear underwear with a cotton panel to facilitate air circulation
   h. Measure VS, especially temperature, and assess for resolution of symptoms
   i. Teach preventive measures: use underwear with cotton crotch to facilitate air circulation; avoid fabrics such as nylon that retain moisture and heat; when intercourse is resumed, void beforehand (to prevent bladder trauma) and after (to wash contaminants from area of urinary meatus)

IV. THROMBOEMBOLIC DISEASE

A. Overview

1. May occur during pregnancy and postpartum; consists of venous thromboembolism (including deep vein thrombosis and pulmonary embolism), and **thrombophlebitis** (thrombus formation in response to inflammation in vein wall)
2. Three general causes of thromboembolic disease are called Virchow's triad (hypercoagulability of blood, venous stasis, and injury to blood vessel wall)
3. Contributing factors in pregnant women
   a. Increased amounts of blood-clotting factors in postpartum period
   b. Postpartum thrombocytosis (increased number and adhesiveness of circulating platelets)
   c. Release of thromboplastin substances from placental tissue and fetal membranes
   d. Increased amounts of fibrinolysis inhibitors

NCLEX® **B. Predisposing factors**

1. Maternal factors such as obesity, cigarette smoking, increased maternal age, multiparity, anemia, or hypothermia
2. Anesthesia or surgery (such as cesarean birth) resulting in trauma to leg (incorrect positioning or prolonged time in stirrups), venous stasis, immobility
3. Disorders such as diabetes mellitus, heart disease, endometritis, varicosities or injury to leg, and history of deep vein thrombosis (DVT)

C. Types of thromboembolic disorders

1. Superficial thrombophlebitis (more common in postpartum period)
2. DVT
   a. More frequently seen in women with a history of thrombosis
   NCLEX® b. Increased incidence in women with obstetric complications such as hydramnios, preeclampsia, and operative birth
3. Septic pelvic thrombophlebitis
   a. Develops in conjunction with infections of reproductive tract
   b. More common in women with a cesarean birth
   c. DVT and septic pelvic thromboemboli predispose clients to pulmonary embolization

D. Nursing assessment

1. Superficial thrombophlebitis
   a. Symptoms become apparent about third or fourth postpartum day
   b. Tenderness in portion of vein, cord-like vein
   c. Local heat and redness is present; may have low-grade fever
   d. Pulmonary embolism is extremely rare
2. Deep vein thrombosis
   a. Frequently occurs in women with history of thrombosis
   b. NCLEX® Characterized by edema of ankle and leg; increased calf circumference by more than 2 cm (0.8 inch)
   c. NCLEX® Initial low-grade fever followed by chills and high fever
   d. Pain located in lower leg, popliteal or inguinal area, or lower abdomen depending on which vein is involved
   e. NCLEX® Homans sign may or may not be positive, but pain results from calf pressure
   f. Peripheral pulses may or may not be decreased
   g. NCLEX® May result in pulmonary embolism; signs include dyspnea and chest pain, diagnosis may be verified by VQ (ventilation quotient) scan, blood gas studies, or x-ray
3. Septic pelvic thrombophlebitis
   a. Infection ascends upward along the venous system, and thrombophlebitis develops in uterine, ovarian, or hypogastric veins
   b. Usually unresponsive to antibiotics
   c. Characterized by abdominal or flank pain with guarding
   d. Occurs on second to third postpartum day with fever and tachycardia
   e. Intermittent fever and chills may persist
   f. Pulmonary embolism may result; signs include dyspnea and chest pain; diagnosis may be verified by V/Q scan, blood gas studies, or x-ray

E. Implementation

1. Evaluate regarding need for support hose during labor and postpartum period
2. NCLEX® Encourage early ambulation following birth; women who have had a cesarean birth should perform regular leg exercises to promote venous return
3. NCLEX® If diagnosis of DVT is made, monitor for signs of pulmonary embolism
4. NCLEX® Monitor for signs of bleeding related to heparin or sodium warfarin therapy, and keep protamine sulfate (antagonist for heparin) available; keep vitamin K available if receiving warfarin
5. Keep legs elevated and use moist heat application if prescribed
6. Obtain clotting times as prescribed in client who is on anticoagulant therapy
7. Maintain bedrest as prescribed; if client can get up, educate client to avoid either standing or sitting for long periods of time; advise client against crossing legs or ankles
8. Review need for client to wear support stockings, if prescribed, and to plan for rest periods with legs elevated
9. Promote increased fluid intake
10. Promote comfort
    a. Administer nonaspirin analgesic for pain
    b. Elevate extremities on pillow to decrease venous aching
    c. Promote adequate rest and sleep
11. NCLEX® Perform serial bilateral calf measurements daily to compare for any increase in swelling
12. NCLEX® Report to healthcare provider any heavy vaginal bleeding, generalized petechiae, bleeding from mucous membranes, hematuria, or oozing from venipuncture sites as adverse effects of anticoagulant therapy

V. POSTPARTUM PSYCHIATRIC DISORDERS

A. Overview

1. **Postpartum psychiatric disorders** is one diagnosable syndrome in DSM-5 with three subclasses: adjustment reaction with depressed mood, peripartum major mood episodes, and postpartum mood episodes with psychotic features
2. *Adjustment reaction with depressed mood* is also known as postpartum, maternal, or baby blues; may be associated with rapid alteration in estrogen, progesterone, and prolactin levels after birth
   a. Characterized by mild depression interspersed with happier feelings
   b. NCLEX® Typically occurs within 2 to 4 days after baby's birth and is self-limiting, lasting from 1 to 10 days, more severe in primiparas
   c. NCLEX® New mothers feel overwhelmed, unable to cope, fatigued, anxious, irritable, and oversensitive; episodic tearfulness occurs without any reason

3. *Peripartum major mood episodes*, also known as postpartum depression
   a. Develops in about 10–20% of postpartum women across studies
   b. May occur anytime in first postpartum year, most often occurs around fourth week, just before start of menses, or upon weaning
   c. Risk factors: history of major depression, depression during pregnancy, history of postpartum depression or bipolar illness, stressful life events, primiparity, ambivalence about pregnancy, lack of social support or stable relationship with parents or partner, dissatisfaction with self (including body image and eating disorders), age (adolescence increases risk), complications of delivery, and loss of newborn

   NCLEX®
   d. Symptoms: signs of clinical depression, sadness, frequent crying, insomnia, appetite change, difficulty concentrating and making decisions, feelings of worthlessness, obsessive thoughts of inadequacy as a person/parent, lack of interest in usual activities, lack of concern about personal appearance; possible irritability and hostility toward new baby

   NCLEX®
   e. Treatment: individual or group psychotherapy and antidepressants, most frequently selective serotonin reuptake inhibitors (SSRIs) and tricyclic antidepressants (TCAs); all are excreted into breast milk but most are considered safe with breastfeeding (exception is fluoxetine because of long drug half-life)
4. *Postpartum mood episodes with psychotic features* (postpartum psychosis)
   a. Most serious although rare disorder; becomes evident within first few days after birth and progresses rapidly; of concern because of risk of infanticide or suicide

   NCLEX®
   b. Symptoms: sleep disturbances (even while infant is sleeping), confusion (irrational or disorganized thinking, bizarre behaviors), hallucinations or delusions (thinking that infant is evil, a changeling, or would be better off dead), depersonalization (seeming unaware or distant from events and people in environment), and psychomotor disturbances (stupor, agitation with hyperactivity, and possible rapid and incoherent speech)
   c. Risk factors: previous postpartum psychosis, history of bipolar disorder, family history of postpartum psychosis and bipolar disorder

   NCLEX®
   d. Treatment: admission to inpatient psychiatric hospital, antipsychotic medications, sedatives, social support, psychotherapy, assessment for suicide risk, and provisions for safety of infant
5. *Posttraumatic stress disorder (PTSD)*, also called posttraumatic stress syndrome (PTSS)
   a. Development of characteristic symptoms following distorted perception of birth-related events or exposure to traumatic events, such as emergency cesarean delivery, surgery, medical interventions with inadequate anesthesia, or loss of infant
   b. Symptoms include feelings of numbness, being dazed and unaware of environment, intrusive thoughts and flashbacks to event, difficulty thinking or sleeping, irritability, and avoiding others and reminders of traumatic event
   c. Preventive measures may include intervening when possible to prevent traumatic birth experiences, providing competent and concerned care, assessing anxiety and fears on admission and providing information to dispel myths, debriefing client and family after stressful or traumatic event, and assessing for early signs of trauma

B. Nursing assessment

1. History of previous psychological problems; assessment using Edinburgh Postnatal Depression Scale (score above 12 likely to occur with postpartum depression) or Beck's Revised Postnatal Depression Predictors Inventory

NCLEX®

2. Adequacy of coping skills and self-esteem

NCLEX®

3. Presence of mood swings, emotional distress, restlessness, irritability, guilt, extreme anxiety about the baby, anorexia, inability to complete activities of daily living, or trouble concentrating or expressing self
4. Specific symptoms of each postpartum psychiatric disorder listed previously

C. Implementation

NCLEX®

1. Observe client with baby, by herself, and with family and friends; arrange home visits, especially for early-discharge families
2. Telephone follow-up at 2–3 weeks' postpartum to see if mother is having difficulties; recognize early signs of problems
3. Seek client referral to psychiatrist for evaluation of psychological status

NCLEX®

4. Support positive parenting behaviors
5. Encourage client to plan how she will manage at home; provide concrete suggestions about practical assistance with childcare, meeting other demands of daily life, and how to cope with adjustment to motherhood

NCLEX®

6. Refer client to social services if indicated, support groups, and possible online support (such as Postpartum Support International)

Check Your NCLEX–RN® Exam I.Q.

You are ready for testing on this content if you can:

- Identify signs and symptoms of complications in the postpartum period.
- Implement nursing interventions to prevent postpartum complications or assist the client to recover from them.
- Perform client teaching about postpartum complications and their management.
- Evaluate the client and family response to therapy for postpartum complications.

PRACTICE TEST

1 The nurse determines that the client who is at greatest risk for postpartum hemorrhage is the one who delivered which infant?

1. A 2608-gram (5-lb, 12-oz) infant
2. A 2722-gram (6-lb) infant after a 2-hour labor
3. A 3261-gram (7-lb, 3-oz) infant after a 9-hour labor
4. A 3574-gram (7-lb, 14-oz) infant after a 12-hour labor

2 The nurse is preparing for beginning-of-shift rounds on assigned postpartum clients. After reviewing the assignment, the nurse plans to assess for hematoma formation in which client, who is at greatest risk for this complication?

1. A 17-year-old client who gave birth to a small-for-gestational-age infant
2. A 26-year-old client with gestational diabetes and forceps delivery of a large-for-gestational-age infant
3. A 35-year-old client having twins
4. A 40-year-old client having her first baby

3 The clinic nurse receives a telephone call from a 7-day postpartum client who states she is having increased vaginal bleeding and asks if it is serious and what could be the cause. The nurse suspects which most common etiology of late-postpartum hemorrhage?

1. Uterine atony
2. Disseminated intravascular coagulopathy (DIC)
3. Retained placental fragments
4. Laceration

4 The postpartum nurse would use which therapeutic measure to help prevent a urinary tract infection (UTI) in an assigned client who has just delivered an infant?

1. Promote bedrest for 12 hours postdelivery.
2. Discourage voiding until the bladder regains the sensation of being full.
3. Encourage fluids to 3000 mL per day.
4. Encourage the intake of orange, grapefruit, or apple juice.

5 A newly postpartum client is going into hypovolemic shock as a result of uterine inversion. Which initial order should the nurse expect to implement to restore fluid volume?

1. Administer oxygen at 3–4 L/min via nasal cannula.
2. Administer an oxytocic drug via IV.
3. Monitor heart rate every five minutes.
4. Increase the IV infusion rate.

6 A client who previously had an infant by cesarean delivery has successfully delivered an infant by vaginal birth. During postpartum recovery, she suddenly reports severe pain in the abdomen and between her scapulae. There is minimal amount of vaginal bleeding. What is the nurse's priority action?

1. Put the client in Trendelenburg position.
2. Continue to assess for uterine atony.
3. Maintain the rate of IV fluids.
4. Notify the healthcare provider promptly.

7 The nurse interprets that a postpartum client has early postpartum hemorrhage if the amount of vaginal bleeding in the first 24 hours postdelivery exceeds how many mL? Provide a numeric answer.

Fill in your answer below:
Answer: _____ mL

PRACTICE TEST

8. To minimize the risk of early-postpartum hemorrhage in a client who just had a cesarean birth, the postanesthesia care nurse should include which measure in the plan of care? Select all that apply.

1. Maintain an IV rate of 125 mL/hr.
2. Assess the uterus for firmness every 15 minutes.
3. Assess abdominal dressing for drainage.
4. Monitor urinary output.
5. Monitor the drainage on the client's peri-pad.

9. A client has been taking methylergonovine maleate for uterine subinvolution but it has not been effective. Which procedure does the clinic nurse anticipate will be ordered to correct the cause of this late-postpartum hemorrhage?

1. Dilatation and curettage
2. Laparotomy
3. Hysterotomy
4. Hysterectomy

10. The partner of a 4-day postpartum woman calls the nursing unit saying that she is happy one minute and cries the next. He states, "She never was like this before the baby was born." What is the best initial response by the nurse?

1. Make a suggestion to ignore the mood swings, as they will go away.
2. Provide reassurance that this is normal in the postpartum period because of hormonal changes.
3. Advise contacting a psychiatrist immediately; this is the first step in postpartum psychosis.
4. Instruct the partner in signs and symptoms of postpartum psychiatric disorders.

11. The postpartum nurse who is reviewing the client assignment determines that which client is at greatest risk for early postpartum hemorrhage?

1. A client with an infant weighing 2468 grams (5 lb, 7 oz)
2. A client who is 17 years old
3. A client with endometritis
4. A client with uterine atony

12. While performing a postpartum assessment, the nurse notices the client's lochia is very heavy. What should be the nurse's first response?

1. Palpate and massage the uterus.
2. Elevate the head of the bed to Fowler position.
3. Reevaluate in 10 minutes to see if the problem has corrected itself.
4. Place the client in modified Trendelenburg position.

13. The postpartum nurse would use which measure that would be most effective in detecting development of thrombophlebitis?

1. Monitoring the client's temperature
2. Asking if the client has calf pain when getting out of bed
3. Asking if the client has pain during leg massage
4. Assessing for petechiae on the lower extremities

14. What would the postpartum nurse expect to document about the client's lochia and location of uterine fundus on the second day after delivery?

1. Yellowish-white lochia with no clots, fundus three fingerbreadths below the umbilicus
2. Dark red lochia with small clots, fundus midline and two fingerbreadths below the umbilicus
3. Pinkish-brown lochia with no clots, fundus midline and four fingerbreadths below the umbilicus
4. A large amount of bright red lochia with large clots, fundus midline and at the umbilicus

15. The clinic nurse working with women during the postpartum period would interpret that which behaviors exhibited by a client are typical during this time? Select all that apply.

1. The mother experiences feelings of depression as she assumes responsibility for her new baby.
2. The mother does not take care of herself, but attends well to her infant.
3. The mother is receptive to learning about her baby.
4. The mother does not sleep or eat well, but tries to take care of herself.
5. The mother talks to the newborn and looks often at the newborn's face.

16 The nurse is assigned to a postpartum client diagnosed with a right labial hematoma. What instruction should the nurse plan to include in the client's care at this time?

1. A warm pack will be used to increase comfort and to decrease blood loss.
2. Witch hazel pads will be applied to reduce discomfort.
3. She needs to give informed consent for surgery to incise and drain the hematoma.
4. A cool pack will help to decrease bleeding and reduce the swelling.

17 A postpartum client develops thrombophlebitis in her right calf and is started on heparin therapy. Which nursing intervention would be most appropriate at this time? Select all that apply.

1. Encourage the client to ambulate to reduce lower-extremity swelling.
2. Encourage the client to take aspirin for leg pain.
3. Instruct the client to remain on bedrest to reduce the possibility of embolism.
4. Inform the client that she will experience numbness in her leg for several months.
5. Explain that the client should use a soft toothbrush and only an electric razor.

18 A postpartum client receiving heparin asks whether she can continue to breastfeed. What is the best response for the nurse to give?

1. She should stop breastfeeding immediately.
2. She can continue to breastfeed, but must assess the baby daily for ecchymotic spots.
3. Heparin will not affect the breastfeeding and requires no special precautions for the infant.
4. She should alternate breastfeeding and bottle-feeding.

19 During a home visit, a 10-day postpartum client reports development of a reddened, swollen, and tender breast. What should the nurse include in a response to the client?

1. These symptoms suggest an inflammatory or infectious process and require immediate healthcare provider notification.
2. She should mention it to her healthcare provider at her 2-week checkup because it will be abnormal if it continues after 2 weeks.
3. This is normal breast engorgement and should subside within another week.
4. She has to stop breastfeeding immediately until the swelling and redness resolve on their own.

20 A client has developed disseminated intravascular coagulopathy (DIC) following a placenta previa. Which nursing action is important at this time? Select all that apply.

1. Assess Homans sign hourly.
2. Frequently monitor her vaginal bleeding.
3. Administer antibiotics.
4. Monitor reflexes hourly.
5. Monitor results of D-dimer blood tests.

21 The postpartum nurse is caring for a client with thrombophlebitis. The nurse monitors the client for which symptoms of complications? Select all that apply.

1. Confusion
2. Sudden high fever
3. Dyspnea
4. Diaphoresis
5. Sudden onset of chills

ANSWERS & RATIONALES

1 **Answer: 2 Rationale:** A rapid (precipitous) labor and delivery can cause exhaustion of the uterine muscle and prevent contraction of the uterus after delivery, which controls the amount of bleeding. A 2608-gram (5-lb, 12-oz) infant is of normal size while delivery of a large infant is a predisposing factor for postpartum hemorrhage. A labor of 9 hours and 12 hours with birth of infants of normal size does not increase risk of postpartum hemorrhage. **Cognitive Level:** Analyzing **Client Need:** Physiological Adaptation **Integrated Process:** Nursing Process: Diagnosis **Content Area:** Maternal–Newborn **Strategy:** First, eliminate options that are similar (normal-size infants and 9- and 12-hour labors) because they identify infants of similar size who were delivered within reasonably similar time frames. Choose the 2722-gram (6-lb) infant because of the very short duration of labor (2 hours).

2 **Answer: 2 Rationale:** A hematoma is a collection of blood in the pelvic tissue caused by damage to a blood vessel wall without tissue laceration. A client with gestational diabetes is more prone to have a large infant that could cause tissue trauma during delivery. This client was also delivered with forceps, which is another high-risk factor for developing a postpartum hematoma. Delivery of a small-for-gestational-age infant and increasing maternal age do not increase risk of hematoma formation. A large newborn, rather than the number of newborns, determines risk for hematoma formation. **Cognitive Level:** Analyzing **Client Need:** Physiological Adaptation **Integrated Process:** Nursing Process: Assessment **Content Area:** Maternal–Newborn **Strategy:** The core issue of the question is knowledge that large fetal size at delivery is a risk factor for hematoma formation. Evaluate each option carefully, considering the client with diabetes mellitus is more likely to have a large-for-gestational-age infant.

3 **Answer: 3 Rationale:** Retained placental fragments are a cause of late-postpartum hemorrhage (which occurs anytime after the first 24 hours postdelivery). The retained fragments undergo necrosis, forming fibrin deposits and then polyps, which eventually detach from the myometrium, causing hemorrhage. Uterine atony, DIC, and lacerations are causes of early postpartum hemorrhage. **Cognitive Level:** Analyzing **Client Need:** Physiological Adaptation **Integrated Process:** Nursing Process: Diagnosis **Content Area:** Maternal–Newborn **Strategy:** Specific knowledge of how to discriminate etiology of early- and late-postpartum hemorrhage is needed to answer this question. Use nursing knowledge and the process of elimination to make your selection.

4 **Answer: 3 Rationale:** Adequate fluid intake (up to 3000 mL/day) prevents urinary stasis, dilutes urine, and flushes out waste products, all of which help to prevent UTI. Bedrest is of no value in preventing UTI, although urinary stasis can actually increase risk. The client should attempt to void every few hours, rather than waiting to regain a sense of a full bladder. While intake of juices is healthy, it is the large volume, not the type, of fluid consumed that aids in flushing out wastes. **Cognitive Level:** Applying **Client Need:** Physiological Adaptation **Integrated Process:** Nursing Process: Implementation **Content Area:** Maternal–Newborn **Strategy:** The core issue of the question is knowing how to decrease risk for UTIs. Recall that the risk can be diminished by decreasing risk of urinary stasis and increasing fluid intake as well as foods and beverages that yield acidic urine (cranberry juice, ascorbic acid in high doses).

5 **Answer: 4 Rationale:** Increasing the rate of IV fluids is an effective initial measure necessary to replace lost fluid volume that occurs in uterine inversion caused by hemorrhage. Blood products might also be necessary but generally take some time to obtain from the blood bank. Oxygen would be given to increase perfusion to tissues but does not restore circulating volume. An oxytocic drug will help to limit further bleeding but will not restore circulating volume. Monitoring heart rate will not limit the condition because it is an assessment rather than an intervention. **Cognitive Level:** Applying **Client Need:** Physiological Adaptation **Integrated Process:** Nursing Process: Planning **Content Area:** Maternal–Newborn **Strategy:** The core issue of the question is fluid volume replacement. Eliminate each of the incorrect options because they do not replace fluids, although they might be helpful in a specific way.

6 **Answer: 4 Rationale:** A common risk associated with vaginal delivery after cesarean is uterine rupture. Pain in the abdomen and between the scapulae can occur when the uterus ruptures. The hemorrhage is concealed and blood accumulates under the diaphragm, leading to scapular pain. This is an emergency and requires immediate medical intervention, which is initiated by calling the healthcare provider. The client may be put in *modified* Trendelenburg position, not Trendelenburg position, to manage shock. Uterine atony is not the problem, and an action rather than an assessment is required. IV fluids would be increased rather than maintained. **Cognitive Level:** Applying **Client Need:** Physiological Adaptation **Integrated Process:** Nursing Process: Implementation **Content Area:** Maternal–Newborn **Strategy:** Note the core issue of the question is recognition of internal hemorrhage due to uterine rupture. Eliminate the incorrect options because they fail to initiate or provide effective treatment for this medical emergency.

7 **Answer: 500 Rationale:** The traditional definition of early postpartum hemorrhage after a vaginal birth is greater than 500 mL in the first 24 hours. **Cognitive Level:** Analyzing **Client Need:** Physiological Adaptation **Integrated Process:** Nursing Process: Assessment **Content Area:** Maternal–Newborn **Strategy:** The core issue of the question is an understanding of criteria for postpartum hemorrhage. Use nursing knowledge and the process of elimination to make your selection.

8 **Answer: 2, 5 Rationale:** Assessing the uterine fundus every 15 minutes helps ensure that uterine contraction is taking place. Early detection of a boggy uterus can lead to actions that will prevent hemorrhage. Monitoring the drainage on the client's peri-pad will directly detect early postpartum hemorrhage. While maintaining the IV rate helps maintain normal hydration, it will not help to prevent or detect early-postpartum hemorrhage. Assessing the abdominal dressing for drainage is appropriate but will not help to detect early-postpartum hemorrhage. Monitoring urine output is appropriate for the client but reduced urine output is not a specific indicator of early-postpartum hemorrhage. **Cognitive Level:** Applying **Client Need:** Physiological Adaptation **Integrated Process:** Nursing Process: Implementation **Content Area:** Maternal–Newborn

Strategy: Note that the critical word in the question is *hemorrhage*. Use the process of elimination to make selections. Note that none of the incorrect options addresses a direct assessment of postpartum hemorrhage.

9 **Answer: 1 Rationale:** Late-postpartum hemorrhage most frequently occurs due to retained placental tissue. Dilatation and curettage is the vaginal procedure of choice to remove retained tissue from the uterus. Laparotomy, hysterotomy, and hysterectomy are abdominal surgeries but they are not used to treat this condition. **Cognitive Level:** Analyzing **Client Need:** Physiological Adaptation **Integrated Process:** Nursing Process: Planning **Content Area:** Maternal–Newborn **Strategy:** Consider first that the client is bleeding, and determine the most likely cause, retained placental fragments. Then visualize each of the surgeries described and use the process of elimination and nursing knowledge to choose the one that will effectively treat the condition.

10 **Answer: 2 Rationale:** Before providing further instructions, the nurse should explain that these are signs of postpartum blues, which is a normal process related to hormonal changes. Telling the partner to ignore the mood swings fails to address the client's concern. In this case, the partner is the client. Advising the partner to consult a psychiatrist immediately is an excessive response. Teaching the client about various postpartum psychiatric disorders is unnecessary and excessive. **Cognitive Level:** Applying **Client Need:** Psychosocial Integrity **Integrated Process:** Communication and Documentation **Content Area:** Maternal–Newborn **Strategy:** The core issue of the question is recognition and appropriate instruction regarding mood changes in the postpartum period. Use nursing knowledge and the process of elimination to make your selection.

11 **Answer: 4 Rationale:** Uterine atony accounts for 80–90% of all early (within first 24 hours) hemorrhage. Infants weighing between 2268 and 3175 grams (5 and 7 lb) would not overly distend the uterus and thus not cause increased risk of postpartum hemorrhage. The client's age does not increase the incidence of postpartum hemorrhage. Endometritis could cause late-postpartum hemorrhage, not early-postpartum hemorrhage. **Cognitive Level:** Analyzing **Client Need:** Physiological Adaptation **Integrated Process:** Nursing Process: Diagnosis **Content Area:** Maternal–Newborn **Strategy:** First, recall the causes of early postpartum hemorrhage, which might help you to select the correct option easily. Alternatively, eliminate endometritis first because it is a different postpartum complication, then the 2468-gram (5-lb, 7-oz) infant because of small size, and finally the age of 17 years because it is irrelevant.

12 **Answer: 1 Rationale:** Excessive bleeding must be evaluated and managed immediately to prevent excessive loss of blood and shock. The nurse should palpate the uterus to determine whether it is boggy, then massage the uterus. Elevating the head of the bed will not address the possible complication of early postpartum hemorrhage. Waiting represents a failure to act and will only cause the client harm. Bleeding should be addressed immediately. A modified Trendelenburg position is the classic shock position, but the nurse should first try measures to reduce bleeding and thus prevent onset of shock. **Cognitive Level:** Applying **Client Need:** Physiological Adaptation **Integrated Process:** Nursing Process: Implementation **Content Area:** Maternal–Newborn **Strategy:** The core issue of the question is knowledge of measures to reduce postpartum bleeding. With this in mind, eliminate options that delay action or focus on positioning, since these will not correct a boggy uterus.

13 **Answer: 2 Rationale:** Calf pain upon dorsiflexion of the foot (such as when getting out of bed) indicates a positive Homans sign, a sign of thrombophlebitis. Thrombophlebitis may cause a mild temperature elevation, but monitoring temperature is not the most direct or effective measure to assess thrombophlebitis. The legs (especially the calves) should not be massaged with risk of thrombophlebitis because doing so could dislodge a potential clot. Petechiae are not a clinical sign of thrombophlebitis. **Cognitive Level:** Analyzing **Client Need:** Physiological Adaptation **Integrated Process:** Nursing Process: Assessment **Content Area:** Maternal–Newborn **Strategy:** Specific knowledge of assessment of thrombophlebitis is needed to answer this question. First, eliminate the option with leg massage, which is contraindicated. Next, eliminate petechiae because the problem is not evidenced by bleeding into skin tissue. Finally, choose calf pain over monitoring for temperature because it is a more specific sign than mild fever.

14 **Answer: 2 Rationale:** The fundus should be midline, two fingerbreadths below the umbilicus, with dark red lochia, which might contain small clots (lochia rubra). Yellowish-white color with no clots explains lochia alba, which does not occur until about 10 days' postpartum. Pinkish-brown lochia with no clots describes lochia serosa, which usually occurs between days 4 and 9 of postpartum. A large amount of bright red lochia with large clots describes findings that occur with subinvolution. **Cognitive Level:** Analyzing **Client Need:** Physiological Adaptation **Integrated Process:** Nursing Process: Assessment **Content Area:** Maternal–Newborn **Strategy:** Specific knowledge of changes in lochia during the postpartum period is needed to answer this question. Use nursing knowledge and the process of elimination to make your selection.

15 **Answer: 3, 5 Rationale:** Typical behavior during the postpartum period includes accepting responsibility for infant care. Typical behavior during the postpartum period includes activities that demonstrate maternal–newborn bonding. Feelings of depression indicate potential psychiatric problems and require additional investigation. Lack of self-care indicates potential psychiatric problems and requires additional investigation. An inability to eat or sleep well requires investigation as to the cause, as both are especially important during the postpartum period. **Cognitive Level:** Analyzing **Client Need:** Psychosocial Integrity **Integrated Process:** Nursing Process: Assessment **Content Area:** Maternal–Newborn **Strategy:** The core issue of the question is healthy adaptation to life with a new infant. Choose the options that indicate the greatest resemblance to healthy behavior and adaptive coping.

16 **Answer: 4 Rationale:** Applying a cool pack will minimize swelling, bleeding, and discomfort. A warm pack is incorrect because it will increase engorgement at the site via vasodilation. Witch hazel will not decrease the swelling in the area. Labial hematomas do not necessarily need to be drained; they usually resolve on their own. **Cognitive Level:** Applying **Client Need:** Physiological Adaptation **Integrated Process:** Nursing Process: Implementation **Content Area:** Maternal–Newborn **Strategy:** The core issue of the question is knowledge of heat and cold applications to aid in reabsorption of hematoma. Use basic nursing knowledge and the process of elimination to make your selection.

17 **Answer: 3, 5 Rationale:** Bedrest is recommended following a diagnosis of thrombophlebitis, to help prevent development of a pulmonary embolus. The client receiving full anticoagulant therapy with heparin should be placed on bleeding precautions to reduce the risk of bleeding. These precautions include using a soft toothbrush and electric razor rather than a straight razor. The client should not ambulate because it could lead to pulmonary embolus if the blood clot dislodges. The client should be started on heparin therapy and therefore should avoid aspirin and nonsteroidal anti-inflammatory drugs that will potentiate the action of heparin. The client should not experience any residual effects in the extremities. **Cognitive Level:** Analyzing **Client Need:** Physiological Adaptation **Integrated Process:** Nursing Process: Implementation **Content Area:** Maternal–Newborn **Strategy:** The core issue of the question is knowledge of measures to prevent complications of thrombophlebitis and heparin therapy. Note that two options are opposites, which may suggest that one of them is correct. Use knowledge that activity can cause thrombi to travel as emboli to the lungs to choose bedrest over activity. Recall the adverse effects of heparin to choose measures that reduce the risk of bleeding.

18 **Answer: 3 Rationale:** Heparin does not pass to the breast milk. Thus, heparin will not affect breastfeeding and requires no special infant precautions. A woman can continue to breastfeed while on heparin. The infant does not need to be assessed for ecchymoses. It is unnecessary to alternate breastfeeding with bottle-feeding. **Cognitive Level:** Applying **Client Need:** Physiological Adaptation **Integrated Process:** Nursing Process: Implementation **Content Area:** Maternal–Newborn **Strategy:** Specific knowledge of acceptable medication to use while breastfeeding is needed to answer this question. Use nursing knowledge and the process of elimination to make your selection.

19 **Answer: 1 Rationale:** These symptoms are suggestive of mastitis and require prompt attention by the client's healthcare provider. It is not therapeutic to wait for the symptoms to resolve on their own. These symptoms are not characteristic of normal breast engorgement. Breastfeeding does not have to be stopped if mastitis is present. **Cognitive Level:** Analyzing **Client Need:** Physiological Adaptation **Integrated Process:** Nursing Process: Assessment **Content Area:** Maternal–Newborn **Strategy:** The core issues of the question are recognition of mastitis and applying knowledge of appropriate intervention. Use nursing knowledge and the process of elimination to make your selection.

20 **Answer: 2, 5 Rationale:** DIC is a disorder of widespread microvascular clotting that can result in bleeding once clotting factors are consumed. Vaginal bleeding can be excessive if a coagulation disorder is present. A D-dimer test monitors fibrinogen level, platelet count, fibrin degradation products, and various coagulation times, all of which are altered during DIC. Homans sign is associated with thrombophlebitis, not with DIC. Antibiotics will not affect a clotting disorder. DIC does not affect a client's reflexes. **Cognitive Level:** Analyzing **Client Need:** Physiological Adaptation **Integrated Process:** Nursing Process: Assessment **Content Area:** Maternal–Newborn **Strategy:** The core issue of the question is knowledge that DIC can be evidenced by bleeding once clotting factors have been consumed. When answering questions about DIC, look for options that address bleeding in some way.

21 **Answer: 1, 3, 4 Rationale:** Confusion can occur because of decreased oxygenation to the brain resulting from loss of adequate gas exchange in the affected area of the lung. Classic symptoms of pulmonary embolus include sudden onset of dyspnea, chest pain, anxiety, diaphoresis, elevated pulse, and hypotension. The client would not experience high fever or chills; these are more indicative of infection. **Cognitive Level:** Analyzing **Client Need:** Physiological Adaptation **Integrated Process:** Nursing Process: Assessment **Content Area:** Maternal–Newborn **Strategy:** Specific knowledge of manifestations of pulmonary embolism is needed to answer this question. Use nursing knowledge and the process of elimination to make your selection.

Key Words to Review

cystitis p. 824
disseminated intravascular coagulopathy (DIC) p. 820
early-postpartum hemorrhage p. 820
endometritis/endomyometritis p. 822
hematoma p. 820
late-postpartum hemorrhage p. 820
mastitis p. 823
pelvic cellulitis/parametritis p. 822
peritonitis p. 822
postpartum psychiatric disorders p. 825
pyelonephritis p. 824
subinvolution p. 820
thrombophlebitis p. 824
urinary tract infection p. 824
uterine atony p. 820

References

Davidson, M., London, M., & Ladewig, P. (2016). *Olds' maternal newborn nursing and women's health across the lifespan* (10th ed.). New York, NY: Pearson Education.

Ladewig, P., London, M., & Davidson, M. (2014). *Contemporary maternal–newborn nursing care* (8th ed.). Upper Saddle River, NJ: Pearson Education.

London, M., Ladewig, P., Davidson, M., Ball, J., Bindler, R., & Cowen, K. (2014). *Maternal and child nursing care* (4th ed.). Upper Saddle River, NJ: Pearson Education.

Lowdermilk, D., Perry, S., Cashion, M., & Alden, K. (2016). *Maternity and women's health care* (11th ed.). St. Louis, MO: Elsevier.

Postpartum Support International. Available at http://www.postpartum.net.

Complicated Newborn Care

52

In this chapter

Cross Reference

Other chapters relevant to this content area are

Reproduction, Family Planning, and Infertility	**Chapter 8**
Uncomplicated Antenatal Assessment and Care	**Chapter 9**
Uncomplicated Labor and Delivery Care	**Chapter 10**
Uncomplicated Postpartum Assessment and Care	**Chapter 11**
Uncomplicated Newborn Care	**Chapter 12**
Maternal and Newborn Medications	**Chapter 34**
Complicated Antenatal Care	**Chapter 49**
Complicated Labor and Delivery Care	**Chapter 50**
Complicated Postpartum Care	**Chapter 51**
Basic Life Support	**Chapter 68**

I. GENERAL NURSING CARE OF HIGH-RISK NEWBORN

A. Assessments that identify high-risk newborns

1. Prenatal and intrapartal risk factors
   - **a.** Limited access to prenatal healthcare, no healthcare, or low socioeconomic status of mother
   - **b.** Maternal factors such as age, parity, and medical conditions such as heart disease, hypertension, diabetes, hyperthyroidism, and renal disease
   - **c.** Exposure to environmental dangers, including illegal drugs and toxic chemicals
   - **d.** Conditions related to pregnancy and associated complications, such as multiple gestation pregnancy, fetus that is small for gestational age (SGA) or large for gestational age (LGA), life-threatening congenital anomalies, maternal and fetal infection, preterm or post-term birth
   - **e.** Complications of pregnancy such as abruptio placentae, oligohydramnios, placenta previa, preeclampsia, premature rupture of membranes, preterm labor, and uterine rupture

NCLEX® 2. Apgar scores: an Apgar score of less than 6 at 1 minute or 7 at 5 minutes indicates unsatisfactory transition to extrauterine life and requires careful monitoring

NCLEX® 3. Changes in physical assessment are often vague, so thorough assessment is essential (see Box 52–1)

NCLEX® 4. Early or late gestational age
   a. Preterm: 36 weeks, 6 days or earlier
   b. Late preterm: 34 weeks, 0 days though 36 weeks, 6 days
   c. Early term: 37 weeks, 0 days though 38 weeks, 6 days
   d. Full term: 39 weeks, 0 days though 40 weeks, 6 days
   e. Late term: 41 weeks, 0 days though 41 weeks, 6 days
   f. Post-term: 42 weeks, 0 days and beyond

B. General planning and implementation for all high-risk newborns

1. Constantly monitor infant for subtle changes in condition and intervene promptly when necessary

NCLEX® 2. Decrease risk of hospital-acquired infections; provide each neonate with own supplies; hand hygiene is most important method of preventing infection

NCLEX® 3. Conserve infant's energy and decrease physiological stress by organizing care and minimizing interruptions; monitor each neonate for signs of stress

4. Provide appropriate stimulation for infant growth and development; high-risk neonates have same developmental needs as healthy neonate

5. Monitor oxygen saturation using pulse oximeter (sensor placed on skin)
   a. Place sensor on palm of hand, sole of foot, or wrap around finger
   NCLEX® b. Assess skin integrity at sensor site every 4 hours and rotate site every 12 hours
   NCLEX® c. Pulse oximeter reading of 88–92% reflects safe clinical range

6. Arterial blood gas (ABG)
   a. Direct measurement of amount of oxygen (O_2), carbon dioxide (CO_2), and pH in a sample of arterial blood via arterial puncture or **umbilical arterial line (UAL)**
   b. Compare oxygen saturation at time of blood sample to correlate values
   NCLEX® c. Apply pressure to arterial puncture site for 3–5 minutes

7. Blood glucose monitoring: warm foot to increase circulation prior to heelstick (preferred site)

8. Umbilical lines
   a. An umbilical arterial line (UAL) is inserted into an umbilical artery primarily to obtain ABG
   b. An **umbilical venous line (UVL)** is inserted into umbilical vein to give IV fluids and medications and to obtain blood for lab tests
   NCLEX® c. Assess all neonates with umbilical lines closely for blue discoloration or blanching on lower extremities or buttocks, which could indicate an embolus or vasospasm and may necessitate removal of line
   d. Assess closely for line placement, bleeding from umbilicus, or disconnected tubing; position infant in a side-lying position for close monitoring

9. Oxygen administration
   NCLEX® a. Administered by **oxygen hood** (hood placed over infant's head), nasal cannula, **continuous positive airway pressure (CPAP)** (pressurized air), or endotracheal tube (ET)
   NCLEX® b. Warm and humidify O_2 prior to administration to decrease insensible fluid loss and heat loss
   NCLEX® c. Monitor amount of O_2 being administered and O_2 saturation and/or ABGs; administer minimum amount of O_2 to meet infant's O_2 needs to prevent complications

Box 52–1

Critical Neonatal Assessment Indicators

The appearance of any of these signs in a neonate could indicate the presence of a serious complication:

- Respiratory: bradypnea or tachypnea, respiratory distress, weak or absent respiratory effort
- Cardiovascular: bradycardia or tachycardia, murmur
- Neuromuscular: lethargy, temperature instability, tremors, unusual behaviors such as lip-smacking
- Gastrointestinal: poor feeding tolerance, poor suck/swallow reflex
- Skin color: cyanosis (acrocyanosis is normal for first 24–48 hours after delivery), jaundice (especially within first 24 hours)
- Obvious major anomalies

10. Gavage tubes
  a. Used to decompress stomach or administer formula, breast milk, or oral medications
  b. It is preferred to insert tube orally instead of nasally because infants are obligate nose-breathers
NCLEX® **c.** A 5 Fr. or 8 Fr. tube is commonly used; measure tube from earlobe to nose and then to tip of xyphoid process; insert tube and secure placement
NCLEX® **d.** Check placement of tube prior to administering any feeding or medication; administer feedings over 3–5 minutes to avoid dumping syndrome; offer a pacifier during feeding

11. Parenting the high-risk newborn
  a. Parents are initially in a state of shock and disbelief and may grieve loss of "perfect baby"
  b. Assess bonding
  c. Explain equipment and infant's condition
  d. Present positive, realistic attitude and establish trust
NCLEX® **e.** Encourage parents to touch infant and perform caretaking activities as infant's condition allows
  f. Encourage parents to verbalize feelings
  g. Provide pictures of infant to parents prior to transfer to neonatal intensive care unit (NICU)
  h. Teach parents care of infant in preparation for discharge

II. PROBLEMS RELATED TO MATURITY

A. *Preterm (premature) infant*

1. Description: infant born before completion of 37th week of pregnancy
  a. Prognosis and severity of complications related to level of maturity: the earlier infant is born, the greater chance of complications
  b. Earliest age of viability is 23–24 weeks' gestation; major problem is variable immaturity of all systems, depending on length of gestation
NCLEX® **c.** Major complications are related to **respiratory distress syndrome (RDS)** (disorder caused by lack of surfactant), difficulty regulating body temperature, infection, and hemorrhage
  d. Generally ready for discharge near their due date

2. Risk factors
NCLEX® **a.** Maternal risk factors: age, smoking, poor nutrition, placental problems (placenta previa, placental abruption, preeclampsia/eclampsia), previous preterm delivery, cervical insufficiency
  b. Fetal risk factors: multiple gestation pregnancy, infection
  c. Other risk factors: low socioeconomic status, environmental exposure to harmful substance

3. Respiratory assessment
  a. Insufficient surfactant allows alveoli to collapse with each expiration
  b. Inadequate number and maturity of alveoli makes adequate alveolar gas exchange difficult
  c. Skeletal muscles weak so may not be able to reposition head and body to maintain patent airway
NCLEX® **d.** Signs of respiratory distress typically develop within 1 to 2 hours after delivery (see Box 52–2)

Memory Aid

Remember respiratory distress in a premature infant by the mnemonic SIN:

S Substernal retractions
I Inspiratory grunting
N Nasal flaring

4. Respiratory interventions
NCLEX® **a.** Attempt to prevent RDS by administering antenatal steroids or postnatal lung surfactant replacement therapy
  b. Maintain respirations at 30–60/min, assess every 1–2 hours and as needed
  c. Assess oxygenation status and ABG results
  d. Auscultate breath sounds; suction as needed

Box 52–2

Signs of Neonatal Respiratory Distress

- Tachypnea
- Intercostal and/or subcostal retractions
- Nasal flaring
- Expiratory grunting
- Seesaw respiratory movements
- Diminished breath sounds
- PaO_2 less than 50 mmHg
- PCO_2 above 60 mmHg
- Increasing exhaustion
- Cyanosis (late finding)

e. Monitor for signs of respiratory distress
f. Supportive respiratory care may range from humidified oxygen administration (mild cases) to use of continuous positive airway pressure (CPAP) in moderate cases, to mechanical ventilation (severe cases)

5. Assessment of thermoregulation
   a. Lack of subcutaneous fat to insulate body and small muscle mass
   b. Large body surface area in proportion to body weight, so more likely to lose heat quickly
   c. Absent sweat or shiver mechanisms
   d. Increased insensible fluid loss
   e. Increased risk of hypothermia
6. Interventions to assist thermoregulation
   a. Maintain **neutral thermal environment** (temperature that prevents heat loss)
   NCLEX® b. Place infant under radiant warmer or incubator and maintain set skin temperature of 96.8–97.8°F (36–36.5°C); compare skin probe temperature to axillary temperature
   NCLEX® c. Warm equipment and linens before contact with infant
   d. Prevent cold stress: warm and humidify oxygen without blowing it over infant's face, keep skin dry, keep infant out of drafts, avoid placing on cold surfaces (x-ray plates, scales, treatment tables), wrap in blankets and keep head covered
   e. Assess for consequences of cold stress: hypoglycemia, hypoxia, pallor, lethargy, metabolic acidosis
7. Immunologic system: low resistance to infection
   a. Lack of immunoglobulins from mother (usually cross placenta in third trimester)
   b. Difficulty localizing infection and poor white blood cell (WBC) response
   c. Skin surface (line of defense against infection) is easily excoriated and likely to be be interrupted for therapeutic procedures
   d. Monitor carefully for signs of infection and document
   e. Report immediately sudden onset of apnea and bradycardia when coupled with metabolic acidosis; could indicate bacterial sepsis, especially if infant has a central line
8. Hepatic and hematologic systems
   a. Glycogen stores in liver lower before birth and are quickly used after birth, increasing risk for hypoglycemia
   b. Increased risk of hyperbilirubinemia caused by difficulty in eliminating bilirubin released by normal breakdown of red blood cells (RBCs); monitor for jaundice
   c. Immature production of clotting factors resulting in increased risk of bleeding disorders
   d. Low iron stores (deposited in liver in greater amounts during last trimester) lead to anemia
   e. Prolonged drug metabolism related to immature liver
   f. Interventions include monitoring for jaundice and preventing excess blood sampling to reduce anemia
9. Gastrointestinal (GI) system
   NCLEX® a. Weak suck/swallow reflex until 33–34 weeks' gestation and poor gag/cough reflexes increase risk of aspiration
   b. Increased risk of **necrotizing enterocolitis (NEC)**, a neonatal disorder related to immature GI system and hypoxia
   c. Increased basal metabolic rate and increased oxygen requirements may cause fatigue during sucking
   d. GI immaturity leads to problems with ingestion, digestion, and absorption
10. Feeding
   NCLEX® a. Feed according to abilities, often determined by gestational age and development; most common feeding methods are bottle, breast, and gavage
   b. Assess tolerance of feedings (absence of abdominal distention and emesis)
   c. Monitor suck/swallow reflex to assess risk of aspiration; if poor, gavage feed as indicated
   NCLEX® d. Use a soft, yellow single-hole nipple ("preemie nipple") to slow flow of milk and reduce excess energy expenditure; burp frequently
   e. Monitor intake and output (I&O), daily weight; assess for dehydration
   f. Monitor for hypoglycemia
11. Renal system
   a. Reduced glomerular filtration rate that directly correlates to lower gestational age
   b. Risk of dehydration increases because of limited ability to concentrate urine effectively and blunted response to ADH
   c. Prolonged drug excretion time because immature kidneys; this may require spacing doses further apart (e.g., every 24 hr instead of every 12 hr)
   d. Monitor urine output and, when possible, avoid use of nephrotoxic drugs

12. Neuromuscular system
    a. Immature control of vital functions; increased risk for apnea
    b. Increased risk of **intraventricular hemorrhage (IVH)**, which is bleeding into ventricles of brain
    c. Possible disorganized sleep–wake cycles
    d. Poor muscle tone and weak or absent reflexes
    e. Weak, feeble cry
    f. Provide appropriate type and amount of visual, tactile, and auditory stimulation according to gestational age and avoid detrimental environmental stimuli when possible
13. General nursing care
    a. Organize care to minimize stress
    b. Provide skin care with special attention to cleanliness and careful positioning to prevent skin breakdown
    c. Assess apical heart rate for 1 min every 1–2 hours
    d. Monitor potential bleeding sites (umbilicus, injection sites)
    e. Monitor overall growth and development; check daily weight, measure length and occipital frontal circumference (OFC) weekly
    NCLEX® f. Monitor closely for medication side effects caused by decreased ability to metabolize and excrete medications
    g. Provide appropriate stimulation such as cuddling and touch to promote healthy development

B. Potential complications related to prematurity

1. RDS, which usually appears during first 24–48 hours after birth and peaks around 72 hours
    a. Predisposing factors include fetal hypoxia and postnatal hypothermia
    b. Protection against RDS can be achieved with prenatal betamethasone to mother to accelerate fetal lung maturity and artificial surfactant in infant's airway after delivery to keep alveoli from collapsing and causing atelectasis
2. **Bronchopulmonary dysplasia (BPD)**, a chronic pulmonary disease requiring mechanical ventilation and high oxygen levels in first weeks of life
3. **Retinopathy of prematurity (ROP)**
    a. Etiology: prolonged exposure to high concentrations of O_2 causes hemorrhage within retina and leads to retinal detachment and loss of vision
    NCLEX® b. Preventable with cautious administration of O_2; acceptable oxygenation is determined by gestational age: 28 6/7 weeks or less = 83–93%; 29–33 6/7 weeks = 85–95%; 34 weeks or greater = 90–98%
    c. All premature infants who receive O_2 should be screened for ROP by an ophthalmologist at times specified by gestational age at birth (range from 4 to 9 chronological weeks postbirth)
    d. Treatment of acute ROP may be delayed because many cases regress spontaneously; current treatments for acute stage include laser photocoagulation and cryotherapy
4. Intraventricular hemorrhage (IVH)
    a. Etiology: rupture of thin, fragile capillaries within ventricles of brain leading to increased intracranial pressure
    b. Prematurity and hypoxia are primary risk factors
    c. Assessment: neurologic changes such as hypotonia and lethargy, bulging fontanels, increasing OFC, bradycardia, apnea
    d. Prenatal interventions include preventing premature birth, administering antenatal steroids, transport to tertiary care center, and cesarean birth
    e. Postnatal preventive interventions include careful resuscitation, slow correction of acid–base imbalances, preventing large fluctuations in BP, and correction of coagulation abnormalities
5. Necrotizing enterocolitis (NEC)
    a. Etiology: intestinal ischemia related to shunting of blood to brain and heart in response to fetal or neonatal distress
    b. Assessment: abdominal distention, poor feeding, vomiting, blood in stool
    c. Treatment involves nothing by mouth (NPO), IV fluids, total parenteral nutrition, antibiotics until intestines healed, or surgery, if indicated
6. Apnea and bradycardia
    a. Preterm neonates are at risk for apnea related to immature regulation of vital functions; if apnea is prolonged, eventually bradycardia occurs
    b. Infants almost always experience respiratory arrest before cardiac arrest; by supporting respiratory function, heart rate should return to normal range
    NCLEX® c. If apnea occurs, first stimulate respirations with gentle tactile stimulation; if unsuccessful, reposition neonate, and finally, support respirations with a manual resuscitation bag if necessary

C. Postmaturity

1. Refers to an infant born after completion of 42 weeks of gestation and who has characteristics of postmaturity syndrome
   a. Characteristics are caused by combination of advanced gestational age, placental aging (with decreasing placental function), and continued exposure to amniotic fluid
   b. Placental insufficiency increases risk of fetal asphyxia that results in passage of meconium in utero and increased risk of **meconium aspiration syndrome (MAS)**, inhalation of meconium into lungs
   c. Other common disorders of postmature newborn include hypoglycemia (depleted nutritional and glycogen stores), polycythemia in response to hypoxia, congenital abnormalities (unknown cause), seizures (hypoxic-ischemic cerebral insult), and cold stress (decreased subcutaneous fat)
2. Nursing assessment
   a. Alert, wide-eyed appearance, which may be normal or indicate chronic intrauterine hypoxia
   b. Dry, cracking, parchment-like skin without vernix or lanugo
   c. Long fingernails, profuse scalp hair
   d. Hypoglycemia related to metabolism of glycogen to meet energy needs in utero
   e. Minimal subcutaneous fat, giving appearance of long, thin body
   f. Skin, nails and umbilical cord have yellow/green staining caused by meconium

NCLEX®

3. Interventions are supportive in nature
   a. Monitor cardiopulmonary status because stress of labor can lead to hypoxia in utero and asphyxia at birth
   b. Provide warmth to counteract cold stress
   c. Monitor blood glucose frequently and initiate feeding early (1–2 hours of age) or provide IV glucose as prescribed
   d. Obtain central hematocrit to accurately determine polycythemia

III. PROBLEMS RELATED TO SIZE

A. Small for gestational age (SGA)

1. Defined as birth weight below 10th percentile; growth charts based on local population should be used; may be born preterm, at term, or post-term
2. SGA infants may also have **intrauterine growth restriction (IUGR)**, which is decreased growth potential of fetus in relation to gestational age

NCLEX®

3. SGA/IUGR infants are more commonly seen when mothers smoke or have either chronic or gestational hypertension
4. Causes of IUGR are many and include factors relating to mother, maternal disease, environment, placental factors, and fetal factors
   a. Symmetric (proportional) IUGR is caused by long-term maternal conditions, maternal substance use (alcohol, tobacco, drugs), or fetal genetic abnormalities
   b. Asymmetric (disproportional) IUGR is associated with acute compromise of uteroplacental blood flow
5. Nursing assessment focuses on most common complications: fetal hypoxia, aspiration syndrome, hypothermia, hypoglycemia, and polycythemia
6. Interventions

NCLEX®

   a. Assess for presence of meconium during labor and delivery; thoroughly suction airway immediately after delivery if present
   b. Maintain patent airway, assess for respiratory distress, and provide supplemental oxygen as prescribed
   c. Assess temperature and provide neutral thermal environment; avoid cold stress
   d. Assess for and treat hypoglycemia (SGA newborn has high metabolic rate)
   e. Initiate oral feeding with breast milk or formula at age of 1 hour after assessing suck, swallow, and breathe reflexes; supplement with IV intake or gavage feedings as prescribed

NCLEX®

   f. Weigh daily and assess changes in weight (aim is weight gain)

B. Large for gestational age

1. Defined as birthweight above 90th percentile at any gestational age; often associated with being an infant of diabetic mother (IDM)
2. Risks
   a. Birth injury: trauma to head, upper body, and nerves; shoulder dystocia; fractured clavicle; and nerve palsies
   b. If preterm, risk for RDS
   c. If post-term, risk for meconium aspiration

3. Nursing assessment
   a. Macrosomia (large body size and high birthweight)
   b. Signs of birth trauma related to cephalopelvic disproportion (CPD)
NCLEX® c. Hypoglycemia, especially in an IDM
NCLEX® 4. Interventions: monitor VS, screen for hypoglycemia and polycythemia, address parental concerns about visual signs of birth trauma, and facilitate nutritional intake and parent–infant bonding

IV. PROBLEMS RELATED TO BIRTH TRAUMA

A. Facial paralysis

1. Temporary problem caused by pressure on facial nerve during delivery
NCLEX® 2. Nursing assessment: face on affected side is unresponsive when neonate cries, eye remains open, forehead does not wrinkle
3. Self-resolves within hours or days of delivery; permanent paralysis is rare
NCLEX® 4. Assess and support ability to feed orally

B. Erb-Duchenne paralysis

1. Brachial paralysis of upper portion of arm that is most commonly associated with stretching or pulling head away from shoulder during difficult delivery
NCLEX® 2. Nursing assessment: flaccid arm with elbow extended and hand rotated inward; Moro reflex absent on affected side; grasp reflex intact
3. Interventions
NCLEX® a. Intermittent immobilization using a brace or splint or pinning sleeve to mattress
   b. Position arm for 2–3 hours at a time with arm abducted 90 degrees, shoulder externally rotated, elbow flexed 90 degrees, and wrist supinated with palm angled slightly toward face ("Statue of Liberty" pose)
   c. Reposition every 2 to 3 hours but avoid positioning on affected side
   d. Delay range of motion until 10th day to prevent further damage

NCLEX® **C. Fractures**

1. Etiology
   a. Clavicle is bone most frequently fractured during delivery
   b. Other bones fractured during delivery are skull, humerus, and femur
   c. CPD is often a predisposing factor
NCLEX® 2. Nursing assessment (fractured clavicle): limited range of motion, crepitus over affected bone, and absence of Moro reflex on affected side
NCLEX® 3. Interventions (fractured clavicle): instruct parents to handle affected arm gently; usually self-resolves

D. Asphyxia

1. Inadequate tissue perfusion that fails to meet metabolic needs of tissues resulting from circulatory, respiratory, and biochemical factors
2. Etiology
   a. Common factors include nonreassuring fetal heart rate (FHR) pattern during labor (late decelerations, bradycardia), prolonged labor, difficult delivery, prematurity, passage of meconium in utero
   b. Initial goal is to identify neonates at risk so resuscitation can begin immediately if necessary
3. Nursing assessment
   a. Fetal scalp pH during labor; 7.20 or less is considered ominous sign of fetal asphyxia
NCLEX® b. Infant color, heart rate, respirations/respiratory effort at birth; time of first gasp, cry, and onset of sustained respirations
   c. Passage of meconium prior to or during delivery
4. Interventions
   a. At delivery, hold neonate in head-down position and thoroughly suction mouth and nares
   b. Place neonate under prewarmed radiant warmer and dry infant quickly with warm blankets
NCLEX® c. Stimulate respiratory effort by rubbing back and feet
NCLEX® d. If respirations inadequate, place neonate in "sniffing" (neutral) position; inflate neonate's lungs with positive pressure using bag and mask with 21% oxygen (room air) for term infant and ranges from 21% to 100% based on clinical assessment of preterm infant
NCLEX® e. Once breathing established, check heart rate (HR), which should increase to over 100 beats/min; if absent or less than 60 beats/min after 30 seconds of positive pressure breathing, begin cardiac compressions; compress lower third of sternum with both thumbs (or two fingertips) at rate of 100–120 beats/min; see also Chapter 68

f. Administer prescribed resuscitative medications, primarily epinephrine, after 30 seconds of assisted ventilation and compressions if neonate's heart rate is not more than 60 beats/min

NCLEX®

g. Administer naloxone as prescribed if mother received narcotics near time of delivery, but only if needed after initial resuscitation attempts are made

h. If hypovolemic shock develops, administer normal saline at 10 mL/kg body weight through umbilical vein as prescribed

V. GENERAL CARE OF NEONATE WITH RESPIRATORY DISTRESS

A. Common causes of neonatal respiratory distress

1. RDS, typically in preterm infants with deficient surfactant
2. Meconium aspiration syndrome (MAS), typically in term and post-term infants
3. **Transient tachypnea of the newborn (TTN)** from delayed absorption of fluid in lungs from delivery; typically in term and post-term infants

NCLEX®

B. Nursing assessment for RDS

1. See Box 52–2 again for respiratory system manifestations
2. Pallor and cyanosis
3. Poor muscle tone
4. Hypothermia

C. Interventions for RDS

1. Monitor respiratory rate and effort and general color
2. Maintain neutral thermal environment due to increased O_2 demand if neonate is hypothermic
3. Administer warmed, humidified O_2 as prescribed or other adjuncts to maintain effective respirations and oxygenation
4. Monitor oxygen saturation and ABG results to ensure effective oxygenation at lowest concentration to reduce complications of oxygen therapy
5. NCLEX® Provide for adequate nutrition; withhold oral feedings if respiratory rate is higher than 60 breaths/min because of increased risk of aspiration; notify healthcare provider
6. NCLEX® Position neonate side-lying or supine with neck slightly extended (sniffing position)
7. Suction prn to maintain a patent airway (possibly every 2 hours or more)
8. Support bonding with infant and encourage parental participation in care according to infant condition
9. Ensure premature infant receiving oxygen therapy is scheduled for eye exam to rule out retinopathy according to gestational age timetable

D. Meconium aspiration syndrome

1. Definition: aspiration of meconium into tracheobronchial tree during first few breaths after delivery in a term or post-term neonate
2. Etiology
   a. Prenatal asphyxia causes increased fetal intestinal peristalsis, relaxed anal sphincter, and passage of meconium into amniotic fluid, which may be aspirated into lungs during first few breaths after delivery
   b. Meconium in lungs produces a ball-valve action (air is allowed in but cannot be exhaled) and is irritating to airway; as lungs become hyperinflated, pulmonary perfusion decreases, leading to increasing hypoxia
   c. Can lead to persistent pulmonary hypertension (PPHN) of the newborn
3. Nursing assessment
   a. May demonstrate signs of fetal distress during labor and delivery
   b. NCLEX® Immediate signs of respiratory distress at delivery (cyanosis, tachypnea, retractions, nasal flaring, grunting) and diminished breath sounds
   c. Overdistended, barrel-shaped chest
   d. Yellow staining of skin, nails, and umbilical cord
4. Interventions
   a. NCLEX® Suction oropharynx then nasopharynx after neonate's head is born, and while shoulders and chest are still in birth canal, to remove as much meconium as possible before baby's first breath
   b. NCLEX® If meconium is thick in amniotic fluid, place neonate under radiant warmer, visualize glottis, and suction any meconium from trachea before stimulating respirations
   c. Administer O_2 to maintain adequate PaO_2 and O_2 saturation
   d. Anticipate need for mechanical ventilation, high-frequency ventilation, or **extracorporeal membrane oxygenation (ECMO)**, which is used for prolonged heart–lung bypass to allow lungs to heal
   e. Perform chest physiotherapy routinely

E. Transient tachypnea of the newborn

1. Respiratory state resulting from incomplete reabsorption of fetal lung fluid in full-term or late-preterm newborn; usually resolves within 24 to 48 hours
2. May be more frequent in infants with cesarean birth who have not experienced mechanical squeezing that occurs during vaginal delivery
3. Nursing assessment
   a. Expiratory grunting, nasal flaring, retractions, mild cyanosis
   NCLEX® b. Tachypnea by 6 hours of age (often in first 1–2 hours); respiratory rate may climb to 100 breaths/min or more
4. Interventions: administer O_2 as needed to maintain PO_2 and O_2 saturation within normal limits and provide supportive care

VI. CONGENITAL INFECTIONS

A. TORCH (see also Chapter 9)

1. Toxoplasmosis
   a. Overview: caused by protozoan *Toxoplasma gondii*; contracted by mother's ingestion of raw or undercooked meat or contact with feces of infected cats; maternal–fetal transmission occurs during pregnancy
   b. Often results in spontaneous abortion if contracted during first trimester
   c. Severe neonatal disorders associated with congenital infection include seizures, coma, microcephaly, and hydrocephalus
   NCLEX® d. Advise pregnant client to practice good hand hygiene, avoid eating raw meat, avoid exposure to cat litter during pregnancy, and have toxoplasma titer checked prenatally if cats live in household
2. Other infections, usually hepatitis B (HBV) but also syphilis, gonorrhea, varicella, HIV, and parvovirus B19, can lead to IUGR, preterm labor, and possibly direct invasion of brain and other fetal tissues, depending on organism
   a. Hepatitis B is transmitted from mother to neonate in about 90% of cases either transplacentally or by contact with blood and body fluids
   NCLEX® b. Infants of mothers with positive HbsAg should receive hepatitis B immune globulin and the first dose of hepatitis B vaccine within first 12 hours of life
   NCLEX® c. Infants of mothers with positive HbsAg should also receive second dose of hepatitis B vaccine at 1 month and third dose at 6 months
3. Rubella
   a. Overview: also called German measles; up to 20% of women of childbearing age are not rubella immune; a rubella titer of 1:8 or greater indicates immunity
   b. Of fetuses exposed during first trimester, 80–90% will be affected by either spontaneous abortion or congenital anomalies
   c. Nursing assessment: clinical signs of congenital infections are congenital heart disease, IUGR, or fetal undergrowth and hearing loss
   NCLEX® d. Intervention: infants born with congenital rubella syndrome are infectious and should be isolated
4. Cytomegalovirus (CMV)
   a. Respiratory or sexual transmission; neonate can contract during delivery through an infected birth canal
   b. Most common cause of congenital viral infection; most (90–95%) are asymptomatic at birth; remaining 5–10% may experience hemolytic anemia and jaundice, hydrocephaly or microcephaly, pneumonitis, deafness, and fetal or neonatal death
   c. Disease is usually progressive through infancy and childhood
5. Herpes simplex virus (HSV) type 1 or type 2
   a. Maternal symptoms include vesicles on genitalia that are usually painful; fetal symptoms include fever or hypothermia, jaundice, seizures, poor feeding; 50% develop vesicular skin lesions
   NCLEX® b. Virus can be lethal to fetus and is transmitted during delivery; cesarean birth is indicated if mother has active lesions at time of delivery

B. Sexually transmitted infections (STIs) (see also Chapter 9)

1. Syphilis
   a. Overview: caused by *treponema palladium*, a spirochete that crosses placenta after 16 weeks' gestation and infects fetus; Langhans' layer in chorion prevents fetal infection early in pregnancy until this layer begins to atrophy between 16 and 18 weeks' gestation
   b. There is no increased risk of anomalies, but spirochete may cause inflammatory and destructive changes in liver, spleen, kidneys, and bone marrow

NCLEX® c. If syphilis is untreated during pregnancy, 25% will end in stillbirth and 40–50% of neonates will have symptomatic congenital syphilis

NCLEX® d. Assessment: clients with syphilis have a positive rapid plasma reagin (RPR) test

2. Gonorrhea
   a. Causative organism is *Neisseria gonorrhea*
   b. Neonate can be exposed to organism during birth, which can result in sepsis or ophthalmia neonatorum, possibly leading to permanent blindness
   c. Penicillin is treatment of choice

NCLEX® d. Eye prophylaxis with erythromycin ointment within 4 hours after birth decreases risk of ophthalmia neonatorum

3. Chlamydia
   a. Overview: most common STI; caused by *Chlamydia trachomatis*
   b. Can be transmitted to neonate during delivery and cause neonatal conjunctivitis and pneumonia

NCLEX® c. Eye prophylaxis with erythromycin ointment shortly after birth can prevent neonatal conjunctivitis

4. Candidiasis
   a. Overview: a neonatal oral yeast infection commonly called thrush; most commonly caused by vaginal *Candida albicans*; occurs more commonly in sick newborns and those receiving antibiotics or steroids
   b. Neonate may contract thrush during birth process or from contaminated hands or feeding equipment

NCLEX® c. Nursing assessment: white patches on oral mucosa, gums, and tongue that cannot be manually removed and may bleed when touched; occasional difficulty in swallowing

NCLEX® d. Interventions: antifungal medications to affected area (feed sterile water prior to administration to rinse out milk); nystatin to mucosa, gums, and tongue after a feeding, using medicine dropper or swab; Gentian violet swabbed over mucosa, gums, and tongue (avoid staining skin, clothes, and equipment)

5. HIV/AIDS

NCLEX® a. Overview: human immunodeficiency virus infection with transmission across placenta, during childbirth, or through breast milk or contaminated blood

   b. Effect on fetal growth and development can be determined by serial ultrasounds, nonstress testing after 32 weeks' gestation, and biophysical profiles
   c. Newborns will test positive for HIV for up to 18 months because mother's antibodies are present in newborn blood
   d. Measures to prevent transmission to newborn include early identification of HIV in pregnancy, limiting exposure of newborn to maternal blood and body fluids, and use of antiviral medication
   e. Nursing assessment: typically asymptomatic at birth, failure to thrive with developmental delays, hepatomegaly, splenomegaly, lymphadenopathy, recurrent infections, persistent thrush, chronic diarrhea

NCLEX® f. Interventions: standard precautions; specific isolation not required; promote comfort; bottle-feeding to prevent HIV transmission in breast milk; thorough cord care and skin care before invasive procedures to prevent infection (no circumcision until HIV status known); prevent exposure to infections; provide all routine vaccines (no live virus vaccines until HIV status known); give skin and mouth care; administer antiretroviral drugs as prescribed for first 6 weeks or longer; HIV culture is recommended at 1 month and after 4 months of age

C. Sepsis

1. Overview: generalized infection caused by bacteria (often beta-hemolytic streptococci) that spread rapidly through bloodstream; aided by immature neonatal immune system and lack of IgM immunoglobulin (necessary to protect against bacteria; does not cross placenta)
2. Etiology

NCLEX® a. Maternal beta-hemolytic streptococcal vaginosis is most common cause of neonatal sepsis and meningitis; obtain cervical culture prior to delivery; if positive, antibiotics given during intrapartum period decrease risk of transmission

   b. Perinatal events such as long difficult labor, prolonged rupture of membranes, resuscitation and other invasive procedures, and aspiration of amniotic fluid, mucus, or formula
   c. Hospital-acquired: caused by infected healthcare workers or equipment
3. Assessment
   a. Symptoms often vague initially
   b. Temperature instability, especially hypothermia

c. Feeding intolerance as evidenced by decreased intake, abdominal distention, vomiting, poor sucking
d. Subtle behavior changes, "infant just doesn't look right," lethargy, seizure activity, pallor
e. Progressive respiratory distress
f. Hyperbilirubinemia
g. Tachycardia initially, followed by periods of apnea and bradycardia

4. Interventions

NCLEX®

a. Obtain cultures (blood, urine, cerebral spinal fluid) before antibiotics are initiated
b. Administer antibiotics as prescribed
c. After 72 hours of treatment, antibiotics may be discontinued if final culture reports are negative and symptoms have subsided; antibiotics are generally continued for 10–14 days if final culture reports are positive
d. Observe for changes in vital signs, such as fever, tachycardia, irregular respirations or periods of apnea
e. Stimulate respirations as needed by rubbing chest or foot gently; administer oxygen as prescribed
f. Maintain warmth using radiant warmer as needed
g. Monitor intake (sucking reflex may be poor) and output; obtain daily weight

VII. COLD STRESS

A. Overview

1. Neonates produce body heat by nonshivering thermogenesis; this process requires increased O_2 and glucose consumption to burn brown fat
2. Subcutaneous fat acts as an insulator and helps conserve body heat
3. A flexed position decreases exposed surface area and conserves body heat
4. Cold stress can cause infant to develop hypoglycemia, hypoxemia, and metabolic acidosis

B. Etiology

1. Hypothermia because of large surface-area-to-mass ratio

NCLEX®

2. Large amount of heat lost from head
3. All newborns are at risk for hypothermia, especially preterm and SGA infants

C. Interventions

1. Maintain neutral thermal environment
   a. Reduce or eliminate heat loss by avoiding drafts (convection), placement near cold objects such as outside walls (radiation), or contact with cold objects (conduction)
   b. Postpone initial bath until temperature has stabilized
   c. Dry infant immediately after delivery and when bathing
2. Place newborn under temperature-controlled warmer or on mother's abdomen immediately after delivery
3. Wrap infant in blanket to conserve heat and place infant on warm padded surfaces for procedures
4. Assess body temperature hourly for first 4 hours after birth, then every 4 hours until 24 hours old, then as indicated by agency protocol; keep axillary temperature 97.6–99.2°F (36.4–37.3°C)
5. If axillary temperature is less than 97.6°F (36.4°C):
   a. Put hat on infant's head
   b. Wrap newborn with warm blankets
   c. Assess oxygenation status and assess for hypoglycemia

NCLEX®

   d. Rewarm infant slowly to prevent hypotension and apnea
6. Chronic hypothermia could be an early sign of sepsis

VIII. HYPERBILIRUBINEMIA

A. Etiology

1. Bilirubin is formed by breakdown of hemoglobin from RBCs; direct (conjugated) is water-soluble and easier to eliminate, and indirect (unconjugated) is fat-soluble so it can more easily cross blood–brain barrier and is harder to eliminate
2. **Kernicterus** is a potential complication of hyperbilirubinemia (high bilirubin level); bilirubin is deposited in basal ganglia of brain and causes permanent impaired neurologic function

B. Physiological jaundice

1. Healthy newborn has twice as much bilirubin as an adult because of higher concentration of circulating RBCs; immature liver has impaired ability to conjugate bilirubin during transition from fetal to neonatal circulation; a shorter lifespan of fetal RBCs is also a factor

2. Factors that increase risk of physiological jaundice include dehydration, infection or sepsis, and resolution of enclosed hemorrhage (cephalohematoma, large amount of bruising from difficult delivery)

NCLEX® 3. Physiological jaundice usually begins after first 24 hours of life

C. Pathologic jaundice

1. Rh incompatibility (hemolytic anemia)
   a. RBCs from Rh-positive fetus enter Rh-negative maternal bloodstream late in pregnancy and after separation of placenta at delivery, causing maternal antibody formation and destruction of fetal RBCs (erythroblastosis fetalis)
   b. In subsequent pregnancy with fetus of same blood type, maternal antibodies attack fetal RBCs, causing hemolysis and anemia
   c. $Rh_0(D)$ immune globulin prevents development of antibodies, but cannot reverse reaction once it occurs
   d. Hydrops fetalis is most severe hemolytic reaction, causing severe anemia, cardiac decompensation, edema, ascites, hypoxia, and possible fetal death
2. ABO blood type incompatibility (hemolytic anemia)
   a. Type O mother carries type A, B, or AB fetus
   b. Maternal antibodies cross placenta, enter and attack fetal RBCs, causing hemolysis and fetal anemia
   c. Reaction tends to be less severe than with Rh incompatibility

NCLEX® 3. Pathologic jaundice begins within first 24 hours of life

D. Nursing assessment

1. Determine mother's blood type and Rh factor; if mother is Rh-negative or type O blood, determine infant's blood type and Rh factor

NCLEX® 2. Evaluate results of Coombs' tests
   a. Indirect Coombs' determines presence of antibodies (sensitization) in maternal blood; a positive test indicates presence of antibodies
   b. Direct Coombs' determines presence of maternal Rh antibodies in fetal blood; cord blood is generally used; a positive test indicates presence of antibodies

3. Golden-colored amniotic fluid indicates severe hemolytic disease

NCLEX® 4. Assess for jaundice (in natural light) by gently pressing on forehead, nose, or sternum; in dark-skinned infants, assess oral mucosa, posterior hard palate, sclera, palms of hands, or soles of feet

Memory Aid

Remember that natural light is best for assessing jaundice; apply slight pressure to blanche the forehead (preferred), tip of nose, or gum line and watch for yellow discoloration when pressure is released.

5. When evaluating jaundice, keep in mind it progresses in cephalocaudal direction from head to trunk, arm, and abdomen, and then to lower extremities
6. Evaluate results of bilirubin levels
   a. Bilirubin can be assessed noninvasively with a transcutaneous bilirubinometer

NCLEX® b. Total serum bilirubin levels higher than 13–15 mg/dL indicate hyperbilirubinemia

7. Other findings may include enlarged liver and spleen, anemia, and dark, concentrated urine

E. Interventions

1. Provide early and frequent feedings to stimulate peristalsis and excretion of bilirubin
2. Keep newborn well hydrated to maintain circulating blood volume
3. **Phototherapy** (exposure of infant to bright light to reduce serum bilirubin)
   a. Undress infant to maximize amount of skin exposed to phototherapy light; genitalia can be covered to prevent soiling

NCLEX® b. Cover infant's closed eyes when under phototherapy light; remove eye covers every shift to assess for conjunctivitis, drainage, and corneal abrasion from irritation of eye patches

c. Remove infant from under light and remove eye covers for feeding to aid visual stimulation and promote bonding

NCLEX® d. Change infant's position every 2 hours and assess for skin breakdown

e. Assess for loose green stools as bilirubin is excreted through intestines
f. Increase fluid intake to prevent dehydration from phototherapy light

NCLEX® g. Assess temperature every 2 hours and monitor for hypothermia or hyperthermia

h. Monitor bilirubin levels

4. **Exchange transfusion**
   a. Used to quickly decrease high bilirubin level by exchanging infant's circulating blood volume with donor blood; also removes anti-Rh antibodies and fetal cells coated with antibodies from infant's blood and corrects anemia

   NCLEX® b. Type O Rh-negative blood is used to decrease risk of transfusion reaction

   NCLEX® c. Warm blood to room temperature to prevent cardiac arrest

   d. Give calcium gluconate, as prescribed, after each 100 mL

   NCLEX® e. Assess vital signs before procedure, every 15 minutes during procedure and postprocedure

   f. Record time and amount of blood withdrawn, time and amount injected, medications given

   g. Assess for dyspnea, listlessness, bleeding, cyanosis, bradycardia or arrythmias, hypoglycemia

IX. HYPOGLYCEMIA

A. Etiology

1. Definition: blood glucose (BG) less than 40 mg/dL in first 3 days of life or less than 45 mg/dL after first 3 days of life (normal is 40–60 mg/dL at 1 day old and 50–90 mg/dL after 1 day old; may vary by agency)
2. BG levels are assessed with a heelstick
3. Newborns at risk: IDM, SGA, premature, and infants experiencing cold stress, hypothermia, or delayed feedings
4. Poor prognosis if hypoglycemia is not treated
5. BG usually stabilizes within 48 to 72 hours

B. Nursing assessment

NCLEX® 1. Tremors, jitteriness

2. Lethargy, apathy, limpness, decreased muscle tone
3. High-pitched or weak cry
4. Apnea, irregular respirations, increased respiratory rate
5. Poor feeding, poor sucking, vomiting

C. Interventions

NCLEX® 1. Check BG on all infants at risk by 1 hour of age (30 minutes if IDM) and any symptomatic newborn

NCLEX® 2. Treat hypoglycemia by breastfeeding immediately or giving formula (avoid glucose water to prevent rebound hyperglycemia followed again by hypoglycemia)

3. Do not feed a lethargic infant orally because of increased risk of aspiration; give lethargic infant or any infant with BG less than 25 mg/dL dextrose 10% via IV
4. If treated for hypoglycemia, reassess BG level before next feeding; assess for feeding problems

X. INFANT OF A DIABETIC MOTHER

A. Etiology

1. Hormones secreted during pregnancy (human placental lactogen, or HPL) increase maternal resistance to insulin, increasing insulin requirements; in diabetic clients, pancreas cannot secrete additional insulin and BG levels increase
2. Maternal insulin cannot cross placenta but glucose can; fetal glucose levels rise; fetal pancreas secretes more insulin, which metabolizes additional glucose and acts as a growth hormone; increased insulin needs decreased surfactant production

B. Nursing assessment

NCLEX® 1. LGA; birth trauma more likely

2. Maternal dystocia related to CPD
3. Enlarged internal organs: cardiomegaly, hepatomegaly, splenomegaly

NCLEX® 4. Hypoglycemia

5. Hypocalcemia
6. Hyperbilirubinemia
7. RDS

NCLEX® 8. False-positive lecithin to sphingomyelin (L/S) ratio

9. Increased risk for congenital anomalies, particularly cardiac and spinal defects

C. Interventions

1. Assess for birth trauma

NCLEX® 2. Assess BG hourly during first 4 hours after birth, then at 4-hour intervals until risk period has passed (about 48 hr) or according to agency protocol

3. Treat hypoglycemia with early feedings or breast milk, formula, or supplemental glucose IV as prescribed if oral feedings do not maintain normal BG levels

XI. SUBSTANCE ABUSE

A. Fetal alcohol spectrum disorder (FASD)

1. A group of physical, behavioral, and cognitive malformations often found in infants exposed to alcohol in utero; a leading cause of preventable, nongenetic intellectual disability
2. Set of five categories that includes the former fetal alcohol syndrome (FAS): FAS with confirmed history of maternal alcohol intake (MAI); FAS with phenotypic features but no confirmed history of MAI; partial FAS with confirmed history of MAI; alcohol-related birth defects (ARBD); and alcohol-related neurodevelopmental disorder (ARND)
3. Nursing assessment
   a. Small for gestational age and often have restricted weight, length, and head circumference
   b. Facial features: epicanthal folds, broad nasal bridge, flattened midface, short upturned or beak-like nose, maxillary hypoplasia, thin upper lip
   NCLEX® c. CNS: irritable, hyperactive, hypotonia, microcephaly, high-pitched cry
   d. Other abnormalities of heart (septal and valvular defects), eyes (optic nerve hypoplasia), ears (conductive and sensorineural hearing loss), kidneys, and skeletal system (especially involving joints such as congenital dislocated hips)
4. Interventions
   NCLEX® a. Reduce environmental stimuli; provide consistency in staff and keep numbers of personnel and visitors at any one time to a minimum
   NCLEX® b. Swaddle to increase feeling of security
   c. Implement measures to reduce heat loss
   d. Maintain nutrition and hydration; provide extra time and patience during feedings
   e. Monitor VS closely, and assess for seizure activity and/or respiratory distress

B. Neonatal abstinence syndrome (NAS)

1. Etiology
   a. Repeated intrauterine absorption of drugs from maternal bloodstream causes fetal drug dependency
   b. Increased risk of spontaneous abortion, preterm labor, stillbirth
   c. Degree of drug withdrawal depends on type and duration of addiction and maternal drug levels at delivery
2. Nursing assessment
   NCLEX® a. Hyperactivity, jitteriness
   b. Absence of "step" reflex and "head-righting" reflex
   c. Shrill, persistent crying
   d. Frequent yawning and sneezing; nasal stuffiness
   e. Respiratory distress
   f. Sweating
   NCLEX® g. Feeding difficulties (regurgitation, vomiting, and diarrhea), increased need for nonnutritive sucking
   h. Developmental delays
3. *NCLEX®* Interventions
   a. Perform neonatal abstinence scoring per agency protocol
   b. Monitor temperature for hyperthermia
   c. Assess pulse, respirations, and oxygen saturation every 15 minutes until stable
   d. Position infant on side to facilitate drainage of secretions and avoid aspiration of vomitus or secretions
   e. Provide small, frequent feedings, especially if vomiting, regurgitation, or diarrhea are present
   f. Monitor I&O; measure daily weight and increase calorie content of formula as needed
   g. Suction as needed to maintain patent airway
   h. Decrease environmental stimuli, swaddle for comfort

> **Memory Aid**
> Remember that infants are jittery during withdrawal. Create a soothing environment by keeping the room darkened and quiet.

   i. Use soothing techniques such as swaddling with hands near mouth (reduces injury and disorganized behavior), non-nutritive sucking with pacifier, rocking, cuddling, soft voice tones when speaking, and gentle vertical rocking of infant who is out of control
   j. Obtain meconium drug screening with first stool as prescribed
   k. Administer medications as prescribed: oral morphine, methadone, deodorized tincture of opium; and phenobarbital (sedative) to decrease hyperirritability

Check Your NCLEX–RN® Exam I.Q.

You are ready for testing on this content if you can:

- Identify signs and symptoms of neonatal complications after delivery.
- Implement nursing interventions to prevent neonatal complications or assist the client to recover from them.
- Teach mother about neonatal complications and their management.
- Evaluate the client and family response to therapy for neonatal complications.

PRACTICE TEST

1 The following neonates are admitted to the nursery. The nurse should withhold the scheduled initial feeding on which newborn?

1. A neonate with a sustained heart rate of 118 beats/min
2. A neonate with an axillary temperature of 97.5°F (36.4°C)
3. A neonate with a sustained respiratory rate of 68 breaths/min
4. A neonate who is small for gestational age (SGA)

2 The nurse hears the parents of a 26-week gestation newborn tell family members, "We'll be ready to bring the baby home in a few weeks." What is the most therapeutic response by the nurse?

1. "I'm glad he's doing so well."
2. "He probably won't be ready to come home for a few months."
3. "A therapist could help you resolve your feelings of denial."
4. "Do you have the nursery ready yet?"

3 While observing parents whose newborn is in the neonatal intensive care unit, the nurse interprets that teaching has been effective when the parents perform which activity?

1. Wear gloves every time they touch their baby.
2. Attach family pictures to the side of the isolette.
3. Bring a 2-year-old sibling to visit.
4. Turn off the cardiac monitor when at the newborn's bedside.

4 The nurse is developing a plan of care for an infant born at 28 weeks' gestation. What would be a realistic goal for this infant to achieve within 1 week?

1. Drinking from a bottle
2. Recognizing the parents
3. Maintaining respiratory rate at 30–60 breaths/minute
4. Maintaining body temperature in a bassinet

5 The nurse is making client assignments for the shift. Which baby could be appropriately assigned to an LPN/LVN?

1. An infant being admitted with hypoglycemia
2. An infant scheduled to receive blood this shift
3. A stable premature infant being fed every 2 hours
4. An infant with rising bilirubin levels

6 A newborn is receiving phototherapy for the treatment of hyperbilirubinemia. The nurse evaluates that teaching has been effective when the parents demonstrate which behaviors? Select all that apply.

1. Cover the infant with a loose blanket while under the bililights.
2. Continue breastfeeding during the jaundice.
3. Limit the infant's intake due to loose green stools.
4. Cover the infant's eyes before placing him under the bililight.
5. Keep the genitalia covered to prevent soiling.

7 Which data would be most important for the nurse to note as part of an initial assessment of a newborn's history?

1. Mother received morphine sulfate 4 mg IV 20 minutes before delivery.
2. Mother reports drinking a glass of wine with dinner each night.
3. Mother's age is 14.
4. Mother's blood type is O negative.

PRACTICE TEST

8 The parents of a preterm neonate ask why their baby gets cold so easily. The nurse responds with which explanation about preterm neonates?

1. Able to shiver to produce body heat
2. Have minimal body fat to retain body heat
3. Have blood vessels that are deep under the skin surface
4. Lose heat faster because they lie in a fetal position

9 While feeding an infant, the nurse notices white, adherent patches on the infant's gums and buccal cavity. Which action should the nurse take at this time?

1. Document this normal finding.
2. Further evaluate for yeast infection.
3. Verify that vitamin K was given at delivery.
4. Assess for maternal history of herpes simplex.

10 Which assessment data would alert the nurse that a newborn infant is experiencing dehydration? Select all that apply.

1. Urine-specific gravity 1.006
2. Urine volume 2 mL/kg/hr
3. Low serum sodium
4. Sunken anterior fontanel
5. Poor skin turgor

11 A newborn male is admitted to the nursery 15 minutes after delivery. His skin is mottled and mucous membranes are blue; he is active and is wrapped in a blanket. The nurse should make which assessment as a priority?

1. Umbilical cord for bleeding
2. Infant's temperature
3. Visible deformities
4. Patent airway

12 Which nursing intervention is appropriate in the care of an infant with respiratory distress syndrome (RDS)?

1. Maintain a neutral thermal environment.
2. Perform a complete gestational-age assessment.
3. Perform chest physiotherapy twice a day.
4. Suction meconium from airway as needed.

13 A 26-week-gestation neonate has received 80–100% oxygen via mechanical ventilation for 2 weeks and has received several blood transfusions for anemia. The nurse should plan for which intervention needed by the infant?

1. Begin phototherapy.
2. Arrange for eye exam by ophthalmologist prior to discharge.
3. Wean supplemental oxygen rapidly.
4. Administer surfactant via endotracheal tube.

14 The nurse is caring for a neonate born to a mother who is HIV positive. Which sign in the newborn should be evaluated further?

1. Absence of tears
2. White bumps on nose
3. Enlarged liver
4. Fine, red rash over trunk

15 An infant of a diabetic mother (IDM) is admitted to the newborn nursery. Which nursing intervention has highest priority at this time?

1. Clean the umbilical cord.
2. Administer vitamin K intramuscularly.
3. Complete a gestational-age assessment.
4. Assess the infant's blood glucose level.

16 A father asks how the bilirubin lights make the newborn's bilirubin level go down. What is the best reply by the nurse?

1. "The lights prevent more bilirubin from being released into your baby's body."
2. "Exposing the skin to the air helps get rid of the jaundice. The bililights really just keep the baby warm while this occurs."
3. "The bililights help convert the bilirubin to a form the baby can get rid of."
4. "The bililights release a substance in the body that attacks the bilirubin and destroys it."

17 The nurse assesses a newborn and obtains the following information: Left arm limp and extended; left hand internally rotated; positive grasp reflex bilaterally; no response on left side to Moro reflex. What is the most appropriate nursing intervention for this infant? Select all that apply.

1. Assess for congenital hip dysplasia.
2. Avoid positioning infant on left side.
3. Provide passive range of motion exercises after 24 hours
4. Prepare supplies for a cast application.
5. Immobilize the arm by securing the infant's sleeve to the shirt.

18 A neonatal nurse is attending a high-risk delivery and is told that the mother received morphine sulfate IV 30 minutes ago. The nurse should be prepared to give which medication to the infant immediately after delivery?

1. Naloxone
2. Regular insulin
3. Double dose of vitamin K
4. Magnesium sulfate

19 The maternal–newborn nurse determines that which infant is at greatest risk for infection?

1. 38 weeks' gestation, small for gestational age (SGA)
2. 39 weeks' gestation, diagnosed with caput succedaneum
3. 38 weeks' gestation, cesarean delivery for breech presentation
4. 41 weeks' gestation, infant of a diabetic mother (IDM)

20 An infant with fetal alcohol spectrum disorder is about to be discharged home with foster parents. Place in order the priority of the nurse in teaching the following topics to the foster parents.

1. Toy safety
2. Infection prevention
3. Feeding methods
4. Immunizations

Fill in your answer below:

Answer: ____________________

PRACTICE TEST

ANSWERS & RATIONALES

ANSWERS & RATIONALES

1 **Answer: 3 Rationale:** Feeding a baby with a respiratory rate greater than 60 breaths/min orally increases the risk of aspiration. A heart rate of 118 is slightly below the normal range of 120–160 beats/min, but it is not a contraindication to feeding the infant. A hypothermic or SGA infant is at risk for hypoglycemia and requires a consistent source of glucose. **Cognitive Level:** Analyzing **Client Need:** Physiological Adaptation **Integrated Process:** Nursing Process: Diagnosis **Content Area:** Maternal–Newborn **Strategy:** Simply recall that breathing and swallowing cannot be done at the same time. This will help you to select the infant with an elevated respiratory rate as the one who is at risk if given feedings orally.

2 **Answer: 2 Rationale:** Families are often in a state of denial with the birth of a sick newborn. It is important for nurses to gently encourage the parents to be realistic by sharing truthful information. Agreeing with the parent's statement (by being glad the infant is doing well) prolongs the state of denial and makes it more difficult for the parents to see the situation realistically. Some parents do benefit from professional counseling, but nurses still need to provide support when working with families. It is not important if the nursery is ready yet, and this question distracts from the real issues this family is facing at this time. **Cognitive Level:** Applying **Client Need:** Psychosocial Integrity **Integrated Process:** Communication and Documentation **Content Area:** Maternal–Newborn **Strategy:** Use knowledge of therapeutic communication techniques to answer the question. The correct response is one that provides factual information about the infant's status while respecting the parent's potentially vulnerable status.

3 **Answer: 2 Rationale:** The act of taping family pictures to the sides of the isolette promotes bonding and infant stimulation. Parents should wash their hands when they enter the unit but do not need to wear gloves when in contact with their infant. Young children often harbor organisms that could be transmitted to vulnerable newborns, so they should not have contact until the infant is moved out of the neonatal intensive care unit. The cardiac monitor should not be turned off unless specifically allowed by staff. **Cognitive Level:** Analyzing **Client Need:** Physiological Adaptation **Integrated Process:** Nursing Process: Evaluation **Content Area:** Maternal–Newborn **Strategy:** The wording of the question tells you that the correct answer is an option that contains an appropriate action on the part of the parents. Use nursing knowledge and the process of elimination to make a selection.

4 **Answer: 3 Rationale:** A healthy respiratory rate for all newborns is 30–60 breaths/min. Drinking from a bottle, recognizing parents, and maintaining body temperature in a bassinet are not timely goals for a 28-week-gestation infant at 1 week of age. **Cognitive Level:** Applying **Client Need:** Physiological Adaptation **Integrated Process:** Nursing Process: Diagnosis **Content Area:** Maternal–Newborn **Strategy:** Specific knowledge of expected fetal development by gestational age is needed to answer this question. Use nursing knowledge and the process of elimination to make your selection.

5 **Answer: 3 Rationale:** An LPN/LVN is qualified to perform certain procedures and care for stable clients. An LPN/LVN is not qualified to admit a client, administer blood, or make nursing decisions for clients whose status is changing (such as rising bilirubin levels). The infants identified in these options require assessment and care by a registered nurse. **Cognitive Level:** Applying **Client Need:** Management of Care **Integrated Process:** Nursing Process: Planning **Content Area:** Maternal–Newborn **Strategy:** Specific knowledge of scope of practice by RNs and LPNs/LVNs is needed to answer this question. Use this knowledge and the process of elimination to make your selection.

6 **Answer: 2, 4, 5 Rationale:** Breastfeeding is not contraindicated with hyperbilirubinemia. It is important to protect the infant's eyes from the bililight to prevent permanent damage. It is acceptable practice to keep the genitalia covered to prevent soiling from urine or feces. The infant should be unclothed to allow as much skin exposure to the bililight as possible. Increased fluid intake will aid excretion of bilirubin and loose green stools are an indication that bilirubin is being excreted. **Cognitive Level:** Applying **Client Need:** Physiological Adaptation **Integrated Process:** Nursing Process: Evaluation **Content Area:** Maternal–Newborn **Strategy:** The core issue of the question is knowledge of hyperbilirubinemia and its treatment with phototherapy. Use specific nursing knowledge about hyperbilirubinemia and the process of elimination to make your selection.

ANSWERS & RATIONALES

7 **Answer: 1 Rationale:** Opioid analgesics cross the placenta and, if given close to delivery, can cause respiratory depression in the newborn, making this the priority item. Maternal drinking, young maternal age, and maternal Rh-negative status might warrant further investigation and follow-up, but the priority at delivery is to establish and maintain an airway. **Cognitive Level:** Analyzing **Client Need:** Physiological Adaptation **Integrated Process:** Nursing Process: Assessment **Content Area:** Maternal–Newborn **Strategy:** Note that critical words in the stem of the question are *most important*. This tells you that some or all of the options are correct, but you must select the priority option. Use nursing knowledge and the process of elimination to make your selection.

8 **Answer: 2 Rationale:** Preterm infants have minimal adipose tissue, so they lose heat more quickly through their skin. In general, infants are not able to shiver to produce body heat when they are cold. The skin is thin, with blood vessels near the surface, which increases heat loss through the skin. Because they are weak and neurologically immature, they aren't able to lay in a tight fetal position, allowing greater exposure of the body to the air, which results in heat loss. **Cognitive Level:** Applying **Client Need:** Physiological Adaptation **Integrated Process:** Communication and Documentation **Content Area:** Maternal–Newborn **Strategy:** The wording of the question tells you that the correct option must be a true statement. Use knowledge about the physical characteristics of premature infants and the process of elimination to make your selection.

9 **Answer: 2 Rationale:** The primary sign of an oral yeast infection, or thrush, is the presence of white patches in the mouth that tend to bleed if they are touched. The presence of white adherent patches in the mouth is not a normal finding. The presence of white patches is unrelated to whether vitamin K was given at delivery. Maternal history of herpes simplex is not relevant. **Cognitive Level:** Applying **Client Need:** Physiological Adaptation **Integrated Process:** Nursing Process: Diagnosis **Content Area:** Maternal–Newborn **Strategy:** The core issue of the question is the significance of white patches in the infant's mouth. First recall this is not a normal finding. Then recall that vitamin K aids in blood clotting to determine it is unrelated. Finally, recall that herpes simplex (cold sores) would present as vesicles, not white patches.

10 **Answer: 4, 5 Rationale:** Signs of dehydration in a newborn infant include dry mucous membranes, sunken fontanels, and poor skin turgor. A urine-specific gravity of 1.006, urine volume of 2 mL/kg/hr, and low serum sodium are expected findings in a newborn infant. **Cognitive Level:** Analyzing **Client Need:** Physiological Adaptation **Integrated Process:** Nursing Process: Diagnosis **Content Area:** Maternal–Newborn **Strategy:** Specific knowledge of manifestations of dehydration is needed to answer this question. Use nursing knowledge and the process of elimination to make your selection.

11 **Answer: 4 Rationale:** The highest priority after delivery is to maintain and support respiratory function. This infant is demonstrating initial signs of respiratory deficiency. Once airway and breathing are assessed, the nurse may check the umbilical cord for bleeding, measure temperature, and, finally, check for visible deformities. **Cognitive Level:** Analyzing **Client Need:** Physiological Adaptation **Integrated Process:** Nursing Process: Diagnosis **Content Area:** Maternal–Newborn **Strategy:** Follow the ABCs of resuscitation (airway, breathing, and circulation) to select the correct answer to this question. Airway and breathing are assessed before circulation (bleeding).

12 **Answer: 1 Rationale:** Infants use additional oxygen and glucose when faced with cold stress. Infants with RDS are already compromised, so it is important to keep environmental temperatures stable to minimize their oxygen and glucose requirements. A complete assessment could increase oxygenation requirements even further. Chest physiotherapy might or might not be needed. There is no specific evidence in the question that meconium is present. **Cognitive Level:** Analyzing **Client Need:** Physiological Adaptation **Integrated Process:** Nursing Process: Implementation **Content Area:** Maternal–Newborn **Strategy:** Note that the core issue of the question is care of an infant with respiratory distress. First, eliminate complete gestational assessment because of the word *complete*. Choose temperature control over chest physiotherapy or suctioning the airway because there is no evidence in the question that these are needed.

13 **Answer: 2 Rationale:** This infant has been receiving high levels of oxygen for 2 weeks, and is at risk for retinopathy of prematurity (ROP). All preterm infants who receive oxygen should have a thorough eye exam done by an ophthalmologist prior to discharge. It is important to administer the minimum amount of oxygen to infants to decrease the risk that this condition will develop. Phototherapy is indicated for treatment of high bilirubin levels. Oxygen should be weaned as tolerated but this may or may not be rapidly. Artificial surfactant may be administered within the first several days of life to decrease the risk of respiratory distress syndrome (RDS). **Cognitive Level:** Applying **Client Need:** Physiological Adaptation **Integrated Process:** Nursing Process: Planning **Content Area:** Maternal–Newborn **Strategy:** The core issue of the question is knowledge of the effects of long-term oxygen therapy for a neonate. Use nursing knowledge and the process of elimination to make your selection.

14 **Answer: 3 Rationale:** Hepatosplenomegaly (enlarged liver and spleen) can be an early sign of HIV infection in an infant.

The absence of tears, the presence of milia on the nose, and a fine red rash over the trunk are assessment data that are within normal limits for a neonate. **Cognitive Level:** Applying **Client Need:** Physiological Adaptation **Integrated Process:** Nursing Process: Diagnosis **Content Area:** Maternal–Newborn **Strategy:** The core issue of the question is discriminating normal findings from abnormal findings in a newborn whose mother is HIV-positive. Use nursing knowledge and the process of elimination to make your selection.

15 **Answer: 4 Rationale:** An infant of a diabetic mother is at risk for hypoglycemia, and blood glucose should be monitored closely after delivery and treated if necessary. Cleaning the umbilical cord, administering vitamin K, and completing a gestational-age assessment are important but are not the highest priority. **Cognitive Level:** Applying **Client Need:** Physiological Adaptation **Integrated Process:** Nursing Process: Implementation **Content Area:** Maternal–Newborn **Strategy:** Note the critical word *priority* in the stem of the question. This tells you that multiple options are technically correct, but you must decide which has the greatest importance at this time. Note the connection between the word *diabetic* in the stem and the word *glucose* in the correct option to help you make a selection.

16 **Answer: 3 Rationale:** Phototherapy assists the body in converting unconjugated bilirubin to conjugated bilirubin, which is water-soluble and easier for the body to eliminate. The statements that light prevents more bilirubin from being released, that the bililight just keeps the baby warm while air corrects the jaundice, and that bililights release a substance that destroys the bilirubin are all inaccurate explanations. **Cognitive Level:** Applying **Client Need:** Physiological Adaptation **Integrated Process:** Communication and Documentation **Content Area:** Maternal–Newborn **Strategy:** The core issue of the question is knowledge of how phototherapy assists in lowering the bilirubin levels of a jaundiced newborn. Use nursing knowledge and the process of elimination to make your selection.

17 **Answer: 2, 5 Rationale:** The infant should not be positioned on the affected side. The arm may be secured by pinning the infant's sleeve to the shirt or by using a brace or splint. Congenital hip dysplasia is characterized by a clicking sound with hip rotation, while this infant has Erb-Duchenne's paralysis (Erb's palsy) of the left arm. Passive range of motion is delayed until the 10th day to prevent further damage. Occasionally a splint may be applied, but a cast is not indicated. **Cognitive Level:** Analyzing **Client Need:** Physiological Adaptation **Integrated Process:** Nursing Process: Implementation **Content Area:** Maternal–Newborn **Strategy:** The core issue of this question is recognition of and appropriate intervention for an infant with Erb's paralysis. Note the wording of the question indicates more than one option may be correct. Use nursing knowledge and the process of elimination to make your selections.

18 **Answer: 1 Rationale:** Opioid analgesics (narcotics) such as morphine cross the placenta and can cause respiratory depression in a neonate when given shortly before delivery. Naloxone is the drug of choice to reverse respiratory depression in the neonate caused by narcotics. Insulin would be given to treat hyperglycemia. Double doses of vitamin K are not given. Magnesium sulfate is given to the mother to prevent eclampsia. **Cognitive Level:** Applying **Client Need:** Pharmacological and Parenteral Therapies **Integrated Process:** Nursing Process: Planning **Content Area:** Maternal–Newborn **Strategy:** The core issue of the question is knowledge of adverse effects of morphine sulfate. Use nursing knowledge and the process of elimination to make your selection. The wording of the question tells you that there is only one correct option.

19 **Answer: 1 Rationale:** SGA infants often experience intrauterine growth restriction related to decreased blood flow to the placenta, which increases their risk for infection. In comparison, the infants born at 39 weeks with caput succedaneum, born at 38 weeks by cesarean for breech presentation, and born at 41 weeks from a diabetic mother are at less risk for infection. **Cognitive Level:** Analyzing **Client Need:** Physiological Adaptation **Integrated Process:** Nursing Process: Diagnosis **Content Area:** Maternal–Newborn **Strategy:** The wording of the question tells you the correct answer is the infant who is at greatest risk for infection. Recall the relative risk for infection in each neonate listed to answer this question. Use nursing knowledge and the process of elimination to make your selection.

20 **Answer: 3, 2, 4, 1 Rationale:** Infants with fetal alcohol syndrome have an increased risk of feeding difficulties related to hyperactivity. Nutrition is a key concern for this infant for proper growth and development. Infection prevention is the second priority concern, since this will help to maintain healthy physiological condition. The immunization schedule has third priority because it is also related to prevention of communicable diseases and infection. Although toy safety is important, it is the fourth priority because newborns are not developed sufficiently to play with toys. **Cognitive Level:** Analyzing **Client Need:** Physiological Adaptation **Integrated Process:** Nursing Process: Planning **Content Area:** Maternal–Newborn **Strategy:** Use Maslow's hierarchy of needs to guide priority setting. Physiological needs come first, followed by safety needs, then psychosocial needs.

ANSWERS & RATIONALES

Key Terms to Review

bronchopulmonary dysplasia (BPD) p. 837
continuous positive airway pressure (CPAP) p. 834
exchange transfusion p. 845
extracorporeal membrane oxygenation (ECMO) p. 840
intrauterine growth restriction (IUGR) p. 838
intraventricular hemorrhage (IVH) p. 837
kernicterus p. 843
meconium aspiration syndrome (MAS) p. 838
necrotizing enterocolitis (NEC) p. 836
neutral thermal environment p. 836
oxygen hood p. 834
phototherapy p. 844
preterm (premature) infant p. 835
respiratory distress syndrome (RDS) p. 835
retinopathy of prematurity (ROP) p. 837
transient tachypnea of the newborn (TTN) p. 840
umbilical arterial line (UAL) p. 834
umbilical venous line (UVL) p. 834

References

Davidson, M., London, M., & Ladewig, P. (2016). *Olds' maternal newborn nursing and women's health across the lifespan* (10th ed.). New York, NY: Pearson Education.

Ladewig, P., London, M., & Davidson, M. (2014). *Contemporary maternal–newborn nursing care* (8th ed.). Upper Saddle River, NJ: Pearson Education.

London, M., Ladewig, P., Davidson, M., Ball, J., Bindler, R., & Cowen, K. (2014). *Maternal and child nursing care* (4th ed.). Upper Saddle River, NJ: Pearson Education.

Lowdermilk, D., Perry, S., Cashion, M., & Alden, K. (2016). *Maternity and women's health care* (11th ed.). St. Louis, MO: Elsevier.

Test Yourself

Are you ready for the NCLEX-RN® or course exams? Access the NEW web-based app that provides students with thousands of practice questions in preparation for the NCLEX experience.

Fluid and Electrolyte Imbalances

53

In this chapter

Cross Reference

Other chapters relevant to this content area are

I. CONCEPTS OF FLUID AND ELECTROLYTE BALANCE

A. Fluid transport

1. Body fluid compartments: fluid constantly moves between these to maintain body fluid balance
   a. Intracellular fluid (ICF): fluid within cells; two-thirds of body fluid is ICF
   b. Extracellular fluid (ECF): fluid outside of cells; made up of two components, interstitial fluid (surrounding cells) and fluid within vascular space (blood vessels [BVs])
   c. ICF is most stable and is fairly resistant to major fluid shifts
   d. Vascular fluid is least stable; it is quickly lost or gained in response to fluid intake or losses
   e. Interstitial fluid is reserve fluid, replacing fluid either in BVs or cells, depending on need
2. Osmosis
   a. Water moves through a semipermeable membrane (allows passage of water and small particles, but not large particles) from an area of lower concentration (fewer particles, more water) to an area of higher concentration (more particles, less water) until concentrations are equalized (see Figure 53–1)
   b. Osmosis is a major force in body fluid movement and intravenous (IV) fluid therapy; water moves through semipermeable membranes of cells and capillaries by osmosis

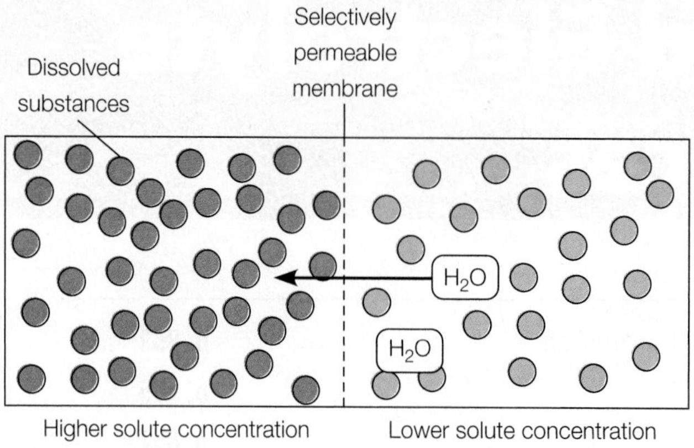

Figure 53–1

Osmosis. Movement of water across a semipermeable membrane to equalize concentrations of solutes.

3. Osmolality and osmotic pressure
   a. Osmolality and osmolarity refer to concentration of a solution, which creates its osmotic pressure (pulling power of a solution for water)
   b. Osmolality is concentration of solute (particles) measured per *kilogram* (kg) of water, while osmolarity is concentration of solute (particles) measured per *liter* (L) of solution (solvent does not have to be water)
   c. Because body fluid solvent is water and one liter of water weighs one kilogram, labels *kg* and *L* can be used interchangeably in discussing human fluids
   d. The higher the osmolality of a solution, the greater its pulling power for water
   e. Serum osmolality is concentration of particles (major particles are sodium and protein) in plasma: normal is 280–300 mOsm/kg or mmol/kg water; concentrations are labeled as isotonic, hypotonic, and hypertonic
   f. Isotonic: having same osmolality as normal plasma (see Table 53–1 for examples of IV solutions that are isotonic; also see Chapter 31)
   g. **Hypertonic**: having higher osmolality than normal plasma; water is pulled from cells into BVs, which increases vascular volume and decreases cell water (see Table 53–1 for examples of hypertonic IV solutions; also see Chapter 31)
   h. **Hypotonic**: having lower osmolality than normal plasma; water is pulled out of BVs into cells, which decreases vascular volume and increases cell water (see Table 53–1 for examples of hypotonic IV solutions; also see Chapter 31)
4. Diffusion
   a. Particles (such as electrolytes) move from an area of higher concentration (more particles, less water) to lower concentration (fewer particles, more water) until equalized

Table 53–1 Tonicity of Typical IV Solutions

Tonicity	Examples of IV Solutions	Comments
Isotonic	0.9% sodium chloride (normal saline [NS], 0.9% NaCl) Ringer's solution Lactated Ringer's solution (LR) 5% dextrose in water (D_5W)	Same osmolality as normal plasma; no osmotic pressure difference is created, so fluids remain primarily in ECF; isotonic IV fluids replace ECF losses and expand vascular volume quickly D_5W is isotonic in bag but has hypotonic effect in body after dextrose is metabolized; two-thirds of water goes to body cells
Hypotonic	0.45% sodium chloride (½ NS) 0.225% sodium chloride (¼ NS)	Provides free water and small amounts of sodium and chloride to cells
Hypertonic	5% dextrose in 0.45% sodium chloride (D_5 ½ NS) 5% dextrose in 0.225% sodium chloride (D_5 ¼ NS) 5% dextrose in 0.9% sodium chloride (D_5NS) 3% sodium chloride (3% NaCl) 5% sodium chloride (5% NaCl) 10% dextrose 50% dextrose	D_5 ½ NS and D_5 ¼ NS are hypertonic in IV bag and provide dextrose and some water to cells D_5NS is isotonic after dextrose is metabolized 3% and 5% NaCl: used to treat specific problems; administered in carefully controlled, limited doses to avoid vascular volume overload and cell dehydration; also used to pull excess fluid from cells and promote osmotic diuresis

b. Urea, glucose, and albumin are large particles that do not pass easily through semipermeable membranes

B. Capillary fluid movement

1. Hydrostatic pressure: pushing force of a fluid; generated in BVs by heart's pumping action and varies within vascular system
2. Oncotic pressure (also called colloid osmotic pressure, or COP): pulling force exerted by colloids (such as albumin, other plasma proteins) in bloodstream to attract water
3. Starling's law of the capillaries: filtration (net fluid movement into or out of capillary) is determined by difference between forces favoring filtration and those opposing it (like a tug of war—pushing and pulling)

C. Chemical regulation of fluid and electrolyte balance

1. Antidiuretic hormone (ADH): synthesized by hypothalamus and secreted by posterior pituitary to regulate water (see also Chapter 60); released and inhibited in a feedback loop
2. Aldosterone: produced by adrenal gland that causes renal retention of sodium and excretion of potassium; water follows sodium because of osmosis, so aldosterone has an indirect effect on water; released and inhibited in a feedback loop as part of the renin-angiotensin-aldosterone (RAA) system
3. Glucocorticoid (cortisol): produced and released by adrenal gland and increased during stress; promotes renal retention of sodium and water
4. Atrial natriuretic peptide (ANP): released when cardiac atria are stretched by high blood volume or BP; causes direct vasodilation of BVs, suppresses RAA system, decreases ADH release, and increases glomerular filtration rate (GFR) in kidneys; all these actions promote fluid excretion
5. Thirst mechanism: occurs with fluid losses or increases in serum osmolality; stimulated by receptors in hypothalamus; stimulates ADH and aldosterone release to promote water reabsorption; thirst is depressed after age 60 as an age-related change
6. Fluid losses occur via kidneys (approx. 1500 mL/day), skin (400 mL/day), perspiration (100 mL), lungs (350 mL/day), and feces (150 mL/day); fluid losses that are not measureable are called insensible losses

II. HYPOVOLEMIA (DEHYDRATION)

A. Overview

1. Fluid intake is inadequate for bodily needs; goal is to replace fluid and eliminate cause of deficit
2. Types of fluid loss: isotonic, hypotonic, hypertonic (see Table 53–2)
   a. Isotonic dehydration involves equal losses of all fluid components and is most common type of fluid volume deficit

Table 53–2 Comparison of Isotonic, Hypertonic, and Hypotonic Dehydration

Type of Dehydration	Description	Causes
Isotonic	Fluid and solutes are lost in proportional or equal amounts; serum osmolality remains normal, and no osmotic force is created Intracellular water is not disturbed, and fluid losses are primarily ECF (especially vascular), which can quickly lead to shock Primarily an ECF loss that requires ECF replacement, with emphasis on vascular volume	Hemorrhage Gastrointestinal losses (mild nausea and vomiting, gastric suction, etc.) Fever, environmental heat, and diaphoresis Burns (especially large burns) Diuretics Third space fluid shifts
Hypertonic	More water than solute (primarily sodium) is lost, creating a fluid volume deficit and a relative solute excess Solute (sodium or glucose more commonly) can also be gained in excess of water, creating a similar imbalance Serum osmolality is elevated, resulting in hypertonic ECF that pulls fluid into BVs from cells by osmosis and causes cells to shrink and become dehydrated	Inadequate fluid intake (those unable to respond to thirst, nausea, anorexia, dysphagia) Severe or prolonged isotonic fluid losses (vomiting, watery diarrhea, diabetes insipidus) Increased solute intake (salt, sugar, protein) without proportional fluid increase, such as concentrated enteral feedings, hyperglycemia, excess salt or sugar ingestion, excess osmotic diuretic use
Hypotonic	More solute than water is lost Fluid moves into cells, causing cellular swelling	Chronic illness Malnutrition Excess hypotonic fluid replacement

Box 53–1

Causes of Third Spacing

Injury or inflammation
(increases capillary permeability; allows fluid, electrolytes, and proteins to leak from BVs)

Massive trauma

Crush injuries

Burns

Sepsis

Cancer

Intestinal obstruction

Abdominal surgery

Malnutrition or liver dysfunction
(lowers albumin, thus reducing capillary oncotic pressure)

Starvation

Cirrhosis

Chronic alcoholism

High vascular hydrostatic pressure
(pushes more fluid out of BVs)

Heart failure

Renal failure

Other forms of vascular fluid overload

   b. Hypertonic dehydration involves greater losses of ECF volume than electrolytes, leading to an increased plasma osmolality; fluid shifting occurs as body tries to compensate to restore balance
   c. Hypotonic dehydration involves greater losses of electrolytes, leading to a decreased plasma osmolality; fluid shifting occurs as ECF volume decreases

3. Third spacing
   a. Occurs when fluid is deposited into extracellular spaces that do not normally hold large amounts of fluid but in which fluids can accumulate; fluid is useless because it is not available as reserve fluid or to transport nutrients
   b. Common locations for third space fluid accumulation include tissue spaces (edema), abdomen (ascites), pleural spaces (pleural effusion), and pericardial space (pericardial effusion); see Box 53–1 for causes of third spacing

NCLEX® **B. Nursing assessment**

1. See Table 53–3 for signs of hypovolemia
2. Presence of risk factors: age (very young or old), acute or chronic illness, vigorous exercise or heat injuries, dysphagia, malnutrition, and medications (diuretics, chemotherapy agents that cause vomiting)
3. Low urine volume: less than 1–2 mL/kg/hour in children; less than 30 mL/hour (240 mL/8 hours) or 0.5 mL/kg/hour for adults

Table 53–3 Fluid Volume Imbalances: Quick Summary of Assessment Findings

Hypovolemia (Dehydration)	Hypervolemia (Fluid Overload)
Thirst (unreliable in older adults, children who cannot express needs)	Peripheral edema
Low urine output; concentrated, dark urine	Increased urine output that is dilute (if normal kidney function)
Acute weight loss	Acute, rapid weight gain
Dry mucous membranes, tongue	Tense or bulging fontanels (before age 18 months)
Dry skin and decreased turgor; skin "tenting"	Distended neck veins (high central venous pressure); delayed peripheral vein emptying
Decreased tearing and dry conjunctiva; sunken eyeballs	S_3 heart sound in adults
Sunken or depressed fontanels in infants	Possible hepatomegaly and splenomegaly from venous congestion
Flat neck veins (low central venous pressure); poor peripheral vein filling	Tachypnea, dyspnea, lung crackles, and other signs of pulmonary edema
Hypotension (late sign); postural or frank	Full or bounding peripheral pulses; warm extremities; brisk capillary refill
Tachycardia (earlier sign); weak, thready pulse	Mental status changes (headache, confusion, lethargy; seizures possible)
Delayed capillary refill	
Tachypnea (usually without dyspnea)	
Weakness, dizziness, lightheadedness, syncope	
Mental status changes (irritability, restlessness, lethargy, confusion, drowsiness, seizures, or coma)	

4. Concentrated, dark urine with specific gravity higher than 1.035 (normal 1.010–1.030); note that if diabetes insipidus is causing fluid loss, urine will be pale, dilute, and high in volume
5. Low-grade fever (higher fever can occur in severe dehydration)
6. Mental status changes
   a. Often first signs noted in older adults; tend to cause alarm in parents of infants and small children
   b. Serious sign of significant fluid loss; if fluid loss is severe, client can progress to seizures and coma
7. Acute weight loss (an important sign in infants and young children)
   a. 1 liter (L) water = 1 kg (2.2 lb)
   b. Monitoring weight is considered more accurate than monitoring intake and output (I&O) because of difficulty in keeping accurate records *NCLEX®*
8. Laboratory findings: normal or high hematocrit (Hct) and blood urea nitrogen (BUN), high urine-specific gravity (>1.030) except in diabetes insipidus (<1.010); possible elevated serum osmolality (>300 mOsm/kg), hypernatremia over 150 mEq/L

NCLEX®

C. Therapeutic management

1. Oral replacement therapies if deficit is mild, thirst is intact, and client can drink; during initial rehydration, avoid fluids with sugar or salts, which can worsen fluid loss, and caffeinated beverages, which have diuretic effect
2. Parenteral replacement therapies: IV fluid replacement depending on type of fluid loss (isotonic, hypertonic, hypotonic)
3. Monitor vital signs (VS), urine output (UO), mental status, IV site, I&O, and daily weight
4. Provide comfort measures such as mouth care and lip moisturizer; avoid giving client hard candy or chewing gum with sugar, which have drying effect
5. Provide measures to prevent **hypovolemia** (insufficient or reduced fluid volume) and dehydration
   a. Provide additional plain water boluses periodically during enteral feedings
   b. Implement measures to control nausea and vomiting (N/V), diarrhea, and high fever
   c. Recognize acutely ill clients who are at risk for dehydration and initiate measures to provide adequate fluids by oral, enteral, or parenteral routes
6. Medication therapy as needed: antiemetics, antidiarrheals, ADH (vasopressin), antipyretics for fever

D. Client teaching

1. Awareness of predisposing or risk factors; contact healthcare provider if illness lasts more than 24 hours, if client is an older adult, very young, or has a chronic illness (such as diabetes or heart, kidney, or liver disease)
2. Measures to help prevent fluid deficit and dehydration (frequent fluid intake during day in hot weather even if not thirsty; avoid highly salty fluids and excess table salt; avoid caffeine)
3. Specific measures that treat underlying cause

III. HYPERVOLEMIA (FLUID OVERLOAD)

A. Overview

1. A state in which rate of fluid intake or retention exceeds rate of fluid loss; goal is to restore balance
2. Types of **hypervolemia** (fluid volume excess or fluid overload)
   a. Isotonic: caused by renal or heart failure, excess fluid intake, high corticosteroid or aldosterone levels
   b. Hypotonic (**water intoxication**): caused by repeated plain water enemas or repeated plain water nasogastric (NG) tube or bladder irrigations, overuse or excessive speed of hypotonic IV fluid infusions, excessive plain water intake (such as in extreme dieting), syndrome of inappropriate ADH (SIADH) secretion, or psychogenic polydipsia
   c. Hypertonic: caused by excessive salt intake

NCLEX®

B. Nursing assessment (see again Table 53–3)

1. Predisposing risk factors: age (very old or young), surgery, chronic illess (especially cardiac or renal failure), medications such as long-term glucocorticoids
2. Signs of pulmonary edema
   a. Tachypnea and dyspnea, irritated cough (often early sign of fluid in alveoli)
   b. Hacking cough that eventually becomes moist and productive (clear to white sputum); a late sign of fluid in alveoli and larger airways
   c. Labored breathing (seen as intercostal and substernal retractions, nasal flaring, and expiratory grunting in infants)
   d. Moist crackles on lung auscultation (first in bases bilaterally and progress upward as hypervolemia worsens)

e. Decreased O_2 saturation due to inadequate or mismatched ventilation and perfusion as a result of hypervolemia
f. Cyanosis (a late sign of hypoxemia)

3. VS (reflect normal or increased cardiac output): normal heart rate, full or bounding peripheral pulses, warm extremities, brisk capillary refill
4. Third space fluid accumulations may be present (ascites, pleural effusion, pericardial effusion)
5. A weight gain of 1.4 kg (3 lb) or more can occur over 2–5 days
6. Hct and BUN are decreased because of hemodilution (plasma has more water than normal), possible significant decreases in serum osmolality (<280 mOsm/kg) or serum sodium (<125 mEq/L); chest x-ray may show pleural effusions

NCLEX®

C. Therapeutic management

1. Restrict fluid intake (as low as 1000–1500 mL per 24-hour period) and restrict sodium (helps decrease water retention); keep IV access with saline lock instead of infusing IV fluids
2. Involve client in dividing fluid allowances over 24 hours; plan for more fluids during meals and with oral medications
3. Promote excretion (diuretics, cardiac glycosides in heart failure to increase cardiac output and renal perfusion)
4. Increase protein intake in clients who have low serum protein levels to increase capillary oncotic pressure (and pull fluid into BVs for excretion)
5. Monitor cardiac and respiratory status
6. Monitor fluid I&O carefully, ice chips count as fluid intake (1 cup ice chips equals ½ cup water); improved UO indicates response to therapy
7. Monitor daily weights (same time, same clothing, same scale); a change of 1 kg (2.2 lb) equals a 1 liter water loss or gain
8. Assess for peripheral edema (differentiate dependent, or stasis, edema from more generalized edema related to heart, kidney, or liver problems)
9. Observe for developing or worsening water intoxication (hypotonic fluid overload), often associated with neurologic changes
10. Monitor for overcorrection, in which signs of dehydration begin to appear
11. Evaluate follow-up electrolytes, BUN, serum osmolarity for return to normal values
12. Use an infusion pump to help prevent inadvertent administration of excess fluid
13. Institute measures to prevent hypervolemia: irrigate NG tube and bladder with normal saline rather than plain water; avoid repeated plain tap water enemas; mix infant formula according to package directions; do not use a water bottle as a pacifier for infants

D. Client teaching

1. Risk factors for hypervolemia
2. Weigh self (adult) daily and report a gain of more than 0.9 kg (2 lb) per week
3. Elevate extremities and change position frequently if peripheral edema present
4. Dietary education: sodium-restricted diet and use of alternative seasonings (natural, sodium-free herbs and spices); clients taking potassium-sparing diuretics and/or ACE inhibitors (which cause potassium retention) should not use salt substitutes because most contain potassium; avoid adding salt while cooking or at table; assess sodium content by reading food/OTC drug labels

IV. HYPONATREMIA

A. Overview

1. **Hyponatremia**: a serum sodium (Na^+) level below 135 mEq/L (normal range 135–145 mEq/L)
2. Usually associated with hypervolemia, which can then be referred to as dilutional hyponatremia or water intoxication (excess fluid that dilutes serum Na^+); can also occur in euvolemia (normal volume) and hypovolemia states (see Table 53–4)
3. Predisposing conditions (see Box 53–2)

NCLEX®

B. Nursing assessment

1. Common signs relate to shift of water into cells and role of Na^+ in nerve impulse transmission and muscle contraction (see Table 53–5)
2. Decreased BUN and Hct if concurrent hypervolemia
3. Dietary: prolonged NPO status; excess infusion of nonelectrolyte solutions, causing free water accumulation

C. Therapeutic management

1. Focuses on restoring normal levels, preventing complications, and treating underlying problems

Table 53–4 Hyponatremia in Various Fluid Volume States

Euvolemic State	Hypervolemic State	Hypovolemic State
Description		
Decrease in fluids in both intravascular and interstitial spaces Results in a normal serum osmolality Use of sodium-free solutions that dilute the ECF	High-glucose states that pull water from cells, leading to cellular dehydration as seen in diabetic ketoacidosis (DKA) Fluid loss from ECF is greater than solute loss, leading to increased serum osmolality	Glucose in isotonic solutions is oxidized, leading to cellular swelling Loss of solute from ECF is greater than excess of water, resulting in a decreased serum osmolality
Clinical presentations		
SIADH, medications, hypothyroidism, psychiatric disorders	CHF, cirrhosis, nephrotic syndrome, and renal failure	GI fluid loss, diuretic therapy, osmotic diuresis, adrenal insufficiency, burns, sweating, hypotonic dehydration
Treatment		
Water restriction, correct underlying cause, treat SIADH with demeclocycline (unlabeled use), and increase dietary salt intake	Water restriction, treat existing disease states, loop diuretics such as furosemide, and restrict dietary salt intake	NS to correct ECF deficits, in crease dietary salt intake; hypertonic saline to raise Na^+ level

Box 53–2

Causes of Hyponatremia

- Loss of sodium
- Renal losses through excretion, diuretics, renal disease (salt-wasting nephropathy)
- GI losses through vomiting, diarrhea, suctioning, tap water enemas (TWEs), GI surgery, bulimia
- Skin losses through perspiration, environmental heat and humidity, burns, tissue destruction
- Conditions that increase extracellular water
- Hormone regulation of ADH and aldosterone, leading to fluid shifts and water gain
- Disorders that add to increased volume, such as CHF, cirrhosis, and nephrotic syndrome
- Conditions such as psychiatric disorders that involve compulsive water drinking
- Disorders such as tumors, SIADH, and adrenal insufficiency that affect hormonal response, leading to increased secretion
- Hyperglycemic states such as diabetic ketoacidosis (DKA) that cause cellular dehydration
- Prolonged or excessive use of hypotonic fluid administration
- Conditions that lead to inadequate dietary intake of sodium
- Prolonged use of fluids without sodium replacement
- Anorexia and other eating disorders

Table 53–5 Sodium Imbalances: Quick Summary of Assessment Findings

	Hyponatremia ($Na^+ < 135$ mEq/L)	Hypernatremia ($Na^+ > 145$ mEq/L)
Cardiovascular	Bounding pulse, tachycardia, hypotension (↓ ECV), hypertension (↑ ECV)	Tachycardia, hypertension, ↓ cardiac contractility
Integument	Pale, dry skin and mucous membranes (↓ ECV), edema and weight gain (↑ ECV)	Dry and sticky mucous membranes; rough, dry tongue; flushed skin
Renal	↑ UO with low specific gravity (<1.010)	Thirst, ↑ UO as kidneys try to eliminate Na^+
Neuromuscular	Lethargy, agitation, dizziness, weakness, headache, confusion, seizures	Twitching, tremor and hyperreflexia, agitation and CNS irritability, hallucinations, seizures, coma
Gastrointestinal (GI)	Anorexia, N/V, diarrhea, hyperactive bowel sounds, abdominal cramping	Watery diarrhea, nausea, thirst

Box 53–3

Sodium Food Sources

The following foods are considered adequate sources of sodium:

- Processed food products (highest sources of sodium in diet)
- Lunch meats
- Ham, bacon, and pork products (high sodium levels)
- Dill pickles, corned beef, and products that are "pickled" in brine solutions
- Potato chips and other salted snack foods
- Butter, cheese, and milk
- Condiments such as ketchup, mustard, soy sauce, relishes
- Anchovies, mackerel, and other saltwater fish products

NCLEX® 2. Encourage inclusion of high Na^+ foods in diet (refer to Box 53–3 for Na^+ food sources)
3. For hyponatremia with normal fluid volume (euvolemia) or hypertonic dehydration, use water restriction and treat underlying cause
4. Use isotonic saline (NS) for wound or other irrigations
5. Client may require salt and fluid restrictions, and possibly dialysis if clinical picture indicates
6. Continue to monitor laboratory results; aim is to raise Na^+ level no more than 25 mEq/L in the first 48 hours with a rate not to exceed 1–2 mEq/L/hr
7. Keep accurate I&O records

NCLEX® 8. Obtain daily weights; a weight loss of more than 0.5 pound in 24 hours is considered to be caused by fluid loss

NCLEX® 9. Monitor for resolution of signs of hyponatremia, including CNS changes such as confusion, lethargy, and seizures

NCLEX® 10. Protect client from injury and maintain a safe environment if client experiences neurologic changes due to hyponatremia
11. Medication therapy: loop diuretics, LR or NS (isotonic dehydration) or 3% or 5% hypertonic saline (severe deficits)

D. Client teaching

1. Predisposing factors: age (older adults and very young), environmental conditions (heat and humidity)
2. Dietary education: high-sodium foods
3. Preventing a recurrence: observe for and report early signs and symptoms of hyponatremia such as abdominal cramps, muscle weakness, and nausea
4. Observe for changes in mental status, especially if client already has cardiac, renal, or endocrine problems that might exacerbate hyponatremia

V. HYPERNATREMIA

A. Overview

1. **Hypernatremia**: a serum Na^+ level greater than 145 mEq/L (normal range 135–145 mEq/L)
2. Sodium excess always exists in a **hyperosmolar** (osmotic pressure greater than normal plasma pressure) state
3. Sodium excess can exist in hypovolemic, euvolemic, and hypervolemic states (see Table 53–6 for a summary of this disorder)
4. Predisposing clinical conditions
   a. Disturbances in water regulation such as decreased intake, increased insensible loss, or watery diarrhea
   b. Water loss due to fever, hyperventilation, diuretic therapy, burns, diabetes insipidus
   c. Increased Na^+ intake either from food or sodium-containing fluids, or rarely saltwater drowning

NCLEX® **B. Nursing assessment**

1. Common signs relate to water shifting from cells into vascular space (cellular dehydration) and sodium's role in nerve impulse transmission and muscle contraction (see again Table 53–5)
2. Risk factors: age (very young or old), OTC or prescribed medications, high Na^+ diet or excessive use of salt as flavoring

NCLEX® **C. Therapeutic management**

1. Focuses on restoring normal levels, preventing complications, and treating underlying problems
2. Decrease Na^+ intake depending on severity to 2 grams, 1 gram, or 500 mg/day

Table 53–6 Hypernatremia in Various Fluid Volume States

Euvolemic State	Hypervolemic State	Hypovolemic State
Description		
Decrease in water that leads to elevated serum sodium Does not present with contracted volume unless severe water loss occurs	Greater gain of sodium in relation to fluids, leading to elevated serum sodium	Greater loss of water than sodium, leading to elevated serum sodium
Clinical conditions		
Increased fluid loss via skin or lungs (hyperventilation)	Administration of hypertonic saline solutions or $NaHCO_3$, hyperaldosteronism or hypertonic dehydration	Renal losses (osmotic diuresis), insensible loss (sweating and/or fever), GI losses (diarrhea) Young and older adult clients are most at risk
Treatment		
Free water replacement either orally or by fluid-hydrating IV solutions	Remove sodium source, administer diuretics, and replace water	NS to correct intravascular volume deficit, then hypotonic fluids can be used to restore Na^+ level

3. Refer client to a dietitian to evaluate dietary intake for hidden sources of Na^+
4. Maintain safe environment because of CNS irritability and risk of seizure activity; initiate seizure precautions
5. Assess I&O and daily weight
6. Medication therapy: loop diuretics (sodium excess), IV fluids as needed

D. **Client teaching**
1. Awareness of predisposing factors in older adults: limited mobility, multiple medication profile, and restricted access to fluids
2. Report recurrence of early signs of hypernatremia to healthcare provider
3. Dietary education (*NCLEX®*)
   a. Na^+ content of foods and sources of hidden Na^+, read all labels for Na^+ content before use
   b. Follow a low-sodium diet; do not routinely add salt before tasting foods
   c. Use herbs, lemon juice, spices, and vinegar instead of salt or salt substitutes

VI. HYPOKALEMIA

A. **Overview**
1. **Hypokalemia**: a serum potassium (K^+) level below 3.5 mEq/L (normal range 3.5–5.1 mEq/L)
2. Has widespread effects on body, and if severe or not corrected quickly, death can result from cardiac and respiratory arrest
3. Predisposing factors
   a. Increased secretion of aldosterone leading to excretion of K^+ from renal tubules (adrenal adenomas, cirrhosis, nephrosis, heart failure and hypertensive crisis, Cushing's syndrome, diabetes insipidus)
   b. Excessive loss of K^+ by diuretics and a variety of other medications
   c. GI loss by N/V, diarrhea, prolonged NG tube suctioning, new ileostomy, laxative, or enema overuse
   d. Heat-induced diaphoresis
   e. Diuretic phase of renal failure; possible effects of hemodialysis or peritoneal dialysis
   f. Reduced intake (K^+ restricted diets), NPO status without sufficient IV replacement, starvation, malnutrition, alcoholism, anorexia, high glucose levels (leading to diuresis), large ingestion of black licorice (causes aldosterone effects)

NCLEX® B. **Nursing assessment (see Table 53–7)**

NCLEX® C. **Therapeutic management**
1. Restore normal levels, prevent complications, and treat underlying problems
2. If client also has hypocalcemia and/or hypomagnesemia, correct all electrolyte levels together
3. Assess for metabolic alkalosis (irritability, paresthesias); hypokalemia is present in alkalosis
4. Monitor client for possible effects related to hypokalemia and for response to therapeutic treatment
   a. VS, especially BP (hypokalemia can lead to orthostatic hypotension) and respiratory rate, depth, and pattern
   b. Serum electrolyte levels
   c. ECG changes and heart rate and rhythm pattern
   d. I&O and possibly daily weight

Table 53–7 Potassium Imbalances: Quick Summary of Assessment Findings

	Hypokalemia (K^+ <3.5 mEq/L)	Hypernatremia (K^+ >5.1 mEq/L)
Cardiovascular	Weak, thready pulse with variable rate; pedal pulses difficult to palpate; ECG changes (ST segment depression, flattened T wave, onset of U wave, ventricular dysrhythmias, heart block); digitalis toxicity is potentiated	Irregular, slow heart rate, ↓ BP, ECG changes (narrow, peaked T waves, widened QRS complexes, prolonged PR intervals, flattened P waves, frequent ectopy, ventricular fibrillation and standstill)
Respiratory	↓ breath sounds; weak, shallow respirations; dyspnea	Unaffected until level is very high, leading to muscle weakness and paralysis and causing respiratory failure
Neuromuscular	Anxiety, lethargy, depression, confusion, paresthesias, weakness, leg cramps	Muscle twitching (early) and cramps, irritability, anxiety; a late sign is ascending flaccid paralysis involving arms and legs
Gastrointestinal (GI)	Nausea, diarrhea or constipation (from ↓ peristalsis), polydipsia	Hyperactive bowel sounds, diarrhea, nausea
Other	Renal: polyuria and nocturia, ↓ urine specific gravity	Not applicable

5. Monitor therapeutic drug level for clients taking digoxin and serum K^+ levels for clients taking loop and thiazide diuretics
6. Protect client from injury and maintain a safe environment (hypokalemia causes weakness)
7. Dietary interventions to promote normal K^+ levels
   a. Encourage high-fiber diet and increased fluid intake, if not on fluid restriction, to prevent constipation
   b. Provide adequate dietary sources of K^+; see Box 53–4 for good food sources of K^+
   c. Avoid foods such as black licorice that, when eaten in large quantities, can cause hypokalemia
8. Oral replacement (note: K^+ supplements should never be given unless client's UO is at least 0.5 mL/kg/hour); usual dose is 20 mEq; higher doses may be indicated
9. Administer parenteral K^+ carefully
   a. Verify additive K^+ in solution prior to hanging infusion
   NCLEX® b. Always use an infusion pump, paying attention to rate, intake and output
   c. Do not exceed an infusion rate of 5–10 mEq/hr unless there is moderate hypokalemia
   d. Dilute K^+ in a solution that provides no more than 1 mEq/10 mL
   e. If more than 20 mEq/hr is given, monitor cardiac rhythm; check serum level every 4 to 6 hours
   f. Monitor IV site closely; K^+ is irritating to BVs and can lead to infiltration, phlebitis, and tissue necrosis
   NCLEX® g. Never administer K^+ by IV push or intramuscular routes because of risk for fatal dysrhythmias

D. Client teaching

1. Report signs and symptoms of hypokalemia to healthcare provider
2. Take K^+ supplements (including powder form) with at least .1 kg (4 oz) fluid or with food
3. Never crush or break K^+ tablets or capsules
4. Take K^+ after meals to prevent GI upset
5. Do not use salt substitutes when taking K^+ supplements
6. NCLEX® Report signs of hyperkalemia to healthcare provider; get serum K^+ levels drawn as scheduled

Box 53–4

Potassium Food Sources

The following foods are considered adequate sources of potassium:

- Vegetables such as spinach, broccoli, carrots, green beans, tomato juice, acorn squash, and potatoes
- Fruits such as bananas, cantaloupe, apricots, oranges, and raisins
- Milk, milk products, yogurt, and meat
- Legumes, nuts, and seeds
- Whole grains

VII. HYPERKALEMIA

A. Overview

1. **Hyperkalemia**: a serum K^+ level greater than 5.1 mEq/L (normal range 3.5–5.1 mEq/L)
2. Actual hyperkalemia (K^+ level in ECF is elevated) is caused by excessive K^+ intake or decreased K^+ excretion
3. Relative hyperkalemia (movement of K^+ from ICF to ECF without a true body increase of K^+) is caused by massive cell damage, transcellular shifting, medications, and Addison's disease (effects of decreased aldosterone)

NCLEX®
B. Nursing assessment (see again Table 53–7)

NCLEX®
C. Therapeutic management

1. Decrease K^+ intake: implement prescribed K^+ restrictions; do not administer K^+ supplements; refer client to dietitian to evaluate hidden dietary intake of K^+
2. Promote K^+ excretion: increase urinary output and monitor adequate renal function
3. Monitor serum K^+ levels; report abnormals; assess cardiac status and signs of hyperkalemia and metabolic acidosis
4. When possible, determine and treat underlying cause
5. Dialysis may be performed for intractable conditions to prevent development of potentially lethal problems
6. Monitor for response to therapeutic treatment
7. Sodium polystyrene sulfonate (to reduce K^+ levels) can be given orally or as an enema with an osmotic agent (sorbitol) to reduce risk of constipation
8. Intravenous medications: calcium gluconate, sodium bicarbonate, or regular insulin and dextrose (usually 50%) solution (shifts K^+ from ECF to ICF)
9. K^+ wasting diuretics (loop diuretics and thiazide and thiazide-like diuretics)

D. Client teaching

1. Recognize predisposing factors
2. Avoid foods that are high in K^+, read food and medication labels, and avoid salt substitutes

VIII. HYPOCALCEMIA

A. Overview

1. **Hypocalcemia**: a serum calcium (Ca^{++}) level less than 8.5 mg/dL (normal range 8.5–10.5 mg/dL) or decreased availability of ionized Ca^{++}
2. Result from decreased physiologic availability of Ca^{++}, decreased Ca^{++} intake or absorption, or increased Ca^{++} excretion (see Box 53–5)
3. Other risk factors
   a. History of Crohn's or small bowel dysfunction
   b. Increased incidence of fractures; osteoporosis and/or osteopenia
   c. Immobility
   d. Excessive use of dietary phosphorus supplements
   e. Lactose intolerance unless alternative products are used
   f. Foods that limit absorption of Ca^{++} (oxalates such as spinach and rhubarb, phytates such as bran and whole grains, and tannins as in tea)
   g. Medications (loop diuretics, antiepileptics, citrate-buffered blood products, phosphates, corticosteroids, bisphosphonates, antacids, and heparin)

Box 53–5

Clinical Conditions That Lead to Hypocalcemia

- Hypoparathyroidism or post-thyroidectomy
- Hypomagnesemia
- Alkalotic states
- Multiple blood transfusions
- Hypoalbuminemia
- Acute pancreatitis
- Hyperphosphatemia
- Vitamin D deficiency
- Malabsorptive states
- Renal disease
- Alcoholism
- Neonatal hypocalcemia
- Gram-negative sepsis
- Medullary thyroid carcinoma
- Burns

Table 53–8 Calcium Imbalances: Quick Summary of Assessment Findings

	Hypocalcemia (Ca^{++} <8.5 mEq/L)	Hypercalcemia (Ca^{++} >10.5 mEq/L)
Cardiovascular	↓ BP; ECG changes include prolonged QT interval and lengthened ST segment; cardiac arrest	Hypertension, shortened ST segments and QT interval on ECG, cardiac dysrhythmias such as heart block; cardiac arrest
Neuromuscular	Paresthesias in hands and feet; muscle cramps, positive Chvostek sign (twitching of cheek) and Trousseau sign (spasm of arm when BP cuff inflated); ↑ deep tendon reflexes (DTRs), ↑ irritability and apprehension; mental status changes (depression, memory impairment, delusions, hallucinations), seizures	Headache and confusion, subtle changes in personality to acute psychosis, fatigue, ↓ DTRs; impaired memory and bizarre behavior, lethargy, or coma (seizures are rare)
Renal	↓ serum Ca^{++} levels are associated with renal failure, along with other electrolyte disturbances	Polyuria and polydipsia due to altered renal function; ↓ ability of kidneys to concentrate urine; renal colic from development of kidney stones due to high Ca^{++} levels; renal failure may occur
Gastrointestinal (GI)	Possible hyperactive bowel sounds and diarrhea, intestinal cramps	Anorexia, N/V; abdominal pain; constipation, hypoactive bowel sounds
Musculoskeletal	Possible bone fractures from demineralization; bone pain; chronic deficit may retard growth and cause rickets in children and osteomalacia and osteoporosis in adults	Pathologic bone fractures; bone thinning, deep bone pain

NCLEX®

B. Nursing assessment

1. See Table 53–8
2. Other systems: laryngospasm can occur, leading to respiratory compromise, airway failure, and respiratory arrest; development of cataracts; dry, brittle nails and dry hair; increased bleeding or bruising

C. Therapeutic management

1. Treatment focuses on restoring normal levels, preventing complications, and treating underlying problems

NCLEX®

2. Replacement therapies
   a. Calcium gluconate (more common) or calcium chloride IV (less common; irritating to vein)
   b. Daily oral doses of elemental Ca^{++}, usually 1.0–3.0 grams/day
   c. Calcitriol, vitamin D supplements, or phosphorus-binding antacids based on need
   d. Thiazide diuretics may be used to decrease urinary excretion of calcium
3. Continue monitoring client (laboratory values and clinical condition) for treatment effectiveness
   a. Continuous ECG monitoring, especially during calcium gluconate or calcium chloride therapy
   b. Continually reassess neurologic, respiratory, and cardiac status

NCLEX®

4. Protect client from injury and maintain a safe environment
   a. Be prepared for emergencies that may result from hypocalcemia, such as tetany, seizures, laryngospasm, and respiratory and cardiac arrest
   b. Initiate seizure precautions and maintain a quiet environment
   c. Closely observe respiratory and airway status; have emergency tracheostomy kit available and IV calcium gluconate at bedside after thyroidectomy (if inadvertent removal of parathyroid gland)
   d. Observe for signs of tetany in clients receiving multiple blood transfusions
   e. Observe for signs of bleeding or increased bruising
5. Monitor for possible hypercalcemia resulting from replacement therapy
6. Encourage foods high in Ca^{++}, such as dairy products

D. Client teaching

1. Predisposing factors
2. Paresthesias, tingling and numbness in extremities are early warning signs of tetany
3. Report onset of signs of tetany or seizures immediately to healthcare provider
4. Take oral replacements as prescribed
5. Avoid overuse of antacids and/or laxatives containing phosphorus
6. Increase intake of foods rich in Ca^{++} (dairy products)
7. Vitamin D and protein are important to keep Ca^{++} within normal limits

8. Use appropriate substitutes for milk and dairy products if lactose intolerant
9. Avoid foods high in phosphorus

IX. HYPERCALCEMIA

A. Overview

1. **Hypercalcemia**: a serum Ca^{++} level greater than 10.5 mg/dL (normal range 8.5–10.5 mg/dL); symptoms may not appear until serum Ca^{++} level is higher than 12 mg/dL
2. Predisposing clinical conditions (see Box 53–6)
3. Other risk factors: excessive dietary intake of Ca^{++}-rich foods; excessive use of Ca^{++}-containing antacids

NCLEX® **B. Nursing assessment (see again Table 53–8)**

NCLEX® **C. Therapeutic management**

1. Decrease Ca^{++} intake: limit milk and dairy products; eliminate use of calcium carbonate antacids until Ca^{++} levels return to normal
2. Promote calcium excretion
   a. Prescribed loop diuretics, such as furosemide or bumetanide, promote increased UO so that more Ca^{++} will be excreted
   b. Maintain hydration of 3000–4000 mL (3–4 L) of fluid/day; oral fluids should be high in acid ash, such as cranberry or prune juice
   c. Give 0.9% NaCl IV at 300–500 mL/hr up to 6 liters as prescribed until volume status restored, then 0.45% NaCl may be used; watch for fluid overload as a complication, especially with preexisting cardiac or respiratory disease
   d. Corticosteroids such as prednisone for 5–10 days to decrease GI absorption of Ca^{++}
   e. Chronic management of hypercalcemia is effective only with parathroidectomy for primary hyperparathyroidism
3. Continued monitoring of client: strict I&O, daily weight, serum Ca^{++} and phosphate levels, possible ECG monitoring
4. Treatment of hypercalcemic crisis
   a. 0.9% NaCl at 300–500 mL/hr initially and up to 6 liters until intravascular volume restored or calcium level is 8–9 mg/dL
   b. Bisphosphonates, such as pamidronate IV to inhibit bone resorption; returns Ca^{++} to normal within 24 to 48 hours with effects lasting for weeks in most clients
   c. Salmon calcitonin may temporarily lower Ca^{++} level by 1–3 mg/dL in clients with severe hypercalcemia
   d. Phosphorus IV to decrease Ca^{++} because of inverse relationship in emergency situations only
5. Dialysis: during oliguric/anuric stage, severe renal dysfunction can lead to life-threatening fluid and electrolyte imbalances
6. Prevent injuries and maintain safe environment
   a. Monitor for pathologic fractures in clients with long-term hypercalcemia
   b. Assist client with mobility to prevent injury and maintain safety

D. Client teaching

1. Predisposing factors
2. Take agents containing phosphorus or other medications as prescribed
3. Notify healthcare provider if symptoms worsen or flank pain develops (risk of kidney stones); strain urine for kidney stones if indicated
4. Avoid foods and OTC antacids that are high in Ca^{++}

Box 53–6

Clinical Conditions That Lead to Hypercalcemia

- Hyperparathyroidism
- Metastatic cancer
- Use of thiazide diuretics
- Sarcoidosis
- Immobility
- Hypophosphatemia
- Hyperthyroidism (thyrotoxicosis)
- Renal tubular acidosis
- Milk-alkali syndrome
- Familial hypocalciuric hypercalcemia
- Lithium therapy
- Vitamin D intoxication

NCLEX®

5. Increase fluid intake to 2–3 L in 24 hours, especially fluids high in acid-ash such as prune or cranberry juice
6. Increase dietary fiber and fluid to prevent constipation
7. Do not take large doses of vitamin D supplements

X. HYPOMAGNESEMIA

A. Overview

1. **Hypomagnesemia**: a serum magnesium (Mg^{++}) level less than 1.4 mEq/L (normal range 1.4–2.1 mEq/L)
2. Usually occurs with decreased intake, decreased GI absorption, increased renal or GI losses, or redistribution of body magnesium
3. Predisposing clinical conditions
   a. Chronic alcoholism is most common cause
   b. Prolonged IV therapy without Mg^{++} supplementation; in parenteral nutrition therapy, Mg^{++} moves into cells from bloodstream, leading to low serum Mg^{++} levels
   c. Increased intestinal (lower GI) losses: prolonged diarrhea, draining intestinal fistulas, and ileostomy
   d. Increased renal excretion: loop diuretics, hyperaldosteronism that leads to volume expansion, diabetes that leads to osmotic diuresis

NCLEX®

B. Nursing assessment

1. Clinical manifestations usually appear when serum Mg^{++} level drops below 1 mEq/L
2. Cardiorespiratory: laryngeal stridor, tachydysrhythmias, and increased susceptibility to digitalis toxicity (possibly enhanced by concurrent hypokalemia)
3. ECG complex changes: diminished voltage of P wave; broad, flat, or inverted T waves; depressed ST segments; prolonged QT interval; possible prominent U wave
4. Neuromuscular: mood changes, such as apathy, depression, and confusion; muscle twitching, tremors, hyperreactive reflexes; seizures and tetany if severe
5. GI: diarrhea, N/V, and anorexia (from concurrent hypokalemia)

NCLEX®

6. Signs and symptoms are similar to hypokalemia or hypocalcemia (all are cations and may occur together); positive Chvostek sign (twitching of cheek when stimulated) can occur

Memory Aid

Rember the *Ch* in *Ch*vostek and in *ch*eek to help remember how Chvostek sign is manifested.

NCLEX®

C. Therapeutic management

1. Identify risk factors: malabsorption and/or GI dysfunction, renal disease, diabetes, alcohol intake, and medications such as diuretics
2. Monitor client with continuous IV fluid therapy without Mg^{++} replacement
3. Monitor client taking a diuretic for increased renal excretion of Mg^{++}
4. Institute ECG monitoring and seizure precautions
5. Monitor for stridor and/or difficulty swallowing
6. Keep bed rails partially raised if client is confused; take other safety precautions as needed

NCLEX®

7. Monitor DTRs in clients receiving IV solutions containing Mg^{++}; depressed DTRs indicate a rebound elevated Mg^{++} level
8. Monitor I&O and ensure UO of at least 30 mL/hr (120 mL every 4 hours) during therapy to avoid rebound hypermagnesemia if renal insufficiency is present
9. Medication therapy: oral Mg^{++}-containing antacids or magnesium oxide; parenteral magnesium sulfate or chloride
10. Dietary therapy: for mild hypomagnesemia, encourage foods high in Mg^{++}, such as legumes, whole-grain cereals, nuts, dark green vegetables, seafood, bananas, oranges, and chocolate

D. Client teaching

1. Predisposing factors
2. Increase intake of foods high in Mg^{++} and hard water or mineral water (high in Mg^{++})
3. Take 300–350 mg magnesium daily with an extra 150 mg for pregnant or lactating women

XI. HYPERMAGNESEMIA

A. Overview

1. **Hypermagnesemia**: serum Mg^{++} level greater than 2.1 mEq/L (normal range 1.4–2.1 mEq/L)
2. Predisposing factors
   a. Decreased renal excretion of Mg^{++}, such as with decreased UO or renal failure
   b. Increased Mg^{++} intake, such as with overuse of Mg^{++}-containing antacids, cathartics, or enemas; total parenteral nutrition (TPN); or hemodialysis using hard water dialysate
3. Predisposing clinical conditions: untreated diabetic ketoacidosis (glucose carries cations across cell membranes); adrenal insufficiency (Addison's disease), which causes fluid and electrolyte shifts; Mg^{++} treatment in preeclampsia of pregnancy; lithium ingestion; and volume depletion

NCLEX®

B. Nursing assessment

1. Neuromuscular symptoms (most common): decreased DTRs and depressed neuromuscular activity; symptoms are similar to those seen in hyperkalemia
2. Cardiovascular: hypotension, bradycardia, bradyarrhythmias, flushing and sensation of warmth, possible cardiac arrest
3. ECG may show prolonged PR interval, widened QRS complex, and elevated T wave
4. CNS: somnolence, weakness and lethargy, respiratory depression, and coma

NCLEX®

C. Therapeutic management

1. Decrease Mg^{++} intake; withhold Mg^{++}-containing drugs (antacids) and enemas
2. Promote Mg^{++} excretion using diuretics (in stable renal function)
3. Provide rehydration to promote increased UO and Mg^{++} excretion; monitor I&O
4. Emergency treatment includes IV calcium gluconate to antagonize effect of Mg^{++} and counteract cardiac and respiratory symptoms
5. Dialysis, especially in clients with renal failure; if hemodialysis is not feasible, peritoneal dialysis is an option
6. Promote client safety

D. Client teaching

1. Predisposing factors such as antacid use, laxative use, diabetic instability, and renal failure
2. Signs and symptoms of hypermagnesemia to report
3. Avoid foods high in Mg^{++} such as legumes, whole-grain cereals, nuts, dark green vegetables, and cocoa

XII. HYPOCHLOREMIA

A. Overview

1. **Hypochloremia**: a serum chloride (Cl^-) level less than 95 mEq/L (normal range 95–108 mEq/L)
   a. Decreases in Cl^- usually are accompanied by decreases in Na^+, K^+, and/or a reduction in hydrochloric acid
   b. Chloride is excreted with cations during massive diuresis and when HCO_3^- is elevated
2. Predisposing clinical conditions
   a. Hyponatremia, metabolic alkalosis, hypokalemia, prolonged D_5W IV therapy
   b. Chronic lung disease accompanied by high pCO_2 and HCO_3^- levels that result in decreased serum Cl^-
   c. Diabetic ketoacidosis because of increased anion gap
   d. Vomiting (loss of HCl), GI suctioning, excess perspiration, diarrhea, and fistulas
   e. Disease states such as Addison's disease, anorexia, salt-wasting renal nephropathy, SIADH, and hypervolemic states such as congestive heart failure (CHF) and cirrhosis
   f. Medications that promote electrolyte loss, are diuretics, or promote alkalosis

B. Nursing assessment

1. Neuromuscular: tremors and twitching
2. Respiratory: slow and shallow breathing
3. Cardiac: hypotension if severe Cl^- and ECF losses
4. Seldom a primary problem; usually associated with hyponatremia, hypokalemia, metabolic alkalosis or hypokalemic alkalosis

C. Therapeutic management

1. Administer oral salt tablets or if levels are critical, IV infusion of Cl^- (as NaCl or KCl)
2. Monitor I&O because excess water intake can cause dilutional hypochloremia and hyponatremia
3. Monitor BP (if hypochloremia is caused by ECF volume loss) and ABG results (if occurring as response to acid–base imbalance)

4. Maintain safety precautions: keep bed rails up and assist with ambulation if client has muscle tremors and/or decreased BP
5. Diet therapy: foods high in Cl^-, such as salt, canned or processed foods, dates, bananas, cheese, spinach, milk, eggs, celery, crabs, fish, olives, and rye

D. Client teaching

1. Predisposing factors
2. Include in diet Na^+ and processed foods that are also high in Cl^-
3. *NCLEX®* Replace electrolytes as well as fluid if activity level is increased and client perspires excessively

XIII. HYPERCHLOREMIA

A. Overview

1. **Hyperchloremia**: a serum Cl^- level greater than 108 mEq/L (normal range 95–108 mEq/L)
2. Predisposing clinical conditions
   a. Fluid and electrolyte imbalances such as hypernatremia, metabolic acidosis, and dehydration
   b. Drugs that promote Cl^- retention, such as IV saline, certain diuretics, salicylate intoxication, and others
   c. Diabetes insipidus, hyperaldosteronism (increased sodium and chloride reabsorption) hyperparathyroidism associated with hypercalcemia
   d. Renal changes that manifest as renal tubular acidosis or acute renal failure

B. Nursing assessment

1. Neuromuscular: weakness and lethargy; can progress to significant CNS damage
2. Respiratory: deep, rapid, vigorous breathing that can lead to unconsciousness (attempt to compensate for acidotic state due to loss of bicarbonate)
3. Cardiac: dysrhythmias due to retained Cl^- and result in acid–base imbalance
4. Fluid volume disturbances: dehydration, retention of salt and water due to drug administration, and a greater Na^+ loss than Cl^- loss
5. Increased Cl^- sweat levels are seen in diabetes insipidus, hypothyroidism, malnutrition, acute renal failure, and genetic disorders such as cystic fibrosis and glucose-6-phosphate-dehydrogenase (G6PD) deficiency
6. Electrolyte imbalances associated with elevated Cl^- levels: elevated K^+ and Na^+ levels and decreased HCO_3^- levels

C. Therapeutic management

1. Decrease Cl^- intake; stop all chloride-containing agents used as treatment measures
2. Promote Cl^- excretion by administering diuretics
3. Monitor VS, I&O, acid–base, respiratory, and cardiac status
4. Promote client safety
5. Hypotonic IV solutions such as 0.45% NaCl or D_5W to correct dehydration or IV diuretics to promote Cl^- loss

D. Client teaching

1. Predisposing factors
2. Avoid foods high in Cl^- and processed foods (high in both Na^+ and Cl^-); maintain adequate hydration

XIV. HYPOPHOSPHATEMIA

A. Overview

1. **Hypophosphatemia**: serum phosphate level of less than 2.5 mg/dL (normal range 2.5–4.5 mg/dL)
2. May be associated with increased Ca^{++} levels (hypercalcemia)
3. Predisposing factors
   a. Complication of refeeding after severe malnourishment (high mortality rate) or TPN with inadequate phosphorus
   b. Poor dietary intake or decreased absorption from vitamin D deficiency, malabsorption disorders, and starvation
   c. Prolonged use of aluminum- and Mg^{++}-based antacids (bind to phosphorus)
   d. Losses from severe vomiting and diarrhea; prolonged gastric suction or renal excretion
   e. Respiratory alkalosis (stimulates glycolysis to enhance phosphorus movement into cells)

B. Nursing assessment

1. Hematologic effects (anemia from RBC fragility), impaired granulocyte functioning (immunosuppression), bruising and bleeding from platelet dysfunction and destruction
2. Neuromuscular: slurred speech, confusion, apprehension, seizures, coma

3. Cardiac: chest pain, dysrhythmias related to decreased oxygenation, heart failure and shock from decreased myocardial contractility
4. Respiratory: alkalosis from an increased rate/depth of breathing in response to hypoxemia; respiratory muscle fatigue leading to respiratory failure
5. GI: hypoactive bowel sounds, anorexia, dysphagia, vomiting, gastric atony and ileus related to reduced gastric motility

C. Therapeutic management

1. Administer phosphorus via oral supplements or IV replacement; monitor infusion site for infiltration (possible tissue necrosis)
2. Avoid use of phosphorus-binding antacids
3. Assess for difficulty speaking and weakening hand grasps or respiratory efforts (have airway available)
4. Investigate episodes of bleeding and/or bruising
5. Monitor for other electrolyte imbalances, especially with N/V and/or diarrhea
6. Assess orientation and neurologic status with each set of VS; incorporate seizure precautions into care
7. Carefully monitor fluid I&O
8. Increase intake of foods high in phosphorus, such as red and organ (brain, liver, kidney) meats, fish, poultry, eggs, milk and milk products, legumes, whole grains, and nuts
9. Reduce dietary sources of oxalates (spinach and rhubarb) and phytates (bran and whole grains), which bind phosphates in GI tract and reduce absorption

D. Client teaching

1. Predisposing factors and signs and symptoms of hypophosphatemia
2. Avoiding phosphorus-binding antacids
3. Increase intake of foods high in phosphorus

XV. HYPERPHOSPHATEMIA

A. Overview

1. **Hyperphosphatemia**: serum phosphate level of greater than 4.5 mg/dL (normal range 2.5–4.5 mg/dL)
2. Predisposing factors
   a. Disorders such as acute kidney injury and chronic renal failure, hypoparathyroidism
   b. Hypocalcemia from antacids, diuretic agents, steroids
   c. Cellular release from rhabdomyolysis (breakdown of striated muscle, releases cellular phosphorus) or chemotherapy for malignant tumors
   d. Excessive intake of phosphorus or its supplements, increased GI absorption, or vitamin D excess
   e. Massive transfusions (phosphorus can leak from cells during blood storage)
   f. Large milk intake

NCLEX® **B. Nursing assessment**

1. Most signs relate to development of hypocalcemia or soft tissue calcification (calcium phosphate deposits in nonosseous sites such as kidney and heart)
2. Metastatic calcification includes oliguria, corneal haziness, conjunctivitis, irregular heart rate
3. ECG changes and conduction disturbance, tachycardia
4. Paresthesias (especially lips and fingertips), muscle spasms, and tetany (positive Chvostek and Trousseau signs) from decreased Ca^{++} that accompanies increased phosphorus
5. Anorexia, N/V

NCLEX® **C. Therapeutic management**

1. Restrict dietary phosphorus; avoid medications or enemas with phosphorus
2. Administer phosphate binding agents
3. Perform renal dialysis in clients with renal failure
4. Treat concurrent hypocalcemia
5. Monitor renal function carefully, particularly UO, BUN, creatinine
6. Monitor I&O; keep clients well hydrated, but avoid carbonated beverages (high in phosphates)

D. Client teaching

1. Purpose of phosphate binders; take with or after meals to maximize effectiveness; use bulk laxative or stool softener to combat constipating effect
2. Avoid OTC phosphorus in laxatives, enemas, and vitamin-mineral supplements
3. Avoid or limit foods high in phosphorus and carbonated beverages, which have low nutrient value and are also high in phosphates

Check your NCLEX–RN® Exam I.Q.

You are ready for testing on this content if you can:

- Describe the pathophysiology and etiology of fluid and electrolyte imbalances.
- Discuss expected assessment data and diagnostic test findings for fluid or electrolyte imbalance.
- Discuss therapeutic management of a client experiencing a fluid or electrolyte imbalance.
- Discuss nursing management of a client experiencing a fluid or electrolyte imbalance.
- Identify expected outcomes for the client experiencing a fluid or electrolyte imbalance.

PRACTICE TEST

1 A 10-month-old infant is admitted to the emergency department with a 102°F (38.9°C) rectal temperature and a history of vomiting and diarrhea for 48 hours. For which signs should the nurse assess?

1. Bulging fontanels, tearless cry, and low urine output
2. Sunken eyes, lethargy, and dry, furrowed tongue
3. Weight loss, dilute urine, and peripheral edema
4. Dry skin, thready pulse, and neck vein distention

2 Which assessment of an adult client is a reliable indicator that therapy for fluid overload is achieving the desired outcome? Select all that apply.

1. Full, bounding peripheral pulses
2. Flat neck veins with the head of the bed elevated
3. Hand veins emptying longer than 20 seconds
4. S_3 heart sound clearly audible on auscultation
5. Lung sounds are clear

3 The nurse concludes that which sign reliably indicates that ascites fluid is being effectively mobilized in response to therapy? Select all that apply.

1. Weight gain of 0.45 kg (1 lb) in 24 hours
2. Increase in urine output
3. Drop in blood pressure
4. Hand veins fill slowly
5. Abdominal girth has decreased by 2.5 cm (1 in.) in 24 hours

4 What instruction should the nurse include in an education program to prevent dehydration for a high school hiking club that is planning a 12-mile hike in early summer?

1. Take water and commercial sports drinks to sip often along the way.
2. Drink large amounts of water, at least 0.47 L (16 oz) every hour, while hiking.
3. Take salt tablets every 3 to 4 hours, and drink plenty of water while in the heat.
4. Stop every 4 hours along the way, and drink a few ounces of water while resting.

5 Which postoperative client would be at risk for developing a sodium imbalance?

1. A client who has just had a tonsillectomy
2. A client who has a primary cesarean delivery for failure to progress in labor
3. A client who has a transurethral resection of the prostate (TURP)
4. A client who has a right knee arthroscopy

6 The nurse is caring for a client who has a sodium level of 128 mEq/L. As part of the care, the nurse should restrict which item for this client?

1. Sports drinks containing electrolytes
2. Eggs and cheese products
3. Salt on the diet tray
4. Water

7 The nurse is caring for a client who has a sodium level of 149 mEq/L. The nurse anticipates that this client would benefit from which therapy?

1. Cough suppressant
2. 3% saline solution
3. 5% dextrose in water solution
4. Lactulose

8 The community health nurse makes a home visit to a client newly discharged from the hospital with resolving hypernatremia. During the initial interview, what information should the nurse follow up on to determine an effective plan of care?

1. The client lives on the second floor of an apartment building that has an elevator.
2. The client needs to walk 100 feet each day to reach the mailbox for the apartment building.
3. The client performs self-monitoring of blood glucose once a day.
4. The client uses antacids on a frequent basis for gastrointestinal complaints.

9 The nurse is caring for a client who has sustained partial- and full-thickness burns over 30% of his body 18 hours ago. The nurse assesses for which fluid and electrolyte imbalances at this time? Select all that apply.

1. Hyperkalemia
2. Hypokalemia
3. Hypervolemia
4. Hypercalcemia
5. Hypovolemia

10 The nurse concludes that a history of which condition places a client at risk for possible hypokalemia?

1. Chronic obstructive pulmonary disease (COPD)
2. Cirrhosis
3. Addison's disease
4. Chronic renal failure (CRF)

11 Which healthcare provider prescription for potassium chloride (KCl) should the nurse question for a client with severe hypokalemia?

1. Infuse 1000 mL normal saline with 20 mEq KCl IV over 8 hours.
2. Give KCl 20 mEq PO daily after meals.
3. Infuse 1000 mL normal saline with 40 mEq KCl IV at 200 mL/hour.
4. Give 20 mEq KCl IV over 10 minutes.

12 Which treatment option does the nurse anticipate will be most appropriate for a client with a potassium level of 3.5 mEq/L?

1. Give sodium polystyrene sulfate (Kayexalate) per rectum.
2. Use salt substitutes in the diet.
3. Administer oral potassium chloride (KCl).
4. Continue to monitor and offer foods high in potassium.

13 The nurse includes in the plan of care to periodically monitor which item for a client who is at risk for developing hypocalcemia? Select all that apply.

1. Blood urea nitrogen (BUN) and creatinine levels
2. Constipation
3. Serum albumin level
4. Fluid overload related to intravenous saline therapy
5. Serum magnesium level

14 A client with hypocalcemia is taking supplemental vitamin D. When the client asks the purpose of this therapy, what explanation should the nurse give?

1. It directly opposes calcitonin.
2. It prevents renal disease in clients with hypocalcemia.
3. Calcium is absorbed in the intestines only under the influence of activated vitamin D.
4. The only way to obtain vitamin D is with oral supplementation.

15 Which medication reported by a client during a nursing history could be associated with the development of hypocalcemia?

1. Phenytoin
2. Calcium carbonate
3. Calcitriol
4. Hydrochlorothiazide

16. The family of a client with hypercalcemia states that the client is "not acting like himself." The nurse focuses assessment on which manifestation?

1. Personality change
2. Anxiety
3. Seizure activity
4. Carpal spasms

17. The nurse assessing a client for signs of hypocalcemia would conclude that this electrolyte imbalance exists after noting which finding?

1. Negative Chvostek sign
2. Positive Trousseau sign
3. Positive Kernig sign
4. Hypoactive bowel sounds

18. The nurse should review a client's electrolyte levels to detect a possible increase in magnesium if the client has which condition? Select all that apply.

1. Cushing's syndrome
2. Diabetes
3. Addison's disease
4. Splenomegaly
5. Dehydration

19. The nurse concludes that a client does not have an increased magnesium level based on which finding?

1. Hypotension
2. Bradycardia
3. Supraventricular tachycardia (SVT)
4. Flushing and sweating

20. A client with end-stage renal disease is experiencing hypermagnesemia. The nurse explains that which treatment will decrease the magnesium level most effectively?

1. Dialysis
2. Diuretics
3. Fluid restriction
4. High-volume IV fluids

21. The nurse reviews the laboratory test results for a client with preeclampsia, expecting to find which value?

1. Sodium 148 mEq/L
2. Sodium 125 mEq/L
3. Magnesium 3.1 mEq/L
4. Magnesium 1.2 mEq/L

22. A client admitted to the hospital with a 13.6-kg (30-lb) weight gain over the past month has moon facies. Admission laboratory results indicate low serum potassium and magnesium, and high serum chloride and sodium levels. The nurse interprets that which disorder is most consistent with these electrolyte abnormalities?

1. Addison's disease
2. Cushing's syndrome
3. Rhabdomyolysis
4. Syndrome of inappropriate ADH (SIADH)

23. A home health nurse is making a visit to an older adult client with a history of heart failure (HF). The client was prescribed diuretics twice a day and a low-sodium diet. The nurse should be most concerned about which current laboratory result?

1. Sodium 145 mEq/L
2. Chloride 90 mEq/L
3. K^+ 4.2 mEq/L
4. HCO_3^{2} 27 mEq/L

24. Which finding in a client's history would alert the nurse to assess for signs of hypophosphatemia?

1. Alcohol abuse
2. Oliguric phase of acute tubular necrosis
3. Short-term gastric suction
4. Occasional use of aluminum-containing antacids

25 Which concurrent electrolyte imbalance should the nurse anticipate while caring for a client with hyperphosphatemia?

1. Potassium 2.8 mEq/L
2. Sodium 131 mEq/L
3. Calcium 6.8 mEq/L
4. Magnesium 3.4 mEq/L

26 The nurse would report to the charge nurse that an assigned client has hyperkalemia after noting that the serum potassium level drawn that morning was greater than how many mEq/L? Provide a numerical answer.

Fill in your answer below:
Answer: ___ mEq/L

ANSWERS & RATIONALES

1 **Answer: 2 Rationale:** The client's history suggests dehydration. Sunken eyes, altered mental status and behavior, and dry, furrowed tongue are reliable signs of dehydration in infants. Bulging fontanels, peripheral edema, and neck vein distention are seen with fluid overload. **Cognitive Level:** Applying **Client Need:** Physiological Adaptation **Integrated Process:** Nursing Process: Assessment **Content Area:** Adult Health: Endocrine and Metabolic **Strategy:** The core issue of the question is the ability to correlate a clinical picture with risk for hypovolemia. Use nursing knowledge of signs of dehydration and the process of elimination to make a selection.

2 **Answer: 2, 5 Rationale:** Flat neck veins with the head of the bed elevated are an indicator of the absence of venous congestion. With fluid overload, crackles can often be auscultated in lung fields. Absence of crackles is consistent with normal fluid balance. Venous congestion results from fluid volume excess, and causes full, bounding pulses, delayed hand vein emptying, and S_3 heart sounds. **Cognitive Level:** Applying **Client Need:** Physiological Adaptation **Integrated Process:** Nursing Process: Evaluation **Content Area:** Adult Health: Endocrine and Metabolic **Strategy:** The core issue of the question is knowledge of signs of fluid overload and normal findings. Use nursing knowledge and the process of elimination to make a selection.

3 **Answer: 2, 5 Rationale:** Ascites is a form of third space fluid in the abdomen. Therapy is aimed at moving third space fluid back into the circulation, where it can be eliminated by the kidneys. When this fluid is drawn back into the vascular space (leading to a rise in BP and venous pressure), the kidneys increase the urine output to eliminate the excess fluid. Loss of fluid results in loss of weight and abdominal girth decreases. Weight gain, drop in BP, and slow filling of hand veins do not indicate effective therapy. **Cognitive Level:** Analyzing **Client Need:** Physiological Adaptation **Integrated Process:** Nursing Process: Evaluation **Content Area:** Adult Health: Endocrine and Metabolic **Strategy:** The core issues of the question are recognition of ascites as a third space fluid and knowledge of effective mobilization of that fluid. Recall that mobilized fluid must be eliminated via the kidneys to assist in making a selection.

4 **Answer: 1 Rationale:** Drinking a combination of water and sports drinks is helpful. Sports drinks provide carbohydrates, water, and electrolytes. Drinking large amounts of only water fails to replace electrolytes, which can lead to water intoxication. Salt tablets are no longer recommended because too much salt has a hypertonic effect, causes diuresis, and can actually worsen fluid loss. Those who exercise in hot climates need to continuously replace both fluid and electrolyte losses. A few ounces of fluid every 4 hours are insufficient. **Cognitive Level:** Analyzing **Client Need:** Physiological Adaptation **Integrated Process:** Nursing Process: Implementation **Content Area:** Adult Health: Endocrine and Metabolic **Strategy:** The core issue of the question is knowledge of measures to prevent fluid and electrolyte imbalance during exercise. Use nursing knowledge and the process of elimination to make a selection.

5 **Answer: 3 Rationale:** A TURP procedure can place a client at risk for developing hyponatremia in the postoperative period due to increased fluid irrigation used during and after surgery. Clients with a TURP procedure have a CBI (continuous bladder irrigation) as a routine part of their postoperative care. A tonsillectomy, cesarean delivery, and an arthroscopy do not place a client at risk for development of sodium imbalances because they do not require lengthy fluid and dietary restrictions or excessive fluid irrigation. **Cognitive Level:** Applying **Client Need:** Physiological Adaptation **Integrated Process:** Nursing Process: Diagnosis **Content Area:** Adult Health: Endocrine and Metabolic **Strategy:** The core issue of the question is knowledge that procedures and surgeries requiring use of water for irrigation can lead to dilutional hyponatremia. Use nursing knowledge and the process of elimination to make a selection.

6 **Answer: 4 Rationale:** Hyponatremia can also be referred to as dilutional hyponatremia or water intoxication. Water restriction would be an important part of the treatment plan when caring for a client who has hyponatremia. Restrictions of electrolyte-rich solutions, eggs, cheese products, and salt on the diet tray are not indicated because the client is experiencing a sodium deficit. **Cognitive Level:** Analyzing **Client Need:** Physiological Adaptation **Integrated Process:** Nursing Process: Implementation **Content Area:** Adult Health: Endocrine and Metabolic **Strategy:** The core issue of the question is effective treatment measures for hyponatremia. Use nursing knowledge and the process of elimination to make a selection.

7 **Answer: 3 Rationale:** Clients with hypernatremia are thirsty and need water replacement to balance their increased sodium levels. Cough medication and lactulose can further increase sodium levels and should not be administered unless there is sufficient clinical information to warrant their use. Three-percent saline is a hypertonic solution that would also increase serum sodium levels and should not be given to this client. **Cognitive Level:** Analyzing **Client Need:** Physiological Adaptation **Integrated Process:** Nursing Process: Implementation **Content**

Area: Adult Health: Endocrine and Metabolic **Strategy:** The core issue of the question is knowledge of measures that effectively treat hypernatremia. Use nursing knowledge and the process of elimination to make a selection.

8 **Answer: 4 Rationale:** The nurse should investigate what type of antacids are used because some may be high in sodium, such as sodium bicarbonate. Elevator use and 30.5-m (100-ft) walking distance would not cause or aggravate a sodium imbalance, although it is helpful data for mobility status. Self-monitoring of blood glucose suggests that the client might have diabetes, but this does not relate to increases in serum sodium levels. **Cognitive Level:** Applying **Client Need:** Physiological Adaptation **Integrated Process:** Nursing Process: Assessment **Content Area:** Adult Health: Endocrine and Metabolic **Strategy:** The core issue of the question is knowledge of factors that can lead to elevated serum sodium levels. Use nursing knowledge and the process of elimination to make a selection.

9 **Answer: 1, 5 Rationale:** During major burn injury, potassium shifts from the intracellular fluid to the extracellular fluid because of cell death, leading to high serum levels of potassium. Hypokalemia is not seen in burn clients during the time of fluid shifting secondary to trauma. The client with burns is more likely to be hypovolemic than hypervolemic and more likely to be hypocalcemic than hypercalcemic at this time because of fluid and electrolyte loss caused by altered capillary integrity. **Cognitive Level:** Applying **Client Need:** Physiological Adaptation **Integrated Process:** Nursing Process: Assessment **Content Area:** Adult Health: Endocrine and Metabolic **Strategy:** The core issue of the question is knowledge that burn injury increases the risk of hyperkalemia. Use nursing knowledge and the process of elimination to make a selection.

10 **Answer: 2 Rationale:** In clients with cirrhosis, increased amounts of aldosterone are secreted, which leads to sodium retention and potassium excretion from the kidneys; these clients are likely to become hypokalemic. Clients with COPD are likely to develop hyperkalemia due to retention of acids, which leads to loss of hydrogen ions and retention of potassium as an alternate cation. Clients with Addison's disease (hypofunction of adrenal gland) are likely to develop hyperkalemia because of high sodium loss. Clients with CRF are likely to develop hyperkalemia because of inadequate potassium excretion. **Cognitive Level:** Analyzing **Client Need:** Physiological Adaptation **Integrated Process:** Nursing Process: Diagnosis **Content Area:** Adult Health: Endocrine and Metabolic **Strategy:** The core issue of the question is the ability to discriminate predisposing factors for hypokalemia from factors for hyperkalemia. Use nursing knowledge and the process of elimination to make a selection.

11 **Answer: 4 Rationale:** Potassium is never given as a bolus when it is administered intravenously. KCl should never be given rapidly or by IV push because serious arrhythmias or cardiac arrest can occur. All of the other prescriptions (normal saline infusion with 20 mEq KCl, KCl 20 mEq PO, and normal saline with 40 mEq KCl) are within a safe and therapeutic range. **Cognitive Level:** Analyzing **Client Need:** Pharmacological and Parenteral Therapies **Integrated Process:** Nursing Process: Planning **Content Area:** Adult Health: Endocrine and Metabolic **Strategy:** The core issue of the question is knowledge of safe and unsafe methods of administering potassium as replacement therapy in hypokalemia. Use nursing knowledge and the process of elimination to make a selection.

12 **Answer: 4 Rationale:** A serum potassium level of 3.5 mEq/L is at the low end of the normal range. With a low normal level, it is better to continue to monitor the client and offer foods that are good sources of potassium. Kayexelate reduces the potassium level and is contraindicated in this client. In the absence of additional medical history, it is not advisable to use salt substitutes or oral KCL as sources of additional potassium. **Cognitive Level:** Applying **Client Need:** Physiological Adaptation **Integrated Process:** Nursing Process: Planning **Content Area:** Adult Health: Endocrine and Metabolic **Strategy:** The core issue of the question is knowledge of treatment measures depending on the severity of hypokalemia. First, recognize that this is a value at the low end of normal, and then select the mildest intervention of the choices provided. Note the critical word *most*, which indicates that some options may be plausible, but one is better than the others.

13 **Answer: 3, 5 Rationale:** A client who is at risk for developing hypocalcemia requires monitoring of serum albumin (provides information relative to physiologically available calcium) level. Decreased magnesium levels are usually seen concurrently with low serum calcium levels. Assessing BUN and creatinine or constipation would be useful for a client at risk for hypercalcemia. Assessing for fluid overload would be important for a client being treated with fluid therapy for hypercalcemia. **Cognitive Level:** Applying **Client Need:** Physiological Adaptation **Integrated Process:** Nursing Process: Planning **Content Area:** Adult Health: Endocrine and Metabolic **Strategy:** The core issue of the question is the ability to choose assessments to detect hypocalcemia. Use nursing knowledge and the process of elimination to make a selection.

14 **Answer: 3 Rationale:** Calcium is absorbed in the intestines only under the influence of vitamin D, which is activated in the kidneys. Parathyroid hormone, not activated vitamin D, directly opposes calcitonin. Vitamin D does not prevent renal disease in hypocalcemia, but renal disease prevents activation of vitamin D, thereby reducing the body's ability to absorb calcium. There are other ways besides supplementation to obtain vitamin D in the body, such as exposure to sunlight. **Cognitive Level:** Applying **Client Need:** Pharmacological and Parenteral Therapies **Integrated Process:** Nursing Process: Implementation **Content Area:** Adult Health: Endocrine and Metabolic **Strategy:** The core issue of the question is knowledge of the purpose and effects of vitamin D in a client with hypocalcemia. Use nursing knowledge and the process of elimination to make a selection.

15 **Answer: 1 Rationale:** Antiepileptics such as phenytoin alter vitamin D metabolism and lead to hypocalcemia. Calcium carbonate and calcitriol represent calcium sources, and the inclusion of these in a treatment plan would lead to increased serum calcium levels. Hydrochlorothiazide is incorrect because thiazide diuretics can lead to calcium retention. **Cognitive Level:** Applying **Client Need:** Physiological Adaptation **Integrated Process:** Nursing Process: Assessment **Content Area:** Adult Health: Endocrine and Metabolic **Strategy:** The core issue of the question is knowledge of medications that increase the risk of hypocalcemia. Use nursing knowledge and the process of elimination to make a selection.

16 **Answer: 1 Rationale:** Clinical manifestations of hypercalcemia include personality changes. Anxiety, seizures, and carpal spasms are manifestations of hypocalcemia. **Cognitive Level:** Applying **Client Need:** Physiological Adaptation **Integrated Process:** Nursing Process: Assessment **Content Area:** Adult Health: Endocrine and Metabolic **Strategy:** The core issue of the question is knowledge of manifestations of

hypercalcemia. Use nursing knowledge and the process of elimination to make a selection.

17 **Answer: 2 Rationale:** Clinical manifestations of hypocalcemia include a positive Trousseau sign, which is presence of carpopedal spasm. A positive Chvostek sign (twitching of muscles of cheek) would be associated with hypocalcemia, but this client has a negative sign. Kernig sign is an indication of meningeal irritation. Hypoactive bowel sounds are a sign of hypercalcemia. **Cognitive Level:** Applying **Client Need:** Physiological Adaptation **Integrated Process:** Nursing Process: Assessment **Content Area:** Adult Health: Endocrine and Metabolic **Strategy:** The core issue of the question is knowledge of manifestations of hypocalcemia. Use nursing knowledge and the process of elimination to make a selection.

18 **Answer: 3, 5 Rationale:** Addison's disease, known also as adrenal insufficiency, can cause increased magnesium levels resulting from volume depletion. Dehydration can lead to an elevated magnesium level because of hemoconcentration. Cushing's syndrome is hyperfunction of the adrenal gland and could lead to low magnesium levels from fluid overload. Diabetes mellitus could lead to low magnesium levels if osmotic diuresis is present from hyperglycemia. Splenomegaly is an unrelated finding. **Cognitive Level:** Applying **Client Need:** Physiological Adaptation **Integrated Process:** Nursing Process: Assessment **Content Area:** Adult Health: Endocrine and Metabolic **Strategy:** The core issue of the question is knowledge of risk factors for hypermagnesemia. Use nursing knowledge and the process of elimination to make a selection.

19 **Answer: 3 Rationale:** SVT is seen with decreased magnesium levels, as are premature ventricular contractions and ventricular fibrillation. Hypotension, bradycardia, and flushing and sweating are associated with hypermagnesemia. **Cognitive Level:** Analyzing **Client Need:** Physiological Adaptation **Integrated Process:** Nursing Process: Assessment **Content Area:** Adult Health: Endocrine and Metabolic **Strategy:** The core issue of the question is the ability to discriminate signs of hyper- and hypomagnesemia. Use nursing knowledge and the process of elimination to make a selection.

20 **Answer: 1 Rationale:** Either hemodialysis or peritoneal dialysis is used to remove excess magnesium in the client with renal failure. Diuretics will not be effective if the kidneys are not functional. Fluid restriction will be part of the treatment for end-stage renal disease but will be ineffective alone in decreasing magnesium level. High-volume IV fluid replacement is contraindicated in renal failure. **Cognitive Level:** Applying **Client Need:** Physiological Adaptation **Integrated Process:** Nursing Process: Implementation **Content Area:** Adult Health: Endocrine and Metabolic **Strategy:** The core issue of the question is knowledge of effective therapies for increased magnesium levels. Note the critical words *end-stage renal disease*, which lead you to look for a treatment that does not involve functional kidneys. Use nursing knowledge and the process of elimination to make a selection.

21 **Answer: 4 Rationale:** A decreased magnesium level can occur in toxemia of pregnancy, preeclampsia, and eclampsia, causing seizures. A magnesium level of 3.1 mEq/L is an increased level, the opposite of the concern for this client. Sodium is not the electrolyte of concern in a client with preeclampsia. **Cognitive Level:** Applying **Client Need:** Physiological Adaptation **Integrated Process:** Nursing Process: Assessment **Content Area:** Adult Health: Endocrine and Metabolic **Strategy:** The core issue of the question is knowledge of conditions that are consistent with decreased magnesium levels and the ability to determine a reduced level. Use nursing knowledge and the process of elimination to make a selection.

22 **Answer: 2 Rationale:** Cushing's syndrome causes low potassium and magnesium levels and an increase in sodium and chloride levels. The moon facies is also a sign of excess corticosteroids. Addison's disease causes low sodium and increased magnesium and potassium levels. Rhabdomyolysis is associated with high phosphate levels. SIADH is associated with hyponatremia. **Cognitive Level:** Analyzing **Client Need:** Physiological Adaptation **Integrated Process:** Nursing Process: Assessment **Content Area:** Adult Health: Endocrine and Metabolic **Strategy:** The core issue of the question is the ability to synthesize electrolyte results with a clinical picture in a client with Cushing's syndrome. Use nursing knowledge and the process of elimination to make a selection.

23 **Answer: 2 Rationale:** The decreased chloride level is of greatest concern because it can be associated with dilutional hypochloremia from fluid overload. The client's history of HF places the client in a higher risk category for fluid retention. The sodium, potassium, and bicarbonate levels are within normal range and are reassuring. **Cognitive Level:** Analyzing **Client Need:** Physiological Adaptation **Integrated Process:** Nursing Process: Assessment **Content Area:** Adult Health: Endocrine and Metabolic **Strategy:** The core issue of the question is the ability to determine abnormal electrolyte levels. Use nursing knowledge and the process of elimination to make a selection.

24 **Answer: 1 Rationale:** Poor nutritional intake, such as occurs in clients with alcoholism, can lead to hypophosphatemia. During oliguria, the kidneys are unable to excrete phosphorus, leading to hyperphosphatemia. Clients with prolonged (not short-term) gastric suction are more likely to experience hypophosphatemia. Prolonged or continuous use of aluminum-containing antacids (not occasional use) leads to hypophosphatemia. **Cognitive Level:** Analyzing **Client Need:** Physiological Adaptation **Integrated Process:** Nursing Process: Assessment **Content Area:** Adult Health: Endocrine and Metabolic **Strategy:** The core issue of the question is knowledge of risk factors for hypophosphatemia. Use nursing knowledge and the process of elimination to make a selection.

25 **Answer: 3 Rationale:** Calcium and phosphorus have an inverse relationship in the body. For this reason, when phosphorus levels are high, calcium levels are low. Potassium, sodium, and magnesium do not have an inverse relationship with phosphorus. **Cognitive Level:** Analyzing **Client Need:** Physiological Adaptation **Integrated Process:** Nursing Process: Assessment **Content Area:** Adult Health: Endocrine and Metabolic **Strategy:** The core issue of the question is knowledge that hypocalcemia accompanies hypermagnesemia. To answer the question correctly, you must also be able to recognize abnormal laboratory values. Use nursing knowledge and the process of elimination to make a selection.

26 **Answer: 5.1 Rationale:** Hyperkalemia exists when the serum potassium level rises above the upper limit of normal, which is 5.1 mEq/L. **Cognitive Level:** Analyzing **Client Need:** Physiological Adaptation **Integrated Process:** Nursing Process: Diagnosis **Content Area:** Adult Health: Endocrine and Metabolic **Strategy:** The core issue of the question is knowledge that hypocalcemia accompanies hypermagnesemia. To answer correctly, you must also be able to recognize abnormal laboratory values. Use nursing knowledge and the process of elimination to make a selection.

Key Terms to Review

hypercalcemia p. 865
hyperchloremia p. 868
hyperkalemia p. 863
hypermagnesemia p. 867
hypernatremia p. 860
hyperosmolar p. 860
hyperphosphatemia p. 869
hypertonic p. 854
hypervolemia p. 857
hypocalcemia p. 863
hypochloremia p. 867
hypokalemia p. 861
hypomagnesemia p. 866
hyponatremia p. 858
hypophosphatemia p. 868
hypotonic p. 854
hypovolemia p. 857
water intoxication p. 857

References

Berman, A., Snyder, S., & Frandsen, G. (2016). *Kozier & Erb's fundamentals of nursing: Concepts, process, and practice* (10th ed.). New York, NY: Pearson Education.

Ignatavicius, D., & Workman, L. (2016). *Medical-surgical nursing: Patient-centered collaborative care* (10th ed.). Philadelphia: Saunders.

Kee, J. (2017). *Pearson's handbook of laboratory and diagnostic tests* (8th ed.). New York, NY: Pearson Education.

LeMone, P., Burke, K., Bauldoff, G., & Gubrud, P. (2015). *Medical surgical nursing: Clinical reasoning in patient care* (6th ed.). Hoboken, NJ: Pearson Education.

Lewis, S., Dirksen, S., Heitkemper, M., & Bucher, L. (2014). *Medical surgical nursing: Assessment and management of clinical problems* (9th ed.). St. Louis, MO: Elsevier Science.

Test Yourself

Are you ready for the NCLEX-RN® or course exams? Access the NEW web-based app that provides students with thousands of practice questions in preparation for the NCLEX experience.

Acid–Base Imbalances

54

In this chapter

Cross Reference

Other chapters relevant to this content area are

Common Laboratory Tests	Chapter 46
Fluid and Electrolyte Imbalances	Chapter 53

I. NORMAL ACID–BASE BALANCE

A. Nature of acids and bases

1. An **acid** is a substance that releases a hydrogen (H^+) ion when dissolved in water
2. A **base** is a substance that will bind to an H^+ ion when dissolved in water
3. Weak acids do not completely separate in water; they only release some H^+ ions
4. A weak base accepts H^+ ions less easily, but it is extremely valuable in preventing major alterations in **pH** of extracellular fluid (ECF)

B. Chemical buffer systems in body

1. A **buffer** prevents major changes in ECF by releasing or accepting H^+ ions
2. The major chemical buffers (found in blood) include bicarbonate–carbonic acid buffer system, phosphate buffer system, and protein buffer system
3. Chemical buffers are present in both intracellular fluid (ICF) and ECF
4. Buffers are found in all body tissues, including bone
5. Chemical buffers act within seconds to neutralize acids and bases and keep pH within narrow normal range of 7.35–7.45
6. Bicarbonate–carbonic acid buffer system
   a. Consists of a water solution that contains a weak acid, carbonic acid (H_2CO_3), and a bicarbonate salt, usually sodium bicarbonate ($NaHCO_3$)
   b. Normally, body maintains pH by keeping ratio of bicarbonate (**HCO_3^-**) to H_2CO_3 at a proportion of 20:1; this ratio is changed if pH goes up or down
   c. Once compensation occurs, ratio becomes stable again
   d. Bicarbonate–carbonic acid buffer system is linked to both respiratory and renal systems
   e. H_2CO_3 is respiratory compensatory component; it can dissociate into carbon dioxide (CO_2) and water, with CO_2 being exhaled by lungs
   f. HCO_3^- is the primary renal compensatory component; it can be excreted by kidneys or retained with excretion of H^+ ions
   g. This function is illustrated by the following equation:
      $CO_2 + H_2O \leftrightarrow H_2CO_3 \leftrightarrow HCO_3^- + H^+$

7. Phosphate buffer system buffers both ICF and ECF to maintain a normal pH
8. Protein buffer system acts similarly to bicarbonate–carbonic acid buffer system; it releases or accepts H^+ readily and can exist as either an acid or a base; major intracellular buffer
9. Hemoglobin-oxyhemoglobin buffer system helps to maintain pH within normal range in both arterial and venous blood, which have different amounts of CO_2

C. Physiological buffers in body

1. Pulmonary regulation
   a. Lungs control respiratory carbonic acid buffer system and compensate for acid–base disturbances that are metabolic in nature (e.g., lactic acidosis that occurs with exercise)
   b. Lungs increase or decrease respiratory rate (RR) and depth in response to amount of CO_2 in ECF
   c. Respiratory system is extremely sensitive to changes in pH; begins compensatory efforts within seconds to minutes but becomes quickly exhausted and is not as efficient as renal compensation
   d. Older adults have reduced gas exchange and less alveolar membrane so CO_2 retention and increased H^+ ion concentrations may be a problem
2. Renal regulation
   a. Kidneys control metabolic buffer $NaHCO_3^-$ by excreting an acidic urine or an alkaline urine
   b. Work within several hours to days but are powerfully effective by eliminating either acids or bases
   c. Kidneys control HCO_3^- in ECF by either reabsorbing or excreting H^+ ions; they also combine ammonia (NaH_3) with hydrochloric acid (HCl) to form ammonium (NH_4Cl), which is excreted by kidneys; approximately 50% of excess H^+ can be excreted by this mechanism
   d. Kidneys can also excrete weak acids into urine, such as from cellular metabolism; thus urine is normally acidic (average pH 6)
   e. Renal function decreases with age, so older adults do not excrete H^+ ions or synthesize HCO_3^- as efficiently, making their acid–base imbalances more difficult to correct

NCLEX®

3. **Compensation** occurs when body uses regulatory mechanisms to return pH to normal by transforming acids and bases within body; pH becomes normal, but there are abnormal amounts of CO_2 and/or HCO_3^-
   a. A primary metabolic disturbance triggers respiratory compensation
   b. A primary respiratory disturbance activates blood buffers and causes metabolic compensation by kidneys
   c. Complete compensation means that buffers have achieved homeostasis and pH is fully corrected
   d. Partial compensation means that buffers are working to restore homeostasis
   e. Decompensation refers to a worsening state of acid–base imbalance
4. Correction of acid–base imbalance occurs when lungs and/or kidneys eliminate offending substance(s) from body, and both CO_2 and HCO_3^- levels (not just pH) are returned to normal

D. Indicator measures of acid–base status

1. pH: the negative logarithm of H^+ ion concentration in mEq per liter

NCLEX®

   a. Normal pH in arterial blood is 7.35–7.45; in venous blood, it is 7.32–7.42
   b. A pH less than 7.35 is labeled acidotic; acidosis has depressant effect on central nervous system (CNS)
   c. A pH greater than 7.45 is labeled alkalotic; alkalosis has excitatory effect on CNS

Memory Aid

The pH is like the center of a seesaw; it wants to stay balanced.

2. **$PaCO_2$** (partial pressure of arterial CO_2): measurement of CO_2 pressure being exerted on plasma; directly related to amount of CO_2 being produced
   a. $PaCO_2$ is regulated by lungs and indicates amount of H_2CO_3 that is available to act as a buffer
   b. $PaCO_2$ indicates whether condition is a respiratory disturbance

NCLEX®

   c. Normal value of $PaCO_2$ is 35–45 mmHg
   d. Values less than 35 mmHg indicate alkalosis
   e. Values greater than 45 mmHg indicate acidosis

Memory Aid

Carbon dioxide (CO_2) acts as an acid in the body. It is also the indicator of how the respiratory system is functioning.

3. HCO_3^- (bicarbonate): measurement of HCO_3^- in plasma and is directly related to attraction and release of H^+ ions from H_2CO_3
   a. HCO_3^- is regulated by kidneys and indicates body's ability to buffer H^+ ions (acid) by combining to form H_2CO_3
   b. HCO_3^- indicates whether condition is a metabolic disturbance
   c. *NCLEX®* Normal value of HCO_3^- is 22–26 mEq/L in arterial blood gas
   d. Values less than 22 mEq/L indicate acidosis
   e. Value greater than 26 mEq/L indicate alkalosis

Memory Aid

Bicarbonate (HCO_3^-) acts as a base in the body. It is also the indicator of how the metabolic system is functioning.

4. **PaO_2** (partial pressure of oxygen): measurement of amount of pressure exerted by oxygen on plasma
   a. Range of normal values for PaO_2 is 80–100 mmHg for adults under age 60 years; for every year above 60, there is an expected decrease in PaO_2 of 1 mmHg
   b. If PaO_2 drops dramatically, then O_2 saturation also decreases greatly
5. **SaO_2**: percentage of hemoglobin saturated with O_2; since most O_2 is carried on hemoglobin, total O_2 concentration is measured using hemoglobin saturation (SaO_2)
   a. A relationship between PaO_2 and SaO_2 influences binding affinity and dissociation of O_2 and hemoglobin (oxyhemoglobin dissociation curve)
   b. Acidosis causes a shift toward right on oxyhemoglobin dissociation curve (decreased affinity); O_2 is more easily released to tissues
   c. Alkalosis causes a shift toward left on oxyhemoglobin dissociation curve (increased affinity); O_2 is held more tightly and is less available to tissues
   d. Other factors that affect O_2 affinity include body temperature and transfusion of banked blood
6. Electrolyte interactions
   a. *NCLEX®* HCO_3^- is a direct reflection of kidneys' ability to compensate for pH changes; a decreased HCO_3^- level is consistent with acidosis, and an increased HCO_3^- level is consistent with alkalosis
   b. Base excess (BE) indicates amount of HCO_3^- available in ECF, and normal values range from −3.0 to +3.0 in adults; values above +3.0 indicate metabolic alkalosis, while values below −3.0 indicate metabolic acidosis
   c. Serum anion gap (AG) (normal range 10–12 mEq/L) calculates concentrations of anions (HCO_3^-, chloride [Cl^-], proteins, phosphates, and sulfates) and cations (sodium [Na^+], potassium [K^+], magnesium [Mg^{++}], calcium [Ca^{++}]) by using the following equation:
      $Na^+ - [Cl^- + HCO_3^-]$
   d. Increased AG of more than 12 mEq/L indicates metabolic acidosis (AG acidosis); however, a normal AG can exist with a metabolic acidosis (non-AG acidosis) when there is a decrease in HCO_3^- balanced by an increase in Cl^-
   e. Decreased AG of less than 10 mEq/L occurs with low albumin levels or in conditions in which there is an increase in unmeasured cations (multiple myeloma, lithium toxicity, or nephrotic syndrome)
   f. Potassium (K^+) helps to maintain acid–base balance by exchanging for H^+ ions across cell membranes; in acidosis, K^+ comes out of cell and allows H^+ in to reduce circulating acids; in alkalosis, K^+ goes into cell and allows H^+ to come out to increase circulating acids
   g. Chloride levels are used to evaluate clients who are at risk for metabolic alkalosis to determine cause of alkalosis and thus corrective treatment

E. Arterial blood gas (ABG) analysis (see Table 54–1 for normal values)

1. *NCLEX®* Follow a systematic approach (see Figure 54–1)
2. Interpret pH: a pH less than 7.35 indicates acidosis, while a pH greater than 7.45 indicates alkalosis
3. Identify primary cause—respiratory or metabolic
   a. Examine first $PaCO_2$ value and then HCO_3^- value
   b. If $PaCO_2$ is abnormal and direction of change in value is inversely related to direction of change in pH, then primary problem is respiratory
   c. If HCO_3^- is abnormal and direction of change in value is same as direction of change in pH, then problem is metabolic

Table 54–1 Normal Arterial Blood Gas Values

	Normal Reference Ranges		
Serum Laboratory Value	**Adult**	**Child**	**Infant**
pH (arterial)	7.35–7.45	7.37–7.43 (c) 7.35–7.41 (a)	7.36–7.42
PCO_2 (mm Hg)	35–45	35–41 (c) 38–44 (a)	30–34
HCO_3^- (mEq/L)	22–26	18–25 (c) 23–25 (a)	17.2–23.6
PO_2 (mm Hg)	80–100	80–100	80–100
SaO_2 (%)	95–100	95–100	95–100
Anion gap base excess	10–12 mEq/L +3 to −3(+/−2 mEq/L)	10–12 mEq/L +3 to −3(+/−2 mEq/L)	10–12 mEq/L +3 to −3(+/−2 mEq/L)

c, children; a, adolescents

Memory Aid

Interpret ABGs by looking first at pH, then at CO_2, then at HCO_3^-. Determine first whether there is acidosis or alkalosis, then evaluate whether the imbalance is respiratory (CO_2) or metabolic (HCO_3^-) in origin. The cause will be the value that *matches* or correlates with the change in the direction of the pH.

4. Determine presence of compensation
   a. Determine if $PaCO_2$ and HCO_3^- are decreased or increased as body attempts to maintain ratio of HCO_3^- to H_2CO_3 at 20:1
   b. Partial compensation exists when pH remains abnormal but parameter that did not originally alter pH now changes (e.g., pH indicates an acidotic state and CO_2 is high, indicating respiratory origin, but HCO_3^- is also increased, indicating use of buffer systems to bring pH back into line)

Memory Aid

The pH is like a seesaw, with CO_2 and HCO_3 as riders on opposite ends. When one side goes up, the other tries to go up to compensate. When one side goes down, the other side tries to go down to compensate and bring the pH back toward normal.

   c. Full or complete compensation occurs when buffer system brings pH back to a value of 7.35–7.45 (e.g., respiratory acidosis exists as indicated by an elevated $PaCO_2$; however, pH is normal and HCO_3^- is increased)

Memory Aid

If CO_2 and HCO_3^- are both abnormal, again look to see which value has a change that *matches* the direction of the change in pH (e.g., CO_2 acts as an acid; HCO_3^- acts as a base). This match will be the primary imbalance, while the other system is compensating. If the pH is back in normal range, the value will be a number that is nearer to the side of the primary imbalance (e.g., 7.43 is nearer to alkalosis than acidosis, while 7.36 is nearer to acidosis than alkalosis). Remember that the body does not overcompensate!

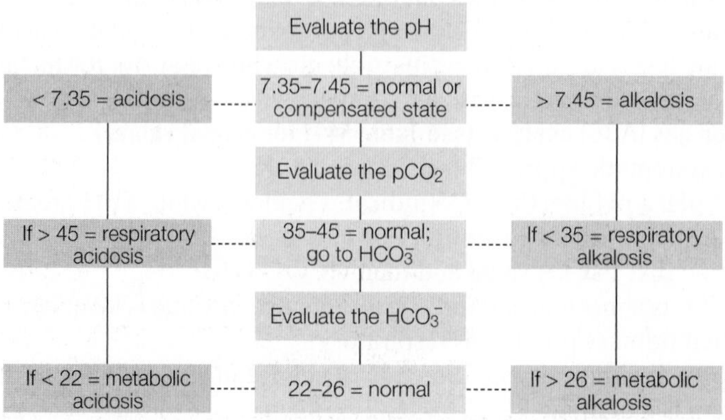

Figure 54–1

Interpreting ABGs: If CO_2 and HCO_3^- are both abnormal, look to see which one has a change that *matches* the change in the pH (CO_2 acts as an acid; HCO_3^- acts as a base). This match will be the primary imbalance, while the other system is compensating.

F. Assisting with obtaining an ABG specimen

1. Determine site of specimen collection (radial or femoral artery, intra-arterial line) and obtain baseline vital signs (VS)

NCLEX®

2. Perform Allen test prior to radial artery puncture
   a. Ask client to rest affected hand facing upward and observe color of palm
   b. Ask client to make tight fist (forcing blood from hand)
   c. Compress radial and ulnar arteries with direct pressure using index and middle finger of hand (obstructs blood flow to hand)
   d. Have client clench and unclench fist several times and then relax hand in a slightly flexed position (hand should look blanched)
   e. Release pressure on ulnar artery and note whether fingers and palm become flushed within 5 seconds (indicates adequate collateral circulation from ulnar artery, making it safe to use radial artery for puncture)
   f. If palm and fingers remain pale, use other extremity for arterial puncture
3. Assist with specimen preparation by preparing heparinized syringe and placing ice in collection bag prior to blood draw; prepare specimen labels
4. Note on laboratory requisition any factors that could affect results, such as body temperature and O_2 or ventilator settings; also mentally note client's activity level in last 20 minutes
5. Explain procedure and provide emotional support during blood draw, which may be uncomfortable

NCLEX®

6. After procedure, immediately apply firm pressure for a full 5 minutes, and longer if client takes drugs that interfere with coagulation (e.g., anticoagulants, aspirin); arrange for specimen to be sent immediately for analysis

II. RESPIRATORY ACIDOSIS

A. Overview

1. In **respiratory acidosis**, CO_2 is retained and pH is decreased (Table 54–2)

NCLEX®

2. Occurs in response to hypoventilation, such as with respiratory depression, inadequate chest expansion, airway obstruction, or interference with alveolar–capillary exchange

B. Nursing assessment

1. See Table 54–2 for clinical manifestations

NCLEX®

2. Diagnostic findings: pH decreased below 7.35, $PaCO_2$ elevated above 45 mmHg, and hyperkalemia

Table 54–2 Overview of Acid–Base Imbalances

Primary Abnormality	Compensation	Common Etiologies	Clinical Manifestations
Respiratory acidosis pH < 7.35 $CO_2 \uparrow > 45$	$HCO_3^- \uparrow$ to raise pH	COPD, sedative or barbiturate overdose, chest wall abnormalities, pneumonia, atelectasis, respiratory muscle weakness, hypoventilation	RR ↑ and shallow to attempt to blow off CO_2, hypotension, heart block, peaked T waves, prolonged PR interval, weak and thready pulse, tachycardia, warm and flushed skin, headache, papilledema, decreased LOC, drowsiness, coma
Respiratory alkalosis pH $\uparrow > 7.45$ $CO_2 \downarrow < 35$	$HCO_3^- \downarrow$ to lower pH	Hyperventilation caused by hypoxia, fever, fear, pain, exercise, anxiety, or pulmonary embolus; mechanical ventilation, septicemia (respiratory center stimulation), brain injury, encephalitis, salicylate poisoning	↑ myocardial irritability, ↑ heart rate, ↑ sensitivity to digitalis preparations, dyspnea, chest tightness, dizziness, anxiety, panic, tetany, seizures, blurred vision
Metabolic acidosis pH $\downarrow < 7.35$ $HCO_3^- \downarrow < 22$	$CO_2 \downarrow$ to raise pH	DKA, lactic acidosis, starvation, severe diarrhea, renal tubule acidosis, renal failure, GI fistulas, shock	Hypotension, dysrhythmias, peripheral vasodilation, cold clammy skin, deep rapid respiratory pattern (Kussmaul respirations), drowsiness, headache, confusion, lethargy, weakness, coma, nausea and vomiting, diarrhea, abdominal pain
Metabolic alkalosis pH $\uparrow > 7.45$ $HCO_3^- \uparrow < 26$	$CO_2 \uparrow$ to lower pH	Severe vomiting, excessive nasogastric suctioning, diuretic therapy, hypokalemia, excess licorice intake, excessive $NaHCO_3$ use, excessive mineralocorticoids	↑ heart rate, dysrhythmias secondary to hypokalemia, hypotension, premature ventricular contractions, atrial tachycardia, hypoventilation, respiratory failure, dizziness, irritability, nervousness, confusion, tremors, muscle cramps, tetany, hyperreflexia, parasthesias in fingers and toes, seizures

3. Compensation
   NCLEX® a. Increased rate and depth of respirations to blow off CO_2
   b. Kidneys eliminate H^+ ions and retain HCO_3^- (urine pH less than 6)
   c. HCO_3^- levels rise when body is compensating for acidosis

C. Collaborative management

1. Treatment is aimed at correcting underlying cause and improving ventilation
2. Use pulmonary hygiene measures to clear respiratory tract of mucus and purulent drainage
3. NCLEX® Provide adequate fluid intake to liquefy secretions
4. NCLEX® If indicated, administer supplemental O_2 cautiously to a client with chronic respiratory acidosis
   a. Note that clients with chronic acidosis have compensated and are adjusted to living with higher $PaCO_2$ levels
   b. Remember that low O_2 level contributes to respiratory drive in these clients
   c. O_2 administration at higher levels can lead to a decreased ventilatory drive and can cause further hypoxia
   d. Low-flow oxygen is expected treatment
   e. Collaborate with healthcare provider and respiratory therapist to manage chronic respiratory disease
5. Mechanical ventilation may be required to improve respiratory status; CO_2 is decreased gradually to prevent alkalosis and seizures from occurring
6. NCLEX® Assess RR and depth
7. NCLEX® Position to facilitate maximum lung expansion (upright as tolerated)
8. NCLEX® Assess apical pulse for tachycardia and irregularities; assess color of skin, nail beds, and mucous membranes
9. NCLEX® Assess LOC
10. Monitor ECG for dysrhythmias
11. Monitor results of ABGs and serum electrolytes, especially potassium
12. Administer medications as prescribed
    a. Bronchodilators to decrease bronchospasm; inhalation medications may be administered by respiratory therapists per agency policy
    b. Antibiotics to treat infections in respiratory tract
    c. Respiratory agents to decrease viscosity of pulmonary secretions, such as acetylcystine (Mucomyst)
    d. Anticoagulants and thrombolytics to prevent or treat pulmonary emboli
    e. Medications are usually administered via IV in acute situations and then changed to oral route as client's condition stabilizes
13. Provide oral hygiene frequently and adequate fluid intake
14. Keep partial side rails up, bed at lowest level, and call bell within client's reach
15. Maintain a calm, quiet environment; if client is confused, orient frequently to person, place, and time
16. Satisfactory outcomes include ABGs improved to client's baseline, decreased anxiety, improved breathing with less effort, freedom from injury, absence of cardiac dysrhythmias, improved LOC, and decreased rate but increased depth of respirations

D. Client education

1. Preventive measures for clients at risk
2. NCLEX® Deep breathing techniques
3. Report signs of infections, shortness of breath, fatigue, and increased pulse rate to healthcare provider

III. RESPIRATORY ALKALOSIS

A. Overview

1. NCLEX® In **respiratory alkalosis**, pH is elevated and $PaCO_2$ is decreased (Table 54–2)
2. Occurs with hyperventilation and leads to a decreased level of CO_2; sometimes called an H_2CO_3 deficit
3. Other causes can include infection, excessive mechanical ventilation, and respiratory center stimulation from fever, salicylate intoxication, and trauma to CNS

B. Nursing assessment

1. NCLEX® See Table 54–2 for clinical manifestations
2. NCLEX® Diagnostic findings: high pH (over 7.45), low $PaCO_2$ (under 35 mmHg), hypokalemia, and hypocalcemia (as pH increases, calcium binding occurs in plasma and calcium levels decrease)
3. Compensation
   a. Kidneys conserve H^+ and excrete HCO_3^- (urine pH greater than 6)
   b. Low HCO_3^- indicates body is attempting to compensate

C. Collaborative management

1. Treat underlying cause
2. Assist client to breathe more slowly; if needed, have client rebreathe CO_2 by using a rebreather mask or a paper bag
3. NCLEX® Give oxygen therapy if client is hypoxic
4. Medicate as needed with anti-anxiety drugs or sedatives to control hyperventilation associated with anxiety
5. NCLEX® Monitor VS and ABGs, protect from injury, and provide support and reassurance
6. NCLEX® Satisfactory outcomes include decreased RR, absence of numbness and tingling in extremities, return of ABGs to normal or client's baseline, and diminished anxiety; additionally, client remains free from injury

D. Client education

1. Relaxation techniques
2. Benefits of stress management classes as indicated
3. NCLEX® Keep aspirin and other salicylates out of reach of children and follow current poison control guidelines if exposure occurs

IV. METABOLIC ACIDOSIS

A. Overview

1. In **metabolic acidosis**, pH decreases and HCO_3^- decreases (see Table 54–2)
2. NCLEX® Occurs when there is a loss of HCO_3^- or when acids other than carbonic acid (H_2CO_3) accumulate in ECF
3. Rarely occurs spontaneously; is accompanied by other problems, such as gastrointestinal (GI) conditions (starvation, malnutrition, and chronic diarrhea), renal (kidney failure), diabetic ketoacidosis (DKA), hyperthyroidism, trauma, shock, increased exercise, severe infection, and fever

B. Nursing assessment

1. NCLEX® See Table 54–2 for clinical manifestations

Memory Aid

Acidosis of any origin tends to be a CNS depressant.

2. NCLEX® Diagnostic findings
   - **a.** pH less than 7.35, HCO_3^- less than 22 mEq/L, and hyperkalemia frequently seen
   - **b.** ECG may show tall, tented T-wave changes related to high K^+ levels
   - **c.** AG calculation increases and BE decreases
3. Compensation
   - **a.** Lungs eliminate CO_2; kidneys conserve HCO_3^-
   - **b.** Urine pH less than 6
   - **c.** $PaCO_2$ decreases when compensation is occurring

C. Collaborative management

1. Treatment is aimed at correcting underlying problem
2. Provide hydration to restore water, nutrients, and electrolytes
3. Alkalotic IV solution (sodium bicarbonate or sodium lactate) may be indicated to correct acidosis
4. Mechanical ventilation is used only if other treatment modalities are ineffective
5. Monitor ABGs, serum electrolytes, and ECG (for conduction problems)
6. NCLEX® Monitor VS (especially RR and depth), I&O, daily weights, LOC, and GI function
7. NCLEX® Protect from injury
8. NCLEX® Administer IV fluids and medications as prescribed, based on underlying cause
   - **a.** If cause is secondary to DKA, implement hydration with normal saline, regular insulin, and possibly potassium
   - **b.** If diarrhea is cause, treat with hydration and antidiarrheal agents
   - **c.** Administer $NaHCO_3$ cautiously and only when HCO_3^- levels are very low (below 16–18 mEq/L); can cause metabolic alkalosis and hypokalemia; titrate closely to avoid further acid–base imbalances
9. Satisfactory outcomes: client is free from injury and has no dysrhythmias, ABGs return to normal, fluid volume deficits are corrected, LOC returns to normal, and GI upset is relieved

D. Client education

1. Seek healthcare for prolonged diarrhea
2. Importance of preventing occurrences of DKA (for clients with diabetes) and how to manage DKA should it occur

V. METABOLIC ALKALOSIS

A. Overview

1. In **metabolic alkalosis**, there is an increased pH and increased HCO_3^- (see Table 54–2)

NCLEX®

2. Occurs when there is a loss of H^+ ions (e.g., because of vomiting or nasogastric suctioning) or an increase in HCO_3^- level (such as with ingestion of bicarbonate-based antacids)

B. Nursing assessment

1. See Table 54–2 for clinical manifestations

Memory Aid

Alkalosis of any origin tends to have an excitatory effect on the CNS.

NCLEX®

2. Diagnostic findings
   a. pH greater than 7.45 and HCO_3^- above 26 mEq/L; BE increases
   b. Hypokalemia, hypocalcemia (as pH increases, Ca^{++} binding occurs and serum Ca^{++} levels decrease), hyponatremia, and hypochloremia
   c. Urine chloride levels reveal whether client is chloride responsive (under 10 mEq/L) or chloride resistant (over 10 mEq/L)
3. Compensation
   a. Lungs retain CO_2; kidneys conserve H^+ and excrete HCO_3^-
   b. $PaCO_2$ increases with compensation
   c. Urine pH greater than 6

C. Collaborative management

1. Treatment aimed at correcting underlying problem
2. Provide sufficient Cl^- to enhance renal absorption of Na^+ and excretion of HCO_3^-
3. Restore normal fluid balance and monitor I&O

NCLEX®

4. Assess LOC and VS, especially RR and depth
5. Administer medication and IV fluids as ordered
   a. Normal saline-based IV fluid replacement
   b. Potassium supplementation if hypokalemic
   c. Histamine-2 receptor antagonists such as famotidine to reduce secretion of H^+ ions and loss of H^+ ions from GI drainage
   d. If client is chloride responsive, administer acetazolamide to increase renal bicarbonate excretion
   e. If client is chloride resistant, then correct K^+ and Mg^{++} deficits with appropriate supplementation

NCLEX®

6. Protect from injury
7. Monitor ECG for conduction abnormalities
8. Monitor results of ABGs and serum electrolytes
9. Satisfactory outcomes: client is free from injury, ABGs return to normal, hypertension is corrected, electrolytes are restored to normal, cardiac conduction is normal, and client states ways to prevent reoccurrence

D. Client education

1. Take antacids correctly to prevent excessive dosing
2. Signs and symptoms to report to healthcare provider for those at risk, especially older adults
3. Signs and symptoms of hypokalemia to report to healthcare provider

VI. MIXED ACID–BASE DISORDERS

A. Identification and treatment of primary disorder

1. A **mixed acid–base disorder** occurs when two or more independent acid–base disorders occur at same time
2. pH depends on type and severity of each simple disorder

3. Respiratory acidosis and alkalosis cannot occur concurrently; it is impossible to have hyperventilation and hypoventilation at same time
4. Treatment is aimed at correcting underlying cause of each disorder
5. When identifying acid–base imbalances, mathematical formulas can be used to assess degree of expected compensation
6. AG and urine pH values will also help determine which imbalance is occurring

B. Chronic and superimposed acid–base disturbances

1. Mixed metabolic acidosis and respiratory acidosis
   a. Clients with acute pulmonary edema
   b. Clients with cardiac arrest as a result of buildup of lactic acidosis and CO_2 retention due to inadequate ventilation
   NCLEX® c. pH values decrease and are more pronounced because of decreasing HCO_3^- level coupled with increasing CO_2 level
2. Mixed metabolic alkalosis and respiratory acidosis
   NCLEX® a. Clients with chronic obstructive pulmonary disease (COPD) and who have treatment with potassium-wasting diuretics, severe vomiting, or development of diarrhea
   b. Clients with COPD who have a quick improvement in ventilation
   c. pH values tend to become balanced because of an increase in both HCO_3^- and $PaCO_2$ values
3. Mixed metabolic acidosis with respiratory alkalosis
   a. Clients with a rapid correction of metabolic acidosis
   NCLEX® b. Clients with salicylate intoxication
   c. Clients with Gram-negative septicemia
   d. pH values tend to become balanced because of decreases in both HCO_3^- and $PaCO_2$
4. Mixed metabolic alkalosis and respiratory alkalosis
   a. Postoperative clients with severe hemorrhage
   b. Clients who have massive transfusions
   c. Clients with excessive nasogastric (NG) drainage
   d. pH values increase and are more pronounced because of increasing HCO_3^- coupled with decreasing CO_2 levels
5. Mixed metabolic acidosis and metabolic alkalosis
   NCLEX® a. Seen in clients with gastroenteritis, vomiting, and diarrhea
   b. If imbalance is present in same proportion, there is usually no change in values (pH, HCO_3^-, and $PaCO_2$) even though there is volume depletion
6. Chronic and acute respiratory acidosis
   NCLEX® a. Chronic respiratory conditions with an acute condition superimposed can lead to increased $PaCO_2$ levels, causing further pulmonary dysfunction and leading to serious consequences that can compromise both treatment and expected response to treatment
   b. Clients with both a chronic and a superimposed acute respiratory acid–base imbalance should be closely monitored by a pulmonologist
   c. Respiratory therapist should be part of collaborative healthcare team plan during client's treatment

C. Collaborative management

1. Treatment focuses on correcting underlying causes of disorder
2. Mixed disorders must be treated before acid–base balance can be restored
3. A collaborative team approach (including a pulmonologist, respiratory therapist, nurses, and dietitian) is needed to assist client in restoring acid–base balance, increasing activity tolerance, and improving physiological function
4. *NCLEX®* Monitor VS, LOC, and oxygen saturation
5. Monitor ABGs, pulmonary function tests, CXR, ECG, hemoglobin and hematocrit, and electrolytes
6. *NCLEX®* Protect from injury
7. Ensure adequate fluid intake
8. *NCLEX®* Implement therapeutic measures such as O_2 therapy and medications to resolve underlying causes of imbalances
9. Satisfactory outcomes: client remains free from injury, ABGs return to normal or baseline, cardiac conduction is normal, fluid balance and electrolyte levels are restored, LOC is improved, and client is able to report ways to prevent problem from recurring

D. Client education

1. Clients with chronic respiratory conditions should report exacerbations to healthcare provider

2. Clients who experience fluid losses through emesis or diarrhea are at increased risk for acid–base imbalance and should notify healthcare provider if condition is not self-limiting (lasts more than 2 or 3 days)
3. Clients with diabetes are at risk for metabolic acidosis due to high glucose levels and should closely monitor serum glucose and use measures to maintain euglycemia
4. Clients who have renal problems are prone to develop acid–base imbalance due to alterations in electrolyte levels; closely monitor renal status to identify potential disturbances and allow for intervention

Check Your NCLEX–RN® Exam I.Q.

You are ready for testing on this content if you can:

- Use knowledge from the biological and physical sciences to assess acid–base status.
- Apply concepts of pathophysiology to acid–base imbalances.
- Identify signs and symptoms of acid–base imbalances.
- Describe interventions to treat acid–base imbalances.
- Evaluate the client's response to treatments for acid–base imbalances.

PRACTICE TEST

1 A client has been admitted for dehydration after fasting for 5 days. For which acid–base imbalance should the nurse assess this client?

1. Metabolic acidosis
2. Metabolic alkalosis
3. Respiratory acidosis
4. Respiratory alkalosis

2 A client is admitted to the hospital after vomiting for 3 days. What arterial blood gas (ABG) results should the nurse expect?

1. pH 7.30; $PaCO_2$ 50; HCO_3^- 27
2. pH 7.47; $PaCO_2$ 43; HCO_3^- 28
3. pH 7.34; $PaCO_2$ 50; HCO_3^- 28
4. pH 7.48; $PaCO_2$ 30; HCO_3^- 23

3 A client is admitted to the hospital with a diagnosis of respiratory acidosis secondary to overdose of barbiturates. Which assessment findings would the nurse anticipate? Select all that apply.

1. Slow, shallow respirations
2. Tetany symptoms
3. Increased deep tendon reflexes
4. Palpitations
5. Headache

4 A client is admitted with a diagnosis of renal failure. What arterial blood gas (ABG) result should the nurse expect to see with this client?

1. pH 7.49; $PaCO_2$ 36; HCO_3^- 30
2. pH 7.30; $PaCO_2$ 35; HCO_3^- 18
3. pH 7.31; $PaCO_2$ 50; HCO_3^- 23
4. pH 7.43; $PaCO_2$ 48; HCO_3^- 30

5 A client is admitted to the hospital with atelectasis and reports of chest pain. For which acid–base imbalance should the nurse assess this client?

1. Respiratory alkalosis
2. Metabolic acidosis
3. Metabolic alkalosis
4. Respiratory acidosis

6 A client is admitted to the hospital with respiratory acidosis. The nurse considers that which condition could be an etiology for this state? Select all that apply.

1. Severe diarrhea for several days
2. Diabetic ketoacidosis
3. Obesity
4. Diuretics
5. Sedative overdose

7 The nurse should assess for which signs and symptoms in a client who has metabolic acidosis? Select all that apply.

1. Weight gain
2. Rapid, deep respirations
3. Drowsiness
4. Decreased respiratory rate and depth
5. Melena

8 Which client medication should the nurse review first for its potential interaction in a client admitted to the hospital in a state of alkalosis?

1. Warfarin
2. Metformin
3. Digoxin
4. Ibuprofen

9 A client is admitted to the hospital with sudden onset of severe abdominal pain. Which arterial blood gas (ABG) value should the nurse expect to see with this client?

1. $PaCO_2$ 48
2. HCO_3^- 18
3. pH 7.32
4. SaO_2 90

10 A client is admitted to the hospital with an acid–base imbalance. Arterial blood gas (ABG) results are pH 7.33; $PaCO_2$ 49; HCO_3^- 28. How should the nurse interpret these results?

1. Respiratory acidosis, uncompensated
2. Metabolic alkalosis, uncompensated
3. Partially compensated respiratory acidosis
4. Partially compensated metabolic acidosis

11 A client is admitted to the hospital with numerous episodes of muscle weakness and twitching. Arterial blood gas (ABG) results are pH 7.44; $PaCO_2$ 49; HCO_3^- 30. How should the nurse interpret these findings?

1. Uncompensated metabolic acidosis
2. Compensated respiratory alkalosis
3. Uncompensated respiratory alkalosis
4. Compensated metabolic alkalosis

12 The nurse should suspect that a client who frequently uses which medication is at risk for developing metabolic alkalosis?

1. Calcium carbonate
2. Ibuprofen
3. Aspirin
4. Acetaminophen

13 The nurse is admitting a client who has metabolic alkalosis. The nurse plans to assess for manifestations of which electrolyte imbalance? Select all that apply.

1. Hypernatremia
2. Hypochloremia
3. Hypermagnesemia
4. Hypocalcemia
5. Hypokalemia

14 A client's arterial blood gas (ABG) results are pH 7.48; $PaCO_2$ 30; HCO_3^- 23. How should the nurse interpret these results?

1. Compensated respiratory alkalosis
2. Uncompensated metabolic alkalosis
3. Uncompensated respiratory alkalosis
4. Compensated metabolic alkalosis

15 The nurse determines that a client with a nasogastric tube on low suction for 5 days is at risk for developing which acid–base imbalance?

1. Respiratory acidosis
2. Metabolic alkalosis
3. Metabolic acidosis
4. Respiratory alkalosis

16 The following arterial blood gas (ABG) results are on the client's chart: pH 7.50; $PaCO_2$ 36; HCO_3^- 30. How should the nurse interpret this report?

1. Partially compensated metabolic alkalosis
2. Compensated respiratory alkalosis
3. Uncompensated metabolic alkalosis
4. Uncompensated respiratory alkalosis

17 A client admitted to the hospital has these arterial blood gas (ABG) results: pH 7.50; $PaCO_2$ 40; HCO_3^- 29. Which question should the nurse ask the client to help determine an etiology for these results?

1. "Have you had diarrhea lately?"
2. "Do you have a history of COPD?"
3. "How long have you had nausea and vomiting?"
4. "Do you smoke?"

18 A client's arterial blood gas (ABG) results are pH 7.36; $PaCO_2$ 50; HCO_3^- 28. What should these results indicate to the nurse?

1. Compensated respiratory acidosis
2. Compensated metabolic acidosis
3. Uncompensated metabolic acidosis
4. Uncompensated respiratory acidosis

19 Which statement by the client indicates that discharge teaching for respiratory alkalosis is understood?

1. "I will not take so many antacids anymore."
2. "I will take a stress management class."
3. "I will not take my furosemide without taking my potassium supplement."
4. "I will tell the doctor the next time I have diarrhea for so long."
5. "I am more aware of how my breathing changes when I get nervous."

20 A client is admitted with severe diarrhea. Arterial blood gas (ABG) results are pH 7.33; $PaCO_2$ 42; HCO_3^- 20. The nurse concludes this client has which acid–base imbalance?

1. Uncompensated metabolic acidosis
2. Compensated respiratory acidosis
3. Compensated metabolic acidosis
4. Uncompensated respiratory acidosis

ANSWERS & RATIONALES

1 **Answer: 1 Rationale:** A prolonged fasting state can lead to dehydration. During fasting, the body reverts to cellular breakdown to maintain energy, and lactic and pyruvic acids build up in the body. This accumulation of acids leads to the development of metabolic acidosis. Metabolic and respiratory alkalosis are incorrect because alkalosis would not occur. Respiratory acidosis is incorrect because the primary disturbance is not respiratory. **Cognitive Level:** Applying **Client Need:** Physiological Adaptation **Integrated Process:** Nursing Process: Assessment **Content Area:** Adult Health: Endocrine and Metabolic **Strategy:** Note the critical word *fasting* that indicates this is a metabolic rather than respiratory problem, which eliminates respiratory acidosis and alkalosis. Choose metabolic acidosis because metabolic by-products are acidic in nature, not alkaline.

2 **Answer: 2 Rationale:** Vomiting leads to the loss of hydrochloric acid from gastric acids. Hydrogen ions must leave the blood to replace this acidity in the stomach. Metabolic alkalosis occurs and is reflected by elevated pH and HCO_3^- and normal $PaCO_2$. The ABG with the pH of 7.30 is incorrect because it reflects respiratory acidosis with partial compensation (decreased pH and elevated $PaCO_2$ and HCO_3^-). The ABG with the pH of 7.34 is incorrect because it reflects a mixed acid–base imbalance (metabolic alkalosis with respiratory acidosis) with a normal pH and elevated $PaCO_2$ and HCO_3^-. The ABG with the pH of 7.48 is incorrect because it reflects respiratory alkalosis (increased pH, decreased $PaCO_2$, and normal HCO_3^-). **Cognitive Level:** Applying **Client Need:** Physiological Adaptation **Integrated Process:** Nursing Process: Assessment **Content Area:** Adult Health: Endocrine and Metabolic **Strategy:** Note the critical word *vomiting*, and recall that stomach contents are rich in acid. Loss of acid would raise the pH (eliminating options with pH of 7.30 and 7.34) and lead to increased free circulating HCO_3^-, eliminating the ABG with the pH of 7.48.

3 **Answer: 1, 5 Rationale:** Clients with respiratory acidosis from ingestion of barbiturates would have slow and shallow respirations, leading to hypoventilation. Headache is associated with respiratory acidosis because the increased CO_2 level causes cerebral vasodilation, which leads to headache. Tetany symptoms, increased deep tendon reflexes, and palpitations are associated with respiratory alkalosis. **Cognitive Level:** Applying **Client Need:** Physiological Adaptation **Integrated Process:** Nursing Process: Assessment **Content Area:** Adult Health: Endocrine and Metabolic **Strategy:** Recall that barbiturates are central nervous system (CNS) depressants, while palpitations, tetany, and increased deep tendon reflexes indicate CNS excitation. Choose slow shallow respirations as consistent with CNS depression, and choose headache because of the dilating effect of retained CO_2 on cerebral blood vessels.

4 **Answer: 2 Rationale:** Clients with renal failure have difficulty synthesizing HCO_3^- in the renal tubules secondary to the renal failure. These clients also retain K+ and subsequently develop metabolic acidosis. The ABG with the pH of 7.30 reflects uncompensated metabolic acidosis. The ABG with the pH of 7.49 is incorrect because it reflects metabolic alkalosis (increased pH and HCO_3^-) and normal $PaCO_2$. The

ABG with the pH of 7.31 is incorrect because it reflects respiratory acidosis (decreased pH, increased $PaCO_2$) and normal HCO_3^-. The ABG with the pH of 7.43 is incorrect because it reflects a mixed acid–base imbalance metabolic alkalosis with a respiratory acidosis (normal pH and increased $PaCO_2$ and HCO_3^-). **Cognitive Level:** Applying **Client Need:** Physiological Adaptation **Integrated Process:** Nursing Process: Assessment **Content Area:** Adult Health: Endocrine and Metabolic **Strategy:** First, recognize renal failure as a metabolic condition in which there is an impaired ability to eliminate metabolic acids and wastes, leading to acidosis. With this in mind, eliminate options that have elevated or normal pH. Then choose the option with the HCO_3^- of 18 rather than 23 because 18 is low while 23 is normal.

5 **Answer: 4 Rationale:** A client with atelectasis has collapsed alveoli that retain CO_2, which can lead to respiratory acidosis. The client most likely would have hypoventilation as a respiratory pattern, which would further contribute to the development of respiratory acidosis. Respiratory and metabolic alkalosis are incorrect because the client would not be in an alkalotic state. Metabolic acidosis is incorrect because the primary disturbance is respiratory. **Cognitive Level:** Applying **Client Need:** Physiological Adaptation **Integrated Process:** Nursing Process: Assessment **Content Area:** Adult Health: Endocrine and Metabolic **Strategy:** The critical word in the stem of the question is *atelectasis*. Recall that this term is associated with respiratory problems to eliminate options referring to metabolic disorders. Choose respiratory acidosis over alkalosis, recalling that CO_2 retention characterizes many respiratory conditions, leading to acidosis (since CO_2 acts as an acid in the body).

6 **Answer: 3, 5 Rationale:** Obesity can lead to chest wall abnormalities and hypoventilation, which can lead to respiratory acidosis. Sedative overdose depresses the central nervous system, which leads to hypoventilation and respiratory acidosis. Prolonged diarrhea can lead to the development of metabolic acidosis. DKA leads to the development of metabolic acidosis. Diuretic administration leads to the development of metabolic alkalosis. **Cognitive Level:** Analyzing **Client Need:** Physiological Adaptation **Integrated Process:** Nursing Process: Diagnosis **Content Area:** Adult Health: Endocrine and Metabolic **Strategy:** Note the term *respiratory acidosis* in the stem of the question. First, evaluate each option to determine whether it would lead to acidosis and alkalosis. Then, differentiate between respiratory and metabolic acidosis to choose correctly. Note the wording of the question suggests that more than one option is correct.

7 **Answer: 2, 3 Rationale:** Clients who have metabolic acidosis develop Kussmaul's breathing (rapid and deep respirations). Drowsiness occurs because of the CNS depressant effect of acidosis. Weight gain is not an associated finding with metabolic acidosis. Shallow breathing is associated with the development of metabolic alkalosis. Melena (blood in stool) is not associated with metabolic acidosis. **Cognitive Level:** Applying **Client Need:** Physiological Adaptation **Integrated Process:** Nursing Process: Diagnosis **Content Area:** Adult Health: Endocrine and Metabolic **Strategy:** The critical words in the stem of the question are *metabolic acidosis*. Recall that in metabolic abnormalities, the respiratory system helps to compensate; this will help to eliminate weight gain and melena. Choose rapid breathing over slower shallower breathing because this option assists the body to "blow off" acid in the form of CO_2. Finally, choose drowsiness, recalling that acidosis causes CNS depression, whereas alkalosis causes CNS excitation.

8 **Answer: 3 Rationale:** Alkalosis, especially respiratory alkalosis, makes the client more sensitive to the effects of digoxin; toxicity can develop even at therapeutic levels. A serum digoxin level should be obtained, and the client evaluated for potential digoxin toxicity. Warfarin affects clotting factors. Metformin can cause the development of lactic acidosis. Ibuprofen can cause gastric irritation. **Cognitive Level:** Applying **Client Need:** Physiological Adaptation **Integrated Process:** Nursing Process: Planning **Content Area:** Adult Health: Endocrine and Metabolic **Strategy:** Specific knowledge of medications that are affected by alkalosis is needed to answer this question. Use nursing knowledge and the process of elimination to make your selection.

9 **Answer: 2 Rationale:** Acute pain usually leads to hyperventilation, which causes CO_2 to be blown off, leading to an increased pH and decreased CO_2 level. If the client has not compensated, the bicarbonate level will be normal. If the client is compensating, then the bicarbonate level will decrease in an attempt to restore the pH. A $PaCO_2$ of 48 is incorrect because it reflects a slight elevation; if the client were in severe pain, the level would likely be lower as the client would have increased respirations. A pH of 7.32 is incorrect because the pH is slightly acidotic. An SaO_2 of 90 is incorrect because the oxygen saturation should be within normal limits. **Cognitive Level:** Analyzing **Client Need:** Physiological Adaptation **Integrated Process:** Nursing Process: Assessment **Content Area:** Adult Health: Endocrine and Metabolic **Strategy:** Visualize a picture of the client in pain. This person is most likely to have an increased respiratory rate, which blows off CO_2 and decreases the bicarbonate level as a compensatory mechanism. This will help you to easily choose the correct option.

10 **Answer: 3 Rationale:** The pH is low, indicating acidosis; the $PaCO_2$ is elevated, indicating a respiratory basis; and the HCO_3^- is elevated, indicating that compensatory mechanisms are partially working. Uncompensated respiratory acidosis is incorrect because compensation is taking place due to increased HCO_3^- level. Uncompensated metabolic alkalosis is incorrect because the client is not alkalotic. Partially compensated metabolic acidosis is incorrect because the primary disturbance is respiratory. The change in the $PaCO_2$ level is greater than the change in the HCO_3^- level, which indicates a respiratory disturbance. **Cognitive Level:** Analyzing **Client Need:** Physiological Adaptation **Integrated Process:** Nursing Process: Diagnosis **Content Area:** Adult Health: Endocrine and Metabolic **Strategy:** First, eliminate the option with alkalosis because the pH of 7.33 indicates acidosis. Next, note that both the CO_2 and HCO_3^- levels are abnormal, indicating that the body is attempting to compensate (eliminating uncompensated). Choose correctly from the remaining options, noting the elevated CO_2 "matches" a respiratory acidosis and the HCO_3^- (an alkaline substance) is rising to try to compensate.

11 **Answer: 4 Rationale:** The pH is just below the high limit and the HCO_3^- is elevated, indicating a metabolic problem. The $PaCO_2$ is elevated, indicating compensation, so the correct interpretation is compensated respiratory alkalosis. Uncompensated metabolic acidosis is incorrect because the client is not acidotic. Compensated respiratory alkalosis is incorrect because the CO_2 would be decreased rather than elevated. Uncompensated respiratory alkalosis is incorrect

because the primary disturbance is metabolic and the CO_2 is elevated rather than decreased. **Cognitive Level:** Analyzing **Client Need:** Physiological Adaptation **Integrated Process:** Nursing Process: Diagnosis **Content Area:** Adult Health: Endocrine and Metabolic **Strategy:** Note that the pH is within normal range, which indicates that the condition is compensated, thus eliminating acidosis options. Note the high HCO_3^- is a metabolic indicator (not respiratory), and is consistent with a pH near the high end of normal, to help you choose the compensated respiratory alkalosis option.

12 **Answer: 1 Rationale:** Excessive use of oral antacids can lead to metabolic alkalosis. Use of ibuprofen and acetaminophen is not associated with the development of metabolic alkalosis. Overdoses of aspirin can be associated with the development of respiratory alkalosis, and eventually can lead to metabolic acidosis. **Cognitive Level:** Applying **Client Need:** Physiological Adaptation **Integrated Process:** Nursing Process: Assessment **Content Area:** Adult Health: Endocrine and Metabolic **Strategy:** Knowledge of medication side effects is needed to answer this question. First, eliminate ibuprofen and acetaminophen because they are similar (nonopioid analgesics). Then, eliminate aspirin because acid would not lead to alkalosis. Alternatively, recall that calcium carbonate is an antacid, which in excess could lead to metabolic alkalosis.

13 **Answer: 2, 4, 5 Rationale:** Clinical manifestations of metabolic alkalosis are associated with the presence of tetany-like symptoms. Clients should be monitored for the presence of these symptoms because they usually correlate with low levels of calcium. Hyponatremia (not hypernatremia), hypochloremia, and hypokalemia can occur with metabolic alkalosis. Hypomagnesemia (not hypermagnesemia) can occur with hypocalcemia. **Cognitive Level:** Applying **Client Need:** Physiological Adaptation **Integrated Process:** Teaching and Learning **Content Area:** Adult Health: Endocrine and Metabolic **Strategy:** Specific knowledge of the association between metabolic alkalosis and various electrolytes is needed to answer this question. Use nursing knowledge and the process of elimination to make your selection.

14 **Answer: 3 Rationale:** The client's pH is high, indicating alkalosis. The $PaCO_2$ is abnormal, indicating a respiratory basis. The HCO_3^- is normal, indicating that compensation has not started. Compensated respiratory alkalosis is incorrect because the HCO_3^- level would decrease with compensation. Uncompensated metabolic alkalosis is incorrect because the primary disturbance is respiratory, as indicated by the decrease in the CO_2 parameter. Compensated metabolic alkalosis is incorrect because the primary disturbance is respiratory, as indicated by the decrease in the CO_2 parameter. **Cognitive Level:** Analyzing **Client Need:** Physiological Adaptation **Integrated Process:** Nursing Process: Diagnosis **Content Area:** Adult Health: Endocrine and Metabolic **Strategy:** Note that the pH is high, so the condition is not compensated, eliminating compensated states. Choose respiratory because a low CO_2 correlates with a high pH, whereas HCO_3^- at the lower end of the normal range does not correlate with a high pH.

15 **Answer: 2 Rationale:** A client who has prolonged nasogastric suction is apt to have higher levels of bicarbonate because of hydrogen ion loss. Bicarbonate excess leads to a metabolic disturbance and the development of metabolic alkalosis. Respiratory and metabolic acidosis are incorrect because the client will not experience acidosis. Respiratory alkalosis is incorrect because the primary disturbance is caused by retained levels of bicarbonate (not elimination of carbon dioxide) in the body. **Cognitive Level:** Applying **Client Need:** Physiological Adaptation **Integrated Process:** Nursing Process: Diagnosis **Content Area:** Adult Health: Endocrine and Metabolic **Strategy:** Eliminate respiratory imbalances first because nasogastric suction is a metabolic problem. Choose alkalosis, recalling that pancreatic juices are rich in bicarbonate and are not neutralized because the nasogastric suction eliminates hydrochloric acid that would neutralize the alkaline pancreatic secretions.

16 **Answer: 3 Rationale:** The pH indicates alkalosis; HCO_3^- is high, indicating a metabolic origin, and the $PaCO_2$ is normal, which indicates that compensation has not taken place. Partially compensated metabolic acidosis is incorrect because with compensation, the $PaCO_2$ level would be increased. Compensated and uncompensated respiratory alkalosis options are incorrect because the primary disturbance is metabolic, as reflected by the increased bicarbonate level. **Cognitive Level:** Analyzing **Client Need:** Physiological Adaptation **Integrated Process:** Nursing Process: Diagnosis **Content Area:** Adult Health: Endocrine and Metabolic **Strategy:** First, note that the pH is high, and so the imbalance cannot be compensated. Then note that HCO_3^- is the abnormally high value (not CO_2), so the imbalance must be metabolic rather than respiratory. Choose uncompensated over compensated metabolic alkalosis because the CO_2 (normally 35–45) has made no attempt to rise to compensate for the high HCO_3^-.

17 **Answer: 3 Rationale:** ABG results reflect elevated pH, indicating alkalosis, and normal $PaCO_2$ and an increased HCO_3^-, indicating metabolic alkalosis. Vomiting is a common cause of this condition. The presence of diarrhea is associated with metabolic acidosis. COPD is associated with respiratory acidosis. Smoking can be associated with respiratory acidosis if it leads to respiratory disease. **Cognitive Level:** Analyzing **Client Need:** Physiological Adaptation **Integrated Process:** Nursing Process: Assessment **Content Area:** Adult Health: Endocrine and Metabolic **Strategy:** An ability to interpret ABGs and specific knowledge of manifestations of metabolic alkalosis are needed to answer this question. Use nursing knowledge and the process of elimination to make your selection.

18 **Answer: 1 Rationale:** The pH is just within normal range, so the blood gas results are either normal or compensated. However, the $PaCO_2$ is high, indicating a respiratory problem, and thus the ABGs cannot be normal. The HCO_3^- is also high, which along with a normal pH indicates complete compensation. The metabolic acidosis options (compensated or uncompensated) are incorrect because the primary disturbance is respiratory, as reflected by the correlation between an elevated $PaCO_2$ and a pH toward the low end of normal. Uncompensated respiratory acidosis is incorrect because the HCO_3^- level would be normal if no compensation is taking place. **Cognitive Level:** Analyzing **Client Need:** Physiological Adaptation **Integrated Process:** Nursing Process: Assessment **Content Area:** Adult Health: Endocrine and Metabolic **Strategy:** Because the pH is within normal range, eliminate the uncompensated options. Choose respiratory over metabolic acidosis because the pH is near the acidic end of the range and the high CO_2 correlates with acidosis, whereas a high HCO_3^- would correlate with an alkalotic state.

19 **Answer: 2, 5 Rationale:** Respiratory alkalosis is caused by hyperventilation, which can be caused by stress and anxiety, as examples. It is important that clients who are prone to develop respiratory alkalosis be aware of how to manage causative factors. Antacids and diuretics are associated with metabolic alkalosis. Diarrhea is associated with metabolic acidosis. **Cognitive Level:** Analyzing **Client Need:** Physiological Adaptation **Integrated Process:** Teaching and Learning **Content Area:** Adult Health: Endocrine and Metabolic **Strategy:** The critical word in the question is *respiratory*. Eliminate each of the incorrect options that would correlate better with a metabolic condition than with a respiratory one. Alternatively, consider that a common cause of respiratory alkalosis is hyperventilation, which is often caused by anxiety, and managed with stress management.

20 **Answer: 1 Rationale:** The pH and HCO_3^- are decreased, indicating metabolic acidosis. The $PaCO_2$ is normal, indicating that compensatory mechanisms have not started working. Compensated or uncompensated respiratory acidosis is incorrect because the primary disturbance is metabolic, as indicated by the low bicarbonate level. Compensated metabolic acidosis is incorrect because with compensation, a decrease in $PaCO_2$ to restore balance would be expected. **Cognitive Level:** Analyzing **Client Need:** Physiological Adaptation **Integrated Process:** Nursing Process: Diagnosis **Content Area:** Adult Health: Endocrine and Metabolic **Strategy:** First, correlate diarrhea with a metabolic problem to eliminate compensated respiratory acidosis and uncompensated respiratory acidosis. Then, note that the pH is not within normal limits to choose uncompensated metabolic acidosis over compensated metabolic acidosis.

Key Terms to Review

acid p. 877
base p. 877
buffer p. 877
compensation p.878
HCO_3^- p. 877
metabolic acidosis p. 883
metabolic alkalosis p. 884
mixed acid–base disorder p. 884
$PaCO_2$ p. 878
PaO_2 p. 879
pH p. 877
respiratory acidosis p. 881
respiratory alkalosis p. 882
SaO_2 p. 879

References

Berman, A., Snyder, S., & Frandsen, G. (2016). *Kozier & Erb's fundamentals of nursing: Concepts, process, and practice* (10th ed.). New York, NY: Pearson Education.

Ignatavicius, D., & Workman, L. (2016). *Medical-surgical nursing: Patient-centered collaborative care* (10th ed.). Philadelphia: Saunders.

Kee, J. (2017). *Pearson's handbook of laboratory and diagnostic tests* (8th ed.). New York, NY: Pearson Education.

LeMone, P., Burke, K., Bauldoff, G., & Gubrud, P. (2015). *Medical surgical nursing: Clinical reasoning in patient care* (6th ed.). Hoboken, NJ: Pearson Education.

Lewis, S., Dirksen, S., Heitkemper, M., & Bucher, L. (2014). *Medical surgical nursing: Assessment and management of clinical problems* (9th ed.). St. Louis, MO: Elsevier Science.

Smith, S., Duell, D., Martin, B., Aebersold, M., & Gonzalez, L. (2017). *Clinical nursing skills: Basic to advanced skills* (10th ed.). New York, NY: Pearson Education.

55 Respiratory Disorders

In this chapter

Cross Reference

Other chapters relevant to this content area are

I. OVERVIEW OF ANATOMY AND PHYSIOLOGY

A. Respiratory system structures

1. Upper respiratory tract (conducting airways): nose (filters, humidifies, and heats inspired air), paranasal sinuses (contribute to mucus production and voice resonance), pharynx (air and food passage, immune function of adenoids), larynx (vocal cords for speech and epiglottis for closure of trachea during swallowing), and epiglottis (prevents food and liquids from entering trachea)
2. Lower respiratory tract (conducting airways and gas exchange airways): trachea (connects upper and lower respiratory tract), right and left mainstem bronchi, bronchioles, alveolar ducts, and alveoli (basic units of gas exchange), lungs (lined with visceral pleura and located within pleural cavity lined with parietal pleura)
3. Accessory structures (contribute to breathing mechanics and/or provide support and protection): rib cage (12 pairs of ribs and sternum), intercostal muscles (located between ribs), and diaphragm (flattens/contracts during inspiration via phrenic nerve to enhance chest expansion)

B. Respiratory system functions

1. Primary function is gas exchange; **respiration** (process of O_2 and CO_2 exchange) involves ventilation, perfusion, diffusion, and nervous system control
2. Secondary functions: assist with smell; aid in maintaining temperature, fluid, and acid–base balance (through exhaled air); form speech
3. Ventilation: passage of gases between atmosphere and lungs during inspiration and expiration; adequacy is influenced by tissue properties, airway resistance, body position, disease processes, lung compliance, and lung volumes and capacities (see Box 55–1)
   a. **Pulmonary ventilation**: total volume of gas exchange between atmosphere and lungs
   b. **Alveolar ventilation**: volume of air that undergoes gas exchange
4. **Perfusion**: blood flow through pulmonary capillary bed in pulmonary and bronchial circulation to respiratory system structures
5. **Diffusion**: movement of air and O_2 from atmosphere into alveoli; O_2 crosses into pulmonary capillaries; CO_2 diffuses out of pulmonary capillaries into alveoli
   a. Variables that influence gas exchange (see Table 55–1)
   b. Ventilation–perfusion relationship: adequate gas exchange requires alveolar ventilation of about 4 L/min balanced with alveolar capillary perfusion of about 5 L/min (see Figure 55–1); normal ventilation–perfusion (V/Q) ratio: 4:5
6. Nervous system control of breathing: initiates within medulla oblongata (inspiration, expiration, breathing pattern) and pons (rate, depth) of brainstem

II. DIAGNOSTIC TESTS AND ASSESSMENTS

A. Radiologic studies

1. Chest x-ray: visualizes structures, fluid, and air in thoracic cavity; anterior–posterior and lateral views are most common; appropriate use of lead shielding reduces overall exposure to x-rays

Box 55–1

Lung Volumes and Capacities

- Tidal volume (V_T): total air volume inspired and expired during one breathing cycle.
- Inspiratory reserve volume (IRV): maximum air volume inspired with forced inspiration (i.e., movement of air from atmosphere into respiratory system) following normal inspiration.
- Expiratory reserve volume (ERV): air volume that can be expired with force following normal expiration.
- Residual volume (RV): air volume remaining in lungs following forced expiration.
- Total lung capacity (TLC): maximum capacity of air volume of lungs. $TLC = IRV + V_T + ERV + RV$
- Inspiratory capacity (IC): maximum air volume that can be inhaled following a normal exhalation. $IC = V_T + IRV$
- Vital capacity (VC): maximum air volume that can be exhaled after a maximum inhalation. $VC = IRV + V_T + ERV$
- Functional residual capacity (FRC): residual air volume in lungs after a normal exhalation. $FRC = ERV + RV$

Table 55–1 Variables That Influence Gas Exchange

Variable	Example
Partial pressure of gas	Supplemental oxygen increases partial pressure of inspired air
Surface area	Loss of lung tissue by surgery or disease decreases surface area available for gas exchange
Molecular weight and gas solubility	CO_2 is more soluble in membranes and diffuses more quickly than oxygen
Thickness of membrane	Membrane is thickened by some disease processes, such as pneumonia, pulmonary edema; a thicker membrane impedes effective air exchange

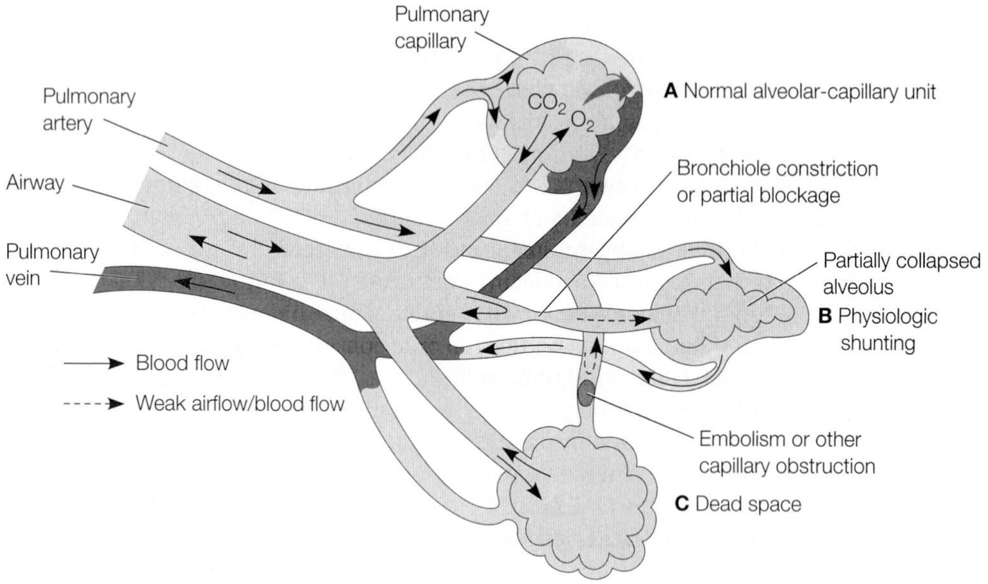

Figure 55–1

Ventilation–perfusion relationships. (**A**) Normal alveolar-capillary unit with an ideal match of ventilation and blood flow. Maximum gas exchange occurs between alveolar wall and blood. (**B**) Physiological shunting: a unit with adequate perfusion but inadequate ventilation. (**C**) Dead space: a unit with adequate ventilation but inadequate perfusion. In the latter two cases, gas exchange is impaired.

2. Computed tomography (CT): provides a cross-sectional view of tissue; detects lesions not seen on x-ray; performed with or without contrast media (check allergies to iodine or contrast medium)
3. Magnetic resonance imaging (MRI): images similar to CT identify subtle changes in tissue structure; ensure metal objects are removed; clients with metal implants may be ineligible for MRI
4. Pulmonary angiogram: outlines pulmonary vasculature; radioactive contrast is injected via central venous catheter into right side of heart and pulmonary artery; identifies tumors and circulation abnormalities (congenital, thromboembolism); assess for allergy to iodine or contrast media
5. Ventilation–perfusion scan: radioactive isotope injected to identify areas of ventilation and perfusion within lungs; also called VQ (ventilation quotient) scan

B. Pulse oximetry

NCLEX® 1. Intermittent or continuous monitoring of arterial **oxygen saturation** (SpO_2 or percentage of O_2 bound to hemoglobin) using light sensors and photo detector; normal is 95% or greater if no lung disease; target SpO_2 is 90% or greater with lung disease

2. Uses a probe with sensors attached to a finger, earlobe, nose, or toes; avoid extremity with intra-arterial catheter or noninvasive BP cuff

NCLEX® 3. Accuracy is reduced with poor peripheral blood flow, shivering or excessive movement, dark nail polish or artificial nails

C. Pulmonary function test

1. Uses a spirometer to measure lung volumes and capacities during forced breathing techniques
2. Differentiates restrictive from obstructive lung disease; assesses effects of bronchodilator therapy; see also Chapter 47

D. Bronchoscopy (see Chapter 47)

E. Thoracentesis (see Chapter 47)

F. Laboratory tests

NCLEX® 1. Arterial blood gases (ABGs): arterial blood specimen that identifies oxygenation status, acid–base balance, and compensatory mechanisms; see Table 55–2 for normal values and refer to Chapter 54 for additional information

Table 55–2 Normal Arterial Blood Gas Values

Arterial Blood Gas Parameter	Normal Value
pH	7.35–7.45
PCO_2	35–45 mmHg
HCO_3^-	22–26 mEq/L
PO_2	80–100 mmHg

2. Sputum analysis: specimen obtained for microbiology (Gram stain, culture and sensitivity) or cytology analysis
   a. Sample obtained by expectoration, suctioning, thoracentesis, lung needle biopsy, or transtracheal aspiration; have client rinse mouth prior to obtaining expectorated specimen
   b. *NCLEX®* Specimens for acid-fast bacilli (mycobacterium tuberculosis or TB) may be obtained on three different days; collect specimen after a long sleep period (early morning) because of greater concentration
3. Skin testing: detects allergic reactions to specified antigens (type I hypersensitivity), tuberculosis-causing organisms (type IV hypersensitivity), or fungi
   a. Administer by intradermal route; circle injection site with a long-lasting marker; diagram forearm injection site on chart
   b. *NCLEX®* For purified protein derivative (PPD) test for TB: measure area of induration (if present), *not* reddened area 48–72 hours after placement; an uncertain reading at 48 hours may be reread at 72 hours
   c. *NCLEX®* Induration of 5–10 mm indicates exposure to TB; follow-up with chest x-ray and possible sputum culture is indicated
   d. Two-step method is now used initially for healthcare workers, in which first negative test is repeated in 1 week
   e. *NCLEX®* When performing skin tests to detect type I allergies, ensure that antihistamines, which could interfere with test results, are discontinued 72 hours prior to testing

III. COMMON NURSING TECHNIQUES AND PROCEDURES

A. Airway management: goal is to maintain patent airway

1. Head and jaw position
   a. Upper airway obstruction is often caused by foreign object or loss of local muscle tone
   b. *NCLEX®* Open airway using head-tilt and anterior chin-lift maneuver
   c. *NCLEX®* In clients with suspected neck injury, open airway by anterior chin displacement and/or jaw thrust; do *not* perform head tilt
   d. Perform Heimlich maneuver in conscious clients with suspected foreign-body obstruction of airway
2. Oropharyngeal airway: maintains airway patency by preventing posterior tongue displacement; for use in unconscious clients only (possible vomiting or laryngeal spasms); must be sized for each client; maintain head and jaw position also
3. Nasopharyngeal airway: maintains airway patency via nasal route in semiconscious client or when oral placement is not feasible; must be sized for client; maintain head and jaw position even when airway is in place
4. Endotracheal (ET) intubation: a long, cuffed ET tube is inserted with a laryngoscope by specially trained personnel for long-term airway management or connection to a mechanical ventilator; see Chapter 27
5. Tracheostomy: surgical placement of cuffed airway into trachea of clients who cannot maintain an airway or require prolonged mechanical ventilation; see Chapter 27
6. Cricothyrotomy: emergency surgical opening of cricothyroid membrane to maintain patent airway when other methods fail or are not feasible
7. Techniques for airway clearance
   a. Oropharyngeal suctioning: nonsterile procedure to remove secretions from upper airway; alert clients may be taught to self-suction
   b. Nasotracheal suctioning: sterile procedure to remove secretions from tracheal area; may be performed to obtain sterile sputum specimen
   c. Tracheobronchial suctioning: sterile procedure using individual suction catheters or in-line suction catheter for clearing secretions via ET tube
   d. *NCLEX®* Limit suctioning to 10 seconds per catheter pass (5 in children) to reduce risk of inadequate oxygenation and cardiac dysrhythmias from hypoxia

B. Body positioning

1. Lung ventilation and perfusion are gravity-dependent; changes in body position from supine (0 degrees) to varying degrees of head elevation or lateral positioning activates reflexive cardiovascular changes that produce fluid shifts in lungs and chest blood vessels

NCLEX®

2. Acute respiratory failure: elevate head of bed at least 45 degrees to increase chest expansion and mobilize fluid from chest to more dependent areas

NCLEX®

3. Unilateral lung disease: position by using gravity to promote ventilation–perfusion matching; position with unaffected lung in dependent position ("good lung down")
4. Acute respiratory distress syndrome (ARDS): prone positioning may be used for clients on maximal mechanical ventilation with unresponsive hypoxemia
   a. Allows previously nondependent air-filled alveoli to become dependent, increasing perfusion to air-filled alveoli and may improve ventilation–perfusion matching
   b. Use caution to avoid unintentional dislodgment of ET tube during position changes

C. Oxygen (O_2) administration (see also Chapter 26)

NCLEX®

1. Nasal cannula: typical O_2 flow of 1–6 L/min will provide O_2 concentrations of 24–44%; clients with chronic obstructive pulmonary disease (COPD) should receive low flow oxygen, about 1–2 L/min, to prevent respiratory depression
2. Face mask: provides O_2 concentration of 40–60%, but flow should be greater than 5 L/min to prevent rebreathing of exhaled CO_2 trapped by mask
3. Face mask with O_2 reservoir (partial rebreather): flow of O_2 into reservoir bag allows rebreathing of one-third of exhaled air along with O_2
4. Nonrebreather mask: used for clients who require higher O_2 concentrations (95–100% O_2 with high flow rates)
5. Venturi mask: delivers O_2 in precise concentrations; used in clients with COPD and chronic CO_2 retention

D. Pulmonary hygiene

1. Pursed-lip breathing: client exhales through pursed lips, which slows exhalation and reduces airway collapse, thus enhancing respiration
2. Coughing
   a. Coughing adequate for airway clearance requires higher airway pressures
   b. Augmented coughing: caregiver places hand below xiphoid process and thrusts downward on abdomen as client ends inspiration

   NCLEX®

   c. Huff coughing: client attempts sequential coughing while saying "huff"; maneuver keeps glottis open during coughing; beneficial in clients with COPD
3. Chest physiotherapy (CPT) (see Box 55–2): mobilizes bronchial secretions into larger airways for removal by coughing or suctioning; useful for clients with more than 30 mL secretions per day, secretions with artificial airway, and/or atelectasis; see also Chapter 27

E. Mechanical ventilation

1. Purpose: maintain adequate gas exchange via ET or tracheostomy tube
2. Indications: ineffective breathing pattern or hypoxia (e.g., dyspnea, cyanosis, altered mental status, absent breath sounds, tachycardia with no underlying cardiac disease); O_2 saturation less than 80%, pH less than 7.35, $PaCO_2$ greater than 50 mm Hg, V_T less than 5 mL/kg, or minute volumes less than 10 L/min
3. Types of positive pressure ventilators
   a. Volume-cycled: deliver air until a preset volume of air is delivered; allows for pressure and time limits to be set; most common type used
   b. Pressure-cycled: delivers air until a preset pressure limit is reached on inspiration

Box 55–2

Chest Physiotherapy (CPT)

- Client is dressed in a lightweight shirt
- Percussion is performed with a cupped hand striking chest over a portion of lung; if done properly, a popping sound will be heard
- Postural drainage facilitates removal of secretions that are loosened during percussion; for drainage, various head-down positions drain all lung segments
- Positioning for bronchial drainage can be achieved by child standing on his head, hanging upside down on monkey bars, and other playground activities that are fun for child
- Avoid performing CPT immediately after eating

c. Flow-cycled: cycled by a preset inspiratory flow rate
d. Time-cycled: delivers air for a preset time interval

4. Modes of ventilation
   a. Synchronized intermittent mandatory ventilation (SIMV): delivers a preset volume synchronized to client's inspiratory effort; client can breathe spontaneously between ventilator breaths; commonly used, especially for ventilator weaning
   b. Assist control ventilation (ACV): delivers a preset volume with each ventilator breath and those initiated by client; risk is hyperventilation if client has frequent spontaneous respirations
   c. High-frequency ventilation (jet ventilation): delivers small gas volumes at a rapid rate for hemodynamically unstable clients and other who cannot tolerate mechanical ventilation
   d. Positive end expiratory pressure (PEEP): maintains positive pressure to keep alveoli open during exhalation to increase gas exchange; expressed in terms of centimeters of pressure (e.g., 5 cm); used in conjunction with other ventilation modes
   e. Continuous positive airway pressure (CPAP): maintains positive pressure in airways; is delivered during spontaneous breathing by snug-fitting mask; biPap is a variation that delivers one pressure on inspiration and maintains a lower pressure during expiration to aid oxygenation

NCLEX®

5. Key ventilator settings
   a. Rate: number of breaths/min delivered by ventilator; number that is combined with mode often in clinical practice (e.g., SIMV of 6/min)
   b. FiO_2: fraction of inspired O_2 or O_2%; amount of O_2 in air inhaled via ventilator; expressed as a decimal instead of a percentage (e.g., FiO_2 of .40 vs. 40%)
   c. Tidal volume (V_T): amount of air delivered with each breath; often expressed in milliliters or liters (e.g., 700 mL or 0.7 L)
   d. Pressure limit: maximum pressure allowed in airway; if exceeded, ventilator breath will terminate; often exceeded during coughing or when client needs suctioning

NCLEX®

6. Key ventilator alarms
   a. High pressure alarm: indicates pressure in airway exceeds preset pressure limit; assess client for obstruction of tube or tubing or need for suction
   b. Low pressure alarm: indicates low pressure in airway; assess client for leak or disconnect from system
   c. Never turn off ventilator alarms, which indicate potential threats to client's ventilation; if source of alarm cannot be identified and corrected quickly, call for assistance and maintain client respirations using manual resuscitation bag
   d. Implement agency measures to control alarm fatigue; ignoring alarms (especially those that go off frequently) poses a threat to client safety

NCLEX®

7. Nursing care
   a. Position client for maximum alveolar ventilation and comfort; implement standard agency measures to avoid accidental extubation
   b. Monitor for any changes in respiratory status or effort; suction as needed to maintain airway patency
   c. Maintain ventilator settings as prescribed and know how to troubleshoot ventilator alarms; never turn off ventilator alarms
   d. Monitor ABGs and maintain continuous SpO_2 monitoring
   e. Complete a thorough physical assessment, especially cardiac, neurologic, and respiratory systems
   f. Administer antibiotics, neuromuscular blocking agents, and sedatives as prescribed
   g. Maintain nasogastric suction to prevent aspiration
   h. Supply nutritional support as prescribed
   i. Perform frequent oral care to enhance client comfort and reduce risk of ventilator-acquired pneumonia
   j. Provide emotional support to client and family; provide alternative communication method (word or picture board, white board, paper and pen)
8. Potential complications: pneumothorax, GI stress ulcers, hypotension from increased intrathoracic pressure leading to decreased venous return, increased intracranial pressure, infection, ventilator dependence
9. Weaning methods to return client to breathing independently
   a. SIMV: systematically reducing number of ventilator breaths/min as tolerated until client is breathing without ventilator assistance
   b. T-piece: removal of ventilator and attachment to a T-piece delivering oxygen and possibly CPAP to allow independent breathing for short, preset time periods; times are extended according to client tolerance
   c. Pressure support ventilation: amount of preset pressure delivered by ventilator and/or number of preset breaths delivered is systematically reduced according to client tolerance

F. Respiratory isolation

1. Standard precautions include hand hygiene, gloves, and protective face gear to be used whenever there is possible contact with blood, body fluids or secretions, mucous membranes, nonintact skin, or parenteral devices

NCLEX®

2. Droplet precautions (transmission-based precautions)
   a. In addition to standard precautions, mask should be worn when near client who has known or suspected pathogen transmitted by droplet route
   b. Limit client transport within facility; when transport is necessary, place mask on client
   c. Limit contamination of equipment and/or environment
   d. Place client in private room or with a cohort (client with same diagnosis)
3. Airborne precautions (transmission-based precautions): use same principles as droplet precautions but use fit-tested N95 respirator and place client in private room with negative air pressure; door to room is kept closed; see Chapter 7 for additional information on transmission-based precautions

IV. NURSING CARE OF CLIENT HAVING LUNG SURGERY

NCLEX®

A. Preoperative period

1. Reduce anxiety with preoperative teaching about procedure and postoperative course and care
2. Assess client's support systems and ability to care for self after surgery
3. Administer preoperative medications, such as antibiotics, opioid analgesics, and anti-anxiety agents, as prescribed
4. Obtain baseline vital signs (VS), oxygen saturation (SpO_2), and mental status for comparison postoperatively

B. Postoperative period

1. Perform baseline assessments for VS, SpO_2, and mental status as for all postoperative clients
2. NCLEX® Maintain patent airway
3. NCLEX® Position client for optimal ventilation and perfusion; note any specific surgeon's prescriptions for positioning; typical positions include being tilted slightly to either side; with pneumonectomy, avoid complete lateral turning to either side, which changes pressure dynamics within chest and could lead to mediastinal shift
4. Be prepared to initiate respiratory support (intubation, emergency tracheostomy, mechanical ventilation) as needed
5. Provide standard care to client with a chest tube, if present; see also Chapter 27
6. Maintain sterility of operative dressing
7. NCLEX® Maintain client safety and prevent risk of postoperative infection
8. Administer prescribed antibiotics, bronchodilators, corticosteroids, inhalation agents, or other medications
9. Administer analgesics as prescribed; adequate pain management facilitates chest expansion and optimal ventilation
10. NCLEX® Assess for and report possible surgical complications to maintain oxygenation
    a. Change in level of consciousness (LOC) ranging from restlessness and agitation to lethargy or unresponsiveness
    b. Increase in respiratory rate, unequal chest expansion, decreased breath sounds, and/or use of accessory muscles for breathing
    c. Loss of water seal drainage in closed chest drainage system
    d. Greater than desired volume of chest drainage (75–100 mL drainage over 1 hour is an average acceptable upper limit); orders should specify volume of acceptable chest tube drainage; should decrease over first 24 hours
11. Teach client and family about postdischarge home care, follow-up care, and available community health resources; home oxygen therapy and assistance with daily activities may be needed if client has significant reduction in respiratory reserve because of lung resection

V. CHRONIC OBSTRUCTIVE PULMONARY DISEASE (COPD)

A. Overview

1. A disease characterized by slowly progressive airway obstruction, with periods of remission and exacerbation; clients may or may not return to previous baseline with each exacerbation
2. Typically includes components of two underlying disorders, although one or the other may predominate in a single client

a. **Chronic bronchitis:** chronic airway inflammation resulting from inhaled irritants with a chronic productive cough lasting 3 or more months in 2 consecutive years; key features are persistent airway edema, excess mucus production, and inadequate airway clearance
b. **Emphysema:** inflammation (often from cigarette smoking) leads to destruction of alveolar walls, alveolar ducts, and underlying tissue supports for pulmonary capillary bed; key features are loss of alveolar tissue and elastic recoil, air trapping on exhalation, inadequate gas exchange

3. Key risk factors include cigarette smoking (primary cause), air pollution, occupational exposure to noxious dusts and gases, airway infection, and genetic risk (alpha$_1$-antitrypsin deficiency)

NCLEX® 4. Assessment
a. Exertional dyspnea that progresses to dyspnea at rest and use of accessory muscles as disease advances
b. Chronic cough with sputum production
c. Diminished breath sounds, crackles and wheezing upon auscultation
d. Persistent tachycardia related to inadequate oxygenation
e. Respiratory infection is a frequent **trigger** (initiator) for exacerbation of symptoms
f. **Barrel chest**, noted by increased A-P diameter of chest, and pursed lip breathing (to aid exhalation) in emphysema
g. Chronic fatigue and inability to perform routine activities without dyspnea as disease progresses
h. ABGs: worsening hypoxemia (decreased PaO_2) as disease progresses; carbon dioxide ($PaCO_2$) is elevated in later stages (respiratory acidosis)
i. Chest x-ray: possible hyperinflated lungs and flattened diaphragm; evidence of respiratory infection
j. Pulmonary function tests: low VC and forced expiratory volume (FEV_1); increased residual volume with emphysema

5. Collaborative management
a. Goals are to improve ventilation and promote patent and effective airway
b. Remove environmental pollutants and encourage smoking cessation
c. Monitor VS and oxygen saturation

NCLEX® d. Administer low-flow oxygen as prescribed (not to exceed 2L/min) to enhance oxygenation without increasing risk of respiratory failure (low PaO_2 becomes stimulus for respiration instead of elevated CO_2)

NCLEX® e. Position client with head of bed elevated to optimize breathing; teach client tripod position (leaning forward with arms resting on knees or overbed table) to reduce work of breathing

f. Ensure delivery of prescribed therapies such as nebulizer therapy or chest physiotherapy

NCLEX® g. Encourage clients to eat a nutrient-dense diet (high-calorie, high-protein), with smaller, more frequent meals if dyspnea and fatigue interfere with eating

NCLEX® h. Provide adequate hydration (up to 3,000 mL/day), if not contraindicated, to prevent thick secretions that are hard to expectorate

i. Assist with and supervise activity according to client's level of fatigue; encourage client to sit down or lean against wall for support if dyspnea occurs while ambulating
j. Administer prescribed medications, which may include rapid-acting (beta-agonist) bronchodilators, anticholinergics, corticosteroids, mucolytics, and, if infection is present, antibiotics
k. Provide immunization against pneumonia (one-time or every 5 years) and influenza (yearly)

6. Client education
a. Smoking cessation methods; avoid occupational or environmental pollutants

NCLEX® b. Energy conservation techniques (alternate activity with rest periods)

c. Maintain adequate nutrition with emphasis on higher protein intake (carbohydrates produce carbon dioxide as an end product of metabolism)
d. Prescribed medication therapy, including oral medication and use of metered-dose inhaler
e. Follow up regularly with healthcare provider, receive recommended immunizations, and give information (if referred) about structured pulmonary conditioning program

VI. PLEURAL EFFUSION

A. Overview

1. Accumulation of fluid in pleural space that indicates underlying pulmonary disease or abnormality
2. Transudative type: associated with increased hydrostatic pressure (heart failure) or decreased oncotic pressure from low albumin level (chronic renal or liver disease)
3. Exudative type: fluid shift associated with increased capillary permeability from inflammatory processes such as pulmonary tumors, infection, or emboli

4. Empyema: pleural fluid containing pus associated with infections such as pneumonia, lung abscess, and tuberculosis
5. Chylothorax: accumulation of lymph fluid in pleural space from lymph vessel disruption; produces fat malabsorption from GI tract

NCLEX® **B. Assessment**

1. Worsening dyspnea with diminished or absent breath sounds on affected side from lung compression
2. Dullness to percussion on affected side
3. Chest wall pain that increases with inspiration and is sharp in quality (pleuritic pain)
4. Nonproductive dry cough because of bronchial irritation
5. Fever, night sweats, and weight loss with empyema
6. Visible on chest x-ray; mediastinal shift is possible if greater than 250 mL effusion
7. Diagnostic thoracentesis: differentiates source of pleural fluid; may also be used to drain fluid

NCLEX® **C. Collaborative management**

1. Goal is to identify and treat underlying cause; assist with thoracentesis
2. Monitor respiratory and oxygenation status; auscultate lung sounds
3. Position for comfort with head of bed elevated; provide supplemental O_2 PRN
4. Provide adequate nutrition with focus on adequate protein intake
5. Medication therapy: analgesics, antipyretics, antibiotics if indicated; possible IV lipids if chylothorax present
6. Prepare client for possible pleurectomy (stripping parietal pleura away from visceral pleura to trigger inflammation and adhesion of pleural layers) or pleurodesis (instilling sclerosing agent into pleural space via thoracotomy tube to trigger inflammation and adhesions)

D. Client education

1. Explain underlying cause of pleural effusion
2. Teach client/family to monitor for changes in respiratory and oxygenation status
3. Instruct about purpose of diagnostic and therapeutic procedures

VII. PNEUMOTHORAX AND HEMOTHORAX

A. Overview

1. Pneumothorax: air accumulation in pleural space with loss of negative intrathoracic pressure and collapse of lung tissue
   a. Spontaneous: rupture of air-filled bleb allows air to leak from alveoli into pleural space; may seal leak with minimal client symptoms or progress until client is symptomatic
   NCLEX® b. Tension: blunt trauma or excessive pressure from mechanical ventilation causes air accumulation in pleural space; increased pressure can decrease venous return to heart and cause mediastinal shift; requires emergency chest tube placement to relieve increasing intrathoracic pressure and restore adequate cardiac output
   c. Traumatic: disruption of pleura, bronchi, or lung tissue caused by blunt trauma (closed pneumothorax) or penetrating trauma (open pneumothorax) with air accumulation in pleural space
2. Hemothorax: blood accumulation in pleural space; clinical manifestations and treatment are same as for pneumothorax

NCLEX® **B. Assessment**

1. Tachypnea and dyspnea
2. Diminished or absent breath sounds on affected side
3. Possible tracheal deviation toward unaffected side if tension pneumothorax
4. Unequal chest expansion (reduced on affected side)
5. Subcutaneous emphysema (crepitus) palpable at site
6. Sucking sound at site of chest wound (open pneumothorax)
7. Tachycardia and possible hypotension
8. Chest x-ray reveals pneumothorax; ABG shows decreased PaO_2

NCLEX® **C. Collaborative management**

1. Monitor respiratory and oxygenation status
2. Provide supplemental O_2 as indicated
3. Apply occlusive dressing over open chest wound and leave untaped on one side (prevents air trapping and tension pneumothorax)
4. In very mild cases or small spontaneous pneumothorax, no chest tube is required
5. If pneumothorax is significant, a chest tube is inserted and attached to water seal drainage; see care of client with a chest tube previously discussed in Chapter 27

6. Maintain infection control practices
7. Medication therapy: analgesics and possibly antibiotics

D. **Client education:** purpose of chest tube, activity limitations, and pain management

VIII. ATELECTASIS

A. **Overview**

1. **Atelectasis** is an incomplete expansion or collapse of lung tissue resulting from obstruction of air passages by pulmonary secretions, exudates, or a foreign body
2. Airway obstruction increases intra-alveolar pressure, causing alveolar collapse
3. Surface area available for gas exchange is decreased
4. Common complication among postoperative or immobilized clients

NCLEX® B. **Assessment**

1. If small, diminished or absent breath sounds in affected area may be only sign
2. Possible low-grade fever or other signs of infection
3. Possible tachycardia, tachypnea, dyspnea, and other signs of hypoxemia (if more severe)
4. Physical inactivity caused by immobility or pain
5. Chest x-ray reveals affected area

NCLEX® C. **Collaborative management**

1. Primary goal is prevention
2. Deep breathing and coughing exercises; incentive spirometry hourly while awake
3. Frequent position change (every 2 hours)
4. Supplemental oxygen as indicated
5. Monitor respiratory and oxygenation status
6. Chest physical therapy as indicated
7. Ambulation as soon as feasible with client condition
8. Maintain adequate hydration and nutrition
9. Medication therapy: analgesics and antipyretics

D. **Client education:** diaphragmatic and abdominal breathing techniques, nonpharmacologic pain control measures

IX. PNEUMONIA

A. **Overview**

1. Acute inflammation of lung parenchyma (alveoli and respiratory bronchioles)
2. Classified as viral versus bacterial, community-acquired versus healthcare facility–acquired, atypical, aspiration or pneumocystis
3. Causative agent can be infectious (bacteria, viruses, fungi, and other microbes) or noninfectious (aspirated or inhaled substances)
4. Spread of microbes in alveoli activates inflammatory and immune response
5. Antigen–antibody response damages mucous membranes of bronchioles and alveoli, resulting in edema
6. Microbe cellular debris and exudate fill alveoli and can impair gas exchange

NCLEX® B. **Assessment**

1. Fever: low grade with viral infection; higher with bacterial infection; possible chills
2. Cough with sputum production
3. Rhonchi and wheezes on lung auscultation
4. Pleuritic-type pain in chest
5. Tachypnea, possible dyspnea with use of accessory muscles
6. Mental status changes if sufficient hypoxemia develops
7. Elevated white blood cell count (higher with bacterial infection than viral)
8. Chest x-ray: shows affected lung area(s)

NCLEX® C. **Collaborative management**

1. Maintain patent airway; monitor respiratory and oxygenation status
2. Elevate head of bed to reduce respiratory effort
3. Provide oxygen as prescribed to treat hypoxemia
4. *NCLEX®* Provide pulmonary hygiene measures (coughing and deep breathing, repositioning, incentive spirometer)
5. *NCLEX®* Provide small, frequent meals with high-calorie, high-protein foods (client tires easily with simultaneous effort to breathe and eat)
6. *NCLEX®* Encourage increased fluids up to 3 liters per day, if no contraindications, to reduce viscosity of sputum

7. Provide for adequate physical rest
8. For all hospitalized clients, institute measures to prevent pneumonia (encourage ambulation and mobility; practice infection control measures such as hand hygiene and proper disposal of expectorated secretions; initiate aspiration precautions for clients at risk)
9. Medication therapy: antibiotics or other indicated anti-infectives, analgesics, and antipyretics

D. Client education

1. Immunization against influenza and pneumococcal pneumonia
2. Activity limitations and importance of rest for healing
3. Effects and dosages of medications
4. Avoid pollutants and irritants such as smoke
5. Symptoms to report: return of fever, worsening respiratory status

X. INFLUENZA

A. Overview

1. Acute highly contagious viral respiratory infection; also called *flu*
2. Major strains of virus are influenza A, B, and C; H1N1 (swine) flu results from a more recent type A virus
3. In some countries, H5N1 subtype of influenza A (avian flu) has infected humans who have been in contact with infected birds and also have underlying chronic illness; not currently known to be transmitted from person to person
4. Viruses are capable of antigenic drift (small, continuous changes as virus makes copies of itself), which creates a need to produce new flu vaccines each year
5. Prevention of infection is key; yearly vaccination is recommended for those over age 50, those who are immunosuppressed or have chronic illness, and healthcare personnel (a contraindication to vaccination is egg allergy)
6. Other preventive measures include diligent hand hygiene, disinfecting contaminated surfaces, and avoiding crowds during flu season and infected individuals

NCLEX® **B. Assessment**

1. Sore throat and cough that becomes productive; cough can persist for weeks after other symptoms resolve
2. Coryza (nasal congestion and runny nose) and possible tachypnea
3. Fever and chills
4. Weakness and fatigue
5. Headache and muscle aches

NCLEX® **C. Collaborative management**

1. Provide significant periods of rest during acute febrile phase of illness
2. Elevate head of bed as needed for comfort and to ease breathing
3. Provide adequate hydration to prevent dehydration and thick respiratory secretions
4. Assess respiratory rate, pattern, and lung sounds
5. Institute droplet precautions for hospitalized clients with suspected or diagnosed flu
6. Administer prescribed antipyretics, analgesics, and, in unvaccinated clients, medications to control severity such as amantadine, rimantadine, oseltamivir, zanamivir, or ribavirin

D. Client education

1. Importance of yearly vaccination to prevent future infection
2. Infection control measures to prevent spreading infection to others
3. Signs and symptoms of complications (such as pneumonia) to report

XI. PULMONARY TUBERCULOSIS

A. Overview

1. Lung infection caused by *Mycobacterium tuberculosis*, an acid-fast, Gram-positive bacillus (although intestines, kidney, peritoneum, liver, joints, and brain can also be affected)
2. Transmitted via airborne droplets *NCLEX®*
3. Infection usually results from frequent close contact with an infected individual
4. Inhaled bacilli inhabit respiratory bronchioles and alveoli, and may spread to other areas if not contained by encapsulation in lungs by cell-mediated immune defenses
5. Eventual activation of cell-mediated immunity produces a granuloma lesion
6. Liquefied necrotic material from Ghon tubercle portion of granuloma lesion allows passage of infectious particles into major airways for exhalation into air
7. Treatment is aimed at preventing transmission and controlling symptoms and progression of infection

NCLEX® **B. Assessment**

1. Early symptom is nonproductive cough (especially in early morning), followed by frequent cough with copious purulent or blood-tinged sputum
2. Chest tightness or dull ache in chest may accompany cough
3. Late-afternoon low-grade fever and night sweats
4. Anorexia and weight loss
5. Fatigue and lethargy
6. History may indicate recent exposure to infected individual
7. Positive tuberculin skin test (indicates exposure or inactive dormant disease)
8. Appearance of characteristic Ghon tubercle on chest x-ray
9. Positive QuantiFERON-TB Gold blood test (enzyme-linked immunosorbent assay) or positive acid-fast bacillus sputum cultures (cultures provide definitive diagnosis of infection)

NCLEX® **C. Collaborative management**

1. Monitor respiratory and oxygenation status
2. Provide adequate nutrition and hydration
3. Institute standard precautions (Centers for Disease Control [CDC] Tier 1) and airborne precautions (Tier 2, transmission-based precautions); see also Chapter 7
   a. Use a private room with negative air pressure that has 6–12 full air exchanges per hour and is vented to outside or has own air filtration system
   b. Wear specially fitted mask (N95 respirator) whenever entering client's room; fit-test mask with each use
   c. Provide visitors with appropriate masks
   d. Wear gown as well as mask if client does not reliably cover mouth during coughing or sneezing to reduce risk of transmission to others
   e. Provide client with a surgical mask if client must be transported to another department; choose shortest and least busy route and alert department ahead of time about client's status; schedule tests for least busy times of day
4. Administer antimicrobial therapy as prescribed
5. Provide supplemental O_2 as indicated
6. Obtain periodic sputum cultures following onset of antimicrobial therapy (three negative sputum cultures are needed to be considered noninfectious)
7. Medication therapy; see Chapter 45

D. Client education

1. NCLEX® Explain mechanisms of transmission and infection control measures, including diligent hand hygiene, coughing into tissues and disposing of them in a closed bag
2. No special precautions need to be taken with clothing, books, personal objects, or eating utensils because inanimate objects do not easily spread these bacteria
3. NCLEX® Teach principles of antimicrobial therapy, including need to take medication exactly as prescribed for full course of therapy (usually 6–12 months) to prevent recurrence and/or development of drug-resistant organisms
4. Teach client about adverse effects of medications; see also Chapter 45
5. Provide adequate nutrition for healing (high protein, iron, vitamin C) and rest periods to reduce fatigue

XII. PULMONARY EMBOLISM (PE)

A. Overview

1. Embolus (most commonly from deep vein thrombosis) travels through right side of heart and lodges in branch of pulmonary artery, impeding blood flow
2. Causes **ventilation–perfusion mismatch**, a clinically significant imbalance between volume of air and volume of blood circulating to affected area of lungs; leads to impaired gas exchange
3. Risk factors include immobility, hypercoagulability, trauma to endothelial layer of blood vessels, and long bone fractures (fat emboli)
4. If obstructed area is large enough, can lead to pulmonary infarction
5. Severe impairment of gas exchange can be rapidly fatal

NCLEX® **B. Assessment**

1. Restlessness, anxiety, agitation, apprehension
2. Vital signs: tachycardia, tachypnea, hypotension, low-grade fever
3. Dyspnea, shortness of breath, and chest pain
4. Cough and possible hemoptysis

5. Mental status changes with possible decreasing level of consciousness (LOC)
6. Possible diaphoresis, pallor that may progress to cyanosis
7. Recent history of thromboembolism and/or long bone fractures
8. Lung crackles upon auscultation
9. S_3 and/or S_4 gallop; atrial fibrillation may result in mural thrombi (thrombi that form on atrial walls) that may be source of PE if they arise from right atrium
10. Diagnostic tests: chest x-ray may be normal or show pulmonary infiltration; pulmonary angiogram reveals site of PE; ventilation–perfusion scan indicates areas of mismatch; abnormal ABGs reveal significantly low PaO_2

NCLEX® **C. Collaborative management**

1. Remain with client and elevate head of bed
2. Provide supplemental oxygen as prescribed or per protocol
3. Assess vital signs and respiratory status, including lung sounds
4. Maintain IV access and provide circulatory support as needed
5. Provide reassurance to client (and family) and explain procedures and therapies
6. Initiate anticoagulant and/or thrombolytic therapy as prescribed
7. Administer opioid analgesics and anti-anxiety agents as prescribed
8. Surgical procedures may include embolectomy or, if there is a recurrent known source, insertion of a vena cava filter

D. Client education

1. Prevention of thromboembolism
2. Avoid immobility as much as feasible
3. Teach signs/symptoms of venous occlusion
4. Instruct client/family regarding anticoagulant therapy as indicated

XIII. LUNG CANCER

A. Overview

1. Lung cancer is a malignancy affecting bronchi and peripheral lung tissue
2. Bronchogenic carcinoma accounts for most primary lung lesions; lungs are also a common site for metastasis from other organs
3. Tumors can be differentiated by cell type: small-cell (oat cell) carcinoma, adenocarcinoma, squamous cell carcinoma, and large-cell carcinoma
4. Cigarette smoking is leading cause; cancer risk increases with length of smoking exposure; secondhand smoke (passive smoking) is also a risk
5. Contributing factors: genetic tendency (abnormality often seen on chromosome 3) and inhaled environmental substances such as air pollution, arsenic, asbestos, iron, radon, and aromatic hydrocarbons
6. All forms of bronchogenic carcinoma tend to grow aggressively, invade local tissue, and cause widespread metastasis to organs such as brain, bones, and liver

NCLEX® **B. Assessment**

1. Chronic cough with or without hemoptysis
2. Dyspnea and wheezing (often unilateral) from airway obstruction
3. Diminished or absent breath sounds over affected area
4. Localized dull aching chest pain (mediastinal involvement) or pleuritic pain (pleural invasion)
5. Swallowing difficulty (pressure of tumor on esophagus)
6. Hoarseness (pressure of tumor on trachea)
7. Systemic signs such as anorexia, weight loss, fatigue, and weakness
8. Possible enlarged lymph nodes
9. Mass visible on chest x-ray, CT scan, or MRI
10. Sputum or bronchoscopy washings for cytology reveal tumor cells

NCLEX® **C. Collaborative management**

1. Monitor respiratory status, including rate, pattern, breath sounds, dyspnea, oxygen saturation, sputum production and hemoptysis; assess for tracheal deviation
2. Place client in high Fowler position to optimize oxygenation
3. Provide humidified oxygen as prescribed
4. Provide rest periods and supervise and assist with activity, such as ambulation
5. Administer prescribed bronchodilators, corticosteroids, and analgesics
6. Provide psychological support for client and family

7. Provide preoperative and postoperative care for client having surgical removal of tumor, including maintenance of chest tubes (see also Chapter 27)
   a. Lobectomy: removal of a lobe of lung
   b. Segmentectomy (segmental resection): removal of a segment or segments of a lung
   c. Wedge resection: dissection and removal of a defined area in lung
   d. Pneumonectomy: removal of entire lung (no chest tube placement)
8. Provide care for client undergoing nonsurgical therapies (see also Chapter 65): chemotherapy, radiation therapy, laser therapy, immunotherapy

D. **Client education:** treatment plan, pain management, active range of motion exercises postoperatively to shoulder on affected side, assistance with coping skills, need for home oxygen therapy, possible need for assistance with activities of daily living during recovery period

XIV. CANCER OF LARYNX

A. Overview

1. Many laryngeal tumors are benign; most common form of malignant tumor is squamous cell carcinoma
2. Primary etiologies include long-term cigarette smoking and alcohol ingestion
3. Contributing factors: chronic laryngeal irritation caused by singing, air pollution, and environmental hazards
4. Tumor growth occurs in glottis, supraglottis, and subglottis; symptoms are specific to site of tumor
5. Chronic laryngeal irritation leads to precancerous lesions, leukoplakia, and erythroplakia
6. Carcinoma may develop at site of precancerous lesions
7. Most common site for laryngeal metastasis is lungs
8. Treatment depends on stage of disease and general condition of client; may include radiation therapy or brachytherapy (placement of a radioactive source next to tumor), chemotherapy, or surgery (radical neck dissection or laryngectomy)

NCLEX®

B. Assessment

1. Hoarseness and/or change in voice characteristics
2. Palpable jugular nodes
3. Pain when swallowing
4. Unexplained earache
5. Diagnostic test results: laryngeal biopsy findings, x-ray visualization, MRI or CT findings, barium swallow visualization

NCLEX®

C. Preoperative care for laryngectomy

1. Provide standard preoperative care as for any surgical client
2. Educate client and family about long-term implications, including loss of voice, swallowing difficulties, altered route for nutrition, and permanent tracheostomy
3. Establish a means for communicating with client after surgery (such as written means, eye or hand signals)

NCLEX®

D. Postoperative care for laryngectomy

1. Maintain airway patency and respiratory status; elevate head of bed, provide humidified oxygen as prescribed, and routine tracheostomy care
2. Provide standard postsurgical pain management
3. Provide prescribed hydration and nutritional support (IV, enteral feedings, and oral when allowed)
4. With total laryngectomy, there is full separation of trachea from upper airway and pharyngeal structures, eliminating the risk of aspiration (see Figure 55–2A)
5. Teach client and family how to care for tracheostomy and feeding tube (if applicable)
6. Explain that swallowing may not be automatic after surgery and that client will need to purposefully initiate swallowing
7. Use communication devices such as writing supplies or picture or word board or use speech rehabilitation methods (see section to follow)
8. Provide emotional support to client and family; make appropriate referrals

E. Speech rehabilitation

1. Tracheoesophageal puncture (TEP): most common method (see Figure 55–2B)
   a. Small fistula is created between posterior trachea and anterior esophagus
   b. A small, one-way valve is inserted into fistula; using a finger to occlude trachea forces exhaled air through valve into esophagus and hypopharynx, creating vibration and sound
2. Esophageal speech: client swallows air and uses controlled burping to form words, using muscles of mouth and tongue; takes practice and fluent speech might not be restored

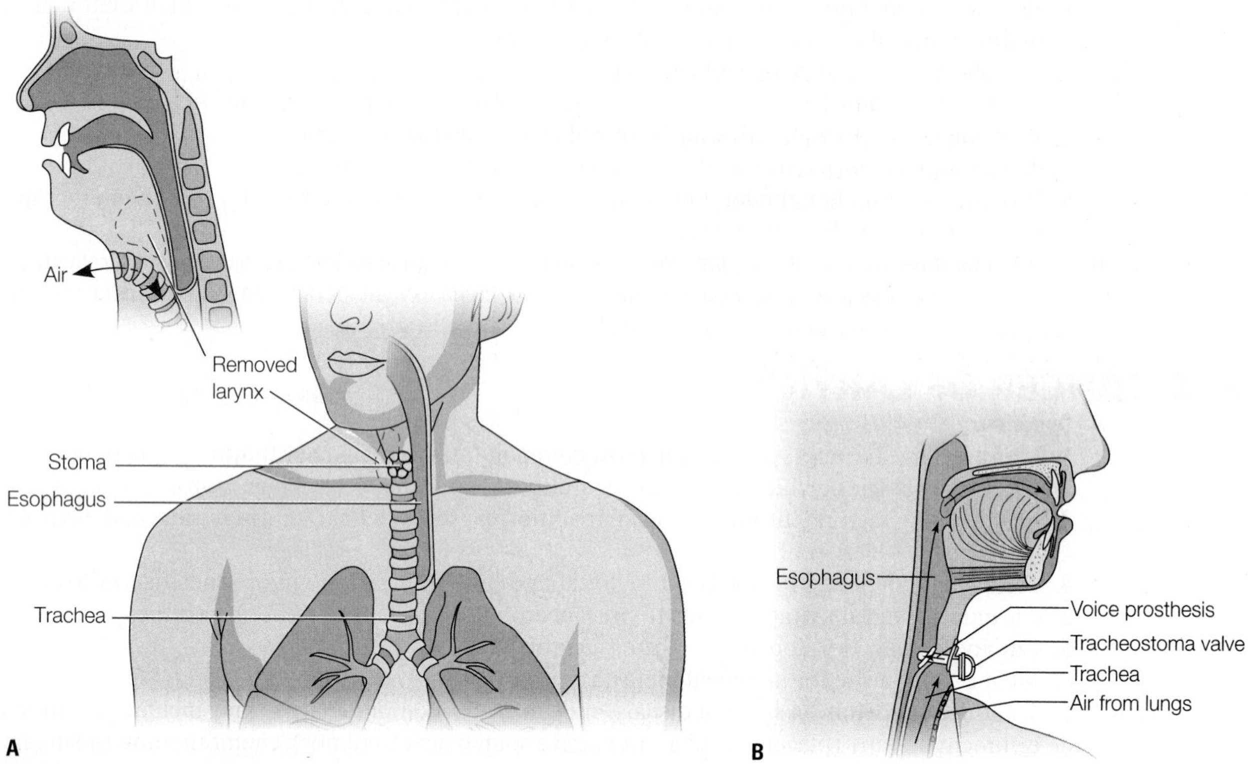

Figure 55–2 Laryngectomy. (**A**) Permanent tracheostomy eliminates connection between trachea and esophagus; (**B**) Transesophageal prosthesis with one-way valve for air movement allows speech when stoma is occluded.

3. Speech generator (electrolarynx): one type is held against throat while mouth is used to form words; in another, plastic handpiece of generator is placed into mouth, which forms words from audible tone generated

F. **Client education:** includes smoking cessation, changes in body image, care of tracheostomy, how to use method chosen for speech production, nutritional access device if indicated, pain management, and signs of tumor spread

XV. CHEST TRAUMA

A. Overview

1. Alteration of breathing mechanics and/or gas exchange caused by respiratory system trauma
2. Blunt trauma: injury to chest wall without disruption of pleura
   a. Rib fractures or flail chest
   b. Soft tissue rupture: diaphragm, trachea, bronchi, and major blood vessels
   c. Tension pneumothorax
   d. Contusion: lungs, heart
   e. Mechanism of injury commonly involves motor vehicle collisions, falls, and assaults
3. Penetrating trauma: injury involves disruption of pleura
   a. Internal wounds communicate with external atmosphere
   b. Open air-sucking wounds
   c. Pneumothorax and hemothorax
   d. Tissue wounds: heart, lungs, major blood vessels
   e. Mechanism of injury commonly involves firearms, knives, motor vehicle collisions, falls, or assaults
4. Flail chest
   a. Multiple rib fractures in two or more places (separated from bony skeleton)
   b. Chest wall unstable with paradoxical chest expansion (flail segment moves inward with inhalation and outward with exhalation)
   c. Ventilation–perfusion mismatch
   d. Possible underlying lung injury
5. Rupture of diaphragm
   a. Abdominal contents dislocate upward into thoracic cavity
   b. Decrease in diaphragmatic control of breathing

NCLEX®

B. Assessment

1. Varies with cause
2. Chest pain, may be severe such as with flail chest, or worse on inspiration (such as with fractured ribs)
3. Shallow breathing with splinting
4. Possible unequal chest expansion
5. Tachycardia, tachypnea, hypotension
6. Crepitus over chest
7. Chest x-ray findings show white opacifications (pulmonary contusion), site of fracture, or accompanying pneumothorax or hemothorax
8. ABGs reveal hypoxemia

NCLEX®

C. Collaborative management: same as pneumothorax and hemothorax

1. Ventilation support with O_2 therapy; be prepared to initiate mechanical ventilation
2. Maintain IV access
3. Possible placement of chest tube with water seal drainage
4. Medication therapy: opioid analgesics, patient-controlled or epidural analgesia may be appropriate

D. Client education

1. Techniques for pulmonary hygiene
2. Pain management: patient-controlled analgesia or oral analgesics
3. Prevention of thromboembolic phenomena
4. Measures to decrease anxiety

XVI. ACUTE RESPIRATORY DISTRESS SYNDROME

A. Overview

1. Syndrome characterized by acute respiratory failure, diffuse alveolar membrane injury, and accumulation of fluid in interstitial lung spaces (interstitial edema)
2. Occurs as a secondary response or complication of some other health problem or injury, such as sepsis, shock, trauma, burns, fluid overload, aspiration, coagulopathy, neurologic insult, ingestion or inhalation of drugs or toxins
3. Interstitial edema compresses terminal airways, leading to reduced lung compliance, reduced lung volume, respiratory acidosis, and hypoxemia (from shunting of unoxygenated blood) that is unresponsive to increasing amounts of oxygen

NCLEX®

B. Assessment

1. Early tachypnea followed by dyspnea
2. Diminished breath sounds
3. Worsening ABGs and hypoxemia that persists, even with increasing levels of prescribed oxygen
4. Pulmonary infiltrates seen on chest x-ray and decreased lung compliance with PFTs

NCLEX®

C. Collaborative management

1. Identify and manage underlying triggering condition
2. Administer oxygen as prescribed and track effects of oxygen therapy on ABGs
3. Be ready to assist if client is intubated and placed on mechanical ventilation
4. Maintain head of bed elevation in high Fowler position; prone positioning may be used occasionally for clients with severe ARDS receiving mechanical ventilation
5. Provide standard pulmonary hygiene measures and ensure client receives respiratory treatments as prescribed
6. Medications may include diuretics, corticosteroids, and possibly anticoagulants

D. Client education

1. Provide simple explanations of course of illness, treatments, and procedures; be prepared to repeat explanations to anxious client and family
2. Energy conservation measures while client is recovering
3. Follow-up care for initial triggering insult and ongoing respiratory care

XVII. ASTHMA

A. Overview

1. Common chronic disorder beginning in childhood characterized by bronchial constriction, hyperresponsive airways, and airway inflammation
2. Has multiple etiologies, including genetic predisposition, viral illnesses, allergens, and environmental exposures

NCLEX®

3. Episodes are caused by one or more specific initiators (known as a trigger), which include exercise, environmental allergens (e.g., pet dander, dust, mold, pollen, smoke, fragrances, cockroach feces), recurrent respiratory viral infections, hormonal influences, allergic disease such atopic eczema or gastroesophageal reflux disease, weather changes, air pollutants, food additives, and stress
4. Pathophysiology includes activation of IgE, sensitized mast cells, release of inflammatory mediators (histamine, leukotrienes, prostaglandins), and release of proinflammatory cytokines
5. Bronchial constriction, airway swelling, and mucus production are responsible for airway narrowing, decreased perfusion of alveolar capillaries, air trapping, and hypoxemia
6. Inability to control episodes can lead to status asthmaticus, a medical emergency that can lead to respiratory failure

NCLEX®

B. Assessment

1. Severe **dyspnea** (difficulty breathing), **tachypnea** (rapid respirations) with use of accessory muscles
2. Wheezing with expiration; intensity of wheezing is not related to severity of airway obstruction; clients with severe airway obstruction may not be able to move enough air to produce wheezing sound
3. Cough
4. Feelings of chest tightness
5. Prolonged expiration
6. Mild to greatly diminished breath sounds; may be related to atelectasis or narrowed airway lumens
7. Tachycardia and increased blood pressure (BP)
8. Extreme restlessness, anxiety, agitation
9. Hyperresonant sound on lung percussion
10. Decreased PaO_2, mild respiratory alkalosis during episode
11. Elevated eosinophil count
12. Increased residual volume, decreased VC, FEV_1 and peak expiratory flow rate (PEFR)

NCLEX®

C. Collaborative management

1. Acute episodes are managed with "rescue medications": rapid-acting inhaled beta-agonists (bronchodilation), anticholinergics (relief of bronchospasm), bronchodilators, and systemic corticosteroids
2. Long-term control to prevent attacks may include long-acting beta-agonists, leukotriene modifiers, corticosteroids, nonsteroidal anti-inflammatory drugs (for general anti-inflammatory action), anti-allergy medications (to prevent reaction to triggers), and monoclonal antibody
3. Assess respiratory and oxygenation status
4. Administer supplemental O_2 as needed and be prepared to initiate mechanical ventilation if indicated
5. Observe characteristics of sputum
6. Be prepared to establish IV access
7. Identify, avoid, and remove precipitating factors
8. Teach client relaxation techniques during nonacute periods
9. Diagnostic testing during nonacute period includes chest x-ray, pulmonary function studies, allergy skin testing, serum eosinophils, and IgE
10. Provide emotional support to client and family
11. Allergy desensitization therapy if appropriate

D. Client education

1. Identify asthma triggers and eliminate when possible (environment, food)
2. Teach client and family proper use of metered-dose inhaler and oral medications; teach proper cleaning of inhalation devices to prevent yeast infection with inhaled corticosteroids
3. Instruct client/family about use of peak-flow meter for self-assessment of asthma status (decrease may indicate impending exacerbation or infection)
   a. Goal is to remain in green zone (80–100% of personal best)
   b. Use action plan for medications when PEFR is in yellow zone (50–80%)
   c. Use action plan and seek healthcare when in red zone (less than 50%)
4. Teach to recognize asthma symptoms requiring emergency intervention
5. Encourage general health measures such as adequate nutrition, fluid intake, sleep, and exercise (specific program may be recommended)

XVIII. CYSTIC FIBROSIS (CF)

A. Overview

1. Multisystem disorder of exocrine glands, leading to increased production of thick mucus in bronchioles, small intestines, and pancreatic and bile ducts

2. Increased viscosity of secretions obstructs small passageways of these organs and interferes with normal pulmonary and digestive functioning
3. Respiratory problems are most serious threat to life; thick, sticky secretions pool in bronchioles, cause atelectasis, and serve as a medium for bacterial growth; chronic hypoxemia can ultimately lead to pulmonary hypertension and cor pulmonale
4. Pancreatic ducts become clogged with thick secretions and prevent pancreatic enzymes from reaching duodenum, impairing digestion and absorption
5. Small intestines, without aid of pancreatic enzymes, are unable to absorb protein, fats, and fat-soluble vitamins; thus, signs of vitamin deficiency can develop and growth and puberty are retarded
6. Skin has high concentrations of sodium and chloride, leading to child tasting "salty" when kissed; client is at risk for dehydration and fluid and electrolyte imbalances, especially with high environmental temperature or fever
7. Usually diagnosed in infancy and early childhood

NCLEX®

B. Assessment

1. Quantitative **sweat chloride test** (pilocarpine iontophoresis) analyzes Na^+ and Cl^- content in sweat; a chloride concentration greater than 60 mEq/L (or greater than 40 mEq/L in infant less than 3 months of age) is diagnostic of CF
2. Possible newborn screening with immunoreactive trypsinogen analysis or direct DNA analysis
3. A 72-hour fecal fat analysis determines amount of fat, trypsin, or both in stool sample (food intake must be recorded during specimen collection period)
4. Chest x-ray (atelectasis, obstructive emphysema) and pulmonary function studies (reduced function because of abnormal small airways)
5. History usually reveals frequent bouts of respiratory infections
6. Observe for respiratory impairment (i.e., cough, presence and color of sputum, dyspnea, retractions), color of nailbeds and mucous membranes, O_2 saturation; auscultate breath sounds for equality, crackles, wheezes, or any increased effort during breathing; observe for clubbing of fingers and toes; **digital clubbing**, an indication of hypoxia, produces nails with increased rounding and a loss of normal angle at base of nail
7. Assess nutritional status by plotting measured height and weight on growth charts; assess skin turgor and mucous membranes for hydration status; record diet history and activity tolerance; signs of malabsorption include bulky, frothy, foul-smelling stools called steatorrhea and unusually protruberant abdomen and thin extremities; often first sign of CF is meconium ileus, where intestine is blocked with thick, tenacious secretions in newborn period and neonate is unable to pass first meconium stool

NCLEX®

C. Collaborative management

1. Respiratory: ensure pulmonary hygiene is performed; auscultate breath sounds before and after treatments; encourage coughing and deep breathing exercises and physical activity as tolerated; administer prescribed antibiotics and bronchodilator(s)
2. Digestive: provide high-calorie (150% above normal recommendations), high-protein diet and snacks; give infants a predigested formula as prescribed; administer pancreatic enzymes with all meals and snacks; individualize to achieve stools as near normal as possible (but no more than two to three per day); administer fat-soluble vitamins; determine food preferences to encourage acceptance of diet; weigh daily; avoid pulmonary treatments immediately after meals to decrease risk of vomiting
3. Medications: antibiotics for pulmonary infection and purulent secretions, pancreatic enzymes for fat absorption, vitamin supplementation, mucolytics to decrease viscosity of sputum, bronchodilators to improve lung function; see Chapter 36 for overview of commonly ordered respiratory care medications

D. Child and family education

1. Avoid exposure to respiratory infections; report immediately any fever, increase in cough, or change in sputum
2. Chest percussion and postural drainage must be performed three to four times daily; nonadherence will result in increased infections and hospitalizations; see Box 55–2 for instructions on CPT and postural drainage (p. 896)

NCLEX®

3. High-calorie, high-protein diet is essential; give pancreatic enzymes with all meals and snacks; may need extra salt in hot weather
4. Physical activity and exercise loosen secretions and promote lung expansion

5. Provide information on community resources, such as Cystic Fibrosis Foundation, American Lung Association; provide social service consults, home-health referrals with visiting nurses and respiratory therapists
6. Provide information on recommended follow-up and importance of adhering to vaccination schedules, including annual influenza vaccine after age 6 months
7. Provide written information on medications, breathing exercises, CPT, and postural drainage
8. Suggest clergy, mental health services, respite care, and families of other children with CF to assist with psychological and emotional coping with chronic, progressive illness

XIX. *BRONCHOPULMONARY DYSPLASIA (BPD)*

A. Overview

1. A chronic obstructive pulmonary disorder occurring in infants as a sequela to prolonged O_2 therapy and mechanical ventilation
2. Premature infants with BPD have usually survived respiratory distress syndrome (RDS) at birth; term infants who develop BPD also generally had serious respiratory problems that required ventilatory assistance
3. High O_2 concentrations and mechanical ventilation damage bronchial epithelium and alveoli; thickened alveolar walls, scarring, and fibrosis lead to atelectasis, poor airway clearance of mucus, and poor gas exchange; chronic low oxygenation results in decreased lung compliance and altered function

NCLEX® **B. Assessment**

1. Diagnosed by chest x-ray, which reveals lung changes and air trapping with or without hyperinflation
2. ABGs reveal hypercapnia (increased CO_2) and respiratory acidosis
3. Respiratory signs include tachypnea, tachycardia, nasal flaring, retractions, decreased air movement, crackles, occasionally wheezing, and barrel chest
4. Pallor, activity intolerance, and poor feeding result from chronic hypoxia

NCLEX® **C. Collaborative management**

1. Infants with BPD are cared for in intensive care units and require an artificial airway; avoid pressure or trauma to ET tube and infant's airway
2. Perform suctioning, turning, and weighing carefully to ensure adequate O_2 saturation levels are maintained
3. Monitor respiratory status continuously; infant's condition can worsen in a short period of time
4. Monitor for fluid overload because of increased risk for pulmonary edema; weigh daily; maintain strict intake and output (I&O)
5. Strict hand hygiene; avoid exposure to respiratory infections
6. Cluster nursing care to minimize O_2 requirements and caloric expenditure
7. Plan quiet stimulation and activities to foster normal infant development and parental bonding with extended and often repeated hospitalizations of infants with BPD
8. Medications
   a. Bronchodilators open airways and increase lung compliance
   b. Corticosteroids reduce airway edema and inflammation
   c. Diuretics remove excess fluid from lungs and help prevent pulmonary edema
   d. Antibiotics may be given prophylactically

D. Client and family education

1. Infants are discharged with multiple needs; assess family's understanding and ability to follow treatment regimen
2. *NCLEX®* Teach parents cardiopulmonary resuscitation (CPR), use of home monitoring equipment and O_2 therapy; infants are usually discharged with a tracheostomy when O_2 concentration requirements are low
3. *NCLEX®* Review infection control practices such as hand hygiene and avoidance of family members with respiratory infections; teach warning signs of illness
4. Teach safety precautions regarding O_2 therapy and tracheostomy care; see Box 55–3 for instructions on home tracheostomy care; before discharge, notify utility companies, emergency services, and telephone companies of a technology-dependent infant or child
5. Review basic care—feeding, bathing, playing, holding—with parents; allow parents an opportunity to care for child in hospital before discharge; after basic care is mastered, medical treatment plan is developed with assistance of parents
6. Make referrals to community agencies for supplies, medications, nutrition, parental support, and stimulation programs to foster growth and development

Box 55–3

Tracheostomy Home Care and Oxygen Therapy

Discharge instructions for child with tracheostomy (trach):

- Keep small toys, talcum powder, plastic bibs and bedding, and any small particles away from child to decrease risk for aspiration or occlusion of trachea
- Be sure child wears cloth bib loosely over trach when eating to prevent food particles from entering tube
- Be careful when bathing to keep water from entering trachea; showers are not recommended
- Cover trach loosely when outside in strong wind or cold to prevent tracheal spasms
- Observe skin around trach daily for redness, breakdown, or signs of infection
- Change trach ties weekly; be sure to use nonfraying material; always have assistance to change ties
- Clean area around trach daily with half-strength saline and cotton applicators
- Suction trach tube when needed to remove secretions from airway; use sterile gloves and limit suctioning to 5 seconds; insert suction catheter only to length of trach tube and apply intermittent suction while withdrawing catheter
- Allow child to rest between suctioning if catheter is passed more than once
- Notify healthcare provider if tracheal secretions are increased or become purulent or fever develops
- Keep emergency bag with extra suction catheters and trach tubes available
- Notify utility companies and emergency medical services that child in the home requires emergency equipment
- Do not allow smoking in the home of child with oxygen therapy
- Keep oxygen tanks away from any heat source; keep a fire extinguisher nearby

XX. *LARYNGOTRACHEOBRONCHITIS* (LTB)

A. Overview

1. Inflammation, edema, and narrowing of larynx, trachea, and bronchi; may be preceded by a recent upper respiratory infection (URI)
2. Most common croup syndrome, usually caused by parainfluenzae virus, influenzae A and B, respiratory syncytial virus (RSV), and mycoplasma pneumoniae
3. Inflammation and narrowing of airways cause inspiratory stridor and suprasternal retractions as child struggles to inhale air; increased production of thick secretions and edema further obstruct airway and cause hypoxia and CO_2 accumulation, and lead to respiratory acidosis and failure

NCLEX®

B. Assessment

1. Onset is gradual after URI
2. Child awakens with low-grade fever, hoarseness, seal bark or brassy cough, and inspiratory stridor
3. Child is agitated, restless, has a frightened appearance, sore throat, and rhinorrhea
4. Signs can progress to worsening tachypnea, dyspnea, inspiratory and expiratory stridor, retractions and use of accessory muscles, pallor progressing to cyanosis, apneic periods, and possibly cessation of breathing
5. Pulse oximetry is used to detect hypoxemia (via SpO_2 or O_2 saturation); anteroposterior (AP) and lateral upper airway x-rays may be prescribed

NCLEX®

C. Collaborative management

1. Monitor child's respiratory effort continuously to ensure a patent airway; observe for diminished breath sounds, circumoral cyanosis, diminishing noisy breathing, and drooling
2. Quiet respiratory effort is a sign of physical exhaustion and impending respiratory failure
3. Provide cool humidity and supplemental O_2; oral or IV fluids prevent dehydration and help liquefy secretions
4. Assist child to assume upright position or any position of comfort; promote a calm, quiet environment; keep parents nearby to reduce child's stress/crying
5. Keep emergency intubation equipment available at bedside; readily respond to call bell or requests for assistance
6. Assess parental and child's anxiety level; provide emotional support

7. Medications
   a. Bronchodilators decrease mucosal constriction and laryngeal edema; nebulized racemic epinephrine has a rapid onset with improvement of symptoms, although relapse may occur within 2 hours
   b. Corticosteroids decrease inflammation and edema
   c. Antibiotics if source of infection is bacterial
   d. Antipyretics (acetaminophen, ibuprofen) as needed to treat fever

D. Child and family education

1. Assess parental anxiety and ability to adhere to medical therapy
2. Symptoms are usually worse at night and may recur for several nights; instruct parents that child can be cared for at home if able to take fluids by mouth and has no stridor at rest
3. NCLEX® Cool-mist humidifier and parental presence can be initial treatment of crisis; comforting measures include cuddling, rocking, singing, and any calming measures until breathing becomes easier
4. NCLEX® Instruct parents to seek medical attention immediately if breathing becomes labored, child seems exhausted or very agitated, or if symptoms do not improve after cool-air humidity treatment
5. Teach parents to keep child from contact with large groups of people and practice infection control measures

XXI. EPIGLOTTITIS

A. Overview

1. Inflammation and swelling of epiglottis, primarily affecting children ages 2–8
2. Epiglottis covers larynx during swallowing to prevent food from entering trachea
3. Bacteria, usually *Haemophilus influenzae*, cause epiglottis to become cherry red, swollen, and so edematous that it obstructs airway; secretions pool in pharynx and larynx above epiglottis; child has a sore throat and is unable to swallow; complete airway obstruction can occur within 2 to 6 hours
4. Onset is sudden in a previously healthy child; Hib vaccine has reduced incidence of epiglottitis, although causative organisms may also be streptococcus and staphylococcus

NCLEX® **B. Assessments**

1. Child awakens with sudden onset of high fever (102°F [38.9°C]), extremely sore throat, and pain on swallowing
2. Child is very anxious, restless, looks ill, and insists on sitting upright leaning on arms, with chin thrust out and mouth open (tripod position; opens airway)
3. Dysphonia (muffled voice), dysphagia (difficulty swallowing), drooling of saliva, and distressed respiratory effort are classic signs
4. Tachypnea, dyspnea, use of accessory respiratory muscles, nasal flaring, inspiratory stridor, and absence of spontaneous cough; can progress to respiratory distress
5. Fever and tachycardia
6. Edematous, inflamed cherry-red epiglottis is most reliable diagnostic sign
7. Examination of throat is contraindicated unless emergency intubation equipment and trained personnel are available; physical manipulation of hypersensitive and irritated airway muscles may result in spasm and complete obstruction
8. Lateral neck x-ray confirms an enlarged epiglottis; portable x-rays are completed in exam room with child on parent or caregiver's lap to minimize stress and maximize comfort and calm behavior

NCLEX® **C. Collaborative management**

1. Assess continuously for respiratory distress and decrease in respiratory effort; monitor respiratory status and oxygen saturation; report changes in status
2. Never leave child unattended; support child in position of comfort; encourage parent or caregiver to hug and cuddle child
3. Constitutes a medical emergency; have equipment available for resuscitation or for endotracheal intubation or tracheotomy to maintain patent airway
4. Ensure NPO status
5. NCLEX® Do not take temperature by mouth, obtain throat culture, or try to visualize posterior pharynx because this could lead to epiglottis spasm and airway occlusion
6. NCLEX® Keep client positioned upright; provide cool humidified oxygen to aid in oxygenation and reduce airway edema
7. Implement measures to keep child calm; do not leave child alone or restrain child that is agitated
8. Initiate IV therapy for hydration once airway is established and child is calmer
9. Medication therapy includes nebulized (racemic) epinephrine for severe case, antibiotics (IV followed by oral), analgesics, and antipyretics such as acetaminophen or ibuprofen, and possible corticosteroids

D. Client and family education
1. Provide emotional support and explain all procedures calmly; encourage parents to cuddle and comfort child
2. Teach parents importance of completing antibiotic regimen after discharge; explain medications, how to administer, and any side effects to be expected
3. Discuss importance of Hib vaccine and reassure parents that recurrence of epiglottitis is uncommon

XXII. BRONCHIOLITIS

A. Overview
1. Inflammation of bronchioles with edema and excess accumulation of mucus; air trapping and atelectasis result from increased airway resistance because of small obstructed bronchioles
2. A major cause of hospitalization of high-risk infants
3. Respiratory syncytial virus (RSV) is primary causative organism, which is spread by contact with respiratory secretions and contaminated objects; RSV is not airborne but can live for several hours on nonporous surfaces
4. RSV bronchiolitis is most prevalent during first 2 years of life, with most occurrences in spring and winter; bronchiolitis usually begins with a mild URI; as disease progresses, gas exchange is compromised, hypoxemia results, and metabolic acidosis develops
5. Useful preventive measures are breastfeeding, avoiding exposure to cigarette smoke, hand hygiene, and for high-risk infants, monthly intramuscular injection of monoclonal antibody palivizumab from November through March

NCLEX® **B. Assessment**
1. Initial clinical manifestations include sneezing, coughing, rhinorrhea, eye drainage, intermittent fever, and possible wheezing
2. Progressive symptoms with worsening infection include tachypnea, retractions, anorexia, thick nasal secretions, and increasingly labored breathing; older infants may have a frequent, dry cough
3. Auscultation of lungs reveals wheezing or crackles
4. Nasopharyngeal washing to obtain respiratory secretions identifies causative virus; chest x-ray may be normal or indicate hyperinflation or nonspecific inflammation

NCLEX® **C. Collaborative management**
1. Assess respiratory status hourly; provide humidified O_2 to ease respiratory effort; use pulse oximetry to assess O_2 saturation
2. Clear nasal passages with bulb syringe; elevate head of bed
3. Cluster nursing care to allow for rest; assess anxiety level of parents and provide support; maintain a calm environment
4. IV fluids may be needed if oral intake is compromised; monitor strict I&O; weigh daily to assess fluid loss
5. Maintain strict hand hygiene and contact precautions; caregivers should not care for other high-risk children
6. Medications: possible ribavirin via inhalation; bronchodilators and corticosteroids are sometimes used

D. Child and family education
1. Explain disease process and provide support to lessen anxiety
2. Encourage parents to assist in care of infant; explain all procedures and treatments
3. Teach parents to use bulb syringe as needed to keep nasal passages clear
4. Teach parents to provide frequent oral fluids
5. Instruct parents to notify healthcare provider if child refuses to eat or breathing becomes worse
6. Instruct parents to use humidifier in child's bedroom
7. Teach parents to avoid smoking in child's vicinity
8. Teach parents to practice strict hand hygiene and keep child away from individuals with upper respiratory infections; RSV can reoccur

XXIII. *FOREIGN BODY ASPIRATION*

A. Overview
1. Inhalation of an object into respiratory tract, intentional or otherwise
2. Peak age for foreign body aspiration is children under 3 years old
3. Foreign bodies usually lodge in right main bronchus (which is shorter and wider than left); obstruction may be partial or complete and causes atelectasis, air trapping, and hyperinflation distal to site of obstruction

NCLEX®
4. Severity is determined by type and shape of object and small diameter of infant's airway; round objects such as hot dogs, round candy, nuts, and grapes do not break apart and are more likely to occlude airway; latex balloons are particularly hazardous; objects with irregular shapes may irritate airway and partially obstruct airflow
5. Failure to remove a foreign object is usually fatal; a delay in removal may cause aspiration pneumonia

NCLEX®
B. Assessment
1. Sudden coughing and gagging is first sign, and objects in upper airway may be expelled by coughing
2. Partial obstruction may cause symptoms of respiratory infection for days or even weeks; child may have hoarseness, croupy cough, wheezing, and dyspnea
3. If obstruction is complete, child will demonstrate stridor, cyanosis, difficulty swallowing and speaking
4. A child who cannot speak, is cyanotic, and collapses requires immediate attention for complete airway obstruction
5. Fluoroscopy and chest x-ray reveal foreign body in respiratory tract

NCLEX®
C. Collaborative management
1. Assess respiratory status to determine severity of problem and degree of obstruction; continuously monitor and provide assistance if obstruction worsens
2. If total airway obstruction occurs, perform back blows and chest thrusts for infants and Heimlich maneuver in children older than 1 year
3. Keep NPO; foreign body is usually removed in surgery
4. Position for comfort and to optimize airway; provide emotional support to parents and child and alleviate anxiety
5. After removal of object, assess for additional obstruction that may result from laryngeal edema and tissue swelling
6. Medications: antibiotics may be administered if secondary infection is suspected, or if purulent secretions are present in airway, with or without signs of pneumonia

D. Child and family education
1. Teach parents about hazards of aspiration and importance of childproofing home
2. Review age-appropriate foods and discuss most frequently aspirated objects: coins, hot dogs, balloons, nuts, popcorn, grapes, round candy, peanut butter
3. Discuss toy safety and avoidance of toys with small, removable parts; caution against allowing child to run and play with objects in mouth
4. Teach parents CPR and techniques of chest thrusts, back blows, and abdominal thrusts

Check Your NCLEX–RN® Exam I.Q.

You are ready for testing on this content if you can:

- Identify basic structures and functions of the respiratory system.
- Describe the pathophysiology and etiology of common respiratory disorders.
- Discuss expected assessment data and diagnostic test findings for selected respiratory disorders.
- Discuss collaborative management of a client experiencing a respiratory disorder.
- Discuss nursing management of a client experiencing a respiratory disorder.
- Identify expected outcomes for the client experiencing a respiratory disorder.

PRACTICE TEST

1 What should the nurse include when teaching health maintenance strategies to the client with COPD? Select all that apply.

1. Yearly influenza immunizations
2. Immunization against pneumonia
3. Limitation of physical activity
4. Oral fluid restriction
5. Adequate caloric intake

2 The nurse who is explaining the pathophysiology of COPD to a client includes which manifestations that can result from alveolar destruction? Select all that apply.

1. Decreased surface area for gas exchange
2. Increased dead space air
3. Development of pulmonary emboli
4. Chronic dilation of bronchioles
5. Airway collapse related to loss of elasticity

3 What explanation should the nurse give to a client and family regarding the development of COPD in a young adult?

1. Hereditary deficiency of alpha-1-antitrypsin
2. Onset of smoking during childhood
3. Heavy secondary smoke exposure during childhood
4. Use of smokeless tobacco during childhood

4 A client who develops acute respiratory distress syndrome (ARDS) is exhibiting hypoxemia unresponsive to oxygen therapy. In explaining the client's condition to the family, the nurse would incorporate which concept?

1. Blood is shunted past alveoli with no ventilation.
2. The individual has difficulty expelling air trapped in the alveoli.
3. There is excess surfactant production by the alveoli.
4. Thick secretions block the airways.

5 What intervention should the nurse identify as the priority for the client who is unable to adequately clear the airway because of a tumor mass?

1. Providing supplemental oxygen
2. Keeping the head of the bed elevated
3. Coughing, deep breathing, and hydration maintenance
4. Preparing for insertion of a tracheostomy tube

6 When assisting with psychological issues for the client with lung cancer, which epidemiologic factor should the nurse keep in mind?

1. The 5-year survival rate for lung cancer tends to be low.
2. Symptoms are usually recognized early during lung cancer progression.
3. Tumor growth usually begins in a bronchus, then migrates upward in the tissue.
4. Risk of lung cancer is associated with length of exposure to cigarette smoking.

7 What pharmacologic treatment would the nurse administer aimed at prevention of pulmonary embolism?

1. Streptokinase
2. Vitamin K
3. Enoxaparin
4. Protamine sulfate

8 A client is hospitalized with a diagnosis of pneumonia. Which findings, based on the nurse's knowledge, are indicative of a deteriorating clinical state? Select all that apply.

1. Increased respiratory rate
2. Tachycardia
3. Agitation
4. Cyanosis
5. Increased urinary output

9 For the hospitalized client, which manifestation would the nurse assess to be a symptom of pulmonary embolism?

1. Slow increase in heart rate and respiratory rate
2. Cyanosis of the upper torso
3. Abrupt onset of dyspnea and apprehension
4. Significant bilateral wheezing

10 A client underwent a thoracentesis a few hours earlier. What finding should the nurse report immediately to the healthcare provider?

1. Oozing of blood from the puncture site
2. Onset of crepitus
3. Diminished sounds in the affected lung base
4. Fever that is gradually elevating

PRACTICE TEST

11 The nurse assisting the client with obstructive pulmonary disease should use which statement to explain why dyspnea occurs?

1. "Decreased surfactant causes many of your alveoli to collapse."
2. "You have difficulty breathing in enough air."
3. "Your airways open wider on inspiration, and trap air on expiration."
4. "Your lung compliance is decreased."

12 A client is admitted to the hospital with a medical diagnosis of viral pneumonia. The nurse should assess for which frequent manifestations? Select all that apply.

1. Presence of Ghon's tubercle on chest x-ray
2. Nonproductive cough
3. Normal or near-normal white blood cell count
4. High fever that is intermittent
5. Profuse pleural diffusion on chest x-ray findings

13 The nurse would question a prescription for ipratropium for a client with asthma if the client had which concurrent medical history?

1. Glaucoma
2. Cushing's syndrome
3. Warfarin therapy
4. Fluid retention

14 A client newly diagnosed with asthma has infrequent acute episodes. The nurse should teach the client that which medication is most effective for providing quick relief in acute episodes?

1. Corticosteroid via metered-dose inhaler as needed
2. Beta-agonist via metered-dose inhaler
3. Anti-inflammatory via metered-dose inhaler
4. Daily use of a bronchodilator inhaler

15 The nurse caring for a client diagnosed with acute respiratory distress syndrome (ARDS) should consider that, in this client, impaired gas exchange is mostly likely related to which factor?

1. Air trapping in the alveoli
2. Accumulation of exudative fluid into the alveoli
3. Shunting of blood around nonventilated alveoli
4. Excessive alpha-1-antitrypsin

16 A child with laryngotracheobronchitis (LTB) is being treated in the emergency department. What should the nurse plan to do to ease respiratory distress? Select all that apply.

1. Place the child in a high-Fowler position.
2. Administer racemic epinephrine.
3. Administer corticosteroids.
4. Administer intravenous antibiotics.
5. Ask parent to help keep child calm.

17 The parents of an infant with bronchiolitis ask the nurse why their baby's room has a sign on the door that says "Contact Precautions," and why the nurses wear gowns and gloves when they hold him. What is the nurse's best response?

1. "Extra precautions prevent the virus from spreading to other babies."
2. "Your baby is very ill, and we don't want to have another baby catch what he has."
3. "It's because we need to protect your baby from other illnesses."
4. "We always wear gowns when babies are coughing."

18 What should be a priority nursing intervention for a child with bronchiolitis?

1. Keep the child well stimulated.
2. Maintain strict intake and output.
3. Encourage visitors.
4. Encourage oral fluids, if tachypneic.

19 When taking the nursing history of a child with cystic fibrosis, what piece of information about the child's newborn period would the nurse expect the mother to report?

1. That the child required resuscitation in the delivery room
2. That labor was longer than 24 hours
3. That the child had a meconium ileus
4. That labor was less than 4 hours

20 The parents of a child with asthma are learning about performing postural drainage exercises. The nurse should teach them to perform which action before performing the exercises?

1. Administer the child's bronchodilator.
2. Change the child's clothes.
3. Administer the child's antibiotic.
4. Suction the child's throat.

21 If treatment for acute epiglottis is effective, what should the nurse expect to record about the child?

1. Pale lips and mucous membranes
2. Maintains tripod position
3. Tachypneic and dysphonic
4. Clear bilateral breath sounds

22 The parents of a child with bronchopulmonary dysplasia (BPD) are receiving home instructions on tracheostomy care. With regard to suctioning, the nurse should advise the parents that each suction pass should take no longer than _____ seconds. Provide a numerical answer.

Fill in your answer below:
Answer: _____ seconds

23 A young toddler is being discharged after an emergency admission for foreign body aspiration. The parents ask what they can do to prevent another accident. What advice is appropriate for the nurse to give the parents?

1. Watch the child very carefully.
2. Teach the child not to eat nonfood items.
3. Keep small objects and toys out of the child's reach.
4. Keep the child under continuous observation while awake.

24 The nurse wears gloves when assessing a child with respiratory syncytial virus (RSV). After removing the gloves, what should be the nurse's next action?

1. Discard the gloves in the laundry basket.
2. Inspect the gloves for holes or fraying.
3. Remind the parents to wear gloves.
4. Perform careful hand hygiene.

25 A 6-year-old child is hospitalized following an acute asthmatic episode. Which statement by the parents indicates that further teaching is needed?

1. "Next time, we'll be sure he takes his cromolyn before soccer."
2. "After this episode, he will need to quit the swim team."
3. "We think this was an exercise-induced asthma episode."
4. "We need to make sure he has his inhaler at all times."

26 The nurse is preparing to administer respiratory medications to a child hospitalized with asthma. By which most frequently used route will the medication be administered?

1. Aerosol
2. Intravenous
3. Subcutaneous
4. Oral

27 The nurse anticipates using postural drainage as a treatment modality for which condition?

1. Epiglottitis
2. Foreign body aspiration
3. Cystic fibrosis
4. Bronchopulmonary dysplasia

28 The nurse teaches a mother how to attach a spacer to the metered-dose inhaler for a young child. How should the nurse explain the purpose of the spacer?

1. Makes the device look less intimidating to a small child
2. Makes it unnecessary to shake the inhaler before administering the drug
3. Concentrates the medication in the upper respiratory tract
4. Reduces the risk for oral yeast by depositing medication more deeply into the airways

29 The nurse documents which expected finding after auscultating the lungs of a child with bacterial pneumonia?

1. Wheezes
2. Crackles
3. Apnea
4. Retractions

30 An infant with respiratory syncytial virus (RSV) is receiving ribavirin. While caring for this infant, what actions should the nurse avoid? Select all that apply.

1. Maintaining contact precautions
2. Clearing nasal passages with a bulb syringe
3. Wearing contact lenses
4. Staying in the room with the door closed
5. Caring for the other high-risk children

ANSWERS & RATIONALES

1 **Answer: 1, 2, 5 Rationale:** Clients with COPD are highly susceptible to respiratory infections such as influenza, so they should be immunized yearly. Clients with COPD are highly susceptible to respiratory infections such as pneumonia so they should be immunized as prescribed by their healthcare provider. Clients with COPD use a large amount of calories because of labored respiratory function; increased caloric intake is necessary to maintain a healthy weight. Clients with COPD should undergo a progressive rehabilitation program to increase their activity tolerance. Fluid restriction is not needed with COPD unless there is fluid retention from another etiology. **Cognitive Level:** Applying **Client Need:** Health Promotion and Maintenance **Integrated Process:** Teaching and Learning **Content Area:** Adult Health: Respiratory **Strategy:** The critical words in the stem of the question are *health maintenance*. This phrase indicates that you should focus on the option that prevents a health problem rather than diagnoses or treats it. When there is more than one correct answer, consider each option as a true/false statement.

2 **Answer: 1, 5 Rationale:** The impaired gas exchange occurring with COPD is caused by the loss of alveolar surface area available for gas exchange. The loss of elasticity in the airway of a client with COPD can be airway attributed to repeated infections and inflammation, which leads to airway collapse. Airway collapse can cause alveolar destruction because of either over- or underinflation of alveolar sacs. Destruction of alveoli is not related to increased dead space air, pulmonary emboli, or chronic dilation of bronchioles. With COPD, there is progressive narrowing of bronchioles. **Cognitive Level:** Analyzing **Client Need:** Physiological Adaptation **Integrated Process:** Communication and Documentation **Content Area:** Adult Health: Respiratory **Strategy:** The core issue of the question is the nature of the pathophysiology of COPD. Use general nursing knowledge and the process of elimination to make a selection. When more than one answer is correct, consider each option as a true/false statement.

3 **Answer: 1 Rationale:** Onset of the physiological changes compatible with COPD is most often associated with a hereditary deficiency of alpha-1-antitrypsin, an enzyme that protects lung tissue against loss of elasticity. Onset of smoking during childhood, heavy secondary smoke exposure during childhood, and use of smokeless tobacco during childhood are not typically associated with early onset of the physiological alterations of COPD. **Cognitive Level:** Applying **Client Need:** Physiological Adaptation **Integrated Process:** Communication and Documentation **Content Area:** Adult Health: Respiratory **Strategy:** The core issue of the question is sharing with a client and family the correct basis of the current health problem. Use nursing knowledge and the process of elimination to make a selection.

4 **Answer: 1 Rationale:** One of the primary alterations occurring with ARDS is the collapse of alveoli and therefore loss of ventilation in those areas. Air does not become trapped in hyperinflated alveoli in ARDS; instead, alveoli collapse. Surfactant production decreases with ARDS, a factor that impairs adequate gas exchange. One of the primary alterations occurring with ARDS is the collapse of alveoli and therefore loss of ventilation in those areas; thick secretions blocking the airways are not a consideration. **Cognitive Level:** Applying **Client Need:** Physiological Adaptation **Integrated Process:** Teaching and Learning **Content Area:** Adult Health: Respiratory **Strategy:** The core issues of the question are an understanding of the disease process and how to select appropriate concepts for family teaching. Use nursing knowledge and the process of elimination to make a selection.

5 **Answer: 3 Rationale:** Coughing, deep breathing, and adequate hydration are essential for achieving effective airway clearance. The provision of supplemental oxygen is important, but it is not related to the ability to clear secretions from the airway. Elevating the head of the bed might help the client to cough more forcefully, but head elevation alone is not an effective maneuver for clearing secretions. Insertion of a tracheostomy is not a primary treatment to maintain airway clearance. **Cognitive Level:** Analyzing **Client Need:** Physiological Adaptation **Integrated Process:** Nursing Process: Implementation **Content Area:** Adult Health: Respiratory **Strategy:** The critical word in the stem of the question is *priority*, which tells you that more than one option could be correct, and you must choose the most important one. Use nursing knowledge and the process of elimination to make a selection.

6 **Answer: 1 Rationale:** The nurse should help the client and family to approach the diagnosis of lung cancer from a realistic perspective. Five-year survival rates tend to be low because symptoms can be ignored or attributed to other causes early in the disease. Symptoms of lung cancer are usually recognized as needing treatment late in the course of the disease. Tumor growth does typically begin in a bronchus and progress upward, but this information has no relation to the client's psychological adaptation to the disease. The risk of lung cancer is associated with multiple causes, with exposure to cigarette smoking being just one factor. **Cognitive Level:** Applying **Client Need:** Psychosocial Integrity **Integrated Process:** Communication and Documentation **Content Area:** Adult Health: Respiratory **Strategy:** The core issue of the question is the knowledge of the interrelationship between prognosis and the communication approaches used by the nurse. Use nursing knowledge and the process of elimination to make a selection.

7 **Answer: 3 Rationale:** Administration of anticoagulants is an effective intervention to prevent pulmonary embolism. Thrombolytic drugs may be used to dissolve a clot that is already formed. Vitamin K facilitates clotting and counteracts the effect of anticoagulants. Protamine sulfate facilitates clotting and counteracts the effect of anticoagulants. **Cognitive Level:** Applying **Client Need:** Pharmacological and Parenteral Therapies **Integrated Process:** Nursing Process: Implementation **Content Area:** Adult Health: Respiratory **Strategy:** The core issue of the question is knowledge of medication to reduce risk of pulmonary embolus. Use nursing knowledge and the process of elimination to make a selection.

8 **Answer: 1, 2, 3, 4 Rationale:** Increased respiratory rate, tachycardia, and agitation are early signs of respiratory distress, and can be interpreted by the nurse as deteriorating clinical state. Cyanosis develops later in the progression of respiratory distress, but is still an indication of client deterioration. Increased urinary output is the opposite of what the nurse would expect in a client with respiratory distress whose condition is deteriorating. **Cognitive Level:** Analyzing **Client Need:** Physiological Adaptation **Integrated Process:** Nursing Process: Assessment **Content Area:** Adult Health: Respiratory **Strategy:** The critical word in the stem of the question is *deteriorating*, which indicates that the nurse should be assessing for both early and late manifestations of respiratory distress. In an adult, cyanosis is always a late sign, but it occurs early in children. Use nursing knowledge and the process of elimination to make a selection. When there is more than one correct answer, consider each option as a true/false statement.

9 **Answer: 3 Rationale:** Symptoms associated with pulmonary embolism typically have a sudden onset. The client often feels panic because of the sudden dyspnea. Increase in heart rate is abrupt, not slow, with a pulmonary embolism. Cyanosis of the upper torso is associated with embolism of a central vein other than the pulmonary vasculature. Bilateral wheezing is more often associated with asthma than with pulmonary embolism. **Cognitive Level:** Applying **Client Need:** Physiological Adaptation **Integrated Process:** Nursing Process: Assessment **Content Area:** Adult Health: Respiratory **Strategy:** The critical words in the stem of the question are *symptom* and *pulmonary embolism*. They tell you that the question is seeking an answer that is a correct assessment. Use nursing knowledge and the process of elimination to make a selection.

10 **Answer: 2 Rationale:** The finding of crepitus at any time is associated with pneumothorax, and should be reported immediately to the healthcare provider. Oozing of blood from the thoracentesis puncture site is not uncommon, and does not require emergency intervention, as would crepitus. Diminished breath sounds in the affected lung base would occur with atelectasis. Fever might or might not be related to the thoracentesis. **Cognitive Level:** Analyzing **Client Need:** Physiological Adaptation **Integrated Process:** Nursing Process: Assessment **Content Area:** Adult Health: Respiratory **Strategy:** The core issue of the question is the ability to recognize and prioritize complications that need to be reported to the healthcare provider. Use nursing knowledge and the process of elimination to make a selection.

11 **Answer: 3 Rationale:** The primary physiological alterations occurring with COPD are alveolar air trapping and alveolar hyperinflation, which lead to alveolar rupture and loss of area available for gas exchange. Decreased surfactant production is associated with ARDS, and is not a primary alteration of COPD. The difficulty that a COPD client has with breathing in is related to alveolar air trapping and hyperinflation; newly inhaled air has no place to enter. Lung compliance is decreased, but this is due to the alveolar air trapping and hyperinflation. **Cognitive Level:** Applying **Client Need:** Physiological Adaptation **Integrated Process:** Teaching and Learning **Content Area:** Adult Health: Respiratory **Strategy:** The core issues of the question are knowledge of the underlying changes associated with COPD and how to communicate that information effectively to a client or family. Use nursing knowledge and the process of elimination to make a selection.

12 **Answer: 2, 3 Rationale:** Viral pneumonia is considered less serious for the client because symptoms are not as apparent compared with bacterial pneumonia. Viral pneumonia is associated with a nonproductive cough and normal or near-normal white blood cell count. Ghon's tubercles are seen on x-ray in clients with tuberculosis. Viral pneumonia is associated with low-grade fever. The client with viral pneumonia will display normal or minimal chest x-ray findings. **Cognitive Level:** Analyzing **Client Need:** Physiological Adaptation **Integrated Process:** Nursing Process: Assessment **Content Area:** Adult Health: Respiratory **Strategy:** The critical words in the stem are *most frequent*. With this in mind, you must compare options in terms of their frequency. Use nursing knowledge and the process of elimination to make a selection. When there is more than one correct answer, consider each option as a true/false statement.

13 **Answer: 1 Rationale:** Anticholinergics such as ipratropium are contraindicated in clients with angle-closure glaucoma because they can inhibit flow of aqueous humor and raise intraocular pressure. Cushing's syndrome, warfarin therapy, and fluid retention would not lead the nurse to question a prescription for ipratropium. **Cognitive Level:** Applying **Client Need:** Pharmacological and Parenteral Therapies **Integrated Process:** Nursing Process: Implementation **Content Area:** Adult Health: Respiratory **Strategy:** The core issue of the question is knowledge of contraindications to medication therapy. Use nursing knowledge and the process of elimination to make a selection.

14 **Answer: 2 Rationale:** Clients with mild and infrequent asthma symptoms are treated with a short-acting beta-agonist inhaler for quick relief in acute episodes. Corticosteroids as oral or inhaled medication are used for clients with more severe and frequent episodes of asthma. Clients with mild and infrequent asthma symptoms are treated with regular *daily* administration of an anti-inflammatory inhaler. Bronchodilators as oral or inhaled medication are used for clients with more severe and frequent episodes of asthma. **Cognitive Level:** Applying **Client Need:** Physiological Adaptation **Integrated Process:** Nursing Process: Planning **Content Area:** Adult Health: Respiratory **Strategy:** The core issue of the question is knowledge of the rapid management of symptoms in a client with asthma. Use nursing knowledge and the process of elimination to make a selection.

15 **Answer: 3 Rationale:** A primary physiological alteration occurring with ARDS is shunting of blood around nonventilated alveoli. Alveoli collapse in ARDS, preventing air from entering the alveoli, and ventilation decreases. The development of ARDS is not associated with the accumulation of exudative fluid in the alveoli or excessive alpha-1-antitrypsin.

Cognitive Level: Applying **Client Need:** Physiological Adaptation **Integrated Process:** Nursing Process: Diagnosis **Content Area:** Adult Health: Respiratory **Strategy:** The core issue of the question is knowledge of pathophysiology in the development of ARDS. Use nursing knowledge and the process of elimination to make a selection.

16 **Answer: 1, 2, 5 Rationale:** The best position is semi- to high-Fowler position. Epinephrine is a bronchodilator used to increase the diameter of the airways. Calming the child will ease respiratory function; crying and anxiety will cause an escalation in respiratory distress. Corticosteroids may be used, but will not ease respiratory distress immediately. Antibiotics may be used, but will not ease respiratory distress immediately. **Cognitive Level:** Analyzing **Client Need:** Physiological Adaptation **Integrated Process:** Nursing Process: Implementation **Content Area:** Child Health **Strategy:** The core issue of the question is the expected plan of care for a client with laryngotracheobronchitis. Use nursing knowledge and the process of elimination to make a selection. When there is more than one correct answer, consider each option as a true/false statement.

17 **Answer: 1 Rationale:** RSV is the cause of bronchiolitis in most cases; RSV can live for several hours on nonporous surfaces, and can be transferred by the hands; gown and gloves will prevent the nurse from spreading the RSV to other clients. The nurse's statement should be therapeutic and not cause the parents additional stress. The infant with RSV does not need to be protected from other illnesses; the objective is to protect the virus from spreading to other children. Nurses do not always wear gowns and gloves when infants are coughing. **Cognitive Level:** Analyzing **Client Need:** Physiological Adaptation **Integrated Process:** Nursing Process: Implementation **Content Area:** Child Health **Strategy:** The core issue of the question is the ability of the nurse to explain the rationale and use of isolation techniques. Use nursing knowledge and the process of elimination to make a selection.

18 **Answer: 2 Rationale:** Maintaining strict I&O will provide immediate notification of signs of dehydration; children with bronchiolitis could already have a history of poor fluid intake when initially seen by medical personnel. The child with bronchiolitis should be kept quiet, with limited stimulation and visitors. Limited visitors will prevent over-stimulation and promote a quiet environment. If the child is tachypneic, oral fluids present a risk of aspiration; fluids would be provided intravenously. **Cognitive Level:** Analyzing **Client Need:** Physiological Adaptation **Integrated Process:** Nursing Process: Implementation **Content Area:** Child Health **Strategy:** The core issue of the question is knowledge that a client with bronchiolitis has a priority need for hydration. Use nursing knowledge and the process of elimination to make a selection.

19 **Answer: 3 Rationale:** Meconium ileus in the newborn period is often the first indication of cystic fibrosis. Requiring resuscitation in the delivery room, a labor lasting more than 24 hours, and a labor lasting less than 4 hours are not indications that a child may have cystic fibrosis. **Cognitive Level:** Applying **Client Need:** Physiological Adaptation **Integrated Process:** Nursing Process: Assessment **Content Area:** Child Health **Strategy:** The core issue of the question is knowledge of the association between meconium ileus and cystic fibrosis in the neonate. Use nursing knowledge and the process of elimination to make a selection.

20 **Answer: 1 Rationale:** Bronchodilators open the airways and afford easier removal of secretions. Changing the child's clothes prior to the postural drainage exercises is unnecessary. Administering the child's antibiotic before the postural drainage is not necessary. Suctioning of the child's throat could be done after the procedure, if necessary. **Cognitive Level:** Analyzing **Client Need:** Physiological Adaptation **Integrated Process:** Nursing Process: Implementation **Content Area:** Child Health **Strategy:** The core issue of the question is knowledge of the proper sequence of actions when a client undergoes chest physiotherapy. Use nursing knowledge and the process of elimination to make a selection.

21 **Answer: 4 Rationale:** Clear breath sounds indicate an ability to clear the airway and decreased mucosal swelling and obstruction. Pale lips and mucous membranes could indicate hypoxia. Tripod position is a clinical manifestation of a child in distress due to epiglottitis. Tachypneic and dysphonic findings are symptoms of the disease. **Cognitive Level:** Analyzing **Client Need:** Physiological Adaptation **Integrated Process:** Nursing Process: Evaluation **Content Area:** Child Health **Strategy:** The core issue of this question is correctly identifying when an appropriate outcome measure has been achieved. Use nursing knowledge and the process of elimination to make a selection.

22 **Answer: 5 Rationale:** Tracheostomy suctioning can be stressful to the child and increases risk for hypoxia, infection, and mucosal damage. Each pass of the suction catheter should be limited to no more than 5 seconds. The child should be allowed to rest between passes with supplemental oxygen, if needed. **Cognitive Level:** Applying **Client Need:** Physiological Adaptation **Integrated Process:** Nursing Process: Implementation **Content Area:** Child Health **Strategy:** The critical issue of this question is the appropriate length of time for suctioning without impairing the respiratory status of a child. Use nursing knowledge and the process of elimination to make a selection.

23 **Answer: 3 Rationale:** Toddlers are naturally inquisitive, and explore things with their hands and mouths. Small objects and foods should be kept out of reach. Toddlers should be supervised but this may not be sufficient to prevent aspiration of another object if the environment has not been cleared of unsafe objects. It is developmentally inappropriate to attempt to teach a toddler to stop normal hand-to-mouth activity. While toddlers need to be observed and supervised, it may not be possible to monitor them continually. **Cognitive Level:** Applying **Client Need:** Safety and Infection Control **Integrated Process:** Nursing Process: Implementation **Content Area:** Child Health **Strategy:** The core issue of the question is the best method to provide a safe environment for a toddler, while understanding the normal patterns of growth and development. Use nursing knowledge and the process of elimination to make a selection.

24 **Answer: 4 Rationale:** Hand hygiene is the most important infection control practice, and decreases the spread of RSV and other organisms. Gloves worn when assessing a child with RSV should be discarded in the trash basket. Defects in gloves should be noted before they are worn to assess a client. A teaching activity is not as timely immediately after glove removal because the nurse is still engaged in

ANSWERS & RATIONALES

infection control activities. **Cognitive Level:** Applying **Client Need:** Safety and Infection Control **Integrated Process:** Nursing Process: Implementation **Content Area:** Child Health **Strategy:** The core issue of the question is basic principles of infection control using medical asepsis. Use nursing knowledge and the process of elimination to make a selection.

25 **Answer: 2 Rationale:** Swimming is recommended for children with asthma because prolonged expiration under water is beneficial. Cromolyn is used prophylactically to prevent exercise-induced asthma. When an asthma episode occurs in conjunction with high-level physical activity, it is considered to be an exercise-induced episode. Immediate access to a rescue inhaler is recommended. **Cognitive Level:** Analyzing **Client Need:** Physiological Adaptation **Integrated Process:** Nursing Process: Evaluation **Content Area:** Child Health **Strategy:** The core issue of the question is an understanding of the relationship of exercise to episodes of asthma. Use nursing knowledge and the process of elimination to make a selection. When the stem of a question is negative, look for the option that is wrong.

26 **Answer: 1 Rationale:** Aerosol therapy such as a nebulizer is frequently used during hospitalization to administer medications. An advantage is that this route delivers medication directly to the airways. The intravenous route is not frequently used to administer respiratory medications to a child hospitalized with asthma. Some respiratory drugs can be administered subcutaneously but aerosol is most direct. Oral respiratory medications take time to be effective. **Cognitive Level:** Applying **Client Need:** Pharmacological and Parenteral Therapies **Integrated Process:** Nursing Process: Implementation **Content Area:** Child Health **Strategy:** The core issue of the question is an understanding of medication routes used in children, specifically those with respiratory problems. Use nursing knowledge and the process of elimination to make a selection.

27 **Answer: 3 Rationale:** Chest physiotherapy and postural drainage for children with cystic fibrosis help loosen pulmonary secretions and facilitate removal from airways. This treatment would not be helpful in a child with epiglottitis, foreign body aspiration, or bronchopulmonary dysplasia. **Cognitive Level:** Applying **Client Need:** Physiological Adaptation **Integrated Process:** Nursing Process: Planning **Content Area:** Child Health **Strategy:** The core issue of the question is the purpose of doing chest physiotherapy in a child with cystic fibrosis. Use nursing knowledge and the process of elimination to make a selection.

28 **Answer: 4 Rationale:** Steroids given via metered-dose inhaler on oral mucosa increase the risk for yeast infection. A spacer avoids the mucous membranes and works directly on the airways. The purpose of the spacer is not related to the appearance of the inhaler. Use of a spacer on a metered-dose inhaler does not change the need to shake the medication before administration. It is desirable for the medication to penetrate into the lower respiratory tract to be most effective. **Cognitive Level:** Applying **Client Need:** Safety and Infection Control **Integrated Process:** Teaching and Learning **Content Area:** Child Health **Strategy:** The core issue of the question is the rationale for using a spacer. Use nursing knowledge and the process of elimination to make a selection.

29 **Answer: 2 Rationale:** Excess fluid in the alveoli is a manifestation of bacterial pneumonia. The sound produced by fluid in the airways is crackles. Wheezes are often typical of pneumonia caused by RSV, or conditions where the air passages are narrowed, such as asthma. Apnea is a pause in respirations, which is under the control of the central nervous system. Retractions are asymmetrical chest wall movements that are seen in any client having respiratory difficulty. **Cognitive Level:** Analyzing **Client Need:** Physiological Adaptation **Integrated Process:** Communication and Documentation **Content Area:** Child Health **Strategy:** The core issue of the question is the type of adventitious breath sound that is expected in bacterial pneumonia. Eliminate apnea because the focus is respiratory, not the central nervous system. Eliminate retractions next because they are seen rather than heard. Choose crackles over wheezes, recalling that the infection process leads to fluid accumulation, not to bronchoconstriction.

30 **Answer: 3, 5 Rationale:** Ribavirin is an antiviral drug used to treat RSV, which causes crystallization of soft contact lenses, and is associated with conjunctivitis. Because RSV is easily transferred, it is advisable that the nurse caring for the child with the virus not care for other high-risk children. Strict hand hygiene and contact precautions will help prevent transfer of the virus. Clearing the nasal passages with a bulb syringe will promote breathing; infants are nose breathers and are not able to blow their noses. Staying in the room with the door closed will help prevent the transfer of RSV. **Cognitive Level:** Applying **Client Need:** Safety and Infection Control **Integrated Process:** Nursing Process: Planning **Content Area:** Child Health **Strategy:** The core issue of the question is providing care for a client with RSV. Because the stem of the question is negative, the correct answers address actions that should not be taken by the nurse. When more than one answer is correct, consider each option as a true/false statement.

ANSWERS & RATIONALES

Key Terms to Review

alveolar ventilation p. 893
atelectasis p. 901
barrel chest p. 899
bronchopulmonary dysplasia (BPD) p. 910
chronic bronchitis p. 899
diffusion p. 893
digital clubbing p. 909
dyspnea p. 908
emphysema p. 899
epiglottitis p. 912
foreign body aspiration p. 913
laryngotracheobronchitis p. 911
oxygen saturation p. 894
perfusion p. 893
pulmonary ventilation p. 893
respiration p. 893
sweat chloride test p. 909
tachypnea p. 908
trigger p. 899
ventilation–perfusion mismatch p. 903

References

Ball, J., & Bindler, R., & Cowen, K. (2015). *Principles of pediatric nursing: Caring for children* (6th ed.). Hoboken, NJ: Pearson Education.

Berman, A., Snyder, S., & Frandsen, G. (2016). *Kozier & Erb's fundamentals of nursing: Concepts, process, and practice* (10th ed.). New York, NY: Pearson Education.

Ignatavicius, D., & Workman, L. (2016). *Medical-surgical nursing: Patient-centered collaborative care* (10th ed.). Philadelphia: Saunders.

LeMone, P., Burke, K., Bauldoff, G., & Gubrud, P. (2015). *Medical surgical nursing: Clinical reasoning in patient care* (6th ed.). Hoboken, NJ: Pearson Education.

Lewis, S., Dirksen, S., Heitkemper, M., & Bucher, L. (2014). *Medical surgical nursing: Assessment and management of clinical problems* (9th ed.). St. Louis, MO: Elsevier Science.

Smith, S., Duell, D., Martin, B., Aebersold, M., & Gonzalez, L. (2017). *Clinical nursing skills: Basic to advanced skills* (10th ed.). New York, NY: Pearson Education.

Test Yourself

Are you ready for the NCLEX-RN® or course exams? Access the NEW web-based app that provides students with thousands of practice questions in preparation for the NCLEX experience.

Cardiovascular Disorders

56

In this chapter

Cross Reference

Other chapters relevant to this content area are

Cardiovascular Medications	**Chapter 37**
Common Laboratory Tests	**Chapter 46**
Common Diagnostic Tests and Procedures	**Chapter 47**
Fluid and Electrolyte Imbalances	**Chapter 53**

I. OVERVIEW OF ANATOMY AND PHYSIOLOGY OF CARDIOVASCULAR SYSTEM

A. Structures of heart

1. Hollow muscular organ enclosed in a protective sac, has four chambers—two atria and two ventricles—divided by septum into right and left sides
2. Heart wall has three layers: *epicardium*, fibrous outside protective layer; *myocardium*, middle layer of specialized cardiac muscle; *endocardium*, endothelial lining of chambers
3. *Pericardium*: protective sac encasing heart
4. Valves of heart
   a. Atrioventricular (AV) valves (tricuspid on right and mitral on left) separate and control blood flow between atria and ventricles
   b. Semilunar valves (pulmonic on right and aortic on left) separate ventricles from pulmonary artery and aorta, respectively, and control blood flow from heart
   c. S_1, first heart sound ("lub"), is heard when AV valves close during systole
   d. S_2, second heart sound ("dub"), is heard when semilunar valves close during diastole
5. Coronary circulation
   a. Left anterior descending (LAD) artery supplies anterior left ventricle (LV), anterior ventricular septum, and LV apex; circumflex artery supplies left atrium and lateral and posterior LV
   b. Right coronary artery (RCA) supplies right atrium and ventricle, inferior LV, posterior septal wall, and sinoatrial (SA) and atrioventricular (AV) nodes

B. Functions of heart

1. Circulation: right side circulates deoxygenated blood to lungs; left side pumps oxygenated blood throughout body to perfuse tissues
2. Coronary arteries branch off aorta to supply oxygenated blood to heart
3. Cardiac conduction system transmits electrical impulses, stimulates depolarization and cardiac muscle contraction; cells have electrophysiologic properties: *automaticity* (able to initiate an electrical impulse), *excitability* (able to respond to a stimulus), and *conductivity* (able to transmit impulses from one cell to another); see Table 56–1
4. Cardiac cycle: one complete heartbeat; includes two parts—systole (ventricular contraction) and diastole (relaxation and ventricular refilling)
5. **Cardiac output (CO)**: volume of blood in liters ejected by heart each minute; indicator of pumping function of heart; normal adult CO is 4–8 L/min

$$CO = HR \times SV$$

   a. Heart rate (HR): number of complete cardiac cycles per minute
   b. **Stroke volume (SV)**: volume of blood ejected from LV with each cardiac cycle; SV and ultimately CO are influenced by preload, afterload, and contractility
   c. **Preload**: degree of myocardial fiber stretch at end of ventricular diastole; influenced by ventricular filling volume and myocardial compliance
   d. **Afterload**: resistance that ventricles must overcome to eject blood into systemic circulation; directly related to arterial blood pressure (BP)
   e. **Contractility**: strength of contraction regardless of preload; decreased by hypoxia and some drugs (e.g., beta-blockers and calcium channel blockers); increased by drugs (e.g., digoxin and dopamine)

Table 56–1 Functions within Cardiac Conduction System

Area	Function
Sinoatrial (SA) node	Natural pacemaker; generates heart rate normally at 60–100 beats/min
Internodal pathways	Carry impulse from SA node to AV node; depolarization results in myocardial contraction of both atria
AV node	Slows electrical impulse; allows atria to fully empty before transmitting impulse to depolarize ventricles; when SA node is not functioning, AV node can initiate an impulse at rate of 40–60 beats/min
Bundle of His	Short branch of conductive cells connecting AV node to bundle branches at intraventricular septum
Bundle branches	Right (RBB) and left (LBB) split off on either side of intraventricular septum; carry impulses to Purkinje fibers
Purkinje fibers	Terminal branches of conduction system; initiate rapid depolarization wave causing ventricular contraction; when SA and AV nodes fail, can initiate impulses at rate of 20–40 beats/min

6. Autonomic nervous system: responds to chemoreceptors, baroreceptors, and stretch receptors
   a. Sympathetic: produces norepinephrine; results in increased HR, myocardial contractility, peripheral vasoconstriction, and arterial BP
   b. Parasympathetic: produces acetylcholine, results in decreased HR and contractility

C. Fetal circulation

1. Ductus venosus
   a. Umbilical vein carries oxygenated blood from placenta to fetus; blood bypasses liver through ductus venosus
   b. At birth when umbilical cord is clamped and cut, blood flow from maternal circulation ceases and ductus venosus closes; blood flows into liver
2. Foramen ovale
   a. Oxygenated systemic blood enters right atrium; flows from right to left atria through foramen ovale
   b. Blood bypasses lungs, which are nonfunctional
   c. Blood flows from left atria to LV and out to aorta
   d. Foramen ovale closes after birth with change in pressure in cardiac chambers
3. Ductus arteriosus
   a. A fistula that allows blood flowing through pulmonary artery to enter aorta; this is normal and desired in fetus
   b. Closes after birth with first few breaths so neonate's heart can circulate oxygenated blood to body

D. Structure and function of blood vessels

1. Distribute blood to body tissues
2. Arterial and venous walls have three layers: tunica intima, tunica media, and tunica adventitia; amount of pressure in vessel determines thickness of walls and amount of connective tissue and smooth muscle
3. Arterial system consists of high-pressure vessels, beginning with aorta, then arteries, arterioles, and ending with capillaries; delivers blood to various tissues and contributes to temperature regulation
4. Venous system begins after capillaries; consists of venules and veins (large-diameter, thin-walled vessels) under much less pressure; some veins, most commonly in legs, contain valves to regulate one-way flow; system returns blood from capillaries to right atrium and acts as a reservoir for blood volume

E. Regulation of BP

1. Autonomic nervous system
2. Baroreceptors in aortic arch and carotid sinus; chemoreceptors
3. Antidiuretic hormone (ADH)
4. Renin-angiotensin-aldosterone (RAA) system; angiotensin I is converted to angiotensin II, a powerful vasoconstrictor
5. Others: temperature (cold results in vasoconstriction, heat results in **vasodilation**), substances such as nicotine (vasoconstrict) and alcohol (vasodilate), diet (sodium and fat intake), and factors such as age, gender, ethnicity, weight, physical health, and emotional state

II. DIAGNOSTIC TESTS AND ASSESSMENTS

A. Laboratory tests (see also Chapter 46)

NCLEX®

1. Serum cardiac enzymes: myoglobin, troponins, creatinine kinase (CK), and lactic dehydrogenase (LDH); increase with cell death (**infarction**); serial testing over days detects trend and determines peak time and extent of injury
2. Serum drug levels:

NCLEX®

   a. Digoxin: therapeutic range is 0.5–2.0 ng/mL; signs of toxicity include nausea and vomiting (N/V), anorexia; abdominal pain, bradycardia, other dysrhythmias, and visual disturbances (blurred or yellow-green vision or halos)
   b. Quinidine: therapeutic range is 2–6 mcg/mL; signs of toxicity include tinnitus, hearing loss, visual disturbances, N/V, dizziness, widened QRS, ventricular dysrhythmias
3. Electrolytes: normal levels of sodium (135–145 mEq/L or mmol/L), potassium (3.5–5.1 mEq/L or 3.5–5.0 mmol/L), calcium (8.5–10.5 mg/dL or 2.2–2.58 mmol/L), and magnesium (1.6–2.5 mg/dL or 0.65–1.05 mmol/L) are essential for proper cardiac function; cardiac disorders and medications can alter electrolyte balance; see Chapter 53 for detailed information

NCLEX®

   a. Potassium (K^+): hypokalemia such as with diuretic therapy increases risk of digoxin toxicity, ventricular dysrhythmias; hyperkalemia from renal disease or excess potassium supplements can lead to ventricular dysrhythmias and asystole

↓ K^+ = dig Tox

NCLEX®
b. Sodium (Na^+): hyponatremia with long-term diuretic therapy; hypernatremia could occur with excess saline IV infusion
c. Calcium: cardiac effects of hypocalcemia include ventricular dysrhythmias, prolonged QT interval and cardiac arrest; hypercalcemia shortens QT interval and causes AV block, digoxin hypersensitivity, and cardiac arrest
d. Magnesium: cardiac effects of decreased magnesium include ventricular tachycardia and fibrillation, while increased magnesium causes bradycardia, hypotension, prolonged PR and QRS intervals

4. Serum lipid profile: a measurement used to determine risk of developing atherosclerosis (see also Chapter 46)
   a. Includes total serum cholesterol (<200 mg/dL or <5.2 mmol/L) triglycerides (<200 mg/dL or 0.45–1.69 mmol/L), and lipoproteins

NCLEX®
   b. High-density lipoproteins (HDL): transport cholesterol to liver for excretion ("good" cholesterol); normal is 60 mg/dL (1.5 mmol/L) and above

NCLEX®
   c. Low-density lipoproteins (LDL): transport cholesterol to peripheral tissues ("bad" cholesterol) and increases risk of heart disease; normal is under 130 mg/dL (<3.5 mmol/L)

B. **Electrocardiography** (see also Chapter 47)
1. A graphic recording of electrical activity of heart; diagnoses areas of myocardial ischemia, injury, and necrosis (MI); hypertrophy, electrolyte imbalance, and effects of antidysrhythmic drugs
2. Resting electrocardiogram (ECG): represents a single recorded picture of electrical activity of heart
3. Holter monitoring: continuous ambulatory ECG monitoring over time (usually 24 hr) with small, timed, portable ECG recording device
4. Stress test: continuous multilead ECG monitoring during controlled and supervised exercise, usually on treadmill

C. **Echocardiography**: ultrasound to evaluate structure and function of heart chambers and valves

D. **Phonocardiography**: a graphic recording of heart sounds with simultaneous ECG; not painful

E. **Coronary angiography and arteriography** (see also Chapter 47): an invasive procedure during which contrast medium is injected into coronary arteries and flow is recorded to assess structure of arteries

F. **Cardiac catheterization**
1. Insertion of a catheter into heart chambers and coronary vessels to detect abnormalities of heart structure and function (see also Chapter 47)

NCLEX®
2. Client preparation, nursing care during procedure, and postprocedure nursing care are summarized in Box 56–1

G. **Radionuclide tests**
1. Safe, nonpainful methods of evaluating LV muscle function and coronary artery blood distribution; radionuclide contrast is injected via venipuncture; encourage client to drink fluids postprocedure to facilitate excretion of contrast; assess venipuncture site for bleeding or hematoma; may be used in conjunction with stress testing
2. Allows visualization of ventricles through several cardiac cycles; calculate **ejection fraction (EF)**, portion of blood ejected during systole compared to total ventricular filling volume, (normal EF = 55–70%)
3. MUGA (gated pool imaging or multigated acquisition) scan
4. Thallium imaging: used to assess myocardial **ischemia** (decreased supply of oxygenated blood) during stress testing
5. PET (positron emission tomography) scan: evaluates cardiac metabolism and assesses tissue perfusion

H. **Electron beam computed tomography (EBCT)**: detects calcium deposits in arteries; a coronary artery calcium (CAC) score greater than 400 indicates high need for preventive treatment

I. **Electrophysiology studies (EPS)**: invasive procedure to investigate nature of cardiac rhythm disturbances; delivers a programmed electrical stimulus to determine source of dysrhythmias or conduction defects; aids in determining treatment (medication therapy, cardiac ablation, pacemaker, implantable cardioverter debribrillator [ICD], or surgery)

J. **Hemodynamic monitoring**
1. Measurement of heart pressures and calculation of hemodynamic parameters
2. Central venous pressure (CVP) monitoring: monitors fluid volume status and right heart function in clients who do not have pulmonary artery (PA) pressure monitoring
   a. Long catheter is inserted with tip lying in superior vena cava at juncture with right atrium
   b. Measures right heart filling pressure; does not measure left heart pressures

NCLEX®
   c. Normal CVP is 2–8 cm H_2O or 2–6 mmHg; decreased CVP indicates hypovolemia; increased CVP indicates hypervolemia or right heart failure

Box 56–1

Care of the Client Undergoing Cardiac Catheterization

Client Preparation

➤ Obtain written consent

➤ Assess client history of allergies to iodine or contrast medium

➤ Explain that client will be awake and may experience various sensations during procedure, including flushing sensation as dye is injected or fluttering feeling as catheter passes through heart

➤ Explain postprocedure routine (see Postprocedure Nursing Care)

➤ Prepare insertion site by shaving and cleansing with antiseptic

➤ Nothing by mouth (NPO) except sips of water with cardiac medications as indicated for 6–8 hours

➤ Initiate IV site with fluids as prescribed

➤ Administer preprocedure medications as prescribed

Nursing Care during Procedure

➤ Procedure is performed in cardiac catheterization laboratory by cardiologist; nurse monitors ECG and vital signs (VS) continuously, administers moderate sedation as prescribed, and provides emotional support

Postprocedure Nursing Care

➤ Maintain client on bedrest (often 6–12 hr) with affected extremity straight; do not elevate head of bed more than 15 degrees if femoral insertion site used

➤ Maintain pressure dressing at insertion site or external vice-type compression device (if applied postprocedure)

➤ Monitor BP, heart rate, distal pulses, color and temperature of extremity, and assess for bleeding or hematoma formation at site (with leg site, check under client for bleeding) per agency protocol (routinely q 15 minutes for 1 hour, q 30 minutes for 2 hours, q hour for 4 hours, or q 8 hours for associated procedure of percutaneous transluminal coronary angioplasty [PTCA])

➤ Report signs of chest pain, dysrhythmias, bleeding, hematoma formation, or other changes; report significant changes in VS, pulses, and color or temperature of extremity immediately to healthcare provider; bleeding may be felt by client as warmth around insertion area

➤ If bleeding occurs, restore manual pressure to site (manual pressure also applied immediately postprocedure, often for up to 20 minutes because of heparin use during procedure)

➤ Maintain IV and encourage oral fluids as prescribed to eliminate contrast medium, which can be nephrotoxic

➤ Monitor I&O to determine whether client is becoming dehydrated from increased urine output because of contrast excretion

3. PA pressure monitoring: appropriate for critically ill clients requiring accurate assessments of left heart pressures
   a. PA (Swan-Ganz) catheter has tip in pulmonary artery
   b. Pressure measurement obtained after catheter tip is wedged in small pulmonary artery (called pulmonary capillary wedge pressure, or PCWP); is a good indicator of left-ventricular end diastolic pressure (LVEDP)
   c. Allows calculation of CO and other hemodynamic parameters at frequent intervals

NCLEX®

4. Nursing responsibilities in hemodynamic monitoring: position transducer at level of right atrium (left midaxillary line, fourth intercostal space—phlebostatic axis); level CVP or PA catheter transducer to this point each shift and before each measurement; maintain catheter patency with a constant small amount of fluid delivered under pressure

K. **Doppler ultrasound**: a noninvasive test that detects blood flow and emits an audible signal; can determine blood flow when arterial palpation is difficult or impossible because of occlusive disease; a palpable pulse and a Doppler pulse are not equivalent, so document clearly

L. **Plethysmography**: records volume changes in an extremity associated with cardiac contractions or in response to pneumatic venous occlusion; can detect and quantify vascular disease by changes in pulse contour, BP, or arterial and venous blood flow

M. **Digital subtraction angiography**: computer-aided visualization of blood vessels after IV injection of contrast medium

N. **Venography**: injection of radiopaque contrast into veins, with serial x-rays taken to detect deep-vein thrombosis and incompetent valves

O. **Angiography**: injection of radiopaque contrast into arteries to detect plaques, occlusions, injury, and so on; similar to care for postcardiac catheterization

P. **Ankle-brachial index**: commonly used parameter for overall evaluation of extremity status; ankle pressure normally is same or higher than brachial systolic pressure

Q. **Computed tomography**: computer-aided visualization of arterial wall and its structures; used to diagnose abdominal aortic aneurysm (AAA) and postoperative vascular complications such as graft occlusion and hemorrhage

R. **Magnetic resonance imaging (MRI)**: uses magnetic fields rather than radiation; used with angiography to detect abnormalities, especially in clients who cannot have contrast injected

III. COMMON NURSING TECHNIQUES AND PROCEDURES

A. Blood pressure (BP) measurement

1. BP is primarily a function of CO and systemic vascular resistance (SVR); arterial BP equals CO multiplied by SVR
2. Have client sit with arm bared, supported, and at heart level; ensure no smoking or caffeine intake 30 minutes prior
3. Take BP in both arms initially using appropriate-sized cuff (rubber bladder should at least encircle arm by 80%)
4. If averaging two or more readings, separate measurements by at least 2 minutes
5. If both client's arms are inaccessible (from combination of IV lines, dialysis shunt, mastectomy, burns, etc.), obtain readings from thigh or calf, auscultating popliteal or posterior tibial arteries, respectively

B. Dysrhythmia monitoring

1. Continuous ECG monitoring in one lead with portable telemetry unit; indicated for high-risk clients who have cardiac disease, take cardiac medications, or are undergoing surgery or diagnostic or therapeutic procedures
2. Lead placements (ECG continuous monitors have three leads or five leads)
   a. Placement of leads with three-lead monitor are below right clavicle (right arm—white lead), below left clavicle (left arm—black lead), and at lowest rib, left midclavicular line (left leg—red lead)
   b. Placement of leads with five-lead monitor are same as three-lead with fourth lead placed at lowest rib, right midclavicular line (right leg—green lead) and fifth lead on site of one of six chest leads (V leads—brown lead)

NCLEX®
3. Preparation of client: explain procedure and reassure that client will not receive electrical impulses or shocks; identify proper placement, cleanse skin with soap and water, shave hairy areas, use alcohol or skin prep as per agency policy, dry with cloth or gauze, and apply fresh electrodes

NCLEX®
4. ECG patterns originating in sinus node
   a. See Table 56–2 for descriptions of sinus rhythm (normal), sinus tachycardia, sinus bradycardia, and sinus arrhythmia

   NCLEX®
   b. Nursing and therapeutic interventions: with sinus arrest, tachycardia, or bradycardia, assess for signs of inadequate CO and tissue perfusion, including changes in BP, activity tolerance, and level of consciousness (LOC); identify and treat cause of sinus tachycardia; atropine and possible pacemaker indicated for symptomatic or extreme low rates (<50)
5. ECG patterns originating in the atria

   NCLEX®
   a. See again Table 56–2 for descriptions of premature atrial contractions (PAC), paroxysmal supraventricular tachycardia (SVT), atrial flutter, and atrial fibrillation

   NCLEX®
   b. Nursing and therapeutic interventions: carotid massage, synchronized cardioversion, antidysrhythmia medications including beta-blockers, calcium channel blockers, and digoxin; anticoagulant therapy to reduce the risk of thrombus
6. ECG patterns originating from the AV node
   a. See again Table 56–2 for descriptions of first-degree heart block, second-degree heart block (Mobitz type I or Wenckebach and Mobitz type II), third-degree (complete) heart block and junctional escape rhythm

(*Text continues on p. 932.*)

Table 56–2 Selected Cardiac Rhythms and Dysrhythmias

Rhythm/ECG Appearance	ECG Characteristics	Management
Supraventricular Rhythms		
Normal sinus rhythm (NSR) 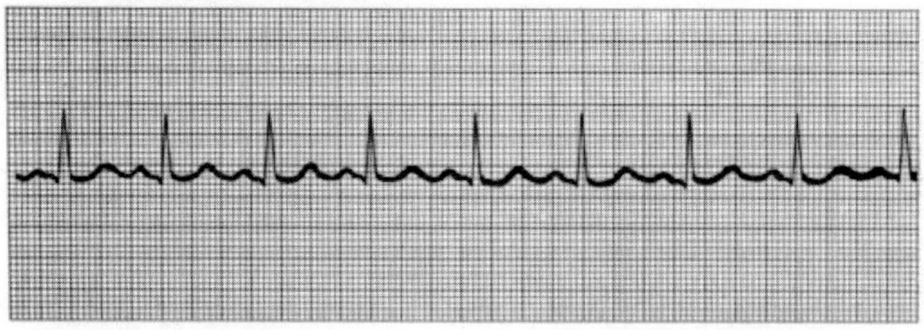	Rate: 60–100 beats/min Rhythm: regular P:QRS ratio: 1:1 PR interval: 0.12–0.20 sec QRS complex: 0.06–0.10 sec	None; normal heart rhythm
Sinus arrhythmia 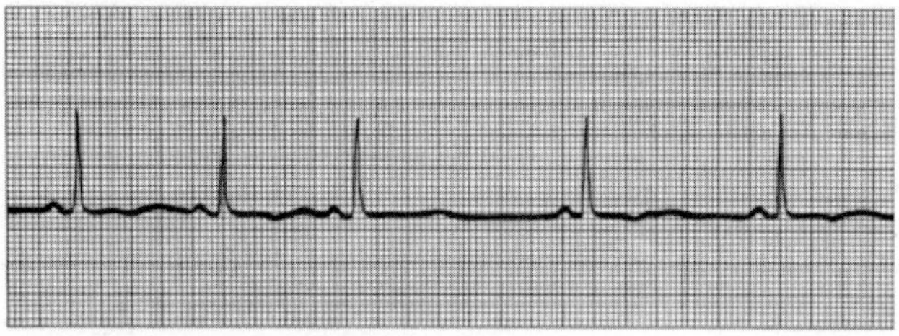	Rate: 60–100 beats/min Rhythm: irregular, varying with respirations P:QRS ratio: 1:1 PR interval: 0.12–0.20 sec QRS complex: 0.06–0.10 sec	Generally none; considered a normal rhythm in the very young and very old
Sinus tachycardia 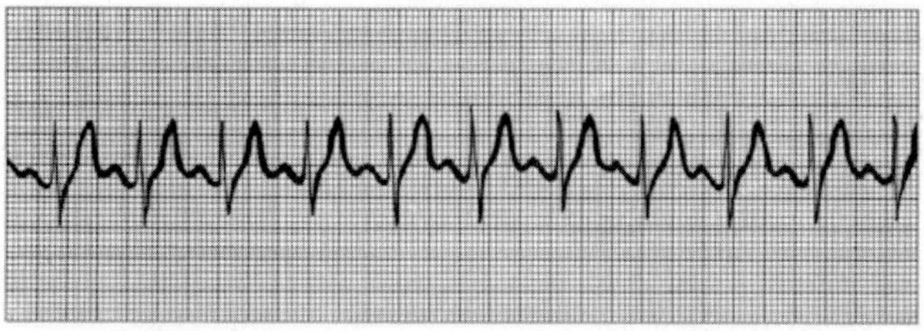	Rate: 101–150 beats/min Rhythm: regular P:QRS ratio: 1:1 (with very fast rates, P wave may be hidden in preceding T wave) PR interval: 0.12–0.20 sec QRS complex: 0.06–0.10 sec	Treat only if client is symptomatic or client is at risk for myocardial damage; treat underlying cause (e.g., hypovolemia, fever, pain); beta-blockers or verapamil may be used
Sinus bradycardia 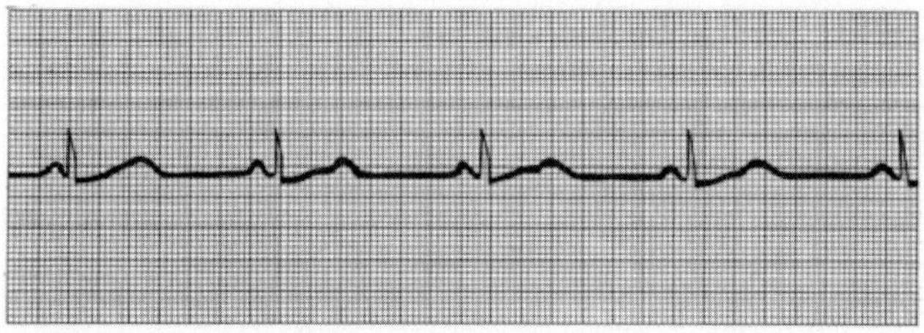	Rate: less than 60 beats/min Rhythm: regular P:QRS ratio: 1:1 PR interval: 0.12–0.20 sec QRS complex: 0.06–0.10 sec	Treat only if symptomatic; intravenous atropine or isoproterenol and/or pacemaker therapy may be used
Premature atrial contractions (PAC) 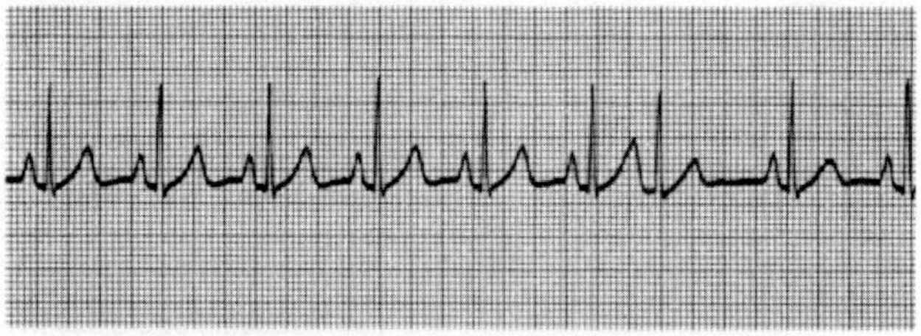	Rate: variable Rhythm: irregular, with normal rhythm interrupted by early beats arising in atria P:QRS ratio: 1:1 PR interval: 0.12–0.20 sec but may be prolonged QRS complex: 0.6–0.10 sec	Usually requires no treatment; advise client to reduce alcohol and caffeine intake, to reduce stress, and to stop smoking; beta-blocker therapy may be prescribed
Paroxysmal supraventricular tachycardia (PSVT) 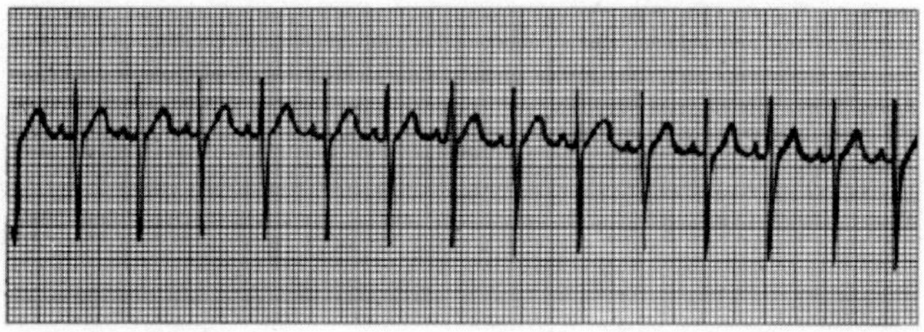	Rate: 100–280 beats/min (usually 150–200 beats/min Rhythm: regular P:QRS ratio: P waves often not identifiable PR interval: not measured QRS complex: 0.06–0.10 sec	Treat if symptomatic; treatment may include vagal maneuvers (Valsalva, carotid sinus massage); oxygen therapy; adenosine or a beta-blocker; temporary pacing or synchronized cardioversion

(*continued*)

Table 56–2 Selected Cardiac Rhythms and Dysrhythmias (*continued*)

Rhythm/ECG Appearance	ECG Characteristics	Management
Atrial flutter 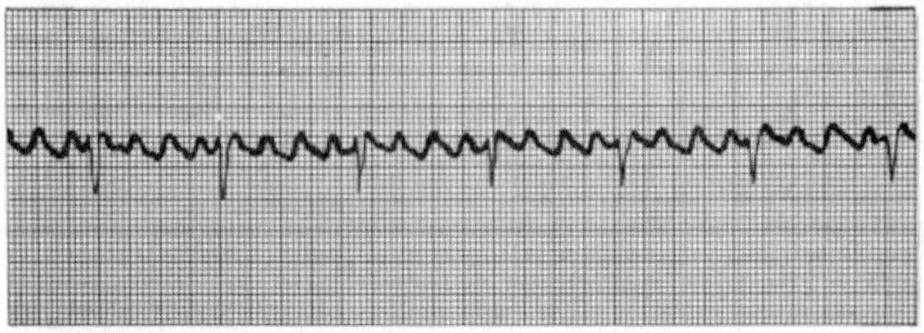	Rate: atrial 240–360 beats/min; ventricular rate depends on degree of AV block; usually <150 beats/min Rhythm: atrial regular, ventricular usually regular P:QRS ratio may be 2:1, 4:1, 6:1, or may vary PR interval: not measured QRS complex: 0.06–0.10 sec	Synchronized cardioversion; medications to slow ventricular response, such as beta-blocker or calcium channel blocker, followed by class I antidysrhythmic or amiodarone
Atrial fibrillation 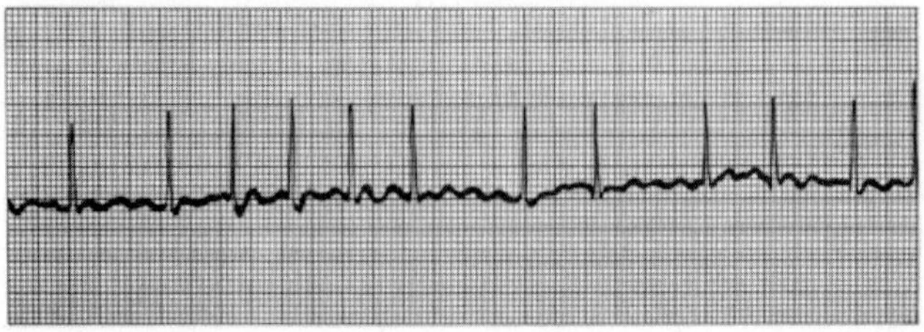	Rate: atrial 300–600 beats/min (too rapid to count); ventricular 100–180 beats/min in untreated clients Rhythm: irregularly irregular P:QRS ratio is variable PR interval: not measured QRS complex: 0.06–0.10 sec	Synchronized cardioversion; medications to reduce ventricular response rate: metoprolol, diltiazem, digoxin; anticoagulant therapy to reduce risk of clot formation and stroke
Junctional escape rhythm 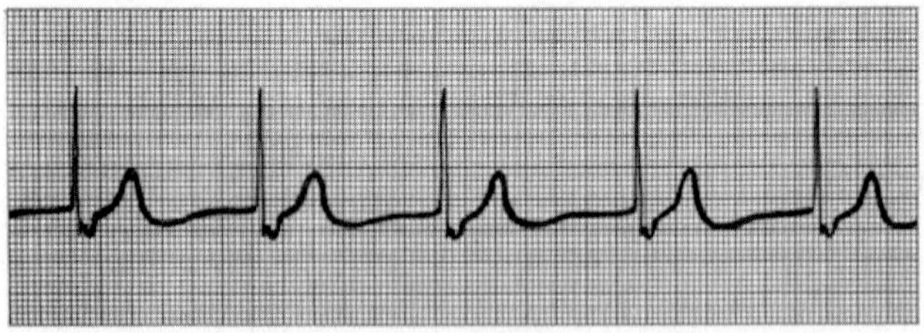	Rate: 40–60 beats/min; junctional tachycardia 60–140 beats/min Rhythm: regular P:QRS ratio: P waves may be absent, inverted, and immediately preceding, hidden in, or following QRS complex PR interval: less than 0.10 sec if P wave present QRS complex: 0.06–0.10 sec	Treat cause if symptomatic
Ventricular Rhythms *Premature ventricular contractions (PVCs)* 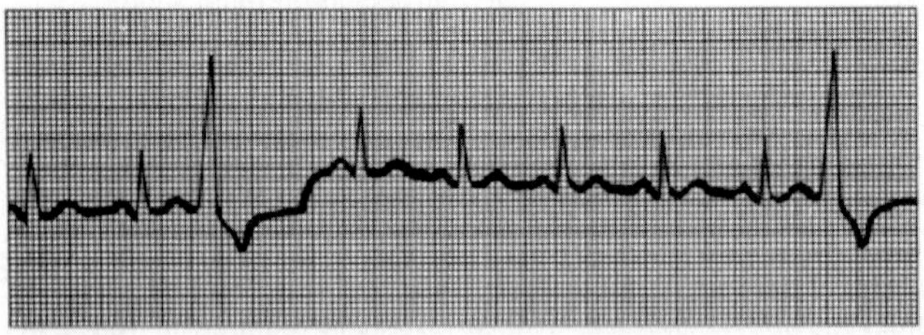	Rate: variable Rhythm: irregular; PVC interrupts underlying rhythm and is followed by compensatory pause P:QRS ratio: no P wave noted before PVC PR interval: absent with PVC QRS complex: wide (>0.12 sec), bizarre in appearance; differs from normal QRS complex	Treat if symptomatic or in presence of severe heart disease; advise against stimulant use (caffeine, nicotine); drug therapy includes class I and III antidysrhythmics and possibly addition of beta-blocker
Ventricular tachycardia (VT or V tach) 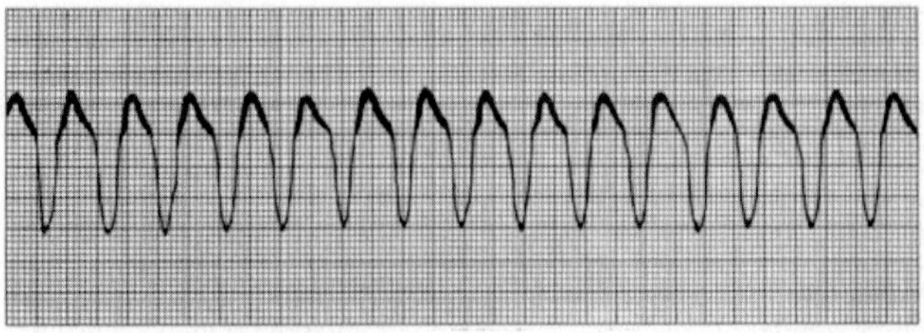	Rate: 100–250 beats/min Rhythm: regular P:QRS ratio: P waves usually not identifiable PR interval: not measured QRS complex: 0.12 sec or greater; bizarre shape	Treat if VT is sustained, symptomatic, or associated with organic heart disease; treatment includes DC cardioversion or IV procainamide, lidocaine or a class III antidysrhythmic, if hemodynamically unstable; surgical ablation or antitachycardia pacing with implanted cardioverter/defibrillator (ICD) for repeated episodes

Table 56–2 Selected Cardiac Rhythms and Dysrhythmias (*continued*)

Rhythm/ECG Appearance	ECG Characteristics	Management
Ventricular fibrillation (VF or V fib) 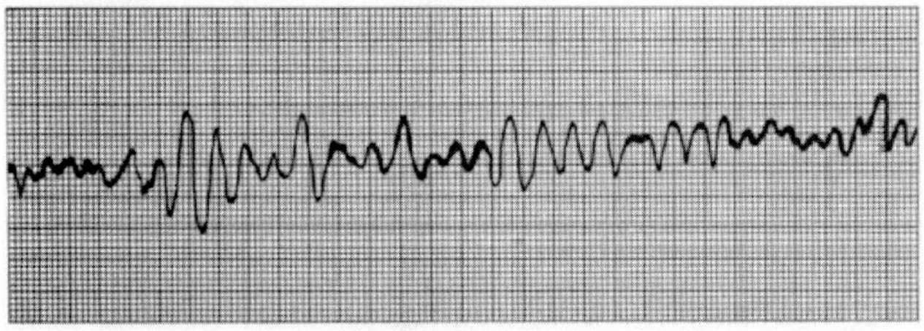	Rate: too rapid to count Rhythm: grossly irregular P:QRS ratio: no identifiable P waves PR interval: none QRS: bizarre, varying in shape and direction	Immediate cardioversion/ defibrillation
Atrioventricular Conduction Blocks *First-degree AV block* 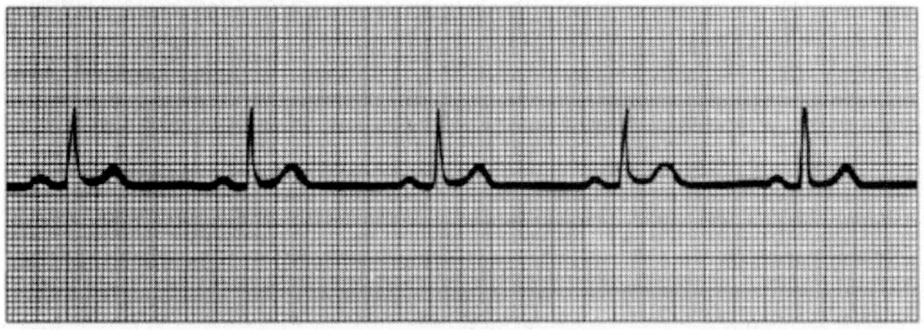	Rate: usually 60–100 beats/min Rhythm: regular P:QRS ratio: 1:1 PR interval: >0.20 sec QRS complex: 0.06–0.10 sec	None required
Second-degree AV block, type I (Mobitz I, Wenckebach) 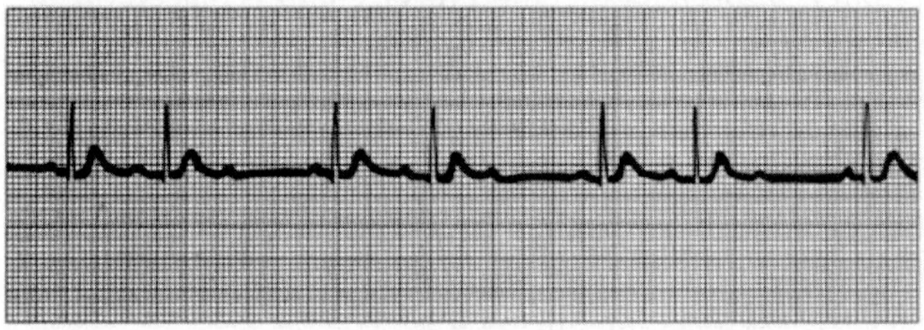	Rate: 60–100 beats/min Rhythm: atrial regular; ventricular irregular P:QRS ratio: 1:1 until P wave blocked with no QRS following PR interval: progressively lengthens in a regular pattern QRS complex: 0.06–0.10 sec; sudden absence of QRS complex	Monitoring and observation; rarely progresses to a higher degree of block or requires treatment
Second-degree AV block, type II (Mobitz II) 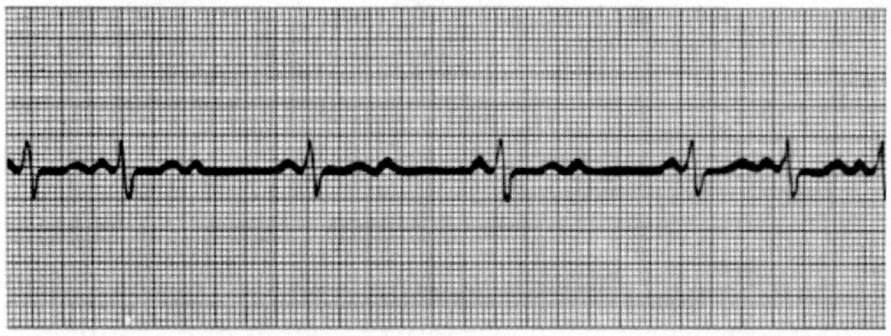	Rate: atrial 60–100 beats/min; ventricular less than 60 beats/min Rhythm: atrial regular; ventricular irregular P:QRS ratio: typically 2:1, may vary PR interval: constant PR interval for each conducted QRS complex QRS complex: 0.06–0.10 sec	Atropine or isoproterenol; pacemaker therapy
Third-degree AV block (complete heart block) 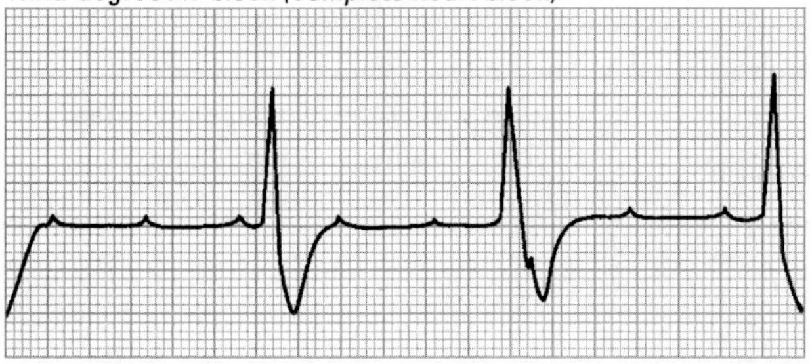	Rate: atrial 60–100 beats/min; ventricular 15–60 beats/min Rhythm: atrial regular; ventricular regular P:QRS ratio: no relationship between P waves and QRS complexes; independent rhythms PR interval: not measured QRS complex: 0.06–0.10 sec if junctional escape rhythm; > 0.12 sec if ventricular escape rhythm	Immediate pacemaker therapy

Source: LeMone P., Burke, K. Bauldoff, G., & Gubrud, P. (2015). *Medical surgical nursing: Clinical reasoning in patient care* (6th ed.). New York, NY: Pearson Education; pp. 898–900, Table 30–7.

NCLEX® b. Nursing and therapeutic interventions include monitoring and observation; atropine, isoproterenol or pacemakers for symptomatic heart block (external or transthoracic, temporary, or permanent)

7. ECG patterns originating from ventricles

NCLEX® a. See again Table 56–2 for descriptions of premature ventricular contractions (PVC), ventricular tachycardia (VT), and ventricular fibrillation (VF)

NCLEX® b. Nursing and therapeutic interventions: for PVCs monitor for signs of decreased CO; instruct client to avoid caffeine and nicotine; with VT, assess immediately to determine LOC and if client has stable BP and pulse; if stable, treat with amiodarone, procainamide, lidocaine, and cardioversion; if client becomes unconscious or unstable or has pulseless VT or VF, immediate defibrillation is required

C. Percutaneous transluminal coronary angioplasty (PTCA)

1. An invasive nonsurgical procedure that increases coronary blood flow by dilating coronary artery using a balloon-tipped catheter inserted into narrowed segment; may also include insertion of an expandable intracoronary stent (see next section)
2. A variation of this procedure is *laser-assisted angioplasty*, in which a laser probe is advanced into artery instead of a balloon-tipped catheter; artery reopens after heat from laser vaporizes plaque; this procedure can also be used to treat small occlusions in arteries of legs

NCLEX® 3. Client preparation, nursing care during procedure, and postprocedure nursing care are same as for cardiac catheterization, outlined previously in Box 56–1

D. Coronary artery stents

1. Devices used in conjunction with PTCA procedure that spring open in area of occlusion when balloon is inflated; once opened, they remain against arterial wall to promote long-term patency; devices may be made of plain metal or may be drug-eluting
2. Client preparation and postprocedure care is same as for cardiac catheterization and PTCA
3. A risk of stent placement is acute thrombosis (stent is a foreign object in body); client is placed on antiplatelet therapy according to protocols based on type of stent inserted
4. Complications of stent placement include migration or occlusion of stent, dissection of coronary artery, and bleeding from anticoagulant therapy

E. Coronary artery bypass grafting (CABG)

1. Arteries occluded with plaque are surgically "bypassed" with saphenous veins, mammary arteries, or less frequently, artificial grafts; indicated for myocardial ischemia not managed by medical treatment; client is typically maintained on cardiopulmonary bypass machine during surgery
2. Client preparation
   a. Ensure that all standard preoperative care is provided and that consents are signed
   b. Perform routine preoperative teaching, including turning, deep breathing and coughing (with splinting of sternal incision), use of incentive spirometer (IS) to prevent respiratory complications, and leg exercises and sequential compression devices (SCDs) to prevent thrombus formation
   c. Explain postoperative course, including respiratory support on ventilator with an endotracheal tube; suctioning; surgical incisions (sternal and one or both legs or arms), chest tubes, multiple IV lines, tubes, drains, and monitors with alarms and noises; pain management, communication techniques, visiting policies, and expected length of hospitalization and recovery period
   d. Encourage client and family to share questions and concerns; provide support to client and family; provide preoperative tour of postsurgical cardiac intensive care unit if feasible

NCLEX® 3. Immediate postoperative care in cardiac surgical critical care unit
   a. Continuously monitor cardiac rhythm, pulmonary artery, CVP, and arterial line waveforms and pressures; titrate vasoactive IV medications to keep arterial pressure within target range (avoiding hypotension and possible graft closure or hypertension and possible bleeding from graft sites)
   b. Provide frequent monitoring of other VS, neurologic status, lung sounds, UO, drainage from mediastinal and other tubes, and general assessments as per protocol
   c. Monitor client respiratory status on ventilator and during weaning protocol, usually within first 24 hours postoperative
   d. Keep epicardial pacing wires grounded using agency-specified caps if not attached to temporary pacemaker (prevents microshock)
   e. Provide effective pain management using IV medications per protocol; sternotomy pain can interfere with pulmonary hygiene efforts and lead to atelectasis and pneumonia; differentiate incisional pain from pain of cardiac origin
   f. Monitor fluid and electrolyte balance; measure daily weight starting on first postoperative day; client gains fluid weight during surgery

4. Within 1–2 days client is transferred to a step-down/telemetry unit where care continues
   a. Monitor client for signs of decreased CO; assess ECG via continuous monitoring; I&O; full assessments with lung sounds and heart sounds every 4 hours initially, then at least every 8 hours
   b. Assess and treat postoperative pain
   c. Monitor indicators of CO with client's increasing activity; watch for signs of activity intolerance (increase in pulse rate by 10–15 beats/min or drop in systolic BP of 10–20 mmHg) and have client sit or lie down if these occur
   d. Monitor respiratory status and encourage deep breathing, IS, and coughing when sternotomy incision is splinted for comfort and sternal stability
   e. Maintain standards of general postoperative care (wound assessment and management, monitoring fluid and electrolyte balance, monitoring for infection)
   f. Instruct client (and appropriate family) about new medication regime, activity plan for home (progressive return of activity over time), diet (low-fat and low-sodium), cardiac rehabilitation, resumption of sexual activity (usually allowed when client can walk up two full flights of stairs or one block without shortness of breath [SOB] or chest pain; client should be rested, not after a heavy meal or alcohol consumption)
   g. Instruct about symptoms to report to healthcare provider after discharge including chest pain, SOB, decrease in activity tolerance, fever, redness, swelling or drainage from surgical incisions, or signs of depression (can occur up to 6 months after cardiac surgery, and client should notify healthcare provider for further assessment and treatment)
5. Newer procedures that may be an alternative to traditional CABG surgery for selected clients include minimally invasive coronary artery surgery (reduced recovery time) and transmyocardial revascularization (laser drills tiny holes into myocardium to provide collateral circulation)

F. Pacemakers

1. Permanent pacemakers are inserted to treat permanent cardiac conduction defects; generator box is implanted under chest wall and wires are threaded into blood vessel and through right atrium for implantation in right ventricle (RV) (commonly), or pacing can be dual-chambered (right atrium and ventricle)
2. Pacemaker function is programmed at time of insertion and can be reprogrammed externally using a programmer held above skin over generator box; pacemaker function can be monitored periodically after discharge using transtelephonic monitoring (device is placed over implanted generator box and attached to telephone for transmission of signal)
3. Client preparation: obtain informed written consent; bedrest is required for 24 hours after procedure and activity is gradually increased to prevent dislodging leads

NCLEX®

4. Postprocedure nursing care
   a. Monitor ECG continuously to ensure that pacing impulses are captured (e.g., pacer spike is followed by QRS with ventricular pacing) and that client rhythm is sensed (pacemaker does not fire when client rhythm is present); report abnormalities promptly
   b. Monitor pacemaker site for signs of bleeding or infection; monitor temperature each shift
   c. Dressing should remain clean and dry with no swelling, warmth, redness, or tenderness of incision
   d. Minimize right arm and shoulder movements immediately postprocedure to ensure that pacemaker wire remains in contact with ventricular wall
5. Client teaching after permanent pacemaker insertion
   a. Count 1-minute pulse rate daily and notify provider if rate is less than preprogrammed rate (could indicate battery failure or malfunction)
   b. Carry medical identification and pacemaker identification card
   c. Protective measures include avoiding contact sports, wearing loose clothing over generator site, using mobile phone on opposite side of pacemaker, avoiding use of electrical devices directly over generator site (most appliances can be used safely), and moving away (5–10 feet) from electrical devices if client experiences any unusual symptoms and counting pulse rate
   d. Avoid devices that could be alarmed by implanted pacemaker such as airport security scanners and store antitheft apparatus
   e. Follow up with healthcare provider regularly; know and report signs of infection (during healing) or pacemaker malfunction (pulse below preset rate, dizziness, return of previous symptoms)
6. Temporary pacemakers are used to treat heart block that occurs suddenly or as temporary reponse to cardiac surgery or myocardial infarction
   a. May be placed transvenously with external pacemaker box used to set milliamps of energy and rate

b. Monitor cardiac rhythm for lack of capture and watch for site infection as risks
c. External pacemaker can also be used as initial measure; noninvasive and easy to use but may be uncomfortable to client

IV. CORONARY HEART DISEASE AND ANGINA PECTORIS

A. Overview

1. **Coronary heart disease** (CHD) is a buildup of atherosclerotic plaque that narrows lumen one or more coronary arteries and restricts blood flow to myocardium
2. Resulting inadequate myocardial oxygen supply ultimately leads to disorders such as hypertension, angina pectoris, cardiac dysrhythmias, myocardial infarction, and heart failure
3. Development of collateral coronary circulation over time can mediate effects of progressive blockage (an advantage of older adults over younger adults)
4. Risk factors for **atherosclerosis** (local accumulation of lipid and fibrous tissue along intimal layer of artery) leading to heart disease
   a. Nonmodifiable risk factors include age, gender, family history, and ethnic background
   NCLEX®
   b. Modifiable risk factors include smoking, obesity, stress, elevated cholesterol, diabetes mellitus, and pre-existing hypertension

B. Nursing assessment

1. Generally asymptomatic until occlusion is sufficient to cause myocardial ischemia (usually greater than 75% of major arteries or 50% of left main coronary artery)
2. Classic symptoms of heart disease include dyspnea, palpitations, syncope, cough, fatigue, and onset of chest pain

NCLEX®

3. Chest pain, also called **angina pectoris**; may occur in three forms
   a. *Stable angina*, a predictable symptomatic response to increased activity; pain occurs with same amount of exertion or emotion and a stable pattern of onset, severity, duration (usually less than 5 mins), and alleviating factors (rest and/or nitroglycerin)
   b. *Unstable angina* (preinfarction angina) has less predictability and increasing severity; pain may occur at rest, and pain episodes increase over time in number, severity, and duration (may last longer than 15 mins); may not be relieved by rest and/or nitroglycerin
   c. *Prinzmetal angina* caused by arterial spasm often awakens client from sleep
4. Angina pectoris may change in pattern and progress to MI; because it is difficult to differentiate unstable angina from MI symptomatically, they are grouped together under classification of acute coronary syndrome for prompt protocol-based assessment and treatment

C. Therapeutic management

1. Diagnostic studies (ECG, stress testing), cardiac enzyme and troponin levels (should be negative if no MI), and cardiac catheterization
2. Interventional cardiology procedures PTCA and intracoronary stent placement

NCLEX®

3. Care of client experiencing chest pain
   a. Do not leave client alone; have other caregivers obtain needed supplies or contact healthcare provider
   b. Assess pain (OPQRST mnemonic for onset, provoking or palliating factors, quality, radiation, severity, and timing); document findings
   c. Have client lie down with head of bed in semi-Fowler position
   d. Apply oxygen as per protocol (usually 2 L/min) and 12-lead ECG; administer prescribed medications (usually nitroglycerin); initiate IV access in case emergency medications are needed
   e. Monitor VS frequently, including BP after each nitroglycerin dose, and assess pain after each dose until relieved; medication protocol may prevent additional dose if BP < 90 or 100 mmHg systolic

D. Client teaching

1. Modifiable risk factors that apply to client and measures to reduce them (low-fat diet, aerobic exercise, smoking cessation, stress management)
2. Triggering events for chest pain and strategies for prevention
3. Potential barriers to adhering to plan of care and measures to counteract them
4. Follow-up care and symptoms to report to healthcare provider

V. MYOCARDIAL INFARCTION (MI)

A. Overview

1. MI occurs when there is a sudden, severe deprivation of blood supply to a portion of heart

NCLEX®

2. Affected cells first experience ischemia, then injury, and finally cell death (necrosis); MI can be differentiated from angina because cell necrosis with release of cardiac cell enzymes does not occur

with angina; each type of change has corresponding changes on ECG (T-wave inversion, ST elevation, and Q waves, respectively); Q waves are only seen after actual MI

3. Life-threatening condition; requires immediate access to emergency cardiac care for increased chance of favorable recovery; "time is muscle"

NCLEX®

B. Nursing assessment

1. Chest pain unrelieved by nitroglycerin or rest often indicates MI; may be a crushing substernal pain; may radiate to jaw, neck, back, or left arm (some clients, especially diabetic clients and women, report no pain—silent MI)
2. Other symptoms may include diaphoresis, cool mottled skin, nausea and vomiting, fear, anxiety and sense of impending doom, dyspnea and shortness of breath, palpitations and dysrhythmias, hypertension or hypotension
3. ECG (12-lead): ST elevation, accompanied by T-wave inversion in leads that monitor affected area of heart; these changes resolve as treatment progresses; new pathologic Q wave in affected leads develops as a permanent change if ischemia not reversed before cell death occurs
4. Lab findings: elevated troponins (early or late diagnosis); elevated CK-MB isoenzymes over 5% (early diagnosis); or elevated LDH with "flipped" isoenzymes (late diagnosis)

NCLEX®

C. Therapeutic management

1. Assess pain status frequently with pain scale or other appropriate tool to estimate changes in pain level; pain is usually first presenting sign of new or extended MI
2. Assess hemodynamic status including BP, HR, LOC, skin color, and temperature frequently (every 5 minutes during pain; every 15 minutes postpain) during acute phase to evaluate CO; continue to monitor frequently (every 1 to 2 hours) for first 24 hours post-MI
3. NCLEX® Emergency treatment usually includes MONA: morphine, oxygen, nitrates, and aspirin that is chewed and swallowed (see Memory Aid)
4. Monitor continuous ECG to detect dysrhythmias (PVCs and tachycardia common); perform 12-lead ECG immediately with new pain or changes in level or character of pain to identify ischemia and injury
5. Monitor respirations, breath sounds, and I&O to detect early signs of heart failure as a complication
6. Monitor O_2 saturation and administer O_2 (usually via nasal cannula at 2–4 L/min) as prescribed to increase oxygenation to heart

Memory Aid

Remember MONA as a key treatment approach to MI:
***M** orphine* to relieve chest pain
***O** xygen* to increase oxygenation
***N** itrates* to vasodilate coronary blood vessels and increase blood supply
***A** spirin* (chewed and swallowed) as an antiplatelet agent to interfere with thrombus formation

7. Provide for physiological rest to decrease O_2 demands on heart
8. Keep client NPO or progress to liquid diet as ordered; maintain IV access for medications as needed
9. Provide care in specialized cardiac critical care unit; provide a calm environment and reassure client and family to decrease stress, fear, and anxiety
10. Report significant changes immediately to healthcare provider to ensure rapid treatment of complications
11. Interventions in recovery phase: maintain bedrest (with bedside commode) for 24–36 hours and gradually increase activity as prescribed while closely monitoring CO, ECG, and pain status; reinforce importance of reporting any new pain immediately; progress diet from NPO or liquids to soft, low-fat, and low-sodium diet as prescribed
12. Administer nitroglycerin as prescribed to dilate coronary vessels and increase blood flow
13. Administer morphine sulfate as prescribed to relieve chest pain
14. Administer anticoagulants (IV heparin) and aspirin (antiplatelet) as ordered to prevent additional clot formation; monitor PTT to maintain heparin at therapeutic level (often 60–80 seconds)
15. Administer thrombolytic therapy if no contraindications (recent hemorrhagic stroke, surgery, childbirth, trauma); common drugs include alteplase recombinant, tissue plasminogen activator, or streptokinase; they dissolve clot, stop progress of MI, and decrease myocardial damage; monitor frequently for signs of bleeding

16. Monitor neurologic status frequently for changes; alteplase recombinant and streptokinase are not clot-specific and will dissolve other clots—can cause thrombolytic (hemorrhagic) stroke, a life-threatening complication
17. Administer beta-blockers post-MI as ordered to decrease cardiac work and decrease O_2 demands on heart
18. Administer antidysrhythmic drugs as prescribed or by emergency protocol
19. Surgical interventions: PTCA, CABG, stent placement (see previous discussion)

D. Client teaching

1. Include appropriate family members whenever possible
2. Cardiac rehabilitation program if prescribed
3. Explain modifiable risk factors (coronary heart disease) and develop a plan with client, including supportive resources to change lifestyle to decrease these factors
4. Medication regime as prescribed; identify side effects to report (provide written instructions for later reference)
5. Importance of immediate reporting of chest pain or signs of decreased CO
6. *NCLEX®* Bleeding precautions if client is on anticoagulant therapy: use soft toothbrush, electric razor, avoid trauma or injury; wear or carry Medic-Alert identification

VI. HEART FAILURE

A. Overview

1. Inability of heart to pump adequate blood (CO) to meet metabolic needs of body, leading to insufficient perfusion to major organs and peripheral tissues
2. Can be classified as acute or chronic; client with chronic heart failure (HF) can have an acute exacerbation
3. Multiple causes include myocardial damage from MI, incompetent valves, inflammatory conditions of heart, cardiomyopathy, hypertension, and pulmonary hypertension (right-sided failure, called **cor pulmonale**)
4. Compensatory phase (early): CO falls → sensed by baroreceptors → stimulate sympathetic nervous system → release norepinephrine → increase in HR and vasoconstriction → increase in filling pressures → increase in SV and CO (because $CO = HR \times SV$, CO is increased); compensatory mechanisms increase cardiac metabolic demands and over time decrease cardiac function and ability to compensate
5. Depending on cause, HF presents initially as right-sided failure or left-sided failure; other side becomes affected as it progresses
   a. Left HF: LV has reduced capacity to pump blood into systemic circulation, causing decreased CO and stasis or "backup" of fluid into pulmonary circulation
   b. Right HF: RV has reduced capacity to pump blood into pulmonary circulation, causing stasis or "backup" of fluid in venous circulation
6. Onset of HF
   a. Acute, with significant overload in lungs (**pulmonary edema**, characterized by acute restlessness, anxiety, increased crackles and gurgling respirations, tachypnea, tachycardia, accessory muscle use and nasal flaring, pink frothy sputum, cool clammy skin, pallor progressing to cyanosis, decreased SO_2 and PO_2)
   b. Chronic, with fatigue and activity intolerance as main features; clients with advanced chronic HF require careful management to prevent acute exacerbations

NCLEX® **B. Nursing assessment**

1. Presenting symptoms
   a. Left HF: dyspnea on exertion (often first clinical sign), orthopnea, paroxysmal nocturnal dyspnea, crackles, new S_3 (ventricular gallop) as early sign; pulmonary edema is acute life-threatening left heart failure
   b. Right HF: lower-extremity edema; **jugular venous distention (JVD)** is visible more than 3-4 centimeters above clavicle with client supine with 45-degree head elevation; abdominal discomfort and nausea occur from fluid congestion in abdominal organs
   c. Both sides: unexplained fatigue or altered mental status, decreased exercise tolerance
2. Diagnostic findings
   a. Elevated atrial natriuretic factor or hormone (ANF or ANH) and B-type natriuretic peptide (BNP) elevate in HF but are not singly diagnostic since they can elevate also in women and those over age 60
   b. Chest x-ray may show cardiomegaly or vascular congestion
   c. Echocardiogram shows decreased ventricular function and ejection fraction
   d. CVP elevated in right HF; PA diastolic pressure and LVEDP elevated in left HF

C. Therapeutic management

1. Acute phase
   a. Monitor and record BP, pulse, respirations, ECG, and CVP or PCWP (if appropriate) to detect changes in CO
   NCLEX® b. Raise head of bed to decrease pulmonary congestion and improve gas exchange
   c. Auscultate heart and lung sounds frequently: increasing crackles, increasing dyspnea, decreasing lung sounds, or new S_3 heart sound indicate worsening HF
   d. Administer O_2 as prescribed to improve gas exchange and increase oxygenation of blood; monitor SO_2 and arterial blood gases (ABG) to assess effectiveness
   e. Administer prescribed medications on time
   f. Monitor serum electrolytes to detect hypokalemia secondary to diuretic therapy
   g. Monitor accurate I&O to evaluate fluid status (may require urinary catheter for accurate measurement of urine output)
   h. If fluid restriction is prescribed, spread fluid throughout day to reduce thirst
   NCLEX® i. Encourage physical rest and organize activities with frequent rest periods to reduce cardiac work
   j. Provide a calm, reassuring environment to reduce anxiety, thus decreasing O_2 consumption and demands on heart
2. Chronic HF
   a. Educate client and family about rationale for therapeutic regime
   b. Establish baseline assessment for fluid status and functional abilities: it is baseline "normal" for some clients with HF to have bilateral crackles in bases, some amount of peripheral edema, or to be unable to walk more than a specific number of feet before tiring
   NCLEX® c. Monitor daily weights to evaluate changes in fluid status
   d. Assess at regular intervals for changes in fluid status or functional activity level
3. **Medication therapy**
   a. Angiotensin-converting enzyme (ACE) inhibitor such as lisinopril or angiotensin II receptor blocker (ARB) to reduce afterload and thus increase CO (primarily used in ongoing management); monitor for hypotension, especially orthostatic hypotension
   NCLEX® b. Diuretic to decrease preload and pulmonary congestion, which decreases cardiac work and increases CO; carefully monitor potassium levels for hypokalemia or hyperkalemia, depending on whether potassium-losing or potassium-sparing diuretic is used
   c. Vasodilators including nitroglycerin to reduce preload; monitor for hypotension
   d. Low-dose beta-blockers to inhibit sympathetic nervous system activity and improve CO; typically used in conjunction with ACE inhibitor for best effect
   NCLEX® e. Digoxin to improve contractility and correspondingly increase stroke volume and CO; take apical pulse for 1 full minute and withhold if heart rate is less than 60 and notify prescriber
   f. Morphine to sedate and aid vasodilation during acute pulmonary edema; decreases cardiac work; monitor for hypotension or respiratory depression
   g. Other: vasodilators such as milrinone or inotropic agents such as dopamine and dobutamine are used in critical care settings when decompensation of CO includes hypotension; monitor BP and IV site frequently

D. Client teaching

1. Include family members or others in teaching as appropriate
2. NCLEX® Weight monitoring: measure and record daily weights (with same amount of clothing before breakfast but after voiding) and report unexplained increase of 1.36–2.26 kg (3–5 lb)—most sensitive indicator of increased fluid overload
3. NCLEX® Diet: sodium restriction to decrease fluid overload; increase intake of potassium-rich foods if taking potassium-losing diuretics; restriction of high-potassium foods and salt substitutes if taking potassium-sparing diuretics; do not restrict water intake unless directed (this will not decrease fluid retention)
4. Medication regime: follow all medication instructions; although frequent urination is bothersome, regular diuretic therapy prevents fluid overload and acute exacerbation; take radial pulse for 1 full minute before taking digoxin; withhold dose and call prescriber if pulse is lower than 50 or 60 as instructed (variability exists) or is higher than 100 or 120 per prescriber
5. Activity: plan paced activity to maximize available CO
6. Symptoms: report promptly any chest pain, new onset of dyspnea on exertion, paroxysmal nocturnal dyspnea
7. Other: report even minor changes to prescriber or home care nurse because they may be early signs of decompensation

VII. INFLAMMATORY DISORDERS OF HEART

A. Endocarditis (infective, subacute bacterial)

1. Inflammation of inner layer of heart; usually involves cardiac valves
2. Caused by microorganisms in blood: risk factors include IV drug use, structural heart or valve defects (which increase number of platelet and fibrin strands in endothelium)
   a. Acute endocarditis: sudden onset with *Staphylococcus aureus* being most common organism
   b. Subacute endocarditis: gradual onset with *Streptococcus viridans* or other less virulent bacteria
3. Microorganisms in bloodstream colonize on fibrin and platelet strands in endothelium, multiply and develop new strands; seen as "vegetation" attached to endothelium, particularly valves, causing damage; segments of vegetation may break off and travel to extremities, manifested as petechiae (pinpoint hemorrhagic spots)

NCLEX®

4. **Nursing assessment**
   a. Acute: spiking fever and chills; signs of HF (see previous section); WBC elevation
   b. Subacute: fever of unknown origin; cough; dyspnea; anorexia; malaise; normal WBC; anemia; and elevated erythrocyte sedimentation rate (ESR)
   c. Both: positive blood cultures; new cardiac **murmurs** (abnormal heart sounds heard during systole or diastole) or change in existing murmur; petechiae on trunk, conjunctiva, or mucous membranes as embolic complications from segments of vegetation circulating in body; splinter hemorrhages (streaks) in nail beds; Janeway lesions (purple-red macular lesions on palms and soles); Roth's spots (small, whitish "cotton wool" spots on retina)

NCLEX®

5. **Therapeutic management**
   a. Manage IV therapy; assess for any signs of infection
   b. Assess appropriateness of home infusion therapy; client may require inpatient treatment in a subacute care facility if home infusion therapy is contraindicated (such as IV drug abuse)
   c. Provide periods of rest and moderate periods of exercise to prevent venous stasis
   d. Use antiembolism stockings to prevent thrombus formation
   e. Provide for diversional activity; client is restricted from resuming normal activity for 4–6 weeks
   f. Antibiotics given by IV route are needed for 6 weeks
6. **Client teaching**
   a. Role in home infusion therapy
   b. After one episode of endocarditis, client is susceptible to repeated infections because of lesions on endocardium; tell future caregivers about infection
   c. Symptoms to report to healthcare provider, such as fever, anorexia, malaise
   d. Gentle, thorough oral care because infectious organisms can easily enter bloodstream through gums with vigorous brushing or oral treatments
   e. Need for prophylactic antibiotics before invasive procedures and routine dental care

B. Pericarditis

1. Inflammation of pericardial sac, either acute or chronic
2. Acute pericarditis: may have multiple causes, including infection (viral most common), post-MI status (Dressler's syndrome), neoplasms, trauma, uremia, connective tissue diseases, or endocrine diseases
3. Chronic pericarditis: leads to fibrous thickening of pericardium, constricting movement of myocardium, and restricting diastolic filling

NCLEX®

4. **Nursing assessment**
   a. Acute: substernal pain, radiating to neck, aggravated by breathing (particularly during inspiration) or coughing; friction rub (scratchy, high-pitched sound on auscultation); elevated WBC; fever; malaise; ECG changes including ST and T-wave elevations followed by inverted T waves when ST returns to baseline
   b. Chronic restrictive pericarditis: increasing dyspnea, fatigue leading to progressive signs of heart failure

NCLEX®

5. **Therapeutic management**
   a. Assess and relieve chest pain
   b. Administer O_2 as ordered and monitor SO_2

NCLEX®

   c. Monitor for complications, especially **cardiac tamponade** (medical emergency; excess fluid collection in pericardial sac that interferes with heart filling and function); signs include JVD with clear lungs, elevated CVP, narrowing pulse pressure, decreased CO, and muffled heart sounds
   d. Report significant changes immediately
   e. Position client for comfort: high Fowler, sitting and leaning forward, or side-lying
   f. Provide for periods of rest and limit activity to decrease cardiac workload

g. Medication therapy: analgesics for pain, nonsteroidal anti-inflammatory drugs (NSAIDs) followed by corticosteroids if needed, antibiotics (after blood culture and sensitivity results are known) if caused by infection; avoid anticoagulants because of risk of tamponade
h. Pericardiocentesis: aspiration of fluid from pericardial sac to determine cause or as emergency treatment for tamponade

6. **Client teaching**
   a. Disease process and medication management
   b. Take anti-inflammatory drugs with food, milk, or antacids to reduce gastric distress
   c. Risk for repeat episodes of pericarditis; report similar pain or dyspnea promptly

VIII. VALVULAR DISORDERS

A. Overview

1. Defects in cardiac valve structure or function that interfere with proper cardiac circulation
2. **Stenosis**: heart valve leaflets are fused together; opening is narrow, stiff, and unable to open or close properly
3. **Regurgitation**: there is improper or incomplete closure of heart valves, resulting in backflow of blood
4. Multiple causes including rheumatic heart disease (most common), congenital, MI, endocarditis
5. Calcium deposits or scar tissue from endocarditis or MI may cause valve stiffening in stenosis

NCLEX®

B. Nursing assessment

1. Heart sounds: valve dysfunctions have distinctive characteristic changes in heart sounds (see Table 56–3)
2. Symptoms and severity depend on extent of valve dysfunction, from asymptomatic to severe HF, and on type of valve dysfunction (stenosis or regurgitation); see Table 56–3

NCLEX®

C. Therapeutic management

1. Refer again to Table 56–3
2. Monitor heart sounds to assess for changes
3. With signs of decreased CO, restrict activity to decrease demands on heart
4. Monitor for signs of endocarditis
5. Report changes to healthcare provider

Table 56–3 Heart Valve Disorders

Valve Disorder	Specific Assessment	Planning and Implementation
Mitral stenosis	Murmur: low-pitched rumbling diastolic Common in young women Atrial dysrhythmias, especially atrial fibrillation (A-fib)	Monitor closely during pregnancy Administer diuretics and digoxin as prescribed Maintain sodium-restricted diet Anticoagulant therapy if A-fib present Prepare for surgery
Mitral regurgitation (insufficiency)	Murmur: high-pitched blowing systolic Clients generally asymptomatic A-fib common with low incidence of embolization	Administer diuretics, nitrates, and ACE inhibitors as prescribed Maintain sodium-restricted diet
Mitral prolapse	Murmur: systolic click Most clients asymptomatic May have PVCs and palpitations, syncope, weakness, and anxiety	Administer beta-blockers as prescribed for syncope and palpitations Monitor for signs of infective endocarditis Administer prophylactic antibiotics with invasive procedures
Aortic stenosis	Murmur: harsh systolic Late-course symptoms: angina; S_3 and S_4; syncope	In symptomatic client, restrict activity to decrease myocardial oxygen consumption Monitor for signs of infective endocarditis Administer prophylactic antibiotics with invasive procedures Prepare for surgery: symptomatic aortic stenosis has poor prognosis without surgical intervention
Aortic regurgitation (insufficiency)	Murmur: blowing diastolic Widened pulse pressure Palpitations; tachycardia and PVCs	Medical management same as aortic stenosis Prepare for surgery, which is the only effective long-term therapy for aortic regurgitation

6. Medication therapy is determined by symptoms; may include antidysrhythmics, anticoagulants (atrial fibrillation), antibiotics (endocarditis), and drugs to treat HF as needed
7. Surgery: valve repair or replacement (see section that follows)

D. Client teaching

1. Management of anticoagulants (warfarin) to prevent thrombus formation, including monitoring PT/INR and regulation (moderate steady intake) of vitamin K in diet (green leafy vegetables)
2. Relationships among valve disorders, surgical valves, and increased risk for bacterial endocarditis
3. Methods to prevent endocarditis

E. Valvular repair or replacement of dysfunctional valve

1. Repair
   a. *Valvuloplasty*: reconstruction including repair or removal of calcification or vegetation
   b. *Annuloplasty*: narrowing a dilated valve with a prosthetic ring or purse-string sutures, or enlarging a stenosed valve with a balloon
2. Replacement: valve is completely replaced
   a. Mechanical (prosthetic) valves: more durable and longer lasting; subject to mechanical failure; risk of thrombosis requires lifetime anticoagulation with warfarin; infections are harder to treat
   b. Bioprosthetic (tissue) valves: may deteriorate over years and require replacement; not associated with thrombus formation, so long-term anticoagulation is not necessary; infections are easier to treat

NCLEX® 3. Client preparation and postprocedure nursing care: (same as for cardiac surgery, discussed previously)

4. Provide instructions for preventing infection, including precautions such as prophylactic antibiotic therapy prior to invasive procedures (e.g., dental care), twice daily gentle oral care to prevent bacteria from entering the bloodstream through gums; provide instruction on managing anticoagulation therapy if mechanical valve inserted

IX. CARDIOMYOPATHY

A. Overview

1. An abnormality of heart muscle that leads to functional changes in heart
2. Cause is unknown if primary; secondary cardiomyopathy may occur because of ischemia, infectious disease, exposure to toxins, connective tissue or metabolic disorders, or nutritional deficiencies
3. Three types: dilated, hypertrophic, and restrictive
   a. Dilated cardiomyopathy (most common): enlargement of all four chambers, starting with enlarged ventricles, followed by decreased contractility; CO progressively decreases
   b. Hypertrophic cardiomyopathy: unexplained progressive thickening of ventricular muscle mass causing increased pulmonary and venous pressures; CO progressively decreases
   c. Restrictive cardiomyopathy (least common): excessively rigid ventricular walls do not stretch during diastolic filling, creating back pressure and right HF as well as reduced SV and, consequently, lowered CO

B. Nursing assessment

1. Fatigue with all types
2. Dilated: weakness, signs of left HF, S_3 (ventricular gallop heard immediately after S_2 with left-ventricular failure or mitral regurgitation) and S_4 (atrial gallop heard immediately before S_1 with coronary heart disease, left-ventricular hypertrophy, or aortic stenosis)
3. Hypertrophic: exertional dyspnea, syncope, angina, signs of HF, S_4, sudden death often first sign in asymptomatic individuals
4. Restrictive: dyspnea, right-sided HF, S_3 and S_4, emboli formation

C. Therapeutic management

NCLEX® 1. Monitor indicators of level of HF (VS, lung sounds, edema, dyspnea, activity tolerance)

NCLEX® 2. Encourage rest and minimize stressful situations to reduce cardiac workload

3. Provide counseling and psychological support because of poor prognosis
4. Medications such as digoxin are used to treat signs of HF
5. Anticoagulation therapy is used with restrictive cardiomyopathy to prevent emboli
6. Beta-blockers, calcium channel blockers, antidysrhythmics, or implanted dual-chamber pacemaker or ICD may be needed with hypertrophic type; surgical excision of part of ventricular septum may also be done

D. Client teaching

1. Instruct client to avoid alcohol because of its cardiac-depressant effects
2. Assist clients in planning to pace activities to reduce cardiac workload

3. Instruct client in medication and dietary management of HF
4. Explain anticoagulation therapy and monitoring if appropriate to prevent emboli formation
5. Provide usual postsurgical teaching after pacemaker or IACD insertion or surgery on septum

X. HYPERTENSION

A. Overview

1. BP of 140 mmHg or higher systolic, or 90 or greater diastolic, based on average of three or more readings done on separate occasions
2. Hypertension can be primary (essential) or secondary; risk factors for primary hypertension include family history, age, race (more common in African Americans), high sodium intake (or low potassium, calcium, and magnesium intake), obesity, stress, excessive alcohol intake, and insulin resistance (with resulting hyperinsulinemia and effects on vascular smooth muscle and sympathetic nervous system)
3. Classified by stage: prehypertension (120–139 systolic or 80–89 diastolic), stage 1 (140–159 systolic or 90–99 diastolic), or stage 2 (160 or higher systolic or 100 or higher diastolic)
4. A hypertensive crisis or emergency occurs when BP is 180/120 or higher; treatment is required within 1 hour to prevent cardiac, vascular, and renal damage

NCLEX®

B. Nursing assessment

1. Past history of cardiovascular, cerebrovascular, renal, or thyroid diseases, diabetes, smoking, or alcohol use
2. Family history of hypertension or cardiovascular disease
3. Often silent with absence of symptoms if no target organ damage
4. Possible fatigue, nocturia, dyspnea on exertion (DOE), palpitations, angina, headaches, weight gain, edema, muscle cramps, or blurred vision may be caused by target organ damage
5. Possible retinal vessel changes, diminished or absent peripheral pulses, bruits, murmurs, and S_3 and S_4 heart sounds
6. Possible cardiomegaly on x-ray or left-ventricular hypertrophy on ECG

NCLEX®

C. Therapeutic management

1. Tell client numeric BP readings for ongoing record-keeping
2. Accurately record I&O and daily weights of hospitalized clients
3. Medication therapy
   a. A stepped-care approach is often used to guide treatment; this begins with lifestyle changes and adds medications based on response to previous therapy
   b. Medications follow a treatment algorithm for hypertensive stage and include thiazide-type diuretics, ACE inhibitors, angiotensin receptor blockers (ARBs), beta-blockers, calcium channel blockers, and, if needed, vasodilators

D. Client teaching

1. Hypertension is usually asymptomatic, and symptoms will not reliably indicate BP levels

NCLEX®

2. Lifestyle modification
   a. Sodium restriction
   b. Weight reduction and aerobic exercise (30 minutes/day on most days of week)
   c. DASH (dietary approaches to stop hypertension) diet: includes prescribed number of servings of following foods: grains and grain products (7–8/day); vegetables (4–5/day); fruits (4–5/day); low-fat or nonfat dairy foods; meats, poultry, and fish (2 or fewer 3-oz servings/day); nuts, seeds, and dry beans (4–5/week); fats and oils (2–3/day); and sweets (4–5/week, should be low in fat)
   d. Limit alcohol intake (1 oz ethanol daily or less if lighter weight or woman)
   e. Relaxation and stress management techniques
   f. Stop smoking

NCLEX®

3. Prevent **orthostatic hypotension** (a drop in BP of 10–20 mmHg with upright posture) by rising out of bed or chair slowly
4. Avoid hot baths and strenuous exercise within 3 hours of taking vasodilators
5. Adhere to treatment plan, even if asymptomatic, to reduce risk of target organ damage

E. Hypertensive crisis

1. Hypertensive emergency with BP greater than 180/120 mmHg
2. Risk factors include poor BP control or abruptly stopping medication therapy; populations at risk include African American men, pregnant women with preeclampsia, or diagnosis of collagen or renal disease
3. Signs and symptoms include headache, confusion, restlessness, papilledema (swelling of optic nerve), blurred vision, and sensory or motor deficits

4. Hypertensive crisis is treated using parenteral vasodilators such as sodium nitroprusside; goal is to reduce BP by no more than 25% in minutes to 1 hour, and then toward 160/100 within 2 to 6 hours to prevent organ ischemia caused by rapid reduction in BP; monitor BP every 5 to 30 minutes during this time

XI. PERIPHERAL ARTERIAL DISEASE

A. Overview

1. Disorders that impede arterial peripheral blood flow; primarily caused by atherosclerosis but also by trauma, embolism, thrombosis, vasospasm, inflammation, or autoimmunity
2. By the time symptoms appear, vessel is about 75% narrowed
3. Femoral-popliteal area is most common site in nondiabetic clients; those with diabetes most often develop disease in arteries below knees
4. Chronic arterial obstruction leads to inadequate tissue oxygenation, causing **intermittent claudication**, ischemic muscle pain precipitated by a predictable amount of exercise and relieved by rest

NCLEX®

B. Nursing assessment

1. Intermittent claudication, an early sign of disease
2. **Rest pain**, which may awaken client at night; pain is usually in distal extremity (toes, arch, forefoot, heel) and is relieved when foot is placed below heart level; indicates more advanced disease
3. Extremities may be cool, pale, and numb with a cyanotic color on elevation
4. Bruits may be auscultated
5. Diminished or absent peripheral pulses
6. Thickened and opaque nails (trophic change)
7. Skin on legs may be shiny with sparse hair growth (trophic change)
8. Ulcers may be present on lower extremities in areas affected by reduced circulation
9. Diagnostic testing: digital subtraction angiography (DSA), angiography, Doppler ultrasound, plethysmography
10. See Table 56–4 for a comparison of arterial and venous vascular disease

NCLEX®

C. Therapeutic management

1. Assess and record strength of pulses
2. Encourage smoking cessation
3. Change position at least hourly and avoid crossing legs
4. Encourage client to exercise and walk to point of pain; stop walking when pain occurs and resume when pain stops to build exercise tolerance and stimulate growth of collateral circulation
5. Assess pain on a 0-to-10 scale and provide analgesics as ordered
6. If an ulcer develops, healing will be slow unless arterial blood flow is improved through surgery
7. If surgery is indicated, provide appropriate postoperative care
8. Angioplasty

NCLEX®

   a. Monitor **neurovascular status** (color, motion, sensitivity, temperature, and presence of distal peripheral pulses) to affected extremity every 15 minutes for 4 hours, every 30 minutes for 4 hours, then every 1 to 4 hours after sheath removal
   b. Notify healthcare provider if client experiences weak or thready pulses, coolness, numbness, or tingling in extremity
   c. Monitor sheath site for external and subcutaneous bleeding

Table 56–4 Comparison of Arterial and Venous Vascular Disease

Assessment	Arterial Disease	Venous Disease
Color	Pale	Ruddy; cyanotic if dependent
Edema	None or minimal	Usually present
Nails	Thick and brittle	Normal
Pain	Worse with elevation and exercise; may be sudden or severe; rest pain; claudication	Better with elevation; possible Homan's sign, dullness or heaviness
Pulses	Decreased, weak, or absent	Normal
Temperature of extremity	Cool	Warm
Ulcers	Dry and necrotic	Moist; malleolar

Box 56–2

Client and Family Education for Peripheral Arterial Disease

- Stop smoking.
- Lose weight and eat a low-fat diet.
- Do not cross legs while sitting.
- Elevate feet at rest, but not above heart level.
- Do not stand or sit for long periods of time.
- Do not wear restrictive clothing.
- Keep affected extremity warm but never apply direct heat.
- Inspect feet daily and keep them clean and dry.
- Avoid walking barefoot; wear proper-fitting shoes.
- Avoid mechanical or thermal injury to the legs and feet; have nail care performed by podiatrist.
- Begin and maintain an exercise and walking program.
- Notify healthcare provider of any changes in color, sensation, temperature, or pulses in extremities.

d. Instruct client to notify nurse and apply manual pressure to site if warm or wet sensation is felt at site
e. Keep affected extremity immobilized for at least 6 hours by reminding client to keep extremity still, or lightly immobilize ankle with sheet tucked under both sides of mattress
f. Maintain a pressure dressing and sand bag at site

9. Bypass grafting
   a. Provide standard postoperative care
   b. Assess for occlusion of graft: severe ischemic pain, loss of pulses, decreasing ankle-brachial index, numbness, tingling or coolness of extremity
10. **Endarterectomy** (opening artery and removing obstructing plaque) or amputation in severe cases; use same principles of care as for other procedures
11. Medication therapy: aspirin inhibits platelet aggregation; pentoxifylline decreases blood viscosity and increases blood flow; cilostazol inhibits platelet aggregation and enhances vasodilation; clopidogrel and ticlopidine prevent thrombi formation with recent MI or stroke

D. Client teaching

NCLEX®

1. See Box 56–2
2. Teach relaxation techniques because stress increases vasoconstriction

XII. ARTERIAL EMBOLISM

A. Overview

1. Arterial emboli usually develop in heart from atrial fibrillation, MI, HF, or prosthetic valves
2. Thrombi become detached and are carried from left heart into arterial system where they may lodge and cause obstruction
3. Symptoms may be abrupt and depend on size and location of embolus
4. Ischemia will progress to necrosis and gangrene within hours if untreated

NCLEX® **B. Nursing assessment: the "six Ps"**

1. Pain
2. Pallor (pale color) and pulselessness (diminished or absent pulses)
3. Parasthesias (altered local sensation) and paralysis (weakness or inability to move extremity)
4. **Poikilothermia** (body temperature that varies with environment, is usually decreased)

NCLEX® **C. Therapeutic management**

1. Assess peripheral pulses and neurovascular status every 2 to 4 hours
2. Place affected extremity in a neutral position with no restrictive bedding or clothing
3. Assess level of pain using a 0-to-10 scale
4. Change position every 2 hours to improve collateral circulation
5. Assess for and report unusual bleeding from anticoagulant therapy
6. Monitor lab values, including aPTT, PT, and INR levels
7. An emergency embolectomy should be performed within 4–5 hours to prevent permanent damage

8. If necrosis or infection is present, surgery is required for definitive treatment
9. Medication therapy (if no necrosis present): thrombolytic therapy with streptokinase; tissue plasminogen activator or anticoagulant therapy with heparin; warfarin therapy at home

D. Client teaching

1. Pre- and postoperative teaching if embolectomy is performed
2. Measures to promote peripheral circulation and maintain tissue integrity (refer back to Box 56–2)

XIII. BUERGER'S DISEASE (THROMBOANGIITIS OBLITERANS)

A. Overview

1. Inflammatory disease of small- and medium-sized veins and arteries accompanied by thrombi and sometimes vasospasm; may occur in upper or lower extremities but is most common in leg or foot
2. Etiology is uncertain but is currently thought to involve an autoimmune reaction (occurs mostly in young men who are heavy smokers); higher incidence of HLA-B5 and 2A9 antigens suggest a genetic link
3. Inflammation occurs; microthrombi form; both can lead to vasospasm, and this process ultimately obstructs blood flow

NCLEX® **B. Nursing assessment**

1. Initially, a bluish cast to a toe or finger and a feeling of coldness in affected limb is common
2. Rest pain, possibly severe
3. Excessive sweating in feet is possible from overactive sympathetic nerves, even though feet feel cold
4. Intermittent claudication and other symptoms similar to those of chronic obstructive arterial disease often appear gradually after occlusion
5. Ischemic ulcers and gangrene are common complications of progressive Buerger's disease

NCLEX® **C. Therapeutic management**

1. Arrest progress of disease by smoking cessation
2. Take measures to promote vasodilation (similar to other arterial disorders)
3. Provide for pain relief
4. Provide emotional support
5. Medication therapy: analgesic pain medications, calcium channel blockers to ease vasospasm, pentoxifylline to reduce blood viscosity
6. Surgical treatment includes sympathectomy (to vasodilate or eliminate vessel spasm) or arterial bypass grafting when larger arteries are involved

D. Client teaching: stop smoking; take measures to promote peripheral circulation and maintain tissue integrity (refer back to Box 56–2)

XIV. RAYNAUD'S DISEASE

A. Overview

1. Localized, intermittent episodes of vasoconstriction of small arteries of hands and, less commonly, feet, causing pallor, coolness, and cyanosis; primarily affects young women
2. Vasospastic attacks tend to be bilateral and symmetrical and usually begin at tips of digits, causing pallor, numbness, and sensation of cold
3. Attacks are triggered by exposure to cold, emotional stress, caffeine ingestion, and tobacco use

NCLEX® **B. Nursing assessment**

1. Classic triphasic color changes (pallor, cyanosis, and rubor) in hands with accompanying reduction in skin temperature
2. Intensity of pain increases as disease progresses
3. Skin of fingertips may thicken and nails may become brittle

C. Therapeutic management

NCLEX®

1. Keep hands warm and free from injury
2. Avoid stressful situations
3. In severe cases, a **sympathectomy** (surgical dissection of nerve fibers to relieve symptoms) may be performed
4. Medication therapy: analgesics for pain and possibly vasodilators and calcium channel blockers (vasospasm)

NCLEX® **D. Client teaching**

1. Keep hands warm: wear gloves when outdoors, in air-conditioned environments, or when handling cold food

2. Avoid injury to hands
3. Lifestyle changes: stop smoking; employ stress relief such as biofeedback

XV. AORTIC ANEURYSM

A. Overview

1. Localized dilation or outpouching of weakened area in aorta, classified by region as thoracic or abdominal or as dissecting (layers of blood vessels separated by a layer of blood)
2. More common in abdominal aorta below level of renal arteries but can occur in thoracic area
3. Growth rate is unpredictable; large aneurysms tend to rupture, a life-threatening emergency
4. Major risk factor is atherosclerosis

NCLEX®

B. Nursing assessment

1. Thoracic aneurysms are often asymptomatic, with first sign being rupture
   a. Symptoms may include pain in back, neck, and substernal area that may occur only when lying supine
   NCLEX® b. Possible dysphagia and dyspnea, stridor, or cough when pressing on esophagus or laryngeal nerve
2. Abdominal aneurysms may also be asymptomatic until rupture
   a. Client may report a "heartbeat" in abdomen when lying down
   NCLEX® b. Possible pulsating abdominal mass; do not palpate (risk of rupture)
   c. Moderate to severe abdominal or lumbar back pain may be present (severe pain may be a sign of impending rupture)
   d. Client may experience claudication
   e. Cool or cyanotic extremities may be noted
   f. Systolic bruit may be heard
3. NCLEX® Dissecting aneurysms present with sudden, severe, and persistent pain described as "tearing" or "ripping" in anterior chest or back
   a. Pain may extend to shoulder, epigastric area, or abdomen
   b. Pallor, sweating, and tachycardia are evidenced
   c. Initially, client may have an elevated BP that may be different in one arm than other
   d. Possible syncope and paralysis of lower extremities

NCLEX®

C. Therapeutic management

1. Diagnosed by chest x-ray, transesophageal echocardiography, aortography, ultrasound, and CT scan or MRI
2. Hematomas into scrotum, perineum, flank, or penis indicate retroperitoneal rupture
3. Surgery may be performed on an emergency or elective basis (not usually performed if less than 5 cm); involves excision of aneurysm with insertion of synthetic graft
4. Preoperatively mark and assess all peripheral pulses for comparison postoperatively
5. Postoperatively assess neurovascular status and assess for complications, such as graft occlusion, hypovolemia (renal failure), respiratory distress, cardiac dysrhythmias, paralytic ileus, and paraplegia (paralysis); use overbed cradle
6. Medication therapy: antihypertensives and diuretics to control BP; postoperative anticoagulant therapy with heparin during hospitalization and warfarin after discharge

D. Client teaching

1. If under medical care, get routine physical exams to monitor status of aneurysm
2. Signs and symptoms of impending rupture (see assessment of dissecting aneurysms above)
3. Monitor BP and report increases immediately; take medications as ordered
4. Postoperative teaching
   a. Do limited lifting for 4–6 weeks after surgery (no heavy lifting at all)
   b. Monitor incision site for bleeding and infection
   c. Self-assessment of neurovascular status of and pulses in extremities
5. Clients with a synthetic graft may require prophylactic antibiotics before invasive procedures

XVI. THROMBOPHLEBITIS

A. Overview

1. Formation of a thrombus (clot) associated with vein inflammation; classified as superficial or deep
2. Etiology: Virchow's triad (at least two of three conditions must be present for thrombosis to occur): stasis of venous flow, hypercoagulability of blood, and damage to inner lining of vein (endothelial layer)
3. If detachment occurs, emboli travel through veins to heart and into pulmonary circulation

NCLEX® **B. Nursing assessment**

1. History of thrombophlebitis, pelvic or abdominal surgery, obesity, neoplasm (hepatic and pancreatic), HF, atrial fibrillation, prolonged immobility, MI, pregnancy and/or postpartum period, IV therapy, hypercoagulable states (polycythemia, dehydration, or malnutrition)
2. Superficial
   a. Palpable, firm, subcutaneous, cordlike vein
   b. Surrounding area warm, red, tender to touch
   c. Edema may or may not be present
   d. Most common cause in arms is IV therapy; in legs it is often related to varicose veins
3. Deep
   NCLEX® a. Unilateral edema, pain, warm skin, and elevated temperature
   b. If inferior vena cava is involved, both legs will be edematous
   c. If superior vena cava is involved, both upper extremities, neck, back, and face may become edematous or cyanotic
   NCLEX® d. If calf is involved, **Homans sign** may be present (pain when client dorsiflexes foot, especially when leg is raised, nonspecific sign)
4. Diagnostic studies: Doppler ultrasonic flowmeter, MRI, and lung scan

NCLEX® **C. Therapeutic management**

1. Provide analgesics for pain relief
2. Elevate affected leg higher than heart to promote venous drainage
3. Apply warm, moist compresses, intermittent or continuous, to affected extremity; never massage affected extremity to reduce risk of embolism
4. Measure and monitor limb circumference when edema is present
5. Monitor status of peripheral pulses
6. Keep bed covers from touching affected limb by using an overbed cradle to avoid pressure and subsequent skin breakdown
7. Maintain strict bedrest
8. Instruct client to report any pink-tinged sputum and monitor for tachypnea, tachycardia, shortness of breath, chest pain, and apprehension, which may indicate a pulmonary embolism
9. Medication therapy: anticoagulants, thrombolytics, analgesics (NSAIDs to reduce pain and relieve inflammation)

D. Client teaching

1. Prevention in general postoperative clients: early ambulation postoperatively, use of sequential compression devices, possible low-dose anticoagulant therapy with enoxaparin
2. Enhance circulation by avoiding prolonged sitting or standing, sitting with crossed legs or ankles, and restrictive clothing
3. Stop smoking
4. Anticoagulant therapy (warfarin) if prescribed

XVII. VENOUS INSUFFICIENCY

A. Overview

1. Inadequate venous return over time causes venous hypertension, which stretches veins and damages valves, reducing blood return
2. Risk factors include thrombus formation, prolonged standing or sitting (teachers, waitresses, nurses, office workers), pregnancy, and obesity

NCLEX® **B. Nursing assessment**

1. Past history of thrombophlebitis, hypertension, varicosities
2. Past history of long periods of sitting and/or standing
3. Edema of lower legs, may extend to knee
4. Thick, coarse, brownish skin around ankles and feet
5. Stasis ulcers, usually in malleolar area
6. Refer back to Table 56–4 for a general comparison of signs of arterial and venous disorders

NCLEX® **C. Therapeutic management**

1. Bedrest with legs elevated above heart level
2. Avoid long periods of standing
3. Wear elastic support or compression hose (apply *before* getting out of bed and placing leg in a dependent position); remove at night
4. Never push hosiery down around leg—will further impair circulation

5. Treat venous stasis ulcer(s)
   a. Open lesions: hydrocolloid dressing possibly covered with compression wraps; possible topical ointment, such as low-dose hydrocortisone, zinc oxide, or an antifungal
   b. Unna boot or other compression wrap that is changed every 1 to 2 weeks and usually applied over a base dressing
   c. Severe ulcers may need surgical debridement
6. Medication therapy
   a. Topical agents to skin ulcers, such as hydrocortisone, antifungals, or zinc oxide
   b. Oral or IV antibiotics may be prescribed (infected ulcer or cellulitis)

D. Client teaching

1. Elevate legs for at least 20 minutes four times a day
2. Keep legs above level of heart when in bed
3. Avoid prolonged sitting or standing and do not cross legs when sitting
4. Do not wear tight, restrictive pants, socks, or boots; avoid girdles and garters that restrict circulation in upper leg
5. Wear support stockings as instructed

XVIII. VARICOSE VEINS

A. Overview

1. A vein or veins in which blood has pooled, producing distended, tortuous, and palpable vessels; valve leaflets become defective
2. As vein swells, increased hydrostatic pressure pushes plasma through stretched vessel walls and edema may occur

NCLEX®

B. Nursing assessment

1. Reports of aching, heaviness, itching, swelling, and unsightly appearance to leg(s)
2. Dilated, tortuous, superficial veins along upper and lower leg
3. Superficial inflammation may develop along path of varicose vein
4. Positive Trendelenburg test (evaluates valve competence; veins fill from proximal rather than distal end after sitting up from supine position with legs raised)

NCLEX®

C. Therapeutic management

1. Analgesics as needed
2. Improve venous circulation as described for venous insufficiency
3. Assess pulses and neurovascular status of lower extremities
4. Apply support stockings
5. Elevate feet above heart level when lying down
6. Prevent skin breakdown; teach proper skin care and importance of avoiding trauma to legs
7. Sclerotherapy: injection of sclerosing agent into varicosed vein, usually in healthcare provider's office (palliative but not curative; elastic bandages often worn for several weeks)
8. Vein ligation surgery involves ligation (tying-off) of entire vein (usually saphenous) and dissection and removal of incompetent tributaries
   a. Perform hourly circulation checks postoperatively in postanesthesia area
   b. Elevate extremity to a 15-degree angle to prevent stasis and edema
   c. Apply compression-gradient stockings from foot to groin
9. Medication therapy: no specific medications are used

D. Client teaching: prevention as for venous insufficiency; lose weight if necessary

XIX. HEART DEFECTS THAT INCREASE PULMONARY BLOOD FLOW

A. Heart conditions in which blood flows from left side of heart to right, resulting from problems with septal wall or communication between arteries; leads to signs of HF

B. Atrial septal defect (ASD) (see Figure 56–1A)

1. Defect in atrial septal wall allowing blood to flow from left atrium to right atrium, called a left-to-right shunt; caused by failure of foramen ovale to close
2. NCLEX® May be located near lower end of septum (ostium primum or ASD1), near central septum (ostium segundum or ASD2), or near junction of right atrium and superior vena cava (sinus venosus defect or ASD3)
3. Assessment: often asymptomatic if defect is small; dyspnea, fatigue, other signs of decreased CO, poor growth, and soft systolic murmur in pulmonic area, splitting S_2
4. Therapeutic intervention includes surgical closure or patch of defect, transcatheter device closure during cardiac catheterization

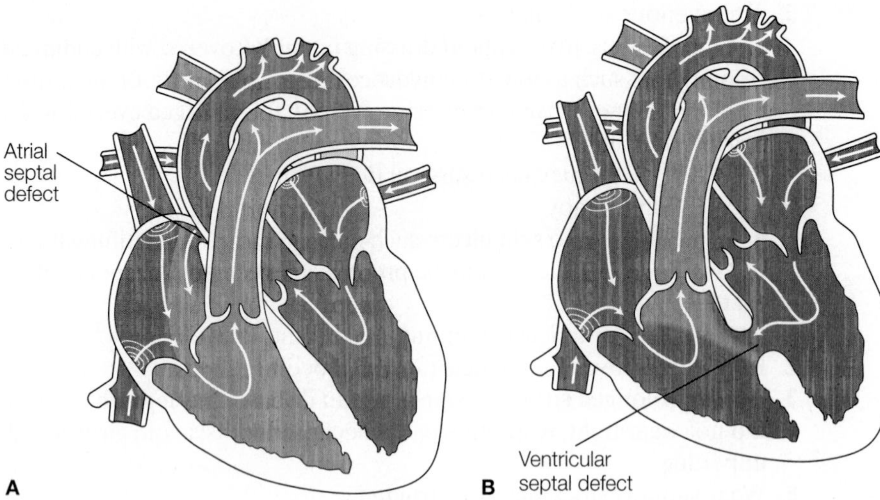

Figure 56–1

Heart defects with increased pulmonary blood flow. (**A**) Atrial septal defect; (**B**) ventricular septal defect.

NCLEX®

5. Nursing management of child with a heart defect that increases pulmonary blood flow (see Table 56–5)
6. Child and family education
   a. Purpose of tests and procedures
   b. Ways to support nutrition, reduce stress on heart, promote rest, and support growth and development during preoperative period
   c. Signs of HF and infection
   d. Prepare parents and child for surgery by visiting intensive care unit, explaining equipment and sounds
   e. Prepare older child for postoperative experience, including coughing and deep breathing and need for movement

C. Ventricular septal defect (VSD) (see Figure 56–1B)

1. Defect in ventricle septal wall allowing blood to flow from LV to RV (**left-to-right shunt**) because of higher pressure in LV
2. Shunting of blood causes an increased load on RV and increases pulmonary blood flow

Table 56–5 Nursing Management of Child with a Heart Defect That Increases Pulmonary Blood Flow

Problem	Nursing Management
Anxiety and inadequate coping	1. Assess coping mechanisms of family. 2. Provide family with information about condition. 3. Refer family to American Heart Association.
Possible delayed growth and development	1. Treat child as normally as possible. Teach parents that children are more comfortable when they know what to expect. 2. Promote mental development activities as appropriate for age and condition.
Risk for infection	1. Limit exposure to individuals with infections. 2. Promote good pulmonary hygiene—change position, use percussion and postural drainage. 3. Possibly use prophylactic antibiotics when undergoing surgical or dental treatments to prevent subacute bacterial endocarditis.
Inadequate nutrition	1. Offer small, frequent meals. 2. Use soft nipple for infant to ease stress of sucking. 3. Organize nursing care to allow for rest.
Impaired gas exchange	1. Promote good pulmonary hygiene. 2. Monitor intake and output. Limit fluids as prescribed. 3. Administer diuretics as prescribed. 4. Change position every 2 hours.

NCLEX®

3. Assessment: tachypnea, dyspnea, poor growth, reduced fluid intake, palpable thrill, systolic murmur at left lower sternal border; ECG and radiology detect larger septal defects; signs of HF

NCLEX®

4. Therapeutic management (see Table 56–5)
   a. May spontaneously close during first year if small or moderate in size
   b. Surgical patching if failure to thrive occurs
   c. Preoperative nursing care involves promoting oxygenation and growth and development (see Table 56–5)
   d. Postoperative nursing care continues with activities of preoperative care, providing analgesics for pain relief, and maintaining sterile dressing on incision
5. Child and family education (same as for ASD)

D. Atrioventricular (AV) canal defect

1. Occurs because of failure of endocardial cushions (fetal growth centers for mitral and tricuspid valves and AV septum) to close
2. Many infants also have trisomy 21 (Down syndrome)
3. Assessment: depends on severity of defect; may include a characteristic holosystolic murmur, tachycardia, tachypnea, signs of HF, poor growth, recurrent respiratory infections, and respiratory failure
4. Therapeutic management
   a. Treatment of HF and pulmonary artery banding to reduce blood flow to lungs before surgery
   b. Surgery by age 3 months with placement of patches or possible valve replacement to prevent pulmonary vascular disease
5. Child and family education (same as for ASD)

E. Patent ductus arteriosus

1. Failure of ductus arteriosus to close within early weeks of life
2. Leads to persistent shunting of blood from aorta to pulmonary artery for recirculation to lungs
3. Assessment
   a. Characteristic "machinery" murmur during systole and diastole and thrill in pulmonic area
   b. Tachycardia, tachypnea, dyspnea, full bounding pulses, widened pulse pressure, signs of HF; may be asymptomatic if very small
4. Therapeutic management
   a. Ibuprofen or indomethacin (prostaglandin inhibitors) to stimulate closure in premature infants if signs of HF have not developed
   b. Surgical closure by open thoracostomy or during cardiac catheterization
5. Child and family education (same as for ASD)

XX. HEART DEFECTS THAT DECREASE PULMONARY BLOOD FLOW

A. Heart conditions that cause blood to contain inadequate O_2 by decreasing pulmonary blood flow; skin and mucous membrane color is usually pale to blue; include pulmonic stenosis, tetralogy of Fallot, and pulmonary atresia (see Figure 56–2)

B. Pulmonic stenosis (Figure 56–2A)

1. Narrowing of pulmonic valve obstructs blood flow into pulmonary artery, leading to right ventricular hypertrophy
2. Stenosis in subvalvular area can occur as heart muscle grows

NCLEX®

3. Assessment
   a. Mild stenosis: may be asymptomatic with normal growth
   b. Moderate stenosis: dyspnea and fatigue on exertion
   c. Severe stenosis: signs of HF and chest pain on exertion
4. Therapeutic management: balloon dilation of valve during cardiac catheterization; surgical valvotomy if other defects such as VSD are present; surgical resection if narrowing is above valve area (leads to regurgitation that is not significant)
5. Nursing care focuses on managing reduced cardiac output, reduced ability to tolerate activity and exercise, possible delays in growth and development, and risk for bacterial infection in blood and sites of blood shunting that promote bacterial growth (see Table 56–6)
6. Child and family education: condition does not increase in severity in most cases; lifelong prophylaxis against infective endocarditis may be needed

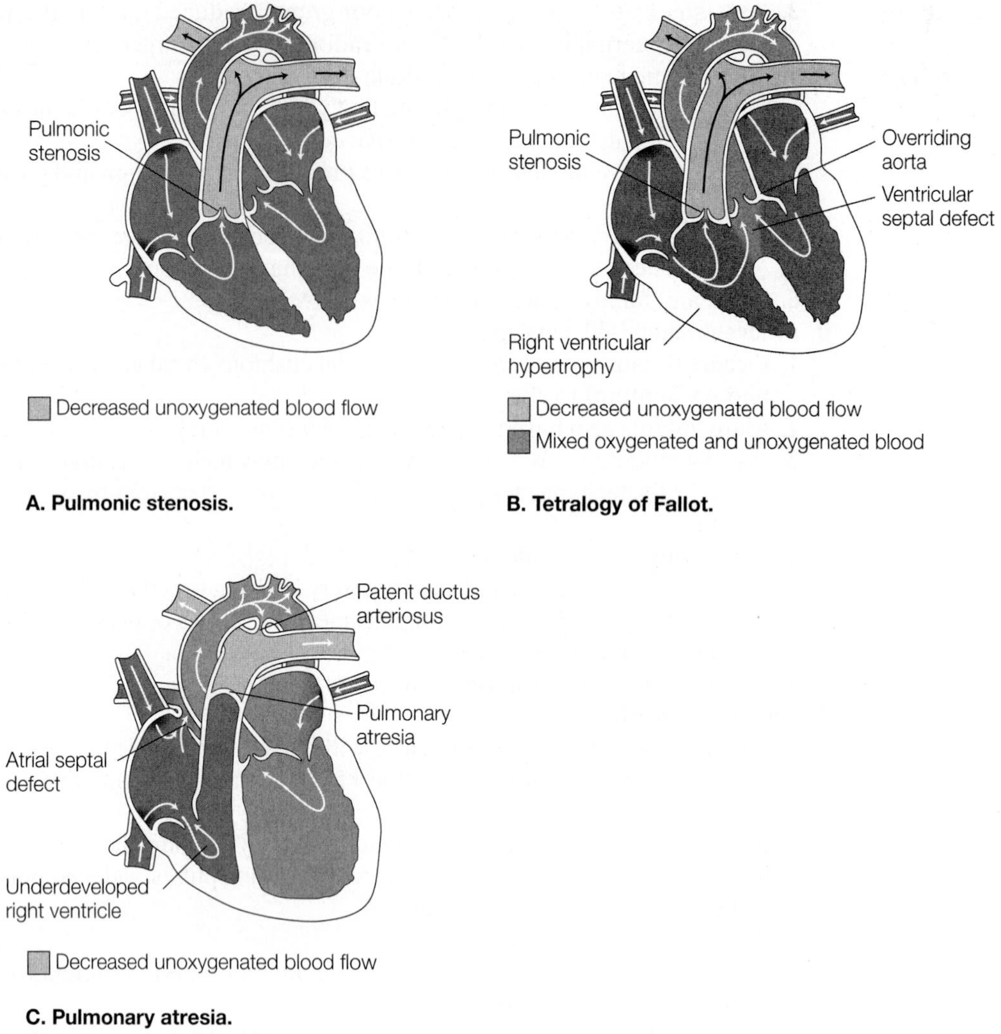

Figure 56–2
Heart defects with decreased pulmonary blood flow.

C. Tetralogy of Fallot (Figure 56–2B)

1. Four defects that combine to allow blood flow to bypass lungs and enter left side of heart, called a **right-to-left shunt**
   a. Four defects: pulmonic stenosis, right-ventricular hypertrophy, ventricular septal defect, and overriding aorta
   b. ASD occurs at times as a fifth defect
   c. Deficient O_2 in tissues leads to acidosis
   d. Hypercyanosis (TET) spells occur, which are transient periods when there is an increase in right-to-left shunting of blood
2. Deoxygenated blood enters systemic circulation, accounting for cyanosis

NCLEX®

3. Assessment
   a. TET spells: hypoxia, pallor, and tachypnea; precipitated by crying, defecation, and feeding; older children assume a squatting position to decrease blood return from lower extremities; treatment involves placing child in knee-chest position and administering morphine or propranolol and oxygen
   b. Clubbing of digits and **polycythemia** (excess number of RBCs), metabolic acidosis
   c. Poor growth, exercise intolerance
   d. Right-ventricular hypertrophy and systolic murmur in pulmonic area
4. Therapeutic management
   a. **Prostaglandin E_1 (PGE_1)**: to maintain open ductus arteriosus
   b. Palliative surgery to improve oxygenation includes modified Blalock-Tassig shunt
   c. Corrective surgery includes patching VSD and relieving pulmonary stenosis

Table 56–6 Nursing Management of Child with Decreased Pulmonary Blood Flow Defect

Problem	Nursing Management
Inadequate tissue perfusion	1. Monitor hemoglobin and hematocrit levels. 2. Keep child calm. Do not allow long periods of crying. 3. When hypercyanosis occurs, assist child to squatting or knee-chest position. 4. Administer oxygen and morphine as ordered during these spells.
Risk for infection	1. Limit exposure to individuals with infections. 2. Promote good pulmonary hygiene—change position, percussion, and postural drainage. 3. Use prophylactic antibiotics when undergoing surgical or dental treatments to prevent subacute bacterial endocarditis.
Inadequate nutrition	1. Offer small, frequent meals. 2. Use soft nipple for infant to ease stress of sucking. 3. Organize nursing care to allow for rest.
Possible impaired gas exchange	1. Limit activity. 2. Maintain clear airway. 3. Monitor electrolytes.
Possible decreased cardiac output	1. Assess vital signs. 2. Monitor for signs of congestive heart failure. 3. Note peripheral edema. 4. Weigh child daily. 5. Maintain strict I&O measurement. 6. Administer diuretics as ordered. 7. Administer oxygen as ordered. 8. Palpate liver every 4 to 12 hours (indicates right-sided failure). 9. Administer digoxin as ordered: a. Assess for apical pulse—monitor for bradycardia or arrhythmias. b. Be consistent in measurement of medication and time of administration. c. Do not repeat dose if child vomits.
Risk for injury	1. Monitor hemoglobin and hematocrit. 2. Observe for signs of thrombus formation.

NCLEX®

5. Nursing care focuses on managing reduced cardiac output, reduced ability to tolerate activity and exercise, possible delays in growth and development, and risk for bacterial infection in blood and sites of blood shunting that promote bacterial growth (see Table 56–6)
6. Child and family education
   a. Promote nutrition in light of weak suck
   b. Discuss activities to promote oxygenation
   c. Symptoms of respiratory infections
   d. Treatments and procedures child will undergo

D. Pulmonary (tricuspid) atresia (Figure 56–2C)

1. Absence of tricuspid valve; prevents blood flow from right atrium to RV; may be accompanied by other defects such as pulmonic stenosis or transposition of great arteries
2. Blood flows to left side of heart through ASD or patent foramen ovale; deoxygenated blood mixes with oxygenated blood in left side of heart

NCLEX®

3. Assessment: cyanosis at birth, tachypnea, continuous murmur from PDA in pulmonic area, signs of HF, pulmonary edema, hepatomegaly, hypoxic spells, clubbing, polycythemia, and growth delays

4. Therapeutic management: immediate PGE_1 to maintain PDA, digoxin, diuretics, and surgical correction
5. Nursing care as outlined in Table 56–6

XXI. MIXED AND OTHER CONGENITAL HEART DEFECTS

A. Mixed heart defect: transposition of great arteries (see Figure 56–3)

1. Pulmonary artery originates from LV; blood travels from LV to pulmonary artery, then to lungs, and then back into left atrium
2. Aorta originates from RV; blood leaves RV by aorta, travels to body cells, and returns to right atrium by way of vena cava
3. There are two closed circulation pathways
4. Survival depends on foramen ovale remaining open to mix oxygenated and deoxygenated blood
5. *NCLEX®* Assessment: progressive cyanosis leads to hypoxia and then acidosis; signs of heart failure, tachypnea, poor feeding, failure to grow; echocardiogram identifies misplacement of arteries
6. *NCLEX®* Therapeutic management
   a. PGE1 to maintain open ductus arteriosus; palliative and corrective surgical interventions
   b. Nursing activities to promote nutrition and reduce respiratory congestion (see Table 56–6)
7. Child and family education
   a. Home care requirements related to nutrition, rest, and oxygenation
   b. Preparation for procedures and treatments
   c. Safe administration of cardiac drugs and diuretics

B. Mixed heart defect: truncus arteriosus

1. Failure to develop separate pulmonary artery and aorta, leading to a single vessel that connects to both ventricles; usually accompanied by VSD
2. Mixing of oxygenated and deoxygenated blood leads to hypoxemia and arterial desaturation
3. Assessment: cyanosis, severe HF, dyspnea, retractions, fatigue, clubbing, polycythemia, bounding peripheral pulses, widened pulse pressure, poor feeding, poor growth, frequent respiratory infections, cardiomegaly
4. *NCLEX®* Therapeutic management: repeated surgeries to correct defect; administration of diuretics and digoxin; nursing care as per Table 56–6

C. Mixed heart defect: total anomalous pulmonary venous return

1. Pulmonary veins lead into right atrium or vessels leading to right atrium rather than left atrium
2. Mixed blood must pass through foramen ovale or VSD to provide systemic circulation
3. Assessment: mild cyanosis that increases during feedings, HF, precordial bulge
4. *NCLEX®* Therapeutic management: PGE_1 to maintain PDA, digoxin and diuretics to treat HF, balloon atrial septotomy to increase blood flow until surgical correction can be done; nursing care as per Table 56–6

D. Defects obstructing systemic blood flow: aortic stenosis

1. Stricture or narrowing of aortic valve that obstructs blood flow into systemic circulation; valve may have two leaflets (bicuspid) instead of three (tricuspid)
2. Overall effect is increased workload of LV
3. Assessment: often asymptomatic with normal growth and development; signs of HF if there is significant stenosis; characteristic systolic murmur with transmission to neck; occasional chest pain with exercise, although exercise intolerance is less common

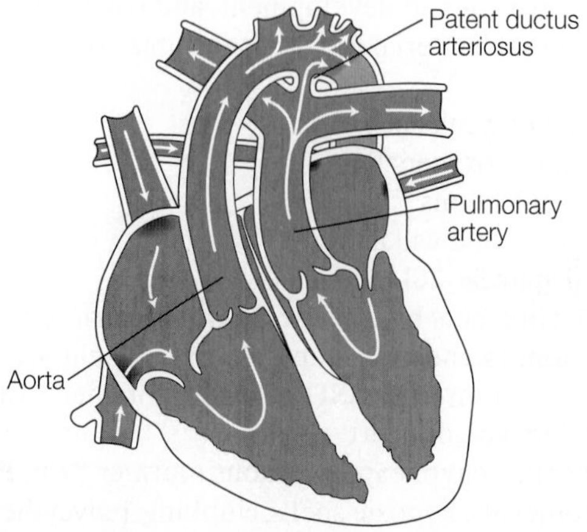

Figure 56–3

Mixed heart defect: Transposition of great arteries.

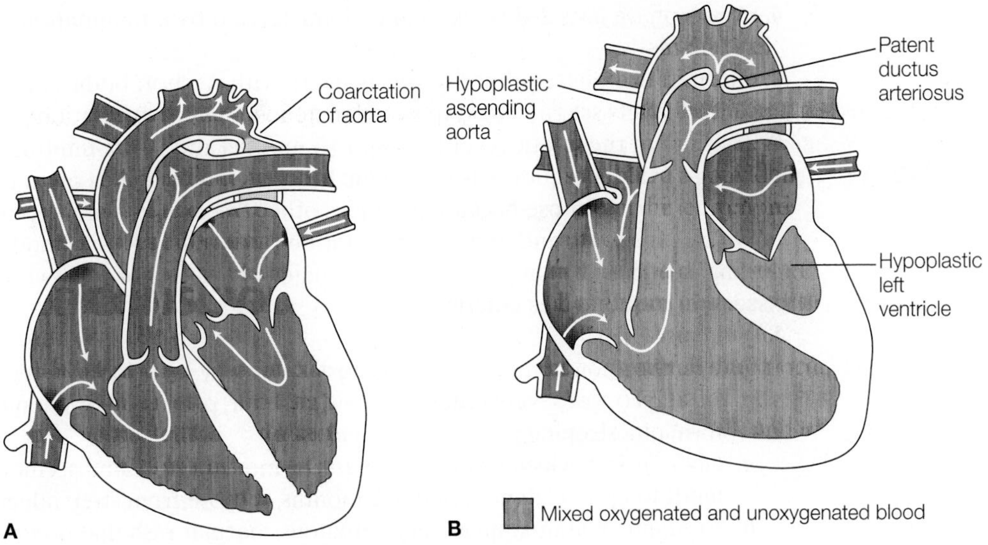

Figure 56–4

Defects obstructing systemic blood flow. (**A**) Coarctation of aorta; (**B**) hypoplastic left heart syndrome.

NCLEX®

4. Therapeutic management: balloon dilation during cardiac catheterization; palliative surgical aortic valvotomy; valve replacement may ultimately be required (usually once adulthood reached), with lifelong anticoagulant therapy and endocarditis prophylaxis

E. **Defects obstructing systemic blood flow: coarctation of aorta** (see Figure 56–4A)

1. Narrowing of descending aorta that restricts blood flow leaving heart, often near ductus arteriosus; progressive disorder that leads to HF

NCLEX®

2. Assessment: may be asymptomatic; BP difference of 20 mm between upper and lower extremities, brachial and radial pulses full, femoral pulses weak, headache, vertigo, epistaxis, exercise intolerance, left-ventricular hypertrophy, dyspnea, cerebrovascular accident (CVA) secondary to hypertension in upper circulation

NCLEX®

3. Therapeutic management
   a. Balloon cardiac catheterization and surgical resection and patch of coarctation
   b. Possible prophylaxis for endocarditis when undergoing surgical or dental procedures
   c. Prior to correction, monitor BP in upper and lower extremities
   d. Rebound hypertension occurs in immediate postoperative period
4. Child and family education
   a. Tests and procedures child will undergo
   b. Signs and symptoms of worsening condition
   c. Administration of cardiac and vasoactive drugs
   d. Need for prophylactic antibiotics for all surgical and dental procedures

F. **Defects obstructing systemic blood flow: hypoplastic left heart syndrome** (see Figure 56–4B)

1. Abnormally small LV and aortic arch with major resistance to aortic blood flow and inadequate oxygen supply; accompanying hypertrophy of RV
2. Absent or stenotic mitral and aortic valves
3. Assessment
   a. Tachypnea, chest retractions, dyspnea, cyanosis
   b. Decreased pulses, poor peripheral perfusion
   c. Increased right-ventricular impulse
   d. Other signs of HF
4. Therapeutic management: PGE_1 given to prevent closure of patent ductus arteriosus; palliative surgery; transplant may be performed; low survival rate

XXII. RHEUMATIC FEVER

A. **Overview**

1. Systemic autoimmune inflammatory disease involving heart, joints, and possibly CNS and connective tissue
2. Follows 2–6 weeks after a group A beta-hemolytic streptococcal infection
3. May be an autoimmune reaction against microorganisms; strep organisms cannot be cultured out of lesions of rheumatic fever

4. Acute phase lasts 2–3 weeks and is characterized by inflammation of connective tissue in heart, joints, and skin
5. Proliferative phase primarily affects heart, with Aschoff bodies developing on heart valves; cardiac valve leaflets scar and lead to valvular stenosis and regurgitation
6. Episode of rheumatic fever lasts up to 3 months and is self-limiting
7. NCLEX® Long-term consequence is rheumatic heart disease, which is often manifested in valvular damage
8. Difficult to diagnose because it mimics other diseases; diagnosis is usually based on **Jones criteria**, which lists major and minor manifestations according to likelihood of rheumatic fever infection; diagnosis is based on presence of two major or one major and two minor criteria

NCLEX®
B. Assessment using Jones criteria

1. Major criteria
   a. Inflammation of multiple joints; most frequently large joints—knees, elbows, and wrists
   b. Carditis (most severe criteria): a new murmur, pericardial friction rub, changes on ECG; tachycardia in form of a sleeping pulse greater than 100
   c. CNS: chorea, which involves involuntary movement of limbs; emotional lability and slurred speech; tends to have a latent period of 2 months or more from strep infection
   d. Erythema marginatum is a erythematous, macular rash that occurs primarily on trunk and proximal limbs; frequently associated with carditis
   e. Subcutaneous nodules (nontender) on skin over flexor surfaces of joints and vertebrae
2. Minor criteria: fever (spiking temperature), arthralgia; elevated ESR, C-reactive protein, and decreased RBC count; prolonged PR and/or QT interval on ECG
3. Supporting evidence (of recent streptococcal infection): history of same, history of scarlet fever, positive throat culture for streptococcus, elevated antistreptolysin O (ASO) titer

C. Therapeutic management

1. Bedrest until ESR returns to normal
2. Aspirin and prednisone as ordered; anti-inflammatory agents to reduce inflammation; aspirin will also promote relief from painful joints
3. Monitor client for cardiac function
4. Give penicillin as ordered in either an oral daily dose or monthly long-acting injection after recovery from rheumatic heart disease to reduce risk of recurrence of strep infection; erythromycin given if client is allergic to penicillin
5. NCLEX® Design nursing activities to promote rest and to encourage diversional activities that do not stress heart; maintain bedrest with bathroom privileges
6. Child and family education
   a. Pathology of disease and rationale for bedrest
   b. Diversional activities that allow for mental stimulation without physical activity
   c. Planning for home care of child

XXIII. KAWASAKI'S DISEASE

A. Overview

1. A multisystem disorder involving **vasculitis** (inflammation of tunica intima lining of arteries and veins)
2. Also called mucocutaneous lymph node syndrome
3. Unknown cause but generally affects young children; most frequently affected are boys under 2 years of age
4. Three phases of disease
   a. Acute phase is characterized by fever, conjunctival hyperemia, swollen hands and feet, rash, reddened throat, and enlarged cervical lymph nodes
   b. Subacute phase is characterized by cracking lips, desquamation of skin on tips of fingers and toes, cardiac disease, and thrombocytosis
   c. Convalescent phase has lingering signs of inflammation
5. Significantly increased platelet count
6. Possible cardiac pathology, including dysrhythmias, HF, and MI

NCLEX®
B. Nursing assessment

1. Phase one (days 1–10): fever lasting longer than 5 days and unresponsive to antipyretics, conjunctivitis, crusted and fissured lips, swelling of hands and feet, erythema, **lymphadenopathy** (a condition that causes swollen glands and can be caused by infection or cancer)
2. Phase two (days 10–25): fever diminishes, irritability, anorexia, desquamation of hands and feet, arthritis and arthralgia, cardiovascular manifestations

3. Phase three (days 26–40): drop in ESR and diminishing signs of illness

C. Therapeutic management

1. Administer aspirin 80–100 mg/kg/day as ordered while temperature is elevated
2. Administer intravenous immune globulin (IVIG) as ordered to reduce risk of coronary artery lesions and aneurysms
3. Nursing management *NCLEX®*
   a. Promote comfort
   b. Small, frequent feedings; encourage fluids
   c. Passive range of motion to extremities
   d. Cool baths and gentle oral care
   e. Monitor for complications: aneurysms; side effects of aspirin therapy (bleeding, GI upset); side effects of IVIG therapy (elevated BP, facial flushing, tightness in chest)
   f. Monitor temperature
   g. Monitor eyes for conjunctivitis

D. Child and family education

1. Safe administration of aspirin therapy
2. Keep skin clean and avoid soaps and lotions
3. Offer liquids high in calories, low in acids
4. Low-cholesterol diet
5. Call healthcare provider if child refuses to walk
6. Monitor temperature in morning and at night prior to giving aspirin

Check Your NCLEX–RN® Exam I.Q.

You are ready for testing on this content if you can:

- Identify basic structures and functions of the cardiovascular system.
- Describe the pathophysiology and etiology of common cardiovascular disorders.
- Discuss expected assessment data and diagnostic test findings for selected cardiovascular disorders.
- Discuss therapeutic management of a client experiencing a cardiovascular disorder.
- Discuss nursing management of a client experiencing a cardiovascular disorder.
- Identify expected outcomes for the client experiencing a cardiovascular disorder.

PRACTICE TEST

1 A client has been admitted to the emergency department with reports of chest pain for the past 2 hours. There are no clear changes on the 12-lead electrocardiogram (ECG). The nurse should expect which laboratory tests to be more specific indicators of a myocardial infarction (MI)? Select all that apply.

1. Elevated potassium level
2. Decreased myglobin level
3. Elevated creatinine kinase level
4. Decreased white blood cell count
5. Elevated troponin level

2 A client scheduled for discharge after coronary artery bypass grafting (CABG) reports new onset of anorexia and nausea. The client's new medications include digoxin, metoprolol, and furosemide. The nurse plans to report this finding to the healthcare provider after checking the result of which laboratory test drawn earlier in the morning?

1. Potassium level
2. Sodium level
3. Creatinine kinase level
4. Digoxin level

3 The registered nurse (RN) has finished reviewing the 0700 shift report on a telemetry unit. Which client would be best for the RN to assign to the licensed practical/vocational nurse (LPN/LVN)?

1. A client 7 days postcardiac surgery with a sternal incisional infection, requiring irrigation and dressing changes
2. A client just admitted from the emergency department (ED) for observation to rule out myocardial infarction
3. A client who has undergone successful valve replacement and will be discharged this morning
4. A client who is scheduled for a percutaneous transluminal coronary angioplasty (PTCA) at 10:00 a.m.

PRACTICE TEST

PRACTICE TEST

4. A client with hypertension is being treated with metoprolol, hydrochlorothiazide, and captopril. Other scheduled medications include docusate and a multivitamin. The client's current BP is 124/86 mmHg and pulse rate is 48. Which scheduled medication doses should the nurse administer? Select all that apply.

1. Metoprolol
2. Captopril
3. Hydrochlorothiazide
4. Docusate
5. Multivitamin

5. The nurse has finished reviewing the shift report on a cardiac unit. The nurse should plan to see which assigned client first?

1. A client with hypertrophic cardiomyopathy who is reporting dyspnea
2. A client who had a cardiac catheterization and will be ambulating for the first time
3. A client taking antibiotics for endocarditis who has sudden dyspnea and anxiety
4. A client who is recovering from coronary artery bypass grafting (CABG) surgery with a temperature of 101°F (38.3°C)

6. The nurse is discharging to home a client with a new diagnosis of atrial fibrillation. The nurse should explain that onset of which symptom is most important to report to the healthcare provider?

1. Irregular pulse
2. Fever
3. Fatigue
4. Hemoptysis

7. The nurse is caring for a client with a history of renal failure and a new myocardial infarction. The nurse who is reviewing laboratory findings should call the healthcare provider to report which result?

1. Potassium level of 5.0 mEq/L
2. Sodium level of 145 mEq/L
3. Calcium level of 7.0 mg/dL
4. Digoxin level of 0.8 ng/mL

8. The nurse is caring for a client who had a permanent pacemaker inserted because of a complete heart block. The nurse determines that which client outcome indicates a successful procedure?

1. Client ambulating in the hall within 4 hours of the procedure without dyspnea or chest pain
2. Client's ECG monitor demonstrates normal sinus rhythm
3. Heart rate of 80 beats per minute, BP 112/74 mmHg
4. Client's ECG monitor shows paced beats at the rate of 72 per minute

9. The nurse is caring for a client with a diagnosis of aortic stenosis who has surgery scheduled in 2 weeks. The client reports episodes of angina and passing out recently at home. What would be the nurse's best explanation about recommended activity at this time?

1. "It is best to avoid strenuous exercise, stairs, and lifting before your surgery."
2. "Take short walks three times daily to prepare for postoperative rehabilitation."
3. "There are no activity restrictions unless the angina reoccurs; then please call the office."
4. "Gradually increase activity before surgery to build stamina for the postoperative period."

10. A client who has just undergone cardiac angiography has a catheter insertion site that has no bleeding or hematoma. Vital signs and distal pulses remain normal and intravenous fluids have been discontinued. The client refuses any food or fluids and asks the nurse to be left alone to rest. What is the nurse's best response?

1. "You are recovering well from the procedure and resting is a good idea."
2. "It is important for you to walk, so I will be back in 1 hour to walk with you."
3. "It is important to drink fluids after this procedure. I will bring you some water, and I encourage you to drink."
4. "You should do leg exercises to keep good circulation to your legs. After your exercises, you can rest."

11 A client undergoes ligation of varicose veins. The nurse includes in the plan of care which important interventions to address concerns with peripheral tissue perfusion? Select all that apply.

1. Teach client to remove compression stockings for at least 1 hour per day.
2. Teach client to flex lower extremities four times a day.
3. Teach client that numbness is common after vein ligation.
4. Encourage client to briskly rub lower extremities to improve circulation.
5. Explain the need to walk and lie down, while avoiding sitting soon after surgery.

12 A client's angiogram demonstrates the final stage of atherosclerosis. The nurse concludes that this client's pathophysiology includes which late-developing element?

1. Presence of atheromas
2. Fatty deposits in the intima
3. Lipoprotein accumulation in the intima
4. Inflammation of the arterial wall

13 When working with a client with peripheral arterial disease (PAD), the nurse assesses for which signs and symptoms that would be consistent with tissue ischemia? Select all that apply.

1. Peripheral edema
2. Thickened toenails
3. Leg pain while walking
4. Brownish discoloration to the skin on the leg
5. Cooler skin temperature on affected extremity

14 In providing community education on prevention of peripheral arterial disease (PAD), the nurse should include which major risk factors? Select all that apply.

1. Dysrhythmias
2. Low-protein intake
3. Exposure to cool weather
4. Cigarette smoking
5. Hypertension

15 When teaching a client with an aneurysm about signs and symptoms that may indicate impending rupture, the nurse first considers which client data?

1. Medication therapy the client is receiving
2. Client's usual blood pressure
3. Age and gender of the client
4. Size and location of the aneurysm

16 The nurse should conclude that an important outcome of care for a female client with hypertension has been met when the client is able to do which of the following?

1. Return to usual activities of daily living (ADLs)
2. Implements actions to counteract two modifiable risk factors
3. Maintain a blood pressure lowered by 10%
4. Discontinue temporary lifestyle modifications

17 Which suggestions should the nurse include when conducting health teaching for clients with arterial insufficiency? Select all that apply.

1. Avoid long periods of sitting and standing.
2. Keep the legs and feet in a raised position.
3. Decrease ambulation to decrease pain.
4. Apply moist heat twice a day.
5. Increase distances walked to build collateral circulation.

18 A client with endocarditis develops sudden leg pain with pallor, tingling, and a loss of peripheral pulses. What should be the nurse's initial action?

1. Elevate the leg above the level of the heart.
2. Wrap the leg in a loose blanket.
3. Notify the healthcare provider about the findings.
4. Perform passive ROM exercise to stimulate circulation.

19 In coordinating care for a client with venous stasis ulcers, the nurse explains to unlicensed assistive personnel that which intervention is most important for ulcer healing?

1. Surgical debridement
2. Meticulous cleaning of the ulcers to prevent infection
3. Leg exercises to increase collateral circulation
4. Elevation of the extremities to increase venous return

20 Which client assigned to the nurse is most at risk for developing a deep vein thrombosis (DVT)?

1. A 30-year-old client who is 1 week postpartum
2. A 63-year-old client post-CVA on anticoagulant therapy
3. A 40-year-old woman who smokes and uses oral contraceptives
4. A 41-year-old female who underwent laparoscopic cholecystectomy

21 The nurse is caring for a 2-month-old child with transposition of the great arteries. Which nursing intervention has highest priority?

1. Providing comfort for parents
2. Maintaining proper caloric intake
3. Reducing stressors for infant
4. Documenting vital signs

22 During the acute phase of rheumatic fever, what is a priority action of the nurse?

1. Encourage ambulation at least four times per day.
2. Assess for early signs of endocarditis.
3. Maintain hydration by encouraging sips of water.
4. Manage pain with routine opioid analgesics.

23 A 6-year-old boy has been diagnosed with coarctation of the aorta. Lately, he has been complaining when he comes in from recess. The school health nurse should question the child about which signs or symptoms?

1. Weakness and pain in legs
2. Blurred vision
3. Increased respiratory rate
4. A bruise on the shin

24 A toddler with Kawasaki disease is going home on aspirin therapy. What should be the priority element in parent teaching at the time of discharge?

1. Monitor child for gastrointestinal bleeding
2. Avoid contact with other children
3. Report if child experiences tingling of extremities
4. Maintain a low-calorie diet

25 A toddler requires supplemental oxygen therapy for a heart defect that decreases pulmonary blood flow. In planning for home care, the nurse would discuss which information with the parents?

1. Need to maintain child on bedrest
2. Promoting mobility while providing supplemental oxygen
3. Symptoms of oxygen toxicity
4. How to draw blood for arterial blood gases

26 The nurse should assess for which manifestations in a client with suspected arterial embolism to the left hand? Select all that apply.

1. Pain
2. Pale skin
3. Bounding radial pulse
4. Parasthesias
5. Pitting edema

ANSWERS & RATIONALES

1 **Answer: 3, 5 Rationale:** An elevated creatinine kinase level is consistent with myocardial damage from acute MI. An increased troponin level (T or I) indicates myocardial damage from acute MI. Elevated potassium is not indicative of MI. Myoglobin level would increase with MI, but is not specific to myocardial tissue, so is not used for diagnosis. WBC count would increase, not decrease, and would not be specific to MI. **Cognitive Level:** Analyzing **Client Need:** Physiological Adaptation **Integrated Process:** Nursing Process: Assessment **Content Area:** Adult Health: Cardiovascular

Strategy: The core issue of the question is the ability to correlate indicators of myocardial damage with a client situation. Evaluate each option carefully, and use nursing knowledge of appropriate laboratory tests and the process of elimination to select answer choices. Note the wording of the question suggests more than one option is likely to be correct.

2 **Answer: 4 Rationale:** Nausea and anorexia are signs of digitalis toxicity, making the digoxin level high priority for assessment. The potassium, sodium, and creatinine kinase levels would not explain the client's symptoms and therefore are not priorities to assess before telephoning the healthcare provider. **Cognitive Level:** Applying **Client Need:** Physiological Adaptation **Integrated Process:** Nursing Process: Diagnosis **Content Area:** Adult Health: Cardiovascular **Strategy:** The core issue of the question is the ability to correlate early signs of digoxin toxicity with a need to check digoxin level in a client with cardiac disease. Evaluate each option carefully, and use nursing knowledge and the process of elimination to make a selection.

3 **Answer: 1 Rationale:** A stable client with complex dressings is an appropriate assignment for an LPN/LVN because the task is within the scope of practice for an LPN/LVN. Initial assessment (new admission from the ED), the assessment of a client before and after a complex procedure (PTCA), and discharge teaching are all responsibilities of the RN and may not be delegated to an LPN/LVN. **Cognitive Level:** Analyzing **Client Need:** Management of Care **Integrated Process:** Nursing Process: Diagnosis **Content Area:** Adult Health: Cardiovascular **Strategy:** Evaluate each option carefully, and use nursing knowledge and the process of elimination to make a selection.

4 **Answer: 2, 3, 4, 5 Rationale:** The captopril does not lower the heart rate and may be safely administered to maintain control of the hypertension. The hydrochlorothiazide does not lower the heart rate and may be safely administered to maintain control of the hypertension. Docusate is a stool softener and may be safely administered to the client. Straining at stool could cause the client to use the Valsalva maneuver, which could temporarily lower the heart rate further. A multivitamin would not adversely affect the client's pulse rate and may be safely administered. The client's heart rate is bradycardic, and metoprolol, a beta-blocker, decreases the heart rate. The dose of this medication should be withheld. **Cognitive Level:** Analyzing **Client Need:** Physiological Adaptation **Integrated Process:** Nursing Process: Planning **Content Area:** Adult Health: Cardiovascular **Strategy:** The core issue of the question is which medication(s) could be responsible for the client's bradycardia and acting accordingly. Evaluate each option carefully, and use nursing knowledge and the process of elimination to make selections. The wording of the question suggests more than one option may be correct.

5 **Answer: 3 Rationale:** A client with endocarditis is at risk for thrombus formation, and chest pain and anxiety are signs of pulmonary embolism (PE), which is a life-threatening complication requiring immediate attention. Dyspnea is a chronic symptom with hypertrophic cardiomyopathy, which requires assessment. A temperature of 101°F (38.3°C) requires additional assessment. A client who is ambulating for the first time will be assessed by the nurse. However, the client who needs to be assessed for PE is the most emergent. **Cognitive Level:** Analyzing **Client Need:** Management of Care **Integrated Process:** Nursing Process: Planning **Content Area:** Adult Health: Cardiovascular **Strategy:** The key to determining the answer to priority-setting questions is to evaluate which client is most unstable or has the greatest risk for developing a complication. Evaluate each option carefully using these methods, and use nursing knowledge and the process of elimination to make a selection.

6 **Answer: 4 Rationale:** Chest pain, dyspnea, and hemoptysis are common symptoms of pulmonary embolism and any of these would be important to report immediately. Irregular pulse is expected with atrial fibrillation. Fever is not associated with atrial fibrillation and is not necessarily included in discharge teaching. However, it could be a sign of illness that could increase the workload of the heart, and therefore it would be the second-most important item to report if it occurred. Fatigue may accompany atrial fibrillation in some individuals. **Cognitive Level:** Analyzing **Client Need:** Physiological Adaptation **Integrated Process:** Nursing Process: Implementation **Content Area:** Adult Health: Cardiovascular **Strategy:** The core issue of the question is knowledge of signs and symptoms of complications to report to the healthcare provider in the presence of atrial fibrillation. Evaluate each option carefully, and use nursing knowledge and the process of elimination to make a selection.

7 **Answer: 3 Rationale:** Renal failure is a common cause of hypocalcemia, and a value of 7.0 mg/dL is below the normal range of 8.5–10.5 mg/dL. The potassium level is within the upper limit of its normal range of 3.5–5.1 mEq/L. The sodium level is within the upper limit of its normal range of 135–145 mEq/L. Digoxin is within the therapeutic range of 0.5–2.0 ng/mL. **Cognitive Level:** Applying **Client Need:** Physiological Adaptation **Integrated Process:** Nursing Process: Implementation **Content Area:** Adult Health: Cardiovascular **Strategy:** The core issue of the question is knowledge of normal and abnormal values that are important to report in a client with an acute cardiac problem and a history of renal failure. The best strategy in questions such as these is to pick the value with the most abnormal number and/or one that relates to the underlying disorder(s).

8 **Answer: 4 Rationale:** Paced beats indicate that the pacemaker is functioning. The client is not allowed to ambulate for 24 hours to prevent dislodging of the electrodes. Normal sinus rhythm does not reflect pacemaker function. Pulse and BP do not reflect pacemaker function. **Cognitive Level:** Applying **Client Need:** Physiological Adaptation **Integrated Process:** Nursing Process: Evaluation **Content Area:** Adult Health: Cardiovascular **Strategy:** Evaluate each option carefully, and use nursing knowledge and the process of elimination to make a selection.

9 **Answer: 1 Rationale:** Symptomatic aortic stenosis has a poor prognosis without surgery. Restricting activity limits myocardial oxygen consumption. Since the incidence of sudden death is high in this population, it is prudent to decrease the strain on the heart while awaiting surgery. The client should not take short walks at this time. Activity restrictions are recommended to reduce myocardial oxygen consumption. The client should not attempt to increase activity preoperatively to build stamina. **Cognitive Level:** Analyzing **Client Need:** Physiological Adaptation **Integrated Process:** Nursing Process: Implementation **Content Area:** Adult Health: Cardiovascular **Strategy:** The core issue of the question is the level of activity that will minimize the client's risk of complications or sudden death until surgery. Evaluate each option carefully, and

use nursing knowledge and the process of elimination to make a selection.

10 **Answer: 3 Rationale:** The contrast used in angiography is nephrotoxic, and a client should have adequate fluids after the procedure to eliminate the dye. Stating the client is recovering well gives false reassurance to a client who could be at risk if fluids are not taken in. The client should lie with the affected leg extended for 6–8 hours. Leg exercises are not recommended because exercise could disrupt the clot that formed at the insertion site. **Cognitive Level:** Analyzing **Client Need:** Physiological Adaptation **Integrated Process:** Communication and Documentation **Content Area:** Adult Health: Cardiovascular **Strategy:** The core issue of the question is knowledge of the correlation between lack of fluid intake and risk of kidney complications following angiography. Evaluate each option carefully, and use nursing knowledge and the process of elimination to make a selection.

11 **Answer: 1, 5 Rationale:** Compression stockings exert pressure on the veins of the lower extremities, promoting venous return back to the heart. Stockings are removed for at least an hour per day to allow for inspection and ensure blood flow through small, superficial vessels. Sitting does not aid in venous return, so the client is encouraged to walk and then lie down soon after surgery to enhance tissue perfusion. Flexing the extremities does not aid tissue perfusion, although it maintains joint range of motion. Numbness is a temporary or rarely permanent complication of surgery. Briskly scrubbing the extremities will not aid tissue perfusion. **Cognitive Level:** Applying **Client Need:** Physiological Adaptation **Integrated Process:** Nursing Process: Planning **Content Area:** Adult Health: Cardiovascular **Strategy:** The core issue of the question is measures to improve tissue perfusion for a client following vein ligation. Using principles of blood flow, choose the option that will aid circulation. Evaluate each option carefully, and use nursing knowledge and the process of elimination to make a selection.

12 **Answer: 1 Rationale:** The final stage of the atherosclerotic process is the development of atheromas, which are complex lesions consisting of lipids, fibrous tissue, collagen, calcium, cellular waste, and capillaries. The calcified lesions may rupture or ulcerate, stimulating thrombosis. Fatty deposits in the intima occur earlier in development of atherosclerosis. Lipoprotein accumulation along the intima occurs earlier in development of atherosclerosis. Inflammation of the arterial wall occurs earlier in development of atherosclerosis. **Cognitive Level:** Applying **Client Need:** Physiological Adaptation **Integrated Process:** Nursing Process: Diagnosis **Content Area:** Adult Health: Cardiovascular **Strategy:** Note the critical words *final stage*. Evaluate each option carefully, and use knowledge of pathophysiology and the process of elimination to make a selection.

13 **Answer: 2, 3, 5 Rationale:** Trophic changes from hypoxia and tissue malnutrition in PAD consist of thickened toenails, hair loss on the extremity, and thin shiny skin. Leg pain (also called intermittent claudication) is a primary manifestation of peripheral arterial disease. Intermittent claudication is muscle pain caused by interruption in arterial flow, resulting in tissue hypoxia. Because of insufficient blood supply, expected temperature of the skin of the affected extremity would be cooler than normal. Peripheral edema on the affected leg would be consistent with venous disease. Brownish discoloration to the skin on the leg would be consistent with venous disease, while pale-colored skin is consistent with arterial disease. **Cognitive Level:** Applying **Client Need:** Physiological Adaptation **Integrated Process:** Nursing Process: Assessment **Content Area:** Adult Health: Cardiovascular **Strategy:** The critical words in the question are *peripheral arterial disease*, which direct you to look for manifestations that are abnormal and that are consistent with arterial but not venous disease. Evaluate each option carefully, and use nursing knowledge and the process of elimination to make a selection.

14 **Answer: 4, 5 Rationale:** Cigarette smoking promotes vasoconstriction and is a major risk factor for PAD. Hypertension is a major risk factor for development of PAD. The presence of dysrhythmias is not a risk factor for PAD. Low protein intake is not a risk factor for PAD, although hyperlipidemia from high fat intake or familial tendency is a risk factor. Exposure to cool weather is not a risk factor for PAD, although it could worsen the symptoms when disease is already present. **Cognitive Level:** Applying **Client Need:** Physiological Adaptation **Integrated Process:** Teaching and Learning **Content Area:** Adult Health: Cardiovascular **Strategy:** Note the critical word *prevention* to focus on the option that contains information that will affect the likelihood of developing peripheral arterial disease. Evaluate each option carefully, using nursing knowledge and the process of elimination to make a selection.

15 **Answer: 4 Rationale:** Aneurysms vary by size and location. Signs of rupture depend on the location of the aneurysm. Dissection can occur anywhere but most often occurs in the ascending aorta where pressure is the highest. The medication the client is receiving is vague and is not directly related to risk of aneurysm rupture. The BP relates to whether the aneurysm may rupture, not to the associated signs and symptoms. The age and gender of the client are unrelated to the size and symptoms of aneurysm rupture. **Cognitive Level:** Analyzing **Client Need:** Physiological Adaptation **Integrated Process:** Nursing Process: Diagnosis **Content Area:** Adult Health: Cardiovascular **Strategy:** With the critical words *signs and symptoms* in mind, choose the option that most directly relates to the core issue of the question. Evaluate each option carefully, and choose size and location as the only option that could affect the specific list of signs and symptoms that would relate to aneurysm rupture.

16 **Answer: 2 Rationale:** An important outcome in care of the hypertensive client is the ability to identify and counteract personal risk factors that the client has the ability to change. Modifiable risk factors for hypertension include smoking, hypercholesterolemia, diabetes mellitus, sedentary lifestyle, obesity, stress, and alcohol use. Returning to ADLs is not likely to be an issue. Lowering BP by 10% may or may not be sufficient. Discontinuing lifestyle modifications is contraindicated because the BP could rise again. **Cognitive Level:** Applying **Client Need:** Physiological Adaptation **Integrated Process:** Nursing Process: Evaluation **Content Area:** Adult Health: Cardiovascular **Strategy:** The core issue of the question is the ability to identify an indicator that is a positive effect of care for the hypertensive client. Evaluate each option carefully, and use nursing knowledge and the process of elimination to make a selection.

17 **Answer: 1, 5 Rationale:** The client should avoid long periods of standing or sitting to promote adequate blood flow. The client with arterial insufficiency should engage in a walking program as prescribed by the healthcare provider to build collateral circulation and slow progression of the disease. The legs and feet should be below heart level to increase

peripheral circulation. Decreasing ambulation inhibits development of collateral circulation and will not help in disease management. Moist heat is helpful for venous problems, but direct heat to the extremity affected by arterial insufficiency could place the skin at risk for burns because of preexisting local hypoxia and friable tissue. **Cognitive Level:** Applying **Client Need:** Physiological Adaptation **Integrated Process:** Nursing Process: Implementation **Content Area:** Adult Health: Cardiovascular **Strategy:** A critical word in the stem of the question is *arterial*, which indicates that correct options are beneficial to the client with impaired circulation to the legs. Discriminate between options that are useful in arterial versus venous disease, and recall that when there are options that are opposite (activity level), only one of them can be correct.

18 **Answer: 2 Rationale:** The client is exhibiting symptoms of acute arterial occlusion. Without immediate intervention, ischemia and necrosis will result within hours. The nurse should first wrap the leg to maintain warmth and protect it from further injury. The leg should not be elevated above heart level because doing so would worsen the tissue ischemia. The nurse should quickly notify the healthcare provider after taking an action that will benefit the client's status. Passive range of motion will increase ischemia by increasing tissue demand for oxygen. **Cognitive Level:** Analyzing **Client Need:** Physiological Adaptation **Integrated Process:** Nursing Process: Implementation **Content Area:** Adult Health: Cardiovascular **Strategy:** The core issue of the question is recognizing the complication of acute arterial occlusion and then determining which action should be taken first. Choose an option that is client focused rather than healthcare provider focused, if one is available. In this case, the nurse can protect the client from further injury by wrapping the leg loosely in a blanket.

19 **Answer: 4 Rationale:** The client with venous ulcers must keep the legs elevated above the level of the heart as much as possible to enhance venous return, which improves overall circulation to the lower extremities. Surgical debridement may or may not be indicated. Asepsis is important, but no ulcer will heal unless the edema and stagnant tissue metabolites can be reduced. The client with a leg ulcer should avoid exercise to prevent further damage to tissues at risk. **Cognitive Level:** Analyzing **Client Need:** Physiological Adaptation **Integrated Process:** Nursing Process: Planning **Content Area:** Adult Health: Cardiovascular **Strategy:** The critical words in the stem of the question are *most important*, indicating that more than one option, or all options, may be helpful, but one is better than the others. Note that the nurse is talking to an ancillary caregiver. Consider that the correct option is one that is within the scope of practice of that caregiver in making a selection.

20 **Answer: 3 Rationale:** A major risk factor for DVT is oral contraceptive use in women who smoke. Being 1 week postpartum does not place a client at risk since mobility is usually restored. Anticoagulant therapy is used to prevent development of thrombi. Laparoscopic surgical procedures are associated with more rapid recovery times with reduced immobility, keeping this client at lower risk for DVT. **Cognitive Level:** Applying **Client Need:** Physiological Adaptation **Integrated Process:** Nursing Process: Assessment **Content Area:** Adult Health: Cardiovascular **Strategy:** The critical words in the question are *most at risk*, indicating the correct option is the one that contains the most severe or greatest number of risk factors for DVT. With this in mind, evaluate each option and use the process of elimination to make a selection.

21 **Answer: 3 Rationale:** The open ductus arteriosus will allow a small amount of mixing of oxygenated and unoxygenated blood. Stress will increase the cardiac workload (and thus decrease cardiac output) and therefore avoiding stress is a priority for the nurse. Providing comfort to parents meets a secondary need rather than a primary need using Maslow's hierarchy. Maintaining caloric intake is a physiological priority that can be considered after ensuring airway, breathing, and circulation. Documenting vital signs is a routine activity and not a priority when compared to actual care activities. **Cognitive Level:** Analyzing **Client Need:** Physiological Adaptation **Integrated Process:** Nursing Process: Planning **Content Area:** Child Health **Strategy:** Use Maslow's hierarchy of needs to review each option and choose the one that most closely relates to the ABCs and thus cardiac workload. Use this knowledge and the process of elimination to make a selection.

22 **Answer: 2 Rationale:** The main complication of rheumatic fever is carditis. The nurse must assess for early signs of bacterial endocarditis. The client should be encouraged to rest during the acute phase. Hydration needs may not be sufficiently met with sips of water. Opioid analgesics may not be necessary, although nonsteroidal anti-inflammatory drugs (NSAIDs) are likely to be prescribed. **Cognitive Level:** Applying **Client Need:** Physiological Adaptation **Integrated Process:** Nursing Process: Planning **Content Area:** Child Health **Strategy:** The core issue of the question is the ability to set priorities for a client with rheumatic fever. Omit ambulation because of the words *at least*, knowing that rest is encouraged. Likewise, eliminate hydration because of the word *sips*. Choose assessing for endocarditis over opioid analgesics knowing that NSAIDs are likely to be effective in managing pain and inflammation from rheumatic fever.

23 **Answer: 1 Rationale:** Decreased circulation to lower extremities would contribute to muscle fatigue and pain in the legs. Blurred vision is not related to coarctation. Many children returning from recess may have increased respiratory rate secondary to play activities. A bruise on the shin is not of special concern if it is related to a play-related fall, since risk of bleeding is not a concern in coarctation. **Cognitive Level:** Applying **Client Need:** Physiological Adaptation **Integrated Process:** Nursing Process: Assessment **Content Area:** Child Health **Strategy:** The core issue of the question is knowledge of signs of exercise intolerance in a 6-year-old client with a cyanotic heart defect. Use principles of gas exchange and knowledge of normal and abnormal findings after exercise to make a selection.

24 **Answer: 1 Rationale:** Aspirin prevents platelet agglutination. Gastrointestinal bleeding is often a side effect of aspirin therapy. It is not necessary to avoid contact with other children. Tingling of extremities is not a related concern in Kawasaki disease, although ringing in the ears could be a sign of salicylate toxicity. A low-calorie diet is not indicated. **Cognitive Level:** Applying **Client Need:** Pharmacological and Parenteral Therapies **Integrated Process:** Nursing Process: Implementation **Content Area:** Child Health **Strategy:** The core issue of the question is knowledge of adverse drug effects of salicylate therapy for the child with Kawasaki disease. Use this knowledge and the process of elimination to make a selection.

25 **Answer: 2 Rationale:** Allowing mobility is helpful to promote growth and development in the toddler. Strategies should be discussed to promote mobility while maintaining the supplemental oxygen. Bedrest is unnecessary. Signs of oxygen toxicity are not the priority based on the information in the question. Drawing arterial blood gases is unnecessary. **Cognitive Level:** Applying **Client Need:** Physiological Adaptation **Integrated Process:** Nursing Process: Planning **Content Area:** Child Health **Strategy:** The core issue of the question is home care needs of a toddler receiving oxygen therapy. Use principles of needs related to normal growth and development to help select the correct option.

26 **Answer: 1, 2, 4 Rationale:** The client would exhibit pain, pallor of the affected skin, diminished or absent radial pulse, parasthesias (altered local sensation), paralysis (weakness or inability to move extremity), and poikilothermia (cooler temperature) because of reduced circulation to the area. The client would not have a bounding radial pulse (opposite finding is true) or pitting edema, indicating a fluid volume excess or heart failure. **Cognitive Level:** Analyzing **Client Need:** Physiological Adaptation **Integrated Process:** Nursing Process: Planning **Content Area:** Adult Health: Cardiovascular **Strategy:** The core issue of the question is knowledge of assessment findings in arterial embolism. Visualize a clot in the local circulation and use that image to determine the effect of the blockage on circulation to the affected area.

Key Terms to Review

afterload p. 924
angina pectoris p. 934
atherosclerosis p. 934
cardiac output (CO) p. 924
cardiac tamponade p. 938
contractility p. 924
coronary heart disease p. 934
cor pulmonale p. 936
ejection fraction (EF) p. 926
endarterectomy p. 943
Homans sign p. 946
infarction p. 925
intermittent claudication p. 942
ischemia p. 926
Jones criteria p. 954
jugular venous distention (JVD) p. 936
left-to-right shunt p. 948
lymphadenopathy p. 954
murmurs p. 938
neurovascular status p. 942
orthostatic hypotension p. 941
poikilothermia p. 943
polycythemia p. 950
preload p. 924
prostaglandin E_1 (PGE_1) p. 950
pulmonary edema p. 936
regurgitation p. 939
rest pain p. 942
right-to-left shunt p. 950
stenosis p. 939
stroke volume (SV) p. 924
sympathectomy p. 944
vasculitis p. 954
vasodilation p. 925

References

Ball, J., & Bindler, R., & Cowen, K. (2015). *Principles of pediatric nursing: Caring for children* (6th ed.). Hoboken, NJ: Pearson Education.

Berman, A., Snyder, S., & Frandsen, G. (2016). *Kozier & Erb's fundamentals of nursing: Concepts, process, and practice* (10th ed.). New York, NY: Pearson Education.

Ignatavicius, D., & Workman, L. (2016). *Medical-surgical nursing: Patient-centered collaborative care* (10th ed.). Philadelphia: Saunders.

LeMone, P., Burke, K., Bauldoff, G., & Gubrud, P. (2015). *Medical surgical nursing: Clinical reasoning in patient care* (6th ed.). Hoboken, NJ: Pearson Education.

Lewis, S., Dirksen, S., Heitkemper, M., & Bucher, L. (2014). *Medical surgical nursing: Assessment and management of clinical problems* (9th ed.). St. Louis, MO: Elsevier Science.

Smith, S., Duell, D., Martin, B., Aebersold, M., & Gonzalez, L. (2017). *Clinical nursing skills: Basic to advanced skills* (10th ed.). New York, NY: Pearson Education.

Neurologic Disorders

57

In this chapter

Cross Reference

Other chapters relevant to this content area are

Neurologic and Musculoskeletal Medications	Chapter 38
Common Laboratory Tests	Chapter 46
Common Diagnostic Tests and Procedures	Chapter 47

I. OVERVIEW OF ANATOMY AND PHYSIOLOGY OF NERVOUS SYSTEM

A. Cells in nervous system (NS)

1. Neurons: basic anatomical and functional units in NS; composed of cell body, axon, and dendrites
2. Glial cells: nourish, support, and protect brain neurons; consist of astrocytes, oligodendrocytes, ependymal cells, and microglia in brain, and Schwann cells in peripheral nervous system

B. Central nervous system (CNS)

1. Consists of cerebrum, cerebellum, brainstem, and spinal cord
2. Cerebrum (largest brain structure), enables individuals to reason, function intellectually, express personality and mood, and interact with environment
   a. Includes two hemispheres; each has a frontal, temporal, parietal, and occipital lobe; each lobe has specific functions
   b. Right hemisphere generally controls left side of body and vice versa; usually one hemisphere is considered dominant
   c. Frontal lobe performs high-level cognitive function, has memory storage, influences somatic motor control, controls voluntary eye movements, and controls motor aspect of speech in **Broca's area**, located in dominant hemisphere (usually left)
   d. Temporal lobe has primary auditory receptive areas and auditory association area (**Wernicke's area**); usually found on dominant side and is responsible for interpreting speech; interpretive area integrates somatic, auditory, and visual data (impacts perception, learning, memory, emotions, and intellect)
   e. Parietal lobe holds primary sensory cortex and sensory association areas that define and localize sensations such as size, shape, weight, texture, and consistency; processes visual–spatial stimuli; controls spatial orientation
   f. Occipital lobe is visual center for eyes; controls eye reflexes and interpretation of sight
3. Diencephalon
   a. Thalamus relays sensory impulses to cortex, including pain, and is part of reticular activating system
   b. Hypothalamus regulates temperature, stress response, emotions, sleep–wake cycle, hunger, water metabolism, and pituitary gland secretions
4. Cerebellum lies posterior to pons; responsible for muscle movement and tone, coordination and balance
5. Brainstem has three major divisions: midbrain (visual and auditory relay centers, motor coordination), pons (respiratory centers and breathing), and medulla (heart rate, respiration, vasomotor tone, vomiting, sneezing, swallowing, and coughing); most cranial nerves originate in brainstem
6. Spinal cord: neuron and synapse networks that run most of length of vertebral column
   a. Divided into four areas: cervical area (C1 to C7) near neck; thoracic area (T1 to T12) near chest; lumbar area (L1 to L5) near lower back; sacral area (S1 to S4) in sacrum
   b. Sensory tracts (dorsal roots) carry afferent impulses from periphery to dorsal root ganglia for transmission to brain, including pain, temperature, touch, proprioception, and stimuli from visceral organs
   c. Motor tracts (ventral roots) carry efferent impulses from spinal cord to somatic fibers that innervate voluntary striated, smooth, and cardiac muscle, and that regulate glandular secretions

C. Peripheral Nervous System (PNS)

1. Consists of 31 pairs of spinal nerves, 12 pairs of cranial nerves, and autonomic NS (sympathetic nervous system [SNS] and parasympathetic NS)
2. Each pair of spinal nerves has dorsal and ganglion roots that exit spinal cord via an intervertebral foramina; they carry input between specific areas called dermatomes and spine
3. Cranial nerves (CN): 12 pairs arise from brain; three are pure sensory nerves, five are pure motor nerves, and four are mixed sensory and motor nerves; olfactory nerve (CN I) and optic nerve (CN II) arise from cerebrum; CN III and IV arise in midbrain; CN V to VIII arise in pons; CN IX to XII arise in medulla (see Table 57–1 for an overview of cranial nerves)
4. Autonomic NS: a collection of motor nerves that regulates activities of viscera, smooth muscles, and glands; two branches (sympathetic and parasympathetic) work antagonistically
   a. SNS is active during times of stress, such as flight-or-fight response; it increases heart rate (HR) and blood pressure (BP) and vasoconstricts peripheral blood vessels (BVs)
   b. Parasympathetic nervous system is a conservation, restoration, and maintenance system; it decreases HR and increases gastrointestinal (GI) activity

D. Neurotransmitters: assist with transmission of impulse from one neuron to next; include acetylcholine, norepinephrine, dopamine, and serotonin

Table 57–1 Overview of Cranial Nerves

Cranial Nerve Name	Type of Nerve	Physiological Functions
Olfactory (I)	Sensory	Ability to smell
Optic (II)	Sensory	Visual fields, visual acuity
Oculomotor (III)	Motor	Extraocular movements (EOM)
Trochlear (IV)	Motor	EOM
Trigeminal (V)	Mixed	Movement of eyelids, ability to clench jaw
Abducens (VI)	Motor	EOM
Facial (VII)	Mixed	Movement of eyelids, facial symmetry
Acoustic (VIII)	Sensory	Hearing ability
Glossopharyngeal (IX)	Mixed	Gag, swallow, and cough reflexes; voice quality
Vagus (X)	Mixed	Gag, swallow, and cough reflexes; voice quality
Spinal Accessory (XI)	Motor	Neck strength and shoulder shrug
Hypoglossal (XII)	Motor	Tongue movement

E. Blood supply

1. Brain can only use glucose for energy; a lack of glucose for 5 or more minutes leads to irreversible brain damage; brain receives 750 mL/min of blood or 15–20% of resting cardiac output
2. Cerebral arteries are thinner, have more internal elasticity, and less smooth muscle than other arteries; two sets of arteries (anterior and posterior circulation) supply brain
   a. Anterior circulation, fed by internal and external carotids, delivers blood to area at base of cerebrum called circle of Willis, which feeds smaller arteries that supply anterior, middle, and posterior cerebrum
   b. Posterior circulation, fed by vertebral arteries, delivers blood to posterior fossa; then join to form one basilar artery to supply cerebellum, midbrain, pons, and medulla
   c. Meninges are supplied by external carotid artery branches entering brain at base of skull
3. Venous system of brain is unique
   a. Vessel walls are thinner than other veins of body; do not follow path of arteries
   b. Because these veins have no valves, drainage depends on venous pressure and gravity
   c. Dural sinuses collect blood from brain and empty it into jugular veins

F. Blood–brain barrier

1. A network of endothelial cells in wall of capillaries and astrocyte projections in close proximity that do not have pores between them
2. Does not allow nonspecific filtering process that occurs in rest of body; molecules enter brain by active transport, endocytosis and exocytosis, creating a highly selective barrier that guards neurons
3. Movement of substances across barrier depends on particle size, lipid solubility, chemical dissociation, and protein-binding potential
4. Barrier is very permeable to water, oxygen (O_2), carbon dioxide (CO_2), other gases, glucose, and lipid-soluble compounds

G. Protective structures

1. **Meninges**: covers brain and spinal cord to protect and support; divided into three layers
   a. Dura mater: outer tough, membranous tissue that surrounds and extends into brain tissue
   b. Arachnoid membrane (middle layer): network of delicate, elastic tissue containing BVs of varying sizes
   c. Pia mater: inner membrane that covers entire brain with tiny BVs that extend into gray matter
   d. Within meninges, there are important potential spaces (epidural, subdural, subarachnoid) where bleeding can occur
2. Skull: includes 8 fused cranial bones and 14 facial bones; encloses brain in a protective vault
3. Spine: flexible column that encloses spinal cord, formed from stacking of 7 cervical, 12 thoracic, 5 lumbar, and 4 sacral vertebrae
4. Cerebrospinal fluid (CSF) and ventricular system
   a. CSF is a clear, colorless, odorless solution that fills ventricles and subarachnoid space of brain and spinal cord; acts as a shock absorber; contains electrolytes, glucose, protein, O_2, and CO_2 dissolved in solution
   b. Ventricular system is composed of four ventricles (one in each hemisphere, one midline in thalamic area, and one anterior to cerebellum and subarachnoid space)

II. DIAGNOSTIC TESTS AND ASSESSMENTS OF NERVOUS SYSTEM

A. Assessment of NS

1. Assess circumstances of injury and admission, pertinent family and social history

NCLEX®

2. Assess chief complaint: use mnemonic APQRST

Memory Aid

Remember the mnemonic APQRST to recall all important points to assess whenever a client has an acute-onset symptom:
A—any associated symptoms with chief complaint
P—what provokes (makes worse) or palliates (makes better) symptoms
Q—quality of pain
R—region and radiation
S—severity of pain on a scale of 0 to 10
T—timing: when it stops and starts, whether it is intermittent or constant, its duration

3. Health information: including past medical history, current medications, recent surgeries or other treatments, alcohol or illegal drug use
4. Mental status exam

NCLEX®

   a. A screening mental status exam includes orientation to person, place, and time; appearance and behavior; mood; speech pattern; thought and perception (insight, thought, content, judgment)
   b. To conduct this exam, client must be awake, alert, and able to understand and respond to questions
   c. A client with an altered **level of consciousness (LOC)** may have a range of behaviors; see Table 57–2 for terms used to describe LOC
   d. Acute confusion or delirium should be recognized and treated by eliminating the cause; try to avoid confusing delirium with dementia (a chronic problem)
5. Cranial nerves (CN): can be assessed as described in Table 57–3
6. Motor function
   a. Inspect all body muscles for size, tone, movement, and strength
   b. Compare left and right side for symmetry and equality
   c. Assess for tremors (rhythmic movements) and fasciculations (twitching)
   d. Criteria for grading muscle strength (see Box 57–1, p. 967)

NCLEX®

7. Cerebellar examination: balance and coordination are under cerebellar control
   a. Gait: have client walk normally and then on heels and toes; perform Romberg test (equilibrium) by having client stand with feet together and eyes closed for 20 seconds while examiner stands by to prevent falling; there should be minimal swaying
   b. Coordination: observe client's ability to touch own nose and then touch one of examiner's fingers, then own nose again; next, observe client's ability to touch each finger to thumb of same hand; finally, observe client's ability to run heel down shin on each side while lying in supine position

Table 57–2 Terms Used to Describe Level of Consciousness

Term	Description
Alert	Client is awake and responding purposefully to voice and other stimuli in environment; often clients who are alert are oriented to person, place, and time, but a client can be alert but disoriented to person, place, and/or time
Lethargic	Client is drowsy but can be easily awakened; may drift back to a state of drowsiness when verbal or tactile stimuli stops
Stuporous	Client can be aroused for a short time with the use of vigorous tactile stimuli (such as rubbing arm) or painful stimuli; may attempt to grab or pull away (withdraw) from source of stimuli
Comatose	Unable to be aroused with verbal, tactile, or painful stimuli; does not withdraw from painful stimuli but may have slight nonpurposeful movement in stimulated area; in deep coma, client is unconscious, with no movement, and no neurologic reflex activity

Table 57–3 Cranial Nerve Assessment Tests

Cranial Nerve (CN)	Assessment
CN I (olfactory)	Assess ability to identify common odors
CN II (optic)	Use Snellen chart to assess vision
CN III, IV, and VI (oculomotor, trochlear and abducens)	EOM: have client follow finger through cardinal fields of gaze Ptosis (III): a droopy eyelid PERRLA: assess pupils equal, round, and reactive to light and accommodation Nystagmus: pupil movement is choppy Doll's eyes: in comatose client, doll's eyes is present when eyes stay center while head moves left and right; absent when eyes move with head
CN V (trigeminal)	Jaw clench: palpate masseter and temporal muscles when client's jaw is clenched; note differences on left or right Compare light, dull, and sharp sensations on both sides of face Corneal reflex: on an unconscious client, a wisp of cotton is touched to cornea; normal response is to blink Lids (V, VII): stroke each lid to elicit a blink response
CN VII (facial)	Facial symmetry: note droopiness of nasal labia fold, lower eyelid, or corner of mouth when asking client to grin, raise eyebrows, and sniff; assess accuracy of tasting sweet, sour, and salty items on anterior two-thirds of tongue
CN VIII (acoustic)	Assess hearing of each ear with a ticking watch or whispering; cold caloric testing: irrigating ear in cold water causes a slow movement of eyes toward irrigated side with a rapid return to midline; this is called oculovestibular reflex and indicates an intact brainstem
CN IX and X (glossopharyngeal and vagus)	Swallow reflex: assess whether client can swallow water or has dysphagia (difficulty swallowing) Gag reflex: assess gag by touching back of both sides of throat; a unilateral loss may be noted Hoarseness: assess client's voice for hoarseness Cough reflex: assess whether client's cough is strong, weak, or absent Assess sweet, salty, and sour taste on posterior third of tongue
CN XI (spinal accessory)	Neck strength: have client turn head against resistance Shoulder shrug: have client shrug shoulders against resistance
CN XII (hypoglossal)	Tongue deviation: have client stick out tongue and move it side to side against resistance; if there is a weakness, tongue will go to stronger side

Box 57–1

Criteria for Grading Muscle Strength

0 = No contraction

1 = Trace of contraction

2 = Active movement with gravity

3 = Active movement against gravity

4 = Active movement against gravity and resistance

5 = Normal power

Note: Findings are recorded as a fraction with 5 (highest possible score) as the denominator; for example, normal finding is 5/5.

8. Sensory function
   a. Have client close eyes; touch client on all dermatomes with objects that are sharp, dull, light to touch, and that vibrate (over bony prominence); client should be able to identify location and type of touch
   b. Position sense (kinesthesia): have client close eyes and move client's finger or toe up or down and ask client to describe movement
   c. Stereognosis: have client identify with eyes closed an object placed in hand
   d. Graphesthesia: have client with closed eyes identify a number or letter traced on palm of hand
   e. Two-point discrimination: have client close eyes; touch client beginning on finger pads with two simultaneous pinpricks and ask how many pinpricks were felt

9. Reflexes
   a. Assess deep tendon reflexes (patellar, biceps, brachioradialis, triceps, and Achilles) with a reflex hammer; see Box 57–2 for scoring criteria

Box 57–2

Standard Criteria for Grading Reflexes

0 = absent or no response

1 = hypoactive; weaker than normal (+)

2 = normal (++)

3 = stronger than normal (+++)

4 = hyperactive (++++)

b. Assess superficial abdominal reflex by lightly stroking abdomen from side to midline; normally, side stroked will contract
c. Assess cremasteric reflex by lightly stroking inside of thigh on a male client to raise testicle on that side
d. Assess Babinski reflex by stroking lateral aspect of sole of foot from heel to ball, curving medially in ball; positive response is dorsiflexion of big toe and fanning of other toes; normal in infants but abnormal in adults (normal adult response is curling of toes, called a negative Babinski)

10. Speech is usually described from interview
   a. Clear: normal, fluent speech
   b. **Dysarthria**: ineffective articulation of speech; may be a motor deficit of tongue and speech muscles
   c. **Aphasia**: a language disorder classified by type
   d. Expressive, motor, nonfluent, or Broca's aphasia: inability to express oneself using motor aspects of speech
   e. Receptive, fluent, sensory, or Wernicke's aphasia: inability to comprehend spoken words
   f. Global (mixed expressive and receptive) aphasia: inability to express or comprehend language

NCLEX®

11. Specialized tests for meningeal irritation
   a. **Kernig sign**: positive or present when client feels resistance or pain when leg is raised with knee flexed; indicates meningeal irritation, such as in meningitis
   b. **Brudzinski sign**: positive or present when there is involuntary flexion of knees or hips when head is flexed while in supine position; commonly found also in meningitis

Memory Aid

Recall that the words *Kernig* and *knee* both begin with *K*, while *Brudzinski* and *brain* both begin with *B*. This will aid in recalling how to conduct each test.

B. Diagnostic studies of NS (see also Chapter 47)

NCLEX®

1. Lumbar puncture (LP): collects CSF for analysis via needle aspiration; normal CSF is colorless, clear, with no blood or bacteria (white cells 0–5 cells/mm^3), glucose 40–80 mg/dL, and protein 16–45 mg/dL; following LP, position head elevated with water-based contrast and flat with oil-based contrast; assess site for leakage of CSF and for signs of infection
2. Cerebral angiography: outlines vascular structure of brain; detects arteriovenous (AV) malformations and/or aneurysms; use standard measures associated with use of contrast media (assess for allergy to iodine or contrast; encourage fluids postprocedure to aid in excretion)
3. Computed tomography (CT) with or without contrast: detects bleeding, hydrocephalus, and ischemic strokes older than 48 hours; see precautions noted above
4. Magnetic resonance imaging (MRI): detects soft tissue changes (necrotic tissue, tumors, edema, congenital or degenerative disorders); implanted sources of metal contradict use of this procedure

NCLEX®

5. Electroencephalography (EEG): measures brain waves with multiple scalp electrodes; aids in diagnosing epilepsy, encephalitis, and dementia disorders; also an important criterion in determining brain death
   a. Teach client that test will not deliver electric shock
   b. Shampoo hair preprocedure for cleanliness and postprocedure to remove residual electrode gel
   c. Withhold antiepileptics and other medications as prescribed for 12–24 hours prior
   d. Have client eat regular meals to avoid hypoglycemia that could affect results
6. Electromyography (EMG) and nerve conduction studies: differentiate between peripheral nerve and muscle disorders; measures conduction velocity of muscles between two points; performed at rest, with movement, and with electrical stimulation

7. Ultrasound
   a. Carotid Doppler scan: noninvasive ultrasound that detects carotid occlusions and stenosis
   b. Transcranial Doppler ultrasonography (TCD): a portable, noninvasive technique that measures intracranial blood flow velocity; assesses vasospasm, transient ischemic attack (TIA), headache, subarachnoid hemorrhage (SAH), head injury, and AV malformations
8. Radiography: x-rays of skull can identify suture separation in infants, fractures, bony defects, erosion and calcifications; x-rays of spine can identify fractures, dislocation of vertebrae, compression, narrowed spinal canal, and degenerative processes

III. ALTERED LEVEL OF CONSCIOUSNESS (LOC)

A. Overview

1. A change in arousal or alertness and/or a change in cognition (thought processes, memory, perception, problem solving, and emotion); often first sign of a change in neurologic status
2. Causes for unconsciousness vary from primary CNS disorders (such as damage to RAS or cerebrum) to dysfunction of other organ systems
3. Metabolic disorders may alter cellular environment enough to inhibit neuronal activity
4. The term **coma** is reserved for those who have long periods (hours to months) of unconsciousness; neurologic origin results from damage to both hemispheres of brain, damage to brainstem, or both

NCLEX®

B. Nursing assessment

1. Except for cases of damage to brainstem, changes in LOC and brain function deterioration follow a predictable pattern from higher functions to primitive functions
2. Early changes in cerebral function can include confusion, forgetfulness, disorientation (time, then person, then place), agitation, poor problem-solving ability, or any change in behavior
3. Changes of lethargy and stupor result from greater cerebral deterioration
4. Midbrain deterioration: a change from purposeful movements to decorticate posturing (see Figure 57–1A), small reactive pupils, and positive doll's eyes (positive oculocephalic reflex; eyes do not turn when head is moved and stay fixed in original direction); decorticate posturing is characterized by elbows, wrists, and fingers flexed while arms are close to sides, and leg extension with internal rotation and plantar flexion
5. Deterioration at level of pons: decerebrate posturing (see Figure 57–1B), fixed pupils, and positive cold calorics test (positive vestibuloocular reflex; sustained deviation of both eyes toward ear being stimulated with cold water); decerebrate posturing is characterized by neck extension, clenched jaws, pronated and extended arms that are close to sides, and legs extended with plantar flexion
6. Fixed pupils, flaccid posturing, and negative cold calorics test indicate involvement of medulla
7. Glasgow Coma Scale assessment includes components of eye opening (scored 1–4), best verbal response (scored 1–5), and best motor response (scored 1–6); total score ranges from 3 to 15; a score of 8 or lower usually indicates coma; see Table 57–4
8. Diagnostic and laboratory test findings
   a. Diagnostic tests: CT and MRI (hemorrhage, tumor, cysts, edema, or brain atrophy), EEGs (unrecognized seizures as cause for altered LOC), cerebral angiography (aneurysm and AV malformations), transcranial Doppler study (blood flow), or LP with CSF analysis (infection)
   b. Laboratory tests: glucose, serum electrolytes, osmolarity, creatinine, liver function, complete blood count (CBC), arterial blood gases (ABGs), and toxicology screens rule out metabolic, toxic, or drug-induced disorders

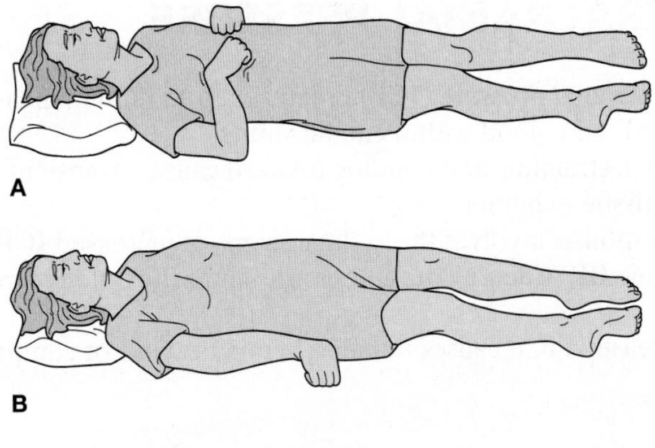

Figure 57–1

Abnormal posturing. (**A**) Decorticate rigidity, (**B**) decerebrate rigidity.

Table 57–4 Glasgow Coma Scoring System

Type of Response Tested	Score	Indicator
Physical (Motor) Response	6	Acts out a simple command
	5	Reacts to a localized discomfort and offensive stimulus
	4	Moves purposelessly or flexes in response to pain
	3	Exhibits abnormal flexion (decorticate posture)
	2	Exhibits abnormal extension (decerebrate posture)
	1	Has no motor response
Verbal Response	5	Has full orientation (time, place, person)
	4	Shows confusion and disorientation
	3	Uses disorganized or inappropriate words; cannot sustain a conversation
	2	Uses sounds instead of words
	1	Makes no verbal response
Eye Response	4	Open when a person approaches (spontaneous response)
	3	Open when a person speaks
	2	Open only when in pain
	1	Open never, even in presence of painful stimuli

Note: Add numbers to find score from 3 (profound coma) to 15 (normal conscious state).

C. Therapeutic management

1. Directed at cause of altered mental status; ongoing care also focuses on maintaining airway, skin integrity, and nutrition and preventing contractures
2. *NCLEX®* Assess for ability to clear secretions; assess breath sounds; maintain patent airway in unconscious client; maintain client with ineffective airway in side-lying position; provide standard care if artificial airway (tracheostomy or endotracheal tube) in place
3. *NCLEX®* Assess swallowing and gag reflex; use measures to prevent aspiration (such as elevated head of bed [HOB]); monitor for and report possible aspiration
4. *NCLEX®* Assess skin integrity every shift; reposition client every 2 hours; implement measures to prevent skin breakdown (client cannot sense discomfort from pressure and shift position); keep linens clean, dry, and wrinkle-free
5. Provide support devices to maintain extremities in functional condition; perform passive range of motion (ROM) regularly
6. Monitor nutritional status and weight; assess need for alternative methods of nutritional support
7. Provide emotional support to client and family
8. *NCLEX®* Provide for alternate means of communication as needed (such as questions with yes and no or other single-word answers)

D. Family teaching

1. Family anxiety is common, especially if prognosis is uncertain
2. Reinforce information from healthcare provider; provide simple explanations about care
3. Encourage family to talk to client
4. Offer support services as needed

IV. INCREASED INTRACRANIAL PRESSURE

A. Overview

1. A prolonged **intracranial pressure (ICP)** greater than 15 mmHg measured in lateral ventricles; exerted by brain tissue, CSF, and blood within cranial vault
2. *NCLEX®* Coughing, sneezing, straining, and bending forward cause a transient increase in ICP that does not cause significant tissue ischemia
3. **Cushing's triad**/response: involves three classic signs of increased ICP: increased systolic BP with unchanged diastolic BP, widening pulse pressure, and reflex bradycardia from stimulation of carotid bodies
4. A prolonged increase in ICP causes tissue ischemia because of compromised cerebral blood flow and perfusion

5. Autoregulation (compensatory mechanism to maintain blood flow) is disrupted and can lead to cellular hypoxia and ischemia
6. Untreated increased ICP leads to herniation and ultimately death
7. Because brain is encased in a closed cavity, expansion of brain can cause increased ICP
8. Cerebral edema is a local or generalized increase in volume of brain tissue because of increased capillary permeability (vasogenic edema), changes in integrity of cell membrane (cytotoxic edema), or increase in interstitial fluids (interstitial cerebral edema); edema is usually proportional to size of injury
9. Hydrocephalus is an increase in CSF volume within ventricular system; it may be noncommunicating (drainage from ventricular system is impaired such as with tumor or mass) or communicating (blood blocks CSF absorption, such as with subarachnoid hemorrhage)

NCLEX® **B. Nursing assessment**

1. Signs of increased ICP include deteriorating LOC, blurred vision, decreased visual acuity, and diplopia from pressure on visual pathways; headache, papilledema, hyperthermia, and vomiting are others; late signs include abnormal posturing, weakness or **hemiplegia** (one-sided paralysis), seizures, and positive Babinski reflex
2. Diagnostic tests usually include CT or MRI; LP is not usually performed because of possibility of brain herniation caused by sudden release of pressure
3. Laboratory tests augment and monitor treatment approaches; serum osmolarity monitors hydration status; ABGs measure pH, O_2, and CO_2 (hydrogen ions and CO_2 are vasodilators that increase ICP)

C. Therapeutic management

1. Increased ICP is a medical emergency with little time for lengthy diagnostic studies; it centers on restoring normal pressure and can be accomplished through medications, surgery, and drainage of CSF from ventricles
2. A drainage catheter, inserted via ventriculostomy into lateral ventricle, can monitor ICP and drain CSF to maintain normal pressure; system is calibrated with transducer leveled 1 inch above ear (height of foramen of Munro); sterile technique is of utmost importance
3. NCLEX® Assess neurologic status every 1–2 hours and report any deterioration; assessment areas include LOC, behavior, motor/sensory function, pupil size and response, vital signs with temperature
4. NCLEX® Maintain airway; elevate HOB 30 degrees or keep flat as prescribed; maintain head and neck in neutral position to promote venous drainage
5. NCLEX® Assess for bladder distention and bowel constipation; assist client when necessary to prevent Valsalva maneuver
6. NCLEX® Plan nursing care so it is not too clustered because prolonged activity may increase ICP; provide for a quiet environment (lights kept low also) and limit noxious stimuli; limit stimulation such as radio, TV, and newspaper; avoid ingesting stimulants such as coffee, tea, cola drinks, and cigarette smoke
7. NCLEX® Maintain fluid restriction as prescribed
8. Maintain body temperature with antipyretics, lightweight bed linens, or hypothermia blanket; take care to avoid shivering, which increases ICP
9. Keep dressings over catheter dry and change dressings as prescribed; monitor insertion site for CSF leakage or infection; monitor client for signs and symptoms of infection; use aseptic technique when in contact with ICP monitor
10. NCLEX® Medication therapy
    a. Osmotic diuretics (mannitol) and loop diuretics such as furosemide are mainstays to decrease ICP; they draw water from edematous tissues into vascular system
    b. Corticosteroids may aid in decreasing ICP, especially with tumors
11. NCLEX® Client education
    a. Teach client at risk for increased ICP to avoid activities that mimic Valsalva maneuver (coughing, blowing nose, straining for bowel movements, pushing against bed side-rails, or performing isometric exercises)
    b. Advise client to maintain neutral head and neck alignment
    c. Encourage family to maintain a quiet environment and avoid upsetting client

V. HEAD INJURY

A. Types of head injuries

1. Open: involve break in skin; include scalp lacerations, skull fractures, interruption of dura mater
2. Closed: do not involve break in skin; include concussions, contusions, and fractures

Box 57–3

Signs of Basilar Skull Fracture

- Battle sign: ecchymosis over mastoid process
- Hemotympanum: blood visible behind tympanic membrane
- Raccoon eyes: bilateral periorbital ecchymosis
- Rhinorrhea: CSF leakage through nose
- Otorrhea: CSF leakage through ear

B. Skull fracture

1. Overview
   - **a.** A break in skull bone with or without intracranial trauma; force of impact increases risk of hematoma formation; disruption of skull can lead to infection and cranial nerve injury
   - **b.** *Linear* fractures are most common of four types; risk of infection and CSF leakage is minimal because dura remains intact; hematoma formation is possible
   - **c.** *Comminuted* and *depressed* skull fractures have a higher risk of brain tissue damage and infection, especially if overlying skin and dura is torn or damaged; risk of secondary brain injury is reduced because energy of impact caused bone fracture instead of being transferred to brain tissue
   - **d.** *Basilar* skull fractures involve base of skull (usually secondary injuries); most are uncomplicated, but CSF leakage and infection can result from disruption of sinuses and middle ear bones
2. Nursing assessment
   - NCLEX® **a.** Clinical manifestations may give clues to area of fracture; basilar skull fracture may produce manifestations listed in Box 57–3
   - **b.** Diagnostic and laboratory tests: plain x-ray films and CT or MRI scans; basilar skull fractures may be difficult to identify on plain x-ray
3. Therapeutic management: treatment depends on type and location of injury
   - **a.** Linear skull fractures generally require bedrest and observation for underlying brain injury; no specific treatment is necessary
   - **b.** Comminuted and depressed skull fractures require surgical intervention within 24 hours
   - **c.** Basilar skull fractures do not require surgery unless there is persistent CSF leakage, but do require regular neurologic assessments for meningitis
   - **d.** Observe client for otorrhea or rhinorrhea
   - NCLEX® **e.** Test clear ear drainage and sinus drainage for glucose; only CSF has glucose; mucous secretions do not
   - NCLEX® **f.** Observe blood-tinged drainage for halo sign; glucose-containing CSF dries in concentric rings on gauze or tissues
   - **g.** Keep nasopharynx and external ear clean; use sterile technique and supplies when cleaning drainage from nose and/or ears
   - NCLEX® **h.** Instruct client not to blow nose, cough, or inhibit sneeze and to sneeze through an open mouth
   - **i.** Use aseptic technique when changing head dressings
   - **j.** Medication therapy: dexamethasone to decrease cerebral edema and antibiotics when there is a risk of infection
4. NCLEX® Client teaching: go to emergency department if client experiences drowsiness or confusion, difficulty waking, vomiting, blurred vision, slurred speech, prolonged headache, blood or clear fluid leaking from ears or nose, weakness in an arm or leg, stiff neck, or seizures

C. Intracranial hemorrhage

1. Overview
   - **a.** An escape of blood into cranium (often because of blunt trauma); hemorrhage may cause a very slow to very rapid neurologic deterioration
   - **b.** Results directly from trauma or from shearing forces on cerebral arteries and veins from acceleration–deceleration injuries; classified by location
   - **c.** Bleeding can be epidural, subdural, or intracranial (see Box 57–4)
2. Assessment
   - **a.** **Epidural hematoma**: client may initially lose consciousness then have a short period of lucidness, followed by rapid deterioration from drowsiness to coma; other manifestations include headache, fixed dilated pupil on affected side, hemiparesis, hemiplegia, and possible seizures; this condition is a surgical emergency

Box 57–4

Types of Intracranial Bleeding

Epidural Hematoma

- Develops between dura and skull
- As hematoma forms, it strips dura away from skull
- Usually develops from a tear in meningeal artery
- Because this is an arterial bleed, it rapidly expands, leading to rapid deterioration in neurologic status

Subdural Hematoma

- Forms between dura mater and arachnoid–pia mater layers of meninges
- Usually involves veins but may involve small arteries as well
- As blood collects, pressure is applied to underlying brain tissue
- May be acute (develops within 48 hours after an acute injury), subacute (2 days to 3 weeks after lesser injury), or chronic (3 weeks to months after a minor injury), or may develop spontaneously

Intracerebral Hemorrhage

- Bleeding into brain tissue
- Can occur anywhere in brain but most commonly in frontal or temporal lobes
- May result from closed head trauma, where shearing forces are applied deep in brain; this type of hemorrhage occurs, for example, in a motor vehicle accident in which client hits head on windshield, resulting in coup and contrecoup injury

b. **Subdural hematoma**: manifestations may develop slowly and may be mistaken for dementia in an older adult; slow thinking, confusion, drowsiness, or lethargy are common; headaches, ipsilateral (same-sided) pupil dilation and sluggishness, and possible seizures are other signs
c. Intracerebral hematomas vary in initial presentation depending on location; headache is common; as hematoma progresses, a decreased LOC, hemiplegia, and ipsilateral pupil dilation occurs; an expanding clot may lead to herniation
d. Diagnostic and laboratory tests: CT and MRI; laboratory values provide baseline client data

3. Therapeutic management
a. Small hematomas reabsorb spontaneously and may be treated conservatively
b. Surgical intervention is needed to drain epidural hematomas and larger subdural hematomas; surgery is less successful with intracerebral hematomas because of widespread tissue damage; supportive care and preventing complications are goals of therapy
c. Assess neurologic signs frequently; clear nose and mouth of secretions; suction airway if necessary
d. Monitor respiratory pattern for rate, depth, and rhythm if client is not mechanically ventilated; prepare for O_2 administration and endotracheal (ET) intubation for respiratory distress
e. Prepare for cranial surgery for deteriorating neurologic condition
f. Provide appropriate preoperative and postoperative care
g. Provide previously discussed measures to manage increased ICP
NCLEX® **h.** Medication therapy: none specific to hematomas; osmotic diuretics and corticosteroids reduce ICP; antiepileptics treat seizures if they occur as a complication

4. Client education: family needs to know of possible surgery to evacuate hematoma

D. Contusion

1. Overview
a. Bruising of brain tissue from blunt trauma or coup/contrecoup injuries
b. Usually involves damage to parenchyma with tears in vessels or tissue, pulling, and subsequent areas of necrosis or infarction

2. Nursing assessment: symptoms vary depending on site of injury; may have decreasing LOC

3. Therapeutic management: monitor neurologic status and look for signs of complications; can have sequelae specific to area of injury

4. Client and family education
a. Teach symptoms of complications that may occur after discharge

NCLEX®

b. Provide written instructions and clear information about when to seek medical care (worsening neurologic status, increasing headache)

E. **Concussion**

1. Overview
   a. Concussion or "mild traumatic brain injury" involves some transient loss of consciousness, usually from blunt head trauma
   b. Usually related to stretching, compression, or shearing of nerve fibers
   c. Postconcussion syndrome occurs after initial head injury; poor concentration and problems with memory may be noted; client may report headache, dizziness, and photophobia; subtle change in personality may be noted

NCLEX®

2. Nursing assessment: symptoms include amnesia of event, headache, and nausea; clients are neurologically intact with a Glasgow Coma Score of 13–15; there are three levels of concussion severity
   a. Grade 1: transient confusion; no loss of consciousness; abnormal mental status less than 15 mins
   b. Grade 2: transient confusion; no loss of consciousness; abnormal mental status more than 15 mins
   c. Grade 3: loss of consciousness for a few seconds, several minutes, or longer
3. Therapeutic management
   a. Treatment is supportive, with close observation for 24 hours in an emergency room or at home under certain circumstances
   b. Clients who had loss of consciousness for more than 5 minutes or amnesia of event are usually admitted for observation to rule out other potential injuries

NCLEX®

4. Client and family education: client may be discharged home with caregivers who have received instructions to continue monitoring and what steps to take if complications arise; share information about postconcussion syndrome (headaches, dizziness, fatigue, irritability, anxiety, insomnia, impaired concentration and memory, noise and light sensitivity)

VI. SPINAL CORD INJURY (SCI)

A. **Overview**

1. Usually caused by trauma; young adults and adolescents are most at risk
2. Disrupts nerve tracts because of cord transection, partial transection, contusion, compression, or lacerations; leads to loss of sensory and motor function at level of injury and below
3. Usually results from excessive force applied to spinal cord and vertebral column; four types of injuries occur:
   a. Hyperflexion compresses vertebral bodies and disrupts ligaments and discs
   b. Hyperextension disrupts ligaments and causes vertebral fractures
   c. Axial loading is an application of excessive vertical force and may cause compression fractures
   d. Excessive rotation tears ligaments and fractures articular surfaces and causes compression fractures (see Figure 57–2)
4. Classified by complete versus incomplete cord injury, cause of injury, and level of injury; in clinical practice, these overlap
5. Levels of injury (named for corresponding level of vertebrae)
   a. Cervical: injury above C4 interferes with respiration and paralysis of all extremities (C4 provides major innervation to phrenic nerve and diaphragm); involvement at C5 to C8 allows some shoulder movement but there is decreased respiratory reserve
   b. Thoracic: depending on specific level, injury may involve loss of sensation and movement of chest, trunk, bladder, bowel, and legs
   c. Lumbar and sacral: loss of sensation and movement to legs; injury results in neurogenic bladder and interference with erection and ejaculation in men
   d. Most frequently involved vertebrae are C5 to C7 (cervical), T12 (thoracic), and L1 (lumbar)

B. **Nursing assessment**

NCLEX®

1. Depends on level of injury, which is defined as lowest area of spinal cord that has intact sensory and motor function
2. Assess respiratory rate, depth, and pattern
3. Assess sensory and motor function
   a. **Paraplegia** is paralysis of lower body; occurs when injury level is in thoracic spine or lower
   b. **Tetraplegia**, formally quadriplegia, is paralysis of arms, trunk, legs, and pelvic portions of body; occurs when level of injury is in cervical spine

NCLEX®

4. Assess other body systems for status and signs of concurrent injury

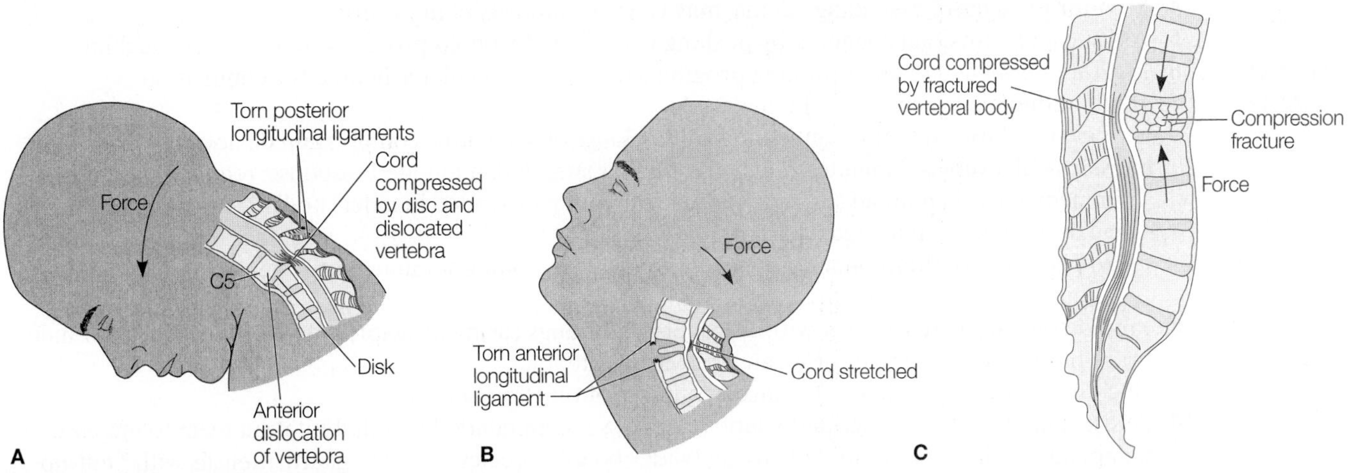

Figure 57–2 Spinal cord injury mechanisms. (**A**) Hyperflexion, (**B**) hyperextension, (**C**) axial loading, a form of compression.

5. Assess for spinal shock (a temporary loss of reflex function): symptoms include bradycardia; hypotension; flaccid paralysis of skeletal muscles; loss of pain, touch, temperature, pressure, visceral, and somatic sensations; bowel and bladder dysfunction; and loss of ability to perspire; spinal shock has resolved once spinal reflexes return
6. Assess for **autonomic hyperreflexia** (an exaggerated SNS response that occurs with injuries at T6 or higher but is seen only after recovery from spinal shock); occurs when stimuli cannot ascend cord; a noxious stimulus triggers massive vasoconstriction below injury, vasodilation above injury, bradycardia, and rapid-onset systolic hypertension with widening pulse pressure
7. Diagnostic and laboratory test findings: x-rays visualize fractures; CT and MRI scans show changes in vertebrae, spinal cord, and tissues surrounding cord; an EMG may be done after acute injury to locate level of injury
8. Incomplete spinal cord injury syndromes
   a. *Central cord syndrome*: loss of motor function more pronounced in upper extremities; varying patterns of intact sensation remain
   b. *Anterior cord syndrome*: sensations of touch, position, and vibration remain intact below level of iniury, while motor function, pain, and temperature sensation are lost
   c. *Posterior cord syndrome*: motor function is intact, but there is loss of position, vibration, and crude touch sensation
   d. *Brown-Séquard syndrome*: Loss of motion function, vibration, proprioception, and deep-touch sensation are lost on same side as cord damage (ipsilateral losses)
   e. *Conus medullaris syndrome*: flaccid lower extremities and bladder and bowel arreflexia; possible intact micturition (voiding) and loss of ability for penile erection if damage is located to upper sacral segment of spinal cord
   f. *Cauda equina syndrome*: arreflexia of bowel, bladder, and lower body reflexes

C. Therapeutic management

1. Acute management involves immobilizing injury to prevent further damage and assessing and stabilizing client
   a. Assess for and maintain a patent airway
   b. Keep head immobilized without flexion, extension, or rotation; maintain manual traction on head if needed by placing hands on head by ears
   c. If client needs to be moved, logroll client without twisting or turning spine; keep head of bed flat so spine remains extended
   d. Stabilize injury with devices such as skeletal traction using Gardner-Wells tongs, halo traction, or surgery as indicated
2. Treat complications: respiratory distress (with measures ranging from oxygen to intubation and mechanical ventilation), atonic bladder (insertion of indwelling urinary catheter), paralytic ileus (preventing constipation by initiating bowel regimen), and cardiovascular instability (with vasoactive drugs as needed)

NCLEX®

3. Monitor vital capacity and respiratory effectiveness; high cervical cord injuries (C4 or above or lower if edema ascends cord) may inhibit respirations, requiring mechanical ventilation

4. Monitor for signs of ascending edema; may cause respiratory compromise
5. Assist client with quad coughing by pushing in and up at xiphoid process when client is coughing
NCLEX® 6. Institute bowel and bladder training programs to restore a regular schedule for elimination
NCLEX® 7. Treat autonomic hyperreflexia immediately
   a. Elevate HOB and remove antiembolism stockings or sequential compression devices
   b. Assess BP every 2–3 minutes while assessing for stimuli that initiated response; remove stimulus immediately when found (offending stimuli are often distended bladder, stool in rectum, or mechanical or thermal stimuli affecting skin)
   c. With severe hypertension unresolved by removing offending stimulus, notify healthcare provider and administer antihypertensives per protocol
8. Provide ongoing care to client with Gardner-Wells tongs (using principles of skeletal traction) or halo brace because of fracture or dislocated cervical vertebrae
9. Encourage client to verbalize feelings about loss of function and care
10. Assist client with techniques and adaptive devices recommended by rehabilitation team to increase independence in activities of daily living (slider board, wheelchair, plate guard, utensils with built-up handles as examples)
11. Encourage self-care and independent decision making
12. Include family and important others in discussions
NCLEX® 13. Medication therapy: corticosteroids (such as methylprednisolone) may control edema of cord; vasoactive drugs treat hypotension or hypertension due to spinal shock or autonomic hyperreflexia; antispasmodics (such as baclofen) treat spasticity; analgesics and tricyclic antidepressants treat pain

D. Client education

1. Teach client and family to promote independence in self-care, such as self-catheterization technique, bowel evacuation, activities of daily living
2. Educate client and family about variety of community resources needed
NCLEX® 3. If client has a halo vest, teach that it raises center of gravity; avoid bending over to reduce risk of falls; neck is immobilized in midline so client must learn to turn entire body to scan environment; eat soft foods and cut food into small pieces and use straw for liquids; driving is prohibited

VII. STROKE (BRAIN ATTACK)

A. Overview

1. A condition in which neurologic deficits result from decreased blood flow to a localized area of brain; onset may be rapid or gradual
NCLEX® 2. Risk factors include hypertension, diabetes mellitus, atherosclerosis, obesity, anticoagulant therapy, oral contraceptive use, and stress
3. Severe and prolonged cerebral blood flow obstruction leads to ischemia and cell death; resulting deficits predict location of stroke; there are four types
   NCLEX® a. Transient ischemic attack (TIA) is a brief period of neurologic deficits that resolve within 24 hours; often a precursor to stroke
   b. Thrombotic (ischemic) stroke is caused by a thrombus (blood clot) occluding a cerebral vessel; thrombi tend to form while BP is low (such as during sleep or rest); thrombosis occurs quickly but deficits progress slowly
   c. Embolic stroke (also ischemic) is caused by a clot that traveled; source of clot is elsewhere in body (such as from heart with atrial fibrillation); has a sudden onset with immediate symptoms
   d. Hemorrhagic stroke or intracranial hemorrhage occurs when a blood vessel ruptures; most often occurs in presence of long-term, poorly controlled hypertension; others include a ruptured intracranial aneurysm, tumors, AV malformations, or anticoagulant therapy as examples; this type is often fatal because of rapidly increasing ICP; onset of symptoms is rapid; loss of consciousness occurs in about half of cases
4. Expected pattern of deficits based on location
   a. Left-brain damage: right-sided **hemiparesis** (one-sided weakness) or hemiplegia, speech and language deficits, impaired left–right discrimination, slow and cautious behavior style, impaired language and math comprehension, and anxiety and/or depression because of awareness of deficits
   b. Right-brain damage: left-sided hemiparesis or hemiplegia, spatial–perceptual deficits, left-sided neglect, quick and impulsive behavior style (safety risk), tendency to deny or minimize problems, impaired judgment and concept of time

B. Nursing assessment

1. Clinical manifestations: vary according to cerebral blood vessel involved

NCLEX®
2. Internal carotid: contralateral motor and sensory deficits of arm, leg, and face; in dominant hemispheric stroke, aphasia; in nondominant hemispheric stroke, **apraxia** (inability to perform known tasks), **agnosia** (inability to recognize), unilateral neglect, and **homonymous hemianopsia** (loss of one half of visual field in each eye)

NCLEX®
3. Middle cerebral artery: drowsiness; stupor; coma; contralateral hemiplegia and sensory deficits of arm and face; aphasia; and homonymous hemianopsia
4. Anterior cerebral artery: contralateral weakness or paralysis and sensory loss of foot and leg, loss of decision-making and voluntary action abilities, and urinary incontinence
5. Vertebral artery: pain in face, nose, or eye; numbness or weakness of face on ipsilateral side; problems with gait; **dysphagia** (difficulty swallowing); and dysarthria (difficulty speaking)
6. Diagnostic and laboratory test findings: CT and MRI demonstrate hemorrhage, tumors, ischemia, edema, and tissue necrosis; cerebral angiography detects abnormal vessel structure, vasospasm, carotid artery stenosis, and loss of vessel wall integrity; ultrasound evaluates blood flow

C. Therapeutic management

1. Measures to take during acute phase include maintain patent airway; administer prescribed oxygen; position client on side with head of bed elevated 15–30 degrees or as prescribed; assess for and take measures to prevent rise in ICP; establish IV access and maintain fluid and electrolyte balance; monitor neurologic status frequently; maintain quiet environment
2. Drug therapy is most common treatment for stroke; if ischemic type, medications could include thrombolytics and/or heparin; others include antiplatelet agents, antihypertensives, diuretics, and possibly antiepileptics

NCLEX®
3. It is imperative not to disrupt a clot that has formed following hemorrhagic stroke to avoid rebleed, which is often fatal
4. Referral to and collaboration with rehabilitation team is crucial
   a. Physical therapist can provide assistance with transfer techniques, gait training, and assistive devices such as walker, cane, splints, or braces
   b. Occupational therapist can provide assistance for techniques and adaptive equipment needed to perform activities of daily living
   c. Speech and language therapist can complete swallowing evaluation, make recommendations about consistency of liquids and foods in diet, and work with client to perform exercises to help regain speech
5. Approach client from unaffected side and place personal objects and those needed for care within line of vision and reach for safety
6. Encourage active ROM on unaffected side and passive ROM on affected side
7. Turn and reposition client with 2 hours on unaffected side and 20 minutes on affected side, or as per agency protocol
8. Monitor lower extremities for thrombophlebitis and use preventive measures such as antiembolism stockings
9. Encourage use of unaffected arm for ADLs
10. Teach client to put clothing on affected side first

NCLEX®
11. Resume diet orally only after confirming successful completion of swallowing evaluation; clients may need thickened liquids and foods with softer textures; this is sometimes called a dysphagia diet and has different levels
12. Assist client to sitting position for meals; instruct to place food at back of mouth on unaffected side (avoids food trapping in affected cheek) and chew on unaffected side of mouth; have client position head and neck forward and slightly flexed (chin tuck) to close glottis and aid in swallowing without aspiration
13. Try alternate methods of communication for clients with aphasia and consult with speech pathologist as needed
14. Accept client's frustration and anger as normal to loss of function

NCLEX®
15. Teach client with homonymous hemianopsia to overcome deficit by turning head side to side to scan visual field fully

D. Client teaching: stroke and stroke prevention, community resources, physical care, need for psychosocial support, medication information, and follow-up care

VIII. INTRACRANIAL ANEURYSM

A. Overview

1. A saccular outpouching of a cerebral artery at site of congenital weakness in BV wall; may be silent until time of rupture
2. May be silent (asymptomatic) or can rupture, which often leads to severe disability or death
3. Major complications after rupture include rebleeding, vasospasm, dysfunction of hypothalamus, hydrocephalus, and seizures

B. Nursing assessment

NCLEX® 1. Signs and symptoms typically occur at time of rupture, which results in subarachnoid hemorrhage

NCLEX® 2. Include sudden severe headache and neck pain, nausea and vomiting (N/V), stiff neck and photophobia (meningeal irritation), cranial nerve defects (ptosis), and stroke syndrome

3. Diagnostic tests: CT scan, bilateral carotid and vertebral angiograms; LP to confirm subarachnoid hemorrhage (and bleeding into CSF) if no suspicion of increased ICP

C. Therapeutic management

1. Nursing care is supportive and is similar to care of a client following a stroke
2. Monitor VS, LOC, pupil response, and motor function frequently per agency protocol

NCLEX® 3. Aneurysm (subarachnoid) precautions (to reduce risk of rupture if identified early or rebleed)
   a. Maintain bedrest in side-lying position or with head of bed elevated 10–15 degrees (does not interfere with arterial circulation and aids in venous return)
   b. Keep room darkened (no bright lights and window shades drawn)
   c. Provide quiet, low-stimulus environment (often no telephone allowed); reading, listening to soft music, and low-volume television may be allowed; gently administer all personal care to minimize stimulation
   d. Visitors are generally limited to family, one or two at a time
   e. Maintain fluid restriction and avoid stimulants such as caffeine
   f. Implement measures to avoid client straining or Valsalva maneuver, such as using stool softeners, exhaling during urination and defecation, wiping nose instead of blowing, avoiding coughing, sneezing with mouth open (avoids closed glottis)
   g. Sedatives may be prescribed to reduce response to environmental stimuli

4. Medication therapy may include antihypertensives, sedatives, or antiepileptics as needed

NCLEX® 5. Provide care after craniotomy (for surgical clipping or removal of aneurysm)
   a. Monitor VS and neurologic status frequently per agency protocol; may be every 30–60 minutes initially and taper as client stabilizes
   b. Monitor for and report signs of increased ICP
   c. Keep head and neck in midline position and avoid extreme neck or hip flexion
   d. Position client as prescribed by healthcare provider (head usually elevated 30 degrees with supratentorial incision, or possibly flat with infratentorial incision)
   e. Monitor head dressing; mark area of drainage at least once every 8 hours; report excessive drainage or saturated dressing
   f. Provide standard care to client with Hemovac or Jackson-Pratt drain; may be in place for 24 hours postsurgery
   g. Maintain fluid restriction (often 1500 mL/24 hours) and monitor I&O
   h. Provide cool compresses or ice packs to eyes as prescribed for periorbital edema and ecchymosis
   i. Provide other standard interventions for postoperative care

6. Monitor for and report sudden neurologic changes or signs mimicking rupture, which could indicate complications of vasospam or rebleed

D. Client education: give rationales for all care and provide information about client status; client may require transfer to rehabilitation center or require home care after hospital discharge

IX. SEIZURE DISORDER

A. Overview

1. A seizure is an episode of excessive and abnormal electrical activity in brain that is manifested by disturbances in skeletal motor activity, sensation, autonomic dysfunction of viscera, behavior, or consciousness
2. Seizures are classified as partial or generalized; partial seizures begin in one area of cortex; generalized seizures involve both hemispheres and deeper brain structures

3. Risk factors in adults include acute febrile state, head injury, infection, metabolic or endocrine disorders, and exposure to toxins
4. Risk factors during infancy include perinatal hypoxia, congenital diseases, infections, metabolic or degenerative diseases, drug withdrawal, and neoplasms
5. Risk factors during childhood include febrile infections, head injury, lead toxicity, drugs, genetic disorders, and neoplasms
6. If seizure activity is chronic (reoccurs within minutes, days, or even years), a diagnosis of epilepsy is made
7. Metabolic needs, O_2 requirements, metabolic by-products, and cerebral blood flow increase dramatically during seizure
8. As long as cerebral blood flow can meet demands of seizure, brain is protected from cellular exhaustion and destruction

B. Nursing assessment

NCLEX® 1. *Simple partial seizures* are limited to one hemisphere; manifestations include altered motor function, sensory signs, or autonomic or psychic symptoms

NCLEX® 2. *Complex partial seizures* originate in temporal lobe and may be preceded by an aura; an impaired LOC and repetitive, nonpurposeful movements such as lip-smacking, picking, or aimless walking are noted; amnesia is common

3. *Generalized partial seizure* is a partial seizure that has spread to both hemispheres and deeper structures of brain
4. *Absence seizure* is a generalized seizure that lasts 5–30 seconds; there is a sudden, brief cessation of motor activity and a blank stare; they may occur occasionally or up to 100 per day; they may be accompanied by eyelid fluttering or automatisms such as lip-smacking; more common in children than adults

NCLEX® 5. **Tonic-clonic** seizures (grand mal) are most common type of seizure
   a. May be preceded by an aura but often occur without warning
   b. Typically start with a loss of consciousness and sharp muscle contractions
   c. Client falls to floor and may have urinary and/or bowel incontinence
   d. Breathing ceases and cyanosis develops during tonic phase (about 15–60 sec); see Figure 57–3A
   e. Clonic phase (60–90 sec) follows with alternating muscle contraction and relaxation in all extremities, hyperventilation, and eyes rolled back in head; see Figure 57–3B
   f. In next phase (postictal period), client is relaxed with quiet breathing and is unconscious and unresponsive; client gradually regains consciousness and may have transient confusion and disorientation; clients often report headache, muscle aches, and fatigue and may sleep several hours
   g. Clients will have amnesia of seizure and events just prior to seizure

NCLEX® 6. *Status epilepticus* is a life-threatening emergency that can occur during seizure activity; it is characterized by continuous cycles of tonic-clonic activity with short periods of calm between them; this cumulative effect can interfere with respiration; client is in great danger of developing hypoxia, hyperthermia, hypoglycemia, and exhaustion if seizure activity is not stopped

NCLEX® 7. During a seizure, observe order of events and duration; for tonic-clonic seizures, be certain to time length of seizure until jerking stops; tonic indicates continuous muscle contraction; clonic indicates alternating contraction and relaxation of muscles; for all other types of seizures, note duration from start of seizure to time that consciousness is regained; describe any precipitating events or unusual behavior; note parts of body involved and whether it begins in a specific body part

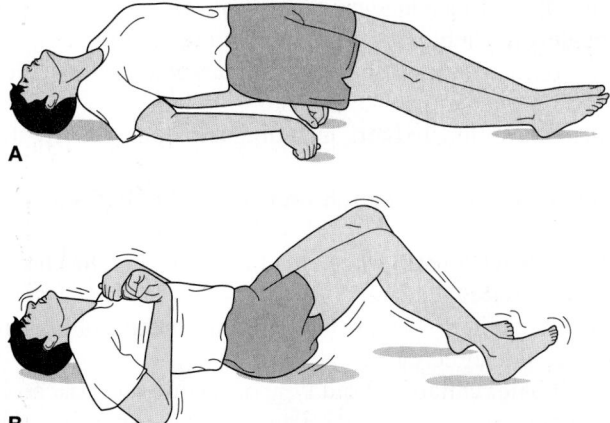

Figure 57–3

Tonic-clonic contractions in grand mal seizures. (**A**) Tonic phase, (**B**) clonic phase.

8. Observe face for any color change, perspiration, and lack of expression; note any sound or cry uttered at beginning of seizure; observe mouth for deviation to one side or other, clenched teeth, tongue-biting, frothing, and/or flecks of blood or bleeding; if able to assess pupils, note any change in size, equality, reaction to light, and accommodation
9. Observe for presence or length of apnea; other general observations may be involuntary urination or defecation
10. Postictally, it is important to note duration of postictal period and LOC; orientation to time, person, place; any alterations in motor ability or speech, and whether client experienced an aura
11. Diagnostic and laboratory tests: complete neurologic examination, EEG, skull x-ray series, CT scan, LP with CSF analysis, blood studies, and electrocardiogram

C. Therapeutic management

1. Provide interventions during seizure to maintain airway patency
   - NCLEX® **a.** Remain with client and turn client to side if necessary in recumbent position to maintain airway and promote drainage of secretions without aspiration
   - **b.** Have O_2 and suction equipment at bedside; administer oxygen as prescribed or have "blow-by" oxygen near client's face; turn client to side to drain secretions from mouth or suction as needed
   - NCLEX® **c.** Do not try to force an object, such as a bite stick, into mouth of client who is seizing, as this may break teeth or cause other injury
2. NCLEX® Provide interventions during a seizure to reduce the risk of injury; do not restrain client but provide an environment that will not create further injury; teach family members how to protect client during seizures
3. Document seizure activity promptly and report it as appropriate
4. Provide support to client that concerns are normal; help client identify leisure activities that are safe; provide information about resources and support groups; provide accurate information about hiring practices and legalities of driving or operating heavy/dangerous equipment
5. Medication therapy
   - **a.** Antiepileptics that raise seizure threshold or limit spread of abnormal electrical activity are mainstay of epilepsy treatment; see also Chapter 38
   - NCLEX® **b.** Some commonly used antiepileptics are phenytoin, divalproex sodium, valproic acid, carbamazepine, gabapentin, and lamotrigine
   - **c.** Diazepam, lorazepam, and sometimes phenobarbital are also used intermittently to stop seizure activity during acute episodes
6. If drug therapy fails to control seizures, surgery to excise tissue involved in seizure activity may be an alternative
7. Promote client's development of a positive self-image, especially if a child; talk with client about his or her feelings; plan strategies to promote acceptance and decrease fear among peers
8. Encourage client and family to express feelings

D. Client teaching

1. Correct misconceptions, fears, and myths about epilepsy
2. Provide information about community and national resources for epilepsy
3. Stress importance of follow-up care
4. Review laws (e.g., driving a motor vehicle) that apply to those with epilepsy
5. Refer for employment or vocational counseling as needed
6. Stress importance of wearing a medical identification
7. Emphasize aura alert so client is aware of impending seizure
8. NCLEX® Stress importance of medication adherence and possible periodic blood draws to measure antiepileptic blood levels
9. Stress importance of avoiding triggers, including inadequate sleep, stress, alcohol use, and strobe lights
10. NCLEX® Avoid alcohol and limit caffeine; take showers instead of baths to avoid risk of drowning if seizure occurs
11. Families need to know what to do when client has a seizure; teach safety measures and when to call emergency medical services
12. Do not use over-the-counter (OTC) drugs without first consulting with healthcare provider (e.g., antihistamines since side effects are increased)
13. Educate adults and older children about type of seizure and past and present medication, and they should be able to give a history of seizure control or number of seizures experienced and their timing

X. PARKINSON'S DISEASE

A. Overview

1. A progressive, degenerative neurologic disease characterized by depletion of dopamine (which inhibits norepinephrine), that leads to excitatory impulses, dysfunction of extrapyramidal system, and classic symptoms of **bradykinesia**, muscle rigidity, and nonintentional tremor
2. Commonly affects older adults and is usually diagnosed between age 50 and 60; disease progressively interferes with movement and self-care, increases risk of falls, and can lead to depression

B. Nursing assessment

1. Clinical manifestations begin subtly with fatigue and a slight resting tremor of hands and fingers (pill-rolling) as initial symptoms; tremors decrease with purposeful movement and during sleep and increase with fatigue
2. NCLEX® Bradykinesia is slow movements caused by muscle rigidity; may also affect face, mouth, and voice, resulting in staring gaze, blank (mask-like) facial expression, difficulty speaking and swallowing, drooling, and monotonous speech
3. Postural disturbance with trunk tilted forward; uncoordinated movements
4. Short-stepped, shuffling, and propulsive gait, leading to increased risk of falls
5. Heat intolerance; excessive sweating of face and neck; absence of sweating on trunk and extremities
6. Constipation
7. Anxiety and depression, possible sleep disturbances

C. Therapeutic management

1. Includes medications, surgery, and rehabilitation to optimize functional level; a team approach is essential to quality care
2. Client should perform active ROM twice a day; provide passive ROM as needed
3. Encourage client to ambulate frequently and avoid prolonged sitting; instruct client to lift feet while walking and keep chin up for better visual field (prevents falls)
4. NCLEX® Have client rock back and forth to initiate movement and avoid sitting in deep, soft chairs; use firm chairs that rock for ease in standing
5. Use assistive devices when recommended; consider velcro instead of buttons and slip-on shoes instead of those with ties
6. Assist client in maintaining posture by teaching to hold hands behind back (keeps neck and spine straight) and lie prone periodically without a pillow
7. Assess communication skills, speech, hearing, and writing (becomes progressively smaller)
8. Consult with a speech pathologist if necessary
9. Assess nutritional status and self-feeding abilities
10. NCLEX® Promote a soft diet that is high-protein, high-fiber, high-calorie, and divided into smaller, more frequent meals; provide increased fluids (2000 mL/day)
11. NCLEX® Medication therapy: monoamine oxidase inhibitors (MAOIs), dopaminergics, dopamine agonists, and anticholinergics; eventually all drugs lose effectiveness; a fluctuating response to drugs is called an on–off response; antidepressants, especially amitriptyline, treat depression; propranolol may be used to treat tremors

D. Client education

1. Preventive measures for malnutrition, falls, and other environmental hazards, constipation, skin breakdown from incontinence, and joint contractures
2. Gait training and exercises to improve ambulation, swallowing, speech, and self-care

XI. MULTIPLE SCLEROSIS

A. Overview

1. Chronic degenerative CNS disorder with demyelinization of nerve fibers in brain and spinal cord, leading to interrupted nerve impulse transmission
2. There are four forms based on rate of progression: benign, relapsing-remitting, primary progressive, and secondary progressive; characterized by periodic exacerbations and remissions
3. Etiology is unknown, but may be an autoimmune response or result from viral infection

NCLEX® B. Nursing assessment

1. Visual disturbances or blindness (retrobulbar neuritis)
2. Sudden, progressive weakness of one or more limbs
3. **Spasticity** of muscles, nystagmus, tremors, and gait instability
4. Fatigue

5. Dysfunction of bowel and bladder (retention, incontinence, urinary frequency or urgency if urinary tract infection develops)
6. Paresthesias and possible decreased perception to temperature, touch, and pain
7. Altered emotional state including depression, apathy, irritability, or even euphoria
8. Abnormal reflexes (may be absent or exaggerated)
9. Diagnostic tests: LP for CSF (clonal IgG bands), MRI, CT scans, muscle testing

C. Therapeutic management

1. Overall goal of care is to maintain as much independent function as possible
2. Institute safety measures because of decreased sensation (risk of burns) or spasticity (risk of falls)
3. *NCLEX®* Include rest periods and energy conservation measures to prevent fatigue
4. Help client to recognize choices in care and set priorities on a day-to-day basis whenever possible to maintain sense of control and independence
5. Assist client with ADLs on an as-needed basis; provide adaptive utensils or other assistive devices as needed
6. *NCLEX®* Maintain fluid intake of at least 2000 mL/day to promote bowel and bladder function and prevent impaction and/or urinary tract infection (UTI)
7. Communicate with client about issues of concern, such as coping skills, sexuality, changing body image, or others identified by client
8. *NCLEX®* Avoid sources of infection; illness can act as a stressor and trigger an exacerbation, as well as fatigue and rapid changes in temperature
9. Medication therapy: immunosuppressants, antivirals, corticosteroids, antibiotics for UTI, interferon-alpha, glatiramer, anticholinergics, and antispasmodics

D. Client education: medications, symptoms, bladder training, intermittent self-catheterization, sexual functioning, avoiding complications, and possible triggers (fatigue, temperature extremes, illness)

XII. MYASTHENIA GRAVIS

A. Overview

1. A chronic progressive disorder of peripheral NS affecting transmission of nerve impulses to voluntary muscles
2. Leads to muscle weakness and fatigue that increases with exertion and improves with rest; eventually leads to fatigue without relief from rest
3. Causes include excessive cholinesterase or insufficient acetylcholine at myoneural junction and interference with binding of acetylcholine to receptor sites
4. *NCLEX®* Onset is usually slow but can be precipitated by emotional stress, hormonal disturbance (pregnancy, menses, thyroid disorders), infections and vaccinations, trauma and surgery, temperature extremes, excessive exercise, drugs that interfere with neuromuscular transmission (opioids, sedatives, barbiturates, alcohol, quinidine, anesthetics), and thymus tumor

B. Nursing assessment

1. *NCLEX®* Mild diplopia (double vision) and unilateral ptosis (eyelid drooping) caused by weakness in extra-ocular muscles; weakness may also involve face, jaw, neck, and hip
2. *NCLEX®* Complications arise when severe weakness affects muscles of swallowing, chewing, and respiration; respiratory distress is manifested by tachypnea, decreased depth, abnormal ABGs, O_2 saturation under 92%, and decreased breath sounds
3. Bowel and bladder incontinence, paresthesias, and pain in weak muscles
4. Myasthenic crisis: sudden motor weakness; dyspnea with risk of respiratory failure, absent cough and swallow reflexes (risk of aspiration), and bowel and bladder incontinence; most often caused by insufficient dose of medication, infection, or stress
5. Cholinergic crisis: severe muscle weakness caused by overmedication; also cramps, diarrhea, bradycardia, facial twitching, and bronchial spasm with increased pulmonary secretions and risk of respiratory compromise
6. ABGs and pulmonary function tests may show respiratory insufficiency
7. Electromyography (EMG) shows decreased amplitude when motor neurons are stimulated
8. *NCLEX®* Tensilon test: diagnosis is confirmed with IV edrophonium chloride, which allows acetylcholine to bind with receptors and temporarily improves symptoms; weakness returns after effects of Tensilon wear off

C. Therapeutic management

1. Focuses on medication management with anticholinesterases (see also Chapter 38): neostigmine and pyridostigmine; others may include corticosteroids, azathiopirine, and cyclosporine as immunosuppressants; and anti-inflammatory drugs

2. Treatment of myasthenic crisis is with anticholinesterase medication, while treatment of cholinergic crisis is with atropine sulfate; differentiate between conditions (if unknown) by administering anticholinesterase drug—if client improves then myasthenic crisis was correct; if client does not improve or worsens, then cholinergic crisis is present and reverse condition with atropine sulfate (antidote)
3. NCLEX® Maintain effective breathing pattern and airway clearance; thoroughly assess for respiratory distress
4. NCLEX® Monitor meals and teach client to bend head slightly forward while eating and drinking to improve swallowing
5. Teach client to avoid exposure to infections, especially respiratory
6. Teach client effective coughing, use chest physiotherapy and incentive spirometry; have oral suction available, teach client and family how to use it; be prepared to intubate if needed
7. NCLEX® Provide adequate nutrition: schedule medications 30–45 minutes before eating for peak muscle strength while eating; frequently offer small amounts of foods that are easy to chew and swallow—soft or semisolid as needed; administer IV fluids and nasogastric tube feedings if client is unable to swallow
8. Promote improved function with referrals to physical and occupational therapy
9. NCLEX® Provide eye care: instill artificial tears; use a patch over one eye for double vision (diplopia); wear sunglasses to protect eyes from bright lights
10. Promote positive body image and coping skills: encourage participation in treatment plan; actively listen to client and encourage expression of feelings; reinforce progress and explain all care

D. Client teaching

1. Plan rest periods and conserve energy; plan major activities early in day; schedule activities during peak medication effect
2. NCLEX® Avoid extremes of hot and cold, exposure to infections, emotional stress, and drugs that may worsen or precipitate an exacerbation (alcohol, sedatives, local anesthetics)
3. NCLEX® Signs of myasthenic crisis (symptoms of disorder caused by inadequate medication related to need) and cholinergic crisis (over medication)
4. Encourage client to wear a Medic-Alert bracelet
5. Instruct in alternative methods of communication if necessary: eye blink, finger wiggle for yes or no; flash cards or communication board; teach to support lower jaw with hands to assist with speech

XIII. GUILLAIN-BARRÉ SYNDROME

A. Overview

1. An acute neuritis of cranial and peripheral nerves, usually preceded by viral infection (upper respiratory or gastrointestinal)
2. Immune system response to infection is exaggerated and is targeted at myelin sheath
3. Outcome is generally excellent if care is appropriate, but recovery is slow (one or more years)

B. Nursing assessment

1. NCLEX® Weakness or paresis or partial paralysis progressing upward from lower extremities (paralysis in Guillain-Barré is "ground to the brain"); about 20% of clients have respiratory paralysis requiring ventilatory support
2. Paresthesias (numbness and tingling) and pain
3. Muscle aches, cramping, and nighttime pain
4. NCLEX® Respiratory compromise and/or failure (dyspnea, diminished vital capacity and breath sounds), decreasing O_2 saturation, abnormal ABGs
5. NCLEX® Difficulty with extraocular eye movements, dysphagia, diplopia, difficulty speaking
6. NCLEX® Autonomic dysfunction (orthostatic hypotension), hypertension, change in HR, bowel and bladder dysfunction, flushing, and diaphoresis
7. Diagnostic tests: nerve conduction test results are diminished, elevated protein in CSF

C. Therapeutic management

1. Supportive care to maintain function of all systems, including respiratory, cardiac, GI, renal, and skin; medications as ordered
2. Plasmapheresis: plasma is removed and separated from whole blood; blood cells are then returned without plasma to remove antibodies that cause disorder; monitor for complications of this therapy, which include bleeding from loss of clotting factors and fluid and electrolyte imbalance
3. NCLEX® Monitor respiratory status: rate, depth, breath sounds; vital capacity; note secretions; check gag, cough, and swallowing ability
4. NCLEX® Monitor cardiac status: HR, BP, dysrhythmias
5. Administer chest physiotherapy and pulmonary hygiene measures

6. Maintain adequate nutrition as appropriate: administer enteral or parenteral nutrition as needed; if client can swallow, assist with small, frequent feedings of soft foods; weigh client weekly; provide mouth care every 2 hours
7. Monitor bowel and bladder function: assess bowel sounds and frequency, amount, color of bowel movements; offer bedpan; check for distention and residuals in client who cannot void spontaneously; perform intermittent catheterization as needed; encourage fluid intake to 3000 mL/day
8. Prevent complications of immobility: encourage use of weak extremities as able; provide assistance with ROM and prescribed exercises; protect immobile extremities with air mattress or special bed and elbow and heel protectors; turn and reposition every 2 hours; elevate extremities to prevent dependent edema; use antiembolism stockings or sequential compression devices
9. Provide eye care for client who cannot close eyelids completely; instill artificial tears, cleanse eyes as needed, use eye shields, and tape eyes closed if needed
10. Provide comfort and analgesics as needed
11. Promote communication with client and family; use alternative means of communication if client is on ventilator or cannot speak because of weak muscles
12. Initiate discharge planning at time of admission
13. Medication therapy: IV immunoglobulins, adrenocorticotropic hormone (ACTH), and corticosteroids or anti-inflammatory drugs; supportive medications include stool softeners, antacids, or H_2-receptor antagonists and analgesics

D. **Client education:** give rationales for all care and provide information about disease progression; encourage client and family to express feelings and participate in care as able

XIV. CRANIAL NERVE DISORDERS

A. Trigeminal neuralgia

1. Overview: a chronic disease of trigeminal nerve (CN V) that causes severe facial pain; affects one or more of three divisions of trigeminal nerve (ophthalmic, maxillary, and mandibular)
2. Nursing assessment
   a. Intermittent intense pain across cheeks or on lips, gums, or nose is characteristic symptom
   NCLEX® b. Some clients may have trigger zones that initiate onset of pain; in others, pain is triggered by light touch, eating, swallowing, talking, shaving, sneezing, brushing teeth, or washing face
3. Therapeutic management
   NCLEX® a. Centered on controlling pain with antiepileptic medications such as carbamazepine
   b. Surgery includes microvascular decompression (removal of blood vessel from posterior trigeminal root), rhizotomy (surgical severing of nerve root), radiofrequency ablation that relieves pain but not sensation or movement, or glycerol injection (can take up to 3 weeks to destroy nerve and relieve pain)
   NCLEX® c. Encourage client to chew on unaffected side
   d. Monitor dietary intake, encouraging soft foods
   NCLEX® e. Avoid triggers for pain, which include firm toothbrush, very hot or cold foods or liquids, or mechanical pressure on cheeks
4. Client teaching: avoidance of triggers

B. Bell's palsy

1. Overview: a sudden onset of unilateral weakness or paralysis of facial muscles; believed to be caused by herpes simplex type 1 and herpes zoster virus; 80% of clients recover completely within a few weeks to months

NCLEX® 2. Nursing assessment
   a. One-sided paralysis of facial muscles causing facial droop with inability to wrinkle forehead, pucker lips, puff out cheeks, raise eyebrows, or close eyelids on affected side
   b. Loss or impairment of taste over anterior portion of tongue on affected side
   c. Increased tearing from lacrimal gland on affected side
3. Therapeutic management
   NCLEX® a. Assist with physical therapy to stimulate facial nerve, gentle massage to maintain muscle tone, moist heat for comfort, and facial exercises
   NCLEX® b. Protect cornea with artificial tears, protective sunglasses or goggles, eye patch at night, and gentle intermittent closure of eye
   NCLEX® c. Medication therapy: a corticosteroid such as prednisone and an antiviral such as acyclovir limit damage to nerve
   d. Assist with body image disturbance, which is often temporary

NCLEX®

4. Client teaching
   a. Wear an eye patch at night and protective glasses or goggles when outside, in dusty conditions, and working with sprays
   b. Chew on unaffected side; after meals, brush teeth and inspect inside of mouth on affected side for food between mouth and teeth
   c. Protect face from cold and wind and use electric razor for shaving

XV. CEREBRAL PALSY

A. Overview

1. A group of permanent disorders of movement and posture caused by nonprogressive disturbance in fetal or infant brain
2. Classified as spastic, athetosis, dystonia, ataxia, or mixed (athetosis and dystonia may be called dyskinetic)
3. Patterns of extremity involvement include hemiplegia, **diplegia** (both legs involved), and quadriplegia (tetraplegia)
4. Causes include brain insult from trauma, hemorrhage, anoxia, or infection before, during, or after birth
5. Muscle growth is usually coordinated with bone growth, but muscle spasticity interferes

B. Nursing assessment

NCLEX®

1. Abnormal muscle tone and coordination: child with spastic cerebral palsy presents with spasticity (hypertonicity of muscle groups); child with athetoid cerebral palsy presents with wormlike movements of extremities; ataxic form of cerebral palsy involves disturbed coordination
2. May display hypertonia or hypotonia and may have varying degrees of tonicity on different extremities
3. Absence of expected reflexes or presence of reflexes that extend beyond expected age suggests cerebral palsy
4. Failure to meet developmental milestones may be first sign of disorder

NCLEX®

5. Physical symptoms include altered speech and difficulty with swallowing and scissoring of legs when walking; visual and hearing deficits may be present
6. Some children experience intellectual disability or develop seizures

C. Therapeutic management

1. Many individuals with CP require increased calorie intake because of spasticity or increased motor functioning and are at risk for inadequate intake because of decreased muscle strength and control

NCLEX®

2. If motor involvement causes child to have poor coordination or if child has seizure activity, ensure a safe environment and use precautions such as protective headgear and a padded bed

NCLEX®

3. Communication can be a problem if there is oral involvement; implement use of a communication board or computer-assisted communication; touch is an excellent way to communicate caring to a child
4. Self-care is a goal for all children; collaborate with occupational therapists for strategies and devices to assist in this area may be necessary

NCLEX®

5. Risk for aspiration is present if oral muscles are involved; use adaptive feeding devices and position upright during feedings to decrease risk
6. Collaborate with multidisciplinary team for speech, nutrition, occupation, and physical therapies; examples of rehabilitation strategies are range-of-motion exercises, stretching exercises, massage, braces, and splinting devices
7. Community-based developmental screenings identify children at risk or those with developmental delays from disorders such as CP; referrals for further assessment help ensure that early intervention is initiated; Denver II is most widely used developmental screening test
8. Provide adequate nutrition and rest

NCLEX®

9. Maintain a safe environment
10. To control spasticity, traditional treatments have included surgery to release tendons to promote mobility, rehabilitation therapies, and oral medications (skeletal muscle relaxants such as baclofen or dantrolene, or benzodiazepines); baclofen may be administered by intrathecal pump

D. Client and family teaching

1. Teach parents physical therapy strategies such as ROM exercises to use at home
2. Child will need to learn self-care skills such as feeding and dressing self and performing hygiene activities
3. Teach parents special feeding techniques and use of adaptive devices such as special silverware and dishes, or how to do gastrostomy tube feedings if indicated

XVI. NEURAL TUBE DEFECTS

A. Overview

1. Results from failure of neural tube to close during embryonic development; surgical closure of defect is performed soon after birth
2. Types of neural tube defects
   a. Myelodysplasia (spina bifida, meningomyelocele): posterior arches fail to fuse, with protrusion of meningeal sac that contains CSF, portion of spinal cord, and nerves; CSF leakage possible; see Figure 57–4
   b. Spina bifida occulta: posterior vertebral arches fail to fuse, but there is no herniation of spinal cord or meninges (fibrous membrane that covers brain and lines vertebral canal); no loss of function
   c. Spina bifida cystica: posterior vertebral arches fail to fuse, with protrusion of meninges through bony spine
   d. Meningocele: posterior vertebral arches fail to fuse, and there is a saclike protrusion at some point along posterior vertebrae; sac contains meninges and CSF
   e. Encephalocele: brain and meninges herniate through defect in skull into a sac
   f. Anencephaly: no development of brain above brainstem

NCLEX®
3. Etiology is uncertain but includes genetics, alcohol use, some medications (valproic acid, carbamazepine for seizures and isotretinoin for acne), and maternal health problems (folic acid deficiency, diabetes mellitus, obesity)
4. Degree of disability is determined by location of defect and number of spinal nerves encased in sac; higher defects are associated with greater neurologic dysfunction

B. Nursing assessment

NCLEX®
1. Prenatal diagnosis can be made by elevations in alpha-fetoprotein (AFP) in fluid obtained by amniocentesis; can also be assessed on prenatal ultrasound

NCLEX®
2. During postnatal period, monitor for leakage of CSF from sac and monitor skin integrity of sac; assess for infection around sac and possible systemic or CNS infection

NCLEX®
3. Assess degree of sensation at or below level of lesion; this can be evidenced by lack of movement or sensation in legs and a **neurogenic** (lacking innervation) bladder or bowel
4. Measure head circumference because there is a high risk of hydrocephalus

C. Therapeutic management

1. Collaborative management: defect/sac is surgically repaired during first 48 hours after birth

NCLEX®
2. Focus preoperative care on maintaining skin integrity of sac and keeping it free of infection; position infant on side or abdomen to achieve this goal; keep sac moist with sterile, saline-soaked dressings; avoid contamination of sac area by urine or feces

NCLEX®
3. Individuals with myelodysplasia have an increased incidence of latex allergies; monitor for this

NCLEX®
4. Neurogenic bladder: frequent, clean, straight catheterization is preferred method of management; maintain home schedule as much as possible

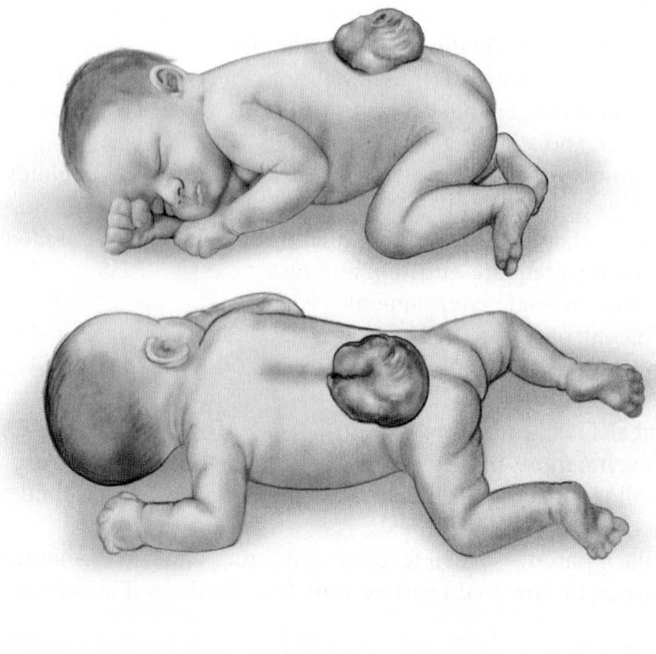

Figure 57–4

Infant with lumbosacral myelomeningocele.

NCLEX®

5. Neurogenic bowel: work with family to develop a bowel management plan using control of high-fiber diet, adequate fluid intake, and pattern for evacuation of bowels; in some cases, laxatives and enemas are used as prescribed by healthcare provider
6. Collaborate with physical therapy to develop modes of transport, such as using braces with crutches or wheelchair
7. Since areas with altered sensation are prone to skin breakdown, teach child and family to reposition frequently and inspect affected areas on a regular basis
8. Medication therapy: antibiotics perioperatively, possible urinary antispasmodics, possible suppository as part of bowel regimen

D. Client and family education

1. Daily care such as positioning, skin care, and range-of-motion exercises
2. Well-balanced diet sufficient in fiber and fluids to promote bowel elimination
3. Measures to manage neurogenic bladder, including clean, intermittent, straight catheterization
4. Associated high risk of latex allergy and possible allergies to certain foods (bananas, avocadoes, kiwi fruit, chestnuts)

XVII. HYDROCEPHALUS

A. Overview

1. A condition characterized by imbalance between CSF production and absorption, resulting in enlarged ventricles and increased ICP; if untreated, can lead to permanent brain damage
2. Etiology: congenital causes include Arnold Chiari malformation associated with myelomeningocele; can be acquired from meningitis, trauma, or intraventricular hemorrhage in premature infants; etiology is idiopathic in up to 50% of cases

B. Nursing assessment

NCLEX®

1. For infants, increased head circumference, split cranial sutures, high-pitched cry, bulging fontanel, irritability when awake, and seizures (see Figure 57–5)

NCLEX®

2. Toddlers and older children may also present with sunset eyes, seizures, irritability, papilledema, decreased LOC, and change in vital signs (increased systolic BP and widening pulse pressure)
3. Older children and adults may report headaches and have difficulty with balance and coordination
4. All clients can present with vomiting, lethargy, and Cheyne-Stokes respiratory pattern
5. Diagnosis confirmed using CT and MRI to reveal location of CSF obstruction

C. Therapeutic management

1. Surgical insertion of a ventriculoperitoneal shunt (tube with consistency of piece of cooked spaghetti) into ventricles with distal end in either the peritoneum or atrium
   a. Preoperatively monitor client for symptoms of increased ICP

NCLEX®

   b. Postoperatively place client flat and on unoperative side; if an infant or child client is held by a caregiver, it is important not to allow head to be elevated

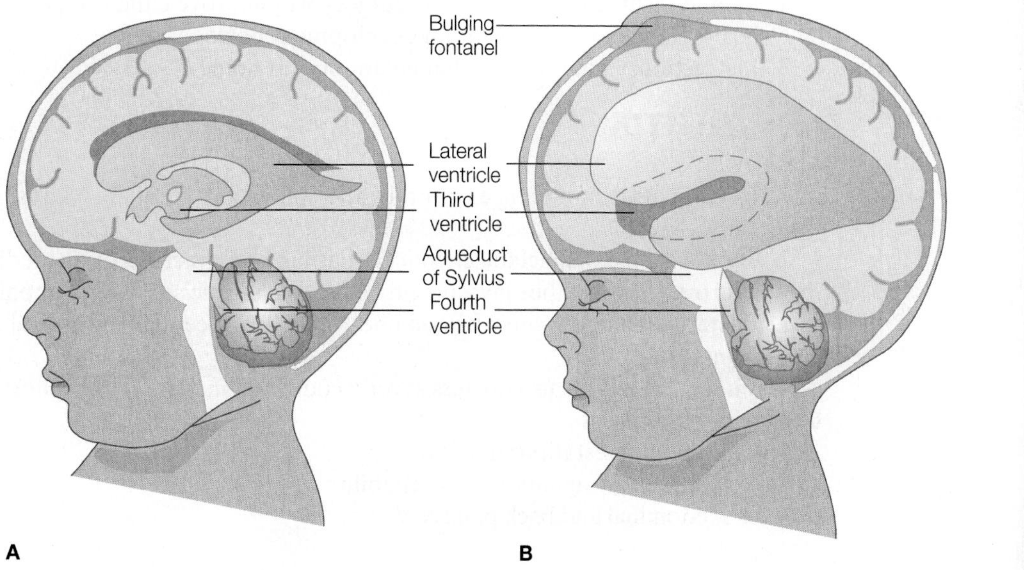

Figure 57–5

Development of hydrocephalus in a young child. (**A**) Normal ventricles, (**B**) enlarged ventricles and bulging fontanel.

NCLEX® c. Postoperatively, monitor client for symptoms of infection; notify healthcare provider if symptoms are present: fever, change in LOC, excessive redness at incision site or along shunt tract, elevated WBC count with leukocytosis, or shift to left

2. Medication therapy: prophylactic antibiotics before and/or after surgery

D. Client and family education

1. Symptoms of shunt infection and malfunction and what actions to take

NCLEX® 2. Signs of shunt malfunction
   a. Infant whose cranial suture lines have not fused; signs include increased head circumference, high-pitched cry, bulging fontanel, irritability when awake, and seizures
   b. Toddlers and older children display vomiting, irritability, and headache; as condition persists, sunset eyes, seizures, papilledema, decreased LOC, and change in VS (increased systolic BP and widening pulse pressure) occur
   c. Older clients have difficulty with balance and coordination
   d. All clients may have lethargy and Cheyne-Stokes respirations

3. Some children with hydrocephalus have brain damage that results in motor, language, perceptual, and intellectual disabilities; parents may need referrals to early-intervention professionals to provide long-term rehabilitation services

NCLEX® 4. Children with hydrocephalus and myelomeningocele have an increased risk of latex allergies; teach parents to avoid nipples, pacifiers, and toys made of latex products

XVIII. CRANIOSYNOSTOSIS

A. Overview

1. Premature closure of cranial sutures in young children; can lead to increased ICP and brain damage
2. There is some relationship between craniosynostosis and several inherited syndromes
3. Etiology is unknown; can be diagnosed by clinical exam and confirmed with skull films, CT scan, and MRI

B. Nursing assessment

1. A bony ridge is palpated along a suture line
2. Compensatory growth of skull in directions parallel to closed suture line creates skull deformities; monitor fontanels in all infants for premature closure of fontanels; monitor head circumference

C. Therapeutic management

1. Medical treatment is surgical correction of skeletal defect

NCLEX® 2. Follow all principles of postoperative care: keep incision dry and intact; monitor for signs of increased ICP, changing LOC, and infection postoperatively

3. Prepare parents and child for child's postoperative appearance; in addition to large, turbanlike bandage, child will have orbital edema and bruising; long-term results of surgery should be discussed, and "before and after" pictures may assist family in mentally preparing for surgery

NCLEX® 4. Fluid restrictions may be ordered in postoperative period; child may be maintained with head of the bed elevated 30 degrees

D. Client and family teaching

1. Should include reassurance that surgery will improve child's appearance and that most children are healthy and have normal brain development postoperatively
2. Instructions about how to change dressing at home

XIX. MENINGITIS

A. Overview

1. Inflammation of meninges of brain and spinal cord frequently caused by infection of meninges and CSF
2. Other risk factors include chemicals, basilar skull fracture, otitis media, sinusitis, mastoiditis, neurosurgery or other invasive procedures, systemic sepsis, and impaired immune function
3. Bacterial meningitis may be complicated by hydrocephalus, cerebral edema, arthritis, and cranial nerve damage
4. Viral meningitis is usually less severe; course of disease is often shorter and more benign

B. Nursing assessment

NCLEX® 1. Clinical manifestations in adults
   a. Restlessness, agitation, and irritability
   b. Abdominal and back pain; N/V

c. Signs of meningeal irritation: **nuchal rigidity** (stiff neck), positive Brudzinski sign (pain, resistance, and hip and knee flexion occur when neck is flexed to chest while lying supine), positive Kernig sign (pain and/or resistance occurs with flexion of knee and hip and straightening of knee in supine position), and **photophobia** (sensitivity of eyes to light)
d. Chills and high fever
e. Severe headaches, confusion, altered LOC
f. Seizures
g. Signs and symptoms of increasing ICP
h. Diagnostic and laboratory test findings: LP with CSF analysis, including Gram stain and culture; blood, urine, throat, and nose cultures identify possible source of infection

NCLEX®
2. Bacterial meningitis in infants and toddlers: poor feeding, vomiting, high-pitched cry, bulging fontanel, fever or hypothermia depending on maturity of infant's neurologic system, and poor muscle tone; children and adolescents present similarly to adults; **opisthotonus** posture (hyperextending head and neck) may relieve some discomfort from meningeal irritation; petechial or purpuric rash will be seen if it is a meningococcal infection
3. Viral meningitis in infants and toddlers: irritability, lethargy, vomiting, and change in appetite; for older child and adult, usually preceded by a nonspecific febrile illness; presents with headache, malaise, muscle aches, N/V, photophobia, and nuchal rigidity or spinal rigidity
4. Diagnosed by analysis of CSF obtained by LP; see Table 57–5

C. Therapeutic management

1. Bacterial meningitis is a medical emergency that, if not treated, can be fatal within days

NCLEX®
2. Treatment of bacterial meningitis focuses on eradicating bacterial infection with antibiotics
3. Surgical treatment may include placement of an Ommaya reservoir to allow **intrathecal** (into subarachnoid space) administration of antibiotics

NCLEX®
4. Monitor respiratory status, administer O_2, and maintain artificial airway
5. Assess neurologic status and vital signs (with temperature) regularly; report changes in neurologic status or presence of cranial nerve dysfunction
6. Assess, prepare for, and report any seizure activity

NCLEX®
7. Provide an environment that will minimize ICP elevation; this can include elevating HOB 15–30 degrees, avoiding neck extension or flexion, and maintaining head in a neutral position; keep environment quiet and subdued; handle client in a gentle manner; assess for signs of increased ICP
8. Administer prescribed medications and maintain fluid restrictions
9. Assess for fluid volume deficits; monitor I&O, daily weights, skin turgor, laboratory values, and urine concentration
10. Medication therapy
    a. Bacterial meningitis is treated for 7–14 days with IV antibiotics sensitive to causative organism

NCLEX®

    b. Preventive care includes Hib vaccine to protect all young children from infection; those who have close contact with clients diagnosed with meningococcal and *H. influenzae* meningitis may receive rifampin prophylactically
    c. Antiepileptics (usually phenytoin) to prevent or control seizures
    d. Antipyretic, antiemetic, and analgesic medications for symptom relief
    e. IV fluid replacement until client can resume oral intake
11. Assess for evidence of pain with all routine assessments; administer nonopioid pain medication as prescribed; however, narcotics (opioids) should be avoided because they mask neurologic signs and increasing ICP; pain relief should promote rest and reduce risk of increased ICP

Table 57–5 Comparison of Cerebrospinal Fluid in Meningitis

	Normal	Viral Meningitis	Bacterial Meningitis
Pressure	5–15 mmHg	Normal or slightly elevated	Elevated
Appearance	Clear	Clear	Cloudy
Leukocytes (mm^3)	0–5	Slightly elevated	Elevated
Protein (mg/dL)	10–30	Slightly elevated	Elevated
Glucose (mg/dL)	40–80	Normal or decreased	Decreased

NCLEX® 12. Clients with bacterial meningitis must be isolated on droplet precautions until at least 24 hours of antibiotic therapy have been completed

NCLEX® 13. Monitor for complications of meningitis (seizures, hearing loss, visual alterations); neurologic sequelae such as intellectual disability, CP, and hydrocephalus may occur in children; a complication of meningococcal meningitis is meningococcemia (overwhelming septic infection with circulatory collapse and tissue necrosis)

14. Viral meningitis is treated symptomatically; usually only infants are hospitalized for viral meningitis

D. Client and family teaching

1. Importance of taking prescribed antibiotics until finished and other medications as ordered
2. Report signs and symptoms of ear, throat, and upper respiratory infections so client can be assessed for meningitis
3. Provide information about disease and its transmission, need for possible droplet precautions and antibiotic therapy, and need for prophylactic treatment for those in contact with client
4. Provide family with information about possible development of sequelae from disease and possible side effects of medications
5. Share information about follow-up as well as rehabilitation services with family

XX. ENCEPHALITIS

A. Overview

1. Inflammation of brain tissue
2. Presenting symptoms vary depending on causative organism and location of infection; classic symptoms include an acute febrile illness accompanied by neurologic signs
3. Etiology is usually a viral organism (herpes simplex type 1 virus, enteroviruses); nonviral agents include bacteria, parasites, fungi, and rickettsiae
4. Infectious process usually begins elsewhere in body
5. Prognosis depends on degree of CNS involvement; permanent neurologic sequelae may result

NCLEX® **B. Nursing assessment**

1. Assess for fever, severe headache, N/V, and signs of an upper respiratory infection
2. Neurologic symptoms include those of nuchal rigidity, photophobia, and positive Kernig and Brudzinski signs
3. Other signs include disorientation, confusion with personality or behavior changes, speech disturbances, motor dysfunction, cranial nerve deficits, and focal or generalized seizures that alternate with periods of screaming, hallucinating, and bizarre movement; LOC can change from stupor to coma

C. Therapeutic management

1. Monitor client's VS, respiratory status, oxygenation, and urine output
2. NCLEX® Provide seizure precautions and have resuscitation materials close to bed; clients are best managed in an intensive care unit (ICU) during acute phase
3. Maintain skin integrity and prevent other complications of immobility through proper positioning, frequent turning, and chest physiotherapy
4. Work with family in planning for discharge; since many clients have neurologic sequelae, family will need support in giving physical and emotional care at home; parents will play an active role in child rehabilitation process; follow-up visits must be coordinated; families may need referral to home care, counseling, social services, and community support groups
5. Medication therapy: if suspected organism is bacterial, appropriate antibiotics will be ordered; acyclovir or other antiviral agents are administered for herpes virus infection

D. Client and family education

1. Information about causative agent and plan of treatment
2. Discharge plans must be started early; because of neurologic sequelae, plans for rehabilitation must be discussed

XXI. REYE SYNDROME

A. Overview

1. An acute metabolic encephalopathy of childhood; fatty degeneration of liver leads to liver dysfunction
2. NCLEX® Characterized by five stages
   a. Vomiting and lethargy
   b. Combativeness and confusion
   c. Coma, decorticate posturing

d. Decerebrate posturing
e. Seizures, loss of deep tendon reflexes, respiratory arrest

NCLEX®
3. While exact etiology is unclear, Reye syndrome usually develops after a mild viral illness such as varicella (chickenpox) and is associated with use of aspirin

B. Nursing assessment

NCLEX®
1. Child presents with an abrupt change in LOC; history reveals child is recovering from a viral disease with sudden onset of vomiting and mental confusion
2. Liver enzymes and ammonia levels are elevated; blood glucose levels are below normal, and prothrombin time is prolonged; bilirubin levels remain normal; liver biopsy shows small fat deposits

NCLEX®
C. Therapeutic management

1. Most children are monitored in an ICU; care is focused on support and on assessing child's physical status, such as monitoring for cerebral edema; enforce fluid restrictions (usually instituted); frequently measure vital signs and neurologic status, which may include Glasgow Coma Scale
2. Monitor lab values for elevated ammonia, acidosis, or hypoglycemia; measure I&O
3. Provide all standard nursing measures to prevent complications of immobility
4. Provide emotional support to family; sudden onset and rapid deterioration in child's condition often overwhelm parents' ability to cope
5. Medication therapy
   a. Controlling cerebral edema is a primary concern; corticosteroids to reduce swelling and barbiturates to induce a coma for severe cerebral edema; mannitol as an osmotic diuretic
   b. Phenytoin may be used to control seizures
   c. Vitamin K may be given to aid in coagulation

D. Child and family teaching

1. Explanations of disease and its cause, treatment plan and prognosis, treatment environment, and medical equipment in use; information helps parents to cope
2. Discharge planning includes rehabilitative needs of child and plans for follow-up
3. Prevent by public education about Reye syndrome and its connection with viral illnesses and administration of aspirin, and that child has better prognosis if symptoms detected early with prompt medical treatment

XXII. AUTISM SPECTRUM DISORDERS (ASD)

A. Overview

1. Set of neurodevelopmental disorders of unknown etiology that begins in early childhood
2. General features include impaired social interactions and communication, repetitive patterns of behavior, and restricted interests, activities, and behaviors
3. There is wide variation among individual presentations
4. Two common types include autism and Asperger syndrome

NCLEX®
B. Nursing assessment

1. Essential features usually become apparent by age 3 years
2. Signs of autism
   a. Inability to relate to people in an age-appropriate way or respond to social and emotional cues; possibly labile emotions
   b. **Stereotypy** (rigid, repetitive, machine-like movement with obsessive behavior) such as banging head, twirling in circles, biting self, or flapping arms or hands
   c. Abnormal responses to sensory stimuli, including aversion to touch, loud noises, and bright lights
   d. Communication difficulties or delays in speech and language development; possible echolalia (compulsive repeating of what is heard)
   e. Ritualistic behaviors such as rigid routines, lining up objects, playing with same toys repeatedly, eating only certain types or colors of foods or foods that are arranged in a specific way
   f. Cognitive development may be delayed, but some children excel in specific areas such art, music, mathematics, or perceptual skills (e.g., puzzle-solving)
3. Signs of Asperger syndrome ("mild autism"): many of same sensory and social issues of autism, but vocabulary and IQ are average to above average
4. Diagnosis is through surveillance at healthcare visits and age-appropriate ASD screening tools

C. Therapeutic management

1. Stabilize environmental stimuli by minimizing unfamiliar sounds and lowering general noise level
2. Orient to environment and provide comfort by encouraging presence and use of favorite toys or objects

3. Assess client's routines, preferences, and habits; maintain consistency with these whenever possible
4. Enhance communication by using short, direct sentences, visual cues, pictures, computers, and other visual aids as appropriate to situation
5. Maintain client safety: monitor client at bathtime and bedtime; prevent contact with harmful objects; use bicycle helmets or mittens to protect client from harm

D. Child and family teaching

1. Anticipatory guidance about possible need for lifelong supervision and support
2. Community-based resources such as childcare, toddler and preschool programs, parent support groups, school-based resources and individualized education plans, family support groups, respite care, and Autism Society of America

Check Your NCLEX–RX® Exam I.Q.

You are ready for testing on this content if you can:

- Identify basic structures and functions of the neurologic system.
- Describe the pathophysiology and etiology of common neurologic disorders.
- Discuss expected assessment data and diagnostic test findings for selected neurologic disorders.
- Discuss therapeutic management of a client experiencing a neurologic disorder.
- Discuss nursing management of a client experiencing a neurologic disorder.
- Identify expected outcomes for the client experiencing a neurologic disorder.

PRACTICE TEST

1 Which assessment finding in a 35-year-old client with an intracranial hematoma should concern the nurse?

1. Hamstring pain when the hip and knee are flexed and then extended
2. Curling of the toes when the bottom of the foot is stroked in upward motion
3. Muscle aches and cramping, especially at night
4. Cogwheel and lead pipe rigidity

2 The nurse should prevent corneal abrasion in a client with myasthenia gravis by performing which nursing intervention?

1. Doing a saline eye irrigation every shift
2. Instilling artificial tears in the eyes every 1–2 hours
3. Ensuring the client's contact lenses are on while awake
4. Providing sunglasses when client is outside

3 The client with newly diagnosed Parkinson's disease states, "I just don't think I can handle having Parkinson's disease." What is the nurse's best first response?

1. "You sound overwhelmed. Can you tell me more?"
2. "I am sure you can. A lot of other people do!"
3. "What do you think will be the hardest thing to handle?"
4. "The entire healthcare team will help you manage the disease."

4 What should the nurse do as a priority when caring for the client with myasthenia gravis to minimize the risk for complications of the disease?

1. Inspect for hemorrhage.
2. Assess for viral pneumonia.
3. Offer to cut the client's food as needed.
4. Provide the client with a bedside commode.

5 A client calls the telephone triage nurse to report fever, nausea, chills, and malaise. The nurse should instruct the client to come immediately to the emergency department after the client shares which additional data?

1. A bad headache
2. A stiff, sore neck
3. A heart rate of 106
4. A roommate with the same symptoms

6 When assessing the client with meningitis, the nurse looks for which manifestation as a frequent first sign of increased intracranial pressure?

1. A rising systolic blood pressure
2. Change in mood or attention level
3. Irregular respiratory rate and depth
4. A bounding radial pulse

7 The nurse is providing instructions to the client hospitalized with bacterial meningitis who will be discharged soon. Which recommendation should have the highest priority?

1. Take all of the antibiotics as directed until completely gone.
2. Eat a high-protein, high-calorie diet.
3. Exercise daily, beginning with active ROM.
4. Get at least 8 hours of sleep per night with frequent rest periods during the day.

8 Which instruction should the nurse give to a client with multiple sclerosis who has urinary retention?

1. "Run water whenever you experience difficulty initiating urination."
2. "Decrease your fluid intake to prevent urgency."
3. "Drink a caffeinated beverage to promote the ability to form urine."
4. "Catheterize your bladder according to the schedule we discussed."

9 What strategy should the nurse suggest to the family of the client with Parkinson's disease as the best approach to helping the client maintain as much functional independence as possible?

1. Assist the client to take a warm bath every morning.
2. Perform passive range of motion (ROM) three times a day.
3. Display an unhurried manner that allows the client sufficient time to respond or act.
4. Obtain assistive devices that will make activities of daily living (ADLs) easier.

10 The home health nurse concludes that more teaching may be necessary after making which observations during the first home visit to a client discharged after a stroke? Select all that apply.

1. A commode is observed at the bedside.
2. A fluid restriction chart is on the refrigerator.
3. A package of psyllium is on the kitchen counter.
4. Hand weights are next to the couch.
5. There is a small scatter rug at the side of the bed.

11 The office nurse should direct a client on the telephone to seek care at the hospital emergency department based on which statement?

1. "My legs are weak and now I'm having trouble getting a good breath."
2. "My shaky hand is no better than last visit. In fact, I think it's getting worse."
3. "The double vision went away when I put my eye patch on."
4. "My headache doesn't seem any better even though I gave up coffee."

12 A 76-year-old woman arrives at the emergency department by ambulance with a possible stroke. Vital signs are pulse 90, blood pressure 150/100, respirations 20. Thirty minutes later, vital signs are pulse 78, blood pressure 170/90, respirations 24 and irregular. The nurse should take which action at this time?

1. Ask the woman to describe any sensations she is feeling.
2. Check the client's serum phenytoin level.
3. Get a prescription to decrease the rate of IV fluids.
4. Offer the client clear liquids to prevent dehydration.

13 A client seen in the neighborhood clinic reports "eye problems" and generalized weakness that became markedly worse after using a friend's hot tub. The client provides long, detailed responses to initial demographic questions. What is the best question for the nurse to ask at this time?

1. "Was the weather the same each time you used the hot tub?"
2. "How do you feel the hot tub is responsible for your worsening condition?"
3. "Could you try to be a little briefer in your answers so I can best help you?"
4. "Can you tell me more about the eye problems?"

14 An abnormal electroencephalogram (EEG) indicates that a 2-year-old client has epilepsy, but the parents say they have never observed a seizure. The pediatric nurse concludes that the child may be experiencing which type of seizure?

1. Absence
2. Myoclonic
3. Jacksonian
4. Grand mal

15 The nurse is providing care for a 13-year-old who was placed in a halo brace within the last 24 hours because of a spinal cord injury. Which assessment is the first priority of the nurse?

1. Loosen the connections on the vest to assess the skin.
2. Assess the pin sites.
3. Ask how the client is able to reposition self in bed.
4. Ask about the client's ability to perform range of motion to legs.

16 The rehabilitation nurse is admitting a client following spinal cord injury. The nurse concludes that the client has developed Brown-Séquard syndrome after detecting which assessment finding in the client?

1. Ipsilateral motor loss above the lesion
2. Contralateral loss of proprioception
3. Hyperanesthesia below the level of the lesion
4. Ipsilateral proprioception loss below lesion

17 The nurse anticipates that the client presenting with increased intracranial pressure would most likely exhibit which set of vital signs?

1. BP 190/84, HR 150, and an irregular respiratory pattern
2. BP 80/50, HR 50, and Kussmaul respirations
3. BP 80/50, HR 150, and Cheyne-Stokes respirations
4. BP 190/84, HR 50, and an irregular respiratory pattern

18 In providing for the safety of the client during a grand mal seizure, the nurse should perform which interventions? Select all that apply.

1. Position the client on his back.
2. Gently place a padded tongue blade between the teeth.
3. Remove nearby objects that could lead to client injury.
4. Apply oxygen immediately via mask.
5. Note the length and progression of the seizure.

19 The community health nurse interprets that clients who live in a swampy bayou area in the southern United States might be at risk of contracting which health problem?

1. Meningitis
2. Parkinson's disease
3. Encephalitis
4. Multiple sclerosis

20 The client recently diagnosed with Guillain-Barré syndrome is drooling and having difficulty swallowing secretions. When the family asks why this occurs, the nurse indicates that which of the following is the cause?

1. Obstructed blood flow to the midbrain
2. Demyelination of cranial nerves responsible for swallow and gag reflex
3. Enlargement of the parotid and salivary glands
4. Deficiency in thiamine and pyridoxine in the central nervous system

21 A 1-year-old child has been diagnosed with cerebral palsy. The child has the spastic form that affects all extremities. What would be an appropriate focus of concern for a child at this age? Select all that apply.

1. Risk of sustaining injury
2. Inadequate ability to try to feed self
3. Impairment of general thought processes
4. Difficulty with producing speech
5. Self-consciousness regarding body image

22 The nurse observes a child starting to have a seizure. After assessing the airway, what should be the highest priority of the nurse?

1. Insert an artificial airway.
2. Observe and record seizure activity.
3. Administer diazepam.
4. Restrain the extremities to protect the child from injury.

23 The nurse has taught the parents of a 6-year-old child with a ventriculoperitoneal (VP) shunt to monitor for shunt malfunction. The nurse determines the parents understand the instructions if they state to notify the healthcare provider for which client manifestation?

1. Bulging soft spot
2. Expanding head size
3. Sunset eyes
4. Altered level of consciousness

24 A child is admitted with a head injury after being in a motor vehicle crash. After noting the presence of clear drainage from the left ear, the nurse should suspect which underlying problem commonly associated with this finding?

1. Linear skull fracture
2. Basilar skull fracture
3. Subdural hematoma
4. Epidural hematoma

25 The nurse has learned that there is a disruption in family dynamics after a child was hospitalized with a severe brain injury sustained in a motor vehicle crash. Which nursing intervention should have the highest priority?

1. Teach the family the importance of using seatbelts.
2. Refer the family to support services in the community.
3. Encourage family to ask questions and express feelings.
4. Explain rules for visiting in the intensive care unit.

ANSWERS & RATIONALES

1 **Answer: 1 Rationale:** Hamstring pain with hip and knee flexion and then extension is called positive Kernig sign; this is common in intracranial hematomas. Curling of the toes with upward stroking on the bottom of the foot is called a negative Babinski; with a hematoma, the nurse should expect a positive Babinski (dorsiflexion of the toes in an adult). Muscle cramps and aching are common in many illnesses. Cogwheel and lead pipe rigidity is specific to Parkinson's disease. **Cognitive Level:** Applying **Client Need:** Physiological Adaptation **Integrated Process:** Nursing Process: Assessment **Content Area:** Adult Health: Neurological **Strategy:** The core issue of the question is knowledge of associated findings with intracranial hematoma. Use nursing knowledge and the process of elimination to make a selection.

2 **Answer: 2 Rationale:** Corneal abrasion in the client with myasthenia gravis is caused by dryness of the cornea from inability to close the eyelids and blink. It can be prevented by application of artificial tears every 1–2 hours. Saline eye irrigations, wearing contact lenses while awake, and wearing sunglasses when outside do not protect against corneal abrasion. **Cognitive Level:** Applying **Client Need:** Physiological Adaptation **Integrated Process:** Nursing Process: Implementation **Content Area:** Adult Health: Neurological **Strategy:** Consider the effect of each intervention on preventing injury to the eye and use nursing knowledge and the process of elimination to make a selection.

3 **Answer: 1 Rationale:** The nurse should first encourage the client experiencing a loss to express his feelings. This answer acknowledges the client's feelings, is open-ended, and promotes further discussion. Stating "I'm sure you can" provides false reassurance and saying "a lot of other people do" draws attention away from the client's concern. Focusing on what will be most difficult to handle does not address the client's feelings. Stating the entire health team will help interrupts the opportunity for the client to share concerns by moving directly to attempted solutions. **Cognitive Level:** Analyzing **Client Need:** Psychosocial Integrity **Integrated Process:** Communication and Documentation **Content Area:** Adult Health: Neurological **Strategy:** The core issue of the question is a therapeutic communication. For communication questions, look first for the option that addresses the client's feelings or concerns.

4 **Answer: 3 Rationale:** When the muscles involved in chewing and swallowing, as well as the diaphragm and intercostal muscles, are weak the client may aspirate or experience poor gas exchange; both increase the risk for pneumonia. Options that protect the airway always have highest priority. The client is not at risk for hemorrhage. The client is not at high risk for viral pneumonia as a complication of the disease, although pneumonia caused by aspiration would be of greater concern. Providing a bedside commode may be an element of routine care. **Cognitive Level:** Analyzing **Client Need:** Physiological Adaptation **Integrated Process:** Nursing Process: Implementation **Content Area:** Adult Health: Neurological **Strategy:** The core issue of the question is the ability to determine a priority complication of myasthenia gravis and to then select the intervention that reduces it. Use nursing knowledge and the process of elimination to make a selection.

5 **Answer: 2 Rationale:** A stiff, sore neck is a sign of meningeal irritation and possible meningitis. The nurse may further inquire if flexion of the neck causes pain and the hip and knee to flex (Brudzinski sign) and how high the fever is. Headache, tachycardia, and being near others with similar symptoms are typical of influenza. **Cognitive Level:** Analyzing **Client Need:** Physiological Adaptation **Integrated Process:** Nursing Process: Implementation **Content Area:** Adult Health: Neurological **Strategy:** The core issue of the question is the ability to recognize clients at risk for or showing early signs of meningitis. Use nursing knowledge and the process of elimination to make a selection.

6 **Answer: 2 Rationale:** The first signs of increased intracranial pressure are often subtle changes in level of consciousness. Rising systolic BP, irregular respiratory rate, and bounding pulse are later signs of increased intracranial pressure. **Cognitive Level:** Analyzing **Client Need:** Physiological Adaptation **Integrated Process:** Nursing Process: Assessment **Content Area:** Adult Health: Neurological **Strategy:** The core issue of the

question is the ability to discriminate early signs of rising intracranial pressure from later ones. Use nursing knowledge and the process of elimination to make a selection.

7 **Answer: 1 Rationale:** It is essential that the client recovering from bacterial meningitis take all of the prescribed antibiotic as directed. Failure to do so puts the client at risk for a relapse of symptoms and contributes to development of bacterial resistance to antibiotics. A high-protein and -calorie diet, adequate exercise, and adequate rest and sleep are important aspects of self-care during recuperation but are not as essential as the completion of antimicrobial therapy. **Cognitive Level:** Applying **Client Need:** Physiological Adaptation **Integrated Process:** Communication and Documentation **Content Area:** Adult Health: Neurological **Strategy:** The core issue of the question is the ability to prioritize completion of antibiotic therapy with bacterial meningitis as essential. Use nursing knowledge and the process of elimination to make a selection.

8 **Answer: 4 Rationale:** Urinary retention in the client with multiple sclerosis is a sequela of impaired conduction of nerves innervating the bladder. Performing self-catheterization will drain the bladder and help prevent urinary tract infection. The client with multiple sclerosis will be encouraged to increase fluid intake to prevent constipation. Because urinary retention is incomplete emptying of the bladder, neither running water nor caffeinated beverages would be useful. **Cognitive Level:** Applying **Client Need:** Physiological Adaptation **Integrated Process:** Communication and Documentation **Content Area:** Adult Health: Neurological **Strategy:** The core issue of the question is knowledge of appropriate methods to manage urinary retention in a client with multiple sclerosis. Use nursing knowledge and the process of elimination to make a selection.

9 **Answer: 3 Rationale:** The essential approach to enhance and encourage self-care abilities is an unhurried one that allows sufficient time for self-expression and for the client to do as much as possible for him- or herself. Passive ROM helps maintain joint mobility but does not foster maintenance of the client's own abilities. A warm bath may be comforting but is not a global approach to self-care. The use of assistive devices is appropriate for the client with Parkinson's disease but does not represent a global approach to maintaining self-care ability. **Cognitive Level:** Applying **Client Need:** Physiological Adaptation **Integrated Process:** Nursing Process: Implementation **Content Area:** Adult Health: Neurological **Strategy:** The critical word in the question is *approach*, which implies a manner of behaving rather than a specific or single action. Use nursing knowledge and the process of elimination to make a selection.

10 **Answer: 2, 5 Rationale:** Fluid restriction may be needed in the period immediately following a stroke, but this is not necessary after discharge to home. Small rugs can increase the risk for falls and should be removed. A bedside commode may be useful if the client has residual limited mobility. Psyllium (as well as increased fluids) may help maintain bowel elimination in a client with reduced mobility. Hand weights may be helpful in increasing upper-extremity strength. **Cognitive Level:** Analyzing **Client Need:** Physiological Adaptation **Integrated Process:** Nursing Process: Implementation **Content Area:** Adult Health: Neurological **Strategy:** The wording of the question indicates that more than one option is likely to be correct and that the correct options will be items of concern. Use knowledge of principles of rehabilitation and the process of elimination to make the correct selections.

11 **Answer: 1 Rationale:** What the client describes is a classic ascending progression of Guillain-Barré syndrome. The muscular weakness may ascend to include the diaphragm. Total respiratory paralysis can occur, requiring ventilatory support. Shaking hands, double vision, and headache refer to chronic problems, not an acute one. **Cognitive Level:** Analyzing **Client Need:** Physiological Adaptation **Integrated Process:** Nursing Process: Implementation **Content Area:** Adult Health: Neurological **Strategy:** Remember the ABCs and prioritize an answer that refers to a possible impaired airway. Use nursing knowledge and the process of elimination to make a selection.

12 **Answer: 3 Rationale:** The client is showing signs of rising intracranial pressure, and reducing the rate of IV fluids prevents hypervolemia that would worsen rising intracranial pressure. Using Maslow's hierarchy, choose physiological actions before psychological ones. A phenytoin level would not be relevant to stroke status. The nurse would want to avoid offering fluids, which would add to the client's volume status. Dehydration is not a concern at this time. **Cognitive Level:** Applying **Client Need:** Physiological Adaptation **Integrated Process:** Nursing Process: Implementation **Content Area:** Adult Health: Neurological **Strategy:** Recognize the inherent pattern in the changing vital signs as increasing intracranial pressure and choose an option that could help to reverse it.

13 **Answer: 4 Rationale:** A more detailed assessment, such as following up on the eye problems, is important in collecting data to meet client needs. A picture of multiple sclerosis may be unfolding. Focusing on the weather is not relevant to the client's situation. The client may not have an understanding of how the hot tub relates to the current condition. Asking the client to be briefer has a slightly judgmental tone. **Cognitive Level:** Analyzing **Client Need:** Physiological Adaptation **Integrated Process:** Communication and Documentation **Content Area:** Adult Health: Neurological **Strategy:** The core issue of the question is selection of an appropriate communication that focuses on assessment. Use nursing knowledge and the process of elimination to make a selection.

14 **Answer: 1 Rationale:** Also known as petit mal seizures, absence seizures may be no more observable than brief staring instances. The parents should be instructed to note and report any change in the child's behavior, no matter how small. Myoclonic movements and Jacksonian or grand mal seizure activity would be very evident to the client's family. **Cognitive Level:** Analyzing **Client Need:** Physiological Adaptation **Integrated Process:** Nursing Process: Assessment **Content Area:** Child Health **Strategy:** The core issue of the question is the ability to discriminate different types of seizures based on presentation (or lack of manifestations). Use nursing knowledge and the process of elimination to make a selection.

15 **Answer: 2 Rationale:** The nurse would want to assess the pin sites for redness, edema, and drainage as a first priority to detect infection as a complication. The nurse would want to ensure that the vest fits snugly to maintain traction. Asking about bed mobility is an important part of routine care to the client to prevent skin breakdown but is not as high a priority at this time as assessing for signs of pin site infection. Assessing ability to perform range of motion is a routine part of care that can be completed once considerations related to the halo traction are addressed. **Cognitive Level:** Applying **Client Need:** Physiological Adaptation **Integrated Process:** Nursing Process: Implementation **Content Area:** Child

Health **Strategy:** The core issue of the question is knowledge of the importance of assessing pin sites for a client who is in a halo vest. Use nursing knowledge and the process of elimination to make a selection.

16 **Answer: 4 Rationale:** Hemisection of the anterior and posterior portions of the spinal cord results in loss of position sense (proprioception) on the same (ipsilateral) side of the body as the trauma, below the level of injury. Ipsilateral motor loss does not occur above the level of a spinal cord injury. Brown-Séquard syndrome does not result in contralateral loss of proprioception. Hyperanesthesia below the level of the injury is seen in anterior cord syndrome. **Cognitive Level:** Applying **Client Need:** Physiological Adaptation **Integrated Process:** Nursing Process: Assessment **Content Area:** Adult Health: Neurological **Strategy:** The core issue of the question is knowledge of characteristics of Brown-Séquard syndrome following spinal cord injury. Use nursing knowledge and the process of elimination to make a selection.

17 **Answer: 4 Rationale:** The brainstem's final effort to maintain cerebral perfusion is seen with an increased systolic blood pressure, bradycardia, and an irregular respiratory pattern known as Cushing's triad. The client would not experience tachycardia. The client would not experience hypotension coupled with Kussmaul respirations. The client would not experience hypotension coupled with Cheyne-Stokes respirations. **Cognitive Level:** Analyzing **Client Need:** Physiological Adaptation **Integrated Process:** Nursing Process: Assessment **Content Area:** Adult Health: Neurological **Strategy:** The core issue of the question is the ability to recognize patterns of change in vital signs that reflect increasing intracranial pressure. Use nursing knowledge and the process of elimination to make a selection.

18 **Answer: 3, 5 Rationale:** The nurse's priority is to protect the client from injury. The nurse would note and then document when the seizure began, how it progressed, when it ended, and associated client findings. To promote drainage, it is more effective to secure an airway by turning the client onto the side rather than the back. Inserting a tongue blade can cause trauma. Oxygen should be available but does not have to be applied. **Cognitive Level:** Applying **Client Need:** Safety and Infection Control **Integrated Process:** Nursing Process: Implementation **Content Area:** Adult Health: Neurological **Strategy:** The core issue of the question is priority concerns for a client experiencing a seizure. Use Maslow's hierarchy of needs, nursing knowledge, and the process of elimination to make a selection.

19 **Answer: 3 Rationale:** Mosquitoes, the vectors that transport encephalitis, are found in large numbers in swampy areas. The risk of acquiring meningitis increases when clients live in overcrowded living conditions. Parkinson's has an uncertain etiology that is not related to insects as vectors. Risk factors for multiple sclerosis include genetics and family history. **Cognitive Level:** Applying **Client Need:** Physiological Adaptation **Integrated Process:** Nursing Process: Assessment **Content Area:** Adult Health: Neurological **Strategy:** The core issue of the question is knowledge of risk factors for encephalitis. Use nursing knowledge and the process of elimination to make a selection.

20 **Answer: 2 Rationale:** Guillain-Barré syndrome is an acute demyelinating disorder that less commonly may present with initial, downward-progressing weakness in the cranial nerves. Impairment of cranial nerves IX and X will affect swallowing. Guillain-Barré syndrome is not caused by obstructed blood flow to the brain. Parotitis could cause enlargement of parotid and salivary glands. Vitamin deficiencies could occur with any condition leading to malabsorption but are not an etiology for Guillain-Barré syndrome. **Cognitive Level:** Applying **Client Need:** Physiological Adaptation **Integrated Process:** Nursing Process: Implementation **Content Area:** Adult Health: Neurological **Strategy:** The core issue of the question is the ability to explain pathophysiology underlying signs and symptoms of Guillain-Barré syndrome. Use nursing knowledge and the process of elimination to make a selection.

21 **Answer: 1, 2, 4 Rationale:** The client could be at risk for sustaining injury because of spasticity. Spasticity as well as age-related factors could lead to difficulty. At this age, a 1-year-old is beginning to speak. This child will have trouble developing language because of the spasticity. Thought processes are difficult to evaluate in a 1-year-old. A 1-year-old client does not have the cognitive development to be self-conscious or develop a body image. **Cognitive Level:** Analyzing **Client Need:** Physiological Adaptation **Integrated Process:** Nursing Process: Diagnosis **Content Area:** Child Health **Strategy:** The core issue of the question is the ability to determine appropriate clinical problems for a client with cerebral palsy while taking into consideration growth and development. Use nursing knowledge and the process of elimination to make a selection.

22 **Answer: 2 Rationale:** Observation and documentation of seizure activity can provide valuable information to help in diagnosis and treatment. Once a seizure is in process, it would be dangerous to attempt to insert an airway. Administration of medication would require a healthcare provider prescription. Restraining the extremities is more likely to inflict injury than prevent it. **Cognitive Level:** Applying **Client Need:** Safety and Infection Control **Integrated Process:** Nursing Process: Implementation **Content Area:** Child Health **Strategy:** The core issue of the question is the ability to provide safe care to a child experiencing a seizure. Use nursing knowledge and the process of elimination to make a selection.

23 **Answer: 4 Rationale:** An altered level of consciousness would be a symptom of shunt malfunction for the older child, whose cranial suture lines have fused and fontanelles have closed. A bulging soft spot, expanding head size, and sunset eyes are signs common at an earlier age before cranial suture lines have fused and fontanelles have closed. **Cognitive Level:** Applying **Client Need:** Physiological Adaptation **Integrated Process:** Nursing Process: Evaluation **Content Area:** Child Health **Strategy:** The core issue of the question is knowledge of early signs of rising intracranial pressure, which is a sign of shunt malfunction. Use nursing knowledge and the process of elimination to make a selection.

24 **Answer: 2 Rationale:** Drainage of cerebrospinal fluid (a clear fluid) from the ear is a symptom of basilar skull fracture. Children with linear skull fractures are often asymptomatic. Subdural and epidural hematomas present with signs of increasing intracranial pressure. **Cognitive Level:** Analyzing **Client Need:** Physiological Adaptation **Integrated Process:** Nursing Process: Diagnosis **Content Area:** Child Health **Strategy:** The core issue of the question is the ability to interpret signs of head injury correctly. Use nursing knowledge and the process of elimination to make a selection.

25 **Answer: 3 Rationale:** It is important for the nurse to learn about family members' perceptions of what is going on and their current needs. The best way to determine this is to encourage

them to ask questions and express their feelings. While families may need education about seatbelts, this can occur at a later time. While families may benefit from community support services, this can occur after the child's likely outcome is better known. Timelines for visitation are appropriate but of less priority than open communication with the family.

Cognitive Level: Analyzing **Client Need:** Psychosocial Integrity **Integrated Process:** Nursing Process: Planning **Content Area:** Child Health **Strategy:** The core issue of the question is the ability to determine priorities for the family of a critically ill child. Select the option that will most closely address the family's current issues and concerns.

Key Terms to Review

agnosia p. 977
aphasia p. 968
apraxia p. 977
autonomic hyperreflexia p. 975
bradykinesia p. 981
Broca's area p. 964
Brudzinski sign p. 968
coma p. 969
Cushing's triad p. 970
diplegia p. 985
dysarthria p. 968
dysphagia p. 977
epidural hematoma p. 972
homonymous hemianopsia p. 977
hemiparesis p. 976
hemiplegia p. 971
intracranial pressure (ICP) p. 970
intrathecal p. 989
Kernig sign p. 968
level of consciousness (LOC) p. 966
meninges p. 965
neurogenic p. 986
nuchal rigidity p. 989
opisthotonus p. 989
paraplegia p. 974
photophobia p. 989
spasticity p. 981
stereotypy p. 991
subdural hematoma p. 973
tetraplegia p. 974
tonic-clonic p. 979
Wernicke's area p. 964

References

Ball, J., & Bindler, R., & Cowen, K. (2015). *Principles of pediatric nursing: Caring for children* (6th ed.). Hoboken, NJ: Pearson Education.

Berman, A., Snyder, S., & Frandsen, G. (2016). *Kozier & Erb's fundamentals of nursing: Concepts, process, and practice* (10th ed.). New York, NY: Pearson Education.

Ignatavicius, D., & Workman, L. (2016). *Medical-surgical nursing: Patient-centered collaborative care* (10th ed.). Philadelphia: Saunders.

LeMone, P., Burke, K., Bauldoff, G., & Gubrud, P. (2015). *Medical surgical nursing: Clinical reasoning in patient care* (6th ed.). Hoboken, NJ: Pearson Education.

Lewis, S., Dirksen, S., Heitkemper, M., & Bucher, L. (2014). *Medical surgical nursing: Assessment and management of clinical problems* (9th ed.). St. Louis, MO: Elsevier Science.

Smith, S., Duell, D., Martin, B., Aebersold, M., & Gonzalez, L. (2017). *Clinical nursing skills: Basic to advanced skills* (10th ed.). New York, NY: Pearson Education.

Test Yourself

Are you ready for the NCLEX-RN® or course exams? Access the NEW web-based app that provides students with thousands of practice questions in preparation for the NCLEX experience.

Renal or Genitourinary Disorders 58

In this chapter

Cross Reference

Other chapters relevant to this content area are

Meeting Nutritional Needs	**Chapter 25**
Renal Medications	**Chapter 39**
Common Laboratory Tests	**Chapter 46**
Common Diagnostic Tests and Procedures	**Chapter 47**
Perioperative Care	**Chapter 48**

I. OVERVIEW OF ANATOMY AND PHYSIOLOGY OF RENAL AND URINARY SYSTEMS

A. Renal structures

1. Kidneys: bean-shaped organs located on either side of spinal column behind peritoneal cavity
2. Adrenal glands: located atop each kidney; influence blood pressure (BP) and sodium (Na^+) and water retention

3. Renal cortex: outer region of kidneys; contains blood-filtering mechanisms
4. Renal medulla: middle region of kidneys; contains renal pyramids (with tubules in apex and calyces) to collect and channel urine to renal pelvis; renal cortex and medulla are referred to as kidney parenchyma
5. Renal pelvis: expansion of upper end of ureters, formed as calyces join together
6. **Nephron**: functional unit of kidneys; selectively secretes and reabsorbs ions; filters fluid, wastes, electrolytes, acids, and bases; contains a **glomerulus** surrounded by Bowman's capsule

B. Function of kidneys

1. Nephrons filter waste products as well as needed materials, such as electrolytes, from blood; necessary substances are returned to blood through reabsorption
2. Filtration: first step in blood processing; water and solutes move from plasma in glomerulus into Bowman's capsule because of pressure gradient
3. Reabsorption: second step in urine formation; molecules move from tubules into blood through tubule cells; active and passive transport mechanisms are used in all parts of renal tubules
   a. Proximal tubules: reabsorb sodium (Na^+) and other major ions
   b. Loop of Henle: reabsorbs through countercurrent mechanism; contents flow in opposite directions
   c. Distal tubules: reabsorb Na^+ in smaller amounts than proximal tubules
   d. Collecting ducts: prevent water from leaving filtrate
4. Tubular secretion: movement of selected substances out of blood into tubular fluid
5. Regulation of urine volume: hormones play a central part in urine regulation
6. Osmolality: osmotic pressure of a solution expressed as a number of osmols of pressure per kg of water; active transport and reabsorption mechanisms are based on osmolality of solutions

C. Renal hormones and enzymes (see Table 58–1)

D. Urinary excretion

1. Ureters: extend from renal pelvis of kidney to urinary bladder; conduct urine
2. Bladder: elastic sac located behind symphysis pubis; stores and excretes urine
3. Urethra: tube that carries urine from bladder to exterior of body
4. Urinary meatus: exterior opening of urethra
5. Urination: an involuntary or voluntary reflex allowing urine to leave body
   a. Micturition reflex: parasympathetic response that stimulates relaxation and contraction of external sphincter, allowing urine to pass
   b. Internal sphincter muscle: helps control urine passage into urethra; relaxes in response to parasympathetic nerve fibers in bladder wall
   c. External sphincter muscle: voluntary muscle that allows urine to pass into urethra; controlled by micturition reflex

NCLEX®

6. Characteristics of normal urine
   a. Color: clear, pale amber
   b. Consistency: 95% water with many dissolved substances
   c. Output: 1000–2000 mL per 24-hour period; kidneys produce a minimum of 30 mL/hour (0.5 mg/kg/hr) under normal circumstances

Table 58–1 Functions of Renal Hormones and Enzymes

Hormone or Enzyme	Function
Antidiuretic hormone (ADH)	Acts in distal tubule and collecting ducts to increase water reabsorption and urine concentration
Atrial natriuretic hormone (ANH)	Secreted by muscle fibers in atria of heart; promotes sodium (Na^+) loss via urine
Aldosterone	Secreted by adrenal cortex; increases Na^+ absorption in tubules and controls potassium (K^+) secretion, leading to osmotic imbalance that causes reabsorption of water; works in conjunction with ADH Increased serum K^+ levels lead to increased aldosterone secretion Increased aldosterone secretion increases Na^+ and water retention and depresses formation of renin
Renin	Enzyme secreted by kidneys; helps regulate Na^+ retention and therefore BP and fluid volume Renin-angiotensin system converts angiotensinogen to angiotensin I in liver Angiotensin I forms angiotensin II in lungs, a vasoconstrictor that stimulates adrenal cortex to produce aldosterone
Erythropoietin	Hormone produced by kidneys in response to low oxygen (O_2) levels in arterial blood; travels to bone marrow and stimulates increased red blood cell (RBC) production

d. Specific gravity: commonly 1.015–1.025 (range 1.010–1.030)
e. Odor: faint ammonia

E. Renal system differences between child and adult

1. Fluid is more important to body chemistry of infants and small children because it constitutes a larger fraction of total body weight
2. During first 2 years of life, kidneys are less efficient at regulating electrolyte and acid–base balance; infants are more prone to fluid volume excess and dehydration
3. Bladder capacity increases from 20–50 mL at birth to 700 mL in adulthood
4. Innervation of "stretch" receptors in bladder wall, which initiates urination and control of bladder sphincters (does not occur before age 2); children under 2 cannot maintain bladder control
5. Urethra is shorter in children and may contribute to frequency of urinary infections in children
6. Kidneys are more susceptible to trauma in children because they do not have as much fat padding

II. DIAGNOSTIC TESTS AND ASSESSMENTS OF URINARY SYSTEM

A. Physical assessment

1. Appearance of meatus: normal position and lack of redness, swelling
2. Voiding pattern: frequency, amount, hesitancy, urgency, dysuria

B. Urine studies

1. Urinalysis: obtained for dipstick results, microscopic examination, or culture; refer to Chapter 46 for normal results and Table 58–2 for significance of color changes
2. Clean-catch specimen: collected in a clean specimen container after cleaning urinary meatus and surrounding tissue; infants and toddlers might be catheterized; parental assistance is needed for school-age, toilet-trained children; adolescents obtain own specimens after instruction
3. Sterile urine specimen: obtained by urinary catheterization only
4. Urine culture: checks urine for bacteria; urine is normally sterile
5. Twenty-four-hour urine specimen: urine is collected over 24 hours for these substances:
   a. **Creatinine**: nitrogenous waste product excreted by muscle tissue; normally found in urine (normal = 15–25 mg/kg in 24 hours)
   b. Creatinine clearance: test to assess how well the kidneys remove creatinine from blood (male = 95–135 mL/min; female = 85–125 mL/min)
   c. Protein: less than 150 mg/24 hours
   d. Urea nitrogen: end product of protein metabolism (normal = 6–17 grams/24 hours)
6. Urine osmolality: osmotic pressure (concentration) of urine; average is 500–800 mOsm/kg water, with an extreme range of 50–1400 mOsm/kg water

C. Renal scan: intravenous (IV) radioactive substance (radionuclide) is injected, and then observed passing through kidneys; evaluates renal structures and blood flow and nephron and collecting system function

Table 58–2 Interpreting Changes in Urine Color

Color	Possible Meaning
Pale yellow	Normal
Yellow	Concentrated urine
Amber	Bile in urine
Orange	Alkaline or concentrated urine
Red-orange	Acidic urine, medication effect
Red	Blood, menses
Pink	Dilute blood
Burgundy	Laxatives
Tea	Melanin, hematuria
Dark gray	Medications, dyes
Blue	Dyes, medications

D. Radiographic studies (see also Chapter 47)

1. Kidney–ureter–bladder (KUB) radiography: shows kidney size, position, and structure as well as ureters and bladder; provides limited diagnostic information
2. Renal angiography: detects abnormalities such as cysts, renal artery stenosis, and renal infarction
3. Renal venography: detects renal vein thrombosis
4. Retrograde cystography: contrast medium instilled into bladder via a catheter, followed by x-ray examination; several films are taken and dye is then drained via catheter; a final picture is taken when bladder is emptied; helps diagnose ruptured or neurogenic bladder and other conditions
5. Voiding cystourethrography: same process as a cystogram except when bladder is filled with contrast dye, urethral catheter is removed; client is allowed to void when urge is felt; films are taken during bladder filling, during **micturition** (voiding), and after voiding

E. Computerized tomography (CT) scan: identifies masses and other lesions; contrast medium may be injected

F. Magnetic resonance imaging (MRI): produces three-dimensional images of renal tissue

G. Ultrasonography: evaluates kidney size, shape, and position

H. Blood studies

1. *Blood urea nitrogen (BUN)*: measures nitrogenous urea in blood from protein metabolism; insufficient excretion causes level to rise and may indicate renal disease; also rises with dehydration, intake of high-protein diet, and other conditions in which excess protein is metabolized
   a. Normal: 8–22 mg/dL (3.6–7.1 mmol/L)
   b. BUN levels best evaluated in conjunction with serum creatinine levels
2. Serum creatinine: a nitrogenous waste in blood resulting from muscle metabolism of creatine; creatinine levels reflect glomerular filtration rate
   a. Measures renal damage more reliably than BUN because severe renal damage is single cause of significant elevation
   b. Normal: 0.6–1.3 mg/dL (44–133 micromol/L)

I. *Intravenous pyelography (IVP)*: series of x-rays of renal pelvis and ureters after injection of a contrast medium; special preprocedure care may be necessary

J. Cystoscopy or cystourethroscopy: insertion of a cystoscope with a fiberoptic light source and telescopic lens into urethra for biopsy of bladder and prostate, lesion resection, calculi collection, or passage of catheter to renal pelvis

K. Percutaneous renal biopsy: client is positioned on abdomen while needle is inserted into kidney to remove tissue; x-ray may be used to guide needle; reveals renal disease, malignant tumors, and other conditions; risks include bleeding, hematoma, arteriovenous fistula, and infection

III. COMMON NURSING TECHNIQUES AND PROCEDURES

A. Urinary catheterization: introduction of a catheter into urinary bladder

1. Indwelling urinary catheter: a retention (Foley) catheter with balloon is inserted and remains in place; see Box 58–1
2. Intermittent catheterization: used for clients with neurogenic bladder dysfunction; may be done by nurse or at home by client after instruction on procedure (Box 58–2)

Box 58–1

Insertion of an Indwelling Urinary Catheter

1. Explain procedure to client and ensure privacy.
2. *Female*: assist client to supine position with knees flexed and thighs externally rotated; drape client.
3. Wearing disposable gloves, cleanse perineal area; remove gloves.
4. Prepare equipment and sterile field; don clean gloves to position sterile drape under client's buttocks, touching only outer margins of drape; remove gloves and apply sterile gloves; drape client with sterile fenestrated drape.
5. Moisten sterile cotton balls with antiseptic solution (per agency policy) and lubricate catheter tip with sterile water-soluble lubricant.
6. Attach syringe prefilled with sterile water to catheter balloon port for inflation after insertion.
7. Use nondominant hand to separate labia minora and expose urinary meatus; assess meatus for swelling, discharge, or redness.
8. Clean meatus three times with antiseptic-moistened cotton balls, using fresh cotton ball each time.

9. Grasp catheter near insertion end with sterile, gloved hand; gently insert catheter into meatus and advance catheter 5 cm (2 in.) until urine flows; do not use forceful pressure; ask client to take deep breaths to relax external sphincter.
10. Advance catheter gently an additional 2.5–3.5 cm (1–1.5 in.) and inflate balloon by injecting contents of prefilled syringe. If client feels pain with balloon inflation, aspirate syringe contents (balloon may be in urethra).
11. Apply slight tension by pulling back on catheter until resistance is felt to confirm balloon placement in bladder.
12. Anchor catheter to client's thigh with nonallergic tape and secure drainage bag to bed frame below level of bladder.
13. *Male*: use same positioning except knees do not need to be flexed and no drape needs to be placed under buttocks.
14. Wearing disposable gloves, wash penis and dry it well.
15. Follow catheter preparatory steps as described above.
16. Grasp insertion end of catheter with sterile, gloved hand; lift penis to 90-degree angle with body and exert slight traction.
17. Insert catheter steadily about 25–30 cm (10–12 in.) until urine begins to flow; ask client to take deep breaths to relax external sphincter on insertion; rotate catheter during insertion if slight resistance is met because of curvature of urethra.
18. Advance catheter an additional 2.5–5 cm (1–2 in.) and inflate balloon by injecting contents of prefilled syringe; secure as described above.

Box 58–2

Client Instructions for Intermittent Urinary Self-Catheterization

- Catheterize as often as needed; may be every 2–3 hours at first, then every 4–6 hours.
- Encourage client to void before procedure if appropriate; use catheter to obtain residual urine if amount voided is less than 100 mL.
- Assemble all supplies and use good lighting.
- Wash hands.
- Clean urinary meatus with towelette or soapy washcloth, then rinse and dry; female clients should clean perineum from front to back.
- Assume comfortable position, such as standing with one foot elevated, semireclining in bed, or sitting on chair or toilet.
- Apply lubricant to catheter tip and place other end of catheter in container to catch urine.
- *Female*: locate meatus using a mirror or touch; separate labia with dominant hand; direct catheter through meatus, then forward and upward.
- *Male*: hold penis with slight upward tension to 90-degree angle and insert catheter.
- Advance catheter 8 cm (3 in.) for females or 18–25 cm (7–10 in.) for males until urine flows.
- Press down on abdominal muscles to promote bladder emptying.
- Hold catheter in place until all urine is drained, then pinch off catheter and withdraw slowly.
- Wash and dry perineal area. For males, replace foreskin if present.
- Wash catheter with soap and warm water, rinse with clear water, and dry outside with paper towel; store in clean container.
- Perform hand hygiene.
- Use catheter for recommended amount of time (often 2–4 weeks) then discard and use new one.
- Notify healthcare provider of cloudy urine, sediment, bleeding, fever, or difficulty passing catheter.
- Drink at least 2000–2500 mL of fluid daily; cranberry and prune juices help to acidify urine to possibly reduce bacterial growth in bladder.

B. Urine collection

1. Twenty-four-hour urine collection
   a. Obtain specimen container with preservative from laboratory
   b. Provide clean receptacle to collect urine (bedpan, urinal, commode, or collection device on toilet) unless client already has an indwelling urinary catheter
   c. Post signs in client's room, chart, and bathroom alerting staff to save urine
   NCLEX® d. Have client void and discard first urine at beginning of collection period; if indwelling catheter used, empty collection bag at start time and discard
   e. During collection period, save all urine in container; place container on ice or refrigerate as indicated; don't contaminate urine with bathroom tissue or feces
   NCLEX® f. Instruct client to empty bladder at end of collection period and save this urine
   g. Send collected urine to laboratory with completed requisition
   h. Document collection of specimen, time started and completed, and any observations
2. Clean catch (midstream)
   a. Ask client to wash genital and perineal area with soap and water from front to back
   b. Instruct to clean meatus with antiseptic towelettes
   c. Female clients: use three towelettes; clean perineal area from front to back; use each towelette once
   d. Male clients: clean meatus with circular motion and distal portion of penis; use each towelette once
   e. For client who needs assistance: nurse may don gloves, clean perineal area, assist client to a comfortable position, and open clean-catch kit
   f. Instruct client to begin voiding, then place specimen container in stream of urine; collect 30–60 mL
   g. Cap container, touching only outside
   h. Label container, place in biohazard bag with requisition, and immediately send to laboratory
   i. Document pertinent data, such as difficulty voiding, strong odor to urine, or sediment

C. *Peritoneal dialysis*: removes toxins from blood of client with renal failure; uses peritoneal membrane as semipermeable dialyzing membrane (see Figure 58–1A)

1. Hypertonic dialyzing solution (dialysate) is instilled through a catheter in peritoneal cavity
2. Excess electrolytes and uremic toxins move by diffusion across peritoneal membrane into dialysate; excess water also moves into solution by osmosis
3. Dialysate is drained after appropriate dwelling time
4. Procedure is performed manually or using a cycler machine; client may also perform continuous ambulatory peritoneal dialysis (CAPD)
5. NCLEX® Possible complications
   a. Peritonitis from bacteria entering peritoneal cavity (use surgical aseptic technique when handling catheter or tubing); critical to prevent because it could require a change in therapy to hemodialysis (see section that follows)
   b. Catheter obstruction (keep all lines unobstructed; add heparin to dialysate per protocol)
   c. Insufficient outflow (reposition client to bring fluid into contact with catheter; allow ambulation if condition permits)
   d. Hypotension and hypovolemia from excess fluid removal (carefully monitor intake and output [I&O] records)
   e. Hyperglycemia (from glucose in dialysate; monitor diabetic clients closely; do not allow fluid to dwell longer than prescribed)
6. NCLEX® Peritoneal dialysis procedure (see Box 58–3, p. 1006)

D. Care of an arteriovenous (AV) fistula

1. An AV fistula provides vascular access to a vein and an artery for hemodialysis; most common sites are radial or brachial artery and cephalic vein
2. NCLEX® Assess circulation at access site by auscultating for bruits and palpating for thrills; lack of bruit may indicate blood clot and requires immediate surgical intervention
3. NCLEX® Avoid using accessed arm for other procedures, such as IV insertion, BP monitoring, or venipuncture
4. Monitor site for bleeding after completion of hemodialysis
5. Home care instructions for client
   a. Keep fistula area clean and dry
   b. Notify healthcare provider of pain, swelling, redness, or drainage in accessed arm
   c. Exercise is beneficial and helps stimulate vein enlargement
   NCLEX® d. Don't allow any treatments or procedures on accessed arm

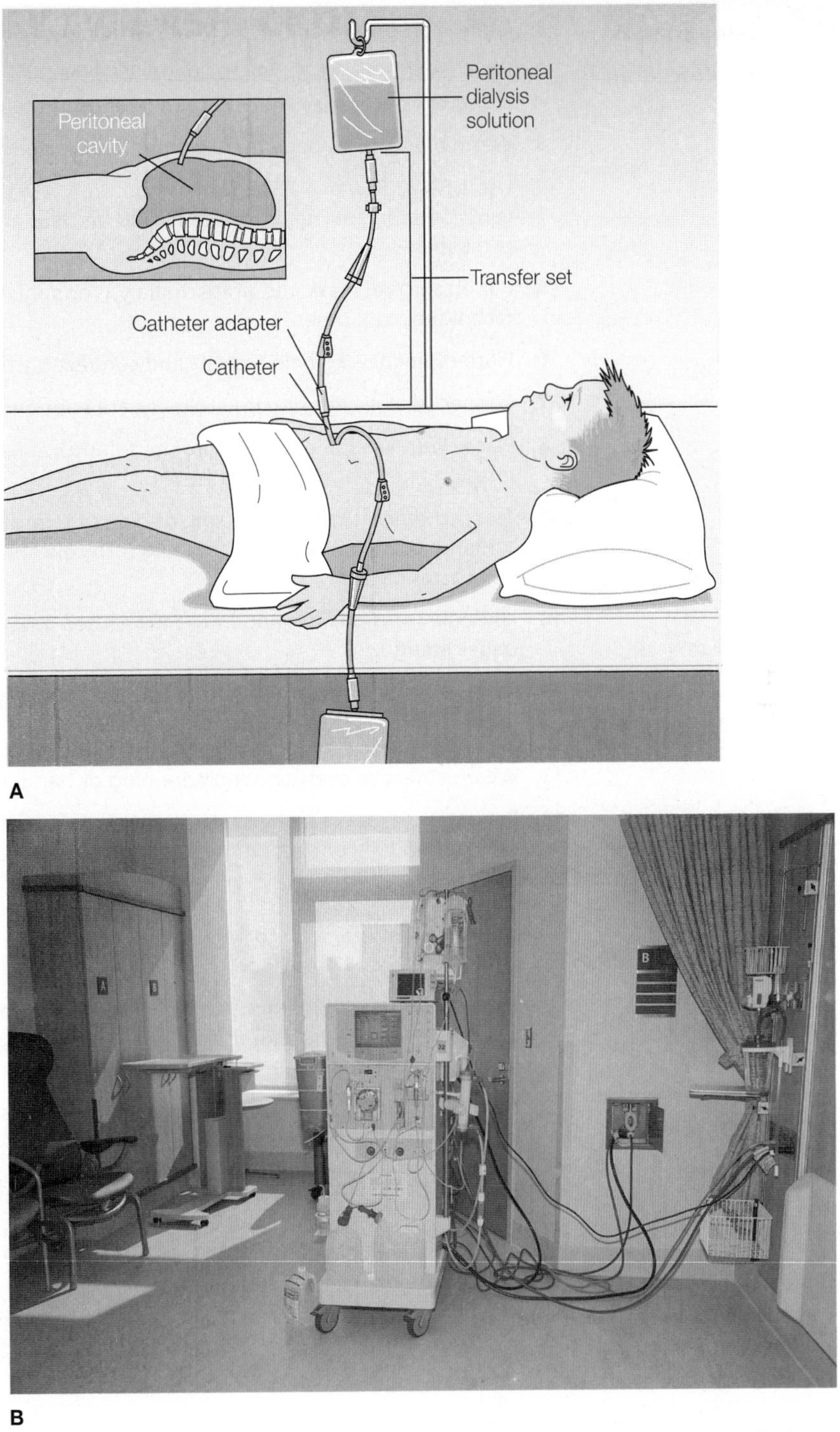

Figure 58–1

(**A**) Peritoneal dialysis; (**B**) hemodialysis.

NCLEX®

e. Avoid excessive pressure to arm; don't sleep on it, wear constrictive clothing or jewelry, or lift heavy objects

f. Avoid showering, bathing, or swimming for several hours after dialysis

E. ***Hemodialysis***: removes wastes from body by filtering client's blood using a machine intermittently connected to client (see Figure 58–1B)

1. Nurses who have undergone specialized instruction and training perform hemodialysis

NCLEX®

2. Before procedure, weigh client and take vital signs (VS); check BP in lying and standing positions (orthostatic BPs); check for scheduled medications that should be withheld until after dialysis (i.e., antihypertensives that could lower BP, drugs that would be dialyzed out of circulation, or once-daily drugs that can be given postdialysis)

NCLEX®

3. Wear protective eyewear, gown, and gloves for protection during hemodialysis procedure

Box 58–3

Peritoneal Dialysis Procedure

1. Explain procedure and check vital signs and weight.
2. Have client urinate, if able, to avoid bladder puncture or discomfort upon initial catheter insertion; perform catheterization if client is unable to void.
3. Warm dialysate to body temperature in a warmer.
4. Use 1.5%, 2.5%, or 4.25% dextrose solution, usually with heparin added to prevent catheter clotting; dialysate should be clear and colorless; add medication as prescribed.
5. Put on surgical mask and prepare dialysis administration set, maintaining strict sterile technique at all times.
6. Place drainage bag below client and connect outflow tubing.
7. Connect dialysis infusion line to dialysate bags and hang on IV pole.
8. Place client in supine position, prime tubing with solution, close clamps, and connect infusion line to abdominal catheter.
9. Test catheter by instilling 500 mL of dialysate into peritoneal cavity; clamp tubing; unclamp outflow line and drain fluid into collection bag; if outflow is brisk, then catheter is patent.
10. Unclamp infusion lines and infuse prescribed amount of dialysate; close clamps when bag is empty.
11. Allow solution to dwell for prescribed time (usually up to 4 hours).
12. Open outflow clamps and allow solution to drain.
13. Wear protective eyewear when draining or handling outflow solution.
14. Repeat cycle for prescribed number of times; when completed, clamp peritoneal catheter and disconnect inflow line while wearing sterile gloves.
15. Apply sterile dressing to catheter site.
16. During procedure, monitor vital signs every 10 to 15 minutes until stable, then every 2 to 4 hours or as prescribed.
17. Observe for signs of peritonitis: fever; persistent abdominal pain and cramping; slow or cloudy dialysate drainage; swelling, redness, or tenderness around catheter; increased WBC count.
18. Check outflow tubing periodically for clots or kinks; have client change position to increase flow.
19. Clients lose protein during peritoneal dialysis and require fewer or no dietary restrictions of protein.
20. Calculate fluid balance at end of each exchange (with manual dialysis), or at end of each session, or every 8 hours, depending on protocol; include oral and IV intake, urine output (UO), and wound drainage in calculations.

4. Dialysis is continued usually for 3–4 hours; monitor partial thromboplastin time (PTT) or other standard laboratory studies as per protocol (heparin is used as an anticoagulant during procedure)
5. At end of treatment, obtain blood samples as prescribed, return blood remaining in dialyzer to client, and remove needles from vascular access device
6. Monitor access device for bleeding and maintain pressure on site as needed

NCLEX®

7. Early in course of hemodialysis, assess for and report disequilibrium syndrome, in which cerebral edema forms from less rapid excretion of wastes behind blood–brain barrier, and subsequent uptake of fluid by brain cells and cerebral edema
    a. Assess client for headache, confusion, restlessness or agitation, nausea and vomiting (N/V), muscle twitching, and possible seizure activity
    b. Stop dialysis procedure and reduce environmental stimuli
    c. Obtain necessary prescriptions for mannitol, albumin, or hypertonic saline
    d. Prevent occurrence by dialyzing for shorter times or at reduced blood flow rates early in therapy

IV. NURSING MANAGEMENT OF CLIENT HAVING RENAL OR BLADDER SURGERY

A. ***Lithotripsy***: also called extracorporeal shock-wave lithotripsy (ESWL); uses high-energy shock waves to break up calculi, restoring normal passage of urine
1. Perform preprocedure teaching: procedure is noninvasive and treatment takes 30 minutes to 1 hour; client will receive a general or epidural anesthetic
2. Postprocedure care
a. Perform baseline assessment and check VS following agency policy
b. Maintain patency of indwelling urinary catheter and monitor I&O

NCLEX®
c. Strain urine for calculi fragments and send these to laboratory for analysis
d. Slight hematuria is common, but report persistent bleeding
e. Encourage ambulation to aid passage of calculi fragments

NCLEX®
f. Increase fluid intake as prescribed to aid passage of calculi fragments
g. Give analgesics as needed; severe pain may indicate presence of new calculi—report such findings immediately

NCLEX®
3. Home care instructions for client
a. Drink 3–4 L of fluid daily up to 1 month after treatment
b. Strain urine during first week and save any calculi fragments; bring these to first follow-up healthcare provider visit
c. Expect blood-tinged urine, mild GI upset, and pain in treated side as calculi fragments pass; bruising on affected side will disappear
d. Report severe pain, persistent blood in urine, inability to void, fever and chills, or N/V
e. Review prescribed medications or dietary regimen

B. **Percutaneous lithotripsy**
1. An invasive method of lithotripsy guided by fluoroscopy during cystoscopy or nephroscopy procedure
2. Uses ultrasonic waves aimed at stones in bladder, ureter, or kidney to shatter them into fragments
3. Explain that client will not have an incision if cystoscopy is used, but will have a small flank incision for nephroscopy
4. Client may have indwelling urinary catheter and may have a nephrostomy tube (if nephroscopy performed) for 1–5 days postprocedure for administration of irrigations to break down stone(s)
5. Monitor for complications of hemorrhage, infection, and possible leakage of fluid into retroperitoneal cavity (may be asymptomatic or lead to back or posterior abdominal discomfort)

NCLEX®
6. Postprocedure instructions include drinking 3–4 L of fluid daily as prescribed and measures recommended after other forms of lithotripsy

C. **Ureterolithotomy, pyelolithotomy, nephrolithotomy**: involve making an incision into ureter, renal pelvis, or renal calyx to remove urinary calculi
1. Preoperative period: explain procedure and postoperative care, including presence of a urinary catheter; administer pre-anesthetic medications as prescribed

NCLEX®
2. Postoperative period
a. Perform baseline and ongoing postoperative assessments (VS, LOC, status of dressing)
b. Monitor UO for amount, color, and clarity; urine may be bright red initially, but bleeding should diminish; cloudy urine may indicate infection
c. Maintain placement and patency of urinary catheters; irrigate gently as prescribed
d. Assess for pain and administer analgesics as needed
e. Increase client's fluid intake, as prescribed, to aid passage of calculi fragments
f. Strain urine for calculi fragments and send them to laboratory for analysis
3. Home care for client
a. Follow agency policy for home incision care

NCLEX®
b. Drink 3–4 liters of fluid daily up to a month after treatment
c. Report bloody, cloudy, or foul-smelling urine
d. Report inability to void, fever, chills, redness, swelling, or purulent drainage from incision
e. Strain urine during first week and save any calculi fragments; bring them to first follow-up visit with healthcare provider
f. Avoid strenuous exercise, sexual activity, heavy lifting, or straining until advised otherwise by surgeon
g. Mild activity aids passage of any retained calculi fragments
h. Review prescribed medications, dietary regimen, and explain catheter care if client is discharged with indwelling catheter

D. Cystectomy with urinary diversion

1. Complete radical **cystectomy** involves removal of bladder and adjacent muscles and tissues
   a. In men, prostate gland and seminal vesicles are removed, which results in impotence
   b. In women, uterus, Fallopian tubes, and ovaries are removed, resulting in sterility
   c. A urinary diversion is created to provide for urine collection and drainage
2. **Urinary diversion**: a procedure that provides an alternative route for urine excretion when normal channels are damaged or defective
   a. Ileal conduit: reroutes urine by connecting ureters to tubular pouch created from a segment of ileum and brought to skin surface to form a stoma; urine drains continuously via pouch
   b. Cutaneous ureterostomy: diverts ureter(s) to abdominal skin surface to form a stoma
   c. Continent urinary reservoir: connects ureters to a reservoir (pouch) created from a portion of ileum; a nipple-like valve is created, which allows client to self-catheterize pouch after full healing and eliminates need to wear a pouch over stoma; see Figure 58–2
   d. Sigmoidostomies: divert urine by connecting ureters to sigmoid colon or to tubular portion of ileum that is connected to sigmoid colon; urine is eliminated with stool; no stoma is required but bowel incontinence could result
   e. Nephrostomy: urine drains through a catheter placed directly into kidney; used when a ureter is blocked or damaged; may be temporary; does not involve bladder
3. Preoperative period
   a. Reduce anxiety through preoperative teaching about procedure and postoperative course and care; client may awaken with nasogastric tube, IV, indwelling urinary catheter, Penrose drain, or other drains
   b. Assess client's support systems and ability to care for self after surgery
   c. Address concerns about possible body image changes and loss of sexual or reproductive function
   d. *NCLEX®* Begin bowel preparations about 4 days prior to surgery
   e. Administer antibiotics (usually erythromycin and neomycin) before surgery to reduce bacteria count in bowel, as prescribed
   f. *NCLEX®* Administer enema on night before surgery to clear fecal matter from bowel as prescribed
   g. Administer preanesthetic medications as prescribed
4. Postoperative period
   a. Perform standard postoperative assessments and care (see also Chapter 48)
   b. *NCLEX®* Monitor amount and character of UO every hour; report output less than 30 mL/hour
   c. Assess urine color and consistency; may be pink or red initially, fading to pink and clearing by third postoperative day; cloudy urine may result from mucus production by bowel tissue
   d. Administer prescribed analgesic and antispasmodic medications as needed
5. Urinary diversion stoma care
   a. *NCLEX®* Assess size, color, and condition of stoma and surrounding skin every 2 hours for 24 hours, and then every 4 hours for 2–3 days (stoma should be bright pink or red and edematous initially; suspect a problem if it is pale, deep red, purple, or bluish in color); slight bleeding during initial cleansing is normal

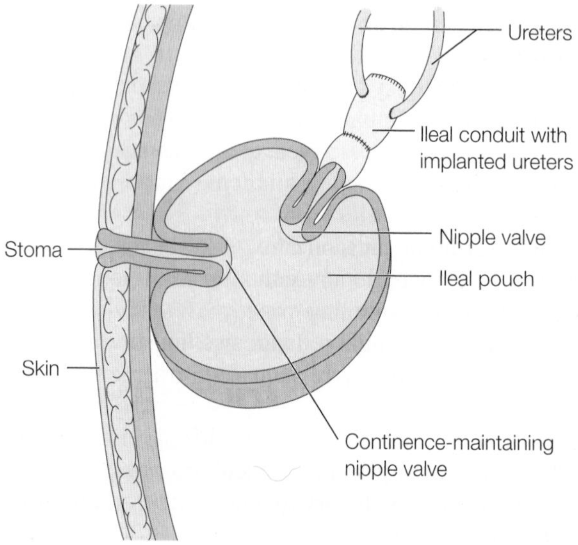

Figure 58–2

A continent urinary diversion. A segment of ileum is separated from the small intestine and formed into a pouch. Nipple valves are formed at each end of pouch by intussuscepting tissue backward into a reservoir to prevent leakage.

b. Observe incision for signs of infection (redness and purulent drainage); change dressing per agency policy or as prescribed
c. Irrigate diversion catheter with 30–60 mL normal saline every 4 hours or as prescribed
NCLEX® d. Collection device should fit snugly around stoma; allow no more than 0.3–cm (⅛-in.) margin of skin between stoma and faceplate
NCLEX® e. Check peristomal skin for breakdown; main cause of irritation is urine leakage; change device and cleanse skin if leakage occurs
f. Cleanse area with warm water and pat dry; apply light coating of karaya powder and thin layer of protective dressing
g. Notify healthcare provider if severe skin excoriation occurs
h. Assess I&O; note changes in urine color, odor, or clarity

NCLEX® 6. Client teaching for home care
a. Instruct client to report fever, chills, flank pain, abdominal pain, cloudy urine, pus (**pyuria**) or blood in urine (**hematuria**), incisional redness, or decline in UO
b. Weakness, incisional pain, and fatigue may persist for some weeks
c. Appliance is often a one-piece unit (faceplate and collection bag) and must be emptied regularly and changed according to product directions
d. Encourage client to change appliance as needed in early morning when urine production is less because of no fluid intake during sleep
e. Expect stoma shrinkage within 8 weeks after surgery; may require smaller pouch opening
f. Instruct in stoma care and provide supplies as needed; refer client to support organization, such as United Ostomy Association

E. **Ureteral stent**: catheter used to maintain patency and promote healing of ureters; may be temporary after surgery or for longer periods in clients with a damaged ureter
1. Stent is positioned during surgery or cystoscopy
2. Nursing care
a. If stent has been brought to surface, secure it and maintain its position
b. Monitor UO, including color, consistency, and odor
c. Observe for signs of infection, obstruction, or bleeding, including fever, tachycardia, cloudy urine, pain, hematuria
d. Maintain fluid intake
e. If stent is semipermanent, instruct client and family in its care

F. ***Nephrectomy***: removal of kidney
1. Preoperative period
a. Provide standard preoperative care (see also Chapter 48)
b. Reduce anxiety through preoperative teaching about procedure and postoperative course and care; client may awaken with nasogastric tube, IV, indwelling urinary catheter, Penrose drain, or other drains
c. Assess client's support systems and ability to care for self after surgery
d. Assess baseline urinary status
2. Postoperative period
NCLEX® a. Provide standard postoperative care (see Chapter 48); be vigilant with pain management and pulmonary hygiene measures because high abdominal or flank incision could cause pain with deep breathing and coughing
NCLEX® b. Assess client's fluid and electrolyte status and urine specific gravity; monitor hemoglobin and hematocrit because of expected blood loss during nephrectomy
NCLEX® c. Monitor for UO of 30–50 mL hourly for adequate renal function; report UO less than 30 mL/hour
d. Observe for signs of urinary infection: fever, redness at surgical site, cloudy urine, or discharge
e. Assess placement, patency, and drainage from wound or urinary catheters, stents, nephrostomy tubes, or drains; do not manipulate nephrostomy tube or irrigate unless prescribed
f. Reinforce surgical dressing as needed; assess under client for bleeding through surgical dressing
g. Monitor for signs of adrenal insufficiency (if adrenal gland removed with kidney), which include large urine output from drop in adrenal hormone levels, followed by possible oliguria and circulatory collapse
3. Client teaching
a. Importance of protecting remaining kidney by preventing trauma, renal calculi, and UTI
b. Maintain fluid intake of 2000–2500 mL/day to prevent dehydration and maintain good urine flow
c. Gradually increase activity; avoid heavy lifting for 1 year; do not participate in contact sports
d. Care of any indwelling tubes and signs of infection to report to provider

G. Renal transplantation

1. Preoperative period
   a. Reduce anxiety by teaching about procedure and postoperative course and care; encourage client to express feelings and ask questions
   b. Assess support systems and ability to care for self after surgery and follow medical regimen
   NCLEX® c. Instruct client that rejection of donated organ is major obstacle in transplantation (see Table 58–3); reassure client that rejection usually isn't life-threatening and client can resume dialysis if needed
   d. Begin administering immunosuppressant drugs; discuss purpose and possible adverse effects; monitor for increased BP and signs of anaphylaxis
   e. Plan for client to undergo dialysis on day before surgery, a cleansing enema, and many laboratory tests
2. Postoperative period
   a. Provide standard postoperative care (see Chapter 48), including pain management
   NCLEX® b. Monitor amount and character of UO hourly; report UO less than 30 mL/hour; maintain urinary catheter patency and closed drainage system
   c. Maintain fluid replacement therapy, calculated to replace urine output over last 30–60 minutes to maintain vascular volume
   d. Monitor VS and hemodynamic pressures closely; possible diuresis post-transplant could lead to hypovolemia and impaired perfusion to kidney
   e. Administer diuretics if prescribed to maintain flow of urine
   NCLEX® f. Assess client's fluid and electrolyte status, BUN and creatinine, and urine creatinine clearance and specific gravity; monitor hemoglobin and hematocrit because of expected blood loss
   g. Assess patency of any wound drainage tubes; reinforce or change dressing as needed; assess for signs of infection
   NCLEX® h. Use special infection control measures: strict aseptic technique with dressing changes or care of drains; limit client's contact with staff and visitors; wear surgical mask when in client's room; monitor WBC count and report high or low results
   NCLEX® i. Observe for signs of tissue rejection: fever; redness, tenderness, and swelling at surgical site; elevated WBC count; decreased UO with increased **proteinuria** (protein in urine); sudden weight gain; hypertension; elevated BP
   NCLEX® j. With a living donor transplant, urine flow should begin immediately after revascularization and connection of ureter to client's bladder; with a cadaver transplant, **anuria** (UO less than 100 mL in 24 hr) could occur for 2 days to 2 weeks, requiring dialysis during this period
   k. Weigh client daily; rapid weight gain may indicate fluid retention
3. Client teaching for home care
   a. Carefully measure and record I&O; notify healthcare provider if UO falls below 600 mL for any 24-hour period
   b. Instruct client how to collect 24-hour urine samples
   NCLEX® c. Advise client to weigh self daily or as prescribed
   d. Drink 2 liters of fluid daily unless advised otherwise

Table 58–3 Renal Transplant Rejection

Description	Manifestations	Management
Hyperacute Occurs within hours of surgery; results from antibody reaction to donor antigens; occurs rarely now because of better histocompatibility assessments	Urine output stops; examination of kidney shows a blue, flaccid appearance	Transplanted kidney must be removed; client must resume hemodialysis until (possibly) another kidney is available
Acute Occurs within days to months after surgery; body mounts an immune system defense against tissue in donor organ	Urine output drops sharply and BUN and creatinine rise; possible fever, graft tenderness, swelling	Increased dosage of immunosuppressant drugs, including steroids and monoclonal antibodies
Chronic Occurs from months to years after surgery; etiology is unclear but may involve immune response to donor tissue	More gradual decline in kidney function, including urine output, BUN, and creatinine; proteinuria may occur	No specific treatment; client must resume hemodialysis caused by loss of graft until or unless another donor kidney is transplanted

NCLEX®
e. Report signs of rejection: redness, warmth, tenderness, or swelling over graft site; fever; decreased UO; elevated BP (obtain and use home BP measuring device)

NCLEX®
f. Avoid crowds and persons with known infections or obviously ill

g. Practice regular, moderate exercise, but avoid heavy lifting or contact sports for at least 3 months; use shoulder but not lap-style seat belts

h. Use and side effects of prescribed medications, including antihypertensives, immunosuppressants, and prophylactic antibiotics

V. RENAL AND URINARY CALCULI

A. Overview

1. Occur when calculi (stones) form in urinary tract (urolithiasis) or more frequently in kidney parenchyma (nephrolithiasis); see Figure 58–3
2. Types of stones: calcium phosphate and/or oxalate (most common type), struvite, uric acid, and cystine (least common type); can be single or multiple and vary in size; stone analysis guides subsequent treatment
3. Calculi can lead to pain, tissue trauma, secondary hemorrhage, and infection
4. Large calculi cause pressure necrosis or lead to obstruction such as hydronephrosis or hydroureter; see section that follows
5. Stone location can be diagnosed by KUB x-ray, IV pyelography, renal ultrasound, and CT scan

NCLEX®
6. Risk factors
   a. Family history
   b. Dehydration: concentrates calculus-forming substances
   c. Urinary stasis, infection, or obstruction (allows solid materials or bacteria to collect and form nucleus of calculus)
   d. Metabolic factors: hyperparathyroidism, renal tubular acidosis, elevated uric acid levels (gout), defective oxalate metabolism
   e. Diet high in vitamin D or calcium, purines, oxalates, protein, or alkali

B. Nursing assessment

NCLEX®
1. Renal calculi cause renal colic on affected side; originates in lumbar region and radiates around side to groin

NCLEX®
2. Fluctuates in intensity but tends to be sharp and severe; N/V, pallor, and diaphoresis sometimes accompany severe pain
3. Other symptoms: possible dull ache in kidney, abdominal distention, fever, and chills
4. Possible reduced urine output if urine drainage from one kidney is obstructed, or alternating periods of urinary retention and frequency
5. Urinalysis may reveal hematuria, pyuria, and crystal fragments
6. Twenty-four-hour urine levels may reveal high calcium, uric acid, and/or oxalate

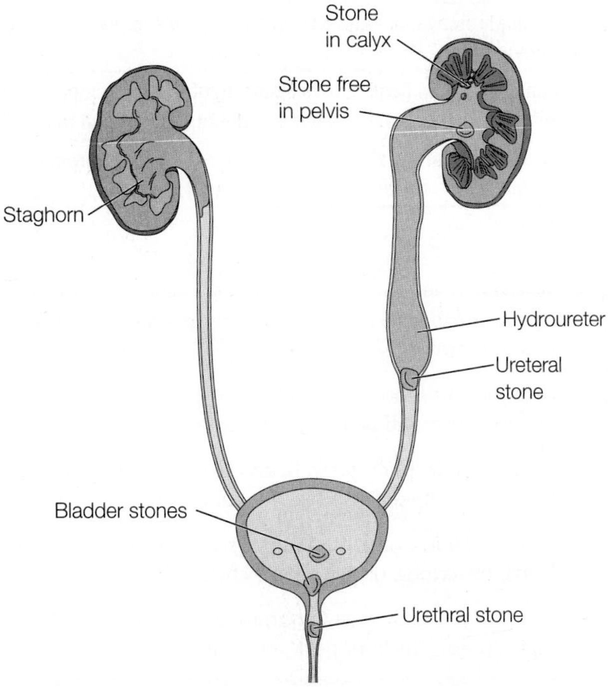

Figure 58–3
Development and location of calculi within kidneys and urinary tract.

C. Therapeutic management

1. Stones that are too large to pass spontaneously (diameter >5 mm), multiple stones, and those that obstruct urinary tract usually require surgery (see Table 58–4)

NCLEX®
2. Treatment for calcium phosphate and/or oxalate stones
   a. Acid-ash diet with limitations of foods high in calcium and oxalates (see Box 58–4)
   b. Increase hydration and exercise

NCLEX®
3. Treatment for struvite stones: acid-ash diet

NCLEX®
4. Treatment for uric acid stones: alkaline-ash and low-purine diet; increase hydration

NCLEX®
5. Treatment for cystine stones: alkaline-ash diet; increase hydration
6. Goal of treatment is to relieve symptoms, remove or destroy calculi, and prevent future stone formation
7. Most calculi (90%) pass out of urinary system without invasive treatment
8. Provide pain relief measures and treat other symptoms as they occur
9. Assess urinary function and monitor I&O

NCLEX®
10. Strain all urine and save stones or stone fragments for analysis

NCLEX®
11. Encourage ambulation and large fluid intake to help client pass calculi (unless obstruction from stone contraindicates overhydration)
12. Record daily weight to assess fluid status and renal function
13. Medication therapy: antimicrobial therapy for infection, analgesics for pain, and diuretics to prevent urine stasis

NCLEX®
D. Client teaching

1. Dietary alterations to prevent recurrence of stones; teach dietary needs related to type of calculus (refer again to Box 58–4)
2. Increase fluid intake to 2500–3500 mL/day
3. Maintain activity at level that will prevent urinary stasis and resorption of calcium from bone
4. If discharged prior to stone passage, collect and strain all urine and bring stones to follow-up visit; observe urine amount and characteristics and report to healthcare provider at follow-up visit also
5. Report increased pain, persistent blood in urine, inability to void, significant decrease in UO
6. Report signs of infection: burning with urination, cloudy urine, or fever
7. Review specific drug information and procedures for self-administration

Table 58–4 Therapeutic Procedures to Treat Urinary Stones

Surgical Procedure	Description
Extracorporeal shock-wave lithotripsy (ESWL)	Procedure that uses externally generated waves to pulverize or shatter urinary stones and calculi, which are then excreted in urine
Ureterolithotomy, pyelolithotomy, or nephrolithotomy	Surgical removal of calculi from affected areas; requires a large flank incision and an extended recovery time
Percutaneous nephrostomy	Small incision in flank allows insertion of an endoscope to visualize renal pelvis; stones are removed with forceps or a basket device, or lithotripsy is used to crush stones
Transurethral uroscopy	Passage of a ureteral catheter via a cystoscope to drain urine proximal to a stone and dilate ureter, allowing stone to pass; or use of a basket catheter passed through cystoscope to remove calculus

Box 58–4

Dietary Considerations with Urinary Calculi

Acid-ash foods: Cranberries, plums, grapes, and prunes; tomatoes; eggs and cheese; whole grains; meat and poultry

Alkaline-ash foods: Legumes, milk and milk products, green vegetables, rhubarb, fruits except those acid-ash fruits noted above

Foods high in calcium: Milk and other dairy products, beans and lentils, dried fruits, canned or smoked fish (except tuna), flour, chocolate, and cocoa

Foods high in oxalates: Asparagus, beets, celery, cabbage, dark green leafy vegetables, fruits, tomatoes, green beans, chocolate and cocoa, beer, cola beverages, nuts, and tea

Foods high in purines: Organ meats, sardines, salmon, herring, venison, and goose; other meats (beef, chicken, pork, veal) also contain purines and should be limited in quantity

E. Hydronephrosis and hydroureter

1. *Hydronephrosis* is a state of urine stasis in kidney from an obstruction to outflow; *hydroureter* is urine stasis in ureter proximal to obstruction with urine "backup" into kidney
2. Can lead to kidney damage and renal scarring if untreated
3. Common causes include calculi (commonly), scar tissue, ureteral obstruction, tumors, and prostatic hyperplasia
4. Nursing assessment: dull flank pain or colicky pain with radiation to groin, hypertension, and headache
5. Therapeutic management
   a. Treat underlying cause
   b. Monitor for decreased urine output (during obstruction) and increased urine output (after obstruction relieved)
   c. Monitor VS frequently as indicators of fluid volume status, daily weight, and electrolyte balance
   d. Administer fluid volume replacement as prescribed
   e. Prepare client for possible surgical correction of obstruction or insertion of nephrostomy tube

VI. URINARY RETENTION

A. Overview

1. Inability to empty bladder leading to bladder distention, poor contractility of detrusor muscle, and further inability to urinate
2. Mechanical obstruction of bladder outlet is most often caused by benign prostatic hyperplasia (BPH) or acute inflammation
3. Detrusor muscle function can be disrupted by surgery or medications (anticholinergics, antidepressants, antipsychotics, anti-Parkinson drugs, antihistamines, and some antihypertensives)

B. Nursing assessment

NCLEX® 1. Firm, distended bladder that may be displaced to one side of midline

NCLEX® 2. Overflow voiding or incontinence may occur, with 25–50 mL of urine eliminated at frequent intervals

NCLEX® 3. Residual urine (postvoiding catheterization) in amounts over 50 mL obtained from bladder catheterization

4. Cystometrography evaluates muscle function

C. Therapeutic management

1. Surgical correction of any condition causing mechanical obstruction to urine flow, including BPH and calculi
2. Palpate bladder for distention at regular intervals
3. Monitor I&O and observe urine characteristics
4. Stimulate relaxation of urethral sphincter by running water, pouring warm water over client's fingers or perineum, or providing warm sitz bath
5. Perform intermittent straight catheterization as prescribed

NCLEX® 6. Evaluate client's medication regime for drugs that cause urinary retention

NCLEX® 7. Medication therapy: cholinergic medications to promote detrusor muscle contraction and bladder emptying; anticholinesterase drugs to increase detrusor muscle tone

D. Client teaching

1. How to perform straight catheterization at home if necessary
2. Recognize and report signs of UTI: burning with urination, cloudy urine, pelvic pain, fever, and strong urine odor

NCLEX® 3. Moderate to high fluid intake and a diet that acidifies the urine; cranberry juice and ascorbic acid (vitamin C) help maintain acidity

4. Use and side effects of prescribed medications

VII. URINARY INCONTINENCE

A. Overview

1. Involuntary urination of varying types
   a. Stress: occurs during times of increased abdominal pressure, such as sneezing, coughing, or lifting
   b. Overflow: occurs because of incomplete bladder emptying; leads to overdistended bladder, with dribbling or voiding small amounts of urine
   c. Urge: occurs soon after a strong urge to void is felt (also called overactive bladder)
   d. Functional: results from a variety of physical, environmental, and psychosocial causes, such as dementia, confusion, depression, sedation, or physical impairment of mobility
   e. Mixed: combination of types

Box 58–5

Teaching Kegel Exercises

- First, sit or stand with legs apart.
- Tense your muscles to pull your rectum, urethra, and vagina up inside, and hold for a count of 3–5 seconds; a pull should be felt at the cleft of your buttocks.
- Try to stop and start your stream of urine.
- Develop a schedule that will help remind you to do these exercises.
- To control episodes of stress incontinence, brace the muscles and use the Kegel maneuver when doing any activity that increases intra-abdominal pressure, such as coughing, laughing, sneezing, or lifting.

2. May be acute or chronic, and cause may be congenital or acquired
3. Occurs with any condition causing higher than normal bladder pressure or reduced urethral resistance
4. Common etiologies: relaxation of pelvic musculature, disruption of cerebral and nervous system control, and disturbances of bladder musculature
5. Risk factors in older clients: decreased bladder capacity, lax pelvic muscles in females, immobility, chronic degenerative diseases, diabetes mellitus, and stroke

B. Nursing assessment

NCLEX®
1. Clinical manifestations: involuntary passage of urine
2. Postvoiding residual urine greater than 50 mL
3. Weak abdominal and pelvic muscle tone in women and possible enlarged prostate in men
4. Cystometrography: reduced muscle function and tone
5. Ultrasonography and cystoscopy identify possible causes of the incontinence

C. Therapeutic management

1. A variety of surgical procedures treat incontinence based on cause, such as suspension of bladder neck and surgical slings
2. Goal is to identify and correct cause of incontinence; if unable to correct underlying problem, client may learn techniques to manage UO

NCLEX®
3. Use behavioral techniques, such as Kegel exercises, limiting fluids such as caffeinated or carbonated beverages or other bladder irritants, voiding before bedtime and upon arising from bed, voiding at predetermined frequencies (such as every hour or two, and slowly increasing time interval as able)

NCLEX®
4. Medication therapy: anticholinergics for stress incontinence (increase bladder capacity, inhibit detrusor muscle contraction), antihistamines (enhance smooth muscle contraction of bladder neck)

D. Client teaching

1. Care of indwelling urinary catheter at home, if required
2. Recognize and report signs of UTI: burning with urination, cloudy urine, pelvic pain, fever, and strong urine odor
3. Moderate to high fluid intake and a diet that acidifies urine
4. Specific drug information and procedures for self-administration
5. Possible need to keep a voiding diary to help diagnose cause(s) of incontinence

NCLEX®
6. Teach behavioral techniques, including Kegel exercises to strengthen pelvic floor muscles (see Box 58–5)
7. Dietary and fluid intake modifications to reduce stress and urge incontinence; consume most fluids during times of day client is most able to remain continent
8. Wear clothing that is easily removed for ease in toileting
9. Use assistive devices, such as raised toilet seats, bedside commode, and urinal or bedpan as needed

VIII. URINARY TRACT INFECTIONS (UTI)

A. Overview

1. Presence of microorganisms in urinary tract leading to inflammation
2. Infections are classified by region and primary site affected
   a. **Cystitis**: inflammation of bladder from infection, other irritant, or urethral obstruction; most common type of UTI
   b. *Urethritis*: inflammation of urethra; may occur with cystitis; most common cause in men is sexually transmitted infection; in women may also occur with use of spermicidal jelly or perfumed feminine hygiene products
   c. *Ureteritis*: inflammation of ureter; may occur with ascending bladder infection or accompany pyelonephritis (see section that follows)

3. *Escherichia coli* is most frequent infective organism
4. Females, especially those who are sexually active or pregnant, are more prone to UTIs because urethra is shorter than in men
5. Noninfectious cystitis results from exposure to radiation, chemical agents, or a metabolic disorder

B. Nursing assessment

NCLEX®
1. Burning, frequency, urgency, small volume of urine with voiding, fever, cloudy urine, strong urine odor, possible hematuria, pain in pelvic area, bladder spasms

NCLEX®
2. Older clients may have nonspecific symptoms, such as nocturia, incontinence, confusion, lethargy, or anorexia
3. Positive urine nitrites or leukocyte esterase
4. Urine cultures and Gram stain determine presence and number of bacteria
5. Blood or urine tests are also done to rule out sexually transmitted infections, which produce similar symptoms

C. Therapeutic management

NCLEX®
1. Increase fluid intake to 3000 mL per day unless contraindicated by other condition

NCLEX®
2. Administer prescribed urinary antimicrobials after obtaining urine culture and sensitivity
3. Encourage intake of acid-ash foods to maintain acidic urine (pH 5.5), unless not recommended by type of antimicrobial (sulfonamide, aminoglycoside, nitrofurantoin)
4. Encourage client to void every 2–3 hours and completely empty bladder to reduce urinary stasis
5. Monitor I&O and observe urine characteristics
6. Medication therapy: antimicrobials to eradicate bacteria; antispasmodics and analgesics to relieve pain, frequency, and burning
7. Corrective surgery if recurrent UTI is caused by structural abnormalities, including ureteroplasty (surgical repair of ureter) for stricture, or placement of ureteral stent (catheter in ureter to provide free flow of urine)

NCLEX® **D. Client teaching**

1. Avoid beverages that irritate bladder: carbonated or caffeinated drinks and alcohol
2. Teach preventive hygiene measures for women: wipe from front to back, keep perineum clean and dry, do not douche, avoid tight-fitting pants; wear undergarment with cotton panel; void after sexual intercourse; avoid harsh soaps, bubble bath, powder, or sprays in perineal area
3. Teach use and side effects of medication; complete full course of antimicrobials
4. Phenazopyridine, a urinary analgesic, turns urine reddish orange; protect clothing and do not mistake color for bleeding (hematuria)
5. Maintain acidic urine with acid-ash diet, which may include cranberry juice or ascorbic acid daily (helps prevent bacteria from clinging to bladder wall)
6. Maintain high fluid intake during treatment; then maintain fluid intake at 8–10 glasses per day or more
7. Practice frequent voiding (every 2–4 hours) to flush bacteria from urethra
8. Take showers rather than baths if recurrent infection is a problem
9. Take protective measures against sexually transmitted infection as a cause

E. Urosepsis

1. Bacteremia caused by Gram-negative microorganisms in urinary tract, most frequently *E. coli*

NCLEX®
2. Indwelling urinary catheter or unrecognized urinary tract infection in older adult are frequent causes
3. Can progress to septic shock if unrecognized or inadequately treated
4. Nursing assessment reveals fever in addition to any previous or underlying signs of infection
5. Treat with IV antibiotic therapy until client has been afebrile for 3–5 days, then follow up with oral antibiotic therapy as prescribed
6. Nursing care is same as for UTI and assessment for septic shock
7. Client teaching focuses on recognition and prompt treatment of UTI

IX. BENIGN PROSTATIC HYPERPLASIA (BPH)

A. Overview

1. Enlargement of prostate gland that occurs as an age-related change in men
2. Enlarging gland causes compression on urethra, leading to partial or complete obstruction to urinary elimination
3. Subsequent urinary retention and stasis increases risk of UTI

NCLEX® **B. Nursing assessment**

1. Weakened force of urinary stream (early sign), urinary frequency, urgency, hesitancy (difficulty starting or maintaining urine stream); possible nocturia

2. Urinary retention, bladder distention, incomplete bladder emptying (increased postvoid residual on bladder scan), postvoid dribbling (overflow incontinence)
3. Dysuria, pain, and hematuria may indicate onset of UTI from urinary stasis

NCLEX®

C. Therapeutic management

1. Encourage large fluid intake of 2000–3000 mL/day unless contraindicated by another condition
2. Prepare to catheterize bladder to relieve urinary retention
3. Administer antiandrogen agents such as finasteride or dutasteride (shrink prostate) or alpha-adrenergic antagonists (terazosin, doxazosin, tamulosin, or alfuzosin) to relieve obstruction and increase urine flow
4. Surgical treatment includes minimally invasive surgery, transurethral resection of prostate (see section that follows), or open prostatectomy

D. Client teaching

1. Popular herbal therapies (such as saw palmetto berry, *Pygeum africanum* bark, *Echinacea purpurea* and *Hypoxis rooperi* roots, and trembling poplar leaves) show no significant reduction in symptoms in recent studies
2. Follow a timed voiding schedule to promote urinary elimination
3. Avoid OTC drugs that promote urinary retention, such as anticholinergics, antihistamines, and decongestants

E. Care of client undergoing transurethral resection of prostate (TURP)

1. Implement standard preoperative and postoperative care (see Chapter 48)
2. Monitor for urinary hemorrhage for 24–48 hours, indicated by bloody urine, large blood clots, decreased UO, increased bladder spasms, and signs of hypovolemia
3. Maintain traction on three-way indwelling urinary catheter with tubing attached to client's leg using urinary catheter attachment device and asking client to keep leg straight (inflated balloon puts pressure against operative site to prevent bleeding)

NCLEX®

4. Maintain continuous bladder irrigation, often for 24–48 hours after surgery
   a. Maintain flow of irrigating solution to keep UO light pink or yellow; monitor and record amount of irrigant used each shift
   b. Assess UO every 1–2 hours per protocol for color, consistency, amount, and presence of blood clots
   c. Assess for and report TURP syndrome caused by systemic absorption of irrigant through bladder wall (hyponatremia, hypertension, decreased hematocrit, bradycardia, nausea, and confusion)
   d. Follow agency policy for irrigating urinary catheter if urine drainage blocked by blood clots; use sterile technique if performed
   e. Calculate true UO by noting entire volume of output for shift and subtracting amount of irrigant used during same time period
5. Explain that client may experience dribbling of urine or small blood clots after catheter removal; full bladder control can take up to 1 year; Kegel exercises may be helpful

X. PYELONEPHRITIS

A. Overview

1. Acute or chronic infection of one or both kidneys; usually begins in renal pelvis and may also affect parenchyma (functional portion of kidney)
2. Kidney becomes edematous and abscesses may develop; tissue destruction primarily affects tubules; with healing, scar tissue replaces normal tissue and affected tubules atrophy
3. Acute form is a bacterial infection, often from *E. coli*, which usually ascends from lower urinary tract
4. Risk factors: pregnancy, urinary tract obstruction, congenital malformation, urinary tract trauma, calculi, diabetes mellitus, asymptomatic bacteriuria or cystitis
5. Chronic form is associated with recurrent acute infections and sometimes with metabolic, chemical, or immunologic disorders
   a. Can result from an autoimmune process leading to inflammation
   b. Acute episodes may contribute to inflammation and scarring associated with chronic form
   c. Fibrosis and scarring are associated with destruction of nephrons and dilation of renal pelvis
   d. May lead to **acute kidney injury** or **chronic kidney disease**
6. **Vesicoureteral reflux** (urine moves from bladder back toward kidneys) is a common risk factor in children; seen also in adults with obstructed bladder outflow

NCLEX®

B. Nursing assessment

1. Clinical manifestations: urinary frequency, dysuria, flank pain, costovertebral tenderness, tachypnea, nausea, fever, chills, malaise, urine that is cloudy, blood-tinged, or malodorous
2. Urine culture: hematuria, pyuria, bacteriuria, leukocyte casts, leukocytosis

NCLEX® **C. Therapeutic management**

1. Encourage sufficient rest with possible temporary bedrest until symptoms subside
2. Encourage large fluid intake up to 3000 mL/day to maintain UO of 1500 mL/day
3. Monitor VS (especially temperature)
4. Provide nonpharmacologic comfort measures such as warm, moist compresses to flank area or warm bath
5. If **oliguria** (UO <400 mL/day) is present, maintain diet low in protein and high in calories and vitamins
6. Observe for edema and signs of acute kidney injury
7. Medication therapy: antimicrobials, urinary antiseptics, analgesics, and possibly antiemetics

D. Client teaching

1. Monitor UO and notify healthcare provider if reduced
2. Take high-calorie, low-protein diet if oliguria is present
3. Hygiene measures to prevent further infections (see previous section on UTI)
4. NCLEX® Finish complete course of antibiotics, even if symptoms resolve

XI. *GLOMERULONEPHRITIS*

A. Overview

1. A group of kidney diseases caused by inflammation of glomerular capillary membrane
2. NCLEX® Most often follows pharyngeal or skin infections with group A-beta-hemolytic streptococcus, but staphylococcal and viral infections and autoimmune processes are other causes
3. Antigen–antibody complexes form during primary infection and become trapped within glomerular membrane, producing an inflammatory response that damages glomeruli and leads to loss of renal function
4. Acute form occurs 2–3 weeks after infection; chronic phase may follow acute phase or develop over time
5. May lead to permanent kidney damage

NCLEX® **B. Nursing assessment**

1. Early symptoms may be mild: pharyngitis, fever, and malaise; weakness and fatigue
2. History of recent upper respiratory or skin infections, pericarditis, or lower UTI
3. Anorexia, N/V, pallor, lethargy, headache
4. Smoky, brown, coffee, or cola-colored urine (hematuria) or proteinuria (may cause ongoing foam in urine)
5. Hypertension and edema (face and extremities) from salt and water retention
6. Pulmonary infiltrates can develop, especially in clients with heart failure
7. Lab tests reveal hypoalbuminemia, **azotemia** (increased BUN and creatinine; retention of nitrogenous wastes in blood), increased antistreptolysin O titer (if streptococcal infection) and erythrocyte sedimentation rate (ESR), decreased creatinine clearance, decreased sodium and phosphate, and increased potassium
8. Diagnostic tests reveal delayed uptake and excretion of radioactive dye in renal scan and positive renal biopsy findings
9. Complications can include kidney failure, heart failure, pulmonary edema, hypertensive encephalopathy, and seizures

C. Therapeutic management

1. NCLEX® Plasmapheresis: removal of damaging antibodies in plasma
2. Dialysis if disease progresses to renal failure
3. NCLEX® Provide appropriate diet: protein restriction if azotemia is present; high CHO to provide energy; K^+ restricted during oliguria; Na^+ restricted for hypertension and edema
4. Maintain fluid restriction; offer ice chips in limited amounts and provide mouth care to relieve thirst; develop fluid intake schedule
5. NCLEX® Encourage restricted activity during acute stage and implement energy conservation measures (short periods of activity, assistance with activities of daily living, limit on number of visitors and length of visits)
6. Monitor VS every 4 hours (tachycardia, hypertension)
7. NCLEX® Monitor I&O and daily weight; auscultate lungs for crackles if indicated
8. Evaluate for signs of renal failure: oliguria, azotemia, and acidosis
9. Medication therapy: antimicrobials (such as penicillin) for infection; prednisone and aggressive immunosuppressive therapy; analgesics for pain relief; and vitamin and electrolyte replacement as needed

D. Client teaching
1. Limit activity during acute phase
2. Dietary changes and importance of maintaining diet
3. Importance of fluid restriction to manage risk for fluid overload as prescribed
4. Nephrotoxic drugs should be avoided to reduce risk of further kidney damage

XII. *NEPHROTIC SYNDROME*

A. Overview

NCLEX® 1. Renal disease characterized by massive proteinuria, hypoalbuminemia, hyperlipidemia, and severe edema of dependent tissues, face, and periorbital areas
2. Seen with any renal condition that damages glomerular capillary membrane: glomerulonephritis, lipoid nephrosis, syphilitic nephritis, amyloidosis, or SLE
3. More likely to resolve without long-term effects in children than in adults, who may experience progressive renal impairment over time

NCLEX® **B. Nursing assessment**
1. Severe generalized edema and facial and periorbital edema more prominent in morning
2. Weight gain from fluid retention
3. Loss of appetite and fatigue
4. Decreased urine output with dark, frothy urine

C. Therapeutic management

NCLEX® 1. Provide nursing care to control edema, including sodium-restricted diet, diuretic therapy, and administration of salt-poor albumin

NCLEX® 2. Provide regular diet with restricted Na^+ if edema is present, and possible fluid restriction as indicated
3. Administer prescribed drugs such as corticosteroids, immunosuppressants, and anti-infectives if there is documented infection
4. Observe for signs of pulmonary edema: tachypnea, dyspnea, crackles in lungs
5. Record total I&O every 4–8 hours and weigh client daily
6. Maintain fluid restriction; offer ice chips and provide frequent mouth care

NCLEX® 7. Provide for adequate rest and energy conservation, especially until edema subsides

NCLEX® 8. Take measures to reduce risk of infection, including hand hygiene, standard infection control practices, limiting invasive procedures, and physical hygiene of client

NCLEX® 9. Medication therapy: immunosuppressants, diuretics, and antihypertensives as needed to lower BP

D. Client teaching
1. Take measures to maintain general health, as disorder may persist for months or years
2. Avoid sources of infection such as people with upper respiratory infections
3. Nutritious diet with no added salt or with sodium restriction during periods of edema
4. Activity as tolerated
5. Use and potential effects of medications
6. Signs, symptoms, and implications of improving or declining renal function

XIII. *POLYCYSTIC KIDNEY DISEASE*

A. Overview
1. Hereditary disease characterized by cyst formation and massive kidney enlargement (see Figure 58–4)
2. Autosomal-dominant form affects adults (symptoms manifest by age 30 or 40 years), while autosomal-recessive form affects infants

NCLEX® 3. As cysts enlarge and multiply, kidneys also enlarge; renal blood vessels and nephrons are compressed and obstructed, and functional tissue is destroyed
4. Clients with this disorder often develop cysts elsewhere in body, including liver, spleen, pancreas, brain, and other organs

NCLEX® **B. Nursing assessment**
1. Flank, lumbar, or abdominal pain; tends to be relieved when lying down and aggravated by activity
2. Microscopic or gross hematuria, proteinuria, **polyuria** (increased UO), and nocturia
3. Signs of UTI and renal calculi when cysts interfere with normal urine drainage
4. Hypertension from disruption of renal blood vessels
5. Palpable, enlarged, and knobby kidney
6. Increasing abdominal girth
7. Signs of chronic kidney disease as the client approaches age 50–60
8. Positive findings in renal ultrasonography, IVP, and CT scan

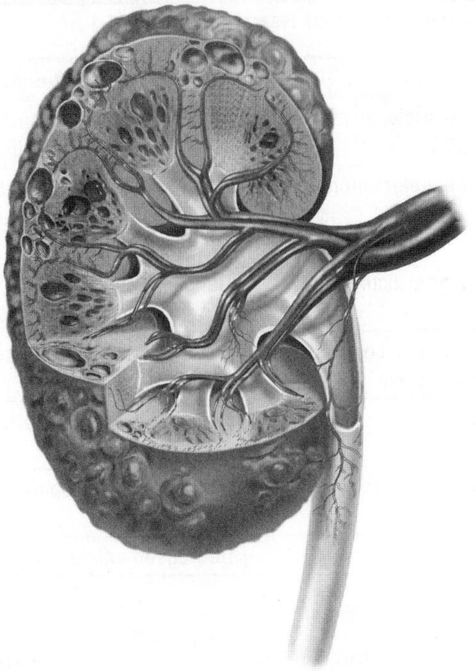

Figure 58–4
Polycystic kidney disease.

Source: © Stocktreck Images, Inc./Alamy Stock Photo

C. Therapeutic management

1. Provide supportive care to help client cope with symptoms; no effective treatment is available
2. NCLEX® Encourage fluid intake of 2000–2500 mL/day to help prevent UTI and calculi
3. Administer antihypertensive agents as prescribed
4. Discuss that hemodialysis and possibly renal transplant will be indicated as disease progresses
5. NCLEX® Provide Na^+-restricted diet to help control edema
6. NCLEX® Medication therapy: ACE inhibitors to control hypertension; diuretics to control edema; and antibiotics if infection develops

D. Client teaching

1. Maintenance of general health because disorder is chronic and progressive
2. How to avoid UTI and to recognize early signs of infection
3. NCLEX® Avoid medications that are potentially toxic to kidneys and check with healthcare provider before taking any new drug
4. Need for genetic counseling and screening of family members for disease
5. NCLEX® Maintain fluid intake of at least 2500 mL/day

XIV. *ACUTE KIDNEY INJURY* (AKI)

A. Overview

1. Sudden loss of kidney function caused by failure of renal circulation or damage to the tubules or glomeruli
   a. Usually reversible, with spontaneous recovery in a few days to weeks
   b. Ischemia is primary cause; it produces irreversible damage to tubules if continues for more than 2 hours
2. Etiologic categories
   a. Prerenal: caused by decreased blood flow to kidneys; readily reversible when recognized and treated early; may be caused by severe dehydration, diuretic therapy, circulatory collapse, hypovolemia, or shock
   b. Intrinsic: caused by ischemia, nephrotoxins, and conditions such as acute glomerulonephritis, vascular disorders, or severe infection; *acute tubular necrosis* (destruction of tubular epithelial cells) often results from ischemia or toxins
   c. Postrenal: caused by any condition that obstructs urine flow such as in BPH, renal or urinary tract calculi, or tumors

NCLEX® **B. Nursing assessment** (see also Table 58–5)

1. Clinical manifestations follow three phases: initiation, maintenance, and recovery; initiation stage has very few manifestations; maintenance phase is characterized by oliguria; recovery stage shows signs of improving UO and renal function
2. Muscle weakness, N/V, and diarrhea may occur

Table 58–5 Clinical Manifestations of Renal Failure

Body System	Clinical Manifestations	Cause of Manifestations
Cardiovascular	Hypervolemia, hypertension, tachycardia, arrhythmias, congestive heart failure, pericarditis	Increased fluid volume, buildup of metabolic wastes, chronic hypertension, change in renin-angiotensin mechanism
Hematologic	Anemia, leukocytosis, decreased platelet function, thrombocytopenia	Decreased production of erythropoietin and RBCs, decreased survival of RBCs, decreased platelet activity; blood loss through dialysis and bleeding
Gastrointestinal	Anorexia, nausea, vomiting, abdominal distention, diarrhea, constipation, bleeding	Buildup of uremic toxins, electrolyte imbalances, changes in platelet activity, conversion of urea to ammonia by saliva
Neurologic	Lethargy, confusion, convulsions, stupor, coma, sleep disturbances, behavioral changes, muscle irritability	Uremic toxins, electrolyte imbalances, cerebral swelling caused by fluid shifts
Dermatologic	Pallor, pigmentation, pruritus, ecchymosis, excoriation, uremic frost	Anemia, decreased activity of sweat glands, dry skin, phosphate deposits on skin
Urinary	Decreased urine output, decreased specific gravity, proteinuria, casts and cells in urine	Damage to nephrons
Skeletal	Osteoporosis, renal rickets, joint pain	Decreased calcium absorption, decreased phosphate excretion

3. Neurologic symptoms such as confusion, agitation, disorientation, seizures, and coma may also be present
4. Hyperkalemia, hyperphosphatemia, and hypocalcemia
5. Metabolic acidosis
6. Anemia
7. Azotemia; elevated creatinine and BUN levels
8. Urinalysis: proteinuria, specific gravity (SG) same as plasma SG; presence of casts, RBCs, WBCs, and renal tubular epithelial cells
9. Positive renal biopsy findings

C. Therapeutic management

1. Monitor VS every 4 hours and I&O every shift
2. Monitor electrolyte status (hyponatremia from fluid retention, hyperkalemia and hyperphosphatemia from inadequate excretion)
3. Maintain fluid restriction as prescribed using mouth care, hard sugarless candy, or ice chips (equal half fluid volume) to reduce thirst; administer medications with meals
4. Supportive therapy with dialysis
5. Observe for oliguria followed by polyuria from diuresis
6. *NCLEX®* Weigh daily and observe for edema
7. *NCLEX®* Monitor for acidosis and complications of electrolyte imbalances, such as hyperkalemia
8. *NCLEX®* Encourage prescribed diet: moderate protein restriction, high in carbohydrates (CHO), restricted potassium (K^+) and sodium (Na^+)
9. Once diuresis phase begins, evaluate slow return of BUN, creatinine, phosphorus, and K^+ to normal
10. Medication therapy
    a. *NCLEX®* Avoid nephrotoxic drugs
    b. Volume expanders restore renal perfusion in hypotensive clients
    c. Loop diuretics reduce toxic concentration in nephrons and establish urine flow
    d. ACE inhibitors control hypertension
    e. Antacids or histamine H_2-receptor antagonists prevent gastric ulcers
    f. Sodium polystyrene sulfonate reduces serum K^+ levels and sodium bicarbonate treats acidosis

D. Client teaching

1. *NCLEX®* Dietary and fluid restrictions, including those that may be continued after discharge
2. Signs of complications, such as fluid volume excess, CHF, and hyperkalemia
3. *NCLEX®* Monitor weight, BP, pulse, and UO as measures of fluid status
4. *NCLEX®* Avoid nephrotoxic drugs and substances: NSAIDs, some antibiotics, radiologic contrast media, and heavy metals; avoid alcohol (increases nephrotoxicity of some materials); consult with healthcare provider before using OTC drugs
5. Recovery of renal function requires up to 1 year; during this period, nephrons are vulnerable to damage from nephrotoxins

XV. *CHRONIC KIDNEY DISEASE* (CKD)

A. Overview

1. Progressive loss of renal function with a glomerular filtration rate (GFR) of 60 mL/minute or less for 3 months or longer
2. Occurs in stages with further declines in GFR but ultimately leads to end-stage renal disease (ESRD)
3. *NCLEX®* Most common causes of CKD are diabetes mellitus, hypertension, glomerulonephritis, autoimmune disorders, polycystic kidney disease, recurrent infection or urinary obstruction, or as sequel to AKI
4. Client develops uremic syndrome because of accumulation of waste products in blood
5. Loss of erythropoietin leads to chronic anemia and subsequent fatigue
6. *NCLEX®* There is inadequate clearance of fluid and electrolytes, leading to fluid and Na^+ retention, as well as hyperkalemia, hypermagnesemia, hyperphosphatemia, and hypocalcemia; metabolic acidosis occurs because of impaired hydrogen ion excretion

NCLEX® **B. Nursing assessment**

1. Early: nausea, apathy, weakness, and fatigue; declining UO leading to oliguria
2. Late: possibly frequent vomiting, increasing weakness, lethargy, and confusion
3. Client may report "restless leg syndrome," paresthesia, and sensory loss
4. Personality changes, such as anxiety, irritability, and hallucinations; seizures and coma possible in late stages
5. Respirations may change to Kussmaul pattern, with declining LOC (acidosis)
6. Skin becomes pale and dry, with yellowish hue; metabolic wastes cause itching and uremic frost (crystallized deposits of urea on skin)
7. Urinalysis shows fixed specific gravity approximately 1.010, equivalent to plasma; presence of proteinuria, hematuria, and casts
8. Elevated creatinine and BUN and decreased creatinine clearance
9. Abnormal electrolyte values as noted above
10. Moderate anemia
11. Decreased platelets
12. Decreased renal size by ultrasonography; positive renal biopsy if caused by cancer

C. Therapeutic management

1. *NCLEX®* Provide diet low in protein (such as 60 grams protein) with supplemented amino acids; restrict fluids as prescribed
2. *NCLEX®* Provide electrolyte replacement or restriction
   - **a.** Na^+ restriction (such as 2 grams daily)
   - **b.** K^+ restriction (such as 2 grams daily)
   - **c.** Replacement of bicarbonate stores to treat acidosis
3. Monitor and plan nursing care for hypertension and heart failure
4. *NCLEX®* Prepare client for dialysis or kidney transplant
5. Monitor I&O and VS
6. Monitor laboratory results: BUN and serum creatinine, pH, electrolytes, and CBC
7. Provide symptomatic relief for N/V
8. Observe for signs of infection
9. *NCLEX®* Provide rest periods to combat chronic fatigue
10. Help client learn about and adjust to diagnosis; support coping strategies and work with client to develop realistic goals
11. *NCLEX®* Medication therapy: limited by kidneys' inability to excrete
    - **a.** Diuretics to reduce volume of extracellular fluid
    - **b.** ACE inhibitors to maintain normal BP
    - **c.** Electrolyte replacement
    - **d.** Phosphate binding agents, such as calcium carbonate
    - **e.** Sodium polystyrene sulfonate if needed to reduce serum K^+ levels
    - **f.** Folic acid, multivitamins, iron supplements, and possibly epoietin alfa to combat anemia
    - **g.** Medications for other health problems may require reduced dosage if excreted via kidneys

D. Client teaching

1. Monitor weight, VS, and UO at home
2. *NCLEX®* Fluid and dietary restrictions (low-Na^+, low-K^+, low-protein) need to be followed carefully

3. Monitor symptoms of uremia

NCLEX® 4. Avoid nephrotoxic drugs and substances: NSAIDs, some antibiotics, radiologic contrast media, and heavy metals

NCLEX® 5. Teach strategies to avoid thirst, yet continue fluid restrictions, such as frequent mouth care, sugarless hard candy, using ice chips instead of liquids, or using a spray bottle instead of a cup to limit fluids ingested

6. Discuss hemodialysis or renal transplant therapies as indicated
7. Suggest ways to combat nausea: antiemetics; mouth care; small, frequent meals
8. Provide referral to mental health counseling or support group

XVI. HYPOSPADIAS AND EPISPADIAS

A. Overview

1. **Hypospadias**: congenital defect in which urinary meatus is not at end of penis but is located on lower or underside of shaft; often accompanied by **chordee**, a downward curvature of penis
2. **Epispadias**: congenital defect in which urinary meatus is not at end of penis but on upper side of penile shaft; less common than hypospadias but is often associated with **exstrophy** of bladder

B. **Nursing assessment**: noted on newborn assessment following birth

C. **Therapeutic management**

1. Does not interfere with voiding but could interfere with reproduction if not repaired before adulthood
2. Document findings carefully and report to healthcare provider
3. **Circumcision** (operation to remove part or all of prepuce) is delayed because prepuce may be used in reconstruction of defect
4. If chordee is present, curvature of penis may be released before hypospadias repair

NCLEX® 5. Surgical correction is usually between 16 and 18 months before toilet training begins

NCLEX® 6. Postoperative care
   a. Penis may have a urethral stent in place and be wrapped with a pressure dressing
   b. Arm and leg restraints may be needed to prevent accidental removal of stent
   c. Encourage increased fluid intake to maintain UO and stent patency
   d. Notify healthcare provider if no UO occurs for 1 hour because there could be kinks in system or occlusion by sediment
   e. Medication therapy includes antibiotics as prescribed, acetaminophen for pain, and anticholinergics such as oxybutynin for bladder spasms

D. **Client and family teaching**

1. Parents need explanation of disorder and surgical repair

NCLEX® 2. Postsurgical discharge teaching
   a. Double-diapering technique to protect stent (inner diaper collects stool and outer diaper collects urine)
   b. Limit activity for approximately 2 weeks; restrict activities that put pressure on site (riding toys, sitting on lap, or straddling child on hip); no tub baths while stent in place
   c. Medication administration, including full course of antibiotic therapy, anticholinergic for bladder spasm; acetaminophen or ibuprofen for pain
   d. Maintain adequate fluid intake
   e. Monitor for signs of infection (strong-smelling urine, redness, fever, pain, change in flow of urine stream)
   f. Call healthcare provider if urine leaks from anywhere but penis (urine will also be blood-tinged for several days)

XVII. EXSTROPHY OF BLADDER

A. Overview

1. Lower portion of abdominal wall and anterior bladder wall are missing, resulting in bladder being open and exposed on abdomen
2. Bladder appears as reddish mass glistening with urine
3. Continuous drainage of urine from ureters may lead to skin excoriation around bladder
4. Exstrophy of bladder can be life-threatening and correction must be initiated as soon after birth as possible

B. Nursing assessment: defect is immediately obvious at birth, with exposed bladder mucosa, defects of external genitalia, and widening of symphysis pubis

C. Therapeutic management

NCLEX® 1. Closure of bladder and anterior abdominal wall are completed during first 48–72 hours of life

NCLEX® 2. Correction is usually a staged surgical correction, with epispadias repair at about 9 months of age (if present) and bladder neck reconstruction with ureteral reimplantation when bladder capacity reaches 80–90 mL

NCLEX® 3. Preoperative nursing care involves covering bladder with sterile plastic wrap and maintaining integrity of surrounding skin using skin sealant to protect from excoriating effects of urine

NCLEX® 4. Postoperative nursing care may involve Bryant's traction to facilitate healing, avoiding abduction of legs (puts stress on surgical area), changing dressings as prescribed; monitoring UO and characteristics, and watching for signs of obstruction, bladder spasms, and urine or blood draining from meatus

5. Emotional support of infant and parents is important; activities to support bonding and help parents accept deformity are a major component of care

D. Client and family teaching

1. Explanation of anomaly as well as instructions for care
2. As soon as possible, parents should participate in care of their infant

XVIII. *CRYPTORCHIDISM*

A. Overview

1. Failure of one or both testes to descend from inguinal canal into scrotum; normal descent of testes occurs late in gestation
2. More frequently seen in premature infants than in full-term infants

NCLEX® 3. Failure to descend exposes testes to body heat, leading to low sperm counts at sexual maturity

4. Undescended testicles are also at greater risk for torsion (twisting of a testis on its blood supply) and trauma; undescended testes have a higher incidence of cancer
5. Frequently associated with an inguinal hernia

B. Nursing assessment: absence of one or both testes in scrotal sac at birth

C. Therapeutic management

1. Often testes descend spontaneously during first year of life; monitor periodically
2. If testes remain undescended, an orchiopexy is performed at 1 year of age; if testes are damaged or absent, a prosthesis is placed in scrotum
3. Nursing care preoperatively is directed at preparing child and family for surgery

NCLEX® 4. Postoperatively, nursing care includes putting cool pack on surgical area, providing analgesics for pain, and monitoring for infection

D. Client and family teaching

1. Explanations of surgical repair
2. Postoperative incision care: clean diaper area after each diaper change; provide sponge bath for 2 days after surgery, then tub bath is allowed; do not apply ointment or OTC product over incision
3. Avoid straddling infant across hip; prevent strenuous activity or straddle toy riding for 2 weeks after surgery to prevent injury and promote healing
4. Use medications (analgesics) as prescribed
5. Symptoms of infection to report include redness, warmth, swelling, and discharge at surgical site

Check Your NCLEX–RN® Exam I.Q.

You are ready for testing on this content if you can:

- Identify basic structures and functions of the renal system.
- Describe the pathophysiology and etiology of common renal disorders.
- Discuss expected assessment data and diagnostic test findings for selected renal disorders.
- Discuss therapeutic management of a client experiencing a renal disorder.
- Discuss nursing management of a client experiencing a renal disorder.
- Identify expected outcomes for the client experiencing a renal disorder.

PRACTICE TEST

1 Which statement made by a client who has chronic kidney disease and is on hemodialysis indicates the need for further teaching?

1. "I will report any increase in my weight of 5 pounds in a 2-day period."
2. "I take my prescribed antihypertensive drugs daily."
3. "I am careful to take precautions in the arm with the AV fistula."
4. "I comply with salt restrictions in my diet by using salt substitutes."

2 What type of renal failure would the nurse expect to see in a client who accidentally self-administered an excessive dose of tobramycin?

1. Prerenal failure
2. Postrenal failure
3. Extrarenal failure
4. Intrarenal failure

3 A client with urinary tract infection (UTI) is prescribed phenazopyridine. Which instruction would the nurse give the client?

1. "This drug will take care of the infection causing your symptoms."
2. "Your urine may turn reddish-orange and may cause staining of your clothes."
3. "Take the drug before meals to minimize GI symptoms."
4. "Always keep this drug and use it at the first symptom of a UTI."

4 A client with a urinary diversion device is at risk for skin breakdown around the stoma. Which interventions will the nurse use with this client? Select all that apply.

1. Change urine collection device every other day.
2. Teach self-catheterization technique.
3. Empty the bag reservoir every 2 hours.
4. Monitor for foul-smelling urine.
5. Ensure appliance wafer is not more than 0.3 cm (1/8 in.) larger than stoma.

5 A client with renal calculi is advised to restrict calcium in the diet. The nurse determines that the client understands the restriction when the client states to avoid which types of foods?

1. Chicken, beef, and salmon
2. Green vegetables, fruit, and legumes
3. Chocolate, smoked fish, and low-fat milk
4. Eggs, meat, and poultry

6 In conducting client teaching with a client who will undergo peritoneal dialysis at home, the nurse includes discussion of what common and significant complication of peritoneal dialysis?

1. Pulmonary embolism
2. Hypotension
3. Dyspnea
4. Peritonitis

7 The nurse is preparing to admit a client with urge incontinence. In writing the nursing care plan, the nurse writes interventions that target which manifestation?

1. Involuntary loss of urine because of an overfilled bladder
2. Loss of urine when coughing or sneezing
3. Inability to empty bladder
4. Inability to inhibit urine flow long enough to reach the toilet

8 A male client who presents to the emergency department with coffee-colored urine and edema states he had a sore throat a few weeks ago. His blood pressure is elevated and urinalysis shows blood and protein in the urine. The nurse interprets that this clinical picture is consistent with which developing health problem?

1. Urinary tract infection
2. Urinary calculi
3. Acute glomerulonephritis
4. Acute prostatitis

9 A critical care nurse learns during intershift report that the assigned client experienced the prerenal type of acute kidney injury following surgery. Which of the following causes should the nurse suspect?

1. Vascular disease
2. Urethral obstruction
3. Hypovolemia
4. Glomerulonephritis

10 Which discharge instructions would the nurse give to address the risk of nephrotoxicity for a client who has been given a prescription for an aminoglycoside antibiotic? Select all that apply.

1. Increase fluid intake to 2000–2500 mL fluid daily.
2. Report sudden weight gain or puffy eyes.
3. Don't be concerned with edema as a normal side effect.
4. Elevated blood pressure is an expected drug effect.
5. Eat a low-protein diet while taking this antibiotic.

11 The nurse caring for a client undergoing a hemodialysis procedure places high priority on evaluating the client frequently for what common complication during the treatment?

1. Hyperglycemia
2. Infection and fever
3. Dialysis dementia
4. Hypotension

12 The nurse is explaining the process of peritoneal dialysis to a client recently diagnosed with chronic kidney disease. Which statement would the nurse include in a discussion with the client?

1. "The solutes in the dialysate will enter the bloodstream through the peritoneum."
2. "The peritoneum is more permeable because of the presence of excess metabolites."
3. "The peritoneum acts as a semipermeable membrane through which wastes move by diffusion and osmosis."
4. "The metabolites will move from the interstitial space to the bloodstream mainly through diffusion and ultrafiltration."

13 Which laboratory data is the most accurate indicator that a client with acute kidney injury has met the expected outcomes?

1. Decreasing blood urea nitrogen (BUN) levels
2. Decreasing serum creatinine
3. Decreasing neutrophil count
4. Decreasing lymphocyte count

14 Which statement made by a client with polycystic kidney disease indicates that the desired outcome has been met?

1. "I know these drugs will make the cysts disappear."
2. "The development of renal failure with this disease is very rare."
3. "I will have my family seek genetic counseling and screening."
4. "I sure am glad that hemodialysis will shrink the cysts."

15 A client is scheduled for a partial nephrectomy. In teaching the client about postoperative care, the nurse uses which rationale to explain why aggressive measures are needed to prevent atelectasis and pneumonia?

1. Nephrectomy involves paralyzing the intercostal muscles.
2. Intraoperative surgical contamination of the pulmonary structures is unavoidable.
3. The client must be maintained in a flat position for 24 hours.
4. The surgery involves an upper abdominal or flank incision.

16 Which statements made by a client who has received a renal transplant indicates that the desired outcome of discharge teaching has been met? Select all that apply.

1. "I will double my prednisone dose if my urine output is less than 300 mL/day."
2. "I will need to avoid crowds and prevent infection."
3. "Now I can eat whatever I want as long as I watch how much salt I use."
4. "Since I have not yet rejected the transplant, I never have to worry about rejection anymore."
5. "I should check my temperature and report increases to the healthcare provider."

17 Which statements by a female client indicate that instruction in ways to prevent urinary tract infection (UTI) was understood? Select all that apply.

1. "I should avoid tub baths and take showers instead."
2. "I should drink 8–10 glasses of fluid per day."
3. "I should only wear nylon underpants."
4. "I should void every 6 hours while I am awake."
5. "I should use powder or talc to aid in keeping the perineal skin dry."

18 A client with chronic kidney disease asks the nurse why he is anemic. What response by the nurse is best?

1. "The increased metabolic waste products in your body depress the bone marrow."
2. "We will need to review your dietary intake of iron-rich foods."
3. "There is a decreased production by the kidneys of the hormone erythropoietin."
4. "It is most likely that you have hereditary traits for the development of anemia."

19 A client with end-stage renal disease (ESRD) is to be admitted to the hospital because of shortness of breath. The serum potassium level is 7.0 mEq/L. What appropriate hospital unit should this client be admitted to?

1. A semiprivate room in a medical surgical unit
2. A private room in a medical surgical unit
3. A nursing unit with continuous cardiac monitoring
4. A nursing unit for ventilator-assisted clients

20 A client with chronic kidney disease has fluid overload. The laboratory report indicates the sodium level to be 120 mEq/L. The nurse should draw which conclusion from this data?

1. An elevated sodium level that must be reported
2. An error in the laboratory analysis
3. A possible hemodilution effect
4. An expected reduction in sodium ions

21 A child has been admitted to the unit with nephrotic syndrome. The mother reports that a cousin had acute glomerulonephritis (AGN) last year and asks how these two diseases compare, since they both affect the kidneys. What information should the nurse include in a response?

1. Both disorders produce smoky-colored urine.
2. Both disorders cause greatly reduced urine output.
3. Both disorders have a genetic basis.
4. Both disorders require treatment with antibiotic therapy.

22 The nurse has told the mother of a child being treated for nephrotic syndrome that it is important to keep the child's skin clean and dry. When the mother asks why, what rationale would the nurse include in a response?

1. The skin is fragile secondary to electrolyte deficiency.
2. Frequent urination may leave moisture on the skin that predisposes to breakdown.
3. Dietary restrictions make fighting infection hard.
4. The condition causes a reduction of gamma globulin in the body.

23 In a child with acute kidney disease, the nurse would help to prevent hyperkalemia by limiting which foods in the child's diet?

1. Grains, cheese, and citrus fruits
2. Potatoes, tomatoes, and oranges
3. Cereals, processed sugars, and wheat
4. Rice, yellow vegetables, and iced tea

24 A child has been admitted with acute glomerulonephritis (AGN). The nurse concludes that which positive laboratory test is the most specific indicator of this disease?

1. Elevated antistreptinolysin O (ASO) titers
2. Elevated erythrocyte sedimentation rate (ESR)
3. Presence of hematuria according to urinalysis
4. Elevated creatinine concentrations

25 The mother of a child at the renal clinic asks why an x-ray is performed since the child has only had one documented urinary tract infection (UTI). What information would the nurse include as the best explanation?

1. It rules out structural abnormalities.
2. It confirms the absence of bacterial colonies after antimicrobial therapy.
3. It determines which kidney was infected.
4. It determines the probability of the infection recurring.

26 The nurse is caring for an adult client with poor urine output. The nurse would report to the healthcare provider if the client had a urine output less than how many milliliters (mL) per hour for 2 consecutive hours? Provide a numerical answer.

Fill in your answer below:
Answer: ______________ mL

ANSWERS & RATIONALES

1 **Answer: 4 Rationale:** Many salt substitutes use potassium chloride. Potassium intake is carefully regulated in clients with renal failure, and the use of salt substitutes will worsen hyperkalemia. Increases in weight do need to be reported to the healthcare provider as a possible indication of fluid volume excess. The control of hypertension is essential in the management of a client with renal failure. An AV fistula does need to be protected from injury that could be caused by constricting clothing, venipunctures, and other items. **Cognitive Level:** Analyzing **Client Need:** Physiological Adaptation **Integrated Process:** Nursing Process: Evaluation **Content Area:** Adult Health: Renal and Genitourinary **Strategy:** The core issue of the question is the ability to determine accurate statements about self-care of clients with renal failure. Specifically, clients need to restrict both sodium and potassium, and salt substitutes are high in potassium. Use nursing knowledge and the process of elimination to make a selection.

2 **Answer: 4 Rationale:** Nephrotoxic drugs, such as aminoglycoside antibiotics (tobramycin), can damage the nephrons and cause intrinsic (within the kidneys) failure. Prerenal causes of renal failure include any condition that reduces the blood flow to the kidney, such as heart failure, shock, and other conditions. Postrenal failure can be caused by conditions that obstruct urine outflow in the lower urinary system. There is no condition called extrarenal failure. **Cognitive Level:** Applying **Client Need:** Physiological Adaptation **Integrated Process:** Nursing Process: Diagnosis **Content Area:** Adult Health: Renal and Genitourinary **Strategy:** The core issue of the question is the ability to associate causes of renal failure with their categories in specific client situations. Use nursing knowledge and the process of elimination to make a selection.

3 **Answer: 2 Rationale:** Phenazopyridine makes the urine reddish-orange in color, and the client should be advised that this might stain the underwear and other clothing. The client should also be reassured that it should not be confused with blood in the urine. Phenazopyridine does not target the cause of the infection. Taking the drug after meals minimizes GI symptoms associated with the use of this drug. Indiscriminate use of a urinary analgesic can mask symptoms and delay initiation of treatment. **Cognitive Level:** Analyzing **Client Need:** Pharmacological and Parenteral Therapies **Integrated Process:** Communication and Documentation **Content Area:** Adult Health: Renal and Genitourinary **Strategy:** The core issue of the question is knowledge of expected adverse effects of phenazopyridine. Use nursing knowledge and the process of elimination to make a selection.

4 **Answer: 3, 5 Rationale:** Emptying the reservoir bag every 2 hours prevents overfilling and possible leakage of urine onto the skin surface. Ensuring that opening is not more than 0.3 cm (⅛ in.) larger than stoma reduces the risk of skin irritation and breakdown from urine on the skin. The urine collection device should be changed as needed to maintain integrity of the system. Self-catheterization is not appropriate for this clinical situation. Monitoring for foul-smelling urine and monitoring for signs of infection are more appropriate interventions for addressing a risk for infection. **Cognitive Level:** Applying **Client Need:** Physiological Adaptation **Integrated Process:** Nursing Process: Implementation **Content Area:** Adult Health **Strategy:** The core issue of the question is knowledge of appropriate care for a client with a urinary diversion. Use nursing knowledge and the process of elimination to make a selection.

5 **Answer: 3 Rationale:** Chocolate, smoked fish, milk products, beans, lentils, and dried fruits are high in calcium. In calcium phosphate and calcium oxalate calculi, dietary management includes an acid-ash diet and limiting foods high in calcium and oxalate. Chicken, beef, and salmon may be consumed as desired. Green vegetables, fruit, and legumes may be consumed as desired. Eggs, meat, and poultry may be consumed as desired. **Cognitive Level:** Analyzing **Client Need:** Physiological Adaptation **Integrated Process:** Nursing Process: Evaluation **Content Area:** Adult Health: Renal and Genitourinary **Strategy:** The core issue of the question is knowledge of high-calcium foods to avoid with renal calculi. Use nursing knowledge and the process of elimination to make a selection.

6 **Answer: 4 Rationale:** Peritonitis is a grave complication of peritoneal dialysis, caused by bacteria that may enter through the catheter or dialysate solution. Hypotension is a common complication of hemodialysis but not peritoneal dialysis. Pulmonary embolism and dyspnea are not common complications of peritoneal dialysis. **Cognitive Level:** Applying **Client Need:** Physiological Adaptation **Integrated Process:** Nursing Process: Implementation **Content Area:** Adult Health: Renal and Genitourinary **Strategy:** The core issue of the question is knowledge of complications of peritoneal dialysis and their relative frequency. Use nursing knowledge and the process of elimination to make a selection.

7 **Answer: 4 Rationale:** Urge incontinence is the unpredictable passage of urine soon after a strong urge to void is felt. Overflow incontinence is involuntary loss of urine because of a full bladder. Stress incontinence is loss of urine when intra-abdominal pressure rises, such as with coughing or sneezing. Urinary retention is an inability to empty the bladder. **Cognitive Level:** Applying **Client Need:** Physiological Adaptation **Integrated Process:** Nursing Process: Planning **Content Area:** Adult Health: Renal and Genitourinary **Strategy:** Use nursing knowledge and the process of elimination to make a selection.

8 **Answer: 3 Rationale:** The symptoms are typical of acute glomerulonephritis. Hematuria and proteinuria are caused by a damaged glomerular capillary membrane, which allows blood cells and proteins to escape into the renal filtrate. A urinary tract infection usually manifests with signs of infection including fever, malodorous urine, frequency, and urgency. Clients with urinary calculi usually present with renal colic. Prostatitis, or inflammation of the prostate gland, has presenting symptoms similar to a urinary tract infection. **Cognitive Level:** Analyzing **Client Need:** Physiological Adaptation **Integrated Process:** Nursing Process: Assessment **Content Area:** Adult Health: Renal and Genitourinary **Strategy:** The core issue of the question is the ability to identify signs and symptoms of glomerulonephritis and associate it with a common etiology. Use nursing knowledge and the process of elimination to make a selection.

9 **Answer: 3 Rationale:** Prerenal type of acute kidney injury is caused by factors such as hypovolemia and decreased cardiac output that reduce renal blood flow and perfusion. Vascular disease may be a factor in the development of intrinsic failure. Urethral obstruction can cause postrenal failure. Glomerulonephritis may be a factor in the development of intrinsic failure. **Cognitive Level:** Applying **Client Need:** Physiological Adaptation **Integrated Process:** Nursing Process: Diagnosis **Content Area:** Adult Health: Renal and Genitourinary **Strategy:** The core issue of the question is the ability to identify causes of prerenal failure. Use nursing knowledge and the process of elimination to make a selection.

10 **Answer: 1, 2 Rationale:** The client should maintain a fluid intake of 2000–2500 mL per day to reduce the risk of nephrotoxicity. To detect nephrotoxicity early, the client should report signs of edema. Edema is not a normal side effect of the medication. To reduce the risk of nephrotoxicity, the client should report hypertension. It is unnecessary to eat a low-protein diet while taking an aminoglycoside antibiotic. **Cognitive Level:** Analyzing **Client Need:** Pharmacological and Parenteral Therapies **Integrated Process:** Nursing Process: Implementation **Content Area:** Adult Health: Renal and Genitourinary **Strategy:** The core issue of the question is the ability to correctly institute client teaching about nephrotoxicity as an adverse effect of aminoglycoside medications. Use nursing knowledge and the process of elimination to make a selection.

11 **Answer: 4 Rationale:** Hypotension is the most common complication during hemodialysis and is related to several factors, including changes in serum osmolality and rapid removal of fluid from the intravascular compartment. Hyperglycemia could occur in peritoneal dialysis because of the glucose composition of the dialysate. Infection and fever should be an ongoing assessment, not just when the client is undergoing hemodialysis. Dialysis dementia is a progressive, long-term complication. **Cognitive Level:** Applying **Client Need:** Physiological Adaptation **Integrated Process:** Nursing Process: Assessment **Content Area:** Adult Health: Renal and Genitourinary **Strategy:** The core issue of the question is the ability to identify important complications associated with hemodialysis. Use nursing knowledge and the process of elimination to make a selection.

12 **Answer: 3 Rationale:** The peritoneum acts as a semipermeable membrane, allowing substances to move from an area of high concentration (the blood) to an area of lower concentration (the dialysate). Metabolic waste products and excess water can be eliminated through osmosis and diffusion, utilizing the peritoneum as the semipermeable membrane. Solutes in dialysis are not intended for absorption into the bloodstream, although glucose in dialysate may do so, raising blood glucose levels in clients with diabetes. Excess metabolites do not make the peritoneum more permeable. How metabolites move from interstitial spaces into the bloodstream is not relevant to the procedure for peritoneal dialysis. **Cognitive Level:** Applying **Client Need:** Physiological Adaptation **Integrated Process:** Communication and Documentation **Content Area:** Adult Health: Renal and Genitourinary **Strategy:** The core issue of the question is the ability to relate accurately the key elements of peritoneal dialysis. Use nursing knowledge and the process of elimination to make a selection.

13 **Answer: 2 Rationale:** Creatinine is the metabolic end product of creatine phosphate and is excreted via the kidneys in relatively constant amounts. It is the most reliable indicator of kidney function. BUN, a measurement of the nitrogen portion of urea, is also excreted in urine and is a good indicator of renal function. However, conditions that increase protein catabolism also cause a rise in BUN levels. Neutrophils and lymphocytes are not used to monitor the return of renal function. **Cognitive Level:** Analyzing **Client Need:** Physiological Adaptation **Integrated Process:** Nursing Process: Evaluation **Content Area:** Adult Health: Renal and Genitourinary **Strategy:** The critical words in the question are *most accurate*. This tells you that more than one response is technically correct, and you must prioritize an option that best answers the question. Use nursing knowledge and the process of elimination to make a selection.

14 **Answer: 3 Rationale:** Adult polycystic kidney disease is an autosomal-dominant disorder, and the client should be advised to have family members screened for the disease. The cysts will not disappear. Eventually, clients with this disease require dialysis or transplantation because of renal failure. The management of clients with polycystic kidney disease is mainly supportive and not curative. **Cognitive Level:** Analyzing **Client Need:** Physiological Adaptation **Integrated Process:** Nursing Process: Evaluation **Content Area:** Adult Health: Renal and Genitourinary **Strategy:** The core issue of the question is knowledge that polycystic kidney disease has a genetic basis. Use nursing knowledge and the process of elimination to make a selection.

15 **Answer: 4 Rationale:** The proximity of the incision to the muscles involved in breathing and coughing makes the client breathe shallowly and avoid coughing because of the fear of pain. This can lead to atelectasis and pneumonia. The intercostal muscles are not paralyzed by nephrectomy. Pulmonary structures are not contaminated during surgery. The client should be turned and repositioned to reduce the risk of atelectasis and pneumonia. There is no need to lie flat for 24 hours. **Cognitive Level:** Applying **Client Need:** Physiological

Adaptation **Integrated Process:** Nursing Process: Implementation **Content Area:** Adult Health: Renal and Genitourinary **Strategy:** The core issue of the question is the ability to correlate location of incision with risks for postoperative complications after nephrectomy. Use nursing knowledge and the process of elimination to make a selection.

16 **Answer: 2, 5 Rationale:** Clients with renal transplant need to be on long-term immunosuppressive drugs that predispose them to infection. The client must verbalize factors that potentially expose him to infection. Self-monitoring of temperature helps the client detect signs of rejection early that can be reported. The client must adhere to medication doses prescribed by the healthcare provider. Dietary restrictions for sodium must be discussed with the healthcare provider and the dietician. The success of transplantation is not guaranteed and the client could experience signs of rejection after discharge. **Cognitive Level:** Analyzing **Client Need:** Physiological Adaptation **Integrated Process:** Nursing Process: Evaluation **Content Area:** Adult Health: Renal and Genitourinary **Strategy:** The core issue of the question is the knowledge that clients who have had organ transplant are greatly at risk for infection because of drug therapy needed to prevent organ rejection. Use nursing knowledge and the process of elimination to make a selection.

17 **Answer: 1, 2 Rationale:** Tub baths can promote migration of bacteria in the lower urinary tract; the client should shower instead. Maintaining an intake of 8–10 glasses of fluid daily will help prevent UTI. Cotton underpants are best, and nylon should be avoided because synthetic fibers retain body moisture and irritate the perineal area, which can promote the growth of bacteria. Emptying the bladder every 2–4 hours while awake is recommended to prevent urinary stasis. Powder or talc can be irritating to perineal skin and should be avoided. **Cognitive Level:** Analyzing **Client Need:** Physiological Adaptation **Integrated Process:** Nursing Process: Evaluation **Content Area:** Adult Health: Renal and Genitourinary **Strategy:** The core issue of the question is knowledge of risk factors for UTIs that must be avoided by clients at risk. Use nursing knowledge and the process of elimination to make a selection.

18 **Answer: 3 Rationale:** Anemia is common in clients with renal failure because of decreased production of erythropoietin by the kidneys and shortened RBC life. Erythropoietin is involved in the stimulation of the bone marrow to produce RBCs. Metabolic wastes do not depress the bone marrow. Anemia is common in clients with renal failure but is not caused by iron deficiency. Heredity does not play a role in anemia associated with renal failure. **Cognitive Level:** Applying **Client Need:** Physiological Adaptation **Integrated Process:** Communication and Documentation **Content Area:** Adult Health: Renal and Genitourinary **Strategy:** The core issue of the question is the pathophysiology of renal failure and associated changes. Use nursing knowledge and the process of elimination to make a selection.

19 **Answer: 3 Rationale:** Clients with potassium levels of 6.5 and greater are predisposed to develop cardiac arrhythmias, muscle cramps, and gastrointestinal symptoms. The client should be admitted to a nursing unit with telemetry or cardiac monitoring capabilities because of the risk of developing life-threatening cardiac dysrhythmias. Typical ECG abnormalities associated with hyperkalemia are prolonged PR interval; wide QRS; tall, tented T wave; and ST segment depression. Major cardiac dysrhythmias common in clients with highly elevated potassium levels include heart block, ventricular standstill, and ventricular fibrillation. A semi-private room may not necessarily have cardiac monitoring. A private room is not necessary. The client does not need to be admitted to a unit with ventilated clients. **Cognitive Level:** Analyzing **Client Need:** Physiological Adaptation **Integrated Process:** Nursing Process: Planning **Content Area:** Adult Health: Renal and Genitourinary **Strategy:** The core issue of the question is knowledge of the significance of a high serum potassium level in ESRD and the appropriate placement of the client to detect possible complications. Use nursing knowledge and the process of elimination to make a selection.

20 **Answer: 3 Rationale:** Clients with renal failure retain sodium, and any decrease in the serum level (normal 135–145 mEq/L) will most likely be caused by hemodilution from the excessive fluid retention. A sodium level of 120 mEq/L is not an elevated level; it is significantly lower than normal. There is no reason to conclude there is a laboratory error. Clients with renal failure retain sodium, and the number of sodium ions would be expected to increase if there was not a corresponding increase in fluid retention. **Cognitive Level:** Analyzing **Client Need:** Physiological Adaptation **Integrated Process:** Nursing Process: Diagnosis **Content Area:** Adult Health: Renal and Genitourinary **Strategy:** The core issue of the question is the ability to accurately interpret laboratory data in a client with renal failure. Use nursing knowledge and the process of elimination to make a selection.

21 **Answer: 2 Rationale:** Both AGN and nephrotic syndrome are characterized by a reduction in urine output. AGN presents with smoky urine while the urine in nephrotic syndrome is clear and frothy. AGN is a postinfectious disease with no genetic basis. Antibiotics are not used in nephrotic syndrome. **Cognitive Level:** Analyzing **Client Need:** Physiological Adaptation **Integrated Process:** Nursing Process: Diagnosis **Content Area:** Child Health **Strategy:** The core issue of the question is knowledge of the similarities and differences between nephrotic syndrome and glomerulonephritis. Use nursing knowledge and the process of elimination to make a selection.

22 **Answer: 4 Rationale:** Nephrotic syndrome involves the loss of protein in the urine. Gamma globulins, which help the body fight infections, are proteins. There is no electrolyte deficiency. The child is oliguric and therefore does not urinate frequently. The only restrictions on the child's intake are fluid and perhaps sodium. **Cognitive Level:** Analyzing **Client Need:** Physiological Adaptation **Integrated Process:** Nursing Process: Implementation **Content Area:** Child Health **Strategy:** The core issue of the question is the ability to relate gamma globulin deficiency in nephrotic syndrome to situations that increase risk of infection, such as unclean or moist skin. Use nursing knowledge and the process of elimination to make a selection.

23 **Answer: 2 Rationale:** Potatoes, tomatoes, and oranges have a high level of potassium content. Although some citrus fruits (such as oranges) are higher in potassium, grains and cheese are not. Cereals, processed sugars, and wheat are not high in potassium. Rice, yellow vegetables, and iced tea are not high in potassium. **Cognitive Level:** Applying **Client Need:** Physiological Adaptation **Integrated Process:** Nursing Process: Implementation **Content Area:** Child Health **Strategy:** The core issue of the question is knowledge of foods that are high in potassium to avoid in the client with renal failure. Use nursing knowledge and the process of elimination to make a selection.

24 **Answer: 1 Rationale:** An elevated ASO titer indicates a recent streptococcal infection, which is a precursor to AGN. An elevated ESR indicates inflammation in the body, but is nonspecific and can be associated with many diseases. Hematuria is simply blood in the urine, which has many possible causes. Creatinine concentrations reflect the functioning of the kidney. **Cognitive Level:** Analyzing **Client Need:** Physiological Adaptation **Integrated Process:** Nursing Process: Diagnosis **Content Area:** Child Health **Strategy:** The critical words in the question are *most indicative*. This tells you that all options are correct, and you must select the response that uniquely identifies glomerulonephritis as the disorder. Use nursing knowledge and the process of elimination to make a selection.

25 **Answer: 1 Rationale:** Radiologic evaluations done after a documented UTI in children reveal structural abnormalities in 1–2% of girls and 10% of boys. X-rays cannot confirm bacterial colonies, determine the site of an old infection, or help predict whether infection will reoccur. **Cognitive Level:** Applying **Client Need:** Physiological Adaptation **Integrated Process:** Nursing Process: Implementation **Content Area:** Child Health **Strategy:** The core issue of the question is knowledge that UTIs are uncommon in children and could result from structural abnormalities that are yet undiagnosed. With this in mind, use the process of elimination to make a selection from the available options.

26 **Answer: 30 Rationale:** The minimal urine output by the kidneys per hour is 30 mL. It is prudent for the nurse to report a drop below this amount if it persists for 2 hours or longer so that corrective treatment can be undertaken. **Cognitive Level:** Applying **Client Need:** Physiological Adaptation **Integrated Process:** Nursing Process: Implementation **Content Area:** Adult Health: Renal and Genitourinary **Strategy:** The core issue of the question is knowledge of minimal hourly urine output based on normal kidney function. Use nursing knowledge to formulate an answer.

ANSWERS & RATIONALES

Key Terms to Review

acute kidney injury p. 1016
anuria p. 1010
azotemia p. 1017
chordee p. 1022
chronic kidney disease p. 1016
circumcision p. 1022
creatinine p. 1001
cryptorchidism p. 1023
cystectomy p. 1008
cystitis p. 1014
epispadias p. 1022
exstrophy p. 1022
glomerulonephritis p. 1017
glomerulus p. 1000
hematuria p. 1009
hemodialysis p. 1005
hypospadias p. 1022
intravenous pyelography (IVP) p. 1002
lithotripsy p. 1007
micturition p. 1002
nephrectomy p. 1009
nephron p. 1000
nephrotic syndrome p. 1018
oliguria p. 1017
peritoneal dialysis p. 1004
polycystic kidney disease p. 1018
polyuria p. 1018
proteinuria p. 1010
pyelonephritis p. 1016
pyuria p. 1009
urinary diversion p. 1008
vesicoureteral reflux p. 1016

References

Ball, J., & Bindler, R., & Cowen, K. (2015). *Principles of pediatric nursing: Caring for children* (6th ed.). Hoboken, NJ: Pearson Education.

Berman, A., Snyder, S., & Frandsen, G. (2016). *Kozier & Erb's fundamentals of nursing: Concepts, process, and practice* (10th ed.). New York, NY: Pearson Education.

Ignatavicius, D., & Workman, L. (2016). *Medical-surgical nursing: Patient-centered collaborative care* (10th ed.). Philadelphia: Saunders.

LeMone, P., Burke, K., Bauldoff, G., & Gubrud, P. (2015). *Medical surgical nursing: Clinical reasoning in patient care* (6th ed.). Hoboken, NJ: Pearson Education.

Lewis, S., Dirksen, S., Heitkemper, M., & Bucher, L. (2014). *Medical surgical nursing: Assessment and management of clinical problems* (9th ed.). St. Louis, MO: Elsevier Science.

Smith, S., Duell, D., Martin, B., Aebersold, M., & Gonzalez, L. (2017). *Clinical nursing skills: Basic to advanced skills* (10th ed.). New York, NY: Pearson Education.

Gastrointestinal Disorders

59

In this chapter

Cross Reference

Other chapters relevant to this content area are

Total Parenteral Nutrition	**Chapter 33**
Gastrointestinal Medications	**Chapter 40**
Common Laboratory Tests	**Chapter 46**
Common Diagnostic Tests and Procedures	**Chapter 47**
Perioperative Care	**Chapter 48**

I. OVERVIEW OF ANATOMY AND PHYSIOLOGY OF GI SYSTEM

A. Gastrointestinal tract

1. Oral cavity and pharynx: consists of mouth, oropharynx and laryngopharynx; passageway for food, fluids, and air
2. Esophagus: extends from pharynx to stomach; enters stomach at gastroesophageal sphincter (also called lower esophageal sphincter, or LES), which prevents reflux
3. Stomach: distensible organ located high on left side of abdomen; has four regions (cardiac, fundus, body, and pyloric); churns gastric contents via peristalsis and mixes food with gastric secretions (including pepsin and hydrochloric acid) to form chyme; produces intrinsic factor for vitamin B_{12} absorption in small intestine
4. Small intestine: extends from pyloric sphincter to ileocecal valve; has three regions: duodenum, jejunum, and ileum; pancreatic enzymes (trypsin, chymotrypsin, lipase, and amylase) and bile enter duodenum near pyloric sphincter to further digest chyme; most absorption occurs in villae of small intestine
5. Large intestine: also called colon; extends from ileocecal valve to anus; has five areas: cecum, appendix, colon (ascending, transverse, and descending), rectum, and anus; major functions are to absorb water, salts, and vitamins (some B vitamins and vitamin K) formed by bacteria in large intestine and eliminate undigestible food and residue

B. Hepatobiliary system

1. Liver
   a. Located in right upper quadrant (RUQ) of abdomen, beneath diaphragm; produces bile, an alkaline, yellow-green fluid containing bile salts (conjugated bile acids), cholesterol, bilirubin (by-product of red blood cell [RBC] destruction), electrolytes, and water
   b. Stores vitamin B_{12} and fat-soluble vitamins (A, D, E, and K)
   c. Stores and releases blood during hemorrhage
   d. Synthesizes plasma proteins to maintain plasma oncotic pressure
   e. Synthesizes prothrombin, fibrinogen, and clotting factors I, II, VII, IX, X
   f. Converts amino acids to carbohydrates through deamination
   g. Stores and releases glucose and copper; stores iron as ferritin
   h. Detoxifies alcohol and certain drugs
2. Biliary tract: composed of gallbladder and associated ducts (cystic, hepatic, and common bile ducts); transports bile formed in liver to bile ducts, gallbladder, and eventually duodenum
3. Gallbladder: saclike organ located on inferior surface of liver; stores and concentrates bile; releases bile into cystic duct and common bile duct in response to presence of fat in duodenum (which leads to secretion of cholecystokinin to contract gallbladder and relax sphincter of Oddi)
4. Pancreas: performs exocrine and endocrine functions; head is located within curve of duodenum, tail touches spleen, and body lies behind stomach
   a. Pancreatic secretions flow into duodenum via pancreatic duct
   b. Endocrine pancreas secretes insulin from islets of Langerhans into bloodstream for carbohydrate metabolism; also secretes glucagon to stimulate glycogenolysis in liver (raising blood glucose) and somatostatin to inhibit pancreatic hormones (insulin and glucagon)
   c. Exocrine pancreas secretes sodium bicarbonate, which neutralizes acidic chyme that enters duodenum and pancreatic digestive enzymes (lipase for fat breakdown, amylase for carbohydrate breakdown, and trypsin, chymotrypsin, and carboxypeptidase for protein breakdown)

II. DIAGNOSTIC TESTS AND ASSESSMENTS OF GI SYSTEM

A. Laboratory tests: serum chemistry study, liver profile, lipid profile, gastrin levels, Schilling test, erythrocyte sedimentation rate (ESR), C-reactive protein (CRP), thyroid function (see Chapter 46)

B. Upper GI series: fluoroscopy study using barium sulfate to diagnose hiatal hernia, tumors, ulcerations, inflammation, varices, or obstruction

1. After client drinks barium, fluoroscopy documents progression of contrast as client is placed in different positions
2. Gastroesophageal reflux (from stomach into esophagus) can be assessed with client in a flat or head-down position
3. Contraindications: complete bowel obstruction, esophageal or gastric perforation, pregnancy, or unstable vital signs (VS)

NCLEX®

4. Possible complications: aspiration of contrast medium, constipation, or partial bowel obstruction

C. Lower GI series: fluoroscopy study using contrast medium (barium enema)

1. Visualizes colon, including appendix, for anatomic abnormalities, polyps, ulcers, tumors, inflammatory bowel disease, fistulas, and diverticula

NCLEX®

2. Scheduling considerations: perform before an upper GI study to prevent residual barium remaining in colon, and colon should also be empty
   a. Clear liquid diet day before test
   b. Magnesium citrate or other bowel prep night before test
   c. NPO after midnight and continue until test is complete
   d. Cleansing enemas may be prescribed before test
   e. Contraindications: perforated colon, uncooperative client
   f. Possible complications: colonic perforation or barium impaction

D. Upper GI endoscopy: *esophagogastroduodenoscopy (EGD)*, gastroscopy

1. Allows direct visualization of esophagus, stomach, and duodenum through lighted endoscope under moderate sedation
2. Used also to directly sample tissues and fluids, to stop areas of active GI bleeding with injection of sclerosing agents or cautery, or to perform GI laser surgery
3. Contraindications: perforated colon, fulminant ulcerative colitis, toxic megacolon, or pregnancy

NCLEX®

4. Possible complications: pulmonary aspiration of GI contents; perforation of esophagus, stomach, or duodenum; bleeding from biopsy site; and reactions to sedatives given during test

NCLEX®

5. Postprocedure nursing considerations: NPO until client is alert and swallowing/gag reflexes have returned (2–4 hours); general safety precautions because of moderate sedation; monitor for bleeding, dyspnea, or dysphagia

E. Colonoscopy

1. Fiberoptic direct visualization of colon from anus to cecum; tissue biopsy can be performed

NCLEX®

2. Possible complications: perforation of colon, bleeding from biopsy sites, oversedation

NCLEX®

3. Special nursing considerations: requires complete bowel prep; monitor VS postprocedure for signs of bleeding and colon perforation
4. A variation is *sigmoidoscopy*: direct visualization of anus, rectum, and sigmoid colon with either a rigid or flexible sigmoidoscope; less extensive study than colonoscopy but similar in procedure, contraindications, complications, and nursing considerations

F. Ultrasonography

1. Noninvasive visualization of abdominal organs using high-frequency sound waves; detects organ size, cyst formation, tumors, and filling defects
2. No contrast medium or radiation is involved, so there are no contraindications and no complications

G. Computed tomography (CT) scan: radiologic procedure (with or without contrast) used to diagnose a variety of conditions (see also Chapter 48)

1. Take usual precautions with use of iodinated contrast medium; contraindicated with pregnancy, unstable VS, morbid obesity, and claustrophobia

NCLEX®

2. Special nursing considerations: encourage clients to drink fluids to promote contrast elimination and monitor for delayed reaction to contrast medium

H. Gastric analysis

1. Stomach contents are aspirated via NG tube; pH is measured in four samples taken 15 minutes apart to measure basal acid output (BAO); a medication such as histamine or pentagastrin is given subcutaneously to stimulate acid output; then four additional samples are taken 15 minutes apart to measure maximal acid output (MAO)
2. Differentiates causes of hypergastrinemia, including **Zollinger-Ellison syndrome** (elevated gastrin levels from pancreatic tumor), chronic antacid ingestion, and atrophic gastritis
3. Preprocedure care includes withholding medications that stimulate gastric secretions for 12–24 hours prior to test, fasting for 8–12 hours prior, and avoiding tobacco or chewing gum for 6 hours prior

NCLEX®

4. Postprocedure care: no special precautions are needed but assess clients who have heart failure, carcinoid syndrome, or hypertension because symptoms may be exacerbated because of histamine use during test

Box 59–1

Common Foods and Substances Affecting Results for Occult Blood in Stool

Causes False-Positive Results	Causes False-Negative Results
➤ Red meat	➤ Vitamin C
➤ Fish	➤ Turnips
➤ Oral iron supplements	➤ Horseradish
➤ Iodine	➤ Beets
➤ Boric acid	➤ Melons
➤ Colchicine	
➤ Drugs irritating to gastric mucosa: aspirin, NSAIDs, corticosteroids	

I. Stool examination

1. Examines fecal specimen for consistency, color, and other targeted tests
2. Stool culture, ova, and parasites: detects bacterial pathogens and parasitic pathogens such as hookworm, tape worm, and protozoa
3. Stool for occult blood: tests stool with a reagent to detect blood that is not visible; see Box 59–1 for substances that cause a false-positive or false-negative result for blood
4. NCLEX® Fecal fat: measures fat content of stool over 24 hours from conditions such as cystic fibrosis, celiac disease, sprue, Crohn's disease (regional enteritis), Whipple's disease, and maldigestion from pancreatobiliary tree obstruction; instruct client to abstain from alcohol and eat a diet that contains 100 grams of fat per day for 3 days before and during stool collection
5. NCLEX® Stool for clostridial toxin: *Clostridium difficile* bacteria release a toxin that causes necrosis of bowel epithelium; infection occurs in people who are immunocompromised or after taking broad-spectrum antibiotics

III. NURSING MANAGEMENT OF CLIENT HAVING GI SURGERY

A. ***Colostomy***: fecal diversion to an external collection device; named for portion of colon from which it is formed: ascending, transverse, descending, or sigmoid; see Figure 59–1

1. Preoperative period
   a. Teach client and family about procedure and postoperative course, including pain relief, breathing exercises, and appearance of stoma (to reduce client anxiety and promote postoperative participation in care); encourage client to verbalize concerns about lifestyle changes; provide appropriate referrals for support (such as United Ostomy Association)
   b. Consult with enterostomal therapist, who will advise surgeon regarding optimal ostomy placement
   c. NCLEX® Carry out preoperative checklist activities and bowel preparation prescriptions, which usually include low-residue diet for 1–2 days before surgery; bowel cleansing with cathartics and enemas as well as oral or parenteral antibiotics (to reduce bacteria count)

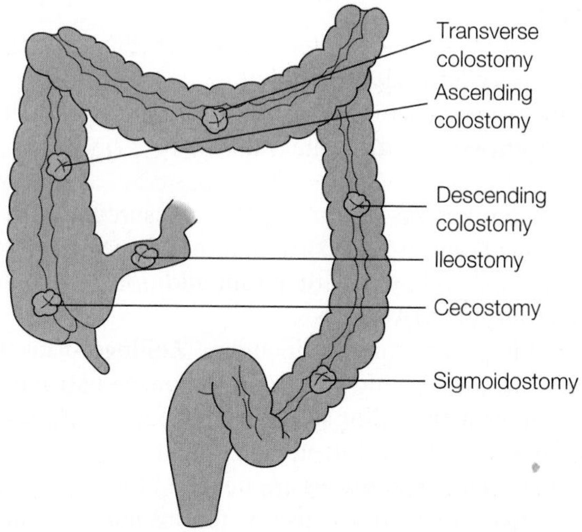

Figure 59–1

Colostomy locations and types.

2. Postoperative period
    a. Routine postoperative care(see also Chapter 48): monitor VS and bowel sounds; assess I&O including drainage from tubes (wound, NG, urinary catheter, etc.); evaluate incision(s) and perianal area; assess LOC and encourage pulmonary hygiene measures

NCLEX®
    b. Assess appearance and drainage from stoma, identify any changes, and notify surgeon if stoma becomes pale, darkened, cyanotic, sunken, stenosed (narrowed opening), or if bleeding increases

NCLEX®
    c. Assess pouch system for proper fit (only 3 mm [⅛ in.] space between stoma and appliance) and signs of leakage; empty when one-third full; assess skin surrounding stoma to be sure it is intact when changing ostomy appliance
    d. Monitor pain control and take appropriate actions if pain is not controlled (check patency of IV access, notify healthcare provider, provide comfort measures)
    e. Encourage ambulation as prescribed to stimulate peristalsis
    f. Resume oral intake as prescribed and monitor for nausea, abdominal distension, and adequacy of bowel sounds

NCLEX®
    g. Begin discharge teaching: possible postoperative complications (infection, bowel obstruction, abdominal abscess) and preventative measures; colostomy care (irrigation depending on stoma location, pouch management, skin care)

B. *Ileostomy*: large intestine is removed and fecal diversion is created at level of ileum
1. Preoperative period: same care as before colostomy surgery
2. Postoperative period
    a. Provide routine postoperative care as per colostomy surgery
    b. Apply ostomy appliance (pouch) over stoma and teach client and family about procedure and nature of effluent (initially dark green, more liquid than colostomy, but will thicken slightly over time and become yellow-brown)

NCLEX®
    c. Protect skin around stoma with a skin barrier from irritating effects of liquid effluent, which contains digestive enzymes and bile salts
    d. Begin educating client and family early about how to manage stoma, appliance, and skin care, and when to report abnormalities in stoma, effluent, or abdomen

NCLEX®
    e. Emphasize importance of nutrition, need for adequate fluid and electrolyte intake, and symptoms of an imbalance; because of liquid effluent, clients are at high risk for dehydration and electrolyte imbalance, especially during hot weather, sustained exercise, or fever

C. Gastrectomy: removal of stomach with anastomosis of esophagus to jejunum (esophagojejunostomy); rarely performed, usually only for extensive gastric cancer or Zollinger-Ellison syndrome unresponsive to medical treatment
1. Preoperative period
    a. Reinforce healthcare provider teaching and obtain signed surgical consent form
    b. Advise client and family what to expect postoperatively, including pain relief, breathing exercises, expected tubes (nasogastric [NG], drains, jejunostomy feeding tube), and ambulation
2. Postoperative period
    a. Assess VS, lung and bowel sounds, I&O including drainage from NG tube, wound drainage (amount and character), effectiveness of pain-control measures

NCLEX®
    b. Do not reposition, irrigate, or check placement of NG tube because of risk of disrupting esophagojejunostomy sutures (check agency policy and surgeon's prescriptions)
    c. Implement standard postoperative care (pain management, progressive activity to ambulation)
    d. Discuss limitations in oral intake and alternate methods to maintain nutrition; may require jejunostomy tube with an elemental (requires no digestion) enteral feeding

NCLEX®
    e. Teach client about postoperative complications, including pernicious anemia (requiring vitamin B_{12} injections monthly), abdominal abscess or infection, and decreased nutrition

D. Gastric resection: portion of stomach removed for diseases such as cancer and peptic ulcer disease refractory to medical management (removing antrum eliminates most gastrin-producing cells)
1. Preoperative period
    a. Insert NG tube if prescribed and connect to suction (may be inserted in operating room)
    b. Provide standard preoperative care for client having abdominal surgery
2. Postoperative period
    a. Provide standard postoperative care for client having abdominal surgery (see also Chapter 48)
    b. Do *not* reposition, irrigate, or check placement of NG tube (unless there is a specific healthcare provider prescription) because of risk of disrupting stomach sutures
    c. Encourage ambulation to promote peristalsis and prevent postoperative complications such as paralytic ileus and obstruction

NCLEX® d. Assess for signs of acute gastric dilation as a postoperative complication (epigastric pain, fullness, hiccups, tachycardia, and hypotension, which results from a malfunctioning NG tube and rapidly improves after tube is flushed (if prescribed by healthcare provider) or replaced (by surgeon or designee)

NCLEX® 3. **Dumping syndrome** is a common complication of gastric resection when pylorus is bypassed; after eating there is rapid emptying of food into jejunum without proper mixing and duodenal digestion

a. Early manifestations: occur 15–30 minutes postprandial (after eating) and include vertigo, tachycardia, syncope, sweating, pallor, and palpitations; believed to be caused by a rapid shift of extracellular fluid into bowel to dilute hypertonic chyme, thereby decreasing blood volume

b. Late manifestations occur 2–3 hours postprandial and include epigastric fullness, distension, diarrhea, abdominal cramping, nausea, and high-pitched bowel sounds; caused by excessive release of insulin in response to a rapid rise in blood glucose due to high-carbohydrate (CHO) bolus entering jejunum

c. Can be minimized by a low-CHO, high-protein, high-fat diet; suggest also that client avoid drinking fluids with meals and lie down after eating; prescribed antispasmodics or sedatives may delay gastric emptying

E. Bariatric surgery

1. Reduces gastric capacity in morbidly obese clients to aid in long-term weight loss
2. Procedures include Roux-en-Y gastric bypass, vertical sleeve gastrectomy, biliopancreatic diversion with duodenal switch, adjustable gastric banding, and vertical banded gastroplasty
3. Client needs to be willing to modify lifestyle to lose weight and maintain weight loss; community support services include American Obesity Association, Overeaters Anonymous, and American Society for Metabolic and Bariatric Surgery
4. Preoperative period
   a. Provide standard preoperative care with special attention to preventing pulmonary and thromboembolic complications (see also Chapter 48)
   b. Be attentive to potential skin integrity irritations (such as in skinfolds), mobility issues, and need for special equipment to accommodate client size and weight (such as bed, mechanical lifts, extended-capacity wheelchair, and friction-reducing devices such as slider boards and pressure-reducing mattress)
5. Postoperative period
   a. Provide standard postoperative care for client having abdominal surgery (see also Chapter 48)
   b. Elevate head of bed and be prepared to use continuous positive airway pressure (CPAP) device as prescribed to maintain adequate respiratory function
   c. Be prepared to monitor cardiac rhythm (increased risk of heart disease) and blood glucose levels (stress from surgery increases cortisol) and provide meticulous wound care (excess adipose can impair immune function and wound healing)

NCLEX® d. Diet progression after surgery includes clear liquids after bowel sounds return until tolerated for 24–48 hours, then full liquids and pureed foods for about another 6 weeks, then a nutrient-dense regular diet with small meals

   e. Diet teaching includes avoiding foods high in sugar, fat, and protein; avoiding alcohol; eating slowly and chewing thoroughly; taking multivitamin and/or mineral supplements as prescribed (often additional B_{12}, calcium, and iron)

F. Billroth I (gastroduodenostomy): a partial gastrectomy in which distal portion of stomach (including antrum) is removed and remainder is anastomosed to duodenum (see Figure 59–2A); gastrin-producing cells in antrum, as well as some parietal cells (acid-pepsinogen secreting cells), are removed

1. Preoperative and postoperative care is same as for any client having gastric surgery
2. Dumping syndrome is a common complication of this procedure

G. Billroth II (gastrojejunostomy): a partial gastrectomy in which lower portion of stomach is removed and proximal remnant is anastomosed to jejunum (see Figure 59–2B); used to treat gastric and duodenal ulcers refractory to medical treatment

1. Preoperative and postoperative care is same as for any client having gastric surgery

NCLEX® 2. Dumping syndrome is a common complication of this procedure

IV. NUTRITIONAL DISORDERS

A. Malnutrition

1. Insufficient amounts, improper proportions, malabsorption, or improper distribution of foods needed to provide body with energy for normal functions

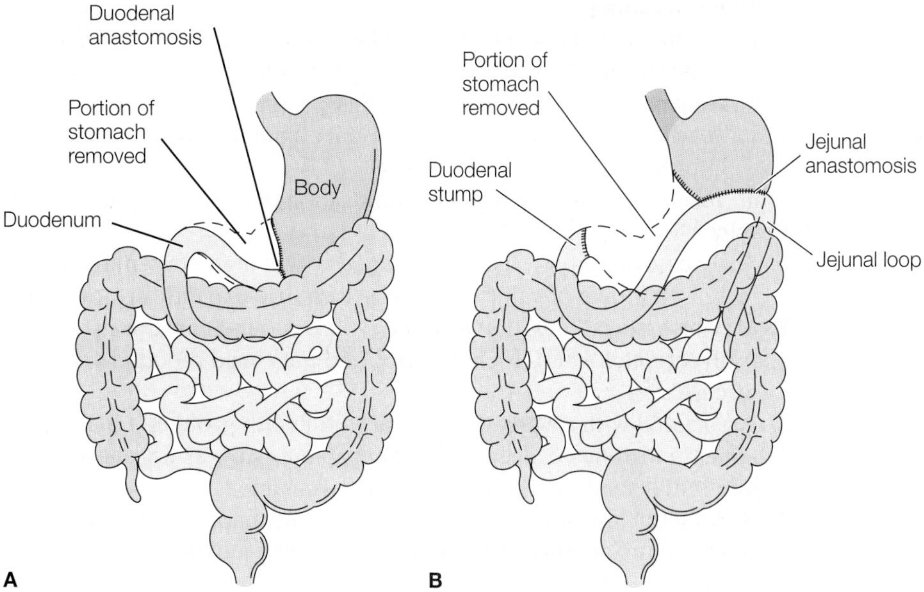

Figure 59–2

Partial gastrectomy. (**A**) Gastroduodenostomy or Billroth I, (**B**) gastrojejunostomy or Billroth II.

2. Can also result from loss of nutrients as in prolonged vomiting
3. When more energy is expended than is consumed, body uses stored forms of energy in a certain order: first CHOs stored as glycogen, then fat stores, and finally protein stores in form of muscle tissue

NCLEX®

4. Malnutrition can result from a variety of conditions (see Table 59–1)
5. Nursing assessment
   a. Body mass index (BMI) estimates total body fat stores in relation to height and weight (weight in kg divided by body surface area)

NCLEX®

   b. Clinical manifestations include cheilosis, glossitis, stomatitis, muscle wasting, anemia, edema, alopecia, spongy bleeding gums, dry scaling skin, subcutaneous fat loss, bone pain, confusion, disorientation, paresthesia, heart failure, and decreased hair pigmentation
   c. Diagnosed by history, physical exam, and laboratory results (protein, iron stores, vitamin levels, serum cholesterol, and electrolytes)

NCLEX®

6. **Therapeutic management**
   a. Ensure that client receives prescribed diet (high-calorie, high-protein), and provide a pleasant dining environment, removing sources of unpleasant odors
   b. Encourage client to eat in a slow, relaxed manner
   c. Provide enteral nutrition if prescribed (see also Chapter 25)
   d. Provide skin care and encourage activity to prevent skin breakdown
   e. Assess for and instruct client about signs and symptoms of infection and to report them to healthcare provider if they occur
   f. Medications generally include pancreatic enzymes, vitamins, minerals, antiemetics, antidiarrheals, antibiotics (for infectious diarrhea), insulin, and possibly total parenteral nutrition (TPN)

Table 59–1 Causes and Conditions Leading to Malnutrition

Type of Cause	Sample Conditions
Insufficient nutrients	Liver failure (liver normally makes blood proteins), starvation, anorexia nervosa or bulimia, severe illness or trauma (increases protein and calorie requirements)
Improper dietary proportions	Fad dieting, unavailability of variety of foods, maldigestion of certain foods because of a loss of enzymes, acid, or hormones
Malabsorption	Rapid GI transit time, gastric resection, partial gastrectomy, intestinal infections, absence of some enzymes (as in celiac disease), decreased production or release of bile
Improper distribution	Diabetes mellitus type I (without insulin, glucose cannot enter cells to be used for energy)
Loss of nutrients	Vomiting and severe diarrhea

7. **Client teaching**

NCLEX®
   a. Reinforce diet teaching provided by dietitian and emphasize need to adhere to diet prescription; safe weight gain is 0 45–0.9 kg (1–2 lb) per week

NCLEX®
   b. Help client choose high-calorie, high-protein foods
   c. Teach client about use of any prescribed medications for digestion, vomiting, diarrhea, or intestinal infections
   d. Teach client about proper administration of enteral or parenteral feedings if prescribed

B. Obesity

1. An excess of adipose tissue associated with a high body mass index (30 kg/m^2 or higher) because of increased intake of calories, decreased calorie expenditure, or both
2. May be associated with *metabolic syndrome* (increased waist circumference, hypertension, elevated triglycerides, low HDL cholesterol, and increased blood glucose) and subsequent coronary heart disease
3. Associated with several other comorbid health problems, including type 2 diabetes mellitus, sleep apnea, gallstones, cancer, and joint problems such as degenerative joint disease of weight-bearing joints; may lead to disability or death over time
4. Risk factors include physical inactivity, ready access to high-fat, high-calorie foods (such as served in fast-food restaurants), tendency to eat excessively large portions, psychological factors, and to some extent genetic tendency

NCLEX®

5. Therapeutic management consists of diet, exercise, medication therapy, and bariatric surgery according to client need; see also Chapter 16 for healthy exercise habits and Chapter 25 for healthy nutrition
   a. Medication therapy may include phenteramine or lorcaserin (appetite suppressants) or orlistat (lipase inhibitor)
   b. Diet therapy is planned to created a deficit of 500–1,000 calories/day to achieve a general weight loss of 0.45–0.9 kg (1–2 lb) per week
   c. Food choices should be low in fat and provide adequate nutrients, minerals, and fiber
   d. Exercise level should be self-monitored by client according to maximum heart rate or perceived exertion because fitness levels differ among clients
   e. Behavioral modification strategies include controlling environment (amount and types of food in home, eating meals in one location such as kitchen, and avoiding eating while reading or using computer), controlling physiological responses to food (eat and chew slowly; eat salad or drink hot beverage before meal; put down food or utensil between bites; stop eating when first feeling full), and controlling psychological responses to food (attractive eating environment, small plates to make portions look larger, nonfood rewards for achieving goals)
   f. Community and social support programs include Overeaters Anonymous, Take Off Pounds Sensibly (TOPS), and others

V. GASTROESOPHAGEAL REFLUX DISEASE (GERD)

A. Overview

1. Backward movement of stomach contents into esophagus without vomiting
2. Caused by relaxation of lower esophageal sphincter (LES), decreased LES tone, increased intra-abdominal pressure, increased gastric volume, motility disorder, or a combination of factors (see Box 59–2 for factors influencing LES tone)
3. Reflux of gastric contents is irritating to esophagus and causes breakdown of mucosal barrier, leading to inflammation and erosion

Box 59–2

Factors Decreasing Lower Esophageal Sphincter (LES) Tone

- Nicotine
- Caffeine (coffee, tea, cola)
- Chocolate
- Fatty foods
- Alcohol
- Peppermint, spearmint
- High levels of estrogen and progesterone
- Tight, restrictive clothing
- Bending, straining
- Hiatal hernia
- Medications: anticholinergics, beta-adrenergic blockers, calcium channel blockers, nitrates, theophylline, diazepam

NCLEX® **B. Nursing assessment**

1. Heartburn or substernal burning pain is most common symptom and is exacerbated by bending over, recumbent position, or straining
2. Other symptoms include regurgitation not associated with vomiting or nausea; bad or sour taste upon awakening; coughing, hoarseness, or wheezing at night; painful and difficult swallowing; belching and flatulence

C. Therapeutic management

NCLEX® 1. Avoid foods and medication that reduce LES tone (see Box 59–2)
NCLEX® 2. Do not eat within 2 hours of bedtime or lie down after eating
3. Avoid restrictive clothing that increases intra-abdominal pressure
NCLEX® 4. Avoid large meals; eat smaller meals more often (such as six small meals/day)
5. Limit amount of liquid intake during meals; drink more fluids between meals
NCLEX® 6. Elevate head of bed for sleeping
7. Stop smoking
8. Prescription and OTC medications
   a. Antacids neutralize stomach acid; treat mild to moderate symptoms
   b. H_2 receptor antagonists: ranitidine, famotidine, nizatidine, and cimetidine
   c. Proton pump inhibitors: omeprazole, lansoprazole, esomeprazole, pantoprazole, and rabeprazole

D. Client teaching

1. Reinforce importance of smoking cessation and avoidance of caffeine
2. Avoid bending over and other activities that increase intra-abdominal pressure, especially after eating
3. Take medications as prescribed
4. Lose weight if overweight to decrease intra-abdominal pressure
5. Raise head of bed using wedge under mattress to reduce nighttime reflux

VI. HERNIAS

A. Diaphragmatic hernia in children

1. Overview
   a. A **hernia** is a protrusion of bowel through an abnormal opening in abdominal wall
   b. Congenital diaphragmatic hernia (CDH) is rare and results when abdominal contents protrude into thoracic cavity through an opening in diaphragm because of incomplete development of diaphragm
   c. Intestines and other abdominal structures enter thoracic cavity
   d. Lung growth may cease; after birth, respiration becomes further compromised by pulmonary hypoplasia and lung compression, including airways and blood vessels
2. Nursing assessment
   a. Clinical findings depend on severity of defect
   b. Fetal ultrasound and/or postnatal chest x-ray show abdominal organs in chest
   NCLEX® c. Diminished or absent breath sounds on affected side, with possible barrel-shaped chest, dyspnea, cyanosis, nasal flaring, tachypnea, and retractions
   NCLEX® d. Bowel sounds may be heard over chest; heart sounds may be heard on right side of chest
   e. Abdomen may appear sunken
3. Preoperative therapeutic management
   a. Assess VS frequently with ongoing respiratory assessment
   b. Elevate head of bed and position on affected side
   c. Maintain patency of NG tube to decompress stomach
   d. Monitor IV fluids
   e. Maintain mechanical ventilation, extracorporeal membrane oxygenator (ECMO), chest tubes
   f. Provide minimal stimulation
NCLEX® 4. Postoperative therapeutic management
   a. Focuses on promoting lung function; monitor for signs of infection and respiratory distress
   b. Continue to support respirations by positioning in semi-Fowler position on affected side; organize care to decrease exertion
   c. Promote nutrition when feeding is resumed
   d. Support family through crisis
5. Client and family teaching
   a. Instruct parents on wound care, prevention of infection, and feeding techniques
   b. Provide written and verbal information on growth and developmental needs
   c. Provide information regarding long-term problems and necessity of regular follow-up visits

B. Hiatal hernia in adults

1. Overview
   a. Diaphragmatic weakness through which a portion of stomach herniates into thoracic cavity
   b. Caused by congenital weakness of diaphragm, trauma, obesity, aging, anything that increases intra-abdominal pressure, or a combination of these factors
   c. May lead to complications such as regurgitation, aspiration of stomach contents, ulceration, hemorrhage, or strangulation or incarceration in chest (leading to necrosis of tissue, mediastinitis, and peritonitis)
2. Nursing assessment
   a. Many cases are asymptomatic
   NCLEX® b. Symptoms include heartburn (pyrosis), substernal burning or pain, feeling of fullness, dysphagia, belching, possible vomiting; these are usually worse when reclining
3. Therapeutic management
   NCLEX® a. Conservative treatment: diet therapy and lifestyle modifications (same as discussed for GERD)
   NCLEX® b. Avoid straining and excessive vigorous exercise
   NCLEX® c. Sleep with head of bed elevated 20–30 cm (8–12 in.)
   d. Support client in decision making about surgical procedure (such as Nissen fundoplication or Hill repair), which is used only when conservative treatment has failed
   e. Provide preoperative and postoperative care as discussed previously for client undergoing gastric surgery
   NCLEX® f. Medication therapy: antacids and H_2 receptor antagonists (see treatment for GERD)
4. Client teaching
   a. Report any increase in symptoms
   b. Do not take antacids within 2 hours of other medications
   c. Avoid alcohol, caffeine, NSAIDs, and any medication containing aspirin
   NCLEX® d. Follow diet recommendations and avoid lying down for an hour after meals

C. Umbilical hernia

1. Overview
   a. A soft, skin-covered protrusion of intestine and omentum (double fold of peritoneum) through a weakness in abdominal wall around umbilicus
   b. In an umbilical hernia, incomplete closure of umbilical ring results in protrusion of portions of omentum and intestine through opening
   c. Defect usually closes spontaneously by age 3 or 4 years; surgical correction is needed if closure does not occur or if incarceration of herniated bowel occurs
2. NCLEX® Nursing assessment
   a. Soft swelling or protrusion around umbilicus, usually reducible using a finger
   b. An incarcerated hernia is one that cannot be reduced and increases risk of bowel ischemia; it produces symptoms such as irritability, tenderness at site, anorexia, abdominal distention, and difficult defecation
3. Therapeutic management
   a. Most umbilical hernias disappear spontaneously by 1 year of age
   NCLEX® b. No surgical repair is needed unless it causes symptoms, persists past 5 years of age, becomes strangulated, or continues to grow
   c. Binding is not effective in reducing or minimizing the protrusion
   d. Monitor for changes in size of hernia
   NCLEX® e. Assess for increased bowel sounds and irreducible mass, which may indicate strangulation
   NCLEX® f. Postoperatively, assess for wound infection, maintain hydration, assess and manage pain, allow for self-expression
4. Client and family education
   a. Signs of strangulation, such as vomiting, pain, and an irreducible mass at umbilicus; signs and symptoms of wound infection
   NCLEX® b. Avoid ineffective and potentially harmful home remedies such as "belly binders"
   c. Any precautions and restrictions, such as tub bathing or strenuous activity if surgery was performed

VII. PEPTIC ULCER DISEASE (PUD)

A. Overview

1. A generic term for ulcers or breaks in mucosal lining of GI tract that come in contact with gastric secretions; can occur in stomach (gastric ulcers, less common), duodenum (duodenal ulcers, more common), or lower esophagus (esophageal ulcers, rare)

2. Gastric ulcer
   a. Results from a disruption in normal protective mechanism that keeps gastric epithelial pH normal
   b. Prostaglandins in gastric mucosa increase resistance to acid; therefore, medications that reduce prostaglandins (such as aspirin, NSAIDs, alcohol), will decrease gastric mucosal resistance
   c. Gastric ulcers are associated with *H. pylori*, gastritis, alcohol, smoking, use of NSAIDs, stress, and an increased incidence of gastric cancer
3. Duodenal ulcer
   a. A chronic break in duodenal mucosa to muscularis mucosae layer; most common type of ulcer
   b. Results from increased gastric acid from increased number of parietal cells, vagal activity, or secretion of gastrin
   c. Associated with chronic *H. pylori* infection, alcohol, smoking, cirrhosis, and stress
4. Other factors that increase risk for PUD include cigarette smoking, family history, blood group O (duodenal ulcer), alcohol use, and increasing age (peaks in sixth decade)

NCLEX® **B. Nursing assessment**

1. Pain: gnawing, burning, aching, hungerlike, in epigastrium
   a. Duodenal ulcers: pain relieved by eating
   b. Gastric ulcers: pain not relieved by food and may be worsened by food intake
2. Tests for *H. pylori* usually positive; ulcer can be visualized by EGD
3. Observe for complications: perforation (pain, signs of peritonitis, shock), pyloric obstruction (vomiting, feeling of fullness), and hemorrhage (hematemesis more common if gastric, tarry stool or melena more common if duodenal, stool positive for occult blood with either type)

C. Therapeutic management

1. Reinforce importance of following treatment plan to reduce symptoms
2. NCLEX® Explain that no foods cause ulcers but some foods aggravate active PUD (coffee, cola, tea, chocolate, foods high in sodium, and foods that are spicy to client) and should be avoided during acute phase; even decaffeinated coffee stimulates gastrin release
3. Provide smoking-cessation information and refer to smoking-cessation program
4. Smaller, more frequent meals (six small meals/day) may be better tolerated
5. NCLEX® Medication therapy
   a. Antacids are used to neutralize acid
   b. H_2 receptor antagonists block histamine-stimulated gastric secretions; proton pump inhibitors suppress the production of hydrochloric acid
   c. Prostaglandin analogs: misoprostol contributes to mucosal barrier, preventing NSAID-induced ulcers
   d. Mucosal barrier fortifier: sucralfate forms protective barrier over ulcer crater and prevents further erosion by acid and pepsin
   e. Treatment for *H. pylori* changes frequently but generally includes antimicrobials such as metronidazole or erythromycin, proton pump inhibitors, and bismuth subsalicylate

D. Client teaching

1. Take medications as prescribed
2. Learn signs of complications: blood in stool, vomiting, increased pain
3. Follow diet recommendations restricting caffeine, alcohol, and nicotine

VIII. IRRITABLE BOWEL SYNDROME (IBS)

A. Overview

1. Common noninflammatory functional bowel disorder characterized by abdominal pain with bloating and constipation, diarrhea, or both
2. May result from increased motor reactivity of bowel to aggravating factors such as stress, anxiety, depression, certain foods and food additives in some clients, drugs, toxins, and hormones

B. Nursing assessment

1. NCLEX® Abdominal pain: relieved by defecation; intermittent and colicky or continuous and dull
2. NCLEX® Change in bowel motility and character: diarrhea and/or constipation, mucus in stool, feeling of incomplete evacuation, and possible bloating, flatulence, or urgency

C. Therapeutic management

1. NCLEX® Dietary fiber 30–40 grams/daily may help regulate bowel and reduce both diarrhea and constipation
2. Assist client to identify and eliminate foods that exacerbate problem
3. NCLEX® Common offenders: fruit, berries, lettuce, lactose, caffeinated drinks, preservatives (sodium sulfite), alcohol
4. Eliminating gas-forming foods (beans, cabbage, nuts, raisins, and apple and grape juices) may help reduce flatulence

5. Encourage relaxation and stress reduction; regular exercise may help control symptoms
6. Medication therapy
   a. No standard pharmacologic treatment; nonprescription probiotics may be helpful
   NCLEX® b. Prescribed medications may include bulk-forming laxatives, antidiarrheal agents if needed, anticholinergics such as dicyclomine or hyoscamine, and selected tricyclic antidepressants or selective serotonin uptake inhibitors (to relieve abdominal pain)

D. Client teaching
1. Information about fiber content of various foods
2. Importance of following prescribed regimen and keeping follow-up appointments; notifying healthcare provider if symptoms worsen
3. Information about programs of relaxation or support groups

IX. CHRONIC INFLAMMATORY BOWEL DISEASE (IBD)

A. Ulcerative colitis
1. Overview
   a. Chronic inflammation of mucosa and submucosa in colon and rectum characterized by periods of exacerbation and remission
   b. Cause is unknown but may be related to stress, genetics, infection, dietary factors (low fiber intake), or antibody formation
   c. Inflammation (at base of crypts of Lieberkuhn, usually in rectum) causes edema and bleeding with ulcer formation
   d. Begins in rectum and can progress proximally, but is usually limited to sigmoid colon and rectum
   e. Scar tissue formation over time reduces elasticity of bowel and reduces ability of colon to absorb nutrients and water

NCLEX® 2. Nursing assessment
   a. Abdominal tenderness, cramping, and diarrhea (10–20 liquid stools per day often containing blood and sometimes mucus); nocturnal diarrhea is common
   b. May report fatigue and malaise resulting from blood loss, lack of sleep, and/or fluid imbalance
   c. Malabsorption may lead to malnutrition, weight loss, dehydration, electrolyte imbalances, anemia, and vitamin K deficiency
   d. Complications include hemorrhage, abscess formation, toxic megacolon, malabsorption, bowel obstruction, bowel perforation, increased risk of colon cancer, and extraintestinal symptoms (arthritis, uveitis)
3. Therapeutic management
   a. Provide standard pre- and postsigmoidoscopy or colonoscopy care
   NCLEX® b. Rest and restricted activity is required to decrease intestinal activity
   NCLEX® c. Diet therapy during acute exacerbation may include NPO status with intravenous fluid and electrolyte replacement or parenteral nutrition if prescribed(see also Chapter 33)
   d. Diet therapy after acute phase may include progression from clear liquids to a low-residue, high-protein diet with vitamins and iron supplementation
   e. Assess bowel sounds, abdominal distention, and stool characteristics (color, consistency, possible blood)
   f. Surgery (proctocolectomy with colostomy or ileostomy) may be needed if IBD not controlled medically
   NCLEX® g. Medications: corticosteroids during exacerbations to decrease bowel inflammation; salicylate compounds (sulfasalazine, mesalamine) to decrease prostaglandin formation and bowel inflammation; immunosuppressants such as azathioprine to decrease immune response; antidiarrheals for symptom management
4. Client teaching
   a. Smoking cessation if appropriate
   NCLEX® b. Avoid foods that exacerbate symptoms: raw vegetables and fruits, whole-grain breads and cereals, seeds, nuts, popcorn, gas-forming foods, alcohol, caffeine, and spices such as pepper
   c. Notify healthcare provider if symptoms increase or there is blood in stool
   d. Provide information about ulcerative colitis support groups
   e. Educate client about exacerbation and remission nature of disease and symptom management
   f. If appropriate, instruct postoperative client in stoma and incision care as described in earlier section

B. Crohn's disease (regional enteritis)
1. Overview
   a. Chronic inflammation of mucosa anywhere in GI tract but most often in terminal ileum; characterized by exacerbations and remissions
   b. Cause is unknown, but possible factors are autoimmune, genetics, infectious agents, and environmental (stress)

c. Lesions extend to all thicknesses of bowel wall; over time, chronic inflammation causes fibrotic changes in bowel wall, narrowed bowel lumen, and possible fistulas, ulcerations, and abscesses
d. Depending on severity and location of lesions, malabsorption may occur as well as losses of protein from lesions themselves

2. Nursing assessment
   NCLEX® a. Diarrhea (five or six liquid to semiformed stools/day) is most common symptom (usually without blood but may contain mucus or pus); depending on location, **steatorrhea** (fatty stool) may occur
   NCLEX® b. Abdominal pain that is cramplike and colicky after meals and is unrelieved by defecation
   NCLEX® c. Other manifestations include abdominal distention, fever, fatigue, malaise, anorexia, dehydration and electrolyte imbalance, malnutrition (more severe than in ulcerative colitis), and weight loss
   d. Complications include abscess and fistula formation, intestinal obstruction, malnutrition, and bowel perforation; hemorrhage is uncommon

3. Therapeutic management ↑Cal ↑Protein
   NCLEX® a. Provide prescribed diet: usually high-calorie, high-protein similar to ulcerative colitis; involve client in making appropriate menu choices
   b. Encourage intake of prescribed nutritional supplements
   NCLEX® c. Weigh daily, maintain calorie count, and monitor I&O
   NCLEX® d. Medications are same as for ulcerative colitis (antidiarrheals, antispasmodics, salicylate-containing compounds, corticosteroids, immunosuppressants)
   e. TPN may be prescribed during periods of severe exacerbation to provide total bowel rest

4. Client teaching
   a. Reinforce information about disease, medications, and diet
   b. Teach client and family signs of complications: increased pain, rectal bleeding, fever, chills, lethargy
   c. If TPN is prescribed, teach client and family about proper catheter care and administration techniques(see also Chapter 33)
   d. Encourage intake of nutritional supplements, such as Ensure, for optimum nutrition

X. DIVERTICULAR DISEASE

A. Overview

1. *Diverticulitis* is an inflammation of diverticula, which are outpouchings in intestinal wall (*diverticulosis* is presence of multiple diverticula)
2. Most diverticula occur in sigmoid colon (see Figure 59–3); incidence increases with age

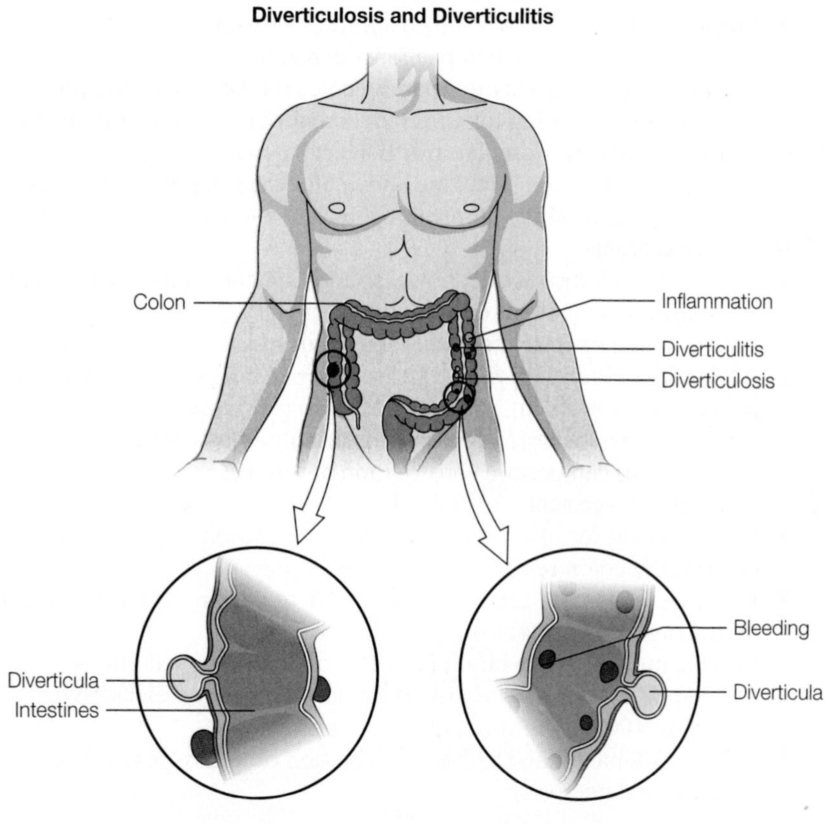

Figure 59–3
Diverticula tend to occur in sigmoid colon.

3. Caused by increased pressure in intestinal lumen and herniation of mucosa through defects in bowel wall; decreased fecal bulk (low-fiber diet) contribute to bowel wall hypertrophy and result in increased intraluminal pressure
4. Diverticula become inflamed when undigested food or bacteria are trapped; abscess formation can occur and diverticulum may rupture, leading to peritonitis

B. Nursing assessment

NCLEX® 1. Pain of diverticulitis is usually in LLQ, ranges from mild to severe, and can be constant or cramping; if perforation occurs, abdominal pain is generalized

NCLEX® 2. Diverticulosis is generally asymptomatic

NCLEX® 3. May note abdominal distention and pattern of constipation alternating with frequent bowel movements

NCLEX® 4. Fever, chills, and tachycardia along with generalized abdominal pain may indicate perforation of diverticulum and onset of peritonitis

5. Diverticular disease is diagnosed with CT scan, ultrasound, or barium enema, but barium enema is contraindicated when diverticulitis is present (risk of rupturing diverticulum)

C. Therapeutic management

NCLEX® 1. Reinforce dietary modifications to reduce complications of diverticulosis
   a. Bowel rest: NPO status, clear liquids or low-residue diet during initial acute phase
   b. Reintroduce fiber in diet after acute phase (inflammation) resolves
   c. Add bran to everyday foods to increase bulk of stool
   d. Avoid gas-forming foods and intake of foods with indigestible roughage (nuts, seeds, and foods with small seeds such as berries and figs) that could become trapped in diverticula and lead to inflammation
   e. Increase fluid intake to 2–3 liters/day unless contraindicated by another condition

2. Assess for signs of bleeding: check stool for occult blood

3. Prepare for possible surgery; colon resection is done in 25% of cases of diverticulitis; temporary or permanent colostomy may be necessary

NCLEX® 4. Medication therapy includes antibiotics to decrease bowel flora and reduce infection, analgesics to relieve pain, anticholinergics as needed for bowel spasm, and bulk-forming laxatives

D. Client teaching: fiber content of various foods, self-administration and side effects of medications, to avoid signs and symptoms of complications of diverticulitis

XI. INTESTINAL OBSTRUCTION

A. Overview

1. Failure of bowel contents to move forward; can be partial or complete
2. Mechanical obstruction results from forces outside of intestines (adhesions, hernia, fibrosis) or blockage in lumen (fecal impaction, edema, tumor, stricture, volvulus, intussusception)
3. Nonmechanical obstruction (paralytic ileus) results from impaired muscle tone or nervous system innervation preventing forward movement of intestinal contents (anesthesia, abdominal surgery, spinal injuries, peritonitis, vascular insufficiency)
4. Peristalsis increases in intestine above blockage, leading to increased secretions, edema, and increased capillary permeability and resulting in fluid and electrolyte imbalances and hypovolemia

B. Nursing assessment

NCLEX® 1. Early in bowel obstruction, bowel sounds may be high-pitched and tinkling proximal to obstruction and hypoactive or silent distal to obstruction

NCLEX® 2. Late in bowel obstruction bowel sounds decrease and become absent

3. Abdominal distention, visible peristalsis, vomiting (with fecal odor), and colicky pain may be present; pain becomes more intense as obstruction progresses

NCLEX® 4. Vital signs may be normal in early obstruction but signs of shock (tachycardia, fever, tachypnea, hypotension) can occur as obstruction progresses

C. Therapeutic management

1. Prepare client for insertion of nasogastric or nasointestinal tube and possibility of surgery: exploratory laparotomy, colon resection, colostomy
2. Prepare client for insertion of nasogastric or nasointestinal tube; monitor amount and characteristics of drainage after insertion
3. Provide mouth care to minimize effect of fecal-type secretions

NCLEX® 4. Provide IV therapy as prescribed to replace fluid and electrolytes

NCLEX® 5. Maintain NPO status until peristalsis returns

NCLEX® 6. Monitor VS including I&O; early detection of hypovolemic shock can prevent complications (bowel ischemia and necrosis)

NCLEX® 7. Monitor level of pain; sudden change in nature of pain may indicate complications (ischemia and necrosis)

NCLEX® 8. Medication therapy: analgesics are generally limited because opioids decrease GI motility, which further compromises bowel

D. Client teaching

1. Instruct client about insertion and maintenance of NG tube or intestinal tube
2. Reinforce instructions for postoperative use of incentive spirometer, coughing and deep breathing (C&DB) exercises, ambulation, activity, and wound care
3. Provide support to client and family in coping with possibility of a colostomy

XII. JAUNDICE

A. Overview

1. **Jaundice** is yellow-orange discoloration of skin and mucous membranes; caused by a disturbance of bilirubin metabolism causing **hyperbilirubinemia** (serum bilirubin greater than 2.5 mg/dL); also known as icterus
2. Associated with diffuse hepatocellular disorders or present in newborns because of impaired bilirubin uptake and conjugation
3. Hyperbilirubinemia and jaundice can result from hemolysis or from disorders of bile ducts (obstruction) or liver cells
4. Obstructive jaundice is classified as extrahepatic (gallstones or tumor, with increased direct bilirubin) or intrahepatic (drug reactions or hepatitis, with increased indirect bilirubin)
5. Hemolytic jaundice is caused by excessive breakdown of red blood cells (RBCs)

NCLEX® **B. Nursing assessment**

1. Recent appetite and color of urine and stool
2. Abdominal swelling, RUQ pain, and hepatomegaly
3. Yellowish discoloration of skin and mucous membranes
4. Scleral icterus (yellowish discoloration of sclera)
5. Pruritus (severe itching) because of accumulation of bilirubin in skin
6. Elevated conjugated bilirubin that causes dark (tea- or cola-colored) urine; may be present before jaundice appears
7. Complete obstruction of flow of bile into duodenum causes light or clay-colored stools
8. Jaundice caused by an infectious process may be accompanied by fever and chills
9. Any client with liver dysfunction or injury may experience nausea, anorexia, and/or fatigue
10. Laboratory findings (see also Chapter 46) vary depending on specific cause, but may include increased indirect bilirubin and direct bilirubin; elevated urine bilirubin; increased alanine aminotransferase (ALT), aspartate aminotransferase (AST), and alkaline phosphatase (ALP)
11. Radiologic procedures can help confirm infiltrative or cholestatic processes; abdominal ultrasound and CT scans can detect tumors, stones, and other focal liver lesions that may be causing jaundice

C. Therapeutic management

1. Aimed at symptom management, keeping client comfortable, and treating cause of jaundice

NCLEX® 2. Often clients are kept NPO pending diagnostic testing and because food increases pain secondary to stimulation of GI tract

NCLEX® 3. Maintain IV hydration and manage pain effectively

NCLEX® 4. Provide cool or tepid baths containing colloidal substances (oatmeal, cornstarch, soybean powder) can reduce or ease pruritus

5. Keep room cool at 68–70°F (20–21.1°C) with 30–40% humidity

NCLEX® 6. Use an emollient lotion rather than one containing alcohol, which is drying

7. Medication therapy: none specific, but topical corticosteroids may provide some relief of itching; bile sequestrants remove excess bile from fat deposits under skin, decreasing pruritus

D. Client teaching

1. Explain diagnostic tests, disease process causing jaundice, and future management
2. Some causes of jaundice are correctable

NCLEX® 3. Advise client with liver problems to avoid alcohol and acetaminophen, since both can cause further liver damage

XIII. HEPATITIS

A. Overview

1. An inflammation of liver; ranges greatly in severity and can be caused by several different viruses, toxins, or disease states
2. Hepatitis occurs in varying levels of severity from asymptomatic or mild cases, in which liver cells regenerate completely in 2–3 months, to more severe forms, in which hepatic necrosis and death may occur in 1–2 weeks

3. Treatment is aimed at reducing demands and allowing rest of inflamed liver to promote liver cell regeneration to prevent further damage
4. Forms of hepatitis (see Table 59–2)
5. Hepatitis A
   a. Sources include contaminated food, water, and shellfish; may also be contracted from contact with infected persons
   b. Highly contagious and easily spread throughout households and daycare centers
   c. Client is most contagious 10–14 days prior to onset of symptoms when fecal shedding of virus is greatest
   d. Usually self-limiting
6. Hepatitis B
   a. Risk increases with multiple sex partners, in men who have sex with other men, and IV drug users; healthcare workers comprise a small percentage of cases
   b. Transmitted also through contaminated blood or blood products; clients who require hemodialysis are also at risk
   c. Can progress to a chronic form of disease; common cause of cirrhosis and hepatocellular carcinoma
7. Hepatitis C
   a. Also called post-transfusion hepatitis; most common cause of chronic hepatitis
   b. Blood transfusions, sexual contact, sharing of contaminated needles, and unintentional needlesticks account for a significant number of cases
   c. Up to 80% of clients develop chronic hepatitis, which is a risk factor for liver failure and hepatocellular carcinoma
8. Hepatitis D is also known as Delta-agent hepatitis, and occurs only in people infected with hepatitis B (depends on HBV virus to replicate)
9. Hepatitis E is often transmitted by infected water supply; uncommon in the United States
10. Acute fulminating hepatitis: rare but rapidly progressive form that leads to bleeding problems, hepatic encephalopathy, ascites, and acute liver failure within 2–3 weeks of onset of symptoms

B. Nursing assessment

NCLEX® 1. A range of symptoms occurs, including anorexia, nausea and vomiting (N/V), malaise, fever, jaundice, and abdominal pain secondary to liver swelling; client may show signs of dehydration if vomiting is severe

NCLEX® 2. Course of acute viral hepatitis is divided into three phases
   a. Prodromal (preicteric) phase (most contagious) occurs before jaundice appears, about 2 weeks after exposure to virus, and includes flulike symptoms (general malaise, GI complaints such as N/V, diarrhea, and anorexia), headache, fatigue, myalgia, joint pain, and low-grade fever; food odors, smoking, or alcohol may trigger nausea
   b. **Icteric** phase is marked by onset of jaundice; occurs about 2 weeks after prodromal phase and lasts 2–6 weeks; includes dark-colored urine and clay-colored stools before appearance of jaundice and pruritis; liver remains enlarged and possibly tender to touch
   c. Recovery (posticteric) phase begins with resolution of jaundice and lasts several weeks, during which symptoms improve, energy levels increase, and serum enzymes normalize

3. Acute infection with hepatitis C is generally asymptomatic, although some clients develop malaise, weakness, and anorexia
4. Diagnostic and laboratory test findings
   a. Antibodies to specific virus (see again Table 59–2)
   b. Depending on cause, elevated ALT, AST, ALP, direct and indirect bilirubin, and gamma-glutamyl transferase (GGT)

Table 59–2 Forms of Hepatitis

Virus	Route of Transmission	Incubation Period	Lab Results	Vaccine Preventable	Carrier State
Hepatitis A (HAV)	Fecal–oral	2–6 weeks	Anti-HAV antibodies	Yes	No
Hepatitis B (HBV)	Blood and body fluids; perinatal	6–24 weeks	Positive HBsAG (surface antigen); anti-HBV antibodies	Yes	Yes
Hepatitis C (HCV)	Blood and body fluids	5–12 weeks	Anti-HCV antibodies	No	Yes
Hepatitis D (HDV)	Blood and body fluids; perinatal	3–24 weeks	Positive HDVAg (antigen); anti-HDV antibodies	No	Yes
Hepatitis E (HEV)	Fecal–oral	3–6 weeks	Anti-HEV antibodies	No	Yes

c. Prothrombin time (PT) is prolonged if liver injury prevents production of adequate proteins necessary for blood coagulation

C. Therapeutic management

NCLEX® 1. Includes both pre- and postexposure prophylaxis for forms A and B as well as symptom management
   a. With cases of hepatitis A, controlling spread of infection is a major nursing focus; includes reporting to local public health department; exposed individuals should receive immune globulin as soon as possible; those at risk should receive vaccine
   b. With cases of hepatitis B, prevention is major health focus; hepatitis B vaccines are begun during neonatal period and are recommended for all infants as part of well-child care

NCLEX® 2. Use standard precautions and meticulous hand hygiene for all forms, but especially for hepatitis A (client, family, and staff)

NCLEX® 3. Hepatitis A precautions include private bathroom and proper bagging, cleansing, and disposal of contaminated items

NCLEX® 4. Provide antiemetic medications as prescribed and encourage a diet high in CHO and low in fat

NCLEX® 5. Abstinence from alcohol is essential

6. If liver function is compromised, protein and salt should be restricted

NCLEX® 7. Encourage a good breakfast; clients tend to become more nauseous later in day

8. Initiate intravenous (IV) fluids as prescribed

9. Assess for signs of dehydration and monitor electrolyte status

NCLEX® 10. Encourage bedrest initially and very gradual increase of activity as tolerated

11. Plan nursing activities to allow for adequate rest

12. Inform clients they may never donate blood

13. Observe for blood in stool or urine, multiple ecchymosis, petechiae, or oozing of blood from gums or minor cuts

14. Medication therapy
   a. Aimed at symptom relief; consists of antiemetics, analgesics, and, if pruritus is present, antihistamines; because most analgesics are metabolized in liver, their use must be limited
   b. IV fluids may be necessary if client is unable to tolerate oral fluids

NCLEX® c. Prophylaxis may be considered if client has known HAV exposure and is early in incubation period

NCLEX® d. Vaccination for hepatitis B is available; given as a series of three intramuscular injections to adults, children, and infants; second and third injections are given at 1 and 6 months after initial injection; efficacy of vaccination approaches 95%

NCLEX® e. Postexposure vaccination for hepatitis B is recommended for clients in contact with infected blood or body fluids, those who have sexual contact with infected individuals, and infants exposed to a caregiver with known HBV infection or born to a mother with known HBsAg
   f. Hepatitis C: combination therapy is used for 12–18 weeks or as long as 48 weeks with interferon alfa-2b and ribavirin therapy
   g. Hepatitis D: there are no medications specific to treatment of HDV
   h. Vitamin K is indicated if PT is prolonged

D. Client teaching

1. Hepatitis A and E: information about disease and prevention of transmission, need for meticulous hand hygiene, and need to avoid sharing of eating utensils, bath towels, and other personal care items that are in contact with body fluids

2. Educate client about safe-sex practices as a general health measure (hepatitis B, C, D) and vaccination and prevention of disease transmission according to type

NCLEX® 3. Avoid alcohol and any drugs that may be hepatotoxic (such as acetaminophen)

4. Instruct client about possibility of developing chronic active hepatitis and importance of follow-up

XIV. CIRRHOSIS

A. Overview

1. **Cirrhosis**: irreversible and chronic liver disease characterized by diffuse inflammation and fibrosis of liver tissue, which cause scarring and obstruction of hepatic blood flow

2. Three classifications: alcoholic, biliary, and postnecrotic
   a. Alcoholic cirrhosis (most prevalent type) is caused by prolonged, excessive alcohol intake with or without malnutrition; directly related to toxic effects of alcohol on liver
   b. Biliary cirrhosis is caused by obstruction of bile canaliculi and ducts and results in necrosis and fibrosis; cause can be autoimmune or result from tumors, gallstones, or chronic pancreatitis
   c. Postnecrotic cirrhosis results from a chronic, severe liver disease such as hepatitis; also caused by inherited metabolic liver disorders such as Wilson's disease

3. Regardless of cause, cirrhosis develops slowly; severity and rate of progression depend on cause and repeated injury to hepatocytes

B. Nursing assessment

NCLEX®

1. See Box 59–3
2. Vital signs: pulse, orthostatic BP measurement, temperature, and weight
3. Decreased ability to metabolize CHOs leads to hypoglycemia and decreased energy (altered glycogenolysis, glyconeogenesis, and glycogenesis)
4. Altered fat metabolism causes increased synthesis of fatty acids and triglycerides leading to fatty liver and hepatomegaly

NCLEX®

5. Altered protein metabolism leads to low albumin levels and subsequent development of edema and ascites; decreased protein also decreases production of clotting factors, which increases risk of bleeding
6. Decreased metabolism of sex steroids (estrogen, progesterone, and testosterone) leads to gynecomastia, loss of body hair, development of palmar erythema and spider angiomata, erectile dysfunction, and menstrual disorders
7. Decreased metabolism of aldosterone results in sodium and water retention and worsening edema and **ascites** (fluid in peritoneal cavity)

NCLEX®

8. Decreased metabolism of ammonia leads to increased serum ammonia levels and hepatic encephalopathy (see section that follows)
9. Decreased stores of vitamins and minerals leads to malnutrition, fatigue, and anemia
10. Obstruction of bile flow leads to hyperbilirubinemia and jaundice, clay-colored stools, dark-colored urine
11. Splenomegaly leads to pancytopenia

Box 59–3

Signs and Symptoms of Cirrhosis

- General malaise
- Skin
  - Pruritis
  - Jaundice and scleral icterus
  - Spider angiomata and telangiectasia
  - Ecchymoses, petechiae, hematomas, and propensity for bleeding
  - Edema
- Gastrointestinal
  - Nausea and vomiting
  - Anorexia, weight loss/malnutrition
  - Pyrosis
  - Clay-colored stools
  - Constipation
  - Flatulence, hemorrhoids
- Abdomen
  - Change in bowel sounds
  - Pain or tenderness in RUQ
  - Hepatomegaly, splenomegaly
  - Ascites (increasing abdominal girth)
  - Abdominal pain (RUQ)
  - Positive fluid wave
  - Shifting dullness
  - Caput medusa
- Neurological
  - Fatigue
  - Disorientation
  - Decreased level of consciousness
  - Encephalopathy
  - Asterixis (flapping tremor of hand from increased ammonia levels)
  - Decreased deep-tendon reflexes (DTRs)
- Pulmonary
  - Decreased breath sounds in bases (may indicate pleural effusion)
  - Crackles (might indicate development of heart failure)
- Reproductive
  - Gynecomastia
  - Testicular atrophy
  - Erectile dysfunction
  - Menstrual irregularities
- Palmar erythema
- Anemia
- Loss of body hair
- Dark urine

12. Fibrosis and scarring continue, resulting in increased portal pressure that causes ascites, hemorrhoids, esophageal varices, caput medusa (superficial abdominal veins)

NCLEX® 13. Involuntary tremor or flapping of hands is called **asterixis** (see Figure 59–4)

NCLEX® 14. Liver biopsy definitively diagnoses type of cirrhosis; may not be necessary if clinical picture supports diagnosis or advisable if client has prolonged PT (risk for bleeding); see also Chapter 47

15. Laboratory findings include varying degrees of increased transaminases, decreased albumin, prolonged PT, hyperbilirubinemia, hyponatremia from excess free water, hypokalemia from diuretic therapy, hypomagnesemia, and elevated serum ammonia

16. Complete blood count (CBC) reflects pancytopenia (anemia, thrombocytopenia, leukopenia)

17. Liver ultrasound may reveal an enlarged fibrofatty liver or a small fibrotic and nodular liver

C. Therapeutic management

1. Abdominal **paracentesis** for only severe ascites; invasive procedure that drains fluid from abdomen via needle; ensure client is sitting in straight-back chair with bowel and bladder emptied before procedure; watch for fluid shifts leading to increased pulse and decreased BP after procedure

NCLEX® 2. Surgical intervention to relieve portal hypertension and prevent reaccumulation of ascitic fluid: insertion of a LeVeen shunt or transjugular intrahepatic portosystemic shunt (TIPS)

NCLEX® 3. Fluid restriction to prevent further accumulation of ascitic fluid

NCLEX® 4. Diet restrictions include decreased protein intake (to prevent encephalopathy) and low sodium intake to prevent worsening of ascites

NCLEX® 5. Weigh daily, and monitor I&O; provide smaller, more frequent meals

NCLEX® 6. Measure abdominal girth each day or shift as prescribed to monitor ascites

NCLEX® 7. Elevate head of bed to reduce upward pressure of ascites on diaphragm; use supplemental O_2 as prescribed; encourage deep breathing; allow activity as tolerated; measure O_2 saturation and ABGs as prescribed

8. Maintain skin integrity; remove moist linens promptly; keep skin clean and moistened with emollient; administer antihistamines as prescribed for itching; encourage activity as tolerated, or reposition every 2 hours

NCLEX® 9. Institute bleeding precautions as needed: prevent constipation, avoid injections, observe for signs of bleeding, encourage use of soft toothbrush, monitor labs (CBC, PT)

10. Assess understanding of illness; identify support system; assess coping skills; offer clergy support; encourage Alcoholics Anonymous for those with cirrhosis secondary to alcohol dependence; provide substance abuse consultation as indicated

NCLEX® 11. Medication therapy includes diuretics such as spironolactone (potassium-sparing) or furosemide (loop), lactulose to reduce absorption of ammonia from GI tract, vitamins (especially B vitamins), vitamin K to treat prolonged PT, antihistamines, and antiemetics

D. Client teaching

1. Lifestyle changes include dietary restrictions, abstinence from alcohol, fluid restrictions; suggest nutrition consultation

2. Reduce intake of foods high in sodium; avoid canned and frozen foods, highly processed cheeses, potato chips, and other salty foods

NCLEX® 3. Limit intake of foods high in protein: eggs, cheese, milk, and meats

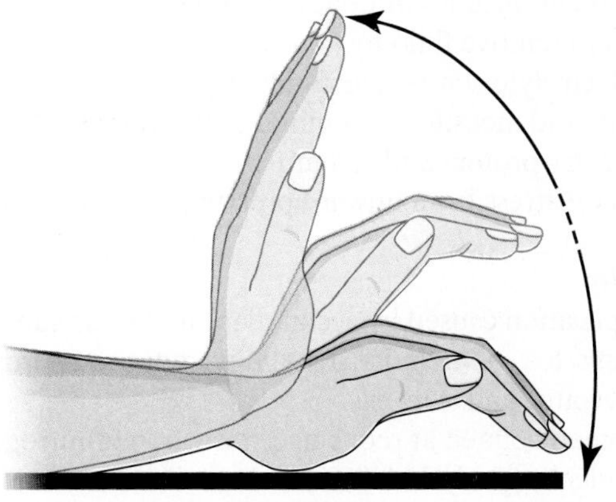

Figure 59–4

Asterixis. A downward-flapping hand tremor noted on dorsiflexion of wrist.

4. Avoid taking any OTC medications without checking with healthcare provider first because many are hepatotoxic (such as acetaminophen)
5. Signs and symptoms that require medical attention after discharge: weight gain, increased abdominal girth, respiratory distress, bleeding gums, blood in the stool or urine, fever, abdominal pain

E. Complications of cirrhosis

1. **Portal hypertension**
   a. An abnormally high BP within portal vein most commonly caused by obstruction to blood flow through liver (liver disease or right heart failure)
   b. Clinical manifestations include all findings described with cirrhosis
   NCLEX® c. Splenomegaly can result from increased pressure within splenic vein, which branches off portal vein
   d. Clients may report irritation from hemorrhoids or may present with bright red rectal bleeding secondary to hemorrhoids
   e. Therapeutic management involves treating cirrhosis
   NCLEX® f. Medication therapy: diuretics (and fluid restriction) and propranolol (a beta blocker) aim to decrease portal venous pressure without causing hypotension
2. **Esophageal varices**
   a. Develop from increased portal pressure; are distended and tortuous blood vessels that can rupture secondary to coughing, sneezing, vomiting, or ingestion of foods high in roughage
   NCLEX® b. Clinical manifestations: vomiting of blood (**hematemesis**) secondary to rupture of esophageal varices is common and can lead to hypovolemic shock (tachycardia, hypotension); if bleeding is slow (oozing varices), melena (blood in stool) and decreasing hemoglobin and hematocrit are present
   NCLEX® c. Therapeutic management: includes stopping bleeding either by **sclerotherapy** (injection of sclerosing drugs) or banding via endoscopy, or by **esophageal tamponade** (direct pressure using Sengstaken-Blakemore or Minnesota tube with esophageal and gastric balloons); keep scissors at bedside to cut tube if tube position changes and airway is compromised; see also Chapter 27
   d. Maintain airway, breathing, and circulation; monitor VS; initiate cardiac monitoring
   e. Start two large-bore IVs with infusion of normal saline (NS) as prescribed
   f. Draw serum laboratory tests (CBC, type and cross-match, chemistries)
   g. Begin gastric **lavage** (irrigation) if prescribed
   h. Keep clients NPO for both sclerotherapy and esophageal tamponade (if elective); explain procedure and give a mild preprocedure sedative as prescribed
   NCLEX® i. Administer vasopressin via IV intermittent or continuous infusion; lowers portal pressure and controls bleeding by causing splanchnic vasoconstriction; use with caution in clients with cardiac disease
   j. Administer propranolol, a beta-blocker that reduces portal pressure, or sandostatin, which decreases splanchnic blood flow to decrease bleeding
3. Ascites
   a. Accumulation of plasma-rich fluid within peritoneal cavity secondary to portal hypertension, increased aldosterone, and decreased oncotic pressure (from decreased circulating albumin levels, called **hypoalbuminemia**); cirrhosis is common cause; kidneys retain sodium and thus water, further increasing third-spaced fluid and anasarca (generalized body edema)
   NCLEX® b. Clinical manifestations: abdominal distention, weight gain, increased abdominal girth, dilated abdominal veins (caput medusa), generalized edema, and respiratory distress if accumulation of ascitic fluid is large
   NCLEX® c. Therapeutic management includes diuretics, shunting devices to treat portal hypertension, and, if needed, paracentesis to remove fluid by aspiration
   d. Monitor fluid and electrolyte status; give fluids as prescribed
   e. Monitor daily weights and measure abdominal girth every 8–24 hours
   f. Restrict intake of dietary protein and sodium
   g. Assess for respiratory distress from upward pressure on diaphragm; monitor VS for hypotension and/or tachycardia
4. **Hepatic encephalopathy**
   a. A neurological complication caused by accumulation of toxic substances (primarily ammonia) in blood
   NCLEX® b. Clinical manifestations: loss of memory, irritability, reduced coordination, confusion, lethargy, sleep disturbances, stupor, coma, and asterixis
   NCLEX® c. Therapeutic management: aimed at reducing production of nitrogenous wastes (urea) and ammonia, correcting fluid and electrolyte imbalances, and eliminating use of sedating drugs and drugs metabolized by liver

d. Perform frequent neurologic assessment to note progression of lethargy
e. Restrict dietary protein as prescribed
f. Monitor for fluid and electrolyte imbalances and implement prescribed treatments
g. Treat cause of liver disease by implementing prescribed therapies
NCLEX® h. Medications may include lactulose to reduce ammonia; neomycin is sometimes used to reduce bacteria in bowel, thus limiting further ammonia production; use with caution because of nephrotoxicity

5. **Hepatorenal syndrome**
   a. Renal failure associated with advanced liver failure and caused by circulatory alterations without primary renal disease; characterized by intrarenal vasoconstriction, oliguria, azotemia, anorexia, and fatigue; associated with a poor prognosis
   NCLEX® b. Clinical manifestations include decreased urine output (UO), hyponatremia, decreased urine osmolality, hypotension, jaundice, ascites, possible GI bleeding, increased BUN and creatinine
   c. Treat fluid and electrolyte imbalances and encephalopathy with aim of restoring renal and liver function
   NCLEX® d. Eliminate nephrotoxic or hepatotoxic drugs (such as neomycin sulfate)
   NCLEX® e. Hemodialysis is used to treat hyperkalemia and fluid overload
   f. Carefully assess I&O and daily weights

XV. CHOLELITHIASIS

A. Overview

1. **Cholelithiasis** (gallstones) can occur anywhere in biliary tree; most are within gallbladder
2. Cholesterol stones (most common form) develop slowly; hard, white, or yellow-brown, radiolucent; can be up to 4 cm in size
3. Pigmented stones form because of an increase in unconjugated bilirubin and calcium with a concurrent decrease in bile salts
4. Increased bile concentration, bile stasis, and hypercholesterolemia contribute to stone formation
5. Risk factors associated with the formation of gallstones are listed in Box 59–4

B. Nursing assessment

NCLEX® 1. Classic manifestations include severe and steady epigastric or RUQ pain that radiates to right scapula or shoulder; sudden onset, lasting 1–3 hours
NCLEX® 2. May occur after a high-fat meal
NCLEX® 3. Other symptoms include nausea and vomiting, heartburn, and flatulence
4. Fever and chills occur with acute cholecystitis
5. Biliary colic or cramping pain occurs when stone is lodged in cystic or common bile duct; if stone blocks duct, edema and inflammation of gallbladder (cholecystitis) occur and may be associated with jaundice
6. Physical exam findings include positive Murphy's sign (palpation of RUQ causes severe pain with inspiration); bowel sounds may be absent
7. Jaundice is not usually seen unless common bile duct is blocked
8. Laboratory findings include elevated WBC count (infection), increased serum bilirubin levels (stone in biliary ductal system causing obstruction), possible electrolyte depletion secondary to vomiting or anorexia; elevated liver function tests (LFTs) with hepatic involvement or damage caused by bile duct obstruction

Box 59–4

Risk Factors for Gallstones

- Increasing age
- Female gender
- Family history (may relate to familial high dietary fat intake and sedentary lifestyle)
- Obesity and hyperlipidemia
- Rapid weight loss (very low calorie diet, bariatric surgery)
- Biliary stasis from pregnancy, prolonged TPN or fasting state
- Use of estrogen-containing medications (oral contraceptives, hormone replacement therapy)
- Comorbid medical diagnoses: Crohn's disease or ileal resection, diabetes mellitus, cirrhosis, sickle-cell anemia
- Native American and Northern European ethnicity

9. Diagnostic tests include ultrasound (identifies stones, gallbladder, and ductal dilatation in nonobese clients), oral cholecystogram (outlines stones for visualization), and gallbladder scans (evaluate for accompanying cholecystitis; also called HIDA, DIDA, or DISIDA scans)

C. Therapeutic management

NCLEX® 1. Extracorporeal shock wave **lithotripsy** uses shock waves to disintegrate stones; oral dissolution therapy may be used postprocedure to dissolve stone fragments; clients may experience biliary colic postprocedure when gallbladder is contracting to pass stone fragments

NCLEX® 2. Endoscopic retrograde cholangiopancreatography (ERCP) uses a fiberoptic endoscope to visualize biliary tree, remove stones, drain bile sludge, and collect biopsies

NCLEX® 3. Laparoscopic cholecystectomy is less invasive than ERCP; abdomen is insufflated with CO_2; laparoscope is introduced through a small incision, and gallbladder is deflated and removed through small abdominal incision

4. Cholecystectomy: surgical removal of gallbladder; occasionally a T-tube is placed in common bile duct to assist passage of bile until edema has decreased; bile collects in a bag by gravity drainage
5. Implement comfort measures, including prescribed analgesics and antiemetics
6. Provide education regarding diagnostic tests and disease process
7. Maintain NPO status preprocedure as prescribed; institute IV fluids as prescribed
8. Provide diet instruction regarding low-fat diet and frequent, small meals
9. Encourage obese individuals to lose weight
10. Monitor fluid and electrolyte balance
11. Medication therapy
    a. Opioid analgesics and antiemetics during acute attack
    b. Cholestyramine for severe pruritus (binds bile salts to hasten excretion through feces)
    c. Ursodiol or chenodiol to dissolve cholesterol stones; ursodiol is often well tolerated but chenodiol frequently causes diarrhea and is hepatotoxic (requiring monitoring of liver enzymes)

D. Client teaching: disease process and gallstone formation; diagnostic procedures and expected outcomes; diet instruction to limit high-fat foods

XVI. CHOLECYSTITIS

A. Overview

1. **Cholecystitis**: acute or chronic inflammation of gallbladder disorder, often caused by gallstones obstructing cystic duct, resulting in a distended and inflamed gallbladder; pain is similar to that of gallstones
2. Acalculous cholecystitis is precipitated by trauma, prolonged TPN, fasting, or surgery

NCLEX® **B. Nursing assessment**

1. Clinical manifestations include all of those previously identified for cholelithiasis
2. Fever, leukocytosis, elevated serum bilirubin (possible jaundice) and ALP, elevated amylase if pancreatic duct is involved
3. Abdominal guarding, rigidity, and rebound tenderness suggest peritoneal involvement
4. Diagnostic and laboratory testing as outlined for cholelithiasis

NCLEX® **C. Therapeutic management**

1. NPO with IV fluids for hydration until the pain subsides
2. Opioid analgesics (usually morphine) are used for pain control
3. IV antibiotics are administered
4. Surgery is postponed until acute infectious process has subsided

D. Client teaching: preoperative teaching; some clients are discharged and return after convalescence for elective cholecystectomy

E. Surgical intervention for disorders of gallbladder

1. Laparoscopic cholecystectomy: removal of gallbladder through a small abdominal incision guided by a fiberoptic endoscope
2. Cholecystectomy: removal of gallbladder through a RUQ abdominal incision
3. Cholecystectomy with T-tube placement (less common): gallbladder is removed and a T-tube is placed within common bile duct to facilitate bile flow through edematous duct postprocedure

NCLEX® 4. Postoperative nursing care
    a. Provide standard postoperative care(see also Chapter 48)
    b. Prevent infection: administer IV antibiotics as prescribed, keep incision clean and dry; perform abdominal assessment for peritonitis every 4 hours; monitor VS, report any temperature over 100°F (38°C)

c. Manage pain effectively to aid in postoperative exercise/ambulation and to promote pulmonary hygiene (incision is near diaphragm)

NCLEX®
d. Maintain clients with T-tube in Fowler position to promote gravity drainage of bile; report bile drainage in excess of 500 mL in first 24 hours; should be less than 200 mL daily in 2–3 days

e. Instruct client that T-tube is removed when bile drainage has subsided and stools have returned to a normal brown color

f. Assess surrounding skin for inflammation secondary to bile leakage

g. Instruct client about proper handling of tube for turning and ambulating

h. Maintain NPO status as prescribed; advance diet as tolerated

i. Provide postoperative discharge teaching (wound care, analgesics, diet, and signs of infection)

XVII. PANCREATITIS

A. Overview

1. Acute or chronic inflammation of pancreas associated with obstruction to flow of pancreatic enzymes, which escape into tissue and cause autodigestion of pancreas
2. Can be mild, severe, or fulminant
3. Acute pancreatitis may occur as a single or recurrent event that resolves, while chronic pancreatitis involves continual inflammation that leads to replacement of normal pancreatic tissue with scar tissue
4. Risk factors include alcohol abuse, obstructive cholelithiasis causing reflux of bile into pancreas, PUD, trauma, hyperlipidemia, bacterial or viral infection, ischemic vascular disease, and hyperparathyroidism
5. Types include acute interstitial edematous pancreatitis, necrotizing pancreatitis, biliary pancreatitis, and alcoholic pancreatitis

B. Nursing assessment: acute pancreatitis

1. Clinical manifestations vary with severity of attack
2. NCLEX® Acute epigastric pain, steady and severe, can occur in umbilical area and radiate to back because of retroperitoneal location of pancreas; it may be temporally associated with ingestion of alcohol or a fatty meal
3. NCLEX® Pain is greater when lying supine and improves with sitting up and leaning forward, flexion of knee, or fetal positioning
4. NCLEX® N/V is common and worsens with oral intake; vomiting does not relieve abdominal pain
5. VS: fever (rarely above 102°F [38.9°C]), hypotension, and tachycardia
6. NCLEX® Leukocytosis, hyperglycemia (as high as 500–900 mg/dL), and elevated amylase (for 48 hours) and lipase (for 5–7 days); increased urinary amylase
7. Abdominal tenderness, rigidity, progressive distention, and decreased bowel sounds
8. NCLEX® Bluish discoloration over flank area (Grey Turner sign) or around umbilicus (Cullen sign)
9. Fulminant disease can progress to hypovolemic shock, ascites, jaundice, and renal failure
10. Laboratory test results include hypocalcemia (if calcium is sequestered by fat necrosis in abdomen, sign of severe pancreatitis), elevated C-reactive protein, hypomagnesemia and hypoalbuminemia in habitual alcohol users, elevated bilirubin and LFTs if liver is involved
11. NCLEX® Diagnostic tests include CT scan (visualizes size of pancreas, fluid collections, abscesses, masses, and areas of hemorrhage or necrosis) abdominal x-ray, and ultrasound; chest x-ray identifies pleural effusion caused by enzymatic irritation from leaking pancreatic fluid

C. Nursing assessment: chronic pancreatitis

1. Recurrent epigastric and LUQ abdominal pain; possible left upper quadrant mass
2. Chronic anorexia and possible N/V, muscle wasting and weight loss
3. NCLEX® Steatorrhea and foul-smelling stools; may increase over time as disease progresses
4. NCLEX® Manifestations of diabetes mellitus as pancreatic function declines

D. Therapeutic management: acute pancreatitis

1. Treatment is aimed at supportive care, preventing further pancreatic autodigestion and preventing systemic complications
2. NCLEX® NPO status with NG tube if there is ileus or protracted vomiting or to decrease gastric secretions that stimulate pancreatic secretions
3. IV hydration to prevent hypotension and shock
4. NCLEX® TPN if needed for prolonged episodes; reverses catabolic state
5. NCLEX® Monitor VS, daily weights, hourly UO, bowel sounds, and stool chart (frequency, color, odor, and consistency)

6. Assess respiratory function; provide pulmonary hygiene measures to prevent pneumonia
NCLEX® 7. Administer pain medications as prescribed and on regular schedule
NCLEX® 8. Provide diet instruction (several small meals; no alcohol allowed) when oral feeding is resumed (usually when amylase level returns to normal and abdominal pain subsides)
NCLEX® 9. Maintain bedrest during acute phase and increase as tolerated
10. Medication therapy: opioids and antiemetics, H_2 receptor blocker or proton pump inhibitors to decrease gastric acidity, antispasmodics such as dicyclomine, anticholinergics to inhibit GI motility and pancreatic enzyme secretion, insulin as required to regulate serum glucose levels, and antibiotics as prescribed for infection

E. Therapeutic management: chronic pancreatitis

1. Provide nutritional supplements, vitamins, and minerals as prescribed
2. Administer pancreatic enzymes as prescribed as function of pancreas declines
3. Monitor insulin or oral antidiabetic therapy if client develops diabetes mellitus
4. Explain that client with onset of signs of acute pancreatitis notify healthcare provider

F. Client teaching

1. Disease process and expected outcomes
2. Nutrition; explain necessity for NPO status during acute phase and rationale for several small meals with no alcohol allowed once diet resumes
NCLEX® 3. Importance of taking enzyme replacement to prevent malnutrition and weight loss

XVIII. CLEFT LIP AND CLEFT PALATE

A. Overview

1. Cleft lip is a congenital anomaly involving one or more clefts in upper lip; degree of cleft varies from a small notch to a complete separation; can range from soft palate involvement alone to hard palate and portions of maxilla in severe cases (see Figure 59–5)
2. Causes include hereditary, environmental, and teratogenic factors
3. Both anomalies occur during embryonic development; cleft lip results from failure of fusion of lateral and medial tissues forming upper lip around 7 weeks' gestation; cleft palate is a failure of fusion of tissues forming palate around 9 weeks' gestation

B. Nursing assessment (defects are readily apparent at birth)

NCLEX® 1. Cleft lip involves a notched upper lip border, nasal distortion, and may include unilateral or bilateral involvement
NCLEX® 2. Cleft palate is a visible or palpable gap in uvula, soft palate, hard palate, and/or incisive foramen with exposed nasal cavities and associated nasal distortion
3. Perform careful physical assessment to rule out other midline birth defects
4. Infants who have cleft lip or palate are more prone to recurrent otitis media

C. Therapeutic management

NCLEX® 1. Depending on severity of defect and infant's general health, cleft lip is often surgically corrected around 3 months of age; cleft palate is generally repaired before age 18 months to protect formation of tooth buds and allow development of more normal speech patterns

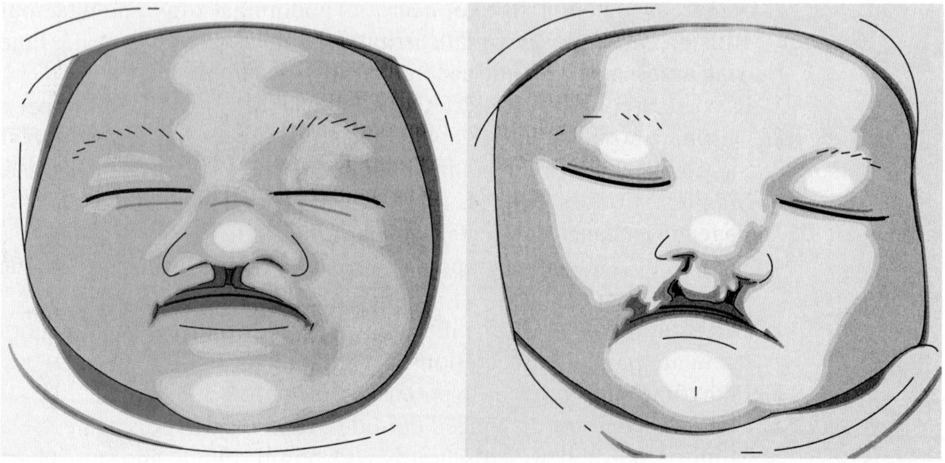

Figure 59–5

Cleft lip. (**A**) Unilateral, (**B**) bilateral.

A B

2. Preoperative nursing care
   a. Assess respiratory status continuously during feedings (risk of aspiration)

   NCLEX®
   b. Feed infant in upright position; feed slowly and burp infant frequently

Memory Aid

Use ESSR: *E*nlarged nipple, *S*timulate suck by placing nipple inside cheek toward back of tongue, *S*wallow, *R*est after each swallow to allow for complete swallowing.

NCLEX®
   c. Use alternate feeding devices such as elongated nipple (lamb's nipple) or breast shield
   d. Assess degree of cleft and ability to suck
   e. Keep suction equipment and bulb suction available at bedside
   f. Encourage parents to verbalize fears, concerns, negative emotions
   g. Facilitate grief responses of shock, denial, anger, and mourning
   h. Encourage touching, cuddling, and bonding; discuss infant's positive characteristics
   i. Provide parents with pictures of other children before and after surgical repair
   j. Refer to community resources and parent support groups
3. Postoperative care
   a. Monitor for respiratory distress; monitor lung sounds and encourage deep breathing without placing stress on suture line

   NCLEX®
   b. No oral temperatures; no straws, pacifiers, metal utensils, or fingers in or around mouth for 7–10 days
   c. Advance feedings as tolerated

   NCLEX®
   d. For cleft lip, resume preoperative feeding techniques; a metal appliance or adhesive strips may be used to prevent tension on surgical site

   NCLEX®
   e. For cleft palate, liquids can be taken from a cup; no straws are allowed; soft foods can be taken from side of spoon; to reduce risk of injury, child is not allowed to feed self

   NCLEX®
   f. Clean lip from suture line outward after feedings and prn; no toothbrushing for 1–2 weeks
   g. Apply antibacterial ointment as prescribed
   h. Use soft elbow restraints to keep infant from putting fingers in mouth or near surgical site
   i. Place infant in side-lying position on unaffected side to avoid excessive contact with bed linens

   NCLEX®
   j. Monitor site for redness, swelling, excess bleeding, purulent drainage, or fever
   k. Assess pain using appropriate tools and provide analgesics and sedatives as scheduled
   l. Provide comfort measures to decrease stress, such as crying, on suture line; encourage rocking, cuddling, and holding
   m. Provide age-appropriate activities for diversion

D. Client and family teaching

1. Precautions to prevent aspiration and phone numbers in case of emergency
2. Provide information on CPR certification

NCLEX®
3. Teach parents safety and care issues regarding use of restraints
   a. Do not apply restraints too tightly
   b. Remove at least every 2 hours and play games to encourage flexion
   c. Remove only one restraint at a time
4. Stress importance of follow-up care and referral appointments
5. Make appropriate and early referrals for speech and language therapy
6. Encourage good dental hygiene and orthodontic follow-up

XIX. PYLORIC STENOSIS

A. Overview

1. Occurs when circular muscle of pyloric canal hypertrophies and impedes gastric emptying into duodenum; inflammation and edema develop and lead to obstruction
2. Risk factors include family history, hypergastrinemia (too much gastrin in blood), use of prostaglandin E to treat patent ductus arteriosus, and oral erythromycin at less than 1 month of age
3. Pyloromyotomy (creation of an incision along anterior pylorus to split muscle) is commonly performed to relieve obstruction

B. Nursing assessment

NCLEX®
1. Previously healthy infant with progressive, projectile, nonbilious vomiting; may become blood-tinged from repeated irritation of esophagus from vomiting

NCLEX® 2. Movable, palpable, firm, olive-sized mass in RUQ
3. Visible, deep, peristaltic waves from LUQ to RUQ immediately before vomiting
4. Irritability, hunger, and crying
5. Sunken fontanels, poor skin turgor, dry mucous membranes, decreased urine output, constipation, jaundice, metabolic alkalosis
6. Laboratory findings: possible increased pH and bicarbonate level (metabolic alkalosis); decreased serum chloride, sodium, and potassium levels; and increased hematocrit and hemoglobin (hemoconcentration)

C. Therapeutic management

1. Assess skin turgor, mucous membranes, and fontanels at least every shift, monitor urine specific gravity, weigh daily
NCLEX® 2. Maintain NPO status prior to surgery, monitor I&O hourly, administer IV fluids and electrolytes as prescribed
3. Maintain NG tube patency and monitor NG output
4. Keep infant warm and quiet
NCLEX® 5. Initiate small, frequent feedings of clear liquids within 4–6 hours after surgery; follow strict diet regimen of gradual advancement of feedings until normal formula feedings have been resumed
6. Continue IV hydration until age- or weight-appropriate amounts of formula are tolerated
NCLEX® 7. Assess incision for redness, swelling, and drainage; immediately report signs of infection to healthcare provider
8. Monitor VS at least every 4 hours
9. Encourage parental involvement and rooming-in

D. Client and family teaching

1. Explanation of disorder and treatment, including all equipment such as NG tube and IV
2. Discharge instructions: report any vomiting, abdominal tenderness, fever, incisional redness, or drainage to healthcare provider
3. Provide verbal and written feeding instructions if child has not returned to full-strength formula feedings prior to discharge
4. Importance of follow-up care with healthcare provider

XX. OMPHALOCELE AND GASTROSCHISIS

A. Overview

1. Omphaloceles are congenital malformations in which intra-abdominal contents herniate through umbilical cord
   a. Viscera is outside of abdominal cavity but inside translucent sac covered with peritoneum and amniotic membrane
   b. May be associated with other congenital anomalies such as cardiac defects or an associated chromosomal anomaly
2. Gastroschisis occurs when bowel (usually small intestine and ascending colon) herniates through abdominal wall defect, usually to right of umbilical cord, and through rectus muscle; there is no membrane covering exposed bowel
   a. Viscera is outside of abdominal cavity and not covered with peritoneal sac
   b. Rarely associated with other major congenital anomalies, but jejunoileal atresia, ischemic enteritis, and malrotation may occur because of defect

B. Nursing assessment

NCLEX® 1. With gastroschisis, there is obvious protrusion of abdominal contents present at time of delivery
NCLEX® 2. With omphalocele, size of sac varies depending on extent of protrusion; rupture of sac results in evisceration of abdominal contents and needs to be prevented
3. Defect may be noted on prenatal ultrasound

C. Therapeutic management

1. Assess body temperature continuously using skin probe; place infant in warmer immediately after birth
NCLEX® 2. Use sterile technique when handling or working with defect
NCLEX® 3. Immediately cover with sterile gauze soaked with warm sterile normal saline, and place infant feet first into a silastic silo to preserve heat and allow visualization of defect
4. Minimize movement of infant and handling of intestines
5. Assess respiratory status continuously during immediate newborn period by placing on cardiac and apnea monitor with pulse oximetry
6. Monitor for circulatory compromise by monitoring temperature, pulses, capillary refill, skin color, and heart rate and respiratory rate

NCLEX® 7. Assess mucous membranes for moisture and skin for elastic turgor; monitor I&O, weigh daily, assess fontanels, monitor electrolytes, maintain IV, and administer fluids and TPN as prescribed
8. Maintain NG tube for decompression and NPO status
NCLEX® 9. Monitor for signs of ileus by auscultating bowel sounds, measuring abdominal girth, assessing bowel movements
10. Anticipate surgical correction as single procedure or in stages depending on severity
11. Assess parents' coping mechanisms and encourage them to verbalize feelings of loss of "perfect" child and guilt that may accompany congenital anomaly; encourage parental participation in infant's care

D. Family teaching
1. Growth and developmental needs and techniques for developmental stimulation
2. Information regarding support groups and other community resources
3. Signs of bowel obstruction and when to notify healthcare provider

XXI. BILIARY ATRESIA

A. Overview
1. A condition that results when extrahepatic bile ducts fail to develop or become closed; can lead to inflammation and fibrotic changes in liver; may also be caused by hepatocellular dysfunction
2. Obstruction of extrahepatic bile ducts prevents normal flow of bile from liver into gallbladder and small intestine, causing bile accumulation in liver
3. Liver becomes fibrotic; cirrhosis and portal hypertension develop, leading to liver failure
NCLEX® 4. Because of lack of bile in intestines, fat and fat-soluble vitamins cannot be absorbed, resulting in malnutrition, fat-soluble vitamin deficiency, and growth failure
5. Treatment involves surgery (hepatoportoenterostomy, Kasai procedure) to temporarily correct obstruction and supportive care
6. Without treatment disease is fatal; liver transplantation is eventually necessary

B. Assessment
1. Healthy-appearing infant at birth
NCLEX® 2. Jaundice occurs within 2 weeks to 2 months, with intense itching of skin
NCLEX® 3. **Acholic** stools: puttylike, clay-colored stools
4. Abdominal distention and hepatomegaly
NCLEX® 5. Increased bruising of the skin, prolonged bleeding time
NCLEX® 6. Tea-colored urine (excretion of bile)
7. Increased bilirubin levels; ultrasound and liver biopsy confirm disorder

C. Therapeutic management
NCLEX® 1. Weigh daily
NCLEX® 2. Administer TPN with or without lipids and fat-soluble vitamins (A, D, E, K) as prescribed
NCLEX® 3. Monitor stool pattern and characteristics of urine
4. Cluster nursing activities to provide rest
5. Provide tepid baths to reduce itching and pat skin dry (not rub) to reduce further skin irritation
6. Establish an open, caring relationship with family

D. Client and family teaching
1. Instruct parents in meticulous skin care
2. Provide verbal and written information regarding nutritional needs
3. Provide instructions on oral antibiotic therapy, which may continue for 1–2 years after surgery (Kasai procedure)
4. Inform parents of the signs and symptoms for which to call the healthcare provider
5. If a transplant is performed, include detailed instruction on immunosuppressant medications

XXII. HIRSCHSPRUNG'S DISEASE

Megacolon

A. Overview
1. A congenital anomaly resulting from an absence of ganglion cells in colon (rectosigmoid area most commonly affected); also known as congenital aganglionic megacolon
2. Believed to be a familial, congenital defect, with higher incidence in children with congenital heart defects and chromosomal abnormalities such as Down syndrome
3. Absence of autonomic parasympathetic ganglion cells results in lack of innervation in affected area, absence of peristalsis, accumulation of intestinal contents, and distention of bowel proximal to defect

B. Nursing assessment

1. Clinical manifestations in newborns include failure to pass meconium stool within 48 hours after birth, abdominal distention, and bile-stained emesis
2. Clinical manifestations in infants include failure to thrive, constipation, abdominal distention, vomiting, and episodic diarrhea
3. Clinical manifestations in toddlers and older children include chronic constipation, foul-smelling or pencil-thin stools, abdominal distention, failure to gain weight, and malnutrition (including anemia and hypoproteinemia)
4. Rectal examination typically reveals an absence of stool
5. Diagnostic tests commonly reveal an enlarged portion of colon and a rectal biopsy confirms absence of ganglion cells

C. Therapeutic management

1. Involves removing aganglionic bowel through an endorectal pull-through procedure or, if severe, by creation of a temporary colostomy that is later closed at 2–6 months of age if diagnosed at birth
2. Preoperatively, assess bowel function and stool characteristics; measure abdominal girth; monitor for vomiting and respiratory distress
3. Monitor electrolytes and urine specific gravity; assess hydration status
4. Prepare child for surgery and administer antibiotics as prescribed
5. Postoperatively, monitor VS, measure abdominal girth, and assess surgical site for redness, swelling, or drainage
6. Assess stoma (if present) for color, bleeding, breakdown of surrounding skin; provide meticulous skin care, use appropriately sized stoma supplies
7. Assess anal area after pull-through for presence of stool, redness, drainage; do not place anything in rectum (such as thermometer or suppository) and place sign over bed alerting staff of this
8. Notify healthcare provider of any fever, unusual drainage, redness, or odor
9. Keep child NPO until bowel sounds return or flatus is passed; maintain NG tube, administer IV fluids as prescribed; monitor daily weights; begin diet with clear liquids and progress as tolerated
10. Assess pain using age-appropriate scales; provide comfort measures and involve parents; provide pain medications on regular basis as prescribed; notify healthcare provider if pain is not managed
11. Involve child in quiet, age-appropriate activities for diversion
12. Encourage parents to share feelings, anxieties, and concerns about disorder and postsurgical care
13. Refer to support groups and make appropriate referrals

D. Client and family teaching

1. Explain surgical repair and recovery process
2. Teach parents how to assess for distention and obstruction and importance of reporting these findings to healthcare provider
3. Encourage preschool and early school-aged children to draw pictures, use dolls, and play to express concerns about bodily appearance, irrigations, and colostomy
4. Teach ostomy care in immediate postoperative period and encourage parents to participate and give return demonstration while in hospital; encourage child to learn and assume care as soon as appropriate

XXIII. APPENDICITIS

A. Overview

1. Inflammation and infection of vermiform appendix in response to obstruction of lumen by hardened fecal material (**fecalith**), foreign bodies, microorganisms, or parasites
2. Normal mucous secretions accumulate in obstructed area and distend appendix, which causes capillary and venous engorgement and increased intraluminal pressure
3. Ischemia occurs and can lead to necrosis and perforation of intestinal wall (ruptured appendix); if perforation occurs, bacteria from bowel contaminate peritoneum and may lead to peritonitis and sepsis

B. Nursing assessment

1. Generalized abdominal or periumbilical pain progressively worsening and then localizing in RLQ at **McBurney's point** (Figure 59–6), anorexia, possible nausea and vomiting, diarrhea, or acute constipation
2. Signs of ruptured appendix include sudden relief of pain, fever, chills, elevated WBC count (15,000–20,000 cells/mm^3), guarding, abdominal distention, rapid shallow breathing, irritability, and restlessness
3. Ultrasound indicates an enlarged incompressible appendix

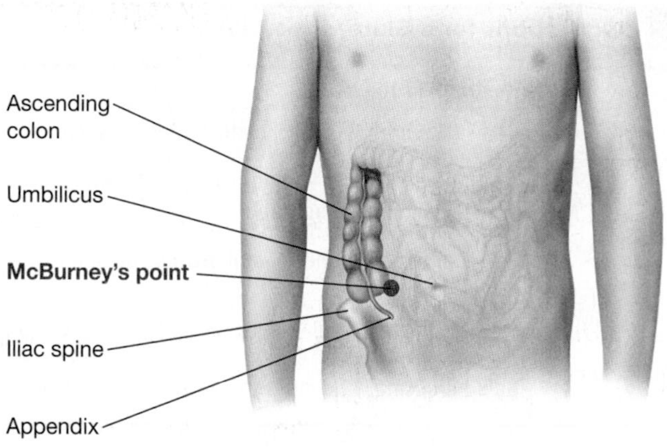

Figure 59–6
McBurney's point in right lower quadrant of abdomen with appendicitis.

C. Therapeutic management

1. Surgical removal (appendectomy) is done as soon as diagnosis made
2. Preoperative nursing care
   a. Explain procedure and postoperative care to client and family
   b. Keep client NPO and prevent dehydration with IV fluids as prescribed
   NCLEX® c. Place client in semi-Fowler or right side-lying position to help localize and prevent spread of any infection (used both preoperatively and postoperatively)
   d. Assess for abdominal distention, auscultate bowel sounds, and observe elimination patterns
   NCLEX® e. Do nothing to stimulate peristalsis, which would hasten perforation; avoid laxatives, enemas, and heat applications
   f. Apply cold packs to client's abdomen to help relieve discomfort
3. NCLEX® Postoperative nursing care
   NCLEX® a. Provide standard postoperative care including pulmonary hygiene and pain management
   b. Monitor VS, assess for abdominal distention, and inspect surgical wound for signs of infection
   c. Encourage ambulation within 6–8 hours after surgery if not contraindicated
   d. Monitor I&O and ensure that spontaneous voiding occurs
   NCLEX® e. If appendix ruptures, postoperative recovery is slowed; child will probably have an NG tube to decompress stomach and a Jackson-Pratt or Penrose drain; antibiotics may be administered

D. Client and family teaching

1. Diagnostic procedures, cause of appendicitis, surgical treatment, and anticipated postoperative care
2. How to assess surgical incision for signs and symptoms of infection
3. Signs to report to healthcare provider, such as fever, increased discomfort, and incision dehiscence (separation)
4. NCLEX® Child should avoid lifting, stretching, and strenuous activities until all follow-up care is completed
5. Provide information on fluids and advancement of diet during recovery period; include symptoms to report to healthcare provider, such as vomiting, abdominal distention, and increased pain

XXIV. CELIAC DISEASE

A. Overview

1. An immunologic disorder characterized by inability to tolerate foods containing gluten, a protein present in wheat, rye, oats, and barley; also known as gluten-sensitive enteropathy
2. NCLEX® Inability to fully digest gliadin and glutenin (protein fractions) leads to accumulation of amino acid glutamine, which is toxic to intestinal mucosa (leading to fatty stools initially and then malabsorption of protein, carbohydrates, calcium, iron, folate, and fat-soluble vitamins as disease progresses)
3. NCLEX® This deficiency in digestion requires lifelong dietary modifications
4. Exact cause is unknown; there may be a genetic predisposition, possibly influenced by environmental factors and an immunologic abnormality
5. NCLEX® Acute episodes (called celiac crises) are characterized by a general flare-up of symptoms; may be precipitated by infections, prolonged fasting, ingestion of gluten, or anticholinergic drugs; can lead to electrolyte imbalance, rapid dehydration, and severe acidosis

Table 59–3 Suggestions for a Gluten-Free Diet

Unrestricted Food Items	Restricted Food Items
Beef, pork, poultry, fish	Items with bread coating using wheat, oats, rye, or barley
Eggs	Any food made from wheat, rye, oats, or barley (bread, rolls, cookies, cakes, crackers, cereal, spaghetti, macaroni)
Milk, cream, cheese	Beer and ale, Ovaltine, instant tea mix, commercially prepared ice cream, malted milk, prepared puddings
Vegetables	Canned baked beans, commercially seasoned vegetable mixes or vegetables with sauce
Fruit	Salad dressings and mayonnaise, ketchup, gravy
Rice, corn, gluten-free wheat flour, puffed rice, corn flakes, cornmeal	

B. Nursing assessment

1. Symptoms typically appear within 3–6 months after introduction of gluten (usually in form of grains) into child's diet
2. NCLEX® Frequent bulky, greasy, malodorous stools with frothy appearance due to steatorrhea
3. Abdominal distention, vomiting, and anorexia
4. Growth retardation with lack of fat deposits and muscle wasting
5. Anemia, irritability, edema
6. NCLEX® In a celiac crisis, severe diarrhea and dehydration ensue; electrolyte imbalances and metabolic acidosis can create life-threatening disease
7. For unknown reasons, some children do not exhibit symptoms until after age 5 with growth retardation and delayed sexual maturation as predominant manifestations
8. Laboratory studies and diagnostic tests: 72-hour fecal fat analysis, biopsy of small intestine, serum IgA antiendomysial antibodies and IgA antitissue transglutaminase antibodies

C. Therapeutic management

1. NCLEX® Nursing care focuses on supporting child and parents in maintaining a gluten-free diet; corn and rice become substitute grains (see Table 59–3)
2. Assess child's growth at each routine visit using a standard growth chart
3. Administer fluids for hydration; serum electrolytes and osmolality may be used as lab indicators of hydration status
4. NCLEX® Monitor I&O, assess skin turgor, mucous membranes, and urine specific gravity
5. Encourage participation in age-appropriate activities
6. Inform parents of organizations such as American Celiac Society, Celiac Sprue Association/United States of America, and Gluten Intolerance Group

D. Client and family teaching

1. Written and verbal instructions on gluten-free diet
2. NCLEX® Read labels of processed foods because most contain gluten as a filler
3. Urgency of seeking medical care in the event of celiac crisis
4. NCLEX® Importance of lifelong adherence to dietary modifications and follow-up health care

XXV. NECROTIZING ENTEROCOLITIS (NEC)

A. Overview

1. An intestinal inflammatory disease that occurs primarily in premature infants characterized by varying degrees of mucosal or transmural necrosis of intestine
2. Usual onset is in first 2 weeks of life but can be later in very low-birth-weight infants
3. Risk factors include intestinal ischemia, bacterial or viral infection, and immaturity of GI tract; occurs most often in terminal ileum and colon
4. Pathology appears to begin when reduced blood flow to bowel leads to bowel wall ischemia, which allows bacteria to enter bowel wall and colonize; can lead to perforation, which leads to need for bowel resection

B. Nursing assessment

1. NCLEX® History may include prematurity, small for gestational age, maternal hemorrhage, preeclampsia, cocaine exposure in utero, exchange transfusions, umbilical catheters, low Apgar scores, or asphyxia

2. Typically, suspected NEC (stage I) consists of nonspecific clinical findings that represent physiologic instability or other common conditions in premature infants:
   a. Temperature instability
   b. Lethargy
   c. Recurrent apnea and bradycardia, with poor peripheral perfusion
   d. Hypoglycemia
   e. Feeding intolerance, vomiting, abdominal distention, increased pregavage gastric residuals
   f. Guaiac-positive stools

NCLEX® 3. NEC (stage II) consists of nonspecific signs and symptoms plus the following:
   a. Severe abdominal distention, tenderness, and edema of abdominal wall
   b. Grossly bloody stools
   c. Palpable bowel loops
   d. Bowel sounds may be absent

NCLEX® 4. NEC (stage III) occurs when infant becomes acutely ill:
   a. Deterioration of VS with evidence of septic shock
   b. Edema and erythema of abdominal wall with RLQ mass
   c. Acidosis (metabolic and/or respiratory)
   d. Disseminated intravascular coagulopathy (DIC)

5. Abdominal x-ray: free peritoneal gas, dilated bowel loops, bowel distention and thickening

C. Therapeutic management

NCLEX® 1. Nursing care focuses on early detection to minimize bowel necrosis
2. Measure abdominal girth frequently
3. Prepare feedings using aseptic technique

NCLEX® 4. Observe tolerance of feedings; assess and maintain optimal hydration status
5. Monitor cardiac and respiratory status
6. Promote and maintain adequate body temperature
7. Administer antibiotics as prescribed
8. Encourage family interaction and promote attachment process
9. Provide developmentally appropriate activities
10. Provide standard preoperative and postoperative care for bowel resection and possible ostomy if perforation or necrosis of bowel occurs

D. Client and family teaching

1. Encourage parents to express concerns about outcomes of surgery

NCLEX® 2. Instruct parents on signs of intestinal obstruction, strictures, poor tolerance of feedings, and impaired healing processes

NCLEX® 3. Instruct parents about care of ostomy and IV central line

XXVI. FAILURE TO THRIVE (FTT)

A. Overview

1. Syndrome in which infant or young child does not eat enough to be adequately nourished
2. Organic FTT results from a physical cause, such as congenital acquired immunodeficiency syndrome (AIDS), cystic fibrosis, celiac disease, congenital heart defects, chronic renal failure, gastroesophageal reflux, malabsorption syndrome, or endocrine dysfunction
3. Nonorganic FTT is called feeding disorder of infancy or early childhood suspected in absence of organic disease
   a. Parental or caregiver risk factors include poverty, depression, substance use, psychosis, developmental delay, social or emotional isolation, and lack of knowledge of infant nurturing and nutrition
   b. Infant may not provide clear cues about hunger and is not easily soothed; preterm and small for gestational age infants are more frequently affected

B. Nursing assessment

NCLEX® 1. Physical findings
   a. Weight often below 5th percentile and weight-for-length is often less than 80%
   b. Delay in developmental milestones
   c. Decreased muscle mass and muscle hypotonia
   d. Abdominal distension
   e. Generalized weakness and **cachexia** (malnutrition accompanied by wasting)

NCLEX® 2. Behavioral indicators include refusal of food, erratic sleep patterns, and disturbed manner, such as being irritable or difficult to soothe

3. Diagnostic tests
   a. Developmental screening
   b. Tuberculin skin test
   c. Bone scan, chest x-ray, ECG, IV pyelogram, upper and lower GI series
   d. Urinalysis, complete blood count, sweat chloride test, stool tests, T_4 test
   e. Bowel and muscle biopsies

C. Therapeutic management

1. Document child's eating patterns and cues given about hunger or satiety
2. Document parent–child interaction patterns such as eye contact, touch, and cuddling
3. Encourage parents to discuss positive and negative feelings of care, procedures, and interaction with child
4. NCLEX® Feed on demand or increase intake as tolerated; try to make mealtimes as stress-free as possible
5. NCLEX® Offer high-protein, high-calorie snacks, and frequent, small portions of a wide variety of foods
6. Document I&O, daily weights, and nutritional assessments
7. Provide consistency in nursing care
8. Upon discharge provide referral to agency that can continue to monitor child's home situation, family stress and behavior patterns, and feeding during meals

D. Client and family teaching

1. Normal growth and development
2. NCLEX® How to recognize and respond to hunger and satiety cues, hold and touch infant during feedings, and establish eye contact with infant or child

XXVII. VOMITING AND DIARRHEA

A. Overview

1. Vomiting is a forceful ejection of gastric contents through mouth that is usually self-limiting and requires no specific treatment unless complications occur (dehydration, electrolyte imbalances, malnutrition, and aspiration)
   a. Can be an associated symptom of an acute infectious disease, increased intracranial pressure, toxic ingestion, food intolerance and allergy, mechanical obstruction of GI tract, metabolic disorder, or psychogenic problem
   b. NCLEX® Color and consistency of emesis suggests etiology: green and bilious suggests bowel obstruction; coffee-ground texture from blood mixing with stomach contents suggests GI bleeding; curdled stomach contents, mucus, or fatty foods several hours after eating suggest poor gastric emptying
   c. NCLEX® Associated symptoms also help to identify etiology: fever and diarrhea with infection; constipation with obstruction; localized abdominal pain with appendicitis, pancreatitis, or PUD; change in level of consciousness or headache with a central nervous system or metabolic disorder; forceful or projectile vomiting with pyloric stenosis
2. **Diarrhea** is defined as frequent, watery, loose stools that has several causes (respiratory infections, GI disorders or infections, stress, food intolerance or sensitivity, effect of medications, and surgical procedures that reduce absorptive surface of intestine)
   a. Can be acute or chronic in nature
   b. Increased intestinal motility and rapid emptying leads to impaired nutrient absorption and excessive excretion of water and electrolytes, leading to dehydration, electrolyte imbalance, hypovolemic shock, and even death in pediatric clients

B. Nursing assessment

1. NCLEX® Assessment of hydration status is highest priority (see Table 59–4 for signs of dehydration)
2. Assess amount, color, consistency, and time of stools and vomitus
3. NCLEX® Assess daily weights (best indicator of fluid balance) and I&O
4. Assess client's activity level
5. Assess for abdominal cramping, fever, and other related symptoms
6. Stool culture for bacteria, ova, parasites, or rotaviruses; stool examination for pH, leukocytes, glucose, and presence of blood; serum electrolytes, BUN, creatinine, and glucose; x-rays, ultrasound, or endoscopy

C. Therapeutic management

1. Priority nursing interventions focus on preventing and managing dehydration
2. NCLEX® Weigh client on admission and daily using same scale at same time of day in same amount of clothing

Table 59–4 Range of Manifestations of Clinical Dehydration

Assessment Parameter	Client Manifestations
Percent of body weight lost	Ranges from mild (up to 5% loss or 40–50 mL/kg) to severe (a 10% or greater loss or 100+ mg/kg)
Level of consciousness	Ranges from alert, restless, and thirsty if mild to lethargic, possibly apprehensive, or comatose state if severe
Vital signs	Pulse ranges from normal to rapid and weak; may need to palpate distal pulses by Doppler if severe BP ranges from normal for age to low for age or may be difficult to detect Temperature ranges from normal to elevated depending on degree and cause Respirations may range from normal to increased rate and/or altered pattern
Skin turgor and mucous membranes	Skin turgor ranges from normal to poor; mucous membranes range from moist to dry or parched
Extremities	Range from warm with normal capillary refill to cool and discolored with delayed capillary refill
Urine	Ranges from normal (initially) to decreased and eventually absent if severe enough
Thirst	Ranges from slightly to greatly increased unless client is lethargic; older adults may also experience reduced thirst as an age-related change (not a reliable sign in this population)
Fontanels in infant	May range from normal to sunken

NCLEX®

3. Monitor and document I&O hourly; weigh infant diapers after voiding and episode of diarrhea; monitor urine specific gravity
4. Monitor VS and avoid rectal temperatures
5. Client is usually NPO to allow bowel rest; administer IV fluids for severe dehydration

NCLEX®

6. Begin oral rehydration for mild to moderate dehydration and as supplement to IV fluid in severe dehydration
   - **a.** Oral rehydration fluids (ORFs) include commercial preparations such as Infalyte, Rehydralyte, and Pedialyte for children
   - **b.** Start with frequent, small amounts of liquids—1–3 teaspoons every 10–15 minutes (target goal for first 2–4 hours of treatment is 50 mL per kg weight); for older children and adults, offer sips to total up to 8 oz in an hour; offer 1 teaspoon every 2–3 minutes if vomiting since some fluid may still absorb
   - **c.** Infants progress from clear liquids to their typical diet, although soy protein formula rather than milk-based formula may be recommended for formula-fed infants
   - **d.** When diet resumes, advise intake of cereals, starches, soups, fruits, and vegetables; avoid simple sugars and carbonated beverages, which could worsen diarrhea
7. Administer antidiarrheals, antibiotics, antiprotozoals as prescribed based on cause
8. Monitor lab tests (electrolytes, hematocrit, pH, serum albumin)
9. Implement measures to reduce fever if needed
10. Cleanse diaper area (infants) or perianal skin with mild soap and water after each stool; avoid harsh astringent wipes that could further irritate reddened skin

NCLEX®

11. Practice standard precautions

D. **Client and family teaching:** causes of vomiting and diarrhea, oral rehydration therapy, skin care, and signs and symptoms requiring medical attention

Check Your NCLEX–RN® Exam I.Q.

You are ready for testing on this content if you can:

- Identify basic structures and functions of the gastrointestinal system.
- Describe the pathophysiology and etiology of common gastrointestinal disorders.
- Discuss expected assessment data and diagnostic test findings for selected gastrointestinal disorders.
- Discuss therapeutic management of a client experiencing a gastrointestinal disorder.
- Discuss nursing management of a client experiencing a gastrointestinal disorder.
- Identify expected outcomes for the client experiencing a gastrointestinal disorder.

PRACTICE TEST

PRACTICE TEST

1 A client has a total gastrectomy. The nurse explains to the client the need for long-term injections of which vitamin?

1. Thiamine
2. Folic acid
3. Cyanocobalamin
4. Niacin

2 A client with diverticular disease undergoes a colonoscopy. During an abdominal assessment, the nurse looks for which sign to indicate a possible complication of the procedure?

1. Diarrhea
2. Nausea and vomiting
3. Guarding and rebound tenderness
4. Redness and warmth of the abdominal skin

3 The client who has ulcerative colitis is scheduled for an ileostomy. When the client asks the nurse what to expect related to bowel function and care after surgery, what response should the nurse make?

1. "You will be able to have some control over your bowel movements."
2. "The stoma will require that you wear a collection device all the time."
3. "After the stoma heals, you can irrigate your bowel so you will not have to wear a pouch."
4. "The drainage will gradually become semisolid and formed."

4 The nurse is conducting dietary teaching with a client who has dumping syndrome. The nurse encourages the client to avoid which foods that the client usually enjoys? Select all that apply.

1. Eggs
2. Cheese
3. Fruit
4. Pork
5. Cookies

5 A client is being evaluated for possible duodenal ulcer. The nurse assesses the client for which manifestation that would support this diagnosis?

1. Epigastric pain relieved by food
2. History of chronic aspirin use
3. Distended abdomen
4. Positive fluid wave

6 The client returning from a colonoscopy has been given a diagnosis of Crohn's disease. The oncoming shift nurse expects to note which manifestations in the client? Select all that apply.

1. Steatorrhea
2. Firm, rigid abdomen
3. Constipation
4. Enlarged hemorrhoids
5. Diarrhea

7 A client is scheduled for a fecal fat exam. In planning client education, the nurse includes that which dietary modification is necessary before the test?

1. Eat a fat-free diet the day before the exam.
2. Eat a high-fat meal right before the exam.
3. Eat a diet containing 35 grams of fat for 36 hours before the test.
4. Eat at least 100 grams of fat for 3 days before and during the test.

8 The client with diverticular disease is scheduled for a sigmoidoscopy and suddenly reports severe abdominal pain. On examination, the nurse notes a rigid abdomen with guarding. What action should the nurse take next?

1. Notify the healthcare provider.
2. Place the client in a more comfortable position.
3. Keep the client distracted until the procedure begins.
4. Tell the client that the test will show what is causing his problem.

9 The nurse is educating the client with gastroesophageal reflux disease (GERD) about ways to minimize symptoms. Which information in the client's history should the nurse address as indicators that need to be changed? Select all that apply.

1. Lifting weights for exercise
2. Being a vegetarian
3. Having a body mass index of 26
4. Taking calcium carbonate tablets
5. Drinking 2–4 cups of coffee daily

10 The client with a duodenal ulcer asks the nurse why an antibiotic is part of the treatment regimen. Which information should the nurse include in the response?

1. Antibiotics decrease the likelihood of a secondary infection.
2. Many duodenal ulcers are caused by the *Helicobacter pylori* organism.
3. Antibiotics are used in an attempt to sterilize the stomach.
4. Many people have *Clostridium difficile*, which can lead to ulcer formation.

11 The nurse should evaluate the results of which laboratory tests while caring for a client who has cirrhosis of the liver? Select all that apply.

1. Prothrombin time
2. Urinalysis
3. Serum lipase
4. Serum troponin
5. Serum albumin

12 The nurse is caring for a client with a history of alcoholism. Which findings would indicate that the client has possibly developed chronic pancreatitis? Select all that apply.

1. Steady weight gain
2. Flank pain on left side only
3. Fatty stools
4. Excessive hunger
5. Constipation and flatulence

13 The nurse caring for a client with hemolytic jaundice anticipates which findings on laboratory test results?

1. Elevated serum indirect bilirubin
2. Decreased serum protein
3. Elevated urine bilirubin
4. Decreased urine pH

14 A client was admitted to the hospital with cholelithiasis the previous day. Which new assessment finding indicates to the nurse that the stone has probably obstructed the common bile duct?

1. Nausea
2. Elevated cholesterol level
3. Right upper quadrant (RUQ) pain
4. Jaundice

15 The nurse caring for a client with uncomplicated cholelithiasis anticipates that the client's laboratory results will show an elevation in which test?

1. Serum amylase
2. Alkaline phosphatase
3. Mean corpuscular hemoglobin concentration (MCHC)
4. Indirect bilirubin

16 In caring for a client 4 days' postcholecystectomy, the nurse notices that drainage from the T-tube is 600 mL in 24 hours. Which is the most appropriate action by the nurse?

1. Clamp the tube q 2 hours for 30 minutes
2. Place the client in a supine position
3. Assess drainage characteristics and notify the healthcare provider
4. Encourage an increased fluid intake

17 The post-cholecystectomy client asks the nurse when the T-tube will be removed. Which response by the nurse would be appropriate?

1. "When your stool returns to a normal brown color, the tube can be removed."
2. "The tube will be removed at the same time as your staples."
3. "When the tube stops draining, it will be removed."
4. "The tube is usually removed the day after surgery."

18 Which assessments made by the nurse could indicate the development of portal hypertension in a client with cirrhosis? Select all that apply.

1. Hemorrhoids
2. Bleeding gums
3. Muscle wasting
4. Splenomegaly
5. Ascites

19 The nurse is caring for a client who has ascites, and the healthcare provider prescribes spironolactone. When the client asks why this drug is being used, what is the best response by the nurse?

1. "This drug will help increase the level of protein in your blood."
2. "The drug will cause an increase in the amount of the hormone aldosterone your body produces."
3. "This medication is a diuretic but does not make the kidneys excrete potassium."
4. "This will help you excrete larger amounts of ammonia."

20 When caring for a client who has cirrhosis, the nurse notices flapping tremors of the wrist and fingers. How should the nurse chart this finding?

1. "Trousseau's sign noted."
2. "Caput medusa noted."
3. "Fetor hepaticus noted."
4. "Asterixis noted."

21 A mother arrives at the pediatric clinic with her 6-month-old infant. While the nurse assesses the child, the mother points to the umbilicus and says: "What am I going to do about this? When he cries, it looks like it's going to burst." What is the best response by the nurse?

1. "It's best if you don't let him cry."
2. "It probably won't rupture unless he gets excessively upset. I wouldn't worry about it at this time."
3. "I know it looks frightening, but it really won't burst."
4. "Put a binder around it, and that will keep it from bursting when he gets upset."

22 A 9-year-old male client with severe esophagitis is 12 hours' status/post-Nissen fundoplication for gastroesophageal reflux. What action by the nurse would be appropriate while providing nursing care?

1. Encourage him to take small amounts of clear liquids every 4 hours.
2. Administer nasogastric or gastrostomy feedings every 4 hours.
3. Ask him to choose a face on the Wong FACES pain rating scale.
4. Insert a pH probe to monitor esophageal acidity.

23 A 10-month-old female infant with biliary atresia is being discharged after a Kasai procedure. Which statement, if made by the parents, indicates that teaching with regard to prognosis has been understood?

1. "We are glad this problem was found so early; now everything will be fine."
2. "We will stop her liver medicine now that she is being discharged."
3. "We are happy to be able to stop that special formula and many of those vitamins."
4. "We know that even though surgery is over, she will likely need a liver transplant."

24 Which laboratory test would the nurse expect to be prescribed for a child with dehydration caused by vomiting and diarrhea? Select all that apply.

1. Serum sodium
2. Urine specific gravity
3. Serum ammonia
4. Serum amylase
5. Blood urea nitrogen (BUN)

25 The nurse is caring for a child with a history of severe diarrhea. Which notation about acid–base imbalance would the nurse expect to find in the medical record?

1. Respiratory acidosis
2. Respiratory alkalosis
3. Metabolic acidosis
4. Metabolic alkalosis

26 A nurse who floats to the infant and toddlers nursing unit asks the pediatric nurse about the notation "ESSR" on the care plan of a client. The nurse explains that this documentation refers to which item?

1. The feeding method for children with gastroesophageal reflux
2. The feeding method for children with cleft lip or palate
3. The procedure for repair of pyloric stenosis
4. The procedure for repair of Hirschsprung's disease

27 A child with Hirschsprung's disease is being discharged after a Soave endorectal pull-through procedure for colostomy closure. Which item should the nurse include in the discharge teaching plan?

1. Stools may be infrequent and uncomfortable for the first few weeks.
2. It will be necessary to perform weekly rectal irrigations for approximately 6 weeks.
3. Report fever, increasing pain or discomfort, or redness of the incision to the surgeon.
4. Stools will be fatty for a week or so and then gradually return to normal.

28 The nurse is obtaining a history from the mother of a child being admitted with flare-up of celiac disease. What item of information should the nurse expect the mother to report?

1. Stools that are fatty
2. An increased appetite with no weight gain
3. Wavelike episodes of abdominal pain just before meals
4. Soft, formed stools

29 The mother of a child undergoing an emergency appendectomy tells the nurse, "If I had brought him in yesterday when he complained of an upset stomach, this wouldn't have happened." What is the best response by the nurse?

1. "It's okay; you got him here just in time before it ruptured."
2. "It is often difficult to predict when a simple complaint will become more serious."
3. "Next time he seems sick, you should bring him in immediately."
4. "Sometimes parents can make a mistake without meaning to do so."

30 The nurse is teaching home feeding guidelines to the mother of a child with nonorganic failure to thrive. Essential information for the nurse to include would be the importance of which item?

1. Restricting eating except at mealtimes
2. Allowing the child to eat alone to minimize distraction
3. Allowing the child to snack on finger foods, such as circular oat cereal and bananas
4. A relaxed mealtime with few limits on behavior

31 The nurse is admitting a child with a diagnosis of "rule out appendicitis." The nurse assesses this client for which manifestations? Select all that apply.

1. Generalized abdominal pain
2. Pain localizing in right lower quadrant
3. Fatty stools
4. Elevated white blood cell count
5. Indigestion

ANSWERS & RATIONALES

1 **Answer: 3 Rationale:** The loss of parietal cells that secrete intrinsic factor results in vitamin B_{12} (cyanocobalamin) deficiency postgastrectomy because intrinsic factor is needed for absorption of vitamin B_{12}. For this reason, clients require vitamin B_{12} injections for life. Thiamine, folic acid, and niacin are other B-complex vitamins. **Cognitive Level:** Analyzing **Client Need:** Physiological Adaptation **Integrated Process:** Teaching and Learning **Content Area:** Adult Health: Gastrointestinal **Strategy:** The core issue of the question is knowledge that gastric surgery results in loss of ability to produce intrinsic factor and subsequent vitamin B_{12} deficiency. Use nursing knowledge and the process of elimination to make a selection.

2 **Answer: 3 Rationale:** Bowel perforation is a possible result of colonoscopy if the colonoscope accidentally pierces the bowel wall. Perforation could lead to symptoms of peritonitis, such as guarding and rebound tenderness. Diarrhea is not considered to be a complication of colonoscopy. Nausea and vomiting could be signs of many GI disorders, but are not complications of colonoscopy. Redness and warmth of abdominal skin would suggest a skin irritation or infection, but is not a complication of colonoscopy. **Cognitive Level:**

Analyzing **Client Need:** Physiological Adaptation **Integrated Process:** Nursing Process: Assessment **Content Area:** Adult Health: Gastrointestinal **Strategy:** The core issue of the question is assessment data that correlates with complications of colonoscopy, such as peritonitis. Use nursing knowledge and the process of elimination to make a selection.

3 **Answer: 2 Rationale:** A client with an ileostomy must always wear a collection device. The client has no control over bowel movements. Bowel irrigation is not performed to eliminate the need to wear a drainage pouch. The drainage tends to be liquid but can become pastelike with intake of specific foods. **Cognitive Level:** Applying **Client Need:** Physiological Adaptation **Integrated Process:** Communication and Documentation **Content Area:** Adult Health: Gastrointestinal **Strategy:** The core issue of the question is knowledge of stool characteristics and associated stoma appliance needs following ileostomy. Use nursing knowledge and the process of elimination to make a selection.

4 **Answer: 3, 5 Rationale:** Dumping syndrome, in which gastric contents rapidly enter the bowel, can occur following gastrectomy. Fruits and cookies containing simple carbohydrates will attract fluid into the GI tract, leading to symptoms of dumping syndrome. Eggs are higher in protein and fat (cholesterol), which will slow GI transit time, avoiding dumping syndrome. Cheese has variable amounts of protein and fat, and these are less likely to trigger dumping syndrome. Pork is high in protein, which slows GI transit time to reduce episodes of dumping syndrome. **Cognitive Level:** Applying **Client Need:** Physiological Adaptation **Integrated Process:** Nursing Process: Implementation **Content Area:** Adult Health: Gastrointestinal **Strategy:** The core issue of the question is knowledge of foods to avoid when the client has dumping syndrome. Use nursing knowledge and the process of elimination to make a selection.

5 **Answer: 1 Rationale:** The pain of a gastric ulcer is dull and aching, occurs after eating, and is not relieved by food as is the pain from a duodenal ulcer. The pancreatic juices that are high in bicarbonate are released with food intake and relieve duodenal ulcer pain when the client eats. Chronic aspirin use is irritating to the stomach. Distended abdomen is a vague sign and is unrelated. A positive fluid wave is consistent with ascites and is unrelated. **Cognitive Level:** Applying **Client Need:** Physiological Adaptation **Integrated Process:** Nursing Process: Assessment **Content Area:** Adult Health: Gastrointestinal **Strategy:** The core issue of the question is expected assessment findings in duodenal ulcer. Recall the effect of pancreatic juices on the duodenal ulcer surface and use the process of elimination to make a selection.

6 **Answer: 1, 5 Rationale:** Steatorrhea is often present in the client with Crohn's disease. Diarrhea is also a key feature, but unlike ulcerative colitis, the loose stool usually does not contain blood and is usually less frequent in number of episodes. A firm rigid abdomen is not a manifestation of Crohn's disease. Constipation is not a manifestation of Crohn's disease. Hemorrhoids are not a manifestation of Crohn's disease. **Cognitive Level:** Applying **Client Need:** Physiological Adaptation **Integrated Process:** Nursing Process: Assessment **Content Area:** Adult Health: Gastrointestinal **Strategy:** The core issue of the question is identification of common symptoms of Crohn's disease. Use nursing knowledge and the process of elimination to make a selection.

7 **Answer: 4 Rationale:** It is suggested that adults consume at least 100 grams of fat per day for 3 days before the test and throughout specimen collection. The client is supposed to take in a high-fat diet, not a fat-free diet, for a specified amount of time before the test. Eating a high-fat meal right before the exam is not a sufficient time frame to ensure valid test results. Eating a diet containing 35 grams of fat for 36 hours before the test is insufficient in amount and time. **Cognitive Level:** Applying **Client Need:** Physiological Adaptation **Integrated Process:** Nursing Process: Planning **Content Area:** Adult Health: Gastrointestinal **Strategy:** The core issue of the question is the ability to provide correct information when teaching a client about proper preparation for fecal fat examination. Use nursing knowledge and the process of elimination to make a selection.

8 **Answer: 1 Rationale:** Perforation of an obstructed diverticulum can cause abscess formation or generalized peritonitis. The manifestations of peritonitis are abdominal guarding and rigidity and pain. Because treatment of this complication is beyond the scope of independent nursing practice, the healthcare provider must be notified. Placing the client in a position of comfort could be attempted after notifying the healthcare provider of the complication. Providing a distraction is not the priority nursing action. Sigmoidoscopy is contraindicated in cases of perforation. **Cognitive Level:** Analyzing **Client Need:** Physiological Adaptation **Integrated Process:** Nursing Process: Implementation **Content Area:** Adult Health: Gastrointestinal **Strategy:** The core issue of the question is the ability to identify the occurrence of peritonitis as a complication of diverticular disease and determine the appropriate course of action. Use nursing knowledge and the process of elimination to make a selection.

9 **Answer: 1, 3, 5 Rationale:** Lifestyle modifications can minimize symptoms of GERD. Anything that increases intra-abdominal pressure should be avoided, such as lifting weights. Obesity or being overweight (body mass index of 26) also aggravates symptoms. Coffee, cola, other sources of caffeine, and chocolate decrease lower esophageal sphincter tone and can increase symptoms of GERD. Being a vegetarian does not increase risk of GERD. Calcium carbonate tablets often aid in symptom relief. **Cognitive Level:** Applying **Client Need:** Physiological Adaptation **Integrated Process:** Nursing Process: Diagnosis **Content Area:** Adult Health: Gastrointestinal **Strategy:** The core issue of the question is ability to identify risk factors that aggravate symptoms of GERD. Use nursing knowledge and the process of elimination to make a selection.

10 **Answer: 2 Rationale:** *Helicobacter pylori* infection is a major cause of peptic ulcers so treatment includes antibiotic therapy to eradicate the microorganisms. Antibiotics do not reduce the likelihood of a secondary infection; they treat the primary infection. Antibiotics are not used to sterilize the bowel, which would upset the normal flora of the GI tract. *Clostridium difficile* is a contagious microorganism that can lead to severe diarrhea. **Cognitive Level:** Applying **Client Need:** Physiological Adaptation **Integrated Process:** Nursing Process: Implementation **Content Area:** Adult Health: Gastrointestinal **Strategy:** The core issue of the question is knowledge of etiology of peptic ulcers, including duodenal ulcers. Use nursing knowledge and the process of elimination to make a selection.

11 **Answer: 1, 5 Rationale:** Many clotting factors are produced in the liver, including fibrinogen (factor I), prothrombin (factor II), factor V, serum prothrombin conversion accelerator (factor VII), factor IX, and factor X. The client's ability to form these factors may be impaired with cirrhosis, putting

the client at risk for bleeding. The prothrombin time will evaluate blood-clotting ability. One function of the liver is to synthesize protein, which may be impaired with cirrhosis. Urinalysis is a general screening measure or can be used to diagnose problems with the urinary tract. Serum lipase is a useful indicator of disorders of the pancreas. Serum troponin is a common laboratory test used to diagnose myocardial infarction. **Cognitive Level:** Applying **Client Need:** Physiological Adaptation **Integrated Process:** Nursing Process: Assessment **Content Area:** Adult Health: Gastrointestinal **Strategy:** The critical word in the question is *cirrhosis*. With this in mind, the correct answers are those that could detect a complication of cirrhosis or disturbed liver function. Use nursing knowledge and the process of elimination to make a selection.

12 **Answer: 3, 5 Rationale:** Steatorrhea (fatty stools) result from a decrease in pancreatic enzyme secretion with pancreatitis. The client with chronic pancreatitis is likely to experience bouts of constipation and flatulence. The client with chronic pancreatitis is likely to experience weight loss rather than weight gain. The pain of pancreatitis is felt in the abdomen and is not limited to the left flank. Manifestations of chronic pancreatitis include nausea and vomiting rather than excessive hunger. **Cognitive Level:** Applying **Client Need:** Physiological Adaptation **Integrated Process:** Nursing Process: Assessment **Content Area:** Adult Health: Gastrointestinal **Strategy:** The core issue of the question is the ability to identify assessment findings that are consistent with the development of chronic pancreatitis. Use nursing knowledge and the process of elimination to make a selection.

13 **Answer: 1 Rationale:** Hemolytic jaundice is caused by excessive breakdown of red blood cells, and the amount of bilirubin produced exceeds the ability of the liver to conjugate it, so there is an increase in indirect bilirubin. Serum protein is not measured to detect hemolytic jaundice. Unconjugated bilirubin is insoluble in water and is not found in the urine. Urine pH is not decreased by hemolytic jaundice. **Cognitive Level:** Applying **Client Need:** Physiological Adaptation **Integrated Process:** Nursing Process: Assessment **Content Area:** Adult Health: Gastrointestinal **Strategy:** The core issue of the question is knowledge of clinical indicators of hemolytic jaundice. Use nursing knowledge and the process of elimination to make a selection.

14 **Answer: 4 Rationale:** Obstruction of the common bile duct results in reflux of bile into the liver, which produces jaundice. Nausea occurs with cholelithiasis and would not be a new symptom to signal obstruction. Alkaline phosphatase increases with biliary obstruction but cholesterol level does not increase. RUQ pain occurs as a common symptom in cholelithiasis. **Cognitive Level:** Analyzing **Client Need:** Physiological Adaptation **Integrated Process:** Nursing Process: Assessment **Content Area:** Adult Health: Gastrointestinal **Strategy:** The core issue of the question is knowledge of clinical indicators of common bile duct obstruction. Think about the pathophysiology of blocked bile drainage and use the process of elimination to make a selection.

15 **Answer: 2 Rationale:** Obstructive biliary disease causes a significant elevation in alkaline phosphatase. Serum amylase would increase in pancreatic disorders. MCHC is one type of red blood cell index used to differentiate among different types of anemia. Obstruction in the biliary tract causes an elevation in direct bilirubin, not indirect bilirubin. **Cognitive Level:** Applying **Client Need:** Physiological Adaptation **Integrated Process:** Nursing Process: Assessment **Content Area:** Adult Health: Gastrointestinal **Strategy:** Think about the body system reflected in each option and use nursing knowledge and the process of elimination to make a selection.

16 **Answer: 3 Rationale:** The T-tube may drain up to 500 mL in the first 24 hours and decreases steadily thereafter. If there is excessive drainage, the nurse should further assess the drainage to be able to describe it accurately and notify the healthcare provider immediately. Clamping the T-tube after the first 24 hours would be contraindicated as it is too soon to do this. Placing the client in a supine position will not alter the flow of T-tube drainage. While increased fluids in general would offset fluid loss from the T-tube, this does not address the significance of the excessive drainage. **Cognitive Level:** Applying **Client Need:** Physiological Adaptation **Integrated Process:** Nursing Process: Implementation **Content Area:** Adult Health: Gastrointestinal **Strategy:** Note the critical word *most* in the question, which indicates the need to prioritize. The core issue of the question is knowledge of appropriate nursing action following notation of excessive T-tube drainage. Use nursing knowledge and the process of elimination to make a selection.

17 **Answer: 1 Rationale:** When T-tube drainage subsides and stools return to a normal brown color, the tube can be clamped 1–2 hours before and after meals in preparation for tube removal. If the client tolerates clamping, the tube will then be removed. The tube is not removed at the same time as the incisional staples. It is not necessary for drainage to completely stop before tube removal. The client may not be ready for tube removal the day after surgery. **Cognitive Level:** Applying **Client Need:** Physiological Adaptation **Integrated Process:** Communication and Documentation **Content Area:** Adult Health: Gastrointestinal **Strategy:** The core issue of the question is the appropriate time frame for use of a T-tube following gallbladder surgery. Use nursing knowledge and the process of elimination to make a selection.

18 **Answer: 1, 4, 5 Rationale:** Obstruction to portal blood flow causes a rise in portal venous pressure, which can lead to development of hemorrhoids. Splenomegaly can occur because of increased pressure in the portal system. Ascites occurs with portal blood flow obstruction because the increased pressure in the blood vessels leads to fluid accumulation in the abdomen because of pressure dynamics. Bleeding gums would indicate insufficient vitamin K production in the liver. Muscle wasting commonly accompanies the poor nutritional intake commonly seen in clients with cirrhosis. **Cognitive Level:** Analyzing **Client Need:** Physiological Adaptation **Integrated Process:** Nursing Process: Assessment **Content Area:** Adult Health: Gastrointestinal **Strategy:** The wording of the question indicates that more than one option is likely to be correct. The core issue of the question is knowledge of associated findings in a client with portal hypertension. Use knowledge of the pathophysiology of the condition and the process of elimination to make appropriate selections.

19 **Answer: 3 Rationale:** Spironolactone is used in clients with ascites who show no improvement with bedrest and fluid restriction. It inhibits sodium reabsorption in the distal tubule and promotes potassium retention by inhibiting aldosterone. Spironolactone does not increase protein levels in the blood. Spironolactone does not increase production of aldosterone. Spironolactone does not aid in excreting ammonia, although lactulose will have this effect. **Cognitive Level:** Applying **Client Need:** Pharmacological and Parenteral Therapies **Integrated Process:** Communication and Documentation

Content Area: Adult Health: Gastrointestinal **Strategy:** The core issue of the question is knowledge of medication effects in a client with ascites. Use nursing knowledge related to pharmacology and the process of elimination to make a selection.

20 **Answer: 4 Rationale:** Asterixis is a flapping tremor of the hands when the arms are extended. Trousseau's sign reflects hypocalcemia. Caput medusa refers to spiderlike abdominal veins that are also commonly found in clients with cirrhosis who have portal hypertension as a complication. Fetor hepaticus is a specific odor noted in liver failure. **Cognitive Level:** Applying **Client Need:** Physiological Adaptation **Integrated Process:** Nursing Process: Assessment **Content Area:** Adult Health: Gastrointestinal **Strategy:** The core issue of the question is knowledge of typical assessment findings in a client with cirrhosis. Use nursing knowledge and the process of elimination to make a selection.

21 **Answer: 3 Rationale:** It is a common finding that when the infant with an umbilical hernia cries, the hernia protrudes but will not rupture. It is unnecessary to try to prevent the infant from crying. An umbilical hernia will not rupture because the infant gets upset and this response does not reassure the parent. The family is instructed not to apply tape, straps, or coins to the umbilicus to reduce the hernia. **Cognitive Level:** Applying **Client Need:** Physiological Adaptation **Integrated Process:** Communication and Documentation **Content Area:** Child Health **Strategy:** The core issue of the question is knowledge of the consequences of umbilical hernia and knowledge of therapeutic communication techniques. Use this knowledge and the process of elimination to make a selection.

22 **Answer: 3 Rationale:** Pain management is a high priority following gastric surgery, and the nurse should use age-appropriate tools to assess for pain. A gastrostomy tube or nasogastric tube placed during surgery is kept in place to maintain gastric decompression, so drinking is not allowed. The child is kept NPO until bowel function returns. The use of a pH probe to measure gastric acidity is not necessary. **Cognitive Level:** Applying **Client Need:** Physiological Adaptation **Integrated Process:** Nursing Process: Implementation **Content Area:** Child Health **Strategy:** The core issue of the question is knowledge of appropriate interventions in the first 24 hours following gastric surgery. Use knowledge that the gastric tube should not be manipulated or used for feeding to eliminate some options. Use nursing knowledge of routine postoperative care and the process of elimination to make a final selection.

23 **Answer: 4 Rationale:** Because the Kasai procedure is palliative, a liver transplant is required in a majority of cases. The Kasai procedure is not curative, and prognosis is best if performed before 10 weeks of age. Its purpose is to achieve biliary drainage and avoid early liver failure. Medications need to be continued after discharge as prescribed. Formula and vitamins need to be continued after the procedure. **Cognitive Level:** Analyzing **Client Need:** Physiological Adaptation **Integrated Process:** Nursing Process: Evaluation **Content Area:** Child Health **Strategy:** The core issue of the question is knowledge of the typical success of surgery with the Kasai procedure in an infant with biliary atresia. Use nursing knowledge and the process of elimination to make a selection.

24 **Answer: 1, 2, 5 Rationale:** Serum sodium would be expected to increase in a client with dehydration because of hemoconcentration. Measuring urine specific gravity provides data about the concentration of urine and provides information regarding hydration. The BUN rises with dehydration and is therefore a general indicator of hydration status, although it also reflects kidney function. Serum ammonia could be elevated in liver disease. Serum amylase could be elevated in pancreatic disorders. **Cognitive Level:** Applying **Client Need:** Physiological Adaptation **Integrated Process:** Nursing Process: Implementation **Content Area:** Child Health **Strategy:** The core issue of the question is dehydration and thus the correct option is one that addresses fluid balance in the body in some way. Use nursing knowledge and the process of elimination to make a selection.

25 **Answer: 3 Rationale:** In severe diarrhea, excess bicarbonate (base) is lost, which predisposes to metabolic acidosis. There is also carbohydrate malabsorption and depletion of glycogen stores, resulting in fat metabolism. Ketoacids are the by-products of fat metabolism, which adds to the metabolic acidosis. Diarrhea is not a respiratory problem, although diarrhea can lead to acidosis. Diarrhea is not a respiratory problem and it does not lead to alkalosis. Diarrhea is a metabolic problem but does not lead to alkalosis. **Cognitive Level:** Analyzing **Client Need:** Physiological Adaptation **Integrated Process:** Nursing Process: Diagnosis **Content Area:** Child Health **Strategy:** The core issue of the question is the ability to correlate acid–base imbalance with a diagnosis of diarrhea. Recall that bicarbonate is a base and that the respiratory system is not directly involved to make a selection.

26 **Answer: 2 Rationale:** ESSR is the abbreviation for the four key steps in feeding the infant or child with cleft lip or palate. These steps are to Enlarge nipple; Stimulate suck reflex; Swallow fluid; Rest after each swallow. ESSR does not refer to a treatment or feeding method used in gastroesophageal reflux, pyloric stenosis, or Hirschsprung's disease. **Cognitive Level:** Applying **Client Need:** Physiological Adaptation **Integrated Process:** Nursing Process: Diagnosis **Content Area:** Child Health **Strategy:** The core issue of the question is knowledge of a feeding technique in cleft lip or palate that reduces the risk of aspiration. Use nursing knowledge and the process of elimination to make a selection.

27 **Answer: 3 Rationale:** It is important that any signs of infection be reported at once. After the Soave procedure, normal bowel function is expected. No rectal irrigations are necessary. Stools are not fatty for a week or so following the Soave procedure. **Cognitive Level:** Applying **Client Need:** Physiological Adaptation **Integrated Process:** Nursing Process: Planning **Content Area:** Child Health **Strategy:** The core issue of the question is knowledge of routine discharge teaching following an abdominal surgical procedure. Use nursing knowledge and the process of elimination to make a selection.

28 **Answer: 1 Rationale:** Acute episodes of celiac disease are characterized by bulky, frothy stools with fat. Anorexia would be expected rather than increased appetite. Pain does not occur in waves prior to mealtimes. Stools are not soft and formed. **Cognitive Level:** Applying **Client Need:** Physiological Adaptation **Integrated Process:** Nursing Process: Assessment **Content Area:** Child Health **Strategy:** The core issue of the question is knowledge of assessment findings in a client with celiac disease. Use nursing knowledge and the process of elimination to make a selection.

29 **Answer: 2 Rationale:** Parents often react to a child's illness with feelings of guilt for not recognizing the severity of the condition sooner. A response that provides emotional support and reduces parental anxiety encourages parents to feel confident in their abilities as caregivers. Telling the parent "it's OK" ignores the parent's feelings. Directing the parent to

seek care immediately next time adds to the parent's stress. Using the word *mistake* adds to the parent's perceived guilt. **Cognitive Level:** Applying **Client Need:** Psychosocial Integrity **Integrated Process:** Communication and Documentation **Content Area:** Child Health **Strategy:** The core issue of the question is the ability to formulate a therapeutic response to a parent who indicates distress about not seeking help earlier for an ill child. Use nursing knowledge of therapeutic communication skills and the process of elimination to make a selection.

30 **Answer: 3 Rationale:** Finger foods are helpful in encouraging children with failure to thrive to increase food intake. The parent should be taught to encourage increased food intake, including between-meal snacks. The child does not need to eat alone; instead, mealtimes should be structured family events. Although a relaxed atmosphere is good, there can be limits on behavior during mealtimes to provide structure. **Cognitive Level:** Applying **Client Need:** Physiological Adaptation **Integrated Process:** Nursing Process: Planning **Content Area:** Child Health **Strategy:** The core issue of the question is the intervention that will help to increase food intake in a child with nonorganic failure to thrive. Use nursing knowledge and the process of elimination to make a selection.

31 **Answer: 1, 2, 4 Rationale:** Manifestations of appendicitis often begin with generalized abdominal pain. As abdominal pain progressively worsens, it tends to localize in the right lower quadrant at McBurney's point. Elevated WBC count can elevate to 15,000–20,000 cells/mm^3 because of the inflammatory response. Fatty stools are not part of the clinical picture. Indigestion is not typical, although the client may have nausea and vomiting, fever, chills, anorexia, diarrhea, or acute constipation. **Cognitive Level:** Applying **Client Need:** Physiological Adaptation **Integrated Process:** Nursing Process: Assessment **Content Area:** Child Health **Strategy:** The core issue of the question is knowledge of manifestations that are consistent with appendicitis. Use knowledge that the affected area is the large intestine to eliminate indigestion (stomach area, too vague) and fatty stools (small intestine absorption problem).

Key Terms to Review

acholic p. 1057
ascites p. 1048
asterixis p. 1049
cachexia p. 1061
cholecystitis p. 1052
cholelithiasis p. 1051
cirrhosis p. 1047
colostomy p. 1034
diarrhea p. 1062
dumping syndrome p. 1036
esophageal tamponade p. 1050
esophageal varices p. 1050
esophagogastroduodenoscopy (EGD) p. 1033
fecalith p. 1058
hematemesis p. 1050
hepatic encephalopathy p. 1050
hepatorenal syndrome p. 1051
hernia p. 1039
hyperbilirubinemia p. 1045
hypoalbuminemia p. 1050
icteric p. 1046
ileostomy p. 1035
jaundice p. 1045
lavage p. 1050
lithotripsy p. 1052
McBurney's point p. 1058
paracentesis p. 1049
portal hypertension p. 1050
sclerotherapy p. 1050
steatorrhea p. 1043
Zollinger-Ellison syndrome p. 1033

References

Ball, J., & Bindler, R., & Cowen, K. (2015). *Principles of pediatric nursing: Caring for children* (6th ed.). New York, NY: Pearson Education.

Berman, A., Snyder, S., & Frandsen, G. (2016). *Kozier & Erb's fundamentals of nursing: Concepts, process, and practice* (10th ed.). New York, NY: Pearson Education.

Ignatavicius, D., & Workman, L. (2016). *Medical-surgical nursing: Patient-centered collaborative care* (10th ed.). Philadelphia: Saunders.

Kee, J. (2017). *Pearson's handbook of laboratory and diagnostic tests* (8th ed.). New York, NY: Pearson Education.

LeMone, P., Burke, K., Bauldoff, G., & Gubrud, P. (2015). *Medical surgical nursing: Clinical reasoning in patient care* (6th ed.). Hoboken, NJ: Pearson Education.

Lewis, S., Dirksen, S., Heitkemper, M., & Bucher, L. (2014). *Medical surgical nursing: Assessment and management of clinical problems* (9th ed.). St. Louis, MO: Elsevier Science.

Smith, S., Duell, D., Martin, B., Aebersold, M., & Gonzalez, L. (2017). *Clinical nursing skills: Basic to advanced skills* (10th ed.). New York, NY: Pearson Education.

60 Endocrine and Metabolic Disorders

In this chapter

Cross Reference

Other chapters relevant to this content area are

Meeting Nutritional Needs	Chapter 25
Endocrine Medications	Chapter 41
Common Laboratory Tests	Chapter 46
Common Diagnostic Tests and Procedures	Chapter 47
Fluid and Electrolyte Imbalances	Chapter 53
Neurologic Disorders	Chapter 57

I. OVERVIEW OF ANATOMY AND PHYSIOLOGY OF ENDOCRINE SYSTEM

A. Components of endocrine system

1. Endocrine glands are anatomical structures that secrete hormones directly into bloodstream to coordinate and regulate functions of target body organs and tissues to maintain homeostasis
2. Hormones: chemical messengers that travel in circulatory system and alter cellular activities by changing enzymes and proteins in target cells
   a. **Receptor**: specially designed link on a target cell membrane or in cytoplasm for a specific hormone to contact and initiate an action response

b. Regulation of secretion: effects on target tissue act as a negative-feedback loop to signal initiating gland to slow or stop secretion

3. Secretion of hormones in endocrine glands is controlled by neuronal stimulation, chemical substances, or other hormones
4. **Hyposecretion** is a condition in which an insufficient amount of hormone is secreted
5. **Hypersecretion** is a condition in which an excessive amount of hormone is secreted

B. Major endocrine system glands (see Table 60–1)

1. Anterior pituitary gland: major role is to produce and release several different hormones, most regulate secretion of other hormones
2. Posterior pituitary gland: regulates fluid balance and facilitates childbirth and prostate gland function
   a. Releases antidiuretic hormone (ADH) and oxytocin, which are produced and stored in hypothalamus
   b. ADH stimulates kidneys to reabsorb water, decreasing urine output (UO) and supporting blood pressure (BP) and blood volume
   c. Oxytocin stimulates uterus to contract for childbirth, mammary glands for milk ejection, and smooth muscles of prostate gland to contract and eject secretions
3. Thyroid gland: determines rate of cellular metabolism and, in children, are responsible for normal development of musculoskeletal and nervous systems
   a. Thyrocalcitonin targets bone and kidney cells to regulate calcium ion concentrations in body fluids
   b. Thyroxine (T_4) and triiodothyronine (T_3) increase production of cellular ATP
4. Parathyroid glands: secrete parathyroid hormone (PTH) to increase serum calcium level
5. Pancreas (islets of Langerhans): regulates blood glucose level
   a. Glucagon (from alpha cells) breaks down stored fat and carbohydrate (CHO) to raise blood glucose
   b. Insulin (from beta cells) transports glucose across cell membranes and lowers blood glucose
   c. Somatostatin (from delta cells) inhibits production of glucagon and insulin
6. Adrenal cortex: hormones play a vital role for survival and affect metabolism of many different tissues
   a. Glucocorticoids stimulate most cells to increase rate of glucose synthesis, glycogen formation, release of fatty acids, and breakdown of fatty acids; exert an anti-inflammatory effect to suppress immune system
   b. Mineralocorticoids: aldosterone stimulates kidneys to increase reabsorption of sodium (Na^+) and water
   c. Small amount of androgens
7. Adrenal medulla: secretes catecholamines in response to physical or psychological stress to stimulate cardiovascular and respiratory systems, increase metabolism, and increase blood glucose
8. Gonads: regulate development of secondary sexual characteristics and reproduction
   a. Ovaries in females produce estrogen for follicle maturation and growth of uterine lining, and progesterone, which stimulates uterus to prepare for implantation and mammary glands for lactation
   b. Testes in males produce androgens (primarily testosterone) for maturation of sperm, and inhibin to provide negative feedback to anterior pituitary gland to stop FSH secretion

Table 60–1 Hormones Produced by Endocrine Glands

Gland		Hormone
Pituitary	Anterior lobe	Adrenocorticotropic hormone (ACTH), follicle-stimulating hormone (FSH), luteinizing hormone (LH), somatotropin or growth hormone (GH), melanocyte-stimulating hormone (MSH), prolactin (PRL), thyroid-stimulating hormone (TSH)
	Posterior lobe	Oxytocin, vasopressin or antidiuretic hormone (ADH)
Thyroid		Triiodothryonine (T_3), thyroxine (T_4), thyrocalcitonin
Parathyroid		Parathyroid hormone
Pancreas		Insulin, glucagon, somatostatin
Adrenal	Cortex	Glucocorticoids (cortisol, corticosterone, cortisone) Mineralocorticoids (aldosterone)
	Medulla	Catecholamines (norepinephrine and epinephrine)
Gonads	Testes	Androgens (primarily testosterone), inhibin
	Ovaries	Estrogen, progesterone

II. DIAGNOSTIC TESTS AND ASSESSMENTS OF ENDOCRINE SYSTEM

A. Computed tomography (CT) scan: with or without contrast; see also Chapter 47

B. Stimulation and suppression tests

1. Stimulation tests involve administering a prescribed amount of hormone to determine ability of a suspected hypofunctioning target gland to respond with increased hormone production
2. Suppression tests involve administering a prescribed amount of a substance that interferes with hormone production to determine whether it effectively interferes with hormone production in a gland suspected of hyperfunction

C. Studies of pituitary gland

1. Serum studies include GH or somatotropin, somatomedin C, GH release post-exercise, insulin-induced hypoglycemia, prolactin level, gonadotropin levels (FSH, LH), and water-deprivation test
2. Radiologic studies include skull x-ray to detect integrity of bone and bone tumors, CT scan and magnetic resonance imaging (MRI) to outline organ structure, tumors, edema, infarcts, blood flow patterns, and BV integrity

D. Studies of thyroid gland

NCLEX®

1. Serum studies include
   a. L-thyroxine (total T_4): measures both free and protein-bound thyroxine; normal is 4.5–10.9 mcg/dL in adults
   b. Free T_4 is amount of thyroxine not bound to globulins; normal values are 0.8–2.7 ng/mL by actual assay or 4.6–11.2 by calculated method
   c. Triiodothyronine (T_3) (normal value 60–181 ng/dL), also called T_3 RIA, T_3 resin uptake (T_3RU)
   d. Additional tests are TSH or thyrotropin (normal value 0.5–5.0 units/mL) and serum calcitonin
2. Radiologic studies include thyroid scan or radioactive isotope uptake study to determine uptake of radionuclide by thyroid gland, and whole-body scan to detect metastasis from a known malignant thyroid tumor

E. Studies of parathyroid glands

1. Serum studies
   a. PTH, which regulates serum Ca^{++} and phosphorus
   b. Total Ca^{++} (including free Ca^{++} and Ca^{++} bound to plasma proteins)
   c. Phosphorus: reported as phosphorus (P) or phosphate (PO_4) and 1,25 dihydroxy vitamin D
2. Radiologic studies include skeletal x-ray and CT scan

F. Studies of adrenal glands

1. Serum cortisol: secreted by adrenal cortex, a larger amount in morning, then decreasing during day
2. Serum and/or urinary aldosterone: a mineralocorticoid secreted by adrenal cortex
3. Serum ACTH stimulation to confirm suspected disease of adrenal cortex
4. Dexamethasone suppression and metyrapone suppression
5. Urinary 17-ketosteroids (17 KS): 24-hour urine is collected to measure amount of 17 KS or metabolites of steroids produced by adrenal cortex and testes

NCLEX®

6. Vanillylmandelic acid (VMA): a metabolite of catecholamines
   a. A 24-hour urine is collected in bottle containing HCL (a strong acid) obtained from lab
   b. Warn client about acid in bottle, to keep face away from opening when removing cap to add urine, and to avoid inhaling odor from bottle
   c. Instruct client to avoid exercise or exposure to stress
   d. Check with lab about specific foods to be avoided during testing period
   e. If possible, client should not take any medication for 7 days before and during testing period
   f. Record BP, height, and weight on lab slip

G. Studies of pancreas

NCLEX®

1. Fasting blood glucose (FBG) levels or fasting plasma glucose; withhold food and insulin for at least 8 hours (water is permitted); adult reference value: 70–110 mg/dL (whole blood: 60–100 mg/dL), older adults: 70–120 mg/dL
2. Oral glucose tolerance test (GTT): tests for gestational glucose intolerance; medications, infection, trauma, bedrest, and stress can alter results; see Chapter 46

NCLEX®

3. Capillary glucose monitoring
   a. Warm extremity to encourage vasodilation; select digit to be used
   b. Cleanse site with soap and water or 70% alcohol; dry with a gauze sponge
   c. Avoid squeezing site to enhance blood flow (causes dilution with tissue fluid)
   d. Avoid touching skin with reagent strip; skin oils may affect results
   e. Elevate digit and apply gentle pressure with dry sterile gauze to site until bleeding stops

NCLEX®
4. **Glycosylated hemoglobin**: prolonged **hyperglycemia** (elevated blood glucose) causes glucose to bind irreversibly to hemoglobin (Hgb) of red blood cell (RBC) for remaining life of RBC; HgbA1c determines control of blood glucose over past 3–5 weeks, generally; see Chapter 46, Table 46–3 for expected values
5. Urine studies
   a. Ketones: metabolic end-product of fatty acid metabolism; body uses fatty acids for energy when there is insufficient supply of glucose; ketones should be absent in urine (negative)
   b. Acetone: metabolite of fatty acid metabolism; should also be absent in urine

III. HYPOPITUITARISM

A. Overview

1. A disorder caused by deficiency of one or more pituitary hormones, often in anterior pituitary; may be inherited or caused by infection, pituitary gland infarction (such as in sickle-cell disease), tumor in brain, cranial irradiation, chemotherapy, brain trauma, and psychosocial deprivation
2. Deficiency leads to inadequate stimulation of target gland to produce hormone, leading to symptoms of hypofunction of target gland
3. Treatment generally involves hormone replacement for target gland
4. Common deficiency in anterior pituitary gland is growth hormone (GH) deficiency

B. Nursing assessment of GH deficiency

1. Normal weight and length at birth
2. Below third percentile on growth chart by 1 year of age; child usually grows at rate less than 5 cm (2 in.) per year
3. Infants: hypoglycemic seizures, hyponatremia, neonatal jaundice, pale optic discs, and, in males, micropenis and undescended testes

NCLEX®
4. Children: youthful facial features, high-pitched voice, delayed dentition, "ripply" abdominal fat, decreased muscle mass and skeletal maturation, delayed sexual maturation, and possible associated slipped capital femoral epiphysis
5. Diagnosed by low levels of IGF-1 (insulin-like growth factor) on screening test; radiologic studies to determine bone age (skeletal maturation) or to rule out other disorders

C. Therapeutic management of GH deficiency

1. Treatment of underlying disorder if present

NCLEX®
2. GH therapy by subcutaneous injection daily or every other day until acceptable height is reached or growth velocity drops to less than 2 cm (1 in.) per year
3. Monitor growth and document on growth chart at periodic health checkups (every 3–4 months)

D. Client and family teaching

1. Importance of optimal nutrition and adequate caloric and iron intake before and during therapy
2. Medication therapy: how to administer injections and information about course of therapy
3. Close monitoring and follow-up is important
4. Child can experience disturbed body image; use age-appropriate communication and style of dress (rather than according to body size)

IV. HYPERPITUITARISM

A. Overview: excessive secretion of GH from anterior pituitary gland that leads to gigantism (in children before long bone epiphyseal closure) or acromegaly (in adults after epiphyseal closure)

NCLEX®
B. Nursing assessment

1. Tall stature if onset in childhood
2. Large hands and feet with prominent jawbone
3. Joint changes consistent with arthritis
4. Deep voice and possible dysphagia
5. Hypertension and organomegaly
6. Skin changes leading to rough, oily texture

C. Therapeutic management

1. Assess for body image changes and provide emotional support to client and family
2. Provide measures to relieve joint pain
3. Possible radiation therapy to pituitary gland
4. Possible hypophysectomy (see next section)

D. Hypophysectomy

1. Transphenoidal hypophysectomy may be used to resect pituitary gland
2. Provide standard preoperative care

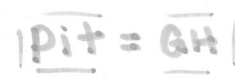

NCLEX® 3. Teach client about measures used to prevent rises in intracranial pressure (ICP) following surgery (see also Chapter 57)

NCLEX® 4. Postoperative care
   a. Monitor vital signs (VS), level of consciousness (LOC), and neurological status
   b. Keep head of bed elevated to approximately 30 degrees
   c. Assess "mustache" dressing taped under nose for drainage and test drainage for glucose to rule out cerebrospinal fluid (CSF) leakage
   d. Assess for postnasal drip, which could also indicate CSF leakage
   e. Monitor intake and output (I&O) and assess for signs of diabetes insipidus (DI; water intoxication) as temporary postoperative complication; see next section
   f. Keep oral mucous membranes moist; drying can occur because nasal packing after transphenoidal surgery can lead to mouth-breathing

5. Client teaching
   NCLEX® a. Avoid activities that raise ICP, such as bending, lifting, sneezing, coughing, blowing nose, and any activity that closes glottis (Valsalva maneuver)
   b. Medication teaching, including analgesics and possible antibiotic postoperatively, and possible hormone replacement therapy if entire gland is surgically removed

V. SYNDROME OF INAPPROPRIATE ANTIDIURETIC HORMONE (SIADH)

A. Overview

1. Excess secretion of ADH from posterior pituitary gland leading to water intoxication and hyponatremia
   a. Usual feedback mechanism does not reduce ADH secretion when there is decreased serum osmolality (indicating increased fluid)
   b. Elevated ADH leads to renal reabsorption of water and suppression of renin-angiotensin mechanism, causing renal excretion of Na^+
   c. Renal excretion of Na^+ leads to water intoxication, cellular edema, and dilutional hyponatremia
2. Causes include certain hormone-secreting malignant tumors; injury, stroke, medications, and activation of limbic system from trauma, pain, stress, and acute psychosis

B. Nursing assessment (NCLEX®)

1. General manifestations of fluid overload, possibly including increased BP, crackles auscultated in lung fields, distended jugular neck veins, taut skin, and intake greater than output
2. Clinical manifestations: headache, fatigue, anorexia, nausea, muscle aches, abdominal cramps, weight gain without edema, progressive altered LOC, seizures, coma, and small amounts of concentrated amber-colored urine
3. Diagnostic and laboratory test findings: high urine osmolality (>1200 mOsm/kg H_2O) and specific gravity (SG) higher than 1.032, low serum osmolality (<275 mOsm/kg), and decreased hematocrit, BUN, and serum Na^+ (dilutional effects)

C. Therapeutic management

NCLEX® 1. Restrict oral fluids, including ice chips, to 800 mL/day or less to prevent further hemodilution
2. Supplement Na^+ intake orally or by hypertonic saline IV infusion
NCLEX® 3. Flush all enteral and gastric tubes with normal saline instead of water to replace Na^+ and prevent further hemodilution
NCLEX® 4. Monitor I&O accurately
NCLEX® 5. Monitor for low serum Na^+ and BUN and concentrated urine
NCLEX® 6. Weigh daily; a weight gain or loss of 1 kg (2.2 lb) indicates a net change of approximately 1 L of fluid
NCLEX® 7. Assess for changes in LOC, mentation, cognition, nutrition, muscle twitching, and comfort
8. Medication therapy: IV hypertonic saline (3%) and demeclocycline; diuretics to eliminate excessive fluid

D. Client teaching

1. SIADH and symptoms to report
2. Medication may be lifelong depending on cause
3. Identify hidden sources of water and fluids, such as ice and ice cream, to prevent accidental excessive intake
   a. Plan meal pattern and maintain fluid limitation and Na^+ prescription
   b. Weigh daily on same scale and report gain of 2 pounds in 1 day

VI. DIABETES INSIPIDUS (DI)

A. Overview

1. Results from excessive loss of water caused by hyposecretion of ADH from posterior pituitary gland or kidneys' inability to respond to ADH
2. Subsequent **polyuria** (excessive UO ranging from 4 to 30 L in 24 hours) can lead to severe dehydration if client does not replace lost water
3. Causes can be neurogenic (insufficient ADH secretion by posterior pituitary gland), nephrogenic (kidneys unable to respond to ADH), and medications (lithium carbonate and demeclocycline can cause kidneys to alter response to ADH)
4. Primary DI results from an inherited or idiopathic malfunction of posterior pituitary gland
5. Secondary DI is caused by tumors, head trauma, infection, stroke, cerebral aneurysm, or surgery on or near pituitary gland

B. Nursing assessment

1. History of head injury, brain surgery, infection, or tumor
2. Obtain a list of current and past medications
3. *NCLEX®* Assess LOC, VS including orthostatic BP, skin turgor, I&O, weight, skin integrity, **polydipsia** (excessive thirst), tenting or sagging skin, bowel sounds, constipation
4. *NCLEX®* Clinical manifestations result largely from dehydration: polyuria; excessive thirst; dry, tented skin; dry mucous membranes; and severe hypotension leading to cardiovascular collapse (if severe water loss is not replaced)
5. *NCLEX®* Diagnostic and laboratory test findings: urine SG less than 1.005, urine osmolality less than 300 mOsm/kg, positive water deprivation test, reduced serum ADH (primary DI), serum sodium greater than 145 mEq/L

C. Therapeutic management

1. Water replacement orally is preferred or intravenous (IV) D_5W as needed to normalize lab values
2. For neurogenic DI, hormone replacement with desmopressin, a synthetic vasopressin; adjunctive medications, such as chlorpropamide, or carbamazepine, may increase ADH release or enhance effect of ADH on renal collecting duct
3. For nephrogenic DI, correct underlying disease or stop causative medication; begin a low-salt, low-protein diet to decrease net excretion of solute
4. *NCLEX®* Monitor I&O hourly; report UO over 200 mL/hour for 2 consecutive hours or 500 mL over 2 hours; assess for continence and provide easy access to bathroom as appropriate
5. *NCLEX®* Weigh daily; report weight loss
6. *NCLEX®* Monitor urine SG and report if it decreases; monitor serum osmolality and Na^+ for increases
7. *NCLEX®* Encourage fluid intake greater than UO; provide fluids within reach at all times; provide IV fluid replacement as ordered
8. Use skin protective barriers with incontinence

D. Client teaching

1. Information about DI, self-administration of medication, and possible need for lifelong medication
2. Wear a Medic-Alert bracelet listing DI and treatments
3. Drink fluid equal to amount of UO, keeping a log of I&O
4. Weigh self daily, on same scale at same time of day, and report weight loss
5. Consult practitioner before taking over-the-counter (OTC) medications

VII. HYPERTHYROIDISM (THYROTOXICOSIS)

A. Overview

1. **Hyperthyroidism**: excessive secretion of thyroid hormone (TH) leads to increased basal metabolic rate, weight loss, heat intolerance, and increased cardiovascular, GI, and neuromuscular function; TH affects metabolism of fats, carbohydrates (CHOs), and proteins
2. Hyperthyroidism can be caused by excess secretion of TSH from pituitary gland, autoimmune reaction (Graves' disease), thyroiditis (inflammation or viral infection of thyroid), tumor, side effects of certain drugs, and excessive dose of thyroid medication

B. Nursing assessment

1. *NCLEX®* Clinical manifestations: range from very minimal to severe depending on amount and time period of hypersecretion
   a. See Table 60–2
   b. Neck goiter and exophthalmos (bulging eyes) are characteristic in Graves' disease form of hyperthyroidism

Table 60–2 Comparison of Signs of Hyperthyroidism and Hypothyroidism

Area of Function	Hyperthyroidism	Hypothyroidism
Cardiovascular	Tachycardia, dysrhythmias, palpitations, hypertension	Bradycardia, dysrhythmias, cardiomegaly, anemia, hypotension
Gastrointestinal	Diarrhea, possible abdominal pain	Constipation
Neurological	Nervousness, insomnia, hand and eye tremors, hyperactive reflexes, emotional lability	Lethargy, somnolence, confusion, memory impairment, hypoactive reflexes, hand and foot paresthesias
Sensory	Possible blurred vision, lacrimation, photophobia, exophthalmos (in Graves' disease)	Periorbital edema
Integumentary	Flushed, moist skin and fine, thin hair	Coarse, dry skin, brittle nails, nonpitting edema, hair loss
Reproductive	Amenorrhea and decreased fertility (females), decreased libido and impotence (males)	Menorrhagia and decreased fertility (females), decreased libido (males)
General metabolic	Hyperthermia, hunger, weight loss, possible fluid volume deficit; high basal metabolic rate	Hypothermia, anorexia, weight gain, systemic edema, and low basal metabolic rate

NCLEX® 2. **Thyroid crisis** or **thyroid storm**: life-threatening emergency occurring in extreme hyperthyroidism
   a. Usually occurs with long-term untreated hyperthyroidism or in clients with hyperthyroidism experiencing a stressor such as infection, trauma, or manipulation of thyroid gland
   NCLEX® b. Common manifestations of thyroid storm are temperature over 102°F (39°C), tachycardia, systolic hypertension, abdominal pain, nausea and vomiting (N/V), diarrhea, agitation, tremors, confusion, and possible seizures
3. Diagnostic and laboratory test findings: elevated serum T_3, T_4, free T_4; decreased TSH; positive RAI uptake scan and thyroid scan depending on cause

C. Therapeutic management

1. Consists of medical treatment or surgical removal of part of thyroid gland (partial or total thyroidectomy)

NCLEX® 2. Ethionamide drugs for life to reduce secretion of thyroid hormone

NCLEX® 3. Ablative therapy with radioactive Iodine 131: thyroid gland absorbs I-131, which destroys some thyroid cells over a period of 6–8 weeks

4. Total or subtotal (partial) thyroidectomy may be indicated based on situation

NCLEX® 5. Nursing care for nonsurgical clients
   a. Keep environment cool and free of distractions and stress as able
   b. Encourage balance of rest with activity periods
   c. With exophthalmos, monitor visual acuity, photophobia, corneal integrity, and ability to close eyes; encourage eye protection measures such as tinted glasses, eye shields, cool moist compresses for irritation, and artificial tears to reduce dryness as needed
   d. Assist nutritional state by weighing client daily; provide diet high in CHOs, protein, and between-meal snacks (variation: six smaller meals may be better than three larger ones); monitor nutritional state with labs such as serum prealbumin, albumin, transferrin, and total lymphocyte count
   e. Assist client to cope with body-image changes with goiter and exophthalmos

NCLEX® 6. Preoperative preparation for thyroidectomy
   a. Teach client about standard postoperative care including pain management and pulmonary hygiene
   b. Instruct client to hold hands behind neck when coughing, sitting, turning, or getting up/back to bed to reduce postoperative pain and neck muscle strain
   c. Instruct client how to self-administer prescribed antithyroid drugs to decrease vascularity and size of thyroid and minimize risk of surgical hemorrhage

7. Postoperative care following thyroidectomy
   NCLEX® a. Provide comfort: analgesics, semi-Fowler position with neck and head supported by pillows to prevent muscle strain, ice collar to wound area for comfort and to prevent edema
   NCLEX® b. Monitor for hemorrhage: tightness of dressing; sanguineous exudate on anterior or posterior neck dressing or on skin of neck, upper chest and upper back, shoulders, and back of neck; auscultate trachea for stridor (indicating edema and narrowed airway); first 24 hours postoperative is time of greatest risk
   NCLEX® c. Promote patent airway: elevate head of bed 30 degrees; assess for respiratory distress; keep oral and sterile suction supplies and emergency tracheostomy tray (with tracheostomy kit and IV calcium gluconate or calcium chloride) within immediate access; maintain humidification of inspired air

if prescribed; encourage deep-breathing exercises and incentive spirometer hourly; cough only if needed to clear secretions

NCLEX®
d. Prevent tetany by early identification of hypocalcemia (serum calcium less than 8 mg/dL) evidenced by numbness or tingling of toes, extremities, and lips; muscle twitches; positive Chvostek and Trousseau signs; see also Chapter 53
e. Maintain patent IV site
f. Assess for laryngeal nerve damage, noting ability to speak loudly, quality and tone of voice (hoarseness may be temporary after surgery)
g. Analgesics to control surgical pain

D. Client teaching

1. Correct self-administration of lifelong medications with medical treatment
2. Hyperthyroidism, hypothyroidism, and symptoms to report; clients with underlying heart disease could experience chest pain and decreased cardiac output from increased workload
3. Postoperative conditions to report, including signs of hemorrhage, hypocalcemia, incisional infection, respiratory difficulty and discomfort

NCLEX®
4. For exophthalmos, use methods to protect eyes and adapt to altered visual field
   a. Have regular eye exams
   b. Call healthcare provider immediately for any change in vision, appearance of eye, eyelid closure, eye pain or exudate, or **photophobia** (sensitivity to light)
   c. Protect eyes with tinted glasses or eye shields because lids do not cover eyes completely and corneal/blink reflex may be delayed
   d. Moisten eyes frequently with artificial tears to prevent dry irritation and corneal infection; use caution not to contaminate eyedropper
   e. Soothe dry-eye irritation with cool, moist compresses
   f. Sleep with head of bed elevated to minimize pressure on optic nerve, and wear eye patches to protect eyes during sleep if lids do not close
5. Surgical client
   a. Surgical procedure and expected outcomes

NCLEX®
   b. Support neck with hands; position neck and head with pillows and maintain semi-Fowler position; avoid hyperextension and sudden, quick movements of head and neck
   c. Wound care

NCLEX®
   d. Avoid/minimize talking and coughing until wound is healed to prevent strain on laryngeal nerve and vocal cords
6. Assist client to cope with lifestyle and self-image changes

VIII. HYPOTHYROIDISM

A. Overview

1. Insufficient secretion of TH, causing decreased metabolic rate and heat production and various effects on body systems
2. Primary hypothyroidism accounts for 99% of all cases, and other causes are thyroiditis, subacute postpartum, external irradiation of gland, iatrogenic, infections, iodine deficiency, congenital, or idiopathic
3. Secondary hypothyroidism, also called central hypothyroidism, is caused by insufficient secretion of TSH from pituitary gland or related to disease of hypothalamus
4. Thyroid gland gradually enlarges, forming a goiter (thickening of gland) in an attempt to secrete more thyroid hormone

NCLEX®
B. Nursing assessment

1. See Table 60–2 again for common manifestations
2. Myxedema (a life-threatening crisis state of hypothyroidism): nonpitting edema in connective tissues throughout body, puffy face and tongue, severe metabolic disorders, hypothermia, cardiovascular collapse, and coma
3. Diagnostic and laboratory test findings: varies according to whether cause is thyroid gland or pituitary; may include decreased T_4 and free T_4, normal T_3, and increased TSH levels; elevated serum lipids

NCLEX®
C. Therapeutic management

1. Medication therapy: thyroid hormone replacement, such as dessicated thyroid, thyroxine, or triiodothyronine
2. Give medication in morning 1 hour before food intake or 2 hours after food intake to facilitate absorption

3. Adjust environmental temperature and use blankets as needed for warmth; chilling increases metabolic rate, cardiac workload, and O_2 demand
4. Pace activities with rest periods; instruct client to report shortness of breath, fatigue, dizziness, or any discomfort
5. Encourage intake of 2000 mL water daily and a high-fiber diet to promote regular bowel movements

D. Client teaching

1. Disorder and its management; report symptoms of hypo- and hyperthyroidism
2. Importance of wearing a Medic-Alert bracelet
3. *NCLEX®* Medication is needed for life and should be taken at same time every morning, 1 hour before a meal or 2 hours after a meal
4. Take same brand of medication because brands vary in bioavailability
5. *NCLEX®* Report weight gain or loss of 2.3 kg (5 lb), activity intolerance, chest pain, heat or cold intolerance, and sleep-pattern disturbance

IX. HYPERPARATHYROIDISM

A. Overview

1. Results from increased PTH secretion from parathyroid gland
2. Increased Ca^{++} reabsorption and increased phosphate excretion lead to hypercalcemia and hypophosphatemia
3. Kidneys increase bicarbonate excretion and decrease acid excretion, leading to metabolic acidosis and hypokalemia
4. Bones increase rate of Ca^{++} and phosphorus release, leading to bone decalcification
5. Hypercalcemia results in Ca^{++} deposits in soft tissues, renal calculi, altered neurological function with muscle weakness and atrophy, altered GI function with constipation, abdominal pain, and anorexia

B. Nursing assessment

1. Polyuria (early sign) and renal calculi
2. Anorexia, constipation, abdominal pain, peptic ulcer disease (from hypercalcemia)
3. Generalized bone pain, pathologic fractures, and muscle weakness and atrophy
4. *NCLEX®* CNS signs (depressed deep-tendon reflexes, **paresthesias** [altered sensations], depression, psychosis)
5. Elevated serum Ca^{++} and PTH; decreased phosphate
6. Possible bone changes on skeletal x-rays and CT scan

C. Therapeutic management

1. *NCLEX®* Decrease serum Ca^{++} level with IV normal saline (NS) infusions, diuretics, and phosphate replacement
2. Possible surgery to remove involved parathyroid glands
3. Promote comfort and safety; client may need to use walker to prevent falls
4. Strain all urine to detect calcium-based urinary stones
5. *NCLEX®* Provide 2000–3000 mL of fluids daily as tolerated and a high-fiber diet
6. Encourage progressive activity as tolerated, pacing activity with rest periods
7. Promote nutrition and fluid and electrolyte balance; weigh daily
8. *NCLEX®* Assess for hypocalcemia to prevent tetany caused by surgery (removal of parathyroid gland) or aggressive excretion of Ca^{++}
   a. Numbness and tingling around mouth and fingertips
   b. Muscle twitching of extremities
   c. Change in voice
   d. Positive Chvostek sign (spasm of facial muscles when cheek touched) and Trousseau sign (spasm of hand when BP cuff inflated)
9. Medication therapy: analgesics to control pain; diuretics and NS by IV infusion to excrete excess calcium; phosphate and calcitonin may be used to inhibit bone reabsorption

D. Client teaching

1. Hyperparathyroidism and appropriate self-administration of medications
2. Symptoms to report, including those indicating hypocalcemia, activity intolerance, and infection

X. HYPOPARATHYROIDISM

A. Overview

1. Low PTH levels causing hypocalcemia, usually caused by surgical removal of all or part of gland
2. Hypocalcemia raises threshold for excitability in nerve and muscle fibers, causing fibers to be easily stimulated; could lead to life-threatening tetany

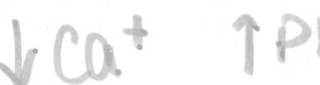

B. Nursing assessment

1. GI symptoms: abdominal pain, N/V, diarrhea, anorexia
2. *NCLEX®* Signs of hypocalcemia (anxiety, headaches, paresthesias [hands, feet, lips], neuromuscular irritability with tremors, muscle spasms, and hyperactive reflexes); positive Chvostek or Trousseau sign
3. *NCLEX®* Possible difficulty swallowing or hoarse voice, sensation of tightness in throat
4. Dry, thin hair, patchy hair loss, ridged fingernails
5. Psychosis, mood disorders (anxiety, irritability, depression)
6. Decreased serum PTH, total calcium, free calcium; increased serum phosphate

C. Therapeutic management

1. *NCLEX®* Supplemental Ca^{++} and vitamin D
2. *NCLEX®* Promote comfort and safety; client may need to use walker to prevent falls
3. Encourage progressive activity as tolerated, pacing activity with rest periods
4. Promote nutrition and fluid and electrolyte balance
5. Medication therapy: Ca^{++} supplement orally or by IV infusion; vitamin D orally to promote intestinal absorption of Ca^{++}

D. Client teaching

1. Disorder and its management, to wear Medic-Alert bracelet listing disease and medications, and self-administration of medication
2. Symptoms to report (see again nursing assessment)
3. *NCLEX®* Diet high in Ca^{++} and vitamin D, identifying minimum daily intake; foods high in calcium are cheese, milk, turnip greens, almonds, collard greens, beans, peanuts, frankfurters, and bologna

XI. CUSHING'S DISEASE

A. Overview

1. Hyperfunction of adrenal cortex (AC), leading to elevated serum glucocorticoids
2. Elevated serum cortisol causes life-threatening changes in physiological, psychological, and metabolic functioning
3. Primary Cushing's disease is caused by a tumor of adrenal cortex, while secondary type is caused by excess production of ACTH

B. Nursing assessment

1. *NCLEX®* See Table 60–3
2. Elevated serum cortisol, Na^{+}, and glucose, and lowered Ca^{++} and potassium (K^{+})
3. Serum ACTH can be elevated or decreased; positive ACTH suppression test
4. Elevated urine 17 KS; normal BUN

C. Therapeutic management

1. Possible radiation therapy to pituitary gland
2. *NCLEX®* Single or bilateral adrenalectomy or hypophysectomy (removal of pituitary gland)
3. Assist client to achieve fluid, electrolyte, glucose, and calcium balance
4. Analyze daily weights and I&O
5. *NCLEX®* Promote safety: uncluttered walking area, adequate lighting, assistive walking devices to prevent falls as needed, and use of stable, nonskid shoes or slippers

Table 60–3 Comparison of Signs of Adrenal Cortex Hyperfunction and Hypofunction

Area of Function	Cushing's Disease (Hyperfunction)	Addison's Disease (Hypofunction)
Fluid balance	Overhydration, hypervolemia, and weight gain	Dehydration, hypovolemia, and weight loss
Electrolytes	Hypernatremia, hypokalemia	Hyponatremia, hyperkalemia
Cardiovascular	Hypertension and possible signs of CHF (from overhydration)	Postural hypotension (from dehydration), tachycardia, dysrhythmias
Integumentary	Thin skin that bruises easily, striae, hirsutism, poor wound healing	Excess melatonin-stimulating hormone, with skin pigmentation (eternal tan), delayed wound healing
Miscellaneous	Hyperglycemia, osteoporosis, emotional lability, abnormal fat deposits (truncal obesity, moon facies, fat pad on back of neck) generalized weakness with muscle wasting, possible amenorrhea, impotence, or decreased libido, susceptibility to infection	Hypoglycemia, anorexia, nausea, vomiting, diarrhea, depression, lethargy, emotional lability, confusion, muscle weakness, muscle and joint pain

6. Assist client to pace activities and rest to prevent fatigue

NCLEX® 7. Prevent infection before and after surgery: use standard precautions, provide aseptic wound care, and promote optimal nutrition
8. Assist client to use effective coping strategies and encourage client to discuss feelings about change in physical appearance
9. Preoperative care: ensure that client understands planned surgical procedure, postoperative routines, and expected outcomes
10. Postoperative care
    - NCLEX® a. Promote effective respirations with hourly coughing and deep-breathing exercises (clients with pituitary removal should avoid coughing)
    - b. Assist with repositioning every 2 hours, and encourage ankle dorsiflexion exercises hourly
    - c. Promote wound healing by minimizing stress on incision line
    - NCLEX® d. After adrenalectomy, client should logroll to side to sit up at bedside and should do the reverse to recline
    - NCLEX® e. Follow principles of postoperative care discussed previously if client underwent removal of pituitary gland
    - f. Elevate head of bed 30 degrees, and use aseptic technique for wound care

NCLEX® 11. Prevent Addisonian crisis: give NS by IV infusion bolus and cortisol per practitioner's order for these symptoms: dry, tenting skin; decreased BP; increased pulse; decreased LOC; anorexia; and weakness
12. Medication therapy: may include metapyrone (directly inhibits cortisol production and secretion by adrenal cortex); octreotide (suppresses ACTH secretion) or mitotane (suppresses function of AC and decreases corticosteroid metabolism, thus decreasing serum cortisol)

D. Client teaching

1. Management of Cushing's disease including medication therapy
2. To wear Medic-Alert bracelet listing disease and medications

NCLEX® 3. Eat a diet high in protein and vitamins B and C to support immune system, and also take supplemental K^+ and Ca^{++}

NCLEX® 4. Wound care and postoperative cortisol replacement for surgical clients (temporary replacement for 1 year or less for unilateral adrenalectomy; lifelong if surgery is bilateral)

XII. ADRENAL INSUFFICIENCY (ADDISON'S DISEASE)

A. Overview

1. Insufficient cortisol level resulting from autoimmune disorder, tuberculosis, septicemia, acquired immunodeficiency syndrome (AIDS), bilateral adrenalectomy, infiltrative diseases, and sudden cessation of long-term high-dose steroid medication
2. Decreased aldosterone and cortisol levels lead to hyponatremia, hyperkalemia, decreased extracellular fluid and intravascular volume, decreased gluconeogenesis, hypoglycemia, and stress intolerance
3. High ACTH level leads to hyperpigmentation

NCLEX® **B. Nursing assessment**

1. See again Table 60–3

NCLEX® 2. Addisonian crisis: a life-threatening response to sudden withdrawal of steroids or exposure to any form of stress, manifested by headache, weakness, confusion, pain (abdomen, back, legs), severe hypotension, circulatory collapse, shock, and coma
3. Decreased serum cortisol, glucose, Na^+, and urine 17 KS
4. Increased serum K^+, BUN, and ACTH levels
5. No increase in cortisol with ACTH stimulation test
6. CT scan can be positive

C. Therapeutic management

NCLEX® 1. Maintain fluid and electrolyte balance: analyze lab values, I&O, and daily weight; encourage 3000 mL of daily oral fluid intake and added Na^+ in diet

NCLEX® 2. Promote safety: appropriate walking assistive devices, adequate lighting, clear area for walking, and appropriate slippers or shoes
3. Medication therapy: hydrocortisone to replace cortisol; fludrocortisone to replace mineralocorticoids as needed

4. For addisonian crisis, monitor VS carefully and neurologic status, provide IV fluids and IV hydrocortisone, and maintain client on bedrest, then resume ongoing care for Addison's disease once crisis resolves

D. Client education

1. Addison's disease and symptoms to report (weight gain, easy bruising or bleeding, weakness, dizziness, lethargy, epigastric discomfort, and change in BP or pulse)
2. Need for lifelong medication and disease management (*NCLEX®*)
3. Need to consult practitioner before taking any OTC medications
4. Self-administration of medication and plan for medication adjustment upward during times of stress
5. Wear Medic-Alert bracelet listing Addison's disease, medications, and contact numbers
6. Diet to promote immune system function and foods high in Na^+ and low in K^+ (see also Chapter 53)

XIII. DIABETES MELLITUS (DM)

A. Overview

1. A group of chronic disorders of endocrine pancreas characterized by hyperglycemia, relative or lack of insulin secretion, or cellular resistance to actions of insulin
2. Type 1: results from autoimmune destruction of beta cells; has a genetic predisposition; can occur at any age but usually occurs in children and adolescents; also characterized by hyperglycemia and **ketosis** (ketones in blood resulting from gluconeogenesis from fats)
3. Type 2: results from compromised ability of beta cells to respond to hyperglycemia, abnormal insulin receptors on cells, and peripheral insulin resistance; has a genetic predisposition, can occur at any age, and is more common in obese clients, older adults, African Americans, and Native Americans
4. Acute complications include hypoglycemia, diabetic ketoacidosis, and hyperglycemic hyperosmolar nonketotic (HHNK) coma, also called hyperosmolar coma (HOC) in type 2
5. Long-term or chronic complications (see Table 60–4)

NCLEX® **B. Nursing assessment**

1. Type 1: polyuria, polydipsia (excess fluid intake, usually from thirst), **polyphagia** (increased food intake), weight loss, malaise, and fatigue
2. Type 2: polyuria, polydipsia, blurred vision, fatigue, paresthesia (numbness, tingling, sensitivity), and skin infections
3. Elevated random and/or fasting blood glucose (BG)
4. Abnormal oral glucose tolerance test; elevated glycosylated hemoglobin (HgbA1c)
5. Glucosuria once renal threshold for glucose is exceeded (often about 180 mg/dL)
6. Positive serum ketones and possible urine ketones or acetone with ketoacidosis
7. Metabolic syndrome (central obesity, hypertension, abnormal lipid panel, FBG greater than 100 mg/dL, and hyperinsulinemia) is a risk factor for developing type 2 DM

C. Therapeutic management

1. Diet (*NCLEX®*)
   a. Follow diet recommended in MyPlate or exchange system diet from American Diabetes Association
   b. Caloric intake is based on individual needs, including activity level, other health problems, and possible weight loss needs for type 2 DM

Table 60–4 Chronic Effects or Complications of Diabetes Mellitus

Body System	Chronic Effect
Neurologic	Somatic neuropathies (paresthesias, pain, and loss of sensation and motor control) and visceral neuropathies (pupil constriction, fixed heart rate, constipation or diarrhea, dysfunction of sweat glands, incomplete voiding, and sexual dysfunction)
Sensory	Cataracts, glaucoma, and diabetic retinopathy
Cardiovascular	Orthostatic hypotension, accelerated atherosclerosis leading to stroke, myocardial infarction (MI), and peripheral vascular disease (PVD), increased blood viscosity, and platelet disorders
Renal	Hypertension, edema, albuminuria, and chronic renal failure
Integumentary	Atrophic changes, foot ulcers or gangrene
Immune	Poor healing, periodontal disease, lung infections, chronic skin infections, urinary tract infections, vaginitis

c. CHO in amounts tailored to individual need, avoiding simple sugars
d. Protein at 10–20% of caloric intake
e. Saturated fat less than 10% of calories with cholesterol intake equal to or less than 300 mg/day
f. Sodium intake 2000 mg/day (lower if client has hypertension)
g. Dietary fiber 20–35 g/day
h. Tailor diet to individual and cultural preferences as possible to improve adherence

NCLEX®
2. Oral antidiabetic medications
a. Used in type 2 DM only and indicated when diet and exercise alone fail to control BG levels
b. Consist of oral sulfonylureas, alpha-glucosidase inhibitors, meglitinides, thiazolidinediones, a biguanide, and combination agents; see also Chapter 41
c. Instruct clients taking oral sulfonylureas that concurrent use of alcohol can cause a disulfiram-type reaction (hypoglycemia, flushing, headache, nausea, and abdominal cramps)
d. Instruct client about risk of metabolic acidosis and to discuss with primary care provider about need to discontinue medicine if severe diarrhea, infection, or dehydration occur
e. Instruct all clients about manifestations of both hyperglycemia and hypoglycemia and appropriate corrective actions

NCLEX®
3. Insulin therapy
a. Used in type 1 DM or when diet, exercise, and oral agents are insufficient to control type 2 DM
b. Different insulin preparations are available to maintain near-normal blood glucose levels; insulin is classified according to source, onset, peak, and duration of action
c. Source: human insulin has a faster onset of action, a shorter peak, and a shorter duration than animal-derived insulin; preferred to pork or beef insulin (higher incidence of allergic reaction)
d. Preparations: include rapid-acting (e.g., Insulin lispro, aspart, and glulisine), short-acting (e.g., regular) intermediate-acting (e.g., isophane suspension, NPH), long-acting (e.g., zinc extended, detemir, glargine), mixtures of NPH and regular, and buffered insulin (for external insulin pumps)
e. Insulin preparations can be combined to mimic pancreatic response to variations in BG levels; for example, rapid- and short-acting insulins are usually given to cover mealtimes, while intermediate- and long-acting insulins maintain basal insulin requirements between meals
f. Insulin regimens combine short-acting, intermediate-acting, and long-acting preparations to maintain target BG levels
g. Only regular insulin may be given IV; insulin preparations are usually given via subcutaneous (subcut) route; a continuous subcut insulin infusion (insulin pump) is also available to deliver a basal rate of insulin and allow for additional bolus doses based on requirements (e.g., before a meal)

4. Encourage an exercise plan that meets needs of growing child or enhances fitness and euglycemia in adult

NCLEX®
5. Promote safety: use appropriate lighting; have client wear protective slippers, socks, and shoes that do not rub or impinge on skin; analyze symptoms, activity tolerance, and coping effectiveness; monitor BG levels; give medication and appropriate food and fluids

NCLEX®
6. Prevent infection through appropriate foot care, aseptic injection technique, and fingerstick glucose monitoring technique
7. Identify appropriate glucose-monitoring protocol and medication administration process depending on client's vision, finances, finger dexterity, living environment, resources, literacy, lifestyle, personal values, work/school environment, and coping status
8. Coordinate continuing care as appropriate for client's school, work, and other schedules, such as health club
9. Promote acceptance and effective coping while living with DM

NCLEX®
10. Promote safety: explain early identification of hypoglycemia; check BG as scheduled; treat hypoglycemia with 15-gram CHO snack, such as 8 oz skim milk, 5 Lifesaver candies, 3 large marshmallows, 6 oz juice; and need to recheck BG after treatment of hypoglycemia

NCLEX®
11. Maintain hydration and avoid hyperglycemia; develop sick-day protocol and exercise protocol with client
12. See Table 60–5 for suggestions on promoting age-appropriate self-care for children with type 1 DM

D. Client teaching

1. Type of DM, symptoms to report, self-administration of medication, fingerstick glucose monitoring, plan for regular exam by practitioner, need to wear Medic-Alert bracelet indicating DM and medication prescription, need for lifelong medication management and lifestyle adjustments

Table 60–5 Developmental Care for Child with Type 1 Diabetes Mellitus

Infants and Toddlers	Preschoolers	School-Age	Teen
Allow toddler to make choices in food selection while monitoring CHO levels Toddler may wish to help with fingerstick by cleaning his or her finger Monitor temper tantrums as a possible sign of hypoglycemia	Allow preschooler to make food choices while monitoring CHO levels Be prepared to substitute snacks at birthday parties and at daycare Encourage guided independence during blood glucose/fingerstick procedure Have appropriate snacks available if needed during sports that require a high energy expenditure	Encourage independence of school-age child in food selection, glucose monitoring, and insulin injections; assess level of knowledge Ensure that school personnel are available and knowledgeable if hypoglycemia should occur during school hours Encourage exercise but have snacks available for child Discourage fast-food or snack-machine selections	Assess teen's body image and sense of identity; assess adherence to other tasks Encourage independence with food selection, blood glucose monitoring, and insulin injections Supervise diabetic tasks if teen is nonadherent to plan Discuss future plans with teen Include diabetic issues, but promote a normal lifestyle

NCLEX®

2. Foot care: keep feet clean and dry; inspect feet daily using mirror to see soles; protect feet by wearing shoes (allow 1.25–1.9 cm [½–¾ in.] toe room) or slippers at all times; avoid snug-fitting socks or stockings; use cotton socks because they wick perspiration away from skin

NCLEX®

3. Sick-day management: maintain food and fluid intake, continue to take insulin; BG monitoring (up to q4h; report >250 mg/dL); monitor urine for ketones
4. Diet plan, including considerations for traveling, sports, attendance at parties, and other alterations in daily routine

NCLEX®

5. Provide these instructions to clients receiving insulin
   a. Storage: store insulin in use at room temperature, away from direct sunlight, and replace after 4 weeks; administration of cold insulin causes subcutaneous atrophy (lipoatrophy) or hypertrophy (lipodystrophy), which alters insulin absorption; store extra vials of insulin not being used in refrigerator
   b. Preparation: note date of expiration; discard vial and use new one if regular insulin appears cloudy; do not shake—may inactivate insulin and/or form bubbles that lead to dosage errors; roll nonregular insulin gently between hands to evenly disperse suspended particles; draw regular (clear) insulin first when mixing it with other types of insulin; only mix insulins of same concentration (e.g., U100 regular and U100 NPH) and from same source
   c. Injection: rotate injection sites to prevent lipoatrophy and lipodystrophy; do not inject insulin in an area that will be involved in exercise, as it will increase rate of absorption, onset, and peak action
   d. Monitor for signs of hypoglycemia; have candy or foods with simple carbohydrates available; if unable to swallow safely because of decreasing level of consciousness, glucagon needs to be administered subcut
   e. Avoid alcohol while taking insulin because it lowers BG levels and can cause hypoglycemia

NCLEX®

6. Teach signs of hypoglycemia (restlessness, irritability, weakness, hunger, nausea, pale diaphoretic skin, shakiness or trembling, headache, confusion, inability to concentrate, deteriorating LOC to coma, seizures), actions to take, causes of hypoglycemia, and methods for prevention
7. Instruct how to prevent and manage acute complications of DM (hyperglycemia, hypoglycemia, diabetic ketoacidosis, and HHNK; and chronic complications of DM (diabetic retinopathy, nephropathy, and neuropathy); see Table 60–6 for comparison of hypoglycemia and hyperglycemia with ketoacidosis

NCLEX®

8. Develop with client a plan for wellness, including exercise
   a. Daily cardiovascular exercise decreases risk for insulin resistance, reduces risk for complications, and improves glucose management
   b. Check BG before exercise; check for urine ketones if fasting BG is 250 mg/dL; call practitioner if ketones are present and avoid exercise
   c. Monitor for signs of hypoglycemia for up to 24 hours after extensive exercise

Table 60–6 Comparison of Hypoglycemia and Hyperglycemia with Ketoacidosis

	Hypoglycemia	Hyperglycemia with Ketoacidosis
Causes	Too much insulin; inadequate intake or missed meals; strenuous exercise without increased intake	Insufficient insulin; infection or other illness may contribute to its development
Symptoms	1. Blood glucose (BG) level drops below normal 2. Diaphoresis, tremors, hunger, weakness, pallor, dizziness, somnolence, coma, seizures, death	1. BG >250 mg/dL 2. Blood pH <7.2; HCO_3^- <15 mEq/L 3. Glycosuria, ketonuria, ↑ serum K^+ and chloride; ↓ serum Na^+, Ca^{++}, Mg^{++}, and phosphate (PO_4^-) 4. Kussmaul respirations, acetone breath, dehydration, weight loss, tachycardia, flushed facial skin, hypotension, decreased LOC, death 5. Reports of stomach ache or chest pain are common; vomiting may occur
Treatment	Depends on severity of symptoms but involves replacement of glucose Mild or moderate: juice or milk, graham crackers, glucose tablets or gel Severe: glucose paste; family may be taught to administer glucagon subcut	Normal saline is given IV until BG ↓ to 250–300 mg/dL; then is changed to 5% dextrose in 0.45% NaCl to avoid rebound hypoglycemia Potassium levels are monitored; initial hyperkalemia may become hypokalemia following fluid and insulin therapy

XIV. DIABETIC KETOACIDOSIS (DKA)

A. Overview

1. Life-threatening metabolic acidosis resulting from persistent hyperglycemia and breakdown of fats into glucose, leading to presence of ketones in blood
2. Can be triggered by emotional stress, uncompensated exercise, infection, trauma, or insufficient or delayed insulin administration
3. Hyperglycemia causes uncompensated polyuria, hemoconcentration, dehydration, hyperosmolarity, and electrolyte imbalance; a significant accumulation of serum ketones leads to acidosis (see Figure 60–1)

NCLEX®

B. Nursing assessment

1. Thirst accompanied by polyuria
2. Nausea and vomiting
3. Malaise and lethargy
4. Warm, dry skin, flushed face
5. Acetone (fruity) odor to breath, Kussmaul respirations (deep, nonlabored, rapid respirations)
6. Serum glucose above 250 mg/dL; plasma pH under 7.35; plasma bicarbonate (HCO_3^-) under 15 mEq/L; positive serum ketones; urine positive for glucose and ketones; possible abnormal serum sodium and chloride levels and hyperkalemia

NCLEX®

C. Therapeutic management

1. Consists of IV fluids (to restore circulating volume and maintain organ perfusion), electrolytes, and regular insulin (to correct hyperglycemia); supportive care as indicated such as NPO status, vasopressors, and respiratory support
2. Insulin
   a. A bolus of IV regular insulin is given followed by a continuous IV drip (0.1 unit/kg body weight) until BG level drops to 250 mg/dL or pH is 7.30
   b. Once this blood level is reached, regular insulin is given on a sliding scale per BG results
   c. Bedside BG monitoring is done every 1–2 hours to evaluate effectiveness of therapy
3. Fluid therapy is needed for excessive dehydration that accompanies DKA
   a. As much as 1–2 L normal saline solution may be given during first hour, then IV rate is decreased to 500 mL/hr as tolerated by cardiac and respiratory systems

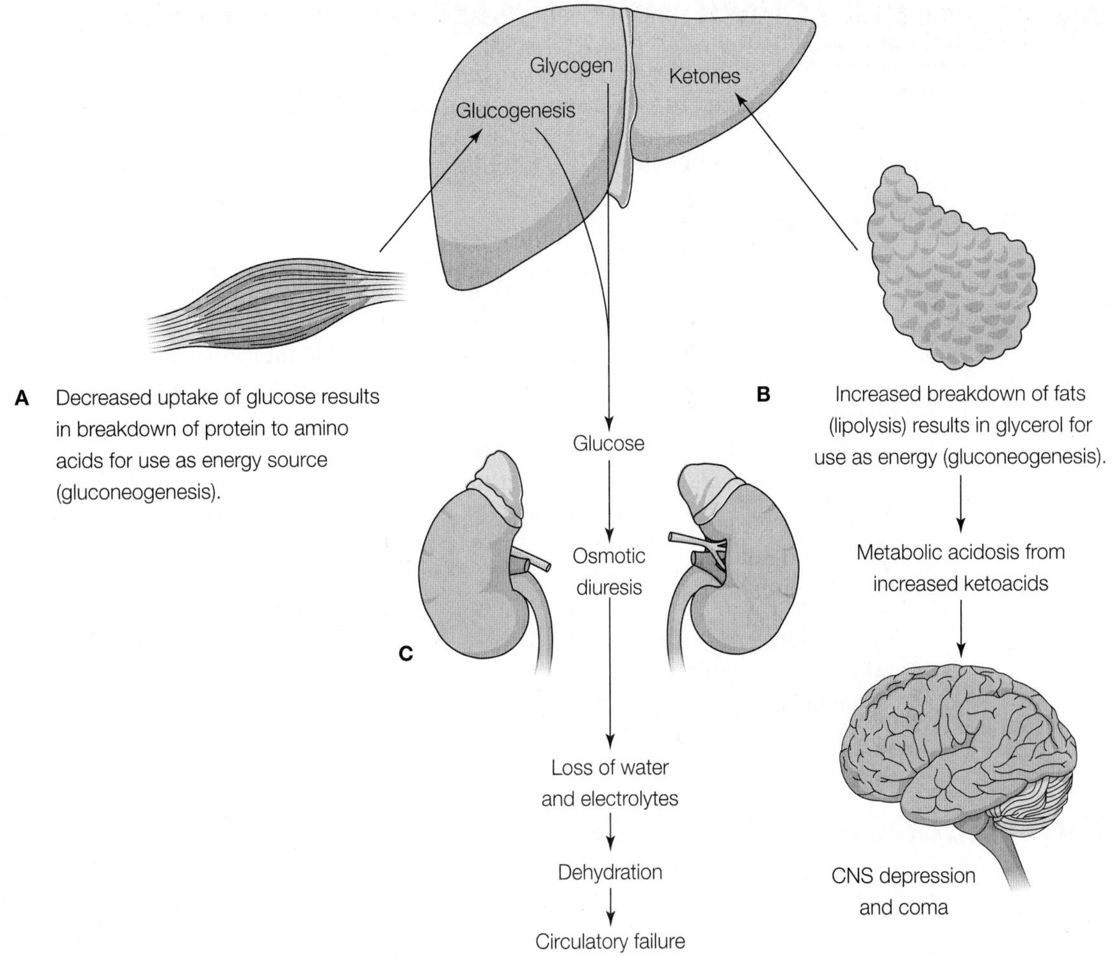

Figure 60–1 Effects of DKA.

b. When BG reaches 250–300 mg/dL, a 5% glucose solution (such as D_5½NS) is added to prevent rebound hypoglycemia and cerebral edema
c. Central venous pressure or hemodynamic monitoring may be needed to evaluate effectiveness of therapy

4. Potassium replacement is generally necessary in DKA
   a. The initial serum (K^+) level is usually elevated
   b. With reversal of acidosis and administration of insulin, K^+ shifts into cells and serum level can drop rapidly
   c. Institute replacement therapy based on serum K^+ level and urine output
   d. Institute cardiac monitoring to detect cardiac changes due to hyper- and hypokalemia and to monitor effects of therapy on serum K^+ level
   e. Replace other electrolytes such as phosphate based on laboratory results; bicarbonate is not given routinely in DKA because rapid correction of acidosis can cause severe hypokalemia
5. Analyze I&O, BG, urine ketones, VS, oxygenation, and breathing pattern
6. Maintain skin integrity; promote healing of impaired skin; prevent infection by repositioning client every 2 hours; provide pressure relief as indicated; manage incontinence and perspiration with skin protective barriers and cleansing; provide appropriate nutrition and oxygen support
7. Promote safety by analyzing VS, client communication, LOC and emotional response, and activity tolerance; implement measures to prevent falls
8. Assist client to verbalize concerns and cope effectively with illness and fears
9. Assist client to update Medic-Alert bracelet information as appropriate

D. **Client education:** nature and causes of DKA (excess glucose intake, insufficient medications, physiological and/or psychological stressors) and any new medications

XV. HYPERGLYCEMIC HYPEROSMOLAR NONKETOTIC SYNDROME (HHNS)

A. Overview

1. Life-threatening hyperglycemia that usually occurs with type 2 DM and triggered by stressors such as medications, infection, acute illness, invasive procedure, or chronic illness
2. A key feature is that sufficient insulin is produced to prevent ketosis or acidosis

NCLEX®

B. Nursing assessment

1. Symptoms gradually occur over 24 hours to 2 weeks
2. Decreased LOC, dry mucous membranes, polydipsia, hyperthermia, impaired sensory and motor function, positive Babinski sign, and seizures
3. Elevated serum Na^+, serum osmolality greater than 340 mOsm/L, serum glucose greater than 600 mg/dL, abnormal serum K^+ and chloride, no serum ketones, and normal serum pH

NCLEX®

C. Therapeutic management

1. Treatment is similar to that used for DKA
2. Determine and treat triggering situation; treat coexisting health deviations
3. Provide IV infusion of NS to replace fluids and Na^+, regular insulin IV until BG drops to 250 mg/dL, and K^+ to replace losses and shifts
4. Monitor I&O, weight, VS, lab values, sensory function, and cognitive function
5. Prevent aspiration by using appropriate feeding precautions, elevate head of bed (HOB) 15–30 degrees during and after feeding for 1 hour; if BP is too unstable to elevate HOB with feeding, then withhold oral feedings

D. Client teaching: HHNS symptoms to report, prevention of triggers, and administration of new or ongoing medications

XVI. PRECOCIOUS PUBERTY

A. Overview

1. A condition characterized by early onset of puberty, usually before age 8 in girls (with breast development or pubic hair) and before age 9 in boys (with pubic hair or genital development)
2. Accompanied by advanced growth rate and bone maturation, causing child to be tall for age, but early fusion of epiphyseal plates leads to eventual short stature as an adult
3. Causes include external sources of hormones (anabolic steroids or estrogen), early activation of hypothalamus to secrete gonadotropin-releasing hormone (GnRH), benign hypothalamic tumors, tumor of pituitary or adrenal gland or ovary

B. Nursing assessment

1. Signs of precocious puberty in females include breast development, pubic hair, axillary hair, and onset of menarche
2. Signs of precocious puberty in males include testicular enlargement, pubic hair, penile enlargement, axillary and chest hair, facial hair, and deepening voice
3. GnRH stimulation test stimulates secretion of FSH and LH; blood samples are obtained every 2 hours; if LH level is higher than FSH level, puberty has occurred
4. Bone age x-rays aid in determining epiphyseal maturation and closure; if bone age is more advanced than chronological age, skeletal growth acceleration is apparent

C. Therapeutic management

1. NCLEX® Support children with precocious puberty by discussing their concerns about body image and sexuality
2. Offer support as family deals with sensitive issues such as premature appearance of secondary sexual characteristics and sexuality
3. NCLEX® Encourage clients to express feelings about body changes; role-playing may help children cope with issues of peer teasing
4. Assure children that friends will go through same body changes
5. If synthetic form of LH-releasing factor is used to slow down or arrest progression of puberty, plan for monthly or daily injections with family
6. NCLEX® Medication therapy: a synthetic form of LH-releasing factor or nafarelin slows or stops progression of puberty and skeletal growth until a more typical age for puberty is reached, which will preserve adult height

D. Child and family education

1. Information about condition and possible referral to pediatric endocrinologist
2. If client is receiving synthetic LH, teach family subcut or intramuscular injection technique, and provide child and family with information about drug side effects as per product literature

XVII. PHENYLKETONURIA (PKU)

A. Overview

1. Inherited autosomal recessive disorder of amino acid metabolism that affects body's use of protein caused by mutation of phenylalanine hydroxylase gene
2. Deficiency in liver enzyme phenylalanine hydroxylase (which breaks down phenylalanine into tyrosine) causes serum phenylalanine metabolite levels to rise, leading to musty body and urine odor (excretion of phenol acids), hyperactivity, hypertonia, hyperreflexive deep-tendon reflexes, irritability, seizures, vomiting, and an eczema-type rash
3. Decreased levels of tyrosine cause a deficiency of pigment melanin, causing most children with PKU to have fair skin that is prone to eczema
4. Continued accumulation of phenylalanine affects protein synthesis and myelinization and results in seizure disorder and untreatable intellectual disability if phenylalanine level is not decreased

B. Nursing assessment

1. Many infants with PKU appear healthy at birth; if treatment is not started to lower phenylalanine level immediately, infant's IQ can drop as many as 10 points within first month and will continue to decline
2. All 50 states require newborn screening
   a. Infant should ingest adequate protein (usually 24 hours of normal feedings of breast milk or formula) prior to testing to avoid false-negative results
   NCLEX® b. Heel blood should be used for specimen; sample should be collected no earlier than 48 hours after birth but no later than 7 days after birth
   c. A normal level is under 2 mg/dL; if level is elevated, a repeat test is performed to validate original results; a level higher than 15 mg/dL is considered dangerous
   d. If infant is discharged before 48 hours, test should be performed within 1 week after discharge from hospital or birthing center by healthcare provider or public health nurse
3. *NCLEX®* Symptoms arise over time and include failure to thrive, vomiting, irritability, and unpredictable behavior in infant; the urine will have a musty odor; the child may experience myoclonic or grand mal seizures

C. Therapeutic management

1. Allow phenylalanines in diet based on weight of child and usually at a level of 20–30 mg/kg body weight or amount prescribed by healthcare provider; consulting with registered nutritionist is essential to aid in food calculations and for family support
2. *NCLEX®* Place infant or child on protein-restricted diet
   a. Encourage use of mature breast milk or modified-protein, phenylalanine-free, hydrolysate formula as a source of infant nutrition to keep phenylalanine level at 2–6 mg/dL
   b. Use special protein foods that are free of phenylalanine
3. Monitor serum phenylalanine levels periodically throughout child's life
4. Maintain restricted phenylalanine diet for life to avoid decline in IQ and neuropsychological abilities; dietary adherence is especially important in early life and for adolescents and women before conception and during pregnancy (to prevent congenital anomalies, including low birth weight, microcephaly, congenital heart defects, and intellectual disability)
5. Parents may be overwhelmed initially by diagnosis and dietary restrictions; emotional support is essential; suggest genetic counseling because each child born to this couple may have a 1 in 4 chance of having PKU

D. Client and family teaching

1. Support parents and teach them disease and its management, including referral to a nutritionist for meal planning
2. Testing may need to be repeated if initial test was done before 48 hours of age or was positive initially
3. *NCLEX®* Review low-phenylalanine diet, including preparation of low-phenylalanine formula; avoid giving child meats, dairy products, and products containing aspartame because they contain large amounts of phenylalanine; it is important to read product labels, which may identify phenylalanine content
4. Offer emotional support and refer older child and parents to a support group for issues and problems related to chronic illness

PRACTICE TEST

Check Your NCLEX–RN® Exam I.Q.

You are ready for testing on this content if you can:

- Identify basic structures and functions of the endocrine system.
- Describe the pathophysiology and etiology of common endocrine disorders.
- Discuss expected assessment data and diagnostic test findings for selected endocrine disorders.
- Discuss therapeutic management of a client experiencing an endocrine disorder.
- Discuss nursing management of a client experiencing an endocrine disorder.
- Identify expected outcomes for the client experiencing an endocrine disorder.

PRACTICE TEST

1 A client recently diagnosed with hypothyroidism demonstrates understanding of prescribed levothyroxine medication when she makes which statement?

Ca+

1. "I should be able to become pregnant in a couple of months."
2. "This medication will help me lose all this excess weight."
3. "I should call the healthcare provider for nervousness, diarrhea, or increased pulse."
4. "This medication should be taken with food, preferably dairy products."

2 The client is post-transsphenoidal hypophysectomy. The client demonstrates understanding of methods for preventing increases in intracranial pressure by stating to perform which activity?

1. Sitting in a soft chair and leaning over slowly to tie shoes
2. Holding breath when reaching down to pick up something from the floor
3. Bending at the knees first before squatting down to reach something on the floor
4. Holding breath while using mouthwash, then leaning head down toward the sink to spit it out

3 The client who is 80 hours post-transsphenoidal hypophysectomy reports numbness on the upper lip and gum, a headache when reclining, and has a tendency to kick around small rugs in the room when walking. What should the home health nurse do next?

1. Explain that these are normal responses and will disappear over 2–3 weeks.
2. Assess neuromuscular function and incisional area and report findings to the surgeon.
3. Immediately arrange for client transportation to the hospital for treatment of increased intracranial pressure.
4. Assess vital signs, fluid volume status, bowel function, and nutrition status.

4 The client with diabetes mellitus requests a medication for headache soon after returning from an early morning x-ray procedure. The nurse observes the client is upset about the headache, angry at missing breakfast, and has moist hands. What priority action should he nurse take at this time?

1. Administer the medication for headache and arrange for a breakfast tray.
2. Check the blood glucose level and be prepared to give 4 ounces of juice immediately.
3. Acknowledge his dissatisfaction, offer to obtain a snack, and give the medication.
4. Administer the headache medication and review the day's lab test results.

5 A 70-year-old client admitted a few hours ago with a blood glucose (BG) of 750 mg/dL is being treated for hyperosmolar hyperglycemic nonketotic syndrome (HHNS) with intravenous regular insulin at 10 units/hour, normal saline with 20 mEq of potassium per liter infusing at 250 mL/hr, and oxygen at 2 L/min. The client has been oriented when stimulated, and BG has dropped to 400 mg/dL. The client now demands to get out of bed and his skin feels cool and moist. What should the nurse do at this time?

1. Interpret this as a sign of hypoglycemia and check his blood glucose.
2. Recognize the client is feeling better and seeks control of his situation.
3. Auscultate breath sounds and assess oxygen saturation.
4. Assess the client for bladder distention or signs of imbalanced body temperature.

6 A client who underwent a colonoscopy after premedication with midazolam returns to the nursing unit. The client is given morphine sulfate 2 mg IV push for abdominal pain associated with BP 140/80, pulse 78, RR 20. Twenty minutes later, the client is lethargic, has weak hand grasps, weak peripheral pulse of 88, BP 120/66, RR 14. How should the nurse interpret these assessment findings?

1. The client is resting with pain relieved.
2. The client is now showing signs of dehydration because of the colon procedure preparation.
3. The client is now fatigued because of anxiety, pain, and fear of outcome of the procedure.
4. The client is experiencing impaired gas exchange because of hypoventilation.

7 The client is scheduled for bilateral adrenalectomy as treatment for an adrenal cortex tumor. What is the nurse's highest priority for this client in the immediate postoperative period?

1. Assess fluid and electrolyte balance, signs of hypoglycemia, and hypotension.
2. Assess for signs of hypoxia, cardiac arrhythmias, and peripheral edema.
3. Monitor the incision integrity, peripheral pulses, and magnesium level.
4. Assess for hyperthermia, bed mobility, pupil reaction, and eye movement.

8 A female client has been taking propylthiouracil (PTU) for 5 months to treat hyperthyroidism. After falling and spraining her ankle, she is treated and is given crutch-walking instructions. She says she will never have enough energy to get around on crutches and is upset about the 4.5 kg (10 lb) she gained this winter. What should be the nurse's first action?

1. Document the client's statements and consult the healthcare provider to order a serum T_4.
2. Discharge the client to home and encourage her to have a TSH level drawn.
3. Encourage the client to rest at home until the sprain is healed, then increase activity.
4. Investigate the availability of a walking splint instead of using the crutches.

9 The client with diabetes mellitus (DM) is going home following angioplasty. The nurse observes that the client walks to the restroom barefoot, although slippers are in reach. What is the priority nursing concern for this client?

1. Potential for falls while walking barefoot
2. Potential for infection from microtrauma while walking barefoot
3. Lack of knowledge about routine postangioplasty care
4. Possible insufficient cerebral perfusion caused by hypoglycemia

10 The client is 6 hours post-thyroid surgery. The unlicensed assistant reports that the client is upset because there is blood on the client's gown. What is the priority action of the nurse?

1. Assess the client's breath sounds and respiratory effort.
2. State that it is normal to have some bleeding and ask the nurse aide to change the gown.
3. Reassure the client that some bleeding is normal, and then assess the client's level of pain.
4. Reinforce the dressing, change the gown, and call the surgeon.

11 A client who was admitted with hyperglycemic hyperosmolar nonketotic syndrome (HHNS) asks how he can prevent recurrence of this illness. The nurse would instruct the client about which helpful prevention measures? Select all that apply.

1. Use sliding-scale insulin to cover periodic snacks that are not part of the dietary plan.
2. Maintain fluid balance by drinking four glasses of water daily.
3. Monitor for signs of infection and treat infection early.
4. Consult primary care provider when fasting blood glucose is elevated.
5. Use stress management techniques because the stress response increases blood glucose.

12 The client who has a long history of type 1 diabetes mellitus is being treated for bronchitis and sinusitis. The nurse observes deep, rapid, unlabored respirations, fruity odor on the client's clothes, and dry skin. Which action should the nurse take next?

1. Assess breath sounds to determine client's response to treatment of the infection.
2. Assess the client for additional signs of hypoglycemia.
3. Encourage the client to rest and to drink 8–10 glasses of fluids daily.
4. Assess blood glucose level for hyperglycemia and check urine for ketones.

13 A female client newly diagnosed with hypothyroidism indicates that she no longer participates in evening social activities, stating, "There is too much walking, and I prefer to go to bed early. I see enough of my friends at work everyday." What is the best interpretation of this statement by the nurse?

1. The client is experiencing social isolation
2. The client is not getting sufficient sleep on a regular basis
3. The client is experiencing fatigue related to the diagnosis
4. The client is at risk for cardiac issues triggered by the diagnosis

14 A recently retired client who lives alone is admitted with myxedema coma, which occurred because of inability to pay for the medication. What is the highest priority of the nurse at the time of admission?

1. Assist the client to chair every 4 hours to promote oxygenation and prevent skin breakdown.
2. Prevent injury related to mental confusion and elevated blood pressure (BP).
3. Prevent skin breakdown and promote nutrition with low-fiber foods.
4. Monitor for signs of decreased cardiac output and airway obstruction.

15 A client with hyperparathyroidism is admitted with cardiac dysrhythmias, including bursts of supraventricular tachycardia (SVT). The client asks why the cardiologist prescribed so much intravenous (IV) fluid and then furosemide. What is the nurse's best explanation?

1. Improve cardiac output
2. Eliminate metabolic wastes
3. Replace missing electrolytes
4. Promote excretion of calcium

16 A client with hypoparathyroidism is to be discharged home after stabilization of fluid and electrolyte levels. Which are critical concepts that the nurse should teach the client prior to discharge? Select all that apply.

1. Importance of keeping follow-up appointments for laboratory tests and with healthcare provider
2. Strategies that will help decrease the risk of falling
3. Significant signs of hypoglycemia to monitor for and report
4. Signs and symptoms of renal calculi to monitor for and report
5. How to plan meals that include increased amounts of calcium and vitamin D

17 A client recently diagnosed with syndrome of inappropriate antidiuretic hormone (SIADH) is receiving continuous enteral nutrition. Considering the impact of the disorder on fluid balance, what action should the nurse take when working with the enteral feeding tube?

1. Discard the 50 mL residual and replace it with 50 mL water.
2. Flush the tube with 50 mL normal saline.
3. Count the flush but not the feeding in planning the fluid limitation.
4. Flush the tube with 50 mL water to maintain patency.

18 A client with a history of Cushing's syndrome is admitted with multiple contusions, lacerations, and blood loss following a motor vehicle accident. Current laboratory values are BUN 30 mg/dL, creatinine 1.0 mg/dL, sodium 148 mEq/L, potassium 4.8 mEq/L, chloride 108 mEq/L, and cortisol 29 mcg/dL. Which problems should the nurse address when initiating the client's plan of care? Select all that apply.

1. Urinary elimination
2. Musculoskeletal disuse
3. Possible difficulty with airway clearance
4. Increased susceptibility to infection
5. Possible dehydration

19 A client who underwent adrenal gland radiation therapy for benign tumors is receiving fludrocortisone acetate for mineralocorticoid and glucocorticoid replacement. What is a priority nursing concern for this client?

1. Risk for fluid overload
2. Risk for infection related to radiation damage
3. Risk for becoming constipated
4. Risk for ineffective respirations

20 The client is being treated for Addison's disease with glucocorticoid replacement medication. The nurse evaluates that the client understands medication therapy when the client makes which statement? Select all that apply.

1. "I should take this medication every evening at bedtime."
2. "My irregular pulse should convert to a regular rate and rhythm."
3. "This medication will help me control my increased blood pressure."
4. "I should call my doctor if I gain 0.9 kg (2 lb)."
5. "I should call my doctor if I feel weak or have a cold."

21 The 8-month-old infant of a newly immigrated family is brought to the endocrine clinic with a musty body odor, seizures, and an eczemalike rash. The infant is diagnosed with phenylketonuria (PKU). What should the nurse consider when planning care for this infant?

1. Need for dietary information about a low-phenylalanine diet
2. Need for admission to a long-term care setting for handicapped infants
3. Preparing the family for the child's early demise
4. Providing instruction on medication management of PKU

22 An adolescent weighing 113 kg (250 lb) has started to experience increased thirst, increased appetite, and frequent urination. After being diagnosed with diabetes mellitus (DM), he is started on oral drug therapy. What information should the nurse give the adolescent about medications as a treatment option?

1. "You might receive a pill now, but you'll get insulin in the future if you don't comply with diet and medication therapy."
2. "Overweight teenagers may develop type 2 diabetes, which can be treated with an oral medication. You may or may not need insulin in the future."
3. "Insulin is used when people with diabetes won't take oral pills, so you can avoid this by taking your medication as ordered."
4. "Your diabetes is mild, so you won't need to take medication for long. You will probably only need to restrict sweets."

23 A mother is quite concerned about her 7-year-old daughter after noticing some breast development and appearance of a small amount of pubic hair. The mother asks the nurse if this is a cause for concern. What would be the nurse's best response?

1. "No. Some girls just develop earlier than boys."
2. "Yes, she may have precocious puberty. Let's talk to the pediatrician because she may need referral to an endocrinologist."
3. "Yes. She probably doesn't want the other children at school making fun of her."
4. "No. This early development may slow down when she reaches 9 years old."

24 The mother of an adolescent with diabetes mellitus tells the nurse that her son likes to eat cheeseburgers and french fries when he goes out with his friends. The son is aware he is exceeding the allowable carbohydrate exchanges on the diabetic diet. How could the nurse best explain why adolescents sometimes make choices that place their health at risk?

1. They want to be like their peers.
2. They have a self-destructive wish.
3. They eat foods with friends that they can't eat at home.
4. They want to show risk-taking behavior.

25 The nurse is assessing a client with a tentative diagnosis of hyperpituitarism. What assessment findings should the nurse observe for in this client? Select all that apply.

1. Short stature if onset is in childhood
2. Large hands and feet with prominent jawbone
3. Joint changes consistent with arthritis
4. Soft, high-pitched voice
5. Hypertension

ANSWERS & RATIONALES

1 **Answer: 3 Rationale:** Nervousness, diarrhea, and increased pulse are indications of excessive effect of the medication, and the dosage may need to be adjusted downward. The client should report these to the healthcare provider. Levothyroxine is not prescribed to affect pregnancy. After the client has reached normal serum T_4 levels, the normal metabolic rate may help the client lose the weight gained during the hypothyroid state, but this is not the purpose of the replacement medication. Usually, the medication should be taken on an empty stomach, 1 hour prior to a meal or 2 hours after a meal. **Cognitive Level:** Analyzing **Client Need:** Pharmacological and Parenteral Therapies **Integrated Process:** Nursing Process: Evaluation **Content Area:** Adult Health: Endocrine and Metabolic **Strategy:** The core issue of the question is knowledge of medications used to manage hypothyroidism. Use nursing knowledge and the process of elimination to make a selection.

2 **Answer: 3 Rationale:** Bending the knees and squatting is preferred to bending at the waist to reach the floor as a means of preventing rises in intracranial pressure (ICP) following pituitary surgery. Holding the breath as well as leaning over will increase ICP. To tie shoes, the client should sit on the couch or bed, bend the knee and place his or her foot on the couch or bed to reach the shoelaces. Alternatively, the client can sit on the floor to tie shoes or can avoid shoes that tie until there is no risk for increased ICP. Clients should be taught to avoid holding the breath for any reason and to avoid leaning forward or bending at the waist to prevent an increase in intracranial pressure. Holding the breath as well as leaning over will increase ICP. **Cognitive Level:** Applying **Client Need:** Physiological Adaptation **Integrated Process:** Nursing Process: Evaluation **Content Area:** Adult Health: Endocrine and Metabolic **Strategy:** The core issue of the question is knowledge of measures to prevent rises in ICP following pituitary surgery. Use nursing knowledge and the process of elimination to make a selection.

3 **Answer: 2 Rationale:** The movement of the small rugs suggests an unsteady gait or foot drop; both this and the headache are signs of increased intracranial pressure. In-depth assessments of neuromuscular function and incision site are needed, and then the surgeon should be consulted immediately. The numbness of the upper lip and gum near the incision as well as a decreased sense of smell are normal but may not resolve for 3–4 months. The client should not be sent to the hospital without assessment and consultation with the surgeon first. General assessments that are part of routine care can be completed once the client's symptoms are addressed. **Cognitive Level:** Applying **Client Need:** Physiological Adaptation **Integrated Process:** Nursing Process: Assessment **Content Area:** Adult Health: Endocrine and Metabolic **Strategy:** The core issue of the question is the ability to accurately interpret the significance of client findings after pituitary surgery and then determine the next action. Use nursing knowledge and the process of elimination to make a selection, recalling that further assessments are often indicated when encountering abnormal data.

4 **Answer: 2 Rationale:** Headache, restlessness, anxiety, sweating, and increased pulse are signs of hypoglycemia. Resolution of symptoms should occur after the client drinks the juice. Treating the headache and obtaining a breakfast tray fail to recognize the client's actual problem. Acknowledging dissatisfaction, obtaining a snack, and giving medication address the client's concerns but do not verify the client's blood glucose as a possible etiology for the symptoms. Treating the headache and checking labs fails to address the immediate risk of hypoglycemia, which can be addressed by checking blood glucose. **Cognitive Level:** Analyzing **Client Need:** Physiological Adaptation **Integrated Process:** Nursing Process: Implementation **Content Area:** Adult Health: Endocrine and Metabolic **Strategy:** The core issue of the question is recognition that the client is at risk for hypoglycemia and the corrective actions that need to be taken. Use nursing knowledge and the process of elimination to make a selection.

5 **Answer: 3 Rationale:** Increased preload caused by the intravenous infusion at 250 mL/hr may exceed the myocardium's workload capacity, leading to signs of decreased cardiac output and congestive heart failure. There is no risk for hypoglycemia while the BG is still elevated to 400 mg/dL. The nurse should seek a physiological basis for the change in client's status rather than seeking control, especially since the skin is cool and moist. Checking for bladder distention or fever represents a failure to directly assess for signs of possible fluid overload. **Cognitive Level:** Analyzing **Client Need:** Physiological Adaptation **Integrated Process:** Nursing Process: Assessment **Content Area:** Adult Health: Endocrine and Metabolic **Strategy:** The core issue of the question is recognition that rapid infusion of fluid in a 70-year-old client could lead to circulatory decompensation. Use nursing knowledge and the process of elimination to make a selection.

6 **Answer: 4 Rationale:** Decreased level of consciousness, weak hand grasp, and peripheral pulses with increased heart rate and decreased BP result from acidosis. These are signs of respiratory acidosis secondary to hypoventilation from the midazolam. Concluding that the client is resting and pain is relieved fails to address the falling respiratory rate and change in level of consciousness. The client is not showing signs of dehydration. Fatigue would not account for the weak peripheral pulse. **Cognitive Level:** Analyzing **Client Need:** Physiological Adaptation **Integrated Process:** Nursing Process: Diagnosis **Content Area:** Adult Health: Endocrine and Metabolic **Strategy:** The core issue of the question is accurate interpretation of a change in client status. A critical word in the stem of the question is *midazolam*. Recall the properties of this medication, and use nursing knowledge and the process of elimination to make a selection.

7 **Answer: 1 Rationale:** During the first 48 hours after adrenalectomy, clients are at risk for adrenal insufficiency and hypovolemic shock. The lack of cortisol production can cause fluid and electrolyte loss and hypoglycemia. Peripheral edema is more likely associated with excess fluid volume but the risk after adrenalectomy is deficient fluid volume caused by sudden decrease in circulating corticosteroids and mineralocorticoids. Incision integrity and peripheral pulses are routine assessments, and magnesium level is not of particular concern at this time. Assessing for hyperthermia, bed mobility are part of routine postoperative assessments, and neurological assessment of pupils and eye movements is not of particular concern after adrenalectomy. **Cognitive Level:** Analyzing **Client Need:** Physiological Adaptation **Integrated Process:** Nursing Process: Assessment **Content Area:** Adult Health: Endocrine and Metabolic **Strategy:** The core issue of the question is knowledge that clients are at risk for adrenal insufficiency following adrenalectomy and how to assess for its occurrence. Use nursing knowledge and the process of elimination to make a selection.

8 **Answer: 1 Rationale:** The client's reports of lack of energy and weight gain are consistent with hypothyroidism, which is diagnosed with a serum T_4. Considering the client's complaints of energy deficit, the recent fall causing the sprain, and information about the thyroid medication, the nurse is obligated to consult the healthcare provider for T_4 evaluation to prevent further injury. Discharging the client ignores the client's concern and a TSH level is expected to be high in hyperthyroidism and may not be of use. Encouraging the client to rest is appropriate after the client's physiological signs have been addressed. Investigating the need for a walking splint is an appropriate action but is not the first priority. **Cognitive Level:** Applying **Client Need:** Physiological Adaptation **Integrated Process:** Nursing Process: Planning **Content Area:** Adult Health: Endocrine and Metabolic **Strategy:** The core issue of the question is the ability to correlate client reports with the underlying emergence of hypothyroidism in response to vigorous treatment of hyperthyroidism. Use nursing knowledge and the process of elimination to make a selection.

9 **Answer: 2 Rationale:** Clients with either diabetic mellitus or other conditions that have arterial insufficiency as a component of the disorder must constantly protect their feet from trauma because they are at risk for undetected minor injury and subsequent infection. The client is not at especially high risk for falls. There is no information that supports a lack of knowledge about routine care after angioplasty. Hypoglycemia is an ongoing potential complication with diabetes mellitus but is not the highest priority at this time. **Cognitive Level:** Analyzing **Client Need:** Physiological Adaptation **Integrated Process:** Nursing Process: Diagnosis **Content Area:** Adult Health: Endocrine and Metabolic **Strategy:** The core issue of the question is interpretation of behaviors that pose risk for complications to the client with diabetes mellitus. Use nursing knowledge and the process of elimination to make a selection.

10 **Answer: 1 Rationale:** Blood on the gown indicates excessive incisional bleeding. Breath sounds, including auscultating over the tracheal area, and respiratory effort should be assessed first to determine if edema is present in the tissues, thus compromising the airway. After thoroughly assessing the client and reinforcing or changing the dressing per protocol, the nurse should inform the surgeon of the amount of bleeding and all other assessment data. Usually, with thyroid surgery, there is minimal bleeding postoperatively and having the nurse's aide change the gown fails to provide proper client assessment. Focusing on the client's pain level does not address the bleeding, which is excessive rather than normal. Reinforcing the dressing and calling the surgeon fails to address the need for assessing the client's airway, which is a critical oversight. **Cognitive Level:** Analyzing **Client Need:** Physiological Adaptation **Integrated Process:** Nursing Process: Implementation **Content Area:** Adult Health: Endocrine and Metabolic **Strategy:** The core issue of the question is possible threat to the airway and breathing with excessive bleeding following thyroid surgery. Use nursing knowledge, the ABCs, and the process of elimination to make a selection.

11 **Answer: 3, 5 Rationale:** HHNS is associated with hyperglycemic response to infection or other disease or illness, some medications, dehydration, stress, or a combination of these factors. The response to stress can increase blood glucose levels so stress management may be helpful as part of overall measures to prevent increased blood glucose. HHNS occurs in clients with type 2 diabetes mellitus, primarily older adults, and thus insulin is not necessarily a part of the ongoing treatment plan (oral antidiabetic agents may be used). Drinking four glasses of water daily is insufficient; six to eight glasses of water are recommended for general health. Consulting a healthcare provider for elevated blood glucose does not demonstrate an understanding of how to prevent HHNS. **Cognitive Level:** Applying **Client Need:** Physiological Adaptation **Integrated Process:** Nursing Process: Implementation **Content Area:** Adult Health: Endocrine and Metabolic **Strategy:** The critical word in the stem of the question is *prevent*. With this in mind, look for options that will reduce the likelihood of the client experiencing a recurrence. Use nursing knowledge and the process of elimination to make a selection.

12 **Answer: 4 Rationale:** Kussmaul respirations, fruity breath odor, and dry skin are signs consistent with diabetic ketoacidosis, which is characterized by hyperglycemia and ketonuria. Assessing breath sounds to determine response to treatment of the infection does not address the client's current problem. Hypoglycemia is the opposite problem of the one the client is experiencing. Rest periods will not help treat hyperglycemia and ketoacidosis, and although fluids are needed, 8–10 glasses daily will not be enough to reverse the dehydration that accompanies diabetic ketoacidosis. **Cognitive Level:** Analyzing **Client Need:** Physiological Adaptation **Integrated Process:** Nursing Process: Assessment **Content Area:** Adult Health: Endocrine and Metabolic **Strategy:** The core issue of the question is recognition that a diabetic client with an infection is at risk for diabetic ketoacidosis and knowing how to assess for this complication. Use nursing knowledge and the process of elimination to make a selection.

13 **Answer: 3 Rationale:** Hypothyroidism is associated with fatigue, weight gain, and decreased activity tolerance. The client states she is able to socialize during the day at work. There is no data to indicate the client is not getting enough sleep. The client's symptoms are not specific to cardiac disease. **Cognitive Level:** Analyzing **Client Need:** Physiological Adaptation **Integrated Process:** Nursing Process: Diagnosis **Content Area:** Adult Health: Endocrine and Metabolic **Strategy:** The core issue of the question is the etiology of the client's symptoms and applying a nursing diagnostic label to the problem. Use nursing knowledge and the process of elimination to make a selection.

14 **Answer: 4 Rationale:** Myxedema is characterized by severely decreased cardiac output, fluid and electrolyte imbalance, acidosis, decreased respiratory function, tongue edema, and hypothermia. The client's airway, breathing, and circulation needs must be attended to first. The client would be on bedrest immediately after admission. The BP would be decreased, rather than elevated, because of reduced cardiac output. The client in myxedema coma has generally lost consciousness. Skin breakdown is a significant risk that needs to be managed concurrently with promotion of oxygenation, but the diet should be high in fiber once the client is stable

enough to eat. **Cognitive Level:** Analyzing **Client Need:** Physiological Adaptation **Integrated Process:** Nursing Process: Planning **Content Area:** Adult Health: Endocrine and Metabolic **Strategy:** The core issue of the question is assigning a priority to client needs during myxedema. Recall that physiological needs take priority before psychosocial needs. Use nursing knowledge about the condition and the process of elimination to make a selection.

15 **Answer: 4 Rationale:** Hyperparathyroidism causes hypercalcemia. Large-volume saline infusion given concurrently with furosemide will stimulate the kidneys to excrete calcium. In acute situations requiring rapid reduction, clients could also be given IV calcitonin and phosphates. IV fluids and furosemide are not given to improve cardiac output, eliminate metabolic wastes, or replace missing electrolytes. **Cognitive Level:** Applying **Client Need:** Physiological Adaptation **Integrated Process:** Nursing Process: Implementation **Content Area:** Adult Health: Endocrine and Metabolic **Strategy:** The core issue of the question is knowledge of methods used to manage hypercalcemia in hyperparathyroidism. Use nursing knowledge and the process of elimination to make a selection.

16 **Answer: 1, 2, 5 Rationale:** Clients should be taught to keep follow-up appointments for laboratory tests and with healthcare providers consistently. Clients with hypoparathyroidism have paresthesias, muscle spasms, and hyperactive reflexes, which place them at risk for falling. Falls prevention measures are important for this client. Clients with hypoparathyroidism have low serum calcium levels and require increased calcium in the diet, and often calcium supplements and increased vitamin D. Hypoglycemia is a primary concern in diabetes mellitus, a disorder of the pancreas. Low serum calcium levels do not predispose the client to renal calculi. **Cognitive Level:** Applying **Client Need:** Physiological Adaptation **Integrated Process:** Teaching and Learning **Content Area:** Adult Health: Endocrine and Metabolic **Strategy:** The core issue of the question is health teaching that is appropriate for a client with hypoparathyroidism. Use nursing knowledge about the disease process, altered calcium levels, safety measures, and the process of elimination to make a selection.

17 **Answer: 2 Rationale:** Clients with SIADH are encouraged to drink fluids high in sodium, so they should have feeding tubes flushed with normal saline. To prevent electrolyte loss, all of the residual that is aspirated from a feeding tube should be returned to the client. Clients with SIADH are usually on a strict fluid restriction to correct water overload; therefore, all fluids (including enteral feeding and flush solution) should be considered when planning fluid restriction. Because of the need for increased sodium, this client should not have the feeding tube flushed with water. **Cognitive Level:** Applying **Client Need:** Physiological Adaptation **Integrated Process:** Nursing Process: Implementation **Content Area:** Adult Health: Endocrine and Metabolic **Strategy:** The core issue of the question is proper fluid use and management in a client with SIADH. Use nursing knowledge about fluid imbalance in this disorder and the process of elimination to make a selection.

18 **Answer: 4, 5 Rationale:** Clients with Cushing's syndrome are more susceptible to infection because of impaired immune function from elevated cortisol level. The BUN and sodium are elevated because of dehydration caused by blood loss, and a potassium and chloride at the higher end of the normal range add further support to this conclusion. The client has no risk factors for problems with urinary elimination. The client's injuries do not predispose the client to be at risk for musculoskeletal disuse. The client is not experiencing any difficulty with the airway. **Cognitive Level:** Analyzing **Client Need:** Physiological Adaptation **Integrated Process:** Nursing Process: Diagnosis **Content Area:** Adult Health: Endocrine and Metabolic **Strategy:** The core issue of the question is the ability to determine priorities of care for a client with Cushing's syndrome who experiences trauma. Use knowledge of pathophysiology and the process of elimination to make a selection.

19 **Answer: 1 Rationale:** Fludrocortisone and other adrenal replacement drugs cause sodium and fluid retention. Clients are at risk for excess sodium and fluid retention leading to fluid overload. The client could be at risk for secondary infection but this is not timely if the client has completed this course of therapy. There is no evidence that the client is at greater risk for developing constipation. The client could have ineffective respirations if fluid overload impairs alveolar ventilation, but the primary problem to address would be the fluid volume status. **Cognitive Level:** Analyzing **Client Need:** Physiological Adaptation **Integrated Process:** Nursing Process: Diagnosis **Content Area:** Adult Health: Endocrine and Metabolic **Strategy:** The core issue of the question is the ability to determine priority concerns for a client receiving mineralocorticoid and glucocorticoid therapy. Use nursing knowledge and the process of elimination to make a selection.

20 **Answer: 4, 5 Rationale:** Glucocorticoid replacement medication can cause fluid and sodium retention, leading to weight gain and fluid volume excess. Doses need to be increased during times of stress and can impair the body's ability to recover from an infection. Therefore, the healthcare provider must be consulted for signs of a cold or infection. Glucocorticoids should be taken in the morning with food. The medication will not affect cardiac rhythm. Glucocorticoids will increase BP and thus are not safe for clients with hypertension. **Cognitive Level:** Applying **Client Need:** Pharmacological and Parenteral Therapies **Integrated Process:** Nursing Process: Evaluation **Content Area:** Adult Health: Endocrine and Metabolic **Strategy:** The core issue of the question is knowledge of adverse effects of drug therapy. Use nursing knowledge and the process of elimination to make a selection.

21 **Answer: 1 Rationale:** A low-phenylalanine diet reduces the amount of toxic metabolites in the body, thus reducing or preventing additional damage. There is no indication of a need to admit the child to a long-term care facility. Infants with PKU have normal life expectancy. No medications are currently being used to treat PKU. **Cognitive Level:** Applying **Client Need:** Physiological Adaptation **Integrated Process:** Nursing Process: Planning **Content Area:** Child Health **Strategy:** The core issue of the question is management of PKU in a newly diagnosed infant. Use nursing knowledge and the process of elimination to make a selection.

22 **Answer: 2 Rationale:** Some adolescents develop type 2 diabetes, especially those who are overweight. They might need to take an oral hypoglycemic with or without accompanying insulin. Warning the client about compliance does not provide the information needed about medication therapy. Insulin is not used for those who won't take oral medication. Sweets and complex carbohydrates will need to be restricted regardless of medication therapy. **Cognitive Level:** Applying **Client Need:** Physiological Adaptation **Integrated Process:** Teaching and Learning **Content Area:** Child Health **Strategy:** The core issue of the question is correct information about medication

therapy for overweight adolescents with new-onset diabetes. Use nursing knowledge and the process of elimination to make a selection.

23 **Answer: 2 Rationale:** The child should be seen by the pediatrician because there might be secretion of sex hormones, and precocious puberty may affect linear growth. Stating that some girls develop earlier than boys ignores the clinical issue. Although she may be teased in school by the other children, the main reason for seeking treatment is health promotion. There is no reason to believe this process will slow down in another year. **Cognitive Level:** Applying **Client Need:** Physiological Adaptation **Integrated Process:** Nursing Process: Planning **Content Area:** Child Health **Strategy:** The core issue of the question is the priority need of a client with suspected precocious puberty. Use nursing knowledge and the process of elimination to make a selection.

24 **Answer: 1 Rationale:** As part of normal psychosocial development, adolescents need to feel like part of their group, even if it means impairing their health. There is no information to support a self-destructive wish. Although some foods may not be allowed at home, it is not likely to be the motivating factor. Displaying risk-taking behaviors is not likely the primary motivation, but rather a secondary event. **Cognitive Level:** Analyzing **Client Need:** Physiological Adaptation **Integrated Process:** Nursing Process: Diagnosis **Content Area:** Child Health **Strategy:** The core issue of the question is knowledge of age-specific concerns of adolescents with diabetes mellitus. Use nursing knowledge and the process of elimination to make a selection.

25 **Answer: 2, 3, 5 Rationale:** The client with hyperpituitarism will exhibit the following: tall stature if onset in childhood, large hands and feet with prominent jawbone, joint changes consistent with arthritis, deep voice and possible dysphagia, hypertension, organomegaly, and skin changes leading to rough, oily texture. The client would not have a soft voice or be short in stature. **Cognitive Level:** Analyzing **Client Need:** Physiological Adaptation **Integrated Process:** Nursing Process: Assessment **Content Area:** Child Health **Strategy:** The core issue of the question is knowledge of assessment findings with hyperpituitarism. Recall the functions of the pituitary gland and then correlate the functions with the logical signs of excess to make the appropriate selections.

Key Terms to Review

glycosylated hemoglobin p. 1075
hyperglycemia p. 1075
hypersecretion p. 1073
hyperthyroidism (Graves' disease) p. 1077
hyposecretion p. 1073
ketosis p. 1083
paresthesia p. 1080
photophobia p. 1079
polydipsia p. 1077
polyphagia p. 1083
polyuria p. 1077
receptor p. 1072
thyroid crisis (thyroid storm) p. 1078

References

Ball, J., & Bindler, R., & Cowen, K. (2015). *Principles of pediatric nursing: Caring for children* (6th ed.). New York, NY: Pearson Education.

Berman, A., Snyder, S., & Frandsen, G. (2016). *Kozier & Erb's fundamentals of nursing: Concepts, process, and practice* (10th ed.). New York, NY: Pearson Education.

Ignatavicius, D., & Workman, L. (2016). *Medical-surgical nursing: Patient-centered collaborative care* (10th ed.). Philadelphia: Saunders.

Kee, J. (2017). *Pearson's handbook of laboratory and diagnostic tests* (8th ed.). New York, NY: Pearson Education.

LeMone, P., Burke, K., Bauldoff, G., & Gubrud, P. (2015). *Medical surgical nursing: Clinical reasoning in patient care* (6th ed.). Hoboken, NJ: Pearson Education.

Lewis, S., Dirksen, S., Heitkemper, M., & Bucher, L. (2014). *Medical surgical nursing: Assessment and management of clinical problems* (9th ed.). St. Louis, MO: Elsevier Science.

Smith, S., Duell, D., Martin, B., Aebersold, M., & Gonzalez, L. (2017). *Clinical nursing skills: Basic to advanced skills* (10th ed.). New York, NY: Pearson Education.

61 Musculoskeletal Disorders

In this chapter

Cross Reference

Other chapters relevant to this content area are

Neurologic and Musculoskeletal Medications	Chapter 38
Common Laboratory Tests	Chapter 46
Common Diagnostic Tests and Procedures	Chapter 47
Fluid and Electrolyte Imbalances	Chapter 53
Cardiovascular Disorders	Chapter 56

I. OVERVIEW OF ANATOMY AND PHYSIOLOGY OF MUSCULOSKELETAL SYSTEM

A. **Skeleton**: consists of bones, joints, and cartilage; provides framework for body; protects soft tissue and vital organs; composed primarily of calcium (as Ca^{++} phosphate and carbonate); points of attachment for muscles

B. **Classification of bones**

1. Two major structural classifications: compact bone (dense) or cancellous bone (spongy)
2. Long bones (e.g., tibia) have a central shaft (**diaphysis**) and two end portions (epiphyseals)
3. Short bones are composed of cancellous bone covered by a thin layer of compact bone (e.g., tarsals)
4. Flat bones have two layers of compact bone separated by a layer of cancellous bone (e.g., skull, ribs, scapula, and sternum)

C. Bone marrow

1. Soft, spongy, highly cellular blood-forming tissue that fills cavities of bones and is site for hematopoiesis (red blood cell [RBC] production) and storage of RBCs
2. Responsible also for production of white blood cells (WBCs) and platelets
3. Becomes predominantly fatty with age, particularly in long bones of limb

D. Axial section

1. Each vertebra is ring-shaped and placed one on top of another, with a padding of cartilage between; vertebral rings have bony projections (processes), which serve as points of attachment for muscles and articulation with bones
2. Twelve pairs of ribs attach to thoracic vertebrae; upper seven opposing pairs attach at front to sternum; three of remaining five pairs attach to rib immediately above by cartilage, and lowest two pairs are unattached

E. Appendicular section

1. Connected to axial skeleton by bones of upper and lower extremities
   a. Shoulder girdle supports arms; humerus is located in upper arm and ulna and radius in forearm
   b. Each innominate bone (hip bone) consists of three parts—ileum, ischium, and pubis; innominate bones unite with sacrum and coccyx of vertebral column to form pelvic girdle, which supports legs

F. Joint articulations

1. Result when two bones are joined together; categorized according to type of motion
2. Composed of fibrous connective tissue and cartilage (dense avascular connective tissue) that covers ends of bones, making movement smooth
3. Joint cavity secretes synovial fluid, which lubricates joint and reduces friction

G. Ligaments: bands of rigid connective tissue that hold joints together, allowing for movement and stability; have a relatively poor blood supply, which significantly prolongs healing process after injury

H. Muscles

1. Primarily function as a source of power and pull against bones to move body
2. Three primary types of muscle: skeletal muscle (striated, voluntary) moves extremities and external areas of body; cardiac muscle (striated, involuntary) is found in heart; smooth muscle (nonstriated, involuntary) is found in walls of arteries and bowel

II. DIAGNOSTIC TESTS AND ASSESSMENTS

A. Radiological tests: x-rays are widely used to assess musculoskeletal problems and effectiveness of treatment; radiological studies other than simple x-rays may be done with or without contrast

B. EMG (electromyogram or myogram): records and evaluates electrical activity of muscles during contraction

1. Two types of EMG are intramuscular EMG (more common) and surface EMG (SEMG)
2. *NCLEX®* Long, small-gauge needles are inserted through skin into muscle; client may feel mild to moderate discomfort during procedure
3. Needles detect electrical activity of muscle and transmit data to EMG machine, which displays electrical activity on an oscilloscope or transmits through an audiotransmitter (microphone)
4. SEMG: electrodes are placed above muscle to detect electrical activity

C. *Arthroscopy*: surgical procedure done under local or general anesthesia to examine internal joint structure using an arthroscope (pencil-sized device with optical fibers and lenses), which is inserted into very small skin incisions; device is connected to a video camera to allow visualization of interior of joint

1. Used to diagnose or treat musculoskeletal disorders such as osteoarthritis, rheumatoid arthritis, infectious types of arthritis, and internal joint injuries like meniscus tears, ligament tears, and cartilage deterioration
2. Arthroscopic surgery can be done during arthroscopy to repair joint tissue, which creates less tissue trauma, less pain, and allows for quicker recovery than traditional joint surgery
3. *NCLEX®* Client education: postprocedure
   a. Take analgesics for comfort and limit activity as directed
   b. Observe site for hematoma or bleeding
   c. Perform neurovascular self-assessment (temperature, color, capillary refill, movement, and sensation) on affected extremity
   d. Report signs of infection: fever, redness and warmth at surgical site, or purulent discharge

D. Arthrogram: contrast media or air is injected into joint cavity to visualize joint structures; client moves joint through a series of movements while a series of x-rays are taken; assess for allergy to contrast media

NCLEX® 1. Client education preprocedure: injection of contrast may lead to a feeling of warmth, nausea, headache, salty taste in mouth, itching, hives, and rash (symptoms are usually temporary and will be treated if necessary)

NCLEX® 2. Client education postprocedure
   a. Temporary discoloration of skin and urine is normal after use of contrast
   b. Perform neurovascular self-assessment on affected extremity
   c. Increase fluid intake to aid in contrast excretion to protect kidneys

E. **CT scan (computerized tomography)**: produces highly detailed, cross-sectional images of bones, joints, and other structures

F. **MRI (magnetic resonance imaging)**: similar uses as CT scan

G. **Bone scan**: creates images of bones using a small amount of radioactive material injected into blood; increased radioisotope uptake is seen with osteomyelitis, osteoporosis, fractures, Paget's disease, and bone cancer

H. **Bone densitometry (bone density)**: uses photon energy beams to measure bone mineral density (BMD) that aids in diagnosis of osteoporosis, predicts fracture risk, and helps evaluate effectiveness of treatment
   1. Noninvasive radiological test that digitally images hip, spine, wrist, finger, tibia, or heel
   2. Takes 30 seconds to 4 minutes per site, and no preprocedure or postprocedure care is required
   3. Client's scores include a T-score (compares client score with that of a normal 30-year-old) and a Z-score (compares client normal to normal in a healthy, age-matched client)
   4. Results are reported in standard deviations (SD) below normal and are expressed as negative numbers; scores within 1 standard deviation are considered normal; a score of −1 SD represents a 12% reduction in bone mass; treatment is initiated at −2.5 SD or lower
   5. Results should be reassessed every 2 years

I. ***Arthrocentesis* (joint aspiration) and analysis:** fluid is removed from joint to reduce swelling and pain and/or obtain fluid for examination using a sterile needle and syringe
   1. Postprocedure complications are uncommon but may include localized bruising, minor bleeding into joint cavity, and loss of pigment at injection site (septic arthritis is a rare but serious complication)

NCLEX® 2. Client education
   a. If cortisone was injected into joint, monitor for inflammation of injected area, atrophy or loss of pigment at injection site, and increased blood glucose
   b. Follow postprocedure activity restrictions and monitor for postprocedure complications; check dressing for excessive bleeding

III. LABORATORY STUDIES

A. **Antinuclear antibodies (ANA)**: sensitive screening blood test used to detect autoimmune disease
   1. ANAs destroy nucleus of cells; suggest presence of autoantibodies (directed against body's own tissue)
   2. Present in clients with a number of autoimmune diseases such as rheumatoid arthritis and others

B. **Calcium (Ca^{++})**: an abundant electrolyte that causes neuromuscular irritability and contractions; adult normal reference range is 8.5–10.5 mg/dL; see also Chapter 53
   1. Decreased calcium levels may be found in osteomalacia, inadequate dietary calcium, renal disease, and hypoparathyroidism
   2. Increased calcium levels may be seen in bone neoplasm, multiple fractures, immobilization, renal calculi, and hyperparathyroidism

C. **Phosphorus** (2.5–4.5 mg/dL is normal reference range); may be measured and compared to calcium level
   1. Decreased levels can be seen with hypercalcemia, starvation, malabsorption syndrome, osteomalacia, and vitamin D deficiency
   2. Increased levels can be seen with healing fractures, metastatic bone tumors, and hypocalcemia

D. **Rheumatoid factor (RF)** (normal is negative or <1:20): screening blood test used to detect antibodies (IgM, IgG, or IgA) in rheumatoid arthritis; elevated RF may indicate diseases other than rheumatoid arthritis

E. **Erythrocyte sedimentation rate (ESR)**: normal is under 20 mm/hr; gender variations exist; nonspecific serologic test that indicates inflammatory process in conditions such as rheumatoid arthritis and osteomyelitis

NCLEX® F. **Uric acid:** normal range is 4.5–6.5 mg/dL in males and 2.5–5.5 mg/dL in females; elevation (hyperuricemia) is seen in gout, poor renal function, excessive purine metabolism, and/or excessive dietary intake of purine foods

IV. COMMON NURSING TECHNIQUES AND PROCEDURES

A. **Crutch-walking**

NCLEX® 1. Crutches need to be fitted properly for client safety; ensure that crutch shoulder rest is at least three fingerwidths (2.5–5 cm or 1–2 in.) below axilla; height of hand bar should be adjusted to allow 30 degrees of elbow flexion (measured with goniometer); see Figure 61–1A

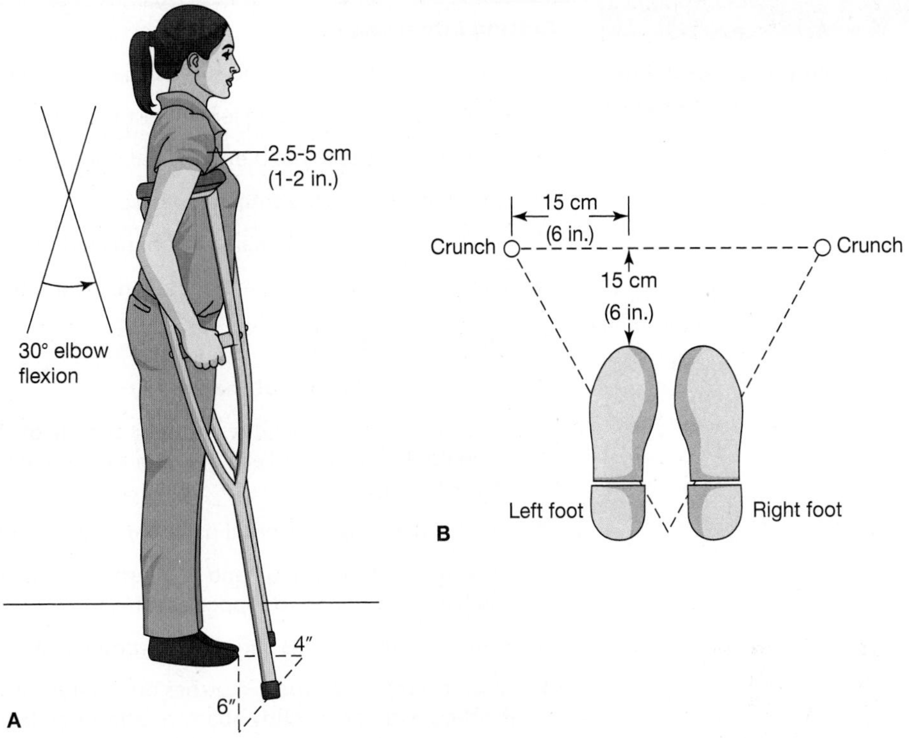

Figure 61–1

Crutch use. (**A**) Correct standing positioning for crutch use; (**B**) tripod position for crutch use.

2. Client stands uses tripod position to maintain posture and balance; crutches are placed 15 cm (6 in.) to the front and 15 cm (6 in.) to the side of foot; see Figure 61–1B
3. Crutch gaits: safe method of walking using crutches, alternating body weight on one or both legs and crutches

NCLEX®

4. See Box 61–1 for crutch-walking techniques

Box 61–1

Instructions for Client on Use of Crutches

Four-Point Alternate Gait

- Slow gait that requires good coordination
- Weight-bearing is on both legs with three points of contact with floor at all times
- Move each foot or crutch separately (right crutch, left foot; left crutch, right foot)

Two-Point Gait

- Faster than four-point gait but requires more balance
- There is partial weight-bearing on each foot
- Arm movements simulate arm movement when walking
- Move left crutch and right foot together; move right crutch and left foot together

Three-Point Gait

- Fast gait in which two crutches and unaffected leg bear weight alternately
- Weaker leg and both crutches move together followed by stronger leg

Swing-To Gait

- Fast gait used by clients with paralysis of legs and hips
- Prolonged use may lead to atrophy of unused muscles
- Advance crutches together, lift body using arms, then swing to meet crutches

Swing-Through Gait

- Fast gait used by clients with paralysis of legs and hips
- Good balance, skill, coordination, and strength required
- Advance crutches together, lift body using arms, swing through and beyond crutches

Box 61–2

Transfer Techniques for Clients with Crutches

Getting Into a Chair

1. Use chair with armrests and support back of chair against a wall for stability.
2. Center back of unaffected leg against chair.
3. Transfer crutches to hand on affected side.
4. Hold crutches by horizontal hand bars.
5. Grasp arm of chair with hand on unaffected side.
6. Lean forward, flex knees and hips, and lower into chair.

Getting Out of a Chair

1. Move forward to edge of chair.
2. Place unaffected leg slightly under or at edge of chair (this position helps client to stand up from chair and achieve balance, since unaffected leg is supported against edge of chair).
3. Grasp crutches by horizontal hand bars using hand on affected side.
4. Grasp arm of chair using hand on unaffected side (body weight is placed on crutches and hand on armrest to support unaffected leg when client rises to stand).
5. Push down on crutches and chair armrest while raising body out of chair.
6. Assume a *tripod position* (crutches out laterally in front of feet, approximately 6 inches, with feet slightly apart, creating a wide base of support) for balance before moving.

5. See Box 61–2 for transfer techniques (getting in and out of a chair) using crutches

NCLEX®

6. See Box 61–3 for negotiating stairs while using crutches

Memory Aid

Use the phrase "good leg up; bad leg down" to help remember which leg to place first when going up and down stairs with crutches.

Box 61–3

Instructions for Clients with Crutches: Negotiating Stairs

Going Up Stairs (stand behind client slightly on affected side for support if needed)

1. Assume tripod position.
2. Transfer weight to crutches and move unaffected leg onto step.
3. Transfer weight to unaffected leg on step and move crutches and affected leg up to step.
4. Repeat steps 2 and 3 until client reaches top of stairs.

Going Down Stairs (stand one step below client on affected side for support if needed)

1. Assume tripod position at top of stairs.
2. Shift weight to unaffected leg.
3. Move crutches and affected leg down onto next step.
4. Transfer weight to crutches and move unaffected leg to that step.
5. Repeat steps 2 and 3 until client reaches bottom step.

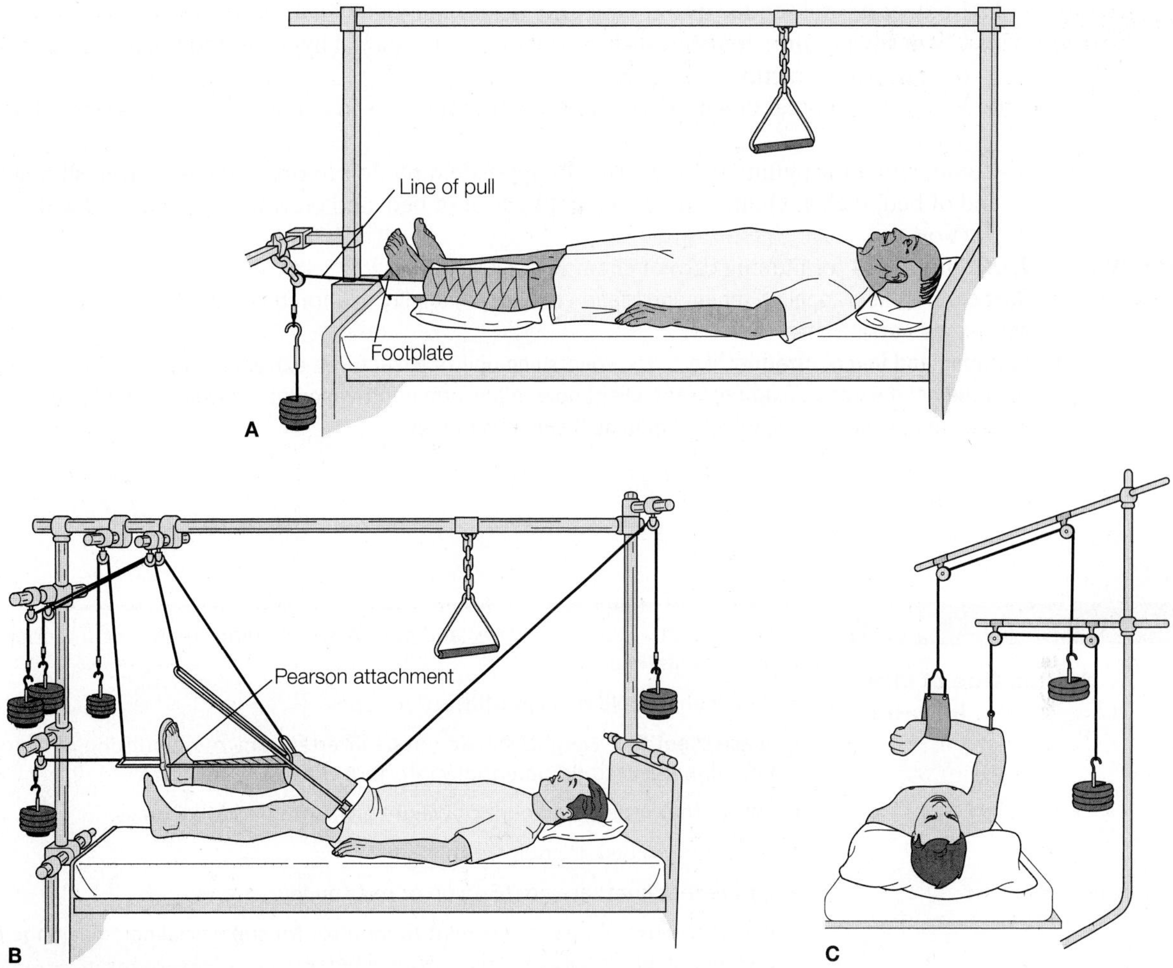

Figure 61–2 Types of traction. (**A**) Skin traction (also called straight traction), such as Buck's traction for hip fracture. (**B**) Balanced suspension traction, often used for fractures of the femur. (**C**) Skeletal traction, in which pulling force is applied directly to bone, such as for a fracture of the humerus.

B. ***Traction***: direct pulling force applied to a fractured extremity that results in realignment of bone; see Figure 61–2)

1. Reduces fracture, lessens muscle spasms, relieves pain, corrects deformities, promotes rest, and allows for exercise
2. Skin and skeletal traction are most commonly used; manual traction is used only briefly under healthcare provider direction to maintain immobility during treatment

NCLEX®

3. Skin traction (using tape, boots, splints)
   a. Generally used for short-term treatment (48–72 hours) and is applied directly to skin; used until skeletal traction or surgery is available to treat fracture
   b. Assists in reduction of a fracture (does not primarily achieve reduction) and helps decrease muscle spasms
   c. Weights range from 2.3 to 4.5 kg (5 to 10 lb)

NCLEX®

4. Skeletal traction (using pins or wires inserted into bones)
   a. Indicated for long-term use
   b. Used to align injured bones and joints or to treat joint contractures and congenital hip dysplasia
   c. Weights are usually 6.8–13.6 kg (15–30 lb) and amounts of weight may be adjusted initially until full fracture reduction is achieved as noted on x-ray
5. Balanced suspension (traction that is a hanging support to immobilize body part in a desired position)
   a. Used with skeletal traction to improve mobility while maintaining alignment of fracture

b. Body part is suspended using splints, ropes, and weights
c. Client can perform activities such as toileting and personal hygiene; bed linens can be changed without disturbing traction alignment
d. Risk for skin breakdown exists over bony prominences in contact with sheets (including back of head)

6. **Countertraction**: pulling force exerted in opposite direction to prevent client from sliding to end of bed, such as client's weight, elevating foot of bed, and elevating head of bed with cervical traction

NCLEX® 7. See Box 61–4 for nursing care of client in traction

NCLEX® C. **Cast care:** a cast is applied for immobilization to ensure stability of a fracture; see Box 61–5 (p. 1105) for associated nursing care

D. **Splinting and immobilization:** like casts, splints immobilize a fractured extremity to ensure stability after closed reduction and external fixation; teach client how to perform neurovascular assessment (color, temperature, pulses, and capillary refill, which should be 3 seconds or less)

Box 61–4

Nursing Care of Client in Traction

- Ensure that all ropes, weights, and pulleys are hanging freely, not shredded or torn, in a straight line.
- Bed linens should be kept off traction ropes.
- Teach client that weights should not be lifted for any reason (lifting of weights alters line of pull and could potentially interfere with bone healing).
- Ensure that ordered amount of weight is maintained at all times.
- Avoid jarring bed or equipment.
- Ensure that knots are not lying on or near pulley.
- Perform neurovascular assessment to monitor for superficial nerve damage (radial, median, ulnar, femoral, sciatic, peroneal nerves).
- Teach client how to perform circulatory assessment on unaffected and affected limb, comparing observations (color, temperature, capillary refill, pulses).
- Perform skin assessment to monitor and prevent skin breakdown on bony prominence and pressure areas.
- Assess client in skin traction for skin breakdown under traction boot or splint caused by friction and shear.
- Ensure that body is always kept in proper alignment to prevent complications such as external rotation of joint, increased pain, and poor healing of fracture.
- Provide pin care using normal saline solution or other agency-approved solution if client is in skeletal traction, and teach client how to monitor for infection at pin sites (fever, localized warmth, redness, swelling, abnormal drainage, and odor).
- Inform client to avoid massaging calves or reddened areas to prevent clot dislodgment caused by venous stasis.
- Encourage client to increase fluid intake (2500 mL/day unless contraindicated) and roughage (fresh fruits and vegetables) in diet to prevent constipation, urinary tract infection, and renal calculi.
- Teach client how to perform deep-breathing and coughing exercises to prevent respiratory complications.
- Encourage client to use overhead trapeze (and unaffected leg if possible) to reposition for comfort, shift weight to prevent skin breakdown, perform exercises, and assist with personal care, toileting, and bed linen changes.
- Encourage client to adhere to exercise regimen to maintain muscle tone, endurance, and prevent bone demineralization.
- Provide diversional activities and encourage social interaction with family and friends to prevent potential isolation.

Box 61–5

Nursing Care of Client in a Cast

- ➤ Teach client that plaster cast should not get wet and that cast padding should not be removed; if cast becomes soiled with feces, clean with a damp cloth or rub baking soda on soiled area to limit odor.
- ➤ Teach client that no foreign objects should be inserted into cast (sticks, food crumbs, etc.) to prevent skin breakdown; teach client how to smooth rough edges.
- ➤ Instruct client to avoid covering a new cast with blanket or plastic for extended periods (air cannot circulate and heat builds up in the cast).
- ➤ Turn client from side to side (using palms, not fingertips) every 2 hours to facilitate drying for first 24–72 hours (use of fingertips causes indentation and pressure areas when cast is dry).
- ➤ Explain that casts made with newer synthetic materials dry more quickly and allow faster mobility (often can bear weight within 30 minutes).
- ➤ Instruct client to apply ice for first 24 hours over fracture site to control edema, ensuring that ice is securely contained so cast does not become wet.
- ➤ Instruct client to elevate extremity above level of heart to promote venous return for first 24 hours after application.
- ➤ Instruct client to perform active range of motion (AROM) to joints above and below immobilized extremity.
- ➤ Teach client about signs and symptoms to report to healthcare provider: increasing pain in immobilized extremity, excessive swelling and discoloration of exposed limb, burning or tingling, sores, or foul odor under cast.

V. NURSING MANAGEMENT OF CLIENT UNDERGOING MUSCULOSKELETAL SURGERY

A. ***Laminectomy***: surgical incision of lamina of vertebrae to relieve symptoms of herniated intervertebral disc or relieve pressure within spinal canal caused by injury to vertebra

1. Provide standard postoperative care (see Chapter 48)

NCLEX®

2. Monitor for signs of nerve root compression
   a. Cervical: assess neurovascular status, hand grips, arm strength, finger mobility, ability to identify touch
   b. Lumbar: assess neurovascular status, leg strength, ability to wiggle toes, and identify touch
3. Assess for nausea, abdominal discomfort, urinary retention (report if unable to void within 8 hours after surgery), amount and character of drainage on dressing (clear liquid may indicate CSF leakage and may be accompanied by headache)
4. With cervical laminectomy, assess for respiratory difficulty or ineffective cough; voice hoarseness may indicate laryngeal nerve damage
5. Use *logroll* technique (turning a client as a unit) to turn and reposition client; maintain proper alignment of spine at all times

NCLEX®

6. Position client so head is flat or minimally elevated to minimize stress on incision: use small pillow under thighs when supine and between thighs when side-lying (lumbar), or use cervical collar and small pillow under neck (cervical)
7. Help client to "rise as a unit" when getting out of bed; client is often allowed to sit on side and dangle legs during evening of surgery and ambulate next day
8. Instruct client that paresthesia (numbness and tingling of extremities) may not be relieved immediately after procedure

B. ***Internal fixation***: fracture immobilization with a metal device (made of screws, pins, and/or plates) that is surgically inserted to realign and maintain a fracture

1. Perform neurovascular assessment regularly; report adverse changes in color, temperature, sensation, or motion promptly
2. Assess and treat postoperative pain promptly; report pain that becomes more severe or is unrelieved by analgesics
3. Perform standard postoperative assessments and care
4. Collaborate with physical therapy to aid client mobility
5. Teach signs of infection to report: elevated temperature, localized pain and warmth, tenderness, chills, malaise, and changes in neurovascular status of affected extremity

C. External fixation: fracture immobilization using a frame connected to pins inserted perpendicular to long axis of bone

1. Assess neurovascular status at least every 4 hours
2. Assess for signs of infection and report promptly; provide pin care as per protocol
3. Perform standard postoperative care assessments and interventions
4. Explain that device allows greater mobility during healing

D. Joint replacement (hip and knee)

1. *Hip replacement* involves implantation of a prosthesis to replace hip joint in conditions such as rheumatoid arthritis, malignant bone tumors, arthritis associated with Paget's disease, juvenile rheumatoid arthritis, and hip fractures
2. *Knee replacement* involves implantation of a prosthesis to substitute for femoral condyles and tibial joint surfaces when knee joint function is severely impaired by degenerative disease or injury
3. Advantages of joint replacement: substantial relief of pain, improved function and quality of life
4. Provide standard preoperative and postoperative nursing care and associated client teaching
5. NCLEX® Provide and teach client about hip dislocation precautions
   a. Position hip and leg to maintain proper alignment, avoiding extremes of internal or external rotation or extreme hip flexion; prescriptions for postoperative positioning generally allow for client to be repositioned to nonoperative side
   b. Prevent hip flexion more than 90 degrees: elevate head of bed only to 30–45 degrees; keep operative leg supported and extended when getting out of bed; avoid low chairs when client sits at bedside; avoid any other position that results in more than 90-degree hip flexion
   c. Prevent adduction: use an abduction pillow; avoid crossing legs, twisting to reach for objects behind, driving a car, or taking tub baths for at least 4–6 weeks
   d. Modify equipment during recovery to avoid 90-degree hip flexion (raised toilet seats, platform under chair, use of reacher device, long-handled shoe horn, and sock puller)
6. Implement measures that reduce effects of immobility and that foster increased mobility with hip replacement: passive range of motion (ROM) and physical therapy exercises beginning on first postoperative day, progressive ambulation maintaining weight-bearing limits on affected side if prescribed, using walker as mobility aid
7. NCLEX® Teach signs and symptoms to report to healthcare provider
   a. Infection: redness, swelling, abnormal drainage, foul odor, and elevated temperature
   b. DVT: pain, sudden swelling in affected extremity, enlargement of superficial veins, skin discoloration, and localized warmth
8. Instruct client that home care management program will include the following:
   a. Ongoing nursing assessment of pain management
   b. Periodic dressing changes and monitoring for infection
   c. NCLEX® Monitoring and adjustment of coagulation status weekly if taking warfarin and less often if taking enoxaparin, a low-molecular-weight heparin
   d. An exercise program assisted by a physical therapist to assess and restore muscle strength and ROM
9. NCLEX® Instruct client to inform all healthcare providers (dentists, etc.) of history of joint replacement surgery so that prophylactic antibiotics can be prescribed as necessary
10. Inform client that periodic x-rays will be required as follow-up throughout lifetime
11. NCLEX® With knee replacement: continuous passive motion (CPM) machine may be put in place immediately after surgery
    a. Ensure that client's limb and knee joint are positioned correctly (limb is centered in device and knee is positioned over area when mechanical flexion and extension occur)
    b. Device should be used at least 8 of every 24 hours and increased as client tolerates it
    c. Note CPM settings (degrees of flexion, number of minutes per cycle) and client's tolerance of device

E. Amputation

1. Common levels of amputation of lower extremity includes toe, foot (part or all), Syme (ankle disarticulation), below knee and above knee
2. Two types of amputation are open (guillotine) and closed (flap)
   a. Open type is used when infection is present and wound is left open; a second surgery is done later to close wound
   b. Closed type involves covering end of wound with flap of skin
3. Provide standard postoperative care
4. Treat postoperative pain with opioid analgesics and provide client teaching about nonpharmacological pain management techniques

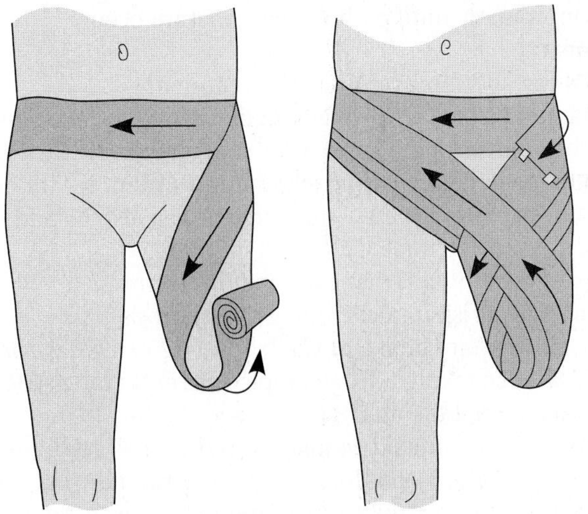

Figure 61–3
Residual limb wrapping in a distal to proximal direction reduces edema and allows conical shape to form in preparation for prosthesis.

5. Assess for and teach client to report signs of infection or complications: redness, elevated temperature, and/or unusual, foul-smelling drainage; abrasions; and any other signs of skin breakdown
6. Assess and maintain placement of residual limb-shrinking devices, such as rigid plaster cast, elastic bandage, shrinker sock, or elastic stockinette, to reduce postoperative edema
7. Use proper technique for wrapping residual limb with elastic bandage, if used (see Figure 61–3)
8. Instruct client to perform upper-extremity active ROM exercises daily
9. Turn and reposition client every 2 hours
10. Assist client to lay prone for 30 minutes three to four times/day (if client is able and if part of standard of care) and avoid elevating or sitting with residual limb on pillows for prolonged amount of time to prevent flexion contractures; limb may be elevated above heart level for first 24 hours after surgery to reduce edema
11. *NCLEX®* Explain that phantom pain may persist in amputated extremity because of irritation of residual nerve endings; this is normal and real; discomfort will be treated with analgesics or other interventions
12. *NCLEX®* Teach client how to care for residual limb
    a. Wash daily using warm water and bacteriostatic soap
    b. Rinse and gently pat dry thoroughly
    c. Expose to air for at least 20 minutes after washing
    d. Avoid use of lotions, alcohol, powder, or oils unless prescribed by health care provider
    e. Change cotton or wool limb sock daily, wash sock using mild soap and dry flat; discard sock that is in poor condition
13. Assist client to cope with changes in body image and participate in physical therapy to aid in rehabilitation

VI. OSTEOPOROSIS

A. Overview

1. **Osteoporosis**: disease characterized by bone demineralization (loss of calcium [Ca^{++}] and phosphate), which causes bone to become more fragile and susceptible to fractures, especially bones such as hip, spine, and wrist
2. Bone resorption happens faster than bone formation
3. Can be classified as either primary or secondary
    a. Primary: aging, postmenopausal status in women (deficient estrogen), low testosterone level in men, decreased calcium intake, vitamin D deficiency
    b. Secondary: immobility, malnutrition (such as with alcoholism), malabsorption, or effects of drugs used to treat another condition (corticosteroids, antithyroid drugs, antiepileptics, and some antacids)

NCLEX® B. Nursing assessment

1. Risk factors include ethnicity (white from European descent or Asian), family history, female sex, being thin with small frame, increasing age, inadequate dietary Ca^{++}, sedentary lifestyle, cigarette smoking, excessive alcohol intake, chronic liver disease, anorexia, malabsorption, and use of certain medications
2. Back pain with activities such as bending, stooping, or lifting, and is aggravated by direct palpation
3. Hip or pelvic pain that is more noticeable with weight bearing; can interfere with balance
4. Physical changes such as reduction in height (vertebral compression), kyphosis of dorsal spine, and evidence of vertebral deterioration and/or reduced bone mineral density (BMD)

5. Client may be asymptomatic until pathological fracture occurs

NCLEX®

C. Therapeutic management

1. Provide client teaching about prevention and treatment
   - **a.** Take adequate amounts of Ca^{++} throughout lifetime to decrease risk
   - **b.** Recommend food sources that provide Ca^{++} and vitamin D: dark green leafy vegetables (such as broccoli, bok choy, collard greens, spinach), sardines, salmon with bone, dairy products (such as milk, cottage cheese, cheese, yogurt); Ca^{++} supplements can also be added to dietary intake
   - **c.** Weight-bearing exercises to force Ca^{++} back into bone
   - **d.** Safety measures to prevent falls that can result in fractures
   - **e.** BMD tests for clients at risk for developing osteoporosis
   - **f.** Recommended daily dietary intake of Ca^{++}: 1000–1200 mg/day for premenopausal women and postmenopausal women taking estrogen replacement therapy (ERT) and 1500 mg/day for postmenopausal women who are not taking ERT
2. Assess home safety and recommend changes to reduce risk for injury that could lead to fracture: hand rails, clear (unobstructed) stairs and floor pathways, firm mattress, and proper use of mobility aids
3. Provide gentle physical care to reduce risk of injury; promote client's use of good body mechanics; assist with proper use of back brace if prescribed
4. Medication therapy
   - **a.** Possible temporary use of hormonal replacement therapy (HRT) after menopause; usually given in form of a pill or skin patch
   - **b.** Calcitonin (available in U.S.): naturally occurring hormone secreted by thyroid gland; currently available as a nasal spray or injection; slows bone loss, increases spinal bone density, relieves pain from bone fractures, and reduces risk for spinal and hip fractures
   - NCLEX® **c.** Bisphosphonates: prevent bone resorption in men and women with glucocorticoid-induced osteoporosis; take dose with a glass of water at least 30 minutes before eating; remain standing or sitting for 30 minutes after dose
   - **d.** Raloxifene: used to prevent or treat osteoporosis; selective receptor modulator (SERM) that prevents bone loss

D. Client teaching

1. In addition to measures noted above, reinforce importance of weight-bearing exercises (jogging, walking, hiking, stair climbing, etc.)
2. Encourage client to stop smoking and avoid excessive intake of alcohol

VII. OSTEOMYELITIS

A. Overview

1. **Osteomyelitis**: acute or chronic infection, usually caused by *Staphylococcus aureus*, occurring from direct or indirect invasion of infectious organisms; see Figure 61–4
2. Long bones are common sites of infection in children, and spine, hip, and foot are common sites of infection in adults
3. Osteomyelitis warrants aggressive immediate treatment with antibiotics or surgery (wound debridement) if infection of bone is extensive

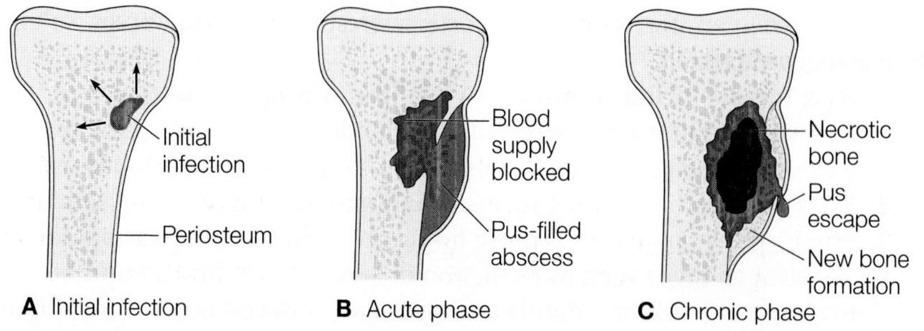

Figure 61–4

Osteomyelitis. (**A**) Site of initial infection. Bacteria enter bone and multiply, initiating inflammatory response. (**B**) Acute phase, with spread of infection to other parts of bone. Pus forms, edema occurs, and vascular supply is compromised. If infection reaches outer margin of bone, periosteum lifts, and ischemia and necrosis can occur. (**C**) Chronic phase. Necrotic bone separates, a new layer of bone forms around necrotic bone, and sinus develops to allow wound to drain.

NCLEX® **B. Nursing assessment**

1. Observe for symptoms of local and/or systemic infection: fever (often above 101°F [38.3°C]) and chills; restlessness; swelling, redness, and warmth at site; bone pain unrelieved by analgesics or rest and aggravated by movement
2. Wound culture, bone scan, CT scan, and MRI diagnose and assess extent of infection

NCLEX® **C. Therapeutic management**

1. Explain all therapies and interventions to client and family
2. Assess pain and evaluate effectiveness of pain management measures diligently
3. Provide ongoing education and emotional support since infection is serious and may require long-term IV antibiotic therapy followed up with oral therapy, hyperbaric oxygen therapy, or surgery
4. NCLEX® Use sterile technique for all dressing changes and manipulation of affected limb; handle extremity very gently
5. NCLEX® Avoid activities that increase circulation to affected area or cause edema, pain, and pathological fractures (exercise, application of heat, or dependent position of extremity)
6. Immobilize affected extremity as prescribed and keep body in proper alignment
7. Monitor temperature at least every 2–4 hours as prescribed
8. Provide cool environment, light clothing, antipyretic medication, antibiotics, and other therapies as prescribed
9. Keep client well hydrated to prevent dehydration from insensible water loss
10. Instruct and assist client with interventions to prevent complications associated with immobility (turn and reposition every 2 hours, coughing and deep breathing exercises, etc.)

D. Client teaching

1. Medication information, including importance of taking antibiotics as prescribed for full course of therapy
2. Importance of rest and nutrient-dense diet with adequate fluids to facilitate healing and prevent constipation and dehydration
3. NCLEX® Importance of limb immobilization during treatment
4. Possible components of long-term management (sterile technique for wound care), medication regimen (including instruction on venous access devices if needed), proper diet, rest, follow-up visits, and laboratory tests
5. Adverse effects of antibiotic therapy such as ototoxicity and nephrotoxicity (aminoglycosides) and hepatotoxicity (cephalosporins)

VIII. MUSCULAR DYSTROPHIES (MDs)

A. Overview

1. Group of genetic childhood disorders characterized by muscle fiber degeneration and progressive muscle wasting
2. Types of MD include Duchenne (most common), Becker, facioscapulohumeral, and Emery-Dreifuss
3. Significant risk factor is family history
4. Each type differs in regard to muscle groups affected, age at onset, rate of progression, and pattern of inheritance

B. Nursing assessment

1. Muscle biopsy confirms diagnosis (shows degeneration of muscle fibers)
2. EMG identifies origin of muscle weakness (muscle destruction, nerve damage)
3. NCLEX® Progressive muscle weakness, hypotonia (loss of muscle mass), delayed development of motor skills such as walking; frequent falls, fatigue when walking, running, or climbing stairs, waddling gait, lordosis, muscle contractures, positive Gowers maneuver to stand (supports body on arms and legs, then pushes off floor and rests hand on knee, and pushes self upright)
4. NCLEX® Ptosis (drooping of the eyelid) and impaired chewing and swallowing may be noted
5. Delayed intellectual development is seen with some forms of MD
6. Enlargement of muscle (pseudohypertrophy) caused by fatty infiltration of muscle
7. Cardiomyopathy or dysrhythmia may be present with Emery-Dreifuss form

C. Therapeutic management

1. Provide support and assist family with decision-making process for home management of condition
   a. Develop home care plan to support as much independence as possible
   b. Modify home environment to support client's maximal functional ability
2. Provide ongoing monitoring of growth and development, nutrition (supplement as needed), physical activity, ability to perform ADLs (provide adaptive aids as needed), and social and coping skills

NCLEX® 3. Assist client and family to cope with progressive and incapacitating nature of disease; refer to local support groups including Muscular Dystrophy Association of America

NCLEX® 4. Encourage family to interact with client based on developmental rather than chronological age

NCLEX® 5. Teach family strategies to prevent skin breakdown (frequent skin care and linen changes if incontinent, turn and reposition at least every 2 hours, use of protective skin barriers, and adequate fluid intake)

6. Perform passive ROM exercises to maintain function in unaffected extremities and prevent or delay contractures in affected extremities
7. Medication therapy: there is no effective drug therapy; corticosteroids are often used to increase muscle strength

D. Client teaching

1. Provide information about healthcare team member roles, including those involved in home care program for client

NCLEX® 2. Teach infection prevention strategies (maintain immunization status, avoid crowds and those who are ill)

NCLEX® 3. Teach injury prevention strategies (body mechanics for caregiver, oxygen safety, emergency backup system if home ventilator in use, emergency evacuation plan in case of fire)

4. Encourage family members to seek genetic counseling (parents, female siblings, maternal aunts, and female offspring)
5. Provide family with information on community support groups and agencies with respite services to prevent role strain

IX. PAGET'S DISEASE (OSTEITIS DEFORMANS)

A. Overview

1. Progressive skeletal bone disorder characterized by excessive local bone resorption (osteoclast activity) followed by rapid bone growth that leads to larger, disorganized, and weaker bone
2. Normal bone marrow is also replaced by vascular, fibrous connective tissue
3. Generally affects femur, tibia, pelvis, vertebrae, and skull

B. Nursing assessment

1. X-ray is most definitive diagnostic test; serum alkaline phosphatase may be elevated; bone scan shows thickened cortex and curved contours
2. Mild case may be undetected because client can be asymptomatic for years

NCLEX® 3. Symptoms include bone pain (most common), increased skin temperature over bone, and other local symptoms
   a. If skull is affected, headache, hearing loss, cranial nerve palsies, and enlarged skull can occur
   b. Pelvis or femur involvement can cause pelvic and hip pain and pathological fractures
   c. Bone deformity can lead to bowing of lower extremities (producing a waddling gait) and collapse of vertebrae (kyphosis and loss of height)

4. Metabolic effects include symptoms of hypercalcemia in immobilized clients and risk of renal calculi from hypercalciuria
5. Complications include pathological fractures (common and may be first indicator of disease) and osteogenic sarcoma (form of bone cancer) rarely

C. Therapeutic management

1. Prognosis is good if treatment is started before major deformity occurs
2. Medication therapy: calcitonin (in U.S.), bisphosphonates (such as pamidronate, alandronate, and tiludronate), zoledronic acid, calcium and vitamin D supplements, and acetaminophen or nonsteroidal anti-inflammatory drugs (NSAIDs) to treat pain from bone deformity, arthritis, or neurological complications
3. Surgery may be indicated to treat severe bone fracture or for hip or knee replacement caused by osteoarthritis
4. If skull is affected, assist with diet modification, dentures, and eating utensils because teeth may become weak from disease
5. Hearing aid may be recommended if hearing loss results from disease
6. Back brace may be prescribed to relieve back pain and provide support
7. Assist client to maintain mobility using correct body mechanics, assistive devices for ambulation, correct body mechanics, and activity or exercise protocols that minimize fatigue and prevent injury

D. Client teaching

1. Explain importance of medication management to interrupt ongoing bone deformity and loss of bone strength

NCLEX®
2. Eat a balanced diet, high in Ca^{++} (1000–1500 mg/day) and vitamin D (at least 400 units/day); vitamin D can be obtained from exposure to sunlight
3. Inform healthcare provider of any history of kidney stones or disease before taking Ca^{++}
4. Participate in an exercise program to maintain skeletal muscle health, ideal body weight, and joint mobility
5. Sleep on a firm mattress if back discomfort is present; if back brace is needed, wear undershirt to prevent skin breakdown under brace and do not drive without brace (safety measure)
6. Modify environment at home to prevent falls that may lead to subsequent fractures

X. FRACTURES

A. Overview

1. A fracture is a break in continuity of a bone caused by trauma (including falls), bone decalcification disorders, or severe twisting
2. May be classified as closed/simple fracture (bone breaks but skin remains intact) or open/compound (broken ends of bone penetrate skin)
3. NCLEX® Other classification of fractures (see Figure 61–5 and Table 61–1)
4. When a bone breaks, healing process occurs in three phases: inflammatory, reparative (new bone forms) and remodeling (ends of fracture unite)

B. Nursing assessment

NCLEX®

1. Deformity: caused by break in continuity of bone and pull of muscles on fragmented bones
2. Edema, erythema, and bruising in affected area
3. Pain and tenderness over affected area; muscle spasms may occur near fractured bone
4. **Crepitation** (grating sensation when broken bone fragments rub together) may be palpable

C. Therapeutic management

NCLEX®

1. Perform frequent neurovascular assessment; report abnormal findings
2. Immobilize joints above and below fracture
3. Cover open fracture wound with sterile dressing
4. Manage fracture pain with prescribed analgesics

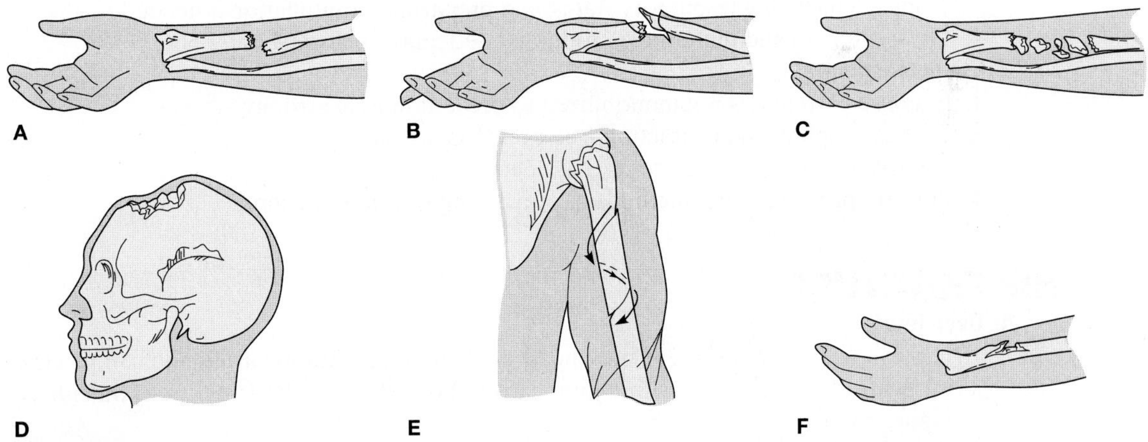

Figure 61–5 Types of fractures. (**A**) Closed, (**B**) open, (**C**) comminuted, (**D**) depressed, (**E**) spiral, (**F**) greenstick.

Table 61–1 Types of Fractures

Type of Fracture	Description
Avulsion	Results from tearing of supporting tendons and ligaments
Comminuted	Broken bone fragments into more than two pieces
Compression	Bone is crushed
Impacted	Ends of broken bone are driven into each other
Depressed	Fracture in which bone structure is broken and pressed inward, such as in skull fracture
Spiral	Break spreads in a spiral fashion along bone shaft; usually caused by sports injuries and child abuse
Greenstick	Incomplete break in bone where one side splinters leaving other side bent or intact; more common in children

5. Elevate fractured extremity to reduce swelling and pain
6. Apply ice to affected extremity
7. Treatment methods for fracture include open or closed reduction, internal or external fixation, and application of a cast or traction
8. Assist in fracture reduction: closed reduction involves nonsurgical external manipulation to realign bones; open reduction involves a surgical procedure to realign bones
9. Fixation of bone fragments
   a. Internal fixation is performed during open reduction surgery and involves placement of screws, pins, plates, or intermedullary rods into bone
   b. External fixation involves insertion of skeletal pins through bone fragments; pins are attached to an external rigid frame; performed often for severe trauma to bone and tissue; principles of skeletal traction care apply
10. Assess and maintain traction as prescribed; see section on nursing care of client in traction
11. Assess and provide care to client with a cast; see section on nursing care of a client in a cast

D. Complications

NCLEX®

1. **Compartment syndrome**
   a. Impairment of circulation within inelastic fascia caused by external pressure (>30 mmHg) that results in tissue death and nerve injury
   b. External pressure can be created by casts, splints, or dressings
   c. Manifestations include unrelieved pain, diminished or absent pulses distal to injury, cyanosis of extremity, tingling or diminished sensation (paresthesia), loss of sensation, pallor, coolness of extremity, and weakness
   d. Treatment is bivalving cast (splitting cast lengthwise and resecuring with elastic wrap) if cast is too tight
2. Infection: wound drainage, fever, pain, and odor; treated with antibiotics

NCLEX®

3. Fat embolism (emergency situation)
   a. Signs include chest pain, dyspnea, tachycardia, decreased O_2 saturation, apprehension, changes in LOC, petechiae on upper trunk and axilla
   b. Immediate treatment includes oxygen therapy, administering IV fluids, maintaining bedrest, monitoring VS including respiratory status, and preparing for intubation if needed
4. DVT: calf pain and tenderness, swelling, or edema; see also Chapter 56

E. Client teaching

1. Exercise extremities not immobilized to prevent muscle atrophy
2. Cast care, splint, and/or traction (see previous discussions)
3. Neurovascular self-assessments that need to be performed
4. Pin care procedure and methods of preventing wound infection

XI. HIP FRACTURE

A. Overview

1. Hip can fracture at different sites: head, neck, and trochanteric areas and can be classified as intracapsular (fracture is within joint capsule) or extracapsular (fracture is outside joint capsule); see Figure 61–6
2. Incidence increases with age; 90% of hip fractures are caused by falls
3. Intracapsular fractures are treated preoperatively with skin traction (to immobilize area and reduce muscle spasms), followed by open reduction with internal fixation (ORIF) with femoral head replacement, or by total hip replacement
4. Extracapsular fractures are treated preoperatively with skin traction or balanced suspension traction, followed by ORIF using hardware (screws, pins, wires, and nail plates)

NCLEX®

B. Nursing assessment

1. Monitor LOC and assess for other injuries if fracture caused by a fall
2. Perform neurovascular assessment on affected extremity (report adverse changes: cool, pale skin, diminished pulses, and delayed capillary refill)

Memory Aid

Use the 5 *Ps* to remember abnormal neurovascular assessment findings: pain, pallor, paresthesia, pulselessness (or decreased pulses), and paralysis (or weakness).

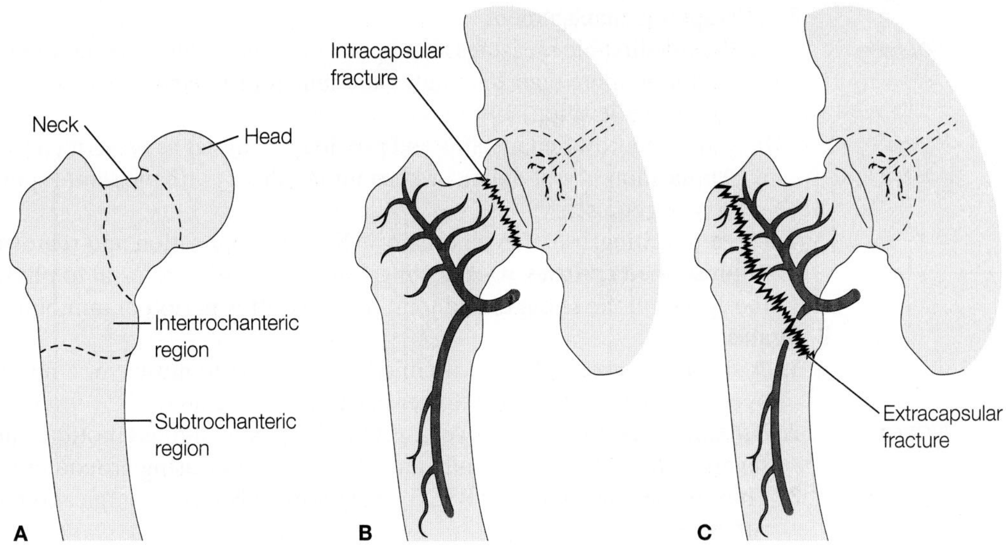

Figure 61–6

Hip fractures. (**A**) Can occur in head, neck, or trochanteric regions of femur. (**B**) An intracapsular fracture affects femur head or neck. (**C**) An extracapsular fracture occurs across trochanteric region. All fractures disrupt blood supply to bone.

3. Extremity of affected hip will be shorter than unaffected extremity and is often externally rotated

NCLEX®

C. Therapeutic management

1. Provide standard preoperative care and teaching; see Chapter 48
2. Monitor preoperative use of skin traction (Buck's traction); assess skin under traction boot/splint for breakdown each shift
3. Provide standard postoperative assessments and care as outlined in Chapter 48, with additional ongoing assessment of neurovascular status of affected leg
4. Maintain procedures to prevent hip dislocation: proper alignment of leg and hip, preventing internal or external rotation and extreme hip flexion, keeping abductor pillow in place
5. Reposition client as prescribed (often to unaffected side)
6. Note and maintain any restrictions on weight bearing; instruct client in use of walker as prescribed
7. Assess pain and administer analgesics as prescribed (patient-controlled analgesia [PCA] may be used postoperatively)
8. Assess and maintain function of wound drains (such as Hemovac or Jackson-Pratt); document amount and character of drainage, which should decrease during first 48 hours postoperatively
9. Implement blood salvage procedures to collect, filter, and auto-transfuse salvaged blood to client
10. Assist client with progressive ambulation schedule prescribed by healthcare provider; collaborate with physical therapist

D. Client teaching

1. Reinforce teaching about postoperative course, pain management strategies, and measures to avoid complications related to immobility and infection

NCLEX®

2. Reinforce postoperative precautions to prevent hip dislocation (no hip flexion greater than 90 degrees, internal rotation of affected hip, or adduction of affected hip); these include such activities as avoiding low chairs, using raised toilet seat, no excessive bending
3. Client may require transfer to subacute unit of skilled nursing facility for further rehabilitation before returning to home or original residence (such as long-term care)

XII. LOCAL MUSCULOSKELETAL INJURIES

A. Sprains

1. A **sprain** is a stretch and/or tear of a ligament surrounding a joint, usually from pulling forces going in opposite directions (such as when stepping onto a very uneven surface or during a fall); classified by degree of ligament injury (1 = mild: overstretching or minimal tear, 2 = moderate: partial tear, 3 = severe: complete tear or ligament rupture)

NCLEX®

2. Nursing assessment: popping sound at time of injury, pain over injured area that increases with movement, rapid swelling, discoloration, loss of joint function, possible adverse neurovascular changes, and increasing joint instability and weight-bearing difficulty with grade 2 or 3 injuries (often ankles and knees are involved)

3. Therapeutic management

NCLEX®

   a. Provide first-aid measures to support joint and reduce edema using *RICE* for first 24–48 hours (*R*est, *I*ce for no more than 20 minutes at a time four to eight times per day, *C*ompression with elastic bandage, *E*levation)
   b. Assess neurovascular status and provide analgesics as prescribed
   c. Application of cast, splint, or knee immobilizer (with moderate sprain) or surgery (with severe sprain) may be required
4. Client teaching: use of analgesics or NSAIDs; application and removal of elastic support bandages; use of prescribed crutches, walker, sling, or cane; possible referral to physical therapy for exercise program to regain muscle strength and joint mobility after period of immobilization

B. Strains

1. A **strain** is a stretch injury with microscopic tears to muscle or a muscle–tendon unit from mechanical overloading (often involves lower back or hamstrings)

NCLEX®

2. Nursing assessment: pain, swelling, muscle spasms, limited motion, and possible muscle weakness; severe strains can cause significant bleeding and bruising around muscle
3. Therapeutic management: RICE, analgesics or NSAIDs, surgical repair if muscle or tendon rupture
4. Client teaching: use of analgesics or NSAIDs; avoid overuse; proper use of body mechanics and warm-up and cool-down exercises

C. Shoulder and knee injuries

1. Rotator cuff injury affects muscles that control arm movement and include tendonitis, bursitis, and partial and complete muscle tears
   a. Signs of rotator cuff injury include shoulder pain that may worsen with movement or when lying on affected side, limited range of motion, and inability to maintain abduction of arm at shoulder (drop-arm test)
   b. Treatment includes joint rest, NSAIDs, moist heat, possible physical therapy, and surgery (if torn rotator cuff)
2. Knee injury results from ligament tears, injury to knee meniscus, or dislocation of patella; often occurs during sports activity that leads to falls or twisting of knee joint
   a. Often affects anterior cruciate ligament (ACL) or medial collateral ligament (MCL)
   b. Signs of knee injury include immediate pain and a tearing or popping sound at time of injury, with knee swelling and loss of joint function
   c. Treatment includes RICE, physical therapy, and possibly surgery
3. Joint dislocation injury leads to bone displacement from normal position and loss of joint articulation; can be partial (called *subluxation*) or complete
   a. Signs of joint dislocation include pain, deformity, and limited motion of affected joint
   b. Treatment for dislocation includes immediate reduction using manual traction followed by short-term joint immobility and gradual return to normal activity; surgery may be needed to realign a joint or prevent complications such as neurovascular injury

Memory Aid

Use RICE for musculoskeletal injuries (rest, ice, compression, and elevation).

XIII. GOUT

A. Overview

1. **Gout**: systemic metabolic disease characterized by elevated serum uric acid level (hyperuricemia) that leads to urate crystals being deposited in joints and other tissues
2. Primary form occurs because of abnormal purine metabolism; secondary form occurs secondary to another health problem
3. Hyperuricemia is caused by increased purine synthesis and/or decreased renal excretion of uric acid; may also be caused by prolonged fasting and excessive alcohol intake
4. May be asymptomatic (elevated uric acid only), intermittent (occasional flare-ups associated with acute symptoms in joints such as great toe or knee), or chronic (with urate crystal deposits under skin and in organs such as kidneys)

B. Nursing assessment

NCLEX® 1. Risk factors: obesity, excessive weight gain, excessive alcohol intake, impaired renal function, hypertension, chemotherapy for leukemia and certain lymphomas, certain thiazide diuretics, aspirin, and tuberculosis medications

NCLEX® 2. Signs with acute flare-up include possible low-grade fever, malaise, inflammation and swelling of affected joint, and excruciating pain

NCLEX® 3. Chronic gout leads to deposits of sodium urate crystals under skin, which are seen as irregularly shaped nodules called *tophi*, and possible renal calculi

NCLEX® **C. Therapeutic management**

1. Encourage client to adhere to activity restriction such as bedrest and immobilize affected extremity during acute exacerbation; keep affected joint in position of mild flexion
2. Prevent any bed linens from touching affected extremity because of extreme tenderness (bed cradle and/or footboard can be used)
3. Monitor uric acid levels to prevent exacerbation and evaluate effectiveness of treatment
4. Restrict foods high in purines (such as liver, kidney sweetbreads, herring, sardines, anchovies, scallops, organ meats, gravy, and beer)
5. Medication therapy: anti-inflammatory agents (such as colchicine, NSAIDs, or corticosteroids), antihyperuricemic agent (such as allopurinol), and/or uricosuric (such as probenecid)

D. Client education

1. Reinforce teaching of therapeutic management above
2. Action, side/adverse effects of medication; take doses with meals to avoid gastric irritation
3. Avoid alcohol when taking medication and limit use if not on medication to avoid flare-ups

NCLEX® 4. Drink at least 2 liters of fluid per day to reduce risk of uric acid stone formation

XIV. DEGENERATIVE JOINT DISEASE (DJD) OR OSTEOARTHRITIS (OA)

A. Overview

1. Slowly progressive deterioration of axial or articulating joints, especially weight-bearing joints and those with repeated stress, such as hands, knees, hips, and back; bone buildup in affected area also occurs
2. Deterioration of articular cartilage causes pain and decreases joint function
3. With progressive damage, bones can ultimately rub against each other, causing more severe symptoms

NCLEX® 4. Risk factors include increasing age (primarily affects middle-age to older adults), obesity (generally causes arthritis of knees), repetitive joint injuries (sports, accidents, or work-related injuries), smoking, and genetics

B. Nursing assessment

1. Disease is diagnosed with physical exam and history of symptoms and confirmed by x-ray

NCLEX® 2. Joint pain occurs with movement and weight-bearing and is relieved by rest in early stage

3. Pain can occur with very little movement or at rest as condition worsens
4. There is limited ROM with progressive loss of joint function over time, which interferes with normal activity, including performing activities of daily living (ADLs)

NCLEX® 5. Other manifestations include joint stiffness after rest periods, crepitation, skeletal muscle disuse atrophy, and occasionally joint swelling

6. Deterioration in spine may cause pain (that can radiate), stiffness, and muscle spasms

NCLEX® 7. Hands may exhibit **Heberden's nodes** (raised bony growths over distal interphalangeal joints) or **Bouchard's nodes** (raised bony growths over proximal interphalangeal joint of hand)

C. Therapeutic management

NCLEX® 1. Assist client in planning scheduled rest periods to relieve stress on joints

2. Encourage participation in prescribed exercise program that limits stress on affected joints but maintains joint flexibility and improves muscle strength
3. Encourage client to lose weight if indicated or maintain normal weight to prevent excessive stress on joints

NCLEX® 4. Instruct client about use of prescribed heat/cold therapy to affected joint for temporary pain relief
   - a. Heat therapy may include hot packs, compresses, moist heat applications, and/or paraffin dips
   - b. Cold therapy may be prescribed when joint is acutely inflamed

5. Assist client with ADLs as needed
6. Joint protection measures to affected areas include maintaining joints in functional position, avoiding flexion of hips or knees, using small pillows (not large) under head or knees, and using any prescribed splints or braces during periods of inflammation

NCLEX®

7. Medication therapy
   a. Acetaminophen or topical agents are generally used first
   b. Anti-inflammatory agents such as NSAIDs may also be used
   c. If NSAIDs are ineffective in controlling inflammation and pain, glucocorticosteroids may be injected directly into joint
8. Surgical treatment options with severe disease may include osteotomy (resection of bone to correct deformity and realign bone) or total joint replacement (hip or knee)

D. Client education

1. Nature of and treatment for disease; principles of good body mechanics
2. Correct use of assistive devices; encourage use as needed
3. Plan daily activities and tasks to allow for scheduled rest periods; limit exercise during periods of severe inflammation
4. Avoid activities that put excessive stress on joints and cause pain; stop exercise if pain occurs

XV. BACK PAIN AND HERNIATED INTERVERTEBRAL DISK

A. Overview

1. Pain may result from degeneration over time, spinal stenosis (narrowing of spinal canal), acute injury such as sprain or strain, repeated minor stress or injury over years, or **herniated intervertebral disk** (herniation of nucleus pulposus)
2. Overall health of back muscles determines degree of risk for injury as well as speed of recovery; lower back is often affected
3. Common locations for injury are at cervical level (C5 to C6 or C6 to C7) and at lumbar level (L4 to L5 or L5 to S1)

NCLEX®

B. Nursing assessment

1. Risk factors include but are not limited to degenerative disc disease, poor muscle tone of lower back, sedentary lifestyle, obesity, poor body mechanics, smoking, and stress
2. Client will report pain (caused by a shift of one vertebra on another or pinching and irritation of spinal nerve root)
3. Pain may be aggravated by muscle spasms of paravertebral tissue or activities that increase intraspinal pressure (e.g., coughing, sneezing, lifting, bending over)
4. Cervical degeneration or injury leading to herniated disk results in upper back pain radiating to scapulae, pectoral muscles, shoulders, arms and hands, and upper-extremity neurological deficits such as weakness, numbness, parasthesias, and decreased biceps and supinator reflexes
5. Lumbar degeneration or injury leading to herniated disk results in lower back pain that can radiate to hip and down affected leg (sciatica); pain may be elicited with straight leg test; deep tendon reflexes may be decreased or absent; bowel or bladder dysfunction can occur

NCLEX®

C. Therapeutic management

1. Conservative treatment includes bedrest if there are no neurological deficits
2. Client should maintain alignment of head, neck, and spine (cervical) or lie on side with hips and knees flexed and a small pillow between knees (lumbar)
3. Heat or cold therapy may be prescribed to reduce muscle spasms (heat) or relieve inflammation or swelling (cold)
4. Cervical or pelvic skin traction may be prescribed to stretch disk interspaces and thereby reduce pain and/or muscle spasms
5. A cervical collar or brace may be prescribed to limit neck movement and maintain head in a neutral or slightly flexed position
6. When pain and inflammation subside, cervical or lumbar back exercises may be prescribed to strengthen local muscles
7. Medication therapy: includes but is not limited to analgesics, NSAIDs, and muscle relaxants; epidural corticosteroid injections may be used if conservative treatment is ineffective
8. Surgical treatment may include laminectomy (discussed earlier in chapter), laminotomy (division of lamina), diskectomy (removal of herniated portion of disk and related tissue), or diskectomy with fusion (insertion of bone graft to fuse vertebrae above and below area of disk removal)

D. Client teaching

1. Use of prescribed medications and/or prescribed heat or cold therapy
2. Importance of adhering to initial activity restrictions (bedrest) and plan for gradual increase in activity
3. Importance of attaining and maintaining body weight within normal range

4. Prescribed exercises to improve muscle strength, flexibility, and tone; client may be referred to physical therapist
5. Importance of using correct posture (including when sitting, standing, and walking) and body mechanics (keep back straight; bend knees when lifting objects; do not lift above elbow level), and avoiding long periods of sitting
6. Need to sleep on a firm mattress (have client demonstrate correct sleeping position)
   a. Cervical problems: avoid prone position; maintain alignment of neck, spine, and hips during sleep
   b. Lumbar problems: side-lying or with hips and knees flexed and a small pillow between knees
7. Need to stop smoking if this is a risk factor for client
8. Use of prescribed brace or corset (if needed) to prevent flexion and extension motions of lower back

XVI. CONGENITAL MUSCULOSKELETAL HEALTH PROBLEMS

A. *Clubfoot*

1. Overview
   a. Foot is twisted and fixed in an abnormal position; may be one or a combination of four deformities: plantar flexion (foot is lower than heel), dorsiflexion (heel is lower than foot), varus deviation (foot turns in), or valgus deviation (foot turns out)
   b. Involves unilateral or bilateral bone deformity, malposition, and soft tissue contracture
   c. Exact cause is unknown but may include abnormal intrauterine position, neuromuscular or vascular problems, and possible familial tendency
2. Nursing assessment
   a. Foot is twisted in a fixed abnormal position, which is easily recognized at birth; may be recognized on prenatal ultrasound
   b. Affected foot is usually smaller and shorter, with an empty heel pad and transverse plantar crease (*NCLEX®*)
   c. When defect is unilateral, affected limb is usually shorter with possible calf atrophy
3. Therapeutic management
   a. Correction is best achieved if begun in newborn period because small bones in foot begin to ossify shortly after birth
   b. Manipulation and serial casting are begun immediately and continued for 8–12 weeks, with foot placed in a cast in an overcorrected position; casts are changed every 1–2 weeks because of rapid growth (*NCLEX®*)
   c. Parents need to perform passive ROM exercises to foot and ankle several times a day for several months once cast is off
   d. Infant may need to sleep in Denis Browne splints (shoes attached to a metal bar to maintain position) or wear corrective shoes for up to 1 year
   e. Surgery is performed when manipulative therapy does not achieve full correction with casting (often between 4 and 12 months of age); involves realigning foot bones and fixating in place with steel pins; foot is casted for 6–12 weeks
   f. Nursing care of child after casting and surgical repair of clubfoot includes neurovascular checks at least every 2 hours; assess for swelling around cast edges; elevate ankle and foot on pillows; monitor for cast drainage; pain management; and appropriate distraction (*NCLEX®*)
4. Client and family teaching
   a. Change diapers often to prevent soiled diapers from soiling cast (*NCLEX®*)
   b. Sponge-bathe infant to keep cast dry (*NCLEX®*)
   c. Evaluate crying episodes carefully because they may be caused by tingling sensation of circulatory compression (*NCLEX®*)
   d. Reinforce need for passive ROM exercises several times a day for several months
   e. Reinforce use of Denis Browne splints or corrective shoes to maintain correction
   f. Discuss options for clothing that accommodates casts
   g. Teach care of a child in a brace or cast (see Box 61–6)

B. Developmental dysplasia of hip (DDH)

1. Overview
   a. Refers to a variety of conditions in which femoral head and acetabulum are improperly aligned
   b. Unilateral in 80% of affected children
   c. Cause is unknown, although certain factors, including family history, increase risk
   d. Prenatal conditions may lead to DDH; these include frank breech position, maternal hormones (relaxin and estrogen may cause laxity of hip joint and capsule, leading to joint instability), twinning, and large infant size

Box 61–6

Child and Family Education for a Child in a Brace or a Cast

Perform Neurovascular Checks

- ➤ Observe fingers or toes for swelling, discoloration, and temperature.
- ➤ Check movement and sensation.
- ➤ Notify healthcare professional with any changes in neurovascular status.
- ➤ Teach parents how to blanch nail bed and watch for capillary refill.

Observe for Infection

- ➤ Monitor for temperature increase.
- ➤ Assess for drainage through cast or brace.
- ➤ Assess for odors coming from beneath cast or brace.
- ➤ Notify healthcare professional of any of above.

Assess and Maintain Skin around Cast or Brace Edges

- ➤ Perform frequent assessment of skin around cast or brace edges for irritation, rubbing, or blistering.
- ➤ Keep edges clean and dry; avoid use of lotions, powders, or oils near cast or brace.
- ➤ Petal cast edges as needed with tape to cover rough edges.
- ➤ Do not allow child to put anything down cast.
- ➤ If child is incontinent, protect cast edges with waterproof tape and plastic.
- ➤ Keep cast or brace clean and dry.

Activity

- ➤ Follow health professional's orders for activity level or restriction of activity.
- ➤ Avoid allowing affected extremity to hang in a dependent position for more than 30 minutes.
- ➤ Encourage frequent rest for first few days following brace or cast application, keeping injured extremity elevated while resting.
- ➤ Keep a clear path for ambulation, removing toys, hazardous floor rugs, pets, or other items over which child might stumble.
- ➤ If in a body cast or brace, assist child to be mobile using a wagon, cart, or large skateboard; do not move or reposition client using bar between lower extremities if present.

Comfort

- ➤ Assess for discomfort and medicate according to healthcare provider's orders.
- ➤ Contact healthcare provider if pain is not relieved by any comfort measures.

Follow-up

- ➤ Encourage compliance with follow-up.
- ➤ Take child to healthcare provider if cast becomes too loose or becomes soft or cracked.

e. Sociocultural methods of childrearing, such as way infants are carried, may promote or decrease extent of involvement; infants held with hips abducted have decreased involvement

2. Nursing assessment in infancy

a. Diagnosis should be made in newborn period; treatment is most successful if begun before 2 months of age

NCLEX® **b.** Shortening of affected limb

c. Allis' sign: child in supine position, thighs flexed to a 90-degree angle toward abdomen, unequal knee height

NCLEX® **d.** Uneven number and placement of skinfolds on posterior thighs

e. Restricted abduction of hips after 6–10 weeks of age

f. Wide perineum in bilateral dislocation

NCLEX®

g. Positive Ortolani up to 2–3 months of age; to assess for this, lie infant supine and flex knees and hips to 90 degrees; place middle fingers over greater trochanter and thumb in internal side of thigh over lesser trochanter; abduct hips while applying pressure over greater trochanter and listen for a clicking sound, which would indicate a positive Ortolani's sign; no sound will be heard with a normal hip

h. Positive Barlow's sign: with fingers in same position, hold knees and hips at 90 degrees, apply backward pressure, and adduct hips; positive Barlow's sign is present if able to feel hips dislocate

NCLEX®

3. Nursing assessment in an older child
   a. Affected leg shorter than other
   b. Telescoping or piston mobility of affected leg
   c. History of delay in walking, presence of limp, and toe walking
   d. Trendelenburg's sign: when child bears weight on affected side, pelvis tilts downward on normal side instead of upward
   e. Waddling gait and lordosis with bilateral dislocation

4. Therapeutic management
   a. Correction involves positioning hip into a flexed, abducted (externally rotated) position to press femur head against acetabulum and deepen its contour
   b. NCLEX® For infants under 3 months, common treatment is a Pavlik harness, an adjustable chest halter that abducts legs; soft plastic stirrups hold hips flexed, abducted, and externally rotated; may or may not be removed for bathing; usually worn for 3–6 months
   c. For infants older than 3 months, skin traction followed by spica cast application may be required
   d. Correction in child older than 18 months requires traction, operative reduction, and rehabilitation

NCLEX®

5. Client and family teaching
   a. Pavlik harness: proper application, sponge bath, assess skin under straps daily for irritation or redness; T-shirt and knee socks should be worn under brace to prevent skin irritation; diaper should be placed under straps and changed without taking harness off
   b. For all abduction devices: modification of car seat, modification of positioning for nursing and eating
   c. Parents need to ensure child has adequate stimulation with toys and activities at appropriate eye level; encourage activities that stimulate upper extremities
   d. Children will catch up with developmental milestones once abduction splint is off

C. Osteogenesis imperfecta (OI)

1. Overview
   a. A connective tissue disorder that primarily affects bones, caused by a biochemical defect in collagen production, although calcium and phosphorus levels are normal
   b. Classified into four types with variable degree of severity
   c. Bones are fragile and can fracture easily because of trauma, but also from pressure of birth or ordinary activity such as walking
   d. OI is genetically transmitted, generally in an autosomal dominant inheritance pattern, although some types are transmitted in a recessive pattern
   e. NCLEX® It is important not to confuse fractures in a child with OI with fractures caused by abuse

2. Nursing assessment
   a. NCLEX® Major clinical manifestations include multiple and frequent fractures, some of which may be present at birth
   b. As child grows older, multiple breaks tend to cause limb and spinal column deformities, interfering with alignment or growth
   c. Other clinical manifestations include blue sclera; thin, soft skin with easy bruising; increased joint flexibility; weak muscles; short stature; and possible conductive hearing loss by adolescence or young adulthood
   d. May have dentinogenesis imperfecta: hypoplastic teeth with opalescent blue or brown discoloration

3. Therapeutic management
   a. Keep floors dry; remove objects that could cause falls
   b. NCLEX® Handle children gently: avoid lifting by a single arm or leg; support trunk and extremities using a blanket when lifting and moving
   c. NCLEX® Never hold by ankles when being diapered, but gently lift by slipping a hand under buttocks
   d. NCLEX® Lightweight leg braces, splints, casting, and physical therapy may be helpful
   e. Surgical insertion of intermedullary rods may be effective in strengthening bones
   f. NCLEX® Nutritional therapy includes a well-balanced diet with additional calcium and vitamins C and D; excess calories should be avoided to maintain weight at recommended levels for age
   g. Medication therapy: bisphosphonates (to increase bone mass)

4. Client and family teaching
   a. Encourage a lifestyle that promotes growth and development yet minimizes risk of trauma
   b. Teach how to support when bathing, dressing, and moving
   c. Encourage exercise, such as swimming, to improve muscle tone and prevent obesity
   d. Explain use of adaptive equipment and possible motorized wheelchairs to promote independent functioning
   e. Suggest genetic counseling
   f. Educational materials and information can be obtained from the Osteogenesis Imperfecta Foundation

XVII. ACQUIRED CHILDHOOD MUSCULOSKELETAL HEALTH PROBLEMS

A. Legg-Calve-Perthes disease

1. Overview
   a. A self-limiting disorder in which there is unilateral or bilateral aseptic necrosis of femoral head caused by decreased circulation to femoral capital epiphysis
   b. Affects children between ages of 2 and 12 years, with average age of 7 years at onset
   c. Cause is unknown but predisposing factors may include family history, mild traumatic injury preceding onset, or breech birth
   d. Consists of four stages: Stage I (avascular stage lasting 3–6 months), Stage II (revascularization stage lasting 1–4 years), Stage III (bone healing with reossification and reduction in pain), and Stage IV (remodeling with absence of pain and improved joint function)

NCLEX®
2. Nursing assessment
   a. Mild pain in hip or anterior thigh and limp; aggravated by increased activity and relieved by rest
   b. Stiffness in morning or after rest
   c. As disease progresses, there is limited ROM, weakness, muscle wasting, possible shortening of affected limb, and positive Trendelenburg sign
3. Therapeutic management
   a. Diagnostic methods include x-rays (anteroposterior and frog-leg radiographs), bone scan, MRI, and arthrography
   b. Initial treatment includes rest to reduce inflammation and restore motion
   NCLEX® c. Goal is to keep head of femur inside of hip socket, which molds head of femur into a spherical shape
   NCLEX® d. Treatment may be conservative: rest; avoid weight bearing on lower extremities; traction and containment with abduction braces (such as Toronto or Scottish Rite braces), leg casts, or leather harness slings
   e. Conservative therapy may be needed for more than 2 years
   f. Surgical correction may be done, which returns child to normal activities in 3–4 months
   NCLEX® g. Assist in selecting suitable activities for a child unable to maintain usual level of physical activity
   NCLEX® h. If surgery is done, postoperative care includes frequent neurovascular checks, pain management, and activity based on surgeon's orders
   i. Assist family with appropriate activities for child during treatment
4. Client and family teaching
   a. Teach purpose, function, application, and care of corrective device and importance of compliance to achieve desired outcome
   b. Stress importance of continuing school activities
   c. Promote normal growth and development with appropriate diversional activities

B. Slipped capital femoral epiphysis

1. Overview
   a. A condition in which upper femoral epiphysis (head) is displaced from femoral neck
   b. Incidence is greatest during prepubertal growth spurt
   c. Occurs more in males, African Americans, and those with predisposing factors such as obesity or endocrine disorders such as hypothyroidism or hypogonadism
   d. Slippage of femoral head occurs at proximal **epiphyseal plate**, and femur displaces from **epiphysis** (rounded end portion of long bones); usually a gradual process, but may result from trauma
2. Nursing assessment
   NCLEX® a. Onset of symptoms may be gradual, with persistent hip pain that is aching or mild, and can be referred to thigh and/or knee, along with limp and decreased ROM and internal rotation of hip; child may hold leg in an externally rotated position to relieve stress and pain in hip joint

NCLEX® **b.** Child with an acute slip presents with sudden, severe pain and cannot bear weight

3. Therapeutic management

NCLEX® **a.** X-ray confirms diagnosis, and bone scan, ultrasound, CT, or MRI may be performed

b. Immediately place client on strict bedrest until surgery; adolescent may use crutches as long as affected leg is non-weight-bearing, but should not sit in a wheelchair, as this may increase slippage

c. Reinforce initial bedrest, as adolescents often do not see value of this measure

d. Provide appropriate diversional activities

e. Prepare for surgery with pinning or external fixation to stabilize femur head

f. Provide standard postoperative care, including frequent neurovascular checks and pain management

g. Provide adequate nutrition for healing

4. Client and family teaching

a. Reinforce ambulation and weight bearing as ordered by surgeon

b. Contact sports are usually restricted until growth is complete

c. Reinforce compliance with follow-up visits until epiphyseal plates are closed

C. *Scoliosis*

1. Overview

a. Lateral or S-shaped curvature of spine often associated with rotational deformity of spine and ribs; may be congenital, idiopathic, or compensatory (spine curves to compensate for unequal leg lengths)

b. Idiopathic scoliosis occurs most often during rapid growth spurt in adolescence, most often in females between 10 and 13 years old

c. Scoliosis is common congenital disorder in which there are musculoskeletal changes, such as CP, MD, and myelomeningocele

2. Nursing assessment

a. Painless and insidious onset is typical

NCLEX® **b.** Parent may first notice that skirts hang unevenly, or that bra straps are adjusted unevenly

NCLEX® **c.** On examination, there is truncal asymmetry, unequal shoulder and hip height, one-sided scapula and rib prominences, and chest asymmetry

d. Screening by school nurses is done in fifth and seventh grades, which is mandated by law in many (but not all) states

e. Scoliometer is used to document clinical deformity found on screening

3. Therapeutic management

a. Prepare adolescent for x-ray, which will identify extent of curvature and give baseline information for follow-up

NCLEX® **b.** With mild scoliosis (spinal curvatures of 10–20 degrees), client is evaluated every 3 months for change, with x-ray every 6 months for change; exercises are prescribed to improve posture and muscle tone and increase flexibility of spine

c. With moderate scoliosis (curvatures of 20–40 degrees), client is prescribed to wear a brace such as a Boston brace (for 23 hours/day) to maintain current degree of spinal curvature with no increase; adherence can be an issue in adolescents who are more concerned with body image or participating in sports

d. Severe scoliosis (curvatures greater than 40 degrees) generally requires surgery for spinal fusion (with segmental instrumentation of spinal cord with hooks, wires, rods, and screws) and possible bone grafting from iliac crests to strengthen fusion

e. Provide standard preoperative care and teaching about what to expect during postoperative period; see also Chapter 48

NCLEX® **f.** Perform standard immediate postoperative care, which includes ROM exercises, logrolling every 2 hours, encouraging coughing and deep breathing and use of incentive spirometer, NPO, strict I&O, frequent VS and neurologic checks, monitoring hematocrit, blood transfusions, pain management, antibiotic administration, and application of antiembolism stockings or sequential compression devices

g. Activity for a client who underwent surgery includes bedrest during recovery period; client is fitted with an anteroposterior plastic shell (thoracolumbar sacral orthosis, or TLSO) that is then worn for several months to stabilize spine

4. Client and family teaching

a. Use of a Boston or other brace: worn for 23 hours a day; off to shower, bathe, and swim; wear T-shirt under brace next to skin for protection; do exercises (such as pelvic tilt and lateral strengthening) several times daily while in brace to prevent worsening of thoracic lordosis

b. Consistent use of brace will provide maximum benefit

c. Slight muscle aches may be noticed when first wearing brace
d. Encourage teens to be as active as possible while in brace
NCLEX®
e. Discharge teaching: must not slump in chairs, bend or twist torso, or lift over 4.5 kg (10 lb); maintain activity restrictions for 6–8 months as prescribed; address self-esteem issues; comply with follow-up visits
f. Additional discharge teaching for surgical client: use of TLSO; limit activity initially to gentle activities such as walking and gentle swimming; for 6–8 months avoid heavy lifting, bending or twisting at waist, or any activities that involve risk of fall or injury (bicycling, sports, skiing, etc.)

Check Your NCLEX–RN® Exam I.Q.

You are ready for testing on this content if you can:

- Identify basic structures and functions of the musculoskeletal system.
- Describe the pathophysiology and etiology of common musculoskeletal disorders.
- Discuss expected assessment data and diagnostic test findings for selected musculoskeletal disorders.
- Discuss therapeutic management of a client experiencing a musculoskeletal disorder.
- Discuss nursing management of a client experiencing a musculoskeletal disorder.
- Identify expected outcomes for the client experiencing a musculoskeletal disorder.

PRACTICE TEST

1 The nurse provides teaching to an adolescent client after removal of a short leg cast. The nurse should include which instructions in discussions with the client? Select all that apply.

1. Wash the skin with undiluted hydrogen peroxide.
2. Vigorously scrub the legs to remove dead skin.
3. Gently wash the leg to remove dead skin over time.
4. Avoid touching the leg for 2 days after cast removal.
5. Use a lubricant to moisten the skin for easier removal of dead skin.

2 Which problem should the nurse choose as a priority focus for a client with Paget's disease?

1. Possible nonadherence to therapy
2. Difficulty falling asleep
3. Reduced mobility from pain
4. Concerns with body image

3 A client with a right arm cast for a fractured humerus states, "I haven't been able to straighten the fingers on my right hand since this morning." What action should the nurse take first?

1. Assess neurovascular status to the hand.
2. Ask the client to massage the fingers.
3. Encourage the client to take the prescribed analgesic.
4. Elevate the right arm on a pillow to reduce edema.

4 A client with an open fracture is at risk for developing osteomyelitis. Which classic symptoms would the nurse assess for to detect development of this complication? Select all that apply.

1. Increased pain at the fracture site
2. Elevated temperature
3. Acute respiratory distress
4. Shortening of the affected extremity
5. Increased swelling at the fracture site

5 An obese client with degenerative joint disease is being treated with aspirin. The nurse concludes that additional client teaching is needed when the client makes which statement?

1. "I take aspirin only when I have extreme pain and stiffness."
2. "I use heat sometimes to help decrease my pain and joint stiffness."
3. "I frequently examine my stools for bleeding."
4. "I started an exercise program to lose weight."

6 A client underwent a lumbar laminectomy earlier today. Which assessment data warrants priority attention by the nurse?

1. Weak cough effort
2. Bowel sounds that are hypoactive
3. Pain rated at 3 on a scale of 0 to 10
4. New-onset numbness and tingling in foot

7 A client had a left above-the-knee amputation today. For the first 24 hours postoperatively, the nurse performs which priority action to properly manage the surgical site?

1. Elevate the residual limb.
2. Loosen the dressing every 4 hours.
3. Maintain the residual limb in a dependent position.
4. Change the dressing as often as needed.

8 A client with a femoral fracture is in Buck's traction. While making rounds, the nurse notices that the client's foot is touching the footboard of the bed. What is the appropriate action by the nurse?

1. Wedge a pillow between the footboard and the client's foot.
2. Praise the client for maintaining countertraction.
3. Center the client on the bed.
4. Ask the client to pull up in bed while holding the weights.

9 A truck driver sees the primary care provider because of persistent back pain. The nurse explains that which client activity documented during the nursing history may contribute to further back injury?

1. Lifting objects close to the body
2. Shifting positions often when sitting for prolonged periods
3. Providing back support with a pillow when sitting
4. Prolonged standing or sitting

10 The nurse is assigned to the care of a client who underwent a lumbar laminectomy. Allowing which activity would be appropriate 4 hours postoperatively?

1. Sitting up in a chair to watch television
2. Sitting at the side of the bed
3. Lying in bed in good alignment with the head of bed flat
4. Using the side-rails for support to get out of bed

11 The nurse is teaching a client with scoliosis about what to expect in the postoperative period following spinal fusion with insertion of hardware. What informational topics should the nurse include in discussions with the client? Select all that apply.

1. The client will be assisted to ambulate on the day after surgery
2. Nursing staff will provide ongoing pain assessment and management
3. The client will be logrolled when being moved in bed
4. It may be necessary to institute tube feedings for a few days
5. The client will be fitted with an orthotic brace to wear for several months

12 The nurse is teaching a postmenopausal client about the use of calcium to reduce the risk of osteoporosis. The client asks: "Why do I have to take vitamin D with my calcium?" What is the nurse's best response?

1. "Vitamin D prevents osteoporosis."
2. "Vitamin D increases intestinal absorption of calcium."
3. "You are most likely to be deficient in vitamin D."
4. "Using calcium and vitamin D supplements together prevents osteoporosis."

13 The nurse is caring for a client with a week-old cast. The client asks why the nurse touches the cast during an assessment. What is the most appropriate response by the nurse?

1. "I am making sure that the cast has dried."
2. "I am evaluating the strength of the cast."
3. "I am feeling for hot spots that might indicate infection."
4. "I am making sure that the cast is not too tight."

14 A client is placed on a continuous passive motion (CPM) machine postoperatively after a total knee replacement. The nurse observes the client's knee is externally rotating during flexion. What should the nurse do next?

1. Move the client up in bed or move the CPM machine toward the foot of the bed
2. Support the knee with sandbags to prevent external rotation
3. Assist the client to sit up in bed in a 45-degree position
4. Do nothing; the client's knee is properly aligned

15 A client in skeletal traction for a right femur fracture reports pain in the affected limb. After assessing that the right foot is pale without a pulse, what should the nurse do next? Select all that apply.

1. Ensure that the leg is not raised above heart level
2. Administer analgesics as ordered
3. Release the traction
4. Recheck the pulse in an hour
5. Document the findings and notify the healthcare provider.

16 A nurse receives a client from the emergency department (ED) in Buck's traction following fracture of the right femur. The nurse documents which information as a priority in the client medical record?

1. Status of skin underneath the traction and over bony prominences
2. Type of pin, wire, or tongs used
3. The effectiveness of pain medication given in the field
4. Medications given in the emergency department

17 A client has been placed in balanced suspension traction after sustaining a fracture. The nurse explains to the family that which of the following is an advantage of this type of traction?

1. It eliminates the risk for skin breakdown.
2. It allows the client to raise the buttocks off the bed for bedpan use and skin care.
3. It is more effective in reducing hip contracture.
4. It requires only one weight to maintain traction.

18 A client taking colchicine for gout reports weakness, abdominal pain, and nausea and vomiting for the past 2 days. How should the nurse interpret these symptoms?

1. Therapeutic effects of the medication
2. Signs of toxicity
3. Expected side effects
4. An allergic response

19 An 87-year-old underweight client who sustained a right hip fracture asks the nurse how long it will take for the fracture to heal. The nurse's response includes consideration of which client factor that influences the rate of bone healing?

1. Frequency of physical therapy
2. Age of the client
3. Weight of the client
4. Early ambulation

20 A client is scheduled to have a closed reduction of a right ankle fracture. The nurse determines the client understands the procedure when the client states that it involves which of the following?

1. Using an arthroscope to realign the bones
2. Realigning the bone using surgery
3. Correcting the bone alignment using manual manipulation
4. Inserting pins, rods, or other implantable devices

21 A child is admitted to the hospital with a diagnosis of osteomyelitis. What data would the nurse likely obtain during a nursing history?

1. History of an upper respiratory infection
2. History of gastroenteritis
3. History of Legg-Calve-Perthes disease
4. History of congenital hip dysplasia

22 Two hours after a child had a cast applied for a fractured radius, the nurse assesses swelling in the hand, which is elevated higher than the heart. Ice has been applied continuously. The child denies any increase in pain but does report numbness and tingling. Which should the nurse do first?

1. Medicate the client for pain again.
2. Elevate the injured extremity even higher.
3. Call the healthcare provider.
4. Provide the child with diversional activities.

23 The pediatric nurse interprets that which infant is least likely to be diagnosed with developmental dysplasia of the hip (DDH)?

1. An infant with a family history of DDH
2. An infant with a birthweight of 4.5 kg (10 lb)
3. The infant carried on the mother's hips
4. The infant who had frank breech position in utero

24 Which intervention would be essential for the nurse to implement to promote a stable respiratory status in an adolescent who recently had a spinal fusion for scoliosis?

1. Logrolling and repositioning every 4 hours
2. Coughing and deep breathing every 2 hours while awake
3. Assessing pain status and ensuring adequate pain relief
4. Encouraging use of incentive spirometry every 4 hours while awake

25 An 8-year-old child presents to the urgent care clinic with ankle pain and difficulty walking, although no injury is recalled. The nurse notes ankle redness, swelling, decreased range of motion, and pain with ankle movement. Temperature is 100.8°F (38.2°C) and heart rate is 140 beats per minute. Which health problem would the nurse suspect?

1. Legg-Calve-Perthes disease
2. Slipped capital femoral epiphysis
3. Fracture of the ankle
4. Osteomyelitis

26 The nurse is preparing to help a client get up from a chair using crutches. Place in order the steps that the nurse outlines to the client to do this procedure correctly.

1. Place unaffected leg slightly under or at the edge of the chair.
2. Grasp the arm of the chair using the hand on the unaffected side.
3. Grasp the crutches by the horizontal hand bars using the hand on the affected side.
4. Move forward to the edge of the chair.
5. Push down on the crutches and the chair armrest while raising the body out of the chair.

Fill in your answer below:

Answer: ______________________

PRACTICE TEST

ANSWERS & RATIONALES

1 **Answer: 3, 5 Rationale:** Dead skin and exudates often collect under the cast, and efforts to remove it should be done gradually. The client can use a lubricant, which will soften dead skin cells for easier removal during cleansing. The use of undiluted peroxide is too harsh for the skin. The client should avoid any vigorous scrubbing of the skin to avoid interfering with skin integrity, which increases the risk for infection. There is no reason why the leg cannot be touched after removal of the cast. **Cognitive Level:** Applying **Client Need:** Physiological Adaptation **Integrated Process:** Teaching and Learning **Content Area:** Adult Health: Musculoskeletal **Strategy:** The core issue of the question is knowledge of skin care following cast removal. Use nursing knowledge and the process of elimination to make a selection.

2 **Answer: 3 Rationale:** Reduced mobility from bone pain is a priority concern of the nurse for a client with Paget's disease. The client needs to remain active to decrease the complications associated with immobility and to maintain the ability to perform self-care activities. There is no information to suggest the client is nonadherent to therapy. Difficulty falling asleep is not a hallmark of Paget's disease. It is possible the client could experience concerns with body image, particularly if signs of the disease are noticeable, but physiological needs would take priority. **Cognitive Level:** Applying **Client Need:** Physiological Adaptation **Integrated Process:** Nursing Process: Planning **Content Area:** Adult Health: Musculoskeletal **Strategy:** The core issue of the question is knowledge of priorities for the client with Paget's disease. Use nursing knowledge and the process of elimination to make a selection.

3 **Answer: 1 Rationale:** This symptom suggests neurologic injury caused by pressure on nerves and soft tissue because of swelling (compartment syndrome). Other symptoms of neurovascular compromise should be assessed and reported to the healthcare provider. Massaging the fingers will not help alleviate the problem. An analgesic will not help with mobility caused by neurologic injury and there is no evidence that the client is experiencing pain. Elevating the limb could worsen the symptoms at a time when circulation is already impaired from swelling, which led to the neurologic injury. **Cognitive Level:** Analyzing **Client Need:** Physiological Adaptation **Integrated Process:** Nursing Process: Implementation **Content Area:** Adult Health: Musculoskeletal **Strategy:** The core issue of the question is knowledge of priority assessments in a client with possible compartment syndrome. Use nursing knowledge and the process of elimination to make a selection.

4 **Answer: 1, 2, 5 Rationale:** Increased pain could indicate development of osteomyelitis. Elevated temperature is a classic symptom seen with osteomyelitis as a systemic response to the invading organism. Increased swelling at the site of the fracture could indicate development of osteomyelitis. Acute respiratory distress is suggestive of fat embolism but not bone infection. The extremity does not shorten with osteomyelitis, although this is a classic finding with hip fracture. **Cognitive Level:** Applying **Client Need:** Physiological Adaptation

ANSWERS & RATIONALES

Integrated Process: Nursing Process: Assessment **Content Area:** Adult Health: Musculoskeletal **Strategy:** The core issue of the question is knowledge of manifestations of osteomyelitis. Use nursing knowledge and the process of elimination to make a selection.

5 **Answer: 1 Rationale:** Aspirin therapy for this condition is continuous and is effective only after a therapeutic level is reached. It should not be taken intermittently. Heat is a beneficial measure to increase client comfort. Aspirin is an antiplatelet agent and the client should monitor for blood in stools as an adverse effect of therapy. Losing weight is beneficial for the client because it decreases the stress on the joints, particularly in the lower limbs. **Cognitive Level:** Applying **Client Need:** Physiological Adaptation **Integrated Process:** Nursing Process: Evaluation **Content Area:** Adult Health: Musculoskeletal **Strategy:** The core issue of the question is knowledge of appropriate self-management techniques for degenerative joint disease. Use nursing knowledge and the process of elimination to make a selection. Note the wording of the question indicates the correct option is an incorrect statement by the client.

6 **Answer: 4 Rationale:** New-onset numbness and tingling in the foot is an adverse neurovascular change that needs to be reported immediately to the healthcare provider. A weak cough effort requires coaching by the nurse, but does not take priority over a complication of surgery. Hypoactive bowel sounds are expected on the day of surgery. Pain that is rated 3 on a scale of 0 to 10 is considered mild pain, and warrants continued routine assessment and management by the nurse. **Cognitive Level:** Analyzing **Client Need:** Physiological Adaptation **Integrated Process:** Nursing Process: Diagnosis **Content Area:** Fundamentals **Strategy:** The core issue of the question is knowledge of priority nursing diagnoses following musculoskeletal surgery. Use nursing knowledge and the process of elimination to make a selection.

7 **Answer: 1 Rationale:** Elevating the limb during the first 24 hours facilitates venous return, decreases swelling, and promotes comfort. The dressing is usually a compression type to mold the residual limb and to decrease the edema associated with inflammation, so loosening the dressing is an inappropriate intervention. Placing the residual limb below heart level increases risk of edema at the surgical site. The dressing would be changed as ordered but is not usually done for the first 24 hours to reduce edema, which could disrupt the surgical incision. **Cognitive Level:** Applying **Client Need:** Physiological Adaptation **Integrated Process:** Nursing Process: Implementation **Content Area:** Adult Health: Musculoskeletal **Strategy:** The core issue of the question is knowledge of postoperative residual limb care and proper positioning to limit development of postoperative edema. Use nursing knowledge and the process of elimination to make a selection.

8 **Answer: 3 Rationale:** The aim in traction is to maintain a constant force to align the distal and proximal ends of a fractured bone. To be effective, traction must have an opposing force (countertraction). Centering the client in bed maintains the line of pull and ensures that countertraction is maintained. Placing a pillow between the foot and the footboard attempts to relieve pressure on the foot but ignores that this position interrupts the proper pull of the traction. The client's current position interrupts traction rather than maintains proper countertraction. Holding the weight interrupts the line of pull of the traction and is contraindicated. **Cognitive Level:** Applying **Client Need:** Physiological Adaptation **Integrated Process:** Nursing Process: Implementation **Content Area:** Adult Health: Musculoskeletal **Strategy:** The core issue of the question is knowledge of proper use of traction. Use nursing knowledge and the process of elimination to make a selection.

9 **Answer: 4 Rationale:** Prolonged sitting or standing aggravates back injury because of the additional stress placed on structures supporting the back. Lifting objects close to the body, shifting positions frequently, and providing back support are appropriate actions to maintain good body mechanics. **Cognitive Level:** Analyzing **Client Need:** Physiological Adaptation **Integrated Process:** Nursing Process: Assessment **Content Area:** Adult Health: Musculoskeletal **Strategy:** The core issue of the question is knowledge of risk factors and aggravating factors of low back pain. Use nursing knowledge and the process of elimination to make a selection.

10 **Answer: 3 Rationale:** Prescriptions after lumbar laminectomy include being kept flat or with head of bed slightly elevated to minimize stress on the suture line. The client is repositioned side to side using logrolling technique to maintain alignment of the vertebral column at all times. Sitting up in a chair or on the side of the bed is usually done the evening of the surgery or the first day following surgery, and it is for brief periods only. Using the side-rails to get out of bed causes shifting of the vertebral column. **Cognitive Level:** Applying **Client Need:** Safety and Infection Control **Integrated Process:** Nursing Process: Implementation **Content Area:** Adult Health: Musculoskeletal **Strategy:** The core issue of the question is knowledge of postoperative activity that will not cause harm to the surgical area following laminectomy. Recall principles of proper body mechanics and use the process of elimination to make a selection.

11 **Answer: 2, 3, 5 Rationale:** The nursing staff will provide ongoing pain assessment and management as for any postoperative client. Logrolling is important when moving the client in bed to maintain alignment of the spine. The client will be fitted with a thoracolumbar sacral orthosis (TLSO) brace or shell to wear to maintain spinal stability for several months postoperatively. The client remains on bedrest during recovery period from surgery. Tube feedings are not necessary after spinal fusion. **Cognitive Level:** Analyzing **Client Need:** Physiological Adaptation **Integrated Process:** Teaching and Learning **Content Area:** Adult Health: Musculoskeletal **Strategy:** The core issue of the question is knowledge of factors that aggravate low back pain. Use nursing knowledge and the process of elimination to make a selection.

12 **Answer: 2 Rationale:** A combination of calcium and vitamin D is recommended for the prevention of osteoporosis. Vitamin D increases the intestinal absorption of calcium and mobilizes calcium and phosphorus into the bone. Vitamin D alone does not prevent osteoporosis. While some older adults may be deficient in Vitamin D, a postmenopausal state does not necessarily cause the deficiency. Lifestyle modifications, such as smoking cessation and exercise, may also help reduce the risk of osteoporosis. **Cognitive Level:** Applying **Client Need:** Health Promotion and Maintenance **Integrated Process:** Communication and Documentation **Content Area:** Adult Health: Musculoskeletal **Strategy:** The core issue of the question is knowledge of risk factors for and prevention of osteoporosis. Use nursing knowledge and the process of elimination to make a selection.

13 **Answer: 3 Rationale:** A complication of cast application is skin breakdown underneath the cast, which can lead to infection and subsequent heat in the infected area. A bad odor in the area may also be noted. A plaster cast dries in 24–48 hours and a fiberglass cast dries in 30 minutes to 1 hour. Evaluating cast strength is not part of nursing assessment and palpating the

cast would not accomplish this anyway. If a cast is too tight, symptoms associated with neurovascular compromise will be noted, which include pain, paresthesia, pallor, diminished pulse distal to the cast, and paralysis. **Cognitive Level:** Applying **Client Need:** Physiological Adaptation **Integrated Process:** Communication and Documentation **Content Area:** Adult Health: Musculoskeletal **Strategy:** The core issue of the question is knowledge of various complications of casts. Use nursing knowledge and the process of elimination to make a selection.

14 **Answer: 1 Rationale:** The client's knee will externally rotate if there is insufficient space between the client's hip and the machine. The knee should be upright, facing the ceiling, as the machine moves the leg back and forth. Sandbags will not prevent external rotation because the issue is the position of the client relative to the CPM machine. Raising the head of bed will not correct external rotation of the leg. Taking no action places the client at risk for injury. **Cognitive Level:** Applying **Client Need:** Physiological Adaptation **Integrated Process:** Nursing Process: Implementation **Content Area:** Adult Health: Musculoskeletal **Strategy:** The core issue of the question is knowledge of appropriate care of the client using CPM. Use nursing knowledge and the process of elimination to make a selection.

15 **Answer: 1, 5 Rationale:** Pain and absent pulse indicate impaired circulation to the affected limb, which requires treatment to prevent damage to nerves and tissues, and necrosis requiring loss of limb (worst case). The nurse needs to ensure that the leg is not above heart level so no further damage occurs. Findings should always be documented and the healthcare provider needs to be notified of the complication, so further medical assessment and treatment can be done. Pain caused by tissue ischemia will not be relieved by analgesics. Releasing the traction would be contraindicated. Rechecking the pulse in an hour is delayed and also fails to assist the client, whose symptoms will not reverse without treatment. **Cognitive Level:** Applying **Client Need:** Physiological Adaptation **Integrated Process:** Nursing Process: Implementation **Content Area:** Adult Health: Musculoskeletal **Strategy:** The core issue of the question is knowledge of adverse neurovascular changes to a client in a cast. Recall principles of gravity and blood flow to aid in answering the question. Use nursing knowledge and the process of elimination to make a selection.

16 **Answer: 1 Rationale:** It is essential to monitor the condition of the skin under traction, as well as bony prominences, because these areas are at risk for breakdown due to continuous friction and pressure from the skin traction device. Skeletal tractions use pins, wires, or tongs to aid in realignment. Buck's traction is a type of skin traction. Effectiveness of medication given in the field is not pertinent to the client's status after admission from the ED. Evaluating effectiveness of analgesia is appropriate, but the most essential documentation for a client with skin traction is the condition of the skin underneath the straps. **Cognitive Level:** Analyzing **Client Need:** Physiological Adaptation **Integrated Process:** Communication and Documentation **Content Area:** Adult Health: Musculoskeletal **Strategy:** The critical word in the question is *priority*, which indicates that more than one or all options are correct and that the most essential ones are correct. Use nursing knowledge about skin traction and the process of elimination to make selections.

17 **Answer: 2 Rationale:** Balanced suspension allows for ease with bedpan use and skin care without disturbing the line of traction. In this type of traction, the client's injured extremity is lifted off the bed and a straight pull is accomplished by the application of several forces and several weights. Skin breakdown is not eliminated with this type of traction because any immobile client can be at risk. Because the extremity is lifted with the traction, the hip is flexed, making hip contracture possible. The number of weights is determined by the total pounds necessary to reduce the fracture. **Cognitive Level:** Applying **Client Need:** Physiological Adaptation **Integrated Process:** Nursing Process: Implementation **Content Area:** Adult Health: Musculoskeletal **Strategy:** The core issue of the question is knowledge of balanced suspension traction as a type of skeletal traction. Use nursing knowledge and the process of elimination to make a selection.

18 **Answer: 2 Rationale:** The symptoms described are signs of toxicity. The client should be instructed to stop the medication and be seen for follow-up treatment. The expected therapeutic effect of colchicine is to diminish the joint pain associated with the acute attack. The combination of symptoms is too severe to be expected as side effects of the medication. The symptoms are not consistent with an allergic response. **Cognitive Level:** Applying **Client Need:** Pharmacological and Parenteral Therapies **Integrated Process:** Nursing Process: Diagnosis **Content Area:** Adult Health: Musculoskeletal **Strategy:** The core issue of the question is knowledge of actions and adverse effects of colchicine. Use nursing knowledge and the process of elimination to make a selection.

19 **Answer: 2 Rationale:** Age, site of the fracture, and blood supply to the affected area all affect the rate of bone healing. Younger and healthy clients will have faster bone healing than older adults and those with chronic illnesses. Although physical therapy will assist in mobility, it does not directly enhance bone healing. The weight of the client, unless accompanied by malnutrition, does not have a direct bearing on bone healing. The healthcare provider determines when ambulation is allowed and thus it is not a client factor. **Cognitive Level:** Applying **Client Need:** Physiological Adaptation **Integrated Process:** Nursing Process: Implementation **Content Area:** Adult Health: Musculoskeletal **Strategy:** The core issue of the question is knowledge of possible threats to bone healing in an identified client. Use nursing knowledge and the process of elimination to make a selection.

20 **Answer: 3 Rationale:** In a closed reduction procedure, the healthcare provider applies traction and manipulates the bone until the broken ends are realigned. Arthroscopy is a surgical procedure for treating some types of joint problems. Open reduction is a realignment of bone with surgery. Internal fixation devices are surgically inserted during an open reduction to immobilize the fracture during the healing process. **Cognitive Level:** Applying **Client Need:** Physiological Adaptation **Integrated Process:** Nursing Process: Evaluation **Content Area:** Adult Health: Musculoskeletal **Strategy:** The core issue of the question is knowledge of various approaches to correct bone fracture. Use nursing knowledge and the process of elimination to make a selection.

21 **Answer: 1 Rationale:** The history of a child with osteomyelitis may include a recent upper respiratory infection (which may include an ear infection or sinus infection), skin infection, or blunt trauma to a bone. A recent history of gastroenteritis would not lead to osteomyelitis. Legg-Calve-Perthes disease is an aseptic necrosis of the femoral head that leads to pain and limping but osteomyelitis is a bone infection. Congenital hip dysplasia affects mobility but does not lead to osteomyelitis. **Cognitive Level:** Analyzing **Client Need:** Physiological Adaptation **Integrated Process:** Nursing Process: Assessment **Content Area:** Child Health **Strategy:** The core issue of the question

is knowledge of risk factors for osteomyelitis. Use nursing knowledge and the process of elimination to make a selection.

22 **Answer: 3 Rationale:** The client's symptoms are compatible with compartment syndrome, which can lead to neurologic damage. This is a medical emergency, and the healthcare provider should be called immediately. Pain medication is not indicated based on the client's data and would not correct the current underlying problem. Elevating the arm further would worsen circulation to the area, which is already impaired. The nurse can provide diversional activities while waiting for definitive orders from the healthcare provider. **Cognitive Level:** Analyzing **Client Need:** Physiological Adaptation **Integrated Process:** Nursing Process: Implementation **Content Area:** Child Health **Strategy:** The core issue of the question is recognition of a complication, compartment syndrome, that can lead to neurologic damage. The correct answer is the one that provides for definitive treatment of the problem, which in this case is in the practice realm of the healthcare provider.

23 **Answer: 3 Rationale:** The infant who is carried with the hips abducted is at decreased risk for developing DDH. A family history of DDH would possibly increase the incidence of this defect. A large infant size at birth has been associated with DDH. Breech position is associated with increased incidence of DDH. **Cognitive Level:** Analyzing **Client Need:** Physiological Adaptation **Integrated Process:** Nursing Process: Diagnosis **Content Area:** Child Health **Strategy:** The core issue of the question is recognition of which situation allows the infant to keep the hips abducted. Evaluate each option according to this criteria to make a selection.

24 **Answer: 3 Rationale:** Pain must be managed properly in the child after spinal fusion in order for the client to participate in respiratory exercises. Logrolling and repositioning, as well as coughing, deep-breathing, and use of incentive spirometry should be done every 2 hours around the clock with this postoperative client. **Cognitive Level:** Analyzing **Client Need:** Physiological Adaptation **Integrated Process:** Nursing Process: Implementation **Content Area:** Child Health **Strategy:** The core issue of the question is the ability to prioritize nursing activities. While the ABCs are quite important, they must be timely. Also, the client cannot meet goals for the respiratory portion of ABCs unless pain relief is achieved. With this in mind, choose pain relief as the correct answer.

25 **Answer: 4 Rationale:** The symptoms described are symptoms of osteomyelitis. This disease can result from a penetrating wound, but it also may result from an infection elsewhere in the body that traveled to the bone. Osteomyelitis may follow an upper respiratory infection, which is common in school-age children. Legg-Calve-Perthes disease affects the femoral head, not the ankle. Slipped capital femoral epiphysis affects the hip. An ankle fracture is generally associated with injury. **Cognitive Level:** Analyzing **Client Need:** Physiological Adaptation **Integrated Process:** Nursing Process: Assessment **Content Area:** Child Health **Strategy:** The issue of the question is the ability of the nurse to analyze assessment data and compare it to typical data of childhood musculoskeletal problems. Note that the temperature is elevated to help choose the option related to infection.

26 **Answer: 4, 1, 3, 2, 5 Rationale:** The client moves first to the edge of the chair to move the center of gravity forward before trying to stand. Placing the unaffected leg slightly under or at the edge of the chair is done second to provide support to help the client to stand up from the chair and achieve balance. Grasping the crutches by the horizontal hand bars using the hand on the affected side is done third to provide support for the affected side before arising. Grasping the arm of the chair using the hand on the unaffected side is done fourth so that the body weight is supported on the armrest of the unaffected leg when the client rises to stand. Pushing down on the crutches and the chair armrest while raising the body out of the chair is done fifth, once the body is fully positioned and supported. **Cognitive Level:** Analyzing **Client Need:** Physiological Adaptation **Integrated Process:** Nursing Process: Implementation **Content Area:** Child Health **Strategy:** Visualize the procedure and think about principles of joint support and balance to complete the ordered steps.

Key Terms to Review

References

Ball, J., & Bindler, R., & Cowen, K. (2015). *Principles of pediatric nursing: Caring for children* (6th ed.). Hoboken, NJ: Pearson Education.

Berman, A., Snyder, S., & Frandsen, G. (2016). *Kozier & Erb's fundamentals of nursing: Concepts, process, and practice* (10th ed.). New York, NY: Pearson Education.

Ignatavicius, D., & Workman, L. (2016). *Medical-surgical nursing: Patient-centered collaborative care* (10th ed.). Philadelphia: Saunders.

LeMone, P., Burke, K., Bauldoff, G., & Gubrud, P. (2015). *Medical surgical nursing: Clinical reasoning in patient care* (6th ed.). Hoboken, NJ: Pearson Education.

Lewis, S., Dirksen, S., Heitkemper, M., & Bucher, L. (2014). *Medical surgical nursing: Assessment and management of clinical problems* (9th ed.). St. Louis, MO: Elsevier Science.

Smith, S., Duell, D., Martin, B., Aebersold, M., & Gonzalez, L. (2017). *Clinical nursing skills: Basic to advanced skills* (10th ed.). New York, NY: Pearson Education.

Test Yourself

Are you ready for the NCLEX-RN® or course exams? Access the NEW web-based app that provides students with thousands of practice questions in preparation for the NCLEX experience.

Integumentary Disorders

62

In this chapter

Cross Reference

Other chapters relevant to this content area are

Meeting Basic Human Needs	**Chapter 26**
Integumentary Medications	**Chapter 42**
Common Laboratory Tests	**Chapter 46**
Common Diagnostic Tests and Procedures	**Chapter 47**

I. OVERVIEW OF ANATOMY AND PHYSIOLOGY OF INTEGUMENTARY SYSTEM

A. ***Epidermis***: outer layer of skin made up of epithelial cells; protects body and internal structures from harm by providing a barrier to external environment

B. ***Dermis***: middle layer of skin composed of flexible connective tissue, containing lymph vessels, blood vessels, nerve fibers, hair follicles, and sweat and sebaceous glands

C. **Subcutaneous tissue**: lies beneath dermis; made up of adipose (fat) tissue and helps connect skin to structures below subcutaneous tissue

D. **Appendages: include hair, nails, and glands**

1. Hair: composed of primarily dead cells; pads scalp and protects from external objects; helps maintain body temperature
2. Nails: primarily made up of dead cells; nail structure begins in epidermis and extends across and protects nail bed

3. Glands
    a. Apocrine: sweat glands located in axilla, anus, and genital area; function unknown
    b. Eccrine: sweat glands located on forehead, hands, and soles of feet; maintain a stable body temperature through perspiration when body is overheated
    c. Sebaceous: oil glands located throughout body that secrete sebum to lubricate skin, decrease water loss, and aid in killing bacteria on skin surface

E. Skin functions

1. Sensitivity to pressure, pain, touch, and temperature
2. First line of defense against infectious organisms
3. Thermoregulation through sweating, shivering, and subcutaneous insulation
4. Protects underlying tissues and organs from injury
5. Synthesizes vitamin D
6. Excretes water, salt, and electrolytes
7. Regenerates itself by shedding old cells and replacing with new cells

F. Pediatric variations in skin

1. Newborns are covered by lanugo—fine, soft hair that is shed in first month of life
2. Newborns have thin skin with little subcutaneous fat
    a. Allows rapid heat loss and problems with thermoregulation
    b. Leads to increased absorption of harmful chemical substances
3. Newborn skin contains more water than skin of older children
4. Dark-colored areas called Mongolian spots may be present on sacrum or buttocks of Native American, Asian, African American, or Latino infants

II. DIAGNOSTIC TESTS AND ASSESSMENTS OF INTEGUMENTARY SYSTEM

A. **Skin culture**: noninvasive procedure in which a skin sample is obtained with a sterile applicator; used to identify viral, bacterial, or fungal causes of skin lesions

B. **Skin scraping**: noninvasive procedure in which epithelial cells are scraped off and examined microscopically to identify viral, bacterial, fungal, or parasitic causes of skin lesion

C. **Skin biopsy**: invasive procedure in which a skin sample is removed for histological analysis

1. Requires informed consent
2. Apply pressure to site until bleeding stops; suture may be required
3. Used to identify tumors or persistent dermatitis

D. Wood's light examination

1. Uses ultraviolet light and a special type of glass (Wood's glass) to examine skin for superficial skin infections
2. Does not cause discomfort, but alert client that room is darkened during procedure

E. **Diascopy:** a technique in which a glass slide is pressed on area of skin lesion to eliminate erythema resulting from increased local blood flow and allow better visualization of lesion

F. Past medical history

1. Note previous problems with skin, hair, scalp, or nails; discuss duration of symptoms, associated symptoms, treatments used, and results
2. Medical disorders: discuss all body systems (cardiovascular, respiratory, hepatic, endocrine/metabolic, hematological) that may manifest as a skin disorder
3. *NCLEX®* Note allergies to medications, foods, environment, and so on; note allergies to tape, latex, povidone-iodine, alcohol, and other substances
4. Nutrition: note dietary changes, new foods introduced, and fluid intake
5. External exposure: note new products exposed to skin, such as soaps, lotions, sun, and chemicals
6. Activity: note daily physical activity and exercise routine
7. Sleep and rest: note number of hours of sleep each night and any rest periods
8. Coping: discuss skin disorders and how skin is affected when stress is experienced (called flares); note coping behaviors used and results
9. Current medications: list current medications and onset and dose of medications
10. *NCLEX®* Recent surgeries or treatments: note phototherapy, radiation therapy, or other therapy that may affect skin
11. *NCLEX®* Current problem: elicit data about current problem; for skin rash, obtain detailed data such as when rash began, how it has changed, medications or ointments used, and results of treatment

Box 62–1

Characteristics of Suspicious Skin Lesions

The ABCDE rule is a useful aid in teaching clients how to monitor for changes in moles or other suspicious skin lesions, and when to seek evaluation for possible removal by healthcare provider.

A = *Asymmetry*: one half of mole or suspicious lesion does not match other half

B = *Border*: irregular instead of smooth

C = *Color*: not uniform (more than one color shade)

D = *Diameter*: larger than 6 mm (approximate size of pencil eraser)

E = *Evolving*: changing in size, shape, or color

G. Physical examination

1. Note color (pink, yellow, white, purple, bruising, etc.)
2. *NCLEX®* For suspicious moles or lesions, document color, size, shape, symmetry, and border (see Box 62–1); note location and palpate texture, consistency, and mobility
3. Inspect hair for color, amount, distribution, lesions, and hygiene
4. Inspect nails for color, growth pattern, and thickness; inspect nail bed for inflammation or trauma
5. Note texture, temperature, and moisture of skin
6. Palpate skin turgor for hydration status
7. Palpate lower extremities (tibia and ankle) for edema
8. Palpate hair for texture (coarse, fine) and nails for texture and capillary refill

III. TYPES OF SKIN LESIONS

A. Vascular skin lesions

1. Spider angioma: a flat, bright red spot with radiating blood vessels (BVs) at edges
   a. Commonly found on upper body; varies in size from a tiny dot up to 1.5–2 cm
   b. Caused by dilation of BVs commonly seen with high estrogen levels, pregnancy, liver disease, and/or vitamin B deficiency
2. Petechiae
   a. *NCLEX®* Flat red spots, approximately 1–2 mm in diameter, that do not blanche with pressure
   b. *NCLEX®* Caused by broken capillaries, possibly caused by anticoagulant effect, liver disease, vitamin K deficiency, or septicemia
3. *NCLEX®* Purpura: purple or blue-appearing patch that varies in size and shape; caused by a bleeding disorder or broken BVs and may appear throughout body
4. Ecchymosis: irregular flat lesion of varying size that does not blanche
   a. Color changes from purple to greenish yellow during healing; in black skin appears as a darkened area; in brown skin can vary from deep purple to blue in color
   b. Caused by bleeding into tissue because of trauma, liver disease, hemophilia, or vitamin deficiency (C or K)
5. Venous star: flat blue lesion ranging from 3 to 25 mm in size radiating outward from center; caused by increased pressure within superficial vein, and appear often on anterior trunk or on legs near varicose veins

NCLEX® **B. Primary skin lesions** (see Table 62–1)

C. Secondary skin lesions (see Table 62–2, p. 1133)

D. Miscellaneous skin lesions

1. Skin tags: benign **papules** that are flesh-colored or soft brown
2. Keratoses: overgrowth and thickening of cornified epithelium that can be either benign (seborrheic) or premalignant (actinic); may be removed with electrocautery or liquid nitrogen
3. Lentigines: benign **macules** of brown or black color that have a defined border
4. Photoaging: areas of skin with decreased elasticity that are mottled, pigmented, or wrinkled; may lead to benign or malignant skin lesions
5. Telangiectases: single dilated capillaries or terminal arteries
6. Keloids: irregularly shaped raised and progressively enlarging scars from excess collagen growth during scar formation in connective tissue repair
7. Nevi: flat or raised macules or papules with well-defined borders; also known as moles

Table 62–1 Primary Skin Lesions

Macule, Patch 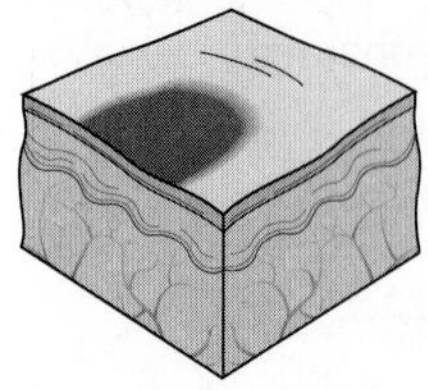	Flat, nonpalpable change in skin color. Macules are smaller than 1 cm, with a circumscribed border. Patches are larger than 1 cm and may have an irregular border. **Examples** Macules: freckles, measles, and petechiae, Patches: Mongolian spots, port-wine stains, vitiligo, and chloasma.	Wheal 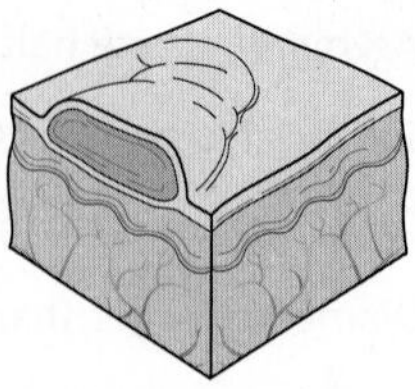	Elevated, often reddish area with irregular border caused by diffuse fluid in tissues rather than free fluid in a cavity, as in vesicles. Size varies. **Examples** Insect bites and hives (extensive wheals).
Papule, Plaque 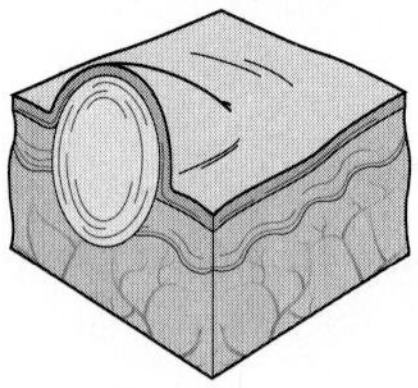	Elevated, solid, palpable mass with circumscribed border. Papules are smaller than 0.5 cm; plaques are groups of papules that form lesions larger than 0.5 cm. **Examples** Papules: elevaled moles, warts, and lichen planus. Plaques: psoriasis, actinic keratosis, and lichen planus.	Pustule 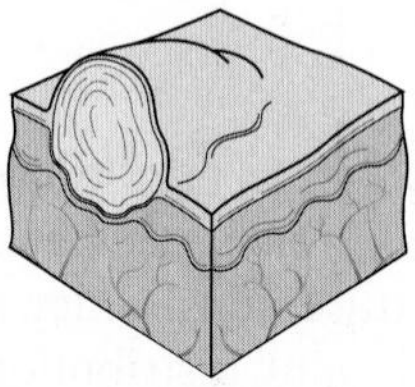	Elevated, pus-filled vesicle or bulla with circumscribed border. Size varies. **Examples** Acne, impetigo, and carbuncles (large boils).
Nodule, Tumor 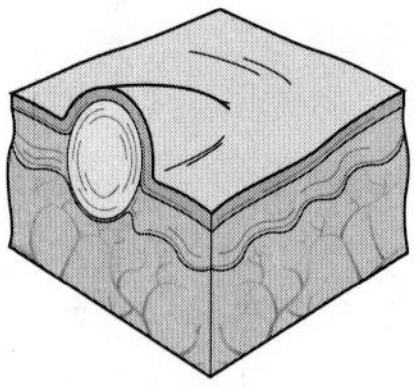	Elevated, solid, hard or soft palpable mass extending deeper into the dermis than a papule. Nodules have circumscribed borders and are 0.5 to 2 cm; tumors may have irregular borders and are larger than 2 cm. **Examples** Nodules; small lipoma squamous cell carcinoma, fibroma, and intradermal nevi, Tumors; large lipoma, carcinoma, and hemangioma.	Cyst 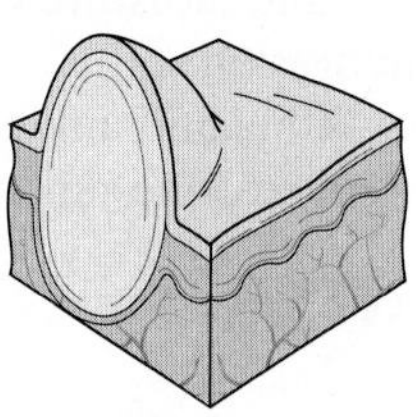	Elevated, encapsulated, fluid-filled or semi-solid mass originating in the subcutaneous tissue or dermis, usually 1 cm or larger. **Examples** Varieties include sebaceous cysts and epidermoid cysts.
Vesicle, Bulla 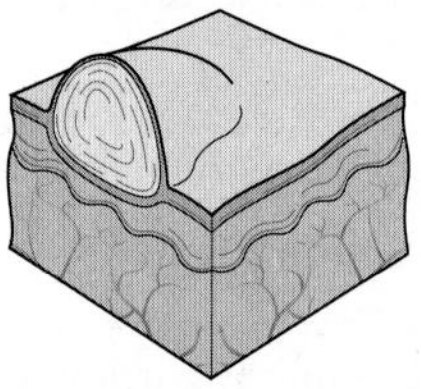	Elevated, fluid-filled, round- or oval-shaped palpable mass with thin, translucent walls and circumscribed borders. Vesicles are smaller than 0.5 cm; bullae are larger than 0.5 cm. **Examples** Vesicles: herpes simplex/zoster, early chickenpox, poison ivy, and small burn blisters, Bullae; contact dermatitis, friction blisters, and large burn blisters.		

Source: LeMone, P., Burke, K., Bauldoff, G., & Gubrud, P. (2015). *Medical surgical nursing: Clinical reasoning in patient care* (6th ed.). Hoboken, NJ: Pearson Education, Table 15-4, p. 386.

IV. DERMATITIS

A. *Atopic dermatitis (eczema)*

1. A chronic relapsing inflammatory skin disorder that may begin in infancy or anytime through adulthood; type I hypersensitivity disorder
2. Etiology may involve a combination of genetic predisposition and defective lipid skin barrier that allows penetration of allergens, irritants, and organisms; possible associated allergic conditions are asthma and food allergies
3. Triggers include stress, changes in temperature and humidity, allergens (foods before age 3 and inhalants such as pollen, mold, dust mites and dander in older children), irritants (soaps, detergents, rough or wooly clothing) and autoantigens to human proteins

NCLEX®

4. Assessment: patches with papules, **vesicles**, exudate, crusts, and excoriation
   a. Infancy and childhood: red papules (raised lesions) associated with **pruritus** (itchiness); **xerosis** (dry skin that may crack,); dry, thickened, scaly, papular patches on extremities, hands, feet, and neck folds and around mouth, eyes, and ears
   b. Adolescents and adults: exudation often caused by external irritation or secondary infection; characterized by **lichenification** (large, dry, thickened lesions or **plaques**) on flexor folds, face, neck, back, upper arms, and dorsal aspects of hands and feet

Table 62–2 Secondary Skin Lesions

Atrophy 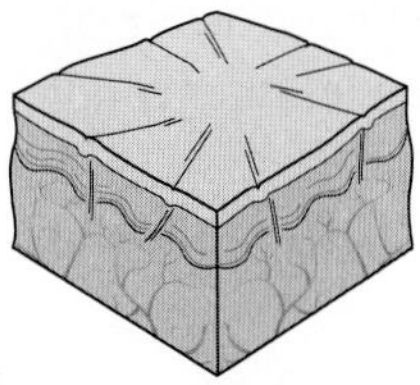	A translucent, dry, paper-like, sometimes wrinkled skin surface resulting from thinning or wasting of the skin due to loss of collagen and elastin. **Examples** Striae, aged skin.	Ulcer 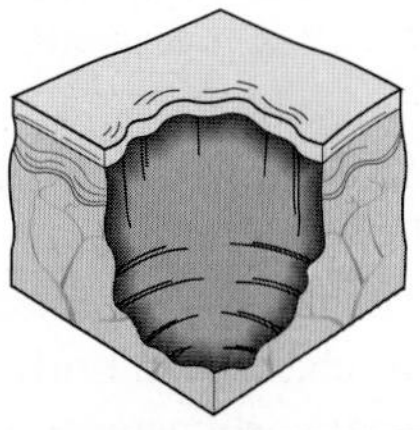	Deep, irregularly shaped area of skin loss extending into the dermis or subcutaneous tissue. May bleed. May leave scar. **Examples** Decubitus ulcers (pressure sores), stasis ulcers, chancres.
Erosion 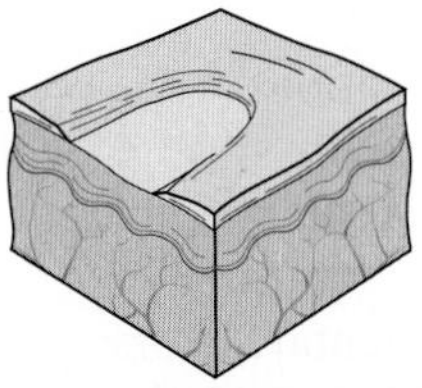	Wearing away of the superficial epidermis causing a moist, shallow depression. Because erosions do not extend into the dermis, they heal without scarring. **Examples** Scratch marks, ruptured vesicles.	Fissure 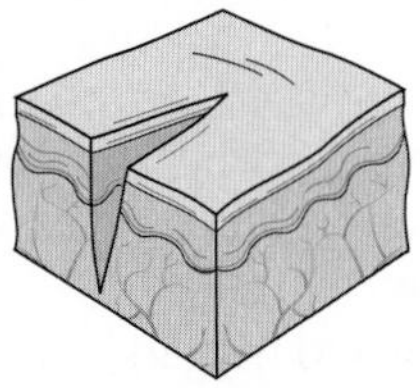	Linear crack with sharp edges, extending into the dermis. **Examples** Cracks at the corners of the mouth or in the hands, athlete's foot.
Lichenification 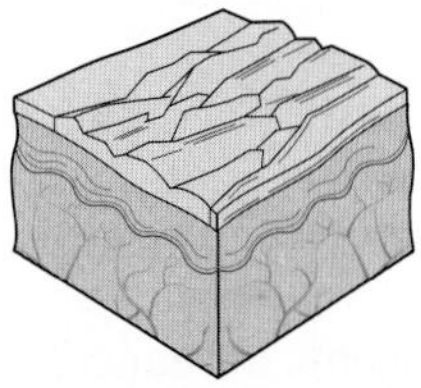	Rough, thickened, hardened area of epidermis resulting from chronic irritation such as scratching or rubbing. **Example** Chronic dermatitis.	Scar 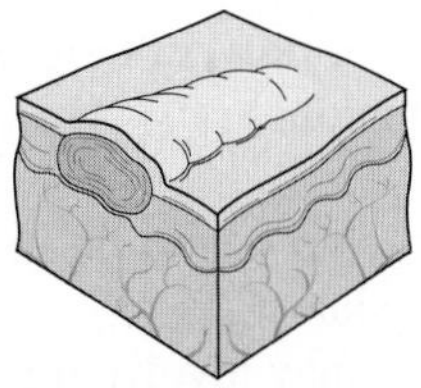	Flat, irregular area of connective tissue left after a lesion or wound has healed. New scars may be red or purple; older scars may be silvery or white. **Examples** Healed surgical wound or injury, healed acne.
Scales 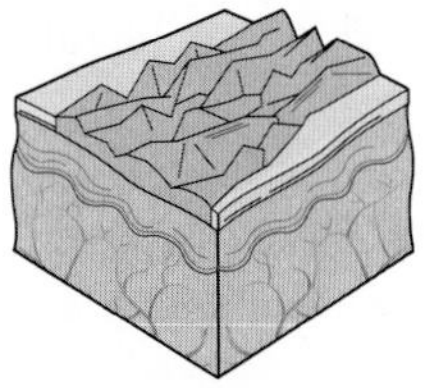	Shedding flakes of greasy, keratinized skin tissue. Color may be white, gray, or silver. Texture may vary from fine to thick. **Examples** Dry skin, dandruff, psoriasis, and eczema.	Keloid 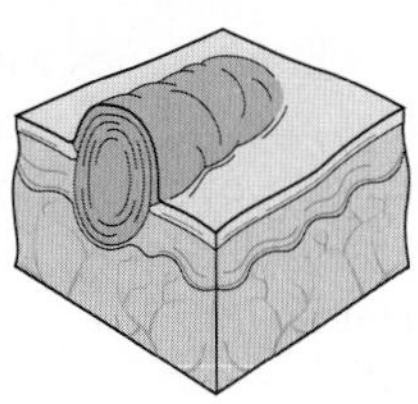	Elevated, irregular, darkened area of excess scar tissue caused by excessive collagen formation during healing. Extends beyond the site of the original injury. Higher incidence in people of African descent. **Examples** Keloid from ear piercing or surgery.
Crusts 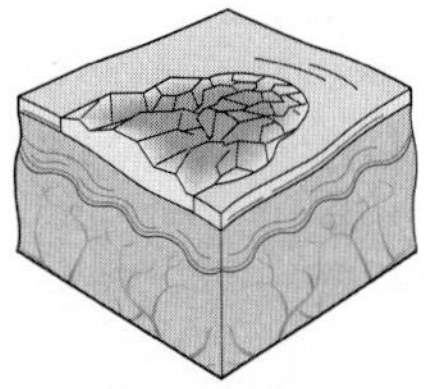	Dry blood, serum, or pus left on the skin surface when vesicles or pustules burst. Can be red-brown, orange, or yellow. Large crusts that adhere to the skin surface are called scabs. **Examples** Eczema, impetigo, herpes, or scabs following abrasion.		

Source: LeMone, P., Burke, K., Bauldoff, G., & Gubrud, P. (2015). *Medical surgical nursing: Clinical reasoning in patient care* (6th ed.). Hoboken, NJ: Pearson Education, Table 15-5, p. 387.

5. Diagnosed by history and physical examination; skin tests or radioallergosorbent tests (RAST) may identify food allergies in allergic type; skin cultures diagnose secondary skin infection

NCLEX®

6. Therapeutic management
   a. Identify and control triggers, keep skin dry and lubricated, and treat flare-ups promptly to reduce risk of secondary infection
   b. Recommend use of humidifier in winter to counteract dry air and air conditioner in summer to limit unnecessary sweating
   c. Have client bathe or shower with tepid to warm water using mild soap only on soiled skin areas; avoid bath additives such as baking soda, bubble bath, or bath oils

   NCLEX®

   d. Pat, rather than rub, skin dry, and immediately apply emollient to retain moisture; reapply three to four times daily or whenever skin feels dry; avoid perfumed or scented lotions

e. Apply topical medications in a thin layer only to affected areas immediately after bath and apply emollient over medication
f. Use antibacterial soaps for handwashing
g. Keep fingernails clean and short; place cotton gloves or socks over hands of infants or young children to prevent scratching

NCLEX®

h. Avoid excessive bathing, woolen or constricting clothing, rough fabrics, wet diapers, and other conditions that can promote itching or trap perspiration
i. Provide support to client and family during flare-ups and reassurance that lesions do not usually scar unless excessively scratched with secondary infection
j. Support client who has changes in body image or self-esteem because of skin lesions

7. Medication therapy: topical corticosteroids to reduce inflammation during flare-ups, immunomodulators, antihistamines (control itching), and topical or oral antibiotics (skin infection only)
8. **Client teaching**
a. Effective hygiene practices and appropriate use of creams, ointments, or other medications
b. Dry skin increases pruritus, which leads to scratching and excoriation
c. Identify foods that exacerbate rash and avoid them; with infants, introduce one new food at a time to see if a flare-up occurs

NCLEX®

d. Avoid known or suspected triggers, such as contact allergens, pets, or other environmental factors; avoid sunburn
e. Use antihistamines before naps or bedtime if itching leads to sleep deprivation
f. Follow treatment plan to prevent flare-ups and secondary infections
g. Condition is not contagious

B. Seborrheic dermatitis

1. A chronic inflammatory skin condition in areas of active sebaceous glands, such as face, scalp, body folds, sternal area, and axilla
2. Etiology is unknown, but may involve hormonal influence, nutrient deficiency, neurogenic influence, sebaceous gland dysfunction, or fungal infection
3. Assessment
a. Lesions with yellow or white plaques with scales (often yellow or orange) and crusts; skin may be oily or flaky and dry, pruritic, and may be at risk for secondary infection
b. Common sites include scalp, eyebrows, nose, ears, sternal area, and axillae
c. Seen more frequently in cold weather, and may be triggered by decreased humidification and decreased exposure to sunlight
4. Therapeutic management
a. Skin care, medications, and client teaching as discussed for atopic dermatitis
b. If scalp is involved, use selenium sulfide 2.5% suspension or other medicated shampoo if recommended by healthcare provider

C. *Contact dermatitis*

1. Overview
a. Skin inflammation caused by an external irritant or an allergic reaction mediated by IgE; epidermal reaction is caused by T-lymphocytes; location of rash helps provide clues to offending substance or antigen
b. Common irritants include chemicals, dyes, metals, poisonous plants (ivy, sumac, oak), and latex; allergic contact dermatitis affects only those previously sensitized and is a delayed hypersensitivity reaction
2. Assessment

NCLEX®

a. Acute: papules, vesicles, bullae with surrounding erythema; crusting, oozing, and pruritis may be present
b. Chronic: erythematous base, thickening with lichenification, scaling, and fissuring

3. Therapeutic management
a. Identify and remove causative agents
b. Topical emollients in combination with mid- to high-potency corticosteroids
c. Drainage of large vesicles may be necessary without removing tops
d. Apply wet dressings to oozing, pruritic lesions to aid in drying and debridement; cool tap water, Burow's solution 1 to 40, saline 1 tsp/pint water, and silver nitrate solution can be used
e. Suppress inflammation with antibacterial solution

NCLEX®

f. May use topical corticosteroid creams but do not use on face
g. Oatmeal baths are helpful to decrease itching
h. Antihistamines may help decrease itching and edema; calamine lotion may aid drying

D. Exfoliative dermatitis

1. An inflammatory skin disorder in which there is excessive shedding or peeling of skin
2. Causes may be idiopathic (about 50%), preexisting skin disorder (other types of dermatitis or psoriasis), reactions to medications, and some cancers (such as lymphoma)

NCLEX®

3. Skin manifestations include scaling, erythema, pruritus, and peeling of skin
4. Systemic manifestations include weakness, malaise, fever, chills, weight loss
5. Primary treatments are therapeutic baths and topical medications

E. Dermatitis from poison ivy, poison oak, and poison sumac

1. An inflammatory reaction following contact with urushiol in these plants
2. Skin manifestations include papulovesicular lesions and severe pruritus in skin areas in contact with plant oils

NCLEX®

3. Therapeutic management consists of cleansing skin thoroughly to remove plant oils (oil is clear and difficult to see, which accounts for possible accidental contamination of other skin areas), application of topical anti-itch products, and possible topical oral or systemic corticosteroids for severe cases

V. PSORIASIS

A. Overview

1. A chronic, inflammatory skin disorder of keratin synthesis leading to raised, reddened, round plaques covered by silvery white scales
2. Possible etiologies include autoimmune reaction, genetic predisposition, trauma, infection, stress, and hormonal influence
3. Various forms exist; psoriasis vulgaris is most common, but psoriatic lesions can develop at sites of skin injury (scratch, sunburn) or with use of certain medications
4. Can lead to arthritis with joint changes that resemble rheumatoid arthritis in some clients

B. Assessment

NCLEX®

1. Dry, scaly rash that may appear as silvery scales or plaques usually found on scalp, knees, or elbows; may involve hands and feet
2. Nails, if affected, are thickened, ridged, and have yellow discoloration
3. Diagnosed by clinical presentation, skin biopsy (if atypical manifestations or for differential diagnosis), or ultrasound (to detect changes in dermis)

NCLEX®

C. Therapeutic management

1. Topical medications such as corticosteroids, coal tar preparations (or shampoos if scalp is affected), calcipotriene (a vitamin D derivative), tazarotene (a synthetic retinoid), and keratinolytics (salicylic acid and sulfur)
2. Systemic medications for severe cases include methotrexate, cyclosporine, and acitretin (teratogenic; contraindicated during pregnancy)
3. Phototherapy for generalized psoriasis (more than 30% of body surface) with ultraviolet-B (UVB) three times weekly in gradually increasing exposure times (measured in seconds) or with PUVA (topical psoralen with ultraviolet-A light) ; eye shielding is needed during treatment
4. Photochemotherapy involves use of a light-activated form of oral methoxsalen, followed by exposure to UVA 2 hours later; treatments are given two to three times per week for 10–20 treatments; exposure to direct light is avoided for 8–12 hours (treatment causes tanning); exposure to light is encouraged if UVA treatment not given
5. Skin care is similar to that described previously for dermatitis
6. Assist client to cope with changes in body image if lesions are large or visible to others; clients may isolate themselves, withdraw from roles and responsibilities, and feel powerless

D. Client teaching: involves skin care, avoiding skin injury (from scratching or dryness), use of prescribed medications, avoiding stress as a trigger, and manifestations of treatment complications to report (skin excoriation, increased erythema, increased skin peeling, or blister formation)

VI. SKIN CANCERS

A. Premalignant condition: *actinic keratosis*

1. Macules on skin caused by chronic sun exposure and photoaging; clients with light complexion are at highest risk; about 20% progress to squamous cell carcinoma

NCLEX®

2. Assessment: erythematous, rough macules a few millimeters in diameter; may be shiny or scaly and appear singly or in groups; commonly seen on face, dorsa of hands, forearms, and upper trunk
3. Prevention includes protection from ultraviolet (UV) sun rays by use of clothing and sunscreens; these measures may also slow or stop progression to carcinoma

NCLEX® 4. Therapeutic management: cryosurgery (freezing) or 5-fluorouracil cream; biopsy and removal of lesion is recommended if changes suggesting malignancy occur; refer back to Box 62–1

B. Nonmelanoma skin cancers

1. Include basal cell carcinoma, squamous cell carcinoma, and other rarer skin tumors
2. Common risk factors include environmental exposure (UV radiation, occupational exposures to coal tar, pitch, creosote, arsenic compounds, or radium) or host factors such as family history, severe sunburn as a child, and skin pigmentation (at greater risk if fair skin, freckles, blond or red hair, or blue or green eyes)
3. Assessment of basal cell carcinoma (five types)
   - NCLEX® **a.** Nodular (most common): small, firm papule (pearly white, pink, or flesh-colored) often on head or neck
   - **b.** Superficial: papule or plaque often on trunk and extremities; second most common; associated with erythema, ulcerations, and well-defined borders
   - **c.** Pigmented: usually found on head or neck; can concentrate melanin
   - **d.** Morpheaform: found on head or neck, forms fingerlike projections (usually ivory- or flesh-colored), and often resembles a scar; can invade and destroy adjacent tissues
   - **e.** Keratotic: found on preauricular or postauricular groove; contains both basal and squamous cells that keratinize; likely to recur after removal and is type most likely to metastasize
4. Assessment of squamous cell carcinoma
   - **a.** Firm red **nodule** initially that may be crusted with keratin "pearls"; may ulcerate, bleed, and cause pain as it grows, with induration (hardness) in skin around lesion
   - **b.** Occurs most often on sun-exposed areas such as forehead, helix of ear, top of nose, lower lip, and back of hands; more aggressive growth and spread than basal cell carcinoma
5. Therapeutic management
   - **a.** Focuses on removal using surgical excision, Mohs' surgery (thin layers of tumor are sequentially shaved off and examined), curettage (scraping away) with electrodessication (low-voltage abrasion of tumor base), cryotherapy, photodynamic therapy, laser surgery, or topical chemotherapy
   - NCLEX® **b.** Educate clients regarding importance of monitoring lesions and early identification of new lesions; suggest monthly self-assessment of skin and periodic screening by healthcare provider based on symptoms
   - NCLEX® **c.** Encourage skin protection from UV light by using sunscreen with SPF 15 or higher, wearing hat and other protective clothing, and minimizing sun exposure between 10:00 a.m. and 4:00 p.m. (strongest UV sun rays)
   - NCLEX® **d.** Postoperative instructions include how and when to change dressing (per provider recommendation), proper hand hygiene and aseptic technique when caring for wound, protecting operative site from trauma and irritation, and signs of infection to report

C. Malignant melanoma

NCLEX® 1. Less common skin cancer arising from melanocytes; responsible for large majority of skin cancer deaths because of tendency to metastasize
2. Risk factors include moles; fair skin with freckling, blond hair or blue eyes; having a close relative with history of melanoma; use of immunosuppressant medications; excess exposure to UV radiation (sunlight, tanning apparatus); age over 50 years; xeroderma pigmentosus (rare inherited disease with reduced ability to repair skin damage from sun)
3. Consists of four different types, but each is characterized by a radial and/or vertical growth phase; metastasis occurs during vertical growth phase
4. Assessment
   - **a.** Lesions often found on trunk of men and extremities of women
   - NCLEX® **b.** Client reports mole that changes (70% of time) according to ABCDE rule (refer again to Box 62–1)
   - **c.** Characteristics vary by type but are generally darker (tan, brown, or black) than other skin cancers
   - **d.** Diagnosis is with skin biopsy; other tests such as bloodwork, CT scan, x-rays, or MRI may be done to diagnose metastasis
5. Therapeutic management
   - **a.** Surgery (with wide excision) is preferred treatment, but others include chemotherapy, immunotherapy, and radiation therapy
   - **b.** Maintain medical and surgical asepsis when changing surgical dressing or caring for incision
   - **c.** Encourage adequate nutrition with sufficient calories, protein, and vitamins
   - **d.** Assist client to cope with diagnosis of cancer and possibility or reality of metastasis

D. Kaposi's sarcoma

1. A rare skin cancer of endothelial lining of small BVs, seen most often on face, nose, and ears
2. May be related to infective agent such as a retrovirus (e.g., human immunodeficiency virus [HIV]) or other client with immunosuppressed state

NCLEX®
3. Assessment
   a. Vascular lesions (macules, papules, nodules) that can affect skin and viscera
   b. Over time, lesions enlarge and converge, forming large masses; underlying tissue becomes involved with invasion of lymphatic tissue, which may lead to lymphedema (primarily affecting genitalia and lower extremities)
   c. As disease progresses, tumor may interfere with internal organ function and may even cause bleeding to point of hemorrhage (a late sign)
   d. Initially Kaposi's sarcoma may be symptom-free; however, pain may be experienced in later stages

NCLEX®
4. Therapeutic management
   a. Isolated lesions may be removed by excision, cryotherapy, and/or local radiation for comfort and/or cosmetic treatment
   b. Medication therapy: single agent or combination chemotherapy

VII. BACTERIAL INFECTIONS

A. Impetigo

1. Overview
   a. A contagious superficial skin infection often caused by *Staphylococcus aureas* and/or *group-A beta-hemolytic streptococcus*; initially appears as a vesicle or **pustule** surrounded by edematous skin and erythema; as it progresses to exudative stage, vesicles rupture, leaving a honey-colored crusted lesion
   b. Most commonly seen in children but occasionally affects adults; common sites are on face, around mouth, or on neck, extremities, or hands
   c. Causative factors may include inadequate hygiene or secondary infection of another skin injury (such as a rash or bite); tends to occur more often during hot, humid months
2. Assessment: presence of characteristic skin lesions (either single lesion or several lesions that have coalesced), erythema, client reports of pruritus and/or burning sensation, possible local lymph node enlargement
3. Therapeutic management

NCLEX®
   a. Encourage frequent and thorough hand hygiene with warm, soapy water to prevent spreading bacteria to others
   b. Initiate contact precautions immediately if child is hospitalized, in addition to standard precautions
   c. Provide or recommend daily bathing with antibacterial soap
   d. Apply warm compresses to site as prescribed two to three times per day to soften crusts, following by washing with warm water and mild soap to remove crusts
   e. Medication therapy: topical or systemic antibiotic therapy, if topical treatment used, do not contaminate medication tube with fingers (squeeze medication onto cotton swab)

NCLEX®
   f. Teach parents (or clients) not to share utensils, dishes, towels, or toiletries with others; wash client's laundry and linens separately from others in hot water and detergent
   g. Keep fingernails short to prevent scratching and spread of bacteria

B. Folliculitis, furuncles, and carbuncles

1. Folliculitis: a superficial bacterial infection of hair follicle, often caused by *Staphylococcus aureus* or *Pseudomonas aeruginosa*; more often seen in males; can be aggravated by shaving, particularly skin on face (beard), legs, and axilla
2. Furuncle (boil): an **erythemic**, warm, tender inflammation of hair follicle that extends down hair shaft into dermis; often caused by *Staphylococcus* organism; common sites are nares, neck, axilla, and genital area
3. Carbuncle: an inflammatory lesion formed when several furuncles coalesce to form one larger infected skin lesion; common sites are hair follicles in back of neck, upper back, and lateral thighs; *Staphylococcus* is a common causative organism
4. Assessment
   a. Folliculitis: hair follicle is surrounded by an erythemic, pruritic, mildly tender pustule
   b. Furuncle: deep, firm, red nodule from 1 to 5 cm in diameter that changes into a large, painful cystic nodule with purulent drainage
   c. Carbuncle: swollen and painful mass that has multiple openings to skin surface; possible malaise and low-grade fever

5. Therapeutic management
   a. Cleanse site with warm water and antibacterial soap two to three times a day maintaining standard precautions
   b. Warm, moist heat may be applied to site for comfort
   c. Teach client about contributing factors such as inadequate hygiene, poor nutrition, prolonged skin moisture, skin trauma, and tight, heavy fabrics on upper legs
   d. Instruct client who uses razors to throw away old razor and use clean, sharp razor
   e. Avoid use of irritating lotions or creams at site
   f. Some lesions may require incision and drainage; culture and sensitivity of drainage is performed
   g. Medication therapy: topical mupirocin applied three times a day for simple folliculitis; for more severe cases, oral antibiotics are prescribed

C. *Cellulitis*

1. Overview
   a. Bacterial infection of dermal and subcutaneous tissues with lesions appearing in various stages, ranging from vesicles, bullae, abscesses, and plaques
   b. Most commonly seen in adults, with group-A beta-hemolytic *Streptococcus pyogenes* and *Staphylococcus aureus* being most frequent organisms
   c. Cellulitis occurs because of a break in skin integrity (abrasion, laceration, etc.); may also occur secondary to a skin lesion

NCLEX®

2. Assessment
   a. Erythemic, swollen, tender-to-touch area of skin at site of entry of bacteria
   b. Associated symptoms include fever, chills, malaise, anorexia, and regional lymphadenopathy

NCLEX®

3. Therapeutic management
   a. Rest and elevation of affected part; apply moist heat to site for comfort
   b. Culture and sensitivity of tissue site for severe cases
   c. For necrotic tissue, surgical excision and debridement are recommended along with antibiotic therapy
   d. Hospitalization is needed if cellulitis is on face or covers a large area; otherwise, management is done at home
   e. Medication therapy: antibiotic therapy

D. Methicillin-resistant *Staphylococcus aureus* infection

1. An infection of skin, hair follicle, or wound by *Staphylococcus aureus* microorganism that is resistant to treatment with methicillin (a penicillin antibiotic)
2. Is highly contagious; can range from mild infection to one that is severe
3. MRSA infection of skin may be diagnosed by skin swab
4. Place hospitalized client on contact precautions and admit to a single bed room
5. Treatment is with another antibiotic to which microorganism is susceptible

VIII. VIRAL INFECTIONS

A. Herpes simplex virus (type 1, type 2)

1. Overview
   a. A viral infection manifested by vesicles on oral mucosa (mouth or lips), which is HSV type 1, or in genital mucosa (HSV type 2); HSV infection can occur at any age
   b. Spread by direct contact with contaminated body fluids; incubation period is 2–14 days
   c. Primary infection: initial outbreak in which blisters occur on mucosa or lips; malaise and fever are also common symptoms
   d. Recurrent infections: outbreaks are commonly precipitated by stress and illness; symptoms are usually milder than primary outbreak, with a prodrome of tingling, itching, or a burning sensation at site prior to outbreak of lesions
   e. Latency period: virus remains dormant in body during this time

NCLEX®

2. Assessment
   a. Primary symptoms include malaise, fever, and vesicles appearing on mucosa
   b. Secondary symptoms include prodrome of tingling, burning sensation prior to outbreak of vesicles on mucosa; latency period is asymptomatic
3. Therapeutic management
   a. Advise rest
   b. Teach and encourage appropriate hand hygiene to prevent spread of virus (*NCLEX®*)
   c. Comfort measures such as petroleum jelly or lip balm may be used for oral lesions

NCLEX®
d. To prevent spreading virus, teach client to avoid close contact with others while lesions are present; to prevent HSV type 2, advise use of latex condoms even if asymptomatic to prevent spreading genital lesions
e. Medication therapy: over-the-counter (OTC) medications, such as acetaminophen or camphophenique for comfort as needed; prescribed antiviral medications such as acyclovir, famciclovir, or valacyclovir may reduce further viral replication and diminish symptoms if started within 24–48 hours after initial onset of lesions

B. Herpes zoster (shingles)

1. Overview
   a. Viral infection in clients with a history of chickenpox, manifested by vesicles on skin; commonly seen in older adults or immunocompromised clients
   b. Reactivation of dormant varicella virus in dorsal root ganglia of sensory spinal or cranial nerves
   c. May be transmitted to those who have not had been immunized against chickenpox and have not had disease

NCLEX®
2. Assessment
   a. A cluster of skin vesicles appears unilaterally on skin along path of one sensory nerve dermatome on trunk or face
   b. Associated symptoms are tingling, itching, burning, and pain at site of lesions, fatigue, malaise, fever, and headache; touch and warmth aggravate pain
3. Therapeutic management
   NCLEX®
   a. For hospitalized clients, maintain standard precautions; if infection is disseminated or if client is immunocompromised, add contact and airborne precautions until lesions are crusted over per CDC recommendations
   b. Provide comfort measures including air mattress, bed cradle, cool environment, and wet dressings or soaks (Burow's solution) on lesions two to three times a day
   NCLEX®
   c. Oatmeal baths, available OTC, are soothing and help to dry lesions; astringent compresses may also be prescribed
   d. Teach client to rest, to avoid scratching or rubbing affected skin, and to wear loose, lightweight cotton clothing (avoid heavy fabrics such as wool)
   e. To prevent viral spread to others, take care to avoid persons at risk
   f. Monitor lesions for secondary bacterial infections and monitor neurovascular and cranial nerve status (complication is palsy of cranial nerve VII or Bell's palsy)
   g. Shingles vaccine is recommended for adults age 60 years or older with normal immune system function to reduce risk of shingles and possible long-term postherpetic neuralgia
   NCLEX®
   h. Medication therapy: topical or oral antiviral medications such as acyclovir, famciclovir, and valacyclovir; acetaminophen and ibuprofen may be used for discomfort

C. Warts

1. Elevation in epidermal skin layer, commonly seen in children and young adults, caused by papillomavirus; virus may be transmitted from person to person by touch and is commonly seen on hands and feet
2. Assessment: painless, flesh-colored nodule on skin surface that has a rough surface with an irregular border; there are several types of warts
   a. Common wart—commonly seen on hands or extremities, but can occur anywhere on body; often appear to have a "black seed" in center of lesion; may appear intermittently and last approximately 6–12 months without treatment
   b. Flat wart—a nodule 1–3 mm in diameter; may appear in clusters on back of hand or forehead
   c. Filiform wart—a tiny, thin, projected nodule commonly seen on face, nose, or eyelids
   d. Plantar wart—a hard nodule (approximate size of a pencil eraser) found on bottom of foot; commonly projects into foot from constant pressure applied while walking; discomfort or pain at site is common
3. Therapeutic management
   a. Sometimes no treatment is necessary for warts because viral lesions will resolve on their own
   NCLEX®
   b. OTC wart removal products include salicylic acid (17%) and retinoic acid
   c. Laser therapy may be used for selected warts (large or located in genital area)
   d. Warts that are treated may reappear in same site or on other areas of skin

IX. FUNGAL INFECTIONS

A. Candidiasis

1. Superficial infection of skin and mucous membranes caused by *Candida albicans* if local immunity is disturbed; also called yeast infection or thrush (oral infection)

2. Common sites include perineal area, vagina, under breasts, axilla and oral mucous membranes

NCLEX® 3. Risk factors include moist, warm, or interrupted skin integrity; systemic antibiotics; pregnancy; birth control use; poor nutrition; diabetes mellitus or chronic illnesses; and immunosuppression

NCLEX® 4. Assessment: lesions are bright red, smooth macules with a macerated appearance and a scaling, elevated border; characteristic "satellite" lesions are small, similar-appearing macules outside main lesion; oral lesions consist of reddish or white milky plaques that may be associated with a burning sensation or decreased taste

5. Diagnosis is made by culture of scrapings or by microscopic examination of scaling with potassium hydrochloride (KOH) preparation

6. Therapeutic management
   - NCLEX® a. Avoid sharing linens or personal items
   - NCLEX® b. Use clean towel and washcloth daily
   - c. Dry all skinfolds; avoid frequent immersion of hands in water
   - d. Wear clean cotton underwear daily
   - e. For vaginal candida, avoid tight clothing and pantyhose, bathe more frequently, and dry genital area thoroughly; may need to treat sexual partner at same time to avoid reinfection or have partner use condoms until resolved; avoid douching and change perineal pads frequently
   - f. For balanitis (inflammation of glans and prepuce of penis), carefully retract foreskin and perform careful cleaning and drying of glans
   - g. For oral candidiasis, provide frequent mouth care with nonirritating products and offer nonirritating foods and tepid fluids
   - h. Encourage weight loss for obese clients and euglycemia in diabetic clients to decrease risk of infection
   - NCLEX® i. Medication therapy: antifungals (topical, shampoo, or vaginal suppository depending on site) or nystatin powder or ointment; systemic medications require monitoring of liver function tests (risk of hepatotoxicity)

B. Tinea infections (dermatophytoses)

1. Overview
   - a. A fungal infection of scalp (tinea capitus), trunk (tinea corporis), groin or upper thighs (tinea cruris or "jock itch"), or feet (tinea pedis or "athlete's foot"); may also be called ringworm
   - b. For most clinical purposes, classification by anatomic site is preferred
   - c. All species of dermatophytes (fungi that grow in nonliving, keratinized portions of skin) can be causative agent; generally more prevalent in hot and humid climates
   - d. Can affect all age groups, but children are more often affected
   - NCLEX® e. Can be spread human-to-human, animal-to-human, and soil-to-human by direct contact; other risk factors include prolonged use of topical steroids or immunosuppression

2. Assessment
   - NCLEX® a. Tinea capitis: scaly, pustular bald areas with nondistinct margins; may be lighter than skin color or have erythema or yellow greasy scales; may have areas where hair has broken off
   - b. Tinea corporis: classic lesions are annular (ringlike), scaly, or erythematous plaques with an expanding and slightly elevated border, sharp margins, and a clearing center
   - c. Tinea cruris: scaly, erythematous annular lesions on groin or thighs that could spread to abdomen or buttocks; usually penis and scrotum are spared
   - d. Tinea pedis: dry, red, scaly patches or plaques on plantar or lateral surfaces of foot or between toes; secondary bacterial infection between toes is noted by peeling macerated skin with fissures
   - e. Diagnosis is by microscopic examination of skin scrapings using KOH wet mount, Wood's light (helps identify some types), or fungal cultures

3. Therapeutic management
   - a. Avoid contact with suspected lesions
   - b. Thoroughly clean environment to remove fungal scales that are shed from skin
   - c. Avoid sharing towels, hair accessories, brushes, hats, or other items that can transmit fungal scales
   - NCLEX® d. Search out infected animals/pets and treat appropriately
   - e. Keep involved areas clean, dry, and exposed to air when possible
   - f. If feet are involved, wear light cotton socks and change frequently throughout day; wear sandals or open-toed shoes when possible; avoid plastic or occlusive shoes
   - g. Use selenium sulfide shampoo to wash hair or body to reduce spores
   - h. Carefully dry skin, such as between toes, after showering or bathing
   - i. Apply drying or dusting powers, topical antiperspirants
   - j. Put socks on before underwear to avoid spreading from foot to groin

k. Monitor for signs of superimposed bacterial infection such as pain, increased inflammation, pustules, or purulent exudates

NCLEX®

l. Medication therapy: topical drugs for superficial infections; oral antifungal drugs as prescribed; eradication is slow and treatment may take 2–8 weeks

X. INFESTATIONS, STINGS, AND BITES

A. Pediculosis

1. Overview
   a. An infestation of skin or hair by species of blood-sucking lice capable of living as external parasites on human host
   b. ***Pediculosis capitis*** is head louse, size of a sesame seed, clear in color when hatched but becomes grayish-white to red/brown after maturing; commonly found in occipital area, at nape of neck behind ears, and sometimes in eyelashes or eyebrows
   c. Head lice infestation is very common among school-age children and is spread by sharing items such as combs, brushes, hats, scarves, and bedding
   d. *Pediculosis pubis*, also known as "crabs," infests genital area and is a common sexually transmitted infection because it spreads by sexual contact
   e. Nits (white eggs) attach to hair shaft by a cementlike or cocoonlike structure and are difficult to remove; adult lice are tan or gray, move quickly, and are difficult to see
   f. All contacts of infested client should be examined and treated if necessary

NCLEX®

2. Assessment
   a. Intensive pruritis is most common symptom that may result in excoriations
   b. Head lice may resemble dandruff flakes, but are not easily brushed off
   c. Papular urticaria may be found at neck or pubic area
3. Therapeutic management
   a. Nits must be mechanically removed daily; a 50/50 white vinegar/water solution may loosen nits; olive oil may also be used; a nit comb removes nits from hair shafts (best effect by back-combing hair); lice may also be removed by fingers or tweezers
   b. To treat eyelashes, apply petrolatum to lashes twice daily for 10 days; lice may suffocate or slide off, or may need manual removal while wearing gloves

NCLEX®

   c. Educate children and parents about mode of transmission (person to person) and preventive measures, such as not sharing combs, brushes, hats, scarves, helmets, headphones, bedding, towels, or sleeping bags
   d. Coats and hats should be hung separately and not touch each other

NCLEX®

   e. All family members need to be examined and treated at same time
   f. Each family member should use own comb or brush and grooming items
   g. Soak personal hair items or any item in contact with hair in boiling water for 10 minutes or OTC pediculocide for 1 hour
   h. Shaving hair is not found to be helpful

NCLEX®

   i. Machine-wash all bedding and washable clothing in hot water with detergent daily for 1 week; dry for 20 minutes in dryer using hot setting
   j. Seal items such as nonessential bedding or clothes and items that cannot be washed or dry-cleaned (such as toys) in air-tight plastic bags for 2 weeks to kill lice
   k. Upholstered furniture or pillows may be ironed with a hot iron
   l. Vacuum mattresses, rugs, upholstered furniture, and stuffed animals frequently; discard collection bag and replace with a new one after each vacuuming

NCLEX®

   m. Medication therapy: permethrin, pyrethrin, or lindane shampoo is left on 5–10 minutes and then washed off; lindane can be repeated in 1 week, but is neurotoxic and should not be used on open skin or by young children, nursing or pregnant women, or clients with known seizure disorders; for pediculosis pubis, a cream or lotion may be applied and left on for several hours

B. *Scabies*

1. Overview
   a. A contagious parasitic skin infestation caused by mite *Sarcoptes scabiei var hominis*; impregnated mite burrows into skin, lays eggs, and remains in burrow for life (approximately 30 days); eggs hatch in 3–4 days and mature, migrate to skin surface, mate, and repeat cycle
   b. Spread by skin-to-skin or sexual contact; easily transmitted within a household and among those in close quarters, such as schools or institutions; mites can live in clothing fibers and can be transmitted by contact with infected clothing or bed linens

c. Diagnosis is usually made by clinical presentation of burrows, vesicles, and nodules; client is infectious throughout infestation

2. Assessment

NCLEX®

a. Presents as a generalized pruritic papular rash with possible flesh-colored, raised burrows (threadlike linear ridges with a pinpoint vesicle at one end)

b. Increased warmth of skin and nocturnal itching (often 10–14 days after exposure) are classic symptoms, since mites tend to have increased movment at night; exposure to hot water or steam can also increase pruritis

3. Therapeutic management

a. Close family members and personal contacts must be treated also, even if there are no apparent signs or symptoms

NCLEX®

b. All bed clothing, linens, and unwashed worn clothing should be washed and dried in a hot dryer to kill mites

NCLEX®

c. Mites and eggs may be killed by placing items in airtight plastic bags for at least 4 days since mite cannot live away from host more than 3 days; mites can live 24–36 hours in room conditions and longer in humid environments

d. Relief from itching may not occur for 3–6 weeks after treatment because of hypersensitivity of skin to debris left in burrow

NCLEX®

e. Scabicide lotions/creams should be applied according to product directions to entire body but avoiding eyes and mucous membranes, using a toothbrush to get under fingernails and toenails; lotion is showered off 8–12 hours later

f. Permethrin lotion or malathion is treatment of choice; a second application 1 week later is recommended

g. Crotamiton is less toxic but is also slightly less effective; therefore, application for two nights is advised

NCLEX®

h. Lindane cream or lotion (see precautions previously noted); treatment may be repeated after 1 week

i. An oral antihistamine may be needed to relieve itching

j. May require emollients and midpotency corticosteroids after using scabicide to suppress hyperreactivity caused by mites; antibiotics may be needed if secondary infection occurs

C. Bee and wasp stings

1. Stings that contain poison cause local tissue inflammation and destruction noted by a **wheal** and flare reaction

2. Allergic reaction can occur from previous sensitization or toxic reaction from large inoculation of poison; IgE-mediated hypersensitivity to insect venom may be confirmed by skin testing

NCLEX®

3. Therapeutic management

NCLEX®

a. Remove stinger promptly by gently scraping it; do not squeeze with a tweezer to avoid pinching sac containing venom; then cleanse wound

NCLEX®

b. Apply ice pack—alternate 10 minutes on and 10 minutes off

c. Elevate and rest affected part

d. If client has allergic response (swelling of lips and tongue, hives, pruritus), maintain adequate airway and provide or activate emergency care

NCLEX®

e. Persons with known sensitivity should wear medical ID tag, prevent reexposure and be able to use EpiPen or anaphylactic kit

f. Instruct to use insect repellants when outdoors or in infested areas

g. Educate client on risks of increasing severity of responses in future; desensitization with immunotherapy may be considered in severe cases

D. Scorpion stings

1. Caused by injection of venom into skin by scorpion tail, leading to local inflammation and pain; mild systemic reactions may occur and are treated supportively with wound care and analgesics

2. Venom from bark scorpion is neurotoxic and potentially fatal; client should be transported to emergency department for treatment with antivenom and supportive care

E. Spider bites

1. Venom from certain spiders can be toxic to humans, including brown recluse spider, black widow spider, and tarantula

2. Black widow spider bite is recognized by a small red papule and onset of acute pain shortly after bite; because venom is neurotoxic, ice should be applied immediately to inhibit systemic absorption of venom; client should seek emergency care

3. Brown recluse spider bite causes reddened skin followed by a blister at site; leads to an open ulceration and tissue necrosis about a week later and may take months to heal

a. Ice should be applied immediately to site and intermittently for up to 4 days to reduce risk of tissue necrosis and possible systemic symptoms
b. If ulceration leads to infection, topical antiseptics and antibiotics may be required

4. Tarantula bite causes pain, inflammation, redness, and swelling at site; ejected tarantula hairs can irritate skin and cause asthma-like symptoms if inhaled
   a. Remove hairs using sticky tape and irrigate area well; elevate and immobilize affected extremity
   b. Client may require antihistamines or corticosteroids, tetanus prophylaxis, and possible treatment of muscle spasms (from systemic absorption of venom) with muscle relaxants

XI. URTICARIA

A. Overview

NCLEX®
1. **Urticaria** is an itchy rash with single or multiple superficial raised, pale macules with red halo; subsides rapidly, with no scars or change in pigmentation, but may reoccur

NCLEX®
2. IgE-mediated response with massive histamine release from mast cells in superficial dermis
3. Can be caused by multiple agents such as drug reaction, food or food-additive allergy, inhalant, contact or ingestion allergy, transfusion reaction, insect bite or sting, bacterial, viral, fungal, or helminthic infection, collagen vascular disease, lupus, heat, cold, sunlight (solar urticaria), or emotional stress
4. True urticarial lesions do not remain in same area of skin longer than 24 hours; lesions that are present 72 hours or longer suggest cutaneous vasculitis as a possible cause
5. Chronic urticaria persists over 6 weeks; not mediated by IgE; also associated with fever, chills, arthralgia, myalgia, and headache

B. Assessment

NCLEX®
1. Single or multiple raised, blanched, central wheals surrounded by red flare that is intensely pruritic; may occur anywhere on body
2. Variable size of 1–2 mm to 15–20 cm or larger
3. Resolves spontaneously in less than 24–48 hours

C. Therapeutic management

1. Cool, moist compresses help to control itching

NCLEX®
2. Avoidance of trigger if etiology is known; there is risk of life-threatening reaction on reexposure
3. Antihistamine if accidentally reexposed
4. Subcutaneous administration of epinephrine 1:1000 for intense itching
5. Cyprohepadine 4 mg every 6 hours for cold urticaria
6. Corticosteroids for pressure urticaria
7. Topical sunscreens and hydroxyzine for solar urticaria

XII. ACNE AND OTHER BENIGN SKIN CONDITIONS

A. *Acne*

1. Overview
   a. A chronic inflammatory disorder of pilosebaceous hair follicles resulting in comedones, papules, inflammatory pustules, nodules, **cysts**, and occasional scarring
   b. Has many contributing factors including androgenic influence to increase sebum production, hormonal influence around time of menstrual cycle, inflammation, abnormal keratinization of follicular epithelium, oily skin, genetic predisposition, and proliferation of *propionibacterium acnes*
   c. More common in males; earliest skin changes of acne may be seen in prepubescent years
2. Assessment
   a. Lesions may occur on forehead, cheeks, nose or extend over upper chest, shoulders, or back
   b. Inspection shows closed comedones (whiteheads) and open comedones (blackheads)
   c. With more extensive involvement, papules and pustules develop that lead to nodules and cysts, an eventual scar formation that is pitted, atrophic, or hypertrophic (keloid)
   d. Grades of acne (see Box 62–2)
3. Therapeutic management
   a. Intended to control disease and is not curative
   b. Use a gentle antibacterial soap and wash affected areas with fingertips
   c. Avoid cosmetics containing oil and use moisturizing lotions only on dry patches of skin
   d. Instruct not to pick lesions, which would increase scarring
   e. Six to eight weeks of treatment is usual before obvious improvement occurs
   f. Explain that diet does not cause acne and that flare-ups may result from increased sweating, heat, humidity, and emotional stress

Box 62–2

Stages and Grades of Acne

Stages of Acne

Mild: few to several papules, no nodules, on face and neck only

Moderate: several to many papules and pustules; few to several nodules on face, back, chest, or upper arms

Severe: numerous and extensive papules and pustules; many nodules with acne-induced scarring

Grades of Acne

Grade 1: comedonal—closed and open

Grade 2: papular—over 25 lesions on face and trunk

Grade 3: pustular—over 25 lesions with mild scarring

Grade 4: nodulocystic—inflammatory nodules and cysts with extensive scarring

NCLEX®
g. Topical retinoids are usually prescribed for all types of acne
h. For mild acne, combination therapy of a topical retinoid plus one or more of the following: benzoyl peroxide, topical antibiotics, or azelaic acid
i. For moderate acne, topical agents and oral antibiotics such as tetracycline for a specified period of time and then antibiotic is discontinued
j. For severe acne, isotretinoin may be prescribed for up to 20 weeks but is teratogenic so pregnancy must be avoided; see also Chapter 42
k. Antiandrogens such as oral contraceptives and spironolactone inhibit sebum production

B. Lentigo

1. Overview
   a. Benign lentigo is a brown macule resembling a freckle except that border is usually irregular
   b. Lentigo maligna (premelanoma) is a brown or black mottled, irregularly outlined, slowly enlarging lesion with atypical melanocytes; usually occurs on face; one-third progress to melanoma but transition may take 10–15 years
   c. Senile lentigo (liver spot) is flat and occurs often on sun-exposed skin of white older adults
2. Therapeutic management consists of client teaching
   NCLEX® a. Report changes in existing skin lesions for evaluation by a healthcare provider
   b. Inspect skin routinely and seek professional advice for changes
   NCLEX® c. Use sunscreens, hats, and protective clothing while in sunlight to avoid overexposure
   d. Lentigo maligna: should follow up with a dermatologist for evaluation and removal

C. *Vitiligo*

1. Overview
   a. An acquired, slowly progressive depigmentation in small or large areas of skin caused by a decrease in active melanocytes
   b. Type A: nondermatomal and widespread involvement in 75% of cases
   c. Type B: dermatomal and segmental; 50% of cases begin between ages 10 and 30
2. Assessment
   a. Loss of pigment with increased sunburning of areas; more often occurs around eyes, mouth, and anus
   b. May be pruritic and associated with premature graying
3. Therapeutic management
   a. Avoid sun exposure, which may increase differentiation between normal and abnormal skin
   b. Consider use of skin dyes or cosmetics for blending purposes
   c. Localized areas may be treated with midpotency corticosteroids
   d. Oral systemic corticosteroids are effective in arresting disease progression
   e. Depigmenting of normal skin may be achieved using hydroquinone cream

XIII. *PRESSURE ULCERS*

A. Overview

1. Ischemic lesions of skin and underlying tissue caused by external pressure over an extended period of time, leading to impaired flow of blood and lymph
2. Common and serious complication affecting frail, disabled, acutely ill, or immobile clients

3. Most common sites are over bony prominences, such as elbows, hips, heels, outer ankles, and base of spine; over 95% of ulcers develop on lower part of body
4. Causes include an uneven application of pressure over a bony site: high pressure applied for 2 hours (produces irreversible tissue ischemia and necrosis), shearing forces that develop when a client slides toward floor or foot of bed, frictional forces that develop when pulling a client across a bed sheet, and moisture from incontinence or perspiration

B. Assessment

NCLEX® 1. Stage pressure ulcers according to their characteristics; see Box 62–3
NCLEX® 2. Assess for risk factors (see Box 62–4) and use pressure ulcer risk assessment scales such as Braden scale or Norton scale (see also Chapter 26)
3. Assess ulcer routinely for location, dimensions, stage, exudate, visible necrotic tissue, or abnormal pathways in wound (sinus tract, tunneling, undermining)
4. Diagnostic and laboratory test findings: culture of wound, WBC with differential; if no progression of ulcer healing, albumin levels may be obtained to determine dietary needs

C. Therapeutic management

NCLEX® 1. Reposition client every 2 hours; encourage active range of motion (ROM) exercises and perform passive ROM as needed; ensure underlying bed sheet is free of wrinkles
2. Control fecal and urine incontinence by checking client frequently and changing bed pad as needed; cleanse skin and dry well; use a moisture barrier cream or ointment to protect skin
3. Avoid massage over bony prominences or areas that do not blanche with applied pressure
NCLEX® 4. Provide relief of pressure on wound; use support devices such as padding (gel pads), flotation pads, mattress overlays, and specialized beds (air-fluidized, oscillating, or kinetic) as indicated
NCLEX® 5. Ensure optimal nutritional status—adequate protein intake; encourage oral high-calorie and high-protein supplements and oral zinc, vitamins A and C, and iron to aid in tissue healing
6. Clean wound with each dressing change to remove dead tissue, excess fluid, and debris; monitor healing and document

Box 62–3

Pressure Ulcer Stages

Stage 1: Nonblanching erythema, warmth, and tenderness

Stage 2: Skin breakdown limited to dermis, excoriation, blistering, drainage, more sharply defined erythema, variable skin temperature, local swelling, and edema

Stage 3: Ulcer formation into subcutaneous tissues, crater formation, slough, eschar, and/or drainage

Stage 4: Ulcers extend beyond deep fascia into muscle or bone, decayed area may be larger than visible wound, osteomyelitis or sepsis may be present, granulation tissue and epithelialization may be present at wound margins

Box 62–4

Risk Factors for Pressure Ulcers

Immobility

Malnutrition, hypoalbuminemia, or vitamin C deficiency

Low body weight

Fecal and/or urinary incontinence

Bone fracture

Low diastolic blood pressure (affects perfusion)

Age-related skin changes such as thinning of epidermis, loss of dermal vessels, and altered barrier properties or diminished perception of pain or pressure

Reduced immunity and slowed wound healing

Disorders such as anemia, infections, peripheral vascular insufficiency, dementia, malignancies, diabetes mellitus, or cerebrovascular accident (CVA or stroke)

Dry skin

Edema

7. Use agency protocols for pressure ulcer management
8. Avoid using antiseptics and harsh skin cleansers that may harm tissue; provide gentle but thorough skin care
9. Avoid use of agents that delay wound healing such as topical corticosteroids, hydrogen peroxide, povidone iodine, and hypochlorite

NCLEX®
10. Assess site every 8–12 hours; carefully document healing (e.g., "healing stage III ulcer" rather than "stage II ulcer" if ulcer was stage III and exhibits healing)

NCLEX®
11. Use appropriate type of dressing, which may include hydrocolloid, alginate, hydrofibers, hydrogel, transparent adhesive, wet-to-moist, or vacuum-assisted closure (see also Chapter 26)

D. Medication therapy

1. Antibiotics such as clindamycin or gentamycin may be prescribed for complications such as cellulitis, osteomyelitis, or sepsis
2. Vitamin C 500 mg twice daily and zinc sulfate supplements aid healing

NCLEX®
3. Enzymatic debriding agents such as collagenase, fibinolysin-desoxyribonuclease, or sutilains are used with a moisture barrier to protect surrounding tissue

E. Client education

1. Need for frequent evaluation of clients with a history of pressure ulcers, especially if they have limited mobility
2. Nutritional requirements (adequate protein, vitamins, minerals, and calories) and meal planning
3. Early identification of skin redness to prevent breakdown
4. Skin cleansing routine and possible use of padded undergarments to wick moisture away from skin
5. Repositioning techniques and frequency
6. Need to evaluate and ensure continence and access to bathroom facilities
7. Use of pressure-relief devices such as mattress overlays, seat cushions, or special mattresses

XIV. FROSTBITE

A. Overview

1. Cold injury from prolonged exposure to freezing temperatures leading to tissue and blood vessel damage
2. Most commonly affected areas are exposed to environment and/or have less underlying supportive tissue to provide warmth, such as fingers and toes, face, nose, and ears

B. Assessment

1. Superficial frostbite: numbness, itching, and prickling sensations, local edema and skin color that is white, reddened, or cyanotic
2. Deeper frostbite: skin paresthesias and stiffness; skin becomes white or yellow during thawing, with burning pain, lost skin elasticity, edema, and development of blisters, necrosis, and possible gangrene

C. Therapeutic management

1. When providing advice to client in the field, recommend applying firm pressure of warm hand(s) to affected area or place affected hands under axillae; if feet are frostbitten and wet, remove footwear, dry feet, and apply dry socks and footwear if available

NCLEX®
2. For hospitalized client, rewarm affected areas in a circulating bath at a temperature of 104–105°F (40–40.6°C) for 20–30 minutes

NCLEX®
3. Handle affected area gently and avoid rubbing area, which could further traumatize underlying tissue
4. When rewarming is complete, place client on bedrest with affected part elevated
5. Administer analgesic and anti-inflammatory agents as prescribed; anticipate that client will experience significant pain with rewarming
6. Provide wound care as prescribed using loose, sterile nonadherent dressings
7. Assess for compartment syndrome as appropriate to area affected
8. Administer prescribed analgesics, antimicrobial agents, and tetanus prophylaxis as needed
9. Anticipate possible need for wound debridement, whirlpool therapy, and possible amputation if necrosis leads to gangrene

XV. BURN INJURY

A. Overview

1. A break in skin integrity leading to tissue loss or injury caused by heat, chemicals, electricity, or radiation

NCLEX®
2. Types of burn injury: thermal, chemical, electrical, and radiation

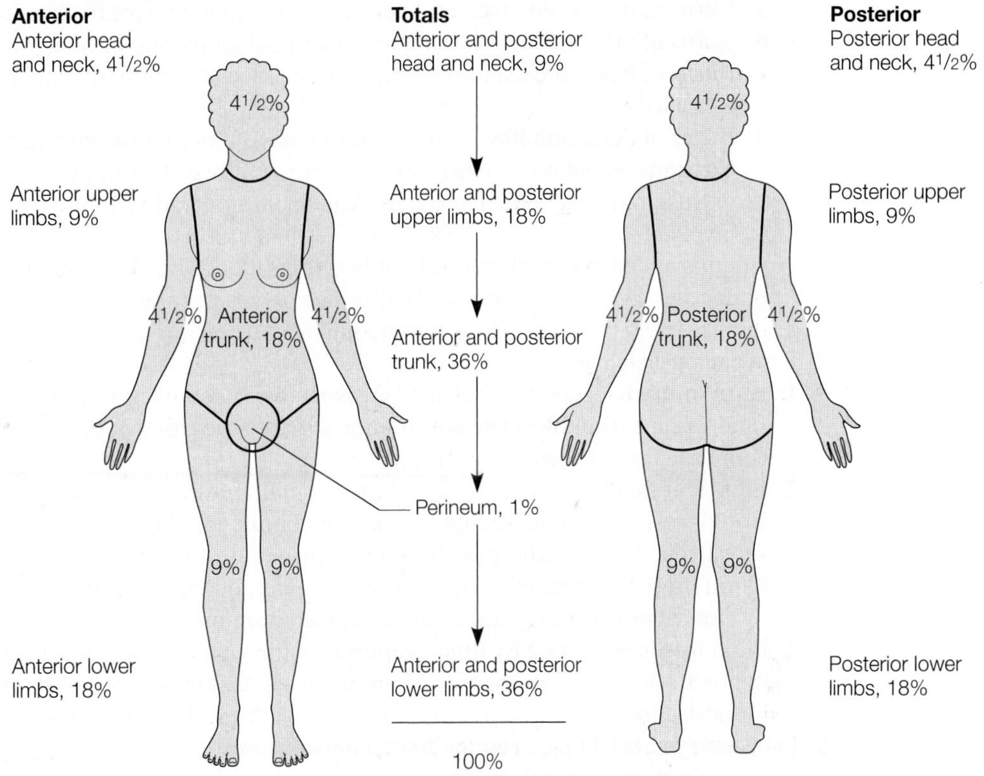

Figure 62–1
Calculating burn injury using the Rule of Nines.

a. Thermal burn (most common): results from dry heat (flames) or moist heat (steam or hot liquids); can also lead to inhalation injury if head and neck area is affected
b. Chemical burn: caused by direct contact with either acidic or alkaline agents; alters tissue perfusion and leads to necrosis
c. Electrical burn: severity depends on type and duration of current and amount of voltage; electricity follows path of least resistance (muscles, bone, blood vessels, and nerves)
d. Radiation burn: usually associated with sunburn or radiation treatment for cancer; usually superficial injury but extensive exposure can lead to tissue damage and multisystem injury

3. Burn size: small burns generate a bodily response that is limited to area of injury, while large burns are more extensive (25% or more of total body surface area [TBSA] in an adult or 10% or more TBSA for child) and lead to a systemic bodily response

NCLEX®
4. An estimate of burn size is calculated using Rule of Nines (see Figure 62–1) or Lund and Browder method; each chart accounts for 100% of TBSA, although Lund and Browder method takes into account client's age when estimating body surface area

NCLEX®
5. Classification of burn depth: made according to depth of damaged tissue (Table 62–3)
6. Severity of burn is classified using American Burn Association criteria as minor burn, moderate uncomplicated burn, and major burn; these categories help determine treatment

Table 62–3 Classification of Burn Injury by Depth of Burn

Classification	Depth of Burn Injury
Superficial thickness	Involves epidermis only and is recognized by characteristics of erythema, absence of blisters for 24 hours, local pain; healing occurs spontaneously in 3–5 days with no scar formation
Superficial partial thickness	Involves epidermis and dermis, characterized by moist areas that are red to ivory in color, blisters form immediately; area is painful because touch and pain receptors are intact; area heals with greater or lesser amounts of scarring within 21–28 days
Deep partial thickness	Involves possibly entire layer of dermis and is more severe than a superficial partial-thickness burn; skin appendages are left intact; area has a dry, waxy, whitish appearance and may be difficult to differentiate initially from full-thickness burns; may heal spontaneously in about 1 month, although skin grafting is often done to close wound, accelerate healing, and reduce scarring and risk of infection
Full thickness	Involves destruction of all skin elements with coagulation of subdermal plexus; muscle and tendons may be involved

a. Burns of hands, feet, face, and perineum are at higher risk for functional impairment
b. Burns of face may be associated with corneal injury and auricular chondritis if ear is involved
c. Burns of head, neck, and/or chest may be associated with inhalation injury and respiratory complications
d. Burns of perineum have higher risk of autocontamination with elimination of urine and feces

NCLEX®

e. Circumferential burns (surrounding an extremity or trunk) pose risk of compartment syndrome in extremities or inadequate chest wall expansion and respiratory insufficiency if thorax is involved

7. Client's age and underlying state of health influence burn outcomes; death rate is higher for children under age 4 years or older adults after age 65 years; comorbid cardiac, respiratory, endocrine, or renal diseases negatively affect client outcome

B. Burn pathophysiology

1. Burn injury triggers local release of vasoactive substances and increase capillary permeability, allowing fluid to shift from blood vessels to interstitial tissues; this begins to reverse after 18–26 hours but is not complete until 2–3 weeks postburn
2. Fluid shift leads to local edema if burn is small but generalized body edema if burn area is large
3. Body's response to decreased circulating volume is same as for hypovolemia, leading to hypovolemic shock (decreasing kidney perfusion and urine output, increasing pulse, decreasing cardiac output and blood pressure, increasing hematocrit from hemoconcentration, possible paralytic ileus from shunting of blood away from GI tract, and depressed immune function)
4. Fluid loss is worsened by fluid evaporation through burn wound; sodium is also lost, leading to hyponatremia, and serum potassium increases as it moves out of damaged or destroyed cells and into bloodstream

C. Burn management during emergent/resuscitative phase

1. Lasts from onset of injury through successful fluid resuscitation; during this phase, it is determined whether client requires care in a burn center based on onset of injury, burn source, and complicating factors
2. Prehospital care begins at scene and continues until arrival in emergency department
   a. Remove client from burn source; assess airway, breathing, and circulation (ABCs) and possible associated inhalation injury or trauma
   b. Specific first-aid measures include to douse flames with water or smother with a blanket, coat, or other similar object; cool a scald burn with cool water; flush chemical burns copiously with water or other appropriate irrigant after dusting away any dry powder if present; remove client from contact with an electrical source only after current has been shut off
   c. Burn care includes covering burns with clean or sterile cloths and removing restrictive clothing nearby
   d. Emergency personnel will initiate intravenous (IV) access and transport to emergency department

NCLEX®

3. Emergency department care continues with priority attention to ABCs
   a. Assess for smoke inhalation injury (singed nasal hairs, eyebrows, or eyelashes; burns on face, neck, or upper chest; edematous and/or reddened oropharynx, stridor, hoarse voice, cough with sooty sputum, increasing dyspnea) and administer O_2 (up to 100% as prescribed until carboxyhemoglobin level approaches normal [1–10%])
   b. Be prepared for possible intubation and mechanical ventilation if severe inhalation injury or carbon monoxide inhalation has occurred
   c. Assess for signs of shock caused by fluid shifts (decreased urine output, increased pulse, falling BP, pallor, cool clammy skin, deteriorating level of consciousness [LOC])

NCLEX®

   d. Assessment also includes brief history of how burn occurred, estimates burn extent and depth, past medical history, medication history including date of last tetanus prophylaxis, and assessment for other concurrent injuries

NCLEX®

4. Fluid resuscitation: modified Brooke formula uses isotonic saline with 5% albumin and lactated Ringer's solution with 2 mL/kg/% TBSA burned for first 24 hours; Parkland (Baxter) formula uses 4 mL/kg/% TBSA burned in first 24 hours (crystalloid only—lactated Ringer's); both formulas give half of 24-hour total in first 8 hours and second half over next 16 hours
5. Goal of fluid resuscitation is to achieve stable vital signs, palpable peripheral pulses, urine output of 30–50 mL/hr, and intact cognition (level of consciousness and thought processes)

NCLEX®

6. For known or suspected inhalation injury, anticipate 100% oxygen therapy via snug nonrebreather face mask until carboxyhemoglobin level drops to 15%; monitor ongoing respiratory status and arterial blood gas results

7. Insert indwelling urinary catheter, monitor urine output, and obtain urine sample for myoglobin or hemoglobin if prescribed
8. Insert nasogastric tube as prescribed; administer prescribed gastric protective agents and assess for paralytic ileus (loss or absence of bowel sounds)
9. Remove rings and jewelry to avoid tourniquet effect from swelling of burn site
10. Initiate and maintain cardiac monitoring for clients with underlying cardiac disease, to detect changes associated with hyperkalemia, and for first 24 hours after an electrical burn

NCLEX®

11. Initiate reverse precautions (protective isolation) with use of sterile gowns, gloves, cap, mask, and shoe covers; obtain a "burn cart" supplied with sterile items for client care, such as sheets, towels, facecloths, and gown
12. Keep client's room temperature warm to avoid chilling with loss of protective skin barrier
13. Protect against pressure injury to skin and underlying tissues by using bed cradle and specialized mattress

NCLEX®

14. Administer prescribed medications: opioid analgesics by IV route, tetanus booster (>5–10 years since last dose), topical antimicrobials, systemic antibiotics
15. Monitor daily weight; anticipate a fluid weight gain of 6.8–9 kg (15–20 lb) in first 72 hours
16. Client education: focuses on brief explanations about injury, treatments, and ongoing nursing care in this phase

D. **Acute phase of burn management**: begins with start of diuresis (usually 48–72 hours postburn) and ends with closure of burn wound

1. Assessment: varies depending on cause, depth, and TBSA of burn; associated symptoms arising from other organ systems may include nausea and vomiting, pain, skin redness, chills, respiratory distress, and hypovolemia

NCLEX®

2. Burn wound management
   a. Wound care consists of cleansing wound (with saline followed by dressing or during hydrotherapy), maintaining open or closed dressing, debridement to remove necrotic tissue or eschar (with enzymes, mechanical removal, or surgical excision), and possible escharotomy

NCLEX®

   b. Premedicate client before dressing changes
   c. Mafenide may be applied in thin layer over open wound and covered with dressing
   d. Sulfadiazine may applied in thin layer over open wound and covered with dressing; use with caution when impaired renal function exists; must be washed off and reapplied every 8–12 hours
   e. Topical or systemic antibiotic therapy may be prescribed as indicated for infection
   f. Escharotomy involves making a lengthwise incision through burn eschar to release constriction and pressure in tissues underlying a circumferential burn to restore adequate circulation; can be done at bedside; assess neurovascular status and control bleeding with pressure after procedure; pack open incision with sterile, moist dressing as prescribed to prevent drying of incised tissue
3. Provide nutritional therapy: progress from NPO to clear liquids to a high-calorie, high-protein diet with vitamins and minerals; continue to maintain hydration status; continue enteral feedings if started based on need
4. Continue protective isolation with strict sterile technique and maintain infection control measures
5. Maintain heated environment to prevent chilling
6. Provide ongoing psychosocial support to client and family
7. Work with interprofessional team to provide physical therapy as needed
   a. Perform prescribed ROM exercises to maintain joint mobility and prevent contractures
   b. Ambulate client as tolerated to reduce hazards of immobility and maintain leg strength
   c. Apply static splints as prescribed to immobilize joint if unable to maintain proper position or during sleep; apply dynamic splints to exercise affected joint; prevent excessive pressure to skin during splint application to prevent additional injury or nerve damage
   d. Apply prescribed elastic bandages or wraps or anti-burn scar support garments to affected areas to reduce scarring during healing; these apply continuous pressure to skin to reduce shear; anti-burn support garments should be worn for 23 hours daily for 18–24 months until burn scar has matured
8. As recovery continues, skin grafting may be required to achieve healing in full-thickness and large, deep partial-thickness burns
   a. Graft materials include biosynthetic materials, synthetic materials, or biological materials, which include own skin from another area of body (autograft), human cadaver skin (allograft or homograft), animal skin (xenograft or heterograft), cultured skin, and artificial skin

PRACTICE TEST

b. Graft site care includes elevation of area, keeping it free from pressure, monitoring healing and attachment of graft to underlying tissue, aspiration of fluid accumulated under site if prescribed using a fine sterile needle and syringe, and monitoring for infection
c. Client teaching related to graft site care includes protecting area from sunlight, use of prescribed lubricant to avoid dryness, and avoiding use of harsh detergents and fabric softeners
d. Donor site care includes nonadherent dressing, biosynthetic dressing, or gauze dressing impregnated with petrolatum per healthcare provider preference; teaching client to avoid scratching area (may itch during healing), other measures as described for graft site care, and that healing occurs in about 7–14 days if cared for appropriately

E. **Rehabilitative phase of burn management:** begins with wound closure and ends when client returns to highest level of health restoration
1. Obtain psychosocial evaluation; provide support and management; assist with referrals for counseling if necessary
2. *NCLEX®* Prevent immobility contractures with exercises or ongoing physical therapy
3. Continue to use preventative measures for scar formation (such as burn garments)
4. Assess home environment for needs and accessibility and assist client in returning to work, family, and social life
5. Medication therapy: ongoing pain management and antibiotic therapy as necessary
6. Client education
   a. *NCLEX®* Environmental safety: use low temperature setting for hot water heater, ensure access to and adequate number of electrical cords/outlets, isolate household chemicals, avoid smoking in bed
   b. Use of household smoke detectors with emphasis on maintenance, especially battery replacement
   c. Proper storage and use of flammable substances
   d. Evacuation plan for family
   e. Care of burn at home and graft site care if applicable
   f. Signs and symptoms of infection
   g. *NCLEX®* Use of sunscreen to protect healing tissue and other protective skin care measures

Check Your NCLEX–RN® Exam I.Q.

You are ready for testing on this content if you can:

- Identify basic structures and functions of the integumentary system.
- Describe the pathophysiology and etiology of common integumentary disorders.
- Discuss expected assessment data and diagnostic test findings for selected integumentary disorders.
- Discuss therapeutic management of a client experiencing an integumentary disorder.
- Discuss nursing management of a client experiencing an integumentary disorder.
- Identify expected outcomes for the client experiencing an integumentarydisorder.

PRACTICE TEST

1 A nurse is teaching a group of young adults about skin lesions. Which item would be appropriate to include in discussions with these clients? Select all that apply.

1. Benefits of suntanning
2. Importance of monthly skin self-inspection
3. Evaluation of skin lesions using the ABCDE method
4. Need to seek professional advice regarding lesions
5. Use of sunscreen with an SPF of 8 or higher

2 A client with psoriasis has a follow-up visit with the healthcare provider. The nurse concludes that the client is receiving first-line therapy after seeing a medical record notation for which treatments? Select all that apply.

1. Emollient
2. Phototherapy
3. Topical corticosteroid
4. Methotrexate
5. Dermabrasion

3 The nurse practitioner documents in a client record that the adolescent has closed comedones. The nurse explains to the client that this means the lesions are what type of skin eruption?

1. Whiteheads
2. Blackheads
3. Pustules
4. Cysts

4 The nurse evaluates that a client understands the clinical management of seborrheic keratosis when he explains the use of which therapy? Select all that apply.

1. Antibiotics
2. Antifungal creams
3. Liquid nitrogen
4. Corticosteroids
5. Electrocautery

5 A client with contact dermatitis asks the nurse how he could have developed the condition. Which etiology should the nurse include in a response to the client?

1. Allergic reaction mediated by IgE
2. Poor hygiene
3. Reactivation of IgA antibodies
4. Side effect of oral medication

6 When explaining the disorder to a client with tinea corporis, the nurse should include which information about this skin disorder?

1. It requires no treatment.
2. It can be passed human to human.
3. It should be exposed to sunlight.
4. It is a malignant skin condition.

7 A client with burn injury asks the nurse what the term “full thickness” means. The nurse should respond that burns classified as full thickness involve tissue destruction down to which level?

1. Epidermis
2. Subcutaneous tissue
3. Internal organs
4. Dermis

8 The client comes to the office for evaluation of a skin rash. What question would the nurse include when obtaining a client history?

1. “Have you ever had a skin rash like this before?”
2. “Do you smoke?”
3. “How long have you had that mole on your left arm?”
4. “Do you have a family history of skin cancer?”

9 The nurse is assessing the client’s skin and wants to evaluate a site for petechiae. What technique can the nurse perform to complete this assessment?

1. Rub the site and watch for bleeding.
2. Apply pressure to the site to evaluate for blanching of the skin.
3. Look for other lesions that are similar to that lesion.
4. Apply a tourniquet in a limb and watch for the development of petechiae.

10 A client has been diagnosed with atopic dermatitis. Which statement made by the client indicates an understanding of its management?

1. “I will avoid excessive use of soap and water and keep my skin well hydrated with emollients.”
2. “I will take daily baths and use strong antibacterial soaps to prevent skin infections.”
3. “I will make sure to expose my skin to the sun at least 1 hour a day.”
4. “I will wait 3 hours after bathing to apply lotion to my skin.”

11 A client diagnosed with psoriasis has been prescribed an antihistamine. The client asks the nurse what this is used for because she does not have nasal allergies and congestion. What is the most appropriate response?

1. “Antihistamines are not used for psoriasis and should not have been prescribed.”
2. “The insert on the package will tell you what the medication is for.”
3. “Let me ask the doctor because I’m not really sure.”
4. “Antihistamines are used to help relieve itching associated with the lesions.”

12 What instructions regarding shampooing the hair would the nurse provide to a client diagnosed with seborrheic dermatitis of the scalp?

1. "Use any brand of shampoo because it does not make a difference in scalp therapy."
2. "Coal tar shampoos are recommended for seborrheic dermatitis of the scalp."
3. "Medicated shampoos are recommended because if not treated successfully, seborrheic dermatitis can cause permanent hair loss."
4. "Daily use of coal tar shampoos will cure seborrheic dermatitis."

13 The nurse should include which instruction when teaching a client measures to reduce the risk of developing basal cell carcinoma?

1. Limit the use of tanning beds.
2. Use sunscreen with SPF protection of 15 or higher when in the sun.
3. Limit exposure of the skin to the sun to between the hours of 10:00 a.m. and 4:00 p.m.
4. Eating a balanced diet is the most important means of preventing skin cancer.

14 The client with cellulitis is being discharged from the hospital. What statement should the nurse include in discharge instructions to the client?

1. "If pustules develop, squeeze the lesions gently each day to remove the pus."
2. "If the lesion looks healed, stop taking the antibiotic so you will not develop resistance."
3. "Monitor for signs of infection such as fever, chills, malaise, and redness or tenderness at the site."
4. "Drainage from the site is an expected finding and is no cause for concern."

15 Which of the following is a priority nursing concern for a client experiencing cellulitis of the arm?

1. Disturbance in normal sleep pattern because of skin infection
2. Client embarrassment and self-isolation because of skin infection
3. Feeling of powerlessness because of inability to control infection
4. Client discomfort or pain related to skin infection of cellulitis

16 The client receives a prescription to treat a skin condition affecting the scalp and neck. The medications prescribed are coal tar shampoo and topical steroids. The nurse concludes that this client has which probable diagnosis?

1. Folliculitis
2. Cellulitis
3. Psoriasis
4. Furuncles

17 A client has just been diagnosed with herpes virus type 2. The nurse should share with the client which item of information?

1. "The initial outbreak of herpes is often the most uncomfortable. Recurrent infections usually present with a tingling and burning sensation prior to outbreak of the vesicle."
2. "Each outbreak of herpes is uncomfortable, with the amount of pain at the genital area worsening each time."
3. "You can only have one outbreak of herpes, so you will never experience another."
4. "You should never experience discomfort with herpes; thus, if you have pain in the genital area, you probably have a sexually transmitted infection."

18 A client presents for removal of a skin lesion after it is determined that he meets all criteria for removal using the ABCDE rule. The nurse interprets this to mean which of the following?

1. The lesion is symmetrical, with a smooth border, a single color, and the diameter has stayed the same.
2. The lesion is symmetrical with an irregular border, a single color, and the diameter has increased.
3. The lesion is asymmetrical with a regular border, two colors, and the diameter is smaller.
4. The lesion is asymmetrical with an irregular border, two colors, and the diameter has increased.

19 The nurse examining the skin of a client notes vascular skin lesions that are flat and bright red in color, with tiny vessels that radiate out from its center. The nurse enters which documentation about these lesions?

1. Petechiae
2. Spider angiomas
3. Venous stars
4. Port wine stains

20 A client presents on admission with pressure ulcers extending into the bone. The nurse documents this ulcer at stage ____. Provide a numerical answer.

Fill in your answer below:
Answer: Stage ___

21 A child was admitted to the emergency department with a thermal burn to the right arm and leg. Which assessment by the nurse requires immediate action?

1. Coughing and wheezing
2. Bright red skin with small blisters on the burn sites
3. Thirst
4. Singed hair

22 A school-age child develops atopic dermatitis secondary to food allergies. What would be a priority concern of the nurse when planning care for this child?

1. Inadequate nutrition
2. Changes in body image
3. Loss of skin temperature regulation
4. Circulation to affected area

23 An infant has a positive family history of allergies. To reduce the risk of the infant developing atopic dermatitis, the nurse teaches the family to do which of the following?

1. Avoid synthetic clothing—use natural fibers like cotton and wool.
2. Keep up with the schedule of childhood immunizations.
3. Avoid contact with infected personnel.
4. Introduce only one new food a week so food allergies can be recognized and eliminated.

24 The parents of an 18-month-old with atopic dermatitis are concerned that a secondary infection that has developed will permanently disfigure their child. How can the nurse best support the parents' feelings?

1. Divert the conversation to another topic.
2. Let them know that they are not being blamed for their feelings.
3. Encourage them to discuss their fears and concerns.
4. Tell them not to worry because scarring is unlikely with eczema.

25 The child has just been admitted to the pediatric burn unit. Currently, the child is being evaluated for burns to his chest and upper legs. He complains of thirst and asks for a drink. What is the most appropriate nursing action?

1. Give a small glass of a clear liquid.
2. Give a small glass of a full liquid.
3. Keep the child NPO.
4. Order a pediatric meal tray with extra liquids.

PRACTICE TEST

ANSWERS & RATIONALES

ANSWERS & RATIONALES

1 **Answer: 2, 3, 4 Rationale:** Monthly skin inspection will aid in detecting skin lesions. Evaluating skin lesions for asymmetry, border, color, diameter, and evolving is important to help detect early changes consistent with skin cancer. Health professionals can accurately diagnose skin conditions as well as determine which ones are benign versus cancerous. Tanning and sun exposure can increase susceptibility to skin cancers. For best protection against ultraviolet light rays, sunscreens should have an SPF factor of 15 or higher. **Cognitive Level:** Applying **Client Need:** Health Promotion and Maintenance **Integrated Process:** Nursing Process: Planning **Content Area:** Adult Health: Integumentary **Strategy:** The wording of the question tells you that more than one option is likely to be correct. Use the process of elimination and knowledge about prevention and assessment of skin lesions to evaluate each option.

2 **Answer: 1, 2, 3 Rationale:** Emollients, phototherapy, and topical corticosteroids are first-line treatments for psoriasis. Methotrexate is used for severe and nonresponsive cases of psoriasis; it is not a first-line form of therapy. Dermabrasion is not a treatment used for psoriasis. **Cognitive Level:** Applying **Client Need:** Physiological Adaptation **Integrated Process:** Nursing Process: Diagnosis **Content Area:** Adult Health: Integumentary **Strategy:** The core issue of the question is knowledge of the sequence of treatments for psoriasis. The wording of the question tells you that more than one option is likely to be

correct. Use the process of elimination and nursing knowledge to make a selection.

3 **Answer: 1 Rationale:** Whiteheads are classified as closed comedones. Blackheads are open comedones. Pustules are a type of primary skin lesion. Cysts are fluid-filled lesions. **Cognitive Level:** Applying **Client Need:** Physiological Adaptation **Integrated Process:** Nursing Process: Assessment **Content Area:** Child Health **Strategy:** The core issue of the question is knowledge of various skin eruptions. The wording of the question tells you that the correct response is also a true statement of fact. Use the process of elimination and nursing knowledge to make a selection.

4 **Answer: 3, 5 Rationale:** Liquid nitrogen or electrocautery may be used to remove the lesions of seborrheic keratosis. Antibiotics, antifungal creams, and corticosteroids are not indicated for treatment of seborrheic keratosis. **Cognitive Level:** Applying **Client Need:** Physiological Adaptation **Integrated Process:** Nursing Process: Evaluation **Content Area:** Adult Health: Integumentary **Strategy:** The core issue of the question is knowledge of treatments for seborrheic keratosis. The wording of the question tells you that more than one option is likely to be correct. Use the process of elimination and nursing knowledge to make a selection.

5 **Answer: 1 Rationale:** Contact dermatitis is an inflammatory response of the skin following prior sensitization to an antigen with production of a specific IgE antibody. Skin manifestations occur with subsequent exposures. Contact dermatitis is not caused by poor hygiene, reactivation of IgA antibodies, or as a side effect of an oral medication. **Cognitive Level:** Applying **Client Need:** Physiological Adaptation **Integrated Process:** Nursing Process: Assessment **Content Area:** Adult Health: Integumentary **Strategy:** The core issue of the question is the ability to correctly describe contact dermatitis. The wording of the question tells you the correct answer is also a true statement. Use the process of elimination and nursing knowledge to make a selection.

6 **Answer: 2 Rationale:** Fungal infections such as tinea corporis may be transmitted by direct contact with animals and other persons. Tinea corporis does require treatment. Tinea corporis is not treatable by sunlight. Tinea corporis is not malignant. **Cognitive Level:** Applying **Client Need:** Physiological Adaptation **Integrated Process:** Nursing Process: Implementation **Content Area:** Adult Health: Integumentary **Strategy:** The core issue of the question is knowledge of the characteristics of infection with tinea corporis. The wording of the question tells you the correct statement is the correct answer. Use the process of elimination and nursing knowledge to make a selection.

7 **Answer: 2 Rationale:** A full-thickness burn involves all skin layers, including the epidermis and dermis, and may extend into the subcutaneous tissue and fat. A full-thickness burn extends deeper than just the epidermal skin layer. Full-thickness burns do not involve internal organs. A full-thickness burn can extend deeper than the dermis skin layer. **Cognitive Level:** Applying **Client Need:** Physiological Adaptation **Integrated Process:** Nursing Process: Implementation **Content Area:** Adult Health: Integumentary **Strategy:** The core issue of the question is knowledge of the various depths of burn injury. The critical words *down to* indicate that the correct option is the deepest level of involvement possible. Use the process of elimination and nursing knowledge to make a selection.

8 **Answer: 1 Rationale:** The most important questions would be aimed at obtaining information about the chief complaint, which in this case is the skin rash. Questions about smoking involve general health and could be asked at a later time. Questions about a skin mole involve a different skin condition and could be asked at a later time. Although important for general health screening, family history of skin cancer is unrelated to the current skin problem. **Cognitive Level:** Applying **Client Need:** Physiological Adaptation **Integrated Process:** Nursing Process: Assessment **Content Area:** Adult Health: Integumentary **Strategy:** The core issue of the question is appropriate questions to ask when obtaining a nursing history about a skin disorder. The wording of the question tells you the correct statement is the correct answer. Use the process of elimination and knowledge of health assessment to make a selection.

9 **Answer: 2 Rationale:** When assessing petechiae, pressure is applied to the site but will not produce blanching of the skin. For other types of lesions, blanching may occur. The site should not be rubbed to try to elicit bleeding. Identifying similar lesions will not aid in assessing current petechiae. Tourniquets interrupt arterial and venous circulation and are not used to assess petechiae. **Cognitive Level:** Applying **Client Need:** Physiological Adaptation **Integrated Process:** Nursing Process: Assessment **Content Area:** Adult Health: Integumentary **Strategy:** The core issue of the question is knowledge of nursing assessment techniques for the skin. The wording of the question tells you the correct statement is the correct answer. Use the process of elimination and nursing knowledge to make a selection.

10 **Answer: 1 Rationale:** Skin care for atopic dermatitis should include keeping the skin well hydrated, which is aided by the use of emollients. The client should avoid using harsh soaps. Sun exposure will not aid in keeping skin hydrated and could exert a drying effect. Emollients should be applied immediately after bathing. **Cognitive Level:** Applying **Client Need:** Physiological Adaptation **Integrated Process:** Nursing Process: Evaluation **Content Area:** Adult Health: Integumentary **Strategy:** The core issue of the question is knowledge of appropriate care to the skin when the client has eczema. The wording of the question tells you the answer is a true statement. Use the process of elimination and nursing knowledge to make a selection.

11 **Answer: 4 Rationale:** Antihistamines are useful to help relieve itching associated with psoriasis. Antihistamines are often prescribed as part of treatment for psoriasis. It is not helpful to answer a question by referring a client to product literature. The nurse should have a basic understanding of the actions of antihistamines. **Cognitive Level:** Applying **Client Need:** Physiological Adaptation **Integrated Process:** Nursing Process: Implementation **Content Area:** Adult Health: Integumentary **Strategy:** Recall the nature of the condition and the client's symptoms to choose the correct response. The wording of the question indicates a true statement is the correct answer. Use the process of elimination and nursing knowledge to make a selection.

12 **Answer: 2 Rationale:** Coal tar shampoos are useful in controlling symptoms of seborrheic dermatitis of the scalp. Over-the-counter shampoos may not control symptoms. Permanent hair loss may not occur. Seborrheic dermatitis cannot be cured. **Cognitive Level:** Applying **Client Need:** Physiological Adaptation **Integrated Process:** Nursing Process: Implementation **Content Area:** Adult Health: Integumentary **Strategy:** The core issue of the question is knowledge of care and treatment of seborrheic dermatitis. The wording of the

question tells you a true statement is the correct answer. Use the process of elimination and nursing knowledge to make a selection.

13 **Answer: 2 Rationale:** Protecting the skin with sunscreen SPF 15 or higher is recommended to help prevent basal cell carcinoma. Avoiding the use of tanning beds is recommended to help prevent basal cell carcinoma. Avoiding the sun during the peak hours of 10:00 a.m. to 4:00 p.m. is recommended to help prevent basal cell carcinoma. While a balanced diet is important for general health, other factors such as ionizing radiation play a key role in development of basal cell carcinoma. **Cognitive Level:** Applying **Client Need:** Health Promotion and Maintenance **Integrated Process:** Nursing Process: Implementation **Content Area:** Adult Health: Integumentary **Strategy:** The core issue of the question is knowledge of behaviors that can reduce the risk of developing basal cell carcinoma. The wording of the question tells you the correct option is a true statement. Use the process of elimination and nursing knowledge to make a selection.

14 **Answer: 3 Rationale:** Infection may be manifested by fever, chills, malaise, erythema and tenderness at the site. Squeezing pustules is not recommended. Antibiotics should be taken for the full prescribed course of therapy. Infection may be manifested by drainage at the site, especially if it is cloudy. The healthcare provider must be notified if signs of infection occur. **Cognitive Level:** Applying **Client Need:** Physiological Adaptation **Integrated Process:** Nursing Process: Implementation **Content Area:** Adult Health: Integumentary **Strategy:** The core issue of the question is recognition of signs of infection that are important to note after being treated for cellulitis. The wording of the question tells you the correct option is a true statement. Use the process of elimination and nursing knowledge to make a selection.

15 **Answer: 4 Rationale:** Clients with cellulitis experience pain at the local site. Controlling the pain is the priority for this client. The client's sleep may be disturbed by pain but this would not be the priority problem. There is insufficient information to determine whether the client is engaging in self-isolating behavior because of cellulitis. Cellulitis can be treated with appropriate antibiotic therapy, so powerlessness is not a concern. **Cognitive Level:** Analyzing **Client Need:** Physiological Adaptation **Integrated Process:** Nursing Process: Diagnosis **Content Area:** Adult Health: Integumentary **Strategy:** Recall that pain relief is a high priority for many clients and is included in the physiological needs on Maslow's hierarchy. Use the process of elimination and nursing knowledge to make a selection, considering that physiological needs take priority over psychosocial needs in most cases.

16 **Answer: 3 Rationale:** Current treatments for psoriasis include coal tar shampoo and topical steroids. Folliculitis, cellulitis, and furuncles are bacterial infections of the skin and would be treated with antimicrobial therapy. **Cognitive Level:** Analyzing **Client Need:** Physiological Adaptation **Integrated Process:** Nursing Process: Diagnosis **Content Area:** Adult Health: Integumentary **Strategy:** The core issue of the question is knowledge of the uses of medication therapy for psoriasis. The wording of the question tells you the correct option is a true statement. Use the process of elimination and nursing knowledge to make a selection.

17 **Answer: 1 Rationale:** The initial outbreak of herpes is the most uncomfortable or painful. Recurrent episodes present with a prodrome of symptoms, such as tingling and burning. The pain of herpes does not increase over time. Repeated episodes may occur during periods of stress. Herpes is characterized by discomfort with each outbreak. **Cognitive Level:** Applying **Client Need:** Physiological Adaptation **Integrated Process:** Nursing Process: Implementation **Content Area:** Adult Health: Integumentary **Strategy:** The core issue of the question is knowledge of the characteristics and presentation of this type of viral infection. The wording of the question tells you the correct option is a true statement. Recall that the first outbreak is the most severe to make a selection.

18 **Answer: 4 Rationale:** To meet all the criteria for removal of a lesion, the lesion will be asymmetrical (A) with an irregular border (B), have color change or more than one color (C), along with an increased diameter (D), and be evolving in size, shape, or color (E). A lesion that is symmetrical, with a smooth border, a single color, and unchanged diameter does not meet any criteria for suspicious lesions. The lesion that is symmetrical and of one color does not meet all of the criteria for suspicious lesions. The lesion with a regular border and small diameter does not meet all criteria for suspicious lesions. **Cognitive Level:** Applying **Client Need:** Physiological Adaptation **Integrated Process:** Nursing Process: Assessment **Content Area:** Adult Health: Integumentary **Strategy:** The core issue of the question is knowledge of criteria that determine the need to remove a skin lesion. The wording of the question tells you the correct option is a true statement. Use the process of elimination and nursing knowledge to make a selection.

19 **Answer: 2 Rationale:** Spider angiomas are red lesions with vessels radiating from the center. Petechiae appear as red "freckles" or dots. A venous star is a flat blue lesion with radiating linear veins. A port wine stain is a flat, irregular-shaped lesion that does not have radiating vessels. **Cognitive Level:** Applying **Client Need:** Physiological Adaptation **Integrated Process:** Communication and Documentation **Content Area:** Adult Health: Integumentary **Strategy:** The core issue of the question is knowledge of various types of skin lesions. The wording of the question tells you the correct option is a true statement. Use the process of elimination and nursing knowledge to make a selection.

20 **Answer: 4 Rationale:** Stage 4 ulcers result in full-thickness skin loss with extensive damage to the muscle and bone. **Cognitive Level:** Applying **Client Need:** Physiological Adaptation **Integrated Process:** Communication and Documentation **Content Area:** Adult Health: Integumentary **Strategy:** The core issue of the question is knowledge of various stages of ulcer development. The wording of the question guides you to a decision. Use nursing knowledge to supply an answer.

21 **Answer: 1 Rationale:** Coughing and wheezing may indicate that the child has inhaled smoke or toxic fumes. Maintaining airway patency is the highest nursing priority in this situation. Skin color changes are expected. Thirst may be present but does not require immediate nursing action. Singed hair warrants attention because of the risk of inhalation injury, but is not as high priority as actual respiratory symptoms. **Cognitive Level:** Analyzing **Client Need:** Physiological Adaptation **Integrated Process:** Nursing Process: Diagnosis **Content Area:** Child Health **Strategy:** The core issue of the question is the ability to determine that the client's airway could be in jeopardy. Use the ABCs whenever a question deals with burn injury as a first method to determine priority setting.

22 **Answer: 2 Rationale:** Atopic dermatitis is a chronic inflammatory skin disorder. School-age children are very aware of their own and others' skin appearance. Children with atopic

dermatitis will feel different from other children, and this may affect their body image. Food allergies do not lead to inadequate nutrition; just the food or foods that initiate the allergic response need to be avoided. Atopic dermatitis does not affect the skin's ability to maintain temperature. Atopic dermatitis does not affect blood flow to the area. **Cognitive Level:** Analyzing **Client Need:** Psychosocial Integrity **Integrated Process:** Nursing Process: Diagnosis **Content Area:** Child Health **Strategy:** The core issue of the question is recognition of key concerns of a child with atopic dermatitis. The wording of the question tells you the correct option is a true statement. Use the process of elimination and nursing knowledge to make a selection.

23 **Answer: 4 Rationale:** Infants with atopic dermatitis frequently have food sensitivities. Slow introduction of new foods allows the parents to recognize food sensitivities and eliminate the offending item from the diet. The mother is taught to avoid scratchy clothing such as wool. Childhood immunizations would be given as scheduled but do not reduce risk. Atopic dermatitis is not an infectious disease. Avoiding infectious personnel is appropriate for all children but does not prevent development of atopic dermatitis. **Cognitive Level:** Applying **Client Need:** Physiological Adaptation **Integrated Process:** Nursing Process: Implementation **Content Area:** Child Health **Strategy:** The core issue of the question is appropriate client teaching to reduce risk of developing atopic dermatitis. Recall the risk factors and use the process of elimination to make a selection.

24 **Answer: 3 Rationale:** The nurse should encourage parents to identify and discuss their feelings and concerns. Changing the topic is not therapeutic. Merely not blaming parents does not give them the opportunity to discuss what is important to them. Giving false reassurance by telling them not to worry is inappropriate. **Cognitive Level:** Applying **Client Need:** Psychosocial Integrity **Integrated Process:** Communication and Documentation **Content Area:** Child Health **Strategy:** The core issue of the question is the ability to use basic communication techniques in responding to the concerns of a parent. Choose the option that directly addresses the client's or family's issues and concerns.

25 **Answer: 3 Rationale:** Until a complete assessment and treatment plan are initiated, the child should be kept NPO. A complication of major burns is paralytic ileus, so until that has been ruled out, the client should not receive clear liquids, full liquids, or a meal tray with extra liquids. **Cognitive Level:** Analyzing **Client Need:** Physiological Adaptation **Integrated Process:** Nursing Process: Diagnosis **Content Area:** Child Health **Strategy:** The core issue of the question is the need to avoid fluid intake during the acute phase of burn injury when hemodynamics could be unstable. Use nursing knowledge to recall that fluid resuscitation needs to be done parenterally.

Key Terms to Review

acne p. 1143
actinic keratosis p. 1135
atopic dermatitis (eczema) p. 1132
candidiasis p. 1139
cellulitis p. 1138
contact dermatitis p. 1134
cysts p. 1143
dermis p. 1129
epidermis p. 1129
erythemic p. 1137
lichenification p. 1132
macules p. 1131
nodule p. 1136
papules p. 1131
pediculosis capitis p. 1141
plaques p. 1132
pressure ulcers p. 1144
pruritus p. 1132
pustule p. 1137
scabies p. 1141
urticaria p. 1143
vesicles p. 1132
vitiligo p. 1144
wheal p. 1142
xerosis p. 1132

References

Ball, J., & Bindler, R., & Cowen, K. (2015). *Principles of pediatric nursing: Caring for children* (6th ed.). Hoboken, NJ: Pearson Education.

Berman, A., Snyder, S., & Frandsen, G. (2016). *Kozier & Erb's fundamentals of nursing: Concepts, process, and practice* (10th ed.). New York, NY: Pearson Education.

Ignatavicius, D., & Workman, L. (2016). *Medical-surgical nursing: Patient-centered collaborative care* (10th ed.). Philadelphia: Saunders.

LeMone, P., Burke, K., Bauldoff, G., & Gubrud, p. (2015). *Medical surgical nursing: Clinical reasoning in patient care* (6th ed.). Hoboken, NJ: Pearson Education.

Lewis, S., Dirksen, S., Heitkemper, M., & Bucher, L. (2014). *Medical surgical nursing: Assessment and management of clinical problems* (9th ed.). St. Louis, MO: Elsevier Science.

Smith, S., Duell, D., Martin, B., Aebersold, M., & Gonzalez, L. (2017). *Clinical nursing skills: Basic to advanced skills* (10th ed.). New York, NY: Pearson Education.

Eye, Ear, Nose, and Throat Disorders

63

In this chapter

Cross Reference

Other chapters relevant to this content area are

Dosage Calculation and Medication Administration	Chapter 29
Eye and Ear Medications	Chapter 43
Common Laboratory Tests	Chapter 46
Common Diagnostic Tests and Procedures	Chapter 47

I. OVERVIEW OF ANATOMY AND PHYSIOLOGY OF EYE AND EAR

A. Layers of Eye

1. Outer protective layer, also called fibrous coat; consists of transparent cornea and white sclera
2. Middle vascular layer, also called uveal tract; contains pigmented iris surrounding pupil, which regulates amount of light entering eye, and ciliary body that surrounds lens and produces aqueous humor to maintain intraocular pressure (IOP) (flows from posterior to anterior chamber and drains into Schlemm's canal); also contains choroid that has blood vessels to supply eye tissues

3. Inner layer, the retina: thin, semitransparent layer containing blood vessels, optic nerve fibers, and photoreceptors called rods and cones, responsible for vision in dim light and perception of fine details, respectively; contains optic disc (blind spot) where optic nerve meets eyeball, and macula lutea (lateral and temporal to optic disc) that has central depressed portion called fovea centralis, which has keenest color vision
4. Other eye structures include gel-like vitreous within vitreous body, which maintains eye shape and transmits light; aqueous humor to fill anterior and posterior eye chambers; canal of Schlemm to allow drainage of excess aqueous humor into circulation, maintaining intraocular pressure; and transparent lens behind iris and in front of vitreous body that bends light rays to fall on retina and can adjust to focus on far or near objects

B. Eye functions

1. Eye receives light waves through cornea; waves are refracted by aqueous humor, lens, and vitreous humor as they are transmitted to retina; retinal images formed by light rays are inverted and reversed by biconvex lens
2. Rods and cones of retina translate light waves into neural impulses for relay to optic nerve and then to brain's occipital lobes for interpretation as vision
3. Fusion of images from each eye into a single image is called binocular vision

NCLEX® **C. Age-related changes of eye that affect vision**

1. Decreased ability of pupil to dilate, which reduces night vision and increases light needed for reading and small motor tasks, such as sewing
2. Development of **presbyopia**, a decreased elasticity of lens that makes focusing for near vision more difficult and results in farsightedness
3. Lens becomes discolored and opacified, which reduces color perception (especially green, blue, and violet)
4. Decreased eye motility and senile enophthalmos (sinking in) of eyes limits peripheral vision upward, downward, and to sides
5. Degenerative changes to choroid, retina, and optic nerve reduce depth perception and ability to see lines of demarcation (stair edges, door frames)

D. Ear structures

1. External ear: outer visible ear or auricle and external auditory canal
2. Middle ear: tympanic membrane; malleus, incus, and stapes bones; and window membranes
3. Inner ear: semicircular canals, cochlea, distal portion of cranial nerve VIII (vestibulocochlear nerve)

E. Ear functions

1. Hearing: sound is transferred from tympanic membrane to malleus, incus, and stapes and through cochlea; vibrations are changed by transduction into action potentials that are sent to brain as neural impulses
2. **Proprioception** (balance): sensation about body's position in space is transferred to brain after changes in body position trigger fluid movement and bending of hair cells in vestibular structures

F. Age-related changes of ear that affect hearing

1. External auditory canal narrows; cerumen glands atrophy and produce thicker, drier cerumen
2. Tympanic membrane is less flexible, and ossicle joints calcify
3. Cochlear hair cell degeneration and loss of auditory neurons in organ of Corti lead to **presbycusis**, an age-related sensorineural hearing loss characterized by decreased ability to hear high-frequency sounds; results in difficulty hearing and localizing normal speech

II. DIAGNOSTIC TESTS AND ASSESSMENTS OF EYE AND EAR

A. Fluorescein angiography: injection of sodium fluorescein into arm blood vessel (BV), followed by serial imaging of retinal vessels to detect disorders such as diabetic retinopathy, tumors, retinal bleeding, and macular degeneration

1. Preprocedure care
   a. Assess for allergies and/or history of reactions to dye
   b. Ensure client has given informed consent
   c. Give prescribed mydriatic medication 1 hour prior to test to dilate pupil

NCLEX®

2. Postprocedure care
   a. Encourage rest and increased fluid intake (aids in dye excretion)
   b. Teach client that dye causes temporary yellow skin discoloration in injected area and temporary green discoloration of urine that resolves when dye is fully excreted
   c. Teach client to avoid sunlight or other bright light sources for several hours until pupil dilation returns to normal

B. Corneal staining: instillation of dye into conjunctival sac to highlight irregularities caused by trauma, abrasions, or ulcers; damaged corneal epithelium appears green when viewed through a blue filter

1. Ensure that contact lenses are removed prior to procedure, if worn
2. Tell client to blink to distribute dye evenly over cornea
3. Wipe excess dye from cheeks and instruct client not to rub eyes

C. *Tonometry*: measurement of IOP to detect glaucoma by determining resistance of eyeball to an applied force

NCLEX®
1. Normal IOP ranges from 12 to 21 mmHg
2. Eye may be anesthetized, and client stares forward
3. Contact tonometry: most accurate; measures force of a flattened cone needed to flatten a small area of cornea; eye is anesthetized
4. Noncontact: measures deflection of a puff of air directed at cornea; no anesthetic needed

NCLEX®
5. Tell client not to rub eyes after test if anesthetic was used to avoid possible corneal scratches or injury

D. Physical assessment of eye and vision

1. Acuity of distance vision: measures vision using Snellen chart hung 20 feet away
   a. Client reads chart lines with one eye covered, moving downward from row that is most clear to last line that is completely read
   b. Findings are recorded as a fraction: numerator is client's distance from chart (20 feet) and denominator is number identified at end of smallest line read, which corresponds to distance at which normal eye can read that line; normal vision is 20/20; a larger denominator indicates myopia (nearsightedness)
   c. Red and green lines on Snellen chart can provide a quick test of color blindness

NCLEX®
2. Acuity of near vision: measures vision using a Rosenbaum chart or a card with newsprint 12–14 inches from client's eyes; impairment indicates hyperopia (farsightedness) in a young client or presbyopia in an adult after approximately 45 years of age
3. Refraction test: uses Snellen chart to assess visual acuity while client reads through various strengths of corrective lenses; used to prescribe correction for *myopia* (nearsightedness), *hyperopia* (farsightedness), and *astigmatism* (irregular corneal surface inhibiting light rays from focusing clearly on retina)

NCLEX®
4. Visual fields: measures peripheral vision, often called confrontation test
   a. Client and examiner face each other; client looks into examiner's eyes; both cover own eye on same side
   b. Examiner raises a finger or small object at arm's length midway between client and examiner and brings it in from periphery into line of vision; procedure is repeated from above and below on same side
   c. Client states "now" when able to see object; examiner should see object at about same time (test assumes examiner has normal peripheral vision); test is repeated on other eye
5. Color vision
   a. Tested for driver's license, employment requiring color discrimination, or with history of difficulty distinguishing colors; sensitive for red/green blindness, but not for blue

NCLEX®
   b. Involves picking colored numbers or letters out of plates with multiple colors in background (such as an Ishihara chart) or noting green and red lines on Snellen chart; results recorded as a fraction of correct identifications divided by total number shown
6. Extraocular muscle movements
   a. Client's eyes follow a small object through six cardinal positions of gaze: to right, upward and right, down and right, left, upward and left, and down and left

NCLEX®
   b. Client should have parallel eye movement and absence of **nystagmus**, involuntary rhythmic oscillating eye movements (vertical, horizontal, rotary, or mixed)
   c. As last step, client follows finger as it moves in to bridge of nose; eyes should sustain convergence to within 5–8 centimeters
7. Outer eye structures
   a. Sclera is white in color, although dark-skinned clients may have slight yellow cast or pigmented dots; yellow discoloration (or heightened yellow) can indicate jaundice
   b. Cornea is normally transparent, smooth, and shiny; opacities or specks may indicate prior injury
   c. Pupils should be round, equal in size, and constrict in response to direct light or to light shone in opposite pupil (consensual response); should constrict and converge when looking at object over examiner's shoulder and then shifting gaze to an object 4–6 inches from own nose (accommodation)
8. Ophthalmoscopy
   a. Used to examine retina, optic disk, optic blood vessels, fundus, and macula

NCLEX®
   b. As light shines on pupil, reflection of light on retina causes a red glare (red reflex); absence of red reflex may indicate lens opacity

E. Otoscopic examination

NCLEX®

1. Tilt client's head slightly away, pull pinna up and back in an adult (down and back in a child) to straighten external auditory canal, and insert speculum while visualizing canal
2. Normal findings
   a. Pink, intact external canal with no lesions and variable amount of cerumen and fine hairs; absence of inflammation, deviations, or foreign bodies
   b. Tympanic membrane should be transparent, opaque, pearly gray, slightly concave, intact, and free of lesions or perforations

F. Whisper test

1. Have client occlude one ear at a time with a finger; stand 1–2 feet away from client on side of unoccluded ear
2. Whisper numbers or a statement and ask client to repeat; perform again with other ear; alternatively, a ticking watch can be held 5 inches from each ear
3. Note whether it is necessary to stand closer or raise voice to be heard

NCLEX®

G. Rinne test

1. Place stem of an activated tuning fork on mastoid bone and ask client to signal when sound is no longer heard
2. Quickly place vibrating end of tuning fork in front of ear close to ear canal and have client indicate when sound is no longer heard
3. With no conductive hearing loss, sound is heard twice as long by air conduction as by bone conduction
4. With conductive hearing loss, bone conduction is greater than air conduction in affected ear

NCLEX®

H. Weber test

1. Especially valuable when hearing in one ear is reported as better than other
2. Place stem of vibrating tuning fork on midline of forehead or vertex of head (skull) and ask whether sound is heard equally in both ears or if one side is better than other
3. Sound that lateralizes to one ear indicates conductive hearing loss in that ear or sensorineural hearing loss in opposite ear

I. Audiometry: quantifies hearing deficits by presenting various sound frequencies to each ear by either sound or bone conduction; speech audiometry identifies intensity at which speech is identifiable

J. Tympanometry: indirectly monitors compliance and impedance of middle ear to sound transmission after neutral, positive, and negative air pressure is applied to external auditory meatus

K. Tests of vestibular function

1. Romberg test: stand close to client to ensure safety; ask client to close eyes while feet are together and arms are resting at sides; observe for a normal slight sway; significant sway is a positive test
2. Past pointing test
   a. Client sits facing examiner, closes eyes, and points both index fingers at examiner; examiner places own index fingers under client's as a reference point; then client raises both arms and then lowers them to original spot with eyes closed
   b. With normal response, client can return to reference point easily; with vestibular dysfunction, fingers deviate to left or right
3. Gaze nystagmus test: observe client's eyes as they look straight ahead, 30 degrees to each side, upward, and downward; with vestibular problems, eyeballs exhibit nystagmus
4. Hallpike maneuver: client lies supine and rotates head to side for 1 minute; positive for positional vertigo or induced dizziness if nystagmus occurs

L. Electronystagmography (ENG)

1. A vestibular test to evaluate clients who have dizziness, vertigo, or problems with balance by assessing oculomotor and vestibular systems
2. It differentiates *nystagmus* (eye oscillations) that are normal, drug-induced, or caused by lesion somewhere in central or peripheral vestibular pathway
3. Preprocedure instructions include NPO status for 3 hours prior to test, no caffeine for 24–48 hours prior to test, discontinue unnecessary medications 24 hours prior to test, and to bring prescription eyeglasses to exam
4. During procedure:
   a. Electrodes are placed on skin around eyes to record changing electrical fields during eye movement
   b. Client is asked to look at lights, focus on a moving pattern or point, and close eyes
   c. Client's chair may be rotated during test to further assess vestibular function
   d. Client's ears are irrigated with cool and warm water (note this can induce nausea and vomiting [N/V])
5. Post-procedure care involves giving clear liquids slowly because of risk of N/V and assisting with ambulation as needed

III. COMMON NURSING TECHNIQUES AND PROCEDURES FOR EYE AND EAR

A. Ocular medications

NCLEX®

1. Eye drops
   a. Ensure that medication is sterile and treat each eye separately, if both are being medicated, to prevent cross-contamination
   b. Follow procedure as outlined in Chapter 29
   c. Wait 2–5 minutes between drops as per manufacturer's directions
2. Eye ointments: as per procedure outlined in Chapter 29
3. Medicated eye disk
   a. Position client with head tilted back and expose lower conjunctival sac
   b. Press tip of index finger of gloved hand against convex part of disk; place disk horizontally in sac between iris and lower eyelid
   c. Pull lower eyelid out and up over disk and ask client to blink until disk is not visible and have client press fingers against closed lids without moving eyes or disk to secure disk in position
   d. To remove disk, expose lower conjunctival sac and use thumb and index finger to pinch and lift disk

B. Ocular irrigation

1. Position client with head tilted toward side to be irrigated and place waterproof pad and curved basin under affected side
2. Cleanse eyelids and lashes with gloved hand and moistened cotton ball, discarding each cotton ball after one wipe
3. Draw up prescribed irrigant into sterile irrigation set or bulb syringe
4. Using nondominant hand to hold eyelids open, hold syringe 2.5 cm (1 in.) above eye and push fluid gently into conjunctival sac (fluid flows across eye from inner to outer canthus)

NCLEX®

5. Avoid flushing directly onto eyeball to avoid damage to cornea

C. Eye patches and shields

1. Have client close both eyes during application of patch or shield

NCLEX®

2. Position patch and secure with two strips of tape extending from midforehead to lateral cheekbone (medial top to lateral bottom) on same side
3. Do not use pressure unless specifically prescribed, and then use two to three pads and extra tape
4. Change only with healthcare provider prescription
5. Apply shield alone or over eye patch to protect eye from pressure or other type of irritation

NCLEX®

6. Place shield on bony prominences of cheek, nose, and brow; secure with transparent tape in same manner as for eye patch

D. Eye prosthesis (artificial eye) care

1. Allow client to perform own artificial eye care if preferred; some prostheses are permanently implanted; others are removable
2. Remove prosthesis by retracting lower eyelid and exerting pressure just below eye to break suction and lift it from socket; can also use rubber bulb syringe or medicine dropper bulb to create suction effect
3. Cleanse with normal saline (NS) or tap water according to client's routine
4. Irrigate eye socket with NS using aseptic technique if prescribed (such as for infection)
5. Cleanse edges of eye socket and surrounding area with moistened gauze
6. Reinsert by retracting upper and lower eyelids and slipping prosthesis into eye socket comfortably under upper eyelid
7. Store prosthesis in labeled container with NS or tap water

E. Otic medications

1. Use clean technique unless tympanic membrane is damaged, then use sterile technique
2. Follow procedure as outlined in Chapter 29

F. Otic irrigation

1. Assist client to a sitting or lying position with head tilted toward affected ear; place a waterproof pad and drainage receptacle under affected ear
2. Check that temperature of irrigant is 98°F (37°C)
3. Determine that tympanic membrane is intact before beginning an otic irrigation

NCLEX®

4. Straighten ear canal and gently insert syringe tip into auditory meatus; direct solution slowly and steadily along wall of canal (not center, which could damage tympanic membrane); use no more than 50–70 mL at one time

5. After solution drains, dry outside of ear with cotton balls and place a dry one in auditory meatus lightly to absorb remaining excess fluid
6. Assist client to a side-lying position on affected side to aid drainage; assess for discomfort

G. Hearing aid prosthesis care

1. There are several types of hearing aids available; they improve quality of hearing with conductive hearing loss but only intensify distortions heard with sensorineural hearing loss (they may be useful in signaling client of danger, enabling client to hear alarms, for example)
2. Wash hands before handling an external hearing aid
3. Ensure battery is functional and inserted correctly; have client keep extra battery on hand
4. Do not drop hearing aid or twist cord

NCLEX®

5. To insert a hearing aid: inspect to ensure it is intact, turn down volume, insert ear mold first into ear canal, then secure rest of device; once in place, turn up volume slowly until comfortable, and check for structural problems or placement problems if feedback occurs
6. Remove a hearing aid after turning it off and lowering volume; remove earmold by rotating it forward slightly and pulling outward
7. After removal, clean a detachable earmold with mild soap and water, rinse and dry well; avoid excessive wetting or use of alcohol, which can cause damage; wipe nondetachable earmolds with a damp cloth

NCLEX®

8. Avoid using aerosol sprays, oils, or cosmetic products near hearing aid because earmold opening could become clogged
9. Remove battery to prevent corrosion and leakage if aid will not be used for more than 24 hours; store in a safe place away from moisture and heat

IV. NURSING MANAGEMENT OF CLIENT HAVING EYE SURGERY

A. Preoperative care

1. Reduce anxiety by teaching about procedure and postoperative course and care
2. Assess client's support systems, ability to care for self after surgery, and environmental safety (such as hand rails, absence of throw rugs)
3. Shampoo or scrub around eyes if prescribed; remove eye makeup; store contact lens or eyeglasses (needed to aid vision in other eye) so they are available after surgery

NCLEX®

4. Administer preanesthetic medications and eye drops as prescribed, which commonly include **mydriatic** eye drops (to dilate pupils) and **cycloplegic** eye drops (to paralyze ciliary muscles); see Chapter 43 for overview of commonly prescribed eye medications

B. Postoperative care

1. Perform baseline assessments as for all postoperative clients (vital signs [VS], level of consciousness [LOC], status of dressing); changes may be minimal if surgery done under local anesthesia
2. Maintain eye patch or shield in place to prevent eye injury and instruct client not to rub or touch area

NCLEX®

3. Elevate head to 30–45 degrees and have client lie on back or unaffected side (to reduce IOP) after surgery to treat cataracts or glaucoma; use small pillows at sides of head to immobilize head when lying on back

NCLEX®

4. Position client with repair of detached retina as prescribed so that area of detachment is dependent/inferior (to maintain pressure on repaired retinal area and improve its contact with choroid)
5. Instruct and assist client to avoid activities that increase IOP, such as coughing, sneezing, vomiting, or straining at stool; if it is necessary to cough or sneeze, client should do so with mouth open and use tissues

NCLEX®

6. Maintain client safety: orient to environment, keep articles and call bell on unaffected side, use side-rails with bed in low position, and assist with ambulation
7. Give antibiotic, anti-inflammatory, and other prescribed topical (eye) or systemic medications
8. Give analgesics as prescribed, avoiding or using caution with opioids to prevent postoperative nausea and vomiting (N/V) and constipation; discomfort may be described as achy or scratching; avoid morphine, which can cause miosis

NCLEX®

9. Assess for and report immediately possible surgical complications to preserve sight:
   a. Sudden sharp eye pain, possibly indicating hemorrhage, sudden rise in IOP, or other ocular emergency
   b. Hemorrhage, with blood noted in anterior chamber of eye
   c. Retinal detachment, with client sensations of light flashes, floaters, or shade being drawn over eye
   d. Corneal edema, noted by a cloudy appearance to cornea
10. Teach client and family about postdischarge care (see Box 63–1)
11. Refer to community health agency for assistance with home care if needed

Box 63–1

Client Education Following Eye Surgery

Include the following points in discharge instructions for client and family after eye surgery:

- Leave eye shield in place until surgeon's office visit on day after surgery; then use eye shield at night during sleep for eye protection as prescribed
- Avoid rubbing, scratching, touching, squeezing, or putting pressure on surgical eye
- Avoid activities that increase intraocular pressure, such as sneezing, coughing, vomiting, straining, moving rapidly, bending, or lifting more than 2.3 kg (5 lb)
- Maintain sedentary lifestyle for approximately 2 weeks or as prescribed by surgeon; avoid heavy work, such as gardening, mowing lawn, or moving furniture
- Avoid reading until allowed by surgeon, and then read in moderation during healing
- Use measures to prevent constipation, such as adequate fiber and fluid intake, maintaining mobility as able, and possible use of stool softener
- Wear sunglasses with side shields when out of doors (photophobia commonly occurs)
- New corrective lenses (if needed) will not be prescribed until vision stabilizes, which may take several weeks; make and keep all recommended follow-up appointments with healthcare provider
- Use proper techniques for applying and removing eye patch or shield and for instilling eye drops
- Understand medication names, dose, schedule, side effects, purpose, and anticipated duration of use
- Symptoms to report to healthcare provider include new, increased, or severe eye pain or pressure; decreased vision; redness; cloudiness; drainage; floaters or light flashes; and halos around brightly lit objects

V. NURSING MANAGEMENT OF CLIENT HAVING EAR SURGERY

A. Preoperative care: principles same as before eye surgery

1. Complete a baseline assessment of hearing for comparison postoperatively
2. *NCLEX®* Shampoo or scrub around ear if prescribed; complete usual preoperative activities and checklist; administer preanesthetic medications as prescribed

B. Postoperative care

1. Perform baseline assessments as for all postoperative clients (VS, LOC, bleeding or drainage from dressing, pain, recovery from anesthesia)
2. *NCLEX®* Implement standard postoperative interventions (pain control, mobility, prevention of postoperative complications)
3. *NCLEX®* Keep client on bedrest for 24 hours with head either elevated or flat (depending on prescription) and lying on nonoperative side (operative ear upward) for 12–24 hours
4. Change internal or external dressings if prescribed; wipe away discharge from ear with dry sterile dressing material
5. *NCLEX®* Assess for N/V; administer antiemetics prn to prevent vomiting, which can disrupt surgical site by increasing pressure in middle ear
6. *NCLEX®* Assess for dizziness and vertigo; avoid unnecessary movements or turning in bed; provide antivertigo medications; provide assistance when client is allowed to ambulate to reduce falls
7. Assess client's hearing postoperatively and compare to baseline; use alternate communication means as needed
8. Remind client that decreased hearing immediately after surgery may be caused by edema and drainage at operative site; permanent hearing loss may be expected if cochlea is involved or no middle ear reconstruction is done
9. *NCLEX®* Teach client and family about postdischarge care (see Box 63–2)

VI. STRABISMUS

A. *Strabismus* overview

1. Misalignment of eyes; two types are esotropia (inward deviation or "crossed eyes," most common type) or exotropia (outward deviation or "wall eyes")
2. Caused by lack of coordination of eye muscles from muscle imbalance or paralysis

Box 63–2

Client Education Following Ear Surgery

Include the following points in discharge instructions given to client and family after ear surgery:

- Keep outer ear dressing clean and dry; change it as prescribed if needed; do not remove inner ear dressing until allowed by surgeon; do not insert small objects to clean external ear canal
- Whenever possible, avoid activities that increase middle ear pressure, such as blowing nose, sneezing, coughing, straining
- If necessary, cough or sneeze with mouth open; wipe nostril with tissue or blow nose one nostril at a time with mouth open; avoid drinking through a straw for 2–3 weeks; avoid air travel until allowed by surgeon
- Use measures to prevent constipation, such as adequate fiber and fluid intake, maintaining mobility as able, and possible use of stool softener
- Do not shower or shampoo hair until allowed by surgeon (usually 1 or more weeks)
- Keep ear dry for 6 weeks with use of petrolatum-coated cotton ball placed in external auditory canal as prescribed; if used, change it daily; do not swim or dive until allowed by surgeon (when full healing occurs)
- Reduce risk of infection by avoiding those with respiratory infections
- Understand medication names, dose, schedule, side effects, purpose, and anticipated duration of use (antibiotics, antiemetics, antivertigo agents)
- Symptoms to report to healthcare provider include persistent postoperative headache, increased drainage or bleeding from site, fever, new or increased ear pain or dizziness, and decreasing hearing

3. Can be congenital or acquired; considered normal until 4 months of age; leads to amblyopia if untreated early

B. Assessment

1. Symptoms may occur only when tired; include squinting when reading, tilting head or closing one eye to see, and difficulty in picking up objects from impaired depth perception, headaches, diplopia, and possible photophobia
2. Cover–uncover test: client fixes gaze ahead, focusing on a distant object; cover one eye with an opaque card while observing uncovered eye for movement; remove card while observing eye just uncovered for movement; this test screens for deviation in eye alignment and eye muscle weakness (weakness is seen as movement of "lazy eye" when it attempts to refocus during cover test)
3. Corneal light reflex (Hirschberg test): assesses parallel symmetry of eyes; examiner shines a penlight directly onto corneas of both eyes, holding penlight about 31 cm (12 in.) away from client's nasal bridge while client focuses on a distant object; light should be reflected at same spot in both eyes; an asymmetric light reflex indicates a deviation in alignment of client's eyes

C. Therapeutic management

NCLEX®

1. Includes occlusion therapy ("good eye" is patched 1–2 hours daily, forcing client to focus with weaker eye, thus strengthening eye muscles), corrective lenses in eyeglasses, eye drops to cause blurred vision in "good eye," eye muscle exercises
2. Surgical treatment
   a. Surgery on rectus muscles of eyes can correct muscle imbalance if conservative treatment fails
   b. Congenital strabismus should be corrected before 24 months of age to prevent amblyopia

D. Client and family teaching

1. Provide explanation of eye patching to parents
2. Preoperative teaching about maintaining NPO status prior to surgery and general preoperative and postoperative care

VII. AMBLYOPIA

A. *Amblyopia* overview

1. Reduction in vision in one or both eyes, usually with one eye having poorer vision than the other, causing loss of binocular vision; also known as "lazy eye"
2. Results from anything causing visual deprivation to eye, including untreated strabismus (most common), congenital cataract, or uncorrected refractive errors

B. Assessment
1. Diagnosed with vision testing by optometrist or ophthalmologist
2. Nursing assessments depend on age of child

NCLEX®
   a. Manifestations of visual impairment for infants include lack of tracking objects or lights with eyes and poor or no eye contact
   b. Signs of visual impairment in toddlers and older children are excessive tearing, rubbing, and squinting of eyes; frequent blinking; and holding objects close to eyes to see them or to read
3. Vision changes may be accompanied by dizziness and headache
4. Diagnosis is confirmed by corneal light reflex and cover–uncover tests

C. Therapeutic management

NCLEX®
1. Medical treatment options include corrective lenses in eyeglasses, occluding unaffected eye with a patch 2–6 hours daily (occlusion therapy), eye muscle exercises, atropine 1% one drop per day in unaffected eye
2. Treatment is discontinued when vision has improved, but 20/20 visual acuity is rarely attained
3. Treatment is most successful when done by age 5–6 years
4. Untreated amblyopia can lead to permanent visual impairment

D. Client and family teaching: how to patch unaffected eye while maintaining skin integrity; therapy and long-term benefits; need to complete treatment

VIII. GLAUCOMA

A. *Glaucoma* overview
1. Damage to optic nerve caused by increased IOP, usually because of an imbalance between aqueous humor production and drainage, can be of two types: primary open-angle glaucoma (POAG) or primary angle-closure glaucoma (PACG)
2. Risk factors are family history, older age, African American race, eye trauma, prolonged corticosteroid use, thin cornea, myopia, and disorders such as diabetes, cardiovascular disease, and migraines
3. POAG: most frequent form; angle of anterior chamber between iris and cornea is normal; flow of aqueous humor to canal of Schlemm is obstructed; usually bilateral process
4. PACG: less common form, often unilateral, although other eye can be affected at a later time
   a. Anterior chamber narrows because of corneal flattening or bulging of iris
   b. When iris thickens (pupil dilation) or lens thickens (during visual accommodation), angle can close completely, blocking outflow and causing sudden elevation of IOP

NCLEX®
   c. Damage to retinal neurons and optic nerve can occur, with rapid vision loss if not treated quickly

B. Assessment

NCLEX®
1. Open-angle (POAG)
   a. Loss of peripheral vision, mild headaches, difficulty adapting to dark, seeing halos around lights, and difficulty focusing on near objects
   b. Symptoms may be vague and unnoticed for a time; vision deteriorates over time with rising IOP

NCLEX®
2. Angle-closure (PACG)
   a. Triggered by pupil dilation (from high emotions, darkness, and other causes)
   b. Symptoms include severe eye and face pain, N/V, malaise, colored halos around lights, and episodes of sudden decline in vision; possible reddened eye, cloudy cornea (edema), and fixed midpoint pupil
3. Diagnosed by history; presenting symptoms; tonometry (IOP >21 mmHg); ophthalmoscopy; **gonioscopy** (measurement of anterior chamber angle; differentiates open-angle from angle-closure glaucoma)

C. Therapeutic management

NCLEX®
1. Acute glaucoma: medical emergency; vision loss can occur within 1–2 days if untreated; administer prescribed medications such as osmotic diuretics or carbonic anhydrase inhibitors such as acetazolamide to lower IOP (see Chapter 43); surgery may be needed

NCLEX®
2. Chronic glaucoma: provide medication therapy and client education
3. Provide pre- and postoperative care as previously outlined if eye surgery is needed; surgical procedures to facilitate drainage of aqueous humor can include trabeculectomy, laser trabeculoplasty, iridectomy, or laser iridotomy
4. Medication therapy
   a. **Miotic** drugs that constrict pupils
   b. Carbonic anhydrase inhibitors to decrease production of aqueous humor
   c. Beta-adrenergic blockers to constrict pupils and reduce production of aqueous humor

D. Client teaching

NCLEX® 1. Drug therapy is needed for life; nonadherence can lead to permanent vision loss; review specific drug information and procedures for self-administration
2. Avoid OTC drugs unless approved by healthcare provider; avoid mydriatics such as atropine that dilate pupils
3. Obtain Medic-Alert card or bracelet specifying type of glaucoma
NCLEX® 4. Use safety precautions at night (lighting, hand rails) to compensate for reduced pupil dilation because of miotics and remove obstacles in environment for safety
5. Report eye pain, halos around lights, or visual changes to healthcare provider
6. Follow general instructions following eye surgery; see previous discussion

IX. CATARACTS

A. *Cataracts* overview

1. Progressive clouding or opacification of eye lens that interferes with transmission of light to retina and reduces ability to see images clearly
NCLEX® 2. Risk factors: see Memory Aid

Memory Aid

Use the mnemonic CATARACT to recall risk factors for cataracts: **C**ongenital, **A**ging, **T**oxicity (such as corticosteroids), **A**ccidents (eye injury), **R**adiation, **A**ltered metabolism (diabetes mellitus), **C**igare**T**te smoking

3. Fibers and proteins of lens degenerate; opacity often begins at periphery of lens and moves to center
4. Partial opacity is termed *immature cataract*; opacity of entire lens is termed *mature cataract*
5. Opacity tends to occur bilaterally but at different rates, with one maturing faster than other

B. Assessment

NCLEX® 1. Decline in close and distance vision, blurred vision, changes in color vision (loss), glare, halos around lights, object distortion, white or cloudy gray pupil
2. Diagnosed by history and physical exam, results of visual acuity tests and slit-lamp exam; absence of red reflex with ophthalmoscopy

C. Therapeutic management

1. Provide emotional support because impaired vision is anxiety-producing
2. Identify and correct safety concerns in environment related to impaired vision
3. Surgical removal of lens is sole treatment option and is accompanied by lens implant in most cases; indicated when vision or activities of daily living (ADLs) are affected or if cataract is causing secondary problems such as uveitis or glaucoma
4. Reinforce explanations about surgical extraction of lens
   a. Extracapsular extraction: removal of lens nucleus and cortex, leaving posterior capsule intact to support lens implant; currently most popular method (see Figure 63–1)
   b. Intracapsular extraction: removal of entire lens and surrounding capsule; requires contact lenses or akaphic corrective lenses (rare)
NCLEX® 5. Surgery is done on one eye at a time, on an outpatient basis using local anesthesia
6. Lens implant rapidly restores binocular vision and depth perception
7. Provide preoperative and postoperative care as outlined in previous section; complications are rare (less than 1%) but include loss of vitreous humor, corneal edema, increased IOP, hemorrhage, inflammation or infection, retinal detachment, or lens displacement
8. Medication therapy: includes postoperative eyes drops (combined antibiotic, anti-inflammatory, and/or corticosteroid eye drops or ointment) and mild analgesic such as acetaminophen
9. Assess client's ability to care for self after surgery and obtain support services as needed

D. Client teaching

1. Adaptive strategies to compensate for changes in vision and depth perception if surgery is not currently indicated or desired
2. Postoperative instructions: avoid lifting, strenuous activity, sleeping on operative side, getting water in eye, or rubbing or scratching eye
3. Protect eye using sunglasses with side shields during day and eye shield at night
NCLEX® 4. Postoperative medication use, such as acetaminophen for general discomfort, prescribed eye drops, and others as needed by individual client

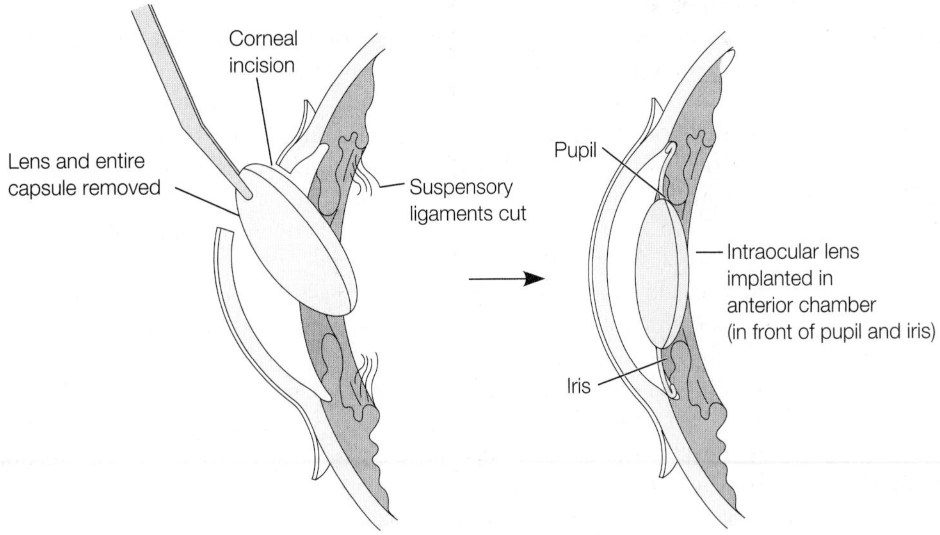

Figure 63–1

Extracapsular cataract extraction removes lens and anterior capsule, with lens implantation within the intact posterior capsule.

5. Insertion and care of postoperative contact lenses if prescribed
6. *NCLEX®* Permanent eyeglasses will be prescribed several weeks after surgery when healing is complete and vision has stabilized
7. Report signs of postoperative complications such as eye pain, adverse changes in vision, headache, nausea, or eye itching or redness

X. DETACHED RETINA

A. Overview

1. Separation of sensory layer of retina from choroid (pigmented vascular layer)
2. Retina may tear and fold back onto itself or remain intact and be pulled away from choroid by shrinking of vitreous humor
3. Most frequently an age-related condition with shrinkage of vitreous humor, which pulls on retina at points of attachment, such as the optic disk, macula, and periphery of eye; other causes are trauma, inflammation, tumor, or complication of eye surgery (lens removal)
4. With a retinal break or tear, fluid enters defect, possibly leading to further rapid tearing and separation due to pressure
5. Incomplete area of detachment can progress slowly or can enlarge quickly and become complete
6. *NCLEX®* Will lead to permanent blindness if untreated so considered a medical emergency

B. Assessment

NCLEX®

1. Initial: presence of floating spots (floaters) and/or flashing lights
2. Progressive blurring of vision; visual field deficits corresponding to area of damage; sense of curtain or veil coming down, up, or across field of vision; painless
3. Ophthalmic exam shows area of gray opaque retina, with possible accompanying tears, holes, or folds

C. Therapeutic management

1. Surgical repair (see Box 63–3)

Box 63–3

Surgical Procedures for Detached Retina

- Laser photocoagulation or cryotherapy (using supercooled probe): both create a local inflammation that will locally adhere retina onto the choroid
- Scleral buckling: holds retina and choroid together with an implant or encircling strap or "buckle"
- Pneumatic retinopexy: injects inert gas into vitreous with adjustment of client's head position to push detached portion of retina back into contact with choroid; silicone oil may also be injected
- Surgical instrument manipulation to move detached segment of torn retina into place, followed by laser therapy or injection of gas or silicone oil to create a bond

2. Preoperative care
   a. NCLEX® Protect eye from further damage: bedrest, cover both eyes with eye patches to limit movement and prevent eye stress, instruct client not to bend forward or make sudden or jerking head movements
   b. NCLEX® Position client with detached area dependent/inferior so gravity pushes detachment closer to choroid (e.g., with left eye superior temporal detachment, keep client supine with head turned toward left)
   c. NCLEX® Protect client from injury by keeping bed low, side-rails up, call bell within reach; talk to client before approaching bed, assist with self-care
   d. Provide support to alleviate anxiety associated with sudden loss of vision; reassure client most detachments are successfully treated (often on outpatient basis); reinforce explanations about surgical repair
   e. Provide preoperative care as described in previous section
3. Postoperative care
   a. Provide standard postoperative care as described in previous section
   b. NCLEX® Stress importance of maintaining prescribed position (affected eye inferior or dependent to maintain contact between retina and choroid)
   c. Usually includes antibiotic, anti-inflammatory, and analgesic medications

D. Client teaching: as previously described for head positioning, activity restrictions (no bending or lifting), use of eye shield, signs to report, and when to follow up with healthcare provider

XI. MACULAR DEGENERATION

A. Overview

1. Degeneration of macular area (center area) of retina, which normally receives light from center of visual field and has greatest visual acuity
2. Most common type is age-related macular degeneration (AMD), a leading cause of vision loss in clients over age 60 in developed countries
3. Causes of AMD are unknown, although associated factors include aging, smoking, race, and genetics; inflammation and interaction of genes with immune system may play a role
4. Possible nutritional protective factors against AMD include omega-3 fatty acids in fish and vegetables high in lutein and zeaxanthin (carotenoids in vegetables such as spinach, kale, and broccoli)
5. In AMD, there is gradual failure of outer layer of retina (pigmented epithelium that attaches retina to choroid layer and removes cellular wastes); in this process, photoreceptor cells are lost
6. There are two types of macular degeneration
   a. Nonexudative ("dry") form: bilateral and gradual but progressive loss of vision occurs because of accumulation of pale yellow cellular waste deposits called *drusen*, leading to slow atrophy and degeneration of macula (most common form)
   b. Exudative ("wet") form: involves formation of new weak blood vessels that are prone to leakage in potential space between choroid and retina; retina elevates from choroid, which distorts vision and may lead to permanent central vision loss (less common form)

B. Assessment

1. NCLEX® Clinical manifestations include loss of central vision with intact peripheral vision, drusen on macula, visual distortion of images (i.e., straight lines may appear crooked or wavy) (see Figure 63–2), and difficulty with activities requiring focused and close central vision (i.e., sewing, needlepoint, reading)
2. Diagnostic tests: vision testing, fundoscopy (examination of eye fundus); fluorescein angiography (for wet form only); and electroretinography (ERG) to measure retinal responses to light

C. Therapeutic management

1. Progression of nonexudative AMD while in early or intermediate stages may be slowed by vitamins C, E, beta-carotene (vitamin A), and zinc
2. Exudative AMD may be treated by:
   a. Drugs that inhibit new blood vessel growth, such as bevacizumab and ranibizumab (improves vision and prevents vision loss in advanced AMD)
   b. Laser photocoagulation
   c. Photodynamic therapy in which a light-activated drug is injected into vein and circulates to retinal blood vessels; a low-intensity light shone on retina activates drug to eventually occlude blood vessel and stop leakage; it is possible for disorder to recur in another area

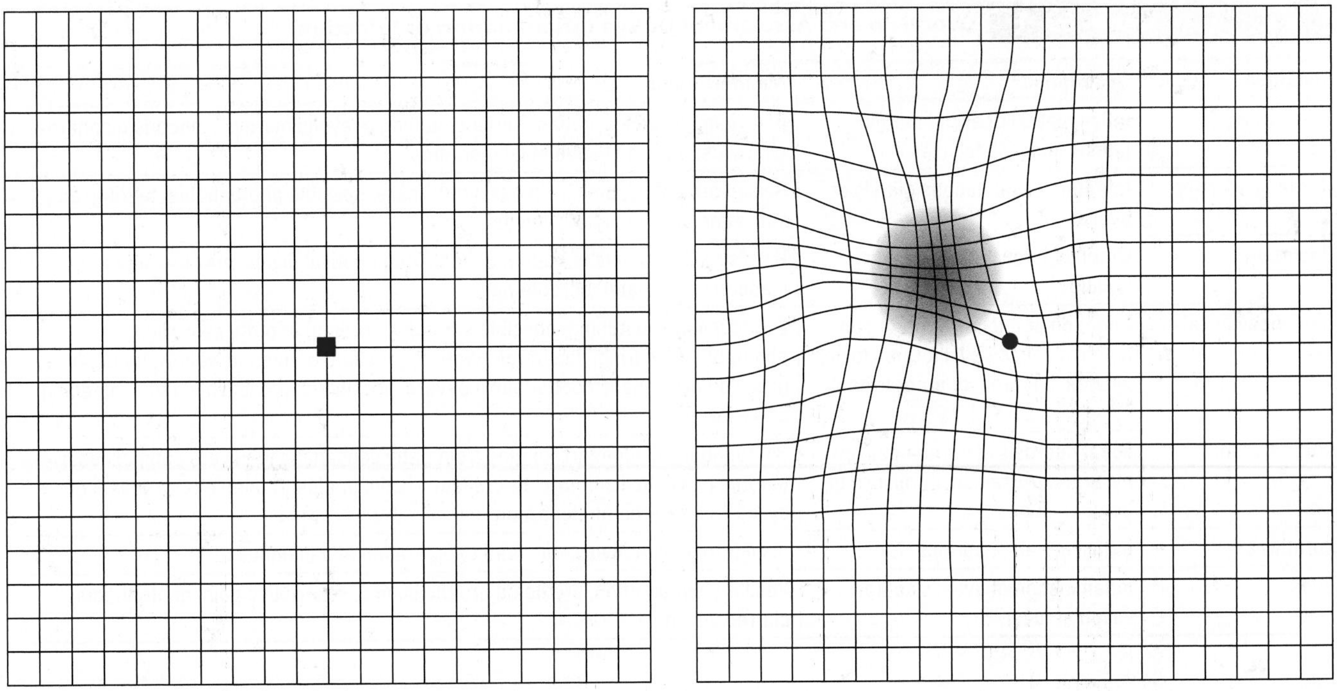

A B

Figure 63–2 Vision changes with macular degeneration. (**A**) Amsler grid with normal vision; (**B**) Amsler grid with possible central vision changes caused by macular degeneration.

NCLEX®

3. Nursing care
   a. Standard nursing measures to prevent falls and other injuries caused by impaired vision
   b. Standard measures to assist those with impaired vision
   c. Obtain home safety evaluation before discharge to minimize risk of injuries and falls in home setting

NCLEX®

D. Client teaching

1. Need for regular eye examinations to determine disease progression
2. Use of Amsler grid for self-monitoring of central vision (available from eye care professionals or on Internet)
3. Measures to maintain safety at home and adapt to visual changes
   a. Obtain aids to enhance vision and promote safety (e.g., magnification devices, enhanced lighting)
   b. Determine availability of large-print books and newspapers and audio books
4. Postprocedure self-care for photodynamic therapy includes use of dark glasses and protective clothing as well as avoiding bright indoor light for a few days

XII. EYE INFECTIONS OR INFLAMMATIONS

A. Overview and assessment (see Table 63–1)

NCLEX®

B. Therapeutic management

1. Medications: topical or systemic antibiotics or antivirals, antihistamines, and corticosteroids
2. Promote infection control through diligent hand hygiene; teach client and family that conjunctivitis can be highly contagious
3. Cleanse eye with warm water and remove any crusting or exudate before instilling eye drops or eye ointment
4. Reduce pain or discomfort with warm compresses, dark sunglasses, and analgesics (acetaminophen and/or codeine)
5. If corneal perforation is suspected, have client lie supine, close eye, and cover with dry, sterile dressing to avoid loss of eye contents until surgery is done

C. Client and family teaching

1. Teach client or caregivers to instill antibiotic drops or ointment into conjunctival sac

NCLEX®

2. Give instructions on measures to limit spread of infection to other eye or other people, including not to share face cloths or towels, not to rub eyes or wear contact lenses during infection, not to cross-contaminate infection to other eye, and discard eye makeup and purchase new after infection clears

Table 63–1 Overview and Assessment of Eye Inflammation or Infection

Condition	Description	Manifestations
Blepharitis	Inflammation of eyelid margin glands and lash follicles	Red-rimmed eyes; irritation, burning, itching of eyelid margins; mucous discharge with crusting and scaling of lid margins
Hordeolum or sty	Infection of sebaceous glands of eyelid	Raised area of lid, pain, redness, tenderness, possible photophobia, tearing, and sensation of foreign body in eye
Chalazion	Granulomatous eyelid cyst or nodule	Hard swelling, painless, reddened local conjunctival tissue, may be due to inadequately treated hordoleum
Conjunctivitis (also called pink eye)	Infection or inflammation of conjunctiva caused by allergen, toxin, viruses, bacteria, or other irritant	Eye redness and itching; possible scratchy, burning, or gritty sensation; photophobia, tearing, discharge (watery, purulent, or mucoid; yellow, white, or green color); usually not painful; if severe, possible conjunctival edema, bleeding, or perforation
Corneal ulcer	Local necrosis of cornea caused by infection, trauma, or misuse of contact lenses	Photophobia, discomfort ranging from gritty sensations to severe pain, excessive tearing; possible discharge; decreased vision; unable to open eye or spasm of eyelid; visible area of ulceration
Keratitis	Inflammation of cornea	Similar to conjunctivitis; can lead to ulceration and blindness
Uveitis	Inflammation of uveal tract (e.g., vascular layer)	Pupillary constriction, erythema around limbus, severe eye pain, photophobia, blurred vision

XIII. EYE INJURY

A. Overview and assessment

1. Corneal abrasion (disruption of superficial cornea from drying, contact lenses, eyelashes, or foreign bodies such as dust, dirt, or fingernails): pain, photophobia, tearing
2. Burns (from chemicals, heat, radiation, explosion): eye pain, decreased vision, swollen eyelids, burns, reddened and edematous conjunctiva, possible corneal haziness or cloudiness, ulcerations
3. Blunt trauma (caused by sports injuries, motor vehicle accidents, falls, physical assault): includes lid ecchymosis (black eye), conjunctival hemorrhage (painless erythema), hyphema (bleeding into anterior chamber with eye pain, decreased vision, and seeing a reddish hue), and orbital fractures (diplopia/double vision, pain with upward eye movement, limited eye movements, sunken appearance to eye, and decreased sensation on affected cheek)

NCLEX® **B. Therapeutic management**

1. If chemical burn present, irrigate eye with copious amounts of normal saline (preferred) or water (if necessary) until pH of eye is in range of 7.2–7.4; use topical anesthetic to make irrigation easier; then evaluate vision with and without any corrective eyeglasses
2. Remove loose foreign bodies quickly using a sterile, moistened cotton-tipped applicator or by irrigation to prevent corneal abrasion
3. If no foreign substances are present, first evaluate vision with and without eyeglasses to provide data about extent of injury and for use as a baseline
4. Apply eye patches or sterile gauze dressings over both eyes if severe or penetrating eye injury occurs to reduce eye movements; stabilize any penetrating objects until surgery is done to help preserve vision; institute bedrest

C. Client education

1. Purpose, effects, and use of medications
2. Use of eye patch or shield
3. Avoid activities that increase IOP during healing (lifting, bending, straining); teach how to avoid future injury

XIV. LEGAL BLINDNESS

A. Overview

1. Visual acuity that is no better than 20/200 even with correction in better eye, or a visual field of less than 20 degrees (instead of 180 degrees)
2. Common causes in United States are glaucoma and cataracts, macular degeneration, diabetic retinopathy, and congenital disorders

B. Therapeutic management

1. Assist client with grieving process that accompanies vision loss because of loss of sight and interference with mobility, self-sufficiency, and possibly finances
2. Support client who is experiencing changes in roles and relationships, communication patterns (loss of ability to perceive nonverbal cues), and possibly sexual expression
3. NCLEX® Foster independence in hospital environment
   a. Verbally and physically orient client to room using bed as a reference point
   b. Keep room and hallway free of clutter
   c. Introduce self when entering client's room and state when leaving
   d. Use increased verbal communication: describe activities in environment and provide stimuli such as radio or television; ask client what assistance is needed
   e. Ensure that call bell and other needed articles are within client's easy reach and that client knows their location
   f. Describe location of food on plate using a clock face description (for a client who was previously sighted and knows what a clock face is)
   g. Assist with ambulation, walking slightly ahead and allowing client to hold your arm (not the reverse); describe environment that lies ahead, such as turns or stairs

NCLEX® **C. Client teaching:** measures to minimize risk of injury in home setting and adapt to performing ADLs with impaired vision

XV. HEARING IMPAIRMENT

A. Overview

1. Condition that interferes with ability to receive auditory signals from environment
2. Types of hearing loss
   a. Conductive: occurs when tympanic membrane cannot vibrate freely or when sounds cannot reach middle ear or inner ear; common causes are otitis media, impacted cerumen, foreign body in ear canal, inflammation of external or middle ear, tumor, or otosclerosis
   b. Sensorineural: damage to cochlea or auditory nerve; causes include congenital disorders; damage to inner ear, cranial nerve VIII, or brain; trauma or ototoxic drugs; prolonged exposure to loud noise; infection, Meniere's syndrome, metabolic or circulatory disorders, or presbycusis (aging leads to degeneration of hair cells of cochlea)
   c. Mixed: combination of both (conductive-sensorineural hearing loss)
   d. Central: pathology in brain that interrupts ability to interpret sound, including speech

NCLEX® **B. Assessment of hearing impairment**

1. In infants and young children, language development is affected, making early diagnosis important
2. Infants may not startle to loud noises or turn head to localize sound; toddlers may have speech problems; school-age children may exhibit poor school performance
3. Common signs of hearing loss include turning head, leaning forward, or straining to hear; routinely asking others to repeat statements; not responding to others' speech if not aligned with direction of sound or speaker's face; not hearing telephone or doorbell; responding incorrectly to others; raising volume of television or other device with audio; withdrawal from groups or favoring small groups over large groups
4. Diagnosed by otoscopic examination, tympanography, and audiography

C. Therapeutic management

1. Prevent acquired hearing loss by client education to avoid exposure to loud noises
2. Advocate prompt treatment of otitis media
3. Perform developmental assessment for early identification of infants and children with hearing loss to prevent significant delays in development and school performance
4. If hearing loss is correctable in child, goal is to treat cause, such as removal of foreign body in conductive loss
5. If hearing loss cannot be corrected, interdisciplinary team (otolaryngologist, audiologist, pediatrician, nurse, and speech-language pathologist) works with child and family to obtain appropriate therapies and enhance communication
6. NCLEX® Hearing aids may be prescribed; see previous section on hearing aid care
7. Advocate for clients with hearing impairment and their families; provide support and referrals

D. Client teaching

1. Means of communicating with children or adults who have hearing loss
2. Encourage parents to enroll child in early-intervention program to promote speech development

Box 63–4

Communication with a Hearing-Impaired Client

- ➤ Approach client from within client's line of vision or tap client lightly on shoulder to get attention before speaking
- ➤ Reduce background noise, such as radio or TV, before beginning to speak
- ➤ Avoid covering mouth with hands or other objects while speaking
- ➤ Face client and speak slowly and clearly—pronounce words clearly without overarticulating them; speak using low pitch and normal loudness
- ➤ Use nonverbal cues and written messages to enhance communication
- ➤ Repeat sentences using different words if client has difficulty understanding
- ➤ Ask client to repeat directions or teaching that was done to ensure understanding

XVI. OTOSCLEROSIS

A. *Otosclerosis* overview

1. Probably autosomal dominant disorder of labyrinthine capsule in which abnormal bone growth occurs around ossicles; most common in adolescent or young adult females
2. Causes fixation of stapes (do not vibrate as they should because of stiffening, which reduces sound transmission to inner ear), leading to conductive hearing loss
3. Inner ear involvement leads to sensorineural hearing loss
4. Bilateral involvement may occur, but hearing loss may be more pronounced in one ear

NCLEX® **B. Assessment**

1. Bilateral conductive hearing loss that is progressive and asymmetrical, tinnitus, possible retention of bone conduction (so client has difficulty in ordinary conversation but can use telephone adequately)
2. Reddish or pinkish orange tympanic membrane from increased vascularity (Schwartz's sign)
3. Rinne test results: bone sound conduction equal to or longer than air conduction (abnormal finding) if hearing loss is greater than 25 decibels (dB)
4. Weber test results: lateralization to ear with greater conductive hearing loss

NCLEX® **C. Therapeutic management**

1. Encourage use of a hearing aid(s) to augment sound
2. Administer sodium fluoride as prescribed to slow bone resorption and overgrowth
3. Implement strategies to enhance communication with a hearing-impaired client (see Box 63–4)
4. Surgical intervention
   a. Stapedectomy with fenestration: microsurgical removal of diseased stapes, with drill or laser creation of a hole in footplate, followed by insertion of a steel or synthetic prosthesis to restore hearing
   b. Stapedotomy: insertion of a wire or platinum ribbon prosthesis into a small hole created in stapes footplate

D. Client teaching: referral to appropriate community agencies; postoperative care as previously outlined

XVII. EAR INFECTIONS

A. Overview

1. Otitis externa: infectious, inflammatory, or allergic response in external auditory canal or auricle; also called "swimmer's ear"; more frequent in warm, humid areas
2. **Otitis media**
   a. Acute or chronic infection or inflammation of middle ear; greatest incidence is between 6 and 36 months of age during winter months
   b. Related to dysfunction of eustachian tube, which provides drainage and ventilation of middle ear; when blocked from edema in upper respiratory infection, fluid can accumulate, providing a medium for bacterial growth and infection
   c. Children with facial malformations such as cleft palate and Down syndrome have anatomic variations of their eustachian tubes, making them more vulnerable to otitis media
3. Mastoiditis: infection of mastoid process (temporal bone adjacent to middle ear), usually results from untreated or inadequately treated otitis media

NCLEX® **B. Assessment**

1. Otitis externa: redness, swelling, and exudate in external auditory canal, earache, itching, sensation that ear is "plugged" or "blocked," hearing loss in affected ear

2. Otitis media
   a. Children (acute): ear pain, irritability, diarrhea, fever, and vomiting are common; possible pulling at the affected ear; some children are asymptomatic; otoscopic examination of tympanic membrane reveals a red, bulging, nonmobile tympanic membrane
   b. Adults (acute): severe earache or ear pain (classic), ear pressure, fever, malaise, diminished hearing, dizziness or vertigo, N/V, possible tinnitus (ringing in ears), presence of fluid behind a bulging tympanic membrane
   c. Chronic: slight fever, diminished hearing, chronic ear discharge
3. Mastoiditis: fever, malaise, possible tinnitus and headache, persistent throbbing ear pain worsened by head movement, tenderness behind ear over mastoid process, local cellulitis of skin, drainage from ear, diminished hearing in affected ear

C. Therapeutic management in adults

NCLEX®
1. Apply local heat three times per day for 20 minutes at a time as prescribed
2. Encourage bedrest as applicable to reduce head movements and pain

NCLEX®
3. Administer prescribed antibiotics (otic or systemic), decongestants, antihistamines, analgesics (acetaminophen or aspirin), and antivertigo agents
4. Teach client to use caution while hearing is diminished
5. Provide care to clients undergoing ear surgery as previously outlined
6. Surgical procedures
   a. Myringotomy: surgical perforation of tympanic membrane to allow drainage of middle ear secretions and relieve pain and pressure (otitis media)
   b. Tympanocentesis: insertion of a 20-gauge spinal needle through inferior portion of tympanic membrane to drain secretions, possibly to obtain culture, and relieve pain and pressure (otitis media)
   c. Mastoidectomy: surgical removal of infected mastoid air cells, bone, and pus; radical mastoidectomy involves removal of middle ear structures such as incus and malleus as well as diseased tissue (conductive hearing loss then occurs unless reconstructive surgery is done as well)
   d. Tympanoplasty: surgical reconstruction of ossicles and tympanic membrane of middle ear to help restore hearing

D. Therapeutic management in children

NCLEX®
1. Nursing management of child with tympanostomy tubes: usually surgery is accomplished in a day-surgery center, not an inpatient hospital setting
   a. Teach parents to give acetaminophen for discomfort following myringotomy and insertion of tympanostomy tubes
   b. Parents should follow healthcare provider's directions for postoperative ear care; ear drops are often prescribed
   c. Some healthcare providers require parents to insert earplugs for bathing and swimming and avoid water in ear canal; others do not
   d. Teach parents that ear tubes will spontaneously extrude and fall out; they may note presence of spool-shaped tube in child's ear canal; ear tubes usually fall out in about 1 year
2. Medication therapy
   a. Oral antibiotic therapy for 10–14 days, such as amoxicillin and trimethoprim-sulfamethoxazole
   b. Recurrent or chronic otitis media infections may require prophylactic antibiotics as a 6-month trial
3. Surgical procedures: as described in previous section for adults
4. Client and family teaching: signs and symptoms of otitis media; need to monitor and treat temperature; how to administer medication safely and effectively (complete full course of antibiotic therapy even if feeling better; give doses on time)

XVIII. MÉNIÈRE'S DISEASE

A. *Ménière's disease* overview

1. Inner ear disorder in which excessive endolymphatic fluid accumulates in membranous labyrinth because of malabsorption or blocked endolymphatic duct; also called idiopathic endolymphatic hydrops
2. Impaired reabsorption of endolymph leads to dilation of lymph channels, which causes symptoms
3. Etiology is uncertain but may include heredity, viral influence, immune dysfunction, trauma, or infection

NCLEX®

B. Assessment

1. Recurrent severe attacks of vertigo accompanied by sense of fullness in ears, roaring or ringing tinnitus, nausea, headache, and gradual but progressive sensorineural hearing loss (often unilateral)

2. Attacks may last minutes to hours with possible associated symptoms of hypotension, diaphoresis, and nystagmus
3. Attacks may be triggered by increased sodium (Na^+) intake, vasoconstriction, premenstrual fluid retention, stress, or allergies (sometimes no trigger is identified)
4. Diagnosed by electronystagmography (including caloric testing), Rinne and Weber tests, x-ray, CT scan, evaluation of response to a test dose of an osmotic or loop diuretic

NCLEX® **C. Therapeutic management**

1. Low-Na^+ diet, avoidance of sugars, and, if symptoms are severe, fluid restriction
2. Avoid use of alcohol, caffeine, nicotine
3. Bedrest to control vertigo; assist with ambulation for safety
4. Medication therapy: diuretics, antihistamines to suppress vestibular system, antivertigo and antiemetic drugs
5. Endolymphatic sac decompression: relieves pressure in labyrinth and creates shunt between membranous labyrinth and subarachnoid space for fluid drainage (preserves hearing in most cases, relieves vertigo in approximately 70% of cases, relieves tinnitus and sensations of ear fullness in 50% of cases)
6. Vestibular nerve sectioning: severing of portion of CN VIII that controls balance and sensation of vertigo (relieves vertigo in about 98% of cases)
7. Labyrinthectomy: complete removal of labyrinth, destroying cochlear function, relieving vertigo but causing loss of any minimal remaining hearing as well ("last resort")
8. Cochlear implant: for sensorineural hearing loss
   a. An electrode is implanted in cochlea to receive stimuli from a processor worn on body; used for a client with intact neurons capable of stimulation (see Figure 63–3)
   b. A second type of device, used for clients with no excitable auditory fibers, amplifies and transmits a signal to a receiver implanted in brainstem
   c. Devices do not restore normal hearing but allow perception of sound to alert a client to conversation or dangers in the environment
9. Complications of all inner ear surgical procedures include infection and cerebrospinal fluid (CSF) leakage

D. Client teaching

NCLEX® 1. Follow restrictions in Na^+, sugar, fluid, nicotine, alcohol, and caffeine
2. Take medications as prescribed

NCLEX® 3. Learn signs of an impending attack: fullness in affected ear, increasing tinnitus, headache; lie down in bed in a dark, quiet room if at home when an attack begins, or pull off the road for safety if driving

NCLEX® 4. Avoid sudden movements or position changes; move head slowly and do not get up unassisted during an attack
5. Wear Medic-Alert identification
6. Learn stress-reduction techniques of choice to help reduce severity of attacks

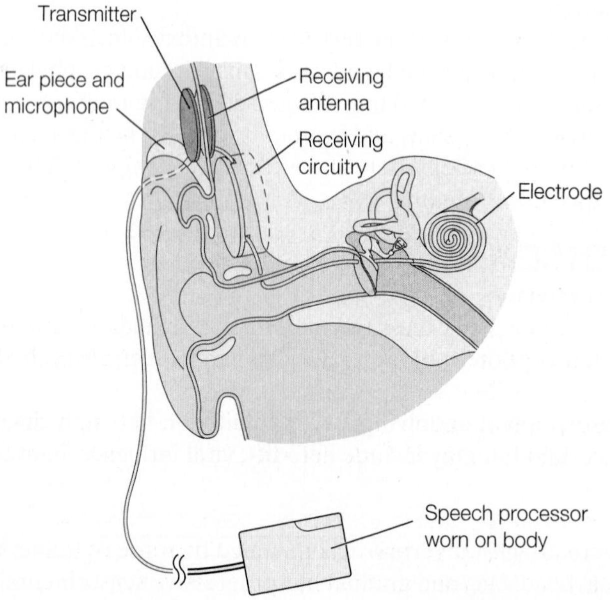

Figure 63–3

Cochlear implant used in sensorineural hearing loss in which excitable auditory neurons remain.

7. If tinnitus persists between attacks, use white noise or ambient sound machine to mask tinnitus and promote sleep; consider use of medication most commonly effective—oral antidepressant nortriptyline taken at bedtime
8. Practice balance training exercises to help brain learn to compensate for damage to vestibular system; exercises consist of moving head up and down, side to side, and tilting left and right; repeat 10 times each twice a day

XIX. EPISTAXIS

A. *Epistaxis* overview

1. Also known as nosebleed; very common in children, especially boys
2. Superficial veins in nares are a common source of bleeding
3. Bleeding can occur from irritation, drying of mucosa from low humidity, increased blood pressure, or picking nose

B. Assessment

1. Assess vital signs of client in emergency department or clinic with uncontrolled epistaxis while simultaneous efforts to control bleeding are being performed
2. If client has had significant blood loss, hemoglobin and hematocrit may be measured

C. Therapeutic management

NCLEX® 1. Teach client or parents to humidify air (especially during winter months and nighttime hours) and have child sleep with head elevated to prevent recurrence
NCLEX® 2. Following an episode of nosebleed, client is prone to rebleeding; client should not bend forward, drink hot liquids, exercise excessively, or take hot baths or showers for 3–4 days following a significant nosebleed
3. If bleeding cannot be controlled using pressure, topical vasoconstrictive agents may be used, such as phenylephrine, epinephrine, or thrombin
4. Cautery may be required with silver nitrate or electrocautery
5. If bleeding cannot be stopped, nose may be packed with absorbent packing material by healthcare provider to stop bleeding

D. Child and family education

NCLEX® 1. Teach client or parents how to stop a nosebleed by applying steady pressure to both nostrils just below nasal bone for 10–15 minutes
2. Instruct client to sit upright and slightly forward for best results when applying pressure to nostrils and to prevent excessive swallowing of blood
3. Instruct client or parents to seek healthcare if bleeding cannot be stopped
4. Teach client to avoid picking at nose or forcefully blowing nose; teach to release sneezes through open mouth covered with tissues

XX. PHARYNGITIS

A. *Pharyngitis* overview

1. An infection of the pharynx, often involving tonsils
2. A common disorder in children age 4–7 years, but rare in infancy
3. About 80% of cases have viral etiology, and symptom relief is indicated
4. Bacterial pharyngitis is most often caused by *group A beta-hemolytic streptococcus* and requires antibiotic therapy

NCLEX® B. Assessment

1. Symptoms include sore throat, difficulty swallowing, drooling caused by sore throat, and inability to swallow saliva; inflammation of pharynx and enlargement of tonsils (with or without exudate), fever, vomiting, cough, lymphadenopathy, and headache; hoarseness or a change in voice quality may be noted
2. A throat culture is necessary to diagnose viral or bacterial etiology of pharyngitis; streptococcal infections can be diagnosed within minutes using a rapid strep test

NCLEX® C. Therapeutic management

1. In viral pharyngitis, relief of symptoms is indicated; offer diet that is easy to swallow (soft or liquids) and soothing to sore throat (no citrus juices or other foods that could cause burning or increased irritation)
2. Saltwater gargles, throat lozenges, or anesthetic sprays promote pain relief
3. Medications: analgesics (acetaminophen); antibiotics for bacterial infections

D. Client and family teaching

1. Stress importance of completing antibiotic therapy to eradicate microorganisms
2. Untreated or inadequately treated streptococcal infections can result in acute rheumatic fever, glomerulonephritis, or other serious sequelae

XXI. TONSILLITIS

A. *Tonsillitis* overview

1. Inflammation of tonsils in posterior pharynx from viral or bacterial infection
2. Causative organism in bacterial infection can be *group A beta-hemolytic streptococcus*, which is particularly virulent

NCLEX®

B. Assessment

1. Diagnosis of etiology is made by throat culture
2. Streptococcal infection can be diagnosed within minutes using a rapid strep test
3. Symptoms
   a. Enlarged, reddened tonsils, with or without exudate; lymphadenopathy
   b. Sore throat, difficulty swallowing because of severe sore throat
   c. Drooling, caused by the inability to swallow saliva secretions
   d. Mouth breathing

NCLEX®

C. Therapeutic management

1. Management for viral tonsillitis is symptom relief: promoting comfort, pain relief with acetaminophen; similar to management of viral pharyngitis
2. Management for bacterial tonsillitis is antibiotic therapy as well as symptom relief
3. Nursing management: offer diet that is easy to swallow (soft or liquids, including ice pops) and soothing to sore throat (no citrus juices or other foods that could cause burning or increased irritation)
4. Use of saltwater gargles, throat lozenges, or anesthetic sprays for pain relief
5. Medication therapy: analgesics (acetaminophen) for comfort and fever; antibiotics as prescribed for bacterial infections

D. Child and family education: importance of completing full course of antibiotic therapy, how to manage symptoms

E. Tonsillectomy

1. Surgical removal of tonsils; may be indicated for recurrent tonsillitis, peritonsillar abcess, or respiratory compromise from airway obstruction
2. Commonly performed in a day-surgery setting, ambulatory surgical setting, or may require an overnight hospital stay
3. Client should not have symptoms of tonsillitis for at least 1 week before surgery
4. Preoperative nursing management: includes client and family preoperative teaching and baseline lab data, including bleeding and clotting times
5. Postoperative nursing management (NCLEX®)
   a. Provide pain control with analgesics and ice collar
   b. Most common complication is excessive bleeding or hemorrhaging from operative site; observe child for frequent or continual swallowing, vomiting bright red blood, and changes in vital signs
   c. Offer clear, chilled fluids or ice pops to relieve pain and reduce inflammation when awake and alert; avoid red-colored fluids because emesis of these fluids could be mistaken for blood
   d. Teach child and parents that a sore throat is to be expected for approximately 1 week postoperatively

F. Client and family education

1. Analgesic medications to be given at home
2. Assess child for signs of complications such as hemorrhage from operative site
3. Ensure adequate fluid intake to prevent dehydration; advance child's diet as tolerated to include soft, nonirritating foods; avoid citrus (acidic) foods and foods that are rough in texture for 10–14 days
4. Avoid strenuous activity for about 1 week; child may return to school in 10 days, when operative site is adequately healed

Check Your NCLEX–RN® Exam I.Q.

You are ready for testing on this content if you can:

- Identify basic structures and functions of the eye and ear.
- Describe the pathophysiology and etiology of common eye and ear disorders.
- Discuss expected assessment data and diagnostic test findings for selected eye and ear disorders.
- Discuss therapeutic management of a client experiencing an eye and ear disorder.
- Discuss nursing management of a client experiencing an eye and ear disorder.
- Identify expected outcomes for the client experiencing an eye and ear disorder.

PRACTICE TEST

1 To communicate effectively with a client who has sensorineural hearing loss caused by presbycusis, the nurse should use which strategies to improve communication with the client? Select all that apply.

1. Approach the client from the front.
2. Use the mouth to exaggerate word pronunciation.
3. Shout initially to get the client's attention.
4. Turn down background noise from radio or TV before speaking.
5. Speak very loudly but in an even tone of voice.

2 A client has completed a full course of antibiotics for acute otitis media. The nurse conducting a follow-up assessment determines whether medication therapy was effective by questioning the client about relief from which most common presenting symptom?

1. Dizziness
2. Impaired hearing
3. Nausea and vomiting
4. Ear pain

3 A client has undergone myringotomy. The nurse working in an ambulatory surgery center would instruct the client to avoid which activity while healing is occurring?

1. Gardening
2. Swimming
3. Softball
4. Bowling

4 A 68-year-old female client tells the ambulatory care nurse during a routine visit that she has recently noticed a decline in her ability to hear. The nurse documents this information on the client's health record, suspecting that this client most likely is exhibiting which disorder?

1. Presbycusis
2. Otitis externa
3. Otalgia
4. Ménière's disease

5 After a client has undergone outpatient surgery for a right-eye cataract removal, the nurse teaches the client to avoid which activities when the client gets home? Select all that apply.

1. Walking about the house unassisted
2. Lying on the right side
3. Picking up objects that are at waist level
4. Washing dishes in the sink
5. Mowing the lawn

6 A client has hearing loss characterized by distortion of sounds that are heard. The client asks the nurse about the benefits of obtaining a hearing aid. The nurse should include in a response that a hearing aid will have which effect for this client?

1. It will intensify the already distorted sounds.
2. It will improve the client's ability to distinguish words from background noises.
3. It will make sounds louder and clearer.
4. It will have no effect on hearing.

7 A client reports ongoing problems with vertigo. The nurse should question the client about which accompanying manifestations to determine whether the client has developed Ménière's disease? Select all that apply.

1. Tinnitus
2. Hearing loss
3. Headache
4. Sense of fullness in the ear
5. Purulent discharge

8 The nurse prepares to initiate client teaching for which medication commonly used to treat Ménière's disease?

1. Meclizine
2. Dexamethasone
3. Acetaminophen
4. Propranolol

PRACTICE TEST

9. A client with glaucoma has been prescribed pilocarpine. Which description should the nurse use when explaining how this medication works?

1. Dilates the pupil
2. Constricts intraocular vessels
3. Constricts the pupil
4. Relaxes ciliary muscles

10. What should be the initial intervention by the nurse for a client in the emergency department who suffered a chemical burn to the eyes?

1. Administer an analgesic as prescribed.
2. Evaluate vision with and without prescription eyeglasses.
3. Administer an antibiotic as prescribed.
4. Irrigate the eyes with normal saline solution or water.

11. The nurse is caring for a client who is in the recovery area following cataract surgery. The nurse should ask the client about which manifestations that would indicate onset of retinal detachment as a postoperative complication? Select all that apply.

1. Increased lacrimation
2. Flashing lights
3. Sudden, severe eye pain
4. Inability to move the eye
5. Loss of part of visual field in the eye

12. A client who was diagnosed with primary open-angle glaucoma has been started on medication therapy with timolol maleate. The nurse assesses for which possible adverse systemic response to the drug?

1. Tachycardia
2. Anxiety
3. Bradycardia
4. Hypertension

13. The daughter of an older adult client diagnosed with nonexudative macular degeneration asks the nurse to explain the disorder. In formulating a response, the nurse should include which characteristics of this condition?

1. Atrophy and degeneration of outer pigmented layer of the retina
2. Scar formation between the retina and the choroid
3. Rapid and severe loss of vision
4. Separation of the retina from the choroids

14. The nurse is evaluating the effectiveness of preoperative teaching for a client who will undergo repair of a detached retina using scleral buckling. The nurse evaluates that the client understands the procedure after the client gives which description of the surgery?

1. Using a piece of silicone to indent the sclera to increase contact between retinal layers
2. Injecting a gas into the vitreous humor to push the detached retina against the choroid
3. Removing the torn segment of retina
4. Replacing the torn segment of the retina with donor retinal tissue

15. The nurse should take which action when a client first comes into the emergency department with blunt trauma to the eye?

1. Irrigate the eye to remove foreign substances.
2. Administer miotics.
3. Place the client in semi-Fowler position.
4. Prevent loss of intraocular contents.

16. Which statement made by a client to the nurse indicates an understanding of home care instructions after cataract surgery?

1. "I should not bend over to pick up objects from the floor."
2. "I can sleep on whichever side I want as long as my head is raised."
3. "I may not watch television for 6 weeks."
4. "I should keep the protective eye shield in place 24 hours a day."

17. The nurse is assessing a client's hearing using the Weber test. The nurse documents the client's result as normal if the client reports which effect after the vibrating tuning fork is placed on the midline vertex of his head?

1. Sound lateralizes to the left ear.
2. Sound lateralizes to the right ear.
3. Sound is absent in both ears.
4. Sound is heard equally in both ears.

18 The nurse has a prescription to irrigate the left ear of an assigned client. The nurse uses which technique to perform this procedure correctly?

1. Direct the stream into the center of the ear canal.
2. Draw up 250 mL of solution.
3. Pack the external ear tightly with cotton balls after instilling the irrigant.
4. Help the client to lie on the left side after the irrigation is finished.

19 Which measures would be beneficial for the nurse to include in collaborative management of a client who has conjunctivitis? Select all that apply.

1. Cold eye compresses
2. Careful hand hygiene
3. Antibiotic therapy
4. Dark sunglasses
5. Opioid analgesics

20 The nurse who is administering an ophthalmic medication to a client should take which action as part of correct procedure?

1. Drop the medication onto the eyeball.
2. Apply pressure to the inner canthus while administering the medication.
3. Rub the closed eyelid with a cotton ball after instillation.
4. Wait 10 seconds between drops.

21 The nurse has administered a dose of antibiotic intramuscularly to a 5-year-old client with tonsillitis. The child cries, asking for a bandage to be placed over the injection site. What is the best action by the nurse?

1. Apply a bandage.
2. Ask the child why he wants the bandage.
3. Explain to the child that a bandage is not necessary.
4. Show the child that the site is not bleeding.

22 What is the most appropriate intervention by the nurse who is caring for an infant with acute otitis media and a fever of 102.7°F (39.3°C)?

1. Provide sponging with cool water to reduce fever.
2. Encourage the baby's intake of solids to maintain adequate caloric intake.
3. Swaddle the baby in layers of blankets to promote comfort and prevent chills.
4. Offer fluids frequently to prevent dehydration.

23 Which priority problem should be a focus of concern for the nurse who is assigned to the care of a child with pharyngitis?

1. The child's anxiety level
2. The risk for an ineffective cough
3. The risk for dehydration
4. The child's growth and development status

24 The nurse recommends a humidified atmosphere for a child with recurrent epistaxis. When questioned by the parent, the nurse explains which benefit of humidity for the child?

1. It helps to liquefy secretions
2. It helps increase the child's oxygen level
3. It helps the child's breathing
4. It helps to prevent dry mucous membranes

25 A 15-month-old child diagnosed with conjunctivitis has been prescribed an antibiotic ointment. In teaching the mother to administer this drug, the nurse should recommend which technique?

1. Wait until the child is asleep to instill the ointment.
2. Mummy the child to prevent accidental injury.
3. Place the ointment on a swab and spread across closed lids.
4. Use sterile gauze to apply the ointment to the lids.

26 The nurse should provide which instructions to a client after fluorescein angiography to diagnose an eye condition? Select all that apply.

1. Encourage reduced fluid intake to limit intraocular pressure.
2. The dye causes temporary green discoloration to urine.
3. Avoid sunlight until pupil size returns to normal.
4. Lie down with eyes closed for 12 hours postprocedure after returning home.
5. Expect headache and blurred vision for approximately 24 hours after the procedure.

ANSWERS & RATIONALES

1 **Answer: 1, 4 Rationale:** The client should be approached from the front so as not to startle the client. An effective method to improve communication with the client is to eliminate background noises that could interfere with hearing. The nurse should use normal pronunciation of words to assist the client's understanding. The nurse should refrain from shouting, which is demeaning and not helpful. The nurse should speak in normal tones to aid hearing; speaking very loudly is not necessarily helpful and can be perceived as demeaning. **Cognitive Level:** Analyzing **Client Need:** Physiological Adaptation **Integrated Process:** Communication and Documentation **Content Area:** Adult Health: Eye, Ear, Nose, and Throat **Strategy:** The core issue of the question is the appropriate strategy for communicating with a client who is hearing impaired. Recall that clients rely on visual cues and can benefit from reduced background noise to aid in answering the question.

2 **Answer: 4 Rationale:** Ear pain is the most common symptom of otitis media that motivates clients to seek healthcare. Secondary or associated symptoms include dizziness, hearing impairment, fever, and nausea and vomiting. **Cognitive Level:** Analyzing **Client Need:** Physiological Adaptation **Integrated Process:** Nursing Process: Evaluation **Content Area:** Adult Health: Eye, Ear, Nose, and Throat **Strategy:** The critical words in the question are *most common*, which tell you it is necessary to prioritize the options by the frequency of their occurrence. Use nursing knowledge and the process of elimination to make this selection.

3 **Answer: 2 Rationale:** Myringotomy is a surgical procedure that perforates the tympanic membrane to allow drainage from the middle ear. Postoperatively, the client should avoid getting water into the ear canal, which could potentially enter the middle ear. Activities such as gardening, softball, and bowling do not risk water getting into the surgical ear and pose no risk to the client. **Cognitive Level:** Applying **Client Need:** Physiological Adaptation **Integrated Process:** Nursing Process: Implementation **Content Area:** Adult Health: Eye, Ear, Nose, and Throat **Strategy:** The core issue of the question is identification of activities that could be harmful to the client while healing is occurring after surgery. Recall that it is necessary to avoid getting the surgical area wet to make the appropriate selection.

4 **Answer: 1 Rationale:** Presbycusis is the most common form of sensorineural hearing loss in older adults. Otitis externa is infection in the external auditory canal and can occur in clients of any age. Otalgia is an earache. Ménière's disease is an inner ear disorder characterized by tinnitus and vertigo that primarily affects middle-age adults. **Cognitive Level:** Applying **Client Need:** Physiological Adaptation **Integrated Process:** Nursing Process: Diagnosis **Content Area:** Adult Health: Eye, Ear, Nose, and Throat **Strategy:** The core issue of the question is the ability to identify age-related changes in hearing in an older adult. Use nursing knowledge and the process of elimination to make a selection.

5 **Answer: 2, 5 Rationale:** The client should avoid lying on the operative side following eye surgery to minimize edema and intraocular pressure. Activities that involved pushing or straining, such as mowing the lawn, can increase intraocular pressure and should be avoided in the postoperative period. Walking unassisted is not a problem given the information in the question. Some clients with severe visual impairment or other health problems may need assistance to move about in the environment. Picking up objects at waist level is acceptable because it does not raise intraocular pressure. Washing dishes in the sink poses no risk to the client as it does not increase intraocular pressure. **Cognitive Level:** Analyzing **Client Need:** Physiological Adaptation **Integrated Process:** Nursing Process: Implementation **Content Area:** Adult Health: Eye, Ear, Nose, and Throat **Strategy:** The core issue of the question is client teaching about safe and unsafe activities following cataract surgery. Recall that it is important to avoid positions in which gravity can lead to increased edema or pressure to make the correct selection.

6 **Answer: 1 Rationale:** When hearing loss is characterized by distortion of sounds, amplification of sound is of little help because it only increases the intensity of distorted sounds. When hearing loss is characterized by distortion of sounds, a hearing aid will not help the client distinguish words from background noises or make words louder and clearer. A hearing aid will have some effect for this client but it will not be helpful. **Cognitive Level:** Applying **Client Need:** Physiological Adaptation **Integrated Process:** Nursing Process: Implementation **Content Area:** Adult Health: Eye, Ear, Nose, and Throat **Strategy:** The core issue of the question is the ability to correlate the types of hearing loss that can be improved with the use of a hearing aid. To do this, reflect on the types of hearing loss and the likely effect of a hearing aid for that condition. Use nursing knowledge and the process of elimination to make a selection.

7 **Answer: 1, 2, 4 Rationale:** Vertigo, tinnitus, hearing loss, and a sense of fullness in the ear are classic symptoms of Ménière's disease. Headache is not part of this clinical picture. Purulent drainage suggests infection. **Cognitive Level:** Applying **Client Need:** Physiological Adaptation **Integrated Process:** Nursing Process: Assessment **Content Area:** Adult Health: Eye, Ear, Nose, and Throat **Strategy:** The core issue of the question is identification of signs and symptoms of Ménière's disease. Recall that this is a disorder of the inner ear, thus making symptoms related to balance as well as hearing important to identify. Use nursing knowledge and the process of elimination to make a selection.

8 **Answer: 1 Rationale:** Antivertigo and antiemetic medications, such as meclizine, are used to control symptoms associated with Ménière's disease. Diuretics are used between acute attacks to reduce the volume of endolymph and prevent attacks. Glucocorticoids such as dexamethasone are not used to treat Ménière's disease. Analgesics such as acetaminophen, which work at the level of the peripheral nervous system, are not part of the treatment plan. Beta-blockers such as propranolol have no role in the treatment of Ménière's disease. **Cognitive Level:** Analyzing **Client Need:** Physiological Adaptation **Integrated Process:** Nursing Process: Planning **Content Area:** Adult Health: Eye, Ear, Nose, and Throat **Strategy:** The core issue of the question is the ability to anticipate medications that will be effective in relieving the symptoms associated with Ménière's disease. To answer correctly, it is necessary to have a core body of knowledge related to pharmacology. Use nursing knowledge and the process of elimination to make a selection.

9 **Answer: 3 Rationale:** Pilocarpine is a miotic agent, which constricts the pupil and thereby increases the flow of aqueous humor and decreases intraocular pressure. Pupil dilation is the opposite effect of pilocarpine. Pilocarpine does not constrict blood vessels within the eye. Pilocarpine does not relax the ciliary muscles. **Cognitive Level:** Applying **Client Need:** Physiological Adaptation **Integrated Process:** Nursing Process: Implementation **Content Area:** Adult Health: Eye, Ear, Nose and Throat **Strategy:** The core issue of the question is the ability to anticipate medications that will be effective in relieving symptoms associated with glaucoma. To answer correctly, it is necessary to have a core body of knowledge related to pharmacology. Use nursing knowledge and the process of elimination to make a selection.

10 **Answer: 4 Rationale:** The immediate priority for clients with chemical burns is flushing the affected eye with copious amounts of normal saline or water. Analgesics, with the exception of topical anesthesia, are not indicated. Evaluation of visual acuity is an appropriate intervention after flushing. Antibiotics may be administered after the initial actions have been taken. **Cognitive Level:** Applying **Client Need:** Safety and Infection Control **Integrated Process:** Nursing Process: Implementation **Content Area:** Adult Health: Eye, Ear, Nose, and Throat **Strategy:** The critical word in the question is *initial*, which indicates more than one or all options could be correct and it is necessary to prioritize the most important or immediate action needed. Whenever there is an injury involving chemicals, the priority action is to remove the offending substance.

11 **Answer: 2, 5 Rationale:** Clients with retinal detachment frequently report flashing lights and loss of vision, commonly described as a veil or curtain being drawn across the eye. Retinal detachment is not associated with increased lacrimation or tearing, eye pain, or change in ocular movements. **Cognitive Level:** Applying **Client Need:** Physiological Adaptation **Integrated Process:** Nursing Process: Assessment **Content Area:** Adult Health: Eye, Ear, Nose, and Throat **Strategy:** The core issue of the question is knowledge of complications of cataract surgery. Use nursing knowledge and the process of elimination to make a selection.

12 **Answer: 3 Rationale:** Medications that end in *-olol* are beta-adrenergic blocking agents. When taken as ophthalmic preparations, they can produce systemic effects such as bradycardia. Tachycardia would be expected if the drug was a beta-adrenergic stimulant, not a beta-blocker. Beta-blockers may also be used to treat adrenergic symptoms associated with anxiety, but this does not relate to glaucoma. The client taking timolol is more likely to experience hypotension as an adverse effect, not hypertension. **Cognitive Level:** Applying **Client Need:** Physiological Adaptation **Integrated Process:** Nursing Process: Assessment **Content Area:** Adult Health: Eye, Ear, Nose, and Throat **Strategy:** The core issue of the question is the ability to identify adverse effects of medication used to treat glaucoma. To answer correctly, it is necessary to have a core body of knowledge related to pharmacology. Use nursing knowledge and the process of elimination to make a selection.

13 **Answer: 1 Rationale:** Nonexudative or dry macular degeneration results from atrophy and degeneration of the outer layer of the retina. In exudative or wet macular degeneration, blood leaks into the subretinal space and scar tissue gradually forms. The resulting loss of vision occurs rapidly and is more profound. Exudative macular degeneration accounts for 90% of all cases of legal blindness. Separation of the retina from the choroid describes retinal detachment. **Cognitive Level:** Applying **Client Need:** Physiological Adaptation **Integrated Process:** Nursing Process: Implementation **Content Area:** Adult Health: Eye, Ear, Nose, and Throat **Strategy:** The core issue of the question is the ability to discriminate correct information to be used in teaching clients and/or families about disease processes. Thus, to answer this question, it is necessary to understand the two types of macular degeneration and how they present in terms of symptoms.

14 **Answer: 1 Rationale:** Scleral buckling involves using a piece of silicone is used to indent the sclera to increase contact between the retinal layers. It is used in conjunction with laser photocoagulation or cryothermy to achieve the best results. A gas is injected into the vitreous humor during pneumatic retinopexy as treatment for detached retina. Scleral buckling does not involve removing the torn segment of retina, which would result in permanent vision loss in that area of the eye. Scleral buckling does not include use of donor retinal tissue. **Cognitive Level:** Applying **Client Need:** Physiological Adaptation **Integrated Process:** Nursing Process: Evaluation **Content Area:** Adult Health: Eye, Ear, Nose, and Throat **Strategy:** The core issue of the question is evaluation of a client's understanding of a surgical procedure. To select correctly, it is necessary to be able to identify how the surgery will be performed. Use nursing knowledge and the process of elimination to make a selection.

15 **Answer: 3 Rationale:** Prevention or reduction of intraocular pressure (that may accompany blunt trauma to the eye) can be accomplished by the use of semi-Fowler position (to reduce edema) and administration of a carbonic anhydrase inhibitor, such as acetazolamide. It is unnecessary to irrigate the eye because no foreign body is present. Constriction of the pupil with miotics is not indicated. Blunt trauma does not cause loss of intraocular contents. **Cognitive Level:** Applying **Client Need:** Physiological Adaptation **Integrated Process:** Nursing Process: Planning **Content Area:** Adult Health: Eye, Ear, Nose, and Throat **Strategy:** The core issue of the question is identification of a correct action in the treatment of eye trauma. Recall that injuries typically cause formation of edema at the site, and thus early actions for an injury may involve proper client positioning to reduce edema formation.

16 **Answer: 1 Rationale:** The client should avoid activities that raise intraocular pressure, such as bending over. The client should sleep on the nonoperative side. Activities involving the eyes are done at the advice of the surgeon. Typically, an eye shield is used at night, and dark protective glasses are worn during the day. **Cognitive Level:** Applying **Client Need:** Physiological Adaptation **Integrated Process:** Nursing Process: Evaluation **Content Area:** Adult Health: Eye, Ear, Nose, and Throat **Strategy:** The core issue of the question is the ability to evaluate client understanding of postoperative instructions after cataract surgery. Evaluate each option in terms of the truth of the statement, since the question contains the critical word *understood*.

17 **Answer: 4 Rationale:** To perform the Weber test, the nurse places a vibrating tuning fork on the midline vertex of the client's head. The sound should normally be heard equally in both ears. Sound that lateralizes to the left side indicates either conductive hearing loss on the left side or sensorineural hearing loss on the right side. Sound that lateralizes to the right side indicates either conductive hearing loss on

the right side or sensorineural hearing loss on the left side. Sound absent in both ears indicates deafness. **Cognitive Level:** Analyzing **Client Need:** Physiological Adaptation **Integrated Process:** Nursing Process: Assessment **Content Area:** Adult Health: Eye, Ear, Nose, and Throat **Strategy:** The core issue of the question is the ability to correctly analyze results of physical assessment techniques. Use nursing knowledge and the process of elimination to make a selection.

18 **Answer: 4 Rationale:** The client should lie on the affected side following the irrigation to allow gravity to further assist in draining the ear canal. The irrigant should be directed along the wall of the external canal, not the center (which could damage the tympanic membrane). Usually, 50–70 mL of solution are used, according to the size of the syringe used for the procedure. A single cotton ball is placed loosely into the external meatus to absorb any remaining irrigant after the procedure. **Cognitive Level:** Applying **Client Need:** Physiological Adaptation **Integrated Process:** Nursing Process: Implementation **Content Area:** Adult Health: Eye, Ear, Nose, and Throat **Strategy:** The core issue of the question is the ability to correctly perform the nursing procedure of eye irrigation. Use nursing knowledge and the process of elimination to make a selection.

19 **Answer: 2, 3, 4 Rationale:** Careful hand hygiene is effective in reducing the risk of transmitting the infection to others. Antibiotic therapy kills the bacteria that are responsible for the eye infection. Dark sunglasses are helpful in reducing photophobia. Warm compresses, not cold, should be used as part of the management of conjunctivitis. Warm compresses help relieve discomfort and reduce inflammation by increasing circulation to the area. Although there is eye discomfort, there is no need for strong analgesics such as opioids. **Cognitive Level:** Applying **Client Need:** Physiological Adaptation **Integrated Process:** Nursing Process: Implementation **Content Area:** Adult Health: Eye, Ear, Nose, and Throat **Strategy:** A critical word in the stem of the question is *useful*, indicating that the correct answer is an option that is either correct or high priority. Use nursing knowledge about care of the client with conjunctivitis and the process of elimination to make selections.

20 **Answer: 2 Rationale:** The nurse should apply pressure to the inner canthus (nasolacrimal duct) during and for at least 30 seconds after instillation, according to agency procedure, to prevent systemic absorption of the medication. The medication should be dropped into the lower conjunctival sac. The eye should not be rubbed after instillation of the medication. The nurse should wait from 1 to 5 minutes between drops, depending on the medication and manufacturer's recommendations. **Cognitive Level:** Applying **Client Need:** Physiological Adaptation **Integrated Process:** Nursing Process: Implementation **Content Area:** Adult Health: Eye, Ear, Nose, and Throat **Strategy:** The core issue of the question is the ability to administer eye medication correctly. Use nursing knowledge and the process of elimination to make a selection.

21 **Answer: 1 Rationale:** It is appropriate to comfort the child following a painful procedure and applying the bandage provides support and comfort. There is no reason to question the child. By fulfilling the child's request, the nurse allows the child to regain some control over the situation. The child may be looking for comfort rather than concerned about bleeding. **Cognitive Level:** Analyzing **Client Need:** Psychosocial Integrity **Integrated Process:** Nursing Process: Implementation **Content Area:** Child Health **Strategy:** The core issue of the question is the best response to a 5-year-old client who is responding to a painful procedure such as an injection. Eliminate options that do not meet the client's immediate need for comfort following the injection.

22 **Answer: 4 Rationale:** A febrile infant is at risk for dehydration from larger-than-normal insensible fluid losses and decreased fluid intake. It is contraindicated to sponge with cool water, which could lead to shivering and higher temperature. Intake of solid food is less important than preventing dehydration. A febrile infant will experience higher fever if blankets are added. **Cognitive Level:** Analyzing **Client Need:** Physiological Adaptation **Integrated Process:** Nursing Process: Implementation **Content Area:** Child Health **Strategy:** The core issue of the question is an appropriate nursing intervention when a client has fever caused by an ear infection. Use nursing knowledge and the process of elimination to make a selection.

23 **Answer: 3 Rationale:** A symptom of pharyngitis is sore throat and difficult swallowing, which could lead to the refusal to drink. Thus, risk for dehydration is an appropriate priority concern. The client may have anxiety because of pain associated with pharyngitis, but this will resolve with treatment of the infection. A risk for an ineffective cough would apply if the client could not clear secretions from the respiratory tract, which is not evident in this question. The child's status related to growth and development is not a concern with this brief health problem. **Cognitive Level:** Analyzing **Client Need:** Physiological Adaptation **Integrated Process:** Nursing Process: Planning **Content Area:** Child Health **Strategy:** The core issue of the question is the ability to determine priority concerns for a client with pharyngitis by selecting a nursing diagnosis. Whenever the airway is involved, first think about the ABCs and then think about hydration/food intake as the next priority of physiological needs using Maslow's hierarchy.

24 **Answer: 4 Rationale:** Humidifying the air can prevent dry mucous membranes and recurrence of epistaxis. Liquefying secretions is not a concern for a client with recurrent nosebleed. Humidification does not increase the oxygen percentage of ambient air, which is 21%. Humidifying the air does not increase the client's ability to breathe with epistaxis. **Cognitive Level:** Applying **Client Need:** Physiological Adaptation **Integrated Process:** Nursing Process: Implementation **Content Area:** Child Health **Strategy:** The core issue of the question is an understanding of the rationale for nursing actions for a client with recurrent epistaxis. Use nursing knowledge and the process of elimination to make a selection.

25 **Answer: 2 Rationale:** Children at 15 months of age cannot understand the necessity of cooperating with medication administration. Mummying the child reduces the risk of injury from the ointment tip and promotes adequate dosing. Applying ointment to the eyes of a sleeping child would increase the child's fears. The ointment is instilled in the lower conjunctival sac, not on the lids. The medication is squeezed from the tube, not applied with gauze. **Cognitive Level:** Applying **Client Need:** Physiological Adaptation **Integrated Process:** Nursing Process: Implementation **Content Area:** Child Health **Strategy:** The core issue of the question is identification of the correct procedure for administering an ophthalmic medication to a child. Use nursing knowledge of this basic procedure and the process of elimination to make a selection.

26 **Answer: 2, 3 Rationale:** The client should know that the dye causes temporary skin discoloration in the injected area and temporary green discoloration of urine that resolves when the dye is fully excreted. The client should avoid sunlight or other bright light sources until pupil dilation returns to normal. Typical instructions after fluorescein angiography include increased fluid intake to aid in dye excretion. Although the client should rest after the procedure, it is not necessary to lie down with eyes closed for 12 hours. Headache and blurred vision are not expected. **Cognitive Level:** Analyzing **Client Need:** Physiological Adaptation **Integrated Process:** Teaching and Learning **Content Area:** Adult Health: Eye, Ear, Nose, and Throat **Strategy:** The core issue of the question is knowledge of postprocedure instructions to a client following fluorescein dye eye examination. Use nursing knowledge and general concepts of procedures that utilize contrast dye to make your selections.

Key Terms to Review

amblyopia p. 1164
cataracts p. 1166
cycloplegic p. 1162
epistaxis p. 1175
glaucoma p. 1165
gonioscopy p. 1165
Ménière's disease p. 1173
miotic p. 1165
mydriatic p. 1162
nystagmus p. 1159
otitis media p. 1172
otosclerosis p. 1172
pharyngitis p. 1175
presbycusis p. 1158
presbyopia p. 1158
proprioception p. 1158
strabismus p. 1163
tonometry p. 1159
tonsillitis p. 1176

References

Ball, J., & Bindler, R., & Cowen, K. (2015). *Principles of pediatric nursing: Caring for children* (6th ed.). Hoboken, NJ: Pearson Education.

Berman, A., Snyder, S., & Frandsen, G. (2016). *Kozier & Erb's fundamentals of nursing: Concepts, process, and practice* (10th ed.). New York, NY: Pearson Education.

Ignatavicius, D., & Workman, L. (2016). *Medical-surgical nursing: Patient-centered collaborative care* (10th ed.). Philadelphia: Saunders.

Kee, J. (2017). *Pearson's handbook of laboratory and diagnostic tests* (8th ed.). New York, NY: Pearson Education.

LeMone, P., Burke, K., Bauldoff, G., & Gubrud, P. (2015). *Medical surgical nursing: Clinical reasoning in patient care* (6th ed.). Hoboken, NJ: Pearson Education.

Lewis, S., Dirksen, S., Heitkemper, M., & Bucher, L. (2014). *Medical surgical nursing: Assessment and management of clinical problems* (9th ed.). St. Louis, MO: Elsevier Science.

Smith, S., Duell, D., Martin, B., Aebersold, M., & Gonzalez, L. (2017). *Clinical nursing skills: Basic to advanced skills* (10th ed.). New York, NY: Pearson Education.

Test Yourself

Are you ready for the NCLEX-RN® or course exams? Access the NEW web-based app that provides students with thousands of practice questions in preparation for the NCLEX experience.

64 Hematologic Disorders

In this chapter

Cross Reference

Other chapters relevant to this content area are

Meeting Nutritional Needs	Chapter 25
Blood and Blood Component Therapy	Chapter 32
Common Laboratory Tests	Chapter 46
Common Diagnostic Tests and Procedures	Chapter 47
Musculoskeletal Disorders	Chapter 61

I. OVERVIEW OF ANATOMY AND PHYSIOLOGY OF HEMATOLOGIC SYSTEM

A. Blood components

1. Plasma: straw-colored liquid portion of blood (50–55%); consists of water (about 92%), amino acids, proteins, carbohydrates, lipids, vitamins, hormones, electrolytes, and cellular wastes; serum is essentially plasma but without fibrinogen and clotting factors
2. Red blood cells (RBCs), white blood cells (WBCs), and platelets comprise remainder of blood; see Chapter 46 for detailed discussion of blood cells
3. Blood volume is approximately 8% of total body weight

B. Normal clotting mechanisms

1. Coagulation is a series of reactions to achieve clot formation and **hemostasis** (cessation of bleeding) in an injured area

2. Involves three mechanisms: vascular constriction and spasm, formation of platelet plug, and activation of clotting factors; fibrin clot is produced through either intrinsic or extrinsic clotting pathway; both pathways end in common coagulation cascade
3. After a clot forms, **fibrinolysis** (clot breakdown) occurs; plasminogen from blood clot is transformed into plasmin, which dissolves fibrin strands of clot; peak action is 7–10 days after clot formation

II. DIAGNOSTIC TESTS AND ASSESSMENTS OF HEMATOLOGIC SYSTEM

A. **Blood studies** (see Chapter 46 for normal references ranges for U.S. and Canada)
1. RBC count
2. Hemoglobin and hematocrit
   a. Hemoglobin (Hgb) measures oxygen-carrying capacity of an erythrocyte
   b. Hematocrit (Hct) is ratio of RBC volume to volume of whole blood
3. RBC indexes
   a. MCV (mean corpuscular volume): estimates size of RBC
   b. MCH (mean corpuscular hemoglobin): measures content of Hgb in RBCs from a single cell
   c. MCHC (mean corpuscular hemoglobin concentration): more accurately measures Hgb content of RBC because it measures entire volume of RBCs
4. Serum ferritin, transferrin, and total iron-binding capacity (TIBC): evaluate iron levels; ferritin measures iron in plasma, which is also a direct reflection of total iron stores; transferrin is major iron-transport protein
5. WBC count
   a. Abnormal elevation of WBC count is referred to as **leukocytosis**
   b. **Leukopenia** is a decrease in number of WBCs
   c. Differential count refers to breakdown of different types of cells
6. Coagulation studies
   a. *Bleeding time*: used to evaluate platelet function; extended bleeding times are seen with **thrombocytopenia** (decreased platelet production) and aspirin therapy, as well anticoagulants and several other drugs

   NCLEX® b. *Prothrombin time (PT)*: measures speed of blood clotting; PT evaluates extrinsic coagulation pathway (factors I, II, V, VII, X); international normalized ratio (INR) is often used instead of PT because it is a standardized value (therapeutic range is often 2–3 depending on condition)

   c. *Partial thromboplastin time (PTT)*: evaluates intrinsic coagulation pathway or fibrin clot formation

   NCLEX® d. *Activated partial thromboplastin time (aPTT)*: modified PTT, preferred because it is quicker to perform; aPTT is used in heparin therapy and when evaluating hemophilia; aPTT is increased in anticoagulation therapy, liver disease, vitamin K deficiency, and disseminated intravascular coagulopathy (DIC)

   e. *Fibrinogen*: soluble plasma protein necessary for clotting that is decreased in DIC and fibrinogen disorders and increased in acute infections, hepatitis, and oral contraceptive use
   f. *Fibrin degradation products (FDP)*: FDP is increased in fibrinolysis, thrombolytic therapy, and DIC
   g. *Fibrin D-dimer*: D-dimer is the most sensitive indicator to differentiate DIC from primary fibrinolysis; elevated in DIC

B. **Bone marrow examination**
1. Specimens may be obtained by aspiration (most common) or biopsy

NCLEX® 2. Sites for bone marrow aspiration may include sternum, iliac crest (most common), and tibia; most common site for bone marrow biopsy is posterosuperior iliac spine (sternum is also used)

3. Position client based on site selected; skin and periosteum are anesthetized to decrease pain with anesthetic such as procaine; marrow aspiration needle is then inserted; after marrow cavity is entered, marrow stylet is removed from needle and a sterile syringe is attached; syringe plunger is drawn back until marrow appears in syringe

NCLEX® 4. During withdrawal of aspirate, client will experience sharp pain, often described as burning

NCLEX® 5. After needle is removed, apply pressure dressing over puncture site, where only minimal bleeding should occur; if client has thrombocytopenia, apply pressure for 3–5 minutes

6. Check agency procedure for handling specimens
7. Most clients experience little, if any, pain or discomfort after procedure; some report tenderness and ache at aspiration site for a few days

NCLEX® **8.** Procedure for a bone marrow biopsy is essentially same as for aspiration; after procedure, assess clients for bleeding from puncture site

C. Lymphangiography: visualization of lymph system radiographically after injection of a dye; used primarily to stage Hodgkin's and non-Hodgkin's lymphoma

D. Lymph node biopsy: obtains lymph tissue for histologic analysis; a closed-needle biopsy can be done at bedside or an open biopsy can be performed in operating room

III. NUTRITIONAL ANEMIAS

A. Overview

1. Several nutrients are needed for hematopoiesis (red blood cell [RBC] production), including iron, protein, vitamins (especially B vitamins, C, and E); a deficiency in key nutrients can lead to **anemia** (decreased production of RBCs)
2. Common nutritional anemias include iron-deficiency anemia, pernicious anemia (vitamin B_{12} deficiency), and folic acid–deficiency anemia
3. Nutritional anemias tend to occur because of inadequate diet, malabsorption of nutrients, or increased need for nutrient; see Table 64–1 for common etiologies of nutritional anemias
4. Iron-deficiency anemia can also be associated with blood loss

NCLEX®

B. Nursing assessment

1. Common manifestations of nutritional anemias
   a. Fatigue and weakness, dizziness
   b. Pallor (earlobes, palms, and conjunctiva)
   c. Smooth, sore, beefy red tongue (**glossitis**)
   d. Cracks in corners of mouth (**cheilosis**)
   e. Possible compensatory changes causing inadequate RBCs, such as increased heart and respiratory rates to increase oxygen transport to cells, or shortness of breath or palpitations with activity
2. Iron-deficiency anemia may also be manifested by brittle spoon-like nails and pica (craving to eat unusual substances such as clay or starch)
3. Diarrhea is common to both vitamin B_{12} and folic acid deficiency
4. Neurologic symptoms such as paresthesias and impaired proprioception are found in vitamin B_{12} deficiency because of its importance for neurologic function
5. Laboratory studies
   a. Iron-deficiency anemia: low RBC count and cells that are **microcytic** (small diameter of RBC) and **hypochromic** (decreased pigmentation of RBC), with an increase in red cell–size distribution width (RDW); low MCV, MCH, and MCHC (analyzed only when Hgb is low); low serum iron level, elevated serum iron-binding capacity, and low serum ferritin levels
   b. Vitamin B_{12} deficiency: macrocytic (megaloblastic) anemia (RBC diameter >8) with increase in MCV and MCHC; gastric secretion analysis reveals achlorhydria (absence of free hydrochloric acid in a pH maintained at 3.5) and positive 24-hour Schilling test (a vitamin B_{12} absorption test that indicates lack of intrinsic factor by measuring excretion of orally administered radionuclide-labeled B_{12})
   c. Folic acid deficiency: macrocytic (megaloblastic) anemia (RBC diameter >8), high MCV with low hemoglobin and low serum folate level

Table 64–1 Risk Factors for Nutritional Anemias

Anemia	Iron-Deficiency Anemia	Vitamin-B_{12} Anemia	Folic Acid–Deficiency Anemia
Dietary deficiency	Inadequate protein, vegetarian diet	Rare; usually affects strict vegetarians only	Chronic undernutrition (chronic alcohol use, possible TPN)
Decreased absorption	Malaborption syndromes, diarrhea (chronic), partial or total gastrectomy	Lack of intrinsic factor following gastrectomy, chronic gastritis, loss of pancreatic secretions	Celiac disease, chronic alcohol use, folate antagonist chemotherapeutic agents (e.g., methotrexate, pentamidine) or antiepileptics
Increased need	Pregnancy and lactation	NA	Infancy, adolescence, pregnancy, hemodialysis
Other	Various types of blood loss, chronic hemoglobinuria	NA	NA

Box 64–1

Foods Useful in Treating Selected Nutritional Deficiencies

Iron-Deficiency Anemia
Organ meats, other meats, beans (black, pinto, and garbanzo), whole-grain breads, brown rice, bran flakes, oatmeal, dried fruits, leafy green vegetables, raisins, and molasses

Vitamin B_{12}–Deficiency Anemia (Pernicious Anemia)
Liver, kidney, muscle meats, eggs, cheese, dairy products, fresh shrimp and oysters, and fortified soy milk

Folic Acid–Deficiency Anemia
Green leafy vegetables, broccoli, asparagus, eggs, milk, yeast, wheat germ, liver, organ meats, fish, and nuts

C. General therapeutic management of nutritional anemias

1. Assess history for causative or contributing factors
2. *NCLEX®* Teach client energy conservation measures (e.g., shower chair, sitting during tasks instead of standing) and to alternate activity with rest periods
3. Encourage adequate rest and sleep (8–10 hours/night) to increase energy levels
4. Assist with activities of daily living (ADLs) as necessary
5. Monitor VS before and after activity and discontinue activity with adverse cardiorespiratory symptoms (change in pulse, respirations, BP, shortness of breath, palpitations, chest pain, dizziness, or vertigo)
6. Monitor for dizziness; recommend position changes be made slowly
7. Provide assistance with activities and ambulation as needed, allowing client independence as much as safely possible
8. Provide frequent oral hygiene with saline gargles and soft toothbrush for glossitis or cheilosis; use lip lubricant as necessary; eating bland and soft foods of moderate temperature may reduce oral discomfort
9. Administer prescribed vitamin replacement therapy and teach client how to self-administer
10. *NCLEX®* Provide dietary teaching about foods to replace dietary deficiency (see Box 64–1)
11. Monitor laboratory studies (e.g., Hgb/Hct, RBC count)
12. Refer to appropriate community resources when indicated (e.g., social services for food stamps, Meals on Wheels)
13. Interventions specific to iron-deficiency anemia
    a. Examine stools for occult blood; endoscopic examination and other diagnostic tests may be done to detect possible sources of bleeding
    b. Assess stool characteristics; may appear greenish black and tarry with iron therapy; iron supplements usually cause constipation and client should take preventive measures (fiber and fluids to 2500–3000 mL/day unless contraindicated by another condition)
14. *NCLEX®* Medication therapy
    a. Iron deficiency: give oral iron preparation on empty stomach with a vitamin C source such as orange juice to increase absorption; liquid form of iron can stain teeth (use a straw or place spoon at back of mouth and rinse mouth thoroughly afterward); give parenteral iron dextran by deep IM route via Z-track method, using separate needles for withdrawing and injecting medication; administer blood products as indicated (see Chapter 32); monitor closely for transfusion reactions
    b. Vitamin B_{12} deficiency: parenteral vitamin B_{12}, 100–1000 mcg subcutaneously daily for 7 days, then once a week for 1 month, then monthly for lifetime is usually prescribed; a nasal form is available; a burning sensation felt after a parenteral dose is temporary
    c. Folic acid deficiency: oral folate, 1–5 mg/day for 3–4 months; folate should be given along with vitamin B_{12} when both are deficient; sufficient folate is necessary during pregnancy to prevent neural tube defects

IV. APLASTIC ANEMIA

A. Overview

1. A form of anemia with decreased production of RBCs, WBCs, and platelets; may be congenital or acquired
2. Congenital aplastic anemia is caused by a chromosomal alteration
3. Acquired form may be caused by radiation, chemical agents and toxins, drugs, viral and bacterial infections, pregnancy, or idiopathic (about 50% of cases)

4. There is a decrease or cessation of production of RBCs, WBCs (leukopenia), and platelets (thrombocytopenia); may result from damage to bone marrow stem cells, bone marrow itself, and replacement of bone marrow with fat; depending on causative factor, condition may be acute or chronic

NCLEX® **B. Nursing assessment**

1. Pallor and fatigue
2. Palpitations and exertional dyspnea
3. Infections of the skin and mucous membranes
4. Purpura (bruising) and bleeding from gums, nose, vagina, or rectum
5. Retinal hemorrhage
6. CBC reveals pancytopenia (decreased RBC, WBC, and platelets) and decreased reticulocyte count
7. Bone marrow examination reveals decreased or absent bone marrow cell activity

C. Therapeutic management

1. Identify and withdraw cause of bone marrow suppression if possible
2. Institute standard interventions for anemia as previously described
3. NCLEX® Institute neutropenic precautions to protect client from infection
4. Limit visitors and potential sources of infection
5. NCLEX® Monitor for evidence of bleeding; avoid invasive procedures including rectal temperatures
6. Prepare for transfusion of leukocyte-poor RBCs
7. Prepare for bone marrow transplantation as indicated
8. Medication therapy: antilymphocyte globulin, antithymocyte globulin, cyclosporine, immunosuppresive agents such as prednisone and cyclophosphamide

D. Client teaching

1. NCLEX® Methods to prevent infection such as avoiding crowds, maintaining good hygiene, hand hygiene, and elimination of uncooked foods from diet
2. NCLEX® Methods to prevent hemorrhage such as using a soft toothbrush, avoiding contact sports, and use of an electric razor
3. NCLEX® Avoid drugs that increase bleeding tendency, such as aspirin
4. Balance activity with adequate rest periods to avoid fatigue
5. Report signs of infection, bleeding, and decreasing tolerance to activity to healthcare provider

V. SICKLE-CELL DISEASE

A. Overview

1. Hereditary, chronic form of hemolytic anemia that predominantly affects clients of African descent
2. Sickle-cell trait (heterozygous state inherited from one parent) is a generally mild condition that produces few, if any, manifestations unless there is very severe hypoxia
3. Sickle-cell anemia (homozygous state inherited from both parents) is an autosomal recessive disorder that results in synthesis of hemoglobin S
4. Hemoglobin S causes RBCs to elongate, become rigid, and assume a crescent, sickled shape when there is decreased O_2 tension in plasma; curved shape causes cells to clump together, obstructing capillary blood flow and leading to ischemia and possible tissue infarction (sickle-cell crisis)
5. Conditions likely to trigger a sickle-cell crisis include hypoxia, low environmental and/or body temperature, excessive exercise, high altitudes, inadequate oxygen during anesthesia, elevated blood viscosity, decreased plasma volume, infection, dehydration, and increased hydrogen ion concentration (acidosis)
6. With normal oxygenation, sickled RBCs resume normal shape; repeated episodes of sickling and unsickling weaken cell membranes, causing them to hemolyze
7. Crisis is extremely painful and can last from 4 to 6 days; consists of vaso-occlusive crisis, splenic sequestration of blood (hypersplenism), hyperhemolytic crisis (rapid RBC destruction), and aplastic crisis (inadequate replacement of RBCs)

NCLEX® **B. Nursing assessment**

1. Fever
2. Painful swelling of hands, feet, and large joints
3. Abdominal pain
4. Pallor and jaundice
5. Fatigue and possible irritability
6. Priapism (abnormal, painful, continuous erection of penis) may occur if penile veins are obstructed
7. Anemia with sickled cells noted on a peripheral smear
8. Hemoglobin electrophoresis to detect presence and amount of hemoglobin S is used for a definitive diagnosis

9. Elevated serum bilirubin levels
10. Elevated reticulocyte count

C. Therapeutic management

1. Blood transfusions to improve oxygenation and reduce sickling
2. Avoid situations that increase risk of tissue hypoxia
3. Use of chemotherapy drug hydroxyurea to increase hemoglobin F and decrease sickling
4. Refer to appropriate agency for genetic counseling and family planning
5. *NCLEX®* Care of client in sickle-cell crisis
   a. Medicate for pain, which is usually severe, with opioid analgesics; an around-the-clock schedule may be prescribed for effectiveness
   b. Administer O_2 to increase oxygenation to cells and reduce sickling effect; keep head of bed elevated to 30 degrees
   c. Provide increased intake of oral and IV fluids to promote hydration to decrease blood viscosity
   d. Cluster care activities to avoid fatiguing client
   e. Keep painful extremities supported and maintain joints in a position of extension
   f. Monitor for complications such as vaso-occlusive disease (thrombosis), hypoxia, CVA, renal dysfunction, priapism leading to impotence, and acute chest syndrome (fever, chest pain, cough, pulmonary infiltrates, and dyspnea)
   g. Manage infection if appropriate
6. Medication therapy
   a. Nifedipine for priapism
   b. Hydroxyurea to increase hemoglobin F and decrease sickling
   c. *NCLEX®* Opioid analgesics during the acute phase of sickle-cell crisis, often in large doses
   d. Broad-spectrum antibiotics to manage acute chest syndrome
   e. Folic acid supplements
7. Splenectomy may be required for client who has recurrent splenic sequestration

D. Client teaching

1. *NCLEX®* Ways to prevent physiological stressors that can lead to sickle-cell crisis
   a. Maintain high fluid intake; avoid conditions that might predispose to dehydration
   b. Avoid low-oxygen environments (high altitudes, airplanes)
   c. Prevent and promptly treat infections
   d. Use stress-reduction strategies
   e. Avoid exposure to cold or overexertion
   f. Avoid physical overexertion
2. Importance of receiving pneumococcal, meningococcal, and annual influenza vaccines because status of spleen increases risk for infection
3. Importance of regular medical follow-up

VI. POLYCYTHEMIA

A. Overview

1. An increased number of circulating RBCs and Hgb concentration in blood; also known as polycythemia vera (PV), or myeloproliferative red cell disorder; can be a primary or secondary disorder
2. Primary
   a. Neoplastic stem cell disorder characterized by increased production of RBCs, granulocytes, and platelets; more common in men of European Jewish descent age 40–70
   b. With overproduction of RBCs, increased blood viscosity leads to congestion of blood in tissues, liver, and spleen
   c. Thrombi form, acidosis develops, and tissue infarction occurs because of diminished blood flow caused by increased viscosity
3. Secondary
   a. Most common form; disturbance is not in RBC development but in excessive erythropoiesis as a physiological response to hypoxia
   b. Chronic hypoxic states may be produced by prolonged exposure to high altitudes, pulmonary diseases, hypoventilation, and smoking
   c. Result of an increased RBC production is increased blood viscosity, which alters circulatory flow

B. Nursing assessment

1. *NCLEX®* **Plethora**: a ruddy (dark, flushed) color of face, hands, feet, ears, and mucous membranes resulting from engorgement or distention of blood vessels

NCLEX® 2. Symptoms associated with increased blood volume, including headaches, vertigo, blurred vision, tinnitus, and distended superficial veins
3. Itching unrelieved by antihistamines
4. Symptoms associated with impaired tissue oxygenation, including angina, intermittent claudication, or dyspnea
5. Erythromyalgia, or burning sensation of the fingers and toes
6. Splenomegaly in majority of those with primary polycythemia vera
7. Epistaxis, gastrointestinal (GI) bleeding
8. Weight loss and night sweats
9. Elevated Hgb, Hct, RBC and WBC counts, basophils, and platelets; decreased MCHC
10. Bone marrow examination shows hypercellularity

C. Therapeutic management

NCLEX® 1. Manage underlying condition (such as COPD) causing chronic hypoxia
2. Periodic phlebotomy to decrease blood volume by 300–500 mL; goal is to keep hematocrit at 45–48% or lower
NCLEX® 3. Hydration to decrease blood viscosity
4. Measures to relieve pruritus, including cool and tepid baths
5. Accurate monitoring of fluid intake and output (I&O)
NCLEX® 6. Nursing measures to prevent thrombotic events, including early ambulation, passive leg exercises when on bedrest, encouraging client to keep legs uncrossed and maintain adequate hydration
7. Medication therapy
   a. Myelosuppressive agents to inhibit bone marrow activity including hydroxyurea, melphalan, and radioactive phosphorus
   b. Allopurinol to manage gout caused by increased uric acid levels (see also Chapter 61)
   c. Antiplatelet agents to prevent thrombotic complications

D. Client teaching

NCLEX® 1. Maintain sufficient hydration; drink at least 3 liters of fluid per day
2. Disease and methods of control, such as smoking cessation
3. Signs and symptoms of complications, including signs of vaso-occlusive states (MI, CVA) and bleeding, which require immediate medical attention
NCLEX® 4. Prevent bleeding states such as by using electric razor and soft-bristled toothbrush, not flossing, and avoiding use of aspirin and aspirin-containing products
5. Importance of a regular medical checkup
6. Avoid products that contain iron
7. Ways to prevent thrombosis

VII. THROMBOCYTOPENIA

A. Overview

1. Platelet count of less than 100,000/mL blood that can lead to abnormal bleeding
2. Decreased circulating platelets may result from three mechanisms: decreased production, increased destruction, or increased sequestration in spleen
3. Cause of decreased platelet production may be inherited or acquired; inherited form is known as idiopathic or immune thrombocytopenic purpura (ITP), and usually follows viral infection such as measles, rubella, or chickenpox
4. Other causes of thrombocytopenia include aplastic anemia, bone marrow malignancy, infection, radiation therapy, drug therapy (such as heparin), or disseminated intravascular coagulopathy
NCLEX® 5. A decrease in number of functional platelets leads to bleeding disorders; high risk for spontaneous bleeding, and hemorrhage if platelet count is below 20,000/mm^3

NCLEX® **B. Nursing assessment**

1. Petechiae (pinpoint hemorrhages on skin and mucous membranes) and purpura (purplish discolored areas) most commonly found in mucous membranes, anterior thorax, arms, and neck
2. Epistaxis, gingival bleeding, menorrhagia, hematuria, and gastrointestinal bleeding (bloody or tarry stools)
3. Signs of internal hemorrhage
4. Decreased hemoglobin and hematocrit if bleeding is present
5. Decreased platelet count; platelet antibodies present if ITP
6. Prolonged bleeding time
7. Bone marrow examination may reveal decreased platelet activity or increased megakaryocytes

C. Therapeutic management

1. Treat underlying cause or remove causative agent in acquired thrombocytopenia

NCLEX®
2. Platelet transfusions if there is active bleeding; little benefit in ITP
3. If medications are not effective, a splenectomy may be done in older child with 1 year of thrombocytopenia

NCLEX®
4. Institute bleeding (thrombocytopenic) precautions when platelet count drops to 50,000 cells/mm^3
   a. Avoid intramuscular or subcutaneous injections
   b. Avoid indwelling catheters
   c. If absolutely necessary, use smallest-gauge needles for injections or venipunctures; apply pressure on injection sites for 5 minutes or until bleeding stops
   d. Discourage straining at stool and vigorous coughing or nose blowing
   e. Avoid rectal manipulation such as rectal temperatures, suppositories, or enemas
   f. Discourage the use of razors; use only electric shavers
   g. Use soft-bristled toothbrush or toothettes and avoid flossing
   h. Pad side-rails if necessary and avoid tissue trauma
   i. Avoid use of aspirin and drugs that interfere with blood coagulation

NCLEX®
5. Monitor for signs of bleeding; test stools for occult blood
6. Monitor CBC and platelet counts
7. Assess neurologic status every shift and PRN
8. Medication therapy
   a. Steroids and immunoglobulins to suppress immune response in ITP
   b. Immunosuppressive agents such as vincristine and cyclophosphamide

NCLEX®
   c. Platelet growth factor such as oprelvekin

D. Client and family teaching

1. Monitor for signs of bleeding and when to contact primary care provider

NCLEX®
2. Bleeding precautions such as using soft-bristled toothbrush, avoiding flossing, preventing tissue trauma and injury (including vigorous sexual intercourse), and using an electric razor for shaving
3. Methods of controlling bleeding and to seek medical assistance if severe

NCLEX®
4. Avoid drugs that contain aspirin and others that interfere with coagulation
5. Medication dosing, schedule, and side effects
6. Importance of regular medical follow-up and platelet monitoring

VIII. HEMOPHILIA

A. Overview

1. A group of hereditary clotting factor disorders characterized by prolonged coagulation time that results in prolonged and sometimes excessive bleeding
2. Hemophilia A and B are **X-linked recessive traits** transmitted by female carriers and displayed almost exclusively in males
   a. *Hemophilia A* (classic hemophilia) is a deficiency in factor VIII (an alpha-globulin that stabilizes fibrin clots); most common form of hemophilia
   b. *Hemophilia B* (Christmas disease) is a deficiency in factor IX (a vitamin-dependent beta-globulin essential in stage 1 of intrinsic coagulation system; influence on amount of thromboplastin available)
3. In clients with hemophilia A and B, platelet plugs are formed at site of bleeding, but clotting factor impairs coagulation response and capacity to form a stable clot
4. *Von Willebrand's disease* is a related disorder caused by deficiency of von Willebrand's factor (vWF) necessary for factor VIII activity and platelet adhesion

NCLEX®

B. Nursing assessment

1. Persistent and prolonged bleeding from small cuts and injuries
2. Subcutaneous **ecchymosis** (purplish color) and subcutaneous hematomas
3. Gingival bleeding
4. GI bleeding, manifested by hematemesis (vomiting blood), occult blood in stools, gastric pain, or abdominal pain
5. Urinary tract bleeding (hematuria)
6. Pain, paresthesia, or paralysis resulting from nerve compression by hematomas
7. **Hemarthrosis** (joint bleeding, swelling, and damage)
8. APTT is increased in all types of hemophilia
9. Bleeding time is prolonged in von Willebrand's disease
10. Decreased factor VIII in hemophilia A, vWF in von Willebrand's disease, and factor IX in hemophilia B

C. Therapeutic management

1. Replacement of deficient coagulation factor(s)

NCLEX® 2. Hemophilia A: cryoprecipitate containing 8–100 units of factor VIII per bag at 12-hour intervals until bleeding ceases; freeze-dried concentrate of factor VIII may also be given

NCLEX® 3. Hemophilia B: plasma or factor IX concentrate given every 24 hours or until bleeding ceases

NCLEX® 4. Von Willebrand's disease: cryoprecipitate containing 8–100 units of factor VIII per bag at 12-hour intervals until bleeding ceases; desmopressin may also be used

5. Supportive treatment for hemarthrosis, including arthrocentesis and physiotherapy
6. Control of topical bleeding with hemostatic agents, pressure, and application of ice
7. Management of complications associated with hemorrhage
8. Refer for genetic counseling and family planning and to National Hemophilia Foundation for support and counseling
9. Monitor for signs of complications, including hemarthrosis and intracranial bleeding

NCLEX® 10. Assist in managing pain associated with hemarthrosis; measures include immobilizing joint, applying ice, and administering analgesics; avoid aspirin and drugs affecting coagulation

11. Control bleeding and maintain hemostasis through direct pressure, applying topical hemostatic agents, and applying ice

D. Client teaching

1. Disease and therapeutic regimen

NCLEX® 2. Signs and symptoms requiring immediate medical attention, such as severe joint pain, trauma or injury, and signs of uncontrolled internal bleeding

NCLEX® 3. Precautions to prevent bleeding, as previously described

4. Wear a Medic-Alert bracelet indicating hemophilia; notify all healthcare providers of condition
5. Maintain good dental hygiene to decrease need for invasive dental procedures
6. Importance of continued follow-up care with healthcare provider
7. Encourage genetic counseling if appropriate

IX. DISSEMINATED INTRAVASCULAR COAGULOPATHY (DIC)

A. Overview

1. A syndrome characterized by abnormal initiation and acceleration of clotting and simultaneous hemorrhage; also called consumption coagulopathy (see Figure 64–1)

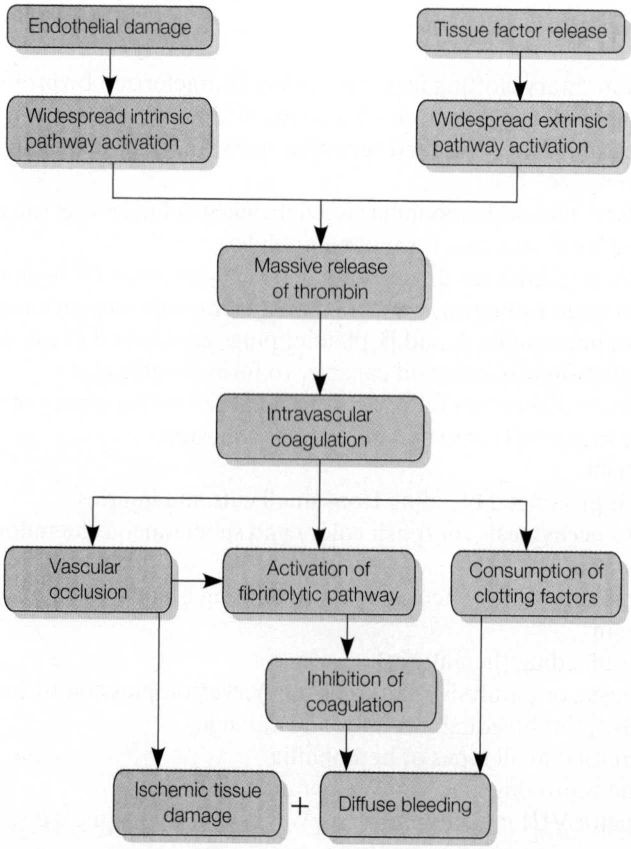

Figure 64–1

Sequence of events in disseminated intravascular coagulopathy.

Box 64–2

Risk Factors for DIC

Venomous snakebite	Acute hemolysis
Tissue necrosis	Neoplasms
Sepsis	Extensive burns
Drug reactions	Vascular disorders
Trauma	Prosthetic devices
Liver disease	Hypoxia
Obstetric complications	

2. Precipitated by conditions such as widespread tissue damage, hemolysis, hypotension, hypoxia, and metabolic acidosis (see Box 64–2)
3. Clotting process initiated either through activation of factor XII, factors II and X, or release of tissue thromboplastin
4. Clotting factors II, V, VIII, fibrinogen, and platelets needed for clotting are consumed more rapidly than they can be replaced
5. Body begins to break down clots with release of fibrin degradation products (FDPs), which are potent anticoagulants used to lyse clots further; anticoagulants worsen bleeding state
6. With depletion of clotting factors and increase in FDPs, stable blood clots no longer form and hemorrhage occurs

B. Nursing assessment

NCLEX® 1. Clinical manifestations (see Box 64–3)

NCLEX® 2. Prolonged aPTT, PT, and thrombin time

Box 64–3

Clinical Manifestations of DIC

Integumentary
- Cool skin
- Pallor
- Purpura
- Ecchymosis
- Petechiae
- Acral cyanosis
- Gingival bleeding
- Bleeding from puncture sites

Gastrointestinal
- Hemoptysis
- Melena
- Occult blood in stool or vomitus
- Abdominal distention
- Abdominal pain

Respiratory
- Dyspnea
- Tachypnea
- Orthopnea
- Decreased breath sounds
- Chest pain

Cardiovascular
- Decreased pulses
- Decreased capillary filling time
- Tachycardia
- Venous distention

Genitourinary
- Hematuria
- Oliguria

Nervous System
- Vision changes
- Dizziness
- Headache
- Irritability
- Anxiety
- Confusion
- Seizures

Musculoskeletal
- Joint pain
- Bone pain
- Weakness

NCLEX® 3. Decreased fibrinogen and platelets
NCLEX® 4. Elevated fibrin degradation products
5. Factor assays (factors V, VII, VIII, X, XIII): reduced
6. D-dimer elevated

C. Therapeutic management

1. Initiate treatment of underlying precipitating medical condition is a priority
2. Supportive treatment includes control of bleeding
3. NCLEX® Life-threatening hemorrhage may be treated with platelets for thrombocytopenia; cryoprecipitate to replace fibrinogen, and factors V and VII; and fresh frozen plasma (FFP) to replace all clotting factors except platelets; see Chapter 32 for administration of blood products
4. Assess client carefully for evidence of bleeding and reduced tissue oxygenation (decreased mental status, circulatory status, oxygen saturation)
5. NCLEX® Institute thrombocytopenic/bleeding precautions (refer to previous discussion on thrombocytopenia)
6. NCLEX® Maintain bedrest with head of bed in low Fowler position as tolerated
7. Monitor I&O hourly
8. Monitor for and treat pain caused by tissue ischemia; handle extremities gently and apply cool compresses to painful joint.
9. Monitor for signs of complications such as renal failure, pulmonary embolism, cerebrovascular accident, and acute respiratory distress syndrome
10. Provide emotional support to anxious or fearful client and family
11. Medication therapy
    a. Heparin and antithrombin III, although their use is controversial, may be used to manage thrombosis
    b. Epsilon aminocaproic acid to inhibit fibrinolysis
    c. NCLEX® Blood products (FFP, platelets, and cryoprecipitate)

D. Client teaching

1. Disorder, its treatments and interventions
2. Report symptoms of complications, including abdominal pain, headache, visual disturbances, and pain
3. Thrombocytopenic/bleeding precautions (see previous client teaching section in thrombocytopenia)

X. NEUTROPENIA

A. Overview

1. Neutrophils constitute about 70% of total circulating WBCs
2. Neutropenia is a neutrophil count of less than 2000/mm^3 (normal >2000/mm^3)
3. Absolute neutrophil count (ANC) is determined using this formula:

$$\frac{\%\text{ neutrophils} + \%\text{ bands}}{100} \times \text{total WBC count} = \text{ANC}$$

4. Caused by either decreased production or increased destruction of neutrophils
5. Because neutrophils play a major role in phagocytosis of microorganisms, neutropenia increases risk for infection
6. Neutropenia may occur as a primary hematologic disorder but may also be caused by drugs (such as cancer chemotherapy), autoimmune disorders, infections, and other medical conditions such as severe sepsis and nutritional deficiencies

NCLEX® **B. Nursing assessment**

1. Clinical manifestations: there are no real symptoms associated with neutropenia; it may not be discovered until client presents with signs of infection
2. Diagnostic and laboratory tests
    a. Absolute neutrophil count less than 1000–1500
    b. Examination of bone marrow cell morphology helps determine etiology

NCLEX® **C. Therapeutic management**

1. If etiology is drug-induced, medication should be discontinued whenever possible
2. Corticosteroids are used if etiology is immunologic
3. If etiology is decreased production, growth factors (granulocyte/macrophage colony–stimulating factor [GM-CSF]) may be used
4. NCLEX® Monitor for signs of infection; monitor temperature elevations
5. Obtain cultures suspected as sites of infection
6. Infections are treated with antimicrobial therapy
7. NCLEX® Enforce strict hand hygiene by all individuals in contact with client

NCLEX® 8. Institute neutropenic precautions; use private room with HEPA filtration if possible; do not allow those with infections to visit; use gloves and masks when entering client's room; prohibit known sources of microorganisms (plants, flowers, fresh unpeeled fruits and vegetables, standing water—such as water pitcher or vase)
9. Avoid invasive procedures whenever possible

D. Client teaching
1. What neutropenia is and rationale for therapeutic interventions
2. Report signs of fever
NCLEX® 3. Strict hand hygiene and reverse-isolation procedure (for client and those who come in contact with client)
4. Maintain good personal hygiene to decrease microbes on skin

XI. LEUKEMIA

A. Overview
1. Malignancy of blood-forming tissues of bone marrow, spleen, and lymph system characterized by unregulated proliferation of WBCs and their precursors
2. Classified by type of WBC affected (granulocyte, lymphocyte, monocyte) and by cell differentiation (acute if majority of cells are primitive or poorly differentiated and chronic if mature or well differentiated)
3. Acute lymphocytic/lymphoblastic leukemia (ALL)
   a. Most common leukemia in children and young adults
   b. Immature granulocytes proliferate and accumulate in bone marrow and may infiltrate central nervous system
4. Chronic lymphocytic leukemia (CLL)
   a. More common in older adults
   b. Abnormal and incompetent lymphocytes proliferate and accumulate in lymph nodes and spread to other lymphatic tissues and spleen; most circulating cells are mature lymphocytes
5. Acute myelogenous/myelocytic leukemia (AML)
   a. All age groups are affected but more common in older adults
   b. There is uncontrolled proliferation of myeloblasts, which are precursors of granulocytes; they accumulate in bone marrow
6. Chronic myelogenous leukemia (CML)
   a. Uncommon in people under age 20; incidence rises with age
   b. Uncontrolled proliferation of granulocytes results in increased circulating blast (immature) cells; marrow expands into long bones and also extends into liver and spleen
   NCLEX® c. In most cases, Philadelphia chromosome, a characteristic chromosomal abnormality, is present
7. Abnormal or immature WBCs do not function properly; abnormal cells continue to multiply, infiltrate, and damage bone marrow, spleen, lymph nodes, liver, kidneys, lungs, gonads, skin, and CNS
8. Normal bone marrow becomes diffusely replaced with abnormal or immature WBCs, interfering with production of cells such as RBCs and platelets; bone marrow becomes functionally incompetent with resulting bone marrow suppression
9. Acute leukemia has rapid onset and progression with a short clinical course; left untreated, death results in days or months; symptoms relate to depressed bone marrow, infiltration of leukemic cells into other organ systems, and hypermetabolism of leukemic cells
10. Chronic leukemia has more insidious onset and prolonged clinical course; usually asymptomatic early in disease; life expectancy may be more than 5 years; symptoms relate to hypermetabolism of leukemic cells infiltrating other organ systems; cells are more mature and function more effectively

NCLEX® **B. Nursing assessment**
1. Fever and night sweats
2. Bleeding such as ecchymoses, gingival bleeding, and epistaxis
3. Lymphadenopathy, splenomegaly, and hepatomegaly
4. Weakness and fatigue
5. Pruritic vesicular lesions
6. Anorexia and weight loss
7. Shortness of breath and decreased activity tolerance
8. Bone or joint pain
9. Visual disturbances
10. Pallor

11. Diagnostic and laboratory tests
    a. Increased WBC (in CLL and CML)
    b. A normal, decreased, or increased WBC (in ALL and AML)
    c. Decreased reaction to skin sensitivity tests (**anergy**)
    d. Bone marrow tests reveal excessive blast cells in AML
    e. *NCLEX®* Philadelphia chromosome found in 90–95% of clients with CML; BCR/ABL gene is present in virtually all clients with CML
    f. Bone marrow biopsy and aspirate is the definitive diagnostic test

C. Therapeutic management

1. *NCLEX®* Induction of remission with chemotherapy and radiation therapy
2. Bone marrow and stem cell transplantation
3. *NCLEX®* Assist in bone marrow biopsy; apply pressure to site for 5 minutes or until bleeding stops; frequently assess site for signs of bleeding up to 4 hours after procedure
4. *NCLEX®* Institute neutropenic and bleeding precautions (see previous discussions)
5. *NCLEX®* Plan activities to prevent fatigue; provide measures for uninterrupted rest and sleep
6. Provide for diversionary activities
7. Maintain adequate nutrition; consult dietitian as needed to meet nutritional needs
8. Assist client in maintaining good personal hygiene and promote good oral hygiene
9. Refer to appropriate agencies such as Meals on Wheels, American Cancer Society (ACS), and Leukemia Society
10. Provide emotional support to client and family; refer to appropriate agency, organization, or professional for counseling and support
11. Administer prescribed drugs and monitor for side effects
12. Monitor laboratory results to evaluate effectiveness of interventions and therapy
13. Prepare client for bone marrow transplant or stem cell transplant if part of treatment plan
14. *NCLEX®* Medication therapy: chemotherapeutic drugs depend on type of leukemia but tend to include alkylating agents, anthracyclines, antimetabolites, plant alkaloids, and others; corticosteroids are also used

D. Client teaching

1. Thrombocytopenic/bleeding precautions; see previous discussion
2. Neutropenic precautions; see previous discussion
3. Maintain oral hygiene; keep oral cavity moist: rinse mouth with saline, lubricate lips and oral mucosa with water-soluble lubricants every 2 hours; avoid alcohol-based mouthwash; use sponge-tipped applicators for oral hygiene if neutrophil and/or platelet counts are low
4. Measures to prevent perirectal complications: wash and clean perineal area thoroughly after each bowel movement
5. Therapeutic plans and interventions

XII. MALIGNANT LYMPHOMAS

A. Overview

1. A group of malignant neoplasms that affect lymphatic system, resulting in proliferation of lymphocytes; can be classified as Hodgkin's lymphoma (Hodgkin's disease) and non-Hodgkin's lymphoma
2. Hodgkin's disease
    a. More common in men than in women; has two peaks, at age 15–35 and over age 50
    b. Etiology unknown but several identified factors contribute to development, including infection with Epstein-Barr virus (EBV), familial pattern, and exposure to toxins
    c. Characterized by presence of Reed-Sternberg cell, a multinucleated and gigantic tumor cell thought to be of lymphoid origin
    d. Originates in a single lymph node or lymph node chain (majority of cases in cervical nodes) and infiltrates spleen, lungs, and liver
3. Non-Hodgkin's lymphoma
    a. Most common form of lymphoma; usually affects older adults; more common in men than in women and in whites than in other races
    b. No known cause but incidence is linked to viral infections, immune disorders, genetic abnormalities, exposure to chemicals, and infection with *Helicobacter pylori*
    c. Has a similar pathophysiology to Hodgkin's disease, although Reed-Sternberg cells are absent and method of lymph node infiltration is different
    d. Often involves malignant B cells; usually originates outside lymph nodes; normal cells are crowded out by malignant cells in affected lymphoid tissues

B. Nursing assessment

NCLEX® **1.** Hodgkin's disease

- **a.** Painless enlarged lymph nodes on one side of neck (cervical or subclavicular region)
- **b.** Fatigue and weakness
- **c.** Anorexia and dysphagia
- **d.** Dyspnea and cough
- **e.** Pruritus and jaundice
- **f.** Severe but brief pain at site after ingestion of alcohol
- **g.** Abdominal pain and bone pain
- **h.** Enlarged lymph nodes, liver, and spleen
- **i.** B symptoms: fever without chills; night sweats, and unintentional 10% weight loss
- **j.** Normocytic, normochromic anemia; neutrophilia, monocytophilia, and lymphopenia
- **k.** Presence of Reed-Sternberg cells in excisional bone biopsy
- **l.** Mediastinal lymphadenopathy seen on chest x-ray, CT scan, and radioisotope studies
- **m.** Mediastinal mass and pulmonary infiltrates may be seen on chest x-ray
- **n.** Absent or decreased response to skin sensitivity testing known as anergy

NCLEX® **2.** Non-Hodgkin's lymphoma

- **a.** Painless lymph node enlargement
- **b.** B symptoms (see above)
- **c.** Abdominal pain, nausea and vomiting
- **d.** Hematuria
- **e.** Peripheral neuropathy, cranial nerve palsies, headaches, visual disturbances, changes in mental status, and seizures
- **f.** Lymphocytopenia
- **g.** X-ray may reveal pulmonary infiltrates
- **h.** Lymph node biopsy helps to identify the cell type and pattern

C. Therapeutic management

1. Hodgkin's disease

- **a.** Lymphangiography to evaluate abdominal nodes
- **b.** Staging laparotomy to obtain specimen of retroperitoneal lymph nodes and remove spleen
- **c.** Staging of disease to determine extent and appropriate therapy; stage I involves single lymph node region; stage IV (for Hodgkin's disease only) indicates diffuse or disseminated involvement of one or more extralymphatic organs, with or without lymph node involvement (liver, lung, marrow, skin)
- NCLEX® **d.** Treatment may include radiation therapy and/or chemotherapy

2. Non-Hodgkin's lymphoma

- **a.** Staging of disease is based on results of CT scans and bone marrow biopsies
- **b.** Combination chemotherapy
- **c.** Radiation alone or in combination with chemotherapy for stage I and II
- **d.** Administration of rituximab, a monoclonal antibody against the CD20 of malignant B lymphocytes, which causes cell lysis and death

NCLEX® **3.** Institute nursing interventions for clients on chemotherapy or radiation therapy

NCLEX® **4.** Assist in balancing activity with periods of rest

NCLEX® **5.** Provide and assist in maintaining good nutritional state

6. Provide measures to diminish the discomfort associated with pruritus

7. Help client to cope with bodily changes such as alopecia, weight loss, and sterility

8. Refer client and family to appropriate agencies for support, such as ACS

NCLEX® **9.** Plan interventions to prevent infection

NCLEX® **10.** Medication therapy: chemotherapy drugs and possible biological therapy agents

D. Client teaching

1. Nature of disease, course of therapy, and associated interventions

2. Medications prescribed, precautions, and side effects

NCLEX® **3.** Symptoms necessitating immediate medical intervention, such as bleeding, infection, or fever

XIII. MULTIPLE MYELOMA

A. Overview

1. A malignancy in which plasma cells proliferate uncontrollably in bone and infiltrate bone marrow, lymph nodes, spleen, and liver

2. Plasma cells are B-cell lymphocytes that produce immunoglobulins (antibodies) once fully developed
   a. Abnormal plasma cells produce M protein or Bence Jones protein (an abnormal immunoglobulin) that can be detected in blood and urine
   b. M protein interferes with normal antibody protein and interferes with humoral immune response
   c. M protein increases blood viscosity and is toxic to kidney tubules, leading to possible renal failure
3. As abnormal cells proliferate, they replace bone marrow and ultimately infiltrate bone (especially vertebrae, ribs, skull, pelvis, femur, clavicle, and scapula), which weakens bone and can lead to pathologic fractures
4. Multiple myeloma may metastasize via bloodstream
5. Etiology is unknown but possible contributing factors are genetic alterations, oncogenic viruses, radiation, inflammatory stimuli, and chronic antigenic stimulation

NCLEX®

B. Nursing assessment

1. Bone pain, which increases and localizes over time
2. Lethargy, confusion, and weakness from hypercalcemia secondary to bone destruction
3. Leukopenia and increased infections from destruction of bone marrow
4. Elevated serum calcium, uric acid, and protein levels
5. Presence of Bence Jones proteinuria
6. Possible signs of renal failure (declining urine output, rising BUN and creatinine)
7. Pathologic fractures; spinal cord compression and possible paralysis if vertebrae are affected
8. Diagnosis confirmed by bone marrow biopsy; staging determined by hemoglobin and calcium levels, amount of proteins present, and bone involvement

NCLEX®

C. Therapeutic management

1. Assess and manage chronic back pain and deep bone pain
2. Assist client to position of comfort and support with pillows; reposition every 2 hours; provide a bed trapeze to assist with repositioning
3. Provide for uninterrupted rest periods
4. Initiate standard safety measures while in bed or during client ambulation to prevent risk of fractures (items close at hand, call bell in reach, nonskid soles on slippers, clear and lit walking pathway)
5. Maintain hydration (at least 2 liters of fluid daily) to counteract effects of hypercalcemia and hyperuricemia
6. Support client during combination chemotherapy followed by stem cell transplant if eligible
7. Maintain neutropenic or thrombocytopenic precautions if indicated
8. Other medication therapy includes bisphosphonate therapy, and vitamin D and fluoride supplements to support bone structure
9. Provide client teaching about nature and course of illness, measures to prevent infection or bleeding, measures to prevent injury, need for hydration, and symptoms to report (increased pain, signs of infection, increased weakness, changes in urine)
10. Provide referrals to home health services, rehabilitation services, social services and hospice service as appropriate

XIV. THALASSEMIA

A. Overview

1. A group of hereditary blood disorders of hemoglobin synthesis (alpha or beta chain of hemoglobin molecule), characterized by mild to severe anemia
2. Most common type is beta-defect thalassemia, also known as Cooley anemia; there are three types of beta-thalassemia:
   a. Thalassemia minor is also known as thalassemia trait and produces mild anemia
   b. Thalassemia intermedia produces severe anemia
   c. Thalassemia major produces anemia that requires transfusions; see Chapter 32 for blood transfusion procedure
3. Commonly seen in those of Mediterranean descent (beta-defect thalassemia); however, may also be seen among African, Asian, and Middle Eastern populations (alpha-defect thalassemia)
4. Condition is autosomal recessive; when both parents carry gene, there is a 25% chance of passing disorder to child; if child acquires one gene, child will be a carrier
5. Thalassemia causes synthesis of defective hemoglobin; RBCs are fragile with shortened lifespan, which leads to anemia and chronic hypoxia

6. Body conserves iron from aged and broken-down RBCs and from transfused RBCs; this leads to **hemosiderosis** (high iron levels), which causes cellular damage and long-term complications, including anemia, splenomegaly, liver enlargement and cirrhosis, gallbladder disease, cardiac complications, delayed sexual maturation, and skeletal changes
7. If untreated, child may die

NCLEX®

B. Nursing assessment

1. Thalassemia can be diagnosed early in infancy when child presents with pallor, failure to thrive (FTT), hepatosplenomegaly, and severe anemia
2. Signs and symptoms of chronic hypoxia such as lethargy, headache, bone pain, exercise intolerance, and anorexia
3. Skeletal changes include enlarged head, prominent forehead and cheek bones, broadened and depressed bridge of nose, enlarged maxilla with protruding front teeth, eyes with mongolian slant and epicanthal fold
4. Hemoglobin electrophoresis shows decreased production of one hemoglobin chain; RBC changes may be detected as early as 6 weeks of age
5. Decreased Hgb, Hct, and reticulocyte count; possible folic acid deficiency

NCLEX®

C. Therapeutic management

1. Administer blood transfusions as prescribed, observing for complications of multiple transfusions
2. Assess for signs of iron overload (hemosiderosis) and hepatitis
3. Observe for signs of infection and prevent infection through good hand hygiene, avoiding those with infection; proper rest and nutrition
4. Administer folic acid as prescribed
5. Work toward fracture prevention by encouraging and providing opportunities for physical activities that do not increase risk of fractures, such as swimming and walking
6. Implement iron chelation therapy (desferoxamine) as prescribed to help eliminate excessive iron
7. Provide support and opportunity for child and family to discuss feelings regarding chronic life-threatening illness
8. Encourage child and family to allow child to live as normal a life as possible

D. Child and family education

1. Nature of disease and its medical management
2. Possible complications, including iron overload, as well as signs of infection
3. Activity restrictions to reduce risk of fractures secondary to excessive iron stores
4. Encourage genetic counseling if appropriate

Check Your NCLEX–RN® Exam I.Q.

You are ready for testing on this content if you can:

- Identify basic structures and functions of the hematologic system.
- Describe the pathophysiology and etiology of common hematologic disorders.
- Discuss expected assessment data and diagnostic test findings for selected hematologic disorders.
- Discuss therapeutic management of a client experiencing a hematologic disorder.
- Discuss nursing management of a client experiencing a hematologic disorder.
- Identify expected outcomes for the client experiencing a hematologic disorder.

PRACTICE TEST

1 The nurse is preparing a care plan for a client with polycythemia vera on ways to maintain nutrition. The nurse should include which measure in the plan?

1. Increase intake of foods high in iron.
2. Encourage small, frequent meals rather than three big meals.
3. Increase the amount of red meats and organ meats in the diet.
4. Encourage the use of hot spices in foods to stimulate appetite.

2 A client with thrombocytopenia presents to the primary care center. During assessment, the nurse notices petechiae. The nurse interprets that which laboratory result best supports the presence of a disorder of hemostasis?

1. Decreased erythrocyte count
2. A platelet count below 150,000/mm^3
3. An elevated lymphocyte count
4. A hemoglobin value of 14 or more

PRACTICE TEST

3 A nurse is admitting a client with a diagnosis of aplastic anemia. Which is the best room for the nurse to assign this client?

1. A semiprivate room with a client whose diagnosis is urosepsis.
2. A regular private room at the end of the hall.
3. A private isolation room equipped with a negative airflow.
4. A semiprivate room with a client whose diagnosis is thrombophlebitis.

4 The nurse is reviewing laboratory results of a client suspected of having disseminated intravascular coagulopathy (DIC). The nurse looks to the results of which test as the more specific marker for DIC?

1. Partial thromboplastin time (PTT)
2. Prothrombin time (PT)
3. Platelet count
4. Fibrin degradation products (FDP)

5 The partner of a client with disseminated intravascular coagulopathy (DIC) expresses concern that the client may be getting the wrong medication after hearing the client was receiving heparin. What is the nurse's best response?

1. "I understand your concern, but the doctors know what they are doing."
2. "Let me make sure that I have not misread the healthcare provider's order."
3. "The drug is being used to stop the abnormal clotting in capillaries and arterioles."
4. "Please ask the healthcare provider why this medication is being given."

6 The nurse is administering oral care to a client with disseminated intravascular coagulopathy (DIC). Which of the following is the most appropriate for this client?

1. Limit flossing to once a day.
2. Use an alcohol-based mouthwash to prevent infection.
3. Use swabs to administer oral care.
4. Encourage toothbrushing at least once a shift.

7 A client with stomatitis and on neutropenic precautions is prescribed to have mouthwashes every 2 hours. The nurse would provide mouthwashes containing which ingredients as most helpful to this client? Select all that apply.

1. Viscous lidocaine
2. Normal saline solution
3. Hydrogen peroxide
4. Diluted baking soda
5. Liquid antacid

8 A client with acute myelogenous leukemia (AML) is scheduled for a bone marrow transplant (BMT). In teaching the client's family about BMT, which statement by the nurse is best?

1. "The client will be in the operating room with the donor so that immediate transplantation can occur."
2. "The specially prepared marrow is infused intravenously to the client."
3. "The client will be brought to the radiology department to transplant the marrow."
4. "A large-bore needle will be inserted into the client's bone marrow where the donor marrow will be infused."

9 A client has undergone a lymph node biopsy. The nurse anticipates that the report will reveal which finding if the client has Hodgkin's lymphoma?

1. Reed-Sternberg cells
2. Philadelphia chromosome
3. Epstein-Barr virus
4. Herpes simplex virus

10 During physical examination, the nurse finds a nontender, moveable cervical node on a client. The nurse makes which interpretation of this finding?

1. Normal, since the node is moveable
2. Abnormal and may suggest presence of malignancy
3. Normal, since the node is nontender
4. Abnormal and a positive indicator of malignancy

11 A client with thrombocytopenia has neurologic checks prescribed every hour. The nurse shares with a curious unlicensed assistant which reason for frequent neurologic assessments?

1. To determine if the coagulopathy is related to a neurologic disorder
2. To monitor for signs of intracranial bleeding
3. To evaluate the effectiveness of pharmacologic interventions
4. To correlate increasing platelet counts with the neurologic status

12 During assessment, the nurse notices a systolic murmur on a client with anemia. The nurse interprets that this finding correlates with which underlying pathophysiological mechanism?

1. Increased quantity and speed of low-viscosity blood through valves
2. Structural abnormality of heart valves from the anemia
3. High viscosity of blood circulating through the cardiac structures
4. Decreased blood flow through the vascular system

13 A client with anemia is unable to tolerate increased periods of activity without onset of fatigue. Which intervention should the nurse implement? Select all that apply.

1. Space interventions during the day.
2. Teach client the basics of good nutrition.
3. Promote active or passive range-of-motion activities.
4. Teach client to change position slowly to prevent dizziness.
5. Encourage defined rest periods during the day.

14 The nurse is teaching a client with hemophilia A about home management. Which strategy should the nurse include in the teaching plan?

1. Increase iron-rich foods in the diet
2. Avoid contact sports
3. Use aspirin when severe pain occurs
4. Minimize joint pain by walking and weight bearing

15 The nurse is obtaining a health history on a client admitted with a diagnosis of "rule out aplastic anemia." Considering the diagnosis, which data is most important for the nurse to elicit during the interview?

1. Recent travel outside the country
2. Exposure to chemicals and drugs
3. History of blood transfusion
4. Medication allergies

16 The nurse is teaching family members about precautions to take in visiting a client who has neutropenia. Which instructions should the nurse include in the discussion? Select all that apply.

1. People who have colds or infectious diseases should not visit.
2. Visitors must wash their hands before and after a visit.
3. Fresh fruits and vegetables will help fortify the client's immune system.
4. Fresh flowers will help to provide a cheerful environment.
5. It is helpful to keep the client's water pitcher full to prevent dehydration.

17 A client has a platelet count of 18,000/mm^3. What intervention must the nurse include in the plan of care?

1. Institute bleeding precautions.
2. Institute neutropenic precautions.
3. Schedule medications by intramuscular route when able.
4. Obtain temperatures rectally.

18 A nurse is assisting the healthcare provider with a bone marrow aspiration on a client with anemia. After the procedure, the nurse should take which action?

1. Apply pressure on the site to stop bleeding.
2. Massage the area to decrease pain.
3. Apply heat to the area to diminish the discomfort.
4. Cover the area with a light dressing.

PRACTICE TEST

19 The white blood cell (WBC) differential on a client indicates a shift to the left. The nurse makes which accurate interpretation of this report?

1. There is an increase in the number of segmented neutrophils.
2. There is an increased number of bands released into the circulation.
3. The number of lymphocytes is decreased overall in the blood sample.
4. The lymphocyte count represents the greatest percent of the WBC count.

20 A client with iron-deficiency anemia is scheduled for a complete blood count. The nurse anticipates that the report will show which characteristics of the red blood cells (RBCs)?

1. Normocytic, normochromic
2. Macrocytic, normochromic
3. Microcytic, hypochromic
4. Normocytic, hyperchromic

21 The nurse in the hematology clinic is reviewing laboratory and assessment data for a 2-year-old being treated for anemia. Which finding is the best indication that the treatment is successful?

1. The child is no longer cyanotic.
2. The reticulocyte count is rising.
3. The child is more active.
4. Stools are black, indicating iron intake.

22 A pregnant woman who has a family history of sickle-cell anemia states she is afraid her baby will be born with the disease. The nurse should provide which information during a discussion with this client?

1. Sickle-cell anemia is a male disease and would be passed on through the man's family.
2. Genetic testing will be needed to determine if her fetus is affected.
3. Both mother and father must carry the defective gene for the child to have sickle-cell anemia.
4. The child only needs one parent to be a carrier in order for the child to be affected.

23 A young child is diagnosed with idiopathic thrombocytopenic purpura (ITP). The child's mother says to the nurse, "I have a friend who has a son with hemophilia. When he bleeds, they give him a 'factor,' which they keep in their home refrigerator. Can we just give my child this factor?" Which response by the nurse would be best?

1. "Your friend's child has a natural deficiency in clotting factors; your child does not."
2. "Factor has a lot of negative side effects, and the doctors would rather not use it on your child."
3. "The amount of factor that would be required to treat your child would be excessive."
4. "That treatment may be tried later if your child does not respond to steroids."

24 The nurse has admitted a child newly diagnosed with anemia of unknown origin. Which clinical problem is of greatest concern?

1. The client's cardiac output will be insufficient
2. The client will become fatigued by increased activity
3. The client has a nutritional deficiency of some type
4. The client may experience pain because of vaso-occlusion

25 The nurse is caring for a child with beta-thalassemia who has received many blood transfusions. The nurse assesses for which problem as a priority at this time?

1. Neutropenia
2. Petechiae
3. Hemosiderosis
4. Hemoglobin S formation

26 A client with folic acid deficiency needs to increase dietary intake of foods that are good sources of this vitamin. The nurse should recommend that the client increase intake of which foods? Select all that apply.

1. Apples
2. Spinach
3. Carrots
4. Wheat germ
5. Liver

ANSWERS & RATIONALES

1. **Answer: 2 Rationale:** Clients with polycythemia experience satiety and fullness resulting from hepatomegaly and splenomegaly. Frequent, small meals will help maintain adequate nutrition. Foods rich in iron are not appropriate because there is an increase in erythrocytes in this condition. Red meats and organ meats may be higher in animal blood content, which is not helpful for this condition. Spicy foods will increase the gastrointestinal symptoms, which also include dyspepsia and increased gastric secretions. **Cognitive Level:** Applying **Client Need:** Physiological Adaptation **Integrated Process:** Nursing Process: Planning **Content Area:** Adult Health: Hematologic **Strategy:** The core issue of the question is knowledge of an appropriate diet for a client with polycythemia. Use nursing knowledge and the process of elimination to make a selection.

2. **Answer: 2 Rationale:** Clients with thrombocytopenia have decreased platelet counts below 150,000/mm^3. The usual presenting manifestation of this condition is the appearance of petechiae, purpura, and ecchymosis. A decreased erythrocyte count, elevated lymphocyte count, or hemoglobin value of 14 or more will not explain the petechiae or support the presence of a clotting disorder. **Cognitive Level:** Analyzing **Client Need:** Physiological Adaptation **Integrated Process:** Nursing Process: Assessment **Content Area:** Adult Health: Hematologic **Strategy:** The core issue of the question is the laboratory test results that best indicate a disorder of abnormal clotting ability. Use nursing knowledge and the process of elimination to make a selection.

3. **Answer: 2 Rationale:** Clients with aplastic anemia usually experience pancytopenia (decreased erythrocytes, leukocytes, and platelets). The client with this type of hypoplastic anemia should therefore have a room where reverse isolation can be instituted. The client with aplastic anemia is susceptible to infection as well as hemorrhage. Respiratory isolation requiring negative airflow is not necessary in the care of clients with aplastic anemia. The client should be admitted to a private room rather than a semiprivate room. **Cognitive Level:** Analyzing **Client Need:** Physiological Adaptation **Integrated Process:** Nursing Process: Planning **Content Area:** Adult Health: Hematologic **Strategy:** The core issue of the question is knowledge of the effects of aplastic anemia on the immune system, which then requires special intervention to prevent infection. Use nursing knowledge and the process of elimination to make a selection.

4. **Answer: 4 Rationale:** In DIC, there is abnormal initiation and formation of blood clots. As clots are formed and then begin to dissolve, more end products of fibrinogen and fibrin are also formed. These are called fibrin degradation products. Although the PT and PTT are prolonged and the platelet count is reduced in DIC, they could also be a result of other coagulation disturbances. Only the increase in FDP would occur because of the widespread accelerated clotting present in DIC. **Cognitive Level:** Analyzing **Client Need:** Physiological Adaptation **Integrated Process:** Nursing Process: Assessment **Content Area:** Adult Health: Hematologic **Strategy:** The core issue of the question is knowledge of trends in changes of laboratory data in DIC. Use nursing knowledge and the process of elimination to make a selection.

5. **Answer: 3 Rationale:** Initially in DIC, there is accelerated coagulation with resulting increase in fibrin and platelet deposits in arterioles and capillaries, resulting in thrombosis. Although it remains controversial, the use of heparin in DIC is aimed at preventing formation of additional thrombi that further complicate the bleeding disorder. Reassuring that the healthcare providers are competent fails to directly address the partner's concern. Rechecking the medication is not necessary at this time. Referring the partner to the healthcare provider fails to acknowledge the concern. **Cognitive Level:** Analyzing **Client Need:** Physiological Adaptation **Integrated Process:** Communication and Documentation **Content Area:** Adult Health: Hematologic **Strategy:** The core issue of the question is the possible role of heparin in the management of DIC. Use nursing knowledge and the process of elimination to make a selection.

6. **Answer: 3 Rationale:** Clients with DIC should be protected from injury that will result in bleeding. An oral swab is least likely to cause tissue injury to the oral cavity during mouth care. Flossing, even once daily, can increase the risk of bleeding from the gums. Mouthwashes containing alcohol should be avoided because they may cause discomfort and tend to dry the mucous membranes. Toothbrushes may be used only if they are soft-bristled, but a swab or toothette is the best option. **Cognitive Level:** Applying **Client Need:** Physiological Adaptation **Integrated Process:** Nursing Process: Implementation **Content Area:** Adult Health: Hematologic **Strategy:** The core issue of the question is appropriate methods of providing mouth care to a client with stomatitis. Use nursing knowledge and the process of elimination to make a selection.

7. **Answer: 1, 2, 4, 5 Rationale:** Viscous lidocaine helps to ease the pain of stomatitis. Normal saline is isotonic and is therefore less irritating to the oral tissues. Diluted solution with baking soda is soothing and acceptable in a mouthwash solution. A solution containing an antacid tends to be soothing for a client with mouth pain due to stomatitis. Hydrogen peroxide is not a good choice because it tends to dry the oral mucosa and further aggravate the discomfort. **Cognitive Level:** Applying **Client Need:** Physiological Adaptation **Integrated Process:** Nursing Process: Implementation **Content Area:** Adult Health: Hematologic **Strategy:** The core issue of the question is a mouth care product that would be irritating to a client with stomatitis. Use nursing knowledge and the process of elimination to make a selection.

8. **Answer: 2 Rationale:** Harvested bone marrow is infused into the recipient intravenously. The transplantation is usually preceded by chemotherapy and radiation therapy. The client does not need to be transported to the operating room for this type of transplant. Bone marrow transplantation is not done in the radiology department. A large-bore needle is inserted into bone marrow when obtaining a bone marrow biopsy, not a bone marrow transplant. **Cognitive Level:** Applying **Client Need:** Physiological Adaptation **Integrated Process:** Teaching and Learning **Content Area:** Adult Health: Hematologic **Strategy:** The core issue of the question is knowledge of bone marrow transplantation as a treatment method. Use nursing knowledge and the process of elimination to make a selection.

9 **Answer: 1 Rationale:** Histological isolation of Reed-Sternberg cells in lymph node biopsy examination is a diagnostic feature of Hodgkin's lymphoma. Philadelphia chromosome is attributed to chronic myelogenous leukemia. Viruses such as the Epstein-Barr virus or herpes simplex virus are much smaller than can be visualized with cytology. **Cognitive Level:** Applying **Client Need:** Physiological Adaptation **Integrated Process:** Nursing Process: Diagnosis **Content Area:** Adult Health: Hematologic **Strategy:** The core issue of the question is knowledge of characteristic findings in the diagnosis of lymphoma. Use nursing knowledge and the process of elimination to make a selection.

10 **Answer: 2 Rationale:** A nontender and movable cervical node may suggest the presence of malignancy and even lymphoma. A movable or nontender cervical node is not normal. Palpable nodes do not confirm the diagnosis of a malignancy; biopsy and histological examination will aid in interpreting the significance of enlarged nodes. **Cognitive Level:** Analyzing **Client Need:** Physiological Adaptation **Integrated Process:** Nursing Process: Assessment **Content Area:** Adult Health: Hematologic **Strategy:** The core issue of the question is the ability to interpret assessment data related to lymph nodes. Use nursing knowledge and the process of elimination to make a selection.

11 **Answer: 2 Rationale:** Neurologic assessment can assist in determining the presence of occult intracranial bleeding from cerebrovascular blood vessels. Neurologic assessment does not determine if the coagulopathy is related to a neurologic disorder. Neurologic assessment is not performed to evaluate the effectiveness of drug therapy. There is no reason to try to correlate increasing platelet counts with the neurologic status. **Cognitive Level:** Applying **Client Need:** Physiological Adaptation **Integrated Process:** Nursing Process: Implementation **Content Area:** Adult Health: Hematologic **Strategy:** The core issue of the question is knowledge that a low platelet increases risk of bleeding, which includes the risk of intracranial bleeding. Use this nursing knowledge and the process of elimination to make a selection.

12 **Answer: 1 Rationale:** The increase in cardiac output and flow are compensatory mechanisms because of the decrease in the quantity of hemoglobin in circulating blood. There is no structural valve deformity. In anemia, there is a decrease in the viscosity of blood as a result of a decrease in the number of red blood cells. In anemia, blood flow is not decreased. **Cognitive Level:** Analyzing **Client Need:** Physiological Adaptation **Integrated Process:** Nursing Process: Diagnosis **Content Area:** Adult Health: Hematologic **Strategy:** The core issue of the question is knowledge of how pathophysiology relates to assessment data in a client with anemia. Use nursing knowledge and the process of elimination to make a selection.

13 **Answer: 1, 4, 5 Rationale:** Because of the imbalance between oxygen demand and supply with anemia, periods of activity should be alternated with periods of rest to decrease hypoxemic episodes and to decrease tissue demand for oxygen. A client with anemia may experience dizziness if there is insufficient oxygenation of red blood cells supplying the brain, so the client should move or change positions slowly. Providing for specific rest periods aids in energy conservation. Teaching basic principles of nutrition to a client with anemia is appropriate but does not directly relate to fatigue. Promoting range of motion would be helpful for a client who has limited mobility, but is not necessary solely because of fatigue. **Cognitive Level:** Applying **Client Need:** Physiological Adaptation **Integrated Process:** Nursing Process: Planning **Content Area:** Adult Health: Hematologic **Strategy:** The core issue of the question is knowledge that anemia causes fatigue and that measures to prevent fatigue need to be incorporated in the plan of care. Use this knowledge and the process of elimination to make a selection.

14 **Answer: 2 Rationale:** Clients with hemophilia should be taught to participate in noncontact sports and to avoid any activities that increase the risk of tissue injury and bleeding. Iron-rich foods are not appropriate in clients with this condition unless there is an accompanying anemia. Clients with hemophilia should never use aspirin because of the risk of bleeding. Joint pain may be caused by hemarthrosis (bleeding in the joints), a situation in which the client should be taught to seek medical care immediately. **Cognitive Level:** Applying **Client Need:** Physiological Adaptation **Integrated Process:** Teaching and Learning **Content Area:** Adult Health: Hematologic **Strategy:** The core issue of the question is an appropriate element of client teaching with hemophilia. Use concepts related to prevention of bleeding and the process of elimination to make a selection.

15 **Answer: 2 Rationale:** Aplastic anemia may be congenital or acquired, but most cases do not have an identifiable etiology. It is known that aplastic anemia may follow exposure to chemicals (e.g., benzene, DDT) or drugs (chloramphenicol, sulfonamides). Recent travel outside the country is not pertinent. Aplastic anemia is not a sequela of blood transfusion. Aplastic anemia is not caused by allergies to medications. **Cognitive Level:** Analyzing **Client Need:** Physiological Adaptation **Integrated Process:** Nursing Process: Assessment **Content Area:** Adult Health: Hematologic **Strategy:** The core issue of the question is knowledge of the possible etiologies of aplastic anemia. Use knowledge about the possible causes of this disorder and the process of elimination to make a selection.

16 **Answer: 1, 2 Rationale:** A client with neutropenia has a compromised immune system and is predisposed to infections, so people who have colds or infections should not visit. Hand hygiene will reduce the risk of infection to the client. Fresh fruits and vegetables carry microorganisms that could lead to infection in a neutropenic client. Fresh flowers are not allowed in the client's room because they tend to harbor bacteria. The client should not have standing water in the room because it can attract and harbor bacteria that could lead to infection in a neutropenic client. **Cognitive Level:** Applying **Client Need:** Reduction of Risk Potential **Integrated Process:** Teaching and Learning **Content Area:** Adult Health: Hematologic **Strategy:** The core issue of the question is knowledge of the components of neutropenic precautions. The wording of the question tells you the correct options are correct statements. Use nursing knowledge and the process of elimination to make a selection.

17 **Answer: 1 Rationale:** A platelet count below 20,000 cells/mm^3 places the client at risk for bleeding and necessitates bleeding precautions be started to decrease this risk. Neutropenic precautions are unnecessary for this client if the pathophysiology affects only the platelet count. The client should receive medications orally or intravenously because the intramuscular route could increase the risk for bleeding during needlesticks. Measuring temperature by the rectal route increases the risk of bleeding and should be avoided.

Cognitive Level: Applying **Client Need:** Reduction of Risk Potential **Integrated Process:** Nursing Process: Implementation **Content Area:** Adult Health: Hematologic **Strategy:** The core issue of the question is appropriate interpretation of a low platelet count and interpreting the appropriate intervention to protect the client from bleeding. Use nursing knowledge and the process of elimination to make a selection.

18 **Answer: 1 Rationale:** Application of direct pressure and pressure dressing should follow the withdrawal of the aspiration needle after a bone marrow aspiration. If the client has thrombocytopenia, pressure should be applied on the site for at least 3–5 minutes or until hemostasis has been achieved. The area should not be massaged. Heat increases local blood flow and could increase the risk of bleeding. Covering the area with a light dressing fails to provide the necessary pressure after the procedure. **Cognitive Level:** Applying **Client Need:** Physiological Adaptation **Integrated Process:** Nursing Process: Implementation **Content Area:** Adult Health: Hematologic **Strategy:** The core issue of the question is knowledge of specific care following bone marrow aspiration that will prevent complications of the procedure. Use nursing knowledge and the process of elimination to make a selection.

19 **Answer: 2 Rationale:** A shift to the left indicates an increase in immature neutrophils or bands. An increase in the number of bands indicates an increase in the production of granulocytes, which could be a compensatory mechanism in response to infection. Segmented neutrophils are mature neutrophils, which is not consistent with a shift to the left. The lymphocyte count does not decrease because of a shift to the left. Lymphocytes do not comprise the greatest percent of the WBC count when there is a shift to the left. **Cognitive Level:** Analyzing **Client Need:** Physiological Adaptation **Integrated Process:** Nursing Process: Assessment **Content Area:** Adult Health: Hematologic **Strategy:** The core issue of the question is the ability to make an accurate interpretation of findings on a laboratory report of WBC count and morphology. Use nursing knowledge and the process of elimination to make a selection.

20 **Answer: 3 Rationale:** The morphologic characteristics of RBCs in iron-deficiency anemia is microcytic and hypochromic. Aplastic anemia, hemolysis, and acute blood loss will reveal RBCs with normocytic and normochromic characteristics. Vitamin B_{12} anemia produces a macrocytic and normochromic morphology. Anemias would be hypochromic rather than hyperchromic. **Cognitive Level:** Applying **Client Need:** Physiological Adaptation **Integrated Process:** Nursing Process: Assessment **Content Area:** Adult Health: Hematologic **Strategy:** The core issue of the question is the pathophysiological changes of RBCs in specific anemias. Use nursing knowledge and the process of elimination to make a selection.

21 **Answer: 2 Rationale:** Reticulocytes are immature RBCs. An increase in the number of reticulocytes indicates the body is producing new RBCs. A child with anemia is not cyanotic but pale. An increase in activity is hard to measure subjectively and would be a late finding. Evidence of iron intake does not ensure an improvement in anemia status. **Cognitive Level:** Analyzing **Client Need:** Physiological Adaptation **Integrated Process:** Nursing Process: Evaluation **Content Area:** Child Health **Strategy:** The core issue of the question is the ability to evaluate outcomes of care for a client with anemia. Use nursing knowledge and the process of elimination to make a selection.

22 **Answer: 3 Rationale:** Sickle cell is inherited as an autosomal recessive disorder, indicating that both parents must carry the defective gene. The disease is not only passed on through the man's family. Genetic testing of the fetus does not need to be done. The child cannot have the disease if only one parent is a carrier. **Cognitive Level:** Applying **Client Need:** Physiological Adaptation **Integrated Process:** Teaching and Learning **Content Area:** Child Health **Strategy:** The core issue of the question is the ability to teach a client about genetics as they relate to sickle-cell disease. Use nursing knowledge and the process of elimination to make a selection.

23 **Answer: 1 Rationale:** Hemophilia is characterized by a deficiency in one or more clotting factors, while ITP is a platelet disorder. Because the child with ITP is not deficient in clotting factors, this treatment would not be beneficial. The side effects of clotting factor therapy are irrelevant to this client's situation. The client's healthcare problem does not require the use of any factor. Clotting factor therapy is not held in reserve while corticosteroid therapy is completed. **Cognitive Level:** Applying **Client Need:** Physiological Adaptation **Integrated Process:** Communication and Documentation **Content Area:** Child Health **Strategy:** The core issue of the question is an understanding of the differences between hemophilia and bleeding disorders caused by platelet problems. Use nursing knowledge and the process of elimination to make a selection.

24 **Answer: 2 Rationale:** Clients with anemia will experience reduced tolerance for activity with even the simplest activities of daily living. There may be insufficient cardiac output, but it will not be related to platelet count. There is no information in the question to indicate that the anemia is secondary to poor diet. There is no vaso-occlusion with anemia. **Cognitive Level:** Analyzing **Client Need:** Physiological Adaptation **Integrated Process:** Nursing Process: Diagnosis **Content Area:** Child Health **Strategy:** The core issue of the question is knowledge of typical pathophysiology and client assessments in anemia and using this information to identify the most important nursing diagnosis. Use nursing knowledge about anemia and the process of elimination to make a selection.

25 **Answer: 3 Rationale:** Frequent blood transfusions will lead to an overload of iron in the body. This iron is stored in tissues and organs and is called hemosiderosis. Blood transfusions do not lower the white count or cause petechiae or hemoglobin S formation. **Cognitive Level:** Analyzing **Client Need:** Physiological Adaptation **Integrated Process:** Nursing Process: Assessment **Content Area:** Child Health **Strategy:** The core issue of the question is identification of a complication of chronic blood transfusion therapy. Use nursing knowledge of thalassemia and the process of elimination to make a selection.

26 **Answer: 2, 4, 5 Rationale:** Green leafy vegetables such as spinach are a good source of folic acid. Wheat germ is a good source of folic acid. Liver and other organ meats are good sources of folic acid. Apples and carrots are not as rich in folic acid as the other food sources listed. **Cognitive Level:** Analyzing **Client Need:** Physiological Adaptation **Integrated Process:** Nursing Process: Implementation **Content Area:** Adult Health: Hematologic **Strategy:** The core issue of the question is knowledge of foods that are rich in vitamin B_{12}. Use nursing knowledge and the process of elimination to make your selections.

Key Terms to Review

anemia p. 1186
anergy p. 1196
cheilosis p. 1186
ecchymosis p. 1191
fibrinolysis p. 1185
glossitis p. 1186
hemarthrosis p. 1191
hemosiderosis p. 1199
hemostasis p. 1184
hypochromic p. 1186
leukocytosis p. 1185
leukopenia p. 1185
microcytic p. 1186
plethora p. 1189
thrombocytopenia p. 1185
X-linked recessive trait p. 1191

References

Ball, J., & Bindler, R., & Cowen, K. (2015). *Principles of pediatric nursing: Caring for children* (6th ed.). Hoboken, NJ: Pearson Education.

Berman, A., Snyder, S., & Frandsen, G. (2016). *Kozier & Erb's fundamentals of nursing: Concepts, process, and practice* (10th ed.). New York, NY: Pearson Education.

Ignatavicius, D., & Workman, L. (2016). *Medical-surgical nursing: Patient-centered collaborative care* (10th ed.). Philadelphia: Saunders.

Kee, J. (2017). *Pearson's handbook of laboratory and diagnostic tests* (8th ed.). New York, NY: Pearson Education.

LeMone, P., Burke, K., Bauldoff, G., & Gubrud, P. (2015). *Medical surgical nursing: Clinical reasoning in patient care* (6th ed.). Hoboken, NJ: Pearson Education.

Lewis, S., Dirksen, S., Heitkemper, M., & Bucher, L. (2014). *Medical surgical nursing: Assessment and management of clinical problems* (9th ed.). St. Louis, MO: Elsevier Science.

Smith, S., Duell, D., Martin, B., Aebersold, M., & Gonzalez, L. (2017). *Clinical nursing skills: Basic to advanced skills* (10th ed.). New York, NY: Pearson Education.

Test Yourself

Are you ready for the NCLEX-RN® or course exams? Access the NEW web-based app that provides students with thousands of practice questions in preparation for the NCLEX experience.

Oncologic Disorders 65

In this chapter

Cross Reference

Other chapters relevant to this content area are

Promoting Healthy Lifestyle Choices	Chapter 16
Meeting Nutritional Needs	Chapter 25
Antineoplastic Medications	Chapter 44
Immunologic and Anti-Infective Medications	Chapter 45
Common Laboratory Tests	Chapter 46
Common Diagnostic Tests and Procedures	Chapter 47
Fluid and Electrolyte Imbalances	Chapter 53
Respiratory Disorders	Chapter 55
Renal or Genitourinary Disorders	Chapter 58
Gastrointestinal Disorders	Chapter 59
Endocrine and Metabolic Disorders	Chapter 60
Hematologic Disorders	Chapter 64

I. OVERVIEW OF CANCER

A. ***Cancer***: mutation of normal cells into abnormally proliferating cells; a neoplasm is an abnormal growth or **tumor** (solid mass functioning independently and serving no useful purpose)

1. **Benign neoplasms**: slow-growing, localized, and encapsulated nonmalignant growths with well-defined borders; are generally easily removed and only cause tissue damage by compressing tissues and interfering with circulation
2. **Malignant neoplasms**: aggressive growths that invade and destroy surrounding tissues; can lead to death unless aggressively treated
3. Invasion occurs when cancer cells infiltrate adjacent tissues surrounding neoplasm
4. **Metastasis** occurs when malignant cells travel through blood or lymph system and invade other tissues and organs to form a secondary tumor

B. **Characteristics of malignant cells**

1. Rapid cell division and growth: regulation of rate of mitosis is lost
2. No contact inhibition: cells do not respect boundaries of other cells and invade their tissue areas
3. Loss of differentiation: cells lose specialized characteristics of function for that cell type and revert back to an earlier, more primitive cell type
4. Ability to migrate (metastasize): cells move to distant areas of body and establish new site malignant lesions (tumors)
5. Alteration in cell structure: cell membrane, cytoplasm, and overall cell shape
6. Self-survival
   a. May develop ectopic sites to produce hormones needed for own growth
   b. Can develop a connective tissue stroma to support growth
   c. May develop own blood supply by secreting angiotensin growth factor to stimulate local blood vessels to grow into tumor

II. RISK FACTORS FOR DEVELOPMENT OF CANCER

A. **Intrinsic or host factors**

1. Age
   a. Increased risk for people over age 65 years
   b. Factors attributed to cancer in older adults include hormonal changes, decreased immune responses, and accumulation of free radicals
2. Gender: certain cancers are more commonly seen in specific genders; for example, breast cancer occurs more often in females
3. Genetics: cancers demonstrating a familial relationship include breast, colon, lung, ovarian, and prostate
4. Race: African Americans experience higher cancer mortality rates than other ethnic groups; disparities in access to treatment appear to play a role

B. **Lifestyle factors**

1. Tobacco
   a. A strong correlation exists between smoking and lung cancer
   b. Other cancers associated with tobacco use include bladder, esophageal, gastric, laryngeal, oropharyngeal, and pancreatic
   c. Smokeless tobacco (snuff and chewing tobacco) increases risk of oral and esophageal cancers
   d. Long-term exposure to secondhand smoke increases risk for lung and bladder cancers
2. Alcohol: serves as a promoter in cancers of liver and esophagus; when combined with tobacco, risks for other cancers are even higher
3. Diet: diets high in fat, low in fiber, and those containing nitrosamines and nitrosindoles (in preserved meats and pickled foods) promote certain cancers such as colon, breast, esophageal, and gastric cancer

C. **Immune disturbance**: some viruses tend to increase risk, such as Epstein-Barr, genital herpes, papillomavirus, hepatitis B, and human cytomegalovirus (CMV)

D. **Geographic location**

1. Risks for cancer vary according to environment and location
2. Rates for specific cancer sites, morbidity, and mortality vary from state to state, nation to nation, and in urban versus rural living

E. **Chemical agents**: over 1,000 chemicals are known to be carcinogenic; exposure in some occupations heightens risk over decades

F. **Miscellaneous factors studied that might correlate with increased incidence of cancer:** stress, occupation involving exposure to carcinogens (such as miners and asbestos workers), viruses

Box 65–1

American Cancer Society's Seven Warning Signs of Cancer

*C*hange in bowel or bladder habits

A sore that does not heal

*U*nusual bleeding or discharge

*T*hickening or lump in breast or elsewhere

*I*ndigestion or difficulty in swallowing

*O*bvious change in wart or mole

*N*agging cough or hoarseness

III. DIAGNOSTIC METHODS, TESTS, AND ASSESSMENTS

NCLEX® **A. American Cancer Society's seven warning signs of cancer** (see Box 65–1; see also Chapter 16 for general recommended health screenings)

B. Grading of cancer

1. Classifies cancer based on degree of abnormality of cells when examined under microscope
2. Grading utilizes a Roman numeral rating of I through IV, with I being least abnormal and IV being most abnormal (see Box 65–2)

Memory Aid

Remember to use CAUTION to recall risk factors for cancer.

C. *Staging*: TNM system is used to classify solid tumors (see Box 65–2)

D. *Tumor markers*

1. Protein substances found in blood or body fluids
2. Released either by tumor itself or by body as a defense in response to tumor (called host response)

Box 65–2

Grading and Staging of Solid Tumors

Grading

Grade I: cells slightly different than normal, well differentiated (mild dysplasia)

Grade II: cells more abnormal, moderately well differentiated (moderate dysplasia)

Grade III: cells clearly abnormal, poorly differentiated (severe dysplasia)

Grade IV: cells anaplastic (immature) and undifferentiated (cell origin difficult to determine)

Staging

T indicates tumor size

T0: no evidence of tumor

Tis: tumor in situ

T1, T2, T3, T4: progressive degrees of tumor size and involvement

N indicates lymph node involvement

N0: no abnormal lymph nodes detected

N1a, N2a: regional nodes involved with increasing degree from N1a to N2a; no metastasis detected

N1b, N2b, N3b: progressive regional lymph node involvement; metastasis suspected

Nx: inability to assess regional nodes

M indicates distant metastasis

M0: no evidence of distant metastasis

M1, M2, M3: increasing degrees of distant metastasis and includes distant lymph nodes

3. Tumor markers may include substances such as oncofetal antigens (e.g., carcinoembryonic antigen [CEA] and alpha-fetoprotein [AFP], certain hormones at high levels (e.g., antidiuretic hormone [ADH], calcitonin, catecholamines, human chorionic gonadotropin [HCG], and parathyroid hormone [PTH]), tissue enzymes, and tissue-specific proteins (e.g., prostatic-specific antigen [PSA] used to identify prostate cancer)
4. Host-response tumor markers include C-reactive protein, interleukin-2, lactic dehydrogenase, serum ferritin, and tumor necrosis factor

E. *Biopsy* and cytology

1. Histologic and cytologic examination of cells collected by needle aspiration of solid tumors, exfoliation from epithelial surface, or aspiration of fluid from blood or body cavities; examples include specimens from Pap smear, bone marrow, or tissue biopsy
2. Tissues for biopsy may be obtained by excisional, incisional, and needle biopsy methods
3. By examining these tissues, tumor name, grade, and stage can be identified

F. Laboratory and diagnostic studies

1. Laboratory studies vary by suspected site
2. Diagnostic studies (other than biopsy) include such tests as x-rays (including mammography), radionuclide and nuclear imaging scans (brain, bone, liver, lung), CT scans, MRI

IV. COMMON TREATMENT TECHNIQUES AND PROCEDURES

A. *Radiation therapy*

1. Use of ionizing rays for therapeutic purposes in cancer therapy
2. Used to eradicate tumor, reduce tumor size, relieve obstruction, or decrease pain
3. Causes lethal injury to DNA so it can destroy rapidly multiplying cancer cells; radiation therapy kills normal cells as well
4. Classified as internal radiation therapy (brachytherapy) or external radiation therapy (teletherapy)

B. External radiation therapy (teletherapy)

1. Radiation oncologist marks specific treatment area using a semipermanent type of ink or tattoo
   a. Treatment is usually given 15–30 minutes per day, 5 days/week, for 2–7 weeks
   b. Client does not pose a risk for radiation exposure to other people
2. Side effects of external radiation therapy
   a. Tissue damage to target area (erythema, sloughing, hemorrhage)
   b. Ulcerations of oral mucous membranes
   c. Gastrointestinal effects such as nausea and vomiting (N/V) and diarrhea
   d. Radiation pneumonia
   e. Fatigue
   f. Alopecia
   g. Immunosuppression

NCLEX®

3. Client teaching for external radiation
   a. Wash marked area of skin with plain water only and pat skin dry; do not use soaps, deodorants, lotions, perfumes, powders or medications on site during duration of treatment; do not wash off treatment site marks
   b. Avoid rubbing, scratching, or scrubbing treatment site; do not apply extreme temperatures (heat or cold) to treatment site; if shaving, use only an electric razor
   c. Wear soft, loose-fitting clothing over treatment area
   d. Protect skin from sun exposure during treatment and for at least 1 year after treatment is completed; when going outdoors, use sun-blocking agents with sun protection factor (SPF) of at least 15
   e. Maintain proper rest, diet, and fluid intake as essential to promoting health and repair of normal tissues
   f. Hair loss may occur; choose a wig, hat, or scarf to cover and protect head (refer to care of client with alopecia later in chapter)

NCLEX®

4. Nursing management of client receiving external radiation
   a. Monitor for adverse side effects of radiation (see preceding section)
   b. Monitor for significant decreases in white blood cell (WBC) and platelet counts
   c. Client teaching (refer to later sections for management of immunosuppression, thrombocytopenia, and anemia)

C. Brachytherapy (internal radiation)

1. Sources of internal radiation are implanted into affected tissue or body cavity, ingested as a solution, injected as a solution into bloodstream or body cavity, or introduced through a catheter into tumor

2. Side effects of internal radiation
   a. Fatigue
   b. Anorexia
   c. Immunosuppression
   d. Other side effects similar to external radiation (see previous section)

NCLEX®
3. Client teaching
   a. Avoid close contact with others until treatment is completed because of radioactivity
   b. Maintain daily activities unless contraindicated, allowing for extra rest periods as needed
   c. Maintain balanced diet; may tolerate food better if consumed in small, frequent meals
   d. Maintain fluid intake to ensure adequate hydration (2–3 liters/day)
   e. If implant is temporary, maintain bedrest to avoid dislodging it
   f. Excreted body fluids may be radioactive; double-flush toilets after use
   g. Radiation therapy may lead to bone marrow suppression (refer to precautions for anemia, thrombocytopenia, and immunosuppression later in chapter)

NCLEX®
4. Nursing management of client receiving internal radiation
   a. Exposure to small amounts of radiation is possible during close contact with persons receiving internal radiation; understand principles of protection from exposure to radiation: time, distance, and shielding
   b. Time: minimize time spent in close proximity to radiation source; a common standard is to limit contact time to 30 minutes total per 8-hour shift; minimum distance of 6 feet used when possible
   c. Distance: maintain maximum distance possible from radiation source
   d. Shielding: use lead shields/aprons and other precautions to reduce exposure to radiation
   e. Place client in private room
   f. Instruct visitors to maintain at least a distance of 6 feet from client and limit visits to 10–30 minutes
   g. Ensure proper handling and disposal of body fluids, ensuring containers are marked appropriately
   h. Ensure proper handling of bed linens and clothing
   i. In event of a dislodged implant, use long-handled forceps and place implant into a lead container; never directly touch implant
   j. Do not allow pregnant women to come into any contact with radiation sources; screen visitors and staff for pregnancy
   k. If working routinely near radiation sources, wear a monitoring device to measure exposure
   l. Educate client in all safety measures
   m. Provide emotional support to client who may feel isolated because of necessary precautions and to family who are concerned for client and unable to assist client at this time

D. *Chemotherapy*

1. Chemotherapy: administration of cytotoxic medications and chemicals to promote tumor cell death; IV route is preferred, but drugs may also be administered by oral, intrathecal, topical, intra-arterial, intracavity, and intravesical routes
   a. Chemotherapy disrupts cell cycle in various phases, interfering with cellular metabolism and reproduction
   b. According to **cell-kill hypothesis**, during each cell cycle a fixed percentage of cells are killed by chemotherapy, leaving some tumor cells remaining; this necessitates repeated doses to reduce number of cells, allowing body's immune system to destroy any remaining tumor cells
2. Classified according to mechanism of action (see Chapter 44 for discussion of specific chemotherapeutic drugs by category); combinations of chemotherapeutic drugs are administered to achieve best results in destroying cancer cells
   a. *Alkylating agents* are non-phase-specific and act by interfering with DNA replication
   b. *Antimetabolites* interfere with metabolites or nucleic acids necessary for RNA and DNA synthesis
   c. *Cytotoxic antibiotics* disrupt or inhibit DNA or RNA synthesis
   d. *Hormones and hormone antagonists* are phase-specific (G1 or first growth stage) and act by interfering with RNA synthesis
   e. *Plant alkaloids* interfere with cell division
   f. *Miscellaneous agents* may be cell-cycle phase-specific or non-phase-specific and interfere with DNA replication

NCLEX®
3. Side effects of chemotherapeutic agents (see also Chapter 44)
   a. **Bone marrow suppression**: decreased WBC count (immunosuppression), platelet count (thrombocytopenia), and Hgb and Hct (anemia)
   b. Gastrointestinal (GI) effects: anorexia, N/V, and diarrhea
   c. **Stomatitis** (inflammation of mouth) and mucositis

d. **Alopecia** (hair loss)
e. Fatigue
f. **Xerostomia** (dry mouth)
g. Other side effects specific to chemotherapeutic agent

NCLEX®
4. Management and client teaching for immunosuppression
   a. Risk for infection is high when WBC count is low
   b. Avoid crowds, people with infections, and small children when WBC is low
   c. Use meticulous personal hygiene to avoid infection
   d. Wash hands before and after eating, after toileting, and after contact with other people and pets
   e. Consume a low-bacteria diet; avoid undercooked meat and raw fruits and vegetables
   f. Be aware of signs and symptoms of infection and report them immediately to primary care provider
   g. Monitor laboratory values: CBC with differential, platelets, BUN, liver enzymes
   h. Assess for infection; monitor vital signs for early indication of infection: fever, tachycardia, and tachypnea
   i. Utilize neutropenic precautions: low-bacteria diet, no fresh plants or flowers in room, no pets, no visitors with infections when WBC level falls below predetermined level (such as 2000/mm^3)

NCLEX®
5. Management and client teaching for thrombocytopenia
   a. Monitor stools and urine for bleeding; stools may be dark or tarry and urine will have pinkish to red tinge
   b. Avoid use of straight razors; use electric shaver only
   c. Avoid contact sports and other activities that may cause trauma
   d. If trauma does occur, apply ice to area and seek medical assistance
   e. Avoid dental work or other invasive procedures unless absolutely necessary
   f. Inform all healthcare providers of chemotherapy and/or radiation treatments
   g. Avoid aspirin and aspirin-containing products
   h. Safety precautions for oral hygiene: use soft toothbrushes and do not floss; avoid alcohol-based mouthwashes
   i. There is a high risk for spontaneous hemorrhage when platelet count is below 20,000; bleeding precautions are necessary for platelet count below 50,000
   j. Assess for bleeding, monitor stools and urine for occult blood
   k. Assess skin for ecchymosis, petechiae, and trauma
   l. Educate client about ways to reduce risk of bleeding and measures that are part of bleeding precautions during times of high risk
   m. Avoid intramuscular (IM) injections and limit venipunctures

NCLEX®
6. Management and client teaching for stomatitis and mucositosis
   a. Use a soft toothbrush; mouth swabs may be needed during acute episode
   b. Avoid mouthwashes containing alcohol; do not use lemon glycerin swabs or dental floss
   c. Consider using chlorhexidine mouthwash to decrease risk of hemorrhage and protect gums from trauma
   d. Assess daily for lesions, infection, bleeding, or irritation
   e. For xerostomia, apply lubricating and moisturizing agents to protect mucous membranes from trauma and infection
   f. May consider using "artificial saliva" and hard candy or mints to help with dryness
   g. Avoid smoking and alcohol, which can further irritate oral mucosa
   h. Teach signs and symptoms of oral infection and to report to healthcare provider
   i. Drink cool liquids, and avoid hot (very warm) and spicy or otherwise irritating foods
   j. Assess oral mucous membranes every 4 hours
   k. Teach and implement proper oral care (see client teaching above)

NCLEX®
7. Management and client teaching for inadequate nutrition and fluid and electrolyte imbalance
   a. Eat frequent, small, low-fat meals
   b. Avoid spicy foods, fatty foods, and extremely hot or extremely cold foods
   c. Perform oral hygiene before and after meals
   d. Take nutritional supplements as prescribed (vitamins, liquid nutrition)
   e. Maintain a daily journal of food and fluid intake
   f. Assess for adequate hydration; for duration of treatment, encourage daily fluid intake of 2–3 liters unless contraindicated
   g. Administer antiemetics *prior* to chemotherapy
   h. Weigh client routinely such as weekly, monitor for weight loss; daily weights are not necessary and could increase client anxiety or depression about weight loss
   i. Monitor lab values indicative of nutritional status (Hgb, Hct, albumin, prealbumin)

j. Monitor for diarrhea or constipation and N/V
k. Encourage adequate nutritional intake with meals that are served attractively and in an environment free of noxious stimuli (bedpan, urinal, perfumes, air fresheners, and other odors)

NCLEX®
8. Management and client teaching for fatigue
a. Fatigue is a normal response to chemotherapy and doesn't necessarily indicate disease progression
b. Continue daily activities as much as possible, allowing for rest periods in between
c. Assist client in self-care needs when indicated
d. Allow for periods of rest; cluster activities

NCLEX®
9. Nursing management and client teaching for alopecia (hair loss)
a. Chemotherapy and radiation therapy may cause hair loss; chemotherapy–induced hair loss is temporary and hair will grow back, usually beginning about a month after completion of chemotherapy, although texture and color of new hair growth may be different; hair loss during radiation therapy to head may be permanent
b. Encourage client to choose a wig *before* hair loss occurs in order to match texture and hair color; an alternative is to wear colorful scarf or turban if client wishes
c. Care of hair and scalp includes washing hair two to three times a week with a mild shampoo; pat hair dry, and do not use a blow dryer
d. Allow client to express feelings concerning altered body image

E. Bone marrow transplant (BMT)
1. BMT is used in treatment of leukemias, usually in conjunction with radiation or chemotherapy
a. *Autologous BMT*: client is infused with own bone marrow harvested during remission of disease
b. *Allogenic BMT*: client is infused with donor bone marrow harvested from a healthy individual
2. Bone marrow is usually harvested from iliac crests, then frozen and stored until transfusion
3. Before receiving BMT, client must first undergo a phase of dose-intensive chemotherapy or radiation therapy to destroy cancer cells, such as leukemic cells; this process also severely suppresses immune system; infection, bleeding, and death are major complications during this conditioning phase
4. After immunosuppression, bone marrow is transfused IV through a central line
5. Side effects of BMT
a. Malnutrition
b. Infection related to immunosuppression
c. Bleeding related to thrombocytopenia
6. Client teaching: refer to previous sections on client teaching for altered nutrition, immunosuppression, and thrombocytopenia
7. Nursing management of client undergoing a BMT
a. Monitor for graft-versus-host disease (in which T lymphocytes in donated marrow identify client tissue as foreign, leading to attack on liver, skin, and GI tract, and resulting in skin rashes and desquamation, diarrhea, GI bleeding, and liver damage)
b. Provide private room for client (will be hospitalized 6–8 weeks)
c. Encourage contact with significant others using telephone, computer, and other means to reduce feelings of isolation
d. Refer to nursing management for imbalanced nutrition, immunosuppression, and thrombocytopenia

F. Other therapeutic interventions
1. Immunotherapy/biologic response modifiers (BRMs); see also Chapter 45
a. Enhances client's immune responses to modify biologic processes responsible for malignant cells
b. Currently considered experimental in use
c. *Monoclonal antibodies*: antibodies are recovered from an inoculated animal with a specific tumor antigen, then given to person with that type of cancer; goal is destruction of tumor
d. *Cytokines*: normal growth-regulating molecules that have antitumor abilities, such as interleukin-2, interferons, hematopoietic growth factors such as erythropoietin, and granulocyte colony–stimulating factors (GCSFs)
e. *Natural killer cells* (NK cells): exert a spontaneous cytotoxic effect on specific cancer cells; they also secrete cytokines and provide resistance to metastasis
2. Gene therapy: investigational; increases susceptibility of cancer cells to destruction by other treatments; insertion of specific genes enhances ability of client's immune system to recognize and destroy cancer cells
3. Photodynamic therapy
a. Used to treat specific superficial tumors such as those of surface of bladder, bronchus, chest wall, head, neck, and peritoneal cavity

b. Photofrin, a photosensitizing compound, is administered IV, where it is retained by malignant tissue
c. Three days after injection, drug is activated by a laser treatment, which continues for 3 more days
d. During IV administration, monitor for chills, nausea, rash, local skin reactions, and temporary photosensitivity
e. Drug remains in tissues 4–6 weeks after injection; direct or indirect exposure to sun activates drug, resulting in chemical sunburn; educate client to protect skin from sun exposure

V. ONCOLOGIC EMERGENCIES: DIAGNOSIS AND MANAGEMENT

A. Spinal cord compression

1. Occurs because of pressure in epidural space of spinal cord from expanding tumor (lung, breast, GI) or lymphoma
2. *NCLEX®* Early symptoms include back and leg pain, coldness, numbness, tingling, paresthesia; progression leads to bowel and bladder dysfunction, weakness, and paralysis
3. Early detection is essential: investigate all reports of back pain or neurologic changes
4. Treatment is aimed at reducing tumor size by radiation and/or surgery to relieve compression and prevent irreversible paraplegia; client may receive corticosteroids to reduce cord edema
5. *NCLEX®* Nursing interventions include early recognition of symptoms, monitoring vital signs, neurologic checks, and medication administration

B. Superior vena cava (SVC) syndrome

1. Compression or obstruction of SVC by a tumor
2. Usually associated with cancer of lung, non-Hodgkin's lymphomas, and Hodgkin's disease
3. Signs and symptoms result from blockage of venous circulation of head, neck, and upper trunk
4. *NCLEX®* Early signs and symptoms are periorbital edema, facial edema, and jugular vein distention (JVD)
5. *NCLEX®* Symptoms progress to edema of neck, arms, and hands; difficulty swallowing; shortness of breath
6. *NCLEX®* Late signs and symptoms are cyanosis, altered mental status, headache, hypotension, and possible seizures
7. Death may occur if compression is not relieved
8. Treatment includes high-dose radiation to shrink tumor and relieve symptoms and possible adjuvant chemotherapy
9. *NCLEX®* Nursing interventions include monitoring vital signs (VS), providing O_2 support, preparing for tracheostomy if necessary, initiating seizure precautions, and administering corticosteroids to reduce edema

C. Disseminated intravascular coagulopathy (DIC)

1. Severe disorder of coagulation, often triggered by sepsis, whereby abnormal clot formation occurs in microvasculature; clotting factors and platelets become depleted, allowing extensive bleeding to occur; tissue hypoxia occurs from occlusion of blood vessels from clots
2. Signs and symptoms are related to decreased blood flow to major organs (tachycardia, oliguria, dyspnea) and depleted clotting factors (abnormal bleeding and hemorrhage)
3. *NCLEX®* Treatment includes anticoagulants to decrease stimulation of coagulation and transfusion of one or more of the following: fresh frozen plasma (FFP), cryoprecipitate, platelets, and packed red blood cells (RBCs)
4. *NCLEX®* Nursing interventions include assessing client, monitoring for bleeding, applying pressure dressings to venipuncture sites, and preventing risk of sepsis

D. Cardiac tamponade

1. Pericardial effusion secondary to metastases or esophageal cancer can lead to compression of heart, restricting heart movement and resulting in cardiac tamponade
2. *NCLEX®* Signs and symptoms are related to cardiogenic shock or circulatory collapse: anxiety, cyanosis, dyspnea, hypotension, tachycardia, tachypnea, impaired LOC, and increased central venous pressure
3. Pericardiocentesis is performed to remove fluid from pericardial sac
4. *NCLEX®* Nursing interventions include administering O_2, maintaining IV line, monitoring VS, hemodynamic monitoring, and administration of vasopressor agents

E. Tumor lysis syndrome

1. Results from death of large numbers of cancer cells and release of intracellular contents into bloodstream
2. While cancer cell death is intended, tumor lysis syndrome can lead to other damaging and potentially fatal conditions if not treated
3. Signs and symptoms include hyperkalemia, hyperuricemia, and hyperphosphatemia
4. *NCLEX®* Nursing interventions include maintaining hydration to clear excess substances via kidneys, monitoring renal function, and administering medications to excrete excess substances such as allopurinol (to reduce uric acid), diuretics, and sodium polystyrene sulfonate or IV glucose and insulin to treat hyperkalemia

F. **Hypercalcemia** (see Chapter 53)
G. **Syndrome of inappropriate antidiuretic hormone (ADH)** (see Chapter 60)

VI. NEUROBLASTOMA

A. Overview

1. Solid tumor outside cranium originating in primitive neurocrest cells, which give rise to adrenal medulla, paraganglia, and sympathetic nervous system cervical chain and thoracic chain
2. In children, most common tumor located outside cranium; usual age at onset is 22 months
3. Prognosis based on client age and staging of tumor; children under 1 year of age have a better prognosis
4. Cause unknown, although environmental factors, such as prenatal drug exposure, may be implicated
5. Oncogenes have been found in neuroblastoma cells; DNA sequence responsible for this is called *N-myc*; high *N-myc* level is associated with rapid disease progression and poorer prognosis
6. Tumor is often silent, leading to late diagnosis and poor prognosis

B. Nursing assessment

NCLEX® 1. Symptoms represent location and stage of disease
   a. A peritoneal tumor may present as an abdominal mass or may be evidenced by bowel and bladder dysfunction; typical signs include weight loss, abdominal fullness, irritability, fatigue, and fever
   b. Mediastinal tumors cause dyspnea and lead to neck and facial edema if tumor is large
   c. Bone metastasis may lead to limp, fever, and malaise; ptosis and ecchymosis of eyes can also occur
2. CT of skull, neck, chest, abdomen, and bone locate tumor
3. Bone marrow aspiration helps to locate mass and determine metastasis
4. Urine testing detects breakdown products of adrenal catecholamines (epinephrine and norepinephrine), which some tumors secrete; these breakdown products are vanillylmandelic acid (VMA) and homovanillic acid (HVA)

C. Therapeutic management

1. Surgery to remove tumor following biopsy
2. Radiation therapy
3. Chemotherapy

NCLEX® 4. If surgery is performed, monitor surgical site for hemorrhage and infection; use temperature as most accurate indicator of infection
5. Monitor skin integrity at radiation site

NCLEX® 6. Monitor mucous membrane integrity; use appropriate nursing interventions to prevent and treat mouth ulcers
7. Minimize exposure to infection as previously discussed
8. Monitor bleeding as previously discussed

D. Client and family teaching

1. Disease process as well as treatment modalities
2. Blood dyscrasias and actions they can take to improve child's condition
3. Need for good nutrition and management of nausea

VII. BRAIN TUMORS

A. Overview

1. Over half of brain tumors in children are **infratentorial** (below tentorium cerebelli in the posterior third of the brain), primarily in cerebellum and brainstem
2. Most adult tumors and some tumors in children are **supratentorial** (above tentorial notch in anterior part of brain) and are mainly in cerebrum
3. Benign brain tumors can also be fatal because of solid skull that allows no room for expansion of tumor and thus causes increased intracranial pressure (ICP)
4. Cause is unknown, although radiation and environmental factors may play a role
5. Supporting cells of brain, such as glias and astrocytes, frequently account for pediatric brain tumors

B. Nursing assessment

1. Symptoms depend on location of tumor and age of client
2. Since an infant's sutures are open, symptoms may be found late

NCLEX® 3. Increased ICP occurs with brain tumors because of presence of the tumor and obstructions in flow of CSF; symptoms related to increased ICP include headache, especially on awakening, and vomiting unrelated to eating

NCLEX® 4. Visual symptoms include diplopia and papilledema

NCLEX® 5. Supratentorial tumors lead to symptoms such as personality changes and seizures

NCLEX® 6. Infratentorial tumor symptoms include ataxia, visual disturbances, delayed or precocious puberty, and growth failures
7. Diagnosis is based on results of MRI, CT scans, and radiographic studies with IV contrast; angiography is done when CT scans are positive
8. Surgery is used for biopsy (diagnosis), to completely remove a tumor, or to **debulk** an unremovable tumor (palliative procedure to surgically remove part of a neoplasm when complete excision is impossible); surgery may also be performed to restore patency of ventricles
9. Laser surgery can be used for more sensitive areas, where greater precision is needed
10. Radiation therapy may be used at the site postoperatively
11. Chemotherapy is commonly used, sometimes intrathecally
12. Complications such as hydrocephalus, seizures, sensorimotor deficits, and endocrine disorders may also need management

NCLEX® 13. Maintain nutritional support; if client vomits from increased ICP, provide hygiene and refeed

NCLEX® 14. Monitor LOC and observe for signs of increased ICP (increasing systolic BP, widening pulse pressure, bradycardia, irregular respirations); regulate fluid status to prevent rises in ICP; observe for seizures and provide nursing care should they occur; protect client from injury and have suction and O_2 available at bedside

NCLEX® 15. Monitor I&O and measure urine specific gravity (to detect diabetes insipidus [DI] or syndrome of inappropriate ADH [SIADH] from pituitary involvement)

NCLEX® 16. Postoperatively, position of head is critical; with an infratentorial incision, head position may be flat with neck slightly extended; with supratentorial incision, head is elevated; surgeon prescribes degree of head elevation, often 30 degrees; keep head and neck midline to promote arterial and venous blood flow

NCLEX® 17. If a ventriculoperitoneal (VP) shunt has been placed to restore ventricle drainage, nursing care includes maintaining suture line and skin integrity over shunt
18. Provide eye care to prevent dryness if client cannot blink or close eyes because of postoperative orbital edema
19. Monitor pain and provide relief; avoid medications that sedate client, which could interfere with assessment of LOC
20. Assess sensory-perceptual status and assist with loss of function
21. Assess surgical site for hemorrhage and infection

C. Client and family teaching

1. Reinforce information provided by healthcare provider about diagnosis and treatment; prepare client and family for craniotomy if indicated, including need to shave head and to expect ecchymosis of eyes (common postoperatively)
2. Teach activities that can reduce pain preoperatively and postoperatively
3. Encourage client and family to talk honestly about diagnosis and their feelings
4. If DI occurs secondary to brain tumor, teach client and family about medication (desmopressin) to control symptoms

VIII. KIDNEY AND BLADDER TUMORS

A. Kidney tumors

1. May involve one or both kidneys; may be either benign or malignant and either primary or metastatic (often from lung or breast cancer, melanoma, or malignant lymphoma)
2. Risk factors include genetics, age over 55 years (other than Wilms tumor), hypertension, exposure to certain occupational chemicals
3. Nursing assessment: gross or microscopic hematuria, palpable abdominal mass, flank pain, fatigue, weight loss, fever without infection, anemia or polycythemia
4. Therapeutic management is primarily surgical with radical nephrectomy (see Chapter 58 for care of client undergoing nephrectomy); chemotherapy has limited success in advanced tumors

B. *Wilms tumor (nephroblastoma)*

1. Overview
   a. Intrarenal tumor that most commonly occurs between 2 and 5 years of age
   b. A small proportion of Wilms tumors show a genetic basis, with family members being at increased risk of development
   c. Tumor may be unilateral or bilateral; bilateral tumors have poorer prognosis
   d. Tumor is often encapsulated until relatively late; it metastasizes to lungs and liver
2. Nursing assessment
   a. Usually asymptomatic

NCLEX® **b.** Most frequent admitting symptom is abdominal mass, which parent often discovers on one side of midline of abdomen

NCLEX® **c.** Pain and hematuria may be present in some children

NCLEX® **d.** Hypertension is present in approximately 25% of children because of increased renin production

e. Diagnosis is made by abdominal ultrasound and intravenous pyelogram (IVP)

f. CT scan and MRI of the lungs are done to detect metastasis

3. Therapeutic management

a. If unilateral tumor is present, surgery is performed to remove affected kidney and assess for metastasis

b. Radiation to abdomen and chemotherapy can be used before and/or after surgery

NCLEX® **c.** Avoid palpating abdomen preoperatively to reduce risk of rupturing capsule and causing tumor spillage; place a sign over child's bed with instruction "No abdominal palpations"

d. Measure abdominal girth daily

NCLEX® **e.** Postoperatively, monitor functioning of remaining kidney by monitoring I&O, daily weight, urine specific gravity, IV infusions, and BP

NCLEX® **f.** Complete pain assessment with VS; provide pain relief with medications and nursing interventions; in addition to incisional pain, pain may result from postoperative shift of internal organs to compensate for loss of kidney

NCLEX® **g.** Assess bowel sounds, abdominal distention, and bowel movements (risk of paralytic ileus)

NCLEX® **h.** Monitor for infection, observing surgical wound and body temperature

4. Client and family teaching

a. Need to avoid unnecessary palpation of abdomen prior to surgical removal

b. Nature of disease, treatment options, and therapeutic and side effects of chemotherapy in use (to parents)

c. Need to protect remaining kidney; signs and symptoms of urinary tract infections; and avoid contact sports, during which injury to kidney might occur

C. Bladder cancer

1. Overview

NCLEX® **a.** Major risk factors in bladder cancer are carcinogens in urine, chronic inflammation or infection of bladder mucosa, and cigarette smoking

b. Other risk factors: exposure to chemicals and dyes used in certain industries, chronic use of phenacetin-containing analgesic; carcinogen from these materials are excreted in urine and stored in bladder between voidings, leading to abnormal cell development

2. Nursing assessment

NCLEX® **a.** Painless hematuria is presenting symptom in a majority of cases; hematuria may be gross or microscopic and is often intermittent

b. Inflammation surrounding tumor may cause signs of UTI, such as frequency, urgency, and dysuria

c. With ureteral tumors, observe for colicky pain from obstruction

d. Neoplasms cause few outward symptoms and may not be discovered until urinary obstruction occurs or a fistula develops

e. Urinalysis shows gross or microscopic hematuria

f. Urine cytology shows abnormal tumor or pretumor cells

g. IVP, ultrasound, CT scan, cystoscopy, or ureteroscopy may show tumors

3. Therapeutic management

a. Radiation therapy

b. Surgical intervention for bladder tumors includes transurethral tumor resection, partial cystectomy with resection of tumor, or complete or radical cystectomy (removal of bladder and adjacent structures)

c. Urinary diversion may also be created (see Chapter 58)

NCLEX® **d.** Monitor urinary status, including I&O, signs of infection, hematuria, and BUN and creatinine levels

e. Monitor UO from all catheters, stents, and tubes for amount, color, and clarity

f. Prepare client for invasive tests to confirm location and size of neoplasm

NCLEX® **g.** Follow guidelines for care before and after surgery, chemotherapy, and radiation treatments

h. Encourage increased fluid intake unless contraindicated

i. Provide analgesics as needed for pain

j. Encourage client to express feelings about potentially life-threatening illness and to ask questions

k. Medication therapy: chemotherapeutic agents may be given IV or by intravesical instillation (into bladder)

4. Client teaching
   a. Explain all nursing and medical interventions, including benefits and possible adverse effects
   b. Reinforce explanations from healthcare provider about diagnosis
   c. Stress importance of compliance with long-term treatment plan and follow-up care
   d. *NCLEX®* Instruct client in methods to prevent infection
   e. For clients with a stoma or indwelling catheter, teach home care procedures and when to consult healthcare provider
   f. *NCLEX®* Teach client with a continent urinary diversion how to catheterize pouch (approximately every 4 hours) and wear a small dressing to protect stoma and clothing
   g. Teach relaxation techniques and other coping mechanisms

IX. BONE TUMORS

A. Osteogenic sarcoma

1. Tumor that arises from a bone cell, probably osteoblast
   a. Most common bone cancer in children; metastasis to lungs is frequent and may be present at time of diagnosis
   b. Most frequently affects metaphysis of long bones
   c. Osteogenic sarcoma usually occurs in adolescent boys; tumor growth is detected at time of rapid bone growth
   d. Most frequently affects distal portion of femur; also affects humerus, tibia, pelvis, jaw, and phalanges
2. Nursing assessment
   a. *NCLEX®* Pain and swelling are initial symptoms
   b. X-rays following traumatic injury may be first indication of disease
   c. Follow-up assessments include CT or MRI imaging to detect areas of metastasis
3. Therapeutic management
   a. Treatment may include radical resection or amputation
   b. Selected clients may have limb-salvaging procedures with prosthetic replacement
   c. Thoracotomy may be performed for metastasis to lung
   d. Chemotherapy may be administered pre- and postoperatively
   e. Emotional support of child and family is important before and after surgery, because of life-threatening disease, and treatment affects body image and mobility
   f. Employ a straightforward approach when amputation is indicated; allow for verbal expression of feelings
   g. *NCLEX®* Postoperative care includes sterile residual limb care and special bandaging as prescribed
   h. *NCLEX®* Elevate residual limb for 24 hours, if prescribed, but avoid prolonged elevation
   i. Maintain body alignment
   j. Perform ROM to joints proximal to amputation
   k. Provide opioid analgesics to relieve postoperative pain as prescribed; be aware that phantom pain can occur in amputated limb because of irritation of residual nerve endings; use opioid analgesics for this type of pain also during postoperative course
   l. Assist with early ambulation; assist with temporary prosthesis use
   m. Teach appropriate use of assistive devices
   n. Encourage early interaction with peers
4. Client and family teaching
   a. Reinforce disease process and treatment options
   b. *NCLEX®* Residual limb care (wash daily; use clean cotton or woolen sock; examine daily for intact skin)
   c. Demonstrate safe use of prosthesis; teach child to monitor condition of residual limb
   d. Phantom limb pain and its management; possibility of phantom limb sensation

B. Ewing's sarcoma

1. Overview
   a. Malignant, small, round cell tumor that usually involves diaphyseal (shaft) portion of long bones; commonly found in femur, pelvis, tibia, fibula, ribs, scapula, humerus, and clavicle
   b. Tumor arises in marrow spaces of bone
   c. Tends to occur between ages 4 and 25
   d. Highly malignant tumor that metastasizes to lung
2. *NCLEX®* Nursing assessment
   a. Pain and soft tissue mass
   b. Secondary symptoms of anorexia, malaise, fever, fatigue, and weight loss

c. Diagnosed with x-rays of affected area
d. Radionuclide bone scans and CT scans of chest assess for metastasis

NCLEX®
3. Therapeutic management
   a. Amputation usually not recommended
   b. Treatment includes extensive radiation along with chemotherapy
   c. Emotional support of child is important, as radiation therapy can affect appearance and mobility of extremity
   d. Encourage mobility of extremity as tolerated
   e. Allow open communication with child and family about disease and prognosis
4. Client and family teaching: disease process and treatment options; skin care related to radiation therapy

X. COLON CANCER

A. Overview

1. Develops in bowel wall or begins as polyps in colon or rectum that deteriorate
2. Metastasizes via circulatory or lymphatic system or by direct extension to other areas of bowel or adjacent organs
3. Can cause abscesses or fistulas, bowel obstruction, hemorrhage or perforation of bowel, leading to peritonitis

NCLEX®
B. Nursing assessment

1. Client may have no signs early in course of disease, making screening tests such as fecal occult blood and colonoscopy so important
2. Anorexia, vomiting, and weight loss; cachexia are late signs
3. Malaise
4. Anemia
5. Abdominal distention and possible guarding
6. Hematest positive or bloody stools with altered bowel pattern
   a. Tumor in ascending colon: diarrhea
   b. Tumor in descending colon: constipation or diarrhea; possible flat, ribbonlike stools from partial obstruction
   c. Tumor in rectum: alternating diarrhea and constipation
7. Abdominal mass (late sign)

NCLEX®
C. Therapeutic management

1. Monitor for development of complications
   a. Bowel perforation: distended abdomen; fever; weak, rapid pulse; and hypotension
   b. Intestinal obstruction: abdominal pain and distention, constipation, vomiting (may be fecal), hyperactive bowel sounds early (attempt to push past obstruction) followed by hypoactive then absent bowel sounds
2. Preoperative or postoperative radiation therapy to shrink tumor and reduce associated symptoms or to prevent recurrence
3. Surgery: bowel resection, ileostomy, or colostomy; see Chapter 59 for highlights of colostomy and ileostomy care
4. Note characteristics of stool following ostomy creation
   a. Ileostomy: liquid stool that is dark green progressing to yellow
   b. Ascending colostomy: liquid stool that is greenish then brown
   c. Transverse colostomy: liquid to semiformed brown
   d. Descending colostomy: semiformed to almost normal brown
5. Provide routine postoperative care including pain management and assessment of stoma and return of bowel function

D. Client teaching

1. Ostomy care
2. Dietary needs with ostomy (foods that loosen or thicken stool; foods that reduce or cause odor of stool)
3. Activity, medications, and follow-up care
4. Signs and symptoms of complications to report (such as infection, delayed wound healing)

XI. LIVER CANCER

A. Overview

1. Most commonly occurs as metastasis from lung, breast, kidney, and GI cancers
2. Primary liver cancer (hepatoma) is caused by tumors arising in liver cells (hepatocellular) or bile duct (cholangiocellular)

3. Tumor can be diffuse, nodular, or single nodule; compresses surrounding cells and can invade blood supply, causing necrosis or hemorrhage
4. May develop as a complication of cirrhosis, hepatitis B or C, aflatoxin (toxin from *Aspergillus* mold exposure), chronic alcohol consumption, and nonalcoholic fatty liver

NCLEX® **B. Nursing assessment**

1. RUQ pain or mass; feeling of fullness in epigastric region
2. Fatigue and general malaise
3. Anorexia and weight loss with possible anemia
4. Later signs can include ascites, fever, jaundice, variceal bleeding, liver failure, and splenomegaly
5. Laboratory findings vary according to degree of liver damage; may include hyperbilirubinemia, prolonged PT, elevated ESR (liver inflammation), hypoalbuminemia (if malnutrition, liver failure), elevated ALP, AST, ALT, and altered blood glucose (due to liver damage); elevated alpha-fetoprotein (AFP) occurs in 70% of those with hepatocellular cancer
6. Ultrasound, CT scan, or MRI may reveal focal liver lesions; biopsy confirms diagnosis

C. Therapeutic management

1. Partial hepatectomy for individuals with solitary lesions and without extrahepatic manifestations; serial AFPs are done postoperatively to assess effect on eradicating cancer
2. Liver transplant may be done for clients meeting established surgical criteria
3. *NCLEX®* Radiation therapy (palliative measure) may shrink tumor or reduce pain or pressure on surrounding structures
4. Chemotherapy as a primary therapy has limited response; sometimes chemotherapy is infused via hepatic arterial pump
5. *NCLEX®* Provide pain control measures and evaluate effectiveness
6. Provide care as outlined for other complications of liver failure or other disorders
7. *NCLEX®* Medication therapy: chemotherapy and other medications commonly used to treat liver disease

D. Client teaching

1. Disease process, expected outcomes, and chemotherapy
2. Etiologic agents that cause or contribute to development of hepatic cancer
3. Refer to prior sections on liver disorders and complications for other teaching points related to liver disease

XII. PANCREATIC CANCER

A. Overview

1. Most involve cancer of ductal epithelium and are adenocarcinomas; usually located in head of pancreas
2. *NCLEX®* Associated with increased age, cigarette smoking, alcohol use, environmental toxins, diet high in fat and/or meat, diabetes mellitus, chronic pancreatitis, and hereditary pancreatitis
3. Metastasis almost always occurs prior to symptoms, with invasion of tumor into posterior wall of stomach, duodenal wall, colon, and common bile duct

B. Nursing assessment

1. *NCLEX®* Slow onset with anorexia, nausea, weight loss, flatulence, and dull epigastric pain
2. Later pain is severe, is worse when lying down, and is unrelated to meals
3. Jaundice, pruritis, clay-colored stools, and dark urine when bile duct is involved
4. *NCLEX®* Classic signs and symptoms with advanced disease include pain, jaundice, and weight loss
5. Some clients may have a palpable abdominal mass or ascites
6. Diarrhea and steatorrhea occur late in disease
7. Development of diabetes mellitus from impaired insulin production
8. Diagnostic tests same as for pancreatitis, jaundice, and cholelithiasis
9. MRI and CT scan reveal a mass; CT-guided needle biopsy confirms diagnosis

NCLEX® **C. Therapeutic management**

1. Most clients do not present for treatment until cancer is too advanced; thus treatment is in many cases aimed at supportive or palliative care
2. ERCP may be performed to place stents within ductal system to facilitate bile drainage
3. Surgical management
   a. Gastrojejunostomy: bypasses duodenum
   b. Choledochojejunostomy: relieves biliary obstruction
   c. Pancreatoduodenectomy (Whipple procedure): surgical removal of head of pancreas, entire duodenum, distal third of stomach, a portion of jejunum, and lower half of common bile duct; see Figure 65–1

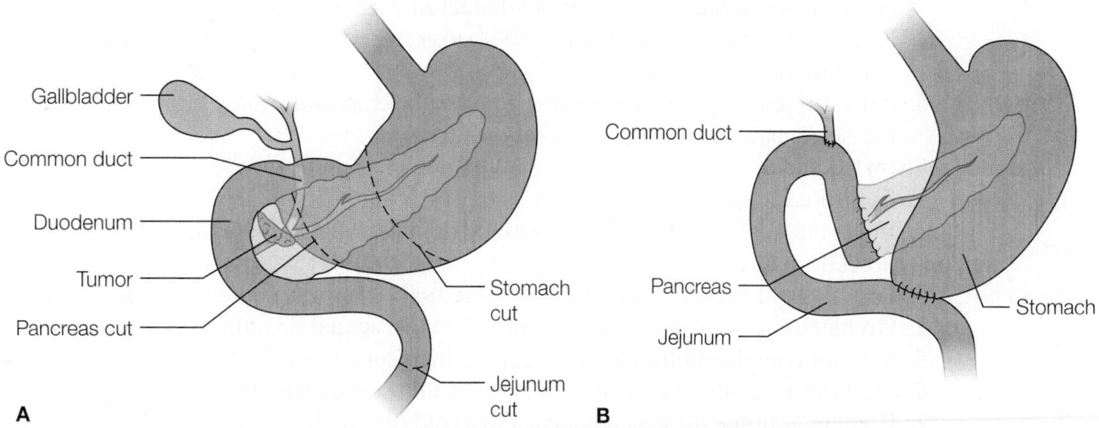

Figure 65–1 Pancreatoduodenectomy (Whipple procedure). (**A**) Dotted lines show areas of resection; (**B**) postresection anastomoses of organs.

4. Chemotherapy and radiation therapy are usually adjuncts to surgery
5. *NCLEX®* Provide supportive care, reinforce information regarding treatment options, and assist with educated decision making
6. Pain management is integral to quality of life; administer analgesics as prescribed and assess effectiveness for appropriate discharge regimen
7. Provide preoperative teaching if client elects to have surgery
8. Provide information about support groups
9. Medication therapy: aimed at controlling symptoms: pain, N/V; chemotherapy is rarely effective and is used most often for palliative treatment

D. **Client teaching:** disease process and poor prognosis; importance of pain control and symptom relief; importance of abstinence from smoking and alcohol

XIII. TESTICULAR CANCER

A. **Overview**

1. Unregulated growth of abnormal cells within testicles
2. Exact cause is unknown, but risk factors include cryptorchidism (undescended testicles at birth), maternal treatment with DES during pregnancy, mumps orchitis, trauma, environmental factors, and age
3. *NCLEX®* Most common cancer among males age 15–35, making sperm banking important to preserve ability to produce offspring
4. Testicular cancer is usually slow-growing and localized, with a good prognosis

NCLEX® B. **Nursing assessment**

1. Painless, hardened area or lump found during testicular self-examination (TSE) is common
2. Dull ache in pelvis or scrotum
3. Testicular pain may occur with associated infection, necrosis, or hemorrhage
4. Weight loss and fatigue
5. Metastatic signs such as respiratory symptoms, GI disturbances, lumbar back pain, lymphadenopathy, and gynecomastia
6. Scrotal ultrasound; CT or MRI scan of chest, abdomen, and pelvis may rule out metastasis
7. IVP to determine kidney involvement
8. *NCLEX®* AFP and beta unit of HCG are tumor markers; elevated levels strongly suggest testicular cancer; markers are measured after surgery to determine residual disease, possibly in lymph nodes
9. Serum lactic dehydrogenase (LDH) is elevated with testicular cancer

C. **Therapeutic management**

1. Prepare client for screening tests to determine type of cancer and stage
2. Provide emotional support for client and family; respond to questions and encourage client to express feelings

3. Prepare client for surgery if indicated (orchiectomy and exploration of adjacent area to identify cancer cell type and stage disease; lymphadenectomy if indicated)
4. Prepare client for chemotherapy after surgery and possible radiation therapy if cancer has spread to lymph nodes

NCLEX®
5. After surgery: provide analgesics, ice packs, and scrotal support to control pain and swelling; monitor for complications, such as bleeding or infection

D. Client teaching

1. Reinforce explanation of type and extent of cancer and plans for treatment
2. Importance of monthly TSE because malignancy may develop in remaining testis; see Chapter 16 for procedure

NCLEX®
3. Possibility of preserving sperm in a bank before surgery to help relieve client's fears about infertility
4. Orchiectomy should have no lasting effects on sexual or reproductive function
5. Signs of complications: bleeding, gaping incision, or purulent drainage from incision
6. Methods to control pain, such as ice bags and scrotal support
7. Remain at home for about 5 days and avoid driving for 1 week
8. Avoid strenuous physical activity for 3 weeks
9. Follow healthcare provider's instructions for resuming sexual activity
10. Importance of follow-up, especially if retroperitoneal lymph nodes were not surgically explored; client will need periodic physical examinations, tumor markers, and CT scans of retroperitoneal nodes for 5–10 years after surgery

XIV. PROSTATE CANCER

A. Overview

1. Unregulated growth of abnormal cells in prostate gland
2. Adenocarcinoma is most common type; high levels of testosterone may play a role; most common after 40 years of age
3. Usually begins in peripheral tissue on back and sides of gland
4. Metastasis via lymph and venous channels is common; bony tissue is major site of distant metastasis—especially pelvic bones and spine

B. Nursing assessment

1. Often no symptoms in early stages; tumor may be found during digital prostate exam

NCLEX®
2. Genitourinary: dysuria, frequency, reduced force of stream, hematuria, nocturia, abnormal prostate found on digital rectal exam
3. Musculoskeletal: back pain, migratory bone pain, bone or joint pain
4. Neurologic: nerve pain, muscle spasms, bowel or bladder dysfunction, bilateral weakness of lower extremities

NCLEX®
5. Systemic: fatigue and weight loss

NCLEX®
6. Diagnostic and laboratory tests: elevated PSA levels, transrectal ultrasound (obtained if PSA results are abnormal), tissue biopsy, bone scan; MRI or CT scans to detect metastasis

C. Therapeutic management

1. Treatment options include hormone therapy, radiation therapy, brachytherapy (radioactive seeds implanted in prostate), prostatic cryosurgery, and conventional surgery
2. Surgical procedures
   a. Orchiectomy decreases androgen production
   b. Radical prostatectomy procedures include removal of gland, capsule, ampulla, vas deferens, seminal vesicles, adjacent lymph nodes, and cuff of bladder neck
   c. Suprapubic prostatectomy: abdominal and bladder incisions to remove prostate tissue; abdominal dressing may leak copious urine; change dressing as needed and maintain continuous bladder irrigation (see next section); risk of hemorrhage and bladder spasms
   d. Retropubic prostatectomy: low abdominal incision without opening bladder; less bleeding and fewer bladder spasms than suprapubic route
   e. Perineal prostatectomy: incision between scrotum and anus (perineal area); minimal bleeding but increased risk of infection; urinary incontinence common; surgery causes sterility; avoid rectal tubes, enemas, and temperatures
   f. Holmium laser: laser treatment; less bleeding, fewer complications, and shorter hospital stay
3. Encourage annual prostate examination for men 40 years old and above
4. Medication therapy: estrogen therapy or luteinizing hormone antagonist (Lupron) given to slow rate of tumor growth and extension

D. Care of client having prostate surgery

NCLEX® **1.** Monitor VS closely for 24 hours, observing for signs of hemorrhage (frank blood in urine, large blood clots, decreased Hgb and Hct, tachycardia, and hypotension)

2. Maintain usual postoperative assessments, including lung and bowel sounds, IV fluid infusions, pain, urine output

NCLEX® **3.** If dressings are present, monitor for drainage and change as needed

NCLEX® **4.** Clients have a urinary catheter following surgery; surgeon may apply traction against prostatic fossa to prevent bleeding; balloon at tip of catheter exerts pressure to prevent hemorrhage (surgeon positions external end of catheter by anchoring it tightly to client's inner thigh to maintain traction; do not reposition catheter)

5. A client who has a large indwelling catheter may feel urge to void, which results from stimulation of micturition center; explain to client this is a normal sensation; efforts by client to void or strain will increase risk of bleeding and aggravate pain

NCLEX® **6.** Continuous bladder irrigation (CBI) postoperatively

- **a.** Purpose is to prevent formation of blood clots
- **b.** If blood clots do form, urinary catheter will become plugged and prevent outflow of urine; obstruction will also cause bladder spasms and pain
- **c.** Titrate flow rate of irrigating solution to maintain outflow light pink (early) or pale yellow (later) in color with no visible clots; it is essential to calculate both intake and output from catheter to determine true urine output; subtract CBI inflow from output for shift or 24-hour period to determine actual urine output
- **d.** Indications that irrigation rate is inadequate (slow) include decreased outflow from catheter; bladder spasms; and dark-colored, "punch-colored," or frankly bloody drainage
- **e.** Maintain sterile technique while changing irrigation bags

7. Monitor client for signs of hemorrhage; bladder spasms and frank bloody output may indicate bleeding

NCLEX® **8.** Irrigating solution used during and after surgery may be absorbed, causing fluid shifts and dilutional hyponatremia, referred to as TURP syndrome

- **a.** Monitor client for signs of hyponatremia and bradycardia and N/V
- **b.** Monitor serum sodium and Hgb and Hct (lowered with dilutional effect)
- **c.** Other signs of volume excess will also be evident, including hypertension and confusion

9. If manual irrigations are prescribed, maintain sterile technique

NCLEX® **10.** Medicate as needed for surgical pain with opioids and use suppositories such as belladonna and opium (B&O) to relieve sudden severe pain caused by bladder spasm

E. Client teaching

1. Reinforce information about illness and treatment plan
2. Methods to deal with urinary incontinence, which occurs temporarily after surgery, but could be permanent if internal or external bladder sphincters have been permanently damaged
3. Care of urinary catheter
4. Teach methods of pain control
5. Impact of surgery on sexual function (temporary or permanent impotence, permanent infertility after radical prostatectomy)
6. Refer client to support groups, such as American Cancer Society
7. Importance of follow-up tests for recurrence of disease
8. Signs of spinal cord compression (back pain and lower-extremity weakness) because of high incidence of metastasis to spinal cord
9. Activity levels as prescribed

XV. CERVICAL CANCER

A. Overview

1. Unregulated growth of abnormal cells in female cervix
2. Most common reproductive system cancer; often seen between ages of 30 and 50
3. May become invasive and spread to tissue outside cervix, uterine fundus, and lymph glands
4. Treatment depends on extent of disease
5. Squamous cell carcinoma accounts for 90% of cervical cancers; have gradual onset; spread by direct invasion of accessory structures

NCLEX® **B. Nursing assessment**

1. Thin, watery, blood-tinged vaginal discharge, which may go unnoticed by client
2. Painless bleeding between periods, often seen after intercourse, douching, or other contact

3. Late symptoms occur as cancer progresses to other organs, including referred pain in back and thighs, hematuria, bloody stools, anemia, and weight loss
4. Early diagnosis is critical because cervical cancer can be cured in early stages
5. Cervical Pap test; abnormal results call for repeat test, colposcopic exam of cervix, and tissue biopsy; diagnosis is based on biopsy results

C. Therapeutic management

NCLEX® 1. Treatment methods consist of chemotherapy, radiation therapy, and surgery
2. Assist client in dealing with psychological effects of illness; provide information and emotional support
3. Explore treatment options with client and family
4. Develop strategies for pain control
5. Maintain skin and tissue integrity during radiation treatment and following surgery

NCLEX® 6. Observe for fistula formation between vagina and bladder or rectum, a possible complication of radiation therapy; signs include voiding or having bowel movement through vagina

NCLEX® 7. Recommend a high-carbohydrate, high-protein diet
8. Medication therapy: chemotherapy for tumors unresponsive to other therapy or that cannot be removed, or as adjunct therapy for metastasis; analgesics for pain control

D. Client teaching

1. Reinforce explanations of diagnostic tests and treatments, allowing client time to express feelings and ask questions
2. Wound and skin care if surgery and/or radiation therapy are performed
3. Importance of regular screening exams and follow-up after treatment is completed

XVI. OVARIAN CANCER

A. Overview

1. Unregulated growth of abnormal cells in the ovaries
2. Most lethal of gynecologic cancers; etiology not understood; risk increases after age 40
3. Often asymptomatic, leading to late diagnosis; usually detected by chance, not through screening
4. May involve one or both ovaries; staged according to tissue involvement
5. Four stages of ovarian cancers: I—limited to ovaries; II—pelvic extension; III—metastasis outside pelvis or positive lymph nodes; IV—distant metastasis

B. Nursing assessment

1. Symptoms are rare until extensive tumor growth is present

NCLEX® 2. Feeling of pelvic pressure or heaviness, vague abdominal discomfort, dyspepsia, bloating, constipation, urinary frequency, and increased abdominal size

NCLEX® 3. Palpable, hard, fixed, firm mass in the area of ovaries during pelvic exam
4. No definitive diagnostic tool is available; diagnosis is made during surgery (exploratory laparotomy)

NCLEX® 5. CA125 antigen level (tumor marker) sometimes aids in detecting ovarian cancer

C. Therapeutic management

NCLEX® 1. Treatment options include surgery, radiation therapy, and chemotherapy
2. Explore treatment options with client and family; surgery is treatment of choice, radiation is used for palliative purposes to shrink tumor
3. Assist client in dealing with psychological effects of illness; provide information and emotional support
4. Develop strategies for pain control
5. Maintain skin and tissue integrity during radiation treatment and following surgery
6. Medication therapy: chemotherapy may be used to achieve remission, but is not a cure

D. Client teaching

1. Reinforce diagnostic tests and treatments, allowing client time to express feelings and ask questions
2. Teach wound and skin care if surgery or radiation therapy is performed
3. Emphasize importance of regular screening exams and follow-up after treatment is completed
4. Teach client not to ignore vague symptoms, such as indigestion, nausea, or urinary frequency

XVII. BREAST CANCER

A. Overview

1. Unregulated growth of abnormal cells in breast tissue

NCLEX® 2. Cause unknown, but many risk factors influence development
   a. Female gender and Caucasian race
   b. Family history of mother or sister with breast cancer
   c. Medical history of cancer of other breast, endometrial cancer, or atypical hyperplasia

d. Menarche before age 12 (early) or menopause after age 50 (late)
e. First birth after 30 years of age, oral contraceptive use (early or prolonged), prolonged use of estrogen replacement therapy
f. Lifestyle factors: high-fat diet, obesity, high socioeconomic status, breast trauma, smoking, ingesting more than two alcoholic drinks daily
g. Exposure to radiation through chest x-ray, fluoroscopy

3. Begins as a single, transformed cell and is hormone-dependent; does not develop in women without functioning ovaries who never received hormone replacement therapy
4. Most often occurs in ductal areas of breasts
5. Noninvasive: does not penetrate surrounding tissues; may be ductal or lobular; usually diagnosed through mammogram or nipple discharge
6. Invasive: penetration of tumor into surrounding tissue; there are five subtypes of invasive cancers, but they have only slight differences in prognosis
7. Staging depends on size of tumor, lymph node involvement, and metastasis to distant sites

NCLEX® **B. Nursing assessment**

1. Lump may be palpable in breast tissue, usually nontender, but may be tender
2. Dimpling of breast tissue surrounding nipple or bleeding from the nipple may be present
3. Possible asymmetry, with affected breast being higher
4. Possible swollen and tender regional lymph nodes
5. Diagnostic and laboratory tests: mammography, ultrasonography, MRI, PET, tissue biopsy, sentinel node biopsy (uses radionuclides to locate sentinel node for removal and analysis rather than a chain of nodes)

C. Therapeutic management

1. Treatment options include surgery, radiation therapy, chemotherapy, and hormonal therapy
2. Explore treatment options with client and family; prepare client for treatment, which is based on stage of disease
3. Radiation therapy is used to destroy remaining cancer cells after surgery or to shrink tumor prior to surgery
4. Various types of mastectomy may be performed
   a. Segmental mastectomy or lumpectomy: removes tumor and a margin of breast tissue surrounding tumor
   b. Simple mastectomy: removal of complete breast but no other structures
   c. Modified radical mastectomy: removal of breast and axillary lymph nodes, but not chest wall muscles
   d. Radical mastectomy: removal of breast, axillary lymph nodes, and underlying chest wall muscles; seldom done anymore
   NCLEX® e. Breast reconstruction: may be performed at time of mastectomy or at a later time; can be accomplished through submuscular breast implant, placing an implant after using a tissue expander, using muscles with intact blood supply from back or abdomen, or creating a free muscle flap with gluteus maximus muscle
5. NCLEX® Assist client in dealing with psychological effects of illness; provide information and emotional support, including information about breast reconstruction surgery
6. Maintain skin and tissue integrity during radiation treatment and following surgery
7. Medication therapy: tamoxifen interferes with estrogen activity for treating advanced breast cancer, and chemotherapy when axillary nodes are involved

D. Nursing management of client undergoing a mastectomy

1. Maintain usual postoperative assessments
2. Begin emotional support before surgery and continue in postoperative period
3. Turn, cough, and deep-breathe to prevent respiratory complications; restrictive surgical dressing may decrease chest expansion
4. Position client on back or unaffected side
5. NCLEX® Maintain Jackson-Pratt drain or Hemovac to drain fluid that accumulates when lymph nodes are removed
6. Note signs of bleeding on dressing and reinforce pressure dressing as needed
7. NCLEX® Encourage early gentle ROM exercise to prevent contractures and lymphedema
8. NCLEX® Use only unaffected arm for IV therapy and venipuncture and to measure BP
9. NCLEX® Position affected arm with each distal joint higher than proximal one before it (shoulder, elbow, wrist, and fingers)

PRACTICE TEST

E. Client teaching

1. Reinforce all diagnostic tests and treatments, allowing client time to express feelings and ask questions
2. Information about mastectomy surgery and what to expect afterward
3. Wound care if surgery is performed, including care of short-term wound drains
4. Discharge instructions postmastectomy *NCLEX®*
   a. Use caution when lifting heavy objects with arm on affected side
   b. Avoid injury and infection on affected side; wear rubber gloves when washing dishes and garden gloves when working outside; use potholders and oven mitts when using warm or hot cooking items
   c. Don't allow procedures, such as BP or venipuncture, on affected side
   d. Availability of support groups for psychosocial support
   e. Avoid heavy lifting for at least 6 weeks or until approved by surgeon
5. Techniques for proper skin care if radiation therapy is performed
6. Encourage client to meet others who have had treatment, if appropriate
7. Postoperative exercises and monthly SBE
8. Self-care during radiation and chemotherapy treatments
9. Importance of regular screening exams and follow-up after treatment is completed

Check Your NCLEX–RN® Exam I.Q.

You are ready for testing on this content if you can:

- Describe the pathophysiology and etiology of common oncologic disorders.
- Discuss expected assessment data and diagnostic test findings for selected oncologic disorders.
- Discuss therapeutic management of a client experiencing an oncologic disorder.
- Discuss nursing management of a client experiencing an oncologic disorder.
- Identify expected outcomes for a client experiencing an oncologic disorder.

PRACTICE TEST

1 A 4-year-old child is receiving postoperative care for surgical resection of a Wilms tumor. In addition to urinary functioning, the nurse should make which priority postoperative assessment?

1. Bowel function
2. Neurologic status
3. Presence of bone pain
4. Activity level

2 A child with a brain tumor has shown symptoms of diabetes insipidus. What should the nurse monitor to provide ongoing assessment of this condition?

1. Blood glucose level
2. Urine specific gravity
3. Adrenocorticotropic hormone (ACTH) levels
4. Serum amylase

3 The nurse determines that the client with Ewing's sarcoma understands instruction about side effects of radiation therapy when the client states to be concerned about which problem?

1. Infection
2. Constipation
3. Metallic taste in mouth
4. Blood in urine

4 A 6-month-old infant being treated with chemotherapy for neuroblastoma feeds poorly and vomits frequently. The nurse would use which assessment to best determine the infant's fluid status?

1. Daily weight
2. Urinary output
3. Specific gravity of urine
4. Hemoglobin and hematocrit

5 A child being treated for acute lymphocytic leukemia (ALL) has a white blood cell (WBC) count of 7,000/mm^3. The nursing care plan identifies measures being taken to reduce the child's exposure to infection. The nurse determines that the plan has been successful when which outcome has been met?

1. Child's WBC count goes up.
2. Child's neutrophil count goes down.
3. Child's temperature remains within normal range.
4. Parents and visitors demonstrate proper hand hygiene.

6 A child with neuroblastoma will be started on total parenteral nutrition (TPN) because of cancer cachexia. The nurse would question which new healthcare provider prescription?

1. Add 10 units NPH insulin to the TPN solution.
2. Monitor blood glucose level every 4 hours.
3. Monitor intake and output (I&O).
4. Begin a regular diet.

7 A child has been diagnosed with a brain tumor, but surgery cannot be scheduled for several days. The mother asks what she can do to ease her child's headaches. What suggestion should the nurse give the mother?

1. Help the child to drink plenty of liquids.
2. Discourage the child from having a bowel movement.
3. Encourage the child to sleep in a semi-Fowler position.
4. Encourage the child to blow the nose when headaches become severe.

8 A child is being treated with corticosteroids for acute lymphocytic leukemia (ALL). On a follow-up visit, the pediatric home health nurse assesses for which side effects of corticosteroid use?

1. Decreased blood pressure
2. Alopecia
3. Weight gain
4. Anorexia

9 A client with squamous cell carcinoma of the lung comes to the emergency department with shortness of breath and respiratory difficulty. The nurse notes cyanosis and edema of the face and arms. Based on these findings, the nurse suspects the client is probably experiencing which oncologic emergency?

1. Spinal cord compression
2. Syndrome of inappropriate antidiuretic hormone (SIADH)
3. Superior vena cava syndrome
4. Sepsis complicated by disseminated intravascular coagulopathy

10 The nurse reads in the medical record that a client's tumor is at stage T2, N0, M0. The nurse should draw which conclusion about the client's status?

1. There is an advanced tumor with metastasis.
2. The client has a measurable tumor with no indication of metastasis or involvement of nodes.
3. There is an advanced tumor with indication of involvement of lymph nodes but no indication of metastasis.
4. The client has an advanced tumor with indication of metastasis but no indication of involvement of lymph nodes.

11 A client with lung cancer is admitted to the oncology clinic for radiation therapy to treat spinal cord compression. The client's spouse asks why radiation is being done. The nurse's response would include that radiation therapy should have which effect?

1. To eradicate the tumor
2. To reduce the size of the tumor
3. To effectively treat all oncologic emergencies
4. Provide an alternative to chemotherapy for the lung tumor

12 A client with esophageal cancer arrives in the emergency department with shortness of breath, tachycardia, hypotension, and cyanosis. Cardiac tamponade is diagnosed. Which intervention would the nurse expect to include in this client's care? Select all that apply.

1. Administer a vasodilator agent intravenously.
2. Insert an intravenous catheter for IV access.
3. Prepare to assist healthcare provider with a thoracentesis.
4. Prepare the client for radiation therapy.
5. Initiate oxygen therapy.

13 The nurse is assigned to a client admitted for cystectomy as treatment for bladder cancer. Which clinical manifestation does the nurse expect to assess during the care of this client?

1. Urge incontinence
2. Postvoid dribbling of urine
3. Painful urination
4. Hematuria

PRACTICE TEST

14 A new nurse on the unit is admitting a severely immunosuppressed client who is receiving radiation therapy. The preceptor determines that the new nurse understands necessary precautionary measures when the new nurse admits the client to which room?

1. A semiprivate room with a client who has pneumonia
2. A private room with contact isolation
3. A private room with neutropenic precautions
4. A private room with no isolation precautions

15 After completing a health risk assessment on an adult client, the nurse determines health education is necessary because of an increased risk for laryngeal cancer caused by which risk factors? Select all that apply.

1. Past infection with Epstein-Barr virus
2. Past exposure to asbestos
3. Cigarette smoking
4. Heavy daily alcohol consumption
5. Recreational use of marijuana

16 A client newly diagnosed with breast cancer is scheduled for lymph node biopsy and asks the nurse why it is necessary when cancer has already been diagnosed. The nurse's response is based on which purpose?

1. It will determine what types of cancer cells are present.
2. It is performed on all females with cancer.
3. It is performed to determine if the cancer has metastasized.
4. It is performed to determine what type of chemotherapy is indicated.

17 A 65-year-old postmenopausal client tells the nurse that she has recently experienced painless vaginal bleeding. What is the appropriate interpretation by the nurse?

1. Not be concerned because postmenopausal bleeding is normal
2. Be concerned because painless uterine bleeding is a sign of uterine cancer
3. Be concerned because the client may develop anemia
4. Not be concerned because the client does not complain of pain

18 A client transferred to the surgical unit after a suprapubic prostatectomy has a three-way urinary catheter. The nurse notices a very dark red output via the catheter. What is the priority nursing intervention?

1. Report the finding to the healthcare provider.
2. Increase the irrigation flow rate.
3. Check the latest hemoglobin and hematocrit count.
4. Chart the observation in the medical record.

19 The nurse who is screening female clients for cancer anticipates which of the following in relation to the early signs of ovarian cancer?

1. Painful urination is a common complaint.
2. Pelvic pain radiating to thighs may occur.
3. Usually no symptoms are seen.
4. Low back pain is a common complaint.

20 A client has stage II ovarian cancer documented as a diagnosis on the medical record. The nurse plans care based on which characteristic of this tumor at this stage?

1. Tumor growth is limited to the ovaries.
2. Tumor growth involves one or both ovaries, with pelvic extension.
3. Tumor growth involves the ovaries and peritoneum, with positive lymph nodes.
4. Tumor growth involves distant metastasis.

21 A client is scheduled for a modified radical mastectomy. When reinforcing the surgeon's explanation of the procedure, the nurse would include that the surgery involves removal of which tissue?

1. Breast tissue and lymph nodes under the arm
2. Entire breast, underlying chest muscles, and lymph nodes
3. Breast tissue but no lymph node resection
4. Tumor and surrounding margin of tissue

22 A client with cervical cancer is going to have internal radiation therapy (brachytherapy). The nurse should provide what explanation about what to expect during this therapy?

1. "The head of bed cannot be raised more than about 15 degrees while the implant is in place."
2. "You will be able to have frequent visitors such as friends and family."
3. "It will be helpful to increase your intake of high-fiber foods during therapy."
4. "You can walk only in your room, not in the hallway, during therapy."

23 The client who underwent prostate cancer surgery is approaching the time of discharge from the hospital. What instruction should the nurse provide to this client as part of discharge teaching? Select all that apply.

1. "Maintain a high fluid intake after you go home."
2. "Call the healthcare provider immediately if you notice blood in your urine."
3. "You may drive yourself home."
4. "Avoid strenuous activity for 4–8 weeks."
5. "Avoid heavy lifting for 2–4 weeks."

24 The nurse should write which interventions in the care plan of a client following left mastectomy for breast cancer? Select all that apply.

1. Use warm, moist compresses on left arm for comfort.
2. Start intravenous lines on left arm only in the antecubital area.
3. Wait for the third postoperative day to begin any arm exercises.
4. Keep left arm elevated above heart level.
5. Take blood pressures on the right arm only.

25 A client has a continuous bladder irrigation running after prostatectomy. During the shift, 600 mL of one bag of irrigant infused and 1500 mL of the next also infused. Upon draining the urine bag three times during the shift, the nurse measures volumes of 800 mL, 1050 mL, and 950 mL. The nurse records the client's true urine output as ______________ mL. Provide a numerical answer.

Fill in your answer below:
Answer: ______________ mL

ANSWERS & RATIONALES

1 **Answer: 1 Rationale:** There is great risk for altered bowel function (adynamic ileus) because of surgery and possible radiation to the abdominal area and use of chemotherapeutic agents. Wilms tumor is an intrarenal tumor, so neurologic status is not a related manifestation. Bone pain is not associated with Wilms tumor. Activity level would not be a specific assessment to make with this diagnosis. **Cognitive Level:** Analyzing **Client Need:** Physiological Adaptation **Integrated Process:** Nursing Process: Assessment **Content Area:** Child Health **Strategy:** The core issue of the question is knowledge that Wilms tumor affects the kidney, and therefore principles related to care after abdominal surgery apply to this client. Use nursing knowledge and the process of elimination to make a selection.

2 **Answer: 2 Rationale:** Diabetes insipidus presents with symptoms of increased urinary output and very dilute urine. Urine specific gravity will measure the concentration of the urine. Blood glucose is unrelated to a pituitary gland problem. ACTH levels are not routinely monitored in any client. Serum amylase would be monitored with a pancreatic disorder such as pancreatitis. **Cognitive Level:** Analyzing **Client Need:** Physiological Adaptation **Integrated Process:** Nursing Process: Assessment **Content Area:** Child Health **Strategy:** The core issue of the question is knowledge of diabetes insipidus as a complication of brain tumor and methods to assess the status of this complication. Use nursing knowledge and the process of elimination to make a selection.

3 **Answer: 1 Rationale:** Bone marrow suppression occurs with radiation therapy, which can lead to risk of infection when white blood cells are affected, bleeding when platelets are affected, and anemia when red blood cells are affected. Diarrhea would be more likely than constipation as a side effect of cancer therapy. Metallic taste in the mouth is not of concern. Hemorrhagic cystitis, noted by blood in the urine, occurs after chemotherapy. **Cognitive Level:** Applying **Client Need:** Physiological Adaptation **Integrated Process:** Nursing Process: Evaluation **Content Area:** Child Health **Strategy:** The core issue of the question is knowledge of bone marrow suppression in a client receiving radiation therapy. Use basic nursing knowledge and the process of elimination to make a selection.

4 **Answer: 1 Rationale:** Weight loss can be directly tied to fluid loss because 1 kilogram of weight is approximately equal to 1 liter of fluid. Although intake and output is commonly

measured, urine output is a less reliable indicator of fluid status than changes in daily weight. Because infant kidneys do not concentrate urine as well as the kidneys of adults, urine specific gravity may not reflect urine concentration or dilution accurately. Hemoglobin and hematocrit could rise and fall with large changes in fluid status but are not specific fluid balance measurements. **Cognitive Level:** Analyzing **Client Need:** Physiological Adaptation **Integrated Process:** Nursing Process: Diagnosis **Content Area:** Child Health **Strategy:** The core issue of the question is the most reliable method of determining fluid balance in an infant who is not feeding well because of neuroblastoma. Use nursing knowledge of fluid balance measurement and the process of elimination to make a selection.

5 **Answer: 3 Rationale:** The reliable outcome measure that indicates the child is infection-free is a temperature that remains in the normal range. An increase in the number of WBCs from the baseline normal value presented could be expected as part of the disease process and might not solely represent a response to infection. A decrease in the neutrophil count could indicate the client is experiencing immunosuppression as a result of therapy. The use of proper hand hygiene is a measure or intervention used to meet a desired outcome but is not an outcome itself. **Cognitive Level:** Analyzing **Client Need:** Physiological Adaptation **Integrated Process:** Nursing Process: Evaluation **Content Area:** Child Health **Strategy:** The core issue of the question is knowledge of an indicator of infection in a client who is immunosuppressed from leukemia. Recall that temperature and WBC counts are frequently used as indicators of infection. Recall that in leukemia the WBCs are abnormal to choose the option related to temperature.

6 **Answer: 1 Rationale:** Only regular insulin is administered in solutions administered by the IV route. Monitoring blood glucose will detect excessive elevations in blood glucose caused by the TPN. Monitoring I&O is appropriate to ensure the client is receiving sufficient nutrition and fluid intake. The child is usually anorexic but will be allowed to eat any food that appeals to him or her. **Cognitive Level:** Analyzing **Client Need:** Physiological Adaptation **Integrated Process:** Nursing Process: Implementation **Content Area:** Child Health **Strategy:** The core issue of the question is knowledge of total parenteral nutrition as a means of providing nutritional support to a client with cancer. Use nursing knowledge about the uses of various preparations of insulin and the process of elimination to make a selection.

7 **Answer: 3 Rationale:** When a client is lying flat, the blood flow to the brain is greater, increasing intracranial pressure. If the client sleeps in a semi-Fowler position, less pressure will develop, which in turn should ease headaches. Excess liquids could aggravate headache. Discouraging bowel movements will reduce straining but is not a helpful measure from a gastrointestinal perspective. Blowing the nose could aggravate headache by further increasing intracranial pressure. **Cognitive Level:** Analyzing **Client Need:** Physiological Adaptation **Integrated Process:** Nursing Process: Implementation **Content Area:** Child Health **Strategy:** Recall principles of gravity to answer this question. When a client lies flat, blood can accumulate to a greater extent in the cranium, resulting in vasodilation, increased pressure, and worsening headache. Placing the client's head in an elevated position allows gravity to drain blood to the heart and thereby keeps intracranial pressure rises to a minimum.

8 **Answer: 3 Rationale:** Clients taking corticosteroids may experience weight gain because of fluid retention as a drug side effect. Corticosteroids may increase blood pressure rather than decrease blood pressure because of retained fluid. Alopecia could result from chemotherapeutic agents used to treat leukemia, but is not a side effect of corticosteroids. Anorexia can be a systemic sign of cancer but would not indicate a side effect of corticosteroid therapy. **Cognitive Level:** Applying **Client Need:** Physiological Adaptation **Integrated Process:** Nursing Process: Assessment **Content Area:** Child Health **Strategy:** The core issue of the question is knowledge of adverse effects of combination agents, specifically steroids in this case, needed to treat cancer in a child. Use nursing knowledge and the process of elimination to make a selection.

9 **Answer: 3 Rationale:** While all identified problems are potential risks to clients with cancer depending on site, edema of the face and arms results from obstruction of blood flow, which is indicative of superior vena cava syndrome. Spinal cord compression would give rise to neurologic symptoms. SIADH would result in general fluid overload. Sepsis and disseminated intravascular coagulopathy would be noted by signs of infection and bleeding, respectively. **Cognitive Level:** Analyzing **Client Need:** Physiological Adaptation **Integrated Process:** Nursing Process: Assessment **Content Area:** Adult Health: Oncology **Strategy:** The core issue of the question is knowledge of various oncologic emergencies. Use nursing knowledge about which body systems are affected by each and then use the process of elimination to make a selection.

10 **Answer: 2 Rationale:** Using the TNM staging system for cancer, a T2 indicates a measurable tumor, N0 indicates no regional node involvement, and M0 indicates no evidence of distant metastasis. An advanced tumor would have a higher number such as T3 or T4, and metastasis would not be associated with a M0 staging. If there was a large tumor and lymph node involvement, there would be a larger number associated with the "T" and there would also be a number rather than a zero associated with the "N." A tumor that was associated with metastasis but not lymph node involvement would have a designation of N0 but would have a number associated with "M." **Cognitive Level:** Analyzing **Client Need:** Physiological Adaptation **Integrated Process:** Nursing Process: Diagnosis **Content Area:** Adult Health: Oncology **Strategy:** The core issue of the question is knowledge of staging for solid tumors. Recall that for an option to be correct, all of the parts of the option must be correct. Note the numeric zeros by the N and the M to choose the option that does not contain metastasis or lymph node involvement.

11 **Answer: 2 Rationale:** Radiation is palliative treatment for spinal cord compression to reduce the tumor size and relieve compression. Radiation therapy will not eradicate the tumor. Radiation therapy is not effective for all oncologic emergencies. Radiation is not a new modality to treat lung cancer. **Cognitive Level:** Applying **Client Need:** Physiological Adaptation **Integrated Process:** Teaching and Learning **Content Area:** Adult Health: Oncology **Strategy:** The core issue of the question is the rationale for using radiation therapy in a client with spinal cord compression secondary to cancer. Recall that radiation therapy is often used as a supplement to shrink tumors to aid in making a selection.

12 **Answer: 2, 5 Rationale:** Inserting an IV catheter for IV access is an immediate intervention for the client with

cardiac tamponade. The client requires immediate oxygen therapy to treat the respiratory symptoms and relieve the cyanosis. Vasopressor agents will be administered to manage hypotension. A pericardiocentesis is performed, not a thoracentesis. Radiation therapy is not indicated for cardiac tamponade. **Cognitive Level:** Analyzing **Client Need:** Physiological Adaptation **Integrated Process:** Nursing Process: Planning **Content Area:** Adult Health: Oncology **Strategy:** The stem of the question indicates that the client has an ineffective airway (shortness of breath and cyanosis). Look for the options that first address airway (oxygen) and circulation (IV access) as correct answers.

13 **Answer: 4 Rationale:** Hematuria is a classic sign of bladder cancer. The client would not experience urge incontinence, which is often associated with urinary tract infection. The client would not experience postvoid dribbling of urine. The client who has bladder cancer does not experience pain during voiding. **Cognitive Level:** Applying **Client Need:** Physiological Adaptation **Integrated Process:** Nursing Process: Assessment **Content Area:** Adult Health: Oncology **Strategy:** Specific knowledge of the risks associated with various cancers in men is needed to answer the question. Use nursing knowledge related to epidemiology of cancer and the process of elimination to make a selection.

14 **Answer: 3 Rationale:** Because of the immunosuppression, the client is at severe risk of infection. Precautionary measures such as a private room and neutropenic precautions must be instituted to protect the client from sources of infection. The client with pneumonia poses a risk of infection. Contact isolation is not necessary. A private room alone does not provide the client with the necessary neutropenic precautions. **Cognitive Level:** Analyzing **Client Need:** Physiological Adaptation **Integrated Process:** Nursing Process: Evaluation **Content Area:** Adult Health: Oncology **Strategy:** The core issue of the question is knowledge of room accommodations required by a client who needs neutropenic precautions. Recall that infection is the risk and use process of elimination to make a selection.

15 **Answer: 3, 4 Rationale:** Cigarette smoking increases the risk of upper airway, esophageal and lung cancers. Drinking large quantities of alcohol daily increase the risk of several cancers. Epstein-Barr virus does not increase the risk of laryngeal cancer. Past exposure to asbestos increases risk of mesothelioma. Recreational use of marijuana is not associated with increased risk of laryngeal cancer. **Cognitive Level:** Analyzing **Client Need:** Physiological Adaptation **Integrated Process:** Nursing Process: Assessment **Content Area:** Adult Health: Oncology **Strategy:** The core issue of the question is risk factors for laryngeal cancer. Consider that alcohol and cigarette smoking are irritants to the upper airway to help choose correctly.

16 **Answer: 3 Rationale:** The lymph node biopsy is performed to assess any metastasis from the primary site of cancer, and a common metastatic site for breast cancer is regional lymph nodes. The biopsy of the tumor itself will determine the type(s) of cancer cells that are present. The lymph node biopsy is performed when indicated regardless of gender. The types of cancer cells determine what cancer chemotherapy drugs will be used. **Cognitive Level:** Analyzing **Client Need:** Physiological Adaptation **Integrated Process:** Communication and Documentation **Content Area:** Adult Health: Oncology **Strategy:** The core issue of the question is knowledge that a biopsy procedure is used to diagnose a primary tumor or to evaluate lymph node involvement or metastasis. Use nursing knowledge and the process of elimination to make a selection.

17 **Answer: 2 Rationale:** The nurse should be concerned because painless bleeding not related to the menstrual cycle is often the only symptom of uterine cancer. Postmenopausal bleeding is not normal. Anemia is not an immediate concern. Pain is often considered to be a late sign related to the diagnosis of cancer. **Cognitive Level:** Analyzing **Client Need:** Physiological Adaptation **Integrated Process:** Nursing Process: Assessment **Content Area:** Adult Health: Oncology **Strategy:** The core issue of the question is the significance of painless vaginal bleeding in a client who is postmenopausal. Use nursing knowledge and the process of elimination to make a selection.

18 **Answer: 2 Rationale:** A very dark red output following prostatectomy may indicate venous bleeding or inadequate dilution of the urine. The three-way urinary catheter is at risk for occlusion. Increasing the irrigation flow will prevent the formation of blood clots and occlusion of the catheter. If the urine does not clear after increasing the rate of bladder irrigation, then it would be appropriate to notify the healthcare provider. Although reviewing the latest hemoglobin and hematocrit may be appropriate, it is not the most pressing intervention the nurse must do for this client. Charting is a routine care activity but further action to clear the urine is indicated immediately. **Cognitive Level:** Analyzing **Client Need:** Physiological Adaptation **Integrated Process:** Nursing Process: Implementation **Content Area:** Adult Health: Oncology **Strategy:** The core issues of the question are interpreting the significance of dark red urine flow following prostatectomy and the ability to choose a corrective action. Interpret that the dark color is due to bleeding and then select an intervention that will reduce clot formation.

19 **Answer: 3 Rationale:** Ovarian cancer generally causes no warning signs or symptoms in the early stages, which is why screening is important. Painful urination, pelvic pain radiating to the thighs, and low back pain are not associated with this health problem. **Cognitive Level:** Applying **Client Need:** Physiological Adaptation **Integrated Process:** Nursing Process: Assessment **Content Area:** Adult Health: Oncology **Strategy:** The core issue of the question is knowledge of early signs of ovarian cancer. Use nursing knowledge and the process of elimination to make a selection.

20 **Answer: 2 Rationale:** In stage II ovarian cancer, tumor growth involves one or both ovaries with pelvic extension. In stage I, tumor growth is limited to the ovaries. In stage III, lymph nodes become positive. In stage IV, there is distant metastasis. **Cognitive Level:** Applying **Client Need:** Physiological Adaptation **Integrated Process:** Nursing Process: Diagnosis **Content Area:** Adult Health: Oncology **Strategy:** The core issue of the question is knowledge of the staging system for ovarian cancer. Use nursing knowledge and the process of elimination to make a selection.

21 **Answer: 1 Rationale:** A modified radical mastectomy involves removal of breast tissue and lymph nodes under the arm. A radical mastectomy includes removal of the entire breast, underlying chest muscles, and lymph nodes. A simple mastectomy involves removal of the breast tissue only, without any lymph node removal. A lumpectomy involves removal of the tumor and a margin of the surrounding tissues. **Cognitive Level:** Applying **Client Need:** Physiological Adaptation **Integrated Process:** Teaching and Learning **Content**

Area: Adult Health: Oncology **Strategy:** The core issue of the question is the ability to discriminate among various types of mastectomy procedures. Use nursing knowledge and the process of elimination to make a selection.

22 **Answer: 1 Rationale:** The head of bed cannot be raised more than about 15 degrees while the implant is in place to reduce the risk of dislodging the device from the effects of pressure and gravity. Visitors are restricted with respect to time and distance to avoid exposure to the radiation. High-fiber foods are discouraged during this time because bowel movements increase intra-abdominal pressure and could increase the risk of dislodging the implant. The client must remain on bedrest to avoid dislodging the device because of the effect of gravity. **Cognitive Level:** Analyzing **Client Need:** Physiological Adaptation **Integrated Process:** Communication and Documentation **Content Area:** Adult Health: Oncology **Strategy:** The core issue of the question is knowledge about internal radiation therapy. Use nursing knowledge and the process of elimination to make a selection.

23 **Answer: 1, 4 Rationale:** Continued increased fluid intake will help the urine to remain dilute and reduce the risk of clot formation. The healing period after prostate surgery is 4–8 weeks, and the client should avoid strenuous activity during this period. Blood in the urine is fairly common after surgery but only needs to be reported if it increases in amount instead of decreasing. The client should not drive for 2 weeks, except for short rides. The client should avoid heavy lifting for 4–8 weeks after surgery while healing continues. **Cognitive Level:** Applying **Client Need:** Physiological Adaptation **Integrated Process:** Teaching and Learning **Content Area:** Adult Health: Oncology **Strategy:** The core issue of the question is knowledge of postdischarge care to a client following prostate surgery. Use nursing knowledge and the process of elimination to make a selection.

24 **Answer: 4, 5 Rationale:** The arm should be elevated above heart level following mastectomy to reduce the risk of edema after lymph node removal on the affected side. Blood pressures and lab draws should be performed on the unaffected side. Warm, moist compresses could enhance edema formation. IV lines should not be used on the affected side at any location. Gentle, simple range-of-motion exercises can be started immediately after surgery. **Cognitive Level:** Applying **Client Need:** Physiological Adaptation **Integrated Process:** Nursing Process: Planning **Content Area:** Adult Health: Oncology **Strategy:** The core issue of the question is knowledge that edema is a risk following mastectomy and of nursing measures that can reduce this risk. Use nursing knowledge and the process of elimination to make a selection.

25 **Answer: 700 Rationale:** The total infused is 600 + 1500 = 2100 mL. The total drained was 800 + 1050 + 950 = 2800 mL. Subtract 2100 from 2800 to obtain 700 mL, the true urine output for the shift. **Cognitive Level:** Applying **Client Need:** Physiological Adaptation **Integrated Process:** Nursing Process: Implementation **Content Area:** Adult Health: Oncology **Strategy:** The principles for intake and output calculation are the same as for any other client. Tally first the intake, then the output, and subtract the difference to determine how much of the output is actually because of urinary drainage. Use knowledge of basic nursing procedures to calculate the answer.

Key Terms to Review

References

Ball, J., & Bindler, R., & Cowen, K. (2015). *Principles of pediatric nursing: Caring for children* (6th ed.). Hoboken, NJ: Pearson Education.

Berman, A., Snyder, S., & Frandsen, G. (2016). *Kozier & Erb's fundamentals of nursing: Concepts, process, and practice* (10th ed.). New York, NY: Pearson Education.

Ignatavicius, D., & Workman, L. (2016). *Medical-surgical nursing: Patient-centered collaborative care* (10th ed.). Philadelphia: Saunders.

Kee, J. (2017). *Pearson's handbook of laboratory and diagnostic tests* (8th ed.). New York, NY: Pearson Education.

LeMone, P., Burke, K., Bauldoff, G., & Gubrud, P. (2015). *Medical surgical nursing: Clinical reasoning in patient care* (6th ed.). Hoboken, NJ: Pearson Education.

Lewis, S., Dirksen, S., Heitkemper, M., & Bucher, L. (2014). *Medical surgical nursing: Assessment and management of clinical problems* (9th ed.). St. Louis, MO: Elsevier Science.

Smith, S., Duell, D., Martin, B., Aebersold, M., & Gonzalez, L. (2017). *Clinical nursing skills: Basic to advanced skills* (10th ed.). New York, NY: Pearson Education.

Immunologic Disorders

66

In this chapter

Cross Reference

Other chapters relevant to this content area are

Blood and Blood Component Therapy	Chapter 32
Immunologic and Anti-Infective Medications	Chapter 45
Common Laboratory Tests	Chapter 46
Common Diagnostic Tests and Procedures	Chapter 47
Respiratory Disorders	Chapter 55

I. OVERVIEW OF ANATOMY AND PHYSIOLOGY OF IMMUNE SYSTEM

A. Basic structures of immunologic system

1. Lymphoid system: consists of lymphoid organs (lymph nodes, spleen, thymus, and tonsils), lymphoid tissues (lymphocytes and plasma cells in mucosa and connective tissues), and bone marrow (myeloid tissue involved in blood cell formation)
2. Central lymphoid organs include thymus gland in mediastinum behind sternum (assists in T-lymphocyte formation) and bone marrow (long bones such as femur and humerus and flat bones of pelvis, ribs, and sternum)
3. Peripheral organs
   a. Tonsils are a group of lymphoid tissue found in palatine area of oropharynx
   b. A lymph node is a small, rounded mass of tissue from which lymph fluid drains; lymph nodes are found throughout body
   c. Mucosa-associated lymph tissue (MALT) consists of a group of lymph tissue found in many organs of body that work together to promote immune response; specific locators identify source of tissue, for example: bronchial-associated lymph tissue (BALT); gut-associated lymph tissue (GALT), also known as Peyer's patches; and skin-associated lymph tissue (SALT)

d. Spleen, located in left upper quadrant of abdomen, is composed of white and red pulp; white pulp is composed of B and T lymphocytes; red pulp is composed of erythrocytes

4. Mononuclear phagocyte system (MPS)
   a. Monocytes are largest component of white blood cells (WBCs) and have one nucleus and very little cytoplasm; considered to be agranulocytes
   b. Macrophages are mature cells of MPS that migrate to different areas of body, becoming specialized cells to perform function of defense
   c. MPS participates in immune response by secreting chemical components and factors (enzymes, complement proteins, and interleukins)

B. Basic functions of immunologic system

1. Thymus gland produces T lymphocytes, which are involved in **cell-mediated immunity**; secretes thymic hormones such as thymosin (stable from birth to age 25 and then gradually decreases as gland atrophies with age)
2. Bone marrow
   a. Provides for analysis of chemical markers that identify specific disease processes
   b. Gives rise to cellular components of blood and stores stem cells
   c. Gives rise to B lymphocytes and humorally mediated responses (**humoral immunity**) that involve production of **antibodies** (specific substances produced in response to specific antigens)
3. Spleen is a site of RBC destruction, a storage site for blood, and a reservoir for B lymphocytes to develop into mature plasma cells; it filters and removes foreign material, worn-out cells, and forms of cellular debris

C. Other immune system participants

1. Natural killer cell (null cell, NK cell) activity is present at birth, increases as individual reaches adulthood, and decreases gradually in old age; null cells do not require prior sensitization and are not considered T or B lymphocytes
2. Cytokines (also referred to as lymphokines and monokines) are soluble protein mediators of immune response; interleukins, tumor necrosis factor, and interferon are examples of these chemical messengers, which are treatment options in boosting immune response

D. Complement system

1. Group of glycoproteins activated in sequential order; provide a link to humoral response
2. IgG and IgM are responsible for activating complement cascade; once activated, complement has been fixed or **complement fixation** has taken place
3. Complement assays diagnose immunodeficiencies and autoimmune diseases
4. There is a classic pathway and an alternate pathway whereby complement system can be activated

E. Biological response modifiers (BRMs)

1. Group of substances that can elicit, modify, and restore biological response between an individual and a tumor cell
2. Examples
   NCLEX® a. **Monoclonal antibodies** (produced by a specific group of identical cells), may be used to treat tumors because of their specific targeting effect
   NCLEX® b. **Colony-stimulating factors** (a group of proteins that stimulate growth of either RBCs or WBCs) prevent or help reduce a client's adverse response to disease; these types of BRMs are used in a variety of hematologic and immunologic diseases

II. NORMAL IMMUNE RESPONSE

A. Defense

1. Nonspecific defenses are external reactions that include anatomic and chemical barriers such as skin and mucous membranes; nonspecific defenses are activated against any foreign substance that body encounters
2. Specific defenses are internal physiological reactions that include both cell-mediated and humorally mediated antibodies; antibodies are unique substances that require activation
3. Immune response is activated in presence of an **antigen**, a protein substance that triggers antibody production

B. Homeostasis: body seeks to maintain a balanced response of circulating and resident lymphocytes to maintain adequate protection

C. Surveillance: body's ability to use memory and recognition to maintain an immune response even if person doesn't remember a specific insult

Table 66–1 Types of Immunoglobulins

Class	Location	Characteristic
IgA	Body secretions, tears, saliva Colostrum and breast milk	Lines mucous membranes; protects body surfaces
IgD	Plasma	Present on lymphocytes
IgE	Plasma, interstitial fluid Exocrine secretions	Allergic response, anaphylaxis; bound to mast cells
IgG	Plasma, interstitial fluid	Crosses placenta; complement fixation; secondary immune response
IgM	Plasma	Complement fixation; primary immune response; involved in ABO antigens

III. TYPES OF IMMUNITY

A. Acquired immunity

1. Long-term response that leads to development of antibodies that offer protection
   a. Individual develops antibodies in response to having a disease process or by a response to artificial antigens such as a vaccine or toxoid
   b. Response can be boosted and maintained via repeated injections
   c. Titer serum levels can be monitored to indicate status of immunity

NCLEX®
2. Passive acquired immunity requires an antibody be introduced to individual, either by maternal transfer (placenta and/or colostrum) or immune serum antibody injection, to promote a specific antigen response

B. Natural immunity: related to a species, race, or genetic trait; an individual is born with natural immunity

C. Humoral immunity

1. Involves recognition of antigens by B lymphocytes
2. B lymphocytes differentiate into plasma cells and memory cells
3. Memory cells lead to a more rapid response by remembering an original insult
4. Plasma cells secrete **immunoglobulins**, a group of glycoproteins, each of which has four polypeptide chains (two heavy and two light chains); the FAB fragment, which is different in each immunoglobulin, denotes specific antigen-binding sites
5. Immunoglobulins are identified as IgA, IgD, IgE, IgG, and IgM; see Table 66–1 for listing and characteristics of immunoglobulins

D. Cell-mediated immunity

1. T lymphocytes recognize a specific **major histocompatibility complex (MHC)**, a group of proteins that participate in autoimmune recognition and tissue rejection, and bind to them to elicit an immune response
2. Protein markers on surface of T cell help define specific function receptor sites; these are called CD antigens or clusters of differentiation; CD markers serve as an important prognostic indicator of immune function and are used to diagnose and manage human immunodeficiency virus (HIV) and acquired immunodeficiency syndrome (AIDS)

NCLEX®
3. Humoral immunity is considered a long-term process whereby T lymphocytes help protect body against bacterial, viral, and fungal infections

NCLEX®
4. Cell-mediated immunity is also responsible for mediation of transplant rejection

IV. COMMON TESTS AND PROCEDURES OF IMMUNE SYSTEM

A. Skin testing

1. A small quantity of allergen is introduced into skin by scratching or intradermal (ID) injection
2. A scratch test is used to test many antigens at a single time; has lower sensitivity than injection, but many allergens can be tested at once and results can be obtained in 30 minutes
3. ID injection is more accurate but leads to higher incidence of systemic reactions
4. Patch test evaluates contact allergens by applying allergen directly to skin and covering with a dressing

NCLEX®
5. Antihistamines that could impair immune response should be discontinued 72 hours prior to skin testing

NCLEX®
6. Immediate positive reaction usually occurs within 10–30 minutes and consists of wheal formation and erythema formation greater than 3 millimeters of a positive control (histamine)

NCLEX®
7. Minor itching at site can be relieved by cool compresses, topical steroids, and topical or oral antihistamines

B. Radioallergosorbent test (RAST)

1. Reveals elevated levels of IgE associated with **atopy** (allergic reactions stemming from hereditary disposition)
2. Allergen is usually planted on a surface such as a paper disk
3. Client blood is then applied to surface and incubated
4. Antibodies specific to an allergen bind to allergen, but others wash away, and level of IgE can be measured
5. More sensitive than skin testing but also more time-consuming and expensive

C. Pulmonary function tests to diagnose asthma (see Chapter 55)

D. Immunoglobulin and complement assays may be positive

E. Eosinophilia may be present with allergic disease

V. HYPERSENSITIVITY REACTIONS

A. ***Hypersensitivity*** is an abnormal exaggerated immune response to a specific substance

B. **The Gell and Coombs Classification of Hypersensitivity Reactions** categorizes a reaction according to type, class, and immunity (see Table 66–2)

C. **Type I:** anaphylactoid reactions

1. Involves an immediate response but responses can also be cumulative; for example, initial or sensitizing dose may not elicit a strong response, but subsequent contacts (even if short term) can cause a stronger response
2. Involves activation of IgE bound to mast cells, with release of histamine
3. Localized hypersensitivity responses as seen in conditions such as asthma, allergic rhinitis (hay fever), conjunctivitis, and atopic dermatitis; general hypersensitivity response is an anaphylactic response

NCLEX®

4. Clinical manifestations range from bronchospasm, wheezing, rhinorrhea, and urticaria to angioedema and finally anaphylaxis; there may be progression from local to systemic reactions; characteristic allergic "gape" (continuous open-mouth breathing) and allergic "shiner" (dark circles under eyes from congestion in small local blood vessels) can be seen in individuals with atopy (localized responses)
5. Diagnostic and laboratory test findings: immunoglobulin titers are predictive of potential allergen response; skin and patch testing determine potential allergens

NCLEX®

6. Therapeutic management
   a. **Antihistamine** medications such as diphenhydramine block chemical release of mediators (histamines)
   b. Mast cell degradation inhibitors such as cromolyn sodium also block chemical response
   c. Decongestants and corticosteroids help minimize immune response; however, in potential anaphylactic reactions, use of epinephrine is warranted; an Epipen may be prescribed for those at profound risk for hypersensitivity reactions and are available in adult and pediatric dosages
   d. Immediately withdraw offending allergen in presence of documented or suspected reaction
   e. Manage client according to ABC (airway, breathing, and circulation) protocol

D. Type II: cytotoxic and cytolytic reactions

1. Involves activation of complement and is considered a form of humoral immunity
   a. Involves production of autoantibodies that destroy own cells or tissues
   b. IgA and IgM are involved with this type of response

NCLEX®

2. Clinical manifestations: range from hemolytic reactions (such as transfusion, erythroblastosis fetalis, hemolytic anemia, and drug-induced hemolysis) to target cell destruction as in Goodpasture syndrome (autoimmune disease affecting pulmonary and renal systems) and other autoimmune disease processes such as myasthenia gravis and Graves disease
3. Diagnostic and laboratory test findings: Coombs blood test can define presence of hemolytic anemia and identify potential ABO incompatibility

Table 66–2 Gell and Coombs Classification

Type	Class	Immunity
I	Immediate hypersensitivity	Humoral
II	Cytotoxic reactions	Humoral
III	Immune complex related	Humoral
IV	Delayed hypersensitivity	Cell-mediated

NCLEX®

4. Therapeutic management
   a. Use proper identification during blood product administration to prevent exposure and sensitization
   b. Detect reactions early by awareness that certain blood types and potential drug interactions can cause antigen complex activation
   c. Remain with client during first 15 minutes of any blood product administration because clients are more likely to experience a reaction during this time
   d. Make sure to follow agency policy and procedure when administering all blood products; see also Chapter 32

E. Type III: immune complex reactions

1. Involves formation of **antigen–antibody complexes** (a binding-together of an antibody and an antigen)
   a. Leads to activation of serum factors, causing inflammation and leading to activation of complement cascade
   b. Rheumatoid arthritis (RA) and systemic lupus erythematosus (SLE) are examples of Type III reactions
   c. Deposits of antigen–antibody complexes in body tissues are not localized and can result in extensive tissue or organ destruction
2. Complement activation impacts vulnerable organs and leads to intravascular changes

NCLEX®

3. Clinical manifestations
   a. Arthrus reaction involves a localized inflammatory response with excess IgG causing edema and necrotic lesions
   b. Serum sickness involves a systemic response leading to deposit and activation of complement throughout body manifested as joint pain, pyrexia, and/or lymphadenopathy
   c. Reactions can be acute or chronic in nature
4. Diagnostic and laboratory test findings: complement assays indicate acute and/or chronic process; erythrocyte sedimentation rate (ESR) is elevated; proteinuria may be found on urinalysis

NCLEX®

5. Therapeutic management
   a. Analgesics, antihistamines and topical steroids may provide symptom relief; disease process is usually self-limiting because of use of human antitetanus serum and availability of antibiotics
   b. Assess for localized inflammatory reactions that may develop at site of serum injections after 1 week; this can be followed by a more systemic response involving both regional as well as generalized lymphadenopathies
   c. If symptoms arise, monitor client for potential complications because organ damage can occur and kidneys can be compromised

F. Type IV: delayed hypersensitivity reactions

1. Form of cell-mediated immunity involving T lymphocytes; considered a delayed response
2. Involve recognition and response of T lymphocytes to foreign substances

NCLEX®

3. Clinical manifestations
   a. Wide range of presentations from tuberculin response, poison ivy, and contact dermatitis to transplant or graft rejection; edema, ischemia, and eventual tissue destruction may ensue
   b. Pyrexia, pain, edema, and failure of transplanted organ characterize transplant rejection
4. Diagnostic and laboratory test findings: purified protein derivative (PPD) test result of induration more than 5 mm identifies type IV hypersensitivity to tubercle bacillus; abnormal test results indicating declining function of transplanted organ are used to diagnose transplant rejection

NCLEX®

5. Therapeutic management
   a. Monitor client for evidence of potential transplant rejection
   b. Medicate client with immunosuppressive drugs to prevent tissue rejection
   c. Identify potential irritants that can cause contact dermatitis and avoid exposure
   d. Teach client to avoid offending irritant if a past exposure has been documented
   e. Use topical and oral medications as indicated to alleviate many symptoms and increase client comfort

VI. ANAPHYLAXIS

A. Overview

1. Sudden, severe allergic reaction mediated by massive histamine release from cells
2. Common causes are drugs, foods (especially nuts and shellfish), latex exposure, insect bites, and stings
3. Can lead to shock state and death if not treated immediately
4. Onset of symptoms can be within minutes to an hour, with more rapid onset associated with severe episode

NCLEX® **B. Nursing assessment**

1. Skin erythema, hives and urticaria, angioedema (swelling of the face, lips, neck, and/or tongue)
2. Dyspnea and wheezing, respiratory obstruction, and difficulty swallowing
3. Syncope, hypotension, shock
4. Circulatory collapse and possible death

NCLEX® **C. Therapeutic management**

1. Maintain patent airway and administer oxygen
2. Administer prescribed subcutaneous epinephrine injection
3. Remove or discontinue causative agent
4. Place in modified Trendelenburg position for shock
5. Administer IV fluids such as normal saline or lactated Ringer's to support circulation
6. Provide antihistamines or corticosteroids as prescribed
7. Provide supportive care to stabilize client and emotional support

D. Client teaching

1. Avoid future contact with allergen
2. Wear Medic-Alert identification listing allergy
3. Tell all future caregivers about allergy and symptoms
4. Learn how to use epinephrine auto-injector pen

VII. AUTOIMMUNE DISORDERS

A. Overview

1. Involves abnormal immune system response whereby body perceives "self" as a threat; mechanisms of action can include cell-mediated, antibody-mediated, and immune complex reactions
2. Genetic component of autoimmune response: **human leukocyte antigens (HLAs)**, genetic markers found on chromosome 6, are involved with diagnosis of many autoimmune diseases and are also used for tissue typing
3. Cell-mediated autoimmunity: associated with an abnormal T-cell response, such as an excess of T-cytotoxic (killer) cells or deficiency of T-suppressor (helper) cells
4. Antibody-mediated autoimmunity: involves development of autoantibodies and complement activation that affects specific receptor sites, causing tissue and organ damage (examples include Graves' disease and myasthenia gravis)
5. Immune complex disease: associated with deposition of immune complexes at serum level; complement activation causes inflammatory reactions and leads to further damage
6. Diagnostic testing for autoimmunity
   a. Autoantibody assays, complement fixation, and complement assays diagnose disorder
   b. Identification of HLA antigens provides indication of genetic inheritance
7. Treatment for autoimmunity
   a. Immunosuppressive agents and corticosteroids suppress abnormal immune response
   b. Symptom management can be achieved with anti-inflammatory agents to minimize pain from tissue damage caused by immune complex deposits
   c. **Plasmapheresis** removes circulating immune complexes; in this treatment, plasma is removed from body, sent through a machine membrane that traps immune complexes, and returned to body
8. Progression of disease
   a. Autoimmune diseases are chronic conditions characterized by acute exacerbations (called flares or flare-ups) and remissions
   b. Splenectomy has been performed as part of therapeutic management of many autoimmune diseases, but its removal is not guaranteed as a form of therapeutic management; alternative therapeutic regimens to splenectomy are chemotherapy and use of biological response modifiers

B. Systemic lupus erythematosus (SLE)

1. Overview
   a. Chronic inflammatory systemic autoimmune disease characterized by deposits of antigen–antibody complexes in connective tissue of blood vessels, lymphatic tissues, and other sites such as kidneys, spleen, GI tract, lungs, brain, heart, musculoskeletal system, skin, and peritoneum
   b. Over time, deposits cause cell and tissue damage and can lead to eventual major organ system failure
   c. Course is mild in most clients with periods of exacerbation and remission, with exacerbations decreasing in number and severity over time, but some clients have more virulent disease
   d. Two forms: discoid and systemic; discoid involves characteristic skin rash without systemic disease while systemic form involves entire system response

e. Exact etiology is uncertain, but may include genetics (certain human leukocyte antigen [HLA] genes), hormonal imbalance (higher risk in women using estrogen-containing oral contraceptives or hormone replacement), and environmental factors (exposure to viruses, silica dust, ultraviolet light exposure, and cigarette smoking)

NCLEX®

2. Nursing assessment
   a. Environmental triggers such as ultraviolet (UV) light, viral or other infection, other stressors, and/or drugs (such as procainamide, hydralazine, and isoniazid)
   b. Painful, swollen joints and muscle pain
   c. Butterfly rash (malar rash) across bridge of nose and cheeks or erythema of face; possible erythema of palms
   d. Weakness, fatigue, and general malaise
   e. Pale or cyanotic fingers and toes, edema in legs and around eyes, possible alopecia
   f. Other symptoms according to target organ involvement such as pleuritis and pleural effusions (lungs), renal failure (kidneys), or anorexia, nausea, abdominal pain, and diarrhea (GI)
   g. Central nervous system (CNS) involvement: photosensitivity, subtle behavioral changes, possible stroke or seizure activity
   h. Hematologic involvement: altered immune responses with anemia (decreased RBC count), leukopenia (noted by infection and fever), thrombocytopenia (low platelet count), and even hemolytic anemia (positive Coombs test)
   i. Pregnancy and use of oral contraceptives can affect estrogen level and may pose an increased risk for disease flare-ups
   j. A positive ANA titer
   k. During flare-ups, decreased complement (C_3 and C_4), elevated ESR and C-reactive protein (CRP), and positive rheumatoid factor (+RF)
   l. Urinalysis may reveal mild proteinuria, hematuria, and blood cell casts during flare-ups if kidneys are involved; creatinine levels may rise as renal involvement progresses

NCLEX®

3. Therapeutic management
   a. Aimed at recognizing flare-ups and preventing further complications; individually adjusted to disease activity
   b. Conservative measures include rest and general supportive pharmacotherapy; aggressive measures include splenectomy and chemotherapy
   c. Collaborate with dietitian to support metabolic needs and immune functions
   d. Plan for rest periods to avoid fatigue and lessen client's stress levels
   e. Avoid environmental triggers such as prolonged UV light exposure that may trigger skin eruptions; consider risk of photosensitivity when planning care
   f. Clients with SLE should try to have a planned pregnancy; alternative birth control methods such as diaphragm and condoms should be used because oral contraceptives can affect estrogen level
   g. Nonsteroidal anti-inflammatory drugs (NSAIDs) and acetylsalicylic acid (aspirin, ASA) are used to control joint pain experienced by most clients
   h. Hydroxychloroquine is used to treat dermatologic symptoms
   i. Glucocorticoids suppress disease activity and provide symptom management during flare-ups; oral or IV route is preferred; tapered dose therapy (pulse dose) is usually initiated to achieve best results to arrive at lowest possible dosage and to prevent side effects
   j. Immunosuppressive agents such as cyclophosphamide and azathiopine may modulate immune response; however, client will be at increased risk for **myelosuppression** (inhibition or destruction of bone marrow) with this regimen and must be monitored accordingly
   k. Gamma globulin can be given IV to promote specific immune function
   l. Plasmapheresis removes immune complexes to help relieve symptoms
4. Client teaching
   a. Likelihood of flare-ups and chronic nature of disease
   b. Self-monitoring of condition to identify potential health problems more quickly
   c. Potential dynamic life changes such as pregnancy and childbearing may influence disease activity
   d. Medication therapy

C. Rheumatoid arthritis (RA)

1. Overview
   a. Systemic disorder involving symmetrical inflammation of synovial membranes and joints that leads to deformities and loss of joint function
   b. Clinical course has periods of remission and exacerbation, but underlying disease process is chronic

c. Thought to be associated with deposits of antigen–antibody complexes and development of rheumatoid nodules
d. RA has a bimodal appearance: there is a juvenile form (JRA) as well as more common adult form

NCLEX®

2. Nursing assessment
   a. Fatigue, general malaise, and anorexia and weight loss
   b. Persistent joint pain lasting more than 3 months that is more evident on motion, but pain at rest can occur
   c. Characteristic morning stiffness lasting more than 1 hour; note onset, duration, and joints involved
   d. Tenderness, swelling, and restricted range of motion in affected joints
   e. With disease progression and less stable joints, characteristic deformities such as swan neck deformity, Boutonniere deformity, subcutaneous nodules, and ulnar deviation or drift (see Figure 66–1) develop
   f. Systemic signs range from fever to splenomegaly and reflect extra-articular findings
   g. Possible joint effusions
   h. +RF is a nonspecific finding because it may be found in healthy population as well
   i. Elevated ESR, CRP, and serum complement
   j. CBC with differential may reveal anemia as well as leukocytosis
   k. X-rays reveal a narrowing of joint spaces and erosive changes at bone margins as disease progresses
   l. Aspiration of synovial fluid reveals turbidity, elevated cell counts, and formation of a poor mucin clot

NCLEX®

3. Therapeutic management
   a. Major treatment goal: help client maintain ability to function
   b. Treatment measures are aimed at decreasing joint pain and swelling
   c. Identify assistive devices needed in client's environment to aid function
   d. Modify client's schedule as needed to incorporate rest periods
   e. Include nonpharmacologic pain relief measures such as imagery and biofeedback
   f. Use heat and cold applications to affected joints to provide relief; individualize these measures to provide maximum comfort
   g. Include foods high in omega-3 fatty acids, since current research shows that these are beneficial to clients who have RA and other diseases such as heart disease; suggested food items include fish oils and salmon

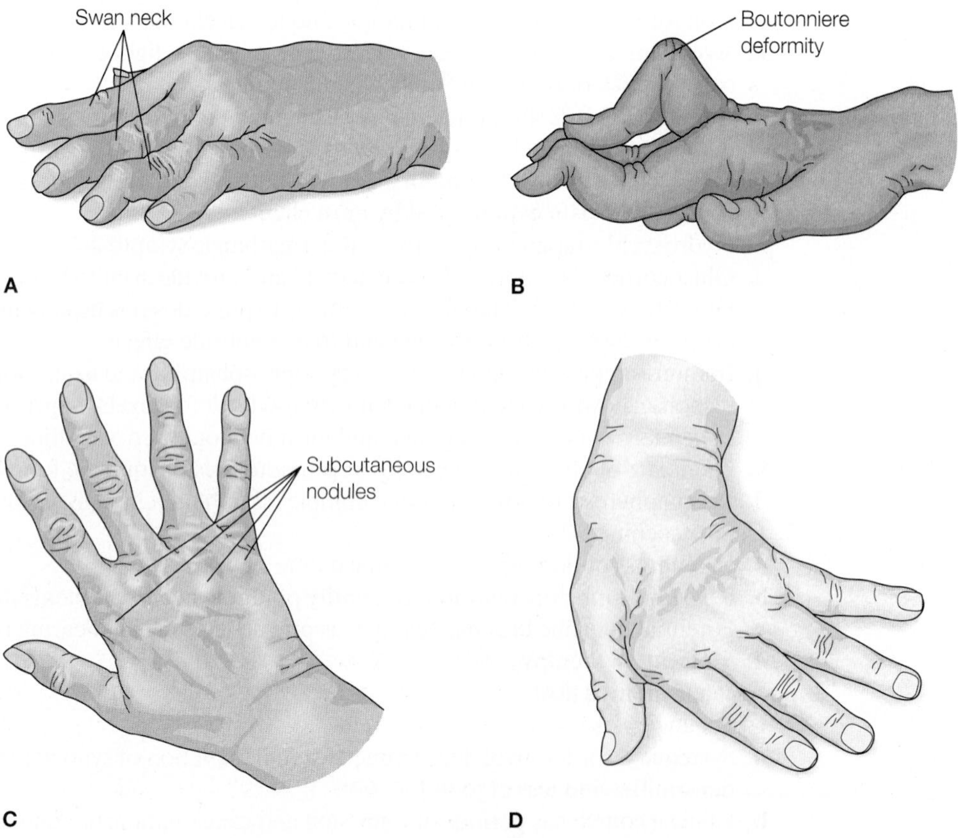

Figure 66–1

Characteristic hand deformities in rheumatoid arthritis. (**A**) Swan-neck deformity; (**B**) Boutonniere deformity; (**C**) subcutaneous nodules; (**D**) ulnar deviation.

h. ASA and NSAIDs decrease joint inflammation and control symptoms
i. Disease-modifying antirheumatic drugs (DMARDs) slow rate of disease progression; examples include antimalarial agent hydroxychloroquine, sulfasalazine, leflunomide, and minocycline
j. Methotrexate, an immunosuppressive agent, has onset of action similar to other DMARDs; dosage is adjusted to get maximum response at lowest dose; may be used in combination with etanercept, a tumor necrosis factor
k. Other immunosuppressive agents such as azathioprine and cyclophosphamide are used in severe, disabling RA or RA refractory to other treatments

4. Client teaching
a. Refer to a rheumatologist to coordinate management of care
b. Occurrence of flare-ups and chronic nature of disease process
c. Importance of adequate symptom management for optimal level of function
d. Importance of client self-monitoring and adherence to treatment plan
e. Potential dynamic life changes that might occur as a result of progression of deformity and loss of function

D. Scleroderma: systemic sclerosis (SS)

1. Overview
a. A multisystem disease with fibrosis (hardening) of visceral organs and skin; leads to inability of involved organs to function with normal motility
b. CREST syndrome is a specific, more limited form of disease

Memory Aid

Remember CREST to identify a form of systemic sclerosis:
*C*alcium deposits
*R*aynaud's syndrome
*E*sophageal dysmotility
*S*clerodactyly (scleroderma digits)
*T*eleangiectasia (spider nevi)

c. Systemic sclerosis morphea is a specific disease form that affects only skin
d. Mild disease may go unrecognized unless it progresses or other medical issues bring it to forefront
e. Has unknown etiology with underlying common factors: inflammation, vasoconstriction, and abnormal immune function and connective tissue

NCLEX®

2. Nursing assessment
a. Skin changes occur in two phases; painless, symmetrical, and edematous changes occur first, then indurative changes lead to hardening and thickening of skin
b. GI tract changes can lead to dysphagia, esophageal reflux, malabsorption, and bowel obstruction
c. Cardiovascular changes: Raynaud's phenomenon (vasospastic disease), secondary bacterial endocarditis, myocardial fibrosis, left-ventricular (LV) dysfunction, and heart failure
d. Respiratory changes can result from lung restriction caused by fibrosis
e. Renal changes lead to uremia, malignant hypertension, and finally renal failure
f. Often seen in conjunction with *Sjögren's syndrome*, an autoimmune disease affecting lacrimal and salivary glands, causing dry mucous membranes
g. Laboratory results: low ANA titer, SCL-70 antibody, elevated ESR, and positive RF
h. Anticentromere antibodies indicate a good prognosis because they are associated with a more limited form of disease
i. Mild hypochromic, microcytic anemia can be seen in some clients
j. Imaging and other studies may detect specific organ system involvement, such as GI, pulmonary, heart, kidney, and skin

NCLEX®

3. Therapeutic management
a. Treatment is aimed at supportive and palliative measures; care should be coordinated by a rheumatologist
b. Dialysis may be indicated if renal function deteriorates
c. If end-organ failure develops, renal or lung transplant may be indicated
d. Develop a support system for client and family members to help them cope with stressors of chronic disease
e. Identify potential complications as they affect client, and coordinate healthcare team approach to manage developing risk situations

f. Protect client's extremities from temperature changes that can exacerbate Raynaud's syndrome; encourage client to use gloves during activities that can affect temperature changes (such as washing dishes)
g. Medication therapy includes calcium channel blockers and peripheral alpha$_1$-adrenergic blocking agents (for symptoms of Raynaud's disease), anti-inflammatory agents (joint pain), H_2 receptor antagonists and proton pump inhibitors (esophageal reflux), angiotensin-converting enzyme (ACE) inhibitors (hypertension), antibiotics (secondary bowel infections caused by decreased motility)
h. O_2 therapy is used to support pulmonary function

4. Client teaching
   a. Importance of adequate symptom management
   b. Chronic nature of disease process
   c. Support client and family members with diagnosis and impact that no known cause exists; provide anticipatory guidance
   d. Client may be referred to a rheumatologist to coordinate care management

E. Polyarteritis nodosa

1. Overview
   a. Collagen disease that leads to inflammation of arteries and subsequent thickening with impaired circulation
   b. Etiology is unknown and often affects middle-aged men
   c. Cardiac and renal sequelae are most serious complications
2. Nursing assessment
   a. Low-grade fever
   b. Weakness and fatigue
   c. Weight loss, abdominal pain, and bloody diarrhea
   d. Elevated ESR
3. Therapeutic management
   a. Provide supportive care, emotional support, and anticipatory guidance
   b. Initiate support services depending on need
   c. Corticosteroids and analgesics manage inflammation and pain
4. Client teaching
   a. Importance of well-balanced diet
   b. Need for follow-up care
   c. Medication therapy
   d. Energy conservation measures

F. Pemphigus

1. Overview: a rare skin disorder of unknown etiology in middle-aged and older adults that begins with lesions on oral mucosa and spreads to generalized body areas
2. Nursing assessment
   a. Bullae that are fragile and appear flaccid; ruptured bullae result in partial-thickness lesions that weep, form crusts, and may bleed
   b. Malaise and pain
   c. Impaired chewing and swallowing
   d. Nikolsky's sign: when skin is rubbed, epidermis separates from underlying skin
   e. Foul-smelling skin discharge
   f. Leukocytosis and eosinophilia
3. Therapeutic management
   a. Oral hygiene and measures to soothe oral lesions
   b. Baths with oatmeal or potassium permanganate for relief of skin symptoms
   NCLEX® c. Medication therapy including topical or systemic antibiotics (secondary infections) and corticosteroids or cytotoxic agents (as immunosuppressants)
   d. Provide general supportive care
4. Client teaching: need for follow-up care and medication therapy

G. Goodpasture syndrome

1. Overview: autoimmune disorder characterized by autoantibody formation that often acts against basement membranes in glomerulus of kidney and alveoli of lungs; etiology is uncertain but smoking is strongly associated with condition
2. Nursing assessment
   a. Pulmonary symptoms include shortness of breath and possible hemoptysis
   b. Renal symptoms include decreasing urine output, edema, weight gain, and hypertension
   c. Cardiovascular effects of fluid retention also include tachycardia

3. Therapeutic management
   a. Provide supportive management of respiratory symptoms, including positioning, pulmonary hygiene measures, oxygen therapy if prescribed, and energy conservation measures
   b. Provide standard care to client with declining renal function (monitoring intake and output, BUN and creatinine levels, and signs of renal failure)
   c. NCLEX® Specific therapies include corticosteroid drug therapy and plasmapheresis to remove autoantibodies
4. Client teaching: nature of disease and its progression, medication therapy, energy conservation measures, when to contact healthcare provider

VIII. PRIMARY IMMUNODEFICIENCY DISORDERS

A. Overview

1. Caused by a primary defect or deficiency involving B lymphocytes, T lymphocytes, complement or phagocytic cells that results in severe recurrent or chronic infection (see Table 66–3 for a listing of selected primary immunodeficiency diseases)
2. Involve specific genetic alterations in immune response seen in infants and young children

B. Nursing assessment

1. Overall immune response is abnormal, leading to opportunistic infections that cause tissue and organ damage to heart and lungs over time because immune response cannot be supported
2. NCLEX® Signs and symptoms of infection and inflammation: fever, chills, cough (nonproductive or productive), difficulty swallowing or breathing, erythema, edema, or drainage
3. Diarrhea either due to overwhelming infection by offending agents or in response to antimicrobial therapy
4. CBC with differential, ESR, antibody titers, ANA, ANC (absolute neutrophil count), and culture and sensitivity of pertinent areas may all provide a baseline and identify potential source(s) of infection
5. Immunoglobulin and complement assay levels provide an overview of immune system function

C. Therapeutic management

1. NCLEX® Therapy is most effective when aimed at infection prophylaxis, early treatment of infections, and replacement of immunologic factors
2. Bone marrow transplant (BMT) and/or thymus transplant may be indicated depending on the severity of presentation
3. Identify clients who present with repeated infections
4. Support family members with impending diagnosis of chronic medical condition
5. Collaborate with healthcare team members to establish treatment goals
6. Refer clients of childbearing families for genetic counseling
7. Assist client and family in decisions regarding lifestyle changes to reduce infection
8. Collaborate with healthcare team members to support the client's ADLs and lifestyle changes during this hospitalization and after discharge
9. Antimicrobial therapy may be started to prevent infection or treat current infection
10. NCLEX® Depending on nature of organism, antifungals may be warranted
11. NCLEX® Gamma globulins may be needed to support and maintain deficient immunoglobulin levels
12. NCLEX® Colony-stimulating factors may be used to boost immune response

D. Client teaching

1. Genetic counseling
2. Antimicrobial therapy, including treatment, response, and need for long-term compliance
3. NCLEX® Importance of prevention and protection from high-risk environments that could lead to further infection

Table 66–3 Selected Primary Immunodeficiency Disorders

Disorder	Immune Cell Problem
X-linked hypogammaglobulinemia	B lymphocytes
Selective IgA deficiency	B lymphocytes
Common variable immunodeficiency	B lymphocytes
DiGeorge's syndrome	T lymphocytes
X-linked immunodeficiency with hyper-IgM	T lymphocytes
Severe combined immunodeficiency syndrome (SCID)	B, T lymphocytes
Graft-versus-host disease	B, T lymphocytes
Wiskott-Aldrich syndrome	B, T lymphocytes

IX. POST-TRANSPLANT (SECONDARY) IMMUNODEFICIENCY

A. Overview

1. State of immunodeficiency caused by drug therapy to prevent rejection of transplanted organs
2. Immunosuppressant drugs have unintended effects of increasing risk of infection or malignancy

B. Nursing assessment

1. Monitor temperature (may not be a reliable indicator of infection in an immunosuppressed client)
2. Monitor WBC count (increased immature WBCs [bands] may indicate infection)
3. Assess for signs of organ transplant rejection (indicates insufficient level of immunosuppression)
4. *NCLEX®* Assess clients for signs of infection, such as respiratory infection, urinary tract infection, or wound infection or communicable disease infections such as tuberculosis or shingles from reactivation of varicella-zoster virus
5. Assess client for **opportunistic infections** (nonpathogenic infections that become pathogenic because of a baseline immunosuppressed state) such as yeast (fungal) infections
6. Assess client for signs of cancer, especially of skin and lips, and lymphoid cancers

C. Therapeutic management

1. *NCLEX®* Initiate neutropenic precautions as indicated by client's immune status
2. Maintain adequate nutrient intake including supplemental feedings for healing and immune function
3. Adhere to agency policy for IV bag and tubing changes (every 24 hours) and IV site changes (every 72–96 hours)
4. Provide or assist with regular mouth care to reduce oral microorganism count
5. Assist or remind client to use meticulous hand hygiene before eating and after using bathroom

D. Client teaching: proper aseptic technique to reduce infection, signs and symptoms of infection and malignancy to watch for and report, and immunosuppressant drug therapy (see also Chapter 45)

X. ACQUIRED IMMUNODEFICIENCY SYNDROME (AIDS)

A. Overview

1. Immune deficiency disorder caused by human immunodeficiency virus (HIV), which infects and destroys T cells, resulting in increased risk of certain infections and developing certain types of cancers
2. Primary HIV infection (transmitted by contact with infected blood or other body fluids) is associated with development of flu-like symptoms that may or may not be recalled by client; a clinical latency period follows lasting from 3 years to more than 15 years (with treatment) or to about 10 years (without treatment) during which client is asymptomatic
3. Groups at high risk of contracting HIV include those who use IV drugs, have unprotected sexual contact, or receive contaminated blood products; other groups at risk include healthcare personnel and infants with perinatal transmission (in utero, during delivery, and/or through breastfeeding)
4. Initial diagnosis of HIV infection can be done using enzyme-linked immunosorbent assay (ELISA) to detect development of antibodies to HIV (results are positive or negative); Western blot is used to confirm HIV infection because it detects both HIV antibodies and individual viral components that cause reactive bands (results are positive or negative)
5. *NCLEX®* Progression from HIV to AIDS is marked by presence of one or more AIDS-defining illnesses such as malignancies, opportunistic infections, and/or neurologic diseases; pulmonary TB, recurrent pneumonia, and invasive cervical cancer are also considered AIDS-defining diseases (see Table 66–4 for a listing of infections and malignancies related to AIDS)
6. Monitoring of disease progression in AIDS includes CD4 lymphocyte counts and viral load testing (such as polymerase chain reaction or RT-PCR assay and bDNA assay) and nonspecific measures such as albumin levels, ESR, and serum chemistries

Table 66–4 AIDS Infections and Malignancies

Classification	Type
Bacterial infection	Mycobacterium avium complex (MAC)
Fungal infection	Candidiasis, cryptococcus neoformans, histoplasmosis
Protozoan infection	Pneumocystis jerovici, toxoplasmosis, cryptosporidium
Viral infection	Cytomegalovirus (CMV)
Cancer	Kaposi's sarcoma, associated lymphomas

7. Other diagnostic tests, such as skin biopsy or imaging studies, may be indicated depending on organ or system involvement and disease progression

B. Nursing assessment

1. Flu-like symptoms such as fever, malaise, joint aches, and anorexia with initial infection
2. Lymphadenopathy can persist for 3 months after initial infection
3. Fatigue
4. Diarrhea
5. Night sweats
6. Oral lesions such as hairy leukoplakia, candidiasis, and gingival inflammation and ulceration
7. Involuntary weight loss and **wasting syndrome** (weight loss of more than 10% ideal body weight associated with cachexia) later in disease process

NCLEX®

8. Signs of opportunistic infections such as oral candidiasis, vaginal candida (yeast) infection, *Pneumocystis jiroveci* pneumonia, histoplasmosis, and viral infections (see Table 66–4 again for full listing)
9. Signs of HIV-associated neurocognitive disorders (HAND) including memory loss, confusion, difficulty concentrating, lethargy, diminished motor speed, and eventual dementia (late signs)
10. Signs of AIDS-associated malignancies such as Kaposi's sarcoma (affecting skin and viscera), lymphomas, and cervical cancer

C. Therapeutic management

1. Assess nutritional status and hydration level, carefully noting baseline weight changes and alterations in taste perceptions
2. Consult with dietitian to analyze client's nutritional requirements and provide high-protein, high-kilocalorie diet to maintain IBW; aggressive nutritional support at time of HIV-positive diagnosis may prevent or deter possible effects of wasting and malnutrition

NCLEX®

3. Provide specific nutrition-related measures, such as small, frequent meals, fluids between meals, and dry crackers to help if mealtime nausea is present
4. Reduce discomfort if oral lesions are present by providing soft, nonspicy and nonacidic foods, and beverages that are neither too warm nor too cold

NCLEX®

5. Explain to client that dairy products, fish, and poultry tend to be better tolerated than red meat when client experiences altered taste
6. Use sorbets as palate cleansers, zinc supplementation, and plastic instead of metal utensils to reduce altered taste perception
7. Premedicate as needed with antiemetics for N/V and appetite stimulants such as oral progesterones for anorexia
8. Monitor for potential fluid losses, especially if diarrhea is present, and electrolyte imbalances, including hyponatremia
9. Assess for interruptions in skin integrity caused by infection or poor healing and provide standard interventions for immobilized client such as repositioning every 2 hours, keeping skin clean and dry, and using mild, nondrying soaps or oils during skin cleansing

NCLEX®

10. Encourage client and family support group to express thoughts and feelings about impact of disease, and explore strategies to manage life issues that will be affected by disease process
11. Administer prescribed antiretroviral medications including nucleoside reverse transcriptase inhibitors (NRTIs), non-nucleoside analogue reverse transcriptase inhibitors (NNRTIs), protease inhibitors, entry inhibitors, and integrase inhibitor; see also Chapter 45
12. Administer medications such as antibacterials and antifungals as prescribed to treat primary and secondary (opportunistic) infections
13. Provide vaccination against preventable illnesses as prescribed by healthcare provider
14. Refer client to home health services, respite services, and/or hospice services according to need
15. Refer client and partner to local support groups for HIV

D. Client teaching

NCLEX®

1. Health promotion measures such as safer sex practices (including nonsexual contact such as hugging, use of latex condoms with spermicidal lubricant, mutual masturbation), not sharing drug paraphernalia or razors, avoiding tattoos, and abstaining from donating blood, organs, or sperm
2. Course of disease and disease progression

NCLEX®

3. Energy conservation measures and adequate time for rest and sleep
4. Health maintenance measures such as cessation of smoking, alcohol use, and recreational drug use if applicable
5. Importance of compliance with long-term treatment regimen and adherence to complex drug regimen; noncompliance could lead to drug resistance over time

6. Need for healthcare provider follow-up to monitor immune status and response to treatment
7. *NCLEX®* Methods to prevention infection and its transmission, including hand hygiene and wearing gloves when handling client's secretions or excretions
8. Signs and symptoms of opportunistic infections and malignancies to report
9. *NCLEX®* Importance of balanced nutrition and adequate nutritional support to maintain immune system function
10. Available community services to assist with life management and support groups

Check Your NCLEX–RN® Exam I.Q.

You are ready for testing on this content if you can:

- Identify basic structures and functions of the immunologic system.
- Describe the pathophysiology and etiology of common immunologic disorders.
- Discuss expected assessment data and diagnostic test findings for selected immunologic disorders.
- Discuss therapeutic management of a client experiencing an immunologic disorder.
- Discuss nursing management of a client experiencing an immunologic disorder.
- Identify expected outcomes for a client experiencing an immunologic disorder.

PRACTICE TEST

1 Which suggestion by the nurse would be most helpful to a human immunodeficiency virus (HIV)-positive client who has altered taste perception?

1. Drink plenty of salty broths and other fluids to stimulate tastebuds.
2. Try zinc supplementation to improve taste perception.
3. Increase intake of meat to at least one serving per day.
4. Avoid using plastic eating utensils.

2 Which suggestion should the nurse give to a client with human immunodeficiency virus (HIV) infection to best alleviate nausea?

1. Drink liquids with meals.
2. Eat high-fat foods.
3. Eat small, frequent meals.
4. Lie down after eating.

3 To enhance meeting the psychosocial needs of a client on transmission-based precautions, the nurse should place highest priority on which intervention?

1. Letting the client sleep to build up stamina
2. Maintaining strict precautions when entering and leaving the room so that the client feels he or she is getting the best care
3. Providing client care within a limited time frame to maintain isolation and keep client safe
4. Providing the client with diversional activities to enhance sensory input

4 A client diagnosed with scleroderma reports painful fingers that change colors (pale to red) when washing dishes. Which suggestion by the nurse might help the client with this symptom?

1. Increase the water temperature.
2. Use gloves during dishwashing.
3. Start physical therapy to increase blood flow to the hands.
4. Take over-the-counter H_2 receptor antagonist medications.

5 A client with systemic lupus erythematosus (SLE) who is taking corticosteroid and immunosuppressive drug therapy has a white blood cell (WBC) count that shows a shift to the left. What should be the priority concern of the nurse at this time?

1. Reduced ability to maintain general health
2. Interrupted skin integrity
3. Fatigue from physiological stressors
4. Increased susceptibility to infection

6 A client is to start taking prednisone for treatment of rheumatoid arthritis (RA). Which client statement indicates that medication teaching was successful?

1. "I will take the medication on an empty stomach to maximize absorption."
2. "I will take the specific dose ordered at the same time every day."
3. "I will not have to limit my sodium intake."
4. "I will not have to adjust my insulin regimen."

7 The nurse assesses the client with rheumatoid arthritis for which characteristic joint changes? Select all that apply.

1. Swan-neck deformity
2. Heberden's and Bouchard's nodes
3. Tophi deposits
4. Charcot's joints
5. Ulnar deviation

8 In establishing a plan of care to manage pain for a client with rheumatoid arthritis (RA), what intervention should the nurse use to increase the client's mobility?

1. Have the client work through pain by continuing exercise in order to establish endurance.
2. Have the client use pain medication only when pain is present.
3. Teach the client that both heat and cold applications may help to relieve pain.
4. Teach the client to flex muscle groups when pain is felt in an extremity.

9 What information should the nurse include when explaining therapeutic measures to a client taking methotrexate for rheumatoid arthritis (RA)?

1. Relief of symptoms will be assessed for within 1 week of starting medication.
2. Fluids should be restricted to prevent possible edema formation.
3. Drug doses will be adjusted for optimum effect at lowest dose once relief has been established.
4. Six months of therapy will be adequate to stop the disease process from progressing.

10 The nurse looks for results of which laboratory measurement that provides a reliable indicator of lymphocyte status in a client with HIV infection?

1. B lymphocytes
2. T-helper cells (CD_4)
3. Natural killer cells (NK)
4. T-cytotoxic cells

11 The nurse who is providing care to a group of clients concludes that the client with which health problem exhibits a type III immune complex–mediated hypersensitivity reaction?

1. Transfusion reaction
2. Goodpasture syndrome
3. Transplant rejection
4. Systemic lupus erythematosus

12 A male client who has acquired immunodeficiency syndrome (AIDS) asks why oral progesterone is being prescribed for treatment. What is the nurse's best response?

1. "It is used to treat the nausea associated with this infection."
2. "It is used as an appetite stimulant to boost nutritional support."
3. "It provides symptomatic relief of constipation."
4. "It is used as an antineoplastic agent for palliative treatment."

13 The nurse should assess for which electrolyte imbalance as a common finding in a client with acquired immunodeficiency syndrome (AIDS)?

1. Hyponatremia
2. Hypernatremia
3. Hyperkalemia
4. Hypocalcemia

14 Which assessment finding by the nurse warrants further investigation to determine if the client has rheumatoid arthritis (RA)?

1. Negative family history
2. Reports of prolonged morning stiffness lasting for 1 hour
3. Occasional use of NSAIDs for aches and pains
4. Reports of pain with movement

15 The nurse teaches a client that which factor might increase risk of developing an exacerbation of systemic lupus erythematosus (SLE)?

1. Pregnancy
2. Hypotension
3. Fever
4. GI upset

16 A client will undergo scratch tests for allergies. In teaching the client about the planned tests, the nurse should include which statement?

1. "This test allows us to rule out one or two specific antigens."
2. "The scratch test is the most sensitive allergy test."
3. "Results can be obtained in 30 minutes."
4. "It involves drawing a small amount of blood for testing."

17 The nurse should anticipate which finding in a client with an immunologic disorder associated with a human leukocyte antigen (HLA)?

1. Acute course
2. Frequent effects on reproductive capacity
3. Strictly genetic determination
4. Chronic and possibly subacute course

18 A client presents with dyspnea, pruritis, and localized swelling of the forearm after being stung by a bee. What is the priority nursing intervention if hypersensitivity reaction is suspected?

1. Remove the stinger from the client's arm
2. Keep the client warm with soft blankets
3. Check the tongue for swelling and listen for stridor
4. Place client in modified Trendelenburg position

19 Medication instruction for the client with rheumatoid arthritis (RA) should include which teaching points? Select all that apply.

1. Aspirin has useful anti-inflammatory effects for RA.
2. Sulfasalazine requires fluid restriction to avoid nausea and vomiting.
3. Acetaminophen may be used to decrease inflammation associated with RA.
4. Penicillamine may be safely used during pregnancy.
5. Nonsteroidal anti-inflammatory drugs (NSAIDs) are first-line agents for RA.

20 The nurse determines that which clinical focus should be a priority early in the care of a client with scleroderma?

1. Interruptions in skin integrity
2. Changes in body image
3. Reduced tolerance for activity
4. Concerns that client may feel hopelessness

21 The nurse is completing a nursing assessment of an infant admitted to the pediatric unit with a diagnosis of sepsis and probable immunodeficiency disorder. What should be the priority nursing assessment for this infant?

1. Skin integrity
2. Temperature
3. Jaundice
4. Respiratory function

22 The nurse is caring for a pediatric client with acquired immunodeficiency syndrome (AIDS). Which event should be reported to the employee health department as an exposure for the nurse?

1. While flushing out the used bedpan, fluid splashes in the nurse's eyes.
2. The nurse does not wear a mask while in the client's room.
3. During the bath, the nurse removes gloves when giving a backrub on intact skin.
4. The nurse is stabbed with a sterile syringe to be used to draw up the client's medications.

23 The pediatric nurse should suspect severe combined immunodeficiency disorder (SCID) when which child is admitted to the hospital nursing unit?

1. A 2-month-old with thrush and low white blood cell counts
2. A 2-year-old with history of recent repeated infections
3. A newborn with positive TORCH titer
4. A newborn admitted with positive ELISA test

24 A 5-year-old child is brought into the clinic after being stung by an insect. The child appears to be going into anaphylaxis. Which nursing action is of highest priority?

1. Assess urinary output to determine renal perfusion
2. Apply cold, wet compresses to the site
3. Position the child's head to maintain an open airway
4. Establish intravenous access for medication delivery

25 A 12-year-old boy tests positive for human immunodeficiency virus (HIV) following factor transfusions for hemophilia. The family is concerned about their ability to manage his care, risk of infection to family members, and whether the child should remain in the home. Which action by the nurse will best promote family coping at this time?

1. Explain to the family that the infection cannot be spread by casual contact.
2. Demonstrate positive acceptance of the child with each contact.
3. Explain that prophylactic drugs will prevent the virus from spreading.
4. Show the family how to wash their hands properly.

26 A child who must undergo skin testing for allergies takes an antihistamine to control symptoms. The nurse explains that the client must discontinue use of the antihistamine for at least ______ days before the skin testing to avoid false-negative results. Provide a numerical answer.

Fill in your answer below:
______ days

PRACTICE TEST | ANSWERS & RATIONALES

ANSWERS & RATIONALES

1 **Answer: 2 Rationale:** Zinc deficiency is associated with taste changes; therefore, supplementation may benefit a client experiencing altered taste perception. Drinking salty broth and fluids will not help with taste changes but may help restore electrolyte balance in clients experiencing diarrhea. Dairy products, fish, and poultry are better protein choices than red meat when taste is altered. Substituting plastic utensils for metal ones is suggested to decrease possibility of taste perception of "metal." **Cognitive Level:** Applying **Client Need:** Physiological Adaptation **Integrated Process:** Nursing Process: Implementation **Content Area:** Adult Health: Immunologic **Strategy:** The core issue of the question is knowledge of measures to minimize taste alterations in a client with HIV infection. Use nursing knowledge and the process of elimination to make a selection.

2 **Answer: 3 Rationale:** Small, frequent meals help lessen nausea because they require less work of digestion and do not overwhelm the client with food odors from a lengthy meal. Drinking liquids can give a sensation of fullness. High-fat foods are more difficult to digest and may distend the stomach. Lying down after eating can encourage reflux. **Cognitive Level:** Applying **Client Need:** Physiological Adaptation **Integrated Process:** Teaching and Learning **Content Area:** Adult Health: Immunologic **Strategy:** The core issue of the question is the ability to provide teaching to minimize nausea in a client with HIV. Use nursing knowledge and the process of elimination to make a selection.

3 **Answer: 4 Rationale:** It is important to assess the psychosocial needs of a client on transmission-based precautions and to intervene to provide sensory stimulation for the client. Isolation procedures can cause clients to become depressed and withdrawn and to sleep excessively. Although it is important to maintain isolation precautions as ordered, attention must be given to include the client's psychosocial needs as part of the plan of care. Limiting contact time may be indicated for infection control, but it does not provide psychosocial support. **Cognitive Level:** Applying **Client Need:** Physiological Adaptation **Integrated Process:** Nursing Process: Planning **Content Area:** Adult Health: Immunologic **Strategy:** The critical word in the question is *psychosocial*. With this word in mind, focus on the intervention that best meets nonphysical needs of the client. Use nursing knowledge and the process of elimination to make a selection.

4 **Answer: 2 Rationale:** Clients who have scleroderma usually have Raynaud's phenomenon, which can be triggered by temperature changes, such as with prolonged contact with water. Use of gloves when washing dishes may prevent temperature changes yet still allow the client to participate in ADLs. Hotter water may increase the risk of scalding and is not suggested. Physical therapy is indicated for treatment of esophageal problems associated with scleroderma. H_2 receptor blockers help to treat esophageal problems associated with scleroderma. **Cognitive Level:** Analyzing **Client Need:** Physiological Adaptation **Integrated Process:** Nursing Process: Implementation **Content Area:** Adult Health: Immunologic **Strategy:** The core issue of the question is recognition of Raynaud's syndrome as part of scleroderma and the ability to select an appropriate intervention for that problem. Use

nursing knowledge and the process of elimination to make a selection.

5 **Answer: 4 Rationale:** While there are many potential areas of concern for a client with SLE, a WBC count with a shift to the left indicates an increased number of immature cells, suggesting infection. This risk is due to the disease process and side effects of corticosteroids and immunosuppressive agents. The client may or may not have a reduced ability to maintain general health. There is no specific indication that the client has an interruption in skin integrity. Fatigue is a common symptom with SLE but does not directly relate to the WBC result. **Cognitive Level:** Analyzing **Client Need:** Physiological Adaptation **Integrated Process:** Nursing Process: Planning **Content Area:** Adult Health: Immunologic **Strategy:** The core issue of the question is the ability to analyze WBC differential count data to determine risk of infection. Use nursing knowledge and the process of elimination to make a selection.

6 **Answer: 2 Rationale:** Corticosteroid therapy is usually done as part of a tapered-dose treatment plan. It is important to take this medication at the same time each day and to become aware of tapered-dose effect. Corticosteroids are usually taken with foods to minimize GI upset. Corticosteroids cause fluid retention, and therefore sodium intake may be restricted. Corticosteroids increase blood glucose, so insulin therapy dosages may have to be adjusted. **Cognitive Level:** Applying **Client Need:** Pharmacological and Parenteral Therapies **Integrated Process:** Nursing Process: Evaluation **Content Area:** Adult Health: Immunologic **Strategy:** The core issue of the question is knowledge of client teaching related to steroid therapy. Use nursing knowledge and the process of elimination to make a selection.

7 **Answer: 1, 5 Rationale:** Swan-neck deformity occurs at the proximal interphalangeal (PIP) joints in rheumatoid arthritis. Ulnar deviation occurs as the joint deteriorates and is a visible finding in clients with RA. Heberden's and Bouchard's nodes are commonly found in clients with osteoarthritis. Tophi (firm, moveable nodules) result from deposits associated with gout. Charcot's joint is considered a neuropathic disorder that falls under the broader category of rheumatism. It is not specific to RA and is more likely to be seen as a complication in clients with diabetes. **Cognitive Level:** Applying **Client Need:** Physiological Adaptation **Integrated Process:** Nursing Process: Assessment **Content Area:** Adult Health: Immunologic **Strategy:** The core issue of the question is identification of signs and symptoms of RA. Use nursing knowledge and the process of elimination to make selections.

8 **Answer: 3 Rationale:** Heat and cold applications can provide analgesia and relieve muscle spasms. The individual client will have to determine whether heat, cold, or alternation of both is most effective. Exercising in the presence of pain may only further exacerbate pain. Pain medication should be taken on a regular schedule if the client has chronic pain so that the pain threshold can be raised and pain relief maintained at a constant level. Flexing of muscle groups is not related to effective pain control. **Cognitive Level:** Applying **Client Need:** Physiological Adaptation **Integrated Process:** Nursing Process: Planning **Content Area:** Adult Health: Immunologic **Strategy:** The core issue of the question is knowledge of measures that relieve the symptoms of RA. Use nursing knowledge and the process of elimination to make a selection.

9 **Answer: 3 Rationale:** Methotrexate treatment takes several weeks to effect relief. Once relief is obtained, the dose is adjusted to achieve maximum response at the lowest dose. If the drug is discontinued, then symptoms of the disease do return. The client should not expect to obtain relief of symptoms within 1 week of starting drug therapy. Fluids are not restricted to prevent possible edema formation. Drug therapy cannot be terminated after 6 months. **Cognitive Level:** Applying **Client Need:** Physiological Adaptation **Integrated Process:** Nursing Process: Implementation **Content Area:** Adult Health: Immunologic **Strategy:** The core issue of the question is knowledge of management principles for RA. Use nursing knowledge and the process of elimination to make a selection.

10 **Answer: 2 Rationale:** CD4 cells are indicative of a client's HIV status. As the disease progresses, the T-helper cells decrease in number and lose their ability to function effectively. B lymphocytes indicate the status of humoral immunity and are not directly associated with HIV infection. NK cells are not directly related to HIV infection. T-cytotoxic cells are not directly related to HIV infection. **Cognitive Level:** Applying **Client Need:** Physiological Adaptation **Integrated Process:** Nursing Process: Assessment **Content Area:** Adult Health: Immunologic **Strategy:** The core issue of the question is knowledge of which laboratory measure will provide information about the status of the immune system of a client with HIV. Use nursing knowledge and the process of elimination to make a selection.

11 **Answer: 4 Rationale:** Systemic lupus erythematosus is an example of a type III hypersensitivity reaction, which involves IgG and IgM with the activation of complement. Transfusion reaction and Goodpasture syndrome are examples of type II cytotoxic hypersensitivity reactions that are involved with the activation of complement. Transplant rejection is a Type IV hypersensitivity reaction. **Cognitive Level:** Applying **Client Need:** Physiological Adaptation **Integrated Process:** Nursing Process: Diagnosis **Content Area:** Adult Health: Immunologic **Strategy:** The core issue of the question is the ability to associate various types of hypersensitivity reactions with their etiologies. Use nursing knowledge and the process of elimination to make a selection.

12 **Answer: 2 Rationale:** In clients with AIDS, oral progesterone provides appetite enhancement. Oral progesterone is not used to treat nausea. Constipation is a side effect of oral progesterone, not an intended effect. Oral progesterone can be used as a palliative treatment with advanced cancers, but it is not the rationale for its use with AIDS. **Cognitive Level:** Applying **Client Need:** Pharmacological and Parenteral Therapies **Integrated Process:** Communication and Documentation **Content Area:** Adult Health: Immunologic **Strategy:** The core issue of the question is the purpose of oral progesterone in a client with AIDS. Use nursing knowledge about anorexia as a symptom of AIDS and the process of elimination to make a selection.

13 **Answer: 1 Rationale:** Hyponatremia is a common finding in clients with AIDS. The incidence of opportunistic infections may contribute to this decrease in sodium. Hypernatremia, hyperkalemia, and hypocalcemia are not usually seen in clients who have AIDS. **Cognitive Level:** Analyzing **Client Need:** Physiological Adaptation **Integrated Process:** Nursing Process: Diagnosis **Content Area:** Adult Health: Immunologic **Strategy:** The core issue of the question is identification of an

electrolyte disturbance that is more common to clients with AIDS. Use nursing knowledge and the process of elimination to make a selection.

14 **Answer: 2 Rationale:** Prolonged morning stiffness is associated with RA. A negative family history does not increase the risk of RA. Occasional use of NSAIDs is not by itself a direct link to the development of RA. Reports of pain with movement are more likely to be associated with degenerative joint disease (osteoarthritis). **Cognitive Level:** Analyzing **Client Need:** Physiological Adaptation **Integrated Process:** Nursing Process: Assessment **Content Area:** Adult Health: Immunologic **Strategy:** The core issue of the question is the ability to identify symptoms that are possibly associated with RA. Use nursing knowledge and the process of elimination to make a selection.

15 **Answer: 1 Rationale:** Pregnancy can be associated with an exacerbation of SLE because of increased estrogen levels. Hypotension, fever, and GI upset do not exacerbate SLE. **Cognitive Level:** Applying **Client Need:** Physiological Adaptation **Integrated Process:** Teaching and Learning **Content Area:** Adult Health: Immunologic **Strategy:** The core issue of the question is risk factors and triggers for SLE. Use nursing knowledge and the process of elimination to make a selection.

16 **Answer: 3 Rationale:** The results of a scratch test can be obtained in 30 minutes. Many allergens can be tested at once because multiple sites on the arm can be used at one time. A scratch test tends to have low sensitivity overall. No blood is drawn for a skin scratch test. **Cognitive Level:** Applying **Client Need:** Physiological Adaptation **Integrated Process:** Nursing Process: Implementation **Content Area:** Adult Health: Immunologic **Strategy:** The core issue of the question is identification of appropriate concepts to teach a client about scratch tests for allergies. Use nursing knowledge and the process of elimination to make a selection.

17 **Answer: 4 Rationale:** Diseases with HLA associations have poorly understood etiologies, are usually chronic in nature, and may have a subacute course. HLA-associated disorders have a chronic course rather than an acute course. HLA-associated disorders have a limited effect on reproductive capacity. Both genetics and environmental influence may be involved in HLA-associated disorders. **Cognitive Level:** Analyzing **Client Need:** Physiological Adaptation **Integrated Process:** Nursing Process: Diagnosis **Content Area:** Adult Health: Immunologic **Strategy:** The core issue of the question is knowledge of diseases associated with the HLA antigen. Use nursing knowledge and the process of elimination to make a selection.

18 **Answer: 3 Rationale:** The priority intervention is to maintain a patent airway in a potential anaphylactic hypersensitivity reaction. Therefore, the nurse should assess for swelling of the tongue and stridor, which could indicate impending respiratory obstruction. The stinger can be removed from the client's arm once concerns about airway, breathing, and circulation are resolved. Keeping the client warm with soft blankets may not be necessary. Placing the client in a modified Trendelenburg position may be necessary if the client goes into shock. **Cognitive Level:** Analyzing **Client Need:** Physiological Adaptation **Integrated Process:** Nursing Process: Implementation **Content Area:** Adult Health: Immunologic **Strategy:** Remember in emergency or near-emergency situations to use the ABCs (airway, breathing, and circulation) to plan priorities of care. Use the process of elimination to make a selection.

19 **Answer: 1, 5 Rationale:** NSAIDs and aspirin decrease inflammation associated with RA. Sulfasalazine may cause nausea and vomiting, but fluids should be encouraged. Acetaminophen is an analgesic, but does not provide an anti-inflammatory effect. Penicillamine cannot be used during pregnancy. **Cognitive Level:** Applying **Client Need:** Pharmacological and Parenteral Therapies **Integrated Process:** Teaching and Learning **Content Area:** Adult Health: Immunologic **Strategy:** The core issue of the question is knowledge of appropriate client teaching related to medications used to treat RA. Use nursing knowledge and the process of elimination to make a selection.

20 **Answer: 1 Rationale:** Skin manifestations are a common finding in clients with scleroderma and therefore require preventative and supportive nursing care as the priority. As the disease progresses, dermatologic effects may lead to changes in body image, but this is not a priority concern. With chronic disease progression, there may be an impact on respiratory and musculoskeletal function, leading to reduced tolerance for activity. Hopelessness is a psychosocial concern that can develop with worsening symptoms later in the disease process. **Cognitive Level:** Applying **Client Need:** Physiological Adaptation **Integrated Process:** Nursing Process: Planning **Content Area:** Adult Health: Immunologic **Strategy:** The core issue of the question is knowledge that scleroderma is primarily a skin disorder in many cases and thus the primary nursing diagnosis needs to address loss of skin as a protective barrier. Use nursing knowledge and the process of elimination to make a selection.

21 **Answer: 4 Rationale:** Respiratory distress is a symptom of sepsis in infants. Assessment of respiratory function has highest priority because without an adequate airway and breathing, the client cannot maintain life. Skin integrity is a routine assessment. The client may experience fever, but temperature measurement is not higher priority than respiratory status. Jaundice may occur in a client with sepsis if liver function is diminished because of hypoperfusion, but airway and breathing take priority. **Cognitive Level:** Analyzing **Client Need:** Physiological Adaptation **Integrated Process:** Nursing Process: Diagnosis **Content Area:** Child Health **Strategy:** Use the ABCs and the process of elimination to make a selection. Airway and breathing typically take priority in situations of high acuity, such as sepsis.

22 **Answer: 1 Rationale:** Body fluid–contaminated liquids may contain the human immunodeficiency virus (HIV) and can be absorbed through the eye mucosa. HIV is not transmitted through the air, so wearing a mask is not necessary. Providing a back rub over intact skin does not create exposure. A needlestick with a sterile needle that has not had contact with the client does not constitute an exposure. **Cognitive Level:** Applying **Client Need:** Safety and Infection Control **Integrated Process:** Nursing Process: Evaluation **Content Area:** Child Health **Strategy:** The core issue of the question is the ability to identify a breach in standard precautions. Use nursing knowledge about transmission of HIV via body fluids and the process of elimination to make a selection.

23 **Answer: 1 Rationale:** The first infection often seen in these children is oral candidiasis (thrush). That symptom, along with the low WBC count, would be a warning symptom of SCID. A 2-year-old is unlikely to have survived this long undiagnosed. A TORCH titer is unrelated. ELISA tests evaluate HIV infection. **Cognitive Level:** Analyzing **Client Need:** Physiological Adaptation **Integrated Process:** Nursing Process:

Diagnosis **Content Area:** Child Health **Strategy:** The core issue of the question is the ability to identify signs and symptoms of SCID. Use nursing knowledge and the process of elimination to make a selection.

24 **Answer: 3 Rationale:** Maintaining an open airway is always the highest priority. With anaphylactic shock, the airway may constrict, mucous membranes swell, and air trapping occurs. Assessing urine output is an important but routine measure to determine kidney perfusion if the client experiences anaphylaxis. Applying cold, wet compresses to the site is a comfort measure that can be completed once the client is stabilized. Establishing intravenous access for medication delivery would be second in priority after ensuring status of airway and breathing. **Cognitive Level:** Analyzing **Client Need:** Physiological Adaptation **Integrated Process:** Nursing Process: Planning **Content Area:** Child Health **Strategy:** Use the ABCs—airway, breathing, and circulation—to answer questions related to anaphylaxis. Airway is always the first priority in life-threatening situations.

25 **Answer: 2 Rationale:** The family has stated multiple concerns, and demonstrating acceptance of the child is the best way to foster acceptance and develop further coping skills. Prevention of transmission, drug therapy, and hand hygiene are all important, but do not target the global concerns of the family. **Cognitive Level:** Analyzing **Client Need:** Psychosocial Integrity **Integrated Process:** Nursing Process: Implementation **Content Area:** Child Health **Strategy:** The core issue of the question is the best nursing action to model acceptance of the child and enhance coping skills of the family. Select the option that is the most global in nature because the family has multiple concerns, and use the process of elimination to make a selection.

26 **Answer: 3 Rationale:** The client needs to discontinue use of antihistamines for 3 days (72 hours) prior to allergy testing to avoid false-negative readings. **Cognitive Level:** Applying **Client Need:** Reduction of Risk Potential **Integrated Process:** Nursing Process: Implementation **Content Area:** Adult Health: Immunologic **Strategy:** The core issue of the question is knowledge of the time frame that antihistamine drugs need to be withheld so as not to interfere with the results of allergy testing. Use specific nursing knowledge to determine the correct answer.

Key Terms to Review

antibody p. 1234
antigen p. 1234
antigen–antibody complexes p. 1237
antihistamine p. 1236
atopy p. 1236
cell-mediated immunity p. 1234
colony-stimulating factors p. 1234
complement fixation p. 1234
human leukocyte antigens (HLAs) p. 1238
humoral immunity p. 1234
hypersensitivity p. 1236
immunoglobulins p. 1235
major histocompatibility complex (MHC) p. 1235
monoclonal antibodies p. 1234
myelosuppression p. 1239
opportunistic infections p. 1244
plasmapheresis p. 1238
wasting syndrome p. 1245

References

Ball, J., & Bindler, R., & Cowen, K. (2015). *Principles of pediatric nursing: Caring for children* (6th ed.). Hoboken, NJ: Pearson Education.

Berman, A., Snyder, S., & Frandsen, G. (2016). *Kozier & Erb's fundamentals of nursing: Concepts, process, and practice* (10th ed.). New York, NY: Pearson Education.

Ignatavicius, D., & Workman, L. (2016). *Medical-surgical nursing: Patient-centered collaborative care* (10th ed.). Philadelphia: Saunders.

Kee, J. (2017). *Pearson's handbook of laboratory and diagnostic tests* (8th ed.). New York, NY: Pearson Education.

LeMone, P., Burke, K., Bauldoff, G., & Gubrud, P. (2015). *Medical surgical nursing: Clinical reasoning in patient care* (6th ed.). Hoboken, NJ: Pearson Education.

Lewis, S., Dirksen, S., Heitkemper, M., & Bucher, L. (2014). *Medical surgical nursing: Assessment and management of clinical problems* (9th ed.). St. Louis, MO: Elsevier Science.

Smith, S., Duell, D., Martin, B., Aebersold, M., & Gonzalez, L. (2017). *Clinical nursing skills: Basic to advanced skills* (10th ed.). New York, NY: Pearson Education.

Test Yourself

Are you ready for the NCLEX-RN® or course exams? Access the NEW web-based app that provides students with thousands of practice questions in preparation for the NCLEX experience.

Communicable or Infectious Diseases

67

In this chapter

Cross Reference

Other chapters relevant to this content area are

Preventing and Controlling Infection	**Chapter 7**
Providing Immunizations	**Chapter 14**
Immunologic and Anti-Infective Medications	**Chapter 45**

I. ANTHRAX

A. Overview

1. Organism: *Bacillus anthracis* (spore-forming bacteria usually seen in cattle, sheep, and goats)
2. Mode of transmission: direct skin contact, inhalation, digestive system

NCLEX®

3. Source: infected animal hides that come in contact with broken skin, airborne spores, or spores impregnated in carrier agent such as a powder (biological weapon); ingestion of contaminated undercooked meat
4. Incubation period: 2–60 days
5. Highly contagious with spores that can survive for years and are resistant to sunlight and temperature

NCLEX® **B. Nursing assessment**

1. Cutaneous form: reddish-brown lesion ulcerates and forms scab surrounded by brawny edema; toxin destroys surrounding tissue
2. GI: internal hemorrhage, abdominal pain, headache, fever, nausea and vomiting, severe diarrhea
3. Pulmonary form: fever, muscle aches and fatigue, rapidly developing respiratory distress and shock

C. Therapeutic management

NCLEX®
1. Ciprofloxacin or doxycycline for 60–100 days for all types
2. Clean contaminated surfaces with 5% hypochlorite solution
3. Provide vaccine to those at occupational high risk (animal workers)
4. Initiate mechanical ventilation as needed and supportive treatment for shock
5. Institute contact and respiratory precautions because of resistant spores

D. Complications: respiratory form more likely to be fatal

II. CHICKENPOX (VARICELLA)

A. Overview

1. Organism: varicella zoster virus
2. NCLEX® Mode of transmission: airborne, direct contact, or contact with contaminated objects (fomites)
3. Source: respiratory secretions and vesicular skin lesions (crusts not infectious)
4. Incubation period: often 13–17 days
5. Communicability: from 1–2 days before onset of rash to crusting over of first set of vesicles (about 6 days)

NCLEX® **B. Nursing assessment**

1. Fever, malaise, and anorexia are initial symptoms
2. Macular rash beginning on scalp and trunk and spreading to extremities; may involve oral mucous membranes or genital and rectal areas
3. Rash rapidly progresses to papules and vesicles that break open and form crusts

NCLEX® **C. Therapeutic management**

1. Prevention: **immunization** with varicella vaccine (see Chapter 14)
2. Maintain airborne and contact precautions in hospital
3. NCLEX® Isolate child in home until vesicles have crusted and dried
4. Skin care: bathe and change clothes and bed linens daily; use oatmeal soaps, soaks, or lotions and calamine lotion or topical antihistamines to prevent scratching of pruritic lesions; encourage child not to scratch; use mittens on young child
5. Administer acetaminophen for fever; avoid aspirin to prevent Reye syndrome
6. Administer acyclovir as prescribed to immunocompromised clients to shorten duration of fever, decrease number of lesions, and reduce symptoms such as itching, anorexia, and malaise
7. Administer prescribed VCZ immune globulin or intravenous immune globulin (IVIG) to immunocompromised child with no history of disease and likely to contract varicella and experience complications of disease

D. Complications: encephalitis, varicella pneumonia, secondary bacterial infections (abscesses, cellulitis, sepsis)

III. DIPHTHERIA

A. Overview

1. Organism: *Corynebacterium diphtheriae*
2. NCLEX® Mode of transmission: direct contact with infected client, carrier, or contaminated objects
3. Source: nasal and respiratory secretions, skin, other lesions
4. Incubation period: 2–5 days, possibly slightly longer
5. Communicability: variable until virulent bacilli absent in three negative cultures; usually 2–4 weeks

NCLEX® **B. Nursing assessment**

1. Low-grade fever, sore throat, malaise, anorexia
2. Foul mucopurulent nasal discharge; may have epistaxis
3. Smooth, adherent, white or gray pseudomembrane on tonsils and pharynx that can interfere with breathing, eating, and drinking
4. Hoarseness, cough, edema of neck (bull neck), lymphadenitis, apprehension, dyspnea with retractions, possible airway obstruction and cyanosis

NCLEX® **C. Therapeutic management**

1. Prevention: diphtheria **vaccine** (see Chapter 14)
2. Maintain droplet precautions (respiratory form) or contact precautions (skin) and bedrest

3. Administer antibiotic therapy and antitoxin as prescribed (do skin or conjunctival test first to rule out sensitivity to horse serum)
4. Provide suction and oxygen as needed to maintain airway
5. Be prepared for emergency tracheostomy if airway obstruction occurs

D. **Complications:** myocarditis, neuritis, toxemia, and septic shock; death possible

IV. ERYTHEMA INFECTIOSUM (FIFTH DISEASE)

A. **Overview**

1. Organism: human parvovirus B19 (HPV)
2. *NCLEX®* Mode of transmission: unknown; possibly respiratory secretions and blood
3. Source: infected individuals; direct contact with contaminated secretions
4. Incubation period: 4–14 days, but possibly up to 20 days
5. Communicability: uncertain, but usually before onset of symptoms

B. **Nursing assessment**

1. *NCLEX®* Rash that occurs in three stages
   a. Erythema of face (mainly cheeks, giving a "slapped cheeks" appearance) that lasts 1–4 days
   b. Symmetrical, maculopapular "lacy" red rash on trunks and limbs (proximal to distal); appears one day after facial rash and lasts 1 week or longer; rash may itch
   c. Rash subsides but can reappear with skin irritation or trauma, as with sunlight, heat, cold, or friction
2. Possible joint swelling of hands, wrists, and knees bilaterally that resolves within 1 or 2 weeks
3. With aplastic crisis, rash is often absent but child has prodromal signs of fever, lethargy, myalgia, and GI symptoms including nausea and vomiting (N/V) and abdominal pain

NCLEX® C. **Therapeutic management**

1. Client is often treated at home
2. Place hospitalized child on respiratory precautions and use care when handling respiratory secretions that can transmit infection
3. Provide antipyretics, analgesics, anti-inflammatory drugs as prescribed
4. Provide supportive care; transfuse blood to clients with aplastic anemia as prescribed

D. **Complications:** self-limited or chronic arthritis, aplastic crisis in clients with hemolytic disease or immune deficiency, myocarditis or encephalitis (rarely), and possible but low risk of fetal death if mother is infected during pregnancy

V. INFECTIOUS MONONUCLEOSIS

A. **Overview**

1. Organism: Epstein-Barr virus (EBV)
2. *NCLEX®* Mode of transmission: direct intimate contact
3. Source: oral secretions
4. Incubation period: 4–6 weeks
5. Communicability: unknown; viral shedding occurs before onset of symptoms until 6 months or longer after recovery

NCLEX® B. **Nursing assessment**

1. Fever, sore throat, and enlarged red tonsils
2. Nausea, abdominal pain, headache, fatigue, and malaise
3. Possible macular rash more prominent on trunk
4. Lymphadenopathy and hepatosplenomegaly

NCLEX® C. **Therapeutic management**

1. Supportive care including rest
2. Assess for abdominal pain, left upper quadrant or left shoulder pain (signs of ruptured spleen)

D. **Complication:** ruptured spleen

VI. INFLUENZA

A. **Overview**

1. Organism: various strains of influenza virus (A, B, C), with newer strains identified by strain, geographic area, and year identified
2. *NCLEX®* Mode of transmission: airborne droplet and direct contact with infected person or contaminated object
3. Source: respiratory secretions and contaminated objects
4. Incubation period: 18–72 hours

NCLEX® **B. Nursing assessment**

1. Prevention: annual influenza vaccine, frequent hand hygiene, avoiding infected individuals, keeping infected individuals home from school or work until free of fever for at least 24 hours (without antipyretic therapy)
2. Sudden onset of high fever, chills, headache, body aches, sore throat, congestion, cough, anorexia, N/V, diarrhea

C. Therapeutic management

NCLEX®
1. Drug prophylaxis within 48 hours with amantadine or rimantadine for unvaccinated individuals exposed to flu
2. Selected additional antiviral drugs may be prescribed to reduce severity and duration of flu symptoms
3. Client is generally treated at home; promote respirations with head of bed elevated, bedrest to prevent fatigue, and frequent rest periods
4. Provide adequate hydration and humidification of air to promote clearance of airway secretions; teach coughing techniques and monitor effectiveness
5. In hospital, implement droplet precautions and place client in private room if influenza is suspected or confirmed; apply mask to client who must be transported within facility
6. Explain measures to reduce transmission such as frequent hand hygiene, controlling respiratory secretions using tissues, wearing mask when coughing or sneezing, and standing 3 feet from others while coughing and sneezing

D. Complications: more likely to occur in young children, older adults, pregnant women, and those with chronic health problems; examples include pneumonia, sinus and ear infections, exacerbation of chronic health problem, and sepsis

VII. LYME DISEASE

A. Overview

1. Organism: *Borrelia burgdorferi* (spirochete)
2. NCLEX® Mode of transmission: bite from ixodid tick (found in wooded areas and survives by attaching to host, where it feeds); not communicable person to person
3. Source: bite from infected tick
4. Incubation period: symptoms appear several days to months after bite

NCLEX® **B. Nursing assessment**

1. First (early localized disease) stage: painless expanding annular red rash (erythema migrans) that starts as red macule or papule and expands to 5–15 cm in diameter; may have partial central clearing (bull's eye) or appear as a bruise in dark-skinned clients; rash occurs in 50% of clients and appears at site of tick bite or elsewhere on body; fever, body aches, headache, and malaise occur
2. Second (early disseminated disease) stage: multiple, smaller erythema migrans lesions appear 3–10 weeks after tick bite; fever, headache, neck pain, joint stiffness, conjunctivitis, and fatigue; possible facial nerve palsy, carditis, and meningitis
3. Third (late disseminated disease) stage: Lyme arthritis in large joints such as knee in 2–12 months, with joint swelling, pain, and tenderness

C. Therapeutic management

NCLEX®
1. ELISA and Western blot tests can detect Lyme disease 4–6 weeks after bite (not effective earlier); treatment is not delayed to wait for test results
2. Antibiotic therapy for 14–21 days (first stage), 21–28 days (second stage), and up to 28 days with possible IV route for third stage with arthritic changes
3. Provide antipyretics and analgesics for fever, headache, and joint aches; provide for rest and caution client against vigorous activity
4. Teach measures to prevent and manage tick bites (see Box 67–1)

D. Complications: if untreated, leads to late disseminated disease with cranial nerve palsies, carditis, encephalitis, meningitis

VIII. METHICILLIN-RESISTANT *STAPHYLOCOCCUS AUREUS* (MRSA)

A. Overview

1. Organism: a strain of staphylococcus aureus that is resistant to antibiotic methicillin; normally found on skin or in nose; presence on skin is called *colonization* and, when symptoms occur, it is called *infection*

Box 67–1

Prevention and Management of Tick Bites

Preventing Tick Bites

- Avoid areas that are likely to contain ticks, such as wooded areas and areas with shrubs or tall grass, especially during summer months; use walking paths instead
- Maintain yard around home by keeping grass short and clearing leaves or brush so they do not accumulate
- Protect body surfaces by wearing long-sleeved shirts, long pants, long socks (to pull up over pants legs), shoes with closed heel and toes, and hat when walking in such areas
- Wear light-colored clothes to make it easier to identify presence of ticks
- Use spray repellent effective against ticks (usually contain diethyltoluamide [DEET] or permethrin) before going outside or entering areas likely to be tick-infested; note cautions on product for infants and small children
- Examine skin and scalp for presence of tick(s) when coming in from outdoors
- Protect pets with commercial tick repellant for animal use; check pets for ticks that could transfer to children or other family members

Managing a Tick Bite

- Remove tick from skin by attaching tweezers to tick where mouthparts are attached and pulling gently upward until tick releases (avoid squeezing tick, which could break off body and leave mouthparts attached to skin)
- Dispose of tick by placing in sealed jar for later inspection by healthcare provider or flush tick down toilet
- Clean area with soap and water

NCLEX® 2. Mode of transmission: skin-to-skin contact, contact with contaminated objects, or infection of preexisting skin lesion or wound not covered by a dressing (community-acquired MRSA or CA-MRSA); during invasive procedures such as surgery or use of medical devices such as IV tubing or artificial joints, as examples (healthcare-associated MRSA or HA-MRSA)
3. Individuals at risk for HA-MRSA have been hospitalized or treated in other healthcare settings (skilled nursing facilities, dialysis centers)
4. Individuals at risk for CA-MRSA include those who live in crowded conditions (such as military recruits, prisoners), childcare workers, daycare attendees, athletes with skin contact such as high school wrestlers, those with poor hygiene practices or compromised immune systems, or those who use contaminated items (such as tattoo equipment)

NCLEX® **B. Nursing assessment**
1. Local skin infection (boils, furuncles, open skin lesions or wounds) with erythema, swelling, warmth, pain at site, possible purulent drainage at site, and fever
2. Signs of a more serious site-specific infection such as respiratory infection or urinary infection, or generalized signs such as muscle aches, rash, headache, fever, chills, malaise, and fatigue

C. Therapeutic management

NCLEX® 1. Prevention: hand hygiene for public and standard precautions for healthcare workers; appropriate cleaning and disinfection of potentially contaminated shared equipment (such as athletic equipment, saunas, pools, hot tubs, and whirlpools); not sharing personal items; adequate personal hygiene
2. Implement contact precautions for hospitalized client with known source of MRSA
3. Obtain culture and sensitivity of skin or wound site, sputum or urine as indicated
4. Administer prescribed antibiotic and teach client to complete full course of therapy

D. Complications: bacteria entering bloodstream can cause cellulitis, endocarditis, osteomyelitis, septic arthritis, pneumonia, sepsis, organ failure, and possible death

IX. MUMPS (PAROTITIS)

A. Overview
1. Organism: paramyxovirus

NCLEX® 2. Mode of transmission: direct contact or via droplets from infected client
3. Source: saliva
4. Incubation period: 2–3 weeks
5. Communicability: greatest immediately before and after swelling begins

NCLEX® **B. Nursing assessment**
1. First 24 hours: fever, headache, malaise, and anorexia
2. Jaw pain and/or ear pain aggravated by chewing
3. Unilateral or bilateral swelling of parotid glands with pain and tenderness

NCLEX® **C. Therapeutic management**
1. Prevention: mumps vaccine (see Chapter 14)
2. Institute droplet precautions during hospitalization
3. Maintain bedrest; encourage fluids and soft, bland foods that require little chewing
4. Comfort measures: analgesics, antipyretics, warm or cool compresses to neck, warmth and local support (snug-fitting underwear) for orchitis

D. Complications: sensorineural deafness, meningitis, or encephalitis, myocarditis or arthritis, hepatitis, epididymo-orchitis, and possible sterility

X. PERTUSSIS (WHOOPING COUGH)

A. Overview
1. Organism: *Bordetella pertussis*
2. NCLEX® Mode of transmission: direct contact or droplet; contact with freshly contaminated articles
3. Source: respiratory tract secretions
4. Incubation period: range of 5–21 days, usually 10 days

NCLEX® **B. Nursing assessment**
1. Catarrhal stage: sneezing, runny nose, lacrimation, low-grade fever, and cough that gradually worsens over 1–2 weeks
2. Paroxysmal stage: coughing occurs frequently at night, with short, rapid coughs followed by inspiration with a high-pitched "whooping" sound; cheeks become flushed or cyanotic; attack often followed by vomiting; lasts 4–6 weeks, then convalescent stage begins

NCLEX® **C. Therapeutic management**
1. Prevention: pertussis vaccine (see Chapter 14)
2. Maintain bedrest during fever; maintain hydration
3. Provide humidity via humidifier or tent; also humidify any oxygen given
4. Reduce environmental triggers for coughing, such as dust, sudden temperature change, smoke, or known allergens
5. Institute airborne droplet and contact precautions during catarrhal stage
6. Administer antimicrobial agents as prescribed and possibly pertussis immune globulin

D. Complications: atelectasis, pneumonia, otitis media, dehydration, hemorrhage (subarachnoid, epistaxis, subconjunctival), hernia and/or prolapsed rectum, seizures

XI. POLIOMYELITIS

A. Overview
1. Organism: three types of enterovirus—abortive or unapparent, nonparalytic, and paralytic—each associated with varying severity of paralysis
2. NCLEX® Mode of transmission: direct contact or transmission by fecal–oral or oropharyngeal routes
3. Source: oropharyngeal secretions and feces
4. Incubation period: usually 7–14 days, with range of 5–35 days
5. Communicability: uncertain; virus present in throat and feces shortly after infection and lasts about 1 week in throat and 4–6 weeks in feces

NCLEX® **B. Nursing assessment**
1. Abortive or unapparent type: fever, uneasiness, sore throat, headache, anorexia, vomiting, abdominal pain (lasts a few hours to a few days)
2. Nonparalytic type: similar to abortive poliomyelitis, but more severe, with pain and stiffness in back, neck, and legs
3. Paralytic type: initially similar to nonparalytic type, followed by recovery and then CNS paralysis

NCLEX® **C. Therapeutic management**
1. Institute contact and enteric precautions
2. Maintain complete bedrest
3. Assess for impending respiratory paralysis (shallow, rapid respirations, dyspnea, difficulty talking, ineffective cough); be prepared for intubation and mechanical ventilation

4. Care of immobilized client: range-of-motion exercises, proper positioning for body alignment; prevent skin breakdown
5. Physical therapy for muscles after acute stage; moist heat to muscles

D. Complications: renal calculi from bone demineralization during immobility, hypertension, respiratory arrest, permanent paralysis

XII. ROCKY MOUNTAIN SPOTTED FEVER

A. Overview

1. Organism: *Rickettsia rickettsii*
2. NCLEX® Mode of transmission: bite of infected tick
3. Source: tick; mammal source such as dog or rodent
4. Incubation period: 2 days to 2 weeks
5. Communicability: contact with tick or infected animal

NCLEX® **B. Nursing assessment**

1. Chills, fever, malaise, myalgia, anorexia, nausea, headache, mental confusion
2. Maculopapular or petechial rash often on extremities (ankles or wrists) that may spread over trunk and face; characteristic locations are palms and soles

NCLEX® **C. Therapeutic management**

1. Prevention: avoid contact with ticks or infected animals; use insect repellents and protective clothing; immunize children at risk; inspect skin for ticks (do not crush on skin if found; remove with tweezers)
2. Provide supportive care
3. Administer antibiotics as prescribed

D. Complication: can be fatal

XIII. ROSEOLA (EXANTHEM SUBITUM)

A. Overview

1. Organism: human herpesvirus type 6
2. NCLEX® Mode of transmission and source: unknown
3. Incubation period: 5–15 days
4. Communicability: unknown, but may extend from febrile stage until rash appears

NCLEX® **B. Nursing assessment**

1. Sudden fever above 38.8°C (102°F) for 3–4 days in child who appears well
2. Appearance of blanchable rose-pink macular or maculopapular rash up to 2 days after fever subsides
3. Nonpruritic rash begins on trunk, then spreads to neck, face, and extremities; lasts 1–2 days
4. May be associated with lymphadenopathy in cervical area and behind ears, cough, runny nose, and infected pharynx

NCLEX® **C. Therapeutic management**

1. Supportive care and antipyretics to control fever
2. Seizure precautions for child at risk of recurrent febrile seizures

D. Complications: recurrent febrile seizures; meningitis and rarely encephalitis; hepatitis

XIV. RUBEOLA (MEASLES)

A. Overview

1. Organism: paramyxovirus
2. NCLEX® Mode of transmission: direct contact with droplets
3. Source: respiratory secretions, blood, and urine
4. Incubation period: 10–20 days
5. Communicability: 4 days before to 5 days after appearance of rash but mainly communicable during prodromal (catarrhal) stage

NCLEX® **B. Nursing assessment**

1. Prodromal stage: fever, malaise, coryza (upper respiratory or cold symptoms), cough, conjunctivitis, and Koplik spots (small, irregular red spots with tiny bluish white center) on oral mucosa 2 days before rash appears until about 2 days after
2. Erythematous maculopapular rash begins 3–4 days after prodromal stage; blanches with pressure; appears on face and spreads downward to feet; discrete areas of rash become confluent (blend together) over time and turn brown; rash lasts 6–7 days; moist desquamation occurs over areas extensively involved

NCLEX® **C. Therapeutic management**

1. Prevention: measles vaccine (see Chapter 14)
2. Isolate child at home until fifth day of rash; institute airborne, droplet, and contact precautions for hospitalized child
3. Maintain bedrest with quiet activity during prodromal stage
4. Provide supportive care: antipyretics for fever (no aspirin, to prevent Reye syndrome), seizure precautions if prone to febrile seizures, cool-mist vaporizer; adequate fluid intake; tepid baths for skin care; warm saline to remove eye crusts; dim lights if photophobia present; possible vitamin A supplementation

D. Complications: otitis media, pneumonia, bronchiolitis, obstructive laryngitis or laryngotracheitis, encephalitis

XV. RUBELLA (GERMAN MEASLES)

A. Overview

1. Organism: rubella virus
2. NCLEX® Mode of transmission: direct contact or contact with objects freshly contaminated with nasopharyngeal secretions, urine, or feces
3. Source: respiratory secretions, virus also present in urine, stool, and blood
4. Incubation period: 2–3 weeks
5. Communicability: 7 days before to about 5 days after appearance of rash

NCLEX® **B. Nursing assessment**

1. Low-grade fever, headache, malaise, anorexia, mild conjunctivitis, coryza, sore throat, and lymphadenopathy lasting 1–5 days in adolescents and adults until 1 day after appearance of rash; children might not have this prodromal stage
2. Discrete pinkish-red maculopapular rash on face and spreading downward to neck, arms, trunk, and legs within 1 day
3. Rash disappears in the order it began and is usually gone by third day

NCLEX® **C. Therapeutic management**

1. Prevention: rubella vaccine (see Chapter 14)
2. Institute airborne, droplet, and contact precautions for hospitalized child
3. Provide antipyretics for fever and comfort measures since illness is benign in children
4. Isolate child from pregnant women

D. Complications: rare, but include arthritis, encephalitis, or purpura; greatest risk is teratogenic effect on fetus (fetal deformity)

XVI. SCARLET FEVER

A. Overview

1. Organism: *Streptococcus pyogenes*, a type of group A beta-hemolytic streptococci
2. NCLEX® Mode of transmission: direct contact, droplets, indirect contact with contaminated objects, ingestion of contaminated milk or food
3. Source: respiratory secretions and carriers
4. Incubation period: 2–4 days with range of 1–7 days
5. Communicability: approximately 10 days during period of incubation and clinical illness; also during first 2 weeks to perhaps months in carrier phase

NCLEX® **B. Nursing assessment**

1. Sudden-onset high fever, headache, chills, malaise, vomiting, abdominal pain
2. Pharyngeal or tonsillar redness, swelling, and enlargement; tonsils are covered with gray-white exudate
3. Tongue is coated with white exudate with red papillae that project upward (white strawberry tongue), followed by sloughing of exudate to leave a red swollen tongue (red strawberry tongue) after 4–5 days
4. Red, pinhead-sized rash appears 12 hours after prodromal stage, which rapidly progresses to generalized rashes in axillae, groin, and neck; desquamation of skin on feet and soles begins at end of first week and may last for 3 weeks or longer
5. Rash is characteristically absent on face, which has flushed appearance with circumoral pallor

NCLEX® **C. Therapeutic management**

1. Initiate respiratory and contact precautions until 24 hours after antibiotic therapy begins
2. Provide supportive care, including bedrest with quiet environment, and comfort measures for sore throat (gargles, lozenges, cool mist, throat sprays)
3. Increase fluid intake while avoiding irritating citrus juices; provide soft diet (no rough foods) during acute phase

D. Complications: otitis media, sinusitis, peritonsillar abscess, glomerulonephritis, carditis, polyarthritis (uncommon)

XVII. SMALLPOX

A. Overview

1. Organism: variola major or variola minor virus

NCLEX®

2. Mode of transmission: inhalation of droplets and direct contact
3. Source: frozen stores in U.S. Centers for Disease Control and Prevention (CDC); other sources unknown but is a potential agent for biological warfare

B. Nursing assessment

1. High fever and malaise, headache, vomiting
2. Vesicular, pustular rash on face and extremities after onset of earlier symptoms

C. Therapeutic management

1. Prevention: immunization with vaccinia (a related poxvirus) for laboratory workers, those at risk for exposure (such as military), or those who have been exposed (before rash appears for up to 4 days postexposure)
2. Supportive care with isolation in a negative-pressure room once lesions break open and spread virus into mouth and throat (highly contagious at this time)

D. Complication: death

XVIII. ZIKA VIRUS

A. Overview

1. Organism: zika virus
2. Mode of transmission: bite of infected *Aedes* species mosquito, via vaginal, anal, or oral sex with infected person (zika present in sperm and vaginal secretions), pregnant woman to fetus
3. Incubation period: unknown, but likely to be a few days to a week
4. Zika remains in blood of infected client for about a week, but might be longer in some clients
5. Greatest concern with zika virus infection is during pregnancy, which can cause microcephaly and other severe fetal brain defects; see CDC website for new information as it emerges

B. Nursing assessment

1. Some clients are asymptomatic or have mild symptoms and may not recognize infection
2. Manifestations include fever, rash, joint pain, conjunctivitis, muscle pain, headache lasting several days to a week
3. Symptoms are similar to those caused by dengue and chikungunya viruses, which are transmitted by same species of mosquitoes

C. Therapeutic management

1. No vaccine or medications are available to treat infection with zika virus
2. Diagnosis: blood or urine sample is evaluated using real-time reverse transcription polymerase chain reaction (rRT-PCR)
3. Prevention includes steps to prevent mosquito bites
   a. Wear long-sleeved shirts and long pants
   b. Use insect repellent with DEET, picardin, IR3535, oil of lemon eucalyptus, or para-menthane-diol
   c. Use air conditioning when possible and close window and door screens to keep mosquitoes outside; keep screens in good repair
   d. Sleep under mosquito net if unprotected and outside or in endemic area
   e. Cover water storage containers (rain barrels, cisterns, or buckets) or clean items that hold water, such as planters, flowerpot saucers, buckets, bird baths, or trash containers weekly (mosquitoes lay eggs near water)
4. Supportive care includes rest, adequate fluid intake to prevent dehydration
5. Use acetaminophen to treat pain and fever; avoid aspirin and NSAIDs until dengue is ruled out if appropriate (to reduce risk of bleeding)

D. Complications: microcephaly and other severe brain defects of infants born to infected mothers

Check Your NCLEX–RN® Exam I.Q.

You are ready for testing on this content if you can:

- Identify basic structures and functions of the immunologic system.
- Describe the pathophysiology and etiology of common infectious diseases.
- Discuss assessment data and diagnostic test findings for selected infectious diseases.
- Discuss therapeutic and nursing management of a client experiencing an infectious disease.
- Identify expected outcomes for a client experiencing an infectious disease.

PRACTICE TEST

1 After conducting client teaching with the mother of a 4-year-old child exposed to chickenpox, the nurse determines additional instruction is needed when the mother makes which statement?

1. "I should monitor my child for Reye syndrome, which is a complication of chickenpox."
2. "My child should not visit my pregnant sister at this time."
3. "During the prodomal period, my child will have pox all over his body."
4. "Chickenpox is a viral infection that can be spread to other children."

2 A mother overhears two nurses discussing the incubation period for a measles outbreak. The mother asks why it is important to know this. The nurse's reply would include which statement about the incubation period?

1. "It describes a period when the child might be contagious."
2. "It determines the severity of the infection."
3. "It varies depending on the age of the child."
4. "It is a time when medications can prevent the development of symptoms."

3 A 2-year-old child hospitalized for a fractured femur breaks out with chickenpox. Which nursing intervention will best prevent secondary skin infections?

1. Calamine lotion to lesions
2. Acetylsalicylic acid
3. Immune globulin for the first 3 days
4. Nalbuphine every 4 hours as needed for pain

4 A child is being treated at home for chickenpox. The visiting home-health nurse notes an elevated temperature. To prevent a common complication of fever, the nurse recommends which of the following?

1. Tepid sponge baths
2. Aspirin as needed for fever control
3. Keep child well covered to prevent chilling
4. Antibiotics as prescribed

5 A child has been diagnosed with mumps and the mother has been given instructions on caring for the child during the acute period. Which statement by the mother indicates a need for additional education?

1. "I can give my child acetaminophen for fever."
2. "My child will be more comfortable if I give him fluids and soft foods."
3. "I should watch my child for headache and vomiting."
4. "I will give my child antibiotics every 4 hours around the clock."

6 A 2-year-old child with rubeola (measles) is brought to the hospital with a rash covering the entire body, photophobia, and stuffy nose that interferes with breathing. What should be the priority clinical concern of the nurse when caring for this child?

1. Interruption in skin integrity
2. Possible embarrassment about rash
3. Possible effect on respiratory status
4. Lack of restful sleep because of symptoms

7 A child is exposed to a playmate who contracted chickenpox. Two days later, the child is brought to the healthcare provider for another problem, and the parents inform the nurse of the exposure. The nurse should teach the parents to watch for signs of upper respiratory illness for how long after the exposure?

1. 5–10 days
2. 10–21 days
3. 21–25 days
4. 28–30 days

8 The home health nurse sees a child with mumps. The mother says that the child is not eating well and asks for suggestions. The nurse most appropriately makes which suggestion?

1. Provide warm, chopped foods.
2. Provide cool table foods with spices.
3. Provide cool fluids with minimum of acids.
4. Provide a regular diet tray at frequent intervals.

9 The mother of a 3-year-old child with measles telephones the clinic nurse and asks what she can do to help decrease the redness and itching. The nurse responds that which action is likely to be helpful?

1. Overdress the child and cause him to perspire.
2. Keep the child out of drafts.
3. Bathe the child in an oatmeal (Aveeno) bath.
4. Provide adequate oral fluids.

10 The clinic nurse is working with a toddler diagnosed with roseola (exanthem subitum) after being seen for fever and a skin rash. The nurse makes which response to the mother who asks how to reduce the risk of infecting other children at home?

1. "There is no way to reduce risk because the route of transmission is unknown."
2. "Do not allow the child to cough or sneeze in the presence of others whenever possible."
3. "Use disposable dishes and eating utensils, and dispose of them in a separate trash bag."
4. "Select one bathroom to be used exclusively by the toddler until the rash clears."

11 A college student was hospitalized following onset of a severe case of pertussis. In preparing for discharge, the nurse would correct which client statement that indicates a misunderstanding about postdischarge care?

1. "Irritants that I breathe, such as smoke or dust, could make me have coughing spells again."
2. "I will try to avoid being around people for a full week after going home so I don't spread this to others."
3. "I will be very careful to wash my hands often."
4. "It will still be important to try to drink a lot of fluids when I go home."

12 A child who may have scarlet fever is being evaluated in the urgent care clinic. The nurse concludes that the client's presentation is not consistent with scarlet fever after noting which finding during assessment?

1. Rash in the axillae and groin
2. Pharyngeal redness and swelling
3. Koplik's spots in the oral mucosa
4. Red strawberry tongue

13 The nurse is assessing a child in the outpatient clinic who has fever, lethargy, and nausea and vomiting. The nurse notes that the child's cheeks have the appearance of being wind-burned or slapped. The nurse suspects which childhood communicable disease?

1. Chickenpox
2. Measles
3. Diphtheria
4. Fifth disease

14 The spouse of a postal worker who contracted cutaneous anthrax asks the nurse whether this communicable disease can be treated. Which response by the nurse is most appropriate?

1. "No, there is only supportive care available for the itching associated with skin lesions."
2. "No, although we will be ready to provide aggressive respiratory support measures if needed."
3. "Yes, the infection can be treated with antiviral agents and immune globulin."
4. "Yes, the infection can be treated with antibiotics such as ciprofloxacin or doxycycline."

15 The nurse is providing health teaching to a group of high school students about infectious mononucleosis. When discussing timing of disease transmission, the nurse explains that the incubation period for this infection is up to ____ weeks. Provide a numeric answer.

Fill in your answer below:
Answer: ____ weeks

16 A young male college student came to the clinic after contracting genital herpes. Which of the following interventions would be most appropriate?

1. Encourage him to maintain bedrest for several days.
2. Monitor temperature every 4 hours.
3. Instruct him to avoid sexual contact during acute phase of illness.
4. Encourage him to use antifungal agents regularly.

ANSWERS & RATIONALES

1 **Answer: 3 Rationale:** The prodromal period is the time between the initial symptoms and the presence of the full-blown disease. The rash would not be apparent during this time. Reye syndrome can occur as a complication of chickenpox. It is advisable to keep infected individuals from having contact with pregnant women. Chickenpox is caused by a virus and can be spread to other children. **Cognitive Level:** Analyzing **Client Need:** Physiological Adaptation **Integrated Process:** Nursing Process: Evaluation **Content Area:** Child Health **Strategy:** The core issue of the question is knowledge of client teaching points related to chickenpox, particularly related to the timing of symptoms. Use nursing knowledge and the process of elimination to make a selection.

2 **Answer: 1 Rationale:** The incubation period is the time between exposure and outbreak of the disease. It is often a period when the child can be contagious without others being aware of the possible exposure. The incubation period has nothing to do with the severity of the infection. The incubation period is constant and does not vary from child to child. Measles can be prevented by vaccination early in life. **Cognitive Level:** Applying **Client Need:** Physiological Adaptation **Integrated Process:** Nursing Process: Implementation **Content Area:** Fundamentals **Strategy:** The core issue of the question is knowledge of the significance of the prodromal period in a communicable disease. Use nursing knowledge and the process of elimination to make a selection.

3 **Answer: 1 Rationale:** Calamine lotion will reduce itching and discomfort and therefore diminish scratching and skin breakdown. Acetylsalicylic acid should not be given to young children with a viral disease because of the relationship to Reye syndrome. Immune globulin will not decrease skin eruptions. Nalbuphine is an opioid analgesic that is not indicated for use in this client. **Cognitive Level:** Applying **Client Need:** Physiological Adaptation **Integrated Process:** Nursing Process: Implementation **Content Area:** Child Health **Strategy:** The core issue of the question is knowledge of various products used in the care of children and which one will reduce the likelihood of itching or pruritus with skin lesions. Use nursing knowledge and the process of elimination to make a selection.

4 **Answer: 1 Rationale:** Tepid baths allow heat to be removed from the body. Aspirin use is avoided because of the risk of Reye syndrome. The child should wear only light clothing to allow heat to escape. Antibiotics are not prescribed because this is a viral infection, not a bacterial infection. **Cognitive Level:** Applying **Client Need:** Physiological Adaptation **Integrated Process:** Nursing Process: Implementation **Content Area:** Child Health **Strategy:** The core issue of the question is an effective measure to prevent febrile seizures as a complication of fever in a child. Use nursing knowledge and the process of elimination to make a selection.

5 **Answer: 4 Rationale:** Mumps is a viral infection and thus antibiotics will not be effective. The other statements are true. Acetaminophen, fluids, and soft foods are helpful, and the mother should watch for vomiting and headache. **Cognitive Level:** Analyzing **Client Need:** Physiological Adaptation **Integrated Process:** Nursing Process: Evaluation **Content Area:** Child Health **Strategy:** The core issue of the question is knowledge of supportive measures for a child with mumps. Use nursing knowledge and the process of elimination to make a selection.

6 **Answer: 3 Rationale:** The child has a stuffy nose, which can impair air exchange. Nursing care involves use of a cool-mist vaporizer and gentle suctioning of the nose to prevent adverse effects on respiratory status. The rash of rubeola does not create a break in skin integrity. A 2-year-old would not be embarrassed about a skin rash. A lack of restful sleep can be problematic for the client, but does not take priority over oxygenation. **Cognitive Level:** Analyzing **Client Need:** Physiological Adaptation **Integrated Process:** Nursing Process: Planning **Content Area:** Child Health **Strategy:** The core issue of the question is the ability to set appropriate priorities of care for a child with a communicable disease. Use nursing knowledge and the process of elimination to make a selection.

7 **Answer: 2 Rationale:** The upper respiratory symptoms may be early prodromal symptoms of chickenpox. The incubation period of chickenpox is 10–21 days. A period of 5–10 days is not a sufficiently long incubation period. An incubation period of 21–25 days or 28–30 days is too long for chickenpox. **Cognitive Level:** Applying **Client Need:** Physiological Adaptation **Integrated Process:** Nursing Process: Assessment **Content Area:** Child Health **Strategy:** The core issue of the question is knowledge of the incubation period for chickenpox. Use nursing knowledge and the process of elimination to make a selection.

8 **Answer: 3 Rationale:** Cool fluids will help decrease the swelling of the glands around the mouth and neck. Acidic foods are too irritating and difficult to swallow, which is why they should be avoided. Warm, chopped foods may be difficult to swallow. Although cool foods may be soothing, spices are likely to be irritating. The child should be given small, frequent meals with soft foods rather than a regular diet. **Cognitive Level:** Applying **Client Need:** Physiological Adaptation **Integrated Process:** Nursing Process: Implementation **Content Area:** Child Health **Strategy:** The core issue of the question is knowledge of foods and beverages that will be helpful to the child with mumps. Use principles of diet therapy that utilize cool, soft, and nonirritating food items to make a selection.

9 **Answer: 3 Rationale:** Soothing the skin with an oatmeal-based substance will decrease the itching and redness. Overdressing the child will increase perspiration and thereby increase the itching. Keeping the child out of drafts has nothing to do with itching. Although drinking adequate fluids is helpful, it does not directly affect the itching. **Cognitive Level:** Applying **Client Need:** Physiological Adaptation **Integrated Process:** Nursing Process: Implementation **Content Area:** Child Health **Strategy:** The core issue of the question is an effective measure to treat itching caused by a communicable disease such as measles. Use nursing knowledge and the process of elimination to make a selection.

10 **Answer: 1 Rationale:** The route of transmission of roseola is unknown. Roseola is not known to be transmitted by the respiratory tract, contact with contaminated articles, or body secretions such as urine or stool. **Cognitive Level:** Analyzing **Client Need:** Physiological Adaptation **Integrated Process:** Teaching and Learning **Content Area:** Child Health **Strategy:** The core issue of the question is knowledge of transmission of roseola. The wording of the question tells you the correct answer

is also a true statement. Use nursing knowledge and the process of elimination to make a selection.

11 **Answer: 2 Rationale:** Pertussis is most infectious early in the course of the disease, so it is not necessary for the client to self-isolate following discharge from the hospital. Coughing bouts may still be triggered by irritants, so these should be avoided. Frequent hand hygiene is a generally helpful measure that should also be continued after discharge. Increased fluid intake is a generally helpful measure that should also be continued in the home setting. **Cognitive Level:** Analyzing **Client Need:** Physiological Adaptation **Integrated Process:** Teaching and Learning **Content Area:** Adult Health: Communicable Disease **Strategy:** The core issue of the question is knowledge of care to a client recovering from pertussis. The wording of the question tells you the correct answer is an incorrect client statement. Use nursing knowledge and the process of elimination to make a selection.

12 **Answer: 3 Rationale:** Koplik's spots are seen with roseola, not scarlet fever. Reddened edematous pharynx, red strawberry tongue, and rash in the axillae and groin are findings consistent with scarlet fever. **Cognitive Level:** Analyzing **Client Need:** Physiological Adaptation **Integrated Process:** Nursing Process: Assessment **Content Area:** Adult Health: Communicable Disease **Strategy:** The core issue of the question is the ability to discriminate between clinical findings associated with scarlet fever and roseola. The wording of the question tells you the correct answer is an incorrect client statement. Use nursing knowledge and the process of elimination to make a selection.

13 **Answer: 4 Rationale:** Fifth disease is characterized by flu-like symptoms such as fever, malaise, nausea, and vomiting, and by the characteristic "slapped cheeks" appearance. A slapped cheeks appearance is not characteristic of chickenpox, measles, or diphtheria. **Cognitive Level:** Analyzing **Client Need:** Physiological Adaptation **Integrated Process:** Nursing Process: Assessment **Content Area:** Child Health **Strategy:** The core issue of the question is the ability to discriminate the classic sign of Fifth disease from other childhood communicable diseases. Use nursing knowledge and the process of elimination to make a selection.

14 **Answer: 4 Rationale:** Anthrax is caused by a bacterium and is therefore amenable to treatment with antibiotics. Antivirals and immune globulin play no role in treating this disease. Inhaled anthrax leads to respiratory symptoms, not cutaneous anthrax. **Cognitive Level:** Analyzing **Client Need:** Physiological Adaptation **Integrated Process:** Communication and Documentation **Content Area:** Adult Health: Communicable Disease **Strategy:** The core issue of the question is knowledge of available treatment methods for anthrax. Use nursing knowledge and the process of elimination to make a selection.

15 **Answer: 6 Rationale:** The incubation period for infectious mononucleosis is up to 6 weeks (with a minimum of 4 weeks). This has important implications for the nurse and client, since the source of the exposure may be difficult to determine after several weeks. **Cognitive Level:** Analyzing **Client Need:** Safety and Infection Control **Integrated Process:** Teaching and Learning **Content Area:** Adult Health **Strategy:** The core issue of the question is knowledge of the incubation period for infectious mononucleosis. Specific knowledge is needed to answer this type of question. Note that the question asks for the number of weeks, which suggests that the number to be provided is not excessively large.

16 **Answer: 3 Rationale:** Herpes is a virus and is spread through direct contact. Bedrest is usually not necessary. Viral infections cause only low-grade fever so temperature measurement is usually not necessary. An antifungal would not be useful since herpes infection is caused by a virus. **Cognitive Level:** Applying **Client Need:** Health Promotion and Maintenance **Integrated Process:** Nursing Process: Implementation **Content Area:** Adult Health: Communicable Disease **Strategy:** Because the priority with this condition is prevention of transmission, select the option that would accomplish this.

Key Terms to Review

immunization p. 1254

vaccine p. 1254

References

Ball, J., & Bindler, R., & Cowen, K. (2015). *Principles of pediatric nursing: Caring for children* (6th ed.). Hoboken, NJ: Pearson Education.

Berman, A., Snyder, S., & Frandsen, G. (2016). *Kozier & Erb's fundamentals of nursing: Concepts, process, and practice* (10th ed.). New York, NY: Pearson Education.

Centers for Disease Control and Prevention. (2016, October 9). *Zika virus*. Available at https://www.cdc.gov/zika/.

Ignatavicius, D., & Workman, L. (2016). *Medical-surgical nursing: Patient-centered collaborative care* (10th ed.). Philadelphia: Saunders.

Kee, J. (2017). *Pearson's handbook of laboratory and diagnostic tests* (8th ed.). New York, NY: Pearson Education.

LeMone, P., Burke, K., Bauldoff, G., & Gubrud, P. (2015). *Medical surgical nursing: Clinical reasoning in patient care* (6th ed.). Hoboken, NJ: Pearson Education.

Lewis, S., Dirksen, S., Heitkemper, M., & Bucher, L. (2014). *Medical surgical nursing: Assessment and management of clinical problems* (9th ed.). St. Louis, MO: Elsevier Science.

Smith, S., Duell, D., Martin, B., Aebersold, M., & Gonzalez, L. (2017). *Clinical nursing skills: Basic to advanced skills* (10th ed.). New York, NY: Pearson Education.

68 Basic Life Support

In this chapter

Cross Reference

Other chapters relevant to this content area are

Respiratory Disorders	Chapter 55
Cardiovascular Disorders	Chapter 56

I. OVERVIEW OF BASIC LIFE SUPPORT

A. ***Basic life support (BLS)*** consists of a set of guidelines for use with respiratory or cardiac arrest

B. **Commonly called *cardiopulmonary resuscitation (CPR)***

1. Mechanical effort to deliver oxygen and blood flow to perfuse brain, heart, and other vital organs

NCLEX®

2. Follows a series of steps referred to as CAB (circulation, airway, and breathing)
3. Major steps include establishing scene safety, recognizing cardiac arrest (lack of responsiveness and absence of visible breathing), activating emergency response system, initiating prompt CPR, and delivering rapid defibrillation using automated external defibrillator (AED)

Memory Aid

Remember the CAB of Basic Life Support!
C—Chest compressions
A—Airway
B—Breathing
The old mnemonic ABC (airway, breathing, circulation) still applies for a client who has not experienced respiratory or cardiac arrest, but whose status is beginning to deteriorate or become unstable.

II. BARRIER MASKS AND DEVICES

A. **Purpose:** provide a barrier against contracting communicable disease such as HIV or hepatitis during resuscitation efforts

B. **Face shield**

1. A clear plastic or silicon sheet that can be placed over victim's mouth
2. Has an opening or tube in center sheet to permit air flow into airway during ventilations
3. Is small and portable; fits on a key ring; but use only if pocket mask is not available

C. **Pocket (face) mask**

1. Rigid plastic device that fits over mouth and nose; more effective than face shield
2. Bulky, costs more than face shield, and may not always be available

D. Bag–mask ventilation

1. Utilizes a combination of a rigid plastic mask with manual resuscitation bag (Ambu bag)
2. Can be attached to oxygen (O_2) source for more effective oxygenation
3. Eliminates risk of communicable disease transmission
4. Is preferred method for providing respiratory support during respiratory insufficiency or arrest
5. *NCLEX®* Ensure that mouth and nose are covered completely and firmly with mask to make an effective seal

III. ADULT BLS FOR HEALTHCARE PROVIDERS

A. Used for resuscitating individuals at age of puberty and older when following American Heart Association healthcare provider guidelines; BLS for laypersons includes using adult CPR guidelines for adults and children age 8 and older

B. Recognition of need for CPR and emergency cardiac care

1. After assessing scene safety, assess client to determine unresponsiveness by tapping or gently shaking shoulder and asking loudly, "Are you okay?"
2. Briefly observe for absence of breathing or abnormal breathing while checking unresponsiveness
3. Call for help or activate emergency medical system (EMS); dial 911 if outside a healthcare facility; use institutional policy for calling a code or inhouse response team if inside a healthcare agency
4. Retrieve an AED if readily available or send someone else to do so
5. Place client on flat firm surface in supine position; deflate air-fluidized mattress if in use

C. Circulation

1. Position self next to left side of victim near head and chest (left side preferred when using AED)
2. Place two or three fingers on Adam's apple and slide fingers into groove between Adam's apple and neck muscle
3. Palpate for carotid pulse for minimum of 5 seconds but not longer than 10 seconds
4. If pulse is present, assess airway and breathing; provide rescue breathing at rate of 10–12 breaths per minute if needed
5. If no pulse is present, begin external cardiac compressions
   a. Using hand closest to client's feet, place heel of hand at nipple line and place second hand on top of first
   b. Place middle finger on notch and index finger next to middle finger
   c. Place heel of opposite hand next to index finger (hand position is now on lower half of sternum); proper positioning is critical for success of CPR and to avoid injuring client
   d. Position own body directly over hands, with shoulders above hands and elbows straight
   e. *NCLEX®* Provide compressions at rate of 100–120/min and at depth of at least 5 cm (2 in.), while allowing chest to recoil completely after each compression (AHA, 2015a)
   f. Use a 30:2 compression to ventilation ratio for either one- or two-rescuer CPR; change positions for "switch" as needed after five cycles of 30:2
6. Do not interrupt chest compressions for more than 10 seconds at a time except for defibrillation or intubation; interruptions for rescue breaths should take less than 10 seconds; "switches" during two-person CPR should take less than 5 seconds
7. When AED is available, continue CPR while AED pads are being initially placed on chest and stop CPR only when AED is analyzing cardiac rhythm

D. Airway

1. Use gloves and barrier device if available
2. *NCLEX®* Open airway using **head tilt–chin lift** method (if no suspicion of neck injury) by lifting chin with two fingers while pushing down on forehead with other hand; kneel parallel to client's sternum
3. *NCLEX®* If head or neck (cervical spine) injury is suspected or has occurred, use **jaw-thrust maneuver** to open airway by lifting mandible on both sides with fingertips while positioning hands on sides of client's face; kneel at client's head

E. Breathing

1. Client with inadequate or absent breathing
   a. If client is not breathing adequately, maintain head tilt–chin lift and give two rescue breaths at rate of 1 second/breath; use breath sufficient to produce a rise in chest
   b. If chest does not rise with breath, reposition airway and try again (incorrect airway position is most common cause of obstructed rescuer ventilations)
   c. If chest still does not rise and fall, perform finger sweep of mouth to check for foreign body; clear airway and try again; remove dentures only if obstructing airway

NCLEX®
   d. Provide one breath every 5–6 seconds or 10–12 breaths per minute; allow time for client to exhale between ventilations; this is called rescue breathing
2. Improper ventilation technique could lead to ineffective ventilations or gastric distention
3. Variations in breathing technique
   a. Use mouth-to-nose ventilation if mouth cannot be sealed, has serious injuries, or cannot be opened for any reason
   b. Use mouth-to-stoma ventilation after temporary tracheostomy or laryngectomy; seal client's mouth and nose to ensure adequate ventilation
4. Client who is breathing
   a. If client is breathing adequately and has suspected or actual head or neck trauma, do not move client
   b. If client is breathing adequately and does not have suspected head or neck trauma, logroll client onto side as a unit (maintaining alignment of spine) and continue to monitor; this position is called recovery position

IV. PEDIATRIC BLS FOR HEALTHCARE PROVIDERS

A. Overview

1. Principles are same as for adult CPR; differences relate to smaller body size and needs of client
2. Use child CPR if client is age 1–8 (NCLEX®)
3. Use infant CPR for clients less than 1 year of age (NCLEX®)

B. Child CPR

1. With single rescuer who has a mobile device, activate emergency response system after determining scene safety and victim unresponsiveness
2. If single rescuer does not have a mobile device, complete five cycles of compressions and breaths (approximately 2 mins time) before activating emergency response and obtaining AED (AHA, 2015b)
3. Circulation (NCLEX®)
   a. Use hand placement as for adult victims
   b. Provide compressions at ratio of 30 compressions to two breaths; when there are two healthcare provider rescuers, may use a 15:2 ratio
   c. Maintain a compression rate of 100–120 per minute (same as for adult) (NCLEX®)
   d. Use heel of one hand or two hands for compressions to child with compression depth of at least one-third of anterior–posterior (AP) diameter of chest (about 5 cm or 2 in. but not deeper than 6 cm or 2.4 in.); use same hand placement as adult
4. Airway open airway using head tilt–chin lift method
5. Breathing
   a. After checking breathing, if needed, provide two rescue breaths initially with visible chest rise (same as for adult client)
   b. After initial two breaths, provide 2 breaths after each 30 compressions with single rescuer (NCLEX®)
   c. Deliver a breath every 3–5 seconds for a total ventilation rate of 12–20 breaths per minute (NCLEX®)

C. Infant CPR

1. Determine unresponsiveness by gently tapping infant, such as rubbing or tapping soles of feet
2. With single rescuer, complete 5 cycles of compressions and breaths (approximately 2 minutes' time) before activating emergency response and obtaining AED
3. Circulation (NCLEX®)
   a. Check brachial or femoral pulse for infant
   b. Provide compressions at ratio of 30 compressions to two breaths
   c. Maintain rate of 100–120 compressions per minute; same as for adult (NCLEX®)
   d. Use middle and ring fingers for compressions to infant at a depth of at least one-third AP diameter of chest (about 4 cm or 1.5 in.)
   e. Determine correct hand placement by placing index finger of hand further from infant's head on sternum just below an imaginary line between nipples; lower middle and ring fingers onto sternum and then lift index finger; provide compressions with middle and ring fingers (with two rescuers use two thumbs with encircling hands technique)
4. Airway open airway using head tilt–chin lift method
5. Breathing
   a. After checking breathing, if needed, provide two rescue breaths initially with visible chest rise (same as for adult client); cover mouth and nose with infant breaths
   b. After initial two breaths, provide two breaths after each 30 compressions with single rescuer (NCLEX®)
   c. Deliver a breath every 3–5 seconds for a total ventilation rate of 12–20 breaths per minute (NCLEX®)

V. AUTOMATED EXTERNAL DEFIBRILLATOR USE

A. Overview

1. **Automated external defibrillator (AED)** is a computerized defibrillator that analyzes cardiac rhythm of client, recognizes rhythm amenable to shock, and uses synthesized voice and flashing lights to indicate if shock is warranted

NCLEX®

2. Apply AED when client has signs of cardiac arrest: unresponsive, absence of respirations, absence of pulse (or signs of circulation for laypeople)
3. Place AED machine near client's left ear to allow room for reaching AED controls easily, applying pads without excessive reaching, and performing CPR without interference

B. Steps of AED operation

1. Position AED on client's left side; open AED and turn power on if not automatic upon opening AED
2. Remove clothing on torso and apply AED electrode pads to client's chest
   a. Attach connecting cables to electrode pads (if not preconnected) before applying to client's chest
   b. Peel off backing and attach electrodes to chest as indicated on pad backing or packaging; placement does not have to be exact but should be within an inch or two of placement shown on package diagram
   c. Apply first pad to upper right side of chest (right of sternum between nipple and clavicle)
   d. Apply second pad to outside of left nipple, with top margin of pad several inches below left axilla (see Figure 68–1)
3. Analyze rhythm

NCLEX®

   a. Do not touch client in any way, and do not allow others to do so; announce loudly to stand clear of client
   b. Do not push button to analyze rhythm until all contact with client has stopped; some machines analyze automatically without activation by button
4. Charge AED and, if indicated, deliver shock

NCLEX®

   a. Stay clear of client while charging; most models charge automatically
   b. Look to see that no one is touching client; announce to stand clear
   c. AED will analyze rhythm and provide direction to either deliver a shock or continue CPR
   d. Push button to deliver shock when instructed to do
   e. If shock is ineffective, leave AED paddles attached and perform CPR for 2 minutes or five cycles; then reanalyze
   f. If shock is effective, follow CPR guidelines according to client need

C. Special circumstances

1. If available, use child pads and a pediatric dose attenuator system for children age 1–8; if not available, use standard AED and pads
2. Use a manual defibrillator for infants less than 1 year of age, if available; if not available, then use an AED with pediatric dose attenuation; if neither is available, an AED without a pediatric dose attenuator may be used

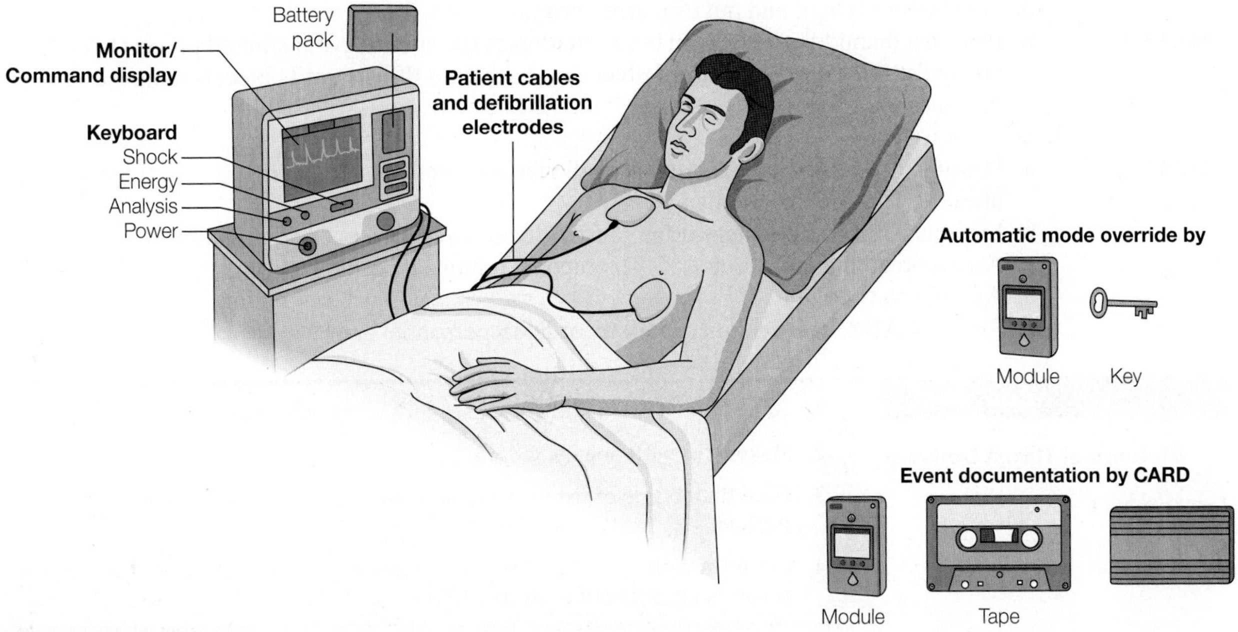

Figure 68–1 Automated external defibrillator attached to client.

NCLEX®

3. Do not use AED on client lying in standing water until client is removed and chest is dried
4. Avoid placing AED electrodes directly over an implantable defibrillator
5. Remove transdermal medication before placing an AED electrode on that site; wipe skin dry and then position electrode
6. Use a prep razor if needed for hairy chest to ensure good contact between client's skin and AED electrodes

VI. FOREIGN BODY AIRWAY OBSTRUCTION

A. Adult or child who is choking

1. Responsive
   a. Ask client, "Are you choking?" (will nod "yes" but will not be able to cough or speak if choking with severe or complete airway obstruction; will also have increasing respiratory distress and developing cyanosis)
   b. Encourage client to cough if crowing noise is heard (partial obstruction)
   NCLEX®
   c. Use **abdominal-thrust maneuver** (see Box 68–1) until client becomes unconscious or blockage is relieved
2. Unresponsive
   a. Place client on back
   b. Proceed to sequence for chest compressions
   c. Open airway for rescue breaths; look in mouth for foreign body; remove if seen and removable
   d. Attempt 2 rescue breaths; check if chest rises
   e. Repeat sequence of compressions and rescue breaths until obstruction is cleared

B. Infant who is choking

1. Responsive
   a. Observe respiratory difficulty in infant
   b. Position client over arm or on lap with head lower than trunk; support head firmly by holding jaw
   c. Deliver five back blows between shoulder blades using heel of hand
   d. Turn client over with head lower than chest and deliver five chest thrusts using same location as for CPR
   e. Check mouth of infant for foreign object after each series, but avoid blind finger sweeps that could push obstruction further into airway
   f. Continue series until relieved or infant becomes unresponsive
2. Unresponsive
   a. Assess unconsciousness of infant
   b. Institute sequence of chest compressions
   c. Assess breathing and observe for foreign object; remove if seen
   d. Attempt ventilation
   e. Repeat CAB sequence until successful or EMS personnel arrive

C. Pregnant or obese client who is choking

1. Responsive
   a. Stand behind client and put own arms around client's chest
   NCLEX®
   b. Place fist on middle of sternum between nipples (be sure to avoid xiphoid process)
   c. Grasp fist with other hand and deliver firm backward thrusts until object is removed or victim becomes unconscious
2. Unresponsive
   NCLEX®
   a. Position victim lying on back; use a small pillow or wedge under right hip of pregnant client to shift uterus to left side of abdomen
   b. Institute chest compressions using ratio of 30 compressions to two ventilations
   c. Assess breathing and observe for obstruction; remove if seen
   d. Attempt to ventilate
   e. Repeat CAB sequence until successful or EMS personnel arrive

Box 68–1

Abdominal Thrust Delivery

1. Stand behind client and encircle client's waist with own arms.
2. Make a fist with one hand.
3. Place thumb side of fist on abdomen above umbilicus but below xiphoid process of sternum.
4. Grasp fist with other hand and give quick inward and upward thrusts until victim becomes unconscious or obstruction is expelled.

Check Your NCLEX–RN® Exam I.Q.

You are ready for testing on this content if you can:

- Recognize and intervene when client requires cardiopulmonary resuscitation or Heimlich maneuver/abdominal thrusts.
- Evaluate and document response to resuscitation efforts.
- Explain emergency interventions to client and family when necessary.

PRACTICE TEST

1 A client is brought to the emergency department awake and alert following a fall from a ladder from a height of 4.6 meters (15 ft). During an initial assessment, the client becomes unresponsive and stops breathing. Which method should the nurse use to open the airway?

1. Head tilt–chin lift
2. Jaw thrust
3. Tongue–jaw lift
4. None; client needs emergency intubation

2 The nurse has begun cardiopulmonary resuscitation (CPR) on a 5-year-old child. The nurse times the rate of ventilation to achieve up to how many breaths per minute? Provide a numeric answer.

Fill in your answer below:
Answer: ________ breaths/minute

3 A nurse has begun to resuscitate a 10-month-old infant. In what location would the nurse check the infant's pulse?

1. Brachial
2. Radial
3. Carotid
4. Temporal

4 The nurse on a surgical nursing unit has just called a code blue using the telephone in the room of an unresponsive adult client who had abdominal surgery. Which action would be appropriate during initiation of CPR?

1. Open the airway using the jaw-thrust method.
2. Deliver one deep breath before checking for a pulse.
3. Depress the sternum at least 5 cm (2 in.) during cardiac compressions.
4. Reevaluate status every 3 to 5 minutes until the code team arrives.

5 The nurse who is doing the documentation during a code blue on an adult client observes an unlicensed assistive person (UAP) doing CPR. The nurse concludes the UAP is using correct procedure after noting that the UAP is depressing the sternum at least how many inches? Provide a numeric answer in inches.

Fill in your answer below:
Answer: ________ inches

6 The nurse is performing cardiopulmonary resuscitation (CPR) on a 10-month-old infant. The nurse times the rate of compressions to achieve a minimum of how many compressions per minute? Provide a numeric response.

Fill in your answer below:
Answer: ________ compressions/min

7 A nurse witnesses an adult male collapse at the airport and an automated external defibrillator (AED) is brought to the scene. The nurse should perform which actions in using the device?

1. Press the electrodes down firmly because the client has a hairy chest.
2. Instruct another person at the scene to keep the airway open during delivery of the electric shock.
3. Initiate CPR after 5 minutes if the AED has not restored a perfusing cardiac rhythm.
4. Quickly wipe up the spilled coffee under the victim's chest before using the AED.

8 A nurse is eating in a restaurant when a woman who is 8 months pregnant at the next table begins to choke. Which hand placement should the nurse use to perform the abdominal-thrust maneuver?

1. Midsternum
2. Lower sternum
3. Midway between umbilicus and xiphoid process
4. Midway between umbilicus and symphysis pubis

9 The long-term care nurse has been called to the aid of a resident who has become unconscious after choking in the dining room. After positioning the client on the back, which action should the nurse take next?

1. Attempt to ventilate the client.
2. Begin cardiopulmonary resuscitation, starting with chest compressions.
3. Perform five abdominal thrusts.
4. Perform five chest thrusts.

10 A nurse enters an adult client's room and says, "Good morning!" while doing initial shift rounds after receiving report. The client does not respond. Put the nurse's actions in order of priority.

1. Call for someone to announce a code blue.
2. Check for a carotid pulse.
3. Gently shake the client's shoulder and ask, "Are you okay?"
4. Begin chest compressions.

Fill in your answer below:

Answer: ______________________

ANSWERS & RATIONALES

1 **Answer: 2 Rationale:** The jaw-thrust maneuver is used whenever head or cervical spine injury is suspected to avoid causing further physiological damage. The head tilt–chin lift method is the standard method for opening the airway when there is no suspected cervical spine injury. The tongue–jaw lift aids in visualizing foreign bodies in the airway. The client does not need emergency intubation. **Cognitive Level:** Applying **Client Need:** Physiological Adaptation **Integrated Process:** Nursing Process: Implementation **Content Area:** Adult Health: Respiratory **Strategy:** Note critical information in the stem, which indicates the client had a traumatic injury and is therefore at risk of cervical spine injury. Next use knowledge of basic CPR procedures to select the option for opening the airway in a client with suspected head or neck injury.

2 **Answer: 20 Rationale:** The proper ventilation rate for a child or infant is 12–20 breaths per minute, which is the same as delivering one breath every 3–5 seconds. The correct answer is 20 based on the words *up to*. **Cognitive Level:** Applying **Client Need:** Physiological Adaptation **Integrated Process:** Nursing Process: Implementation **Content Area:** Child Health **Strategy:** Recall basic CPR procedures to identify the correct rate. Remember that compressions and ventilation rates need to be higher in children than in adults.

3 **Answer: 1 Rationale:** The brachial artery is the correct location for determining whether an infant under 1 year of age has a pulse. The radial artery would not generate enough pulsation in an infant to be reliable and is also more difficult to palpate. The carotid pulse is not as easily located in an infant with a small neck and neck folds. The temporal pulse is not used in CPR for an individual of any age. **Cognitive Level:** Applying **Client Need:** Physiological Adaptation **Integrated Process:** Nursing Process: Implementation **Content Area:** Child Health **Strategy:** First eliminate radial and temporal because they are not used in CPR. Choose brachial over carotid using knowledge of infant anatomy and accessibility of the site.

4 **Answer: 3 Rationale:** In an adult, the sternum should be depressed during CPR to a depth of at least 5 cm (2 in.). The head tilt–chin lift method of opening the airway is used for the client who has no head or neck injury. After determining unresponsiveness while simultaneously checking quickly for breathing, the nurse begins chest compressions. The nurse reevaluates the client's status after approximately 2 minutes. **Cognitive Level:** Applying **Client Need:** Physiological Adaptation **Integrated Process:** Nursing Process: Implementation **Content Area:** Adult Health: Cardiovascular **Strategy:** Use knowledge of basic CPR procedures to answer the question. Recall current guidelines to aid in making the correct selection.

5 **Answer: 2 Rationale:** On an adult client, chest compressions should be done to a depth of at least 5 cm (2 in.) to be effective. **Cognitive Level:** Applying **Client Need:** Physiological Adaptation **Integrated Process:** Nursing Process: Implementation **Content Area:** Adult Health: Cardiovascular **Strategy:** Use the process of elimination and knowledge of basic CPR procedures to answer the question. Recall that compressions are at least 5 cm (2 in.) to answer correctly.

6 **Answer: 100 Rationale:** The rate of compressions for an infant during CPR is 100–120 compressions per minute, making the minimum rate of compressions 100/min. **Cognitive Level:** Applying **Client Need:** Physiological Adaptation **Integrated Process:** Nursing Process: Implementation **Content Area:** Child Health **Strategy:** Use knowledge of basic CPR procedures to answer the question. Memorize the number 100 to answer correctly.

7 **Answer: 4 Rationale:** The client should not be lying in water or other liquid, which could lead to burns or to defibrillating another individual who comes in contact with the liquid during AED shock delivery. The electrodes should not be placed on hairy areas, or the site should be shaved. All people should stand clear of the individual during an AED shock to avoid being defibrillated themselves. CPR is initiated after

1 minute or whenever the series of shocks is terminated, as indicated by client condition. However, 5 minutes is excessive and could lead to permanent brain damage if the client survives. **Cognitive Level:** Applying **Client Need:** Physiological Adaptation **Integrated Process:** Nursing Process: Implementation **Content Area:** Adult Health: Cardiovascular **Strategy:** First, recall hair interferes with good skin contact of any type of electrode to eliminate that option. Next, recall that brain death can occur within 4–6 minutes if CPR is not initiated. Use general principles of electrical safety to choose between the remaining two options.

8 **Answer: 1 Rationale:** In a pregnant client, the abdominal thrust maneuver is performed in a manner that avoids causing injury to the fetus. For this reason, the hand placement is at the midsternum. The lower sternum should be avoided to prevent accidental fracture of the xiphoid process, which could lead to internal injury. Midway between the umbilicus and the xiphoid process is the abdomen, which is contraindicated in the pregnant client. Midway between the umbilicus and the symphysis pubis is the lower abdomen, which is contraindicated in the pregnant client. **Cognitive Level:** Applying **Client Need:** Physiological Adaptation **Integrated Process:** Nursing Process: Implementation **Content Area:** Adult Health: Cardiovascular **Strategy:** Note key information in the question that the client is pregnant. Then use knowledge of basic CPR procedures to answer the question.

9 **Answer: 2 Rationale:** After positioning the client on the back, the nurse would begin cardiopulmonary resuscitation, starting with chest compressions. The nurse would attempt to ventilate after inspecting the mouth. Abdominal thrusts are performed on responsive clients. Chest thrusts are performed in the adult only for pregnant or obese clients. **Cognitive Level:** Analyzing **Client Need:** Physiological Adaptation **Integrated Process:** Nursing Process: Implementation **Content Area:** Adult Health: Respiratory **Strategy:** Remember the ABCs of life support to answer this question. Choose the option that attempts to clear the airway before taking any other actions.

10 **Answer: 3, 1, 2, 4 Rationale:** The first action of the nurse is to establish unresponsiveness. This can be done by shaking the shoulder and asking if the client is okay. The second action of the nurse would be to call for help. The third action of the nurse is to address circulation by checking the client's pulse. If no pulse is present, the nurse should begin chest compressions. The 2015 CPR guidelines use the mnemonic CAB (chest compressions, airway, breathing). **Cognitive Level:** Analyzing **Client Need:** Physiological Adaptation **Integrated Process:** Nursing Process: Implementation **Content Area:** Adult Health: Cardiovascular **Strategy:** Specific knowledge of the sequence of events is needed to answer the question. Using the mnemonic CAB (chest compressions, airway, breathing) will be of assistance once unresponsiveness has been determined.

Key Terms to Review

abdominal-thrust maneuver p. 1270
automated external defibrillator (AED) p. 1269
basic life support (BLS) p. 1266
cardiopulmonary resuscitation (CPR) p. 1266
head tilt–chin lift p. 1267
jaw-thrust maneuver p. 1267

References

American Heart Association (2015a). *CPR and first aid. Emergency cardiovascular care. Part 5. Adult basic life support and cardiopulmonary resuscitation quality.* Available at https://eccguidelines.heart.org/index.php/circulation/cpr-ecc-guidelines-2/part-5-adult-basic-life-support-and-cardiopulmonary-resuscitation-quality/.

American Heart Association (2015b). *CPR and first aid. Emergency cardiovascular care. Part 11. Pediatric basic life support and cardiopulmonary resuscitation quality.* Available at https://eccguidelines.heart.org/index.php/circulation/cpr-ecc-guidelines-2/part-11-pediatric-basic-life-support-and-cardiopulmonary-resuscitation-quality/.

American Heart Association (2016). *Basic life support. Provider manual.* Dallas, TX: Author.

Ball, J., & Bindler, R., & Cowen, K. (2015). *Principles of pediatric nursing: Caring for children* (6th ed.). Hoboken, NJ: Pearson Education.

Berman, A., Snyder, S., & Frandsen, G. (2016). *Kozier & Erb's fundamentals of nursing: Concepts, process, and practice* (10th ed.). New York, NY: Pearson Education.

LeMone, P., Burke, K., Bauldoff, G., & Gubrud, P. (2015). *Medical surgical nursing: Clinical reasoning in patient care* (6th ed.). Hoboken, NJ: Pearson Education.

Smith, S., Duell, D., Martin, B., Aebersold, M., & Gonzalez, L. (2017). *Clinical nursing skills: Basic to advanced skills* (10th ed.). New York, NY: Pearson Education.

Comprehensive Exam

1. A client exposed to *Mycobacterium tuberculosis* starts on chemoprophylaxis. The nurse provides which instruction to the client?

1. "You will take a single drug such as isoniazid by mouth every day for 6–12 months."
2. "You will be on at least two drugs effective against the tubercle bacillus for three months."
3. "You will be on combination therapy in order to prevent development of drug resistance."
4. "You will need to learn to give yourself subcutaneous injections."

2. The nurse delegates an unlicensed assistive person (UAP) to assist a client with a clean urinary catheterization procedure. The client was formerly able to perform the procedure alone but because of arthritis, he is no longer able to do so. Although the UAP has done this procedure before, which direction is most important for the nurse to emphasize to the UAP?

1. Let the client do most of the procedure and report the expected output.
2. Report immediately any unusual observations, such as bleeding.
3. Complete in proper order the steps of the procedure.
4. Perform health teaching while performing the procedure.

3. The surgical unit nurse is assigned to the care of a client who returned from surgery 8 hours ago. Which assessment is of highest priority at this time?

1. Client remembers how to use incentive spirometer.
2. Client remains free of nausea and vomiting.
3. Client has active bowel sounds.
4. Client has been able to void.

4. The clinic nurse is conducting health screenings. Which client assessment findings indicate the need for health education about reducing risk factors for stroke? Select all that apply.

1. Weight 205 lbs and height 5 feet 4 inches
2. Blood pressure 164/92 mmHg
3. Eats bran for breakfast daily
4. Smokes ½ pack of cigarettes per day
5. Serum cholesterol level is 172 mg/dL

5. Which action should the nurse take to maintain medical asepsis when caring for a hospitalized client with diabetes mellitus who requires irrigation of a leg ulcer and insulin injections? Select all that apply.

1. Wash hands before and after performing client care.
2. Wear personal protective equipment during the dressing change.
3. Recap the needle after administering insulin injection.
4. Use sterile gloves to change the dressing for the leg ulcer.
5. Wipe the rubber stopper on the insulin vial before withdrawing dose.

6. Hematologic laboratory test results indicate a client with cancer is in the nadir period following the latest round of chemotherapy. Which drug should the nurse avoid administering to this client at this time?

1. Acetaminophen
2. Ibuprofen
3. Diphenhydramine
4. Guaifenesin

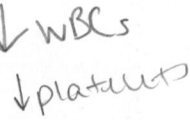

7. The newborn nursery has recently formed a unit operations committee. The nurse who wishes to exert situational leadership in this committee should exhibit which behavior?

1. Ask questions about current unit practices and offer suggestions for revisions.
2. Realize the group needs autonomy early in the process and listen to others' ideas.
3. Refer to the organization's rules, policies, and procedures to direct the group's work.
4. Adjust leadership style during meetings depending on how the group is functioning.

8. The nurse places highest priority on taking which action to reduce the spread of microorganisms when caring for a client at risk for infection?

1. Perform hand hygiene before and after client care.
2. Use clean gloves when implementing client care.
3. Institute transmission-based precautions.
4. Transfer the client to a private room.

9. The nurse should report to the healthcare provider which abnormal laboratory values for a 58-year-old client newly hospitalized with fever and diarrhea? Select all that apply.

1. White blood cell count 12,260 cells/mm^3
2. Sodium 142 mEq/L
3. Potassium 3.9 mEq/L
4. Blood urea nitrogen 38 mg/dL
5. Serum creatinine 0.9 mg/dL

10. A confused client who keeps trying to pull out a central venous access device has been prescribed to have a wrist restraint applied for safety reasons. Which action should the nurse take to apply the restraint correctly?

1. Use a full knot to secure the safety restraint
2. Secure the straps of the safety restraint to the bed frame
3. Ensure that three fingers can slide between the skin and the restraint
4. Secure safety restraint straps so they do not tighten if client pulls on them

11. A postoperative client who will receive enoxaparin subcutaneously wants to know why this drug is being prescribed. What would be the best response by the nurse?

1. "Enoxaparin is almost always used after surgery to reduce the risk of pulmonary emboli."
2. "Enoxaparin is essential after surgery to maintain adequate blood clotting levels."
3. "Enoxaparin injections are given in the abdomen and do not usually cause discomfort."
4. "Enoxaparin helps prevent blood clots in people who have reduced mobility after surgery."

12. The emergency department has experienced a 20% increase in client visits from the same period last year. In an effort to empower staff to reduce staff stress and burnout, the charge nurse should use which approach to demonstrate shared leadership?

1. Assist with formation of self-directed work teams.
2. Encourage the group to try out new evidence-based approaches to care.
3. Suggest that staff excellence be rewarded with professional development opportunities.
4. Provide constructive criticism and assist the nurses to meet their work goals for the shift.

13. While providing a nursing history, a 65-year-old client reports that his sleep patterns are different than when he was younger. The nurse explains to the client that which changes in sleep can occur because of the aging process?

1. The same or less total sleep time but with more rapid eye movement (REM) sleep
2. The same or a little less total sleep time but with less non-REM deep sleep
3. A heavier and deeper sleep and slightly longer total sleep time
4. A light sleep pattern with equal amounts of REM and non-REM sleep

14. A labor and delivery nurse notes a pattern of late decelerations on the fetal monitor. Which priority action should the nurse take at this time?

1. Assist the client to a squatting position
2. Request a prescription to begin an oxytocin infusion
3. Begin oxygen therapy by face mask
4. Ask the client's partner to coach the client with breathing

15. The surgical unit nurse reassesses the condition of a postoperative client who was transferred to the unit 2 hours ago. Which data obtained at this time is of concern to the nurse? Select all that apply.

1. Scant amount of serosanguineous drainage on dressing
2. Brighter red drainage in Jackson Pratt surgical drain
3. Temperature 99.2°F (37.3°C)
4. Urine output 50 mL in last 2 hours
5. Blood pressure 126/78 mmHg

16. After defibrillation, the client continues to be in a pulseless ventricular tachycardia. After administration of procainamide, the nurse should expect to see which therapeutic response?

1. Conversion of rhythm to ventricular fibrillation
2. Conversion of rhythm to atrial fibrillation
3. A reduction in ventricular irritability
4. An increase in level of consciousness

17. The nurse is assigned to a client diagnosed with head and neck cancer who is receiving enteral feedings via gastrostomy tube. When the nurse is called away to care for another client, which task for this client could most appropriately be delegated to the unlicensed assistive person (UAP)?

1. Determining the amount of residual for the tube feeding
2. Giving mouth care and assessing the oral cavity
3. Exploring how the client is currently coping with the diagnosis
4. Administering a bath and changing bed linens

18. A client with uncompensated metabolic acidosis is admitted to the hospital for observation and treatment. Which values should the nurse anticipate when laboratory test results are communicated to the nursing unit?

1. pH 7.40; serum potassium 3.8 mEq/L
2. pH 7.36; serum potassium 3.1 mEq/ L
3. pH 7.24; serum potassium 6.2 mEq/ L
4. pH 7.12; serum potassium 5.0 mEq/ L

19. A client has a BUN of 68 mg/dL and a creatinine level of 6.0 mg/dL. An IV solution of 5% dextrose in 0.9% NaCl with 40 mEq potassium chloride is infusing at 100 mL/hour. Which action would be most appropriate for the nurse to take?

1. Encourage protein restriction in the diet.
2. Ambulate the client more often to promote circulation.
3. Measure and record vital signs every hour.
4. Question the use of potassium in the IV fluids.

20. The emergency department (ED) nurse is notified that a train travelling through the community has derailed and several casualties will be transported to the ED. What should be the first action taken by the nurse?

1. Activate the hospital emergency response plan.
2. Ensure all client treatment areas are well stocked with supplies.
3. Reassign an increased number of staff to the triage area.
4. Begin calling off-duty staff to see if they will come in to work.

21. A 60-year-old client has been prescribed rabeprazole for symptoms of gastroesophageal reflux disease (GERD). The client has trouble swallowing pills. What alternate medication should the nurse plan to request for this client?

1. Omeprazole
2. Pantoprazole
3. Lansoprazole
4. There is no substitute for rabeprazole

22. At the start of the shift one RN and one LPN/LVN were available to care for three newborns in the nursery. Within 2 hours, three newborns were admitted, one requiring Level II care, while parents of two newborns required discharge teaching. The RN is needed full time in the Level II nursery while the newborn is stabilized. The RN determines that what staffing activity is needed to provide appropriate care?

1. The LPN/LVN can complete admission assessments and discharge teaching for five Level 1 newborns.
2. A UAP from the postpartum unit can be reassigned to the nursery to do discharge teaching.
3. The RN can complete admission assessments while continuing to stabilize the Level II newborn.
4. Another RN should be assigned to the nursery to perform admission assessments and discharge teaching.

23. The nurse is working with a client who has chronic diarrhea. In teaching ways to reduce diarrhea, what should the nurse encourage the client to avoid?

To ↓ diarrhea, avoid ______

1. Excessive intake of cheese and eggs — constp
2. Habitually ignoring the urge to defecate
3. Anxiety or anger ~ ↑ peristalsis
4. Lack of exercise

24. The fetal head is determined to be presenting in a position of complete extension. After learning of this, the nurse anticipates which type of delivery?

1. Precipitous labor and delivery
2. Prolonged labor and possible cesarean delivery
3. Normal labor and spontaneous vaginal delivery
4. Short labor with forceps-assisted vaginal delivery

25. The nurse notices that an older adult resident in a skilled nursing home facility has not been eating or drinking as much as usual. Which assessment finding by the nurse would best indicate the presence of dehydration?

1. Clear lung fields with unlabored respirations
2. Tenting and dry, flaky skin
3. Increased drowsiness, mild confusion, and concentrated urine
4. Hand veins that fill within 3 to 5 seconds of being lowered below the heart

26. Following a liver transplant the client is taking prednisone and other immunosuppressive medications to prevent organ rejection. The nurse should instruct the client to make it a priority to report which manifestation to the healthcare provider?

1. Moon face
2. Diminished pigmentation
3. Dysphagia
4. Bleeding

27. The nurse should place highest priority on which nursing intervention when planning to prevent atelectasis in the newly admitted postoperative client?

1. Hourly coughing and deep breathing
2. Assisting the client out of bed
3. Administration of bronchodilators
4. Supplemental oxygen

28. The nurse responds to a voice calling out from a room on the nursing unit. Upon entering the room, the nurse sees a client lying on the floor near the foot of the bed. After attending to the client and notifying the healthcare provider, which notation would be most appropriate to record on the incident/unusual occurrence report?

1. Client fell while walking to bathroom
2. Client found lying on floor at foot of bed
3. Client states nursing staff did not respond to call bell
4. Client was rushing to bathroom to avoid incontinence

29. A client's hemoglobin level is 14 grams/dL. Which interpretation of the laboratory value by the nurse is most accurate?

1. Client has a low value and is malnourished.
2. Client has a normal laboratory value and has no nutritional risk.
3. Client has a low to normal value indicative of a nutritional risk.
4. Client has an elevated value indicative of polycythemia.

30. Which item should the nurse discuss when teaching home care measures to the parents of a child who has bilateral bacterial conjunctivitis?

1. Use of warm, moist, disposable compresses to remove crusting
2. Use of oral antihistamine medication to relieve eye itching
3. Use of ophthalmic corticosteroids to decrease inflammatory response
4. Use of topical anesthetics applied to relieve discomfort

31. After a client has experienced a seizure, the nurse should assist the client into which most appropriate position?

1. On back with head raised 15 degrees
2. On the side
3. On abdomen
4. Upright in chair

32. After correctly positioning a client for a wound dressing change and setting up a sterile field with supplies added, the nurse hears a page to respond to another client who has fallen in the hallway. What is the most appropriate action for the nurse to take at this time?

1. Ensure the client's safety, cover the field with a sterile towel, and respond to the other client.
2. Continue quickly with the procedure, then assist the other client, checking back with the first client as soon as possible.
3. Ensure the client's safety, discard the sterile equipment, and respond to the other client.
4. Explain the situation to the client needing wound dressing change, leave the sterile supplies in place, and attend to the other client.

33. A client recently diagnosed with type 1 diabetes mellitus is learning to use the American Diabetes Association exchange lists. The nurse determines that the teaching has been effective if the client chooses which appropriate exchange for white rice?

1. Egg
2. Tomato
3. Orange
4. Bread

34. The nurse is teaching a group of adults about health screenings for cancer. The nurse should include which item in the discussion? Select all that apply.

1. Genetic screening is helpful in identification of cancer risks.
2. Annual medical exams uncover most tumors.
3. Men should perform breast and testicular self-exams (BSE, TSE) monthly.
4. Annual mammograms are recommended after a total mastectomy.
5. Inspection of the skin for cancer becomes less important as one ages.

35. The nurse observes two unlicensed assistive personnel (UAP) in the corridor on the nursing unit arguing about how to handle a difficult client. What would be the most appropriate approach for the nurse to use to address this conflict between staff members?

1. Let it pass because the coworkers probably did not intend to be critical.
2. Speak privately to the coworkers, telling them about personal reactions to this public encounter.
3. Confront and reprimand the coworkers publicly.
4. Inform each coworker privately that it would be most helpful not to display this behavior again.

36. The school nurse is assessing a muscular 17-year-old female who is coming to the high school health service because of edema, voice changes, and hair loss. What should be the nurse's initial conclusion pending further assessment, based on the client's subjective and objective data?

1. The client is going through a stage of puberty.
2. The client may be using steroids.
3. The client may be abusing barbiturates.
4. The client is using marijuana regularly.

37. A 4-year-old child has been exposed to chickenpox. After providing information about chickenpox, the nurse asks the mother to repeat back the information. Which response by the mother indicates a need for additional information?

1. "During the prodromal period, my child will have chickenpox all over his body."
2. "Chickenpox is a viral infection that can be spread to other children."
3. "I should monitor my child for Reye syndrome, which is a complication of chickenpox."
4. "My child should not visit my pregnant sister at this time."

38. The school health nurse is planning safety education as part of back-to-school night for high school students and their parents. The nurse should plan to address which threat to safety that represents a developmental risk factor for adolescents?

1. Substance abuse as a means of dealing with stress
2. Feelings of being invulnerable to risks that affect others
3. Sports-related injuries that often result from not obeying rules and/or intense competition
4. Polypharmacy, which results in mixing of multiple medications

39. When giving directions to a 24-year-old female with possible appendicitis who is about to undergo a pelvic sonogram, the nurse should make which statement to the client?

1. "Drink nothing for several hours prior to the exam."
2. "You will be given an enema to cleanse the bowel."
3. "Drink plenty of liquids so you will have a full bladder."
4. "Do not take any medications prior to the exam."

40. The nurse is conducting an initial interview with a 10-year-old boy who has been brought to the mental health clinic by his parents. The nurse can establish rapport and credibility with the child by asking the child which question?

1. "Do you have an idea of what you said or did that led your parents to bring you here today?"
2. "Can you tell me a little bit about some of your hobbies or other things that you like to do?"
3. "How do you think you get along with members of your family and friends?"
4. "Do you remember any medical problems or illnesses you had in the past?"

41. The nurse is providing medication instructions to a client. The nurse informs the client that persistent gynecomastia can result from taking which newly prescribed diuretic?

1. Hydrochlorothiazide
2. Furosemide
3. Spironolactone
4. Indapamide

42. As the nursing unit representative to the hospital quality management committee, the nurse has been asked to evaluate the quality of nursing services on the unit. What would be an appropriate quality improvement activity for the nurse to ask team members to participate in?

1. Tracking the number of accidents or incidents on the unit
2. Documenting nursing time and activities spent on direct client care
3. Administering a client and family satisfaction survey
4. Assessing clients and report acuity to shift manager daily

43. When a female client preparing for surgery suddenly bursts into tears, the preoperative holding unit nurse should take which action?

1. Pull the curtain closed and leave the area to provide privacy.
2. Remain with the client in silence as a sign of compassion.
3. Ask the client to share what she is feeling.
4. Continue with the physical preparation of the client.

44. After reviewing the client's health history, the nurse concludes that which item is the most significant factor for development of bronchogenic carcinoma for this client?

1. Asthma
2. Smokeless tobacco
3. Cigarette smoking
4. Air pollution

45. The nurse is setting up the breakfast tray for a client with gastroesophageal reflux disease (GERD) and notices one food that the client should not eat. Which food should the nurse remove from the meal tray?

1. Egg white omelet
2. Dry toast
3. Coffee with cream
4. Skim milk

46. A 50-year-old client with liver disease, heart failure, and chronic obstructive pulmonary disease is experiencing tremors, dizziness, tachycardia, and nausea. The client weighs 68 kg (150 lb), has a prior history of cigarette smoking, and takes theophylline. The nurse explains to the client that which factor may be responsible for these symptoms?

1. History of cigarette smoking
2. Liver disease
3. The client's age
4. The client's weight

47. The nurse has admitted to the surgical unit a client who just underwent open reduction and internal fixation of a severely fractured right radius and ulna. Which nursing care activities would be appropriate for the nurse to delegate to the licensed practical/vocational nurse (LPN/LVN)? Select all that apply.

1. Measure and document vital signs hourly for 4 hours.
2. Observe for drainage on the cast and report if it occurs.
3. Assess neurovascular status of the casted extremity hourly.
4. Elevate the casted arm above heart level with one or two pillows.
5. Administer an opioid analgesic prescribed by the IV push route.

48. Which action should the nurse take that is specific to the care of an assigned client who has tuberculosis?

1. Wearing a particulate respirator mask when taking vital signs
2. Telling the client to cover the mouth with tissues when transported within the hospital
3. Wearing sterile gloves when collecting a sputum specimen
4. Keeping the client's door open to promote ventilation

49. A client has a potassium level of 6.8 mEq/L. Which manifestation should the nurse expect to find when assessing this client?

1. Tall T wave on the cardiac telemetry monitor
2. The absence of bowel sounds, such as in an ileus
3. Muscle cramping of the lower extremities
4. Somnolence with early changes

50. The nurse is preparing to take a client to the electroconvulsive therapy (ECT) treatment suite. The nurse must ensure that which pretreatment process has been completed?

1. The client's legal spouse has signed the consent form.
2. The client is wearing snug-fitting clothing.
3. The client has been NPO.
4. The client has been given ample liquids before the procedure.

51. The nurse should take which action to minimize pain associated with intramuscular (IM) injection of 2 mL of penicillin G benzathine to an adult client?

1. Apply cold compress to site after injection.
2. Divide the dose and inject half into each deltoid.
3. Limit prolonging the time taken to administer the drug by not aspirating.
4. Administer the drug deep IM slowly into a large muscle such as the gluteus.

52. The nurse is assigned to the care of an obese client who has gastroesophageal reflux disease (GERD). Which activity could the nurse appropriately delegate to the unlicensed assistant person (UAP)?

1. Explain to the client the need for weight loss to control symptoms.
2. Explore client concerns about the prescribed regimen for managing GERD.
3. Discuss why it is important to eat several small meals per day.
4. Remind the client to remain upright for at least 2 hours after eating.

53. The nurse is admitting a client with thermal burns to both arms and anterior trunk. The client asks for a drink of water. What is the most appropriate response for the nurse to make?

1. "I'm sorry, you cannot drink anything right now; let me moisten your mouth instead."
2. "I can only give you juice to drink, not water."
3. "I'll get you a drink as soon as I'm finished."
4. "Would you also like me to order you a meal tray?"

54. A mother brings a 3-year-old child to the clinic for a well-child checkup. The child has not been to the clinic since 6 months of age. The nurse determines that which activity is the priority of care for this child?

1. Assess growth and development.
2. Begin dental care.
3. Complete hearing screening.
4. Update vaccinations.

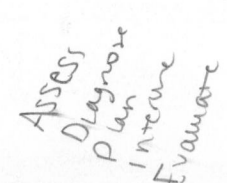

55. A client who has pancreatitis is experiencing pain. After administering an analgesic, the nurse should recommend that the client assume one of which of the following positions to promote comfort? Select all that apply.

1. Supine
2. Prone
3. Left lateral decubitus
4. Sitting up and leaning forward
5. Side-lying with knees pulled up to chest

56. The nurse should be *most* careful to assess for stomatitis as an adverse effect in a client receiving which chemotherapeutic agent?

1. Fluorouracil
2. Cisplatin
3. Doxorubicin
4. Vincristine

57. The nurse will be working with an unregulated care provider (UCP) for the work shift. Prior to delegating tasks to the UCP, the nurse places high priority on completing which activity?

1. Determining that the UCP is competent to perform the required task
2. Providing written directions to the UCP
3. Making sure all the necessary supplies are available at the client's bedside
4. Informing clients that an unlicensed staff member will be assigned to them

58. The nurse detects slight one-sided weakness and further tests muscle strength by asking the client to hold the arms up, as if holding a tray, and then close the eyes. The client's right hand moves downward slightly and turns. The nurse then documents and reports which assessment finding?

1. Pronator drift
2. Nystagmus
3. Hyperreflexia
4. Ataxia

59. When a client has arterial blood gases drawn from the radial artery, the nurse should plan to complete which follow-up action?

1. Hold the site for up to 1 minute.
2. Transfer the blood sample to a heparinized test tube.
3. Pack the sample in ice for transport to the laboratory.
4. Obtain a second specimen after 10 minutes for comparison.

60. The long-term care nurse is aware that a client has dysthymic disorder. What would be the most important nursing intervention to include in the nursing care plan for this client?

1. Provide at least 2 hours of quiet time every morning for the client.
2. Encourage the client to eat in the main dining room with other clients.
3. Include at least three regular meals per day and no snacks.
4. Include at least 2 liters of clear liquids per day in the diet regime.

61. A client who is receiving intravenous heparin by protocol orders has an activated partial thromboplastin time (APTT) level of 140 seconds (control time is 36 seconds). What is the priority action that the nurse should institute?

1. Increase the heparin dose as the APTT level is not therapeutic. Obtain a repeat APTT in 6 hours.
2. Stop the heparin therapy for 6 hours, then restart the therapy at the same unit dose and obtain a repeat APTT in 6 hours.
3. Stop the heparin for 1 hour. Restart it in 1 hour at a decreased rate per protocol. Obtain a repeat APTT in 2–3 hours after restart.
4. Obtain an additional APTT in 1 hour and continue to monitor the client.

62. The nurse has admitted to the intermediate care unit a client who sustained a spinal cord injury at T1 in a motor vehicle crash. Which nursing care activities for this client can the nurse delegate to the unlicensed assistive person (UAP)? Select all that apply.

1. Measure oxygen saturation level every hour.
2. Listen to breath sounds.
3. Provide mouth care.
4. Teach use of incentive spirometer.
5. Use a bladder scanner to detect current urine volume.

63. The nurse has been instructed to have a surgical consent form signed by a client who will be undergoing a surgical procedure. What is the most essential information to include in the discussion prior to the client signing the form?

1. The client's diagnosis
2. Treatment proposed and the cost
3. The technical aspects of the procedure
4. Right to withdraw consent

64. A pregnant client is 7 cm dilated, 100% effaced, and at a +1 station. The fetus is in a face presentation. The nurse concludes that teaching has been effective when the client's husband makes which statement?

1. "Our baby will come out face first."
2. "Our baby will come out with one hip first."
3. "Our baby will come out buttocks first."
4. "Our baby will come out with the back of the head first."

65. A client is scheduled to have a transverse colostomy performed. While doing client teaching, the nurse points to which stoma on the diagram to show the client the location of the stoma? Mark your answer by drawing an "X" on the diagram.

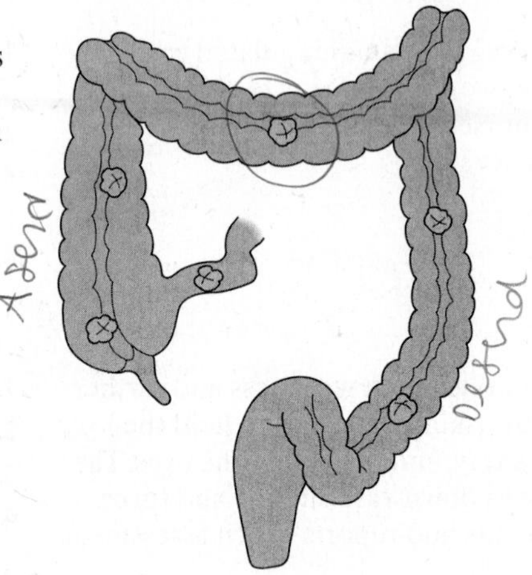

66. A medical unit RN is being floated to the surgical unit for the shift. Which postoperative client would be most appropriate to assign to the float RN?

1. A client who had laparoscopic cholecystectomy and has chronic lung disease
2. A client who underwent hip replacement for rheumatoid arthritis
3. A client who underwent cardiac valve replacement 2 days ago
4. A client who underwent partial thyroidectomy and is at risk for hypocalcemia

67. The medical-surgical unit is understaffed and a nurse from the surgical intermediate care unit has been floated to the unit for the day shift. Which clients should the nurse assign to this RN float nurse? Select all that apply.

1. A client newly admitted with exacerbation of heart failure
2. A client newly diagnosed with type 2 diabetes mellitus
3. A client who underwent emergency appendectomy during the night
4. A client with nephrolithiasis scheduled for lithotripsy later in the morning
5. A client admitted with thyrotoxicosis

68. A nurse teaching a client who has myasthenia gravis about measures to prevent cholinergic crisis should include which suggestion?

1. Space activities evenly over the course of the day.
2. Take care not to exceed recommended medication dose.
3. Eat a well-balanced diet with nutrient-dense foods.
4. Try to avoid individuals who have illnesses such as colds or flu.

69. A client presents to the emergency department with chest pain. Which serum laboratory test does the nurse check off on the laboratory slip as part of a protocol order set to rule out an acute myocardial infarction?

1. LDH^4
2. Troponin
3. Amylase
4. CK-MM

70. The nurse is planning for a multidisciplinary team meeting concerning a client with bipolar disorder in a manic state. In discussing the client's safety needs, the nurse should be sure to include which item?

1. Admission to a two-bed room for companionship
2. The client's risk level for self-harm
3. The benefit of having unrestricted visitors
4. The client's need to participate in several focused activities

71. A nurse is working with a female client newly diagnosed with *Helicobacter pylori* infection. The nurse anticipates that which medication will not be used after learning the client is pregnant?

1. Metronizadole
2. Amoxicillin
3. Clarithromycin
4. Ciprofloxacin — ≠ preg

72. The nurse admitting a client with a history of trigeminal neuralgia should question the client about which manifestation?

1. Facial droop accompanied by numbness and tingling
2. Stabbing pain that occurs with twitching of part of the face
3. Aching pain and ptosis of the eyelid
4. Burning pain and intermittent facial paralysis

73. What would be an appropriate intervention for the nurse to include in a plan of care for an adolescent with a clinical diagnosis of bulimia?

1. Assess for laxative and diuretic possession.
2. Supervise mealtimes to ensure eating.
3. Observe for ritualistic eating patterns.
4. Reward nonpurging behavior with a favorite snack.

74. A client with a strong family tendency toward hypertension denies he will get high blood pressure because he watches what he eats, gets plenty of exercise, and maintains a normal weight. When working with this client, what approach by the nurse may be most useful?

1. Praise and reassure client that these actions will prevent him from becoming hypertensive.
2. Emphasize that the client will eventually develop hypertension because of family history.
3. Recognize healthy lifestyle habits and emphasize importance of early detection to prevent complications.
4. Recommend that the client request antihypertensive medications prophylactically because of family history.

75. A parent asks the nurse what to do with rough edges of her child's cast, which are beginning to excoriate the child's skin. Which response by the nurse describes the appropriate action to take?

1. "Perform good skin care to skin around the cast edges with a protective barrier like petrolatum jelly."
2. "Call the healthcare provider to have the rough edges of the cast cut away."
3. "Tape a soft towel to the cast's edge to provide some protection from the rough edges."
4. "Petal cast edges with adhesive tape, placing strips from just inside the cast over the edge to the outside."

76. A 3-month-old infant is diagnosed with leukemia. What should the nurse anticipate as part of the plan of care for this infant?

1. The infant will be placed in isolation.
2. Leukemia is familial and other children should be assessed.
3. Immunizations will be withheld during exacerbations.
4. The infant will be NPO during chemotherapy.

77. The registered nurse (RN) is assigned to the postpartum unit. Which task could the RN safely delegate to a beginning student nurse?

1. Ambulate a client who had a cesarean delivery 2 days ago.
2. Complete the admission assessment on a newly delivered client.
3. Call the healthcare provider to report a low hemoglobin level.
4. Verify a unit of blood prior to transfusion.

78. A client presents to the emergency department with a stab wound to the right upper abdominal quadrant. The client's vital signs are BP 85/60, pulse 125, and respirations 28 breaths/minute. The nurse should immediately suspect damage to what organ?

1. Stomach
2. Liver
3. Large intestine
4. Kidney

79. The client scheduled for a barium enema expresses concern that the barium will not be evacuated and a bowel obstruction will occur. What response by the nurse to this client would be most appropriate?

1. "Don't worry. The healthcare provider will make sure that all barium is removed before you return to the unit."
2. "You will be given extra fluids and laxatives, and possibly an enema if barium is not expelled within 24 hours."
3. "The barium they are using will not cause an obstruction."
4. "Should I have the test rescheduled for when you are less concerned about it?"

80. The nurse is conducting an educational group on an inpatient unit. One client has not spoken during the group. What would be an effective therapeutic approach by the nurse?

1. Allow the client to remain present but nonparticipative.
2. Explain to the client that everyone in the group needs to participate.
3. Ask group members how they feel about this member not sharing.
4. Stop the group and ask the client to leave.

81. A client is experiencing seizure activity. The nurse should prepare to administer which medication according to protocol?

1. Selegilene
2. Diclofenac sodium
3. Phenytoin
4. Sumatriptan

82. As part of the ongoing assessment of a client who has an electrical burn, a complete blood count (CBC), electrolyte panel, and renal panel were prescribed. The nurse should expect to find which result?

1. Potassium level of 5.9 mEq/L
2. Sodium level of 128 mEq/L
3. Hematocrit of 28 mg/dL
4. White blood cell count of $4000/mm^3$

83. A client with heart failure (HF) has been advised to follow a 2-gram sodium diet. Which statement by the client indicates to the nurse that diet teaching has been effective?

1. "If I stop adding table salt, I shouldn't have any problems."
2. "I need to avoid eating processed foods and canned meats and vegetables."
3. "I can still use a small amount of table salt in cooking."
4. "I mostly have to worry about salty-tasting foods like potato chips."

84. After delivery, a client states she needs to restore the balance between hot and cold forces in her body and refuses to bathe. What is the most appropriate intervention by the nurse?

1. Show her a videotape on postpartum self-care.
2. Recognize her cultural beliefs and respect her wishes.
3. Discuss postpartum complications related to poor personal hygiene.
4. Request a medical social worker consult for this client.

85. While talking with a client the mental health clinic nurse notes that the client rapidly becomes more uncomfortable and anxious. What action should the nurse take?

1. Ask specific, focused questions to elicit detailed information about the source of the client's stress.
2. Encourage the client to try to relax by using guided imagery or other means preferred by the client.
3. Refocus the conversation on a topic that may be less threatening to the client.
4. Ask the client if it would be advisable to stop the interview at this time.

86. The nurse is preparing for discharge a client who will be taking lithium carbonate. Which statement best indicates the client is comfortable with being discharged on a mood-stabilizing medication?

1. "I don't want to take the medicine you will give me, but you said I have to."
2. "I know that if I take my lithium every day, I won't have to come to the hospital again."
3. "I have a hard time taking this medicine and I don't like the shaking, but I will take it every day with meals, have my blood tests done, and come back next month for my check-up."
4. "Even though I don't like taking lithium, I will take it daily, have blood tests done, and enjoy my usual activities. It helps to know that in a few weeks I should feel better."

87. A client has just finished a dose of intravesicular chemotherapy as treatment for bladder cancer. When giving instructions to the unlicensed assistive person (UAP) who will give routine care to this client, what statement should the nurse make?

1. "Be sure the client uses a bedpan for voiding for the next 24 hours."
2. "Double-flush the toilet after each time the client voids."
3. "Ask the client to wipe the toilet seat with a tissue after each bathroom use."
4. "Assist the client to the bathroom and wear sterile gloves for perineal care."

88. The nurse is caring for a young child who has mitt restraints. Which priority action should the nurse take regularly to ensure that the child's needs are met?

1. Check adequacy of circulation and skin condition.
2. Check that the tongue blades in pockets are intact and ends are covered or padded.
3. Ensure that the straps are tied to nonmovable parts of the crib.
4. Check that the call bell is pinned to the child's gown.

89. The client is to undergo an extensive process of allergy testing as an outpatient. The nurse would complete which action as a priority intervention during the initial testing?

1. Have emergency equipment available in the event of an anaphylactic reaction.
2. Instruct the client to wear a t-shirt to ensure easy access to the skin testing sites.
3. Give discharge instructions prior to testing since the client will go home immediately afterward.
4. Set up the room before the client enters the examination area.

90. A client who has been experiencing panic attacks asks why the healthcare provider has prescribed several laboratory tests. The nurse's response should incorporate which information?

1. Laboratory tests can differentiate between true anxiety and anxiety associated with depression.
2. Laboratory tests can determine the specific cause of the panic attacks.
3. Physiologic symptoms associated with panic disorders often mimic medical disorders.
4. Symptoms of panic disorders are usually related to hypochondriasis.

91. A postpartum client is beginning oral contraceptive therapy with norethindrone. The women's health clinic nurse anticipates that which element of the client's history and physical is consistent with this choice of contraceptive?

1. Superficial phlebitis
2. Currently breastfeeding
3. Dysmenorrhea
4. Menarche at age 18

92. The nurse in the emergency department is caring for a client who has fallen 20 feet from a roof. While performing the primary assessment, what is the most important nursing intervention?

1. Maintain cervical spine precautions.
2. Assess for facial lacerations.
3. Remove clothing.
4. Perform a mental status exam.

93. Which breakfast option indicates to the nurse that the client with coronary heart disease requires further diet instruction?

1. Orange juice, shredded wheat, skim milk, toast with jelly
2. Grapefruit juice, oatmeal, 1% milk, bagel with jelly
3. Canned peaches, egg omelet, whole milk, fruited yogurt
4. Applesauce, plain bagel, egg-white omelet, skim milk

94. The nurse would encourage the new mother to use which breastfeeding position to enable optimal control of the newborn's head while giving the mother a full view of the infant's cheeks and jaw?

1. Lying-down position
2. Cradle position
3. Clutch (football) position
4. Across-the-lap position

95. The nurse entering the room to assess an adult client observes sinus rhythm on the cardiac monitor but is unable to palpate a femoral pulse. The nurse should suspect that the client is demonstrating which underlying problem?

1. Pulseless electrical activity (PEA)
2. Ventricular fibrillation
3. Asystole
4. Ventricular tachycardia

96. While teaching a client about the proper administration of dipivefrine, the nurse would provide which instruction?

1. Gently squeeze eyes closed for 30 seconds immediately after instillation of medication.
2. Close, but do not squeeze, eyes immediately after instillation of medication.
3. Do not blink for 30 seconds after instillation of medication.
4. Close the eyes for 1 full minute after instillation of medication.

97. The medical-surgical nursing unit is short-staffed for the shift and a registered nurse (RN) from the pediatric unit has been floated to the nursing unit. Which client should the nurse assign to the float nurse?

1. A 32-year-old client, newly diagnosed with diabetes, who needs dietary and medication teaching
2. A 56-year-old client, newly admitted with Guillain-Barré syndrome, who has severe leg weakness
3. An 86-year-old client with dementia who will be transferred to a skilled nursing facility during the shift
4. A 59-year-old client who will be returning from surgery following transurethral resection of the prostate

98. A client has experienced a near-drowning event in salt water. The nurse anticipates that the client may experience which complication of this trauma?

1. Heart block
2. Renal failure
3. Pulmonary edema
4. Respiratory alkalosis

99. The nurse who reads the results of a client's tuberculin (TB) test notes induration, and the client asks what this means. What is the nurse's best response?

1. "A positive test means that you have been exposed to the TB organism. It does not mean that you currently have active bacteria. Further testing will be needed."
2. "A positive TB test means that you currently have active TB, and you will need to be isolated immediately."
3. "Many false positives occur. You can expect to be retested in 6 months."
4. "A positive TB test means that you are currently infectious and will need to be started on medication immediately."

100. An anxious client begins to yell and interrupt other clients. The client's speech is rapid and pressured. What action should the nurse take?

1. Ask the client to speak more slowly and softly.
2. Instruct the other clients to ignore this client's behavior.
3. Point out to the client that the behavior is a sign of anxiety.
4. Remind the client of the need to use good manners when talking with other people.

101. The nurse suspects that hepatotoxicity is developing in a dark-skinned client who is on an antibiotic. In what area of the body should the nurse assess for jaundice?

1. Palms of the hands or soles of the feet
2. Hard palate of oral cavity
3. Sclera
4. Conjunctivae

102. The nurse on the oncology unit has received intershift reports on four clients. In what order should the nurse assess these clients? All options must be used.

1. Client receiving radiation therapy who has a white blood cell (WBC) count of $4500/mm^3$
2. Client receiving chemotherapy who has a platelet count of $50,000/mm^3$
3. Client who is crying because she has newly learned that her cancer has metastasized
4. Client who has questions about upcoming chemotherapy

Fill in the numerical order of the options below:
Answer: ______________

103. Which nutritional measure should the nurse recommend to help a client with gastroesophageal reflux disease (GERD) to minimize the risk of symptoms?

1. Eat three large meals a day with no snacks.
2. Use a lot of garlic to season food rather than salt.
3. Limit intake of coffee drinks to two or fewer cups a day.
4. Use peppermint candies to take away bitter taste in mouth.

104. A client who is 20 weeks' gestation is concerned about how to tell her 3-year-old son about her pregnancy. Which statement by the nurse would be best when counseling this client?

1. "If he is not pleased with the news of a new baby, you should tell him that you are disappointed in him."
2. "Tell him that he is going to have a lot of responsibilities in helping care for the baby."
3. "Try to provide extra attention to him and include him in plans for the baby."
4. "Tell him that he will have to stay with his grandparents when the baby is born because you will be busy with the baby."

105. A nurse is caring for a client with pneumonia. ABG results are pH 7.49, $PaCO_2$ 32 mmHg, HCO_3^- 28 mEq/L, PaO_2 89 mmHg. How should the nurse interpret these results?

1. Metabolic acidosis, uncompensated
2. Metabolic alkalosis, uncompensated
3. Mixed respiratory and metabolic alkalosis
4. Respiratory acidosis, uncompensated

106. A client experiences severe nausea for up to 2 weeks following her chemotherapy treatment. Which statement indicates a need for further instruction on management of nausea?

1. "I need to call my doctor if I lose more than 10 percent of my body weight."
2. "I should try to eat bland, chilled foods and drink liquids separate from my meals."
3. "I need to lie down for an hour after each meal."
4. "I should call the doctor if my nausea doesn't go away, to see if a different antiemetic could provide better relief."

107. While assessing the chest tube drainage system of a client who underwent thoracotomy, the nurse observes a slight rise and fall in the water level in the water seal. The nurse should take which action?

1. Notify the healthcare provider immediately.
2. Have the client cough.
3. Continue to monitor the system.
4. Reposition the chest tube.

108. During which procedure should the labor and delivery nurse wear protective goggles in addition to gloves?

1. Changing a wet disposable bed pad
2. Assisting during an amniotomy
3. Starting an intravenous line
4. Washing used instruments

109. A client with cancer has a calcium level of 11.8 mg/dL. Which symptom would indicate a need for the nurse to notify the healthcare provider?

1. Increased gastric motility
2. Peaked T waves on 12-lead ECG
3. Muscle spasms
4. Muscle weakness

110. When evaluating the effectiveness of nursing care for an anxious client, it is important to validate that the client understands which of the following?

1. Defense mechanisms should not be used.
2. Some anxiety can be helpful.
3. The client should strive never to experience anxiety.
4. The client should try to avoid the fight-or-flight response.

111. In assessing a hospitalized client 1 hour after receiving hydralazine 20 mg PO, the nurse notes that the BP is 78/42 mmHg. The client has been taking this medication for several years at home without difficulty. Which factor most likely contributed to this episode of hypotension?

1. Dose is excessive for this medication.
2. Fluid intake for previous 24 hours is 1000 mL.
3. Serum potassium is 5.8 mEq/L.
4. Heart rate is 145 beats per minute.

112. A client with a history of heart failure suddenly exhibits shortness of breath, a respiratory rate of 30, crackles auscultated bilaterally, and frothy sputum. After receiving new prescriptions from the healthcare provider, which action should the nurse delegate to the licensed practical/vocational nurse (LPN/LVN)?

1. Start an intravenous line and cap it with a saline lock.
2. Monitor vital signs every 15 minutes.
3. Administer morphine sulfate 2 mg IV push immediately.
4. Insert an indwelling urinary catheter.

113. An 86-year-old client will be undergoing a surgical procedure. Which change should the nurse make in the informed consent process to accommodate for age-related changes in the client?

1. Providing adequate time for client to process information
2. Encouraging family members to make decision for client
3. Encouraging client to sign immediately before forgetting purpose of surgery
4. Providing client with reading material about surgery and postoperative instructions

114. The labor and delivery nurse would make it a priority to assess which two newborn body systems immediately after birth?

1. Gastrointestinal and hepatic
2. Urinary and hematologic
3. Neurologic and thermoregulatory
4. Respiratory and cardiovascular

115. The nurse is caring for the client who is recovering from partial-thickness burns. Which choice of breakfast items indicates the client understands the recommended diet?

1. Two slices of toast with butter, orange juice, skim milk
2. Two poached eggs, hash brown potatoes, whole milk
3. Three pancakes with syrup, two slices of bacon, apple juice
4. One cup of oatmeal with skim milk, ½ grapefruit, coffee

116. An adult client with diabetes insipidus who has been taking desmopressin intranasally comes to the clinic for a regularly scheduled appointment. The nurse assesses the client's mental status and notes some disorientation and behavioral changes. Significant pedal edema is also present. What should be the nurse's next action?

1. Check vital signs and notify the healthcare provider.
2. Have the client return in the morning for reevaluation.
3. Instruct the client to limit salt intake for a few days.
4. Suggest that the client change the route of administration to subcutaneous injections.

117. The nurse is assigned to the care of a hospitalized client receiving radiation therapy for cancer. Which activities needed in the care of a client receiving external beam radiation therapy could be safely delegated to an unlicensed assistive person (UAP)? Select all that apply.

1. Observe the skin site following a treatment session.
2. Document intake from the meal trays.
3. Assess variations in level of fatigue during the shift.
4. Explore how the client is coping with treatment.
5. Assist the client to ambulate in the hall.

118. A 76-year-old woman visits the ambulatory clinic with reports of having difficulty reading and doing needlework due to blurring of images centrally in her line of vision. The peripheral vision assessment by the nurse yields normal findings. The nurse suspects that this client is experiencing which visual problem?

1. Glaucoma
2. Detached retina
3. Cataracts
4. Macular degeneration

119. A female client states that she will not undergo any invasive testing for her "stomach pain." The nurse explains that which test could be completed to assess the abdomen and still meet the client's wishes?

1. Abdominal ultrasound
2. Barium swallow
3. Colonoscopy
4. CT scan with contrast

120. A motorcyclist involved in a motor vehicle crash has sustained trauma to the chest and head and is unresponsive in the emergency department. The client requires emergency surgery but known family members cannot be reached. What action is appropriate at this time regarding informed consent?

1. Keep trying to reach family members by telephone.
2. Have police contact a judge to obtain a court order for surgery.
3. Proceed with surgery despite the absence of a signed consent form.
4. Have the emergency department provider sign the consent form.

121. A client is taking an over-the-counter preparation containing bismuth subsalicylate for diarrhea. For which side effect that is unique to the bismuth portion of this drug should the nurse monitor?

1. Darkening of the tongue
2. Dyspepsia
3. Abdominal pain
4. Diarrhea

122. The nurse is obtaining a nursing history from the mother of a child being admitted with flare-up of celiac disease. Which manifestation should the nurse expect the mother to report?

1. Steatorrhea
2. Increased appetite
3. Excessive sleepiness
4. Soft, formed stools

123. A nurse is discussing the home maintenance regimen with a client who has irritable bowel syndrome. Which statement indicates client understanding?

1. "I'll take an early-evening walk each day after work."
2. "I'll have a cigarette after meals to relax."
3. "I'll chew gum between meals to curb my appetite."
4. "I'll eat a lot of fresh vegetables and fruits."

124. A primigravida client of 16 weeks' gestation states that she has not yet felt fetal movement. What is the nurse's best response?

1. "Your fetus will move any day now. Call me in a week if you don't feel it."
2. "Your fetus will begin moving at about 20 weeks' gestation."
3. "You should have been feeling the movement already."
4. "Your fetus has been moving for the past 9 weeks without you feeling it. You will feel it within a month."

125. The mother of an infant who underwent surgery to repair hypospadias asks the nurse why the infant is diapered as shown. The nurse would respond that this method of diapering will help to do which of the following?

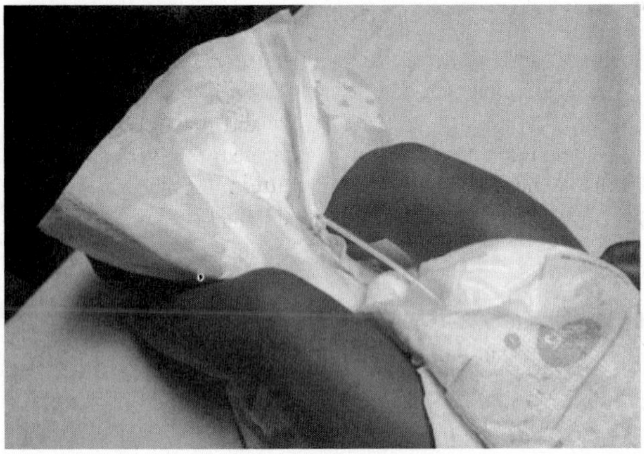

1. Protect the urinary stent that has been put in place.
2. Adequately measure the urinary output.
3. Provide for maximum absorption of urine.
4. Provide optimal protection of perineal skin from infected urine.

---

126. Following the administration of a diphtheria-pertussis-tetanus (DPT) immunization, the nurse notes that the infant has inspiratory stridor. The nurse should take which action?

1. Administer epinephrine per protocol order set.
2. Evaluate for signs of pulmonary edema.
3. Inspect for onset of periorbital edema.
4. Assess the infant again in 5 minutes.

---

127. The nurse is talking with the unlicensed assistive person (UAP) about time management skills and techniques. Which statement would the nurse make if intending to act as a coach?

1. "You must get the vital signs taken on time or you will be disciplined."
2. "You never report morning blood glucose levels on time."
3. "Your timely response to clients' call lights is exemplary."
4. "It may be helpful if you bring in linens to the client rooms when you restock the gloves."

---

128. A nurse is explaining to a woman considering pregnancy how rubella is transmitted. The nurse determines that the teaching session had the desired outcome if the client states that rubella is transmitted by which route?

1. Airborne route
2. Contaminated food
3. Droplet route
4. Direct contact

---

129. A female client has been successfully resuscitated after cardiac arrest. Her arterial blood gas reveals a pH of 7.6. The nurse attributes this result to which of the following?

1. Anaerobic metabolism, which caused lactic acid production
2. Excess sodium bicarbonate, which was administered during the resuscitation
3. Repeat blood gases, which are performed during a code, frequently show acidosis
4. A laboratory error in reporting the blood gas results

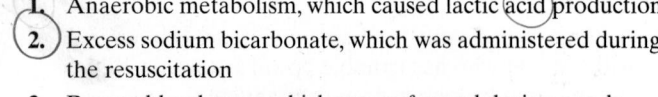

---

130. The nurse would anticipate finding which client characteristic when working with a client who has a pain disorder?

1. A preference to handle pain without medication
2. A lack of understanding of the relationship between pain and stress
3. A need to move slowly to adequately perform roles
4. Evidence of structural damage at the site of pain

---

131. Which high-priority information should be included in the teaching plan for a client being treated with medication therapy for a generalized seizure disorder?

1. Take medication even if there is no seizure activity.
2. Physical dependency may result from extended use of medications.
3. Urine may turn pink to brown but is not harmful.
4. Therapeutic effects of medications may not be seen for 2–3 weeks.

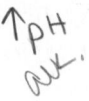

132. The pediatric nurse needs to rearrange client room assignments to accommodate three additional clients scheduled for admission during the shift. Which clients would be best for the nurse to cohort together in the same two-bed room? Select all that apply.

1. An 8-year-old who has encephalitis
2. A 10-year-old who has a white blood cell count of 2800/mm^3
3. A 12-year-old who had an appendectomy for a ruptured appendix
4. An 11-year-old with scarlet fever
5. A 9-year-old receiving chemotherapy for cancer

133. A 32-year-old female client with acquired immunodeficiency syndrome (AIDS) is receiving treatment at an outpatient clinic. The nurse reviewing the dietary assessment record notes that the client has low intake during meals and is progressively losing weight. What dietary interventions would be best for the nurse to suggest to promote weight gain?

1. Have the client keep a food diary and submit it at the next visit so that more information can be obtained regarding food preferences and usual dietary pattern.
2. Tell the client that her weight may fluctuate in response to her menstrual cycle so there is no need to worry for now.
3. Tell the client that additional salt in the diet will help to increase weight.
4. Tell the client that the use of nutrient-dense food and fortified protein shakes will help promote weight gain.

134. The nurse would assess a 76-year-old client for which common medication-related problem that significantly increases the risk for complications of heart and lung disease?

1. Taking over-the-counter meds with prescription meds
2. Sharing medications with family and friends
3. Following directions and taking medications as remembered
4. Polypharmacy resulting from visits to multiple doctors

135. A client with acute respiratory distress syndrome (ARDS) shows no improvement despite increases in the concentration of oxygen administered. What intervention should the nurse attempt that may improve ventilation-perfusion matching?

1. Transfusion of packed red blood cells
2. Infusion of albumin
3. Positioning supine with head elevated 30–45 degrees
4. Prone positioning

136. The nurse is giving general information about antihypertensive medications to a young female client with a history of hypertension. The nurse includes that which type of antihypertensive drug therapy should not be used if the client becomes pregnant?

1. Vasodilator
2. Diuretic
3. Angiotensin-converting enzyme (ACE) inhibitor
4. Calcium channel blocker

137. A nurse from the pediatric intensive care unit has floated to the cardiovascular intermediate care unit for the shift. Which client would the nurse assign to the float nurse for the shift?

1. A client who experienced myocardial infarction 36 hours ago
2. A client in heart failure receiving digoxin and bumetanide
3. A client who just underwent coronary atherectomy
4. A client scheduled for cardiac stent placement later in the day

138. A client is admitted to the preoperative area before undergoing surgery to repair a detached retina. The admitting nurse would take which action first?

1. Position the client properly.
2. Darken the bedside area of the client.
3. Administer the prescribed preoperative analgesic.
4. Cover the affected eye.

139. A client has been admitted to the nursing unit with a 3-day history of severe nausea and vomiting with diarrhea. The client is experiencing fatigue, anorexia, and muscle weakness. Based on this history, which laboratory findings should the nurse expect to find?

1. Calcium 11.6 mg/dL
2. Sodium 144 mEq/L
3. Potassium 2.9 mEq/L
4. Blood urea nitrogen 8 mg/dL

140. An alert hospitalized client has decided to execute an advanced directive and asks for the nurse's help in obtaining the necessary witness signatures. What is the best response by the new nurse who has not witnessed an advanced directive?

1. "Let me contact the nursing supervisor for assistance about this important matter."
2. "Hospital policy prohibits nursing staff from witnessing legal documents."
3. "Anyone on the nursing unit can witness the document for you."
4. "I will be pleased to sign the advance directive as a witness since I am an RN."

141. A client presents to the emergency department with inspiratory and expiratory wheezes and intercostal retractions. The client is prescribed subcutaneous epinephrine after establishing a diagnosis of broncho-spasm secondary to acute bronchitis. The nurse would anticipate seeing the intended effect of the medication within how many minutes?

1. 1 minute
2. 5 minutes
3. 10 minutes
4. 15 minutes

142. A client with diabetes mellitus for the last 3 years has bloodwork drawn prior to a routine health visit. During the visit, the client's glycosylated hemoglobin was found to be 9%. What should the nurse do at this time?

1. Explore the client's general dietary pattern for the past several weeks.
2. Assess for signs of infection and client's intake for the past 2–3 days.
3. Review the client's understanding of diabetic vision screening and foot care.
4. Immediately administer a dose of regular insulin according to sliding scale.

dry synd.

143. A client is admitted to the hospital with a primary diagnosis of hip fracture and a secondary diagnosis of Sjögren's syndrome. Which prescription would be of most concern with regard to the nutritional status of the client?

1. NPO after midnight for surgery with a 7:30 a.m. case
2. IV of lactated Ringer's at 125 mL/hr
3. Maintaining diet as tolerated
4. Restriction of oral fluids to 1000 mL/day

144. The nurse notes on the antepartal history that the client has an android pelvis. The nurse plans to assess this client carefully because of the increased risk of which perinatal event?

1. Occiput posterior position
2. Prolonged labor
3. Precipitous delivery
4. Developing postpartum complications

145. The nurse would use which primary intervention when caring for a client with chronic pain disorder to help the client cope with the disorder?

1. Program of physical exercise
2. Music therapy for expression
3. Patient-controlled analgesia
4. Complete bedrest

146. A client receiving hydroxyamphetamine for primary open-angle glaucoma demonstrates an understanding of serious drug side effects when informing the healthcare provider of which symptom?

1. Stinging on instillation
2. Occasional headache
3. Occasional brow ache
4. Confusion

147. The nurse is seeking employment in a hospital that uses a shared governance model. The nurse should accept a job offer in the hospital that has which attribute?

1. Staff nurses delegate activities to unregulated care providers (UCPs).
2. A unit manager seeks advice from the manager's supervisor.
3. Staff nurses and UCPs make their own work schedules.
4. Procedure manuals are updated by a committee of nurse managers.

148. The nurse observes an unlicensed assistive person (UAP) caring for a client with severe acute respiratory syndrome (SARS). Which action by the UAP indicates the need for intervention and further teaching by the nurse?

1. UAP dons a protective gown, gloves, N95 respirator, and eye protection when entering the room.
2. UAP does not remove the stethoscope, blood pressure cuff, and thermometer being kept in the room.
3. UAP removes all personal protective equipment and washes the hands right before leaving client's room.
4. UAP limits the amount of time in the client's room to 45 minutes at any one time.

149. The nurse examines the white blood cell (WBC) differential for a client who experienced a severe allergic reaction. The nurse anticipates that which value will be elevated?

1. Neutrophils
2. Monocytes
3. Eosinophils
4. Lymphocytes

150. The partner of a client who has dissociative identity disorder with several alters is puzzled about why the children are included in family therapy. What would be the best explanation for the nurse to offer?

1. "Children need to have their experiences confirmed—and to learn to deal with the different personalities."
2. "There is probably a mistake in the referral; your partner is the one who has the problem."
3. "You and your partner should be seen, but it could be traumatizing to the children."
4. "It would be best to ask the children if they would like to participate, and bring them if they want."

151. The nurse assesses the results of a vancomycin blood level drawn just prior to the next scheduled intravenous (IV) dose. The nurse should consult with the prescriber after drawing which conclusion about the result?

1. There is a high serum level, indicating the peak level is too high.
2. This test measures the highest therapeutic concentration and it is low.
3. Toxicity is evident, suggesting the drug's half-life is too short for the frequency prescribed.
4. The drug level is low, indicating the drug dosage and/or frequency should be increased.

152. In a child with acute kidney injury, the nurse would help to prevent hyperkalemia by limiting intake of which foods in the diet?

1. Potatoes, tomatoes, and oranges
2. Grains, cheese, and citrus fruits
3. Cereals, processed sugars, and wheat
4. Rice, leafy green vegetables, and carbonated beverages

153. A 28-year-old female client has recently been diagnosed with systemic lupus erythematosus (SLE). Which approach by the nurse would be most helpful for the overall management of care?

1. Have the client institute advance directives immediately.
2. Discuss with the client lifestyle modifications that will be needed as the disease progresses.
3. Ascertain information about the client's working environment and suggest limiting the work schedule to minimize potential stress.
4. Establish the multidisciplinary healthcare team to help client identify goals.

154. A 78-year-old woman has been brought by ambulance to the emergency department with a fractured lower leg. While examining the client, the nurse notes several bruises in various stages of healing over the torso and on areas of extremities that would be hidden under clothing. Upon questioning, the client reveals that her daughter hits her if she does not give her the check she receives monthly as income or does not follow her directions. What actions should the nurse take at this time? Select all that apply.

1. Tell the client that the matter will be discussed with the daughter.
2. Suggest the client have the check handled by direct deposit.
3. Explain to the client the nurse's legal obligation to report abuse.
4. Ask the client if she has any other family to stay with after discharge.
5. Remain with the client while she provides the report.

155. A pregnant client at 26 weeks' gestation experiences a partial placenta abruptio. She asks, "Will this harm my baby?" What should the nurse include in a response?

1. "It may decrease the amount of nutrients the fetus receives."
2. "It may cause a buildup of urine in the fetus, causing kidney damage."
3. "It may cause the fetus to develop hydrops."
4. "It may cause a fetal anomaly."

156. The nurse assesses a client taking cholestyramine for signs of possible deficiency of which vitamins?

1. Niacin and thiamine
2. Folic acid and vitamin C
3. Vitamins A and D
4. Thiamine and cyanocobalamin

157. The nurse would place highest priority on referring which client to a hospital case manager?

1. A 21-year-old male with a gunshot wound to the arm
2. A 32-year-old male with a fractured tibia
3. A 75-year-old female awaiting a hip replacement
4. A 41-year-old male having same-day surgery for tonsillectomy

158. While making rounds, the nurse observes a client receiving oxygen by the delivery system shown. The nurse concludes the client is using this mode of oxygen therapy because of which primary benefit?

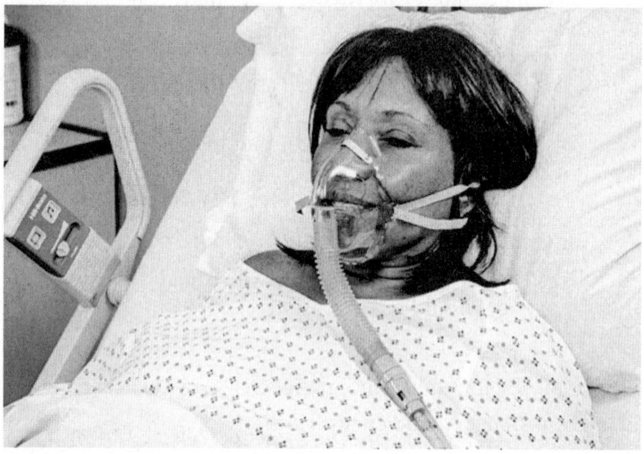

1. Ability to prevent rebreathing of exhaled carbon dioxide.
2. Oxygen concentration can be regulated.
3. Constant humidity can be administered to liquefy pulmonary secretions.
4. Delivery of up to 100% oxygen concentration for clients with COPD.

159. A client diagnosed with hypochondria states an allergy to contrast media used in diagnostic tests and "all" radioisotopes. The nurse explains that the client could undergo which diagnostic procedure without risk of possible allergic response?

1. Magnetic resonance imaging (MRI)
2. Myelogram
3. Ventilation/perfusion (VQ) scan
4. Computed tomography (CT) scan with contrast

160. A client had assumed a new identity and started a new job when he was relocated 400 miles from his home. The mental health nurse interprets that this client's behavior is characteristic of which problem?

1. Amnesia
2. Akathisia
3. Confabulation
4. Fugue state

161. The client is receiving a loading dose of lidocaine 100 mg IV for treatment of ventricular tachycardia. The nurse prepares to take which action next?

1. Start a continuous IV infusion at 1–4 mg/minute.
2. Repeat the dose every 10 minutes for 1 hour or PRN.
3. Begin oral procainamide therapy.
4. Prepare for pacemaker insertion to override the dysrhythmia.

162. The nurse on a cardiac medical unit would delegate which client care activity to an unlicensed assistive person (UAP)?

1. Assist the client to choose low-fat and low-sodium food selections from the dietary menu.
2. Measure client's pulse, blood pressure, and oxygen saturation after ambulation.
3. Explain the need to alternate activity periods with rest.
4. Help the client use nitroglycerin left at the bedside if chest pain occurs.

163. A client recovering from Guillain-Barré syndrome is admitted to the rehabilitation unit for general rehabilitative care. The nurse anticipates that which method will most likely be used to provide nutritional support for the client during this time?

1. Using a gastrostomy tube for feedings due to high risk for malabsorption
2. Maintaining oral intake sufficient to maintain positive nitrogen balance
3. Limiting fresh fruit in the diet, especially fruits with skins
4. Using thickening agents in liquids to prevent aspiration

164. Based on anticipated risks during this period of life, what would be the focus of the nurse who is setting up a health promotion booth for healthy adults in their 30s?

1. Screenings for breast, cervical, uterine, and prostate cancers
2. Chest x-rays for lung cancer
3. Bone density test for osteoporosis
4. Safety education for accident prevention

165. A client admitted with exacerbation of chronic obstructive pulmonary disease (COPD) has a respiratory rate of 18, a dry cough, and arterial blood gases that reveal a pH of 7.29, CO_2 of 50 mmHg, and O_2 of 72 mmHg. The nurse identifies which clinical concern as a priority for this client?

1. Inadequate alveolar ventilation
2. Decreased tolerance for ordinary activity
3. Increased susceptibility to infection
4. Risk for erratic breathing patterns

166. The nurse is caring for a client who has just been diagnosed with Graves' disease. Client education regarding medication therapy needs to include which of the following?

1. Atropine
2. Thyroxine
3. Insulin
4. Propylthiouracil

167. The nurse has delegated to an unlicensed assistive person (UAP) the care of a client who had a right-hemisphere thrombotic stroke with hemiplegia. The nurse would give further direction to the UAP after observing the UAP perform which action?

1. Provide passive range-of-motion exercises to the affected arm and leg.
2. Place a chair for a visitor to the left of the bed.
3. Place the overbed table to the right side of the bed.
4. Sit the client up slowly.

168. The nurse determines that a client who has an infection with which antibiotic-resistant microorganism requires transmission-based droplet precautions?

1. Methicillin-resistant *Staphylococcus aureus*
2. Penicillin-resistant *Streptococcus pneumoniae*
3. Vancomycin-resistant *Enterococcus*
4. Vancomycin-intermediate-resistant *Staphylococcus*

169. The nurse is reviewing the results of a client's recent lipid profile. The nurse notes that the client is experiencing beneficial effects of a heart-healthy diet and exercise after noting an elevation in which laboratory value?

1. High-density lipoprotein (HDL)
2. Low-density lipoprotein (LDL)
3. Total cholesterol
4. Triglycerides

170. The high school nurse concludes that a female student diagnosed with depression may be at risk for suicide after the nurse notes which behavior during the school day?

1. Student states she does not want to eat the school lunch.
2. Student gets up and leaves classroom angrily after reprimand by teacher.
3. Student gives away favorite poster hanging inside of school locker.
4. Student has started wearing clothes that are brown or black in color.

171. A client is advised to take an antiemetic prior to chemotherapy to prevent nausea and vomiting. The nurse explains that anticipatory dosing should be done how long prior to chemotherapy to be effective?

1. 24 hours
2. 3–5 hours
3. ½–1 hour
4. 12 hours

172. The nurse working on a neuroscience unit has just received an intershift report. Which assigned client should the nurse assess first?

1. A client with Parkinson's disease who cries about not being able to get up easily
2. A client with multiple sclerosis who is having noticeable leg spasms
3. A client who had a hemorrhagic stroke and reports a severe headache
4. A client scheduled for a craniotomy in 4 hours

173. Which statement made by a client regarding human immunodeficiency virus (HIV) and acquired immunodeficiency syndrome (AIDS) would the nurse seek to further clarify?

1. "I can get the disease from eating contaminated food products."
2. "Blood tests will tell me if I have a nutritional anemia."
3. "Maintaining adequate fluid and fiber intake will help me."
4. "If I feel sick to my stomach, I should not drink liquids."

174. The registered nurse is assigned to the postpartum unit. Which task could the RN safely delegate to an unlicensed assistive person (UAP)?

1. Ambulate a client who had a vaginal delivery yesterday.
2. Complete the admission assessment on a newly delivered client.
3. Call the healthcare provider to report a low hemoglobin level.
4. Verify a unit of blood prior to transfusion.

175. The client has undergone hypophysectomy using a transphenoidal approach. While changing the mustache dressing, the nurse notes clear exudate with a pale, yellow-colored ring at the edge of the drainage. What should the nurse do next?

1. Document this as serous drainage and continue to monitor the client.
2. Assess for headache and check the glucose level in the drainage.
3. Apply an ice pack to the nasal bridge and a large, fluffy dressing.
4. Report the finding to the healthcare provider.

176. The client is experiencing severe itching with a skin disorder. Which medication, if prescribed, should the nurse administer as an appropriate oral preparation to decrease the itching?

1. Cimetidine
2. Lorazepam
3. Hydroxyzine
4. Bupivacaine

177. A client who is legally blind has been admitted to the nursing unit. Which activities should the nurse delegate to the unlicensed assistive person (UAP)? Select all that apply.

1. Assist the client with meals.
2. Complete the admission interview form.
3. Determine how the vision loss affects the client's daily life.
4. Assist the client to ambulate in the hall.
5. Ask the client what community services are being utilized.

178. A client who has a history of Graves' disease is arriving from surgery. Based on the photo shown, what activity should the nurse instruct the unlicensed assistive person (UAP) to complete?

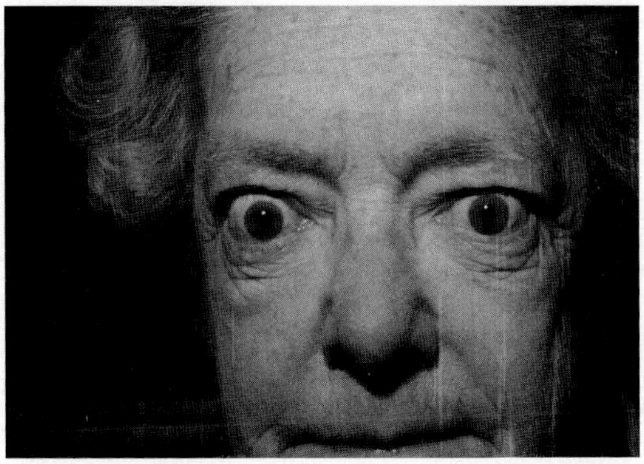

1. Keep the client's room warm to promote eye comfort.
2. Obtain fingerstick blood glucose every 4 hours.
3. Keep the head of the bed flat for 8 hours.
4. Position the client in bed in a manner that provides eye protection.

179. A client with bone cancer receiving chemotherapy has developed bone marrow suppression. Which laboratory report is of highest priority for the nurse to monitor at this time?

1. Calcium
2. Phosphorus
3. White blood cell (WBC) count
4. Prostate-specific antigen (PSA)

180. Which behavior would the nurse conclude is expected in a client who suffers from localized amnesia?

1. Wandering in the neighborhood using a new name
2. Forgetting what happened during a recent assault
3. Awareness of only a few of many alters
4. Feelings of separation from his body

181. A client hospitalized for depression will be discharged to home tomorrow morning. The client asks, "Do I have to take medicine every day? How will I be able to sleep when I go home? Do you think I'll be able to go back to work after being in the hospital?" What is the nurse's best response?

1. "The best approach is to take it one step at a time, so that everything will work out."
2. "I understand you're worried, but you and your spouse will decide tomorrow when you get home."
3. "You seem worried about how you will function after going home. Would you like us to discuss a plan for your daily activities?"
4. "I'll do my best to set up a written plan for discharge that you can take home with you and refer to later."

182. The 39-year-old client is admitted with several prescriptions to correct a state of diabetic ketoacidosis (DKA). The nurse should consult with the healthcare provider after noting which prescription?

1. Begin infusion of sodium chloride 0.9% IV at 200 mL/hr.
2. Insert an indwelling urinary catheter.
3. Administer NPH insulin.
4. Initiate continuous pulse oximetry.

183. The nurse is advancing the diet of a client from clear liquids to full liquids per healthcare provider prescription. Which new beverages from the nursing unit kitchen can the nurse offer to the client because of the advancing diet prescription? Select all that apply.

1. Apple juice
2. Orange juice
3. Coffee with cream
4. Tomato juice
5. Ginger ale

184. The nurse is taking the health history of a 77-year-old man. Which symptom reported by the client would the nurse consider to be the most significant abnormal finding?

1. Hesitation and decreased flow of urine stream
2. Increasing intolerance to spicy foods
3. Increased isolating behaviors after his wife's death
4. Slight dizziness when getting up too quickly after lying down

185. In planning care for a client with a personality disorder, the nurse anticipates that the client will differ from clients with other mental health problems in that this client will exhibit which features?

1. Tend to experience symptoms as egosyntonic.
2. Usually display clinical symptoms.
3. Tend to experience symptoms as egodystonic.
4. Seldom experience addictive behaviors.

186. The home healthcare nurse is visiting an older adult client who is taking a prescribed calcium channel blocker. In conducting dietary teaching, the nurse instructs the client to avoid which fruit that is contraindicated while taking a calcium channel blocker?

1. Oranges
2. Grapefruit
3. Bananas
4. Grapes

187. A client is hospitalized in a state of myxedema coma. Assessment reveals: BP 88/56, HR 66 regular, RR 12, temperature 95.6°F (35.3°C), no urine output since admission to the emergency department 3 hours ago, and unresponsive. Of the following therapeutic measures prescribed, which intervention should the nurse complete first?

1. Initiating prescribed thyroid replacement therapy
2. Obtaining a warming device to counteract hypothermia
3. Inserting an indwelling urinary catheter to monitor urine output
4. Applying oxygen as per protocol order set

188. The nurse must assess every shift the temperature and blood pressure of a client on contact precautions because of wound infection. What is the appropriate nursing action to minimize the spread of microorganisms?

1. Keep the equipment in the client's room.
2. Store the equipment in the soiled utility room between uses.
3. Cleanse the equipment after each use.
4. No special action is required with the equipment.

189. A client presents to the clinic reporting a swollen and painful great toe and says his brother gets the same symptoms from time to time. The healthcare provider suspects gout. What specific laboratory test would the nurse expect to be prescribed to confirm the diagnosis?

1. Calcium
2. Hematocrit
3. Uric acid
4. Sodium

190. A female client has been diagnosed with a dependent personality disorder. Which statement is likely to be her response to the nurse's suggestion that she complete morning care?

1. "I'll have no problem in deciding what to wear."
2. "I think you should wear more makeup."
3. "I think this outfit looks good on me."
4. "What do you think I should wear?"

191. The nurse should question a prescription for which beta agonist to treat respiratory disease in a client with a history of atrial fibrillation accompanied by intermittent tachycardia?

1. Terbutaline
2. Pirbuterol
3. Isoproterenol
4. Metaproterenol

192. A client with osteoporosis who has experienced fractures in the past is now admitted for dizziness and shortness of breath. After being determined to be at risk for falls, which nursing interventions should the nurse delegate to the unlicensed assistive person (UAP)? Select all that apply.

1. Clear the room of unnecessary objects.
2. Inquire if the dizziness has led to any recent falls.
3. Remain with the client during ambulation.
4. Ask the physical therapist to evaluate the client for a walker.
5. Advise the client about the benefits of calcium in the diet.

193. A client is receiving radiation to the head and neck area for treatment of cancer. What interventions should the nurse employ to relieve the client's complaint of a dry mouth?

1. Have client eat prior to radiation therapy.
2. Encourage the client to eat larger portions of food.
3. Advise the client to use mouthwash.
4. Suggest the use of sugar-free candies.

194. The primipara experienced a 22-hour labor with a second stage that lasted 2 hours. When the nurse brings the infant to the mother 30 minutes after delivery, the client tells the nurse to leave the infant in the isolette and shows no interest in holding the newborn. What conclusion about the mother's behavior should the nurse draw at this time?

1. The client is not showing signs of early coping with being a new mother.
2. The client is trying to exert some power over her current situation.
3. The client may be fatigued following such a long labor.
4. The client may be anxious about assuming a role as a parent.

195. The nurse should expect to find a diminished $PaCO_2$ level in the assigned client who has which physical assessment finding?

1. Hyperventilation
2. Hypoventilation
3. Prolonged expiration
4. Stridor

196. A client is scheduled for an ophthalmic examination. Before administering the prescribed epinephrine solution, the nurse should assess for which condition?

1. Hypotension
2. Open-angle glaucoma
3. Angle-closure glaucoma
4. Brow ache

197. The nurse is working on an orthopedic unit. After receiving the intershift report, which client should the nurse assign to the unlicensed assistive person (UAP) for completion of care activities?

1. A client with a newly applied cast who has increasing pain despite medication
2. A client with osteoporosis admitted 2 hours ago who fell and fractured the vertebra at L1
3. A client with a below-knee amputation who is anxious because "the leg feels like it's still there"
4. A client 6 days' post repair of a fractured hip being discharged to a rehabilitation facility near end of shift

198. An adult client arrives at the emergency department reporting chest pain and shortness of breath. The nurse should conclude that which data, if present in the client's history, could indicate the pain may be related to cardiac disease? Select all that apply.

1. History of diabetes and smoking
2. Recent travel out of the country
3. The pain increases with activity
4. The pain is reproducible when taking a deep breath
5. The pain is associated with nausea

199. A client asks the nurse to repeat what the healthcare provider explained about moderate sedation planned for an upcoming procedure. Which statement should the nurse make to the client concerning moderate sedation?

1. "You will be able to breathe and respond appropriately to physical stimuli and words that are spoken."
2. "Your pain threshold will be decreased so you can tolerate the pain."
3. "You will have a patent airway and will be able to remember and comprehend what is happening."
4. "You will not be awake but you will still feel slight pain during the procedure."

200. A client is diagnosed with paranoid personality disorder. Which assessment data does the nurse conclude are consistent with this diagnosis?

1. Delusions and hallucinations
2. Passivity and compliance with rules
3. Jealousy and secretiveness
4. Respect and deference to authority figures

201. A client with cancer who is receiving chemotherapy with nitrogen mustard has swelling at the intravenous (IV) site. The nurse should take which action initially?

1. Continue with infusion after trying to aspirate for a blood return.
2. Stop administration and attempt to aspirate.
3. Flush the line with saline.
4. Obtain a new site for drug administration.

202. The nurse working on an adult medical-surgical unit would assign which client to the licensed practical/vocational nurse (LPN/LVN) under supervision of the RN?

1. A 62-year-old client admitted 8 hours ago with exacerbation of COPD
2. A 25-year-old client with a concussion from an auto crash the prior evening
3. An 81-year-old client with chronic heart failure and emphysema admitted 3 days ago
4. A 54-year-old client newly diagnosed with diabetes mellitus who will be discharged today

203. A client has been referred for dietary teaching regarding the management of hepatitis. The nurse would base development of nutritional goals on which data?

1. The type of hepatitis that the client has, which will affect dietary needs
2. The need to institute tube feedings to allow the liver to rest and regenerate
3. That the diet should be balanced except for limiting dietary fats
4. That the diet should be high in calories and high in protein

204. The nurse caring for a 15-year-old primipara who delivered yesterday identifies that the new mother requires instruction on newborn care. Which is the most appropriate intervention when planning this client's discharge teaching?

1. Show the client a video on newborn care and answer questions.
2. Give her information about a support group for adolescent mothers.
3. Demonstrate care for the newborn and have client give a return demonstration.
4. Give the client printed instructions on newborn care and a contact telephone number.

205. To decrease skin irritation in a child with atopic dermatitis, which instruction should the nurse give the parent?

1. Provide very warm baths (not showers) daily
2. Apply a lotion of choice liberally over entire body
3. Use fabric softener when washing all clothes
4. Use mild soap as needed, avoiding harsh soaps

206. A client taking warfarin comes to the healthcare provider office for a follow-up visit and tells the nurse that he has been taking propoxyphene with aspirin to treat pain related to an old back injury. How should the ambulatory care nurse respond?

1. Ask how long the back pain has been present and assess the need for a referral for pain management.
2. State that it is important to prevent the pain cycle from starting and to continue to take propoxyphene with aspirin as prescribed.
3. Explain that aspirin may interfere with warfarin therapy, and consult with the healthcare provider for an alternative.
4. Explain that continued daily use would help to relieve back pain, but would require an increase in warfarin dose.

207. Which assessment finding would the nurse consider to be unique to developmental dysplasia of the hip in a 5-year-old client?

1. Asymmetry of gluteal and thigh fat folds
2. Positive Ortolani-Barlow maneuver
3. Telescoping of the femoral head into the pelvis
4. Limited abduction of the affected hip

208. The nurse would intervene after noting another nursing staff member perform which action in the care of a child who has had surgery for clubfoot? Select all that apply.

1. Keeping the ankle and foot elevated on a pillow
2. Observing for swelling around cast edges
3. Administering pain medication immediately when it is due
4. Performing neurovascular status checks every 2 hours
5. Covering the cast with heavy blankets

209. An adolescent will undergo a spinal fusion for scoliosis. Which items would be included in the preoperative teaching by the nurse? Select all that apply.

1. Deep-breathing and coughing exercises
2. Use of postoperative pain medications
3. Details of the procedure for spinal fusion and bone grafting
4. Placement of a urinary catheter to drain urine after surgery
5. Use of incentive spirometry

210. The nurse should plan to take which actions when assigned to the care of a client in a state of acute alcohol withdrawal? Select all that apply.

1. Restrict the client to a clear liquid diet.
2. Monitor vital signs, especially blood pressure.
3. Reorient the client during care as needed.
4. Promote a stimulating environment to distract the client.
5. Respond to hallucinations in a factual and caring manner.

211. A hospitalized client experiences chest pain that has not been relieved after one dose of sublingual nitroglycerine (NTG). The nurse measures the blood pressure, which has dropped to 126/84 from 130/90. Using a chest pain protocol order set, which action should the nurse take next?

1. Notify the healthcare provider.
2. Obtain an electroencephalogram (EEG).
3. Give another dose of nitroglycerine.
4. Add a dose of nitroglycerine paste.

212. The nurse working on an adult medical-surgical unit would assign which client to the licensed practical/vocational nurse (LPN/LVN) under supervision of the RN?

1. A 45-year-old client admitted yesterday after a nephrectomy
2. A 78-year-old client with diabetes mellitus and osteoarthritis
3. A 32-year-old client with a fractured pelvis from a motor vehicle crash 3 days ago
4. A 62-year-old client who underwent pelvic exenteration receiving medication via patient-controlled analgesia

213. A nurse on the intermediate care medical unit reports to work and is told to float (report to) the emergency department (ED) because of short staffing. The nurse has never worked in the ED. What should be the initial action by the nurse?

1. Refuse to float, giving a full rationale for the decision.
2. Ask the ED charge nurse to page the nursing supervisor.
3. Identify nursing activities that the nurse can safely perform in the ED.
4. Telephone the hospital risk management department for advice.

214. A mother telephones the clinic nurse, stating that a letter from her child's school advises her to examine the child for nits from *pediculosis capitis*. She asks where she should look for these nits. What areas should the nurse tell the mother to examine?

1. Hair along forehead and above ears
2. In the webs of the fingers and toes
3. Base of hair shafts, especially at nape of the neck
4. In the folds of the elbows and behind the knees

215. Which activity instruction would be appropriate for the nurse to include in the discharge teaching of an adolescent after a spinal fusion?

1. "You will have activity restrictions for 3 months."
2. "Normal stair climbing is allowed."
3. "Limit walking to one-half mile per day."
4. "You can help with limited chores such as vacuuming."

216. The healthcare provider has prescribed vitamin D for a client. The client asks the nurse what the medication is for. What is the most accurate response by the nurse?

1. "Vitamin D decreases absorption of calcium and inhibits mobilization from bone."
2. "Vitamin D helps regulate the serum calcium level circulating in the bloodstream."
3. "Vitamin D helps the kidneys rid the body of excess calcium."
4. "Vitamin D decreases blood levels of calcium and phosphorus."

217. The nurse working on an adult medical-surgical unit would assign which client to the licensed practical/vocational nurse (LPN/LVN) under supervision of the RN?

1. A 45-year-old client who underwent bilateral adrenalectomy the previous day
2. A 66-year-old client being discharged to home following arthroscopy
3. A 24-year-old with hemophilia who fractured a leg after falling from a horse yesterday
4. A 53-year-old client with hypertension and chronic renal insufficiency

218. A client with acquired immunodeficiency syndrome (AIDS) who has *Pneumocystis jiroveci* pneumonia is being admitted to the nursing unit. The nurse instructs staff to use which type of precautions?

1. Standard precautions
2. Airborne precautions
3. Droplet precautions
4. Contact precautions

219. A family member sitting at bedside observes the nurse admitting a client from the postanesthesia care unit (PACU). The family member asks why the area around the surgical wound is orange. Which statement about surgical skin preparation is the best response to the family member?

1. "It reduces the risk of many postoperative complications."
2. "It reduces the risk of postoperative wound infection."
3. "It lessens the chance for decreased tissue perfusion."
4. "It decreases the possibility for dermatitis."

220. A client whose home was lost in a severe flood a week ago seeks treatment at a local mental health crisis center. During the intake interview, which question by the nurse would help to identify the client's perception about the precipitating event?

1. "Do you have many family or friends in the area?"
2. "What has led you to seek help at this time?"
3. "Where have you been living since the flood?"
4. "What have you been doing to cope since the flood?"

221. Following injection of a measles-mumps-rubella (MMR) vaccine, the nurse should make a priority assessment for which possible client manifestation?

1. Wheezing
2. Pain at the site
3. Anxiety
4. Vomiting

222. The nurse working on an adult medical-surgical unit would assign which client to the licensed practical/vocational nurse (LPN/LVN) under supervision of the RN?

1. A 46-year-old client with COPD who will be seen by the pulmonary rehabilitation specialist in 2 hours
2. A 26-year-old client who is in sickle-cell crisis
3. A 59-year-old client with Paget's disease who also has hypertension
4. A 75-year-old client who fractured a hip and is awaiting surgical repair scheduled for mid-morning

223. When assessing the genitourinary system of a 75-year-old male client, what would be the priority question for the nurse to ask this client?

1. "Have you or anyone in your family ever had testicular cancer?"
2. "Do you have any difficulty in starting the stream of urine?"
3. "Did you ever experience an injury as a child leading to testicular torsion?"
4. "Have you recently had signs of or been treated for gonorrhea?"

224. The nurse is teaching a class on newborn care to a group of expectant parents. In explaining why parents need to protect the infant from heat loss, the nurse should discuss which characteristic of the infant's skin that is responsible for heat loss?

1. Lanugo
2. Nonfunctioning sebaceous glands
3. Nonfunctioning apocrine glands
4. Thinner skin

225. Which statement indicates that a client understands appropriate information about premenstrual syndrome (PMS)?

1. "I have PMS all month long."
2. "My partner says having sex more often would help my PMS."
3. "PMS starts about 10 days before my period."
4. "I should drink more coffee when I have PMS."

226. Which symptom should the nurse assess for in a child having a tonic-clonic seizure?

1. Facial expression of inattention and daydreaming
2. Sudden loss of muscle tone and falling
3. Repetitive small-muscle-group activity
4. Muscle rigidity followed by muscle contractions

227. A client who has been admitted to the nursing unit is placed on contact precautions. What action should the nurse take regarding the client's meal trays?

1. Inform the dietary department that disposable meal trays will be needed.
2. Tell unlicensed assistive personnel (UAPs) to place used meal trays in the soiled utility room.
3. Tell the client that the dishes used for meals will be kept in the client's room and washed between meals.
4. Ask UAPs to wash the meal tray items with chlorhexidine before returning tray to the meal cart in the hall.

228. The surgical unit nurse would implement which priority measure for a client on the first postoperative day following abdominal aortic aneurysm repair?

1. Administer anticoagulant therapy.
2. Elevate the legs 15–30 degrees.
3. Maintain sequential compression devices to both legs.
4. Palpate peripheral pulses every 2–4 hours per protocol.

229. The nurse is preparing a client for surgery. Prior to completing the skin preparation, the nurse assesses the surgical site for which of the following?

1. Presence of pustules or abrasions
2. Absence of hair growth
3. Presence of lanugo
4. Absence of pulsation

230. A client with schizophrenia is admitted to the psychiatric unit. As the nurse approaches the client with medication, he refuses it, accusing the nurse of trying to poison him. What is the nurse's best response?

1. "It is not poison, and you must take the medication."
2. "If you won't take this, I will give you an injection."
3. "I'm sorry you think that this medication is poison. You don't have to take it right now if you don't want to."
4. "You may decide if you want to take the medication by mouth or injection, but this medication will help you."

231. The nurse is caring for a client who is prescribed fluphenazine 1 mg daily at bedtime. The nurse should plan to take which action based on common side effects of the medication?

1. Remind him frequently to rise slowly when getting out of bed or from a chair.
2. Assess for dizziness or lightheadedness frequently during the day.
3. Make sugarless hard candy, gum, and water available during the day.
4. Monitor for confusion frequently during daytime waking hours.

232. The nurse working on an adult medical unit would assign which client to the licensed practical/vocational nurse (LPN/LVN) under supervision of the RN?

1. A 46-year-old client who will undergo cardiac catheterization later in the morning
2. A 54-year-old client who has osteoarthritis and low back pain
3. A 62-year-old client admitted the previous evening with chest pain
4. A 79-year-old client who has chronic bronchitis and early Alzheimer's disease

233. A client with venous stasis ulcers is being treated with an Unna boot. The nurse should include which additional interventions in the plan of care? Select all that apply.

1. Assessment of peripheral pulses
2. Keeping legs dependent for pain relief
3. Wet to dry dressings to ulcer twice daily
4. Standing as much as possible
5. Elevating the legs as able

234. The nurse should initiate which priority nursing action after a client has had a full body scan to detect cancer?

1. Pain assessment due to discomfort of the actual procedure
2. Vital signs to assess for possible bleeding
3. Prophylactic antiemetic due to radiation exposure causing nausea
4. Therapeutic communication to reduce possible anxiety caused by outcomes

235. The nurse is teaching a client and family about health maintenance with chronic obstructive pulmonary disease (COPD). The nurse uses which rationale when explaining the importance of nutrition in managing this condition?

1. Proper diet can prevent susceptibility to respiratory infection.
2. Additional calories are needed because of increased work of breathing.
3. Weight gain may occur because of fluid retention.
4. Decreased energy requirements can lead to weight gain.

236. The nurse provides discharge instructions to the client with severe hypertension. The nurse should explain that a hypertensive emergency (crisis) will exist if the diastolic blood pressure (BP) is greater than how many mmHg? Provide a numeric response.

Fill in your answer below:
Answer: __________ mmHg

237. Which statement, if made by a client receiving dietary instruction for atherosclerosis, would indicate a need for further discussion?

1. "Margarine has less fat than butter, so I will no longer use butter."
2. "I will steam, bake, or broil my foods."
3. "American cheese has 76 percent fat calories."
4. "I will increase my consumption of fruits and vegetables."

238. The nurse should use medical aseptic technique when collecting which specimen from a client?

1. Wound culture from an abdominal wound
2. Sputum specimen via a tracheostomy
3. Stool specimen for ova and parasites
4. Urine specimen via straight catheterization

239. Following placement of a central venous access device, which information should the nurse report immediately to the healthcare provider?

1. Discomfort at the insertion site
2. Development of a low-grade fever
3. Increased heart rate and respiratory rate
4. Diminished breath sounds in lung bases

240. The condition of a client diagnosed with schizophrenia has improved and the client is playing a card game with peers. The group begins laughing at a joke told to them. The client jumps up and shouts, "You are all making fun of me!" The nurse concludes that the client is displaying which feature of the disorder?

1. Hallucinations
2. Ideas of reference
3. Delusions
4. Loose association

241. A 70-year-old client with chronic obstructive pulmonary disease (COPD) has a serum theophylline level of 25 mg/dL. What explanation by the nurse helps the client understand this lab result?

1. "Your dose of theophylline needs to be increased."
2. "The level is low because dosing was based on total body weight instead of lean body weight."
3. "The value could be high because of your age. The healthcare provider may decide to decrease the dose."
4. "I suspect that lab value is incorrect. Theophylline levels do not rise that high."

242. The mother of a 2-month-old receiving immunizations for the first time is also a college student. When the mother asks how immunizations relate to what she learned in microbiology class, the nurse states that immunizations interrupt the chain of infection at what link?

1. Mode of transmission
2. Portal of entry
3. Susceptible host
4. Portal of exit

243. A 9-year-old child is being treated with methimazole for Graves' disease. She has not responded to the drug therapy as quickly as expected so a thyroidectomy is being considered. The child's mother asks the nurse, "Why would the healthcare provider seem hesitant to encourage the surgery?" Which response by the nurse is best?

1. "The surgery will leave a scar on the child's neck and will cause problems with her self-esteem."
2. "Removal of the gland may result in permanent hypothyroidism, requiring lifelong hormone replacement."
3. "The convalescent time for this surgery is rather long, since it is 6 months."
4. "Removal of the thyroid gland causes a change in the body's thermoregulation."

244. The nurse in an ambulatory women's health clinic would plan to teach Kegel exercises to a woman with which condition?

1. Menopause
2. Uterine prolapse
3. Urinary tract infection
4. Premenstrual syndrome

245. A client diagnosed with paranoid schizophrenia threatened his parents with a knife and was placed on a 48-hour involuntary admission by the courts and psychiatrist. The nurse explains to the family that once the 48-hour hold is expired, the psychiatrist and court must make which determination?

1. Whether the client is a danger to himself
2. Whether the client is a danger to himself and others
3. Whether the client is willing to take his medications
4. Whether the client is willing to receive outpatient treatment

246. Which statement made by a client receiving ophthalmic corticosteroids indicates a need for further teaching?

1. "I remove my contact lenses before instilling the medication, then put them back in after 30 minutes."
2. "I am not wearing my contact lenses for the duration of the corticosteroid treatment."
3. "I will take my medication for the length of time prescribed by my healthcare provider."
4. "I will return to my healthcare provider to have my eyes examined after treatment is completed."

247. A nurse is teaching a new group of adolescent hospital volunteers about the chain of infection. Which item should the nurse include as an example of how an infection would spread through droplets?

1. Nonsterile surgical instruments
2. Soiled linens
3. Contaminated dressings
4. Sneezing and coughing

248. A 12-year-old client with signs of precocious puberty is 1.7 meters (5 ft 7 in.) tall, has a deep voice, and has started to shave his facial hair. The client says he expects to be over 1.8 m (6 ft) tall and play basketball professionally. What information should the nurse use when explaining that the client will probably not reach that height?

1. It is difficult to reach or exceed 1.8 m (6 ft) in height if neither of the parents is that tall.
2. Growing to more than 1.8 m (6 ft) tall requires a consistently healthy diet with nutrient-dense foods.
3. The early presence of testosterone leads to early closure of the epiphyseal growth plates and shorter adult height.
4. Few children attain heights above 1.8 m (6 ft) and become professional basketball stars.

249. A preoperative client was taught calf-pumping exercises to decrease the risk of thrombophlebitis postoperatively. The nurse concludes that the client understands how to perform these exercises after seeing the client perform which movements?

1. Alternately contracting and relaxing the leg muscles
2. Alternately flexing and extending the knees
3. Raising and lowering the legs
4. Alternately dorsiflexing and plantar flexing the feet

250. The nurse determines that which action would be of *highest* priority when caring for a client who has alcohol-withdrawal delirium?

1. Orienting the client to reality
2. Applying restraints as needed
3. Referring the client to Alcoholics Anonymous
4. Ensuring adequate replacement of fluids and electrolytes

251. The nurse working the evening shift on an adult surgical unit would assign which client to the licensed practical/vocational nurse (LPN/LVN) under supervision of the RN?

1. A 24-year old client who underwent extraction of four wisdom teeth earlier in the day
2. A 54-year-old client who had a laparoscopic cholecystectomy the previous day and will be discharged
3. A 62-year-old client who underwent open reduction, internal fixation of a fractured femur 3 days ago
4. A 48-year-old client returning from PACU following partial gastrectomy

252. The nurse should implement contact precautions with a client who has which health problem?

1. Scarlet fever
2. Measles
3. A wound infection
4. Rubella

253. The nurse is caring for a 68-year-old male diagnosed with benign prostatic hyperplasia (BPH). Which statement by the client indicates the need for further teaching?

1. "My enlarged prostate is what's causing me to get up twice each night to urinate."
2. "Having an enlarged prostate gland does not put me at greater risk for prostate cancer."
3. "I can get urinary tract infections because of an enlarged prostate gland."
4. "I should cut down on the fluids I drink so I won't have to urinate so often."

254. Parents of a 10-year-old boy with mild cerebral palsy who attends school ask the nurse about having their son join a Boy Scout troop that meets after school. What should the nurse consider when formulating a response?

1. The rigors of most Scout events would be physically beyond this child's capability.
2. Scouting can provide children of all abilities opportunities for recreation and socialization.
3. It could be embarrassing for the child to be different from other boys and lower his self-esteem.
4. It is more important that the child conserve his energy for doing schoolwork and homework.

255. The nurse should assess carefully a 79-year-old client who has been receiving haloperidol for signs of which adverse effect?

1. Tardive dyskinesia
2. Fecal impaction
3. Respiratory depression
4. Insomnia

256. A new staff nurse wants to clarify legal responsibilities regarding delegation while working on the unit. To which document would the nurse mentor refer this nurse?

1. Policy manual
2. Job description
3. American Nurses Association (ANA) standards of practice
4. State nurse practice act

257. The nurse is preparing to enter the room of a client with pneumonia caused by penicillin-resistant *Streptococcus pneumoniae* (PRSP). The client has a tracheostomy and requires suctioning. In what order would the nurse put on the following personal protective equipment? All options must be used.

1. Eye protection
2. Gloves
3. Mask
4. Gown

Fill in the correct order of the options below:
Answer: ____________________

258. A nurse is contacted by a neighbor who is upset, saying that she discovered her child eating half a bottle of flavored vitamins. What should the nurse recommend that the neighbor do immediately?

1. Take no action since they are only vitamins.
2. Contact the Poison Control Center.
3. Drive the child to the Emergency Department.
4. Check whether the vitamins were fat-soluble or water-soluble.

259. The nurse is preparing to administer a purified protein derivative (PPD) tuberculin skin test to a client. Before administration, the nurse should take which action?

1. Cleanse the area thoroughly with soap and water.
2. Ensure that the client has not had a positive test result in the past.
3. Determine whether the client can return to the office in 24 hours for the test to be read.
4. Instruct the client not to wash the area for 48 hours.

260. The nurse determines that which outcome criterion would be appropriate for the *initial* nursing care of a client who has acute delirium secondary to drug use?

1. The client will verbalize dependence on drugs.
2. The client will demonstrate adaptive coping strategies for dealing with stress.
3. The client will be oriented to person, place, and time during lucid periods.
4. The client will explore reasons for addictive behaviors.

261. A child is admitted to the nursing unit with acute kidney injury (AKI). When reviewing the client's health record, the nurse concludes that which item in the child's history most likely precipitated the onset of AKI?

1. Past history of chickenpox
2. Severe case of influenza 4 months ago
3. Dehydration on a recent hiking trip
4. Asthma since 3 years of age

262. The nurse concludes client teaching about infection control measures has been effective when a client with tuberculosis makes which statement?

1. "I need to wear a mask when I go to x-ray."
2. "Nurse, can you give me some gloves so I can blow my nose?"
3. "I will need to use paper plates and cups to eat."
4. "I will flush the toilet twice after urinating."

263. The home health nurse is completing a home safety inspection when visiting an older adult woman returning home after hospital discharge. Which safety concerns should the nurse point out to the client's daughter who is managing her care at home? Select all that apply.

1. Scatter rugs are present in entry hall and bottom of stairs
2. Second-floor hallway has nightlights in two different locations
3. Bathroom has a single grab bar that is near toilet
4. Light at top of stairs does not work
5. A stack of magazines are on floor next to client's chair

264. The nurse evaluates that an unlicensed assistive person (UAP) is providing safe care after noting which behavior by the UAP when working with a hospitalized client? Select all that apply.

1. Reminds client to use call bell system when in bed
2. Positions overbed table near the window
3. Adjusts bed to low position before leaving room
4. Assists client to put on nonskid footwear before ambulating
5. Puts all side-rails up before leaving room

265. A client with recently diagnosed Alzheimer's disease tends to become disoriented and confused at night. What initial suggestion can the nurse provide to family caregivers?

1. Lock the windows and the door to the client's bedroom.
2. Provide low-level indirect light in the client's bedroom at night.
3. Keep a television or music playing softly in the client's bedroom.
4. Try to walk in the neighborhood with the client to promote sleep.

Comprehensive Exam Answer Key

1. **Answer: 1 Rationale:** To prevent active tuberculosis after exposure, the client is initiated on a single agent regimen, usually isoniazid. For newly diagnosed active disease, a combination of antitubercular agents is used for at least the first several weeks: isoniazid, rifampin, and pyrazinamide. Combination therapy lessens the risk of drug resistance when treating a client with active disease, but this client has experienced exposure and does not have active disease. Except for streptomycin, which is for intramuscular use, antitubercular agents are administered orally. **Cognitive Level:** Applying **Client Need:** Pharmacological and Parenteral Therapies **Integrated Process:** Teaching and Learning **Content Area:** Pharmacology **Strategy:** The critical words in the stem of the question are *exposed* and *chemoprophylaxis*. Differentiate exposure from infection as the key concept being tested. Recall that while active infection requires multidrug therapy, exposure can be managed with a single agent alone.
2. **Answer: 2 Rationale:** The nurse should ensure the UAP understands the need to report immediately any difficulties during the procedure such as bleeding. The client may or may not be able to do most of the procedure, although the UAP should report the output. Advising the UAP to complete the procedure in the proper sequence should be unnecessary if the UAP is qualified to do the procedure. Health teaching is a function of the nurse, not the UAP. **Cognitive Level:** Applying **Client Need:** Management of Care **Integrated Process:** Communication and Documentation **Content Area:** Leadership and Management **Strategy:** The core issue of the question is the appropriate procedure for the nurse to use when delegating care to a UAP. Remember that the five rights of delegation include the *right direction* to choose correctly.
3. **Answer: 4 Rationale:** Eight hours after surgery, it is most important to ensure that the client has voided. If not, the nurse should assess urine volume using a bladder scanner and contact the healthcare provider for a prescription for catheterization to prevent acute urinary retention. Assessing use of an incentive spirometer is a routine nursing measure. Ensuring the client remains free of nausea and vomiting is a routine measure. Bowel sounds may take up to 24 hours to return depending on the type of surgery, so it is not the most critical assessment 8 hours after surgery. **Cognitive Level:** Applying **Client Need:** Reduction of Risk Potential **Integrated Process:** Nursing Process: Assessment **Content Area:** Fundamentals **Strategy:** The core issue of the question is knowledge of physiological assessment priorities in the perioperative client. Take into account the time period specified in the question to aid in making a selection.
4. **Answer: 1, 2, 4 Rationale:** A client who is 1.6 meters (5 ft 4 in.) and weighs 93 kg (205 lb) meets criteria for obesity (BMI 35.2), which is a modifiable risk factor for stroke. A blood pressure of 164/92 mmHg meets the criteria for hypertension, which is a modifiable risk factor for stroke. Cigarette smoking is an important modifiable risk factor for stroke and many other health problems. Hypercholesterolemia (cholesterol level greater than 200 mg) would also be a risk factor, but this client's level is less than 200 mg/dL. Eating a diet containing fiber helps keep cholesterol levels low and is not a risk factor for stroke. **Cognitive Level:** Analyzing **Client Need:** Health Promotion and Maintenance **Integrated Process:** Nursing Process: Assessment **Content Area:** Adult Health: Cardiovascular **Strategy:** The core issue of the question is knowledge of risk factors for stroke. Recall that these are similar to the risk factors for cardiac disease to help make your selections.
5. **Answer: 1, 2, 5 Rationale:** Washing hands before and after care is a core principle of medical asepsis. Wearing personal protective equipment is a core principle of medical asepsis. Wiping a rubber stopper of a medication vial involves the use of medical asepsis. Recapping a needle is unsafe and unrelated to medical asepsis. Use of sterile gloves involves principles of surgical asepsis rather than medical asepsis. **Cognitive Level:** Applying **Client Need:** Safety and Infection Control **Integrated Process:** Nursing Process: Implementation **Content Area:** Fundamentals **Strategy:** Use knowledge of medical versus surgical asepsis as essential core concepts. Eliminate options that utilize surgical asepsis or are unrelated to the needs of the client.
6. **Answer: 2 Rationale:** Chemotherapeutic drugs that have hematological toxicity may decrease the red blood cell, white blood cell, and platelet counts. Medications that inhibit platelet aggregation, such as ibuprofen and aspirin, should be avoided during the nadir period because they could increase the risk for bleeding. Acetaminophen is the drug of choice for mild pain and fever. Diphenhydramine is often used to dry up sinus drainage or as an antihistamine. Guaifenesin is an antitussive used to reduce cough. **Cognitive Level:** Analyzing **Client Need:** Pharmacological and Parenteral Therapies **Integrated Process:** Nursing Process: Implementation **Content Area:** Pharmacology **Strategy:** The core issue of the question is the ability to determine which drugs could increase the risk of bleeding when a client's blood counts may be low. Use the process of elimination and knowledge of drug actions and adverse effects to make a selection.
7. **Answer: 4 Rationale:** A situational leader recognizes that leadership style depends on how group members are

functioning to complete assigned work and achieve group goals. A democratic or participative leader asks questions, offers suggestions, and guides the group toward achieving group goals. A laissez-faire leader recognizes the group's need for autonomy and takes a more passive role in the group, which abdicates responsibility to others. A bureaucratic leader relies on the organization's rules, policies, and procedures to direct the group's work. **Cognitive Level:** Applying **Client Need:** Management of Care **Integrated Process:** Nursing Process: Implementation **Content Area:** Leadership and Management **Strategy:** The core issue of the question is knowledge of various leadership styles. Use this knowledge and the process of elimination to make a selection.

8. **Answer: 1 Rationale:** Hand hygiene is a core principle of standard precautions. Using gloves is appropriate when there is a risk of exposure to blood, body fluids, secretions, and excretions. However, handwashing should be done after removal of gloves. Not all clients require transmission-based precautions. A client who is at risk for infection does not necessarily require a private room. **Cognitive Level:** Applying **Client Need:** Safety and Infection Control **Integrated Process:** Nursing Process: Implementation **Content Area:** Fundamentals **Strategy:** Use the process of elimination based on nursing knowledge of standard precautions. Elements of transmission-based precautions are not initiated with all clients.
9. **Answer: 1, 4 Rationale:** The white blood cell count is elevated (normal 5000–10,000/mm^3), which is expected because of inflammation or infection associated with fever. The BUN is elevated (normal 8–22 mg/dL), which is expected because dehydration could occur as a result of fluid loss from fever and diarrhea. The sodium level is within the normal limits of 135–145 mEq/L. The potassium level is within the normal limits of 3.5–5.1 mEq/L. The serum creatinine is within the normal limits of 0.8–1.6 mg/dL. **Cognitive Level:** Analyzing **Client Need:** Reduction of Risk Potential **Integrated Process:** Nursing Process: Diagnosis **Content Area:** Adult Health: Immunological **Strategy:** The core issue of the question is the ability to discriminate between normal and abnormal laboratory values. Note the critical symptoms *fever* and *diarrhea*, which could lead you to select elevated white count for infection and elevated BUN with fluid loss from diarrhea.
10. **Answer: 2 Rationale:** The straps of a safety restraint should be secured to the bed frame rather than a movable part such as a side-rail. The nurse should use a half-bow or safety knot instead of a full knot so that the safety restraint can be released quickly if needed. The nurse should be able to slide one to two fingers between skin and safety restraint, which will not interfere with circulation yet be snug enough so it cannot be removed. A properly applied safety restraint allows the straps to remain taut if the client pulls against the restraint. **Cognitive Level:** Applying **Client Need:** Safety and Infection Control **Integrated Process:** Nursing Process: Implementation **Content Area:** Fundamentals **Strategy:** The core issue of the question is the ability to apply a safety restraint correctly to a client. Recall principles of safe application to make a selection.
11. **Answer: 4 Rationale:** Enoxaparin therapy is indicated in many postoperative clients who are immobilized to prevent the development of thromboembolic episodes. Enoxaparin inhibits clot formation that could lead to pulmonary emboli but is prescribed for clients who are likely to be immobilized for a short time following surgery. Enoxaparin is not prescribed to maintain adequate blood clotting levels; it is given to inhibit clotting. While the statement about subcutaneous administration into the abdomen and low risk of discomfort is factual, it does not explain to the client the reason it has been prescribed. **Cognitive Level:** Applying **Client Need:** Pharmacological and Parenteral Therapies **Integrated Process:** Communication and Documentation **Content Area:** Pharmacology **Strategy:** The critical words in the stem of the question are *best answer the question*. This tells you that the correct answer is one that responds to the client's concern, rather than just reciting a fact about the medication. Use nursing knowledge and the process of elimination to answer the question.
12. **Answer: 1 Rationale:** Shared leadership recognizes that there are many leaders within a group so the leader should encourage and assist with formation of self-directed work teams. In transformational leadership, the leader encourages risk-taking such as trying out new care approaches that are evidence- or research-based. A transactional leader uses incentives to promote productivity such as giving rewards for excellent performance. A democratic leader provides constructive criticism and facilitates the group's ability to meet their goals. **Cognitive Level:** Applying **Client Need:** Management of Care **Integrated Process:** Nursing Process: Implementation **Content Area:** Leadership and Management **Strategy:** The core issue of the question is knowledge of various leadership styles. Use this knowledge and the process of elimination to make a selection.
13. **Answer: 2 Rationale:** Older adults typically have a little less total sleep time and less stage 4 non-REM sleep. Older adults do not have more REM sleep because of the aging process, although they may have the same or a little less total sleep time. Older adults tend to have a lighter sleep pattern rather than a heavier and deeper sleep, and they do not have a longer total sleep time. A light sleep pattern with equal amounts of REM and non-REM sleep is characteristic of neonates. **Cognitive Level:** Analyzing **Client Need:** Basic Care and Comfort **Integrated Process:** Nursing Process: Assessment **Content Area:** Fundamentals **Strategy:** The core issue of the question is knowledge of age-related changes in sleep pattern. Use this knowledge and the process of elimination to make a selection.
14. **Answer: 3 Rationale:** Late decelerations occur because of uteroplacental insufficiency, which is decreased blood flow to the fetus through the placenta that occurs during uterine contractions. The initial nursing action is to apply oxygen by mask, usually at 8–10 liters/min, to increase fetal oxygenation. The client should be assisted to a side-lying position to shift the weight of the gravid uterus away from the inferior vena cava. Oxytocin could worsen uteroplacental insufficiency by making contractions even stronger. The laboring client's breathing pattern is unrelated to uteroplacental insufficiency. **Cognitive Level:** Analyzing **Client Need:** Health Promotion and Maintenance

Integrated Process: Nursing Process: Implementation **Content Area:** Maternal–Newborn **Strategy:** The critical word in the stem of the question is *late decelerations*. Use knowledge of the significance of this event and the process of elimination to make a selection.

15. **Answer: 2, 4 Rationale:** Surgical drainage that becomes brighter red rather than darker red is of concern because it could indicate increased bleeding or onset of new bleeding after surgery. A urine output of 50 mL over the course of 2 hours is of concern because it does not meet the minimum average of 30 mL/hr (60 mL total). A scant amount of drainage is very small and is of no concern at this time. A low-grade temperature of 99.2°F (37.3°C) is expected after surgery and warrants ordinary monitoring but is not a cause for concern at this time. A blood pressure of 126/78 mmHg is within normal range and is not of concern. **Cognitive Level:** Analyzing **Client Need:** Reduction of Risk Potential **Integrated Process:** Nursing Process: Assessment **Content Area:** Fundamentals **Strategy:** The core issue of the question is knowledge of normal and abnormal data during the early postoperative period. Use this information and the process of elimination to make a selection.

16. **Answer: 3 Rationale:** Procainamide is an antidysrhythmic medication used to treat ventricular dysrhythmias by suppressing automaticity in the His-Purkinje system. Ventricular fibrillation indicates a worsening dysrhythmia. Conversion to atrial fibrillation is not consistent with the action of procainamide. An increase in level of consciousness would only occur once the ventricular rhythm is terminated. **Cognitive Level:** Applying **Client Need:** Pharmacological and Parenteral Therapies **Integrated Process:** Nursing Process: Evaluation **Content Area:** Pharmacology **Strategy:** The core issue of the question is knowledge that procainamide is an antidysrhythmic that should reduce the irritability of the ventricle, thus making it more amenable to shock therapy.

17. **Answer: 4 Rationale:** The UAP is qualified to complete simple procedures, such as bathing a client and changing bed linens. The nurse should be the one to assess tube feeding residual. While the UAP could possibly administer mouth care to this client, the nurse must assess the oral cavity. UAPs are not trained in therapeutic communication skills and techniques. **Cognitive Level:** Analyzing **Client Need:** Management of Care **Integrated Process:** Nursing Process: Implementation **Content Area:** Leadership and Management **Strategy:** The core issue of the question is an appropriate activity to delegate to an unlicensed assistant. Keep in mind that any activity that involves assessment is retained by the RN, and then choose the option that is procedural in nature.

18. **Answer: 3 Rationale:** A client in metabolic acidosis may also be hyperkalemic. As the hydrogen ions shift from extracellular fluid (ECF) to intracellular fluid (ICF), potassium enters the ECF, leading to an increased serum potassium in addition to the low pH of acidosis. A pH of 7.4 is a normal pH and a serum potassium level of 3.8 mEq/L is also normal. A pH value of < 7.35 is associated with uncompensated acidosis. A serum potassium level of 5.0 is near the upper end of normal but is within normal limits. **Cognitive Level:** Analyzing **Client Need:** Reduction of Risk Potential **Integrated Process:** Nursing Process: Diagnosis **Content Area:** Adult Health: Endocrine and Metabolic **Strategy:** Note the critical word *acidosis* in the question. Use this to eliminate options in which the pH is not low. Focus on the critical word *metabolic* to pick the option that contains a cation with the highest value since hydrogen ions can enter the cell, which in this case is the hyperkalemic value.

19. **Answer: 4 Rationale:** Potassium is contraindicated in clients with renal dysfunction (evidenced by the high BUN and creatinine) because the renal damage interferes with potassium excretion. Although a diet lower in protein could reduce urea as an end product of metabolism, it is not the most important intervention at this time. Ambulating the client is not a priority at this time. The client may not require hourly vital sign monitoring, but might benefit from continuous electrocardiographic monitoring if the potassium level rises. **Cognitive Level:** Analyzing **Client Need:** Reduction of Risk Potential **Integrated Process:** Nursing Process: Implementation **Content Area:** Adult Health: Renal and Genitourinary **Strategy:** Recall the dangers of high potassium and that action needs to be taken immediately to discontinue the IV with the potassium because hyperkalemia could be life-threatening.

20. **Answer: 1 Rationale:** The first action of the nurse who is notified of a disaster (either external or internal) should be to follow agency policy to activate the emergency response plan. Stocking the treatment areas will be accomplished as part of a coordinated response to the disaster after activating the emergency response plan. Reassigning personnel from other work areas will occur as part of work flow once the agency emergency response plan is activated. The command team for the emergency response plan can determine the most appropriate person to begin calling in extra staff to handle the emergency. **Cognitive Level:** Applying **Client Need:** Safety and Infection Control **Integrated Process:** Nursing Process: Implementation **Content Area:** Leadership and Management **Strategy:** The core issue of the question is knowledge of appropriate agency responses to a disaster. Use this knowledge and the process of elimination to make a selection.

21. **Answer: 3 Rationale:** Lansoprazole and esomeprazole capsules may be opened and sprinkled on applesauce or dissolved in 40 mL of juice. Omeprazole must be swallowed whole. Pantoprazole must be swallowed whole. There is an alternative to rabeprazole, which must be swallowed whole. **Cognitive Level:** Applying **Client Need:** Pharmacological and Parenteral Therapies **Integrated Process:** Nursing Process: Planning **Content Area:** Pharmacology **Strategy:** The core issue of the question is knowledge of which medications used for GERD can be opened because they come in capsule form. Use knowledge of pharmacology to answer this question, which tests specific nursing knowledge of drug forms.

22. **Answer: 4 Rationale:** It is an RN's responsibility to do assessments, analyze the data, plan and implement care and teaching, and evaluate the outcomes. A second RN needs to be assigned to the nursery to safely manage the care of the Level I newborns. It is not part of the LPN's scope of practice to complete admission assessments and discharge teaching. It is beyond the scope of UAP

practice to complete discharge teaching. The RN cannot manage all the assessments and stabilize the Level II newborn. **Cognitive Level:** Analyzing **Client Need:** Management of Care **Integrated Process:** Nursing Process: Implementation **Content Area:** Leadership and Management **Strategy:** Recognize that assessment and client education are part of the professional scope of practice. The correct answer would be the option that safely retains these functions for the RN given the change in unit census.

23. **Answer: 3 Rationale:** Anxiety or anger increases peristalsis, leading to subsequent diarrhea, so stress management to deal with situations provoking these emotions is useful. Excessive intake of cheese or eggs can lead to the development of constipation. Ignoring the urge to defecate can lead to the development of constipation. Lack of exercise can lead to the development of constipation. **Cognitive Level:** Applying **Client Need:** Basic Care and Comfort **Integrated Process:** Nursing Process: Implementation **Content Area:** Fundamentals **Strategy:** The core issue of the question is knowledge of ordinary factors that can contribute to diarrhea. Evaluate each option to determine whether it is likely to aggravate diarrhea. Note that anxiety and anger stimulate the sympathetic nervous system, which then increases peristalsis; this will help you to choose correctly.

24. **Answer: 2 Rationale:** The normal attitude of the fetal head is one of moderate flexion. Changes in fetal attitude, particularly the position of the head, present larger diameters to the maternal pelvis, which contributes to a prolonged and difficult labor and increases the likelihood of cesarean delivery. Precipitous labor and delivery may be more likely to occur when the fetal head is small and in normal position. Normal labor and spontaneous vaginal delivery are not as likely to occur when the fetal attitude widens the presenting part in the maternal pelvis, such as with complete fetal head extension. Complete extension of the head may make delivery more difficult, so labor would not be expected to be short, although forceps-assisted delivery may be an option. **Cognitive Level:** Analyzing **Client Need:** Health Promotion and Maintenance **Integrated Process:** Nursing Process: Diagnosis **Content Area:** Maternal–Newborn **Strategy:** The core issue of the question is the significance of moderate flexion of the fetal head. Recognize that changes in the position of the fetal head affect delivery to choose the correct option.

25. **Answer: 3 Rationale:** Mental status changes and concentrated urine are common signs of dehydration in older adults. Clear lung sounds with unlabored breathing are normal findings. Tenting and dry, flaky skin are consistent changes seen with normal aging. Hand veins that fill within 3–5 seconds are normal findings. **Cognitive Level:** Applying **Client Need:** Physiological Adaptation **Integrated Process:** Nursing Process: Assessment **Content Area:** Adult Health: Cardiovascular **Strategy:** Note the critical words in the question are *not eating or drinking* and *dehydration*. With this in mind, look for a physical assessment finding that is consistent with dehydration. Eliminate two options readily because of the words *clear* and *dry*. Choose correctly between the remaining two, recalling that neurological symptoms are often present with altered fluid balance because sodium imbalance may occur simultaneously.

26. **Answer: 4 Rationale:** Liver function includes the regulation of blood clotting and corticosteroids can impair wound healing and irritate the GI tract. Thus, the client should be instructed to report signs and symptoms of bleeding. Moon face is a side effect of corticosteroids but is not the priority from a physiological basis. Diminished pigmentation does not reflect a risk associated with corticosteroid or immunosuppressive medications. Dysphagia is not a concern with corticosteroid or immunosuppressive medications. **Cognitive Level:** Analyzing **Client Need:** Pharmacological and Parenteral Therapies **Integrated Process:** Nursing Process: Implementation **Content Area:** Pharmacology **Strategy:** The core issue of the question is knowledge that the liver is a vascular organ and that some medications used to suppress the immune system to prevent rejection, such as corticosteroids, can lead to bleeding.

27. **Answer: 1 Rationale:** Frequent coughing and deep breathing is an easy maneuver that has great benefit to optimize ventilation in the postoperative client. Getting the client out of bed is an appropriate intervention for preventing or treating atelectasis, but this client is newly arrived on the unit and may not yet be able to get out of bed. Administering bronchodilators may aid in treatment of respiratory difficulty caused by pneumonia resulting from atelectasis. Supplemental oxygen aids in oxygenation but is not sufficient to prevent atelectasis. **Cognitive Level:** Analyzing **Client Need:** Physiological Adaptation **Integrated Process:** Nursing Process: Planning **Content Area:** Adult Health: Respiratory **Strategy:** Note the client in the question has newly arrived to the nursing unit following surgery. The critical words *nursing interventions* help you to eliminate options that require a medical prescription. Choose correctly from the remaining two options because of the word *hourly* and because there is not enough information in the stem to determine whether the client can safely get out of bed at this time.

28. **Answer: 2 Rationale:** The incident/unusual occurrence report should contain factual information about the incident, any injuries sustained, and actions taken and outcomes. To state that the client fell while walking to the bathroom is a judgment, not an observation by the nurse. Documentation of anything the client said should use exact words and should be placed in quotation marks. Stating that the client was rushing to the bathroom to avoid incontinence is either a judgment by the nurse or a report by the client that does not cite the clients words exactly and use quotation marks. **Cognitive Level:** Applying **Client Need:** Management of Care **Integrated Process:** Communication and Documentation **Content Area:** Fundamentals **Strategy:** The core issue of the question is knowledge of legal concepts as they apply to completion of incident or unusual occurrence reports. Use nursing knowledge and the process of elimination to make a selection.

29. **Answer: 2 Rationale:** The laboratory value given is within normal limits (12–16.5 grams/dL). The client is not malnourished. The client is not at nutritional risk. The client does not have polycythemia (high hematocrit). **Cognitive Level:** Analyzing **Client Need:** Reduction of Risk

Potential **Integrated Process:** Nursing Process: Diagnosis **Content Area:** Adult Health: Hematological **Strategy:** The core issue of the question is knowledge of normal and abnormal hematological laboratory values. Use specific nursing knowledge and the process of elimination to make a selection. Note that two options are somewhat similar so you may eliminate both of those initially.

30. Answer: 1 Rationale: Crusting of dried exudate is common with bacterial conjunctivitis and it is important for the child's vision and safety that the crusts are removed. Warm, moist wipes aid in comfort and they need to be disposable to reduce the risk of transmitting the infection to others in the home. Oral antihistamines are not needed to manage bacterial conjunctivitis. Ophthalmic corticosteroids are not used to decrease the inflammatory response, although antibiotics will be used to kill the bacteria. Topical anesthetics are not needed to manage eye discomfort. **Cognitive Level:** Applying **Client Need:** Physiological Adaptation **Integrated Process:** Teaching and Learning **Content Area:** Child Health **Strategy:** Note the critical word *conjunctivitis* in the stem of the question. Recall that this infection is highly contagious. Then determine the correct option by associating the word *disposable* in the correct option with the concept of infection in the stem of the question.

31. Answer: 2 Rationale: After the seizure, the client will be postictal, which is a deep sleeping state. The client could aspirate secretions unless side-lying to promote drainage from the upper airway. Positioning the client on the back increases risk of aspiration. Positioning the client on the abdomen is unrealistic given the client's postictal state. Positioning the client upright in a chair does not promote safety during the client's postictal state. **Cognitive Level:** Applying **Client Need:** Safety and Infection Control **Integrated Process:** Nursing Process: Implementation **Content Area:** Adult Health: Neurological **Strategy:** The core issue of the question is knowledge of a position that will reduce the risk of aspiration following seizure activity. Use nursing knowledge and the process of elimination to make a selection. Recall that the side-lying position is commonly used in any situation in which aspiration is a risk.

32. Answer: 1 Rationale: A client fall is a potential medical emergency; however, the nurse's responsibility is ensuring the safety of the client being attended to. Covering the sterile field protects the contents from contamination. Continuing the procedure ignores the safety of the potentially injured client. Discarding the supplies is wasteful and ignores principles of resource management. Leaving the sterile field unattended could lead to a contaminated sterile field. **Cognitive Level:** Analyzing **Client Need:** Management of Care **Integrated Process:** Nursing Process: Implementation **Content Area:** Leadership and Management **Strategy:** Recall that sterile equipment is considered contaminated if left unattended and therefore must be thrown away to eliminate two options. Then prioritize—the nurse needs to respond to the client who fell rather than continue with the wound dressing change.

33. Answer: 4 Rationale: The American Diabetes Association Exchange Lists divide food into groups with similar content (milk, vegetables, fruit, starch/bread, meat, and fat). Portion sizes are indicated so that foods may be exchanged within the same list. Rice and bread are starches. Egg is a meat on the exchange list. Tomato is a vegetable on the exchange list. Orange is a fruit on the exchange list. **Cognitive Level:** Analyzing **Client Need:** Basic Care and Comfort **Integrated Process:** Nursing Process: Evaluation **Content Area:** Foundational Sciences: Nutrition **Strategy:** First recall the basic food groups that are part of the American Diabetes Association Exchange Lists. Then compare each food choice identified with the list. Eliminate options that are vegetables and fruits first, then pick bread over egg because it is a starch.

34. Answer: 1, 3 Rationale: Genetic screening can identify markers for several types of cancer. Men should perform BSE and TSE monthly as self-checks for cancer. Self-exams as well as regular medical tests and exams uncover tumors. After a total mastectomy, women do not need mammograms. Skin cancer risk increases with age, so skin inspection continues to be important. **Cognitive Level:** Applying **Client Need:** Health Promotion and Maintenance **Integrated Process:** Teaching and Learning **Content Area:** Adult Health: Oncology **Strategy:** Evaluate each option in terms of whether the statement is true or false. The wording of the question indicates correct options will be correct statements. When in doubt, identify alternatives with *most* or *all* in the answer as false.

35. Answer: 2 Rationale: The nurse should speak privately to the coworkers about their behavior and the impact on the nurse overhearing them. This approach also personalizes the discussion between the nurse and the coworkers, which may help to diffuse the situation. It does not help the climate of the unit to let it pass. Reprimanding staff in a public venue is not helpful to deescalate the situation. Speaking to each person separately is somewhat plausible but is not efficient of the nurse's time and energy. **Cognitive Level:** Applying **Client Need:** Management of Care **Integrated Process:** Communication and Documentation **Content Area:** Leadership and Management **Strategy:** Recall that to effectively manage conflict between staff members, address the conflict within an appropriate time frame; do not let it pass unattended. Do not openly and publicly reprimand staff. Finally, address staff members privately but keep in mind what behavior is acceptable on the unit.

36. Answer: 2 Rationale: Edema, voice changes, and hair loss are among the many symptoms associated with steroid use. The student's age, along with symptoms of hair loss and edema, indicate that this is not a stage of puberty. Barbiturates have a depressant effect on the central nervous system, and this is not consistent with this client's presentation. Edema, voice changes, and hair loss are not associated with marijuana use. **Cognitive Level:** Applying **Client Need:** Pharmacological and Parenteral Therapies **Integrated Process:** Nursing Process: Diagnosis **Content Area:** Mental Health **Strategy:** The core issue of the question is knowledge of adverse effects of steroid use. Use this information and the process of elimination to make a selection.

37. Answer: 1 Rationale: The prodromal period refers to the period of time between the initial symptoms and the presence of the full-blown disease. The rash would not be apparent during this time. Chickenpox is a contagious viral illness. Reye syndrome can be a complication of chickenpox, especially with concurrent aspirin use. Pregnant women should not be in the company of those with chickenpox. **Cognitive Level:** Analyzing **Client Need:** Physiological Adaptation **Integrated Process:** Nursing Process: Evaluation **Content Area:** Child Health **Strategy:** The critical words in the stem of the question are *need for additional information*. This tells you that the correct option is an incorrect statement. Use knowledge of this communicable viral infection and the process of elimination to make a selection.

38. Answer: 2 Rationale: Adolescents tend to feel that they are invulnerable and that if anything bad will happen, it will affect others but not themselves. Substance use as a means of dealing with stress is a factor more often related to an adult. Sports-related injuries from not following rules or intense competition are most often associated with school-age children. Polypharmacy tends to be a risk factor that interferes with the safety of older adults. **Cognitive Level:** Applying **Client Need:** Safety and Infection Control **Integrated Process:** Nursing Process: Planning **Content Area:** Child Health **Strategy:** Focus on the developmental level of the client. To answer this question correctly, it is necessary to understand growth and development and apply this knowledge to the needs of the adolescent for safety.

39. Answer: 3 Rationale: A full bladder is necessary to bounce the sound waves off to compare other tissues or structures that are being assessed. It would not be helpful to deprive the client of fluids for several hours because this could lead to dehydration. Enemas are unnecessary before tests involving ultrasound. Withholding medications would be unnecessary. **Cognitive Level:** Applying **Client Need:** Reduction of Risk Potential **Integrated Process:** Teaching and Learning **Content Area:** Adult Health: Gastrointestinal **Strategy:** Recall that fluids are needed to fill the bladder and are not withheld prior to testing. Bowel structures do not interfere with the assessment of structures and an enema is not required. Medications do not have an impact on sound waves, and holding medications is not necessary for any reason.

40. Answer: 2 Rationale: Children at 10 years of age are developmentally egocentric. Asking about interests and hobbies is nonthreatening and likely to foster establishment of rapport. Focusing on behavioral symptoms, such as what brought the client to the clinic, would be more appropriate once rapport has been established. Children often are uncomfortable talking about relationships with friends and family until they get to know a person better. Ten-year-old clients may be unconcerned about past medical problems or may not recall them; such questions do not promote initial rapport between nurse and client. **Cognitive Level:** Applying **Client Need:** Psychosocial Integrity **Integrated Process:** Nursing Process: Assessment **Content Area:** Mental Health **Strategy:** The core issue of the question is knowledge of communication strategies that are likely to be effective in developing a therapeutic relationship. Focus on the age of the child and cognitive developmental level to make a selection.

41. Answer: 3 Rationale: Spironolactone is a potassium-sparing diuretic used to treat hypertension. Gynecomastia is one of its adverse reactions. Adverse reactions usually disappear after the drug is discontinued; however, gynecomastia may persist after discontinuing spironolactone. Persistent gynecomastia is not an adverse reaction of hydrochlorothiazide. Persistent gynecomastia is not an adverse reaction of furosemide. Persistent gynecomastia is not an adverse reaction of indapamide. **Cognitive Level:** Applying **Client Need:** Pharmacological and Parenteral Therapies **Integrated Process:** Teaching and Learning **Content Area:** Pharmacology **Strategy:** The core issue of the question is knowledge of adverse drug effects of spironolactone. Use specific drug knowledge and the process of elimination to make a selection.

42. Answer: 3 Rationale: Client and family satisfaction surveys are a formal set of activities that can be used to remedy deficiencies identified in the quality of direct patient care, administrative, and support services. Incident reports serve as an indicator of risk to the institution. Documentation of time and activities related to direct care may be done as part of time and motion studies. Acuity relates to the need for nursing staff on the unit. **Cognitive Level:** Applying **Client Need:** Management of Care **Integrated Process:** Nursing Process: Planning **Content Area:** Leadership and Management **Strategy:** Note the critical word *services* in the stem of the question. With this in mind, the correct option is one that gathers data from the recipients of services, who are the clients.

43. Answer: 3 Rationale: Asking the client to share her feelings is best because it represents a communication with the client and is open-ended. Leaving the client alone is not the most appropriate initial approach because it does not allow the client to share her concerns. Being silent initially may be interpreted by the client as disinterest rather than compassion. Continuing with physical preparation ignores the client and does not address the client's concerns. **Cognitive Level:** Applying **Client Need:** Reduction of Risk Potential **Integrated Process:** Communication and Documentation **Content Area:** Fundamentals **Strategy:** The core issue of the question is the ability of the nurse to care for the emotional needs of a perioperative client. Since this is potentially an anxiety-producing time for clients, choose the option in which the nurse provides a therapeutic response to the client.

44. Answer: 3 Rationale: Cigarette smoking is the leading cause of lung cancer. History of asthma is not associated with greater risk of lung cancer. Smokeless tobacco is more often associated with oral cancer. Air pollution may be a lesser contributing factor to development of lung cancer. **Cognitive Level:** Analyzing **Client Need:** Health Promotion and Maintenance **Integrated Process:** Nursing Process: Assessment **Content Area:** Adult Health: Respiratory **Strategy:** Eliminate asthma first because it is a health problem, not a risk factor. From there, choose cigarette smoking over the other options because it is highly associated with lung cancer.

45. Answer: 3 Rationale: Foods that reduce lower esophageal sphincter (LES) pressure will increase reflux symptoms. These include coffee, fatty foods, alcohol, and chocolate. An egg-white omelet is high in protein and will not increase symptoms of GERD. Dry toast will not aggravate symptoms of GERD. Skim milk is low in fat so it is helpful for a client with GERD. **Cognitive Level:** Analyzing **Client Need:** Basic Care and Comfort **Integrated Process:** Nursing Process: Implementation **Content Area:** Foundational Sciences: Nutrition **Strategy:** The core issue of the question is knowing that certain types of foods lower LES pressure, and then being able to take it a step further and identify what types of foods those are. Eliminate each option systematically by reasoning that any foods high in fat (such as the cream in the coffee) can have this effect.

46. **Answer: 2 Rationale:** Theophylline is a xanthine bronchodilator. Increased levels of theophylline occur with liver disease and congestive heart failure. Smoking history is not an issue; in fact, smokers metabolize theophylline more quickly and may need increased doses. The client is a middle-aged adult, while older age would be more significant. There is no data about the client's height to calculate a BMI, but the client's weight may not be excessive. **Cognitive Level:** Analyzing **Client Need:** Pharmacological and Parenteral Therapies **Integrated Process:** Nursing Process: Diagnosis **Content Area:** Pharmacology **Strategy:** The core issue of the question is knowledge that adverse effects of xanthine medication such as theophylline are increased in liver disease. Use specific knowledge of drug adverse effects and the process of elimination to make a selection.

47. **Answer: 1, 2, 4 Rationale:** The LPN/LVN is trained to collect data that is then reported to the registered nurse (RN). The LPN/LVN can be expected to take vital signs. The LPN/LVN can observe for and report any drainage on the cast. The LPN/LVN can elevate the casted arm above heart level to prevent edema formation. Assessments such as neurovascular assessments of the casted extremity remain the responsibility of the RN. The RN is responsible for medications that are administered by the direct IV push route. **Cognitive Level:** Analyzing **Client Need:** Management of Care **Integrated Process:** Nursing Process: Implementation **Content Area:** Leadership and Management **Strategy:** Recall that routine procedures and simple data collection can be delegated to the LPN/LVN. With this in mind, eliminate each of the incorrect options systematically.

48. **Answer: 1 Rationale:** Tuberculosis is a respiratory infection, transmitted via airborne droplet nuclei less than 5 microns in size. The nurse should wear a particulate respirator mask when working with the client. The client needs to wear a surgical mask during transport to other departments. Wearing sterile gloves for specimen collection for culture and sensitivity is a general measure that is not specific to a client with tuberculosis. The door to the client's room should remain closed. **Cognitive Level:** Applying **Client Need:** Safety and Infection Control **Integrated Process:** Nursing Process: Planning **Content Area:** Fundamentals **Strategy:** Specific knowledge of the mode of transmission of *Mycobacterium tuberculosis* and the types of transmission-based precautions is needed to select the correct answer. Eliminate the options with gloves and leaving the door open because tuberculosis is transmitted via air currents. Then recall that tuberculosis is transmitted via airborne droplet nuclei less than 5 microns in size to choose wearing the particulate respirator.

49. **Answer: 1 Rationale:** The potassium level is abnormally high (normal 3.5–5.1 mEq/L), indicating hyperkalemia, and can alter the characteristics of the cardiac waveform (tall T waves). With hyperkalemia, diarrhea and abdominal cramping are present, which would be associated with hyperactive bowel sounds. Muscle weakness and flaccidity of muscles are present in hyperkalemia, rather than being in a cramping state. Cerebral functions are stimulated in hyperkalemia so somnolence (sleeping, sluggishness) is not present. **Cognitive Level:** Analyzing **Client Need:** Reduction of Risk Potential **Integrated Process:** Nursing Process: Assessment **Content Area:** Adult Health: Cardiovascular **Strategy:** The core issue of the question is accurate interpretation of the potassium level and its significance. From there, associate the symptoms of hyperkalemia to make a selection.

50. **Answer: 3 Rationale:** The client needs to be NPO before the procedure, which requires administration of anesthesia. The client, not the legal spouse, should sign the consent form. The client should be wearing loose-fitting clothing. Liquids cannot be given before the procedure. **Cognitive Level:** Applying **Client Need:** Reduction of Risk Potential **Integrated Process:** Nursing Process: Implementation **Content Area:** Mental Health **Strategy:** The core issue of the question is knowledge that ECT requires anesthesia, which leads to loss of airway protective reflexes. Use this knowledge to reason that the client must be NPO to prevent the risk of aspiration during the procedure.

51. **Answer: 4 Rationale:** Administering very thick preparations such as penicillin G with benzathine can be painful. To lessen the pain, IM injection into a larger gluteal muscle should be administered over 12–15 seconds to separate the muscle fibers more gradually. Cold compresses to the injection site would delay absorption of the drug. Injection into the deltoid may also result in prolonged discomfort, resulting in limited motion of the upper extremities. Aspiration for blood return with all IM injections is necessary for safety since muscles contain larger blood vessels. **Cognitive Level:** Applying **Client Need:** Pharmacological and Parenteral Therapies **Integrated Process:** Nursing Process: Implementation **Content Area:** Pharmacology **Strategy:** The core issue of the question is knowledge of proper administration technique for thick liquid parenteral medications. Use knowledge of intramuscular injection techniques and knowledge of drug absorption principles to make a selection.

52. **Answer: 4 Rationale:** The only activity that can be delegated to the UAP is the simple direction to the client to remain upright after eating. Teaching about the rationale for weight loss cannot be delegated to a UAP. Exploring concerns about the treatment regimen requires therapeutic communication skills and possibly teaching and is therefore beyond the UAP's role. Explaining rationale for dietary changes constitutes teaching and is beyond the role of the UAP. **Cognitive Level:** Analyzing **Client Need:** Management of Care **Integrated Process:** Nursing Process: Implementation **Content Area:** Adult Health: Gastrointestinal **Strategy:** The core issue of the question is knowledge of the appropriate tasks to delegate to a UAP. Recalling that teaching, counseling, and assessment remain the RN's responsibility assists in eliminating each of the incorrect options.

53. **Answer:** 1 **Rationale:** Clients should remain NPO upon admission to the clinical setting with a major burn. Initial fluid replacement is started via the parenteral route. NPO status is maintained because the client may be in shock, with blood flow directed away from the digestive organs to more vital tissues. In addition, it is possible that the client suffered burn injuries that could cause internal damage to body structures, and aspiration is also a risk initially. The other options are incorrect—fluids and food by mouth would be restricted at this time. **Cognitive Level:** Applying **Client Need:** Basic Care and Comfort **Integrated Process:** Nursing Process: Implementation **Content Area:** Foundational Sciences: Nutrition **Strategy:** The core issue of the question is knowledge that the client who has experienced burn injury is under severe physiological stress and, as such, blood flow is directed away from the digestive tract. Focus on the need to stabilize the client physiologically and provide fluids by the IV route to help you choose correctly.

54. **Answer:** 4 **Rationale:** Every time a child enters the healthcare system, the immunization status should be checked. Some children have uncertain history of immunization because of parental noncompliance or special circumstances such as being refugees. Assessing growth and development is a routine activity that can be completed after priority concerns are addressed. Teaching the parents about dental care as necessary is considered part of routine care. Completing a hearing screen is a routine activity that would be completed according to recommended timetables; it is not the priority concern for this child. **Cognitive Level:** Analyzing **Client Need:** Health Promotion and Maintenance **Integrated Process:** Nursing Process: Planning **Content Area:** Child Health **Strategy:** The critical word in the stem of the question is *priority*. This tells you that more than one option is likely to be a correct nursing action, but that one is more important than the others. Note the age of the child to help you choose immunizations as the priority, especially noting that the child has not received healthcare for 2.5 years, during a time when vaccinations should be kept up to date.

55. **Answer:** 4, 5 **Rationale:** The pain of pancreatitis can be reduced by sitting up and leaning forward, which reduces pressure caused by contact of the inflamed pancreas with the posterior abdominal wall. Pain can be reduced using the fetal position (side-lying with knees pulled up to the chest), which promotes flexion rather than extension of the posterior abdominal wall. The pain of pancreatitis is usually aggravated by lying in a supine position, which increases pressure on the pancreas by the posterior abdominal wall. A prone position is generally not a comfortable position since it promotes extension of the spine and posterior abdominal wall. The left lateral decubitus position would be helpful only if knees were also pulled up to the chest (fetal position). **Cognitive Level:** Applying **Client Need:** Physiological Adaptation **Integrated Process:** Nursing Process: Implementation **Content Area:** Adult Health: Gastrointestinal **Strategy:** The core issue of the question is knowledge of proper positioning techniques to reduce the pain of inflammation from pancreatitis. Use the process of elimination to select the position in which the pancreas is not as likely to be compressed against other body structures.

56. **Answer:** 1 **Rationale:** Although many chemotherapy agents can cause stomatitis, the antimetabolites are commonly known for causing this side effect. Fluorouracil is the only drug listed in this class. Cisplatin is an alkylating agent, which is likely to cause nausea, vomiting, and diarrhea. Doxorubicin is an antitumor antibiotic, which can cause nausea and vomiting as well as cardiac toxicity. Vincristine is a plant (vinca) alkaloid that tends to be more toxic to the nervous system. **Cognitive Level:** Analyzing **Client Need:** Pharmacological and Parenteral Therapies **Integrated Process:** Nursing Process: Diagnosis **Content Area:** Pharmacology **Strategy:** The core issue of the question is knowledge of which antineoplastic agents cause stomatitis as an adverse effect. Use nursing knowledge and the process of elimination to answer the question.

57. **Answer:** 1 **Rationale:** Safe and effective delegation is based on knowledge of the laws governing nursing practice and knowledge about job duties and responsibilities. Nurses must understand the competencies and training of unregulated care providers. It is not necessary to provide written directions when delegating tasks to UCPs as long as verbal directions are clear and expectations are understood. UCPs can deliver supplies to the client's bedside and this is not a priority consideration of the nurse. UCPs are part of the care delivery team and do not require a special introduction. UCPs can introduce themselves to clients. **Cognitive Level:** Applying **Client Need:** Management of Care **Integrated Process:** Nursing Process: Implementation **Content Area:** Leadership and Management **Strategy:** Use knowledge of the five rights of delegation to answer the question. In this case, consider the competence of the UAP as integral to the question.

58. **Answer:** 1 **Rationale:** Pronator drift occurs when a client cannot maintain the hands in a supinated position with the arms extended and eyes closed. This assessment may be done to detect small changes in muscle strength that might not otherwise be noted. Nystagmus is the presence of fine, involuntary eye movements. Hyperreflexia is an excessive reflex action. Ataxia is a disturbance in gait. **Cognitive Level:** Applying **Client Need:** Physiological Adaptation **Integrated Process:** Communication and Documentation **Content Area:** Adult Health: Neurological **Strategy:** Specific knowledge of physical assessment techniques is needed to answer the question. Note the association between the terms *supinated* in the question and *pronator* in the correct answer in response to the client's change in hand position.

59. **Answer:** 3 **Rationale:** Packing the sample in ice will minimize the changes in gas levels during the transportation of the specimen to the lab. The arterial site should be held for 5 minutes, or even longer if the client is receiving anticoagulant therapy. The blood is drawn originally in a heparinized syringe and does not need to be transferred to one. A second specimen is not necessary. **Cognitive Level:** Applying **Client Need:** Reduction of Risk Potential **Integrated Process:** Nursing Process: Implementation **Content Area:** Adult Health: Respiratory **Strategy:** The wording of the question tells you that the

correct answer is also a true statement of fact. Recall specific elements of the procedure to make the correct selection.

60. **Answer:** 2 **Rationale:** For clients with dysthymic disorder, a type of depressive mood disorder, a major concern is social isolation. Encouraging the client to eat in the dining room with others addresses this concern. Quiet time is not necessarily helpful for a client with a form of depression. Regulating food intake to three meals and no snacks is not helpful, especially if the client has an accompanying symptom of poor appetite. Although fluids are necessary to maintain hydration, assigning clear liquids has no value for the client. **Cognitive Level:** Analyzing **Client Need:** Psychosocial Integrity **Integrated Process:** Nursing Process: Planning **Content Area:** Mental Health **Strategy:** The core issue of the question is knowledge of strategies to reduce the risk of isolation in a client with dysthymia. Use nursing knowledge and the process of elimination to make a selection.

61. **Answer:** 3 **Rationale:** The effectiveness of a heparin protocol is monitored by trending APTT results to achieve a therapeutic level. An APTT of 140 is above the therapeutic level of anticoagulation and therefore the infusion should be stopped per protocol, and resumed at a decreased dose in one hour's time with a repeat APTT done in 2–3 hours per protocol. The dose should not be increased, as this would cause serious consequence to the client. Stopping the medication for a total of 6 hours would undermine the anticoagulation control that the healthcare provider is trying to achieve. Ordering another APTT and continuing to run the infusion could also cause serious consequences to the client. **Cognitive Level:** Analyzing **Client Need:** Pharmacological and Parenteral Therapies **Integrated Process:** Nursing Process: Implementation **Content Area:** Pharmacology **Strategy:** The core issue of the question is recognition that this is a critically high value for the APTT and that the action that will maintain client safety is to turn off the heparin for a period of time. Use the process of elimination and knowledge of the effects of heparin on APTT times to answer the question.

62. **Answer:** 1, 3 **Rationale:** The UAP can perform tasks or nursing care activities, such as measuring oxygen saturation level, under supervision of the nurse. The UAP can perform routine tasks or nursing care activities, such as mouth care. The RN retains responsibility for assessment of breath sounds. The RN retains responsibility for teaching. The UAP can perform routine procedures after training, such as the use of a bladder scanner. **Cognitive Level:** Analyzing **Client Need:** Management of Care **Integrated Process:** Nursing Process: Implementation **Content Area:** Leadership and Management **Strategy:** The core issue of the question is the ability to discriminate between what the RN may or may not delegate. Evaluate each option and either choose it because it is a simple procedure or task, or choose not to select it because it involves assessment or teaching.

63. **Answer:** 4 **Rationale:** The client's right to withdraw consent is a necessary part of the consent and it means that coercion was not utilized in obtaining the signature. It is the healthcare provider's responsibility, not the nurse's, to explain the diagnosis. Cost is not part of discussion for informed consent and it would be the healthcare provider who would explain the proposed treatment. Technical aspects of the procedure are not needed by the client, although an overview of the procedure by the healthcare provider should be included. **Cognitive Level:** Analyzing **Client Need:** Reduction of Risk Potential **Integrated Process:** Nursing Process: Implementation **Content Area:** Fundamentals **Strategy:** The core issue of the question is knowledge of the nurse's role in obtaining informed consent. Keep in mind that the nurse reinforces explanations already given by the healthcare provider and use the process of elimination to make a selection.

64. **Answer:** 1 **Rationale:** Presentation refers to the part of the fetus that is coming through the cervix and birth canal first. Thus a face presentation occurs when the face is coming through first. The hip will not be the presenting part. A breech presentation occurs when the buttocks are delivered first. The back of the head, or occiput, isa common presentation at delivery. **Cognitive Level:** Analyzing **Client Need:** Health Promotion and Maintenance **Integrated Process:** Teaching and Learning **Content Area:** Maternal–Newborn **Strategy:** Associate the word *face* in the question with the word *face* in the correct response. The word *presentation* helps you to choose this option over the one containing the word *facing*, which is inappropriate to the context to this question.

65. **Answer:**

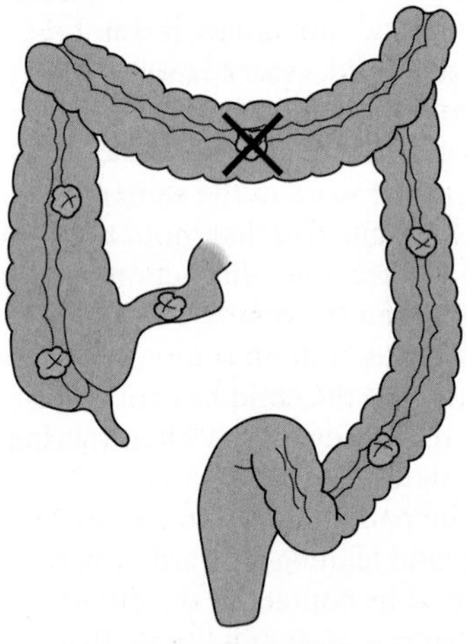

Rationale: The correct area is the center stoma, not the distal one that is nearer to the distal colon and rectum. Coming from the small bowel in the center of the diagram, the stomas represent, in anatomical order, an ileostomy, cecostomy, ascending colostomy, transverse colostomy, descending colostomy, and sigmoidoscopy. **Cognitive Level:** Analyzing **Client Need:** Basic Care and Comfort **Integrated Process:** Teaching and Learning **Content Area:** Adult Health: Gastrointestinal **Strategy:** To answer this question correctly, recall the names of the anatomic portions of the bowel. It will also help you to choose correctly if you recall that the prefix *trans-* means "across." This might help you select the stoma that is halfway across the abdomen.

66. **Answer:** 1 **Rationale:** Laparoscopic surgery is minimally invasive and client recovery times are faster. This client would be best suited to the float from the medical unit,

who should also be familiar with working with clients who have chronic lung disease. Clients who undergo joint replacement typically have protocol-based care that involves collaboration with physical therapy as well. This client would be better assigned to a regular nurse on the unit. A client who underwent cardiac valve surgery 2 days ago should be stable but requires ongoing cardiac monitoring and assessment for early detection of possible postoperative complications. A client who had partial thyroidectomy requires careful airway management and surgical site assessment, which may be better managed by a regular surgical unit nurse. **Cognitive Level:** Analyzing **Client Need:** Management of Care **Integrated Process:** Nursing Process: Implementation **Content Area:** Leadership and Management **Strategy:** The core issue of the question is knowledge of the scope of practice for an RN and similarities in client needs across various care settings. Use nursing knowledge and the process of elimination to make a selection.

67. **Answer: 3, 4 Rationale:** The intermediate care surgical nurse should be most comfortable assuming the care of surgical clients, such as a client post-appendectomy. The client with nephrolithiasis will undergo moderate sedation, and the intermediate care surgical nurse should be familiar with typical preoperative or preprocedure teaching and care. An exacerbation of heart failure is a medical problem that may be better managed by a nurse familiar with these clients. Thyrotoxicosis is a medical problem that may be better assigned to a nurse familiar with the care of clients with medical problems. A client with diabetes will also require extensive teaching and this may be better managed by a nurse on the unit who is more familiar with this client population. **Cognitive Level:** Analyzing **Client Need:** Management of Care **Integrated Process:** Nursing Process: Implementation **Content Area:** Leadership and Management **Strategy:** Note the critical word *surgical* in the description of the work setting of the float nurse. With this in mind, choose the two clients that have procedures that are surgical in nature.

68. **Answer: 2 Rationale:** Cholinergic crisis can result if a client with myasthenia gravis has excessive effects from cholinergic medication used to treat the disorder. For this reason, the client should use caution not to exceed the recommended dose. Spacing activities over the course of the day will help reduce physiological stress, which may then reduce the risk of myasthenic crisis. Eating a well-balanced diet with nutrient-dense foods is sound advice but does not relate to preventing cholinergic crisis. Exposure to illnesses such as colds or flu places the client at risk for infection, which can lead to myasthenic crisis. **Cognitive Level:** Applying **Client Need:** Physiological Adaptation **Integrated Process:** Nursing Process: Evaluation **Content Area:** Adult Health: Neurological **Strategy:** Recall that options that have similarities are not likely to be correct. Examine the options from the viewpoint of neurological stimulation. Eliminate each of the incorrect responses because they reflect abnormally low activity of the nervous system.

69. **Answer: 2 Rationale:** Troponin is a sensitive test that indicates damage to the myocardial cells. The LDH^4 isoenzyme is utilized to determine hepatic function. Amylase is a pancreatic digestive enzyme. A CK-MM isoenzyme elevation would indicate skeletal muscle damage. **Cognitive Level:** Applying **Client Need:** Reduction of Risk Potential **Integrated Process:** Nursing Process: Assessment **Content Area:** Adult Health: Cardiovascular **Strategy:** Specific knowledge is needed to answer this question. Recall that troponin is a newer enzyme that can be measured very early during myocardial damage and is an indicator of myocardial damage and thus myocardial infarction.

70. **Answer: 2 Rationale:** The client's level of risk for self-harm is a major concern and should be a priority focus of discussion during the interdisciplinary team meeting. The client may need a private room if in a manic state, not a two-bed room. The client may need restricted visitors if in a manic state rather than unrestricted visitors. The client should not be overstimulated, making it inadvisable to recommend client participation in several focused activities. **Cognitive Level:** Applying **Client Need:** Psychosocial Integrity **Integrated Process:** Nursing Process: Planning **Content Area:** Mental Health **Strategy:** Critical words in the stem of the question are *safety* and *bipolar disorder*. Use nursing knowledge to associate depression as part of bipolar disorder with the threat to safety with suicide as a form of self-harm. This will lead you to the correct answer.

71. **Answer: 4 Rationale:** Ciprofloxacin is not recommended for *Helicobacter pylori* infection during pregnancy. Metronidazole, amoxicillin, and clarithromycin can be used after consulting with the healthcare provider. **Cognitive Level:** Applying **Client Need:** Pharmacological and Parenteral Therapies **Integrated Process:** Nursing Process: Planning **Content Area:** Pharmacology **Strategy:** The core issue of the question is knowledge of the pregnancy categories of the specific drugs listed. Use the process of elimination to make a selection, realizing that specific drug knowledge is needed to answer the question.

72. **Answer: 2 Rationale:** Trigeminal neuralgia is manifested by spasms of pain that begin suddenly and last anywhere from seconds to minutes. Clients often describe the pain as stabbing or similar to an electric shock. It is accompanied by spasms of facial muscles, which cause closure of the eye and/or twitching of parts of the face or mouth. Facial droop is characteristic of Bell's palsy, a disorder of the facial nerve (cranial nerve VII). Ptosis is drooping of the eyelid on one side and is not part of the presentation of trigeminal neuralgia. Facial muscle paralysis would be the opposite finding of facial muscle spasms. **Cognitive Level:** Applying **Client Need:** Physiological Adaptation **Integrated Process:** Nursing Process: Assessment **Content Area:** Adult Health: Neurological **Strategy:** Note the critical word *neuralgia* in the question, which tells you the pain is of nervous system origin. Recalling that this type of pain is usually sharp, stabbing, and possibly burning may help you to eliminate some incorrect options. Distinguish between spasm associated with this disorder and paralysis (an opposite finding) to discriminate between the final two options.

73. **Answer: 1 Rationale:** Abuse of laxatives and diuretics is a frequent purging behavior for bulimic clients. Supervising mealtimes is more appropriate for a client with anorexia nervosa. The client with bulimia will eat but later purges. The use of ritualistic eating patterns pertains to clients with anorexia nervosa. Food should

never be used as a reward. **Cognitive Level:** Applying **Client Need:** Basic Care and Comfort **Integrated Process:** Nursing Process: Planning **Content Area:** Mental Health **Strategy:** The critical word in the question is *bulimia*. Recall that this disorder has the classic features of bingeing and purging to guide you to the correct answer, which in this question is one that signifies agents that help one to purge.

74. **Answer: 3 Rationale:** Lifestyle modifications and recognition of risk factors are important parts of prevention of long-term complications. Encouraging the client to maintain his current lifestyle and follow up with health screening would be the best plan of action. False reassurance that the client will never be hypertensive is inappropriate. Family history is a very strong risk factor but developing hypertension is not inevitable with lifestyle management. Prophylactic antihypertensive medications are inappropriate. **Cognitive Level:** Analyzing **Client Need:** Health Promotion and Maintenance **Integrated Process:** Communication and Documentation **Content Area:** Adult Health: Cardiovascular **Strategy:** The core issue of the question is lifestyle management to reduce the risk of developing hypertension. Select the option that focuses on prevention while addressing the continued risk that the client faces.

75. **Answer: 4 Rationale:** When a cast is dry, edges that are not smooth or covered by a piece of stockinette should be covered to prevent skin irritation. This can be done by petaling the cast edges with strips of adhesive tape, beginning each strip on the inside of the cast, and folding over the edge to the outside of the cast. Petrolatum jelly is not used around cast edges as it would macerate the skin and cause further skin damage over time. The healthcare provider will not cut away rough cast edges. Placement of towels is unnecessary and could cause excess and uneven pressure on the skin. **Cognitive Level:** Applying **Client Need:** Physiological Adaptation **Integrated Process:** Communication and Documentation **Content Area:** Child Health **Strategy:** The wording of the question indicates that the correct response is a true statement. Visualize each option and eliminate those that are less plausible.

76. **Answer: 3 Rationale:** Immunizations should be withheld during leukemia exacerbations because the immune system is compromised and the client cannot manage an appropriate response to the immunization. There is no need to place the infant in isolation without added evidence of immunosuppression. Assessment of other family members does not apply to the care plan for this client. There is no need to be NPO for chemotherapy, although chemotherapy can lead to nausea and vomiting. **Cognitive Level:** Applying **Client Need:** Physiological Adaptation **Integrated Process:** Nursing Process: Planning **Content Area:** Child Health **Strategy:** The core issue of the question is knowledge that leukemia adversely affects the immune system. With this in mind, the nurse needs to be mindful that immunizations will need to be withheld during an exacerbation. Use nursing knowledge and the process of elimination to make a selection.

77. **Answer: 1 Rationale:** The RN is responsible for delegating tasks appropriately and is responsible for the actions of unlicensed personnel. Ambulating a postoperative client is the only task from those listed that the RN could delegate to a novice student. Completing an admission assessment and calling a healthcare provider to report a low hemoglobin level are critical thinking skills and should be performed by the RN. Verifying a unit of blood must be completed by two licensed nurses, and a student does not yet have a nursing license. **Cognitive Level:** Analyzing **Client Need:** Management of Care **Integrated Process:** Nursing Process: Implementation **Content Area:** Leadership and Management **Strategy:** Note the critical word *beginning* to describe the student nurse. With this in mind, select the delegation assignment that is simple and procedural in nature, and does not require assessment, teaching, or advanced knowledge in nursing.

78. **Answer: 2 Rationale:** The primary organ in the right upper quadrant of the abdominal cavity is the liver. Because of the early shock symptoms, which are presented, it would be expected that this organ has possibly been lacerated, causing extensive uncontrolled internal bleeding. The stomach is located in the left upper quadrant. The large intestine is located more toward the lower half of the abdomen. The kidneys are located in the flank area. **Cognitive Level:** Analyzing **Client Need:** Physiological Adaptation **Integrated Process:** Nursing Process: Assessment **Content Area:** Adult Health: Gastrointestinal **Strategy:** First analyze the client's vital signs to determine that the client's status is consistent with a shock state. Then determine which organs are located in the right upper quadrant. Associate the liver, which is a vascular organ, and the location to determine the correct option.

79. **Answer: 2 Rationale:** The healthcare provider will prescribe laxatives or enemas if the client is potentially not able to expel the barium on his or her own. The nurse should encourage the client to increase fluid intake if possible as well. The client will, in most cases, return to the unit with barium still present in the bowel. This is a common concern for many clients undergoing this procedure, and their concerns should not be ignored. Rescheduling the test would be inappropriate and does not alleviate the concern. **Cognitive Level:** Analyzing **Client Need:** Reduction of Risk Potential **Integrated Process:** Communication and Documentation **Content Area:** Adult Health: Gastrointestinal **Strategy:** Note the critical words *best response* in the stem of the question. This indicates that the correct response is a true statement of fact. Recall that this test can cause constipation from residual barium to aid in selecting the correct option.

80. **Answer: 1 Rationale:** The only respectful therapeutic response here is to allow the client to stay and refrain from participating at this time. Every client does not need to participate in every group session. It is inappropriate to focus the group's attention on one individual because of level of participation. The client should not be asked to leave, which could shame the client and is nontherapeutic. **Cognitive Level:** Applying **Client Need:** Psychosocial Integrity **Integrated Process:** Communication and Documentation **Content Area:** Mental Health **Strategy:** The core issue of the question is knowledge of group process and conduct of a group

meeting. Use knowledge of this treatment modality and the process of elimination to make a selection.

81. **Answer: 3 Rationale:** Phenytoin is an antiepileptic medication that is used to control seizure activity. Selegilene is used to treat Parkinson's disease. Diclofenac is a nonsteroidal anti-inflammatory drug. Sumatriptan is used to treat headaches. **Cognitive Level:** Applying **Client Need:** Pharmacological and Parenteral Therapies **Integrated Process:** Nursing Process: Implementation **Content Area:** Pharmacology **Strategy:** The core issue of the question is knowledge of medications that are effective against seizure activity. Use specific drug knowledge and the process of elimination to make a selection.

82. **Answer: 1 Rationale:** After burn injuries, an elevated potassium level (normal 3.5–5.1 mEq) is expected because of cellular tissue damage with release of intracellular potassium into the bloodstream. The sodium level should not fall. The hematocrit will be elevated (not decreased) due to hemoconcentration. The white blood cell count will be elevated as part of the inflammatory response to injury. **Cognitive Level:** Analyzing **Client Need:** Physiological Adaptation **Integrated Process:** Nursing Process: Assessment **Content Area:** Adult Health: Integumentary **Strategy:** First visualize what happens when cells are destroyed—intracellular contents are released into the circulation. Second, with burn injury fluid is lost through the burn surface and can lead to hemoconcentration. With this in mind, eliminate each option except potassium, which increases for both of the reasons just stated.

83. **Answer: 2 Rationale:** In a 2-gram sodium diet, clients should be taught to read food labels for hidden sodium content and eliminate those foods that are high in sodium. It is not enough to stop adding salt while cooking, which would correspond to the restriction in a 4-gram sodium diet. Adding salt while cooking is not allowed as part of a 2-gram sodium diet. There is more involved with a 2-gram sodium restriction than merely avoiding salty-tasting snacks. **Cognitive Level:** Analyzing **Client Need:** Basic Care and Comfort **Integrated Process:** Nursing Process: Evaluation **Content Area:** Foundational Sciences: Nutrition **Strategy:** The critical words in the question are *low sodium*. With this in mind, first eliminate options that are the least restrictive. Then choose the more comprehensive option of those remaining.

84. **Answer: 2 Rationale:** Clients who have certain cultural beliefs may perceive an imbalance in the hot and cold forces in the body after delivery. They avoid sources of cold, such as wind, cold beverages, and water (even if warmed) to regain balance between these extremes. A client's culture plays a very important part in who they are, and nurses should respect the client's wishes as long as it will not result in harm to the client or others. Showing a video on postpartum care does not demonstrate cultural sensitivity. The nurse should not attempt to have the client comply with bathing by using communications that could frighten the client. A consultation with a medical social worker is unnecessary. **Cognitive Level:** Applying **Client Need:** Health Promotion and Maintenance **Integrated Process:** Culture and Spirituality **Content Area:** Maternal–Newborn **Strategy:** Use principles of culturally competent care to answer this question. If using a multicultural perspective rather than one centered in a Western healthcare approach, you will be able to eliminate each incorrect response easily.

85. **Answer: 3 Rationale:** When a client's level of anxiety markedly increases, the nurse can relieve the anxiety by changing the focus of the discussion. Asking the client for more details will probably further increase the client's anxiety level. Encouraging the client to relax may or may not be effective in reducing the client's anxiety. The client may or may not be prepared to advise whether or not to stop the conversation, and abruptly stopping the interview will probably increase the client's anxiety level. **Cognitive Level:** Applying **Client Need:** Psychosocial Integrity **Integrated Process:** Nursing Process: Implementation **Content Area:** Mental Health **Strategy:** The core issue of the question is the ability to recognize escalating anxiety in a client and determining the best means to effectively reduce it. Use knowledge of therapeutic measures for anxious clients and the process of elimination to make a selection.

86. **Answer: 4 Rationale:** The correct response is one in which the client is honest, has an understanding of how to take the medication and what the side effects are, and knows that the side effect will subside eventually. The client who has no desire to take the medication is not showing feelings of being comfortable with the daily medication routine. Stating that the medication will prevent the client from coming to the hospital again may be unrealistic and it implies that the client is taking it just to avoid such a consequence. The ability to recite memorized actions does not indicate that the client understands the benefits or side effects of the medication. **Cognitive Level:** Analyzing **Client Need:** Pharmacological and Parenteral Therapies **Integrated Process:** Communication and Documentation **Content Area:** Pharmacology **Strategy:** The core issue of the question is which statement *best* indicates correct understanding of lithium as a medication. Use specific drug knowledge and the process of elimination to make a selection.

87. **Answer: 2 Rationale:** For 6 hours after intravesicular chemotherapy, the toilet should be double-flushed to eliminate any small remaining amounts of drug or its metabolites. The client does not need to use a bed pan for voiding, which would require proper handling during cleaning. Wiping the toilet seat with tissue is unnecessary and does not address the biohazardous aspect of chemicals remaining in the toilet. Sterile gloves are unnecessary; clean gloves are appropriate. **Cognitive Level:** Applying **Client Need:** Management of Care **Integrated Process:** Nursing Process: Implementation **Content Area:** Adult Health: Oncology **Strategy:** The core issue of the question is how to prevent unintentional exposure of other people to biohazardous chemicals in the client's urine after intravesicular chemotherapy. With this principle in mind, eliminate ordinary measures that do not provide additional protection. Eliminate next the option with the sterile gloves because only clean gloves are needed.

88. **Answer: 1 Rationale:** It is important that circulation is checked regularly. Typically the restraints are removed, one at a time, every 2 hours to evaluate skin condition

and circulation. Checking that tongue blades are in pockets and ends are covered or padded applies to an elbow restraint. Ensuring that straps are attached to nonmovable parts of the crib is correct, but is the priority response compared to circulation and skin condition. A call bell is a routine part of care but does not become a priority because a client has a restraint. **Cognitive Level:** Applying **Client Need:** Safety and Infection Control **Integrated Process:** Nursing Process: Implementation **Content Area:** Child Health **Strategy:** Focus on the word *priority* in the stem of the question. Recalling that many aspects of restraint care are important, use the ABCs (airway, breathing, and circulation) to focus on the correct option—which addresses the child's circulation to the restrained limb.

89. **Answer: 1** **Rationale:** Emergency airway and resuscitation equipment should be readily accessible whenever allergy testing is administered because of the potential for hypersensitivity response and anaphylactic reaction. Visibility of the tested areas is important but not immediately essential. Because of the potential for a serious reaction, the client will be asked to wait in the office for a period of time to be monitored for any untoward responses. The room should be set up prior to the arrival of the client but it is not a priority. **Cognitive Level:** Analyzing **Client Need:** Reduction of Risk Potential **Integrated Process:** Nursing Process: Planning **Content Area:** Adult Health: Integumentary **Strategy:** Note the critical word *priority* in the stem of the question. This tells you that the correct answer is the most important option and that more than one may be technically correct. Recall that allergic reaction is a risk with skin testing to guide you to the correct answer.

90. **Answer: 3** **Rationale:** Symptoms associated with a number of medical conditions are very similar to the symptoms associated with panic attacks. When a medical condition is present, it should be identified and treated. Laboratory tests cannot differentiate types of anxiety. Laboratory tests cannot determine the etiology of a panic attack. Symptoms of panic disorder are not usually related to hypochondriasis. **Cognitive Level:** Applying **Client Need:** Psychosocial Integrity **Integrated Process:** Communication and Documentation **Content Area:** Mental Health **Strategy:** The core issue of the question is knowledge that physiological symptoms need to be ruled out as having a medical basis before they can be attributed strictly to psychological origins. Use this information and the process of elimination to choose correctly.

91. **Answer: 2** **Rationale:** Norethindrone contains only progestin and no estrogen. Because estrogen may decrease lactation, progestin-only pills are commonly used in lactating women. Superficial phlebitis is not as relevant to the client's status as lactation. Dysmenorrhea would not be an indication to begin norethindrone therapy for a postpartum client. Menarche at age 18 would not be an indication for norethindrone in a postpartum client. **Cognitive Level:** Applying **Client Need:** Pharmacological and Parenteral Therapies **Integrated Process:** Nursing Process: Assessment **Content Area:** Maternal–Newborn **Strategy:** The core issue of the question is which oral contraceptive is safe to use while breastfeeding. Use knowledge of the estrogen component of norethindrone and the process of elimination to make a selection.

92. **Answer: 1** **Rationale:** It is essential that the client's spinal cord be immobilized to prevent further injury and loss of function. Assessing for lacerations is part of the secondary assessment. Exposure of the client is part of the secondary assessment. Performing a full mental status exam is part of the secondary assessment. **Cognitive Level:** Analyzing **Client Need:** Safety and Infection Control **Integrated Process:** Nursing Process: Implementation **Content Area:** Adult Health: Neurological **Strategy:** Focus on the critical words *most important*. Whenever a client has suffered a traumatic injury, the nurse must first address the ABCs and then address neurological status and needs. With this in mind, select spine stabilization as the priority because it safeguards the client.

93. **Answer: 3** **Rationale:** The American Heart Association recommends a diet with reduced saturated fats and cholesterol for clients with coronary heart disease. Canned peaches are high in concentrated sugars, which increase triglyceride levels. Egg yolks are high in cholesterol and whole milk is high in saturated fats. A meal consisting of orange juice, shredded wheat, skim milk, and toast with jelly is low in saturated fat and cholesterol. A meal consisting of grapefruit juice, oatmeal, 1% milk, and a bagel with jelly is low in saturated fat and cholesterol. A meal consisting of applesauce, egg-white omelet, skim milk, and a plain bagel is low in saturated fat and cholesterol. **Cognitive Level:** Analyzing **Client Need:** Basic Care and Comfort **Integrated Process:** Nursing Process: Evaluation **Content Area:** Foundational Sciences: Nutrition **Strategy:** The wording of the question tells you that the correct answer to the question is the one that contains incorrect items. Correlate the words *coronary heart disease* with fat-containing foods to begin the elimination process. Choose the option that contains eggs and whole milk, two sources of fat and cholesterol.

94. **Answer: 3** **Rationale:** The football, or clutch, position provides the mother with more control of the newborn's head and full view of the face. The lying-down position is usually done in bed and does not allow full view of the infant's face. The cradle position often causes the newborn's head to wobble around on the mother's arm and does not allow full view of the infant's face. Placing the client across the lap does not allow full view of the infant's face. **Cognitive Level:** Applying **Client Need:** Health Promotion and Maintenance **Integrated Process:** Nursing Process: Implementation **Content Area:** Maternal–Newborn **Strategy:** Visualize each of the options and systematically eliminate those that do not promote visualization of the face while maintaining control of the head.

95. **Answer: 1** **Rationale:** PEA is associated with what appears to be a normal electrical conduction pattern but there is no mechanical pumping of the myocardium. Ventricular fibrillation, ventricular tachycardia, and asystole will not demonstrate an effective electrical conduction pattern on the cardiac monitor. **Cognitive Level:** Applying **Client Need:** Physiological Adaptation **Integrated Process:** Nursing Process: Assessment **Content Area:** Adult Health: Cardiovascular **Strategy:** Associate the words *unable to palpate* in the stem of the question with the word *pulseless* in the correct option. Otherwise, it is necessary to understand the pathophysiology involved in this question.

96. **Answer: 3 Rationale:** To promote absorption, the client should not blink for 30 seconds after the administration of dipivefrine, an ophthalmic drug used to treat glaucoma. The client should not squeeze the eyes closed, even gently, for 30 seconds because this will inhibit the medication from staying in the eye. The eyes do not need to be closed. It is unnecessary to keep the eyes closed for a full minute. **Cognitive Level:** Applying **Client Need:** Pharmacological and Parenteral Therapies **Integrated Process:** Teaching and Learning **Content Area:** Pharmacology **Strategy:** The core issue of the question is knowledge of proper administration technique for dipivefrine. Use specific drug knowledge that this is an ophthalmic medication and the process of elimination to make a selection.

97. **Answer: 1 Rationale:** Pediatric clients can be diagnosed with diabetes and the float nurse should be familiar with this health problem and could do client teaching. The nurse is not as likely to have recent experience in working with clients with Guillain-Barré syndrome. The client with dementia who is being transferred will require transfer paperwork to be completed, and the pediatric nurse may not be as familiar with these types of forms because of the pediatric population usually worked with. The nurse is not as likely to have recent experience in working with clients who have had prostate gland surgery. **Cognitive Level:** Analyzing **Client Need:** Management of Care **Integrated Process:** Nursing Process: Implementation **Content Area:** Leadership and Management **Strategy:** Review the diagnoses of each of the possible clients and choose the one that the pediatric nurse is most likely to have experience working with.

98. **Answer: 3 Rationale:** Pulmonary edema occurs as a result of fluid shifts caused by the ingestion of the hypertonic salt water. The result is fluid collecting in the interstitial spaces, causing pulmonary edema. Hypoxia, hypovolemia, and acidosis occur as a result of near-drowning incidents. Heart block is not a concern for this client. Renal failure is not the priority concern unless the kidneys are damaged because of persistent ischemia from inadequate ventilation. The client would experience respiratory acidosis, not alkalosis. **Cognitive Level:** Applying **Client Need:** Physiological Adaptation **Integrated Process:** Nursing Process: Diagnosis **Content Area:** Adult Health: Respiratory **Strategy:** Note the critical words *salt water* and consider concepts and dynamics of fluid movement in the body. Because of the hypertonic water entering the client's lungs, envision that the client's own body fluid would move into the alveoli to equalize the tonicity.

99. **Answer: 1 Rationale:** A positive TB test means that the organism is present in the body in either an active or a dormant state. The client can expect to be scheduled for sputum tests for the presence of the bacillus and a chest x-ray to determine the presence of lesions or active disease. Isolation is not instituted until a probable or definitive diagnosis has been made. A positive TB test should not be ignored and further testing should not be deferred for several months. Medications are not instituted until a probable or definitive diagnosis has been made. **Cognitive Level:** Applying **Client Need:** Reduction of Risk Potential **Integrated Process:** Communication and Documentation **Content Area:** Adult Health: Respiratory **Strategy:** Note the presence of the critical word *best*. This tells you that the correct answer is a true statement of fact. Use knowledge of this test and the process of elimination to make a selection.

100. **Answer: 1 Rationale:** Speaking slowly and softly reduces stress-related emotions. Instructing the clients to ignore the behavior will not assist them in reducing anxiety. A client experiencing severe or panic anxiety will be unable to focus on identifying behaviors of anxiety. Reminding a client of the need to use good manners when talking with other clients ignores the client's anxiety and may only increase the symptoms of anxiety. **Cognitive Level:** Applying **Client Need:** Psychosocial Integrity **Integrated Process:** Nursing Process: Implementation **Content Area:** Mental Health **Strategy:** The core issue of the question is knowledge of therapeutic communication techniques with a client whose anxiety is escalating. Select the option that is most likely to have a calming effect on the client from a behavioral perspective.

101. **Answer: 2 Rationale:** Jaundice in the dark-skinned client can best be observed by assessing the hard palate. In dark-skinned clients, palms and soles may appear jaundiced, but calluses on skin surfaces can also make the skin appear yellow. Normally fat may be deposited in the layer beneath the conjunctivae that can reflect as a yellowish hue of the conjunctivae. Fat deposits under the conjunctiva can cause a yellow reflection in the adjacent sclera. **Cognitive Level:** Applying **Client Need:** Pharmacological and Parenteral Therapies **Integrated Process:** Nursing Process: Assessment **Content Area:** Pharmacology **Strategy:** The core issue of the question is how to assess for jaundice in a client with dark skin. Keep in mind that the oral cavity is a good choice to help guide you to a correct response.

102. **Answer: 2, 1, 4, 3 Rationale:** The nurse should assess first the client who has the low platelet count (normal 150,000–450,000/mm^3), who has the greatest threat to physiological status because of risk for bleeding. The second client to assess is the one who has the borderline low WBC count because this is a lesser threat to physiological status. The nurse should assess the client who has questions about chemotherapy third, since the nurse can take some time to answer these questions once potentially unstable clients are attended to. Fourth, the nurse should assess the client who is upset so that the nurse can plan to spend time with this client. **Cognitive Level:** Analyzing **Client Need:** Management of Care **Integrated Process:** Nursing Process: Planning **Content Area:** Leadership and Management **Strategy:** Remember that physiological needs take priority over psychosocial and learning needs. Choose the client with the most serious physiological need first (which is the client with the most abnormal labs) followed by the other client with a physiological concern. Then use time as a means of setting priorities for the remaining clients, since the client who is in psychological distress would benefit from greater interaction time with the nurse.

103. **Answer: 3 Rationale:** A client with GERD should limit (or possibly eliminate) the intake of coffee because this can relax LES pressure and lead to symptoms. Large meals could aggravate the symptoms of GERD. Spicy foods (such as the use of extra garlic) could worsen GERD symptoms. Peppermint relaxes LES pressure, contributing to the development of GERD symptoms: **Cognitive Level:** Applying **Client Need:** Basic Care and Comfort **Integrated Process:** Nursing Process: Planning **Content Area:** Foundational Sciences: Nutrition **Strategy:** Recall that coffee, chocolate, and fatty foods lower LES pressure and therefore increase the risk of reflux. Knowing that these types of food choices need to be limited helps guide you to select the option with coffee. Alternatively, eliminate options that would aggravate the symptoms.

104. Answer: 3 Rationale: The child should be included in planning for the new baby and may need extra time and attention in case they feel threatened by a new sibling. Parents should not show displeasure if the child is not happy about news of a future sibling because they may need time to adjust. Parents should avoid putting too much responsibility on the child. It is unnecessary and not helpful to have the child stay with the grandparents. **Cognitive Level:** Applying **Client Need:** Health Promotion and Maintenance **Integrated Process:** Communication and Documentation **Content Area:** Maternal–Newborn **Strategy:** Use knowledge of growth and development principles and communication skills to make a selection. The correct answer is the option that includes the needs of the child as a client as well as the parents.

105. Answer: 3 Rationale: The pH is elevated, HCO_3^- is elevated, and $PaCO_2$ is low. This indicates that there is a mixed respiratory and metabolic alkalosis. Uncompensated metabolic acidosis is incorrect because the HCO_3^- level alone would be decreased. Uncompensated metabolic alkalosis does not account for the low CO_2 level. Uncompensated respiratory acidosis does not account for the high HCO_3^- level, which constitutes an effort toward compensation. **Cognitive Level:** Analyzing **Client Need:** Reduction of Risk Potential **Integrated Process:** Nursing Process: Diagnosis **Content Area:** Adult Health: Respiratory **Strategy:** Note the critical word *pneumonia* in the question. With this in mind, reason that the disorder is likely to be respiratory in origin, which allows you to eliminate purely metabolic disorders. Consider that both the CO_2 and HCO_3^- are abnormal in an alkalotic direction to choose the mixed imbalance.

106. Answer: 3 Rationale: A client at risk for nausea should not lie down for at least 30 minutes after meals to avoid aspiration. The healthcare provider should be notified of excessive weight loss. Foods and beverages are better tolerated when they are neither hot nor cold and not too spicy. Calling the healthcare provider is a good client action if other measures fail. **Cognitive Level:** Analyzing **Client Need:** Pharmacological and Parenteral Therapies **Integrated Process:** Nursing Process: Evaluation **Content Area:** Pharmacology **Strategy:** The core issue of the question is knowledge of factors that will relieve or aggravate nausea caused by cancer chemotherapeutic agents. Use knowledge of the effect of gravity upon digestion as well as general measures of managing nausea to make a selection.

107. Answer: 3 Rationale: The movement of the fluid, also referred to as tidaling, in the water indicates normal lung expansion and requires only continued monitoring. The healthcare provider should not be called unless the movement ceases. Coughing will increase the movement of the fluid by changing intrathoracic pressure. Repositioning the chest tube will have no effect on the oscillation. **Cognitive Level:** Analyzing **Client Need:** Physiological Adaptation **Integrated Process:** Nursing Process: Assessment **Content Area:** Adult Health: Respiratory **Strategy:** To answer this question it is necessary to have a basic understanding of chest tube function. Beyond that, note the critical word *slight* in the stem of the question, which helps to eliminate notifying the healthcare provider. Eliminate chest tube repositioning because it is not within the scope of nursing practice. Make a final selection, realizing there is no reason to ask the client to cough.

108. Answer: 2 Rationale: According to standard precautions, the caregiver should wear goggles when contamination from splashing is possible, as when the membranes are artificially ruptured (amniotomy). Changing a wet disposable bed pad, starting an intravenous line, and washing used instruments require the use of standard precautions. **Cognitive Level:** Analyzing **Client Need:** Safety and Infection Control **Integrated Process:** Nursing Process: Planning **Content Area:** Maternal–Newborn **Strategy:** The core issue of the question is knowledge of when to use various personal protective equipment items. Recall that amniotomy refers to rupture of the amniotic membrane and then reason that this could involve splash and require the use of goggles.

109. Answer: 4 Rationale: The normal calcium level is 9.0–11.0 mg/dL, making this client hypercalcemic, which can occur as a complication of some cancers. Muscle weakness is a key feature of hypercalcemia due to changes in excitability of cell membranes. Peaked T waves, muscle spasm, and increased gastric motility are signs of hyperkalemia. **Cognitive Level:** Analyzing **Client Need:** Reduction of Risk Potential **Integrated Process:** Nursing Process: Planning **Content Area:** Adult Health: Oncology **Strategy:** The core issue of the question is knowledge of electrolyte imbalance (hypercalcemia in this case) and the associated manifestations. Recall that calcium plays a key role in nervous system function to help guide you to the correct option.

110. Answer: 2 Rationale: Anxiety can be a healthy protective response to an actual threat. Defense mechanisms are unconscious psychological responses designed to diminish or delay anxiety. Anxiety, at times, cannot be avoided and is a healthy adaptive reaction when it alerts the person to impending threats. The client may not be able to avoid a flight-or-flight response, although stress management techniques may lessen the response. **Cognitive Level:** Analyzing **Client Need:** Psychosocial Integrity **Integrated Process:** Nursing Process: Evaluation **Content Area:** Mental Health **Strategy:** The core issue of the question is knowledge that anxiety can exist to a greater or lesser state at any given time, and that some anxiety may be helpful as it increases alertness and performance. Use this background knowledge to select the correct option.

111. Answer: 2 Rationale: Hydralazine is a vasodilator that increases the capacity of the vascular bed to decrease blood pressure. During dehydration preload is reduced because of decreased circulating volume, which lowers the blood pressure further. The normal dose of hydralazine is 5–25 mg PO, so the dose is not excessive. Serum potassium is high but would be unrelated to hydralazine. The increased heart rate is a reflexive response to the low cardiac output to compensate with decreased preload and afterload. **Cognitive Level:** Applying **Client Need:** Pharmacological and Parenteral Therapies **Integrated Process:** Nursing Process: Assessment **Content Area:** Pharmacology **Strategy:** The core issue of the question is knowledge of factors that will compound or worsen a low blood pressure in a client taking an antihypertensive medication. Recall that factors that cause vasodilation or reduce the circulating volume (such as dehydration) can cause a drop in blood pressure. Use the process of elimination to systematically discard options that do not have this causative influence.

112. **Answer: 4 Rationale:** In a client whose condition is deteriorating, the RN should delegate the task that is most procedural in nature (in this case the urinary catheter insertion). The RN should insert the IV line because a new IV medication can be administered immediately after insertion. The LPN is able to collect data such as VS to report to the RN, but in a client whose acuity is changing, it is better for the RN to make these assessments. The RN should administer the IV push medication, which is beyond the scope of practice for an LPN/LVN. **Cognitive Level:** Analyzing **Client Need:** Management of Care **Integrated Process:** Nursing Process: Implementation **Content Area:** Leadership and Management **Strategy:** Use knowledge of the principles of delegation. Eliminate the options that address IV and IV medication because these should be retained by the RN. Choose the catheter over vital signs because the RN would need to interpret the significance of the vital signs, not merely measure them.

113. **Answer: 1 Rationale:** Older clients need time to digest the information and ask questions. Most older clients are able to make decisions for themselves. Encouraging a rapid signature can be considered coercion. Reading materials can be appropriate but is not the best option since clients need more than reading material for an informed consent. **Cognitive Level:** Applying **Client Need:** Reduction of Risk Potential **Integrated Process:** Nursing Process: Implementation **Content Area:** Fundamentals **Strategy:** The core issue of the question is the need for the older adult undergoing surgery to have sufficient time to process information. Choose the option that takes into consideration age-related changes of older adults.

114. **Answer: 4 Rationale:** To begin life, the infant must make the adaptations to establish respirations and circulation. These two changes are crucial to life. The gastrointestinal and hepatic systems, urinary and hematologic systems, neurologic and thermoregulatory systems become established over a longer period of time. **Cognitive Level:** Analyzing **Client Need:** Health Promotion and Maintenance **Integrated Process:** Nursing Process: Assessment **Content Area:** Maternal–Newborn **Strategy:** Use the ABCs (airway, breathing, and circulation) as the strategy for answering this question.

115. **Answer: 2 Rationale:** The eggs provide 24 grams of protein and the whole milk adds protein and calories. Toast and orange juice do not reflect an adequate protein source. Pancakes and apple juice reflect an increased carbohydrate source and bacon is considered a fat, not a protein. Oatmeal and skim milk do not reflect a high-protein, high-calorie meal but rather a low-calorie meal selection with a greater carbohydrate content. **Cognitive Level:** Analyzing **Client Need:** Basic Care and Comfort **Integrated Process:** Nursing Process: Evaluation **Content Area:** Foundational Sciences: Nutrition **Strategy:** First recall that clients with burn injury need to take in foods that are high in protein and calories. With this in mind, compare each option against this need to eliminate each of the incorrect options systematically.

116. **Answer: 1 Rationale:** Signs of overdosage of desmopressin, an antidiuretic hormone, include blood pressure and pulse elevation, mental status changes, and water and sodium retention. Because the medication therapy needs to be interrupted, the nurse should notify the healthcare provider. Having the client return for reevaluation would place the client at risk because of lack of timely treatment. Limiting salt intake would not address the current complication. The route by which the drug is administered is not the issue. **Cognitive Level:** Analyzing **Client Need:** Pharmacological and Parenteral Therapies **Integrated Process:** Nursing Process: Implementation **Content Area:** Pharmacology **Strategy:** The core issue of the question is knowledge that fluid retention is an adverse drug effect and that this client is showing signs of excessive drug therapy. Use drug knowledge and the process of elimination to answer the question.

117. **Answer: 2, 5 Rationale:** Documenting intake from meal trays is a simple nursing procedure that can be delegated to the UAP. Assisting the client to ambulate in the hall is part of routine client care and is within the scope of practice for a UAP. The RN retains responsibility for assessment of the skin following a treatment session. The nurse should assess variations in fatigue over the shift as one means to evaluate the client's overall response to therapy. Engaging in therapeutic communication to explore how the client is coping with treatment is part of the role of the RN. **Cognitive Level:** Analyzing **Client Need:** Management of Care **Integrated Process:** Nursing Process: Implementation **Content Area:** Leadership and Management **Strategy:** Recall that the RN does not delegate assessment, teaching, and counseling and evaluate each of the options in relation to these guidelines.

118. **Answer: 4 Rationale:** Visual difficulty caused by distortions and impairment of central vision is common with macular degeneration. Peripheral vision in most cases is normal. Glaucoma is characterized by loss of peripheral vision, not central vision. Cataracts involve a gradual deterioration of vision with opacity of the lens. A detached retina would be noted by a sudden change in vision with a sense of a curtain falling over the field of vision. **Cognitive Level:** Applying **Client Need:** Physiological Adaptation **Integrated Process:** Nursing Process: Diagnosis **Content Area:** Adult Health: Eye and Ear **Strategy:** Specific knowledge of the various visual disorders is needed to answer the question. Eliminate detached retina and cataracts first because of the client's description. Then choose correctly from the remaining two options because of the nature of the disorder.

119. Answer: 1 Rationale: An ultrasound is the only noninvasive procedure listed because it involves transmission of sound waves through the skin of the abdomen. A barium swallow requires swallowing contrast, which makes it an invasive procedure. A colonoscopy requires insertion of an endoscope. A CT scan with contrast involves injecting a contrast medium into the bloodstream. **Cognitive Level:** Applying **Client Need:** Reduction of Risk Potential **Integrated Process:** Teaching and Learning **Content Area:** Adult Health: Gastrointestinal **Strategy:** The core issue of the question is knowledge of noninvasive diagnostic tests for the gastrointestinal system. Eliminate each of the incorrect options because of the words or suffixes *swallow*, *-oscopy*, and *contrast*. These all imply that the test will be intrusive to the body.

120. Answer: 3 Rationale: Consent is implied if the situation is an emergency and delaying treatment until written consent is obtained could result in further injury or death. Continuing to try to reach family members might be done by police, but the client's treatment should not be delayed until they are contacted. A court order for surgery is not necessary in this situation because consent is implied. It is inappropriate for the emergency department provider to sign the consent because it is unnecessary and the provider is not authorized to do so. **Cognitive Level:** Applying **Client Need:** Management of Care **Integrated Process:** Nursing Process: Implementation **Content Area:** Leadership and Management **Strategy:** The core issue of the question is the ability to take action using legal concepts of informed consent. Compare each option with these principles to choose correctly.

121. Answer: 1 Rationale: The bismuth portion of bismuth subsalicylate can cause the unique side effect of transient darkening of the tongue. Bismuth subsalicylate is administered to treat dyspepsia. Bismuth subsalicylate may help relieve abdominal pain depending on the cause. Diarrhea is not a unique side effect from the bismuth portion of bismuth subsalicylate. **Cognitive Level:** Applying **Client Need:** Pharmacological and Parenteral Therapies **Integrated Process:** Nursing Process: Assessment **Content Area:** Pharmacology **Strategy:** The critical word in the stem of the question is *unique*. With this in mind, use the process of elimination and knowledge of drug components to determine which side effect is caused by bismuth. As an alternative strategy, select darkening of the tongue because it is the only one that is located in the very upper GI tract.

122. Answer: 1 Rationale: Acute episodes of celiac disease are characterized by fatty stools (steatorrhea) because of malabsorption. The client would experience anorexia rather than increased appetite. The client may experience irritability but would not have excessive sleepiness. The client would experience bulky, frothy stools rather than soft, formed stools. **Cognitive Level:** Applying **Client Need:** Physiological Adaptation **Integrated Process:** Nursing Process: Assessment **Content Area:** Child Health **Strategy:** The core issue of the question is the manifestations of celiac disease that occur because of the underlying pathophysiology. Recall that this disorder is characterized by malabsorption of key nutrients to help eliminate incorrect options.

123. Answer: 1 Rationale: Regular exercise can help to normalize bowel function. Cigarette smoking is generally harmful and offsets any perceived benefits of relaxation. Gum chewing increases the amount of air that is swallowed, which can cause gas and is not a helpful measure. An excessive amount of fruits and vegetables may not be helpful in controlling bowel function with irritable bowel syndrome. **Cognitive Level:** Analyzing **Client Need:** Basic Care and Comfort **Integrated Process:** Nursing Process: Evaluation **Content Area:** Adult Health: Gastrointestinal **Strategy:** Use knowledge of healthy lifestyle habits that stimulate normal bowel function as a means of answering this question. Eliminate cigarettes and gum first as least helpful in health promotion. Choose exercise over fresh fruits and vegetables because they could aggravate irritable bowel syndrome.

124. Answer: 4 Rationale: The embryo's muscles spontaneously contract beginning at 7 weeks. The mother perceives sensations of movement anytime from 16 to 20 weeks' gestation. There is no need to call within 1 week (at 17 weeks' gestation) if movement is not felt. Although a primigravida usually perceives movement closer to 20 weeks, it can be felt before 20 weeks' gestation. It is inaccurate to tell the client she should have felt movement already, and this response could also frighten the client. **Cognitive Level:** Applying **Client Need:** Health Promotion and Maintenance **Integrated Process:** Communication and Documentation **Content Area:** Maternal–Newborn **Strategy:** The core issue of the question is knowledge of fetal growth and development. An easy way to remember this information is to equate 4 weeks to be 1 month and then remember movements are felt at 4–5 months (16–20 weeks).

125. Answer: 1 Rationale: A double-diapering technique will help to protect a urinary stent following repair of hypospadias or epispadias. The inner diaper collects the infant's stool, while the outer one collects urine. The double diaper does not assist with measurement of urine. The double diaper is not intended to maximize absorption of urine. The double-diapering technique should help protect against urinary infection. **Cognitive Level:** Applying **Client Need:** Physiological Adaptation **Integrated Process:** Teaching and Learning **Content Area:** Child Health **Strategy:** The core issue of the question is the rationale for a specific diapering technique following surgery to correct hypospadias. Eliminate measuring urine output as least realistic and choose the correct option after determining which option best reflects safety considerations and protection of the surgical area.

126. Answer: 1 Rationale: An inspiratory stridor is indicative of a hypersensitivity reaction to the DPT immunization; epinephrine should be administered per protocol order set to counteract the symptoms of the allergic response. It is unnecessary to assess for signs of pulmonary edema, which is irrelevant. The infant may experience angioedema, but edema would not be restricted to periorbital edema. Reassessing the infant in 5 minutes places the infant at risk for injury or death. **Cognitive Level:** Applying **Client Need:** Pharmacological and Parenteral Therapies **Integrated Process:** Nursing Process: Implementation **Content Area:** Pharmacology **Strategy:** The core issue of the question is recognition that stridor following immunization is a sign of hypersensitivity to the drug. With this in mind, use the process of elimination to select epinephrine as the drug treatment of choice.

127. **Answer:** 4 **Rationale:** To coach is to give direction and suggestions for improvement; suggesting how to accomplish time savings is an example of this. Instructing to get vital signs or face discipline is threatening rather than coaching. The statement about reporting blood glucose levels is a criticism without a suggestion for improvement. The response to call lights is helpful as a statement of positive reinforcement but does not specifically give direction for future actions. **Cognitive Level:** Analyzing **Client Need:** Management of Care **Integrated Process:** Communication and Documentation **Content Area:** Leadership and Management **Strategy:** The critical word in the stem of the question is *coach*. Use the ordinary definition of the word and choose the option that gives suggestions or advice to improve performance.

128. **Answer:** 3 **Rationale:** The nurse would determine that the client understood the information if the client stated rubella is transmitted by the droplet route. Clients with rubella are placed in droplet precautions, as the causative agent is transmitted by particle droplets larger than 5 microns. Contaminated food is a common means of transmission for hepatitis A. Rubella is not transmitted by the airborne route; tuberculosis is an example of an infection requiring airborne precautions. Rubella is not transmitted by direct contact of one person with another. **Cognitive Level:** Applying **Client Need:** Safety and Infection Control **Integrated Process:** Nursing Process: Implementation **Content Area:** Adult Health: Respiratory **Strategy:** Knowledge about the transmission of rubella and the elements of each type of transmission-based precaution is required. Select an option based on nursing knowledge.

129. **Answer:** 2 **Rationale:** A pH of 7.6 indicates an alkalotic state. The administration of sodium bicarbonate to counteract an acidotic state would be the most likely reason for the value. Although blood gases drawn during a code usually show acidosis, this does not explain why the client has an alkalotic pH post-code. There is no reason to assume that the laboratory has made a mistake in reporting the ABG results. **Cognitive Level:** Analyzing **Client Need:** Reduction of Risk Potential **Integrated Process:** Nursing Process: Evaluation **Content Area:** Adult Health: Endocrine and Metabolic **Strategy:** First recall that a pH of 7.6 is alkalotic to eliminate the options indicating normal findings or acidosis. Alternatively associate the high pH with the drug sodium bicarbonate, which raises pH.

130. **Answer:** 2 **Rationale:** Characteristics of a client with pain disorder tend to include an inadequate understanding of the role of stress in exacerbating pain symptoms. Clients often rely on analgesics to manage the pain of a pain disorder. Moving more slowly does not necessarily assist a client with a pain disorder to fulfill expected roles. With a pain disorder, there is no obvious structural damage at the site of pain. **Cognitive Level:** Analyzing **Client Need:** Psychosocial Integrity **Integrated Process:** Nursing Process: Assessment **Content Area:** Mental Health **Strategy:** The critical words in the stem of the question are *anticipate* and *pain disorder*. With this in mind, determine that the core issue of the question is characteristics that are compatible with this disorder. Use nursing knowledge and the process of elimination to make a selection.

131. **Answer:** 1 **Rationale:** The client must understand the need to take medication consistently as a priority item. There is no risk of physical dependency with antiepileptic drug therapy to treat generalized seizures. Teaching that urine may turn pink to brown may be included if appropriate, but is not of highest priority. Effective medication dosing should control seizure activity without waiting 2–3 weeks. **Cognitive Level:** Applying **Client Need:** Physiological Adaptation **Integrated Process:** Nursing Process: Planning **Content Area:** Adult Health: Neurological **Strategy:** The critical words in the stem of the question are *highest priority*. This tells you that more than one option may be factually correct and that you must choose the most important item. Recall that insufficient drug therapy may lead to seizure recurrence to help you select appropriately.

132. **Answer:** 2, 5 **Rationale:** The child with the low white blood cell count (normal 5000–10,000/mm^3) is at risk for infection and may need neutropenic precautions and can be placed with another child who is at risk for infection. The child receiving chemotherapy could become immunosuppressed as an adverse effect of drug therapy and is at risk for infection. The child who underwent appendectomy for a ruptured appendix may have peritonitis and should not be placed with clients who have active communicable diseases. The child with encephalitis has a viral infection and should be isolated from other children. The child with scarlet fever has a bacterial infection and should be placed on droplet precautions in a private room. **Cognitive Level:** Analyzing **Client Need:** Management of Care **Integrated Process:** Nursing Process: Implementation **Content Area:** Leadership and Management **Strategy:** Examine the clients in the question and determine similarities and differences among them. The two that are the most similar and that have the most similar needs from an infection control perspective are the ones who should be placed together.

133. **Answer:** 4 **Rationale:** A client with AIDS may lose weight due to wasting and malnutrition. The client, who may be unable to merely increase caloric intake, should be instructed about nutrient-dense foods and supplements that maximize the quality of dietary intake. Although a food diary would provide helpful information, this allows for a delay in treatment that could result in further weight loss. Stating to expect weight fluctuations with menstrual cycle provides the client with a false belief that her diet and the diagnosis of AIDS does not have an impact on nutritional status. Even though increased salt in the diet can lead to fluid retention and with potential mild weight gain, it ignores the underlying issue of nutritional balance. **Cognitive Level:** Analyzing **Client Need:** Basic Care and Comfort **Integrated Process:** Nursing Process: Implementation **Content Area:** Foundational Sciences: Nutrition **Strategy:** Analyze each of the options and choose the one that has the most direct and positive impact on weight gain. Using this strategy, you can systematically eliminate each of the incorrect options.

134. **Answer: 4 Rationale:** Polypharmacy (use of multiple medications prescribed by multiple healthcare providers) increases the risk of drug interactions and excessive dosing of required medications. This can occur when healthcare providers are not aware of what other practitioners have prescribed. The client should check with the healthcare provider about over-the-counter drugs that may be taken with prescription medications but this does not necessarily increase risk for complications of heart and lung disease. The client should not share medications with family or friends but this does not necessarily affect the course of the underlying heart or lung disease. The nurse should assess the memory of a client who reports medication adherence as remembered, but this is not the most common medication-related problem in older adults. **Cognitive Level:** Analyzing **Client Need:** Health Promotion and Maintenance **Integrated Process:** Nursing Process: Assessment **Content Area:** Pharmacology **Strategy:** The critical words in the question are *common* and *significantly increases the risk* . . . . Note the age of the client and common issues with medication therapy in older adults to choose correctly.

135. **Answer: 4 Rationale:** Placing the client with ARDS in a prone position allows for expansion of the posterior chest wall, which may be effective in enhancing oxygenation. Transfusing red blood cells does not increase oxygenation in ARDS. Transfusing albumin does not increase oxygenation in ARDS. Elevating head of bed should have been done as an initial measure. **Cognitive Level:** Applying **Client Need:** Physiological Adaptation **Integrated Process:** Nursing Process: Implementation **Content Area:** Adult Health: Respiratory **Strategy:** The core issue of the question is an intervention that may increase oxygenation in a client with ARDS. Note the critical words *nursing intervention* to eliminate options that require a healthcare provider prescription. Choose prone position over head-elevated position because it allows for expansion of the back side of the client's lungs and redistribution of blood flow using gravity.

136. **Answer: 3 Rationale:** Because ACE inhibitors can cause fetal harm or death, they should be discontinued as soon as pregnancy is detected. Their effect on breastfeeding infants is unknown. The effect of vasodilators, diuretics, and calcium channel blockers during pregnancy may warrant their use. **Cognitive Level:** Applying **Client Need:** Pharmacological and Parenteral Therapies **Integrated Process:** Teaching and Learning **Content Area:** Pharmacology **Strategy:** The core issue of the question is knowledge that ACE inhibitors need to be avoided during pregnancy because they are harmful to the fetus. Use knowledge of drug therapy and the process of elimination to make a selection.

137. **Answer: 2 Rationale:** The pediatric intensive care nurse is more likely to have experience working with heart failure, since children can experience heart failure secondary to cardiac defects. Myocardial infarction, stent placement, and coronary atherectomy are relevant to the care of adult clients. **Cognitive Level:** Analyzing **Client Need:** Management of Care **Integrated Process:** Nursing Process: Implementation **Content Area:** Leadership and Management **Strategy:** Note the critical words *pediatric intensive care* in the stem of the question. Then determine which client has the health problem that could also be experienced in the pediatric population.

138. **Answer: 1 Rationale:** The priority nursing intervention is one that maintains contact of the retina with the choroid by positioning the client so the detached area falls against the choroid. It is unnecessary to darken the client's immediate environment. A preoperative medication may be prescribed, but has lower priority than maintaining proper position of the head to protect the eye. Both eyes, not just the affected eye, are patched to minimize eye movement. **Cognitive Level:** Analyzing **Client Need:** Physiological Adaptation **Integrated Process:** Nursing Process: Implementation **Content Area:** Adult Health: Eye and Ear **Strategy:** The critical words in the question are *actions* and *first*. This indicates that more than one option may be correct but that one is more important than the others. Use knowledge of pathophysiology to make the correct selection.

139. **Answer: 3 Rationale:** Electrolyte shifts caused by vomiting and diarrhea, in addition to lack of replacement intake, will lead to a risk for hypokalemia (normal range is 3.5–5.1 mEq/L). Calcium levels (normal 9–11 mg/dL) would not be elevated with vomiting. Sodium level (normal 135–145 mEq/L) will be elevated with the loss of potassium but the client's value is still in the normal range. A blood urea nitrogen level of 8 mg/dL is near the low end of the 8–22 mg/dL range, but dehydration should cause this value to rise. **Cognitive Level:** Analyzing **Client Need:** Reduction of Risk Potential **Integrated Process:** Nursing Process: Diagnosis **Content Area:** Adult Health: Gastrointestinal **Strategy:** Critical words in the question are *vomiting* and *diarrhea*. With this in mind, recall that potassium may be lost from the GI tract. Eliminate sodium first because it is within normal range, and then eliminate the calcium levels as less relevant to the question than potassium.

140. **Answer: 1 Rationale:** Advance directives are executed in writing by clients and must be notarized and/or witnessed by specified individuals. Since laws and guidelines can vary from jurisdiction to jurisdiction, the nurse who is not familiar with the jurisdiction's law and agency policy should seek assistance from a nursing supervisor. Hospital policies can vary depending on state or jurisdiction in which the hospital is located. The nurse should verify agency policy before stating that anyone on the unit can witness the advance directive, but this is not as likely to be a true statement. It is not necessarily sufficient for witnessing an advance directive to be a registered nurse. **Cognitive Level:** Applying **Client Need:** Management of Care **Integrated Process:** Nursing Process: Implementation **Content Area:** Leadership and Management **Strategy:** The core issues of the question is knowledge of legal implications of witnessing an advance directive. With this in mind, use the process of elimination to select the most appropriate option from a legal perspective.

141. **Answer: 2 Rationale:** Epinephrine is a beta-adrenergic agent that has beta 2-adrenergic action, causing bronchodilation. The results of subcutaneous epinephrine should be seen in 5 minutes. One minute

is an insufficient amount of time for the drug to work. Ten minutes is an excessively long time frame. Fifteen minutes would be an unacceptable time frame for drug action in a client with respiratory distress. **Cognitive Level:** Applying **Client Need:** Pharmacological and Parenteral Therapies **Integrated Process:** Nursing Process: Planning **Content Area:** Pharmacology **Strategy:** The core issue of the question is knowledge of the time frame for the onset of action with epinephrine. Use specific drug knowledge and the process of elimination to make a selection.

142. **Answer: 1 Rationale:** Glycosylated hemoglobin is elevated due to persistent hyperglycemia. Values greater than 8 percent indicate consistently poor control of blood glucose and warrant assessment of the client's dietary intake over the past several weeks. Assessing the diet for the last 2–3 days is insufficient, while assessing for signs of infection is not warranted. Assessing knowledge of vision screening and foot care are important but unrelated to the laboratory test result. Insulin is administered to treat high blood glucose levels, not glycosylated hemoglobin levels. **Cognitive Level:** Analyzing **Client Need:** Physiological Adaptation **Integrated Process:** Nursing Process: Implementation **Content Area:** Adult Health: Endocrine and Metabolic **Strategy:** Recall that this test is a general indicator of diabetic control over several weeks. With this in mind, eliminate irrelevant options such as infection and foot care. Choose dietary assessment over insulin administration because insulin is based on blood glucose levels.

143. **Answer: 4 Rationale:** Sjögren's syndrome is an autoimmune disease that destroys exocrine glands in the body and leads to a generalized "dryness" of body systems. The restriction of fluids is a concern because fluid intake helps to keep the oral cavity moist. There is no information to suggest that the client has a need for fluid restriction due to other disease processes, so this prescription should be clarified. Placing a client on NPO status after midnight prior to surgery is expected. Initiation of intravenous therapy can be expected. Allowing the client to eat following admission is expected if the client is not immediately going to surgery. **Cognitive Level:** Analyzing **Client Need:** Basic Care and Comfort **Integrated Process:** Nursing Process: Planning **Content Area:** Foundational Sciences: Nutrition **Strategy:** To answer this question correctly, it is necessary to know the underlying pathophysiology of Sjögren's syndrome. From there, analyze each of the options that could exacerbate or worsen the underlying disease state.

144. **Answer: 2 Rationale:** An android pelvic structure is narrow in both the anterior–posterior diameter and the lateral diameter, and can cause a prolonged labor if there is a large fetus or a malpositioned fetus. An occiput posterior position of the fetus is not related to android pelvis. Prolonged labor, rather than precipitous delivery, is of concern. The risk of postpartum complications is not directly related to android pelvis. **Cognitive Level:** Applying **Client Need:** Health Promotion and Maintenance **Integrated Process:** Nursing Process: Diagnosis **Content Area:** Maternal–Newborn **Strategy:** First determine the significance of the critical word *android* in the stem of the question. Eliminate precipitous delivery and complications first because they relate least to risks during labor caused by bone structure. Choose correctly between the remaining options because the prefix *andr-* refers to males and from there determine that it indicates a narrower pelvis.

145. **Answer: 1 Rationale:** Physical exercise, within the client's ability level, reduces muscle tension and pain. Additionally, exercise creates a feeling of greater self-efficacy. Verbal expressions about pain may be more helpful than music therapy, although this would be a distraction. Minimal use of analgesics that achieves acceptable pain level is also indicated, but the client would not use a patient-controlled analgesia. Complete bedrest would not be indicated unless required by incapacitating conditions, but there is no evidence that this is the case in this question. **Cognitive Level:** Applying **Client Need:** Psychosocial Integrity **Integrated Process:** Nursing Process: Implementation **Content Area:** Mental Health **Strategy:** Note that critical words in the question are *chronic pain* and *cope*. This indicates that the correct answer is an activity that will help the client tolerate the pain to a greater extent. Note the word *primary* in the question, which indicates one option is more helpful than the others. With this in mind, choose the option that provides an outlet for the client.

146. **Answer: 4 Rationale:** Confusion and increased heart rate are signs of toxicity or adverse side effects of hydroxyamphetamine. Stinging on instillation, occasional headache, and occasional brow ache are usual side effects of hydroxyamphetamine. **Cognitive Level:** Analyzing **Client Need:** Pharmacological and Parenteral Therapies **Integrated Process:** Nursing Process: Evaluation **Content Area:** Pharmacology **Strategy:** The core issue of the question is knowledge of adverse drug effects. Use specific drug knowledge and the process of elimination to make a selection.

147. **Answer: 3 Rationale:** Shared governance is based on the philosophy that nursing practice is best determined by nurses. Self-scheduling could be part of that model. Delegating to UCPs represents standard nursing practice. Seeking advice is unrelated to shared governance. Procedure manuals updated by nurse managers represents leadership input into decision making for the organization. **Cognitive Level:** Applying **Client Need:** Management of Care **Integrated Process:** Nursing Process: Diagnosis **Content Area:** Leadership and Management **Strategy:** The critical words in the question are *shared governance*. Choose the option that gives the best evidence of some kind of sharing.

148. **Answer: 4 Rationale:** The employee should limit the amount of time in the client's room to minimize exposure; spending up to 45 minutes with each entry is excessive. The employee has applied the correct combination of personal protective equipment. Equipment required for the care of the isolation client should remain in the client's room to limit exposure to other clients on the nursing unit. The employee has followed the correct procedure for exiting the client's room. **Cognitive Level:** Applying **Client Need:** Safety and Infection Control **Integrated Process:** Nursing Process: Evaluation **Content Area:** Leadership and Management **Strategy:** The wording of the question indicates that something was done incorrectly. Use the process of elimination after noting that three options represent correct actions. Only the correct answer identifies an incorrect action.

149. **Answer: 3 Rationale:** Eosinophils are responsible for responding to allergic reactions. Neutrophils are primary responders to infection and tissue injury and inflammation. Monocytes are primary responders to infection and tissue injury and inflammation. Lymphocytes assist in immune responses. **Cognitive Level:** Applying **Client Need:** Reduction of Risk Potential **Integrated Process:** Nursing Process: Assessment **Content Area:** Adult Health: Immunological **Strategy:** The core issue of the question is knowledge of the various components of the WBC differential and their significance. Specific knowledge is needed to answer the question, so take time to review if you have the need.

150. **Answer: 1 Rationale:** All family members are affected by dissociative identity disorder. Children must also find ways to understand and deal with what is occurring to a parent. There is no mistake in the referral. Including the children will be helpful to them, not traumatizing. The ages of the children are not specified but a decision to attend family therapy should not be placed in the children's' hands. **Cognitive Level:** Analyzing **Client Need:** Psychosocial Integrity **Integrated Process:** Communication and Documentation **Content Area:** Mental Health **Strategy:** The core issue of the question is an understanding of the purposes and benefits of family therapy. Use knowledge of family dynamics to choose the correct answer.

151. **Answer: 4 Rationale:** A blood specimen for trough drug level is drawn just prior to administration of the next IV dose; if it is too low, then the dosage and/or frequency of administration need to be increased. A blood specimen for a peak drug level (highest concentration) would be drawn approximately 30 minutes after a dose finished infusing, not immediately prior to a dose. The timing of this blood draw indicates that the test is being done to measure the amount of drug at the lowest therapeutic concentration, not the highest. If toxicity is present, the drug dose may be too high or the drug's half-life may be too long for the prescribed frequency. **Cognitive Level:** Analyzing **Client Need:** Pharmacological and Parenteral Therapies **Integrated Process:** Nursing Process: Diagnosis **Content Area:** Pharmacology **Strategy:** The core issue of the question is the ability to draw correct conclusions about the significance of serum drug-level results. Focus on the words *just prior to* in the stem of the question, which tell you that it is the trough level that is being described. With this in mind, use the process of elimination to find the conclusion that is true of a need to collaborate about the trough level.

152. **Answer: 1 Rationale:** Potatoes, tomatoes, and oranges have a high level of potassium content. The grouping of grains, cheese, and citrus fruits has less potassium content compared to other groupings. The grouping of cereals, processed sugars, and wheat has less potassium content compared to other groupings. The grouping of rice, green leafy vegetables and carbonated beverages has less potassium content compared to other groupings. **Cognitive Level:** Applying **Client Need:** Physiological Adaptation **Integrated Process:** Nursing Process: Implementation **Content Area:** Child Health **Strategy:** The core issue of the question is knowledge of foods that are high in potassium. Eliminate the options with carbonated beverages and sugars first as lower in potassium. Choose the option with potatoes, tomatoes, and oranges because these foods have a greater potassium content.

153. **Answer: 4 Rationale:** A client who receives a diagnosis of SLE will be profoundly affected by the chronic nature of this autoimmune disease process. The establishment of a healthcare team using a multidisciplinary approach will help the client to identify and realize individual goals. Even though the initiation of advance directives is important, it is not the priority concern at this point in time—there is no information provided to suggest that the client requires them immediately. Even though it is important to discuss the progressive effects of the disease, the priority is to establish a multidisciplinary team to assist the client. Telling the client to limit her work pattern may not be financially feasible or physically indicated at this time. **Cognitive Level:** Analyzing **Client Need:** Physiological Adaptation **Integrated Process:** Nursing Process: Planning **Content Area:** Adult Health: Immunological **Strategy:** The core issue of the question is what are initial priorities of care when a client is diagnosed with a chronic illness in which the client's condition is expected to worsen over time. With this in mind, choose the option that calls together the interdisciplinary team so that the client has the fullest range of resources at hand.

154. **Answer: 3, 4, 5 Rationale:** The nurse has a legal obligation to report abuse, including elder abuse. The nurse should remain with the client for support while the client provides information during this report. The nurse should not discuss the situation with the daughter without the client's permission to protect confidentiality. Suggesting the check be handled using direct deposit does not address the underlying issue of physical abuse. It may be appropriate to assess whether the client has any other living options in planning for safety after discharge. **Cognitive Level:** Analyzing **Client Need:** Management of Care **Integrated Process:** Nursing Process: Implementation **Content Area:** Leadership and Management **Strategy:** The wording of the question indicates more than one option is correct. Consider each option as a true or false statement related to care of a client with suspected abuse to aid in choosing correctly.

155. **Answer: 1 Rationale:** One of the major functions of the placenta is provision of nutrients to the fetus across the placenta membrane. An interference with the placenta circulation, such as abruptio placentae, impairs this ability. Another important function is removing metabolic waste from the fetus. While this takes place metabolically the fetus produces and excretes urine independently of the placenta. Hydrops is gross fetal edema related to hemolytic action, not placenta dysfunction. Anomalies usually occur in the first trimester when organogenesis occurs. **Cognitive Level:** Applying **Client Need:** Physiological Adaptation **Integrated Process:** Teaching and Learning **Content Area:** Maternal–Newborn **Strategy:** To answer this question correctly, it is necessary to recall the function of the placenta to deliver oxygen and nutrients to the fetus. Focus on the critical word *partial* to aid in selecting the correct option.

156. **Answer: 3 Rationale:** Clients who are taking cholestyramine, a bile resin, should be monitored for fat-soluble vitamin deficiencies (vitamins A, D, E, and K), as the gastrointestinal side effects of the medication can lead to reduced absorption. Niacin and thiamine are water-soluble B vitamins. Folic acid and vitamin C are examples of water-soluble vitamins. Thiamine and cyanocobalamin are examples of water-soluble B vitamins. **Cognitive Level:** Applying **Client Need:** Pharmacological and Parenteral Therapies **Integrated Process:** Nursing Process: Assessment **Content Area:** Pharmacology **Strategy:** The core issue of the question is knowledge that cholestyramine places the client at risk for deficiency of fat-soluble vitamins. Use the process of elimination and reason that this answer is correct because the action of cholestyramine is to bind onto cholesterol (fat) and prevent its absorption into the GI tract.

157. **Answer: 3** **Rationale:** A hospital case manager is responsible for coordination of care among the client's healthcare providers, ensuring efficient use of services without duplication, providing continuity during transitions across care settings, and acting as a client advocate. Clients who are expected to need services postdischarge (such as older adults) and those with complex health problems or extended recovery times especially benefit from the services of a hospital case manager. A client with a gunshot wound with localized injury is more likely to require care during this episode of injury only, rather than long-term support. A client with a fractured tibia would not be expected to require extensive services across care settings. A client undergoing tonsillectomy has a need for episodic care and follow-up by the surgeon, but does not need a case manager. **Cognitive Level:** Analyzing **Client Need:** Management of Care **Integrated Process:** Nursing Process: Diagnosis **Content Area:** Leadership and Management **Strategy:** Focus on the critical words *case management*. Use the common definition of this method to eliminate each option systematically.

158. **Answer: 2** **Rationale:** Oxygen administered by a Venturi mask can be regulated to deliver precise concentrations between 24 and 50%, which is a benefit for clients who require higher oxygen supplement without mechanical ventilation. The Venturi mask does not prevent rebreathing of carbon dioxide, a nonrebreather mask would do this. Humidity can be provided when administering oxygen via any device. Oxygen concentration of 100% would be administered to clients only in rare circumstances, usually via mechanical ventilation. **Cognitive Level:** Applying **Client Need:** Basic Care and Comfort **Integrated Process:** Nursing Process: Diagnosis **Content Area:** Fundamentals **Strategy:** Specific knowledge is needed to answer the question. Reflect on the various modes of oxygen delivery and note that this type of device can be regulated easily because it is a mask and because the percentage of oxygen can be manipulated easily.

159. **Answer: 1** **Rationale:** MRI is the only diagnostic examination listed that does not possibly require the ingestion or administration of contrast media or radioactive material. A myelogram involves spinal injection of a contrast medium. VQ scanning is done with use of a radioisotope. CT scan with contrast involves the use of contrast dyes or agents. **Cognitive Level:** Applying **Client Need:** Reduction of Risk Potential **Integrated Process:** Communication and Documentation **Content Area:** Adult Health: Immunological **Strategy:** The core issue of the question is knowledge of which tests do and do not require use of some form of contrast media. With this in mind, eliminate each of the incorrect options using basic knowledge of diagnostic tests.

160. **Answer: 4** **Rationale:** Fugue states are characterized by wandering or moving away from one's familiar place with an amnesia for the complete past, including self. The person often assumes a new identity for the duration of the fugue. Amnesia is a more limited state of forgetfulness that does not involve leaving home and beginning a new life. Akathisia is an abnormal condition characterized by restlessness and agitation. Confabulation is replacement of gaps in memory with imaginary information. **Cognitive Level:** Analyzing **Client Need:** Psychosocial Integrity **Integrated Process:** Nursing Process: Diagnosis **Content Area:** Mental Health **Strategy:** The core issue of the question is the ability to correctly interpret a client's behavior as characteristic of a fugue state. Use knowledge of characteristics of this mental health disorder and the process of elimination to make a selection.

161. **Answer: 1** **Rationale:** Lidocaine is given with an initial IV push loading dose to suppress ventricular dysrhythmias and is followed by an infusion of 1–4 mg/min via infusion pump to maintain drug effect. The dose may be repeated one time after 10 minutes under certain conditions, but the total dose should not exceed 3 mg/kg. Oral antidysrhythmic therapy is not indicated at this time. Pacemaker insertion is not indicated at this time. **Cognitive Level:** Applying **Client Need:** Pharmacological and Parenteral Therapies **Integrated Process:** Nursing Process: Planning **Content Area:** Pharmacology **Strategy:** The core issue of the question is knowledge of therapeutic protocols for intravenous antidysrhythmic medications such as Lidocaine. Use drug knowledge and the process of elimination to answer the question.

162. **Answer: 2** **Rationale:** The nurse should delegate the activity that is procedural in nature and is within the scope of training of the UAP, such as measurement of postactivity vital signs. The nurse would not delegate helping a client with therapeutic diet selections because this is not part of the UAP's scope of practice. The nurse would not delegate teaching to a UAP, including the need to alternate activity and rest periods. The nurse does not delegate interventions for assisting the client to manage chest pain. **Cognitive Level:** Analyzing **Client Need:** Management of Care **Integrated Process:** Nursing Process: Implementation **Content Area:** Leadership and Management **Strategy:** Keep in mind the principles of delegation. Recall that the nurse does not delegate assessment, teaching, or medication administration to a UAP.

163. **Answer: 2** **Rationale:** A client who is recovering from Guillain-Barré syndrome will need a diet that promotes positive nitrogen balance in order to counteract the effects of long periods of immobility on the body. There is no evidence to support that the client is experiencing malabsorption at this time. There is no clinical reason to limit fresh fruit, either with or without skins. Even though the client may experience difficulty in chewing and swallowing, this is usually in the acute phase of the disease process. There is nothing specific to suggest that the client is experiencing problems in this area or is at risk for aspiration at this time. **Cognitive Level:** Applying **Client Need:** Basic Care and Comfort **Integrated Process:** Nursing Process: Planning **Content Area:** Foundational Sciences: Nutrition **Strategy:** The critical words in the question are *general rehabilitative care*. This tells you that the client has no specific deficits that would affect nutritional status. With this in mind, choose the option that promotes the best nutrition for this client. Avoid reading into the question.

164. Answer: 4 Rationale: The greatest risks for healthy adults in their 30s relate to unsafe or unhealthy lifestyle behaviors, which may include multiple sexual partners, driving at high speeds, improper diet or erratic dietary patterns, and possibly insufficient sleep. Health screenings are important but the greatest risks for this age group include lifestyle choices. Chest x-rays for lung cancer are not a high-priority consideration for healthy adults in their 30s. Risk of osteoporosis increases after menopause in women. **Cognitive Level:** Applying **Client Need:** Health Promotion and Maintenance **Integrated Process:** Nursing Process: Planning **Content Area:** Fundamentals **Strategy:** Consider the words *healthy* and *30s* in the question and then eliminate incorrect options because they either are not as important for that age group or focus on diseases rather than health promotion.

165. Answer: 1 Rationale: The primary concern for this client with COPD is related to inadequate alveolar ventilation as evidenced by the abnormal blood gas results. The client may be expected to have decreased tolerance of ordinary activity, but this is a secondary concern The client might be at risk for respiratory infection because of underlying respiratory disease, but this can be reduced with influenza and pneumococcal vaccines. The breathing pattern is satisfactory because the rate is within normal limits, and it is not erratic. **Cognitive Level:** Analyzing **Client Need:** Physiological Adaptation **Integrated Process:** Nursing Process: Planning **Content Area:** Adult Health: Respiratory **Strategy:** Compare the data in the question and use that as a means of selecting the priority nursing diagnosis.

166. Answer: 4 Rationale: Graves' disease is caused by elevated levels of thyroid hormone. Clients experience tachycardia, nervousness, insomnia, increased heat production, and weight loss. Medication therapy with an agent such as propylthiouracil will help control the disorder. Atropine is irrelevant because the client would not have bradycardia. Thyroxine is indicated for hypothyroidism, while this client has hyperthyroidism. The pancreas is not affected by Graves' disease. **Cognitive Level:** Analyzing **Client Need:** Pharmacological and Parenteral Therapies **Integrated Process:** Teaching and Learning **Content Area:** Pharmacology **Strategy:** The core issue of the question is that Graves' disease is characterized by excessive function of the thyroid gland. From there, you need to determine which medication will reduce the function of the thyroid. Eliminate drugs not related to thyroid function first as irrelevant, and then choose the drug used for hyperthyroidism rather than hypothyroidism.

167. Answer: 2 Rationale: A client with right-hemisphere stroke has left-sided paralysis or paresis and may have unilateral neglect. Items should not be placed on the left side of the client. Passive range of motion is helpful to maintain joint mobility. The UAP should keep all items on the right side so that the client is aware they exist in the environment. Sitting the client up slowly is appropriate and does not require intervention by the nurse. **Cognitive Level:** Analyzing **Client Need:** Management of Care **Integrated Process:** Nursing Process: Evaluation **Content Area:** Adult Health: Neurological **Strategy:** Recall that the manifestations of stroke appear on the opposite side of the body from the lesion. Use this principle to eliminate the incorrect responses after eliminating actions that are carried out correctly.

168. Answer: 2 Rationale: Transmission-based precautions are required for all these organisms. Only penicillin-resistant *Streptococcus pneumoniae* is transmitted via respiratory droplets. Methicillin-resistant *staphylococcus aureus*, vancomycin-resistant *enterococcus*, and *vancomycin-resistant staphylococcus* are transmitted by direct contact. **Cognitive Level:** Analyzing **Client Need:** Safety and Infection Control **Integrated Process:** Nursing Process: Assessment **Content Area:** Adult Health: Respiratory **Strategy:** Knowledge of droplet precautions is necessary to answer the question. Penicillin-resistant *Streptococcus pneumoniae* suggests a microorganism that causes a type of pneumonia. Clients with pneumonia have increased respiratory secretions and coughing. Using a process of elimination, choose the microorganism that sounds as though it would cause a respiratory infection.

169. Answer: 1 Rationale: HDL is felt to be a beneficial lipoprotein because of its protective function against coronary artery disease. An elevation in this level is healthy and indicates compliance with diet and exercise recommendations. LDL is a fraction of the total cholesterol level that increases the risk of heart disease when the level is elevated. Triglycerides are another major contributor to coronary heart disease. A healthy diet and exercise should lower the client's cholesterol level. **Cognitive Level:** Analyzing **Client Need:** Reduction of Risk Potential **Integrated Process:** Nursing Process: Assessment **Content Area:** Adult Health: Cardiovascular **Strategy:** The core issue of the question is knowledge of which lipid levels should be raised and lowered to achieve cardiovascular health. Recall that HDL has the letter *H* and associate this with the word *healthy* to make the positive association between these.

170. Answer: 3 Rationale: A depressed client who is contemplating suicide may give away prized possessions to others as a token of farewell and possibly to be remembered once suicide has been accomplished. There can be many reasons for a student to refuse to eat a school lunch. Anger is an expected response to being reprimanded, although leaving the classroom might suggest a possible anger management issue. A student could change clothing color preferences for a variety of reasons, including peer pressure, self-exploration, or others, and is not necessarily a signal of impending suicide. **Cognitive Level:** Analyzing **Client Need:** Psychosocial Integrity **Integrated Process:** Nursing Process: Diagnosis **Content Area:** Mental Health **Strategy:** The core issue of the question is the ability to recognize warning signs that a client may attempt suicide. Use this knowledge and the process of elimination to make a selection.

171. **Answer:** 3 **Rationale:** Anticipatory prevention of nausea with antiemetics is effective if medication is taken 30–60 minutes before the event that triggers nausea. Taking medication 24 hours ahead of time is far too long and would allow for the effect to be fully worn off by the time it is needed. Taking a dose 3–5 hours ahead of time could allow the medication to at least partially wear off before the triggering event, such as chemotherapy. Taking the dose 12 hours ahead of time is too early and the drug would not have the intended effect on the client. **Cognitive Level:** Applying **Client Need:** Pharmacological and Parenteral Therapies **Integrated Process:** Nursing Process: Assessment **Content Area:** Pharmacology **Strategy:** The core issue of the question is knowledge of how soon to take medication prior to activities that cause nausea. Recall that many oral drugs act in 30–60 minutes to help you make a selection.

172. **Answer:** 3 **Rationale:** The client who had a hemorrhagic stroke and has a headache could be about to have another bleed. Headache is a classic sign with intracranial bleed, and a second bleed carries a higher mortality rate than the first. A client with psychological distress because of the effects of Parkinson's disease has a psychosocial need that can be addressed once physiological risks are attended to. A client with noticeable leg spasms may need a dose of an antispasmodic drug or a change in drug therapy, but is not an impending medical emergency. The client who will undergo craniotomy in 4 hours requires routine preoperative care, which can be completed once clients with potential complications are assessed. **Cognitive Level:** Analyzing **Client Need:** Management of Care **Integrated Process:** Nursing Process: Implementation **Content Area:** Leadership and Management **Strategy:** When trying to decide priorities among clients who are acutely ill, it may help to analyze the complications each is at risk for or the consequences that could result from the current condition or complaint. The client with the most serious issue or who could experience the most severe complication is the one that takes priority.

173. **Answer:** 1 **Rationale:** Contaminated foods are not a source of HIV/AIDS infection. The nurse should clarify this statement by the client in order to provide accurate information. Blood tests will identify if a client has nutritional anemia, which could occur if the client experiences anorexia, vomiting, or diarrhea as side effects of drug therapy. Adequate fluid and fiber intake represent healthy living habits for any client. Withholding liquids could place the client at risk for dehydration; the client should at least drink sips of fluids frequently and use any prescribed antiemetic. **Cognitive Level:** Applying **Client Need:** Basic Care and Comfort **Integrated Process:** Nursing Process: Assessment **Content Area:** Foundational Sciences: Nutrition **Strategy:** The critical word in the stem of the question is *clarify*. This tells you that the correct answer is an incorrect statement on the part of the client. Use nursing knowledge and the process of elimination to make a selection.

174. **Answer:** 1 **Rationale:** Ambulating a postoperative client is the only task that the RN could delegate that is within the scope of practice for a UAP. Assessment must be performed by the RN and may not be delegated. Reporting a low hemoglobin level must be done by the RN, who can answer any questions from the provider and accept new prescriptions to treat the client. Blood transfusions must be verified by licensed nurses and cannot be delegated to a UAP. **Cognitive Level:** Analyzing **Client Need:** Management of Care **Integrated Process:** Nursing Process: Implementation **Content Area:** Leadership and Management **Strategy:** Use principles of delegation and select the care activity that is the simplest and requires the least amount of high-level judgment, especially since the level of the student is not identified.

175. **Answer:** 2 **Rationale:** Although the halo effect on the dressing suggests the presence of cerebrospinal fluid (CSF), the nurse should first verify this suspicion by testing the drainage for glucose (which would be positive) and assessing for headache. The nurse would be incorrect to conclude the drainage is serous in nature without further assessment. Applying an ice pack does not address the real problem, a probable CSF leak. The nurse should notify the healthcare provider after completing all necessary assessment data. **Cognitive Level:** Analyzing **Client Need:** Physiological Adaptation **Integrated Process:** Nursing Process: Implementation **Content Area:** Adult Health: Neurological **Strategy:** To answer this question correctly, analyze the significance of the findings. Eliminate each of the incorrect responses systematically after noting that a risk after this type of surgery is CSF leak.

176. **Answer:** 3 **Rationale:** Hydroxyzine hydrochloride is an antihistamine that is a competitive inhibitor of the H_1 receptor. It is used to treat various reactions that are mediated by histamine and decreases pruritus associated with release of histamine. Cimetidine is an H_2 histamine antagonist and these agents are not effective against hypersensitivity reactions. Lorazepam is a short-acting benzodiazepine that is indicated for anxiety. Bupivacaine is a local anesthetic for nerve blocks. **Cognitive Level:** Analyzing **Client Need:** Pharmacological and Parenteral Therapies **Integrated Process:** Nursing Process: Planning **Content Area:** Pharmacology **Strategy:** The core issue of the question is knowledge of which drug relieves itching. Use specific drug knowledge and the process of elimination to make a selection.

177. **Answer:** 1, 4 **Rationale:** The UAP can perform routine care activities, such as assisting the client with meals. The UAP is able to assist a client with mobility needs, such as ambulation in the hall. The nurse needs to complete any activity requiring client assessment, such as completing an admission interview form. Assessing how the client's life has been altered by vision loss is part of the nurse's role. The nurse should inquire about community services used, since the client may require referral back to those services upon discharge. **Cognitive Level:** Analyzing **Client Need:** Management of Care **Integrated Process:** Nursing Process: Implementation **Content Area:** Leadership and Management **Strategy:** Recall that UAPs are trained and educated to perform simple care procedures. Use this framework to eliminate each of the incorrect options systematically.

178. **Answer:** 4 **Rationale:** With exophthalmos, the eyelids may not cover and protect the cornea of the eye. Thus,

protecting the eyes from being scratched by the sheets or pillowcase is important while the client is in bed. With Graves' disease, clients usually experience heat intolerance, thus lighter-weight bed linens and a cool room are preferred. Hyperglycemia is not usually associated with Graves' disease. The head of the bed should be elevated 30 degrees to minimize eye pressure. **Cognitive Level:** Analyzing **Client Need:** Management of Care **Integrated Process:** Nursing Process: Implementation **Content Area:** Leadership and Management **Strategy:** The core issue of the question is which need of the client with Graves' disease can be met by the UAP. The need of the client with respect to eye safety can be met using ordinary nursing procedures, so this is the task that may be delegated to the UAP with education.

179. **Answer: 3** **Rationale:** Most chemotherapeutic agents cause some degree of bone marrow suppression, which can result in a decrease in leukocyte, erythrocyte, and platelet counts. The calcium level could increase because of the underlying bone cancer, but this is not related to bone marrow suppression from chemotherapy. An increase in the calcium level could cause a corresponding decrease in the phosphorus level, but this would not be related to chemotherapy and bone marrow suppression. A serum PSA level is a marker of prostate cancer, but would not be affected by bone marrow suppression. **Cognitive Level:** Analyzing **Client Need:** Reduction of Risk Potential **Integrated Process:** Nursing Process: Assessment **Content Area:** Adult Health: Oncology **Strategy:** The critical word in the question is *priority*. With this in mind, you need to determine which lab value has greatest importance in terms of monitoring. The core issue of the question is bone marrow suppression, which could affect production of red blood cells, white blood cells, and platelets. Choose the option that best correlates with this risk.

180. **Answer: 2** **Rationale:** Forgetting what happened during a recent assault is an example of a localized amnesia, which is the inability to recall events in a circumscribed time period. Wandering the neighborhood using a new name can be considered a dissociative response but it is not localized. An awareness of only a few of many alters is not unusual in a client with dissociative identity disorder, but is not a localized amnesia. A feeling of separation from the body is a dissociative response, but is not a localized amnesia. **Cognitive Level:** Analyzing **Client Need:** Psychosocial Integrity **Integrated Process:** Nursing Process: Assessment **Content Area:** Mental Health **Strategy:** Focus on the critical words *expected* and *localized amnesia*. These words indicate that the correct option is one that is consistent with what is assessed in this state. Focus on the word *localized* in the question and the time-bound nature of the correct option to choose correctly.

181. **Answer: 3** **Rationale:** Acknowledging the client's feelings and offering to assist in developing a plan for daily activities addresses the client's concerns but still allows the client to make his own decisions. Focusing on one step at a time so that "everything will work out" disregards and negates the client's feelings. Deferring decisions until tomorrow and to collaboration with the client's spouse disregards and negates the client's feelings. It is not helpful to take away the client's decision-making options by having someone else (the nurse) make a plan for his daily activities, rather than have the client participate in making decisions for himself. **Cognitive Level:** Applying **Client Need:** Psychosocial Integrity **Integrated Process:** Communication and Documentation **Content Area:** Mental Health **Strategy:** The best answer to communication questions is to choose the response that addresses the client's issue or concern. Use the process of elimination and this principle of communication to make a selection.

182. **Answer: 3** **Rationale:** Hyperglycemia is corrected using regular insulin administered by the intravenous route, rather than NPH insulin, which is administered subcutaneously. The nurse should consult with the healthcare provider to question this prescription. The client requires isotonic fluid replacement to correct the severe dehydration that occurs with DKA. Catheter insertion can be done to monitor output to gauge the effectiveness of rehydration. Initiating pulse oximetry is a routine assessment that may be useful as part of the client's overall clinical picture. **Cognitive Level:** Analyzing **Client Need:** Physiological Adaptation **Integrated Process:** Nursing Process: Planning **Content Area:** Adult Health: Endocrine and Metabolic **Strategy:** The critical words in the question are *consult with the healthcare provider*, which suggests that one prescription is inaccurate or requires clarification. Use knowledge of DKA treatment and the process of elimination to make a selection.

183. **Answer: 2, 3, 4** **Rationale:** Orange juice is a liquid that is not clear that can now be offered to the client. Coffee with cream constitute a full liquid that can be offered to the client at this time. Tomato juice is a liquid that is not clear that can be newly offered to the client. Apple juice is a clear liquid that was previously allowed in the diet. Ginger ale is a clear liquid that was allowed while the clear liquid diet was in effect. **Cognitive Level:** Applying **Client Need:** Basic Care and Comfort **Integrated Process:** Nursing Process: Implementation **Content Area:** Foundational Sciences: Nutrition **Strategy:** The wording of the question tells you that the correct answer is a true statement of fact and that more than option is correct. Focus on the critical word *new* to choose only full liquids and not the previously allowed clear liquids.

184. **Answer: 3** **Rationale:** Increased isolation from others following the death of a spouse is not a healthy adaptation, although it can commonly occur, especially if the client is used to engaging in activities as a couple rather than singly. Signs of prostate enlargement (urinary hesitancy and decreased flow of urine stream) are common as part of the aging process. Decreasing tolerance to spicy foods is expected because of decreased acidity and GI motility that are common in the aging process. Circulatory instability can occur when getting up too quickly since autoregulation and vasoconstriction of blood vessels in the legs can be slower as one ages. **Cognitive Level:** Analyzing **Client Need:** Health Promotion and Maintenance **Integrated Process:** Nursing Process: Assessment **Content Area:** Fundamentals **Strategy:** Understanding the expected changes at the various age brackets will allow you to anticipate what is within the normal range of changes and what is not.

185. **Answer: 1** **Rationale:** Clients who are diagnosed with a personality disorder most frequently perceive their personality patterns as ego-syntonic or a natural part of themselves. This is one reason it is difficult to motivate individuals with personality disorders to try to change their maladaptive behavioral patterns. Individuals with personality disorders display problems living rather than clinical symptoms. Clients with a personality disorder tend to perceive their personality patterns as ego-syntonic rather than as ego-dystonic. Personality disorders are associated with concomitant disorders including substance abuse. **Cognitive Level:** Applying **Client Need:** Psychosocial Integrity **Integrated Process:** Nursing Process: Diagnosis **Content Area:** Mental Health **Strategy:** The core issue of the question is the ability to discriminate among various types of mental health disorders using *DSM-IV* criteria. Use this knowledge and the process of elimination to make a selection.

186. **Answer: 2 Rationale:** Grapefruit should be avoided before and after dosing with a calcium channel blocker due to its ability to alter drug effects. Oranges are citrus fruits that do not affect calcium channel blocker therapy. Bananas are high in potassium and are not contraindicated during calcium channel blocker therapy. Grapes do not interfere with the effectiveness of calcium channel blocker drugs. **Cognitive Level:** Applying **Client Need:** Pharmacological and Parenteral Therapies **Integrated Process:** Nursing Process: Implementation **Content Area:** Pharmacology **Strategy:** The core issue of the question is knowledge that grapefruit juice affects the availability of some drugs, such as calcium channel blockers, because of their action on enzyme systems. Use this knowledge and the process of elimination to make a selection.

187. **Answer: 4 Rationale:** Myxedema coma is a severe state of hypothyroidism that is potentially fatal. The nurse should first apply oxygen to increase oxygenation to tissues that may be poorly perfused because of circulatory collapse. The nurse should administer thyroid replacement therapy, which is likely to be prescribed by the intravenous route as soon as an IV line has been inserted. While it is important to rewarm the client, the nurse can use warm blankets initially while a warming device is obtained. Although the urine output is likely diminished in response to the reduction in blood pressure, inserting the urinary catheter to assess urine output can wait until definitive resuscitative measures have been initiated. **Cognitive Level:** Analyzing **Client Need:** Physiological Adaptation **Integrated Process:** Nursing Process: Planning **Content Area:** Adult Health: Endocrine and Metabolic **Strategy:** Consider the pathophysiology of myxedema coma and use the ABCs (airway, breathing, and circulation) to determine the priority of care.

188. **Answer: 1 Rationale:** Equipment for client care is dedicated to the client on contact precautions and is kept in the client's room. The equipment should not be stored in the soiled utility room between uses because it could contain surface microorganisms that could come in contact with personnel. Cleansing the equipment after each use is not practical; it would be more efficient to keep the equipment in the client's room. The equipment does require special action to prevent transmission of infection. **Cognitive Level:** Applying **Client Need:** Safety and Infection Control **Integrated Process:** Nursing Process: Implementation **Content Area:** Fundamentals **Strategy:** The critical word *appropriate* suggests there is only one correct answer. Look for the nursing action that would limit the spread of pathogenic microorganisms.

189. **Answer: 3 Rationale:** Clients with gout usually have an elevated serum uric acid level, which leads to characteristic symptoms when uric acid gets deposited in joints, such as the great toe. The calcium level is not used to diagnose gout. A hematocrit is not useful, although an erythrocyte sedimentation rate or white blood cell count may be elevated. Serum sodium will not be affected in gout. **Cognitive Level:** Applying **Client Need:** Reduction of Risk Potential **Integrated Process:** Nursing Process: Planning **Content Area:** Adult Health: Endocrine and Metabolic **Strategy:** The core issue of the question is knowledge of diagnostic testing for gout. Recall that the word gout contains the letter *u* to associate this with measurement of uric acid, which begins with *u*.

190. **Answer: 4 Rationale:** Clients with dependent personality disorder often try to get others to make decisions for them. It may be difficult for these individuals to make even simple decisions on their own, such as what to wear. They would be disinclined to make critical remarks or suggestions because of their need for the support of others. Complimenting oneself is not a feature of dependent personality disorder. **Cognitive Level:** Analyzing **Client Need:** Psychosocial Integrity **Integrated Process:** Nursing Process: Implementation **Content Area:** Mental Health **Strategy:** The critical word in the stem of the question is *dependent*. Focus on this word and look for an association between that word and the nature of the statement in each option. The option that most closely simulates a response that relies on another is the correct answer to the question.

191. **Answer: 3 Rationale:** Isoproterenol stimulates beta 1 and beta 2 receptors and therefore is contraindicated and should not be used with clients with tachydysrhythmias. Terbutaline, pirbuterol, and metaproterenol are beta 2 stimulants, which should have a selective effect on the lungs, but not the heart, at usual doses. **Cognitive Level:** Analyzing **Client Need:** Pharmacological and Parenteral Therapies **Integrated Process:** Nursing Process: Implementation **Content Area:** Pharmacology **Strategy:** The core issue of the question is knowledge that isoproterenol is contraindicated because it is a cardiac stimulant. Use specific drug knowledge and the process of elimination to make a selection.

192. **Answer: 1, 3 Rationale:** The nurse can delegate ordinary unskilled activities such as clearing the room of unnecessary objects. The nurse can delegate routine aspects of care such as remaining with the client during ambulation. The nurse should interview the client to determine any history of recent falls because the nurse may need to ask follow-up questions based on client responses. The nurse initiates consultation with other health team members, such as physical therapists, or requests such a consultation from the healthcare provider, depending on agency policy. Responsibility for client teaching needs to be retained by the nurse. **Cognitive Level:** Analyzing **Client Need:** Management of Care **Integrated Process:** Nursing Process: Implementation **Content Area:** Leadership and Management **Strategy:** Use the principles of delegation to answer the question.

Eliminate those options that represent assessment, teaching, or interdisciplinary communication or collaboration.

193. Answer: 4 Rationale: Dry mouth can be a common complaint of clients undergoing radiation therapy. Using sugar-free candies or gum will help to stimulate the flow of saliva and ease the discomfort that the client is experiencing without contributing to dental caries or lack of appetite from sugar intake. Eating meals prior to radiation therapy may lead to increased nausea because the client would be lying down after eating the meal. It has no effect on complaints of a dry mouth. Eating larger portions of food will not help to ease complaints of a dry mouth. Furthermore, the client may not be able to increase the size of meals due to side effects experienced as a result of radiation therapy. The use of mouthwash can further cause the mouth to be dry and intensify the client's symptoms. **Cognitive Level:** Applying **Client Need:** Basic Care and Comfort **Integrated Process:** Nursing Process: Implementation **Content Area:** Adult Health: Oncology **Strategy:** The core issue of the question is determining a strategy to relieve dry mouth for a client with cancer that will not contribute to anorexia. Use general principles of nutrition and knowledge of the disease process to make a selection.

194. Answer: 3 Rationale: Although this client is not demonstrating positive signs of bonding at this time, it is important to look at her history before concluding that she is not bonding well with her infant. This client just experienced a long labor and the influence of fatigue on the attachment process should be considered. There is insufficient data at this time to determine the client is not coping with being a new mother. While it is possible that the client may be trying to exert some power in the situation, it is not a plausible explanation given the physiological stress of labor the client has experienced. There is no data at this time to support that the client is anxious about being a new parent. **Cognitive Level:** Analyzing **Client Need:** Health Promotion and Maintenance **Integrated Process:** Nursing Process: Diagnosis **Content Area:** Maternal–Newborn **Strategy:** Compare the nursing diagnoses with the information in the stem of the question. Eliminate each incorrect option based on lack of supporting data in the question.

195. Answer: 1 Rationale: Carbon dioxide is eliminated from the body as exhaled gas. The faster the rate of breathing, the greater the quantity of carbon dioxide eliminated during exhalation. Hypoventilation is the opposite of hyperventilation, and could lead to increased CO_2 levels. Prolonged expiration could be a result of emphysema, which occurs because of air trapping that would lead to retained CO_2. Stridor indicates narrowing of respiratory passages and diminishes the intake of sufficient oxygen. **Cognitive Level:** Applying **Client Need:** Physiological Adaptation **Integrated Process:** Nursing Process: Assessment **Content Area:** Adult Health: Respiratory **Strategy:** Note the stem of the question contains the words *diminished* $PaCO_2$, which indicates that the client is blowing off excessive CO_2. Use knowledge of respiratory disorders to select the option that is consistent with excessive respiration.

196. Answer: 3 Rationale: Ophthalmic epinephrine is used to produce mydriasis for ocular examination. Dilation of pupil further constricts ocular fluid outflow, possibly causing an acute attack of glaucoma in a client with angle-closure glaucoma. Systemic absorption of epinephrine would cause hypertension, so hypotension would not be a contraindication to drug administration. Open-angle glaucoma would not be as greatly affected by epinephrine as angle-closure glaucoma. Brow ache is a typical side effect of adrenergic agonists such as epinephrine. **Cognitive Level:** Applying **Client Need:** Pharmacological and Parenteral Therapies **Integrated Process:** Nursing Process: Assessment **Content Area:** Pharmacology **Strategy:** The core issue of the question is knowledge that angle-closure glaucoma is a contraindication to use of epinephrine for mydriasis during an ocular examination. Use specific drug knowledge and the process of elimination to make a selection.

197. Answer: 4 Rationale: The client that is the most stable and with the fewest needs requiring the nurse's direct care is the 6-day postoperative client awaiting placement in a rehabilitation facility. The nurse can attend to this client's discharge paperwork later in the shift. The nurse needs to assess the pain and neurovascular status of the client with the new cast, since the client could be at risk for compartment syndrome if the cast is too tight. The nurse needs to assess the client with the new spinal fracture because of potential for neurological instability. The nurse would need to teach and counsel the client who has phantom limb sensation. **Cognitive Level:** Analyzing **Client Need:** Management of Care **Integrated Process:** Nursing Process: Implementation **Content Area:** Leadership and Management **Strategy:** Recall the principles of delegation and that clients who need assessment or teaching need to remain under the direct responsibility of the nurse.

198. Answer: 1, 3, 5 Rationale: A history of diabetes and smoking are known modifiable risk factors to cardiac disease. Chest pain that occurs during activity may indicate cardiac ischemia due to the increased tissue oxygen demand. Associated symptoms of nausea and diaphoresis are known warning signs of cardiac ischemia. Travel out of the country is an unrelated factor. Chest pain that increases with breathing, especially taking a deep breath, is most likely of pleuritic or pericardial origin. **Cognitive Level:** Applying **Client Need:** Physiological Adaptation **Integrated Process:** Nursing Process: Assessment **Content Area:** Adult Health: Cardiovascular **Strategy:** The core issue of the question is knowledge of risk factors of cardiac disease leading to chest pain. Eliminate the option with travel as unrelated, recalling that chest pain from cardiac origin is not related to travel. Eliminate the option with the deep breath next because cardiac pain does not correlate with the respiratory cycle.

199. Answer: 1 Rationale: The definition of moderate sedation is that there is a minimal depression of the level of consciousness in which the client is able to maintain a patent airway and respond appropriately to verbal and physical stimuli. The pain threshold is increased so that the client can better tolerate any pain. The client will have a patent airway, but amnesia is induced partially with moderate sedation. The client should be awake during moderate sedation. **Cognitive Level:** Applying

Client Need: Reduction of Risk Potential **Integrated Process:** Communication and Documentation **Content Area:** Fundamentals **Strategy:** The core issue of the question is knowledge of moderate sedation and communication techniques that explain this clearly and accurately. Use knowledge of key features of moderate sedation and the process of elimination to make a selection.

200. **Answer: 3** **Rationale:** Jealousy and secretiveness are part of the clinical manifestations of paranoid personality disorder. They must be considered in planning and implementing care. Delusions and hallucinations are consistent with schizophrenia or other psychotic disorders. Passivity and compliance are behavior traits that are not consistent with paranoid personality disorder. Respect for and deference to authority figures are behaviors that would not be consistent with paranoid personality disorder. **Cognitive Level:** Applying **Client Need:** Psychosocial Integrity **Integrated Process:** Nursing Process: Assessment **Content Area:** Mental Health **Strategy:** The core issue of the question is knowledge of characteristics of paranoid personality disorder. Use nursing knowledge and the process of elimination to make a selection. Note the word *paranoid* in the stem and *secretiveness* in the correct option to help make an association between the two.

201. **Answer: 2** **Rationale:** The question indicates that extravasation may be occurring. The drug administration should be stopped, since failure to do so will further disperse drug into the tissue and worsen tissue damage. Continuing the infusion after trying to aspirate for a blood return could cause the client harm since there is already evidence of swelling at the site. Flushing the line with saline is not advised, since vesicant drug remaining in the tubing could be pushed into the surrounding tissue. Obtaining a new site should be done once the suspicious area has been assessed and treated to ensure the tissue is not damaged. **Cognitive Level:** Applying **Client Need:** Pharmacological and Parenteral Therapies **Integrated Process:** Nursing Process: Implementation **Content Area:** Pharmacology **Strategy:** The core issue of the question is knowledge that nitrogen mustard is an antineoplastic agent and that these drugs may be vesicants. From there, you need to determine what action will reduce the risk of further damage, which is stopping the drug and trying to aspirate it out of tissue.

202. **Answer: 3** **Rationale:** The nurse should delegate the care of the 81-year-old client with heart failure and emphysema. This client was admitted 3 days ago and has a stable medical status. The nurse would want to assess the client recently admitted with exacerbation of COPD. The nurse would want to monitor the neurologic status of the 25-year-old who sustained a concussion less than 24 hours ago. The newly diagnosed diabetic client would require teaching that should not be delegated to the LPN/LVN. **Cognitive Level:** Analyzing **Client Need:** Management of Care **Integrated Process:** Nursing Process: Implementation **Content Area:** Leadership and Management **Strategy:** Recall the principles of delegation. The nurse should not delegate the care of clients who require assessment due to changes in acuity or status and clients who require teaching. Stable clients may be delegated to the LPN/LVN under the RN's supervision.

203. **Answer: 4** **Rationale:** Nutritional goals for a client with hepatitis are aimed at providing a diet that is high in calories (3000–4000 kcal) and high in quality protein (1.5–2.0 grams/kg). The diet should also be adequate in carbohydrates to spare protein and fat, provide concentrated calories, and improve the taste of food. The nutritional management of hepatitis is the same for all types. There is no clinical indication to place the client on tube feedings given the information that is provided. If the gut works, then the usual clinical model is to use it. Dietary fat should not be limited unless the client is experiencing problems with malabsorption (steatorrhea) and there is no evidence to support this. **Cognitive Level:** Applying **Client Need:** Basic Care and Comfort **Integrated Process:** Nursing Process: Planning **Content Area:** Foundational Sciences: Nutrition **Strategy:** The critical word in the stem of the question is *hepatitis*. From this point, analyze that the client recovering from hepatitis needs a high-calorie, high-protein diet for healing to make the correct selection.

204. **Answer: 3** **Rationale:** Having the mother give a return demonstration of newborn care after seeing it demonstrated allows the nurse to evaluate the client's understanding and provide opportunity to reinforce teaching as needed. Showing a video and answering questions is useful but does not allow the nurse to see the client perform care. Information about support groups may be useful but does not address newborn care. Printed instruction and a contact number for use after discharge is useful as a reference once the client has returned home, but does not allow the nurse to see what aspects of newborn care the new mother can perform. **Cognitive Level:** Applying **Client Need:** Health Promotion and Maintenance **Integrated Process:** Teaching and Learning **Content Area:** Maternal–Newborn **Strategy:** Recall principles of teaching and learning, and recall that active participation leads to most effective learning outcomes.

205. **Answer: 4** **Rationale:** In a child with atopic dermatitis, use of a mild soap such as Dove® or Tone® prevents the skin from becoming excessively dry. Very warm water is drying to the skin so should be avoided. Many lotions contain perfumes that are irritating to the skin and there is no need to apply liberally over the entire body. Many fabric softeners contain perfumes that are irritating to the skin and should be avoided. **Cognitive Level:** Applying **Client Need:** Physiological Adaptation **Integrated Process:** Teaching and Learning **Content Area:** Child Health **Strategy:** To answer this question correctly, it is necessary to be familiar with the skin disorder in the picture. Beyond that, eliminate the incorrect options because of the words *hot* and *daily*, *liberally* and *entire*, and *all*.

206. **Answer: 3** **Rationale:** Aspirin can potentiate the effect of warfarin and increase the risk of bleeding. The use of this analgesic, although previously prescribed, is not in the best interest of the client at this time. While a further assessment of pain and referral may be necessary, it is not the priority action that the nurse should take at this time. Telling the client to keep taking the analgesic would potentiate drug interactions and increase the risk of bleeding with combined aspirin and warfarin use. A need to increase the dose of warfarin is incorrect because the two drugs together could enhance bleeding.

Cognitive Level: Applying **Client Need:** Pharmacological and Parenteral Therapies **Integrated Process:** Nursing Process: Implementation **Content Area:** Pharmacology **Strategy:** The core issue of the question is knowledge that drugs containing aspirin can have an interactive effect with warfarin, which increases the risk of bleeding. With this in mind, use the process of elimination to select the option that results in stopping pain therapy with an aspirin-containing drug.

207. Answer: 3 Rationale: Although all signs identified are manifestations of developmental dysplasia of the hip, the only sign that would be present in a 5-year-old would be telescoping of the femoral head into the pelvis. (Other clinical signs in an older child would be lordosis and a waddling gait with a marked limp.) Asymmetry of thigh and gluteal folds can be detected in an infant older than 3 months of age. A positive Ortolani-Barlow maneuver is found in an infant younger than 2–3 months of age. Limited abduction is a sign most often noted in an infant older than 3 months. **Cognitive Level:** Applying **Client Need:** Physiological Adaptation **Integrated Process:** Nursing Process: Assessment **Content Area:** Child Health **Strategy:** Specific knowledge about this disorder is needed to answer the question. Take time to review this disorder if you had difficulty with this question.

208. Answer: 3, 5 Rationale: Postoperative pain medication should not be administered immediately when due; instead, it should be administered on an as-needed basis according to the client's level of pain. The cast should not be covered with blankets because this will interfere with the cast drying and could enhance swelling if excessive heat is retained under the blankets. Keeping the ankle and foot elevated on a pillow will help to reduce edema formation around the cast. The nurse should observe for swelling around cast edges, which could interfere with circulation if excessive. The nurse should assess the neurovascular status of the affected foot as prescribed to ensure adequate circulation to the distal tissue. **Cognitive Level:** Analyzing **Client Need:** Management of Care **Integrated Process:** Nursing Process: Evaluation **Content Area:** Leadership and Management **Strategy:** The core issue of the question is knowledge that a client who underwent repair of clubfoot will have a cast in place. After determining this, evaluate each of the options in terms of its appropriateness as part of management of the client in a cast.

209. Answer: 1, 2, 4, 5 Rationale: It is important for the client to understand deep-breathing and coughing exercises to prevent atelectasis and pneumonia because the client will be immobilized on bedrest after surgery. The use of postoperative medications to manage pain is an important part of preoperative teaching. The client should know that a urinary catheter will be placed to drain urine postoperatively. The client should learn to use an incentive spirometer to aid full lung expansion and prevent development of atelectasis and pneumonia. The healthcare provider, not the nurse, should explain the actual surgical procedure. **Cognitive Level:** Applying **Client Need:** Reduction of Risk Potential **Integrated Process:** Nursing Process: Planning **Content Area:** Child Health **Strategy:** The core issue of the question is knowledge of which information is within the domain of nursing practice and which information needs to be given by the healthcare provider to obtain informed consent. Choose the options that are within the nurse's scope of practice.

210. Answer: 2, 3, 5 Rationale: The nurse should monitor the vital signs of a client with alcohol withdrawal for changes, especially blood pressure, which could elevate rapidly. The nurse should reorient the client as needed during periods of confusion. Responding to hallucinations in a factual yet caring manner provides reality orientation and conveys empathy to the client. There is no need to restrict the client to a clear liquid diet; the client would benefit from nutritional support. A stimulating environment could be nontherapeutic for a client who is likely to be disoriented and may have hallucinations during withdrawal. **Cognitive Level:** Analyzing **Client Need:** Psychosocial Integrity **Integrated Process:** Nursing Process: Planning **Content Area:** Mental Health **Strategy:** The core issue of the question is knowledge of the therapeutic measures for a client experiencing acute alcohol withdrawal. Consider the needs of the client to make appropriate selections.

211. Answer: 3 Rationale: The standard protocol is to administer up to three doses of NTG 5 minutes apart as long as the vital signs remain stable. The healthcare provider should be notified if pain is unrelieved after three doses, but not after the first dose. An electrocardiogram (ECG) may be prescribed, but not an EEG (to measure brain waves). Using NTG paste, a longer-acting form of the medication, is not appropriate at this time. **Cognitive Level:** Applying **Client Need:** Pharmacological and Parenteral Therapies **Integrated Process:** Nursing Process: Implementation **Content Area:** Pharmacology **Strategy:** The core issue of the question is knowledge that nitroglycerine can be repeated to a total of three doses while pain continues and the blood pressure is stable. Use the process of elimination and knowledge of safe drug administration to answer the question.

212. Answer: 2 Rationale: The nurse should delegate the care of the 78-year-old client with diabetes and osteoarthritis. This client has a stable medical status. The nurse would want to assess the client recently admitted following nephrectomy. The nurse would want to assess the 32-year-old who fractured the pelvis. Since pelvic exenteration is done to treat cancer, the nurse would want to assess this client and also address this client's psychosocial needs in coping with the diagnosis and surgery. **Cognitive Level:** Analyzing **Client Need:** Management of Care **Integrated Process:** Nursing Process: Implementation **Content Area:** Leadership and Management **Strategy:** Recall the principles of delegation. The nurse should not delegate the care of clients who require assessment due to changes in acuity or status, as well as clients who require teaching. Stable clients may be delegated to the LPN/LVN under the RN's supervision.

213. Answer: 3 Rationale: Floating nursing staff to areas of greater need is legally acceptable and is commonly used to solve unit-specific staffing issues for one or more shifts. Legally, a nurse must float as assigned unless exempted by union contract or unless the nurse can demonstrate lack of knowledge of how to perform required nursing care activities. The nurse should first identify which activities in the ED would be safe for the nurse to perform. The nurse might refuse to float if unable to provide safe care to clients because of an insufficient skill set for the ED setting, but this would not be the initial action. The nurse may choose to call the nursing supervisor if requested to perform activities beyond the nurse's skill set or those for which the nurse has not been oriented. Telephoning the risk management department would be premature and not part of the usual chain of communication. **Cognitive Level:** Applying **Client Need:** Management of Care **Integrated Process:** Nursing Process: Implementation **Content Area:** Leadership and Management **Strategy:** The core issue of the question is the ability to implement knowledge of concepts related to floating and safe staffing. Use this information and the process of elimination to choose correctly.

214. **Answer: 3 Rationale:** *Pediculosis capitis* is head lice. The nits (eggs) are usually found at the base of hair shafts, most frequently at the nape of the neck or behind the ears. Nits are not as frequently found along the forehead or above the ears. Head lice do not move away from the scalp to lay eggs, so nits are not found in the webs between fingers and toes. Head lice do not lay eggs in the folds of elbows or behind the knees.**Cognitive Level:** Applying **Client Need:** Physiological Adaptation **Integrated Process:** Communication and Documentation **Content Area:** Child Health **Strategy:** Note that the word *capitis* refers to the head to eliminate two options. Discriminate between the other two options by selecting the one where nits would be harder to detect and remove.

215. **Answer: 2 Rationale:** Normal stair climbing is allowed, along with lying down, standing, sitting, walking, and gentle swimming. Activity restrictions should be followed for 6–8 months following a spinal fusion. It is not necessary to limit walking to one-half mile per day; walking is a beneficial form of exercise following spinal fusion. Household chores such as vacuuming or mowing the lawn are not allowed because of the stress on the spine. **Cognitive Level:** Applying **Client Need:** Physiological Adaptation **Integrated Process:** Teaching and Learning **Content Area:** Child Health **Strategy:** To answer this question correctly, it is important to understand the disorder and the limitations in the postoperative period. Consider the needs of the healing spine and use principles of body mechanics to aid in selection.

216. **Answer: 2 Rationale:** Vitamin D helps to regulate the serum calcium level in the blood. Vitamin D increases intestinal absorption of calcium and mobilization from bone. Vitamin D reduces renal excretion of both calcium and phosphorus. Vitamin D does not decrease blood levels of calcium and phosphorus. **Cognitive Level:** Applying **Client Need:** Pharmacological and Parenteral Therapies **Integrated Process:** Teaching and Learning **Content Area:** Pharmacology **Strategy:** The core issue of the question is the purpose and intended effect of vitamin D. Use basic knowledge of nutrition and vitamin therapy and the process of elimination to make a selection.

217. **Answer: 4 Rationale:** The nurse should delegate the care of the 53-year-old client with hypertension and chronic renal insufficiency. This client has a stable medical status. The nurse would want to assess the client recently admitted following adrenalectomy. The nurse would want to provide teaching to the client being discharged to home following arthroscopy and pain management, limitations in activity, and follow-up care. The nurse would want to assess the 24-year-old who has hemophilia and fractured a leg the previous day. **Cognitive Level:** Analyzing **Client Need:** Management of Care **Integrated Process:** Nursing Process: Implementation **Content Area:** Leadership and Management **Strategy:** Recall the principles of delegation. The nurse should not delegate the care of clients who require assessment due to changes in acuity or status, and clients who require teaching. Stable clients may be delegated to the LPN/LVN under the RN's supervision.

218. **Answer: 1 Rationale:** A client with *Pneumocystis jiroveci* pneumonia is not contagious, so the use of standard precautions is sufficient. This type of pneumonia is not transmitted by the airborne route. *Pneumocystis jiroveci* pneumonia is not transmitted by droplets. There is no need for contact precautions. **Cognitive Level:** Applying **Client Need:** Safety and Infection Control **Integrated Process:** Nursing Process: Implementation **Content Area:** Fundamentals **Strategy:** Use the process of elimination based on nursing knowledge of standard precautions, AIDS, and *Pneumocystis jiroveci* pneumonia.

219. **Answer: 2 Rationale:** Wound infection is decreased by skin preparation when debris and transient microbes from the skin are removed. Skin preparation will not prevent complications such as dehiscence and evisceration. Skin preparation will not prevent complications such as pressure ulcers from reduced tissue perfusion. Dermatitis does not result if surgical skin preparation is omitted. **Cognitive Level:** Applying **Client Need:** Reduction of Risk Potential **Integrated Process:** Communication and Documentation **Content Area:** Fundamentals **Strategy:** The core issues of the question are recognition of the family question as relating to surgical skin preparation and knowledge of the purposes and expected results of that prep. Use nursing knowledge and the process of elimination to make a selection.

220. **Answer: 2 Rationale:** A severe flood constitutes a community crisis. To determine the client's perception about what precipitated the mental health crisis, the nurse should inquire about what has led the client to seek help at this time. Asking about family or friends in the area will provide useful background information about social support. Asking about where the client has been living also gathers data about social or community support systems. Asking about what the client has done to cope since the flood identifies positive coping strategies that have been useful to the client until this time. **Cognitive Level:** Analyzing **Client Need:** Psychosocial Integrity **Integrated Process:** Communication and Documentation **Content Area:** Mental Health **Strategy:** The core issue of the question is the use of therapeutic communication when assessing a client in crisis. Focus on the critical words *identify the client's personal perception* to choose the option that is less factual in nature.

221. **Answer: 1 Rationale:** The nurse should assess for signs and symptoms of hypersensitivity reaction following the administration of all vaccines. Wheezing is a sign of hypersensitivity reaction and warrants immediate further assessment and emergency action to prevent possible death. Local discomfort may be expected and is treated if necessary with acetaminophen. Anxiety is not an adverse drug effect, although it may be present before the injection. Vomiting is not associated with administration. **Cognitive Level:** Applying **Client Need:** Pharmacological and Parenteral Therapies **Integrated Process:** Nursing Process: Assessment **Content Area:** Pharmacology **Strategy:** The core issue of the question is knowledge that the MMR vaccine may cause allergic reaction in clients who have hypersensitivity to egg yolks. Use specific drug knowledge and the process of elimination to make a selection.

222. **Answer: 3 Rationale:** The nurse should delegate the care of the 59-year-old client with hypertension and Paget's disease. This client has a stable medical status. The nurse should collaborate and communicate with the pulmonary rehabilitation specialist to formulate the ongoing plan of care. The nurse should assess and care for the client in sickle-cell crisis because of the acuity of the client's condition. The nurse should assess the client awaiting surgery and complete preoperative care and the preoperative checklist. **Cognitive Level:** Analyzing **Client Need:** Management of Care **Integrated Process:** Nursing Process: Implementation **Content Area:** Leadership and Management **Strategy:** Recall the principles of delegation. The nurse should not delegate the care of clients who require assessment due to changes in acuity or status, as well as clients who require teaching. Stable clients may be delegated to the LPN/LVN under the RN's supervision.

223. **Answer: 2 Rationale:** Benign prostatic hyperplasia (BPH) is the most common disorder of the aging male client; signs include urinary hesitancy, diminished urine stream, and incomplete bladder emptying as examples. Testicular cancer is the most common cancer in men between the ages of 15 and 35, but this client is 75 years of age. Testicular torsion occurs at any age but is not of concern when assessing this client. Gonorrhea is highest in occurrence during the sexually active years, and there is no particular reason to inquire about this specific sexually transmitted infection. **Cognitive Level:** Applying **Client Need:** Physiological Adaptation **Integrated Process:** Nursing Process: Assessment **Content Area:** Adult Health: Renal and Genitourinary **Strategy:** The critical words in the stem of the question are *older men*. Recall that the prostate gland undergoes changes in later life to help select the correct option.

224. **Answer: 4 Rationale:** At birth, the infant's skin is thin with little subcutaneous fat. In addition, the infant has a greater proportion of body surface area relative to the amount of water present in the skin. Lanugo is shed within a few weeks of birth and has no relationship to heat loss. Sebaceous glands are immature in the infant but are not related to heat loss or temperature regulation. Apocrine glands are immature in the infant but are not related to heat loss or temperature regulation. **Cognitive Level:** Applying **Client Need:** Health Promotion and Maintenance **Integrated Process:** Teaching and Learning **Content Area:** Maternal–Newborn **Strategy:** Specific information on the functions of the skin is needed to answer the question. Look at the critical word *newborn* and think about the characteristics of newborn skin to help make a selection.

225. **Answer: 3 Rationale:** PMS occurs only during the luteal phase of the menstrual cycle (7–10 days before menstrual flow begins). Because PMS is related to hormones, it cannot occur all month long. Increasing sexual activity does not prevent PMS. Caffeine does not prevent or reduce the symptoms of PMS. **Cognitive Level:** Analyzing **Client Need:** Physiological Adaptation **Integrated Process:** Nursing Process: Evaluation **Content Area:** Adult Health: Reproductive **Strategy:** The critical word in the question is *understands*. This tells you that the correct option is one that contains a true statement. Use knowledge of PMS to successfully eliminate incorrect options.

226. **Answer: 4 Rationale:** Tonic-clonic seizures are characterized by generalized muscle rigidity followed by generalized muscle contractions. Periods of inattention and daydreaming characterize an absence seizure. Sudden loss of muscle tone and falling characterize an atonic seizure. Repetitive small-muscle-group activity characterizes a partial seizure. **Cognitive Level:** Analyzing **Client Need:** Physiological Adaptation **Integrated Process:** Nursing Process: Assessment **Content Area:** Child Health **Strategy:** The core issue is knowledge of the characteristics of tonic-clonic seizure disorder. Use the process of elimination and specific nursing knowledge to answer the question.

227. **Answer: 1 Rationale:** When a client is on contact precautions, items that the client uses must be either kept in the room, disposed of, or subjected to terminal cleaning upon the client's discharge. The nurse should ensure that disposable meal trays are delivered. It is an inappropriate infection control measure to place a used meal tray in the soiled utility room. The client does not have dishes washed in the room between meals. The tray items are not disinfected after each meal. **Cognitive Level:** Applying **Client Need:** Safety and Infection Control **Integrated Process:** Nursing Process: Implementation **Content Area:** Fundamentals **Strategy:** The wording of the question indicates there is only one correct answer. Evaluate each option in terms of infection control and practicality, and then use the process of elimination to make a selection.

228. **Answer: 4 Rationale:** Pulses are assessed frequently to ensure adequate circulation is present and an occlusion or leakage of the graft has not occurred. Pulses should be marked preoperatively so the nurse has a comparison point postoperatively. Anticoagulant therapy is not indicated. Elevating the legs could reduce blood flow to the affected lower extremities. Sequential compression devices are a *routine* aspect of care to help to prevent deep vein thrombosis, but may not be of highest priority for this client. **Cognitive Level:** Applying **Client Need:** Physiological Adaptation **Integrated Process:** Nursing Process: Implementation **Content Area:** Adult Health: Cardiovascular **Strategy:** Note the critical words *first postoperative day*. This tells you that the client condition could change and that diligent assessment and ongoing monitoring is required. Use knowledge of the surgical procedure and routine postoperative care to make a selection.

229. **Answer: 1 Rationale:** Abrasions, pustules, or other skin conditions have to be assessed and documented because these may interfere with wound healing. Lack of hair growth will not interfere with surgical skin preparation.

Presence of lanugo or fine hair will not interfere with the skin preparation. Pulsation is not always visible or available to assess depending on the part of the body being operated on. **Cognitive Level:** Analyzing **Client Need:** Reduction of Risk Potential **Integrated Process:** Nursing Process: Assessment **Content Area:** Fundamentals **Strategy:** The core issue of the question is knowledge that broken areas of skin are at risk for infection and need to be reported to the surgeon. Knowing that this is an important item helps to prioritize this as the item to assess.

230. **Answer: 4** **Rationale:** Providing the client with the choice of how he would like to take the medication, while being firm that he must take it, is the best option. Having a choice gives the client a sense of control and helps to reduce the power struggle. Simply telling the client that the medication is not poison would do little to persuade him to adhere. Stating to take the medication or get an injection provides no choice and implies punishment; at worst the statement could be construed as assault. Because the client needs the medication, it would be inappropriate to say the client does not need to take it. **Cognitive Level:** Analyzing **Client Need:** Psychosocial Integrity **Integrated Process:** Communication and Documentation **Content Area:** Mental Health **Strategy:** The core issue of the question is knowledge of therapeutic communication techniques when working with a client who has schizophrenia. Use nursing knowledge of this disorder and the process of elimination to make a selection.

231. **Answer: 3** **Rationale:** Dry mouth occurs from the anticholinergic effects seen with fluphenazine, and the client should take measures to reduce this as much as possible. Orthostatic hypotension is not a major side effect of fluphenazine so it is unnecessary to tell the client to rise slowly. Dizziness or lightheadedness is not a major side effect of fluphenazine. Confusion is not a side effect of this agent. **Cognitive Level:** Applying **Client Need:** Pharmacological and Parenteral Therapies **Integrated Process:** Nursing Process: Planning **Content Area:** Pharmacology **Strategy:** The core issue of the question is knowledge of drug adverse effects and how to prevent them. Recall that anticholinergic effects are of concern with this medication and use the process of elimination to make a selection.

232. **Answer: 4** **Rationale:** The nurse should delegate the care of the 79-year-old who has chronic bronchitis and early Alzheimer's disease. This client has a stable medical status. The nurse should assess the client undergoing cardiac catheterization and complete the preparation activities for the procedure. The nurse should assess the client with low back pain, especially with a comorbid diagnosis of osteoarthritis. The nurse should assess and monitor the client who had chest pain the previous evening because of the nature of the problem. **Cognitive Level:** Analyzing **Client Need:** Management of Care **Integrated Process:** Nursing Process: Implementation **Content Area:** Leadership and Management **Strategy:** Recall the principles of delegation. The nurse should not delegate the care of clients who require assessment due to changes in acuity or status, as well as clients who require teaching. Stable clients may be delegated to the LPN/LVN under the RN's supervision.

233. **Answer: 1, 5** **Rationale:** Pulses are assessed to ensure adequate circulation with the rigid compression of the Unna boot. Elevating the legs helps promote venous return and is a generally helpful circulatory measure. Dependent position is not necessary to provide comfort. The Unna boot is a rigid dressing that is changed every 1–2 weeks. Excessive standing uses gravity to impede blood return and is not effective. **Cognitive Level:** Applying **Client Need:** Physiological Adaptation **Integrated Process:** Nursing Process: Implementation **Content Area:** Adult Health: Cardiovascular **Strategy:** The core issue of the question is knowledge of the type of condition that requires the use of an Unna boot and then determining an intervention that meets the same need. To answer correctly, you need to determine that the underlying problem is venous in nature and that leg elevation aids in relieving symptoms of venous disease.

234. **Answer: 4** **Rationale:** Anxiety reduction is needed when the client is waiting for the outcome of tests to assist them in processing their feelings and exploring their options based on test results. A body scan does not cause pain. Bleeding is not a risk of the procedure. The dose of radiation is not high enough to cause nausea or vomiting as effects on gastrointestinal tissue. **Cognitive Level:** Applying **Client Need:** Reduction of Risk Potential **Integrated Process:** Nursing Process: Implementation **Content Area:** Adult Health: Oncology **Strategy:** The critical words in the question are *after full body scan*. This tells you the correct option is a key consideration once the procedure is completed. Use knowledge of the procedure to eliminate incorrect options that address physiological needs, and choose the one that focuses on psychosocial needs because of the nature of the diagnostic test.

235. **Answer: 2** **Rationale:** Clients with COPD are hypermetabolic; they require additional calories due to increased energy requirements as a result of increased work of breathing. Even a healthy diet cannot prevent respiratory infection because of the altered immune response in COPD (decreased cell-mediated immunity, altered immunoglobulin production, and impaired cellular resistance). Weight gain from fluid retention is not associated with COPD. The client has increased energy requirements, which can lead to weight loss if nutrient requirements are not met. **Cognitive Level:** Applying **Client Need:** Basic Care and Comfort **Integrated Process:** Teaching and Learning **Content Area:** Foundational Sciences: Nutrition **Strategy:** The wording of the question tells you the correct answer is a true statement of fact. Use general knowledge of nutritional concepts and COPD to eliminate each of the incorrect options.

236. **Answer: 130** **Rationale:** In hypertensive emergency/crisis, the client's diastolic BP is greater than 130 mmHg. In hypertensive urgencies, clients present with a systolic BP greater than 240 mmHg and diastolic BP greater than 120 mmHg. **Cognitive Level:** Applying **Client Need:** Physiological Adaptation **Integrated Process:** Teaching and Learning **Content Area:** Adult Health: Cardiovascular **Strategy:** The core issue of the question is knowledge of the parameters of hypertensive crisis. Use specific knowledge to identify an answer.

237. **Answer: 1** **Rationale:** Atherosclerosis indicates the need to adopt a low-fat diet. Both butter and margarine have

4 grams of fat per serving, making the client's statement incorrect and in need of further clarification. Steaming, baking, and broiling foods are preferred food preparation methods because they do not add fat or calories. American cheese is high in fat. It is important to increase intake of fruits and vegetables, which tend to be lower in fat. **Cognitive Level:** Analyzing **Client Need:** Health Promotion and Maintenance **Integrated Process:** Nursing Process: Evaluation **Content Area:** Adult Health: Cardiovascular **Strategy:** The critical words in the question are *further discussion*. With this in mind, evaluate each of the options in terms of how it relates to a low-fat diet.

238. **Answer: 3 Rationale:** Medical asepsis requires the use of clean, not sterile, technique and this would be appropriate when collecting a stool specimen for ova and parasites. Collecting a wound culture, suctioning a tracheostomy, and catheterizing the client require use of sterile asepsis. **Cognitive Level:** Applying **Client Need:** Safety and Infection Control **Integrated Process:** Nursing Process: Planning **Content Area:** Fundamentals **Strategy:** Knowledge of medical versus surgical asepsis is essential. Look for similarities in the choices. Three options require sterile or surgical aseptic technique, while only one choice requires medical aseptic technique.

239. **Answer: 3 Rationale:** Increased heart rate and/or respiratory rate within minutes to several hours following central venous line insertion are symptoms of a pneumothorax caused by puncture of the pleura. Discomfort at the central line insertion site may require intervention, but the etiology is not the immediate priority. Development of a low-grade fever will require further assessment and possible intervention, but the etiology is not the immediate priority. Diminished breath sounds in lung bases indicate atelectasis and will require intervention, but this is not the immediate priority with the data presented. **Cognitive Level:** Analyzing **Client Need:** Reduction of Risk Potential **Integrated Process:** Nursing Process: Implementation **Content Area:** Adult Health: Respiratory **Strategy:** The critical word in the question is *immediately* to consider the question is addressing an acute complication of central line insertion, which would include pneumothorax. Then consider how pneumothorax would manifest in the client to make a selection.

240. **Answer: 2 Rationale:** Ideas of reference or misinterpretation occur when the client believes that an incident has a personal reference to one's self when, in fact, it is not at all related. A hallucination is the occurrence of a sight, sound, touch, smell, or taste without any external stimulus to the corresponding sensory organ, although they are real to the person. Delusions are false beliefs that cannot be changed by logical reasoning or evidence. Loose association is a vague, unfocused, illogical flow or stream of thought. **Cognitive Level:** Applying **Client Need:** Psychosocial Integrity **Integrated Process:** Nursing Process: Assessment **Content Area:** Mental Health **Strategy:** The core issue of the question is the ability to draw correct conclusions from the behavior of a client with schizophrenia. Use knowledge of the features of this diagnosis and the process of elimination to make a selection.

241. **Answer: 3 Rationale:** With increased age, there is an increased sensitivity to xanthines, although other disease processes can also lead to this elevated value. The dose of theophylline should be decreased to get the blood level to the 10–20 mg/dL range. The dose does not need to be increased. Theophylline doses should be based on lean body weight to prevent entering the medication into the adipose tissue. Theophylline levels can rise to 25 mg/dL. **Cognitive Level:** Analyzing **Client Need:** Pharmacological and Parenteral Therapies **Integrated Process:** Nursing Process: Diagnosis **Content Area:** Pharmacology **Strategy:** The core issue of the question is knowledge that the drug level is high and knowledge of what factors can increase the drug level. Use concepts of the effects of age on pharmacokinetics and the process of elimination to make a selection.

242. **Answer: 3 Rationale:** Immunizations interrupt the chain of infection by generating immunity in a susceptible host by introducing a weakened or killed antigen into the body. Immunizations do not affect the mode of transmission of a pathogenic organism. Immunizations do not affect the portal of entry, which is how a pathogenic organism enters the host. Immunizations do not affect the portal of exit, which is how a pathogenic organism leaves the host. **Cognitive Level:** Applying **Client Need:** Safety and Infection Control **Integrated Process:** Teaching and Learning **Content Area:** Fundamentals **Strategy:** Knowledge of the chain of infection is required. Immunizations change the immunity status of the person receiving them. A susceptible host is the only choice where that is possible.

243. **Answer: 2 Rationale:** Thyroidectomy is an alternative treatment used when medication and iodine-based radiation therapy are unsuccessful. There is great concern about causing hypothyroidism in the client, which would require lifelong hormone replacement. The focus of concern is not a scar on the child's neck. The recovery time is the same as for other surgical procedures (6 weeks) rather than 6 months. The thermoregulation center is in the brain, and is not affected by thyroid gland removal. **Cognitive Level:** Applying **Client Need:** Physiological Adaptation **Integrated Process:** Communication and Documentation **Content Area:** Child Health **Strategy:** Determine the core issue of the question, which is a disadvantage of performing a thyroidectomy in a child. Use knowledge about hyperthyroid state and age-related concepts to eliminate each of the incorrect responses.

244. **Answer: 2 Rationale:** Uterine prolapse is caused by weakened pelvic muscles, which can be strengthened by pelvic floor exercises such as Kegel exercises. Menopause is an age-related hormonal change that is not influenced by Kegel exercises. Urinary tract infections require treatment with anti-infective medications. Premenstrual syndrome is caused by changing hormone levels and would not be affected by Kegel exercises. **Cognitive Level:** Applying **Client Need:** Health Promotion and Maintenance **Integrated Process:** Nursing Process: Planning **Content Area:** Adult Health: Renal and Genitourinary **Strategy:** The core issue of the question is knowledge that Kegel exercises can strengthen the pelvic floor. Evaluate each of the

options to determine which condition could be improved by the use of these exercises.

245. **Answer: 2 Rationale:** Safety is a priority for the client and all those around him. Even if the client is not a danger to himself, he still may want to harm his parents (others). Although a goal is for the client to continue to take his medication, safety is the priority. Although a goal is for the client to remain in treatment, safety is the priority. **Cognitive Level:** Analyzing **Client Need:** Management of Care **Integrated Process:** Nursing Process: Planning **Content Area:** Mental Health **Strategy:** The core issue of the question is safety of all possible clients in the question. Note the association between the word *knife* in the stem and the word *danger* to narrow the possibilities. Make a final choice using the most comprehensive option.

246. **Answer: 1 Rationale:** Clients receiving ophthalmic corticosteroids have an increased risk of infection, so contact lenses should not be removed 30 minutes prior to dose and reinserted 30 minutes after dose. Contact lenses should not be used during ophthalmic corticosteroid therapy. It is important to take medication for the length of time prescribed by the healthcare provider. The client should return for an eye examination after treatment is completed. **Cognitive Level:** Analyzing **Client Need:** Pharmacological and Parenteral Therapies **Integrated Process:** Nursing Process: Evaluation **Content Area:** Pharmacology **Strategy:** The core issue of the question is knowledge that corticosteroids increase risk of infection and how to reduce this risk when taking ophthalmic corticosteroids. Use nursing knowledge and the process of elimination to make a selection.

247. **Answer: 4 Rationale:** Sneezing and coughing are examples of modes of transmission whereby droplet nuclei can be transmitted directly to a susceptible host. Nonsterile surgical instruments could spread infection by contact. Soiled linens could spread infection by contact. Contaminated dressings could spread infection by contact. **Cognitive Level:** Applying **Client Need:** Safety and Infection Control **Integrated Process:** Teaching and Learning **Content Area:** Fundamentals **Strategy:** Look for commonalities among the options in order to eliminate choices, such as inanimate objects that serve as vehicles to transmit infectious microorganisms. Choose the option with coughing and sneezing as means whereby direct transmission occurs.

248. **Answer: 3 Rationale:** The premature secretion of testosterone promotes the closure of the epiphyseal growth plates. Many of these children appear tall around sixth grade, but their friends eventually catch up and surpass them in linear growth. The height of the parents is unrelated to precocious puberty. There is no information that the diet is inadequate, but diet is not directly related to hormonal effects of precocious puberty. Implying there is a low probability about being tall and playing basketball will not be useful in explaining this child's situation. **Cognitive Level:** Applying **Client Need:** Physiological Adaptation **Integrated Process:** Teaching and Learning **Content Area:** Child Health **Strategy:** To answer this question, it is necessary to have an understanding of the underlying pathophysiology. Take time to review this information if you have the need.

249. **Answer: 1 Rationale:** Calf pumping exercises involve contracting and then relaxing the leg muscles in an alternating fashion. Knee flexion and extension do not exercise the calf muscles, including the gastrocnemius muscles. Raising and lowering the legs would involve use of thigh muscles rather than calf muscles. Plantar flexion and dorsiflexion do not sufficiently exercise the calf muscles, although dorsiflexion will cause pain if thrombophlebitis is present. **Cognitive Level:** Analyzing **Client Need:** Reduction of Risk Potential **Integrated Process:** Nursing Process: Evaluation **Content Area:** Fundamentals **Strategy:** The core issue of the question is knowledge of correct implementation of leg exercises in the perioperative period. Use this knowledge and the process of elimination to make a selection.

250. **Answer: 4 Rationale:** When intervening in delirium, highest priority is given to nursing interventions that will maintain life. Fluid and electrolyte loss caused by nausea and vomiting can be a life-threatening condition during alcohol withdrawal, requiring replacement by intravenous therapy. Orienting the client to reality is a routine nursing measure. Restraints should be applied only when there is sufficient evidence of agitation to warrant their use. Referral to Alcoholics Anonymous is appropriate once the client's clinical condition has stabilized. **Cognitive Level:** Analyzing **Client Need:** Physiological Adaptation **Integrated Process:** Nursing Process: Planning **Content Area:** Mental Health **Strategy:** The core issue of the question is knowledge that a state of delirium is characterized by some type of metabolic imbalance. Recall that questions that address priorities of care in unstable clients often focus on physiological needs (in this case the client's internal metabolic state) first. With this in mind, eliminate options that address psychosocial needs first, and then eliminate safety needs.

251. **Answer: 3 Rationale:** The nurse should delegate the care of the 62-year-old who had surgery 3 days ago to repair the fractured femur. This client has a stable medical status. The nurse would want to assess the client who had wisdom teeth extraction because of postsurgical state. The nurse would want to complete discharge teaching with the client who had the cholecystectomy. The nurse would want to assess the client returning to the unit following gastric surgery. **Cognitive Level:** Analyzing **Client Need:** Management of Care **Integrated Process:** Nursing Process: Implementation **Content Area:** Leadership and Management **Strategy:** Recall the principles of delegation. The nurse should not delegate the care of clients who require assessment due to changes in acuity or status, as well as clients who require teaching. Stable clients may be delegated to the LPN/LVN under the RN's supervision.

252. **Answer: 3 Rationale:** A wound infection can be spread by direct contact with the wound. Scarlet fever requires the use of droplet precautions. Measles requires the use of airborne precautions. Rubella requires the use of droplet precautions. **Cognitive Level:** Applying **Client Need:** Safety and Infection Control **Integrated Process:** Nursing Process: Implementation **Content Area:** Fundamentals **Strategy:** Look for commonalities among the options in order to eliminate choices. Note that three options identify diseases that are contagious infections. Choose the wound infection as direct transmission of microorganisms occurs by direct contact with the client.

253. Answer: 4 Rationale: The client should increase his fluid intake (unless contraindicated) to prevent urinary tract infections and lessen dysuria. Nocturia is a symptom that occurs with BPH. Having BPH is a common and benign age-related problem for men, and is not associated with an increased risk for prostate cancer. Urinary tract infections can occur as a result of the urinary stasis that can occur with BPH. **Cognitive Level:** Analyzing **Client Need:** Physiological Adaptation **Integrated Process:** Nursing Process: Evaluation **Content Area:** Adult Health: Renal and Genitourinary **Strategy:** The critical words in the stem of the question are *need for further teaching*. This tells you that the correct answer is an incorrect statement made by the client. Use the process of elimination and knowledge of the disorder to make a selection.

254. Answer: 2 Rationale: Recreational and socialization activities are an integral part of growing up, and all efforts should be made to provide access to programs that provide these, such as Boy Scouts. The child should be able to find activities as a member of the troop that are not beyond his physical abilities. If the child attends school, he is already aware of similarities and differences between himself and other boys, and scouting programs can do much to enhance a child's self-esteem. Recreational activities are necessary during childhood. Emphasis should not be placed on school alone. **Cognitive Level:** Applying **Client Need:** Physiological Adaptation **Integrated Process:** Nursing Process: Diagnosis **Content Area:** Child Health **Strategy:** Consider the word *mild* in the stem of the question and choose the response that is the broadest and most encompassing.

255. Answer: 1 Rationale: Older adults have slower biotransformation and excretion of drugs, causing an increased susceptibility to adverse effects. Haloperidol is a high-potency antipsychotic that can cause tardive dyskinesia, an irreversible adverse effect, and requires careful monitoring by the nurse. Fecal impaction is not related to haloperidol, but is influenced by fiber and fluids in the diet and activity level. Respiratory depression is not of great concern with haloperidol. Insomnia is not of concern with haloperidol. **Cognitive Level:** Applying **Client Need:** Pharmacological and Parenteral Therapies **Integrated Process:** Nursing Process: Assessment **Content Area:** Mental Health **Strategy:** The core issue of the question is knowledge of adverse effects of the drug haloperidol. Use specific nursing knowledge and the process of elimination to make a selection.

256. Answer: 4 Rationale: The state nurse practice act defines the scope of nursing practice in each state. Although there are general principles that apply to all, each state or jurisdiction retains the right to formulate its own regulations about nursing practice, including delegation. Policy manuals are agency-specific and do not address state regulations directly, although they should be congruent with each other. Job descriptions are agency-specific, although they should fall within the parameters of state law. The ANA standards of practice apply to care given to clients. **Cognitive Level:** Applying **Client Need:** Management of Care **Integrated Process:** Nursing Process: Implementation **Content Area:** Leadership and Management **Strategy:** Use knowledge of the source of various regulations to answer the question. If needed, review concepts related to legal governance of nursing practice.

257. Answer: 4, 3, 1, 2 Rationale: The gown is applied first as recommended by the Centers for Disease Control and Prevention. The mask is donned second, as it can be more securely applied with ungloved hands. Eye protection is put on immediately after the mask. Gloves are donned last, so the gloves can be pulled up to cover the cuffs of the gown. **Cognitive Level:** Applying **Client Need:** Safety and Infection Control **Integrated Process:** Nursing Process: Implementation **Content Area:** Fundamentals **Strategy:** Rationalize the ordering based on nursing knowledge of standard precautions and surgical asepsis.

258. Answer: 2 Rationale: The nurse should recommend the neighbor call the Poison Control Center, who will be able to look up the specific vitamin and give precise instructions to the mother. The nurse should not assume that no action should be taken. Driving the child to the emergency department may delay treatment or may be unnecessary. The nurse's recommendation does not depend on whether the vitamins are water- or fat-soluble. **Cognitive Level:** Applying **Client Need:** Safety and Infection Control **Integrated Process:** Communication and Documentation **Content Area:** Child Health **Strategy:** The focus of the question is on how to maintain the client's self-esteem and the location of the concern centers around being at school. With this in mind, select the option that directly addresses the concern.

259. Answer: 2 Rationale: The nurse should determine if the client has had a positive PPD test in the past because if this is true, the client should be evaluated with a chest x-ray. The arm should be cleansed with alcohol and allowed to air before administering the PPD. The test is usually read in 48–72 hours after injection, not 24 hours later. The client may wash the area as usual. **Cognitive Level:** Analyzing **Client Need:** Reduction of Risk Potential **Integrated Process:** Nursing Process: Assessment **Content Area:** Adult Health: Respiratory **Strategy:** The core issue of the question is knowledge of proper procedure and concerns when administering a PPD test. Recall that this is a skin test for tuberculosis to help you recall that assessment of a client's past reaction is a critical first action.

260. Answer: 3 Rationale: Initially, the delirious client is dazed, drowsy, and perceptions will be disturbed, making it difficult for the client to sustain attention to any mental task. Delirium is characterized by alternating periods of confusion with lucidity; therefore, regaining orientation is an appropriate initial outcome criterion. Verbalizing drug dependence may be appropriate once the client has been stabilized. Stress management might be an appropriate outcome criterion to help the client avoid drug use, once the client has been stabilized. Exploring reasons for addictive behavior may be an appropriate outcome criterion once the client has been stabilized. **Cognitive Level:** Applying **Client Need:** Psychosocial Integrity **Integrated Process:** Nursing Process: Planning **Content Area:** Mental Health **Strategy:** The core issue of the question is understanding of the condition of delirium. The critical word in the stem of the question is *initial*. With this in mind, choose the option that shows the beginnings of return of neurological status to normal.

261. Answer: 3 Rationale: Dehydration results in hypovolemia and decreased glomerular filtration, which can precipitate acute kidney injury in infants and children. A past history of chickenpox places a client at risk for shingles but that would occur in later life. A severe case of influenza would not affect renal perfusion, especially 4 months later. Having asthma since the age of 3 years is not related to onset of acute kidney injury. **Cognitive Level:** Analyzing **Client Need:** Physiological Adaptation **Integrated Process:** Nursing Process: Assessment **Content Area:** Child Health **Strategy:** Consider the various etiologies of acute kidney injury. Recall that the kidneys need a minimum glomerular filtration rate to function properly. Use this concept to choose correctly.

262. Answer: 1 Rationale: A client with tuberculosis must wear a surgical mask if transportation to another hospital department is unavoidable. This is an element of airborne precautions necessary to limit the transmission of the microorganism. Removal and disposal of respiratory secretions is important but does not require the client to wear gloves to blow the nose. Tuberculosis is not transmitted via eating utensils. Tuberculosis is not transmitted via urine. **Cognitive Level:** Applying **Client Need:** Safety and Infection Control **Integrated Process:** Nursing Process: Implementation **Content Area:** Fundamentals **Strategy:** Knowledge of how tuberculosis is transmitted is essential. Eliminate options that do not address transmission via the respiratory tract. Make a final selection knowing that clients would not wear gloves to protect themselves from their own infections.

263. Answer: 1, 3, 4, 5 Rationale: Scatter rugs pose a risk for falls in older adults and should be removed. The bathroom should have grab bars near the toilet and in the bath or shower. The stairs should be illuminated to prevent falls so the light bulb needs to be fixed or the light should be replaced. Magazines should be removed from the floor to avoid an accidental fall. Nightlights that illuminate the hallway enhance the client's safety. **Cognitive Level:** Analyzing **Client Need:** Safety and Infection Control **Integrated Process:** Nursing Process: Assessment **Content Area:** Adult Health: Reproductive **Strategy:** Note that more than one option is correct. Evaluate each option as if it was a true or false statement in relation to the question.

264. Answer: 1, 3, 4 Rationale: Reminding the client to use the call bell represents safe practice. Adjusting the bed to the lowest position before leaving the room represents safe practice. Assisting the client to put on nonskid hospital socks or footwear before ambulating reduces the risk of slips and falls. Positioning an overbed table out of the client's reach poses a potential threat to safety if the client cannot reach needed belongings and must get out of bed unattended or reaches excessively and falls. Putting all side-rails up before leaving the room constitutes a physical restraint. Restraints must be prescribed, and the client could fall if trying to climb out of bed when all side-rails are raised. **Cognitive Level:** Analyzing **Client Need:** Safety and Infection Control **Integrated Process:** Nursing Process: Evaluation **Content Area:** Leadership and Management **Strategy:** Note that more than one option is correct. Evaluate each option as if it was a true or false statement in relation to the question.

265. Answer: 2 Rationale: Providing low-level indirect light helps the client recognize surroundings and may help to reorient the client who has confusion at night. Locking the windows may promote general safety but locking the client's door imprisons the client and does not aid in reorientation to environment. Constant stimuli at night, such as from television or music, does not help with orientation and might disturb sleep. Walking in the neighborhood to promote sleep does not address the underlying concern about nighttime confusion. **Cognitive Level:** Applying **Client Need:** Psychosocial Integrity **Integrated Process:** Nursing Process: Implementation **Content Area:** Mental Health **Strategy:** The core issue of the question is knowledge of helpful actions when a client with dementia is confused. Use nursing knowledge of therapeutic processes and the process of elimination to make a selection.

Preparing for the NCLEX-RN® Exam*

SAFE AND EFFECTIVE CARE ENVIRONMENT: MANAGEMENT OF CARE

Management of Care makes up 17–23% of the questions on the NCLEX-RN® exam.

Key Testing Strategies:

- Recognize questions that require priority setting through words in the question such as first, initial, best, most important, essential, and most therapeutic.
- When answering questions related to delegation to caregivers, such as float registered nurses from other clinical specialties, LPNs/LVNs, and unlicensed assistive personnel (UAPs), recall that the task being delegated needs to be part of that caregiver's skill set and that the other rights of delegation must be upheld.
- Immediately eliminate distracters that violate client rights or ethical principles.

Sample Topics for Management of Care Questions

Advance directives/self-determination/life planning	Establishing priorities
Advocacy	Ethical practice
Assignment, delegation, and supervision	Informed consent
Case management	Information technology
Client rights	Legal rights and responsibilities
Collaboration with interdisciplinary team	Organ donation
Concepts of management	Performance improvement (quality improvement)
Confidentiality/information security	Referrals
Continuity of care	Supervision

Essential Rights of Delegation

Review these "rights" in Chapter 5

1. **Right Task:** Nurses determine those activities team members may perform. For each situation, the nurse must consider the client's condition, the complexity of the activity, the UAP's capabilities, and the amount of supervision the nurse will be able to provide.
2. **Right Circumstances:** The nurse evaluates the individual clients and the individual UAPs and matches the two. The nurse assesses the client's needs, looks at the care plan, and considers the setting, ensuring that UAPs have the proper resources, equipment, and supervision to work safely.
3. **Right Person:** The nurse follows organizational policies, which are congruent with state law, in determining the appropriate staff to which to delegate a nursing activity.
4. **Right Direction and Communication:** The nurse needs to communicate the acceptable tasks and activities. The nurse needs to clearly understand the organization's policies and procedures to carry out effective delegation. In turn, staff nurses need to direct UAPs' actions and communicate clearly about each delegated task. Nurses must be specific about how and when UAPs should report back to them. Nurses should feel comfortable asking, Do you know how to do this? Where did you learn? How many times have you done it in the past? Where is your experience documented?
5. **Right Supervision and Evaluation:** Nurse managers must ensure that each unit has adequate staffing and time, identify the task inherent to each staff role, and evaluate the impact of the organization's nursing service on the community. The delegating nurse then must supervise, guide, and evaluate the UAPs' task implementation. The nurse must ensure that UAPs meet expectations and must intervene if they aren't performing well.

*Based on the April 2016 Test Plan

Strategies for Setting Priorities in Clinical Practice

Review these strategies in Chapter 5

Guiding Principles	First Priority	Second Priority
Physiology	**Airway, breathing, and circulation**	
Maslow's Hierarchy of Needs theory	Physiological (primary) needs: air, breathing, circulation, water, food (oxygen therapy, circulatory support, IV hydration, nutrition, critical lab values, treatment of pain)	Safety and security (primary) needs: prevention of falls, reorientation to surroundings, abnormally high or low values that are not critical, may include some client teaching (e.g. insulin administration)
Policies and Procedures	Activities governed by agency policy or procedure that involves strict timelines (e.g., restraints, falls, stat medications)	Activities governed by policy or procedure that directly affect client care (e.g., non-stat, regularly scheduled medications, dressings)
Care activities related to clinical condition of client	Life-threatening or potentially life-threatening occurrences (adverse changes in VS, change in LOC, potential for respiratory or circulatory collapse); often unanticipated	Activities essential to safety: life-saving medications and equipment that protect clients from infections or falls
Medication or IV therapy priorities	Medications that prevent or treat physiological distress (e.g., analgesics, updrafts or inhalers); medications ordered more frequently (e.g., every 4 hours) because late medication delivery could affect next dose; IV therapy for hydration in clients who are NPO because of nonfunctional GI tract	Medications that prevent reoccurrences of symptoms of disease processes (such as digoxin or antibiotics); medications ordered once per shift, routine maintenance of IV therapy or heparin/saline lock care

Ethical Principles and Decision-making

Review these principles in Chapter 4

Autonomy	Beneficence
Accountability	Justice
Fidelity	Veracity
Confidentiality	Nonmaleficence

Informed Consent

Review these guidelines in Chapter 4

- Requirements of client: has mental capacity to consent; it is voluntarily done; and client understands treatment and information presented
- Requirements of healthcare provider (performing treatment, procedure, or surgery): shares information about planned treatment, procedure or surgery, its associated risks and benefits, and alternatives to treatment; gives client opportunity to ask questions and have them answered
- If a client waives right to informed consent, document this in the medical record
- If client is deemed incompetent to make informed decisions about healthcare in court of law, a court-appointed guardian makes these decisions
- Informed consent for minors is obtained from parent or legal guardian, except in emergency situations, when minor is married or emancipated from parents, or has special care needs, such as with sexually transmitted infection or pregnancy

Upholding HIPAA (Health Information Portability and Accountability Act)

Review these guidelines in Chapter 4

- Protect personal identifying information (such as name, social security number, date of birth) and information about diagnosis or treatment
- Share information only with individuals involved directly in client's care, payment for care, and/or management of client's care
- Verify identify of persons asking for client information

- Dispose of confidential documents in accord with agency policy (such as shredder, locked recycle bin)
- Keep contents of medical record out of public view by placing in a secure area and turning computer screens displaying client data away from general view
- Discuss client's care only in areas where cannot be overheard

SAFE AND EFFECTIVE CARE ENVIRONMENT: SAFETY AND INFECTION CONTROL

Safety and Infection Control makes up 9–15% of the questions on the NCLEX-RN® exam.

Key Testing Strategies

- Questions that focus on assessing the home environment of a client may be seeking to determine knowledge of risks to safety in the home, such as risk of falls (e.g., throw rugs, no night lights, handrails, or bathroom safety bars) or risk of fire (e.g., oxygen in the home, frayed electrical cords, lack of smoke detectors).
- When answering a question that addresses an infectious disease, consider that the question may be determining knowledge of precautions to prevent disease transmission, and discriminate the need to use contact, airborne, or droplet precautions.
- When answering a question that addresses a client with a compromised immune system or who is receiving chemotherapy, consider that the question may be determining whether the client has a need for neutropenic precautions (for low white blood cell count) or thrombocytopenic precautions (for low platelet count).

Sample Topics for Safety and Infection Control Questions

Accident/error/injury prevention	Reporting of incident/event/irregular occurrence/variance
Emergency response plan	Safe use of equipment
Ergonomic principles	Security plan
Error prevention	Standard/precautions/transmission-based precautions/surgical asepsis
Handling hazardous and infectious materials	Use of restraints/safety devices
Home safety	

4 Steps to Maintain Client Safety During a Fire

Review these steps in Chapter 6

Remove clients from danger	Contain the fire
Activate the fire alarm	Evacuate the area (do horizontal evacuation if possible before vertical evacuation)

Fall Risk Factors in Older Adults

Review these guidelines in Chapter 17

Intrinsic Age-Related Changes	Intrinsic Disease Related Changes	Extrinsic Risk Factors
Gait (step length and height)	Orthostatic hypotension	Floor surface; waxed, scatter rugs, tears in carpeting
Gait (symmetry and path)	Dehydration	Steps uneven, without hand rails
Balance when sitting	Cardiac arrhythmias and anemias	Edges and curbing without contrasting colors
Balance when standing	Urinary tract and other infections	Dim lighting, bright lights that cause glare
Balance when turning	Osteoporosis and fractures	Bathrooms without grab bars and tub or shower seats
Stability	Hypoglycemia	High-heeled shoes
Cognition	Seizures, TIA, CVA, adverse effects of medication, delirium	Clutter

Principles of Surgical Asepsis

Review these principles in Chapter 7

- All objects used in a sterile field must be sterile.
- Sterile objects that touch unsterile objects become unsterile.
- Sterile items that are out of vision or below waist level are considered unsterile.
- Sterile objects can become unsterile by prolonged exposure to airborne microorganisms.
- Fluids flow in the direction of gravity.
- Moisture that passes through a sterile object exerts capillary action to draw microorganisms from unsterile surfaces above or below to the sterile surface.
- The edges of a sterile field are considered unsterile.
- The skin is unsterile and cannot be sterilized.
- Conscientiousness, alertness, and honesty are essential qualities in maintaining surgical asepsis.

Centers for Disease Control and Prevention (CDC) Precautions

Review these precautions to prevent the spread of microorganisms in Chapter 7

Tier 1: Standard Precautions

Hand hygiene
Gloves
Face protection (mask, goggles, face shield)
Gowns and other protective apparel
Others

Tier 2: Transmission Based Precautions

Airborne Precautions: Use when small ($<5\ \mu$m) pathogen-infected droplet nuclei may remain suspended in air over time and travel distances greater than 3 feet. *Examples: varicella, measles, tuberculosis*

Droplet Precautions: Use with large ($>5\ \mu$m) pathogen-infected droplets that travel 3 feet or less via coughing, sneezing, etc. or during procedures (suctioning). *Examples: Haemophilus influenzae, Neisseria meningitides, others*

Contact Precautions: Use with known or suspected microorganisms transmitted by direct hand-to-skin client contact or indirect contact with surfaces or care items in the environment. *Examples: Clostridium difficile, diphtheria (cutaneous), herpes simplex (mucocutaneous or neonatal), impetigo, pediculosis, scabies, zoster (disseminated, immunocompromised host), viral/hemorrhagic infections (Ebola, Lassa, Marburg), others*

HEALTH PROMOTION AND MAINTENANCE

Health Promotion and Maintenance makes up 6–12% of the questions on the NCLEX-RN® exam.

Key Testing Strategies

- Make note of whether the client's age is identified in the question. If so, the question may be determining ability to apply concepts of normal growth and development.
- Because health promotion often involves client education, be prepared to apply principles of teaching and learning to questions in this area.
- When determining interventions to enhance a client's wellness, consider options that promote healthy nutrition, regular exercise, proper weight maintenance, proper rest, and avoidance of harmful chemicals, such as nicotine, and risk-taking behaviors, such as not wearing a seat belt.

Sample Topics for Health Promotion and Maintenance Questions

Aging process	High-risk behaviors
Ante/intra/postpartum and newborn care	Lifestyle choices
Developmental stages and transitions	Self-care
Health promotion/disease prevention	Techniques of physical assessment
Health screening	

Health Screening for Cancer

Remember to use CAUTION to recognize possible signs of cancer:

Change in bowel or bladder habits	Indigestion or difficulty in swallowing
A sore that does not heal	Obvious change in a wart or mole
Unusual bleeding or discharge	Nagging cough or hoarseness
Thickening or lump in breast or elsewhere	

Source: From the American Cancer Society.

ABCDE Rule for Evaluating a Suspicious Skin Lesion

A = Asymmetry (one half of lesion does not match the other half)

B = Border irregularity (edges are blurred, jagged, or have a notched appearance)

C = Color variation is present or has a dark black color change

D = Diameter is greater than 6 millimeters in size

E = Evolving (color, size, or shape is changing)

Techniques of Physical Assessment

Review these techniques in Chapter 15

- Inspection: utilizes observation to obtain important information about a client's state of health; have adequate lighting to visually inspect the body without distortions or shadows; lighting can be sunlight or artificial
- Palpation: uses the sensation of touch and pressure of the hands and fingers to determine masses, elevations, temperature, organ position, and any abnormal findings; can be light or deep depending on the area of the body being examined
  - Light palpation is 1 cm in depth
  - Deep palpation is about 4 cm in depth
  - Deep palpation should occur after light palpation
- Percussion: a skill in which the finger of one hand touches or taps a finger of the other hand to generate vibration, which in turn produces a specific, diagnostic sound; the sound changes as the practitioner moves from one area to the next
- Auscultation: uses the sense of hearing to identify sounds produced by the body; some sounds can be heard and identified without a stethoscope; others can only be identified in a quiet environment with a stethoscope

Basic Teaching Principles

- Set priorities for client's learning needs.
- Use appropriate timing.
- Organize materials so that learning proceeds from simple to complex.
- Promote and maintain learner attention and participation.
- Build on the client's existing knowledge.
- Select appropriate teaching methods, including discussion, question and answer, role-play, or discovery, or computerized instruction.
- Use appropriate teaching aids: visual aids (drawings, charts, models, printed materials), audiotapes, films or videotapes, programmed instruction, games, and others.
- Provide teaching related to developmental level.

Age-Related Changes

Review these changes in Chapter 17

Skin: Subcutaneous tissue loss and dermal thinning, leading to wrinkling; increase in lentigines (brown age spots); hair thins and loses pigment; nail growth slows and nails may become thicker; skin tissue is more fragile

Sensory/perceptual: Visual acuity changes; ocular changes lead to near vision problems (presbyopia), increased sensitivity to glare, decreased ability to adjust to darkness; cataracts may develop; eyelids lose elasticity; ear canal narrows with calcification of ossicles and increased cerumen, resulting in progressive hearing loss (presbycusis); reduced ability to smell and discriminate odors; sense of taste decreases (especially to sense sweet taste); touch sensation changes with reduced ability to sense heat and cold

Neurologic: Conduction speeds of neuron firing and transmission decrease; memory retrieval is slower; sleep stages 2–4 shorten, leading to a decrease in deep sleep; proprioception decreases

Musculoskeletal: Muscles atrophy; joint cartilage deteriorates; intervertebral disks atrophy, resulting in a loss of height of 1–3 inches

Pulmonary: Chest wall becomes rigid; thoracic muscles weaken; ciliary activity decreases; delivery and diffusion of O_2 to tissues decreases

Cardiovascular: Cardiac output and stroke volume decrease; valves stiffen; conductivity is altered; blood vessels are less elastic, leading to increasing blood pressure

Renal: Decreased glomerular filtration rate and creatinine clearance; possible residual urine or nocturia

Gastrointestinal: Thirst decreases; swallowing time is delayed; possible loss of teeth; decreased saliva; decreased gastric enzymes; weaker intestinal walls

Endocrine: Slowed basal metabolism; insulin levels increase but insulin sensitivity decreases

Genital: Males: prostate enlarges (often benign); decreased sperm protection. Females: vaginal dryness and atrophy

Immune: First sign of infection in an older adult may be a fall; temperature pattern may be lower than younger adult with the same infection

PSYCHOSOCIAL INTEGRITY

Psychosocial Integrity makes up 6–12% of the questions on the NCLEX-RN® exam.

Key Testing Strategies

- For communication questions, select answers that use therapeutic communication techniques and eliminate options that represent communication blocks.
- If a question suggests that a client is at risk for abuse, assess the client without caregivers present and be aware of mandatory reporting laws.
- When responding to a client's communication, look for options that address the client's concern or issue.
- When answering questions of a psychosocial nature when all options seem of equal importance, follow the SEAs: **s**afety, **e**xpressing feelings, and **a**ssisting with problem solving.

Sample Topics for Psychosocial Integrity Questions

Abuse/neglect	Grief and loss
Behavioral interventions	Mental health concepts
Chemical and other dependencies/substance use disorder	Religious and spiritual influences on health
Coping mechanisms	Sensory/perceptual alterations
Crisis intervention	Stress management
Cultural awareness/cultural influences on health	Support systems
End-of-life care	Therapeutic communication
Family dynamics	Therapeutic environment

Components of a Mental Status Exam

General Appearance	Appears stated age? Hygiene? Body odors? Dressed to season? Layered? Cleanliness?
Orientation	Person, place, time, and situation?
Thought Process	Clear, coherent, appropriate to topic? Concentration? Hallucinations or delusions?
Memory	Short-term (What did you have for breakfast?), long-term (Who is the president, and the president before that?)
Judgment	Appropriate? Safe? Impaired? Poor?

Communication Techniques to Avoid

Review these techniques in Chapter 18

Self-disclosure	Giving personal opinions or advice
Inattentive listening	Prying to satisfy personal curiosity
Overuse of medical jargon	Changing the subject

Suicide Precautions

When a client is acutely or actively suicidal, the following precautions should be taken:

- If not already hospitalized, someone should stay with the client until he or she can be admitted to prevent self-harm and maintain the safety of the client.
- Remove all sharp or dangerous objects from the client and the immediate vicinity, including knives or forks, scissors, mirrors, glass, and other objects that could be used for self-harm.
- Remove clothing that could be used as a tourniquet to cause self-harm, including belts of all kinds, neckties, stockings, handbags with long straps, etc.
- Remove all substances that could be ingested to toxic levels, including alcohol, recreational drugs, and medications. Keep client's medications locked.
- Ensure that the client swallows all pills, tablets, or other oral forms of medication, so that they are not kept in the cheek and then stored for later overdose.
- Keep the client in seclusion under one-to-one supervision while actively suicidal; explain in a gentle manner that this is for the client's safety until he or she is able to resist suicidal urges.
- Monitor a client who is not under one-to-one supervision with a nursing unit staff member every 10 to 15 minutes on an irregular schedule of observation.

Ensuring Your Safety on the Psychiatric Unit

1. Never be with a client by yourself. Alert staff to your whereabouts at all times.
2. Always have the ability to exit; do not put yourself in a position where your back is toward a closed-in area without an escape route.
3. Dress in casual clothes. Avoid sexually provocative clothing. Avoid having too much skin exposed.
4. Psychotic clients generally experience three delusional themes: 1) sexual, 2) political, and 3) religious. Avoid these topics unless you are experienced in managing them.
5. Remember that staff members are trained in managing client behavioral problems. Obtain the assistance of more experienced staff members when encountering unsafe situations early in practice.
6. Avoid wearing necklaces or other items that can be used as a weapon to strangle. Wear closed-toe shoes. Do not wear loop earrings (or rings).
7. Remember safety first. Always listen to your primary or gut instinct. Enlist the aid of other staff to help in maintaining control.

Therapeutic Communication Techniques

Review these techniques in Chapter 18

Acknowledging:	Gives nonjudgmental recognition to a client for a certain behavior or contribution, or indicates attention to and care of the client
Clarifying:	Asks for additional information to ensure understanding of the message sent; a statement like "Would you tell me more about what you have just said?" indicates that understanding the client's message is important to the nurse
Focusing:	Focuses the client on information that is pertinent and helps the client expand on that information; this technique directs the client towards information that is important
Giving information:	Provides specific information to a client either with or without the client's request
Offering self:	Offers the nurse's presence without attaching any expectations or conditions about the client's behavior during that time
Restating or paraphrasing:	Ensures the nurse understands the message sent; utilizing this technique the nurse repeats the main thought of the message sent
Reflecting:	Redirects the content of a client's message back to the client for further thought or consideration
Summarizing:	May be used at the end of an interaction to identify material discussed; it helps to sort out relevant information from irrelevant
Using silence:	Allows for quiet time without conversation for several seconds or minutes to allow for reflection about the discussion that just occurred, to reduce tension, or to gather thoughts about how to proceed

PHYSIOLOGICAL INTEGRITY: BASIC CARE AND COMFORT

Basic Care and Comfort makes up 6–12% of the questions on the NCLEX-RN® exam.

Key Testing Strategies

- Use principles of administering basic physiological care to clients when answering questions in this part of the test plan.
- When questions address a client's mobility, select answers that will preserve muscle tone and joint function and prevent contractures or skin breakdown.
- Keep principles of safety in mind when answering questions about the use of assistive devices, such as canes, walkers, and crutches.
- Promote good nutrition by selecting meal choices that are balanced and that address any diet restrictions, such as low sodium or reduced fat.
- Use principles of gravity when considering how to position the clients or when working with clients who have drainage or wound tubes.

Sample Topics for Basic Care and Comfort Questions

Assistive devices	Nutrition and oral hydration
Elimination	Personal hygiene
Mobility/immobility	Rest and sleep
Nonpharmacologic comfort interventions	

Safety Precautions During Oxygen Therapy

Review these precautions in Chapter 26

- Instruct the client and visitors about the danger of smoking when oxygen is in use. If necessary, remove matches, lighters, and ashtrays.
- If oxygen therapy is used at home, instruct family members or caregivers to smoke only outside. If smoking is permitted, teach visitors to use smoking room.
- Avoid materials that generate static electricity such as woolen blankets and synthetic fabrics; instead use cotton fabrics.
- Avoid use of volatile, flammable substances such as acetone in nail polish removers, alcohol, ether, and oils near clients using oxygen.
- Remove any friction type or battery operated gadgets, devices, or toys.
- Make sure electric devices such as radios, razors, and televisions are in good working order to prevent short-circuit sparks.
- Ensure that electric monitoring equipment and suction machines are properly grounded. Disconnect any ungrounded equipment.
- Personnel need to be aware of the location of fire extinguishers and be able to use them properly.
- Know location of oxygen meter turn-off value.

Therapeutic Diets

Review information about these diets in Chapter 25

Regular diet	High-residue/high-fiber diet
Clear liquids	Low-residue/low-fiber
Full liquids	Carbohydrate controlled
Pureed diet	Fat controlled
Dysphagia diet	Protein controlled
Soft diet	Gastric bypass diet
Mechanical soft diet	Restricted diets (gluten, tyramine, others)
Bland diet	

Types of Dressings

Review these dressings in Chapter 26

Dressing Type	Description
Gauze	Plain or impregnated with an antimicrobial • Packs and fills wound • Absorbs drainage • Used for full- and partial-thickness wounds with drainage • May be apply dry, wet-to-moist, and wet-to-wet
Transparent film	Adhesive plastic semipermeable membrane that allows oxygen into wound but is occlusive to liquids and bacteria • Protects wound from contamination and friction
Impregnated nonadherent	Cotton or synthetic material impregnated with saline, zinc-saline, antimicrobials, petrolatum or others • Protects nonexudative partial- and full-thickness wounds • Requires secondary dressing to keep in place, hold in moisture, and protect wound
Hydrocolloid	Adhesive made of gelatin • Is occlusive to microorganisms and liquids and promotes absorption of wound exudates • Enhances autolysis of necrotic tissue within wound bed • Duo-Derm and Tegasorb are examples
Hydrogel	Water or glycerin is primary component of jelly-like sheet, granules, or gels • Maintains moist wound bed and helps liquefy necrotic tissue or slough • Permeable to oxygen and can fill dead spaces in a wound • Secondary nonadhesive dressing is required
Alginate (exudate absorbers)	Nonadherent dressings with granules, ropes, paste or other materials; requires secondary dressing • Purpose is to absorb up to 20 times their weight in drainage
Polyurethane foam	Nonadherent dressings that absorb large amounts of exudates while keeping wound moist • Use secondary dressing or tape around edges to secure it
Clear absorbent acrylic	Absorbs exudate and allows moisture to evaporate • Aids in wound assessment and protects from bacteria and shearing forces

PHYSIOLOGICAL INTEGRITY: PHARMACOLOGIC AND PARENTERAL THERAPIES

Pharmacologic and Parenteral Therapies makes up 12–18% of the questions on the NCLEX-RN® exam.

Key Testing Strategies

- Use knowledge of drug action, intended effects and key side and adverse effects to answer a question about a specific medication.
- For questions addressing medication history, do not forget to ask about over-the-counter and herbal supplements as well as prescription medications.
- Double-check drug dosages and make sure the answer passes the common sense test (e.g., answer for a subcutaneous dose should not be more than 1 milliliter for an adult).
- Look for certain prefixes and suffixes in drug names to help identify the drug if the name is unfamiliar.

Sample Topics for Pharmacologic and Parenteral Therapies Questions

Adverse effects/contraindications/side effects/interactions

Blood and blood products

Central venous access devices

Dosage calculation

Expected actions/outcomes

Medication administration

Parenteral/intravenous therapies

Pharmacologic pain management

Total parenteral nutrition

Calculating Medication Dosages

Formula 1

$$\frac{\text{dose ordered (desired)}}{\text{dose on hand (have)}} \times \text{amount available (quantity)} = \text{amount to give}$$

Formula 2 (ratio and proportion)

$$\frac{\text{dose ordered}}{\text{dose on hand}} = \frac{\times}{\text{quantity available}}$$

Formula 3 (dimensional analysis)

Rule 1: Multiplying one side of an equation by a conversion factor will not change the value of the equation.

Rule 2: Set up the problem so that all labels cancel from the numerator and denominator except the label desired in the answer.

Calculating IV Drip Rates

$$\frac{\text{volume (of fluid)}}{\text{time (in minutes)}} \times \text{drop factor} = \text{flow rate}$$

Steps for Calculating Pediatric Medication Dosages

1. Convert the child's weight from pounds (lb) to kilograms (kg); 1kg = 2.2 lb.
2. Calculate the safe total daily dose in mg/kg or in mcg/kg for a child of this weight as recommended in a standard drug reference book (mg/kg recommended × weight in kg). Then calculate the amount of one dose (total daily dose divided by the number of doses/day).
3. Compare the ordered dose to the recommended dose and determine if the dose is safe.
4. If the dose is safe, calculate the amount of one dose using one of the medication dosage formulas shown. If unsafe, consult prescriber before administering.

Reducing the Risk of Medication Errors

- Question any medication order that is not written clearly, has an unusual dose, or is not in keeping with treatment for client's known health problems.
- Prepare medications in a quiet area away from noise and distractions.
- Check client drug allergies before giving medications; if there is no notation in the allergy section(s) of the medical record, STOP and be sure to obtain allergy history prior to administration. Verify order for a medication that is questionable based on allergy history before administration.
- Be knowledgeable about medications: various names, correct dosage ranges, method of administration, and side/adverse effects.
- Have another nurse check dosage of parenteral medications (such as heparin, digoxin, and insulin) that could pose immediate harm to client if given incorrectly.
- Be aware of drug-food and drug-drug interactions to reduce risk of either ineffective treatment or toxic effects. Sometimes interactions reduce drug's effectiveness and sometimes they heighten its effect.
- Identify client correctly by asking client to state his or her name; checking identification bracelet is the next best method if client is nonverbal. Be especially careful when there are two clients or more in room. Use two unique identifiers per agency policy. If medication bar coding technology is in use, scan medication per agency policy.
- If client questions a medication or states it is different than one taken at home, STOP and recheck medication order and client history. Verify order as necessary before proceeding to administer.
- Carefully and promptly document medication administration.
- Check results of ordered therapeutic drug levels as soon as they are expected to be available and report results promptly.
- Teach clients and significant others/family members about medications well in advance of discharge so they are prepared for safe self-administration following discharge.

Memory Aid for Drugs by Generic Name Prefix, Root, or Suffix*

Syllable in Generic Name	Interpretation	Examples by Generic Name
-ase, -plase	Thrombolytic agent (-ase usually indicates enzyme)	alteplase, anistreplase, reteplase, streptokinase, tenecteplase
-azole	Antifungal antimicrobial	itraconazole, fluconazole, clotrimazole,miconazole
cef-, ceph-	Cephalosporin, antibiotic; check allergy to this class and penicillins	cefazolin, cephalexin, cefotetan, ceftazidime, ceftriazone
-cillin	Penicillin, antibiotic; check allergy	amoxicillin, penicillin, piperacillin, ticarcillin, nafcillin, oxacillin
-cycline	Tetracycline, antibiotic	doxycycline, minocycline, tetracycline
-dipine	Calcium channel blocker, antianginal, antihypertensive	amlodipine, nicardipine, nifedipine, felodipine
-dronate	Bisphosphonate, bone resorption inhibitor	alendronate, etidronate, pamidronate, risedronate
-floxacin	Fluoroquinolone, antibiotic	ciprofloxacin, levofloxacin, norfloxacin, sparfloxacin

Syllable in Generic Name	Interpretation	Examples by Generic Name
-micin, -mycin	Aminoglycoside, antibiotic**	gentamicin, kanamycin, netilmicin, tobramycin
nitr-, -nitr-	Nitrate, vasodilator, antianginal	nitroglycerin, isosorbide dinitrate
-olol, -lol	Beta adrenergic blocker, antihypertensive and/or antianginal	propranolol, atenolol, metoprolol, nadolol, labetalol, timolol
-parin	Anticoagulant, heparin or heparinoid	heparin, dalteparin, enoxaparin
-phylline	Xanthine type of bronchodilator	aminophylline, theophylline
-prazole	GI proton pump inhibitor, antiulcer	omeprazole, lansoprazole
-pril	Angiotensin converting enzyme (ACE) inhibitor, antihypertensive	captopril, enalapril, fosinopril, lisinopril, quinapril
sal-, -sal-	Contains salicylate; check allergy to salicylates or aspirin	salsalate (nonopioid analgesic), sulfasalazine (GI anti-inflammatory)
-sartan	Angiotensin II receptor antagonist, antihypertensive	candesartan, eprosartan, losartan, valsartan
-sone, -lone, pred-	Corticosteroid	prednisone, betamethasone, dexamethasone, cortisone, triamcinolone, prednisolone
-statin	HMG-Coenzyme A reductase inhibitor, lipid lowering agent	atorvastatin, fluvastatin, lovastatin, pravastatin, simvastatin
sulfa-	Sulfonamide, antibiotic; check allergy to sulfa	sulfacetamide, sulfamethoxazole
-terol	Adrenergic type of bronchodilator	albuterol, formoterol, levabuterol, pirbuterol, salmeterol
-tidine	Histamine H2 antagonist (GI), antiulcer	cimetidine, ranitidine, famotidine, nizatidine
-triptan	Vascular headache suppressant, serotonin (5-HT1) agonist	almotriptan, naratriptan, sumatriptan, zolmitriptan
-vir	Antiviral antiinfective	acyclovir, cidofovir, famciclovir, gangciclovir, valacyclovir
-zepam, -zolam	Benzodiazepine, antianxiety, sedative/hypnotic	diazepam, lorazepam, oxazepam, alprazolam, midazolam
-zosin	Peripherally acting anti-adrenergic, antihypertensive	doxazocin, prazosin, terazosin

* This is not an exhaustive list and may not be inclusive of every drug in each category.
** This category does not include erythromycin, azithromycin, or clarithromycin, all of which are a macrolide type of antibiotic.

PHYSIOLOGICAL INTEGRITY: REDUCTION OF RISK POTENTIAL

Reduction of Risk Potential makes up 9–15% of the questions on the NCLEX-RN® exam.

Key Testing Strategies

- Memorize common laboratory values and use them to answer questions about specific laboratory test results.
- Always ask if a female client of childbearing age is pregnant before she has x-rays taken.
- Remove all metal objects before a client has an x-ray.
- Ask routinely about allergies to contrast dyes or iodine before a client undergoes a diagnostic test using injectable contrast material.
- Recall that clients cannot wear or have imbedded metal (prostheses, for example) to be eligible for magnetic resonance imaging (MRI).

Key Assessments in the Immediate Post-surgical Period

Review these assessments in Chapter 48

- Adequacy of airway
- Adequacy of ventilation
- Cardiovascular status
- Level of consciousness
- Presence of protective reflexes (e.g., gag, cough)
- Activity, ability to move extremities
- Skin color (pink, pale, dusky, blotchy, cyanotic, jaundiced)
- Fluid status: intake and output, status of IV infusions (type of fluid, rate, amount in container, patency of tubing), signs of dehydration or fluid overload
- Condition of operative site, dressing and presence of drainage
- Patency of and character and amount of drainage from catheters, tubes, and drains
- Discomfort (i.e., pain) (type, location, and severity), nausea, vomiting
- Safety (e.g., necessity for side rails, call bell within reach)

Sample Topics for Reduction of Risk Potential Questions

- Changes/abnormalities in vital signs
- Diagnostic tests
- Laboratory values
- Potential for alterations in body systems
- Potential for complications of diagnostic tests/treatments/procedures
- Potential for complications from surgical procedures and health alterations
- System-specific assessments
- Therapeutic procedures

Vital Signs by Age

Age	Heart Rate Range & (Avg) in bpm*		Respiratory Rate Range in rpm**		Median Blood Pressure (mm Hg)***	
Newborn (NB)–1 mo	NB	110–170 (120)		30–60	NB	73/55
	1 mo	90–130 (110)			1 mo	86/52
6 months–1 year		80–130 (110)	6 mo	24–36	6 mo	90/53
			1 yr	20–40	1 yr	90/56
2 years		70–120 (100)		20–40		90/56
3–5 years		70–120 (100)		20–30		92/55
6–9 years		70–110 (90)		16–22	6 yrs	96/57
					9 yrs	100/61
10–15 years		60–100 (85)		16–20	10 yrs	100/61
					12 yrs	107/64
					15 yrs	114/65
18 years		60–100 (85)		12–20		121/70

* Beats per minute.
** Respirations per minute; higher when awake; slower during sleep.
*** Blood pressure varies by gender as well as age.

Normal Arterial Blood Gas Values

Review Chapter 54 for additional information on acid base imbalances.

Arterial Blood Gas Parameter	Normal Value
pH	7.35–7.45
PCO_2	35–45 mm Hg
HCO_3^-	22–26 mEq/L
PO_2	80–100 mm Hg

Adult Reference Range for Common Laboratory Tests

Coagulation Studies	*Prothrombin time (PT): 10–13 seconds; 1.5–2.0 times the control in seconds for anticoagulant therapy; Activated partial thromboplastin time (APTT): 20–35 seconds (1.5–2.5 times the control in anticoagulant therapy); Partial thromboplastin time (PTT): 60–70 seconds; 1.5–2.5 times the control in anticoagulant therapy International normalized ratio (INR): 2.0–3.0 for most anticoagulation needs*
Electrolytes	*Sodium (Na^+): 135–145 mEq/L; Potassium (K^+): 3.5–5.1 mEq/L Chloride (Cl^-): 95–105 mEq/L CO_2 combining power: 22–30 mEq/L; 22–30 mmol/L Calcium, total (Ca^{++}): 4.5–5.5 mEq/L, 9–11 mg/dL, 2.3–2.8 mmol/L Calcium (ionized): 4.25–5.25 mg/dL, 2.2–2.5 mEq/L, 1.1–1.24 mmol/L Magnesium (Mg^{++}): 1.5–2.5 mEq/L, 1.8–3.0 mg/dL*
Glucose	*Fasting (FBS): 70–110 mg/dL (serum, plasma); 60–100 mg/dL (whole blood); 70–120 mg/dL (elderly); panic values: < 40 or > 700 mg/dL Fingerstick glucose (self-monitoring device): 60–100 mg/dL*
Hematology	*White blood cells (WBC): 5000–10,000 microliter or 4500–11,500/mm^3 Neutrophils: 1935–7942 (absolute count) or 45–75% Red blood cells (RBC): 4.5–5.3 million or (10^6)/mm^3 (men), 4.1–5.1 million or (10^6)/mm^3 (women) Hemoglobin (Hgb): 13.0–18.0 grams/100 mL (men), 12–16 grams/100 mL (women) Hematocrit (Hct): 37–49 % (men), 36–46 % (women) Platelet count: 150,000–400,000/mm^3 (or microliter)*
Renal Function Studies	*Blood urea nitrogen (BUN): 5–25 mg/dL Serum creatinine: 0.5–1.5 mg/dL*
Therapeutic Drug Levels	*Digoxin: 0.5–2.0 ng/mL; Phenytoin: 10–20 mcg/mL Theophylline derivatives: 10–20 mcg/mL or 10–20 mg/mL*

PHYSIOLOGICAL INTEGRITY: PHYSIOLOGICAL ADAPTATION

Physiological Adaptation makes up 11–17% of the questions on the NCLEX-RN® exam.

Key Testing Strategies

- Think about the underlying pathophysiology when selecting interventions to assist a client with a health problem affecting a particular body system.
- Remember when a client's status is deteriorating rapidly, follow the ABCs—airway, breathing, and circulation.
- When evaluating the condition of a client with a particular health problem, use knowledge of normal findings or the client's usual baselines as a gauge as to the effectiveness of care.

Sample Topics for Physiological Adaptation Questions

Alterations in body systems	Medical emergencies
Fluid and electrolyte imbalances	Pathophysiology
Hemodynamics	Unexpected response to therapies
Illness management	

Symptom Analysis

P What was the provoking incident (aggravating factor[s]) that caused the symptom, if any? Any palliating factors?
Q What is the quality of the symptom? Is it burning, throbbing, aching, stabbing, other?
R Where is the region of symptom? Does it radiate? Does anything relieve the symptom?
S How severe is the symptom? (intensity, quantity)
T What is the timing of the symptom? When does it occur; how long does it last? (pattern, duration)

Glasgow Coma Scale

See Chapter 57 for review of neurologic disorders.

Glasgow Coma Scoring System

Type of Response Tested	Score	Indicator
Physical (Motor) Response	6	Acts out a simple command
	5	Reacts to a localized discomfort and offensive stimulus
	4	Moves purposelessly or flexes in response to pain
	3	Exhibits abnormal flexion (decorticate posture)
	2	Exhibits abnormal extension (decerebrate posture)
	1	Has no motor response
Verbal Response	5	Has full orientation (time, place, person)
	4	Shows confusion and disorientation
	3	Uses disorganized or inappropriate words; cannot sustain a conversation
	2	Uses sounds instead of words
	1	Makes no verbal response
Eye Response	4	Open when a person approaches (spontaneous response)
	3	Open when a person speaks
	2	Open only when in pain
	1	Open never, even in presence of painful stimuli

Note: Add numbers to find score from 3 (profound coma) to 15 (normal conscious state).

Neurovascular Status: Checking the "6 Ps"

Pain: is there pain or discomfort in the extremity?
Pallor: is the skin color paler than normal or baseline?
Polar: is the skin cooler to the touch than normal or baseline in the area?
Paresthesia: are there any unusual sensations, such as numbness or tingling?
Paralysis: is the extremity without movement or weaker than normal or baseline?
Pulse: is the affected pulse (or pulses) diminished or absent?

Nursing Care of the Client in a Cast

See Chapter 61 for review of musculoskeletal disorders.

- Casts made from plaster of Paris should not get wet and cast padding should not be removed; if cast becomes soiled, clean with a damp cloth. Casts made of synthetic material dry more quickly and allow mobility in less than an hour.
- Smooth rough edges to prevent skin injury; explain that no foreign objects should be inserted into the cast (sticks, food crumbs, etc.) to prevent skin breakdown.
- Avoid covering a new plaster cast with blanket or plastic for extended periods (air cannot circulate, and heat builds up in cast).
- Turn client from side to side (using palms, not fingertips) every 2 hours to facilitate drying for the first 24 to 72 hours.
- Apply ice (crushed or small cubes to avoid denting cast) for the first 24 hours over fracture site to control edema, ensuring that ice is securely contained to avoid wetting cast.
- Elevate extremity above the level of the heart to promote venous return for the first 24 hours after application.
- Encourage active range of motion (AROM) to joints above and below immobilized extremity.
- Report to healthcare provider: increasing pain in immobilized extremity, excessive swelling and discoloration of exposed limb, burning or tingling under cast, sores, or foul odor under cast.

Rule of Nines for Calculating Burn Injury

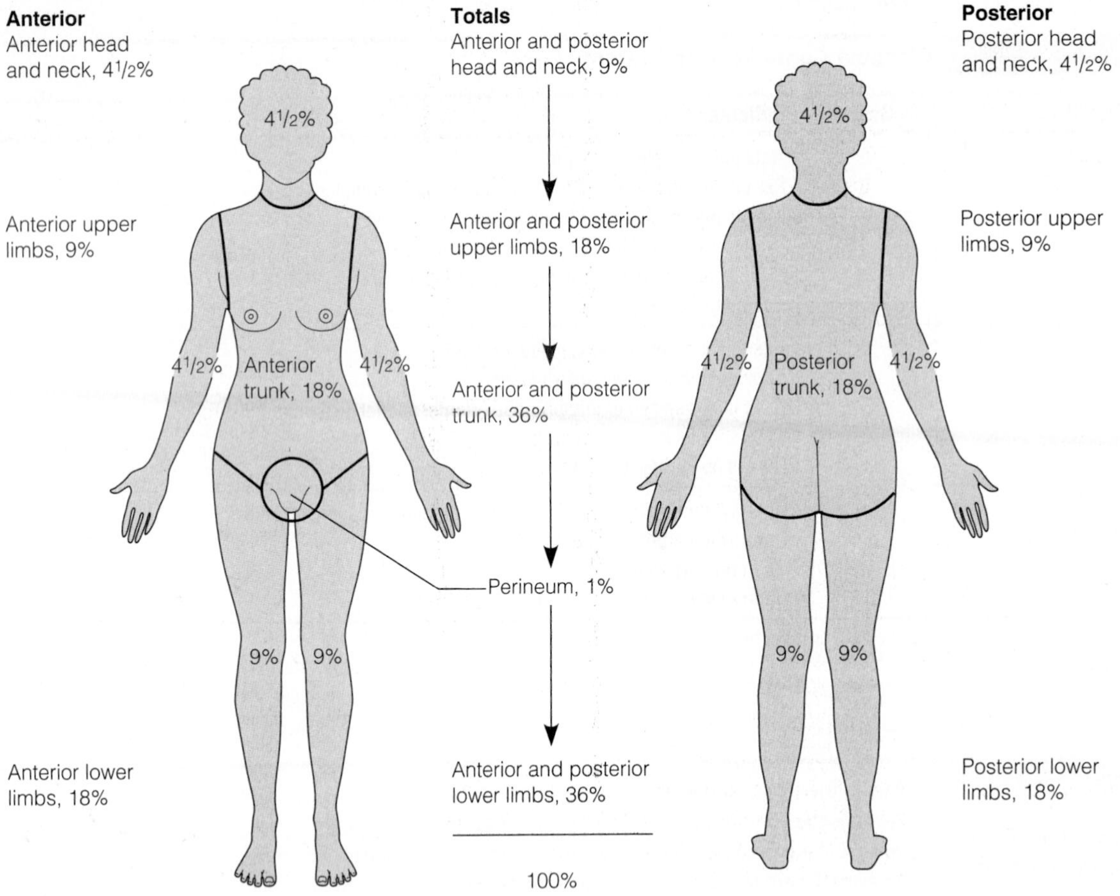

Clinical Manifestations of Chronic Renal Failure

See Chapter 58 for review of renal disorders.

Body System	Clinical Manifestations	Cause of Manifestations
Cardiovascular	Hypervolemia, hypertension, tachycardia, arrhythmias, congestive heart failure, pericarditis	Increased fluid volume, build-up of metabolic wastes, chronic hypertension, change in renin-angiotension mechanism
Hematologic	Anemia, leukocytosis, decreased platelet function, thrombocytopenia	Decreased production of erythropoietin and RBCs, decreased survival of RBCs, decreased platelet activity; blood loss through dialysis and bleeding
Gastrointestinal	Anorexia, nausea, vomiting, abdominal distention, diarrhea, constipation, bleeding	Build-up of uremic toxins, electrolyte imbalances, changes in platelet activity, conversion of urea to ammonia by saliva
Neurologic	Lethargy, confusion, convulsions, stupor, coma, sleep disturbances, behavioral changes, muscle irritability	Uremic toxins, electrolyte imbalances, cerebral swelling caused by fluid shifts
Dermatologic	Pallor, pigmentation, pruritus, ecchymosis, excoriation, uremic frost	Anemia, decreased activity of sweat glands, dry skin, phosphate deposits on skin
Urinary	Decreased urine output, decreased specific gravity, proteinuria, casts and cells in the urine	Damage to the nephron
Skeletal	Osteoporosis, renal rickets, joint pain	Decreased calcium absorption, decreased phosphate excretion

Priority Cardiac Dysrhythmias *Review Chapter 56 for additional information about cardiac dysrhythmias.*

Rhythm/ECG Appearance	ECG Characteristics	Management
Supraventricular Rhythms		
Sinus tachycardia 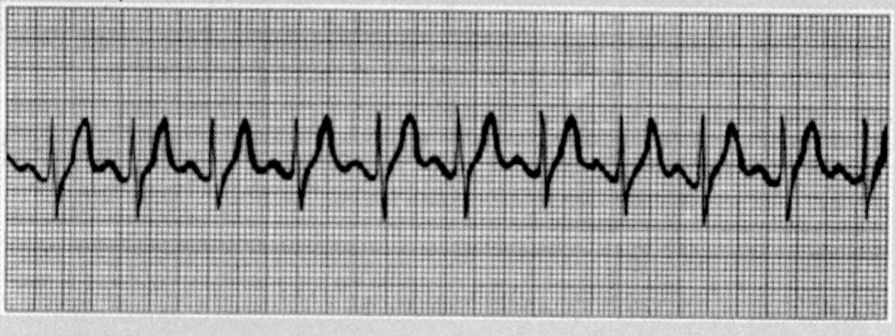	Rate: 101 to 150 bpm Rhythm: regular P:QRS ratio is 1:1 (with very fast rates, P wave may be hidden in preceding T wave) PR interval: 0.12–0.20 sec QRS complex: 0.06–0.10 sec	Treat only if client is experiencing symptoms or is at risk for myocardial damage; treat underlying cause (e.g., hypovolemia, fever, pain); beta blockers or verapamil may be used
Sinus bradycardia 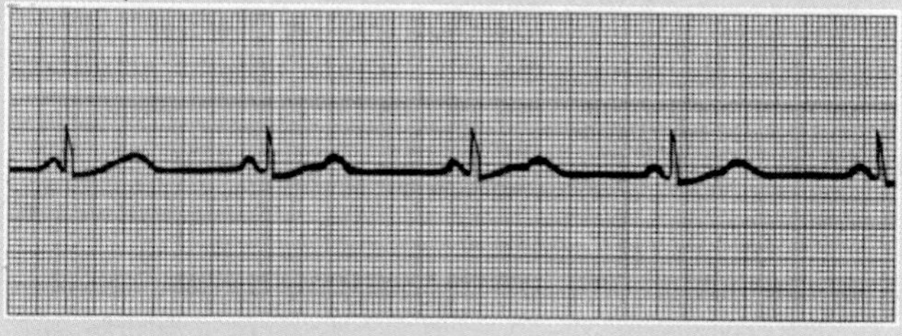	Rate: less than 60 bpm Rhythm: regular P:QRS ratio is 1:1 PR interval: 0.12–0.20 sec QRS complex: 0.06–0.10 sec	Treat only if client is experiencing symptoms; intravenous atropine and/or pacemaker therapy may be used
Atrial fibrillation 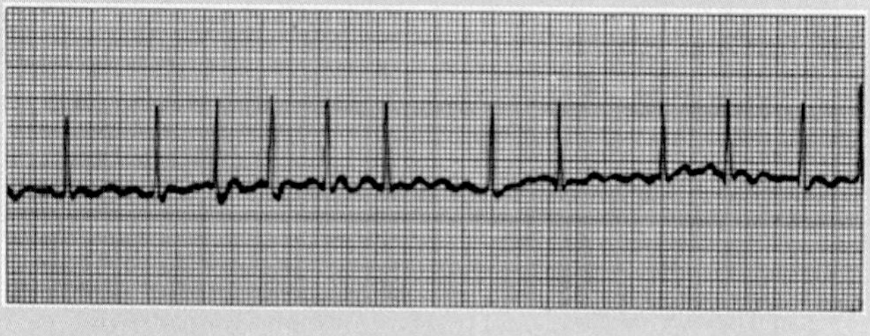	Rate: atrial 300–600 bpm (too rapid to count); ventricular 100–180 bpm in untreated clients Rhythm: irregularly irregular P:QRS ratio is variable PR interval: not measured QRS complex: 0.06–0.10 sec	Synchronized cardioversion; medications to reduce ventricular response rate: verapamil, propranolol, digoxin, anticoagulant therapy to reduce risk of clot formation and stroke
Ventricular Rhythms		
Premature ventricular contractions (PVC) 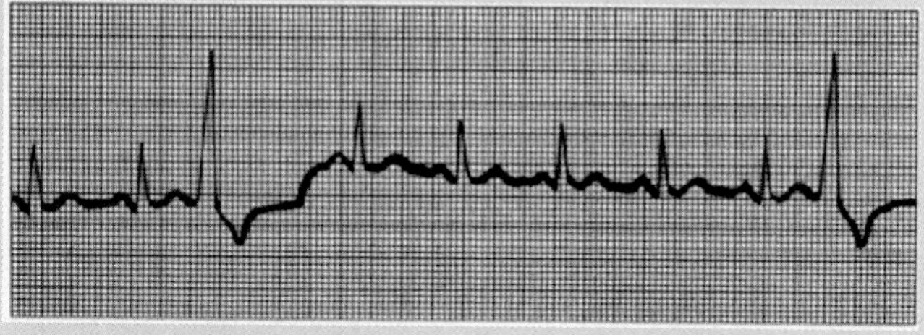	Rate: variable Rhythm: irregular, with PVC interrupting underlying rhythm and followed by a compensatory pause P:QRS ratio: no P wave noted before PVC PR interval: absent with PVC QRS complex: wide (greater 0.12 sec), bizarre in appearance; differs from normal QRS complex	Treat if client is experiencing symptoms; advise against stimulant use (caffeine, nicotine); drug therapy includes intravenous lidocaine, procainamide, quinidine, propranolol, phenytoin, amiodarone
Ventricular tachycardia (VT or V tach) 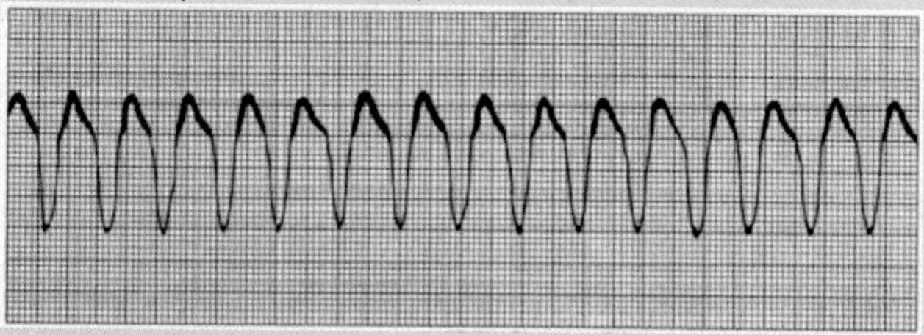	Rate: 100–250 bpm Rhythm: regular P:QRS ratio: P waves usually not identifiable PR interval: not measured QRS complex: 0.12 sec or greater; bizarre shape	Treat if VT is sustained or if client is experiencing symptoms; treatment includes intravenous procainamide or lidocaine and/or immediate defibrillation if the client is unconscious or unstable
Ventricular fibrillation (VF or V fib) 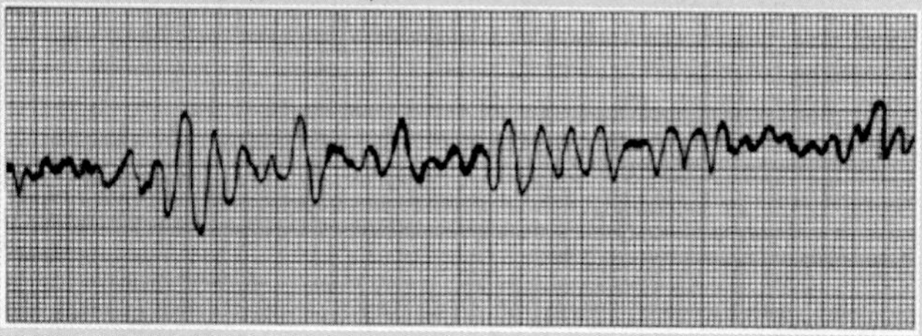	Rate: too rapid to count Rhythm: grossly irregular P:QRS ratio: no identifiable P waves PR interval: none QRS: bizarre, varying in shape and direction	Immediate defibrillation

Index